DATE DUE			

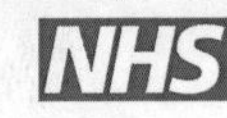
NHS

Library Service
Musgrove Park Hospital

SWNHS
C20118901

ROCKWOOD AND WILKINS'

FRACTURES IN CHILDREN

SIXTH EDITION

ROCKWOOD AND WILKINS'

FRACTURES IN CHILDREN

SIXTH EDITION

EDITORS

James H. Beaty, MD

Professor of Orthopaedics

Department of Orthopaedic Surgery

University of Tennessee-Campbell Clinic

Chief of Staff

Campbell Clinic

Memphis, Tennessee

James R. Kasser, MD

John E. Hall Professor of Orthopaedic Surgery

Harvard Medical School

Orthopaedic Surgeon-in-Chief

Children's Hospital Boston

Boston, Massachusetts

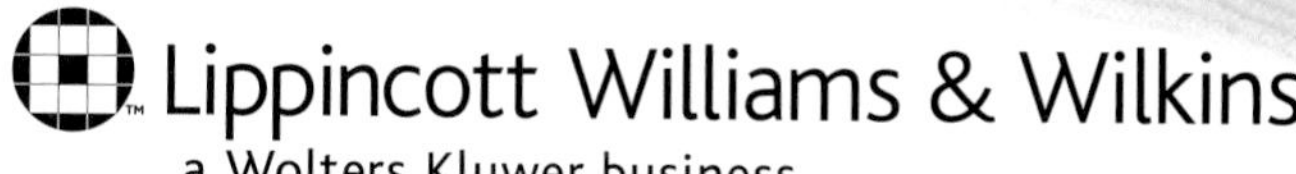

Lippincott Williams & Wilkins

a Wolters Kluwer business

Philadelphia • Baltimore • New York • London

Buenos Aires • Hong Kong • Sydney • Tokyo

Acquisitions Editor: Robert Hurley
Developmental Editor: Keith Donnellan, Dovetail Content Solutions
Managing Editor: Jenny Kim
Project Manager: Alicia Jackson
Senior Manufacturing Manager: Benjamin Rivera
Director of Marketing: Sharon Zinner
Creative Director: Doug Smock
Cover Designer: Mike Pottman
Production Service: Maryland Composition
Printer: RR Donnelley-Willard

530 Walnut Street
Philadelphia, PA 19106 USA
LWW.com

Printed in the USA

Library of Congress Cataloging-in-Publication Data

Rockwood and Wilkins' fractures in children.—6th ed. / editors, James H. Beaty, James R. Kasser.
p. ; cm.
Includes bibliographical references and index.
ISBN 0-7817-5769-X
1. Fractures in children. 2. Children—Wounds and injuries. I. Rockwood, Charles A., 1936- II. Wilkins, Kaye E. III. Beaty, James H. IV. Kasser, James R. V. Title: Fractures in children.
[DNLM: 1. Fractures—Child. 2. Dislocations—Child. WE 175 R6842 2006]
RD101.F74 2006
617.1'5083—dc22

2005028858

Care has been taken to confirm the accuracy of the information presented and to describe generally accepted practices. However, the authors, editors, and publisher are not responsible for errors or omissions or for any consequences from application of the information in this book and make no warranty, expressed or implied, with respect to the currency, completeness, or accuracy of the contents of the publication. Application of the information in a particular situation remains the professional responsibility of the practitioner.

The authors, editors, and publisher have exerted every effort to ensure that drug selection and dosage set forth in this text are in accordance with current recommendations and practice at the time of publication. However, in view of ongoing research, changes in government regulations, and the constant flow of information relating to drug therapy and drug reactions, the reader is urged to check the package insert for each drug for any change in indications and dosage and for added warnings and precautions. This is particularly important when the recommended agent is a new or infrequently employed drug.

Some drugs and medical devices presented in the publication have Food and Drug Administration (FDA) clearance for limited use in restricted research settings. It is the responsibility of the health care provider to ascertain the FDA status of each drug or device planned for use in their clinical practice.

To purchase additional copies of this book, call our customer service department at (800) 638-3030 or fax orders to (301) 223-2320. International customers should call (301) 223-2300.

Visit Lippincott Williams & Wilkins on the Internet: at LWW.com. Lippincott Williams & Wilkins customer service representatives are available from 8:30 am to 6 pm, EST.

10 9 8 7 6 5 4 3 2 1

Although the "science" of pediatric orthopaedics can be garnered from multiple sources, especially since the advent of electronic educational venues, the "art" of treating children with orthopaedic conditions is not so easily learned. Because they taught us so much more than the science of pediatric orthopaedics and inspired us with their willingness to share their knowledge and enthusiasm, we dedicate this edition to some of our special mentors:

Henry H. Banks
Harold B. Boyd
S. Terry Canale
Paul P. Griffin
John E. Hall
Alvin J. Ingram
G. Dean MacEwen

In addition to these individuals, we dedicate this text to all those who invest their time and energy in mentoring young orthopaedic surgeons, passing along traditions and skills that ensure the vitality and excellence of our specialty. Without these teachers of the art of pediatric orthopaedics, the science could not be applied to obtain the best possible outcome for each child we treat.

CONTENTS

SECTION THREE: SPINE

SECTION FOUR: LOWER EXTREMITY

CONTRIBUTING AUTHORS

Alaric J. Aroojis, MS, D OrthDNB(Orth) Lecturer of Orthopaedics, King Edward VII Memorial Hospital, Bombay, India

James H. Beaty, MD Professor of Orthopaedics, Department of Orthopaedic Surgery, University of Tennessee-Campbell Clinic, Chief of Staff, Campbell Clinic, Memphis, Tennessee

John G. Birch, MD, FRCS(C) Professor of Orthopaedic Surgery, University of Texas Southwestern Medical School, Assistant Chief of Staff, Orthopaedics Department, Texas Scottish Rite Hospital for Children, Dallas, Texas

R. Dale Blasier, MD, FRCS(C) Professor of Orthopaedic Surgery, The University of Arkansas for Medical Sciences, Chief of Orthopaedic Trauma, Arkansas Children's Hospital, Little Rock, Arkansas

Robert M. Campbell, Jr, MD The President's Council/Dielmann Chair in Pediatric Orthopaedic Surgery, Professor of Orthopaedics, University of Texas Health Science Center at San Antonio, CHRISTUS Santa Rosea Children's Hospital, San Antonio, Texas

R. Jay Cummings, MD Associate Professor of Orthopaedics, Mayo Graduate School of Medicine, Medical Director, Chairman of Department of Surgery, Chief of Orthopaedics, Nemours Children's Clinic, Jacksonville, Florida

José F. de la Garza, MD Department of Surgery, Universidad Autonoma de Nuevo Leon, Trauma and Orthopaedic Service, University Hospital, Moneterrey, Nuevo Leon, Mexico

John P. Dormans, MD Professor of Orthopaedic Surgery, University of Pennsylvania School of Medicine, Chief of Orthopaedic Surgery, The Children's Hospital of Philadelphia, Philadelphia, Pennsylvania

Robert E. Eilert, MD Rose Brown Professor of Orthopaedic Surgery and Pediatrics, University of Colorado Health Science Center, Chairman, Department of Orthopaedic Surgery, The Children's Hospital, Vice Chairman, Department of Orthopaedic Surgery, University of Colorado Medical School, Denver, Colorado

Mark A. Erickson, MD Associate Professor of Orthopaedics, University of Colorado Health Sciences Center, Chairman of Orthopaedics, The Children's Hospital, Denver, Colorado

John M. Flynn, MD Associate Professor of Orthopaedics, University of Pennsylvania School of Medicine, Orthopaedic Trauma Director, Associate Chief of Orthopaedic Surgery, The Children's Hospital of Philadelphia, Philadelphia, Pennsylvania

Bruce K. Foster, MD, FRACS Clinical Associate Professor of Pediatrics and Orthopaedics, University of Adelaide, Deputy Director and Senior Specialist, Department of Orthopaedic Surgery, Women's and Children's Hospital, North Adelaide, Australia

Joseph R. Furman, MD Children's Hospital Intensive Care Associates, Methodist Children's Hospital, San Antonio, Texas

Daniel J. Hedequist, MD Instructor of Orthopaedic Surgery, Harvard Medical School, Attending Orthopaedic Surgeon, Division of Spinal Surgery, Children's Hospital, Boston, Massachusetts

Stephen D. Heinrich, MD Clinical Professor of Orthopaedic Surgery, Louisiana State University Health Sciences Center, Department of Orthopaedic Surgery, Children's Hospital, New Orleans, Louisiana

Laurie O. Hughes, MD Staff Orthopaedic Surgeon, Arkansas Children's Hospital, Central Arkansas Veteran's Hospital, Little Rock, Arkansas

James G. Jarvis, MD, FRCS(C) Associate Professor of Surgery, University of Ottawa, Chief of Orthopaedic Surgery, Children's Hospital of Eastern Ontario, Ottawa, Ontario, Canada

James R. Kasser, MD John E. Hall Professor of Orthopaedic Surgery, Harvard Medical School, Orthopaedic Surgeon-in-Chief, Children's Hospital Boston, Boston, Massachusetts

Robert M. Kay, MD Associate Professor of Orthopaedic Surgery, Keck School of Medicine at the University of Southern California, Children's Orthopaedic Center, Children's Hospital Los Angeles, Los Angeles, California

Erik C. King, MD Assistant Professor of Orthopaedic Surgery, Northwestern University Feinberg School of Medicine, Attending Physician, Children's Memorial Hospital, Division of Orthopaedic Surgery, Chicago, Illinois

Mininder S. Kocher, MD, MPh Assistant Professor of Orthopaedic Surgery, Harvard Medical School, Assistant Director, Division of Sports Medicine, Department of Orthopaedic Surgery, Children's Hospital Boston, Boston, Massachusetts

Scott H. Kozin, MD Associate Professor of Orthopaedic Surgery, Temple University, Attending Hand Surgeon, Shriners Hospital for Children, Philadelphia, Pennsylvania

R. Mervyn Letts, MD, FRCS(C), FACSC Chief, Department of Surgery, Division of Pediatric Orthopaedics, Children's Hospital of Eastern Ontario, University of Ottawa, Ottawa, Ontario, Canada

Scott J. Luhmann, MD Assistant Professor of Orthopaedic Surgery, Washington University School of Medicine, St. Louis Children's Hospital, Shriners Hospital for Children, Barnes-Jewish Hospital, St. Louis, Missouri

Charles T. Mehlman, DO, MPh Associate Clinical Professor of Pediatric Orthopaedic Surgery, University of Cincinnati College of Medicine, Associate Professor of Pediatric Orthopaedics, Director, Musculoskeletal Outcomes Research, Director of Pediatric Orthopaedic Resident Education, Division of Pediatric Orthopaedics, Cincinnati Children's Hospital Medical Center, Cincinnati, Ohio

Alexander D. Mih, MD Associate Professor of Orthopaedic Surgery, Indiana University School of Medicine, The Indiana Hand Center, Indianapolis, Indiana

James F. Mooney III, MD Chief of Orthopaedic Surgery, Children's Hospital of Michigan, Wayne State University School of Medicine, Detroit, Michigan

Paul J. Moroz, MD, MSc, FRCS(C) Assistant Professor of Orthopaedic Surgery, Faculty of Medicine, University of Ottawa, Pediatric Orthopaedic and Spinal Surgeon, Children's Hospital of Eastern Ontario, Ottawa, Ontario, Canada

Peter O. Newton, MD Associate Clinical Professor of Orthopaedic Surgery, University of California, Director of Scoliosis Program, Children's Hospital, San Diego, California

Karl E. Rathjen, MD Assistant Professor of Orthopaedic Surgery, University of Texas Southwestern Medical School, Staff Pediatric Orthopaedist, Texas Scottish Rite Hospital for Children, Dallas, Texas

John F. Sarwark, MD Professor of Orthopaedic Surgery, Northwestern University Feinberg School of Medicine, Head, Orthopaedic Surgery, The Children's Memorial Hospital, Chicago, Illinois

Timothy Schrader, MD Staff Physician, Department of Orthopaedics, Children's Healthcare of Atlanta-Scottish Rite, Atlanta, Georgia

David L. Skaggs, MD Associate Professor of Orthopaedic Surgery, Keck School of Medicine at the University of Southern California, Associate Director, Children's Orthopaedic Center, Children's Hospital Los Angeles, Los Angeles, California

Anthony A. Stans, MD Chair, Division of Pediatric Orthopaedics, Mayo Clinic, Rochester, Minnesota

Vernon T. Tolo, MD John C. Wilson Jr, Professor of Orthopaedics, Keck School of Medicine at the University of Southern California, Director, Children's Orthopaedic Center, Children's Hospital Los Angeles, Los Angeles, California

Eric J. Wall, MD Associate Professor of Pediatric Orthopaedics, Director of Sports Medicine, Cincinnati Children's Hospital Medical Center, Cincinnati, Ohio

William C. Warner, Jr, MD Associate Professor of Orthopaedic Surgery, University of Tennessee, Staff, Campbell Clinic, Memphis, Tennessee

Peter M. Waters, MD Associate Professor of Orthopaedic Surgery, Harvard Medical School, Associate Chief, Department of Orthopaedic Surgery, Director of Hand and Upper Extremity Surgery, Children's Hospital Boston, Boston, Massachusetts

Roger F. Widmann, MD Associate Professor of Clinical Orthopaedic Surgery, Weill Medical College of Cornell University, Chief of Pediatric Orthopaedic Surgery Service, Hospital for Special Surgery, New York, New York

Kaye E. Wilkins, MD, DVM Professor of Orthopaedics and Pediatrics, University of Texas Health Science Center at San Antonio, San Antonio, Texas

Cory J. Xian, MSc, PhD Affiliate Senior Lecturer of Pediatrics, University of Adelaide, Principal Scientist, Department of Orthopaedic Surgery, Women's and Children's Hospital, North Adelaide, Australia

PREFACE

As with each new edition of this text, we have been amazed and humbled by the amount of information about fractures in children that has appeared since the last edition: innovations in techniques and equipment, findings from clinical outcomes studies and basic science research, new ways of looking at old procedures and philosophies. It is gratifying to see that our specialty remains so committed to continuous learning. Through the hard work of our contributors, we believe we have provided a compendium of information about both "cutting edge" and "tried and true" methods of operative and nonoperative fracture treatment that will allow practitioners to make informed and intelligent decisions for their patients.

Just as the information contained in it is continually being updated, the physical appearance of the text has continued to evolve. Improved formatting has added to the readability of the volume, while retaining the important elements of history, anatomy, diagnosis, x-ray findings, treatment options, and authors' preferred treatment. New formatting and increased use of color have allowed us to better illustrate critical surgical considerations and techniques and to highlight important tables and information in the text.

With this sixth edition of *Rockwood and Wilkins' Fractures in Children,* our goals remain the same as those of the first edition, as expressed by Drs. Rockwood, Wilkins, and King: ". . . to make this volume as comprehensive as possible so that it will serve the orthopaedic resident in training as well as the practicing orthopaedist and contribute to the maintenance of a high standard of fracture care for children."

ACKNOWLEDGMENTS

Without the hard work of many people over several years, this text would not have been possible. The most important contributions were made, as always, by our chapter authors who worked diligently to provide insightful and accurate information and illustrations that provide our readers with the tools necessary for optimal care of children with fractures.

The staff at Lippincott Williams & Wilkins provided their expert guidance and support, as well as encouragement and enthusiasm. Bob Hurley, Jenny Kim, Susan Rhyner, and Eileen Wolfberg were always willing to help when deadlines loomed or problems arose. Keith Donnellan and his crew at Dovetail Content Solutions managed to gather all the pieces we sent and assemble them into useable form, all the while maintaining their calm and good humor.

We also had the invaluable assistance of a number of people from our own institutions in the hands-on phases of preparation of manuscripts and illustrations: from the Campbell Foundation in Memphis, Kay Daugherty (Editorial), Barry Burns (Graphics), and Joan Crowson (Library), and from Boston, Kathryn Macdonald (Editorial) and Alison Clapp (Library).

To our families, we express our appreciation for their understanding and encouragement. Special thanks to our wives, Terry Beaty and Candace Kasser, who through the months of writing, and reading, and proofing provided support and assistance that helped us believe we could actually survive this revision. This finished work is a testament to their steadfast patience and fortitude during the lengthy process of production.

SECTION

ONE

BASIC PRINCIPLES

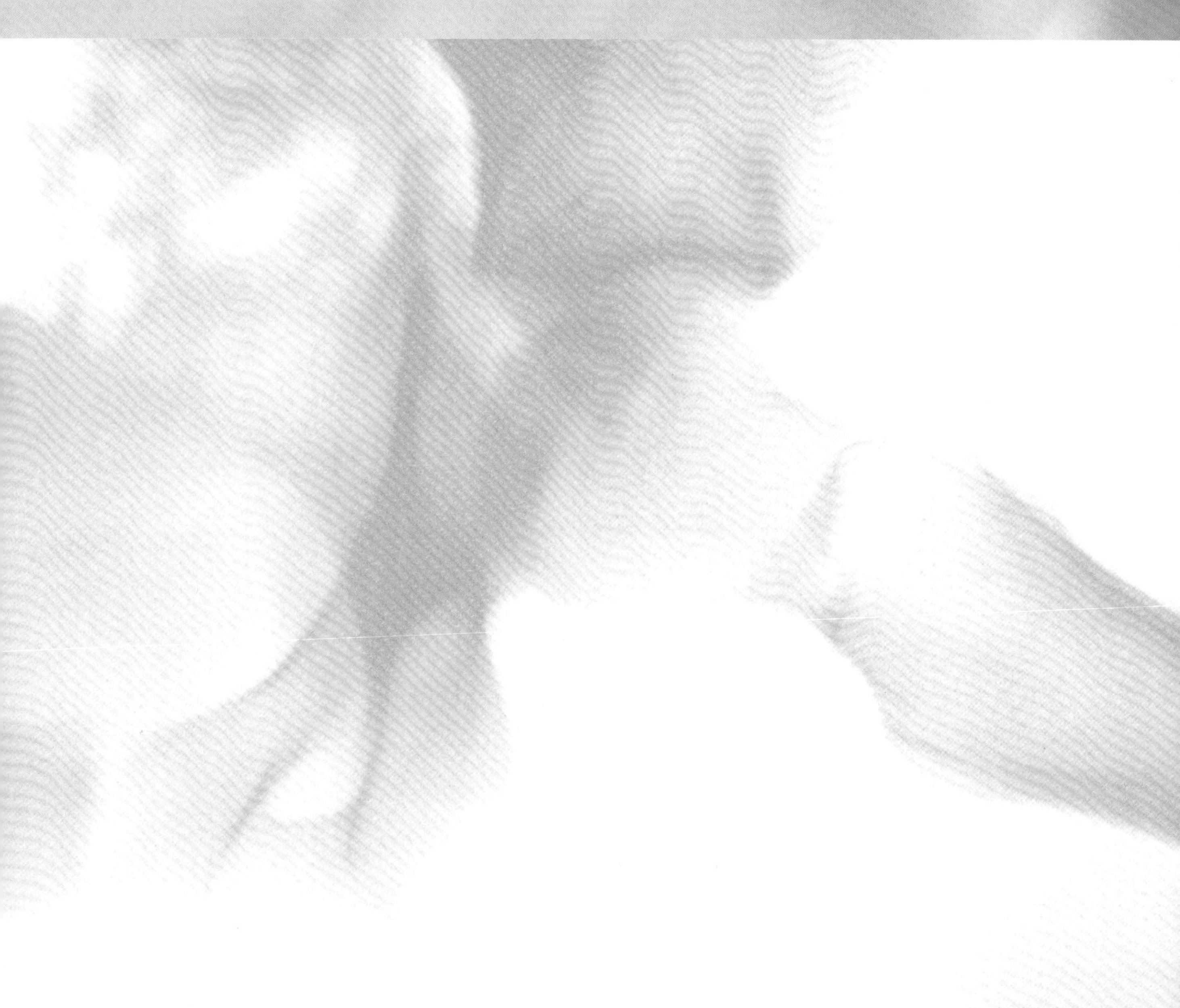

INCIDENCE OF FRACTURES IN CHILDREN

Kaye E. Wilkins and Alaric J. Aroojis

In the years since the production of the first edition of *Fractures in Children*, there have been many changes in how fractures in children are treated in North America and Europe, with more emphasis on operative management. This has not been without some controversy. In most instances, operative management produces better results, but the treating surgeon's decision as to the preferred method of management should be based on the local factors involving that specific patient and the resources available. *The nonoperative management of children's fractures must not become a lost art.*

In addition to changes in the management of children's fractures, there have been changes in the *incidence* and the *etiology* of fractures in North America and Europe.

The importance of studying the incidence of children's fractures is to develop preventative strategies. It is imperative that surgeons who treat fractures in children be involved in applying these strategies in their local communities.

CHANGES IN THE PHILOSOPHY OF TREATING FRACTURES IN CHILDREN

Blount's Nonoperative Axioms

Dr. Walter Blount, in his textbook *Fractures in Children,* emphasized that because of growth children's fractures have a great potential to remodel (1). In fact, he outlined the rules of remodeling as to what amount of angulation would be accepted in children's fractures. He was very opposed to operative intervention, especially intramedullary fixation of femoral shaft fractures in children:

> "The operation is unnecessary, however, and as such must be condemned. It introduces the hazard of an unnecessary anesthetic, unnecessary exposure of bone ends, and trauma to the entire marrow cavity of the femur. There is no reason for doing it" (1).

Complications with Operative Intervention

It was Dr. Blount's experience that nonunions often followed open reductions in children. He went on to delineate the serious other complications that he had seen with open reduction, including death from sepsis. His comment was, "One postoperative osteomyelitis in a lifetime is enough to cure a surgeon of a casual attitude toward open reduction."

This aversion to operative management of children's fractures set the tone for a generation of orthopaedic surgeons.

The Trend toward Minimal Invasion

Certainly, prior to the mid-1950s, when Blount published his textbook (1), operative procedures usually required large incisions and extensive dissection. In the nearly 50 years since the publication of his book, there has been a trend toward more operative intervention with good results. In the methods currently used, the surgery can be done with only minimal invasiveness, and the fixation often is temporary.

Factors Creating the Trend toward Operative Intervention

This trend toward more operative intervention has been the result of four factors: (a) improvement in technology, (b) rapid healing allowing minimal and temporary fixation, (c) the financial and social pressures to limit the hospitalization of children, and (d) the expectation by the public for a perfect outcome in every case.

Improvement in Technology

The use of the image intensifier has greatly improved the ease with which fractures can be reduced and stabilized internally with percutaneous methods. Other technical advances such as computed tomography (CT), magnetic resonance imaging (MRI), and sonographic imaging have expanded the ability to better define the fracture patterns. The use of powered instruments and cannulated implants, coupled with the use of radiographic real time images has greatly facilitated the accuracy of applying fixation devices with percutaneous techniques.

Rapid Healing

Because children heal and remodel rapidly, fixation devices often need to be used for only a short time. Children tolerate all types of casts well for short periods of time, which allows a minimally stabilized fracture to be immobilized with a cast until there is sufficient internal callous to supplement the limited internal fixation.

Minimal Hospitalization

The rising costs of hospitalization have created a trend to mobilize children to an outpatient setting as soon as possible. This has been reinforced by the fact that in two thirds of the families in the United States both parents are wage earners.

There are both social and financial pressures to mobilize the child early. The trend now is to temporarily surgically stabilize these fractures so that the patient can be discharged early.

The Perfect Result

Modern parents have become very sophisticated and now expect a perfect outcome for their child. They inspect the x-rays, question the alignment, and expect the alignment to be perfect or anatomic.

A common statement made by the patient's father is, "He has tremendous potential to be a great athlete." These pressures often direct the treating physician toward operative intervention to obtain a perfect alignment.

Are the Results Better with Operative Intervention?

Yes, for supracondylar humeral fractures.

The superiority of operative treatment of supracondylar fractures of the distal humerus was demonstrated in the report published in 1988 from Toronto, Canada, in which treatment in traction, treatment with a cast alone, and treatment with percutaneous pin fixation were compared (2). The worst results were in patients treated with only a cast. The best results were achieved in those stabilized with percutaneous pin fixation. The universal acceptance of percutaneous pin fixation of these fractures is evidence of the superiority of operative management.

Lower Readmission Rate

Cox and Clarke, in evaluating the fracture management in their hospital in Southampton, England, found a high incidence of secondary hospital treatment for fractures initially managed nonoperatively (3). There was a 12% readmission rate to correct late displacement of fractures of the radius and distal humerus. In addition, 24% of their internal fixation procedures were to salvage unacceptable results of nonoperative management. It was their conclusion that more selective initial operative intervention in radial and distal humeral fractures could decrease the incidence of costly readmissions to the hospital.

Changes from Previous Editions

The trend toward the establishment of surgical intervention can be seen in the changes in the previous editions of this textbook. In the first edition (4), very little mention was made regarding intramedullary fixation of either femoral or radial and ulnar shaft fractures. There was an extensive discussion of methods of traction for femoral shaft fractures and supracondylar fractures. In the fifth edition (5), the reverse was true. There was considerable discussion of intramedullary fixation and very little mention regarding traction techniques.

Phases in the Development of New Operative Techniques

Often, when a new procedure becomes widely used, there is an initial wave of enthusiasm for it. However, with more widespread use, problems become more apparent and modifications are made to the original technique. Thus, it takes a period of time before the technique becomes relatively complication free.

Problems with Specific Operative Techniques

Some of the specific problems that have occurred over the years are: (a) ulnar nerve injury with mediolateral pin fixation of supracondylar fractures (6), (b) high refracture rate with external fixation of femoral shaft fractures (7), and (c) avascular necrosis of the femoral head following the use of interlocking intramedullary nails inserted through the piriformis fossa (8,9).

In the following chapters of this textbook dealing with the specific fractures, the recent changes in operative technique or postoperative management to minimize the development of these problems are discussed.

Nonoperative Techniques Need to Be Maintained

Unfortunately, with this emphasis on operative management, the fact that most children's fractures can be managed by nonoperative techniques has become obscured. As a result, many recent orthopedic trainees are not developing good nonoperative technical skills.

Two articles demonstrated improved results of treating children's fractures by focusing on improvements in nonoperative methods. Chess et al (10) showed that when properly applied, a well-molded short arm cast provides just as good a result as a long arm cast in treating displaced fractures of the distal radial metaphysis. The key to success in using a short arm cast is in a careful molding of the cast at the fracture site so there is the proper cast index of 0.7 or less. Walker and Rang challenged traditional thinking by demonstrating that unstable fractures of the radius and ulna could be treated with a lower frequency of remanipulation if immobilized in elbow extension rather than flexion (11).

It is important to remember that most children's fractures still are treated by nonoperative methods. Therefore, in the present orthopedic training programs there needs to be a continued focus on developing and maintaining nonoperative skills in the treatment of children's fractures. The techniques of appropriate cast application and proper molding need to be preserved in the orthopedic curriculum.

THE PRESENT STATUS OF THE INCIDENCE OF FRACTURES IN CHILDREN

The incidence of children's fractures is extremely variable, depending on the child's age, the season of the year, cultural and environmental climates, and the hour of the day, just to name a few factors. As our culture changes from a primarily rural to an urban setting, the injury patterns may change as well. It is important to develop a general picture of how, when, and why fractures occur in children.

Incidence of Fractures

Earlier Studies Defined the Remodeling Processes

Early reviews primarily developed a knowledge base of fracture healing in children. In 1941, Beekman and Sullivan published an extensive review of the incidence of children's fractures (12). Their pioneering work—still quoted today—included a study of 2,094 long bone fractures seen over a 10-year period at Bellevue Hospital in New York City. The major purpose of their study was to develop basic principles for treating children's fractures.

In 1954, two reports, one by Hanlon and Estes (13) and the other by Lichtenberg (14), confirmed the findings of the previous studies with regard to the general incidence of children's long bone fractures and their ability to heal and readily remodel. These initial reviews were mainly statistical analyses and did not delve deeply into the true epidemiology of children's fractures. In 1965, Wong explored the effect of cultural factors on the incidence of fractures by comparing Indian, Malay, and Swedish children (15). In the 1970s, two other studies, one by Iqbal (16) and another by Reed (17), added more statistics regarding the incidence of the various long bone fractures.

Recent Studies Aimed at Developing Preventive Programs

Landin's 1983 report on 8,682 fractures established a trend in reviewing the incidence of children's fractures (18). He reviewed the data on all fractures in children that occurred in Malmo, Sweden, over 30 years, and examined the factors affecting the incidence of children's fractures. His study remains a landmark on this subject. By studying two populations, 30 years apart, he determined that fracture patterns were changing and the reasons for such changes. His initial goal was to establish data for preventive programs, so he focused on fractures that produced clean, concise, concrete data.

In 1997 Landin updated his work, reemphasizing the statistics from his previous publication (19). He suggested that the twofold increase in fracture rate during the 30 years from 1950 to 1979 in Malmo was due mainly to an increased participation in sports. In 1999, in cooperation with Tiderius and Duppe, Landin (20) studied the incidence in the same age group again in Malmo and found that the rate had actually declined by 9% in 1993 and 1994. The only exception was an increase of distal forearm fractures in girls, which he attributed to their increased participation in sporting events.

Cheng and Shen (21), in their 1993 study from Hong Kong, also set out to define children's fractures by separating the incidences into age groups. They tried to gather epidemiologic data on which to build preventive programs. In 1999 this study was expanded to include almost 6,500 fractures in children 16 and younger over a 10-year period (22). The fracture patterns changed little over those 10 years. What did change was the increased frequency of closed reduction and percutaneous pin fixation of fractures, with a corresponding decrease in open reductions. There also was a marked decrease in the hospital stay of their patients.

In short, the goals for studying children's fractures have changed over the past 60 years. Originally, the goal was to identify the most common bones fractured and how they heal. The goals of present studies are to gather data in an attempt to decrease the incidence of fractures by establishing preventive programs.

Defining the Incidence of Fractures

Variations

Cultural Differences. When one looks at the incidence of specific fractures within a well-defined group of children, the data usually are concise. However, when trying to obtain the global or general incidence of injury or fracture patterns for all types of children, there may be problems. For instance, Cheng and Shen studied children in Hong Kong who lived in confined high-rise apartments (21). Their risk of exposure to injury differed from the study by Reed of children living in the rural environment of Winnipeg, Canada (17). Two separate reviews by Laffoy (23) and Westfelt (24) found that children in a poor social environment (as defined by a lower social class or by dependence on public assistance) had more frequent accidents than more affluent children. In England, children from single-parent families were found to have higher accident and infection rates (25).

Two additional studies in the United Kingdom looked at the relationship of affluence to the incidence of fractures in children. Lyons et al (26) found no difference in the fracture rates of children in affluent population groups compared to those of children in nonaffluent families. On the other hand, Stark et al (27) in Scotland found that the fracture rate in children from nonaffluent social groups was significantly higher than those in affluent families. The differences in the findings may have been due to how their groups were defined as to their level of affluence.

Thus, in the domestic setting where there are many people on public assistance or where there is a higher incidence of disruption of family structure, *social* rather than *physical* factors may have more of an influence on the incidence of injuries.

Climatic Differences. The climate may be a strong factor as well. Children in colder climates, with ice and snow, are exposed to risks different from those of children living in warmer climates. The exposure time to outdoor activities may be greater for children who live in warmer climates. For example, the incidence of chronic overuse elbow injuries in young baseball players (Little League elbow) is far greater in the southern United States than in more northern communities. This is simply because there is greater playing or exposure time.

Difficulties in Comparing Fracture Studies

Defining Age Groups. Another problem with comparing studies is the definition of pediatric age groups. Some use 12 years as a cutoff age; others extend it to 16 or 20.

Inpatient versus Outpatient Studies. Some studies (28–30) report only children admitted to a hospital for fractures, which loads them toward the more serious injuries.

Anatomic Location. Reports vary in the precision of their defined types of fracture patterns. In the older series, reports were only of the long bone involved, such as the radius. More recent series have emphasized a more specific location, separating the radius, for example, into physeal, distal, shaft, and proximal fracture types.

Thus, in trying to define the exact incidence of fractures, it is difficult to compare series because of cultural, environmental, and age differences. In this section, these differences were considered in grouping the results and producing average figures. These data are presented in an attempt to provide a reasonable and accurate reflection of the overall incidence of injuries and fractures in all children.

Frequency of Childhood Fractures

Overall Incidence

In Landin's series from Malmo, Sweden, the chance of a child sustaining a fracture during childhood (birth to age 16) was 42% for boys and 27% for girls (18). When considered on an annual basis, 2.1% of all the children (2.6% for boys; 1.7% for girls) sustained at least one fracture each year. These figures were for all fracture types and included those treated on an inpatient basis and an outpatient basis. The overall chance of fracture per year was 1.6% for both girls and boys in a study from England of both outpatients and inpatients by Worlock and Stower (31).

The chance of a child sustaining a fracture severe enough to require inpatient treatment during the first 16 years of life is 6.8% (21). Thus, on an annual basis, 0.43% of the children in an average community will be admitted for a fracture-related problem during the year.

In a series of 23,915 patients seen at four major hospitals for injury-related complaints, 4,265 (17.8%) had fractures (13,24,28,32). Thus, close to 20% of the patients who present to hospitals with injuries have a fracture.

It is interesting to note that in a follow-up study by Tiderius, Landin, and Duppe (20) in the years 1993 and 1994, 13 years after the termination of the original 30-year study by Landin (18), there was an almost 10% decrease in the incidence of fractures in the 0- to 16-year age group. They attributed this to less physical activity on the part of modern-day children coupled with better protective sports equipment and increased traffic safety (e.g., stronger cars and use of auto restraint systems). The overall incidence of children's fractures is summarized in Table 1-1.

Age Groups

Fractures Show a Linear Increase with Age. Starting with birth and extending to age 12, all the major series that segregated patients by age have demonstrated a linear increase in the annual incidence of fractures with age (Fig. 1-1) (16,18,21,22, 31,33).

TABLE 1-1 Overall Frequency of Fractures

Percentage of children sustaining at least one fracture from 0 to 16 years of age: boys, 42%; girls, 27%

Percentage of children sustaining a fracture in 1 year: 1.6% to 2.1%

Percentage of patients with injuries (all types) who have fractures: 17.8%

Data from references 16,17,19,23,24,27,32,50,52

There seems to be a peak at 12 years, with some decrease until age 16, which is probably related to a significant decrease in the incidence of fractures in girls over age 12. The percentage of injured boys as compared with girls continues to increase in the older age groups.

Early, Soft Tissues Predominate. These fracture statistics differ slightly from the incidence of overall childhood injuries (i.e., all types including soft tissue and cerebral injuries), which peaks early at ages 1 to 2 years (Fig. 1-2) (23). Although there is a high incidence of injuries in children ages 1 to 2, the incidence of fractures is low. Most injuries in children of this age are nonorthopedic entities such as head injuries, lacerations, and

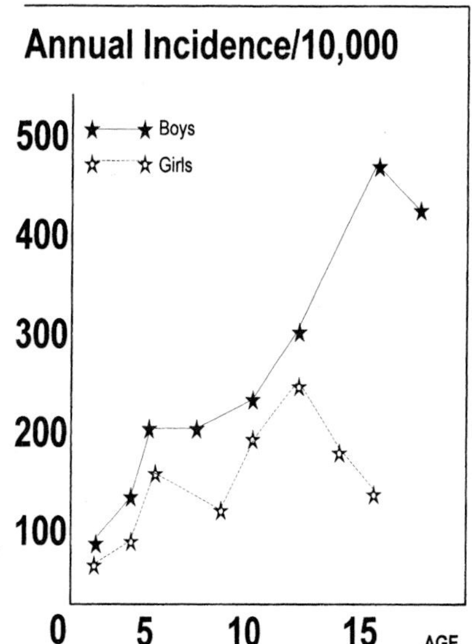

FIGURE 1-1 Incidence of fractures by age. Boys peak at 15 years while girls peak earlier, at 12 years, and then decline. (Reprinted from Landin LA. Fracture patterns in children. *Acta Orthop Scand* 1983;202:13; with permission.)

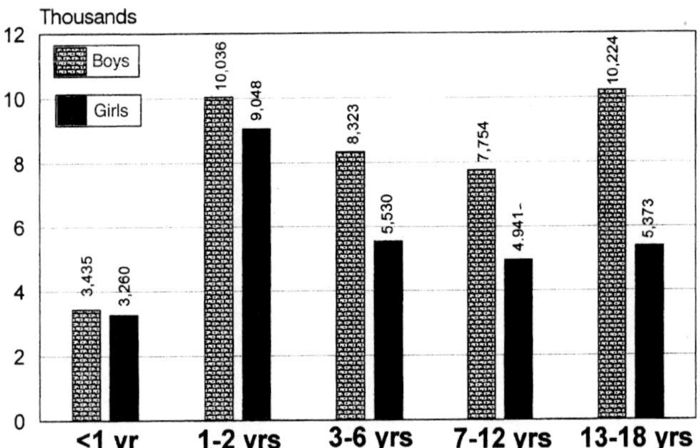

FIGURE 1-2 Injuries per 100,000 children per year. Estimated US injury rates in children by age and sex, 1978. (Reprinted from Rivara FP, Bergman AB, LoGerfo JP, et al. Epidemiology of childhood injuries. *Am J Dis Child* 1982;136:503; with permission.)

abrasions. In fact, the incidence of lacerations in both sexes peaks at this age (34).

Trauma

Nonaccidental. In 1962, Kempe et al (35) called attention to the frequency of fractures and other injuries in young children that were due to nonaccidental trauma. They termed these injuries part of the battered child syndrome. Arkbania et al later defined the specific fracture patterns seen in victims of child abuse (36). The high rate of fractures from nonaccidental trauma has been shown to extend to age 3 (37).

Not all fractures in the first year of life can be attributed to abuse. In a review of fractures occurring in the first year of life, McClelland and Heiple found that fully 44% were from documented accidental and nonabusive etiologies (38). They also noted that 23% of these patients had generalized conditions that predisposed them to fractures. Thus, although nonaccidental trauma remains the leading cause of fractures during the first year of life, other general and metabolic conditions may predispose children to fractures from accidental causes.

Gender

Males Predominate in Late Age Groups. The male predominance of injury and fracture victims has been discussed (Table 1-1; Figs. 1-1 and 1-2). For all age groups, the overall ratio of boys to girls who sustain a single fracture is 2.7:1 (21). In girls, fracture incidence peaks just before adolescence and then decreases during adolescence (17,18,21). In the 10-year study from Hong Kong by Chang et al (22), the male incidence in the 12- to 16-year age group was 83%. The incidence of fractures in girls steadily declined from their peak in the birth to 3-year age group.

In some areas there is little difference in the incidence of fractures between boys and girls. For example, during the first 2 years of life, the overall incidence of injuries and fractures in both genders is nearly equal. During these first 2 years, the injury rates for foreign body ingestion, poisons, and burns have no significant gender differences. With activities in which there is a male difference in participation, such as with sports equipment and bicycles, there is a marked increase in the incidence of injuries in boys (22,34).

Role of Behavior. The injury incidence may not be due to the rate of exposure alone; behavior may be a major factor. For example, one study found that the incidence of auto/pedestrian childhood injuries peaks in both sexes at ages 5 to 8 (39). When the total number of street crossings per day was studied, both sexes did so equally. Despite this equal exposure, boys had a higher number of injuries. Thus, the difference in the rate between the sexes begins to develop a male predominance when behaviors change. The difference in the injury rate between the genders may change in the future as more girls participate in activities with increased physical risk (22,34).

Right versus Left Frequency

In most series, the left upper extremity demonstrates a slight but significant predominance (13,16,18,21,22,34). The ratio of left to right overall averages 1.3:1. In some fractures, however, especially those of supracondylar bones, lateral condyles, and the distal radius, the incidence is far greater, increasing to as much as 2.3:1 for the lateral condyle. In the lower extremity, the incidence of injury on the right side is slightly increased (13,18).

The reasons for the predominance of the left upper extremity have been studied, but no definite answers have been found. Rohl (40) speculated that the right upper extremity often is being used actively during the injury, so the left assumes the role of protection. In a study examining the left-sided predominance in the upper extremity, Mortensson and Thonell (41) questioned patients and their parents on arrival to the emergency department about which arm was used for protection and the position of the fractured extremity at the time of the accident. They found two trends: regardless of handedness, the left arm was used more often to break the fall, and when exposed to trauma, the left arm was more likely to be fractured.

Frequency by Season

Summertime Increase. Fractures are more common during the summer, when children are out of school and exposed to more vigorous physical activities (Fig. 1-3). Five studies from the northern hemisphere have confirmed this summertime increase (21,22,31,40,42).

Hours of Sunshine. The most consistent climatic factor appears to be the number of hours of sunshine. Masterson et al (43), in an eloquent study from Ireland, found a strong positive correlation between monthly sunshine hours and monthly fracture admissions. There also was a weak negative correlation with monthly rainfall. Overall, the average number of fractures in

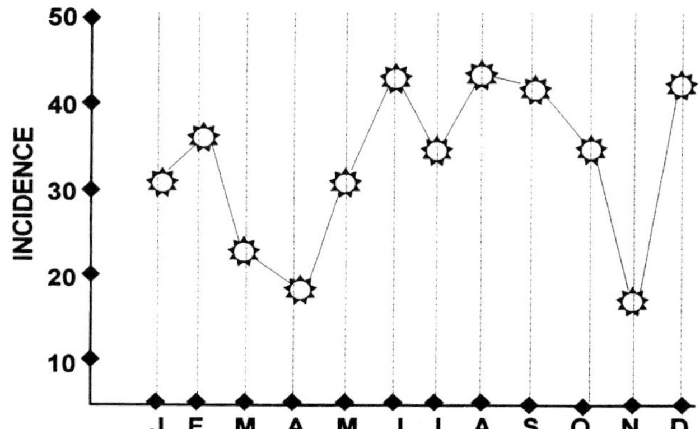

FIGURE 1-3 Distribution of children's fractures on a monthly basis. Note the general increase from May to October. (Reprinted from Reed MH. Fractures and dislocations of the extremities in children. *J Trauma* 1977; 17:353; with permission.)

the summer was 2.5 times that in the winter. In days with more sunshine hours than average, the average fracture admission rate was 2.31 per day; on days with fewer sunshine hours than average, the admission rate was 1.07 per day.

In Sweden, the incidence of fractures in the summer had a bimodal pattern that seemed to be influenced by cultural traditions. In two large series of both accidents and fractures in Sweden by Westfelt (24) and Landin (18), the researchers noticed increases in May and September and significant decreases in June, July, and August. Both writers attributed this to the fact that children in their region left the cities to spend the summer in the countryside. Thus, the decrease in the overall fracture rate probably was due to a decrease in the number of children at risk remaining in the city.

Masterson et al (43) speculated that because the rate of growth increases during the summer, the number of physeal fractures should also increase, as the physes would be weaker during this time. For example, the incidence of slipped capital femoral epiphysis, which is related to physeal weakness, increases during the summer (44). However, Landin, in his study of more than 8,000 fractures of all types, found the overall seasonal incidence of physeal injuries to be exactly the same as nonphyseal injuries (18).

Age may affect the seasonal variation of fractures. In children ages 0 to 3, no seasonal variations are seen. The number of fractures in this age group was consistent throughout the year (37).

Younger Age Groups Unaffected. Thus, it appears that climate, especially in areas where there are definite seasonal variations, influences the incidence of fractures in all children, especially in older children. However, in small children and infants, whose activities are not seasonally dependent, there appears to be no significant seasonal influence.

Time of Day

The time of day in which children are most active seems to correlate with the peak time for fracture occurrence. In Sweden, the incidence peaked between 2 and 3 PM (24). In a well-documented study from Texas by Shank et al (30), the hourly incidence of fractures formed a well-defined bell curve peaking at about 6 PM (Fig. 1-4).

Long-Term Trends

Increase in Minor Trauma. Landin's study is the only one that has compared the changes over a significant time span: his data were collected over 30 years (18). He classified the degree of trauma as slight, moderate, or severe. The incidence of all trauma in both boys and girls increased significantly over the 30-year study period, but the incidence of severe trauma increased only slightly. The greatest increase was seen in the "slight" category. Landin attributed the increase in this category to the introduction of subsidized medical care. Because expense was not a factor, parents were more inclined in the later years of the study to seek medical attention for relatively minor complaints. Physicians, likewise, were more inclined to order x-rays. Thus, many of the minor injuries, such as torus fractures, which were often ignored in the earlier years, were seen more often at medical facilities during the later years.

Likewise, the overall incidence of fractures in Malmo, Sweden, (the same city as Landin's original study) (18) significantly had decreased (10%) in the more recent years (20).

The one fracture type that exhibited a true increase over this period was that of the femoral shaft. This increase was thought to be influenced by new types of play activities and increased participation in sports.

Increase in Child Abuse. The number of fractures due to nonaccidental causes (child abuse) has risen consistently in the past

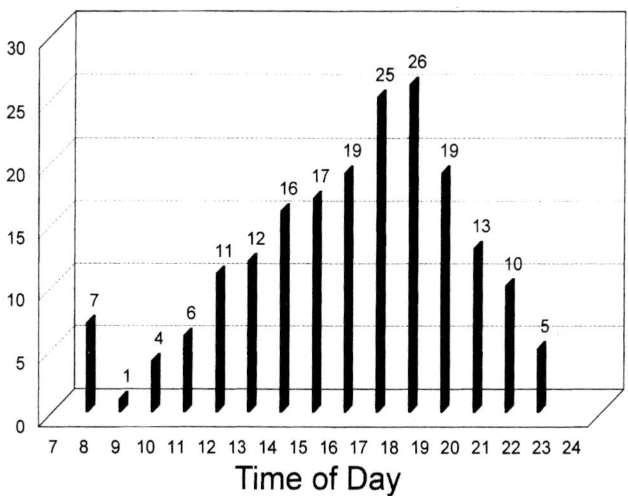

FIGURE 1-4 Incidence of children's fractures per time of day. There is an almost bell-shaped curve with a peak at around 6 PM. (Reprinted from Shank LP, Bagg RJ, Wagnon J. Etiology of pediatric fractures: the fatigue factors in children's fractures. Presented at the National Conference on Pediatric Trauma, Indianapolis, 1992; with permission.)

decades. In the study of fractures in children ages birth to 3 years old by Kowal-Vern et al (37), the number of fractures due to abuse increased almost 150 times from 1984 to 1989. This increase was attributed to a combination of improved recognition, better social resources, and a true increase in the number of cases of child abuse.

Incidences by Specific Fracture Categories

Age Variations

The anatomic areas most often fractured seem to be the same in the major series, but these rates change with age. For example, supracondylar fractures of the humerus are most common in the first decade, with a peak at age 7. Fractures of the femur are most common in children ages 0 to 3. Fractures of the physis are more common just before skeletal maturity. This variation is best illustrated in Cheng and Shen's data (Fig. 1-5) (21).

Landin's Age Patterns

Landin found a similar age variability and divided it into six distinct patterns (Fig. 1-6) (18). When he compared these variability patterns with the common etiologies, he found some correlation. For example, late-peak fractures (distal forearm, phalanges, proximal humerus) were closely correlated with sports and equipment etiologies. Bimodal pattern fractures (clavicle, femur, radioulnar, diaphyses) showed an early increase from lower energy trauma, then a late peak in incidence due to injury from high- or moderate-energy trauma. Early peak fractures (supracondylar humeral fractures are a classic example) were due mainly to falls from high levels.

Locations

Early reports of children's fractures lumped together the areas fractured, and fractures were reported only as to the long bone involved (e.g., radius, humerus, femur) (12–14,16,29,). More recent reports have split fractures into the more specific areas of the long bone involved (e.g., the distal radius, the radial neck, the supracondylar area of the humerus) (16–18,21,31). This change in reporting—from the so-called "lumpers" to the "splitters"—has produced a more accurate picture of the true incidence of each specific fracture type.

Single Bones

In children, fractures in the upper extremity are much more common than those in the lower extremity (13,16). Overall, the radius is the most commonly fractured long bone, followed by the humerus. In the lower extremity, the tibia is more commonly fractured than the femur (Table 1-2).

Specific Areas Fractured

In recent years, five reports produced by so-called splitters divided fracture types into many anatomic areas (16–18,21,31). In trying to reach a global consensus, the author has identified areas common to all the reports but has taken some liberties to do so. For example, distal radial metaphyseal and physeal fractures were combined to form the distal radius. Likewise, the carpals, metacarpals, and phalanges were combined to form the region of the hand and wrist. All the fractures around the elbow, from those of the radial neck to supracondylar fractures, were grouped as elbow fractures. This grouping allows comparison of the regional incidence of specific fracture types in children (Table 1-3).

The individual reports agreed that the most common area fractured was the distal radius. The next most common area, however, varied from the hand in Landin's series (18) to the elbow (mainly supracondylar fractures) in Cheng and Shen's series (21,22).

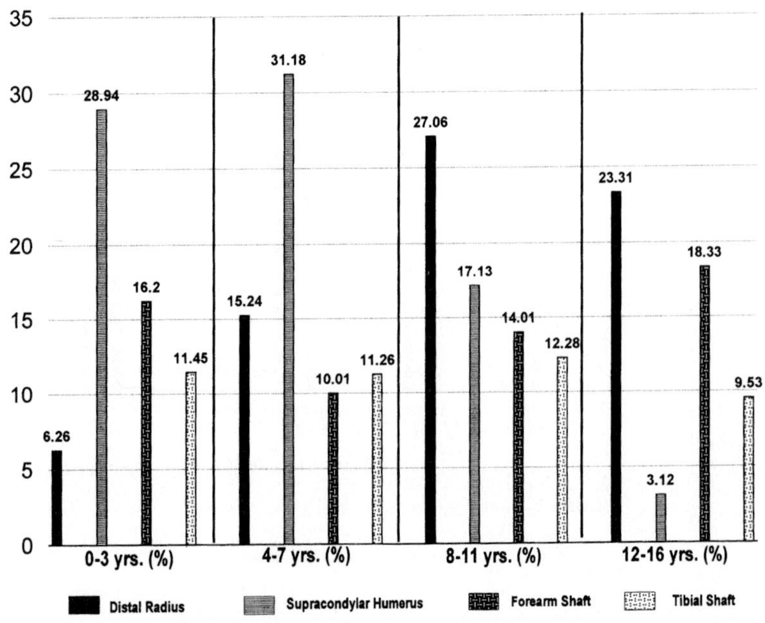

FIGURE 1-5 The frequency of occurrence of the most common fracture areas in children. The frequency of each fracture pattern differs with the various age groups. The figures express the percentage of total fractures for that age group and represent boys and girls combined. (Reprinted from Cheng JC, Shen WY. Limb fracture pattern in different pediatric age groups: a study of 3,350 children. *J Orthop Trauma* 1993; 7:17; with permission.)

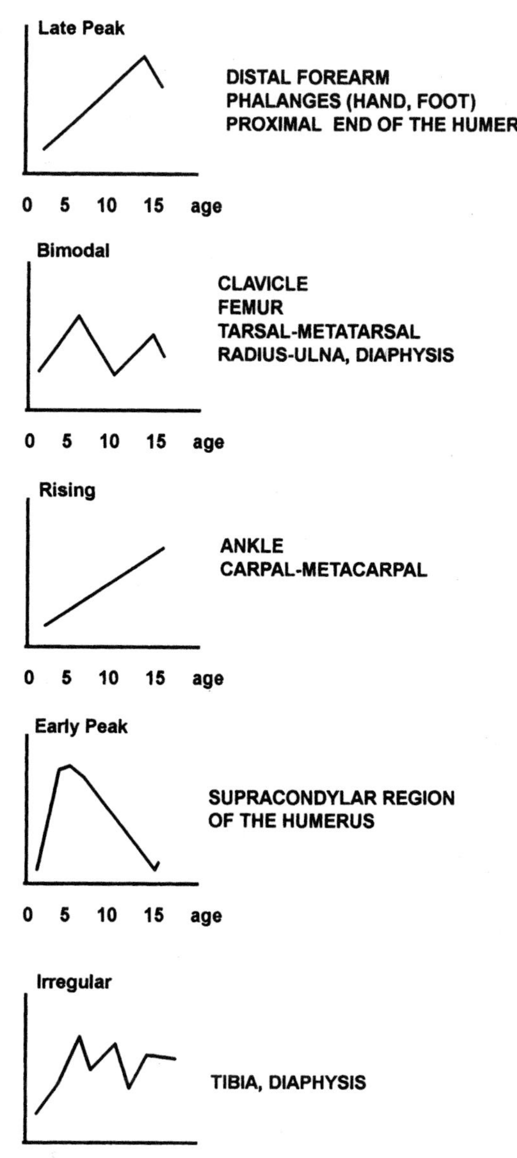

FIGURE 1-6 Patterns of fracture: variations with age. The peak ages for the various fracture types occur in one of five patterns. (Reprinted from Landin LA. Fracture patterns in children. *Acta Orthop Scand* 1983;202: 73; with permission.)

Physeal Injuries

The incidence of physeal injuries overall varied from 14.5% (45) to a high of 27.6% (46). To obtain an overall incidence of physeal fractures, six reports totaling 6,479 fractures in children were combined (17,31,45–48). In this group, 1,404 involved the physis, producing an average overall incidence of 21.7% for physeal fractures (Table 1-4).

Open Fractures

The overall incidence of open fractures in children is consistent. The data were combined from the four reports in which the incidence of open fractures was reported (13,21,31,46). The incidence in these reports varied from 1.5% to 2.6%. Combined, these reports represented a total of 8,367 fractures with 246 open fractures, resulting in an average incidence of 2.9% (Table 1-5).

Regional trauma centers often see patients exposed to more severe trauma, so there may be a higher incidence of open frac-

TABLE 1-2 Incidence of Fractures in Long Bones

Bone	%
Radius	45.1
Humerus	18.4
Tibia	15.1
Clavicle	13.8
Femur	7.6

Data from references 14,23,25,34,35,40.

TABLE 1-3 Incidence of Specific Fracture Types

Fracture	%
Distal radius and physis	23.3
Hand (carpals, metacarpals, and phalanges)	20.1
Elbow area (distal humerus and proximal radius and ulna)	12.0
Clavicle	6.4
Radius shaft	6.4
Tibia shaft	6.2
Foot (metatarsals and phalanges)	5.9
Ankle (distal tibia)	4.4
Femur (neck and shaft)	2.3
Humerus (proximal and shaft)	1.4
Other	11.6

Data from references 19,25,32,42,52.

TABLE 1-4 Incidence of Physeal Fracutres

Total fractures = 6,477

Number of physeal injuries = 1,404

Percentage of physeal injuries = 21.7%

Data from references 15,20,37,40,42,52.

TABLE 1-6 Incidence of Multiple Fractures

Total fractures = 5,262

Total number of multiple fractures = 192

Percentage = 3.6%

Data from references 19,23,25,52.

tures in these patients. The incidence of open fractures was 9% in a report of patients admitted to the trauma center of the Children's National Medical Center, Washington, DC. (28).

Multiple Fractures

Multiple fractures in children are uncommon: the incidence ranges in the various series from 1.7% to as much as 9.7%. In four major reports totaling 5,262 patients, 192 patients had more than one fracture (Table 1-6) (13,16,21,31). The incidence in this multiple series was 3.6%.

Fractures in Weak Bones

Children with generalized bone dysplasias and metabolic diseases that produce osteopenia (such as osteogenesis imperfecta) are expected to have recurrent fractures. In these patients, the etiology is understandable and predictable. However, some children with normal osseous structures are prone to recurrent fractures for reasons that remain unclear. The incidence of recurrent fractures in children is about 1% (49).

Landin and Nilsson (50) found that children who sustained fractures with relatively little trauma had a lower mineral content in their forearms, but they could not correlate this finding with subsequent fractures. Thus, in children who seem to be structurally normal, there does not appear to be a physical reason for their recurrent fractures.

Repeat Fractures

Failure to find a physical cause for repeat fractures shifts the focus to a psychological or social cause. The one common factor in accident repeaters has been a high incidence of dysfunctional families (51). In Sweden, Westfelt found that children who were accident repeaters came from "socially handicapped" families (i.e., those on public assistance or those with a caregiver who was an alcoholic) (24). Thus, repeat fractures are probably due more to behavioral or social causes than physical causes. Landin, in his follow-up article (19), followed children with repeat fractures (four or more) into adolescence and adulthood. He found these children had a significantly increased incidence of convictions for serious criminal offenses when compared with children with only one lifetime fracture.

TABLE 1-5 Incidence of Open Fractures

Total number of fractures = 8,367

Total open fractures = 246

Percentage = 2.9%

Data from references 23,28,37,52.

ETIOLOGY OF FRACTURES

Studies Essential for Prevention

While studying the epidemiology of fractures, it is important to focus on the etiology of fractures and the settings in which they occur. In this age of computerized gizmos and the "need for speed," children often are the victims of the consumer market and unsafe products. Fractures do not occur in a vacuum, and well-researched studies that analyze the physical and social environment in which they occur are extremely valuable. It is a truism that children, unfortunately, learn more from experience than by education, so efforts should be made toward creating a safer environment for play and recreation. Studies that identify risky patterns of use or unsafe playground behavior go a long way in directing specific preventive health measures. Recommendations can be made to manufacturers regarding modification of a product, and education can be imparted to parents, school authorities, health-care professionals, physical trainers, and children.

Three Broad Causes

Broadly, fractures have three main causes: (*a*) *accidental trauma*, (*b*) *nonaccidental injury (child abuse), and* (*c*) *pathologic conditions.* Accidental trauma forms the largest etiologic group. Nonaccidental trauma and fractures resulting from pathologic conditions are discussed in later chapters of this book.

Fractures Resulting from Accidental Trauma

Accidental trauma can occur in a variety of settings, some often overlapping others. However, for purposes of simplicity, fractures can be considered to occur in the following five environments: (a) home environment, (b) school environment, (c) play and recreational activities, (d) motor vehicle and road accidents, and (e) uncommon causes such as ice cream truck, water tubing, and gunshot and missile injuries.

Home Environment

Fractures sustained in the home environment are defined as those that occur in the house and surrounding vicinity. These generally occur in a fairly supervised environment and are mainly due to falls from furniture, stairs, fences, and trees.

Falls from Heights. Falls can vary in severity from a simple fall while running, to a fall of great magnitude, such as from a third story window. In falling from heights, adults often land on their lower extremities, accounting for the high number of lower extremity fractures, especially the calcaneus. Children tend to fall head first, using the upper extremities to break the fall. This accounts for the larger number of skull and radial fractures in children. Femoral fractures also are common in children falling from great heights. In contrast to adults, spinal fractures are rare in children who fall from great heights (52–55).

In one study, children falling three stories or less all survived. Falls from the fifth or sixth floor resulted in a 50% mortality rate (52).

Injury Rate Increases with Age. Injuries also can occur from the unsupervised use of unsafe play equipment, such as trampolines and monkey bars, within the home environment and are considered in detail later. The overall incidence of fractures occurring because of such play activity in the home environment increases with age. Only 15% occur in toddlers, but 56% occur during older years (56).

Social Factors. Interestingly, a Swedish study (57) showed that an increased incidence of fractures in a home environment did not necessarily correlate with the physical attributes or poor safety precautions of the house. Rather, it implicated disruption of the family structure and presence of social handicaps (alcoholism, welfare recipients, etc.) as the true cause for the increase.

School Environment

The supervised environments at school generally are safe, and the overall annual rate of injury (total percentage of children injured in a single year) in the school environment ranges from 2.8% to 9.2% (57–60). True rates may be higher because of inaccurate reporting, especially of mild injuries. In one series, the official rate was 5.6%, but when the parents were closely questioned, the incidence of unreported, trivial injuries was as much as 15% (61). The annual fracture rate of school injuries is low. Of all injuries sustained by children at school in a year, only 5% to 10% involved fractures (59–61). In Worlock and Stower's series of children's fractures from England (56), only 20% occurred at school. A large incidence of injuries (53%) occurring in school are related to athletics and sporting events (59). These injuries are highest in the middle-school children. The peak time of day for injuries at school is in the morning, which differs from the injury patterns of children in general (59).

Play and Recreational Activities

Playground Equipment. Play is an essential element of a child's life. It enhances physical development and fosters social interaction. Noncompetitive sports and recreational activities are enjoyed by all children. Unfortunately, unsupervised or careless use of some play equipment can endanger life and limb. When Mott et al (62) studied the incidence and pattern of injuries to children using public playgrounds; they found that approximately 1% of children using playgrounds sustained injuries. Sixty-five percent of these children were injured by falling from equipment such as climbing frames, slides, swings, and monkey bars. They found that changing playground surfaces from concrete to more impact-absorbing surfaces such as bark reduced the incidence and severity of head injury but increased the tendency for long bone fractures (40%), bruises, and sprains. The correlation of the hardness of the playground surface with the risk of injury has been confirmed in other studies (63,64) Public playgrounds appear to have a higher risk for injuries than private playgrounds, because they usually have harder surfaces and higher pieces of equipment (65).

Swings, climbers, and slides are the pieces of playground equipment associated with 88% of the playground injuries (66).

In a study of injuries resulting from playground equipment, Waltzman et al (67) found that most injuries occurred in boys (56%) with a peak incidence in the summer months. Fractures accounted for 61% of these injuries, 90% of which involved the upper extremity and were sustained in falls from playground equipment such as monkey bars and climbing frames. Younger children (1 to 4 years old) were more likely to sustain fractures than older children. In their study, the surface below the equipment apparently did not influence the type or severity of fracture; with 30 of the 79 fractures occurring on "soft surfaces." Chalmers et al (68) determined the height of the equipment was just as great a risk factor as the surface composition.

Similar observations were made in a study by Lillis and Jaffe (69) in which upper extremity injuries, especially fractures, accounted for most of hospitalizations resulting from injuries on playground equipment. Older children sustained more injuries on climbing apparatus, whereas younger children sustained more injuries on slides.

In a study looking specifically at injuries from monkey bars the peak age group was the 5 through 12-year-old group, with supracondylar humeral fractures being the most common fracture sustained (70).

Newer Play Devices. Other recreational activities enjoyed by children, such as bicycling, skating, skateboarding, and sledding, are important causes of fractures and injuries in children. Several studies have analyzed the incidence and pattern of injuries arising from the unsupervised or careless use of this equipment and have suggested safety precautions and equipment modification to decrease the risk of injury. A disturbing trend is the rekindled enthusiasm toward the use of trampolines, skateboards, and in-line skates over the past decade, and several studies have highlighted their risks and dangers.

Bicycle Injuries. Bicycle injuries are a significant cause of mortality and morbidity for children (71). Bicycle mishaps are the most common causes of serious head injury in children (72). Boys in the 5- to 14-year age group are at greatest risk for bicycle injury (80%). Puranik et al (71) studied the profile of pediatric bicycle injuries in a sample of 211 children who were treated for bicycle-related injury at their trauma center over a 4-year period. They found that bicycle injuries accounted for 18% of all pediatric trauma patients. Bicycle/motor vehicle collisions caused 86% of injuries. Sixty-seven percent had head injuries and 29% sustained fractures. More than half of the incidents occurred on the weekend. Sixteen percent were injured by ejection from a bicycle after losing control, hitting a pothole, or colliding with a fixed object or another bicycle. Fractures mainly involved the lower extremity, upper extremity, skull, ribs, and pelvis in decreasing order of incidence.

Helmet Use Low. More importantly, the study detected that the use of safety helmets was disturbingly low (<2%). Other studies confirm the observation that fewer than 13% to 15% of children wear helmets while riding bicycles (73,74). The Year 2000 Health Objectives called for helmet use by 50% of bicyclists (75). Even as recent as 2003 the use of bicycle helmets was still below 20% (76). Research has shown that legislation, combined with education and helmet subsidies, is the most effective strategy to increase use of safety helmets in child bicyclists (77). As public awareness of both the severity and preventability of bicycle-related injuries grows, the goal of safer bicycling practices and lower injury rates can be achieved (71).

Bicycle spokes and handle bars also are responsible for many fractures and soft tissue injuries in children. D'Souza et al (78) and Segers et al (79) found that bicycle spoke injuries are typically sustained when the child's foot is caught in the spokes of the rotating wheel.

Injuries from Bicycle Parts. Of 130 children with bicycle spoke injuries, 29 children sustained fractures of the tibia, fibula, or foot bone. Several had lacerations and soft tissue defects. D'Souza et al (78) suggested that a mesh cover to prevent the toes from entering between the spokes and a plastic shield to bridge the gap between the fork and horizontal upright can substantially decrease the incidence of these injuries.

Skateboarding. Skateboarding and in-line skating have experienced a renewed surge in popularity over the past three decades. With the increasing number of participants, high-tech equipment development and vigorous advertising, skateboard and skating injuries are expected to increase. There was an initial increase in the early 1980s with a decrease after 1993. Since 1998, there has been an increase in the number of skateboard injuries (80). Because the nature of skateboarding encompasses both high speed and extreme maneuvers, high-energy fractures and other injuries can occur, as highlighted by several studies (81–83). Studies have shown that skateboarding-related injuries are more severe and have more serious consequences than roller-skating or in-line skating injuries (82). In a study of skateboarding injuries, Fountain et al (81) found that fractures of the upper or lower extremity accounted for 50% of all skateboarding injuries. Interestingly, more than one third of those injured sustained injuries within the first week of skateboarding. Most injuries occurred in preadolescent boys (75%) 10 to 16 years of age. Despite traffic legislation, 65% sustained injuries on public roads, footpaths, and parking lots. Several reports (81,84) have recommended safety guidelines and precautions such as use of helmets, knee and elbow pads, and wrist guards, but such regulations seldom are enforced.

Roller Skates and In-Line Skates

Most Injuries Involve the Upper Extremity. In a study of in-line skate and roller skate injuries in childhood, Jerosch et al (85) found that in a group of 1,036 skaters, 60% had sustained injuries. Eight percent of these were fractures, mostly involving the elbow, forearm, wrist, and fingers (78%). Fewer than 20% used protective devices, and most lacked knowledge of the basic techniques of skating, braking, and falling. In a larger study of 60,730 skating injuries in children, Powell and Tanz (83) found that 68% of the children were preadolescent boys with a mean age of 11.8 years. Fractures were the most common injury (65%) and two thirds of these involved the distal forearm. Two and a half percent required hospital admissions; 90% of these admissions were for a fracture. Similarly, Mitts and Hennrikus (86) found that 75% of in-line skating fractures in children occurred in the distal forearm as a result of falls on the outstretched hand. One in eight children sustained a fracture during the first attempt at the sport. The orthopedic community has an obligation to educate the public on the need for wearing wrist guards when using in-line skates or roller skates.

Skate Parks Actually Increase the Injury Rate. It was thought that formal skate parks could decrease the injury rate. However, a study by Sheehan et al (87) demonstrated that dedicated skate parks led to an increase in pediatric fractures referred to the hospital. The authors suggested that there should be closer supervision and training of children and more emphasis on limb protective gear.

Inline Scooters. Since 2000, a substantial increase in injuries related to nonmotorized scooters (kickboards) has been observed among children. Most of the scooter-related accidents were caused by the wheels of the scooter getting caught by uneven ground, whereas most skateboard accidents occurred during attempted trick maneuvers. Protective gear was seldom used (88–90). Scooters seem to have a high incidence of collisions with motor vehicles (89). The recent motorizing of the scooters will only increase the severity of the injuries sustained.

It has been this author's experience that scooters produce unique injuries in the forearm. When the scooter suddenly stops, the rider is thrown forward over the handlebars. As a result, the rider strikes the ground on the dorsum of the wrists producing a volar displacement of the distal radius and ulna.

Trampoline-Related Injuries. Trampolines enjoyed increasing popularity in the 1990s and are a significant cause of morbidity in children. Several studies have noted a dramatic increase in the number of pediatric trampoline injuries (PTIs) during the past 10 years, rightfully deeming it as a "national epidemic" (91,92). Furnival et al (91), in a retrospective study of PTIs over a 7-year period, found that the annual number of PTIs tripled between 1990 and 1997. In contrast to other recreational activities in which males constitute the population at risk, PTI patients were predominantly female, with a median age of 7 years. Nearly a third of the injuries resulted from falling off the trampoline. Fractures of the upper and lower extremities occurred in 45% and were more frequently associated with falls off the trampoline. In another excellent study on PTIs, Smith (92) found that there was virtually a 100% increase in injuries from 1990 to 1995, with an average of more than 60,000 injuries per year. Younger children had a higher incidence of upper extremity fractures and other injuries. In a later study, Smith and Shields (93) came up with some interesting data. Fractures, especially involving the upper extremity, accounted for 35% of all injuries. Interestingly, more than 50% of the injuries occurred under direct adult supervision. More disturbingly, 73% of the parents were aware of the potential dangers of trampolines, and 96% of the injuries occurred in the home backyard. These researchers, along with others (91), rightly concluded that use of warning labels, public education, and even direct adult supervision were inadequate in preventing these injuries and have called for a total ban on the recreational, school, and competitive use of trampolines by children (92,93).

Skiing Injuries. In a study of major skiing injuries in children and adolescents, Shorter et al (94) found more than 90% of injured children were boys 5 to 18 years of age. Sixty percent of the accidents occurred in collisions with stationary objects such as trees, poles, and stakes. Most injuries occurred in the afternoon, among beginners, and in the first week of skiing season. Fractures accounted for one third of the total injuries sustained. The two main factors implicated in skiing injuries are excessive speed and loss of control; effective prevention efforts should target both of these factors.

Snowboarding Injuries. Snowboarding runs a similar risk to skiing. Bladin et al (95) found that approximately 60% of snowboarding injuries involved the lower limbs and occurred in novices. The most common injuries were sprains (53%) and fractures (26%). Compared with skiers, snowboarders had $2\frac{1}{2}$ times as many fractures, particularly to the upper limb, as well as more ankle injuries such as sprains. The absence of ski poles and the fixed position of the feet on the snowboard mean that the upper limbs absorb the full impact of any fall. A recent study (96) has shown that the use of wrist braces can decrease the incidence of wrist injuries in snowboarding.

Motor Vehicle Accidents

This category includes injuries sustained by occupants of a motor vehicle and victims of vehicle-versus-pedestrian accidents.

The injury patterns of children involved in motor vehicle accidents differ from those of adults. In all types of motor vehicle accidents for all ages, children constitute a little over 10% of the total number of patients injured (90,97). Of all the persons injured as motor vehicle occupants, only about 17% to 18% are children. Of the victims of vehicle-versus-pedestrian accidents, about 29% are children. Of the total number of children involved in motor vehicle accidents, 56.4% were vehicle-versus-pedestrian accidents, and 19.6% were vehicle-versus-bicycle accidents (98).

The fracture rate of children in motor vehicle accidents is less than that of adults. Of the total number of vehicle-versus-pedestrian accidents, about 22% of the children sustained fractures; 40% of the adults sustained fractures in the same type of accident. This has been attributed to the fact that children are more likely to "bounce" when hit (98).

Children are twice as likely as adults to sustain a femoral fracture when struck by an automobile, but in adults, tibial and knee injuries are more common in the same type of accident. This seems to be related to where the car's bumper strikes the victim (99,100). Motor vehicle accidents do produce a high proportion of spinal and pelvic injuries (99).

The etiologic aspects of children's fractures are summarized in Figure 1-7 and Table 1-7.

Less Common Etiologies

Ice Cream Truck

Mubarak et al (101) described ice cream truck–related accidents in which children, distracted by ice cream trucks, were struck by an oncoming vehicle, sustaining pelvic and lower limb fractures. The vision of oncoming drivers was often blocked by the large size of the ice cream truck parked by the curb.

Water Tubing

Parmar et al (102) reported serious injuries sustained during water tubing (the pulling of an inner tube behind a power boat).

Gunshot (Missile) Wounds: Definition

Gunshot or missile wounds arise from objects projected into space by an explosive device. The missiles may be single or

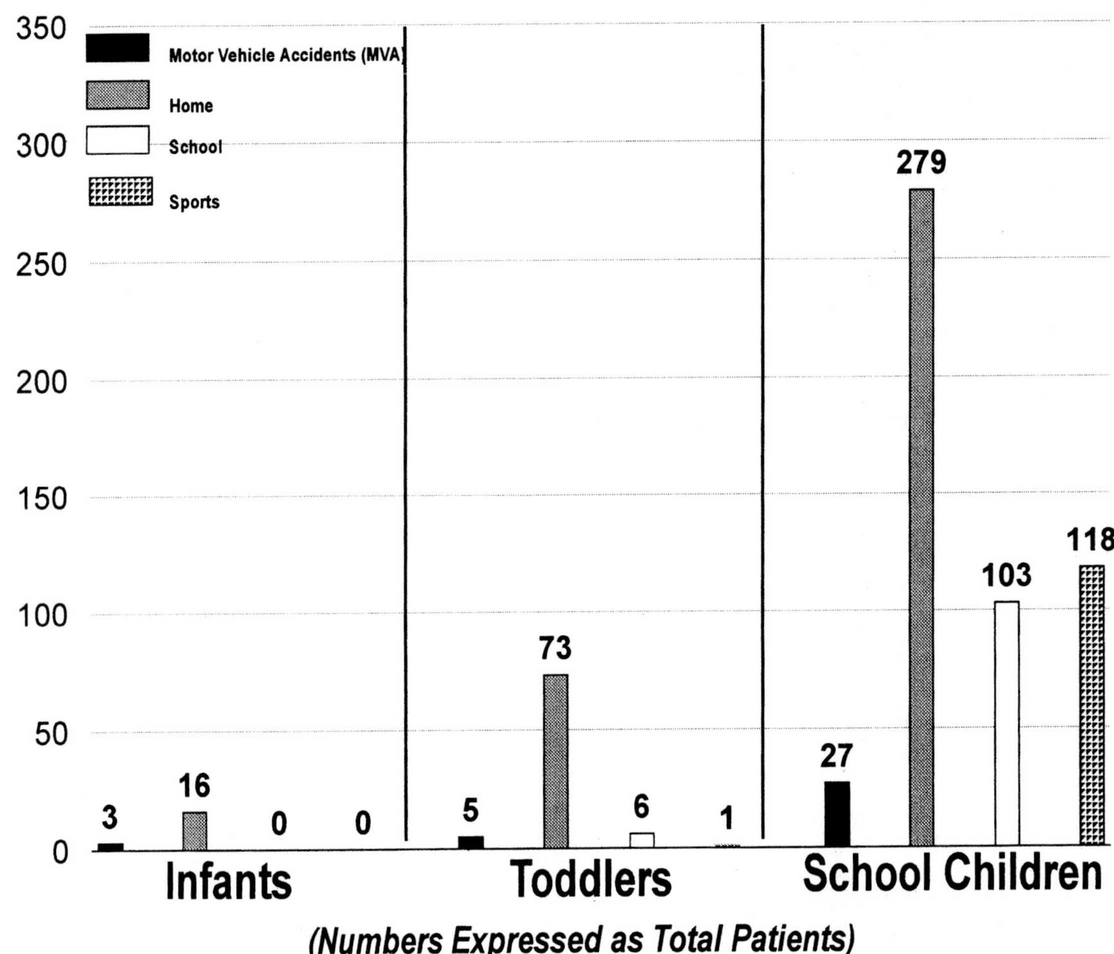

FIGURE 1-7 The incidence of fractures in children expressed as the four common etiologic categories. Most fractures occur at home. The numbers are expressed as total patients per each age category. (Reprinted from Worlock P, Stower M. Fracture patterns in Nottingham children. *J Pediatr Orthop* 1986;6:656; with permission.)

multiple. Single missiles vary from low-velocity handguns to high-velocity assault weapons. Multiple missiles can result from a shotgun blast or shrapnel from war weapons. Missile injuries represent open fractures with varying degrees of soft tissue injury. Gunshot wounds have become increasingly common in children in the United States (103).

Gunshot and Firearm Injuries

In a sad reflection of the changing times and the newly pervasive gun culture, firearms are determined to be second only to motor vehicles as the leading cause of death in youths. In considering the prevalence of firearms in the United States, it has been estimated that there are about 200 million privately owned guns in the United States and that approximately 40% of US households contain firearms of some type (104).

Etiology. In two reports from inner-city hospitals in the United States in the 1990s, most injuries resulted from random violence to innocent bystanders; the prime example was "drive-by shootings" (103,105). Few were self-inflicted, either voluntarily or accidentally. In a 1976 report on patients in a relatively rural setting in Canada, almost all the missile injuries were accidental, having been caused by the patient or a close friend or relative (106).

In the urban setting, handguns and rifles are the most common weapons (103,105,107). In the rural setting, the most common weapon is a shotgun (106). The firepower of these weapons has changed over the years. In one urban hospital reporting gunshot wounds from 1973 to 1983, most of the injuries were from .32- or .38-caliber weapons; only 5% were high-caliber or high-velocity weapons (108). In a later study of gunshot wounds from the same institution from 1991 to 1994, the incidence of injuries from high-caliber and high-velocity weapons (e.g., .357 magnum, AK-47, and other assault rifles) had increased to 35% (94).

In the urban setting, the victims' ages ranged from 1 to 17

TABLE 1-7 Summary of Etiologic Factors in Children's Fractures

Home environment

Injuries

83% of all children's injuries

Fractures

37% of all children's fractures

School environment

Injuries

Overall rate, 2.8% to 9.2% annually

53% related to athletic events

Peak age: middle-school group

Fractures

Occur in only 5% to 10% of all school-related injuries

About 20% of all children's fractures

Motor vehicle accidents (MVA)

Injuries

Children only 10% of all MVAs

Of children's MVAs, only 17% to 18% were occupants; remainder were vehicle/pedestrian or vehicle/bicycle

Fractures

High incidence of femur fractures in vehicle pedestrian accidents in children

Children have a higher incidence of spinal and pelvic fractures with MVAs than with other mechanisms

years, and most of the injuries were in children 12 to 14 (103,105,107,108). In the rural setting, the patients were younger; the average age was 9 years (106).

Of 839 children sustaining gunshot wounds, 274 (32.6%) involved the extremities (103,105,107,108). Of the gunshot wounds that involved the extremities, 51.3% produced significant fractures (103,105,106). No single bone seemed to predominate, although most of the fractures were distal to the elbow (103,105,107,108).

Complications. The two most common complications were growth arrest and infection. Other complications included delayed union and malunion. Considering the magnitude of many of these injuries, the infection rate for extremity wounds was low (about 7.3%). This low rate was probably due to a vigorous and aggressive program of acute wound management (103,105,106). The type of missile did not seem to have any relation to the development of an infection (103).

In Letts and Miller's 1976 series, one sixth of the patients had some type of growth disturbance (106). In a third of their patients, the missile was only in close proximity to the physis. In a 1995 report by Washington et al, the incidence of missiles affecting the physis was exactly the same (103). However, all were a result of a direct injury to the physis by the missile. None of their patients with growth arrest had proximity missile wounds. The higher incidence of growth abnormalities in the 1976 series was due to the larger number of shotgun and hunting rifle injuries, which dissipate more of their energy peripheral to the missile track.

In two of the studies in which patients were followed closely, all of the fractures ultimately healed (103,106).On the other hand, to demonstrate the seriousness of gunshot wounds in children DiScala and Sege (109) found in their review of the children and adolescents who required hospitalization for gunshot wounds, almost half of them were discharged with disability.

Prevention. In an excellent report in 1999, Freed et al (110) analyzed the magnitude and implications of the increasing incidence of firearm-related injuries in children. They suggested a product-oriented approach, focusing on the gun, in an attempt to provide an efficient strategy of gun control and hence reduce the disturbing trend of firearm-related injuries and death among youths. Rather than modifying behavioral or environmental issues, which are more complex, they suggested focusing primarily on strategies that offset the accessibility and design of firearms. In brief, these strategies included: reducing the number of guns in the environment through restrictive legislation, gun buy-back programs, gun taxes, and physician counseling, and modifying the design of guns to make them more child-proof and prevent unauthorized and unintended use.

Falls

Falls can vary in severity from a simple fall while running, to a fall of great magnitude, such as from a third story window. Falls often are classified as the most common cause of injuries. Falls are more likely to be a cause of injury in the younger than in the older child. Falls in the home usually are associated with furniture or stairs; outside the home, most falls involve playground equipment (111,112).

Intrinsic Causes

Nutrition. In a study in Spain, a significant difference in the fracture rate was found when cities with a high calcium content in their water were compared with those with a lower calcium content. With all other factors being equal (e.g., fluoride content, socioeconomic background), children who lived in the cities with a lower calcium content had a higher fracture rate (113).

An increase in the consumption of carbonated beverages has been shown to produce an increased incidence of fractures in adolescents (114).

Bone Density. Bone density may be a factor, but the data are unclear. Landin and Nilsson (115) found that the mineral content of the forearms was lower in children who sustained fractures from mild trauma than in children who had never sustained fractures. It was not significantly different, however, in those sustaining fractures from severe trauma. This study used measurements of bone density of the cortical bone in the forearms. Cook et al (116), using measurements of bone density obtained from trabecular bone in the spine and femoral neck, found no difference between children who had sustained fractures and those who had not.

Premature Infants

Fractures not related to birth trauma reportedly occur in 1% to 2% of low–birth-weight or premature infants during their stay in a neonatal intensive care unit (117). A combination of clinical history, radiographic appearance, and laboratory data has shown evidence of bone loss from inadequate calcium and phosphorus intake in these infants. Correcting the metabolic status of these low–birth-weight infants, with special emphasis on calcium and phosphorus intake, appears to decrease the incidence of repeat fractures and to improve the radiographic appearance of their bony tissues. Once the metabolic abnormalities are corrected, this temporary deficiency seems to have no long-term effects. When premature infants were followed into later years, there was no difference in their fracture incidence compared with that of children of normal birth weight (118).

PREVENTIVE PROGRAMS

One of the major goals of studying the incidence of fractures is to identify problem areas. It is hoped that by targeting these areas, programs can be designed to decrease the risk factors.

National Campaigns

Several safety programs have been started by national organizations. The foremost is the American Academy of Pediatrics, which has committees on accident and poisoning prevention. This group has produced guidelines for athletics (119), playgrounds (120,121), trampolines (122,123), and skateboards (124). The American Academy of Orthopaedic Surgeons has produced a program designed to decrease the incidence of playground injuries. These programs offer background data and guidelines for various activities, but their effectiveness has not yet been fully studied.

Local Community Participation

To be effective, accident prevention programs require local participation and cooperation. They must be broad based, and they require considerable effort by members of the local community. In the United States, one effective program is the New York Health Department's "Kids Can't Fly" campaign, developed in response to the large number of injuries and deaths from children falling out of apartment house windows in the 1970s (125). This extensive program consisted of a good reporting system from hospital emergency rooms, with follow-up by public health personnel; a strong media campaign to educate the public; a door-to-door hazard identification program; and the distribution of low- or no-cost, easily installed window guards to families in high-rise apartments. The city required landlords to provide window guards in apartments where children 10 years or younger lived. The success of this program was demonstrated by a 50% decrease in reported falls after 3 years and a 96% decrease after 7 years (125,126).

Over the past 30 years, Sweden has developed broader based, community-oriented programs to decrease the incidence of all types of childhood injuries (127). The development of these pilot programs has been relatively easy in a country like Sweden because the population is homogeneous, the incidence of poverty is low, and the government is stable. The Swedish program had a three-pronged approach: injury surveillance and prevention research; establishment of a safer environment for children through legislative regulation; and a broad-based safety education campaign. These programs have produced positive results. Schelp demonstrated a 27% reduction in home accidents in the municipality of Falkoping only 3 years after the establishment of a community-wide campaign (128).

One of the most dramatic changes came in the prevention of drowning. In Sweden, 100 children drowned in 1954; by 1988, the number had decreased to 10 (127). In the same time period, there was only a 5% decrease in the number of childhood drownings in the United States. The decrease in drowning did not result from establishing new, sophisticated emergency medical services or intensive care units in hospitals; it came by teaching children to swim and promoting the use of life jackets on toddlers playing near the water. In addition, there was a public education campaign in the media locally and nationally.

Effective prevention programs require local community participation and education. All the articles, lectures, and pamphlets in the world cannot help unless local communities make the necessary changes to decrease accident risks.

REFERENCES

1. Blount WP. *Fractures in children*. Baltimore: Williams & Wilkins, 1955.
2. Pirone AM, Graham HK, Krajbich JI. Management of displaced extension-type supracondylar fractures of the humerus in children. *J Bone Joint Surg [Am]* 1988;70:641.
3. Cox PJ, Clarke NM. Improving the outcome of paediatric orthopaedic trauma: an audit of inpatient management in Southampton. *Ann R Coll Surg Engl* 1997;79:441.
4. Rockwood CA Jr, Wilkins KE, King RE, eds. *Fractures in children*. Philadelphia: JB Lippincott, 1984.
5. Beaty JH, Kasser JR, eds. *Fractures in Children*, Vol III. 5th ed. Philadelphia: Lippincott Williams & Wilkins, 2001.

6. Lyons JP, Ashley E, Hoffer M. Ulnar nerve palsies after percutaneous cross pinning of supracondylar fractures in children's elbows. *J Pediatr Orthop* 1998;18:43.
7. Probe R, Londsey RW, Hadley NA, et al. Refracture of adolescent femoral shaft fractures: a complication of external fixation: a report of two cases. *J Pediatr Orthop* 1993;13:102.
8. Beaty JH, Austin SM, Warner WC, et al. Interlocking intramedullary nailing of femoral shaft fractures in adolescents: preliminary results and complications. *J Pediatr Orthop* 1994;14:178.
9. Mileski RA, Garvin KL, Huurman WW. Avascular necrosis of the femoral head after closed intramedullary shortening in an adolescent. *J Pediatr Orthop* 1995;15:24.
10. Chess DG, Hyndman JC, Leahey JL. Short-arm plaster for paediatric distal forearm fractures. *J Bone Joint Surg [Br]* 1987;69:506.
11. Walker JL, Rang M. Forearm fractures in children: cast treatment with elbow extension. *J Bone Joint Surg [Br]* 1991;73:299.
12. Beekman F, Sullivan JE. Some observations on fractures of long bones in children. *Am J Surg* 1941;51:722.
13. Hanlon CR, Estes WL. Fractures in childhood—a statistical analysis. *Am J Surg* 1954;87:312.
14. Lichtenberg RP. A study of 2,532 fractures in children. *Am J Surg* 1954;87:330.
15. Wong PCN. A comparative epidemiologic study of fractures among Indian, Malay and Swdish children. *Med J Malaya* 1965;20:132.
16. Iqbal QM. Long-bone fractures among children in Malaysia. *Int Surg* 1975;59:410.
17. Reed MH. Fractures and dislocations of the extremities in children. *J Trauma* 1977;17:351.
18. Landin LA. Fracture patterns in children. *Acta Orthop Scand* 1983;54(suppl 202):1.
19. Landin LA. Epidemiology of children's fractures. *J Pediatr Orthop B* 1997;6:79.
20. Tiderius CJ, Landin L, Duppe H. Decreasing incidence of fractures in children—an epidemiological analysis of 1673 fractures in Malmo, Sweden, 1993–1994. *Acta Orthop Scand* 1999;70:622.
21. Cheng JC, Shen WY. Limb fracture pattern in different pediatric age groups: a study of 3350 children. *J Orthop Trauma* 1993;7:15.
22. Cheng JC, Ng BK, Ying SY, et al. A 10-year study of the changes in the pattern and treatment of 6,493 fractures. *J Pediatr Orthop* 1999;19:344.
23. Laffoy M. Childhood accidents at home. *Ir Med J* 1997;90:26.
24. Nathorst Westfelt JA. Environmental factors in childhood accidents: a prospective study in Goteborg, Sweden. *Acta Paediatr Scand* 1982;291:1–75.
25. Fleming DM, Charlton JR. Morbidity and health care utilization of children in households with one adult: comparative observational study. *Br Med J* 1998;316:1572.
26. Lyons RA, Delahunty AM, McCabe M, et al. Incidence of fractures in affluent and deprived areas population based study. *Br Med J* 2000;320:149.
27. Stark, AD, Bennet GC, Stone DH, et al. Association between childhood fractures and poverty: population based study. *Br Med J* 2002;324:457.
28. Buckley SL, Gotschall C, Robertson W Jr, et al. The relationships of skeletal injuries with trauma score, injury severity score, length of hospital stay, hospital charges, and mortality in children admitted to a regional pediatric trauma center. *J Pediatr Orthop* 1994;14:449.
29. Lopez AA, Rennie TF. A survey of accidents to children aged under 15 years seen at a district hospital in Sydney in one year. *Med J Aust* 1969;1:806.
30. Shank LP, Bagg RJ, Wagnon J. Etiology of pediatric fractures: the fatigue factors in children's fractures. Presented at National Conference on Pediatric Trauma, Indianapolis, 1992.
31. Worlock P, Stower M. Fracture patterns in Nottingham children. *J Pediatr Orthop* 1986;6:656.
32. Hindmarsh J, Melin G, Melin KA. Accidents in childhood. *Acta Chir Scand* 1946;94:483.
33. Brinker MR, O'Connor DP. The incidence of fractures and dislocations referred for orthopaedic services in a capitated population. *J Bone Joint Surg [Am]* 2004;86-A(2):290.
34. Rivara FP, Bergman AB, LoGerfo JP, et al. Epidemiology of childhood injuries. II. Sex differences in injury rates. *Am J Dis Child* 1982;136:502.
35. Kempe CH, Silverman FN, Steele BF, et al. The battered-child syndrome. *JAMA* 1962;181:17.
36. Akbarnia B, Torg JS, Kirkpatrick J, et al. Manifestations of the battered-child syndrome. *J Bone Joint Surg [Am]* 1974;56:1159.
37. Kowal-Vern A, Paxton TP, Ros SP, et al. Fractures in the under-3-year-old age cohort. *Clin Pediatr* 1992;31:653.
38. McClelland CQ, Heiple KG. Fractures in the first year of life: a diagnostic dilemma? *Am J Dis Child* 1982;136:26.
39. Routledge DA, Repett-Wright R, Howarth CI. The exposure of young children to accident risk as pedestrians. *Ergonomics* 1974;17:457.
40. Rohl L. On fractures through the radial condyle of the humerus in children. *Acta Chir Scand* 1952;104:74.
41. Mortensson W, Thonell S. Left-side dominance of upper extremity fracture in children. *Acta Orthop Scand* 1991;62:154.
42. Wareham K, Johansen KA, Stone MD, et al. Seasonal variation in the incidence of wrist and forearm fractures, and its consequences. *Injury* 2003;34:219.
43. Masterson E, Borton D, O'Brien T. Victims of our climate. *Injury* 1993;24:247.
44. Andren L, Borgstrom KE. Seasonal variation of epiphysiolysis of the hip and possibility of causal factor. *Acta Orthop Scand* 1958;28:22.
45. Compere EL. Growth arrest in long bones as result of fractures that include the epiphysis. *JAMA* 1935;105:2140.
46. Mann DC, Rajmaira S. Distribution of physeal and nonphyseal fractures in 2,650 long-bone fractures in children aged 0–16 years. *J Pediatr Orthop* 1990;10:713.
47. Bisgard JD, Martenson L. Fractures in children. *Surg Gynecol Obstet* 1937;65:464.
48. Mizuta T, Benson WM, Foster BK, et al. Statistical analysis of the incidence of physeal injuries. *J Pediatr Orthop* 1987;7:518.
49. Dershewitz R. Is it of any practical value to identify accident-prone children? *Pediatrics* 1977;60:786.
50. Landin LA, Nilsson BE. Bone mineral content in children with fractures. *Clin Orthop* 1983;178:292.
51. Jones JG. The child accident repeater, a review. *Clin Pediatr* 1980;19:284.
52. Barlow B, Neimirska M, Gandhi RP, et al. Ten years of experience with falls from a height in children. *J Pediatr Surg* 1983;18:509.
53. Meller JL, Shermeta DW. Falls in urban children: a problem revisited. *Am J Dis Child* 1987;141:1271.
54. Sieben RL, Leavitt JD, French JH. Falls as childhood accidents: an increasing urban risk. *Pediatrics* 1971;47:886.
55. Smith MD, Burrington JD, Woolf AD. Injuries in children sustained in free falls: an analysis of 66 cases. *J Trauma* 1975;15:987.
56. Worlock P, Stower M. Fracture patterns in Nottingham children. *J Pediatr Orthop* 1986;6:656.
57. Nathorst Westfelt JA. Environmental factors in childhood accidents: a prospective study in Goteborg, Sweden. *Acta Paediatr Scand* 1982;291:1–75.
58. Boyce WT, Sprunger LW, Sobolewski S, et al. Epidemiology of injuries in a large, urban school district. *Pediatrics* 1984;74:342.
59. Lenaway DD, Ambler AG, Beaudoin DE. The epidemiology of school-related injuries: new perspectives. *Am J Prev Med* 1992;8:193.
60. Sheps SB, Evans GD. Epidemiology of school injuries: a 2-year experience in a municipal health department. *Pediatrics* 1987;79:69.
61. Feldman W, Woodward CA, Hodgson C, et al. Prospective study of school injuries: incidence, types, related factors and initial management. *Can Med Assoc J* 1983;129:1279.
62. Mott A, Evans R, Rolfe K, et al. Patterns of injuries to children on public playgrounds. *Arch Dis Child* 1994;71:328.
63. Laforest S, Robitaille Y, Lesage G, et al. Playground injuries: surface characteristics, equipment height, and the occurrence and severity of playground injuries. *Inj Prev* 2001;7:35.
64. Mowat DL, Wang F, Pickett W, et al. A case-control study of risk factors for playground injuries among children in Kingston and area. *Inj Prev* 1998;4:39.
65. Petrido E, Sibert J, Dedoukou X, et al. Injuries in public and private playgrounds: the relative contribution of structural, equipment and human factors. *Acta Paediatrica* 2002;91:691.
66. Mack MG, Hudson S, Thompson D. A descriptive analysis of children's playground injuries in the United States 1990–94. *Inj Prev* 1997;3:100.
67. Waltzman ML, Shannon M, Bowen AP, et al. Monkey bar injuries: complications of play. *Pediatrics* 1999;103:58.
68. Chalmers DJ, Marshall SW, Langley JD, et al. Height and surfacing as risk factors for injury in falls from playground equipment: a case-control study. *Inj Prev* 1996;2:98.
69. Lillis KA, Jaffe DM. Playground injuries in children. *Pediatr Emerg Care* 1997;13:149.
70. Mahadev AM, Soon Y, Lam KS. Monkey bars are for monkeys: a study on playground equipment related extremity fractures in Singapore. *Singapore Med J* 2004;45:9.
71. Puranik S, Long J, Coffman S. Profile of pediatric bicycle injuries. *South Med J* 1998;91:1033.
72. Weiss B. Bicycle-related head injuries. *Clin Sports Med* 1999;13:99.
73. Finvers KA, Strother RT, Mohtadi N. The effect of bicycling helmets in preventing significant bicycle-related injuries in children. *Clin J Sport Med* 1996;6:102.
74. Rogers GB. Bicycle helmet use patterns among children. *Pediatrics* 1996;97:166.
75. US Public Health Service. *Healthy People 2000: national health promotion and disease prevention objectives.* Washington, DC: DHSS Publication no. PH58 90-50212, 1990.
76. Hansen KS, Engesaeter LB, Viste A. Protective effect of different types of bicycle helmets. *Traffic Inj Prev* 2003;4:285.
77. Cameron M, Vulcan AP, Furich C, et al. Mandatory bicycle helmet use following a decade of helmet promotion in Victoria, Australia—an evaluation. *Accid Anal Prev* 1996;26:325.
78. D'Souza LG, Hynes DE, McManus F, et al. The bicycle spoke injury: an avoidable accident? *Foot Ankle Int* 1996;17:170.
79. Segers MJM, Wink D, Clevers GJ. Bicycle-spoke injuries: a prospective study. *Injury* 1997;28:267.
80. Kyle SB, Nance ML, Rutherford GW Jr, et al. Skateboard-associated injuries: participation-based estimates and injury characteristics. *J Trauma* 2002;53:686.
81. Fountain JL, Meyers MC. Skateboarding injuries. *Sports Med* 1996;22:360.
82. Osberg JS, Schneps SE, Di Scala C, Li G. Skateboarding: more dangerous than roller skating or in-line skating. *Arch Pediatr Adolesc Med* 1998;152:985.
83. Powell EC, Tanz RR. In-line skate and rollerskate injuries in childhood. *Pediatr Emerg Care* 1996;12:259.
84. Schieber RA, Olson SJ. Developing a culture of safety in a reluctant audience. *West J Med* 2002;176:E1.
85. Jerosch J, Heidjann J, Thorwesten L, et al. Injury patterns in acceptance of passive and active injury prophylaxis for inline skating. *Knee Surg Sports Traumatol Arthrosc* 1998;6:44.
86. Mitts KG, Hennrikus WL. In-line skating fractures in children. *J Pediatr Orthop* 1996;16:640.
87. Sheehan E, Mulhall KJ, Kearns S, et al. Impact of dedicated skate parks on the severity and incidence of skateboard- and rollerblade-related pediatric fractures. *J Pediatr Orthop* 2003;23:440.
88. Chapman S, Webber S, O'Meara M. Scooter injuries in children. *J Paediatr Child Health* 2001;37:567.

89. Mankovsky AB, Mendoza-Sagaon M, Cardinaux C, et al. Evaluation of scooter-related injuries in children. *J Pediatr Surg* 2002;37:755.
90. Schalamon J, Sarkola T, Nietosvaara Y. Injuries in children associated with the use of nonmotorized scooters. *J Pediatr Surg* 2003;38:1612.
91. Furnival RA, Street KA, Schunk JE. Too many pediatric trampoline injuries. *Pediatrics* 1999;103:57.
92. Smith GA. Injuries to children in the United States related to trampolines, 1990–1995: a national epidemic. *Pediatrics* 1998;101:406.
93. Smith GA, Shields BJ. Trampoline-related injuries to children. *Arch Pediatr Adolesc Med* 1998;152:694.
94. Shorter NA, Jensen PE, Harmon BJ, et al. Skiing injuries in children and adolescents. *J Trauma* 1996;40:997.
95. Bladin C, Giddings P, Robinson M. Australian snowboard injury data base study. A four-year prospective study. *Am J Sports Med* 1993;21:701.
96. Ronning R, Ronning I, Gerner T, et al. The efficacy of wrist protectors in preventing snowboarding injuries. *Am J Sports Med* 2001;29:581.
97. Landin LA. Fracture patterns in children. *Acta Orthop Scand* 1983;64(suppl 202):1.
98. Derlet RW, Silva J Jr, Holcroft J. Pedestrian accidents: adult and pediatric injuries. *J Emerg Med* 1989;7:5.
99. Buckley SL, Gotschall C, Robertson W Jr, et al. The relationships of skeletal injuries with trauma score, injury severity score, length of hospital stay, hospital charges, and mortality in children admitted to a regional pediatric trauma center. *J Pediatr Orthop* 1994;14:449.
100. Topoleski T, Schlesinger I, Wexler LM, et al. Motor vehicle injuries in pediatric trauma patients. Presented at the American Academy of Orthopaedic Surgeons Annual Meeting, Orlando, 1995.
101. Mubarak SJ, Lavernia C, Silva PD. Ice-cream truck-related injuries to children. *J Pediatr Orthop* 1998;18:46.
102. Parmar P, Letts M, Jarvis J. Injuries caused by water tubing. *J Pediatr Orthop* 1998;18:49.
103. Washington ER, Lee WA, Ross WA Jr. Gunshot wounds to the extremities in children and adolescents. *Orthop Clin North Am* 1995;26:19.
104. Cook PJ, Ludwig J. *Guns in America*. Washington, DC: Police Foundation, 1996.
105. Stucky W, Loder RT. Extremity gunshot wounds in children. *J Pediatr Orthop* 1991; 11:64.
106. Letts RM, Miller D. Gunshot wounds of the extremities in children. *J Trauma* 1976; 16:807.
107. Valentine J, Blocker S, Chang JHT. Gunshot injuries in children. *J Trauma* 1984;24:952.
108. Ordog GJ, Prakash A, Wasserberger J, et al. Pediatric gunshot wounds. *J Trauma* 1987; 27:1272.
109. DiScala C, Sege R. Outcomes in children and young adults who are hospitalized for firearms-related injuries. *Pediatrics* 2004;113:1306.
110. Freed LH, Vernick JS, Hargarten SW. Prevention of firearm-related injuries and deaths among youth. A product-oriented approach. *Pediatr Clin North Am* 1998;45:427.
111. Gallagher SS, Finison K, Guyer B, et al. The incidence of injuries among 87,000 Massachusetts children and adolescents: results of the 1980–81 statewide childhood injury prevention program surveillance system. *Am J Pub Health* 1984;74:1340.
112. Garrettson LK, Gallagher SS. Falls in children and youth. *Pediatr Clin North Am* 1985; 32:153.
113. Verd VS, Dominguez SJ, Gonzalez QM, et al. Association between calcium content of drinking water and fractures in children. *An Esp Pediatr* 1992;37:461.
114. Wyshak G, Frisch RE. Carbonated beverages, dietary calcium, the dietary calcium/phosphorus ratio, and bone fractures in girls and boys. *J Adolesc Health* 1994;15:210.
115. Landin LA, Nilsson BE. Bone mineral content in children with fractures. *Clin Orthop* 1983;178:292.
116. Cook SD, Harding AF, Morgan EL, et al. Association of bone mineral density and pediatric fractures. *J Pediatr Orthop* 1987;7:424.
117. Amir J, Katz K, Grunebaum M, et al. Fractures in premature infants. *J Pediatr Orthop* 1988;8:41.
118. Dahlenburg SL, Bishop NJ, Lucas A. Are preterm infants at risk for subsequent fracture? *Arch Dis Child* 1989;64:1384.
119. American Academy of Pediatrics, Committee on Pediatric Aspects of Physical Fitness, Recreation and Sports: competitive athletics for children of elementary school age. *Pediatrics* 1981;67:928.
120. Reichelderfer TE, Overback A, Greensher J. Unsafe playgrounds. *Pediatrics* 1979;64: 962.
121. Werner P. Playground injuries and voluntary product standards for home and public playgrounds. *Pediatrics* 1982;69:18.
122. American Academy of Pediatrics, Committee on Accident and Poison Prevention: trampolines. Evanston, Illinois, September 1977.
123. American Academy of Pediatrics, Committee on Accident and Poison Prevention: trampolines II. *Pediatrics* 1981;67:438.
124. American Academy of Pediatrics, Committee on Accident and Poison Prevention: skateboard injuries. *Pediatrics* 1989;6:1070.
125. Spiegel CN, Lindaman FC. Children can't fly: a program to prevent childhood morbidity and mortality from window falls. *Am J Dis Child* 1977;67:1143.
126. Barlow B, Neimirska M, Gandhi RP, et al. Ten years of experience with falls from a height in children. *J Pediatr Surg* 1983;18:509.
127. Bergman AB, Rivara FP. Sweden's experience in reducing childhood injuries. *Pediatrics* 1991;88:69.
128. Schelp L. The role of organizations in community participation—prevention of accidental injuries in a rural Swedish municipality. *Soc Sci Med* 1988;26:1087.

THE BIOLOGIC ASPECTS OF CHILDREN'S FRACTURES

Cory J. Xian and Bruce K. Foster

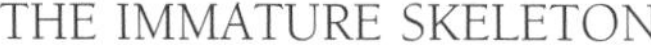

THE IMMATURE SKELETON

Compared with the relatively static, mature bone of adults, the changing structure and function, both physiologic and biomechanical, of immature bones make them susceptible to different patterns of failure. Even the types of fracture patterns within a given bone demonstrate temporal (chronobiologic) variations that may be correlated with progressive anatomic changes affecting the epiphysis, physis, metaphysis, and diaphysis at macroscopic and microscopic levels.

Skeletal trauma accounts for 10% to 15% of all childhood injuries (1–4). Fractures of the immature skeleton differ from those of the mature skeleton (2,3,5). Fractures in children are more common and are more likely to occur after seemingly insignificant trauma. Physeal disruptions make up about 15% of all skeletal injuries in children (2–4,6–8). Damage involving specific growth regions, such as the physis or epiphyseal ossification center, may lead to acute or chronic growth disturbances (2,9–11). The physis is constantly changing, both with active longitudinal and latitudinal (diametric) growth and in mechanical relation to other components. Physeal fracture patterns vary with the extent of chondro-osseous maturation. Salter-Harris type I injuries are common in infants, and types II, III, and IV become more common as the secondary ossification center enlarges and physeal undulations develop. Although joint injuries, dislocations, and ligamentous disruptions are much less common in children, it is more likely that one of the contiguous physes will be damaged. Changing trabecular and cortical structures affect metaphyseal and diaphyseal fracture patterns, and the variable size of the secondary ossification center affects susceptibility to physeal and epiphyseal injuries.

Due to the increasing effort researching into the injury/healing responses in fractures and strategies for enhancing bone and physis repair in children, the options of treatments available for the treatment of skeletal injuries in children are expanding. Most notable is the introduction of growth factors, such as the bone morphogenic proteins (BMPs), for the induction of bone formation in nonunions, large segmental bone, and for the repair of cartilage defects (12), and the research and development of stem-cell–based cell therapy for bone and cartilage regeneration (13) and growth plate repair (14–16). Due to these new developments, it has become necessary for the orthopaedic surgeon to understand the biological aspects of the skeletal injury responses and new treatment options for fracture repair. This chapter covers the basic biology and regulation of bone growth, bone fracture repair responses, physeal injury and physeal bar formation, roles of growth factors and cytokines in regulating injury/repair responses, and future therapeutic strategies for bone/articular cartilage/physis regeneration using growth factors, tissue engineering, stem cells, and gene therapy.

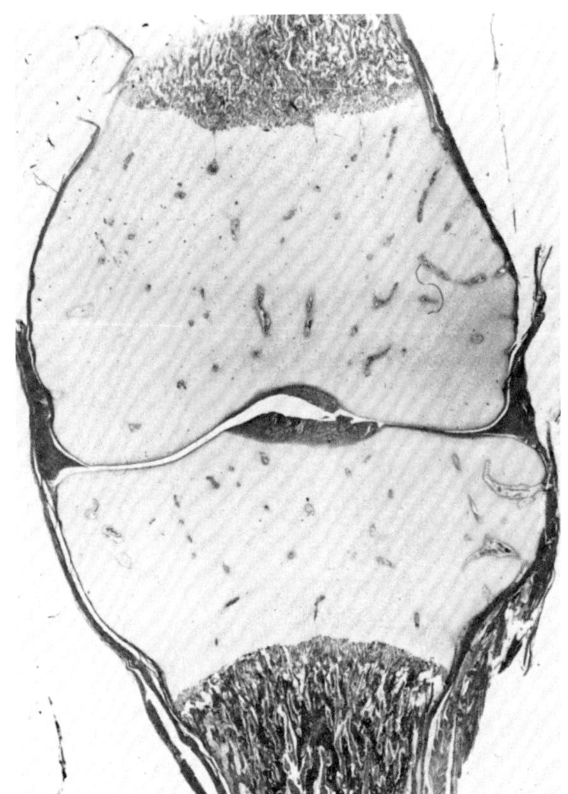

FIGURE 2-1 Chondroepiphyses of the distal femur and proximal tibia. These structures have an extensively developed vascular system (cartilage canals) before secondary ossification.

ANATOMIC REGIONS OF THE CHILD'S BONE

The major long bones of children can be divided into four distinct, anatomic areas: the epiphysis, physis, metaphysis, and diaphysis (17). Each region is prone to certain patterns of injury, and the intrinsic injury susceptibility varies with physiologic and biomechanical changes during postnatal development. The four regions originate and become modified as a result of the basic endochondral ossification process. Subsequently, they are supplemented by membranous bone formation along the metaphyseal and diaphyseal shafts. Finally, the regions are remodeled to create mature cortical and trabecular bone.

Epiphysis

At birth, each epiphysis (except the distal femur) consists of a completely cartilaginous structure at the end of each long bone (Fig. 2-1), the chondroepiphysis. At a time characteristic for each of these chondroepiphyses, a secondary center of ossification forms and gradually enlarges until the cartilaginous area has been almost completely replaced by bone at skeletal maturity. This chondro-osseous transformation is vascular-dependent (Fig. 2-2). Only articular cartilage remains at maturity.

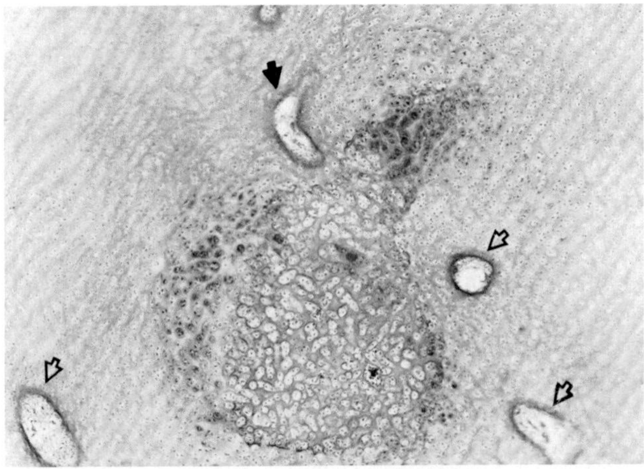

FIGURE 2-2 Early formation of the secondary ossification center within the epiphyseal cartilage. This usually occurs in a region well vascularized by cartilage canals (*open arrows*). One of the canals sends a branch into the hypertrophic cells (*solid arrow*), triggering the ossification process.

As the ossification center expands, it undergoes structural modifications. The region adjacent to the physis forms a distinct subchondral plate parallel to the metaphysis, creating the radiographically characteristic lucent physeal line. The appearance of the ossification centers differ in certain chondroepiphyses, a factor that must be considered when diagnosing fractures of these regions. The ossification center imparts increasing rigidity to the more resilient epiphyseal cartilage as the secondary osseous tissue expands (18).

The external surface of an epiphysis is composed of either articular cartilage or perichondrium (Fig. 2-3). Muscle fibers, tendons, and ligaments may attach directly to the perichondrium, which is densely contiguous with the underlying hyaline cartilage. The perichondrium contributes to the continued centrifugal enlargement of the epiphysis. It also blends imperceptibly into the periosteum. This perichondrial/periosteal tissue continuity contributes to the biomechanical strength of the epiphyseal/metaphyseal junction at the zone of Ranvier.

When the hyaline cartilage of the chondroepiphysis first forms, there are no easily demonstrable histologic differences between the cells of the joint surface and the rest of the epiphyseal cartilage. However, at some point, a finite cell population becomes stabilized and physiologically different from the remaining epiphyseal cartilage. McKibbin (19) established that these two cartilage types are different physiologically and biochemically. If a contiguous core of articular and hyaline cartilage is removed, turned 180°, and reinserted, the transposed hyaline cartilage eventually will form bone at the joint surface, whereas the transposed articular cartilage remains cartilaginous and becomes surrounded by the enlarging secondary ossification center. Normally, articular cartilage does not appear capable of calcification and ossification. As skeletal maturity is reached, a tide mark progressively develops as a demarcation between the articular and calcified epiphyseal hyaline cartilage.

An important aspect of McKibbin's experiment was an explanation of nonunion of certain fractures in which the fragment may be rotated, causing the articular surface to lie against metaphyseal and epiphyseal bone. Union is unlikely in such a situation because the articular surface is incapable of a reparative osteogenic response, an essential component of bone healing.

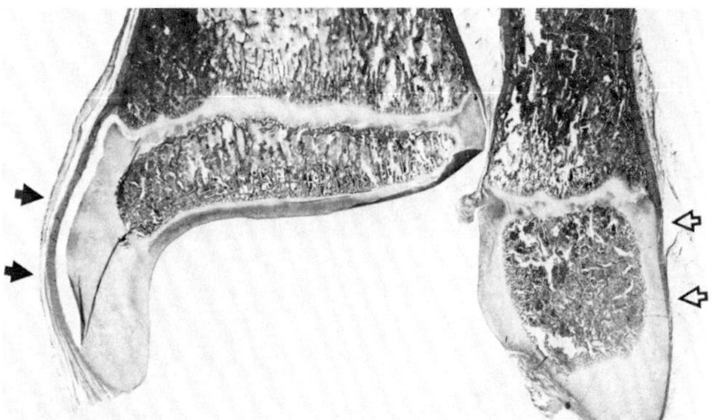

FIGURE 2-3 As the epiphysis matures, the ossification center expands and progressively follows the contours of the chondroepiphysis. The epiphyseal surface is either articular cartilage or perichondrium along the outer surfaces, as in the medial (*solid arrows*) and lateral (*open arrows*) malleoli.

Physis

The growth plate, or physis, is the essential structure adding bone through endochondral ossification (10,20–22). The primary function of the physis is rapid, integrated longitudinal and latitudinal growth. Injuries to this component are unique to skeletally immature patients.

Because the physeal cartilage remains radiolucent, except for the final stages of physiologic epiphysiodesis, its exact location must be inferred from the metaphyseal contour, which follows the physeal contour. The changing size of the secondary ossification center more effectively demarcates the physeal contour on the epiphyseal (germinal layer) side. As this center of ossification enlarges centrifugally to approach the physis, the original spherical shape of the ossification center flattens and gradually develops a contour paralleling the metaphyseal contour. Similar contouring also occurs as the ossification center approaches the lateral and subarticular regions of the epiphysis (Fig. 2-4). The region of the ossification center juxtaposed to the physis forms a discrete subchondral bone plate that the essential epiphyseal blood vessels must penetrate to reach the physeal germinal zone (Fig. 2-5). Damage to this osseous plate in a fracture may cause localized physeal ischemia.

If a segment of the epiphyseal vasculature is compromised, whether temporarily or permanently, the zones of cellular growth associated with these particular vessels cannot undergo appropriate cell division. In contrast, unaffected regions of the physis continue longitudinal and latitudinal growth, leaving the affected region behind (Figs. 2-6 and 2-7). The growth rates of the cells directly adjacent to the affected area are more mechanically compromised than cellular areas farther away. The differential rather than uniform growth results in an angular or longitudinal growth deformity, or both (7,23).

Interruption of the metaphyseal circulation has no effect on chondrogenesis within the germinal zone or the sequential cartilage maturation within the hypertrophic zone of the physis (see Fig. 2-6). However, the subsequent transformation of cartilage to bone (primary spongiosa) is blocked. This causes widening of the affected area, because more cartilage is added to the cell columns but none is replaced by invasive metaphyseal vessels and bone. Once the disrupted metaphyseal circulation is reestablished, this widened, calcified region of the physis is rapidly penetrated and ossified, returning the physis to its normal width. This is the mechanism seen in growth plate fractures and in fractures of the metaphysis. The metaphyseal blood supply is temporarily blocked by separation or impaction, and requires 3 to 4 weeks for restoration. If the circulatory compromise has been caused by a metaphyseal fracture, there also may be a temporary halt to bone formation in the transiently ischemic portion of the metaphysis. This leads to an apparent sclerosis

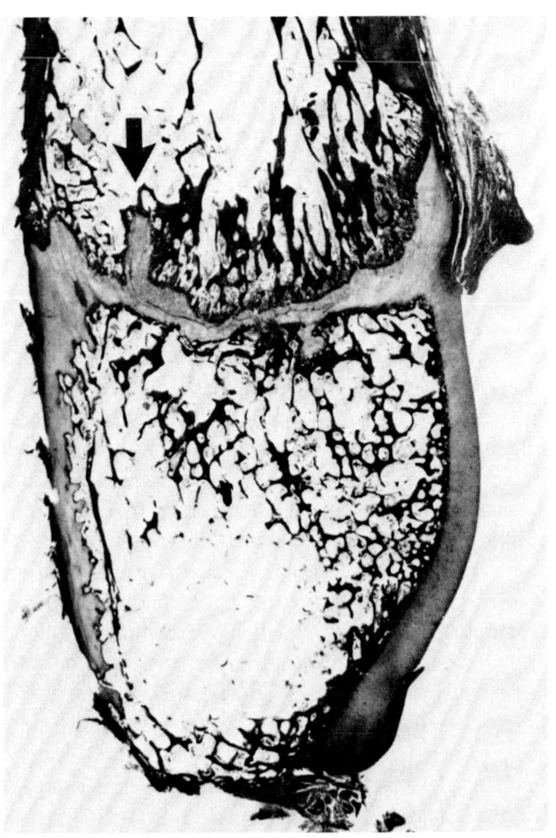

FIGURE 2-4 Distal fibula, showing the variably undulated physis, including a mammillary process (*arrow*). The physeal and epiphyseal cartilage turns proximally at the medial region (lappet formation) to participate in the formation of the distal tibiofibular articulation. Note the difference in the subarticular subchondral bone, which has formed a thick plate, compared with the thin, outer subchondral bone.

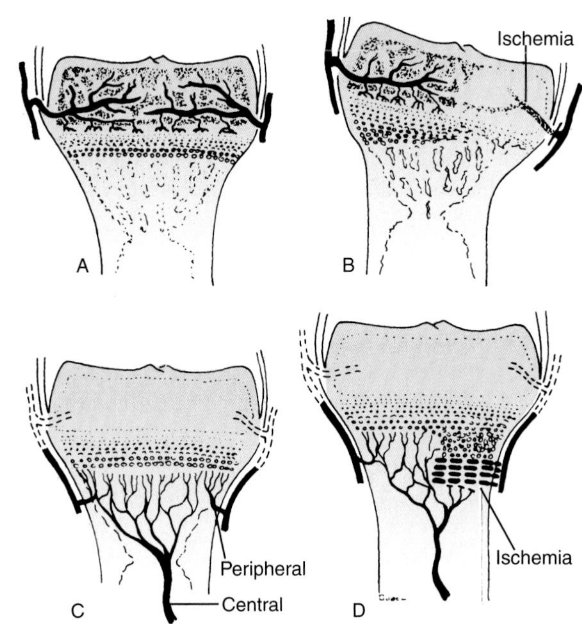

FIGURE 2-6 Patterns of response to ischemia of the epiphyseal **(A,B)** versus metaphyseal **(C,D)** circulatory systems. Metaphyseal ischemia is usually transient; epiphyseal ischemia is usually severe and permanent.

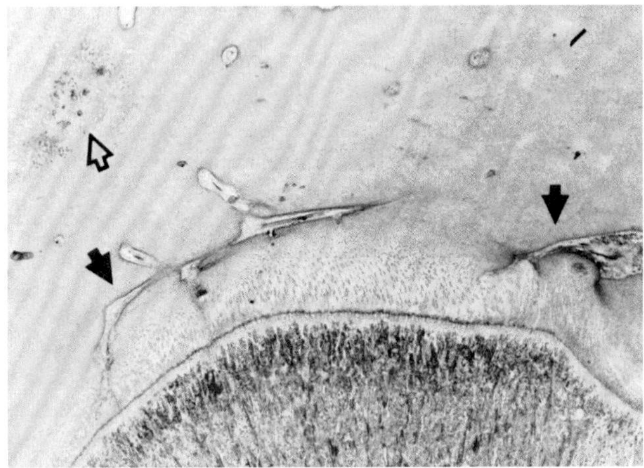

FIGURE 2-5 Epiphyseal circulation (*solid arrows*) in a toddler. These supply the germinal/dividing zones of the physis. The open arrow indicates the early ossification center. As this area enlarges, it will incorporate the epiphyseal vessels.

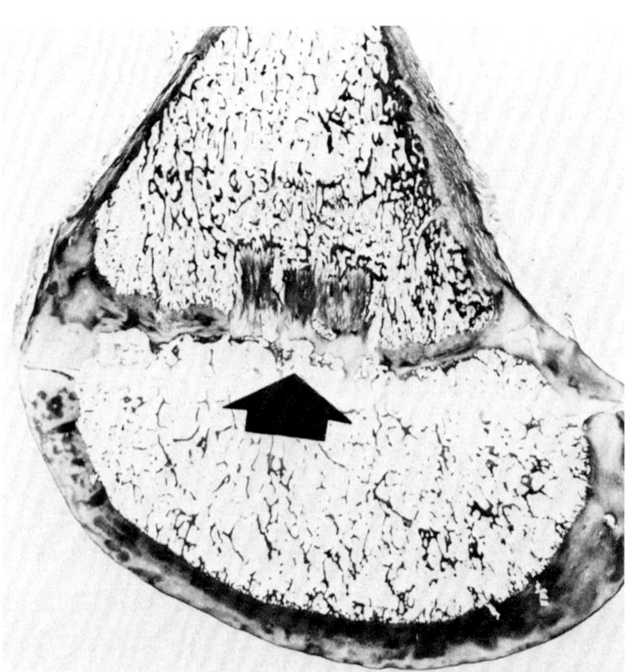

FIGURE 2-7 Histologic section showing an area of central ischemic growth arrest (*arrow*). The infarcted area of cartilage is left behind as the rest of the physis continues longitudinal growth.

when the bone is compared with the adjacent vascularized metaphysis, which undergoes a relative disuse osteoporosis. Compromise of the metaphyseal circulation has minimal, if any, effect on physeal development, particularly when compared with the major detrimental effects of epiphyseal circulatory compromise.

The effects of physeal ischemia have been studied extensively by Trueta and coworkers (24–27). Disrupting the epiphyseal circulation leads to either partial or complete cessation of growth. The central region seems more sensitive to ischemia than the periphery, which may have a variable capacity to recover through continued latitudinal growth (28,29). Ischemic compromise leads to different rates of growth across the affected physis and significant changes in physeal contour (30). Some changes may be caused by venous stasis rather than arterial damage (31).

Metaphysis

The metaphysis is a variably contoured flare at each end of the diaphysis. Its major characteristics are decreased thickness of the cortical bone and increased trabecular bone in the secondary spongiosa. Extensive endochondral modeling centrally and peripherally initially forms the primary spongiosa, which then is remodeled into the more mature secondary spongiosa, a process that involves osteoclastic and osteoblastic activity. Therefore, the metaphyses exhibit considerable bone turnover compared with other regions of the bone, and this factor is responsible for the increased uptake of radionuclides in technetium 99m bone scans (32).

The metaphyseal cortex also changes with time. Compared with the confluent diaphysis, the metaphyseal cortex is thinner and is more porous (trabecular fenestration; Fig. 2-8). These cortical fenestrations contain fibrovascular soft-tissue elements that connect the metaphyseal marrow spaces with the subperiosteal region. The metaphyseal cortex exhibits greater fenestration near the physis than in the diaphysis, with which it gradually blends as an increasingly thicker, dense bone (Fig. 2-9). As longitudinal growth continues, cortical fenestration becomes a less dominant feature, and the overall width of the cortex increases, creating a greater morphologic transition between the juxtaphyseal and juxtadiaphyseal cortices. The metaphyseal region does not develop extensive secondary and tertiary haversian systems until the late stages of skeletal maturation. These microscopic anatomic changes appear to be directly correlated with changing fracture patterns and are the reason why torus

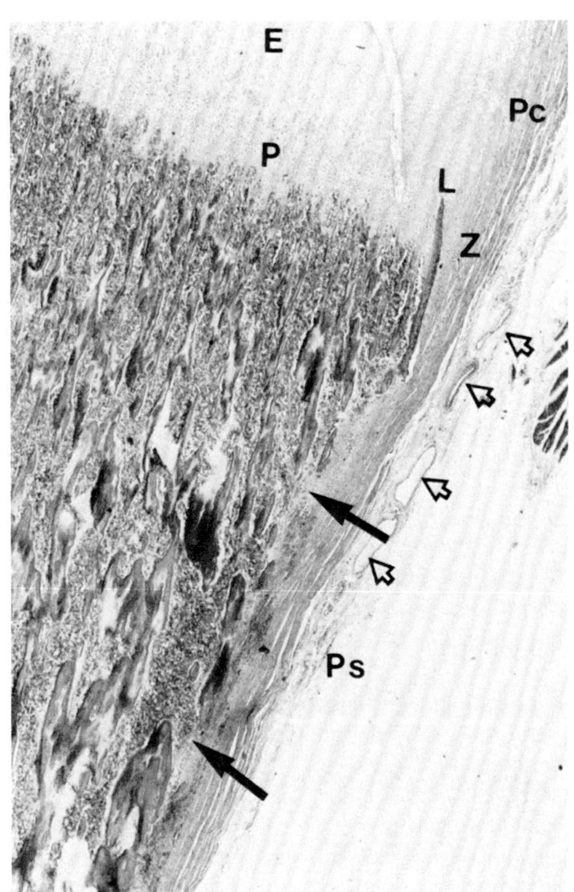

FIGURE 2-8 Cortical fenestration (*solid arrows*) of a metaphysis. Note the interdigitation of periosteal (Ps) tissue with the fenestrations. The periosteum blends into the perichondrium (Pc). Extensive vascularity is often present in this region (*open arrows*). (E, epiphysis; P, physis; Z, zone of Ranvier; L, ring of Lacroix.)

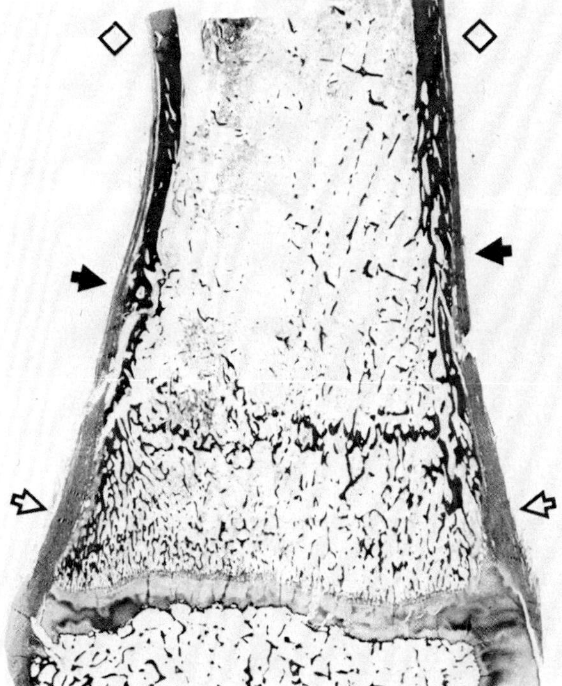

FIGURE 2-9 Section of distal tibia showing the transition (*solid arrows*) of cortical bone from the dense, remodeled diaphysis (diamonds) to the fenestrated metaphysis (*open arrows*). Note the progressive change from a relatively thin periosteum over the diaphysis to a much thicker one at the metaphysis.

(buckle) fractures are more likely to occur than complete metaphyseal or epiphyseal/physeal fractures.

Another microscopic anatomic variation in the metaphysis occurs at the junction of the primary spongiosa and the hypertrophic region of the physis. In most rapidly growing bones, the trabeculae tend to be longitudinally oriented. However, in shorter growing bones, such as the metacarpals and phalanges, trabecular formation is predominantly horizontal. As growth decelerates in adolescence, a similar horizontal orientation may be seen in the major long bones. These variations in trabecular orientation affect the responsiveness of metaphyseal and physeal regions to abnormal stress and predispose to certain fracture modes.

Although the periosteum is attached relatively loosely to the diaphysis, it is firmly fixed to the metaphysis because of the increasingly complex continuity of fibrous tissue through the metaphyseal fenestrations. Such intermingling of endosteal and interosseous fibrous tissues with the periosteal tissue imparts additional biomechanical strength to the region (33). The periosteum subsequently attaches densely into the peripheral physis, blending into the zone of Ranvier as well as the epiphyseal perichondrium. The fenestrated metaphyseal cortex extends to the physis as the thin osseous ring of Lacroix.

The metaphysis is the site of extensive osseous modeling and remodeling, both peripherally and centrally (Fig. 2-10). The metaphyseal cortex is fenestrated, modified trabecular bone on which the periosteum deposits membranous bone to thicken the cortex progressively. Similar endosteal bone formation occurs. As this metaphyseal region thickens, the trabecular bone is progressively invaded by diaphyseal osteon systems, not unlike osteons traversing the fracture site in primary bone healing.

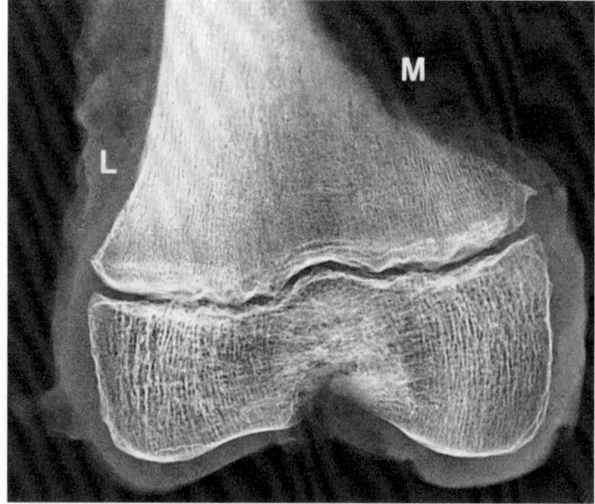

FIGURE 2-10 Extensive modeling and remodeling of the medial (M) versus the lateral (L) cortex of the distal femur may create irregularities that have been misinterpreted as fracture, stress fracture, infection, and tumor. Note the well-formed subchondral bone at the periphery of the epiphyseal ossification center.

This converts peripheral trabecular (woven or fiber) bone to lamellar (osteonal) bone, which has different biomechanical capacities, and thus progressively transforms metaphyseal cortex into diaphyseal cortex as longitudinal growth continues. A torus (buckle) fracture is most likely to occur in a metaphyseal region with a trabecular, fenestrated, compressible cortex.

As in the diaphysis, there are no significant direct muscle attachments to the metaphyseal bone. Instead, muscle fibers primarily blend into the periosteum. The medial distal femoral attachment of the adductor muscles is a significant exception. Because of extensive remodeling and insertion of muscle and tendon in this area, the bone often appears irregular and may be misinterpreted as showing chronic trauma (i.e., a stress fracture), infection, or a tumor.

Transverse Lines of Park and Harris

Many bones exhibit transversely oriented, dense trabecular linear bone patterns within the metaphysis. These lines usually duplicate the contiguous physeal contour. They may appear after trauma, particularly when the child has been immobilized in bed (e.g., traction for femoral fracture), and they also may appear after generalized illnesses or even localized processes within the bone (e.g., osteomyelitis) (34–37). The lines result from a temporary slowdown of normal longitudinal growth after injury or illness, and they often are called Harris or Park growth slowdown or arrest lines (Fig. 2-11). Because of the slowdown, the trabeculae of the primary spongiosa become more transversely than longitudinally oriented, creating a temporary thickening in the primary spongiosa adjacent to the physis. Once the normal longitudinal growth rate resumes, longitudinal trabecular orientation is restored. The thickened, transversely oriented osseous plate is left behind, and will be gradually remodeled as primary spongiosa becomes secondary spongiosa.

Usually, transverse lines are distributed relatively symmetrically throughout the skeleton and occupy identical sites in the corresponding bones on the two sides of the body. They are thickest in metaphyses that grow most rapidly, such as the distal femur and proximal tibia, as more primary spongiosa bone is formed in a transverse orientation in these growing regions (9). In the metaphyses with slowest growth, they may not form at all, or they are exceedingly thin and lie at the very end of the shaft, directly under the provisional zone of calcification. These transverse lines parallel the contours of the physeal provisional zone of calcification. When several transverse lines are present, they tend to be parallel. The lines nearest the end of the shaft ordinarily are the thickest and widest, whereas lines away from the physes tend to be thinner and less distinct and are usually broken and irregular. As remodeling occurs, with migration of the epiphysis away from this region, and with conversion of primary spongiosa to secondary spongiosa, there is a gradual breakup of this transverse trabecular orientation. As they eventually become part of the elongating diaphysis, they disappear completely with endosteal remodeling.

Although the more rapidly growing bones are associated with longitudinally oriented trabeculae in the juxtaphyseal re-

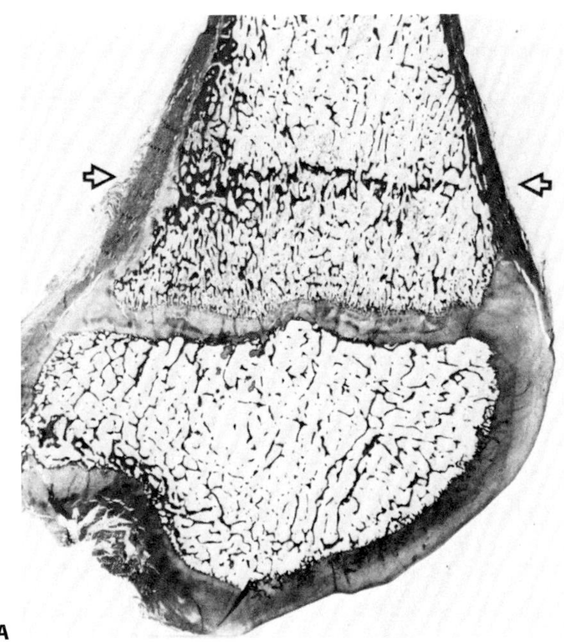

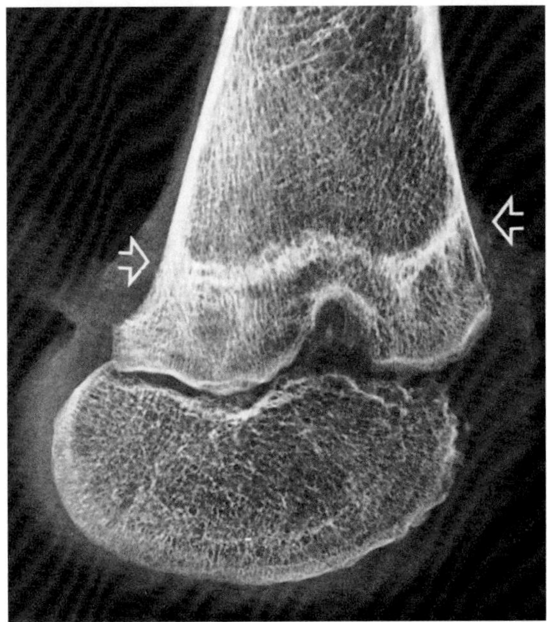

FIGURE 2-11 Histologic section **(A)** and x-ray study **(B)** of a distal femur showing a typical Harris line (*arrows*). This formed during an acute illness and chemotherapy for leukemia. The child then resumed a more normal pattern of growth until her death from leukemia about 14 months later.

gion, slower growing bones, particularly the proximal radius, metacarpals, metatarsals, and phalanges, normally have a greater amount of transversely oriented primary spongiosa (38), making transverse septa a normal finding. These particular bones do not have a sufficient difference in the orientation of trabeculae to manifest transverse lines on x-rays.

In response to administration of bisphosphonate treatment to children with osteogenesis imperfecta, there are some distinct metaphyseal bands in the growing skeleton, which may vary in spacing according to the regimens of treatment, age of the patient, rate of growth, and the location of the metaphysis. The bands may reflect decreased osteoclastic activity occurring in response to drug administration, and the spacing between the bands indicates resumption of osteoclastic activity and linear growth of the bone between treatments. As with growth arrest lines, the migration of these treatment bands varies with the rate of the bone growth of the patient and the particular physis (39).

Useful to Assess Growth After Injury. These biologic marker lines are important in analyzing the effects of a fracture on growth. They can be measured and the sides compared to corroborate femoral overgrowth after diaphyseal fracture and eccentric overgrowth medially after proximal tibial metaphyseal fracture. A line that converges toward a physis suggests localized growth damage that may result in an osseous bridge and the risk of angular deformity.

Diaphysis

The diaphysis constitutes the major portion of each long bone. It is principally a product of periosteal, membranous osseous tissue apposition on the original endochondral model. This leads to the gradual replacement of the endochondrally derived primary ossification center and primary spongiosa; the latter is replaced by secondary spongiosa in the metaphyseal region. At birth, the diaphysis is composed of laminar (fetal, woven) bone that characteristically lacks haversian systems. The neonatal femoral diaphysis appears to be the only area exhibiting any significant change from this fetal osseous state to a more mature bone with osteon systems (lamellar bone) before birth (Fig. 2-12).

Periosteum-mediated, membranous, appositional bone formation with concomitant endosteal remodeling leads to enlargement of the overall diameter of the shaft, variably increased width of the diaphyseal cortices, and formation of the marrow cavity. Mature, lamellar bone with intrinsic but constantly remodeling osteonal patterns progressively becomes the dominant feature (Fig. 2-13).

The developing diaphyseal bone in a neonate or young child is extremely vascular. When analyzed in cross section, it appears much less dense than the maturing bone of older children, adolescents, and adults. Subsequent growth leads to increased complexity of the haversian (osteonal) systems and the formation of increasing amounts of extracellular matrix, causing a relative decrease in cross-sectional porosity and an increase in hardness, factors that constantly change the child's susceptibility to different fracture patterns. Certain bones, especially the tibia, exhibit a significant decrease in vascularity as the bone matures; this factor affects the rate of healing and risk of nonunion.

The vascularity of the developing skeleton constantly

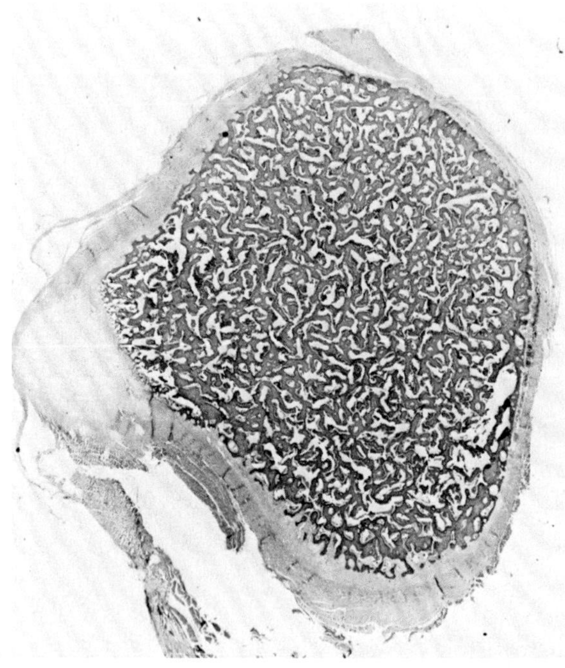

A

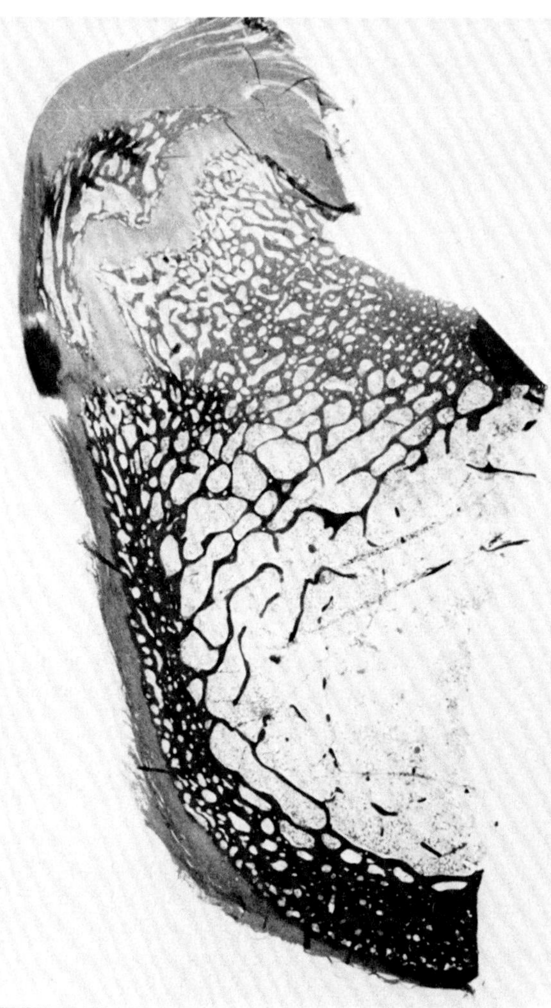

B

FIGURE 2-12 Sections of the femur at the level of the lesser trochanter at birth **(A)** and age 7 years **(B)**. At birth, some cortical thickening and osteon remodeling is evident laterally; the rest of the cortex is irregular. By age 7 years, extensive thickening and remodeling of the cortex has taken place.

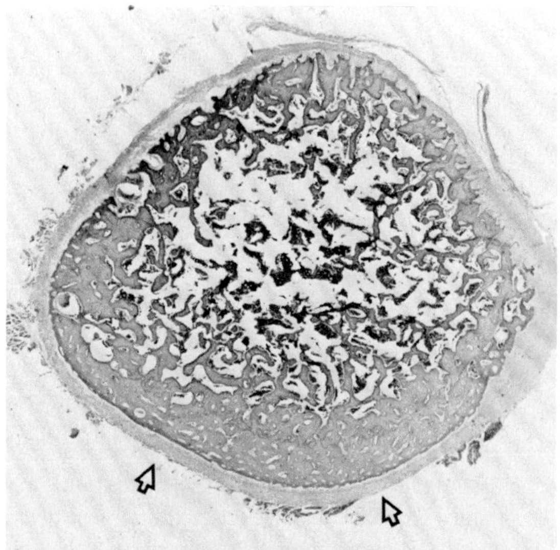

A

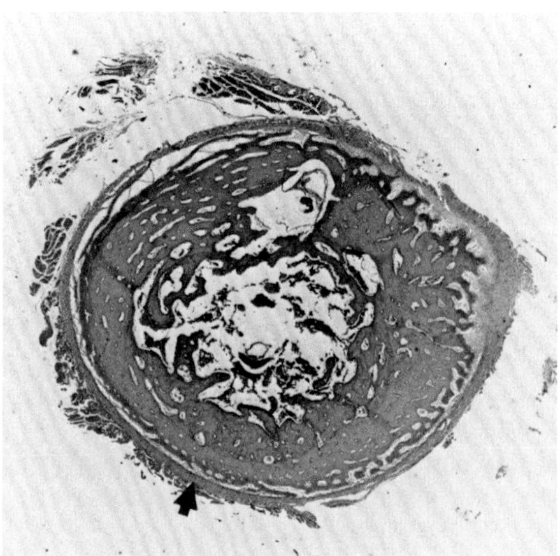

B

FIGURE 2-13 Transverse sections of the tibial diaphysis in a neonate **(A)** and at age 2 years **(B)**. A thick periosteum is evident in **(A)** (*open arrows*), in association with a rapidly forming anterior cortex. At age 2 years, new subperiosteal (membranous) bone is being added to the cortex (*solid arrow*).

changes. In experimental studies, significant chronobiologic changes in flow patterns were found in the developing canine tibia and femur (40–46). In particular, there was a dramatic decrease in tibial circulation with increasing skeletal maturation (45). This also occurs in humans, which helps to explain the increasing delay in fracture healing and the increased incidence of nonunion of the tibia in adolescents and adults. A poor vascular response could impair the early, crucial stages of callus formation.

Other researchers have suggested that adequate vascularity was a major factor in fracture healing (11,47–51), but they did not consider chronobiologic changes in blood flow patterns.

Periosteum

A child's periosteum is thicker, is more readily elevated from the diaphyseal and metaphyseal bone, and exhibits greater osteogenic potential than that of an adult (21). The periosteum is loosely attached to much of the shaft of the bone, but it attaches densely into the physeal periphery (the zone of Ranvier; Fig. 2-14) through intricate collagen meshwork, thereby playing a role in fracture mechanics and treatment of growth mechanism

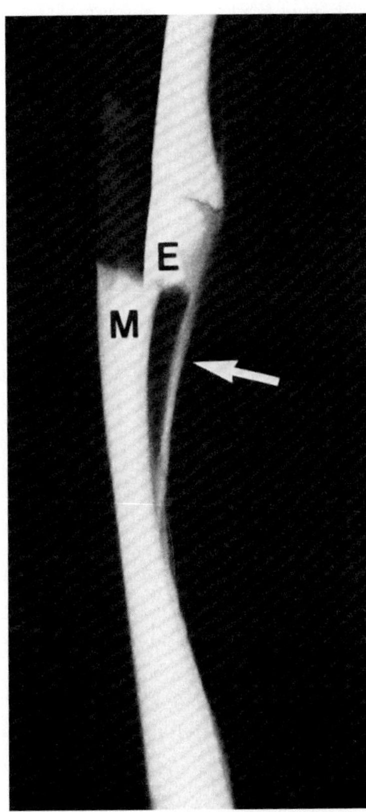

FIGURE 2-14 Simulated type 1 epiphyseal (E) displacement from the metaphysis (M). Note the thick periosteum (*arrow*) and its contiguity with the cartilage of the epiphysis (radiopaque here because of the cartilage and air contrast). In the body, however, the similar soft-tissue radiodensities of cartilage, ligament, muscle, and so forth blend together, making them radiolucent.

injuries (33). The thicker, stronger, more biologically active periosteum affects fracture displacement, reduction, and the rate of subperiosteal callus formation. It also may serve as an effective internal restraint in closed reductions.

Because of its contiguity with the underlying bone, the periosteum is usually injured to some extent in all fractures in children. However, because the periosteum more easily separates from the bone in children, there is much less likelihood of complete circumferential rupture. A significant portion of the periosteum usually remains intact on the concave (compression) side of an injury. This intact periosteal hinge or sleeve may lessen the extent of displacement of the fracture fragments, and it also can be used to assist in the reduction, because the intact portion contributes to the intrinsic stability. Because the periosteum allows some tissue continuity across the fracture, the subperiosteal new bone that forms quickly bridges the fracture gap and leads to more rapid long-term stability. The periosteum may be specifically damaged, with or without concomitant injury to the contiguous bone. Such avulsion injuries may lead to the formation of ectopic bone (52). In contrast, severe disruption of the periosteum, as in an open injury, may impair the fracture healing response. Complete loss of a bone segment, with the periosteal sleeve reasonably intact, may be followed by complete reformation of the missing bone (53).

Histologically, periosteum comprises two tissue layers. While the outer fibroblast layer provides fibrous attachment to subcutaneous connective tissue, muscles, tendons, and ligaments, the inner Cambium layer contains a pool of undifferentiated mesenchymal cells that support bone formation and repair (54). During embryonic and postnatal bone growth, mesenchymal osteoprogenitor cells at the inner layer differentiate directly into bone-forming cells (osteoblasts) and form periosteal bone collar by the intramembranous method (55). Formation of new periosteal bone keeps pace with formation of new endochondral bone. During fracture healing, the mesenchymal cells at the Cambium layer undergo both intramembranous ossification and chondrogenic differentiation with subsequent endochondral ossification (56). Due to the osteochondrogenic potential of these cells from the inner periosteal layer, there has been a lot of interest surrounding the use periosteum as graft tissues or as sources of osteochondroprogenitor cells for repairing cartilage/bone defects or for tissue engineering (57–61).

The periosteum, rather than the bone itself, serves as the origin for most muscle fibers along the metaphysis and diaphysis. This mechanism allows coordinated growth of bone and muscle units; this would be impossible if all the muscle tissue attached directly to the developing bone or cartilage. Exceptions include the attachment of muscle fibers near the linea aspera and into the medial distal femoral metaphysis. The latter pattern of direct metaphyseal osseous attachment may be associated with significant irregularity of cortical and trabecular bone. X-rays of this area often are misinterpreted as showing a neoplastic, osteomyelitic, or traumatic response, even though they exhibit only a variation of skeletal development.

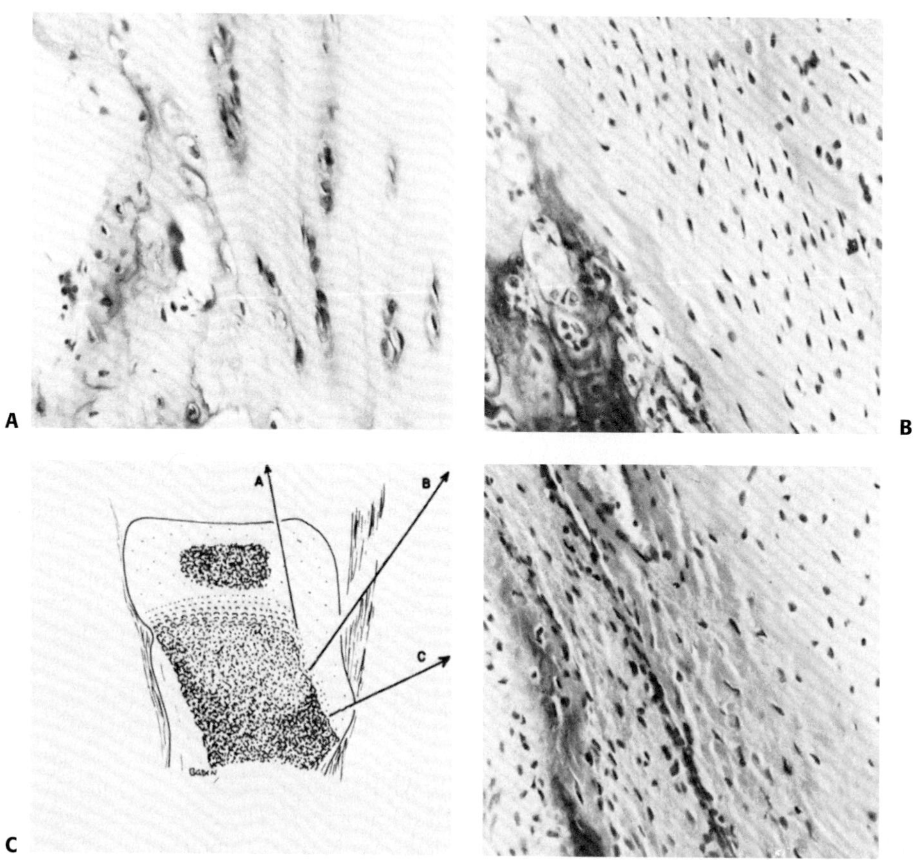

FIGURE 2-15 Histology of a typical apophysis, the tibial tuberosity (tubercle). **A.** Attenuated columnar cartilage adjacent to the main proximal tibial physis. **B.** Fibrocartilage and minimal hypertrophic matrix in the mid-tuberosity region. **C.** Fibrocartilage and membranous ossification in the distal end of the tuberosity.

Apophysis

Because of the differing histologic composition of the tibial tuberosity (fibrocartilage instead of columnar cartilage; Fig. 2-15), failure patterns differ from those in other physes. This area develops primarily as a tensile-responsive structure (i.e., an apophysis). However, the introduction of an osseous secondary ossification center, initially in the distal tuberosity, interposes osseous tissue, which tends to fail in tension and thus may lead to avulsion of part of this ossification center (Fig. 2-16). Healing of the displaced fragment to the underlying undisplaced secondary center creates the symptomatic reactive overgrowth known as an Osgood-Schlatter lesion (62,63). Similarly, in adolescents, excessive tensile stress may avulse the entire tuberosity during the late stages of closure (64).

THE MOLECULAR BONE

Molecules of the Cartilage and Bone Matrices

The Cartilage Matrix

The cartilage matrix is synthesized by chondrocytes. The main constituents of the cartilaginous matrix are collagens (mainly type II) and proteoglycans. Although collagen type II provides structural strength, the proteoglycans have structural and regulatory effects. The structural effects of proteoglycans arise through binding to the collagen components and the water-binding properties that provide resilience to compression. Regulatory effects include growth factor interactions, cell-matrix interactions, and regulation of collagen fibril size. Specific molecules expressed and their functions are listed in Table 2-1.

The Bone Matrix

Except for a small percentage of molecules from the circulation and preexistent matrices that may become entrapped, the bone matrix is almost entirely synthesized by osteoblasts. The composition of the bone matrix was outlined by Buckwalter and associates (65). Briefly, bone matrix is a composite material composed of an inorganic (mineral) portion and an organic portion. The composite structure provides physical strength and resilience to fracture. Bone with deficient inorganic mineral content is pliable, and bone with deficient organic content is brittle.

The composition of living bone is 60% to 70% inorganic components, 5% to 8% water, and the remainder 22% to 35% is organic (66). The inorganic portion is mainly hydroxyapatite, with some carbonate and acid phosphate groups. It has also been suggested that bone crystals do not contain hydroxyl

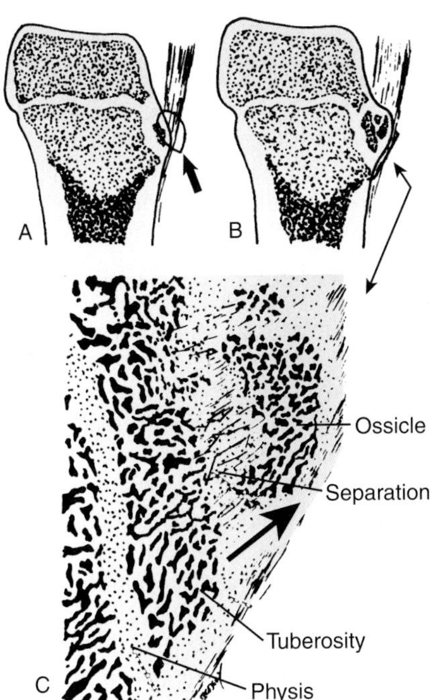

FIGURE 2-16 Avulsion (tension) failure of the developing ossification center of an apophysis. The degree of displacement determines the likelihood of healing and the symptoms and size of the final lump, typical of an Osgood-Schlatter injury.

groups and should be termed apatite rather than hydroxyapatite (65). The organic portion is composed of collagen type I (90%) and noncollagenous proteins. The noncollagenous protein portion includes a number of proteins and proteoglycans that perform structural and regulatory functions. Actual molecules and functions are outlined in Table 2-2 and in the following section.

Matrix Constituents

Although it is not a complete list, the following provides an example of the major proteins found within bone and cartilage matrices.

Collagens. Collagens are a family of proteins coded by at least 19 distinct genes. Members are expressed in most tissues. Collagens have a triple helical region that arises from the repeated winding of three collagen molecules around a common axis. Collagens are synthesized as propeptides that are often glycosylated. Collagen is secreted from cells and is processed in the extracellular space. The processed collagen forms into subunits that then undergo fibrillogenesis (Fig. 2-17). The fact that the final fiber is composed of many individual molecules accounts for the observed dominant negative mutations that can be observed within the collagen family (67). The incorporation of individual molecules containing mutations that affect the packing of the peptides into the triple helix can disturb the structure of the whole fiber. The molecular structures that arise are in the form of fibrils or netlike structures. In reality, the multimeric fibers observed in vivo are often composed of a number of different collagens (68).

TABLE 2-1 Matrix Molecules of Cartilage

Component	Site of Expression Within Physis and Proposed Functions	
Collagens		
Collagen II (fibril)	Predominate collagen of all cartilage; physeal proliferative zone	Imparts strength, site of initial mineralization (78,82,229)
Collagen IX	Proliferative zone of the physis	Associates with the surface of the collagen II fibril (71)
Collagen X (short chain collagen)	Hypertrophic cartilage	Mineralization (75,229,230)
Collagen XI (fibril)	Proliferative and hypertrophic zone of the physis	Collagen fibril size (229)
Proteoglycans		
Aggrecan	Throughout cartilage	Imparts resistance to compression. Forms aggregates with hyaluronic acid and link proteins (81,82,229)
Decorin (DS-PG2)	Within chondrocytes and the Interterritorial capsules of the upper proliferative chondrocytes	Influences collagen fibril size and TGF-β activity (85,86).
Biglycan (DS-PG1)	Territorial capsules of the upper proliferative chondrocytes	TGT-β activity (86)
Fibromodulin	Physeal cartilage	Influences collagen fibril diameter and binding of cells to the matrix (23)
Matrix Gla protein	Cartilage	Inhibits mineralization (89,91,96)

TABLE 2-2 Composition of Bone

Component	Proposed Functions
Collagens	
Collagen I	Imparts strength, site of initial mineralization
Collagen V	Provide the inner core of the collagen fibril (73,232)
Collagen VI	Cell attachment
Collagen XII	Collagen fibril size
Proteoglycans	
Decorin (DS-PG2)	Influences collagen fibril size and TGF-β activity (87,231,233)
Biglycan (DS-PG1)	Influences collagen fibril assembly and TGF-β activity (84,234)
Fibromodulin	Influences collagen fibril diameter and binding of cells to matrix molecules (231)
Osteocalcin (bone Gla protein)	Binds hydroxyapatite (88,92)
Matrix Gla protein	Controls mineralization (88)
Osteonectin	Binds calcium (92)
Osteopontin	Cell attachment (93,94)

Collagen type I is the main collagen found in bone and other tissues. It is composed of two $\alpha1(I)$ and one $\alpha2(I)$ polypeptides. The collagen type I fibers act as sites for initial mineralization and provide tensile strength to the bone. Mutations in the propeptides can cause a variety of phenotypes affecting mineralization and bone fragility, the most severe being osteogenesis imperfecta. In contrast, collagen type II is a triple helical molecule that is composed of three $\alpha1(II)$ polypeptides and is expressed in cartilage, particularly within the proliferative zone of the physis. It is the main fibril-forming collagen in cartilage. Mutations cause Langer-Saldino achondrogenesis and spondyloepiphyseal dysplasia congenita (69,70).

Other collagen types, such as V, IX, and XI, associate with the collagen fibers (71,72). They may influence collagen diameters and interact with other matrix molecules (73). Mutations in types IX and XI can result in a number of clinical manifestations (74). Collagen type X is associated with the matrix of hypertrophic chondrocytes and is involved with the mineralization process of cartilage matrix (75–78). Mutation of collagen X causes spondylometaphyseal dysplasia (32), but the deletion of the encoding gene results in mild changes (32,79).

Proteoglycans. Proteoglycans are present in large amounts within all connective tissues. Proteoglycans are proteins that have either one or a number of polysaccharide chains linked to a protein core. The polysaccharide's glycosaminoglycan side chains are heparin, heparin sulfate, chondroitin sulfate, dermatan sulfate, or keratan sulfate. The glycosaminoglycans differ in the composition of their constituent disaccharide structures. They can combine with other molecules within the matrix to form macromolecular structures (Fig. 2-18) (80).

Proteoglycans are critical components of cartilage and bone (81–84). The proteoglycans present in the physis include large proteoglycans like aggrecan as well as smaller proteoglycans, such as decorin, biglycan, and possibly, fibromodulin. Decorin and biglycan have side chains of dermatan sulfate, and betaglycan has chondroitin and heparin sulfate chains. Fibromodulin has side chains of keratan sulfate. The territorial capsules of the chondrocytes in the upper proliferative region of the physis stain for biglycan, and the interterritorial matrix stains for decorin (85). These proteoglycans have a structural role but are also known to interact with growth factors (83,85–87).

Other Non-collagenous Proteins. Osteocalcin is also known as bone Gla protein. It has three residues of gamma-carboxyglutamic acid that enable it to bind to hydroxyapatite. It is thought to play a role in mineralization of the bone matrix (88,89), but the exact mechanism and function are undetermined (90,91). Osteonectin has the ability to bind calcium and collagen type I, and may enable the process of mineralization that is initiated

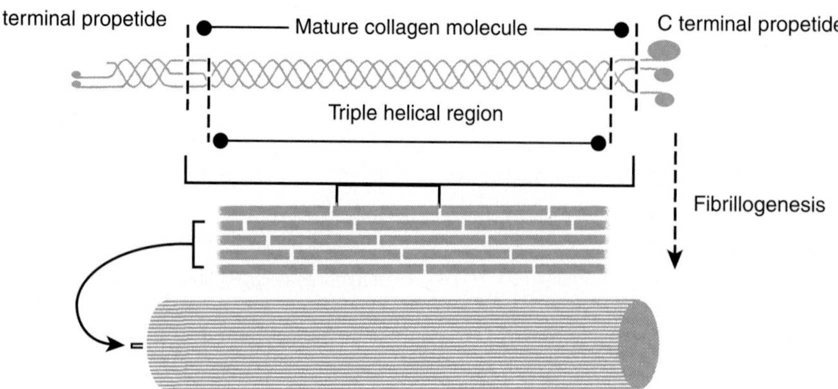

FIGURE 2-17 Collagens are synthesized as a propeptide that is often glycosylated (not shown). The collagen molecule has a triple helical region that arises from the repeated winding of three collagen molecules around a common axis. The processed collagen forms into subunits that then undergo fibrillogenesis.

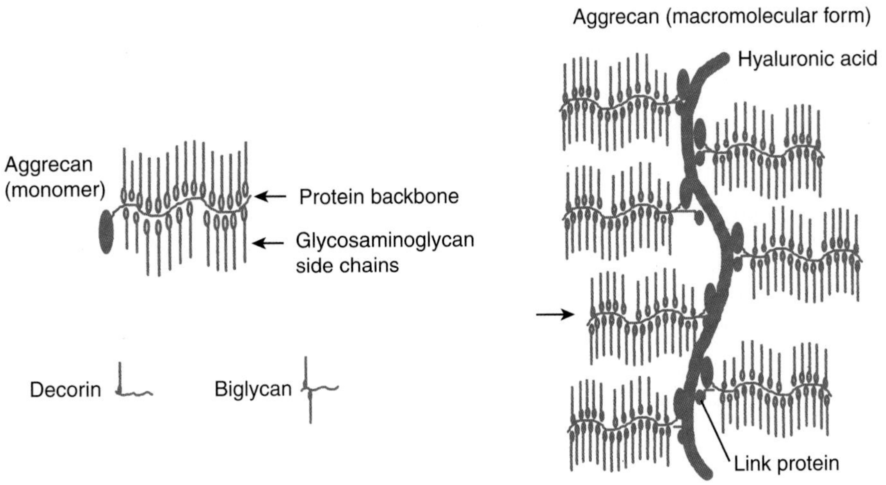

FIGURE 2-18 Proteoglycans are proteins, which have either one or a number of polysaccharide (glycosaminoglycan) chains linked to a protein core. Aggrecan is present in cartilage and has the ability to form macromolecular structures with hyaluronic acid and link protein. Decorin and biglycan are present in bone and cartilage matrix.

on the collagen type I fibers (92). Osteopontin is thought to be critically involved with the binding of osteoclasts (93,94), the cells that degrade the bone and physeal matrix (95). Matrix Gla protein is an inhibitor of calcification. The cartilage of mice lacking this protein undergoes spontaneous calcification (96).

Growth Factors

Within an individual, cell-to-cell communication occurs between neighboring cells and between cells that are separated by up to an almost complete body length. Communication signals take the form of diffusible molecules, which pass between the cells or by cell surface–bound receptor-ligand interactions (97,98). In addition, neighboring cells can pass information between one another via their gap junctions (99). These channels enable the passage of small molecules, including calcium ions, between neighboring cells. Calcium is a key second messenger that provokes a number of cellular events (100).

Hormones are a group of diverse molecules that are secreted by endocrine glands and are transported by body fluids. They coordinate body functions in complex organisms. Hormones can be in the form of amino acid derivatives (e.g., epinephrine), polypeptides (e.g., somatotropin or growth hormone), glycoproteins (e.g., follicle-stimulating hormone), steroids (e.g., testosterone), or fatty acids (e.g., prostaglandins).

Growth factors and hormones may circulate in a free form or be bound to carrier molecules or to the extracellular matrix (101). The binding of growth factors and hormones to other molecules may facilitate their transportation to their target tissues, increase their survival by inhibiting their proteolytic degradation, and control their activities. Many growth factors, including the fibroblast growth factors (FGFs), transforming growth factor-β (TGF-β), and insulin-like growth factors (IGFs), can be bound to the matrix molecules. Cell activation usually requires the factors to bind to their receptors on the cell surface, although a number of hydrophobic hormones pass directly through the outer cell membrane and bind to intracellular receptors (102–105) (Fig. 2-19).

A degree of redundancy often exists in that a gene knockout for one particular growth factor may result in only slight changes in the phenotype observed. A good example is the double mutant of BMP-5 and BMP-7, which is lethal during embryonic development, but a null mutation in either one has little effect (106).

Fibroblast Growth Factors. The biologic effects of the fibroblast growth factors (FGFs) are widespread. FGFs are angiogenic and can influence mitosis, differentiation, migration, and survival in many cell types. FGFs can activate one of four high-affinity FGF receptors (FGFRs). Point mutations of these receptors have been implicated in a number of skeletal deformities including Pfeiffer's syndrome (FGFR1), Crouzon's and Jackson-Weiss syndromes (FGFR2), and achondroplasia (FGFR3) (107), suggesting that FGFR signaling is an essential regulatory component for skeletal growth and development (108).

The ligands activating the FGFRs in the developing skeleton remain largely unknown. To date, the FGF family comprises 22 members including acidic FGF (FGF-1), basic FGF (FGF-2) (109). FGF-1 and FGF-2 are present in the extracellular matrix of bone (110). Recent data reveal that FGF-18 may be a physiological ligand for FGFR-3 in regulating bone lengthening, but it may also signal through another FGFR to regulate osteoblast growth (111).

The FGFs are also complicated by the presence of alternative forms of the specific forms of FGF-1 and FGF-2. FGF-1 is typically 140 amino acids in length, but larger forms of 160 and 154 amino acids have been identified. FGF-2 is normally translated as a 155 amino acid molecule, but through the use of alternative start codons, three higher molecular weight forms have been identified.

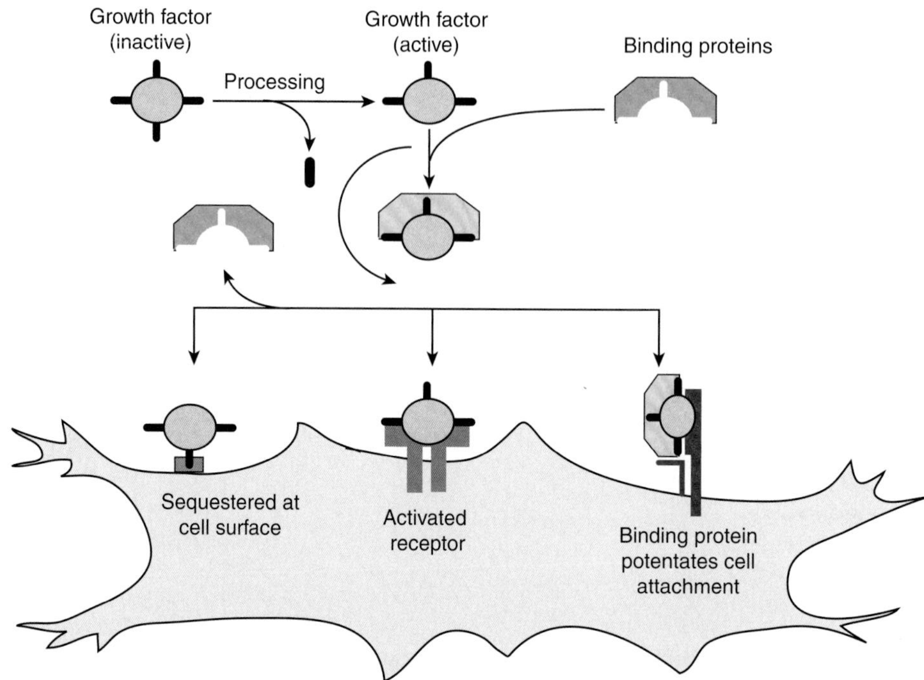

FIGURE 2-19 The figure shows aspects of growth factor interactions. Any particular growth factor will possess only a subset of such interactions. Growth factors may require activation (e.g., TGF-β). Binding proteins may sequester or protect the growth factor. The binding protein may also potentate the binding of the growth factor to the surface receptor (e.g., FGF and heparin). Cells may also sequester the growth factor at the cell surface.

The acidic (FGF-1) and basic (FGF-2) forms of FGFs are well conserved across species. Comparing the amino acid composition of FGF-1 and FGF-2 from different species, Hearn found a 92% sequence identity between human and bovine FGF-1. Only 2/155 and 3/155 amino acids differ in human and bovine, and human and ovine, forms of FGF-2, respectively (112).

Insulin-like Growth Factor. Insulin-like growth factor-1 (IGF-1) is critical for normal bone growth as it has been confirmed by the severe growth retardation in the IGF-1 and its receptor gene knockout mice (113,114). Genetic studies with various mutant, knock out, and congenic mice have revealed that there is a clear relationship between circulating IGF-1 concentrations and bone volume (115). Consistently, delivery of exogenous IGF-1 stimulated growth of growth plate height in normal rats, enhanced chondrocyte maturation and thus longitudinal growth in hypophysectomized rats (116), and stimulated longitudinal and circumferential growth and increased bone mineral density (115).

Cell-surface receptor for IGF-1 has been found present on chondrocytes at all stages of differentiation in growth plate cartilage (117). Expression of IGF-1 mRNA and protein has also been localized in all chondrocyte layers of growth plate (118), suggesting that locally produced IGF-1 acts at the chondrocyte level in a paracrine/autocrine manner to stimulate longitudinal growth. In primary cultures, IGF-1 stimulates proliferation and matrix synthesis in growth plate chondrocytes (119). Consistently, in rodent in vivo studies, infused IGF-1 not only stimulates growth plate chondrocytes at all stages of differentiation, but also promotes chondrogenic differentiation via its effects on resting stem-like cells of the growth plate (116).

In bone, there is a high level of IGF-1 protein deposited in bone matrix, and it has been demonstrated that the vast majority of IGF-1 in bone is derived locally from osteoblastic synthesis (115). Osteoblasts appear to be the major target of IGF-1 as IGF-1 type 1 receptor is present on osteoblasts and IGF-1 stimulates osteoblast proliferation and its recruitment (120). Since IGF-1 is stored within the skeletal matrix and is released during bone resorption, IGF-1 may be a critical coupling factor that keeps bone formation closely linked to bone remodeling (115) (see Bone Remodeling section later).

Transforming Growth Factor-Beta. The transforming growth factor-beta (TGF-β) superfamily is composed of more than 24 members (121). They are subdivided into families including TGF-β, inhibin, decapentaplegic protein/vegetal hemisphere 1 (DPP/Vg1), and müllerian-inhibiting substance. Members of the TGF-β and the DPP/Vg1 families have critical functions in the development of the skeleton, its growth and maintenance, and fracture repair. The bone morphogenic proteins (except for BMP-1) are members of the DPP/Vg1 family and are discussed in the next section.

Previous studies indicated that TGF-β stimulates bone formation when injected into rodent bones, and induces endochondral bone formation in adult non-human primates. Most fracture healing studies have also demonstrated positive effects of TGF-β in stimulating bone repair and its potential usefulness in implant fixation (122).

There are at least nine receptors for TGF-β. However, most of the TGF-β functions are mediated through two receptors termed receptor 1 and 2, which are members of the serine/threonine kinase family (123). TGF-β receptor type 3 is a membrane-bound proteoglycan termed betaglycan. Betaglycan is thought to act as a TGF-β cell surface reservoir and is not involved with signal transduction itself.

Of the five TGF-β family members, four members including three identified in mammals (TGF-β1, -β2 and -β3) and one in amphibians (TGF-β5) are synthesized as large precursor forms that are processed to active forms. Members of the TGF-β family (TGF-β1, TBG-β2) are highly expressed in bone, and like IGF-1, the proteins are sequestered in the matrix. Important in fracture repair, TGF-β1 and TGF-β2 are also released in large quantities during platelet activation. The active form is either a heterodimer or homodimer. It is thought that the pro-region may either help in the folding of the proteins during synthesis or control TGF-β activity. In the case of TGF-β1, the pro-region and a second glycoprotein can also bind to the active factor to form a latent complex. Apart from the presence of the growth factor itself, the presence or absence of the latent complex controls the activity of TGF-β1. The active TGF-β1 complex can be released from the latent complex by extreme pH or by catalytic methods. This is particularly important in fracture repair and bone remodeling. The activation of latent TGF-β is likely to be critical in the induction of fracture repair and osteoblast function.

The active TGF-β molecules may also be bound and their activity controlled by a number of matrix molecules, including betaglycan and decorin (123,124). Betaglycan has the possibility of binding FGFs through the heparin sulfate chains and may present TGF-β in conjunction with FGFs to the cell (123). TGF-β also binds to the small proteoglycans: biglycan, decorin, and fibromodulin (86,87). The small proteoglycans bind TGF-β through the leucine-rich repeats in their protein cores and are thought to sequester TGF-β in the matrix. They also compete with betaglycan in binding TGF-β. Decorin has the ability to negatively regulate the activity of TGF-β (125,126).

Bone Morphogenic Proteins. The bone morphogenic proteins (BMPs) and their orthopaedic relevance and applications have been reviewed previously (12,122,126). The BMPS (except BMP-1) represent a group of related growth factors that have critical roles in the cell proliferation and differentiation of a number of cell types including mesenchymal cells, chondrocytes, and osteoblasts (8,12,122,126–131). They have roles in embryo and fetal development, bone growth, and fracture repair. Several BMPs produce ectopic cartilage or bone when implanted subcutaneously (132–134).

BMPs exist as glycosylated dimers. Like the other growth factors discussed so far, the BMPs have a number of binding proteins both in the extracellular matrix and on the cell surface. A secreted glycoprotein termed noggin can bind and inactivate BMPs (135). Chordin is a similar protein that most likely has a similar function (136). It has been proposed that these proteins control BMP activity and may also serve as a mechanism for establishing gradients of BMPs across the embryo during development. Active BMPs bind to heterotetrameric serine/threonine kinase receptors. The nonactivated receptors exist as type 1 and 2 receptor proteins, with the type 2 receptor being able to autophosphorylate. Once the ligand binds, the two receptors are brought together and the receptor type 1 receptor is phosphorylated. Only after the receptor type 1 is phosphorylated is a cellular response achieved. Intracellular activation is via the intracellular proteins termed SMADs, but other inhibitors can still come into play. Exposure of the cell to a number of other growth factors (including cer-1) can inhibit the activation of the cell by BMPs (126,137).

Angiogenic Growth Factors. The invasion of the metaphyseal vascular supply is crucial to endochondral ossification, and fracture repair does not occur without an adequate vascular supply. Bone fracture disrupts the marrow architecture and blood vessels within and around the fracture site. During fracture healing, regeneration of three normal blood supplies (the medullary, periosteal, and osseous) to the callus and cortical bone need to be coordinated (49).

Angiogenic factors are growth factors that promote neovascularization. They are essential for neovascularization during the normal bone lengthening and fracture repair. Previous studies have shown that the key angiogenic growth factor, vascular endothelial growth factor (VEGF), is essential for blood vessel invasion of the growth plate mineralized hypertrophic cartilage, cartilage remodeling, and bone formation during normal endochondral bone lengthening (138). Endogenous VEGF also plays a key role in bone repair, as blocking VEGF activity inhibited repair of femoral fractures and cortical defects in rodents (139). At the bone fracture site, VEGF activity is essential for appropriate angiogenesis, callus architecture, and mineralization (122). Several studies have demonstrated that local delivery of exogenous VEGF promotes angiogenesis and bone formation at the bone fracture site (122).

Apart from VEGF, several other growth factors are also important angiogenic factors, including FGF-2, TGF-β, platelet-derived growth factor (PDGF). It is probably not by accident that a number of angiogenic factors such as TGF-β and FGF-2 are sequestered in the bone matrix. Angiogenic factors act directly (such as VEGF and FGF-2) or indirectly (such as TGF-β and tumor necrosis factor-α) on endothelial cells, promoting proliferation and migration of the cells into areas in which they are released at the injury site (140). Angiogenic factors acting indirectly by recruiting macrophages and monocytes, in turn, release their own direct-acting angiogenic factors (141). During angiogenesis, while VEGF and FGF-2 induce angioblast differentiation and TGF-β1 enhances smooth muscle cell differentiation from mesenchymal cells, PDGF-B stimulates recruitments of smooth muscle cells and pericytes around nascent vessels (142).

MECHANISMS OF BONE GROWTH

Because bone is rigid, it cannot grow by internal expansion and bone growth is achieved by adding newly synthesized bone to existing bone by two mechanisms: *endochondral ossification* and *intramembranous ossification*. These mechanisms are named by the intermediate structures, which must be passed to form the bone. The production of any particular bone after initial differentiation may involve discrete, juxtaposed, or interspersed areas of each basic pattern. Endochondral-derived bones generally have membranous ossification by appositional bone growth from the periosteum. Similarly, membrane-derived bones may grow and elongate by an endochondral process (21,52).

Endochondral Ossification

Endochondral ossification is the process by which bone forms via a cartilaginous intermediate. The physis (or the growth plate) best reflects this process. Physes are temporary cartilaginous tissue situated between the primary and secondary ossification centers of all long bones. From 9 to 10 weeks' gestational age to skeletal maturity at 15 to 17 years, they are responsible for the longitudinal growth of bone. The physis can be divided into at least three zones. The reserve or resting zone is situated on the epiphyseal side and contains small, spherical cells in groups of two or three cells randomly distributed throughout the zone. These cells are stem cell–like, responsible for generating new chondrocytes of the physis. In the adjacent proliferative zone, chondrocytes undergo mitosis and are organized into columns running parallel to the axis of bone growth. Cells in the proliferative zone mature and eventually increase to five to ten times their volume in the hypertrophic region. Matrix vesicles are also deposited within the longitudinal septa of the physis. Matrix vesicles are membrane-encapsulated structures that are thought to concentrate calcium and phosphate. Enzymes such as alkaline phosphatase convert organic phosphates to inorganic phosphates. The longitudinal septum around the terminal hypertrophic chondrocytes mineralizes, and this mineralized matrix forms the template for new bone deposition in the metaphysis (Fig. 2-20).

Associated with these changes in cellular arrangement and volume, the matrix in the physis also undergoes a continual

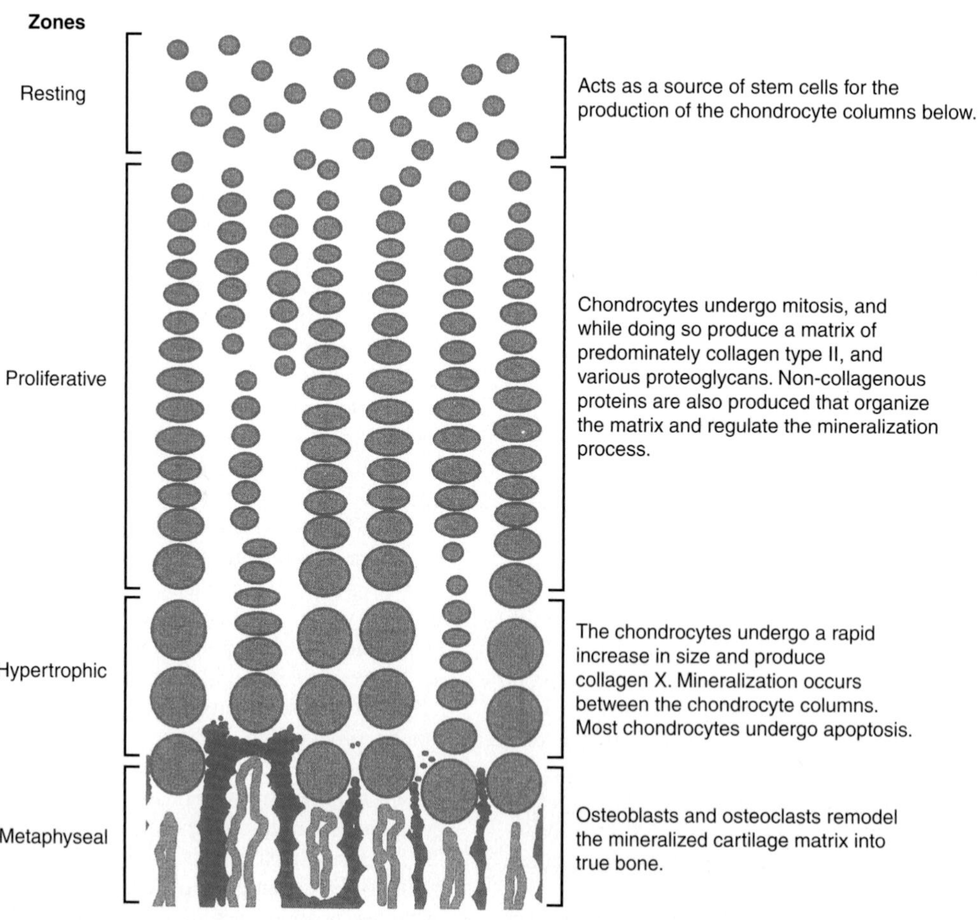

FIGURE 2-20 The figure shows the process of endochondral ossification within the physis. Although not as organized, endochondral ossification follows a similar pattern during fracture repair.

modification in content. The two major macromolecules of cartilage matrix produced by the chondrocytes are the proteoglycans (predominantly aggrecan and with lesser amounts of decorin, biglycan, and fibromodulin) and the collagens (types II, IX, X, and XI). The major change in physeal proteoglycan structure occurs as chondrocytes organize into columns in the proliferative zone. Additional variation occurs in the hypertrophic region, where the glycosaminoglycan sulfation pattern demonstrates differences between the pericellular and extracellular spaces and the appearance of a unique collagen (type X) is observed. The small proteoglycans—decorin, biglycan, and fibromodulin—are also differentially expressed across the physis, although detailed studies of these proteoglycans have not been done (see Table 2-1).

Regulatory Mechanisms in the Physis

The normal process of endochondral bone formation is tightly regulated by endocrine/paracrine/autocrine factors, such as hormones, vitamins, transcriptional factors, and growth factors, and involves coordinated and sequential expression of growth-regulatory factors. Although growth hormone (GH) in the circulation has a global effect on physeal function throughout the body, many locally produced growth factors act locally. Many hormones (such as GH, thyroid hormone, estrogen, glucocorticoids, calcitonin), vitamins (vitamin D3, ascorbate, retinoic acid), morphorgens (Indian hedgehog [IHH], BMPs), growth factors (IGFs, BMPs, FGFs, parathyroid hormone-related peptide [PTHrP], PDGF, TGF-β, VEGF) and their binding proteins (such as IGFBPs, chordin, noggin), and cytokines (tumor necrosis factor-α, interleukin IL-1, and others) have now been shown to have important roles in regulating various processes of the endochondral ossification (Fig. 2-21) (143). Cellular response is determined by parallel processing of the intracellular signals that are induced by a number of active growth factors binding to their specific receptors. Presented below is an outline of the likely actions of a number of key growth factors on endochondral ossification.

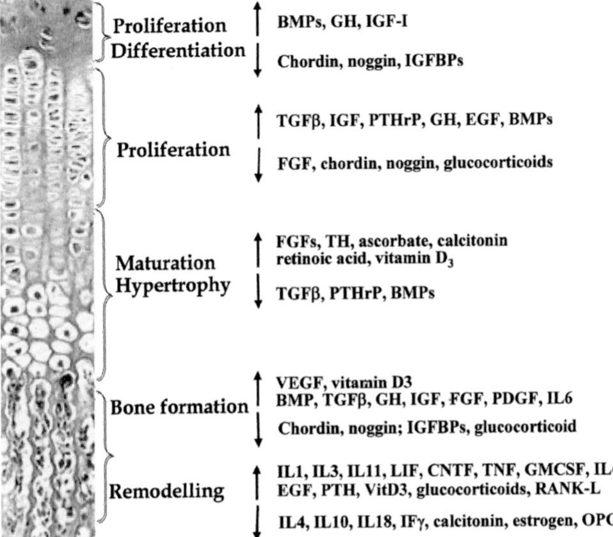

FIGURE 2-21 Systemic and local factors including hormones, vitamins, cytokines, and growth factors that control or influence chondrocyte differentiation, proliferation, and maturation, as well as bone formation and remodeling. See the text for specific actions.

It is well known that growth hormone (GH) and IGF-1 are two major factors regulating postnatal growth. In skeletal tissues, both chondrocytes and osteoblasts synthesize IGF-1, and GH modulates its synthesis in both cell populations. According to the original somatomedin hypothesis, GH stimulates skeletal growth through IGF-1 that is produced in the liver under the influence of GH and secreted into the circulation (145). Upon reaching target tissues, IGF-1 interacts with its receptors and induces a cellular growth signal. However, normal postnatal growth achieved in liver-IGF-1 null mice (in which hepatic IGF-1 expression was abolished specifically) suggests the importance of extrahepatic IGF-1 expression and an autocrine-paracrine role for IGF-1 in normal skeletal growth (146). Therefore, both circulating and locally expressed IGF-1 play important roles in longitudinal bone growth and the maintenance of bone mass, and IGF-1 plays an essential role in longitudinal bone growth in response to GH exposure (147).

GH controls stem cell maturation and this action is at least partially mediated via local production and action of IGF-1 at the stem cell zone (118). GH receptor has been localized in the growth plate chondrocytes particularly in the proliferative zone (148–150), and it is generally accepted that GH acts at both the stem and proliferative phases of chondrocyte differentiation (116). At present, apart from the IGF-1-mediated effects on the stem cells of the growth plate, GH also stimulated proliferation of the prechondrocytes in the resting zone (151) and has some priming effect on these stem cells to promote their differentiation independently of IGF-1, as proposed by the dual effector theory. In addition, there is recent genetic evidence that supports this dual, IGF-1-independent and IGF-1-dependent roles for GH in promoting longitudinal bone growth (152).

Apart from IGF-1 and GH, BMP-2 and BMP-7 also promote proliferation, differentiation, and matrix synthesis in undifferentiated chondrocytes in the resting zone (128,153). It is believed that once the chondrocytes start differentiating, the expression of noggin inhibits the continual outgrowth of the undifferentiated chondrocytes (154). Once the chondrocyte has lost its resting phenotype, IGF-1 may act as a stimulator of proliferation and differentiation (18,155). Epidermal growth factor (EGF) can augment IGF stimulation by increasing the expression of the IGF-1 receptor (156). Although the chondrocytes synthesize large quantities of matrix molecules, they also synthesize FGF-1, FGF-2, TGF-β, VEGF, and a number of the BMPs (53,157,158). These molecules can act in an autocrine or paracrine manner, but many are sequestered into the newly formed cartilage matrix. While FGF-2 in low doses is mitogenic for the chondrocytes (159), as occurs in achondroplasia, constant activation of FGF receptor (FGFR3) inhibits chondrocyte proliferation and accelerates terminal differentiation of chondrocytes (160–162). FGF/heparin sulfate interaction is probable in the differentiation of the physeal chondrocytes because the continuous exposure of FGF-2 inhibits chondrocyte differentiation in vitro and inhibitors of glycosaminoglycan sulfation (including heparin sulfate) restore the differentiation process. Additional sulfate permits glycosaminoglycan sulfation and returns the effect of FGF-2 (163).

Parathyroid hormone (PTH) and parathyroid hormone–related protein (PTHrP) act to maintain the proliferative state of and inhibit the maturation of chondrocytes. It is postulated that two negative feedback loops involving actions of PTHrP regulate the pace of chondrocyte differentiation in the postnatal growth plate (164). The first loop is confined to the proliferative-hypertrophic transition zone and early hypertrophic chondrocytes, which express morphogen Indian hedgehog (IHH), its receptor Patched, and PTH/PTHrP receptor. IHH, which stimulates chondrocyte proliferation and inhibits hypertrophic differentiation, binds Patched in the hypertrophic zone resulting in a stimulated production of PTHrP. PTHrP then acts on its receptor at the proliferating chondrocytes to keep them proliferating and, thereby to delay the production of IHH, thus closing the IHH-PTHrP feedback loop (Fig. 2-22). In the second feedback loop, IHH can bind Patched in the resting stem cell zone, and this may stimulate PTHrP production, which then diffuses to its receptor leading to IHH down-regulation. These two IHH-PTHrP signaling cascade feedback loops limit maturation of proliferative chondrocytes to hypertrophic form (164–166).

Studies have shown that several signaling pathways regulating chondrocyte proliferation and hypertrophic differentiation interact with the IHH-PTHrP feedback loops (Fig. 2-22). Apart from inhibiting chondrocyte proliferation, part of the effects of FGF signaling in positively affecting chondrocyte maturation is mediated by the suppression of IHH expression (167). However, FGF effects on chondrocytes can occur independently of PTHrP/IHH action (168). In the growth plate, expression of the mRNA for BMP-2 and BMP-6 peaks in hypertrophic chondrocytes before mineralization (157). Recent studies have demonstrated that BMPs act on chondrocytes to induce proliferation through the induction of IHH expression by prehypertrophic chondrocytes, suggesting that BMP signaling modulates the IHH/PTHrP signaling pathway that regulates the rate of chondrocyte differentiation (160,169). In addition, in vitro studies have suggested that during embryonic development, signaling of TGF-β2 may act as a critical signal relay between IHH and PTHrP. It mediates the effects of IHH inhibiting hypertrophic differentiation and induces PTHrP expression, maintaining the chondrocytes in proliferative state and slowing down the pace of their maturation (132).

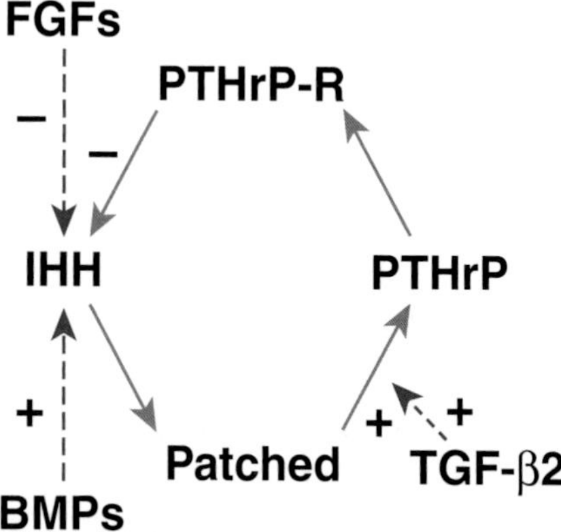

FIGURE 2-22 Schematic representation of an IHH-PTHrP feedback loop controlling the rate of chondrocyte hypertrophic maturation and its modulation by BMPs, TGF-β2, and FGFs in a postnatal growth plate. PTHrP is secreted from hypertrophic chondrocytes and acts on PTHrP receptor on proliferating chondrocytes to keep the chondrocytes proliferating. When PTHrP expression is low, IHH is produced by the maturing cells. IHH binds to its receptor Patched on the hypertrophic cells, resulting in a stimulation of PTHrP expression. Activation of PTHrP receptor by PTHrP in turn represses IHH expression, thus closing a negative feedback loop. FGFs and BMPs interact with this negative feedback loop through their activities in inhibiting and stimulating the production of IHH, respectively. Evidence has suggested that TGF-β2 mediates the function of IHH in stimulating the production of PTHrP.

Although the chondrocytes of the physis will proliferate and form a cartilaginous matrix with only the epiphyseal vascular supply, the metaphyseal vessels are critical for the mineralization process (25). Metaphyseal vascular invasion occurs at the hypertrophic-metaphyseal interface. The endothelial cells invade most likely as a consequence of angiogenic factors present in the matrix or secreted by the chondrocytes themselves. VEGF, TGF-β, and FGFs are known to be present in the growth plate cartilage matrix and are angiogenic. It is interesting that an oversupply of FGF-2 infused into the physis induces vascular invasion from the metaphysis only; even if the FGF-2 is present at the epiphyseal side of the physis, the epiphyseal vessel will not invade (170). Apart from providing the necessary nutrients for the mineralization process, the metaphyseal vessels also bring in osteoblasts, osteoclasts, and other cell types. The osteoclasts degrade the mineralized cartilage matrix while osteoblasts lay down new bone that is also rich in growth factors such as TGF-β, FGF-2, IGF-1, and BMPs.

Membranous Ossification

All axial and appendicular skeletal elements are involved in secondary membranous ossification. The diaphyseal cortex of developing tubular bone is progressively formed (modeled) by the periosteum and modified (remodeled) by the re-formation of osteons. This peripheral periosteal process of membrane-derived ossification is extensive and rapid in fracture healing in infants and young children. The replacement process also may be seen when portions of the developing metaphysis or diaphysis are removed for use as bone grafts.

Intramembranous ossification occurs when osteoprogenitor cells are formed from the overlying tissue, the inner Cambium layer of the periosteum (54) (see Periosteum section earlier). The osteoprogenitor cells continue to differentiate into osteoblasts, which produce and add new bone matrix peripherally that later undergoes mineralization.

Remodeling of Bones

The first bone to be laid down either from the physis at the metaphysis or in the fracture callus is woven bone, which is remodeled to lamellar bone. At the metaphysis, the trabeculae of bone-covered calcified cartilage (primary spongiosa) will be resorbed by osteoclasts and the calcified cartilage template will be replaced by lamellar bone and remodeled into more mature bone trabeculae (secondary spongiosa). The deposited secondary bone trabeculae at the metaphyseal-diaphyseal junction will be further remodeled and incorporated into the diaphysis, in a process in which osteoclasts remove bone from the periphery of the metaphysis and new bone is formed at the endosteal surfaces. Although cancellous bone can be remodeled and obtain its nutrients from the surface, cortical bone is remodeled into a complex structure of osteons that together form the cortical bone. Osteons are tubular structures that interconnect. They consist of layers of ordered lamellar bone around a central canal. The central canal contains blood vessels, lymphatics, and in some cases, nerves (65).

Bone is constantly remodeled by osteoclasts and osteoblasts. The bone is encapsulated by bone-lining cells that have the potential to become activated osteoblasts. The bone-lining cells have slender cellular processes that make contact with the osteocytes within the mineralized bone. Osteocytes are thought to arise from osteoblasts that have become entrapped during bone formation. It has been proposed that the bone-lining cells need to erode the osteoid that covers the underling bone for osteoclasts to bind (171,172). Osteoclasts are bone-degrading cells that are produced from the hematopoietic pathway. Upon activation, they bind to the surface of the bone and secrete enzymes into the space beneath. The space is acidic and contains many proteolytic and bone degrading enzymes (173). The acidic pH and proteases are thought to release and activate the sequestered growth factors IGF-1 and TGF-β, resulting in the recruitment, proliferation, differentiation, and activation of the stromal osteoprogenitor cells and bone-lining cells to become active osteoblasts, synthesizing bone matrix and increasing their survival (Fig. 2-23) (174–177). The newly laid osteoid by osteoblasts is subsequently mineralized to become bone.

It is now generally accepted that the osteoblast activity and osteoclast activity are linked during the bone remodeling. On the one hand, osteoclastic activity release growth factors

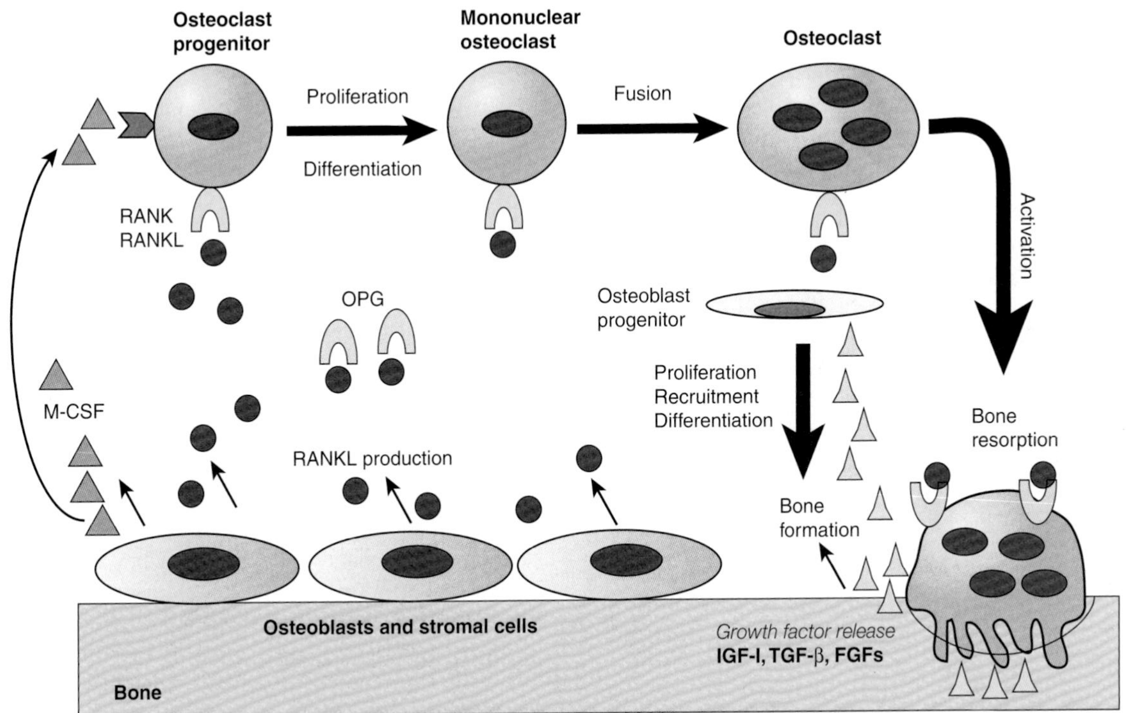

FIGURE 2-23 The linked activities of osteoclast bone resorption and osteoblast bone formation during bone remodeling. Bone-lining cells, osteoblasts or some marrow stromal cells express RANKL, which activates receptor RANK on osteoclast progenitors of the monocyte-macrophage lineage and stimulates the osteoclast differentiation and activation. M-CSF is another essential factor for osteoclast differentiation. However, decoy receptor OPG binds RANKL and antagonizes RANK function and thus inhibits osteoclast formation. Activated osteoclasts secret acid and proteases and erode bone on the surface. During the resorption process, sequestered growth factors, such as IGF-I, TGF-β and FGFs, are released from the bone matrix and activated, which results in the recruitment, differentiation, and activation of the osteoprogenitors to become osteoblasts to initiate bone matrix synthesis and bone formation.

IGF-1 and TGF-β stimulating osteoblastic differentiation and activity as described above (Fig. 2-23), and on the other, cells of the osteoblast lineage provide factors essential for the differentiation of osteoclasts. The discovery of the interaction between the receptor activator of NF-kappaB (RANK) ligand (RANKL) expressed by osteoblasts and its receptor RANK expressed on osteoclast precursors confirms the well-known hypothesis that osteoblasts play an essential role in osteoclast differentiation (Fig. 2-23) (178). It is now known that two hematopoietic factors, namely RANKL and macrophage colony-stimulating factor (M-CSF), together are necessary and sufficient for osteoclast formation (179). Several factors have now been identified that can modulate RANK-induced osteoclastogenesis. Although vitamin D3 metabolite, PTH, PTHrP, PGE2, cytokines IL-1, IL-6, TNF, LIF, and IL-11, and corticosteroids have been shown to induce the expression of RANKL in stromal/osteoblastic cells and thus stimulate osteoclast formation, osteoprotegerin (OPG), a decoy receptor for RANKL, blocks the RANKL-RANK interaction and inhibits osteoclastogenesis (179,180). Recent studies have also shown that lipopolysaccharide and inflammatory cytokines such as TNF-α and IL-1 can also directly regulate osteoclast differentiation and function through a mechanism independent of the RANKL-RANK interaction (181). TGF-β superfamily members and interferon-gamma (INF-γ) are also shown to be important regulators in osteoclastogenesis (182). Estrogens, calcitonin, BMP2/4, TGF-β, IL-17, PDGF, and calcium have been shown to be anabolic or inhibit osteoclastogenesis (179) (Fig. 2-21). In addition, EGF receptor signaling has been shown to be important for the secretion of matrix metalloproteases (MMPs) (183) and maintenance of osteoclast activity (184), both of which are important for the bone remodeling.

The osteocytes may serve as the mechanosensory system that may be associated with bone remodeling. Osteocytes also possess cellular processes that connect osteocytes to one another and to the bone-lining cells above (185). It is possible that the osteocytes are responsible for sensing bone stress; if undue stress is detected, they favor bone deposition, whereas if a lack of stress is detected, they favor bone resorption.

FRACTURE REPAIR

Injuries to the developing skeleton may involve osseous, fibrous, and cartilaginous tissues. Healing of these tissues differs, depending on both the type of tissue and the temporal maturation.

Osseous Healing

The progressive changes of the normal process of osseous fracture healing, whether in the diaphysis, metaphysis, or epiphyseal ossification center, may be grouped conveniently into a series of phases that occur in a reasonably chronologic sequence (19,186). Several factors that influence bone healing have been identified from clinical observation as well as experimental work (36,187), and must be taken into account when treating childhood fractures on a rational basis. However, certain areas of the developing skeleton, particularly the physis and epiphyseal hyaline cartilage, probably do not heal by classic callus formation. In fact, when this type of osseous (callus) repair occurs in these cartilaginous regions, significant growth deformities may result due to formation of an osseous bridge between the secondary ossification center and the metaphysis (see Physeal Healing Patterns section later).

As in adults, there are three basic mechanisms of fracture repair: primary osteonal, secondary osteonal, and nonosteonal. Primary osteonal fracture healing occurs when cortical bone is laid down without any intermediate, and therefore hardly any callus forms; it is only possible if cortical bone is repositioned and fixed in close proximity. Secondary osteonal union occurs if cortical bone is laid down between two segments of fractured cortical bone before callus formation. Nonosteonal union occurs through endosteal and periosteal callus formation (188).

Fracture repair by callus production in the immature skeleton can be divided into three closely integrated, but sequential, phases: the inflammatory phase, the reparative phase, and the remodeling phase (Fig. 2-24). In children, the remodeling phase is temporally much more extensive and physiologically more active (depending on the child's age) than the comparable phase in adults. The remodeling phase is further modified by the effects of the physis responding to changing joint reaction forces and biologic stresses to alter angular growth dynamics. This occurs even when the fracture is mid-diaphyseal.

Cellular Response to Trauma

Inflammatory Phase

Immediately after a fracture through any of the osseous portions of the developing skeleton (diaphysis, metaphysis, or epiphyseal ossification center), disruption of blood vessels leads to activation of the coagulation cascade and formation of a hematoma enclosing the fracture area.

Hematoma Formation

Bleeding of the damaged periosteum, contiguous bone, and soft tissues starts the process of repair through the release of growth factors, cytokines, and prostaglandins. If the fracture is localized to the maturing diaphysis, there is bleeding from the haversian systems, as well as from the multiple small blood vessels of the microcirculatory systems of the endosteal and periosteal surfaces and contiguous soft-tissue anastomoses (189). In the region of the metaphysis, this bleeding may be extensive because of the anastomotic ramifications of the peripheral and central metaphyseal vascular systems. A hematoma accumulates within the medullary canal at the fracture site, beneath the elevated periosteum, and extraperiosteally whenever the periosteum is disrupted during the fracture. In contrast to adults, the periosteum strips away easily from the underlying bone in children, allowing the fracture hematoma to dissect along the diaphysis and metaphysis; and this is evident in the subsequent amount of new bone formation along the shaft.

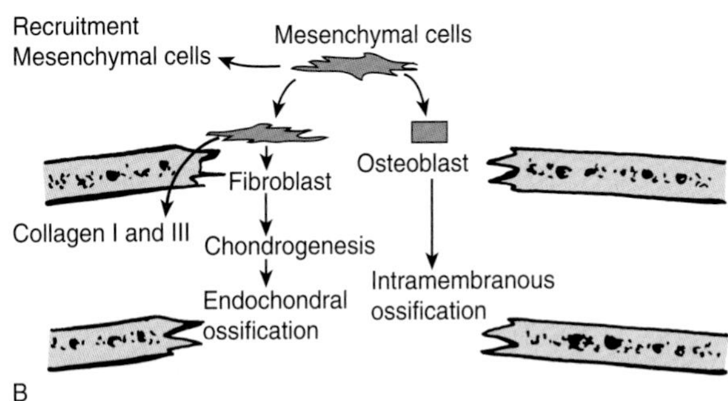

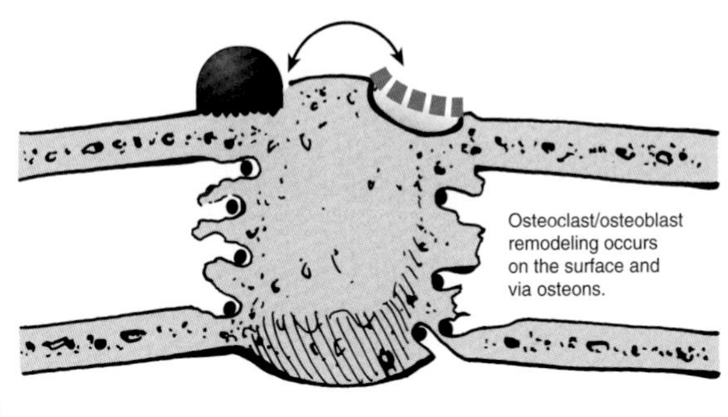

FIGURE 2-24 The figure demonstrates the three phases of fracture repair **(A)** inflammatory phase, **(B)** reparative phase, and **(C)** remodeling phase. The inflammatory cells remove the debris from the fracture site and, together with the fibroblastic cells, develop the site into a matrix that will support the cells that enable new bone to be formed. The mesenchymal cells are recruited by the release of growth factors in the fracture site. The mesenchymal cells may differentiate into osteoblasts that produce bone in a membranous fashion. Alternately the mesenchymal cell may become chondrogenic and produce bone by the endochondral pathway. Remodeling begins with resorption of mechanically unnecessary, inefficient portions of the callus and the subsequent orientation of trabecular bone along the lines of stress.

However, the dense attachments of the periosteum into the zone of Ranvier limit subperiosteal hematoma formation to the metaphysis and diaphysis. Because the perichondrium is densely attached, this type of hemorrhagic response is uncharacteristic of the epiphyseal ossification center, thus limiting its contributions to callus formation and any intrinsic stabilization effect. Further, because of the partially or completely intracapsular nature of some epiphyses, propagation of a fracture into the joint allows decompression of some of the bleeding into the joint, again limiting the potential volume for eventual callus formation.

Coagulation and platelet activation stop the blood loss but also produce both inflammatory mediators and angiogenic factors. Endothelial cells respond and increase the vascular permeability, and allow the passage of inflammatory cells (leukocytes, monocytes, and macrophages), fibroblasts, and stem cells into the fracture site. Neovascularization is also initiated. Angiogenic factors like platelet-derived growth factor (PDGF), VEGF, and TGF-β also promote osteoblast recruitment and activation.

Local Necrosis

The blood supply is temporarily disrupted for a few millimeters on either side of the fracture, creating juxtaposed, avascular trabecular and cortical bone (190) and producing local necrosis. It is likely that the necrosis also results in the release of sequestered growth factors (e.g., IGF-1, TGF-β, FGF-1, and FGF-2) from the bone. These growth factors may help in promoting differentiation of the surrounding mesenchymal cells into bone-forming cells.

The inflammatory response results in the release of several growth factors and cytokines that have important roles in repair. The inflammatory cells remove the debris from the fracture site and, with the fibroblastic cells, develop the site into a matrix that will support the cells that enable new bone to be formed. This initial matrix often contains collagens type I, III, and V.

Organization of Hematoma

The initial cellular repair process involves organization of the fracture hematoma (191). Fibrovascular tissue replaces the clot with a matrix rich in collagens I, III, and V. This matrix allows chondrogenesis or intramembranous bone formation. Such mechanisms eventually lead to mineralization and the formation of the woven bone of the provisional (primary) callus. Initial invasion and cell division are around the damaged bone ends but proceed centrifugally away from the fracture site, thus placing the most mature repair process closest to the fracture site. However, bone formation occurs only in the presence of an intact, functional microvascular supply. If the vascular supply is deficient, then this modulation of cartilaginous to osseous tissue cannot readily occur.

Reparative Phase

The fracture hematoma is the area in which the early stages of healing occur (191). Osteogenic cells proliferate from the periosteum to form an external callus and, to a lesser extent, from the endosteum to form an internal callus. However, when the periosteum is severely disrupted, healing cells must differentiate from the ingrowth of undifferentiated mesenchymal cells throughout the hematoma. By 10 to 14 days in a child, the fracture callus consists of a thick, enveloping mass of peripheral osteogenic tissue that is beginning to be evident radiographically. This new bone is primarily woven (fiber) bone (48,49).

The next step in osseous fracture healing is cellular organization (192). During this stage, the circumferential tissues serve primarily as a fibrous scaffold over which cells migrate and orient to induce a stable repair. This pluripotential mesenchyme is theoretically capable of modulation into cartilage, bone, or fibrous tissue (193). The mesenchymal cells are recruited by the released growth factors within the fracture site. Members of the BMP family, and possibly their inhibitors, are likely to be involved in the recruitment and differentiation of the mesenchymal cells. The mesenchymal cells may differentiate into osteoblasts that produce bone in a membranous fashion or may become chondrogenic and produce bone by the endochondral pathway. Both mechanisms usually are present in a fracture callus, and the degree to which each is present depends on the type of bone, age, degree of fixation, level of bone loss, and trauma. In children, because of the osteoblastic activity, the periosteum contributes significantly to new bone formation by accentuating the normal process of membranous ossification to supplement the cellular organization within the hematoma, which is going through a cartilaginous phase (194,195). The region around the fracture site thus repeats the process of endochondral ossification, in close juxtaposition to membranous ossification from the elevated periosteum. Similar processes occur within the medullary cavity. An integral part of the reparative process at this stage is microvascular invasion, which occurs very readily in children because of the state of vascularity within the bone and surrounding soft tissues (196). Vessels come from the periosteal region as well as from the nutrient artery and endosteal vessels.

Until this healing bone goes through the final stages of maturation, it is still biologically plastic and, if not protected, may gradually deform, especially in an active young child after early release from an immobilization device. Even in a cast, this plasticity may allow deformation from isometric muscle activity.

Clinical union is attained when the fracture site no longer moves and is not painful to attempts at manipulation, although it is by no means restored to its original strength at this time. With time, the primary callus is gradually replaced. This is enhanced in the child because as appositional growth and increasing diameter envelop the original fracture region, the cartilage and woven bone are replaced by mature, lamellar bone, and the fracture is consolidated and essentially returns to most of its normal biologic standards and response to stress.

Remodeling Phase

The last phase (remodeling) begins with resorption of mechanically unnecessary, inefficient portions of the callus and the subsequent orientation of trabecular bone along the lines of stress. The remodeling phase is the longest of the three phases and in children may continue until (and beyond) skeletal maturation in response to constantly changing stress patterns imposed by continued skeletal growth and development. Initially, new bone is laid down by both the fracture callus and subperiosteal tissue. This bone is randomly oriented and cannot withstand all stresses imposed on it. However, as the bone grows diametrically in the diaphyseal or metaphyseal regions, this new bone is gradually and increasingly incorporated into the preexisting cortical bone, aligned in accord with predominant stress patterns, and replaced by physiologic remodeling processes. The degree of remodeling and progressive replacement of fracture callus is greater in younger children, who have an immense capacity for growth and change.

The critical step between the reparative and remodeling phases is the establishment of an intact bony bridge between the fragments. Because this involves the joining of separated segments of hard tissue, the whole system must become immobile. Once the bridge has been established—provided that adequate, continued mechanical protection is given—subsequent biologic failure is unlikely. If the two or more fracture fragments remain connected by the periosteum or related material, as is likely in a child, it is easy to see how reparative activity could be conducted from one side to the other relatively easily and rapidly.

The intact bone must then readapt to functional demands. This is much easier in children, whose skeletons are actively and continually remodeling in response to stress, than in adults, who have more static skeletons. The processes of replacement and repair are continuous and concomitant in the normally developing skeleton. The mechanisms involved in fracture healing essentially are no different than most of the active maturational processes. These processes are much more active in children and are more active in the metaphysis than in the diaphysis.

The fracture remodeling process differs in cortical or cancellous bone. Both involve a process of simultaneous bone removal and replacement by the osteoclasts and osteoblasts through the accompanying blood vessels. In cancellous bone of the metaphysis or the endosteal surface of the diaphysis, the cells are never very far away from blood vessels, and the whole process of apposition and replacement may occur on the surface of the trabeculae. However, in compact bone, the more deeply placed cells require the presence of an adequately functioning perfusion system that must be replaced. This is a much longer sequence of events and is not a major method of bone repair in children, except when the fracture involves densely cortical regions, such as the femoral or tibial shafts. McKibbin (19) presented an extensive discussion of this process, which is sometimes referred to as *primary bone union* because no intermediate cells are involved.

Recently, Gerstenfeld et al (197) have reviewed the molecular, spatial, and temporal aspects of the regulation of bone facture healing in animal models. It is now clear that fracture healing is a specialized postnatal repair process that recapitulates aspects of embryological skeletal development. It is also becoming increasingly evident that the sequential cellular responses in the different phases of bone fracture healing are intricately regulated by many molecules, including (a) M-CSF, IL-1, IL-6, IL-11, RANKL, OPG, INF-γ, TNF, TGF-β1, BMP-2, and growth and differentiation factor GDF-8 after the initial injury and during the inflammatory response; (b) M-CSF, RANKL, OPG, TGF-β2, TGF-β3, BMP-3, BMP-4, BMP-5, BMP-6, BMP-7, BMP-8, GDF-1, GDF-10, VEGF, and matrix metalloproteases MMP-2, MMP-8, MMP-9, MMP-13, MMP-14 during the repair phase; and (c) all the cytokines listed above (except IL-11 and INF-γ), GDF-10, TGF-β1, MMP-9, MMP-13, and all BMP members previously listed in the remodeling phase.

Physeal Healing Patterns

The physis has a limited ability to repair; it primarily heals by increased endochondral bone and cartilage formation, and gradual reinvasion by the disrupted metaphyseal vessels to replace the temporarily widened physis eventually. Very little experimental work, mostly in rats, has been directed at assessing the post-traumatic cellular response patterns of the physis (198–200).

Depending on the level of cellular injury within the physis, *three types of chondro-osseous healing* may occur. First, when the fracture occurs through the cell columns, healing occurs primarily by continued, relatively rapid increases in the number of cells within the columns, causing moderate widening of the physis. Because there are some small epiphyseal vessels in this region, some damaged tissue may be resorbed early in the healing process. These vessels also exhibit a hyperemic response, increasing cellular proliferation rates, especially in the peripheral zone of Ranvier. The metaphyseal response parallels this, in that an increased rate of bone replacement of the hypertrophic cartilage also occurs. Once the level of fracture fibrosis and debris within the physis is encountered, the vessels rapidly invade to reach the rest of the maturing cell columns. These cellular response patterns lead to restoration of normal anatomy within 3 to 4 weeks (201).

Second, when the fracture occurs through the transition of hypertrophic cells to primary spongiosa (the most commonly involved cellular level), there may be marked separation, with the gap filled by hemorrhagic and fibroblastic tissue. This region may progressively form disorganized cartilaginous tissue, which is similar to the initial, disorganized cartilaginous callus around a diaphyseal fracture. Meanwhile, cellular proliferation, cell column formation, hypertrophy, and calcification continue on the epiphyseal side of the disorganized callus, leading to widening of the physis. Vascular invasion of the remnants of hypertrophic, calcified cartilage also rapidly occurs on the metaphyseal side of the fracture. However, once metaphyseal vessel invasion reaches the disorganized cartilaginous callus, vascular-mediated bone replacement is temporarily slowed, because there is no pattern of cell columns to invade in an organized fashion. As the callus cartilage matures and calcifies, the metaphyseal vessels begin to invade and replace the cartilage with bone irregularly (202). This callus may be variably thick, depending on the degree of longitudinal and lateral displacement and periosteal continuity with the physeal periphery. The callus is replaced at different rates, and the invading metaphyseal vessels reach the normal cell columns, which have been maturing in a normal sequence but without osseous replacement. This widened physis is rapidly invaded by the vessels and replaced by primary spongiosa, and normal physeal width is progressively restored.

The callus in the subperiosteal region of the metaphysis contributes to early stability. This region heals by vascular invasion of the callus to form trabecular bone between the original metaphyseal cortex and the subperiosteal membranous bone forming continuously external to the metaphyseal cartilaginous callus. These three microscopic bone regions progressively merge and remodel, strengthening the bone. These initial cellular replacement processes in both metaphyseal and physeal regions probably take 3 to 6 weeks. However, remodeling may continue for months to years, and it enhances the capacity for spontaneous correction of many residual deformities.

Thirdly, when the injury extends across all cell layers of the physis, the repair processes differ slightly. Fibrous tissue initially fills the gap between separated physeal components, whereas typical callus formation occurs in the contiguous metaphyseal spongiosa or epiphyseal ossification center. If large surfaces of nonossified epiphyseal cartilage also are involved, fibrous tissue initially forms in the intervening region. The reparative response shows irregular healing of the epiphyseal and physeal cartilage, with loss of normal cellular architecture. Within the central physeal regions, diametric expansion of cell columns is minimal, so closure of a large defect by physeal cartilage is unlikely. The gap will remain fibrous, but with the potential to ossify. Toward the physeal periphery, diametric expansion is more likely, but still may not lead to closure of large cartilage gaps by progressive replacement of fibrous tissue. This replacement process essentially requires the germinal and hypertrophic cell regions to diametrically expand by cell division, maturation, and matrix expansion. The intervening fibrous tissue may disappear through growth, but only if the gap is narrow. Because blood supply is minimal in this region, the fibrous tissue similarly is not well vascularized, and significant cell modulation, especially to osteoblastic tissue, is less likely in the short term. However, the larger the gap filled with fibrous tissue and the longer the time from fracture to skeletal maturity, the greater the likelihood of developing sufficient vascularity to commence an osteoblastic response and to form an osseous bridge. Further, in young children with minimal epiphyseal ossification, the blood supply to the physeal germinal region is not as well defined, whereas once the ossification center expands and forms a subchondral plate over the germinal region, microvascularity probably increases and the chances for vascularization and ossification of the fibrous region increase. This explains the delayed appearance of the osseous bridge.

If accurate anatomic reduction is performed, a thin gap should be present that should fill in with minimal fibrous tissue, allowing progressive replacement of the tissue by diametric expansion of the physis and contiguous epiphysis. However, if the fragment has been partially or completely devascularized by either the initial trauma or subsequent dissection to effect an open reduction, cellular growth and diametric and longitudinal expansion may not occur. This increases the chances of cellular disorganization, fibrosis, and eventual osteoblastic response. Failure to correct anatomic displacement, especially in Salter-Harris type 4 growth mechanism injuries, increases the possibility of apposition of the epiphyseal ossification center and metaphyseal bone, and thereby enhances the risk of forming an osseous bridge between the two regions. When the defect was large enough and the fracture involved the whole width of the growth plate extending from the metaphysis to the epiphysis, the injured physis will have structural disorganization, formation of vertical septa, and finally formation of a bone bridge. When the bone bridge is large enough, particularly in Salter's type 3 and type 4 injuries, the defect will result in a growth arrest. While growth arrest at the peripheral portions of the physis results in angular deformities, centrally located lesions may cause longitudinal shortening (2).

The cellular and molecular mechanisms for the bone bridge formation at the site of physeal injury site remain largely unknown. Using a proximal tibial drill-hole transphyseal injury model in rats, a recent study from the authors' laboratory characterized the injury-induced responses and cellular mechanisms for the bone bridge formation (Fig. 2-25) (200). At the growth plate injury site, this study demonstrated an early acute inflammatory response (up to day 3 postinjury). Straight after this inflammatory response, the injury site is filled by mesenchymal infiltrate (days 3 to 14) and subsequently is repaired by bone bridge formation (starting from day 7). Histologically, bony bridge trabeculae appeared on day 7 (Fig. 2-25A) and became well-constructed on day 14 with marrow (Fig. 2-25B). Before and during physeal bar formation, there were no new cartilage formation, no collagen-X synthesis at the injury site (Fig. 2-25C), and no expansion of chondrocyte proliferation from adjacent physeal cartilage (Fig. 2-25D), suggesting that the bone bridge formation did not involve endochondral ossification in this rat model. These results are consistent with an earlier study that reported a lack of increased expression of IHH and collagen-2, two molecules typically involved in endochondral ossification (203). Furthermore, Xian et al's (200) study also demonstrated infiltration of marrow-derived fibroblast-like mesenchymal cells starting from day 3 (Fig. 2-25E), presence of osteoblast precursor cells among the mesenchymal infiltrates and their close proximity to bone bridge trabeculae (Fig. 2-25F, Fig. 2-25G), and production of bone matrix protein osteocalcin during formation of bone bridge trabeculae (Fig. 2-25H). These results suggested that bone bridge formation after growth plate injury in this rat model occurs directly via intramembranous ossification through recruitment of marrow-derived osteoprogenitor cells (200).

Remodeling of Bones in Children after Injury

In a growing child, the normal process of bone remodeling in the diaphysis and metaphysis (particularly the latter) may realign initially malunited fragments, making anatomic reduction less important than in a comparable injury in an adult. However, although some residual angular deformities undergo spontaneous correction, accurate anatomic reduction should be the goal whenever possible (3,204,205). Bone and cartilage generally remodel in response to normal stresses of body weight, muscle action, and joint reaction forces, as well as intrinsic control mechanisms such as the periosteum. The potential for spontaneous, complete correction is greater if the child is younger, the fracture site is closer to the physis, and there is relative alignment of the angulation in the normal plane of motion of the joint. This is particularly evident in fractures involving hinge joints such as the knee, ankle, elbow, or wrist, in which corrections are relatively rapid if the angulation is in the normal plane of motion. However, spontaneous correction of angular deformities is unlikely in other directions, such as a cubitus varus deformity following a supracondylar fracture of the humerus. Similarly, rotational deformities usually do not correct spontaneously.

Growth Stimulation

Fractures may stimulate longitudinal growth by increasing the blood supply to the metaphysis, physis, and epiphysis, and at least on an experimental basis, by disrupting the periosteum and its physiologic restraint on the rates of longitudinal growth of the physes (206). Such increased growth may make the bone longer than it would have been without an injury (50,207). Eccentric overgrowth may also occur; this is particularly evident in tibia valgum following an incomplete fracture of the proximal tibial metaphysis.

FIGURE 2-25 Intramembranous ossification mechanism for bone bridge formation at the growth plate injury site. Histologically (Barbara's histology stain), bony bridge trabeculae start to appear on day 7 postinjury **(A)**, and become well-constructed on day 14 with marrow **(B)**. Prior to and during physeal bar formation, there is no new cartilage formation, no collagen-X synthesis (as examined by immunostaining) at the injury site **(C)**, and no expansion of chondrocyte proliferation (as examined by BrdU labeling) from adjacent physeal cartilage **(D)**. Starting from day 3 **(E)** until day 14, there is infiltration of marrow-derived fibroblast-like mesenchymal cells (as examined by vimentin immunostaining), some of which are osteoblast precursor cells displaying positive immunostaining for bone cell differentiation transcription factor cbf-a1 **(F)** and osteoblast/osteoprogenitor maturation marker alkaline phosphatase **(G)**. During bone bridge formation, bone matrix protein osteocalcin is produced by osteoblasts on bone bridge trabeculae (immunostaining) **(H)**. *, injury site; *block arrow*, pointing to adjacent growth plate cartilage; *small arrow*, pointing to bone bridge trabeculae or (*continues*)

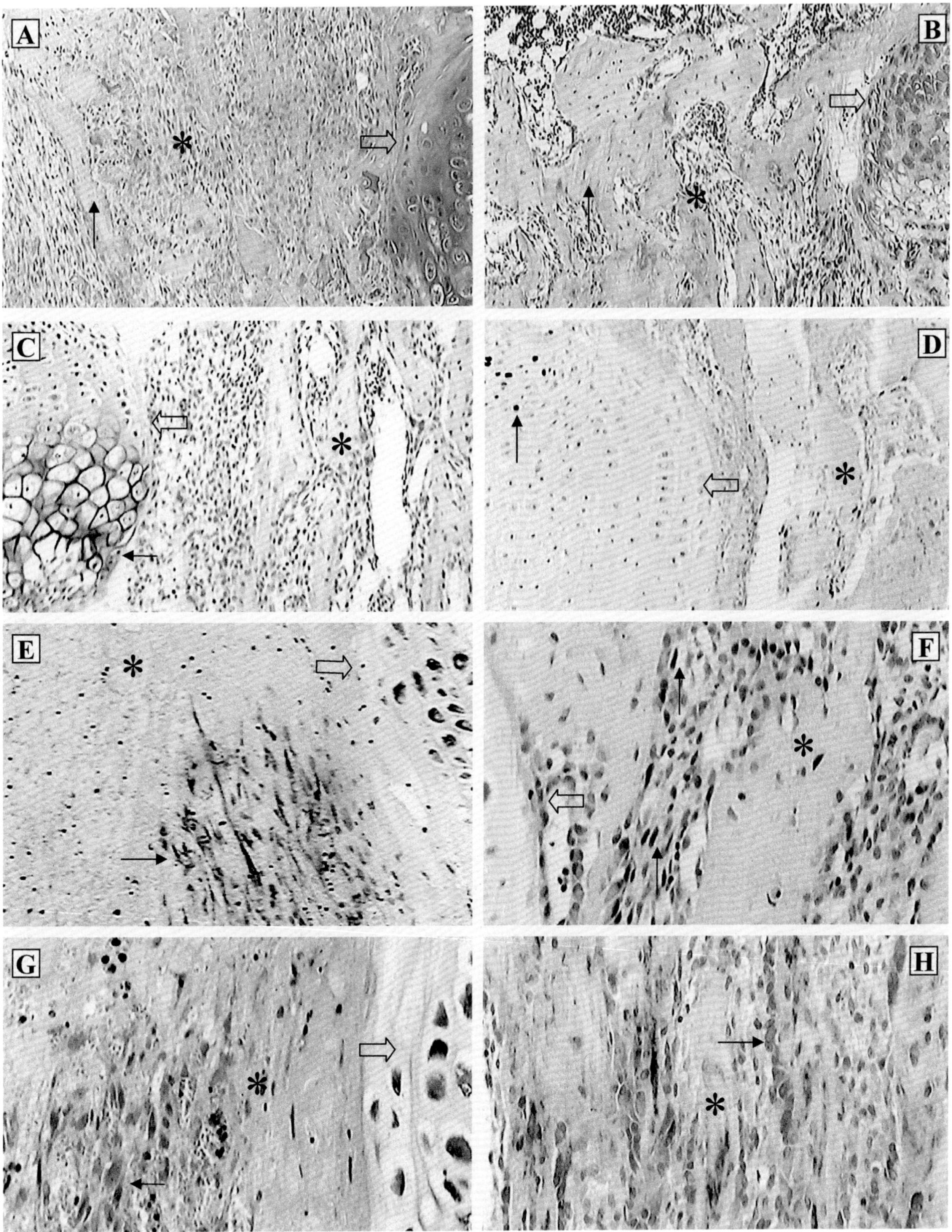

FIGURE 2-25 *(continued)* immunostained positive cells. This photo-composite is derived from the authors' previous study. (From Xian CJ, Zhou FH, McCarty RC, et al. Intramembranous ossification mechanism for bone bridge formation at the growth plate cartilage injury site. *J Orthop Res* 2004;22:417–426; with permission from copyright 2004 Orthopaedic Research Society.)

THE FUTURE OF FRACTURE REPAIR

Bone grafts contain bone growth factors that normally induce bone formation and have the appropriate osteoconductive matrix. Autogenic grafts also contain osteogenic cells. Bone grafts are effective, but there are difficulties in obtaining safe and reliable source tissue. Although the mechanisms of fracture repair are not fully understood, the level of understanding has enabled key molecules or cells to be targeted as therapeutic in controlling and promoting fracture repair. Filler compounds have been developed that stimulate proliferation of mesenchymal cells, and/or enhance their osteoblast or chondrocyte differentiation, leading to formation of new bone or cartilage (osteoinductive or chondrogenic) or enabling the cells to infiltrate and incorporate into bone (osteoconductive) or cartilage. Further studies on repair of bone, articular cartilage, or physis are required to understand the contribution of different cell types (inflammatory, endothelial, chondrocytic, osteoblastic and osteoclastic cells) to the repair process and their associated regulatory molecular pathways. In order to develop the most optimal strategies to treat fracture-associated complications that allow for lower effective doses and fewer side effects, more studies should also be carried out to identify and to test the optimal growth factors, novel factors, inhibitors or their small-molecule mimetics, cell-based therapy including stem cells, and/or gene therapy and their delivery systems.

Growth Factor Therapy

Specific growth factors have been targeted for their ability to promote bone formation. Due to their ability to stimulate proliferation and differentiation of mesenchymal and osteoprogenitor cells, two bone morphogenic proteins (BMP-2 and BMP-7) have shown great promise and acceptance for their ability to promote fracture repair (41,42,128,129,134,208,209). BMP-2 promotes bone formation and repair in critical size defects, fractures and spinal fusions in human, and has been recently approved for clinical use in fracture repair (Wyeth pharmaceuticals) and spinal fusion (Medtronic Sofamor Danek). Like BMP-2, BMP-7 (also called osteogenic protein-1, OP-1) induces ectopic bone formation in vivo and enhances bone repair in preclinical models and clinical studies (122). Clinically, OP-1, delivered with a type-1 collagen carrier, induced bone repair, which was found to be equivalent to autogenous bone graft in a clinical trial of patients with tibial nonunions (210). OP-1 has now been approved for use in the treatment of established nonunions (Stryker Biotech).

A number of other growth factors, such as TGF-β, IGF-1, PDGFs, and FGF-2, also may prove to be useful. TGF-β plays a major role in fracture repair by promoting proliferation and differentiation of the mesenchymal cells. Exogenous TGF-β administration can initiate the repair process and callus formation in uninjured bone (211). The addition of TGF-β to fractures results in a larger, stronger callus (211). It also may be of use in promoting repair in nonhealing bone defects. PDGF also increases callus size but does not improve the fracture mechanically (212). Growth hormone and IGF-1 have also been tested to determine their effects on fracture repair. Although growth hormone produces inconsistent results (213), the administration of IGF-1 increases intramembranous bone formation (214). The FGFs stimulate mitogenesis of mesenchymal cells and osteoblasts, increase the callus size and mineral content, and improve mechanical stability at early stages of fracture repair (215–217). FGF-2 also increases osteoclastic bone remodeling (212). In addition, it is possible that the effects of FGFs (218) and of a number of the other growth factors are a result of the angiogenic properties of such growth factors, as most osteogenic factors also stimulate angiogenesis, if not directly, then indirectly, through production of angiogenic molecules, such as VEGF. The potential synergism between potent pro-angiogenic factors (such as VEGF) and strong osteoinductive factors (such as BMPs) suggest that combination therapies might produce optimum results, particularly for individuals at risk of delayed repair or nonunions (122).

Although there have been many studies and reviews on the use of growth factors for fracture repair (41,42,122,219–222) and some successful clinical applications of BMP-2 and OP-1 in inducing bone formation and repair, more research is required to establish the most effective delivery devices for these growth factors (223). Apart from the requirements of biocompatibility and effectiveness, the growth factor carriers or delivery matrix systems or devices need to make the growth factor delivery cost-effective and practical in their clinical applications to induce bone formation in vivo, which should allow the application of relatively low doses of growth factors for optimal bone or cartilage regeneration in clinical contexts.

Tissue Engineering, Stem Cell and Gene Therapies

In the past decade, there has been an increasing interest in tissue engineering and mesenchymal stem cells for bone reconstruction of nonunion defects and for articular cartilage regeneration. Using tissue-engineering technologies, it is now possible to enhance bone repair and/or replace bone defect; and using the patient's own articular chondrocytes retrieved during arthroscopy and expanded in vitro, it is now possible to repair full-thickness articular cartilage defects with satisfactory clinical results (224). Researchers worldwide are working to prepare the three fundamental components for the successful orthopaedic tissue engineering: (a) appropriate biological or artificial carriers or delivery systems or extracellular matrix scaffolds, and (b) the right set of viable responding cells (such as mesenchymal stem cells) in combination with (c) appropriate soluble inductive signal molecules or growth factors that, once transplanted, will ensure bone repair and/or cartilage regeneration (221).

In particular, due to the capacity of self expansion in vitro, the less stringent ethical and regulatory issues and the lack of immunologic implications, mesenchymal stem cells derived from autologous bone marrow stroma have been the research focus for their potential applications, which have offered a new perspective for bone and cartilage tissue engineering. There have been some excellent advances in understanding the stem cells, their interactions with their matrix, particularly stimuli or signal molecules controlling their proliferation (such as LIF, FGF-2, HGF, Wnt and Dickkopt-1), osteogenic differentiation (such as IHH, Notch-1 and PPARgamma), and chondrogenic differentiation (such as BMP-4 and TGF-β3) (13). However, preclinical and clinical evaluations of the stromal stem cells or their derived osteoblasts or chondrocytes, or the engineered bone or cartilage tissues will yet have to prove their efficacy, biocompatibility, safety, practicality, and reproducibility in bone and cartilage regeneration (225).

Genetic engineering or gene transfer technology has also opened novel treatment avenues for the regeneration or repair of damaged articular cartilage, as gene transfer provides the capability to deliver bioactive proteins or gene products to sites of tissue damage locally and in a sustained manner. Previous research has already convincingly demonstrated the principle of gene delivery to synovium, chondrocytes and mesenchymal progenitor cells, and recent efficacy studies provide optimism that this gene transfer approach can be employed to enhance articular cartilage repair (144).

Regeneration of Injured Growth Plate Cartilage

Biological regeneration of growth plate cartilage remains a great challenge. Foster and colleagues (226) have utilized a sheep tibial growth plate injury model to investigate therapeutic potential of transplanted chondrocytes or periosteum (61), and more recently growth factor OP-1 (15). They unfortunately found that these treatments under the experimental conditions were not preventative of bony bridge formation. Similarly, in a rat tibial physeal fracture model, Gruber et al (227) found that interposed periosteum at the fracture site could not enhance healing of the fractured physis, and in a rabbit tibial physeal injury model, Lee et al (199) observed that BMP-2 gene therapy delivered via adenoviral vectors within muscle implant caused increased osteogenic activity in the injured growth plate. Previous work has demonstrated that implantation of cultured chondrocytes embedded in agarose into growth plate defects resulted in a partial correction of angular deformity and a significant reduction in growth arrest in a rabbit model (228), and muscle-based gene therapy with adenoviral vectors encoding for IGF-1 restored the injured growth plate cartilage (199). More recently, direct transfer of periosteum-derived mesenchymal stem cells embedded in agarose into the tibial growth plate defect resulted in regeneration of the physis, preventing growth arrest or angular deformity of the tibia (14,16). The search for the optimal treatment options to achieve correction of angular deformity and to prevent limb length discrepancy using tissue engineering will continue and is not clinically applicable at this time.

ACKNOWLEDGMENTS

Supported in part by the Bone Growth Foundation (Australia), Channel-7 Children's Research Foundation of South Australia, National Health and Medical Research Council of Australia, Skeletal Educational Association, and the Foundation for Musculoskeletal Research and Education. The authors would like to acknowledge the contribution of Drs. Edward W. Johnstone, John A. Ogden, Timothy M. Ganey, and Dali A. Ogden, writers of the previous two editions, of which parts have been updated and carried forward.

REFERENCES

1. Hanlon CR, Estes WL. Fractures in childhood—A statistical analysis. *Am J Surg* 1954; 87:312–323.
2. Ogden JA. Injury to the immature skeleton. In: Touloukian R, ed. *Pediatric trauma*, 2nd ed. New York: John Wiley & Sons, 1990.
3. Ogden JA. *Skeletal injury in the child*, 2nd ed. Philadelphia: WB Saunders, 1990.
4. Ogden JA. The role of orthopaedic surgery in sports medicine. *Yale J Biol Med* 1980; 53:281–288.
5. Beckman F, Sullivan J. Some observations of fractures of long bones in the child. *Am J Surg* 1941;51:722–738.
6. Mizuta T, Benson WM, Foster BK, et al. Statistical analysis of the incidence of physeal injuries. *J Pediatr Orthop* 1987;7:518–523.
7. Ogden JA, Southwick WO. Electrical injury involving the immature skeleton. *Skeletal Radiol* 1981;6:187–192.
8. Ryoppy S. Injuries of the growing skeleton. *Ann Chir Gynaecol* 1972;61:3–10.
9. Ogden JA. Growth slowdown and arrest lines. *J Pediatr Orthop* 1984;4:409–415.
10. Siffert RS. The effect of trauma to the epiphysis and growth plate. *Skeletal Radiol* 1977; 2:21–30.
11. Warrell E, Taylor JF. The effect of trauma on tibial growth. *J Bone Joint Surg* 1976;58B: 375.
12. Issack PS, DiCesare PE. Recent advances toward the clinical application of bone morphogenetic proteins in bone and cartilage repair. *Am J Orthop* 2003;32:429–436.
13. Otto WR, Rao J. Tomorrow's skeleton staff: mesenchymal stem cells and the repair of bone and cartilage. *Cell Prolif* 2004;37:97–110.
14. Chen F, Hui JH, Chan WK, et al. Cultured mesenchymal stem cell transfers in the treatment of partial growth arrest. *J Pediatr Orthop* 2003;23:425–429.
15. Johnstone EW, McArthur M, Solly PB, et al. The effect of osteogenic protein 1 in an in vivo physeal injury model. *Clin Orthop Rel Res* 2002;395:234–240.
16. Li L, Hui JH, Goh JC, et al. Chitin as a scaffold for mesenchymal stem cells transfers in the treatment of partial growth arrest. *J Pediatr Orthop* 2004;24:205–210.
17. Lacroix P. The organization of bone. Philadelphia: Blakiston, 1951.
18. Treharne RW. Review of Wolff's law and its proposed means of operation. *Orthop Rev* 1981;10:35–44.
19. McKibbin B. The biology of fracture healing in long bones. *J Bone Joint Surg* 1978;60B: 150–162.
20. Ogden JA, Rosenberg LC. Defining the growth plate. In: Uhthoff HK, Wiley JJ, eds. *Behavior of the growth plate*. New York: Raven Press, 1988.
21. Ogden JA. Chondro-osseous development and growth. In: Urist MR, ed. *Fundamental and clinical bone physiology*. Philadelphia: JB Lippincott, 1980.
22. Ogden JA. The development and growth of the musculoskeletal system. In: Albright JA, Brand RA, eds. *The scientific basis of orthopaedics*. New York: Appleton-Century-Crofts, 1979.
23. Calandruccio RA, Gilmer WS. Proliferation, regeneration and repair of articular cartilage of immature animals. *J Bone Joint Surg* 1962;44A:431–455.
24. Trueta J, Cavadias AX. A study of the blood supply of the long bones. *Surg Gynecol Obstet* 1964;118:485–498.
25. Trueta J, Morgan JD. The vascular contribution to osteogenesis. *J Bone Joint Surg* 1960; 42B:97–109.
26. Trueta J. *Studies of the development and decay of the human frame*. Philadelphia: WB Saunders, 1968.
27. Trueta J, Amato P. The vascular contribution to osteogenis III. Changes in the growth cartilage caused by experimentally induced ischaemia. *J Bone Joint Surg* 1960;42B: 571–587.
28. Morscher E. Posttraumatic zapfenepiphyse. *Arch Orthop Unfallchir* 1967;61:128–136.
29. Ogden JA. An anatomical and histological study of the factors affecting development and evolution of avascular necrosis in congenital dislocation of the hip. In: Harris WH, ed. *The hip: proceedings of the Hip Society*, vol 2. St. Louis: CV Mosby, 1974:125–153.
30. Bucholz RW, Ogden JA. Patterns of ischemic necrosis of the proximal femur in nonoperatively treated congenital hip disease. In: Nelson CL, ed. *The hip: proceedings of the Hip Society*, vol 6. St. Louis: CV Mosby, 1978:43–63.
31. Keck SW, Kelly PJ. The effect of venous stasis on intra-osseous pressure and longitudinal bone growth in the dog. *J Bone Joint Surg* 1965;47A:539–544.

32. Jacenko O, LuValle PA, Olsen BR. Spondylometaphyseal dysplasia in mice carrying a dominant negative mutation in a matrix protein specific for cartilage-to-bone transition. *Nature* 1993;365:56–61.
33. Speer D. Collagenous architecture of the growth plate and perichondral ossification groove. *J Bone Joint Surg* 1982;64A:399–407.
34. Acheson RM. Effects of starvation, septicaemia and chronic illness on the growth cartilage plate and metaphysis of the immature rat. *J Anat* 1959;93:123–130.
35. Harris HA. The growth of long bones in childhood with special reference to certain bony striations of the metaphysis and to the role of vitamins. *Arch Intern Med* 1926; 38:785–806.
36. Park EA. Bone growth in health and disease. *Arch Dis Child* 1954;29:269–281.
37. Park EA. The imprinting of nutritional disturbances on growing bone. *Pediatrics* 1964; 33:815–862.
38. Ogden JA, Grogan DP, Light TR. Postnatal skeletal development and growth of musculoskeletal system. In: Albright JA, Brand RD, eds. *The scientific basis of orthopaedics.* New York: Appleton & Lange, 1987.
39. Grissom LE, Harcke HT. Radiographic features of bisphosphonate therapy in pediatric patients. *Pediatr Radiol* 2003;33:226–229.
40. Light TR, McKinstry P, Schnitzer J, et al. Bone blood flow: regional variation with skeletal maturation. In: Arlet J, Ficat RP, Hungerford DS, eds. *Bone circulation.* Baltimore: Williams & Wilkins, 1984.
41. Lind M. Growth factor stimulation of bone healing. Effects on osteoblasts, osteomies, and implants fixation. *Acta Orthop Scand Suppl* 1998;283:2–37.
42. Lind M. Growth factors: possible new clinical tools. A review. *Acta Orthop Scand* 1996; 67:407–417.
43. McKinstry P, Schnitzer JE, Light TR, et al. Relationship of 99mTC-MDP uptake to regional osseous circulation in skeletally immature and mature dogs. *Skeletal Radiol* 1982;8:115–121.
44. McKinstry P, Schnitzer JE, Light TR, et al. Quantitation of regional chondro-osseous circulation in the maturing canine tibia and femur. *Am J Physiol* 1982;1242: H365–H375.
45. Schnitzer JE, McKinstry P, Light TR, et al. Quantitation of regional osseous circulation in the maturing canine tibia and femur. *Surg Forum* 1980;31:509–511.
46. Weinman DT, Kelly PJ, Owen CA. Blood flow in bone distal to a femoral arteriovenous fistula in dogs. *J Bone Joint Surg* 1964;46A:1676–1682.
47. Lockwood R, Latta LL. Bone blood flow changes with diaphyseal fracture. *Trans Orthop Res Soc* 1980;5:158.
48. Rhinelander FW, Phillips RS, Steel WM, et al. Microangiography and bone healing. II. Displaced closed fractures. *J Bone Joint Surg* 1968;50A:643–662.
49. Rhinelander FW. Tibial blood supply in relation to fracture healing. *Clin Orthop* 1974; 105:34–81.
50. Tscherne H, Suren EG. Fehlstellungen, wachstumsstorungen and pseudoarthrosen nach kindlichen frakturen. *Langenbecks Arch Chir* 1976;342:299–304.
51. Wray JB. Acute changes in femoral arterial blood flow after closed tibial fracture in dogs. *J Bone Joint Surg* 1964;46A:1262–1268.
52. Ogden JA, Pals MJ, Murphy MJ, et al. Ectopic bone secondary to avulsion of the periosteum. *Skeletal Radiol* 1979;4:124–128.
53. Boyan BD, Schwartz Z, Park Snyder S, et al. Latent transforming growth factor-beta is produced by chondrocytes and activated by extracellular matrix vesicles upon exposure to 1,25-(OH)2D3. *J Biol Chem* 1994;269:28374–28381.
54. Scott-Savage P, Hall BK. Differentiative ability of the tibial periosteum for the embryonic chick. *Acta Anat (Basel)* 1980;106:129–140.
55. Pechak DG, Kujawa MJ, Caplan AI. Morphology of bone development and bone remodeling in embryonic chick limbs. *Bone* 1986;7:459–472.
56. Poussa M, Ritsila V. The osteogenic capacity of free periosteal and osteoperiosteal grafts. A comparative study in growing rabbits. *Acta Orthop Scand* 1979;50:491–499.
57. Nakahara H, Goldberg VM, Caplan AI. Culture-expanded human periosteal-derived cells exhibit osteochondral potential in vivo. *J Orthop Res* 1991;9:465–476.
58. Niedermann B, Boe S, Lauritzen J, et al. Glued periosteal grafts in the knee. *Acta Orthop Scand* 1985;56:457–460.
59. O'Driscoll SW, Fitzsimmons JS. The role of periosteum in cartilage repair. *Clin Orthop* 2001;391:S190–S207.
60. Stevens MM, Qanadilo HF, Langer R, et al. A rapid-curing alginate gel system: utility in periosteum-derived cartilage tissue engineering. *Biomaterials* 2004;25:887–894.
61. Wirth T, Byers S, Byard RW, et al. The implantation of cartilaginous and periosteal tissue into growth plate defects. *Int Orthop* 1994;18:220–228.
62. Ogden JA, Hempton R, Southwick WO. Development of the tibial tuberosity. *Anat Rec* 1975;182:431–446.
63. Ogden JA, Southwick WO. Osgood-Schlatter's disease and the development of the tibial tuberosity. *Clin Orthop* 1976;116:180–189.
64. Ogden JA, Tross RB, Murphy MJ. Fractures of the tibial tuberosity in adolescents. *J Bone Joint Surg* 1980;62A:205–215.
65. Buckwalter JA, Glimcher MJ, Cooper RR, et al. Bone biology. I: structure, blood supply, cells, matrix, and mineralization. *Instr Course Lect* 1996;45:371–386.
66. Kaplan FS, Hayes WC, Keaveny TM, et al. Form and function of bone. In: Simon SR, ed. *Orthopaedic basic science: American Academy of Orthopaedic Surgeons.* Rosemont, IL: Port City Press, 1994:127–184.
67. Jacenko O, Ito S, Olsen BR. Skeletal and hematopoietic defects in mice transgenic for collagen X. *Ann N Y Acad Sci* 1996;785:278–280.
68. Bateman J, Lamande S, Ramshaw J. Collagen superfamily. In: Comper WD, ed. *Extracellular matrix.* Amsterdam: Harwood Academic Publishers, 1996:22–67.
69. Chan D, Taylor TKF, Cole WG. Characterization of an arginine 789 to cysteine substitution in alpha-1(II) collagen chains of a patient with spondyloepiphyseal dysplasia. *J Biol Chem* 1993;268:15238–15245.
70. Eyre DR, Upton MP, Shapiro FD, et al. Nonexpression of cartilage type II collagen in a case of Langer-Saldino achondrogenesis. *Am J Hum Genet* 1986;39:52–67.
71. Keene DR, Oxford JT, Morris NP. Ultrastructural localization of collagen types II, IX, and XI in the growth plate of human rib and fetal bovine epiphyseal cartilage: type XI collagen is restricted to thin fibrils. *J Histochem Cytochem* 1995;43:967–979.
72. Petit B, Ronziere MC, Hartmann DJ, et al. Ultrastructural organization of type XI collagen in fetal bovine epiphyseal cartilage. *Histochemistry* 1993;100:231–239.
73. Birk DE, Fitch JM, Babiarz JP, et al. Collagen fibrillogenesis in vitro: interaction of types I and V collagen regulates fibril diameter. *J Cell Sci* 1990;95:649–657.
74. Olsen BR. Mutations in collagen genes resulting in metaphyseal and epiphyseal dysplasias. *Bone* 1995;17:45s–49s.
75. Kielty CM, Kwan AP, Holmes DF, et al. Type X collagen, a product of hypertrophic chondrocytes. *Biochem J* 1985;227:545–554.
76. Kirsch T, von der Mark K. Isolation of bovine type X collagen and immunolocalization in growth-plate cartilage. *Biochem J* 1990;265:453–459.
77. Paschalis EP, Jacenko O, Olsen B, et al. The role of type X collagen in endochondral ossification as deduced by Fourier transform infrared microscopy analysis. *Connect Tissue Res* 1996;35:371–377.
78. Poole AR, Matsui Y, Hinek A, et al. Cartilage macromolecules and the calcification of cartilage matrix. *Anat Rec* 1989;224:167–179.
79. Rosati R, Horan GS, Pinero GJ, et al. Normal long bone growth and development in type X collagen-null mice. *Nat Genet* 1994;8:129–135.
80. Fosang A, Hardingham T. Matrix proteoglycans. In: Comper WD, ed. *Extracellular matrix.* Amsterdam: Harwood Academic Publishers, 1996:200–229.
81. Byers S, van Rooden JC, Foster BK. Structural changes in the large proteoglycan, aggrecan, in different zones of the ovine growth plate. *Calcif Tissue Int* 1997;60:71–78.
82. Muir H. The chondrocyte, architect of cartilage. Biomechanics, structure, function and molecular biology of cartilage matrix macromolecules. *Bioessays* 1995;17:1039–1048.
83. Poole AR, Webber C, Pidoux I, et al. Localization of a dermatan sulfate proteoglycan (DS-PGII) in cartilage and the presence of an immunologically related species in other tissues. *J Histochem Cytochem* 1986;34:619–625.
84. Xu T, Bianco P, Fisher LW, et al. Targeted disruption of the biglycan gene leads to an osteoporosis-like phenotype in mice. *Nat Genet* 1998;20:78–82.
85. Bianco P, Fisher LW, Young MF, et al. Expression and localization of the two small proteoglycans biglycan and decorin in developing human skeletal and non-skeletal tissues. *J Histochem Cytochem* 1990;38:1549–1563.
86. Hildebrand A, Romaris M, Rasmussen LM, et al. Interaction of the small interstitial proteoglycans biglycan, decorin and fibromodulin with transforming growth factor beta. *Biochem J* 1994;302:527–534.
87. Schonherr E, Broszat M, Brandan E, et al. Decorin core protein fragment Leu155-Val260 interacts with TGF-beta but does not compete for decorin binding to type I collagen. *Arch Biochem Biophys* 1998;355:241–248.
88. Price PA. Gla-containing proteins of bone. *Connect Tissue Res* 1989;21:51–57.
89. Price PA, Williamson MK. Primary structure of bovine matrix Gla protein, a new vitamin K–dependent bone protein. *J Biol Chem* 1985;260:14971–14975.
90. Ducy P, Desbois C, Boyce B, et al. Increased bone formation in osteocalcin-deficient mice. *Nature* 1996;382(6590):448–452.
91. Hauschka PV, Lian JB, Cole DE, et al. Osteocalcin and matrix Gla protein: vitamin K–dependent proteins in bone. *Physiol Rev* 1989;69:990–1047.
92. Bolander ME, Young MF, Fisher LW, et al. Osteonectin cDNA sequence reveals potential binding regions for calcium and hydroxyapatite and shows homologies with both a basement membrane protein (SPARC) and a serine proteinase inhibitor (ovomucoid). *Proc Natl Acad Sci USA* 1998;85:2919–2923.
93. Hultenby K, Reinholt FP, Heinegard D, et al. Osteopontin: a ligand for the alpha v beta 3 integrin of the osteoclast clear zone in osteopetrotic (ia/ia) rats. *Ann N Y Acad Sci* 1995;760:315–318.
94. Reinholt FP, Hultenby K, Oldberg A, et al. Osteopontin—a possible anchor of osteoclasts to bone. *Proc Natl Acad Sci USA* 1990;87:4473–4475.
95. McKee MD, Nanci A. Osteopontin at mineralized tissue interfaces in bone, teeth, and osseointegrated implants: ultrastructural distribution and implications for mineralized tissue formation, turnover, and repair. *Microsc Res Tech* 1996;33:141–164.
96. Luo G, Ducy P, McKee MD, et al. Spontaneous calcification of arteries and cartilage in mice lacking matrix GLA protein. *Nature* 1997;385:78–81.
97. Levi-Montalcini R, Hamburger V. Selective growth stimulating effects of mouse sarcoma on the sensory and sympathetic nervous system of the chick embryo. *J Exp Zool* 1951; 116:321–362.
98. Wieser RJ, Janik-Schmitt B, Renaver D, et al. Contact-dependent inhibition of growth of normal diploid human fibroblasts by plasma membrane glycoproteins. *Biochimie* 1988;70:1661–1671.
99. Finkbeiner S. Calcium waves in astrocytes-filling in the gaps. *Neuron* 1992;8: 1101–1108.
100. Moolenaar WH, Defize LHK, DeLaat SW. Calcium in the action of growth factors. Calcium and the cell. *Ciba Found Symp* 1986;122:212–231.
101. Pardridge WM. Transport of protein-bound hormones into tissues in vivo. *Endocr Rev* 1981;2:102–123.
102. Cohen S, Ushiro H, Stoscheck C, et al. A native 170,000 epidermal growth factor receptor-kinase complex from shed plasma membrane vesicles. *J Biol Chem* 1982;257: 1523–1531.
103. Evans RM. The steroid and thyroid hormone receptor superfamily. *Science* 1988;240: 889–895.
104. Massague J, Weis Garcia F. Serine/threonine kinase receptors: mediators of transforming growth factor beta family signals. *Cancer Surv* 1996;27:41–64.

105. Neufeld G, Gospodarowicz D. The identification and partial characterization of the fibroblast growth factor receptor of baby hamster kidney cells. *J Biol Chem* 1985;260: 13860–13868.

106. Solloway MJ, Robertson EJ. Early embryonic lethality in Bmp5;Bmp7 double mutant mice suggests functional redundancy within the 60A subgroup. *Development* 1999,126: 1753–1768.

107. Ornitz DM, Marie PJ. FGF signaling pathways in endochondral and intramembranous bone development and human genetic disease. *Genes Dev* 2002;16:1446–1465.

108. Naski MC, Ornitz DM. FGF signaling in skeletal development. *Front Biosci* 1998;3: D781–D794.

109. Ornitz DM, Itoh N. Fibroblast growth factors. *Genome Biol* 2001;2:REVIEWS3005.

110. Hauschka PV, Mavrakos AE, Iafrati MD, et al. Growth factors in bone matrix. Isolation of multiple types by affinity chromatography on heparin-Sepharose. *J Biol Chem* 1986; 261:12665–12674.

111. Liu Z, Xu J, Colvin JS, et al. Coordination of chondrogenesis and osteogenesis by fibroblast growth factor 18. *Genes Dev* 2002;16:859–869.

112. Hearn MTW. Structure and function of the heparin-binding (fibroblast) growth factor family. *Baillères Clin Endocrinol Metab* 1991;5:571–593.

113. Baker J, Liu JP, Robertson EJ, et al. Role of insulin-like growth factors in embryonic and postnatal growth. *Cell* 1993;75:73–82.

114. Liu JP, Baker J, Perkins AS, et al. Mice carrying null mutations of the genes encoding insulin-like growth factor I (Igf-1) and type 1 IGF receptor (Igf1r). *Cell* 1993;75:59–72.

115. Yakar S, Rosen CJ. From mouse to man: redefining the role of insulin-like growth factor-I in the acquisition of bone mass. *Exp Biol Med (Maywood)* 2003;228:245–252.

116. Hunziker EB, Wagner J, Zapf J. Differential effects of insulin-like growth factor I and growth hormone on developmental stages of rat growth plate chondrocytes in vivo. *J Clin Invest* 1994;93:1078–1086.

117. Trippel SB, Van Wyk JJ, Foster MB, et al. Characterization of a specific somatomedin-c receptor on isolated bovine growth plate chondrocytes. *Endocrinology* 1983;112: 2128–2136.

118. Reinecke M, Schmid AC, Heyberger-Meyer B, et al. Effect of growth hormone and insulin-like growth factor I (IGF-I) on the expression of IGF-I messenger ribonucleic acid and peptide in rat tibial growth plate and articular chondrocytes in vivo. *Endocrinology* 2000;141:2847–2853.

119. Trippel SB, Wroblewski J, Makower AM, et al. Regulation of growth-plate chondrocytes by insulin-like growth-factor I and basic fibroblast growth factor. *J Bone Joint Surg Am* 1993;75:177–189.

120. Zapf J, Froesch ER. Insulin-like growth factor I actions on somatic growth. In: Kostyo JL, ed. *Handbook of physiology*. New York and Oxford: Oxford University Press, 1999.

121. Hogan BL, Blessing M, Winnier GE, et al. Growth factors in development: the role of TGF-beta related polypeptide signalling molecules in embryogenesis. *Dev Suppl* 1994; 53–60.

122. Carano RAD, Filvaroff EH. Angiogenesis and bone repair. *Drug Discov Today* 2003;8: 980–989.

123. Massague J. Receptors for the TGF-beta family. *Cell* 1992;69:1067–1070.

124. Yamaguchi Y, Mann D, Ruoslahti E. Negative regulation of transforming growth factor-B by the proteoglycan decorin. *Nature* 1990;346:281–284.

125. Border WA, Noble NA, Yamamoto T, et al. Natural inhibitor of transforming growth factor-beta protects against scarring in experimental kidney disease. *Nature* 1992;360: 361–364.

126. Schmitt J, Hwang K, Winn S, et al. Bone morphogenetic proteins: an update on basic biology and clinical relevance. *J Orthop Res* 1999;17:269–278.

127. Cheifetz S, Li IW, McCulloch CA, et al. Influence of osteogenic protein-1 (OP-1,P-7) and transforming growth factor-beta 1 on bone formation in vitro. *Connect Tissue Res* 1996;35:71–78.

128. Klein Nulend J, Louwerse RT, Heyligers IC, et al. Osteogenic protein (OP-1, BMP-7) stimulates cartilage differentiation of human and goat perichondrium tissue in vitro. *J Biomed Mater Res* 1998;40:614–620.

129. Klein Nulend J, Semeins CM, Mulder JW, et al. Stimulation of cartilage differentiation by osteogenic protein-1 in cultures of human perichondrium. *Tissue Eng* 1998;4: 305–313.

130. Volk SW, Luvalle P, Leask T, et al. A Bmp-responsive transcriptional region in the chicken type X collagen gene. *J Bone Miner Res* 1998;13:1521–1529.

131. Yamamoto N, Akiyama S, Katagiri T, et al. Smad1 and smad5 act downstream of intracellular signalings of BMP-2 that inhibits myogenic differentiation and induces osteoblast differentiation in C2C12 myoblasts. *Biochem Biophys Res Commun* 1997;238: 574–580.

132. Alvarez J, Sohn P, Zeng X, et al. TGFbeta2 mediates the effects of hedgehog on hypertrophic differentiation and PTHrP expression. *Development* 2002;129:1913–1924.

133. Wang EA, Rosen V, D'Alessandro JS, et al. Recombinant human bone morphogenetic protein induces bone formation. *Proc Natl Acad Sci USA* 1990;87:2220–2224.

134. Wang K, Tsai DC, Nam EK, et al. Ectopic bone formation via rhBMP-2 delivery from porous bioabsorbable polymer scaffolds. *J Biomed Mater Res* 1998;42:491–499.

135. Gazzerro E, Gangji V, Canalis E. Bone morphogenetic proteins induce the expression of noggin, which limits their activity in cultured rat osteoblasts. *J Clin Invest* 1998;102: 2106–2114.

136. Piccolo S, Sasai Y, Lu B, et al. Dorsoventral patterning in Xenopus: inhibition of ventral signals by direct binding of chordin to BMP-4. *Cell* 1996;86:589–598.

137. Pearce J, Penny G, Rossant J. A mouse cerberus/Dan-related gene family. *Dev Biol* 1999; 209:98–110.

138. Gerber H-P, Vu TH, Ryan AM, et al. VEGF couples hypertrophic cartilage remodeling, ossification and angiogenesis during endochondral bone formation. *Nat Med* 1999;5: 623–628.

139. Street J, Bao M, deGuzman L, et al. Vascular endothelial growth factor stimulates bone repair by promoting angiogenesis and bone turnover. *Proc Natl Acad Sci USA* 2002; 99:9656–9661.

140. Rappolee DA, Mark D, Banda MJ, et al. Wound macrophages express TGF-a and other growth factors in vivo: analysis by mRNA typing. *Science* 1988;241:708–712.

141. Schultz GS, Grant MB. Neovascular growth factors. *Eye* 1991;5:170–180.

142. Conway EM, Collen D, Carmeliet P. Molecular mechanisms of blood vessel growth. *Cardiovasc Res* 2001;49:507–521.

143. Ballock RT, O'Keefe RJ. The biology of the growth plate. *J Bone Joint Surg Am* 2003; 85-A:715–726.

144. Trippel SB, Ghivizzani SC, Nixon AJ. Gene-based approaches for the repair of articular cartilage. *Gene Ther* 2004;11:351–359.

145. Daughaday WH, Hall K, Raben MS, et al. Somatomedin: proposed designation for sulphation factor. *Nature* 1972;235:107.

146. Sjogren K, Liu JL, Blad K, et al. Liver-derived insulin-like growth factor I (IGF-I) is the principal source of IGF-I in blood but is not required for postnatal body growth in mice. *Proc Natl Acad Sci USA* 1999;96:7088–7092.

147. Sims NA, Clement-Lacroix P, Da Ponte F, et al. Bone homeostasis in growth hormone receptor-null mice is restored by IGF-I but independent of Stat5. *J Clin Invest* 2000; 106:1095–1103.

148. Barnard R, Haynes KM, Werther GA, et al. The ontogeny of growth hormone receptors in the rabbit tibia. *Endocrinology* 1988;122:2562–2569.

149. Edmondson SR, Baker NL, Oh J, et al. Growth hormone receptor abundance in tibial growth plates of uremic rats: GH/IGF-I treatment. *Kidney Int* 2000;58:62–70.

150. Werther GA, Haynes KM, Barnard R, et al. Visual demonstration of growth hormone receptors on human growth plate chondrocytes. *J Clin Endocrinol Metab* 1990;70: 1725–1731.

151. Ohlsson C, Nilsson A, Isaksson O, et al. Growth hormone induces multiplication of the slowly cycling germinal cells of the rat tibial growth plate. *Proc Natl Acad Sci USA* 1992;89:9826–9830.

152. Wang J, Zhou J, Cheng CM, et al. Evidence supporting dual, IGF-I-independent and IGF-I-dependent, roles for GH in promoting longitudinal bone growth. *J Endocrinol* 2004;180:247–255.

153. Erickson DM, Harris SE, Dean DD, et al. Recombinant bone morphogenetic protein (BMP)-2 regulates costochondral growth plate chondrocytes and induces expression of BMP-2 and BMP-4 in a cell maturation–dependent manner. *J Orthop Res* 1997;15: 371–380.

154. Brunet LJ, McMahon JA, McMahon AP, et al. Noggin, cartilage morphogenesis, and joint formation in the mammalian skeleton. *Science* 1998;280:1455–1457.

155. Nilsson A, Ohlsson C, Isaksson OG, et al. Hormonal regulation of longitudinal bone growth. *Eur J Clin Nutr* 1994;48[Supp l]1:S150–S158; discussion S158–S160.

156. Bonassar LJ, Trippel SB. Interaction of epidermal growth factor and insulin-like growth factor-I in the regulation of growth plate chondrocytes. *Exp Cell Res* 1997; 234:1–6.

157. Carey DE, Liu X. Expression of bone morphogenetic protein-6 messenger RNA in bovine growth plate chondrocytes of different size. *J Bone Miner Res* 1995;10:401–405.

158. Chintala SK, Miller RR, McDevitt CA. Basic fibroblast growth factor binds to heparan sulfate in the extracellular matrix of rat growth plate chondrocytes. *Arch Biochem Biophys* 1994;310:180–186.

159. Makower AM, Wroblewski J, Pawlowski A. Effects of IGF-I, rGH, FGF, EGF and NCS on DNA-synthesis, cell proliferation and morphology of chondrocytes isolated from rat rib growth cartilage. *Cell Biol Int* 1989;13:259–270.

160. Kronenberg HM. Developmental regulation of the growth plate. *Nature* 2003;423: 332–336.

161. Legeai Mallet L, Benoist Lasselin C, Delezoide AL, et al. Fibroblast growth factor receptor 3 mutations promote apoptosis but do not alter chondrocyte proliferation in thanatophoric dysplasia. *J Biol Chem* 1998;273:13007–13014.

162. Mancilla EE, De Luca F, Uyeda JA, et al. Effects of fibroblast growth factor-2 on longitudinal bone growth. *Endocrinology* 1998;139:2900–2904.

163. Chintala SK, Miller RR, McDevitt CA. Role of heparan sulfate in the terminal differentiation of growth plate chondrocytes. *Arch Biochem Biophys* 1995;316:227–234.

164. van der Eerden BC, Karperien M, Gevers EF, et al. Expression of Indian hedgehog, parathyroid hormone-related protein, and their receptors in the postnatal growth plate of the rat: evidence for a locally acting growth restraining feedback loop after birth. *J Bone Miner Res* 2000;15:1045–1055.

165. Kronenberg HM, Lanske B, Kovacs CS, et al. Functional analysis of the PTH/PTHrP network of ligands and receptors. *Recent Prog Horm Res* 1998;53:283–301; discussion 301–303.

166. Vortkamp A, Lee K, Lanske B, et al. Regulation of rate of cartilage differentiation by Indian hedgehog and PTH-related protein. *Science* 1996;273:613–622.

167. Minina E, Kreschel C, Naski MC, et al. Interaction of FGF, Ihh/Pthlh, and BMP signaling integrates chondrocyte proliferation and hypertrophic differentiation. *Dev Cell* 2002; 3:439–449.

168. Schipani E, Provot S. PTHrP, PTH, and the PTH/PTHrP receptor in endochondral bone development. *Birth Defects Res Part C Embryo Today* 2003;69:352–362.

169. Zhang D, Schwarz EM, Rosier RN, et al. ALK2 functions as a BMP type I receptor and induces Indian hedgehog in chondrocytes during skeletal development. *J Bone Miner Res* 2003;18:1593–1604.

170. Baron J, Klein KO, Yanovski JA, et al. Induction of growth plate cartilage ossification by basic fibroblast growth factor. *Endocrinology* 1994;135:2790–2793.

171. Meikle MC, Bord S, Hembry RM, et al. Human osteoblasts in culture synthesize colla-

genase and other matrix metalloproteinases in response to osteotropic hormones and cytokines. *J Cell Sci* 1992;103:1093–1099.
172. Meikle MC, McGarrity AM, Thomson BM, et al. Bone-derived growth factors modulate collagenase and TIMP (tissue inhibitor of metalloproteinases) activity and type I collagen degradation by mouse calvarial osteoblasts. *Bone Miner* 1991;12:41–55.
173. Marks SC Jr. Osteoclast biology: lessons from mammalian mutations. *Am J Med Genet* 1998;34:43–54.
174. Erlebacher A, Derynck R. Increased expression of TGF-beta 2 in osteoblasts results in an osteoporosis-like phenotype. *J Cell Biol* 1996;132:195–210.
175. Erlebacher A, Filvaroff EH, Ye JQ, et al. Osteoblastic responses to TGF-beta during bone remodeling. *Mol Biol Cell* 1998;9:1903–1918.
176. Massague J. The transforming growth factor-β family. *J Biol Chem* 1990;6:597–641.
177. McCarthy TL, Centrella M. Local IGF-I expression and bone formation. *Growth Horm IGF Res* 2001;11:213–219.
178. Suda T, Takahashi N, Udagawa N, et al. Modulation of osteoclast differentiation and function by the new members of the tumor necrosis factor receptor and ligand families. *Endocr Rev* 1999;20:345–357.
179. Boyle WJ, Simonet WS, Lacey DL. Osteoclast differentiation and activation. *Nature* 2003;423:337–342.
180. Manolagas SC. Birth and death of bone cells: basic regulatory mechanisms and implications for the pathogenesis and treatment of osteoporosis. *Endocr Rev* 2000; 21:115–137.
181. Kobayashi K, Takahashi N, Jimi E, et al. Tumor necrosis factor alpha stimulates osteoclast differentiation by a mechanism independent of the ODF/RANKL-RANK interaction. *J Exp Med* 2000;191:275–286.
182. Katagiri T, Takahashi N. Regulatory mechanisms of osteoblast and osteoclast differentiation. *Oral Dis* 2002;8:147–159.
183. Miettinen PJ, Chin JR, Shum L, et al. Epidermal growth factor receptor function is necessary for normal craniofacial development and palate closure. *Nat Genet* 1999;22:69–73.
184. Chan SY, Wong RW. Expression of epidermal growth factor in transgenic mice causes growth retardation. *J Biol Chem* 2000;275:38693–38698.
185. Cowin SC, Moss Salentijn L, Moss ML. Candidates for the mechanosensory system in bone. *J Biomech Eng* 1991;113:191–197.
186. Rokhanen P, Slatis P. The repair of experimental fractures during long-term anticoagulant treatment. *Acta Orthop Scand* 1964;35:21–38.
187. Uhthoff HK, Rahn B. Healing patterns of metaphyseal fractures. *Trans Orthop Res Soc* 1981;6:40.
188. Sandberg MM, Aro HT, Vuorio EI. Gene expression during bone repair. *Clin Orthop* 1993;289:292–312.
189. Gotham L. Vascular reactions in experimental fractures: microangiographic and radioisotope studies. *Acta Chir Scand* 1961;284[Suppl]:1–34.
190. Goldhaber P. Osteogenic induction across millipore filters in vivo. *Science* 1966;133: 2065–2067.
191. Potts WJ. The role of the hematoma in fracture healing. *Surg Gynecol Obstet* 1933;57: 318–324.
192. Crelin ES, White AA III, Panjabi MM, et al. Microscopic changes in fractured rabbit tibias. *Conn Med* 1978;42:561–569.
193. Owen M. The origin of bone cells. *Int Rev Cytol* 1970;28:213–238.
194. Ham AW. A histological study of the early phase of bone repair. *J Bone Joint Surg* 1930; 12:827–844.
195. Ham AW. *Histology*, 6th ed. Philadelphia: JB Lippincott, 1969.
196. Chalmers J, Gray DH, Rush J. Observations on the induction of bone in soft tissues. *J Bone Joint Surg* 1975;57B:36–45.
197. Gerstenfeld LC, Cullinane DM, Barnes GL, et al. Fracture healing as a post-natal developmental process: molecular, spatial, and temporal aspects of its regulation. *J Cell Biochem* 2003;88:873–884.
198. Brashear HR Jr. Epiphyseal fractures—a microscopic study of the healing process in rats. *J Bone Joint Surg Am* 1959;41A:1055–1064.
199. Lee CW, Martinek V, Usas A, et al. Muscle-based gene therapy and tissue engineering for treatment of growth plate injuries. *J Pediatr Orthop* 2002;22:565–572.
200. Xian CJ, Zhou FH, McCarty RC, et al. Intramembranous ossification mechanism for bone bridge formation at the growth plate cartilage injury site. *J Orthop Res* 2004;22: 417–426.
201. Rohlig H. Perlost und langenwachstum. *Beitr Orthop Traumatol* 1966;13:603–606.
202. Burger M, Sherman BS, Sobel AE. Observations on the influence of chondroitin sulphate on the rate of bone repair. *J Bone Joint Surg* 1962;44B:675–687.
203. Lee MA, Nissen TP, Otsuka NY. Utilization of a murine model to investigate the molecular process of transphyseal bone formation. *J Pediatr Orthop* 2000;20:802–806.
204. Giberson RG, Ivins JC. Fractures of the distal part of the forearm in children: correction of deformity by growth. *Minn Med* 1952;35:744.
205. Ogden JA, Southwick WO. Adequate reduction of fractures and dislocations. *Radiol Clin North Am* 1973;11:667–682.
206. Crilly RG. Longitudinal overgrowth of chicken radius. *J Anat* 1972;112:11–18.
207. Edvardson P, Syversen SM. Overgrowth of the femur after fractures of the shaft in childhood. *J Bone Joint Surg* 1976;58B:339–346.
208. Margolin MD, Cogan AG, Taylor M, et al. Maxillary sinus augmentation in the non-human primate: a comparative radiographic and histologic study between recombinant human osteogenic protein-1 and natural bone mineral. *J Periodontol* 1998;69:911–919.
209. Takiguchi T, Kobayashi M, Suzuki R, et al. Recombinant human bone morphogenetic protein-2 stimulates osteoblast differentiation and suppresses matrix metalloproteinase-1 production in human bone cells isolated from mandibulae. *J Periodontal Res* 1998; 33:476–485.
210. Friedlaender GE, Perry CR, Cole JD, et al. Osteogenic protein-1 (bone morphogenetic protein-7) in the treatment of tibial nonunions. *J Bone Joint Surg Am* 2001;83-A[Suppl 1]:S151–S158.
211. Joyce ME, Jingushi S, Scully SP, et al. Role of growth factors in fracture healing. *Prog Clin Biol Res* 1991;365:391–416.
212. Nash TJ, Howlett CR, Martin C, et al. Effect of platelet-derived growth factor on tibial osteotomies in rabbits. *Bone* 1994;15:203–208.
213. Bak B. Fracture healing and growth hormone. A biochemical study in the rat. *Dan Med Bull* 1993;40:519–536.
214. Trippel SB. Potential role of insulin-like growth factors in fracture healing. *Clin Orthop* 1998;355:S301–S313.
215. Inui K, Maeda M, Sano A, et al. Local application of basic fibroblast growth factor minipellet induces the healing of segmental bony defects in rabbits. *Calcif Tissue Int* 1998;63:490–495.
216. Kato T, Kawaguchi H, Hanada K, et al. Single local injection of recombinant fibroblast growth factor-2 stimulates healing of segmental bone defects in rabbits. *J Orthop Res* 1998;16:654–659.
217. Wang JS. Basic fibroblast growth factor for stimulation of bone formation in osteoinductive or conductive implants. *Acta Orthop Scand Suppl* 1996;269:1–33.
218. Burgess WH, Mehlman T, Marshak DR, et al. Structural evidence that endothelial cell growth factor is the precursor of both endothelial cell growth factor and acidic fibroblast growth factor. *Proc Natl Acad Sci USA* 1986;83:7216–7220.
219. Einhorn TA, Trippel SB. Growth factor treatment of fractures. *Instr Course Lect* 1997; 46:483–486.
220. Einhorn TA. Enhancement of fracture healing. *Instr Course Lect* 1996;45:401–416.
221. Ramoshebi LN, Matsaba TN, Teare J, et al. Tissue engineering: TGF-beta superfamily members and delivery systems in bone regeneration. *Expert Rev Mol Med* 2002;2002: 1–11.
222. Trippel SB. Growth factors as therapeutic agents. *Instr Course Lect* 1997;46:473–476.
223. Illi OE, Feldmann CP. Stimulation of fracture healing by local application of humoral factors integrated in biodegradable implants. *Eur J Pediatr Surg* 1998;8:251–255.
224. Oakes BW. Orthopaedic tissue engineering: from laboratory to the clinic. *Med J Aust* 2004;180:S35–S38.
225. Lucarelli E, Donati D, Cenacchi A, et al. Bone reconstruction of large defects using bone marrow derived autologous stem cells. *Transfus Apheresis Sci* 2004;30:169–174.
226. Foster BK, Hansen AL, Gibson GJ, et al. Reimplantation of growth plate chondrocytes into growth plate defects in sheep. *J Orthop Res* 1990;8:555–564.
227. Gruber HE, Phieffer LS, Wattenbarger JM. Physeal fractures, part II: fate of interposed periosteum in a physeal fracture. *J Pediatr Orthop* 2002;22:710–716.
228. Lee EH, Chen F, Chan J, et al. Treatment of growth arrest by transfer of cultured chondrocytes into physeal defects. *J Pediatr Orthop* 1998;18:155–160.
229. Sandell LJ, Sugai JV, Trippel SB. Expression of collagens I, II, X, and XI and aggrecan mRNAs by bovine growth plate chondrocytes in situ. *J Orthop Res* 1994;12:1–14.
230. Gibson G, Lin DL, Francki K, et al. Type X collagen is colocalized with a proteoglycan epitope to form distinct morphological structures in bovine growth cartilage. *Bone* 1996;19:307–315.
231. Hedbom E, Heinegard D. Binding of fibromodulin and decorin to separate sites on fibrillar collagens. *J Biol Chem* 1993;268:27307–27312.
232. Fichard A, Kleman JP, Ruggiero F. Another look at collagen V and XI molecules. *Matrix Biol* 1994;14:515–531.
233. Schonherr E, Hausser H, Beavan L, et al. Decorin-type I collagen interaction. Presence of separate core protein-binding domains. *J Biol Chem* 1995;270:8877–8883.
234. Schonherr E, Witsch Prehm P, Harrach B, et al. Interaction of biglycan with type I collagen. *J Biol Chem* 1995;270:2776–2783.

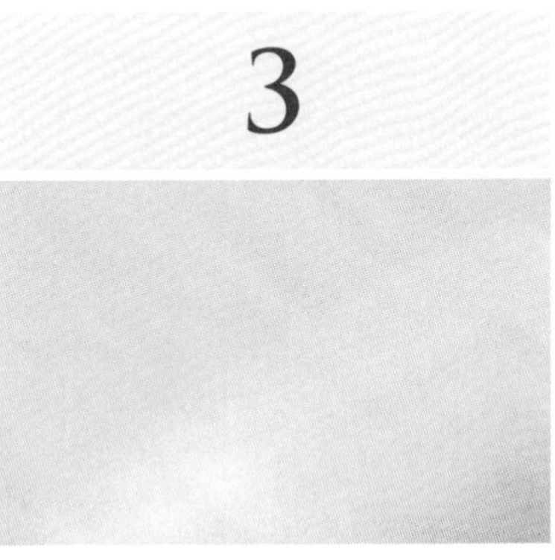

3

PAIN RELIEF AND RELATED CONCERNS IN CHILDREN'S FRACTURES

Joseph R. Furman

Providing pain relief is one of the many important parts of the management of children's fractures. In addition, because having a fracture reduced is not only painful but also frightening to many children, adequate sedation and amnesia are additional welcome elements of good care. However, the correct use of any of the available medications for obtaining these goals must involve an appropriate understanding of proper dose, desired effects, and untoward side effects. The purpose of this chapter is to provide a thorough source of information regarding safe and effective analgesia and sedation for children with fractures. This chapter discusses the concept of sedation and its definitions, the various medications used to achieve the sedation state, and the various medications used to achieve analgesia, including both systemic medications and local anesthetics. Intravenous (IV) regional anesthesia (Bier blocks), hematoma blocks, and femoral nerve blocks (for femur fractures) are discussed in depth. The management of postoperative pain is discussed, along with the treatment of the troublesome side effect of postoperative nausea. The author hopes that the orthopaedic practitioner will find this chapter of significant benefit, not only in the emergency room setting but also in the office and on the hospital ward.

GUIDELINES AND PRINCIPLES OF SEDATION IN CHILDREN

Definitions

Sedation describes a continuum ranging from near wakefulness to complete loss of consciousness (Fig. 3-1). Terms used to describe various stages along this continuum have included conscious sedation, deep sedation, and general anesthesia (1).

Strictly speaking, the term "conscious sedation" means a pharmacologically controlled altered state of consciousness in which patients maintain their ability to respond purposefully to verbal commands. For nonverbal patients or young infants, conscious sedation implies the ability to respond purposefully to physical stimulation, not simply by reflex withdrawal to pain. Unfortunately, most physicians and nurses tend to use the term "conscious sedation" to mean anything short of a general anesthetic. For such reasons, the consensus of the 1996 report by the American Society of Anesthesiologists Task Force on Sedation and Analgesia by Non-Anesthesiologists (2) is that the term "conscious sedation," although in common use, is imprecise. This report recommends replacing the term with the more descriptive term "sedation/analgesia" (see Fig. 3-1).

Whatever the preferred term, the important point to recognize is that the safest level of sedation is that which permits purposeful response to verbal or physical stimulation. It is at this level of sedation that the risk of hypoventilation, apnea, or cardiovascular instability is minimal. Unfortunately, and realistically speaking, such relatively light levels of sedation are totally inadequate for the performance of a painful procedure such as the reduction of a fracture. Also the younger and less cooperative the patient, the less likely that so-called conscious sedation can realistically be achieved at all (3). Therefore, it is very likely that for orthopaedic procedures, children may have to be sedated to levels at which they are not easily responsive to verbal stimulation and, as such, are at increased risk for respiratory and cardiovascular compromise. Even in children in whom light levels of sedation (true conscious sedation) is possible, unintended oversedation may occur without warning. Oversedation may lead to (a) loss of the airway, (b) impaired protective reflexes, leading to the possibility of aspiration of gastric contents, and (c) cardiopulmonary arrest (see Fig. 3-1). It is for these reasons that careful monitoring of sedated patients, as prescribed in standard guidelines (2), is imperative.

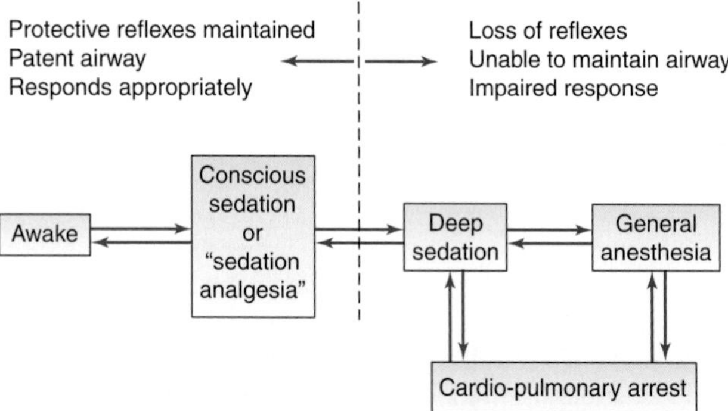

FIGURE 3-1 Sedation and analgesia for procedures is a continuum. (Reproduced with permission from American Society of Anesthesiologists, from ASA 1997 Annual Refresher Course Lectures. *Sedation and analgesia in pediatric patients for procedures outside the operating room.* Richard F. Kaplan, MD, No. 221)

Monitoring

Obviously, the purpose for monitoring sedated patients is to provide timely detection and correction of abnormalities in respiratory and cardiovascular function. The monitoring process begins before the administration of any sedative medications. Monitoring continues unabated until the patient returns to his or her baseline presedation level of consciousness and is ready for discharge. Acceptable discharge criteria are noted later (Table 3-1).

Vital to the monitoring process is the presence of qualified personnel who are competent in the use of monitoring devices and capable of recognizing the clinical signs of airway or hemo-

TABLE 3-1 Recommended Discharge Criteria after Sedation

1. Cardiovascular function and airway patency are satisfactory and stable.
2. The patient is easily arousable, and protective reflexes are intact.
3. The patient can talk (if age-appropriate).
4. The patient can sit up unaided (if age-appropriate).
5. For a very young or handicapped child incapable of the usually expected responses, the presedation level of responsiveness or a level as close as possible to the normal level for that child should be achieved.
6. The state of hydration is adequate.*

* Adequate hydration may be achieved with IV fluids. There is no specific requirement that children be able to tolerate oral fluids before discharge from a treatment facility. Children who are nauseated or actively vomiting should be treated and observed until this problem resolves (see section on treatment of postoperative nausea).

Guidelines for monitoring and management of pediatric patients during and after sedation for diagnostic and therapeutic procedures. *Pediatrics* 1992;89: 1110–1115; with permission.

dynamic instability. Although skill in at least pediatric basic life support is necessary (1,4), training in pediatric advanced life support (PALS) is certainly desirable. In the author's opinion, this training should be considered necessary. The orthopaedic surgeon must always demand, and have available, skilled health professionals, either physicians or nurses, to assist in observing the patient and the monitors during procedures requiring medications that are known to depress respiratory or cardiovascular function. Having one person performing both the surgical procedure and monitoring the patient is a practice that should be strongly discouraged in all but the most desperate circumstances.

Oxygenation, ventilation, and circulation are the three parameters that require careful assessment. Monitoring temperature is usually of minimal importance; the major exceptions, of course, are children who arrive in the hospital either severely hypothermic or febrile.

Monitoring oxygenation requires continuous pulse oximetry and continual visual inspection of the patient. The term "continuous monitoring" refers to a constant measurement undertaken for a period of time without interruption. "Continual monitoring" refers to an assessment taken at frequent, regular intervals.

The value of pulse oximetry as an early detector of impeding hypoxemia has been well demonstrated (5). The problem with relying on visual inspection alone to determine the adequacy of oxygenation is that cyanosis is both a late and variable sign of hypoxemia. Demonstrable cyanosis requires the presence of at least 5 g of desaturated hemoglobin per deciliter. Therefore, for example, a patient with a hemoglobin level of 10 g/dL would theoretically not even appear cyanotic until the oxygen saturation level (SpO_2) plummets to 50%. For this same reason, a severely anemic patient may never develop visible cyanosis even at profound levels of hypoxemia. To add to a potentially confusing situation, the ambient light (especially fluorescent light) in many clinical environments may make any patient appear cyanotic (6). Therefore, pulse oximetry is essential in all heavily sedated patients to detect abnormalities of oxygenation rapidly.

However, the pulse oximeter is not perfect. Factors that affect the accuracy of the pulse oximeter include patient movement (6), direct bright light on the probe (7), and malposition of the probe (8). Correct probe placement, shielding the probe site from bright light, and gentle restraint of the monitoring site should improve the dependability of this all-important monitor.

Monitoring ventilation goes hand in hand with monitoring oxygenation. Monitoring ventilation requires close observation of the patient and either intermittent or continuous auscultation of breath sounds. A sedated child's head may flex forward easily, producing airway obstruction as the child begins to fall asleep (6). Maintaining patients in the so-called sniffing position helps prevent airway obstruction (Fig. 3-2). The sniffing position consists of elevating the patient's head with pads under the occiput, keeping the shoulders flat on the table, and extending the head at the atlanto-occipital joint (9). Children younger than 3 years of age have a relatively large head in proportion to the size of their trunk and do not require padding under the occiput (10).

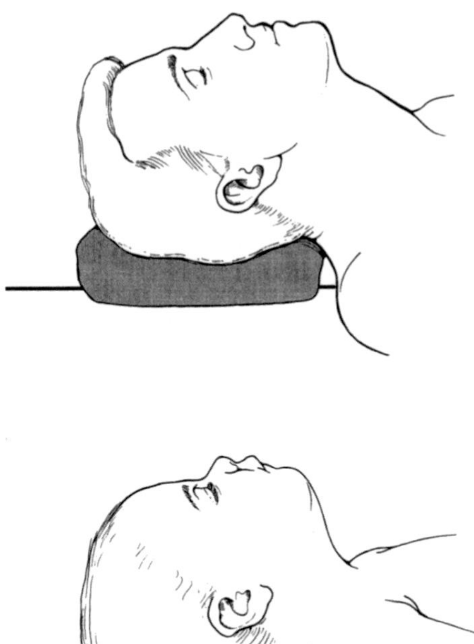

FIGURE 3-2 The sniffing position. In an adult or in an older child, a folded sheet or towel under the occiput, plus moderate head extension at the atlanto-occipital joint, helps to maintain an open airway. In a child younger than 3 years of age, the relatively large head size in proportion to the trunk makes occipital padding unnecessary (10).

Along with continual assessment of the child's head position, any restraining devices should be checked and rechecked to ensure that they are not contributing to either airway obstruction or restriction of chest movement (1).

Auscultation with the precordial stethoscope is valuable in the monitoring of both ventilation (breath sounds) and circulation (heart sounds). Its use is encouraged in the monitoring of deeply sedated patients (1).

Monitoring circulation for most sedated children consists of intermittent determination of heart rate and blood pressure (1). For children, normal values for heart rate and blood pressure vary with age (Tables 3-2 and 3-3). A simple formula for calculating the normal systolic blood pressure and lower limit of normal for systolic blood pressure in children by age is worth memorizing (Table 3-4). Electrocardiographic (ECG) monitoring is especially important for the child with an underlying history of a significant cardiac dysrhythmia or known ECG abnormality such as long QT syndrome, or a history of Wolff-Parkinson-White syndrome. In the absence of monitor artifact, the pulse oximeter provides a continuous assessment of heart rate. Deeply sedated children should have blood pressure and heart rate and respiratory rate measurements determined and recorded at least at 5-minute intervals (1). For children under conscious sedation (sedation/analgesia), the frequency of vital sign determination is at the discretion of the physician (1).

TABLE 3-2 Normal Values for Heart Rate by Age

Age	Range (beats/min)
Newborn	110–150
1–11 months	80–150
2 years	85–125
4 years	75–115
6 years	65–110
8 years	60–110

Rasch DK, Webster DE. *Clinical manual of pediatric anesthesia*. New York: McGraw-Hill, 1994:16; with permission.

TABLE 3-3 Normal Values for Blood Pressure by Age

	Blood Pressure (mm Hg)	
Age	Systolic	Diastolic
Full-term infant	60 (45)	35
3–10 days	70–75 (50)	40
6 months	95 (55)	45
4 years	98	57
6 years	110	60
8 years	112	60
12 years	115	65
16 years	120	65

The numbers in parentheses refer to mean arterial blood pressure.
Steward DJ. *Manual of pediatric anesthesia*. New York: Churchill-Livingstone. 1990:24, and Rasch DK, Webster DE. *Clinical manual of pediatric anesthesia*. New York: McGraw-Hill, 1994:17; with permission.

TABLE 3-4 Calculation of Normal Blood Pressure by Age

80 + (2 × age in years) = normal systolic BP for age

70 + (2 × age in years) = lower limit of normal systolic BP for age

Rasch DK, Webster DE. *Clinical manual of pediatric anesthesia*. New York: McGraw-Hill, 1994:197; with permission.

Monitoring the patient must continue until the patient meets preset discharge criteria (see Table 3-1) (1). Often, when a surgical procedure is over and patients are no longer being actively stimulated, unintentional deep sedation with resulting airway obstruction and apnea may occur. Therefore, it is essential to remain vigilant until the patient recovers completely from the sedative medications. The time to recovery varies depending on the amount and type of sedative medication given, and this point should be taken into account when planning a sedation regimen. The durations of action of particular sedatives and sedative combinations are discussed separately.

Patient Assessment

Only after careful patient assessment can the practitioner decide whether sedation in an emergency room setting, where the airway is uncontrolled and unprotected, is feasible and safe. Administering sedative medications without first evaluating a patient is an invitation for disaster. It is important first to be aware of the child's medical history, previous allergic or adverse drug reactions, current medications, and presence of coexisting diseases before proceeding with deliberate alteration of a patient's state of consciousness (1). In addition to these basic details, the patient with musculoskeletal injuries has to be evaluated for time of last oral intake, hemodynamic status, presence of other injuries, and status of the airway.

Oral Intake Precautions

In the management of elective patients, significant pulmonary aspiration is rare in pediatrics (11). For elective patients, multiple studies support and encourage the liberal intake of clear liquids up until 2 to 3 hours before scheduled surgery in otherwise healthy children (12–15). Acceptable clear liquids are apple juice, water, sugar water, and gelatin. Milk (including breast milk), milk products, and juices with pulp are not clear liquids. For elective patients, most pediatric anesthesiologists now adhere to the so-called 2-4-6-8 rule regarding oral intake. This rule restricts clear fluids to 2 hours before elective surgery, breast milk to 4 hours before elective surgery, baby formula (cow's milk formula) to 6 hours before elective surgery, and solid food to 8 hours before elective surgery (16).

Emergency patients are definitely at risk for aspiration (11).

Sedatives depress the protective reflexes (1). Caution is necessary to avoid the morbidity and possible mortality of aspiration pneumonia.

In trauma patients, the time interval between last oral intake and time of injury is a critical factor in the retention of gastric contents (17). Children injured within 1 to 2 hours after eating present with large gastric volumes (18). Although fasting can reduce an injured child's gastric volume (13), it is not clear how long of a fast is ideal. Also, in the presence of pain and anxiety, and with the administration of opioid pain relievers, all of which may occur in the patient with a fracture, gastric emptying may be radically slowed (19). If the procedure can wait, it is safe to say that a fasting period is in order. Starting IV fluids to prevent dehydration is important. At present, there is no reliable method of assessing the volume of gastric contents, although different methods have been suggested (20). Patient hunger on presentation for surgical treatment is not a good indicator of an empty stomach (13).

In the author's opinion, the safest recommendations regarding sedation of patients with a potential full stomach are as follows:

1. If possible, postpone the procedure, even for as little as 4 hours.
2. Use the lightest effective level of sedation. Titrate sedation to effect, and avoid large bolus doses of medications.
3. Consider the administration of medications to reduce gastric volume (metoclopramide) or to increase gastric pH (histamine-2–receptor blockers). These medications, when indicated, should be administered IV 1 hour before sedative medications are given. The appropriate dose of metoclopramide (Reglan) is 0.15 mg/kg. The usual adult dose for metoclopramide is 10 mg, which should be more than sufficient for any child. Famotidine (Pepcid), a histamine-2–receptor blocker, may be given in a dose of 0.3 to 0.4 mg/kg IV, with a maximum dose of 20 mg.
4. Within 15 minutes of administering sedation, consider the use of oral nonparticulate antacids (Bicitra, sodium citrate) to raise gastric pH. Unfortunately, these medications are not very palatable.
5. Note that pregnancy, morbid obesity, gastroesophageal reflux, bowel obstruction, and increased intracranial pressure all magnify the risk of regurgitation and aspiration of gastric contents. Therefore, additional caution is necessary in managing patients with any of these conditions. Patients with coexisting bowel obstruction should not be sedated, and patients with increased intracranial pressure should not be sedated without the input and knowledge of the attending neurosurgical staff.
6. If treatment cannot wait and the surgical procedure or the patient is not amenable to regional anesthesia, the safest approach is a general anesthetic with a rapid sequence induction and a protected airway (endotracheal tube). This approach is also safest for uncooperative children who urgently need a computed tomography (CT) scan, a magnetic resonance imaging (MRI) scan, or other detailed diagnostic studies.

Hemodynamic Status

The magnitude of blood loss from a child's injuries is not always readily apparent. In children, long bone fractures and head injuries may easily have associated large concealed hemorrhages (21,22). It is important to assess the patient's volume status accurately before administering sedative medications. In a hypovolemic child, sedatives may interfere with catecholamine-mediated compensatory mechanisms and produce profound hemodynamic instability, leading to cardiovascular collapse.

In an injured child, blood pressure monitoring alone does not provide a good indication of the patient's underlying volume status (23,24). Children maintain a normal blood pressure for their age in the face of large intravascular volume deficits (24). More reliable signs of ongoing hypovolemia in children include sinus tachycardia, mottling, cool extremities, poor urine output (less than 1 to 2 mL/kg/h), and altered state of consciousness. Each of these signs can imply poor perfusion of different organ systems (skin, musculoskeletal system, kidneys, and central nervous system [CNS], respectively). Volume replacement, not sedation, should be the initial goal in the management of hypovolemic children.

Coexisting Nonmusculoskeletal Injuries

Serious head injury accounts for 70% of pediatric trauma deaths (23,25). Respiratory depression from sedation, with resultant hypercapnia and hypoxia, may aggravate an underlying closed head injury and worsen its prognosis (22). In addition, any pharmacologic change in the patient's state of consciousness may confuse the neurologic evaluation. Other injuries to major body cavities or injuries associated with major blood loss should be assessed carefully before any sedative medications are administered.

Status of the Airway

A tenuous airway can easily become a completely obstructed airway in a sedated child. There are common problems in children associated with airway obstruction. For example, children with large tonsils and adenoids may have obstructive sleep apnea (26). Obstructive sleep apnea, which is associated with a history of loud snoring and daytime sleepiness, may be acutely exacerbated with the administration of sedative medications (27). Other potentially dangerous problems include micrognathia (short jaw), limited ability to open the mouth, and limited movement of the neck, either congenital or acquired (28).

Treatment Facility

What about the medical facility where the child is receiving treatment? On-site resuscitation equipment, including equip-

TABLE 3-5 Airway Management Equipment

Ventilation face masks* (infant, child, small adult, medium adult, large adult)

Breathing bag and valve set

Oral airways (infant, child, small adult, medium adult, large adult)

Nasal airways (small, medium, large)

Laryngoscope handles

Laryngoscope blades: straight (Miller) No. 1, 2, 3; curved (Macintosh) No. 1, 2, 3

Endotracheal tubes: 2.5–6.0 uncuffed; 6.0–8.0 cuffed

Appropriate-sized stylets for endotracheal tubes (*must be lubricated before insertion*)

Appropriate-sized suction catheters for endotracheal tubes

Yankauer-type suction

Nasogastric tubes (10–18 French)

Nebulizer set-up for treatment of bronchospasm

* The correct-sized ventilation face mask will fit over the child's face from the bridge of the nose to the cleft of the chin. This guideline is also correct when using patient-administered nitrous oxide analgesia.
Guidelines for monitoring and management of pediatric patients during and after sedation for diagnostic and therapeutic procedures. *Pediatrics*, 1992;89:1110–1115; with permission.

TABLE 3-6 Vascular Access Equipment

IV catheters (24–16 gauge)*

Intraosseous bone-marrow needle

IV tubing: pediatric drip (60 drops/mL); pediatric burette-type; adult drip (10 drips/mL)

IV fluids: lactated Ringer's; normal saline

Miscellaneous equipment: tourniquets, alcohol wipes, arm boards

* In resuscitation situations, no more than 90 seconds should be spent attempting to gain peripheral venous access. If attempts have been unsuccessful, then central venous cannulation, intraosseous cannulation, or peripheral venous cutdown should be done according to the expertise of available personnel.
Guidelines for monitoring and management of pediatric patients during and after sedation for diagnostic and therapeutic procedures. *Pediatrics*, 1992;89:1110–1115; with permission.

ment for airway management (Table 3-5) and equipment for vascular access (Table 3-6), must be available for children of all ages and sizes (1). In addition, a positive-pressure oxygen delivery system capable of delivering at least 90% oxygen for at least 60 minutes must also be readily available (1). A working suction apparatus (1) must be easily accessible to handle patient secretions, as well as for unexpected regurgitation and vomiting. These recommendations are essential for patient safety and optimal patient care.

SEDATIVE MEDICATIONS

Having considered the preliminary step of patient assessment, the practitioner must now decide which sedative or sedatives to use. The ideal sedative should be easy to administer, quick in onset, devoid of side effects, and rapid in termination of effects. The abundance of references in the literature extolling the virtues of different sedative drugs and drug combinations is the best indicator that we do not yet have the ideal sedative. Each of the drugs discussed has only some of the properties of an ideal sedative medication. Also, patients demonstrate great variability in response to medications. Treat each patient as an individual; do not expect to be able to fit every child with a fracture into any particular sedation regimen. For patients who cannot be adequately sedated, the orthopaedic surgeon should consult an anesthesiologist for provision of a brief, well-controlled general anesthetic.

Nitrous Oxide

Self-administered 50% nitrous oxide (50% nitrous oxide and 50% oxygen) has been found to be moderately useful in providing sedation and analgesia for the reduction of children's fractures. Evans et al (29) found it to be comparable in efficacy to intramuscular (IM) meperidine (2 mg/kg) and promethazine (1 mg/kg). However, in a different study, Hennrikus et al noted that 46% of their patients experienced significant pain with nitrous oxide alone as a sedative and analgesic for fracture reduction (30). Patients with completely displaced radius and ulna fractures had a statistically higher incidence of failure to achieve analgesia (30). With the addition of a hematoma block (discussed in a subsequent section), Hennrikus et al obtained a 97% incidence of adequate sedation and analgesia (31). This study illustrates the important point that where possible, the use of regional anesthesia, in combination with almost any sedation regimen, is an excellent way to enhance pain relief and minimize the need for systemic sedative and analgesics.

In general, nitrous oxide is a weak sedative and analgesic. It does have the advantages of rapid onset, relative ease of use, and rapid termination of effects (32). Because it diffuses rapidly into enclosed air-filled spaces, its use is contraindicated in patients with bowel obstruction or pneumothorax (32). Nitrous oxide is also contraindicated in patients with altered intracranial compliance (32).

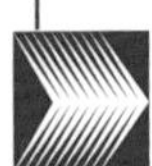

AUTHOR'S PREFERRED TREATMENT

Although nitrous oxide may be a useful part of the sedation armamentarium, this author does not believe that the literature supports the use of nitrous oxide alone as a reliable sedative and analgesic for pediatric orthopaedic procedures.

Ketamine

Ketamine, which is structurally related to phencyclidine, was first synthesized in 1963. Developed to produce the "anesthetic state (analgesia, amnesia, loss of consciousness and immobility)" without total CNS depression, it was approved for general clinical use in 1970 (33,34).

The commercial preparation of ketamine is a racemic mixture of two optical isomers with differing activity (34). Ketamine is typically administered IV or IM (35,36). Rectal (37), oral (38,39), and intranasal (40) routes of administration have been described in the literature.

Ketamine is metabolized in the liver, primarily by *N*-methylation to nor-ketamine. Nor-ketamine has about one-third the sedative and analgesic potency of ketamine. As such, ketamine should be administered cautiously or in reduced doses to patients with impaired hepatic function.

IV ketamine, 1 to 2 mg/kg, produces unconsciousness within 30 to 60 seconds (36). Peak plasma concentrations occur within 1 minute. Return of consciousness occurs within 10 to 15 minutes, although complete recovery may be delayed (36). Dose requirements and recovery times from ketamine are age-related (41,42).

Ketamine has been found to have interactions at multiple binding sites, including *N*-methyl-D-aspartate (NMDA) and non-NMDA receptors, nicotinic and muscarinic cholinergic receptors and opioid receptors (43). Agonist actions of ketamine on opioid receptors play only a minor role in its analgesic effects (43). Naloxone, a narcotic antagonist discussed in the section on opioids, does not reverse the analgesic effect of ketamine (43). The psychotomimetic effects of ketamine, however, may involve interaction with a specific subclass of opioid receptors known as kappa receptors (43). For analgesia, the main site of action is the NMDA receptor. The reader is referred to other sources for further information on this topic (43).

CNS Effects of Ketamine

Ketamine produces a state known as dissociative anesthesia. Dissociative anesthesia refers to a cataleptic state characterized by functional and electrophysiologic dissociation between the thalamo-neocortical and limbic systems (34). Patients keep their eyes open and exhibit a slow nystagmic gaze. Corneal and pupillary reflexes remain intact. Generalized hypertonicity may be present. Even though ketamine has effects on nicotinic acetylcholine receptors in skeletal muscle, this effect is of minor significance, because ketamine increases muscle tone by central mechanisms (43). Patients receiving ketamine may exhibit purposeful movements but not necessarily in response to surgical stimulation (34).

Ketamine's analgesic effect is intense and may outlast its sedative effect (35). In one study of minor surgical procedures with ketamine anesthesia, no additional analgesics were required for 24 hours postoperatively (44). Amnesia persists for about 1 hour after apparent recovery from ketamine (36).

Emergence phenomena are relatively rare in children, although young adults are especially susceptible to this problem (44). Changes in mood and body image, out-of-body experiences, floating sensations, and frank delirium are all possible (34). Emergence phenomena result from misinterpretation of auditory and visual stimuli at the neurologic level (34). Although usually terminating within 24 hours (36), prolonged emergence phenomena lasting as long as 10 to 12 months have been reported in children (45). An increased incidence of emergence reactions is seen in patients older than 16 years, female patients, patients who have received doses of IV ketamine above 2 mg/kg, and patients with a history of abnormal personalities (34). There is no evidence that emergence in a quiet environment decreases the incidence of this problem (34). Benzodiazepines (e.g., diazepam and midazolam) are the most effective treatment for ketamine-induced delirium and hallucinations (34). In fact, the administration of a benzodiazepine 3 to 5 minutes before ketamine is effective in almost entirely eliminating the possibility of emergence delirium (32).

Transient diplopia (33), ataxia (46), and disequilibrium (46) may occur after ketamine use. Early attempts at ambulation should be discouraged (46). Ketamine does not induce seizures and is not necessarily contraindicated in patients with an underlying seizure disorder (34).

Ketamine is contraindicated in patients with increased intracranial pressure or with abnormal intracerebral compliance. Thus, patients who have sustained a head injury as part of their ongoing trauma should not receive this drug (47). Although some reports have actually suggested that there is a neuroprotective effect for ketamine (43), the recommendation that ketamine be avoided in head-injured patients still stands firm for now.

Respiratory Effects of Ketamine

Ketamine can have some potentially troublesome effects on the airway. It causes the production of increased salivary and tracheobronchial secretions, which can lead to coughing, laryngospasm, and airway obstruction. This problem may be especially treacherous in patients with an ongoing respiratory infection. Glycopyrrolate (Robinul), an anti-sialogogue, should be administered 3 to 5 minutes before ketamine (at the same time that the benzodiazepine is given) to ameliorate this problem (32). The dose for glycopyrrolate is 5 to 10 μg/kg, given IV. For large children, a dose of 0.2 mg (200 μg) of glycopyrrolate given IV is sufficient. Unless there is some other strong indication for its use, ketamine should be avoided in patients with ongoing infections of the respiratory tract.

Although ketamine does not usually produce significant depression of ventilation (36), apnea has been reported with its administration (48). Apnea is more likely to occur when the drug is given IV in rapid boluses (48) or in combination with other respiratory depressants (36). However, there are reports of apnea in otherwise healthy children sedated in the emergency department with IM ketamine alone in the usual recommended dosage (49,50).

In addition, ketamine does not protect against aspiration of gastric contents (51,52). In this regard, ketamine is no different from any other sedative and analgesic except maybe for self-administered 50% nitrous oxide in oxygen. Ketamine should never be given in an unmonitored setting, such as a patient's room on a regular hospital ward, or a clinic that does not have appropriate monitoring and resuscitation equipment (see the first part of this chapter).

Cardiovascular Effects of Ketamine

Ketamine stimulates the sympathetic nervous system and leads to the release of endogenous catecholamines. Through such an effect, ketamine produces a dose-dependent increase in heart rate and blood pressure (47); therefore, it is useful in the operating room in patients with mild hypovolemia. As a byproduct of its sympathetic stimulation, ketamine produces bronchodilation, and as such it has been useful in the anesthetic management of patients with asthma (32). However, because ketamine is a direct myocardial depressant, its administration to patients who are profoundly hypovolemic, and whose sympathetic nervous system is already maximally stimulated, will lead to cardiovascular collapse. Any sedation given to a hypovolemic patient must be administered very judiciously and preferably after the volume status is corrected.

Review of Relevant Literature

In 1990, Green et al reviewed a collective experience of nearly 12,000 children sedated with ketamine for various procedures (46,53). In 1998, Green et al (54) published their experience with 1,022 patients aged 15 years and younger sedated with IM ketamine 4 mg/kg for a variety of emergency room procedures, consisting mainly of laceration repairs and fracture reductions. From this group of patients, the authors reported two cases of apnea, four cases of laryngospasm, one case of respiratory depression, and seven cases of partial airway obstruction (e.g., airway malalignment) responding to repositioning of the head. They also reported a 6.7% incidence of vomiting but no cases of aspiration. In an interesting study by Kennedy et al (55), IV ketamine combined with midazolam (Versed) was compared with fentanyl combined with midazolam in the management of pediatric fractures. This particular study is further discussed later.

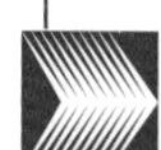

AUTHOR'S PREFERRED TREATMENT

Salient points regarding the safe use of ketamine are summarized in Table 3-7. Monitoring and procedural guidelines for deeply sedated patients (1) should be followed whenever ketamine is used. If given IM, the dose should be limited to 4 mg/kg. If given IV, the total dose should be limited to 2 mg/kg. Glycopyrrolate should be used, and the administration of midazolam (Versed) 0.05 to 0.1 mg/kg should be strongly considered for the prevention of agitation and delirium. There is an increased risk of respiratory depression whenever more than one sedative medication is administered. Also, no reversal drug exists for ketamine.

Benzodiazepines

Initial interest in the use of benzodiazepines developed when these drugs were noted to exert taming effects in animals (56).

TABLE 3-7 Ketamine in Pediatric Sedation

I. Methods of Administration and Dosage
 A. IM: 4 mg/kg
 B. IV: 1–2 mg/kg
 C. PO: 6–10 mg/kg
 D. Rectal: 5–10 mg/kg

II. Contraindications
 A. Altered state of consciousness
 B. Increased intracranial pressure
 C. Active upper respiratory infections (increased quantity of secretions and possible increased risk of laryngospasm)
 D. Full stomach
 E. Prior unfavorable experience with ketamine
 F. Patients >16 yr old (increased incidence of emergence phenomena)

III. Advantages
 A. Provides sedation, amnesia, intense analgesia
 B. Sympathetic-mediated activity may be beneficial for children with asthma.

IV. Disadvantages
 A. Increases production of saliva and tracheobronchial secretions; coadministration of glycopyrrolate 0.01 mg/kg recommended
 B. Potential for loss of the airway from:
  1. Laryngospasm secondary to increased secretions
  2. Aspiration from laryngeal incompetence
  3. Apnea
 C. Emergence phenomena: Rare in young children. No advantage to quiet environment. Midazolam may help, but may contribute to oversedation.

Benzodiazepines provide anxiolysis, hypnosis, centrally mediated (57) relaxation of muscle tone, antegrade and retrograde amnesia, and anticonvulsant activity (58). Benzodiazepines have no analgesic activity and require supplementation for painful procedures (56).

Pharmacology

Midazolam (Versed) is the primary benzodiazepine used for pediatric sedation. It offers several advantages over other benzodiazepines (59). It is water soluble and therefore usually relatively painless on injection (58,59). It does occasionally cause discomfort on injection, although the pain is not as severe as that with diazepam (Valium). At physiologic pH, midazolam becomes highly lipid soluble, facilitating transport into the CNS and onset of sedative effects (59). Initial recovery, which is due to redistribution of the drug away from the CNS, occurs in about 30 minutes. The elimination half-life of midazolam is significantly shorter than that of diazepam (59). On a milligram-per-milligram basis, midazolam is at least two to three times as potent as diazepam (60). Electroencephalographic (EEG) studies indicate that the blood–brain equilibration time is 4.8 minutes for midazolam versus 1.6 minutes for diazepam (61). Therefore, when titrating midazolam for sedation, it is important to wait 5 minutes between doses.

CNS Effects

Anxiolysis and centrally mediated relaxation of skeletal muscle tone are presumed to occur from a benzodiazepine-induced increase in the availability of glycine inhibitory neurotransmitter (56). Facilitating the action of the inhibitory neurotransmitter gamma-aminobutyric acid (GABA) is responsible for the sedative effects of benzodiazepines (56). It remains unclear what the site of action is for the production of amnesia (56).

Midazolam and diazepam produce direct depression of the central respiratory drive (62), and apnea may occur (58,63,64), especially after parenteral administration of these drugs. Although generally considered very safe, orally administered midazolam has been reported to produce airway obstruction in a child with congenital airway anomalies (65). In general, the incidence of respiratory complications increases with the presence of major vital organ disease (64). However, even in healthy adult volunteers, IV sedation with midazolam (0.1 mg/kg) can depress the ventilatory response to hypoxia (66). Concomitant administration of opioids (56,64,67) greatly increases the risk of respiratory complications. Therefore, extra vigilance and careful titration of medications to effect are even more important when using more than one sedative or analgesic medication.

Other Systemic Effects

With careful titration, significant hemodynamic changes are unusual with midazolam (58). Loss of protective airway reflexes is also unlikely under these circumstances (58) as long as the physician pays careful attention to the effects of each incremental dose on the patient's state of consciousness. Caution is always urged if the patient's stomach is full. Slurring of speech is a typical sign of sedation with benzodiazepines (58). Children may also exhibit loss of anxiety, unsolicited smiling, and even laughter.

In reporting their experience with 2,617 children sedated for endoscopic procedures, Massanari et al (68) noted that 36 patients exhibited paradoxical reactions to midazolam, including inconsolable crying, combativeness, and agitation. The authors were able to treat these reactions with flumazenil, a benzodiazepine antagonist, which is discussed below.

Review of Relevant Literature

In children, midazolam can be administered by oral, nasal, sublingual, IV, IM, and rectal routes (32). A liquid oral formulation, whose concentration is 2 mg midazolam/mL, now exists in the United States. It is marketed as Versed Syrup 2 mg/mL and is manufactured by Hoffman-LaRoche. If this formulation is not available at a particular location, then the practitioner can order the parenteral form (usually the 5-mg/mL concentration) to be mixed in 5 to 10 mL of a sweet-tasting syrup (69). Acetaminophen syrup and ibuprofen syrup are useful vehicles for mixing parenteral midazolam, keeping in mind the appropriate pediatric doses of acetaminophen and ibuprofen. The author's preference is to mix the midazolam in 3 to 5 mL of Tylenol syrup. For nasal administration, which the author does not recommend, the parenteral preparation is used with no additives. The reason for discouraging the use of nasal midazolam is because most children find its administration to be very unpleasant: in one study, 84% of children given intranasal midazolam cried in response to administration of the medication (70). Although sublingual administration is a good idea from a pharmacologic point of view (see discussion under morphine), it requires a degree of patient cooperation that may be difficult to obtain in children: an uncooperative child may be unwilling or unable to hold a medication under his or her tongue.

Hennes et al (71) used oral midazolam to allay the anxiety of children requiring laceration repair in the emergency department. Fatovich and Jacobs (72) also noted decreased anxiety in children requiring laceration repair after oral midazolam versus a control group that received only a placebo. For orally administered midazolam, the appropriate dose is 0.5 to 0.75 mg/kg (73) and a waiting period of 10 to 30 minutes is required for onset of effects. The maximum amount of midazolam that should be administered orally has not been determined, but in practice this amount is usually limited to 20 to 25 mg. Analgesic supplementation in the form of local anesthetics, opioids, or both is required for painful procedures. Patients who receive parenteral benzodiazepines must be monitored with pulse oximetry, because oxygen desaturation may occur (74).

Drug Reversal

Flumazenil (Romazicon) reverses the sedative effects of benzodiazepines (75–77). The flumazenil dose for children is 10 μg/kg IV. Flumazenil administration may then be continued at 5 μg/kg/minute until the child awakens, or until a total dose of 1 mg has been given (78). The elimination half-life of flumazenil is 30 minutes, compared with 1 to 2 hours for midazolam. Patients who receive flumazenil should be observed for at least 2 hours before discharge to ensure that resedation from the original benzodiazepine does not occur. In the author's opinion, the use of flumazenil should be limited to situations of relative or absolute benzodiazepine overdose leading to respiratory or hemodynamic compromise. Routinely reversing benzodiazepines is both unnecessary and, in the absence of persistent monitoring, potentially dangerous.

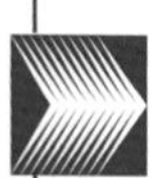

AUTHOR'S PREFERRED TREATMENT

Salient points regarding the use of midazolam and other benzodiazepines are summarized in Table 3-8. Although supplemental analgesia is required for painful procedures, such as the reduction of fractures, the anxiolysis and amnesia that midazolam produces make it an excellent medication for children with orthopaedic injuries. Careful IV titration of midazolam in increments of 0.05 mg/kg may be undertaken, combined with a regional anesthetic block (e.g., Bier block, hematoma block) for pain relief. The author believes that oral midazolam, with its mandatory 10- to 30-minute waiting period, and with its lack of titratability to effect, is probably best reserved for use as a preoperative medication before elective surgical procedures. Also, for emergency patients, IV titration is the best and most efficient way to achieve desirable levels of patient sedation and cooperation. The combination of midazolam and opioids is discussed in the next section.

TABLE 3-8 Benzodiazepines in Pediatric Sedation

I. Method of Administration
   A. Diazepam: 0.1 to 0.3 mg/kg IV or PO. IM administration should be avoided because it is painful.
   B. Midazolam
      1. PO: 0.5–0.75 mg/kg
      2. Nasal: 0.3–0.4 mg/kg*
      3. IM: 0.03–0.1 mg/kg
      4. IV: 0.05–0.1 mg/kg

II. Contraindications
   A. Previous unfavorable experience with benzodiazepines
   B. (?) Early pregnancy (possible teratogenicity)
   C. Altered state of consciousness

III. Advantages
   A. Generally provide excellent sedation and amnesia
   B. Reversible if necessary (flumazenil, 10 μg/kg, up to a total dose of 1.0 mg)

IV. Disadvantages
   A. No analgesic effect
   B. Respiratory depression, especially with parenteral administration
   C. Combination with narcotics may lead to oversedation or respiratory arrest.

* Many children find the intranasal administration of midazolam to be very unpleasant. This method of administering midazolam is not recommended.

Opioids

Opioids include all exogenous substances, natural or synthetic, that bind to specific receptors and produce morphine-like effects (79). There are several types and subtypes of opioid receptors (79,80). Opioids vary in their respective affinity for receptor types, accounting for the difference in side effects. Opioids are classified as pure receptor agonists (e.g., morphine, meperidine, fentanyl), agonist-antagonists (e.g., nalbuphine), or pure antagonists (e.g., naloxone) (79).

Opioid Agonists

All opioid agonists produce dose-dependent respiratory depression and apnea (79). Nausea and vomiting occur because of direct stimulation of the chemoreceptor trigger zone in the floor of the fourth ventricle of the medulla oblongata (79).

Morphine. Morphine is a well-known analgesic. It is usually administered IV or IM, although sublingual and rectal routes have been described (12). Oral morphine is usually used for long-term pain control in patients with severe, chronic pain. Rectal administration of morphine is not recommended because it has been associated with delayed absorption, delayed respiratory depression, and death (12,81). In general, rectally administered medications are absorbed unpredictably (82), and access of the medication to the rectal mucosa may be variably impeded by rectal stool content.

The usual starting dose for IV or IM morphine is 0.05 to 0.1 mg/kg. In infants younger than 3 months old, the dose should be reduced by at least one half because of increased susceptibility to respiratory depression (83). Morphine should be reserved for painful procedures lasting at least 30 minutes (6). Morphine is not very lipid soluble, and its delay in leaving the CNS accounts for a potential duration of action of 3 to 4 hours (6,80). Hypotension secondary to vasodilation, histamine release, or vagally mediated bradycardia can occur even with the administration of small doses of morphine (80). Histamine release along the course of the vein into which the morphine is administered is not by itself an allergic reaction; the overall incidence of true allergic reactions to opioids is very small (79).

Meperidine. The use of meperidine (Demerol) parallels that of morphine. The initial IV or IM dose is 0.5 to 1.0 mg/kg. Again, the dose should be reduced by at least one half in infants younger than 3 months of age (83). Normeperidine, a metabolic breakdown product of meperidine, has been associated with seizures, agitation, tremors, and myoclonus (84,85). Meperidine is not recommended for patients with an underlying seizure disorder. Accumulation of normeperidine is more likely in situations of prolonged meperidine administration. Therefore, meperidine should be used cautiously, if at all, in the treatment of chronic pain (6). As with morphine, meperidine may produce hypotension due to various mechanisms (80). Histamine release has also been reported with meperidine (80).

Fentanyl. Fentanyl is a synthetic narcotic 100 times more potent than morphine and 1,000 times more potent than meperidine on a milligram-per-milligram basis. Fentanyl is highly lipid soluble and rapidly penetrates the CNS (80). When administered in low doses, its duration of action is from 30 to 45 minutes. For sedation, fentanyl is given IV in increments of 0.5 to 1 μg/kg. The maximum total dose is 4 to 5 μg/kg (6). As a preoperative medication, fentanyl is available in an oral raspberry-flavored lollipop known as the Fentanyl Oralet (32). Currently available sizes for the Oralet are 200 μg, 300 μg, and 400 μg. As a preoperative medication, the recommended dose ranges from 10 to 20 μg/kg. Troublesome side effects of this preparation include nausea and vomiting, pruritus, and oxygen desaturation (86).

Reonset of respiratory depression up to 4 hours after fentanyl administration has been reported (87). Glottic closure (88) and muscular rigidity (89–91) can occur, especially, although not exclusively, at higher doses. Respiratory arrest may occur, especially with the co-administration of other sedatives (67). For these reasons, fentanyl should be titrated slowly to effect.

Opioid Agonist-Antagonists

A so-called ceiling effect or limit on the degree of respiratory depression has been demonstrated for various opioid agonist-antagonists, including nalbuphine (92) and butorphanol (93). Nalbuphine and morphine have the same analgesic potency on a milligram-per-milligram basis (83). Nalbuphine has a shorter elimination half-life (94). Opioid agonist-antagonists have no particular advantage over properly dosed opioids (95). The major problem with opioid agonist-antagonists is that their ceiling effect on respiratory depression is often accompanied by a ceiling effect for analgesia (79). Also, agonist-antagonists reduce the analgesic effectiveness of pure agonists (e.g., morphine, meperidine, fentanyl, codeine) if additional analgesia is required (95). In patients receiving opioids on a long-term basis, administration of opioid agonist-antagonists can precipitate acute withdrawal symptoms (95).

Drug Reversal With Opioid Antagonists

Naloxone (Narcan), which has no agonist activity of its own, displaces opioids from opioid receptors (79). Rapid reversal of narcotic effects may precipitate severe hypertension, pulmonary edema, ventricular or supraventricular irritability, seizures, and cardiac arrest (96,97). Dysphoria, nausea, and vomiting may also occur. Acute narcotic withdrawal in this situation reflects sympathetic nervous system stimulation from abrupt reversal of analgesia and sudden perception of pain (80). Therefore, naloxone should be titrated to effect (relief of respiratory depression) in increments of 1 to 5 μg/kg IV. Naloxone has a duration of action of 30 to 45 minutes, and resedation is possible. Close patient observation is required, and supplemental naloxone doses may be necessary. Current dosage recommendations in cases of frank opioid intoxication are significantly higher (98). Caution is always advised against precipitating acute narcotic withdrawal. The first priority in the treatment of narcotic overdose is a patent, well-maintained airway.

Similar to the situation with flumazenil for reversal of benzodiazepines, the author believes that the routine use of naloxone to reverse narcotic sedative medications is unwarranted and, for reasons noted earlier, potentially dangerous. Naloxone use should be reserved for situations of airway compromise brought on by relative opioid overdose, and it should never be used as a way of expediting patient discharge after a procedure requiring sedation.

Review of Relevant Literature

With careful monitoring and judicious administration, combinations of opioids for analgesia and benzodiazepines for amnesia and anxiolysis are probably the most useful sedatives in existence today for the management of children's fractures. Varela et al (99) reported excellent patient and physician satisfaction using IV meperidine and midazolam for IV sedation for the closed reduction of fractures in children. In this investigation, the average meperidine dose was 1.47 mg/kg and the average midazolam dose was 0.11 mg/kg. There were no episodes of apnea or cardiorespiratory complications. These investigators stressed that careful patient monitoring is important, not only during but after the procedure as well. IV morphine 0.1 mg/kg plus midazolam 0.1 mg/kg is another useful sedation mixture for children with fractures, especially when combined with a hematoma block (personal communication, J. Edeen, MD). The hematoma block is discussed later in the chapter. With this particular approach, the midazolam is administered first, followed by the morphine about 5 minutes later. The hematoma block is performed, and the fracture is then reduced. Again, careful patient monitoring as previously outlined is essential to good care.

In the absence of specific contraindications, including tenuous airway status, unstable hemodynamic status, or history of specific allergic reactions, for the performance of painful procedures in children, a combination of a benzodiazepine and a narcotic is probably ideal (67,100,101), as long as the principles of careful titration and close patient monitoring are observed.

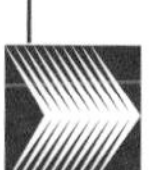

AUTHOR'S PREFERRED TREATMENT

Salient points regarding the use of opioids as well as opioid and benzodiazepine combinations for pediatric sedation are summarized in Tables 3-9 and 3-10. Opioid and benzodiazepine combinations provide amnesia, analgesia, and sedation; the tradeoff is additive respiratory depression and additive depression of protective airway reflexes. In both elective and emergent situations, the practitioner must:

1. Thoroughly evaluate the patient, as discussed earlier in the chapter.
2. Follow standard practice guidelines for deep sedation (1).
3. Pay careful attention to dosing limits (see Table 3-10).
4. Be certain that both flumazenil and naloxone are available. These medications are to be used strictly for the treatment of absolute or relative overdose of benzodiazepines and opioids, respectively. Do not use these medications to expedite discharge from the emergency room.

TABLE 3-9 Opioids in Pediatric Sedation

I. Method of Administration
- A. Morphine: 0.05–0.1 mg/kg IM or IV
- B. Meperidine: 0.5–1.0 mg/kg IM or IV
- C. Fentanyl: In increments of 0.001 mg/kg IV (maximum *total* dose, 0.004–0.005 mg/kg)
- D. Nalbuphine: 0.1 mg/kg IM or IV

Patients younger than 3 mo old should be given no more than half of these doses initially. IV titration to desired effect is the ideal way to administer *all* sedative medications.

II. Contraindications
- A. Altered state of consciousness
- B. Previous unfavorable experience (excludes that medication only)
- C. Sedation for nonpainful procedure

III. Advantages
- A. Provide excellent analgesia
- B. Reversible if necessary (naloxone 0.001–0.005 mg/kg IV *titrated to effect*)

IV. Disadvantages
- A. Risk of respiratory depression and apnea
- B. Increased risk of respiratory depression and apnea when combined with other sedatives
- C. No amnestic effects

V. Additional Side Effects (more likely when used in recurrent doses for treatment of pain)

Nausea, vomiting, pruritus, constipation, decreased gastric motility

TABLE 3-10 Fentanyl and Midazolam in Pediatric Sedation*

I. Method of Administration

IV titration to effect
- A. Midazolam: In increments of 0.05 mg/kg to a maximum of 0.1 mg/kg. Wait 5 min between doses.
- B. Fentanyl: Begin 5 min after last midazolam dose. Give in increments of 0.001 mg/kg to a maximum of 0.003 mg/kg. Wait 2 to 3 min between doses.

II. Contraindications
- A. Altered state of consciousness
- B. Previous unfavorable experience with either medication
- C. Specific contraindications to benzodiazepines or opioids (see Tables 3-8 and 3-9)

III. Advantages
- A. Provides sedation, amnesia (midazolam), and analgesia (fentanyl)
- B. Reversible if necessary (see Tables 3-8 and 3-9)

IV. Disadvantages
- A. Additive respiratory depressant effects
- B. Additive depressant effects on protective airway reflexes with increased risk for regurgitation and aspiration of gastric contents

* An excellent review of the advantages and problems associated with this drug regimen is provided in Yaster M, Nichols DG, Deshpande JK, Wetzel RC. Midazolam–fentanyl intravenous sedation in children: case report of respiratory arrest. *Pediatrics* 1990;86:463–467.

Midazolam and Ketamine Compared With Midazolam and Fentanyl

In a study of 260 children between the ages of 5 and 15 presenting for the emergency room reduction of fractures, Kennedy et al (55) compared the effectiveness of two regimens for sedation and analgesia. For the first reduction attempt in each patient, all of the children initially received midazolam 0.1 mg/kg (maximum dose of 2.5 mg) at 3-minute intervals until either objective signs of onset of drug effect developed (slurred speech, glassy eyes) or three doses of midazolam were given. One minute after the administration of the last dose of midazolam, half the patients began receiving fentanyl, titrated in increments of 0.5 μg/kg until either a decreased response to verbal or painful stimulation was noted, or a maximum dose of 2 μg/kg had been administered. The maximum amount of fentanyl used was 100 μg. The other half of the patients, instead of receiving fentanyl, were given ketamine, titrated in increments of 0.5 μg/kg, using the same criteria as for fentanyl to determine onset of effect. Ketamine titration continued, if necessary, until a maximum amount of 2 μg/kg had been given. All of the patients who were given ketamine also received glycopyrrolate, 5 μg/kg, as an antisialogogue. Additional amounts of midazolam and the study drug were given if analgesia and sedation were judged to be insufficient or if additional reduction attempts were necessary. Treatment failures occurred in patients who experienced significant adverse drug effects or who obtained insufficient sedation and analgesia.

Patient distress was quantified using various behavioral scales; see the article itself for more detailed information about the measurement process. Whereas presedation scores were basically the same for both groups, during fracture reduction, the investigators found a significantly lower score of patient distress for the children receiving midazolam and ketamine than for those receiving midazolam and fentanyl. In general, the ketamine and midazolam combination was favored by parents and by the involved orthopaedic surgeons. On the other hand, however, two patients receiving midazolam and ketamine required brief assisted ventilation with a bag, valve, and mask apparatus, and one patient developed laryngospasm. Vomiting occurred more often in the group taking ketamine, and the patients taking the ketamine had a longer mean time to recovery and discharge.

This detailed study looked very closely at two viable regimens for sedation of children with fractures. Again, with careful monitoring and careful attention to drug titration, practitioners may wish to try both to determine which is more useful in their individual practice. The authors favored the ketamine and midazolam regimen and provided good evidence for their conclusions (55).

Pediatric Cocktail

The so-called pediatric cocktail (DPT) or "lytic" cocktail is a mixture of meperidine (Demerol) and two phenothiazines: promethazine (Phenergan) and chlorpromazine (Thorazine). For multiple reasons, this sedative regimen should be avoided. Prolonged and profound sedation occurs, often far outlasting the procedure for which the sedation was intended. One study reported a mean total recovery time of 19 hours, plus or minus 15 hours, in children receiving DPT in the emergency department (102). Orthostatic hypotension is possible because promethazine and chlorpromazine are alpha-adrenergic blockers (6). Severe respiratory depression and death, both during and after the procedure, have occurred in patients sedated with DPT. All three medications in this mixture lower the seizure threshold, and phenothiazines can produce dystonic reactions (6). There is no reversal agent for phenothiazine overdose.

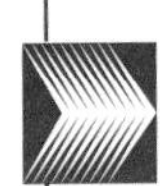

AUTHOR'S PREFERRED TREATMENT

The author strongly believes that the use of the pediatric cocktail should be abandoned (101).

Chloral Hydrate

Of greatest use in sedating children for nonpainful diagnostic procedures such as radiographic studies, chloral hydrate is administered in a dose of 20 to 75 mg/kg orally or rectally. The maximum single dose is 1 g. If more than one dose has to be given, the upper limit for the total dose is either 100 mg/kg or 2 g, whichever is lower.

Although theoretically rectal dosing should be more efficient because of the lack of a first-pass hepatic effect (82), 30 to 60 minutes may elapse before chloral hydrate takes effect no matter how it is administered. Children receiving chloral hydrate must be observed for at least several hours. Respiratory depression is unusual, but children with sleep apnea and adenotonsillar hypertrophy may be particularly vulnerable to airway obstruction after sedation with chloral hydrate (103). At least one death has been reported following its use (104). These problems emphasize that even sedatives thought to have little risk of producing respiratory depression must be administered under properly supervised conditions (1) and with strict adherence to dosage guidelines.

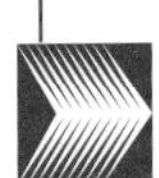

AUTHOR'S PREFERRED TREATMENT

Chloral hydrate is of minimal use in the sedation and treatment of patients with fractures. It provides no analgesia, and it lacks the rapidity of onset and titratability of IV opioids and benzodiazepines. The practitioner should be familiar with this medication, however, because it remains in common use for nonpainful pediatric procedures. Salient features regarding its administration are summarized in Table 3-11.

TABLE 3-11 Chloral Hydrate in Pediatric Sedation

I. Method of Administration
   20 to 75 mg/kg orally or rectally (maximum single dose, 1.0 g; if a second dose is given, the maximum total dose is either 100 mg/kg or 2.0 g, whichever is lower)

II. Contraindications
   A. Compromised hepatic function
   B. History of obstructive sleep apnea*
   C. Previous unfavorable experience with chloral hydrate

III. Advantages
   No specific advantages for sedation and treatment of children with fractures

IV. Disadvantages
   A. Prolonged time to peak effect (as long as 60 min)
   B. Difficult to titrate
   C. Prolonged observation period required

* Caution is required when using any sedative medication in patients with obstructive sleep apnea.

Barbiturates

In general, barbiturates have a lower margin of safety than benzodiazepines (105). In addition, barbiturates seem to lower the pain threshold and are therefore a poor choice for producing sedation in the presence of a painful condition such as a fracture (105). With these points in mind, barbiturates should not be used for sedating children with fractures.

Propofol

Propofol is a substituted isopropylphenol that is a rapid-acting IV anesthetic (36). Because it is virtually insoluble in aqueous solutions, it has to be dissolved in lecithin-containing formulations. The orthopaedist may have seen this whitish medication administered by the anesthesiologist in the operating room, where it has gained the popular name of "milk of amnesia."

Propofol has a fast onset of action, owing to its high lipid solubility, and an extremely short duration of action. Awakening is rapid, with little to no "hangover" effect as seen with other drugs (36). It also has antiemetic effects (32).

However, there are several reasons why this drug should not be used in the management of children with fractures in an emergency room setting. First and foremost, it is easy to lose the airway suddenly in a patient given propofol; therefore, this drug should be administered by an anesthesiologist (106). Second, the drug provides no analgesic effect and therefore has to be combined with an opioid; this in turn will intensify the respiratory depressant effects of propofol. Third, in children the administration of propofol is associated with opisthotonic posturing and myoclonus (32), which is certainly not helpful in the reduction of a fracture. Propofol has vasodilatory and negative inotropic effects, which can lead to hypotension (32). Finally, there is some concern that propofol may be associated with seizures (32), although Momota et al (107) used propofol to stop seizure activity from local anesthetic overdose.

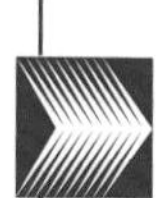

AUTHOR'S PREFERRED TREATMENT

In children with fractures, propofol should be reserved for administration in the operating room as part of a regimen of general anesthesia by an anesthesiologist.

REGIONAL ANESTHESIA IN THE CHILD WITH A MUSCULOSKELETAL INJURY

Within the limitations and guidelines discussed later, the use of regional anesthesia to relieve pain in children with musculoskeletal injuries is reasonable and worthwhile.

Regional Anesthetic Agents

Regional or local anesthetic medications prevent nerve impulse propagation by interfering with the function of the sodium channel on the axonal membrane (108). Commonly used local anesthetics have either an amino amide or amino ester linkage in their molecular structure (109). Amino amide local anesthetics include lidocaine (Xylocaine), bupivacaine (Marcaine, Sensorcaine), mepivacaine, prilocaine, etidocaine, and the relatively new agent ropivacaine. Amino ester local anesthetics include procaine (Novocain), chloroprocaine, tetracaine, benzocaine, and cocaine.

Medications within each group have important intrinsic differences in potency, duration of action, and potential for toxicity (27,109). For example, lidocaine is significantly less toxic a drug than bupivacaine, but it also has a shorter duration of action. An important feature of ropivacaine is that even though its duration of action is similar to bupivacaine, it produces less CNS toxicity and less cardiac toxicity (110). Duration of action for the various local anesthetic medications is also determined in part by the type of regional block performed. For example, single-dose brachial plexus blocks tend to have a far longer duration than do single-dose epidural or subarachnoid blocks (27).

Local Anesthetic Toxicity

At least three types of adverse reactions can occur from local anesthetic agents. Clinically, the most important is systemic toxicity of the CNS and cardiovascular system from relative overdose into the circulation. This type of reaction is not a medication allergy but simply a function of placing too much medication into the bloodstream. In the presence of a major artery, even a few drops of local anesthetic can lead to seizure activity. An example of this problem is seen in the performance of stellate ganglion blocks in the neck for the management of reflex sympathetic dystrophy of the upper extremity, where the vertebral artery can be accidentally entered during administration of the medication.

In most cases, however, the severity of systemic toxicity is directly related to the concentration of local anesthetic in the bloodstream (Table 3-12) (27). Seizures and cardiac arrest may be the initial manifestations of systemic toxicity in patients who rapidly attain a high serum level of medication (111–113). Agents with greater intrinsic potency, such as bupivacaine and etidocaine, require lower levels for production of symptoms (27). Dysrhythmias and cardiovascular toxicity may be especially severe with bupivacaine, and resuscitation of these patients may be prolonged and difficult (27,114).

The prevention and treatment of acute local anesthetic systemic toxicity are outlined in Table 3-13.

Although the potential for CNS toxicity may be diminished with barbiturates or benzodiazepines, given either as premedications or during treatment of convulsions, these measures do not alter the cardiotoxic threshold of local anesthetic agents. With rapid and appropriate treatment, the fatality rate from local anesthetic convulsions should be greatly decreased (27).

It is essential to stay within accepted dose limits when using any local anesthetic (Table 3-14). To aid in dose calculations,

TABLE 3-12 Manifestations of Local Anesthetic Toxicity*

1. Numbness of the lips and tongue, metallic taste in the mouth
2. Lightheadedness
3. Visual and auditory disturbances (double vision and tinnitus)
4. Shivering, muscle twitching, tremors (initial tremors may involve the muscles of the face and distal parts of the extremities)
5. Unconsciousness
6. Convulsions
7. Coma
8. Respiratory arrest
9. Cardiovascular depression and collapse

* With gradual increases in plasma concentration, these signs and symptoms may occur in order as listed. With the sudden development of high plasma concentrations of a local anesthetic agent, the first manifestation of toxicity may be a convulsion, respiratory arrest, or cardiovascular collapse. In young children, or in children who are heavily sedated, subjective evidence of impending local anesthetic toxicity (manifestations 1, 2, 3) may be difficult to elicit.

TABLE 3-13 Prevention and Treatment of Acute Local Anesthetic Systemic Toxicity

Preventive Measures

1. Ensure availability of oxygen administration equipment, airway equipment, suction equipment, and medications for treatment of seizures (diazepam or midazolam, thiopental, succinylcholine).
2. Ensure constant verbal contact with patient (for symptoms of toxicity) and monitor cardiovascular signs and oxygen saturation.
3. Personally prepare the dose of local anesthetic and ensure it is within the accepted dosage range.
4. Give the anesthetic slowly, and fractionate the dose.

Treatment

1. Establish a clear airway; suction if required.
2. Give oxygen by face mask. Begin artificial ventilation if necessary.
3. Give diazepam 0.1–0.3 mg/kg IV in incremental doses until convulsions cease. Midazolam (0.05–0.1 mg/kg) may be used instead, also in increments until convulsions cease.
4. Thiopental in increments of 1–2 mg/kg IV may be used to control the seizures.
5. Succinylcholine (1 mg/kg IV) may be used if there is inadequate control of ventilation with the other medications. Artificial ventilation and possibly endotracheal intubation are required after using succinylcholine.
6. Use advanced cardiac life-support measures as necessary to support the cardiovascular system (more likely with local anesthetics of increased potency, such as bupivacaine).

a simple formula for converting percent concentration to milligrams per milliliter is provided in Table 3-15.

Although rare, true immune-mediated allergic reactions to local anesthetics are possible, more commonly with amino esters than with amino amides (115,116). See other sources for the detailed management of allergic or anaphylactic reactions (117,118).

Local nerve damage and reversible skeletal muscle changes have been reported from the use of local anesthetics (27).

Intravenous Regional Anesthesia

IV regional anesthesia was first described by August Bier in 1908 (119). Although it declined in popularity as brachial plexus blocks were developed, it was revived in 1963, when its safe and successful use for the reduction of forearm fractures in adults was reported (120). Since then, multiple reports have attested to its usefulness in the treatment of upper limb injuries in adults and children (121–127).

The mechanism of action is uncertain. It may involve both direct transport of local anesthetic to major nerve trunks and the blockade of small nerve endings (125).

IV regional anesthesia is reliable, with a higher success rate than other approaches to upper extremity blocks (125). Other advantages include its simplicity, rapidity of onset, and rapidity of recovery. Rapidity of recovery may be considered both an advantage as well as a disadvantage, because, with local anesthetic alone, the analgesic effect is lost once the tourniquet is deflated. A recent report in adults examined the addition of the nonsteroidal anti-inflammatory medication ketorolac (Toradol) to the local anesthetic solution for IV regional anesthesia and found that patients did obtain prolonged analgesia after the tourniquet was released (128). However, no pediatric studies have been performed on this drug combination.

IV regional anesthesia is unsuitable for lesions above the elbow (129). In addition, if the fracture involves the supracondylar area of the humerus, the cuff may limit the degree of hyperflexion needed to produce an adequate reduction. IV regional anesthesia is contraindicated in patients with underlying heart block, known hypersensitivity to local anesthetic agents, and seizure disorders (129). Although not totally contraindi-

TABLE 3-14 Maximum Recommended Doses of Commonly Used Local Anesthetics in Children

	Injection Dose (mg/kg)	
Agent	Plain	With Epinephrine*
Lidocaine† (Xylocaine)	5	7
Bupivacaine‡ (Marcaine, Sensorcaine)	2.5	3
Mepivacaine (Carbocaine)	4	7
Prilocaine§	5.5	8.5

* The addition of epinephrine (vasoconstrictor) reduces the rate of local anesthetic absorption into the bloodstream, permitting use of a higher dose.

† For IV regional anesthesia (Bier blocks), the maximum lidocaine dose is 3 mg/kg. Preservative-free lidocaine without epinephrine should be used for either Bier blocks or hematoma blocks.

‡ Owing to its cardiotoxicity, bupivacaine should never be used for IV regional anesthesia or for hematoma blocks.

§ Of the amide local anesthetics, prilocaine is the least likely to produce CNS and cardiovascular toxicity. However, a byproduct of prilocaine metabolism may lead to severe methemoglobinemia in young children. Prilocaine is, therefore, contraindicated in children younger than 6 months old.

cated, caution is urged when using this technique in patients with underlying hemoglobinopathies such as sickle cell disease.

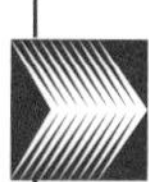

AUTHOR'S PREFERRED TREATMENT

The basic steps involved in performing an IV regional block are as follows:

1. Confirm the immediate availability of a functioning positive-pressure oxygen delivery system, as well as appropriate airway management equipment (see Table 3-5) (1). Also, confirm the immediate availability of medications for the treatment of anesthetic-induced convulsions (see Table 3-12).

TABLE 3-15 Conversion Formula from % Concentration to Milligrams/Milliliter

Percentage concentration × 10 = Number of mg/mL

Examples: 0.25% bupivacaine has 2.5 mg bupivacaine/mL; 2% lidocaine has 20 mg lidocaine/mL

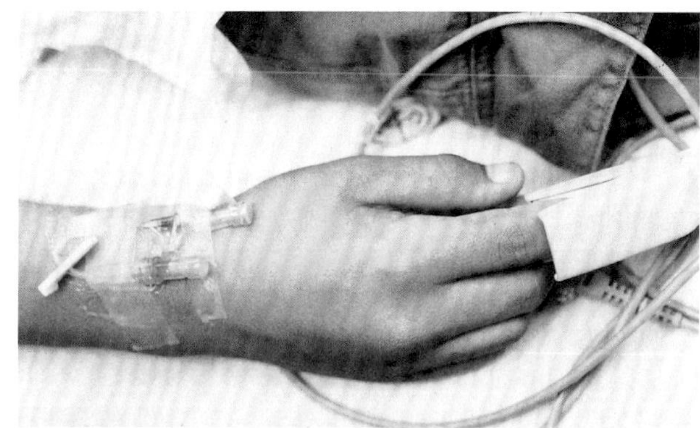

FIGURE 3-3 IV infusion for fluids, sedative medications, and if necessary resuscitative medications has been started in the contralateral hand. A pulse oximeter probe is present on the patient's index finger.

2. Start an IV infusion in the contralateral arm (Fig. 3-3). A patent IV line is of paramount importance in treating the complications of this block. Obtain a baseline set of vital signs, including systolic and diastolic blood pressure. Monitor pulse oximetry as well as the ECG continuously (Fig. 3-4).
3. Select an appropriate tourniquet. An orthopaedic tourniquet that can be fastened securely should be used. Because Velcro may become less adhesive with time, check the tenacity of the tourniquet before use. As an added safety measure, the tourniquet may be covered with strong adhesive tape or an Ace bandage after application. The tourniquet should fully encircle the arm and

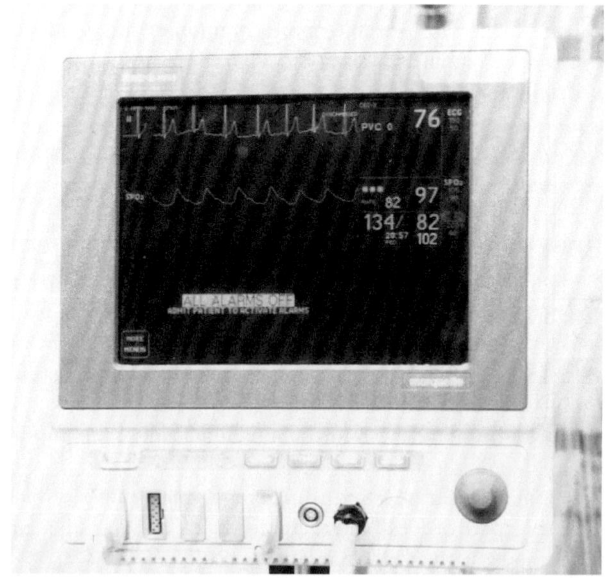

FIGURE 3-4 Continuous display of the electrocardiogram (top waveform) and continuous display of the plethysmographic tracing from the pulse oximeter (second line). Intermittent blood pressure reading is displayed.

overlap back on itself by at least 6 cm (personal communication, K. E. Wilkins, MD). The arm may be minimally padded with cast padding underneath the tourniquet (122). If a pneumatic tourniquet is used, the physician must be familiar with the location of the tourniquet pressure gauge (Fig. 3-5) (123) and valves, because these features vary in location from model to model. Narrow-cuffed double tourniquets may not effectively occlude arterial flow, and their use has been discouraged (129). Tourniquet discomfort should not be a problem during short procedures, but if this develops, a second tourniquet can be applied distally over the anesthetized area of the arm.

4. Palpate the radial pulse of the injured limb.
5. Place and secure a short 22-gauge cannula in a vein on the dorsum of the hand of the fractured limb. A 23-gauge butterfly needle may also be used (Fig. 3-6). Although it may be possible to "thread" a butterfly needle securely into a large vein, butterfly needles may still slip out of the vein more easily than a plastic IV catheter. The author recommends the use of IV catheters whenever possible. If a distal vein is unavailable, a proximal vein or even an antecubital vein can be used, but the use of proximal veins in the arm may result in a less effective block (129).
6. With the tourniquet deflated, exsanguinate the limb by vertically elevating it above the level of the heart for 60 seconds.
7. Rapidly inflate the tourniquet to a pressure of 225 to 250 mm Hg or 150 mm Hg above the patient's systolic blood pressure (130). Check for disappearance of the radial pulse. Cross-clamping the tubing of the cuff after inflation is discouraged (129) because it might prevent detection of a small leak. Constant observation of the cuff pressure gauge is recommended.
8. Lower the extremity and slowly inject the local anesthetic. This injection should be done over a period of 60 seconds. A concentration of 0.5% plain lidocaine (5 mg/mL) is used (Fig. 3-7). Bupivacaine is contraindicated for this block because of its cardiotoxicity. To prevent thrombophlebitis, the local anesthetic solution must be

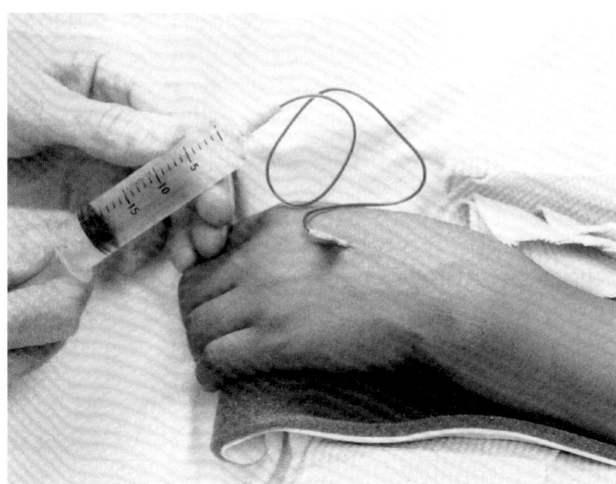

FIGURE 3-6 Venipuncture for administration of local anesthetic has been performed with a butterfly needle. An IV catheter may be more secure than a needle, which can become dislodged from within the vein.

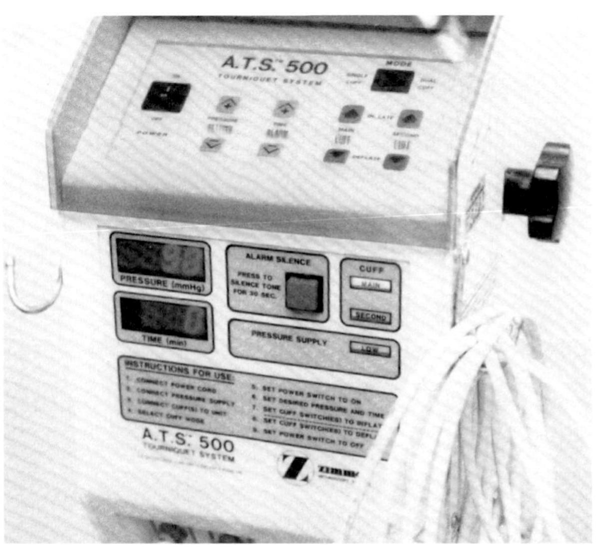

FIGURE 3-5 Tourniquet controls may vary in position from model to model. Be aware of the function of each of the controls to avoid accidental premature deflation of the tourniquet.

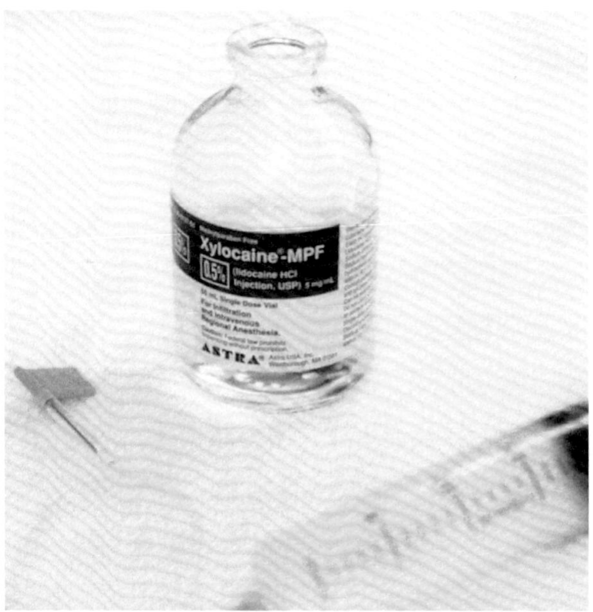

FIGURE 3-7 Preservative-free 0.5% lidocaine without epinephrine for IV regional anesthesia.

free of any additives or preservatives (129). In different studies, the recommended dose of lidocaine has varied from 1.5 to 3.0 mg/kg (121–127). A dose of 1.5 mg/kg appears to be safe and effective and may produce a decreased incidence of complications (122). One study has recommended a maximum lidocaine dose of 100 mg for this block (124). The skin of the extremity becomes mottled as the drug is injected. The patient, unless he or she is very sedated, and the parents, if they are watching, should be warned that the extremity will look and feel strange (personal communication, K. E. Wilkins, MD). Analgesia and muscle relaxation develop within 5 minutes of injection (129). For fractures at the wrist, placement of a regular Penrose drain tourniquet around the distal forearm may improve distribution of the local anesthetic solution at the fracture site (Fig. 3-8) (personal communication, K. E. Wilkins, MD).

9. To improve analgesia for fracture reduction, the last 2 mL of local anesthetic solution may be injected directly into the fracture hematoma (Fig. 3-9) (personal communication, K. E. Wilkins, MD). The technique of local infiltration anesthesia, or hematoma block, is discussed later in this chapter.
10. Perform the surgical procedure (Fig. 3-10).
11. Leave the cuff inflated for at least 15 minutes (129), even if the surgical procedure takes less time.
12. Release the cuff at the end of the operation, or at the end of a 15-minute interval, whichever is longer. Cuff deflation, followed by immediate reinflation, as a method of delaying systemic absorption of local anesthetic is impractical because it cannot be done rapidly enough to prevent significant entry of local anesthetic into the general circulation (129).
13. Monitor the patient closely for at least 15 minutes for any complications related to the block. The treatment of local anesthetic-induced systemic toxicity has been discussed (see Table 3-12).
14. Of course, depending on whatever sedation has been administered, the patient should be monitored until discharge criteria are met (see Table 3-1).

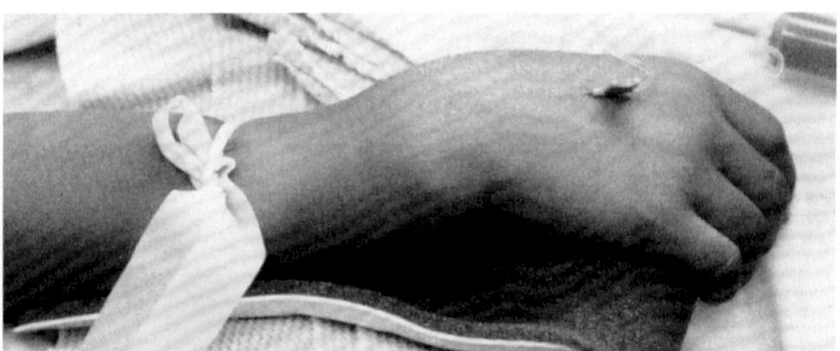

FIGURE 3-8 Penrose drain tourniquet on the forearm to improve distribution of local anesthetic at the fracture site.

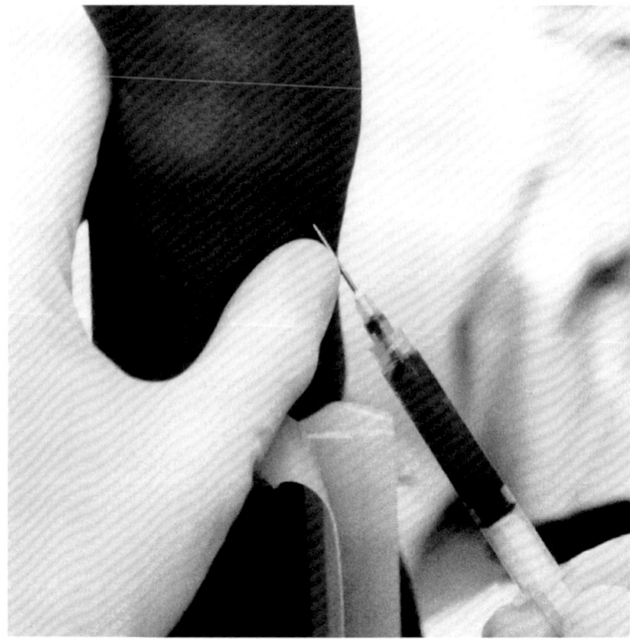

FIGURE 3-9 Hematoma block performed with the last 2 mL of the IV lidocaine solution to enhance analgesia at the fracture site.

An assistant must be present to watch the patient, the tourniquet, and the monitors at all times.

Local Infiltration Anesthesia: Hematoma Block

Hematoma block has been successfully used in the treatment of distal forearm fractures (131,132). This simple technique

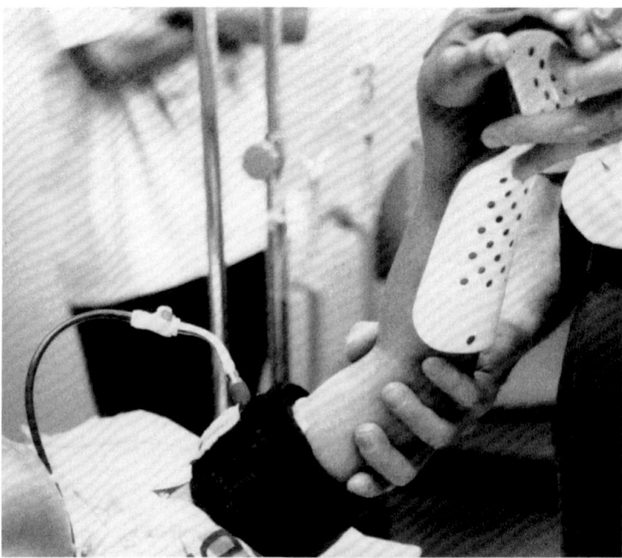

FIGURE 3-10 Fracture reduction under appropriately monitored sedation and IV regional anesthesia.

involves injecting local anesthetic into the fracture hematoma, the location of which is confirmed by aspirating blood into the syringe (see Fig. 3-9). When done alone, 1% lidocaine in a dose of 1 to 2 mg/kg is used (132). As indicated earlier, when combined with a Bier block, the last 1 to 2 mL of local anesthetic solution is used. Although the medication is rapidly absorbed into the circulation, the resulting systemic blood levels of local anesthetic are well below those required for CNS toxicity (132). Hematoma blocks may be used in patients who have received a regional block yet still have residual pain at the fracture site.

Alioto et al (133) described the use of an intra-articular hematoma block for the manipulative reduction of ankle fractures in a population that included both children and adults. The youngest patient in their study group who received a hematoma block was 12 years old. The technique they described consists of a direct injection of 2% lidocaine 1 mg/kg (the authors used 2 mg lidocaine per pound) into the tibiotalar joint space. Absolute sterile technique was used, with the skin overlying the fracture site being prepared with a povidone–iodine preparation. A 22- or 25-gauge needle was used for the injection of the local anesthetic solution. The authors recommended directing the needle in a slightly cephalad direction to avoid injury to the talar and tibial articular surfaces. Aspiration of blood was used to confirm entry into the intra-articular space. The injection was performed only if no resistance was encountered. A minimum of 15 minutes was allowed to pass after the injection, during which time the patient was closely observed and monitored for any evidence of local anesthetic systemic toxicity (see earlier). The injection was considered adequate if the patient was subsequently able to elevate the injured limb off the bed without assistance and perform active ankle dorsiflexion and plantarflexion. The authors found the intra-articular ankle hematoma block to be safe, effective, and well tolerated by patients (133). Although some of their patients tolerated the injection and the subsequent fracture reduction without the use of any other supplemental analgesics or sedatives, most children would probably require the same type of sedation that would be used before performing a Bier block or a hematoma block of the upper extremity.

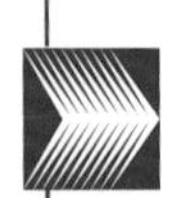

AUTHOR'S PREFERRED TREATMENT

Full aseptic technique, including adequate skin preparation and the use of sterile gloves, is recommended. The incidence of infection from introduction of a needle into the hematoma is greatly decreased if antiseptic precautions are taken (134). The hematoma is localized by aspirating blood into the syringe. The local anesthetic solution is given gradually by alternate injection (barbotage) of a small amount of medication and withdrawal of a small amount of hematoma until all of the medication has been given (Fig. 3-11). In the case of the intra-articular hematoma block at the ankle (133), a slow direct injection is used, with careful ECG monitoring for any evidence of dysrhythmias.

Reported complications with hematoma blocks in the upper extremity include compartment syndrome (135), temporary paralysis of the anterior interosseous nerve (135), and increased incidence of carpal tunnel syndrome (136).

Femoral Nerve Block

Berry (137) has described a technique of rapid analgesia for patients with a fracture of the femoral shaft using 1% lidocaine with 1:200,000 epinephrine or 1.5% lidocaine with 1:200,000 epinephrine deposited at the femoral nerve, just below the inguinal ligament (Fig. 3-12). As always, the anesthetic dose should remain within accepted limits. For lidocaine with epinephrine, 7 mg/kg is the dose limit.

Cooperation and tolerance among young children for regional blocks vary, so careful patient selection is advised.

POSTOPERATIVE ANALGESIA IN THE CHILD WITH A MUSCULOSKELETAL INJURY

Safe and effective postoperative analgesia in children with musculoskeletal injuries can be accomplished with opioids, nonsteroidal anti-inflammatory agents (NSAIDs), or local anesthetic agents.

Simultaneous use of more than one modality may be beneficial to minimize the side effects from any one particular approach (e.g., the use of NSAIDs to decrease the incidence of nausea, vomiting, or even respiratory depression from opioids). The end point is to make patients comfortable while minimizing adverse reactions.

Postoperative Analgesia With Opioids

Opioids have long been the mainstay of postoperative analgesia. It is important for the practitioner to understand the rationale behind different dosage regimens to maximize pain relief for the patient.

Intermittent Dosing

Although commonly used, traditional intermittent as-needed dosing of IM and IV opioids (Table 3-16) makes little pharmacologic sense for control of severe pain (138,139). Wide variations in plasma opioid levels occur, leading to periods of sedation alternating with prolonged periods of no pain relief at all (138). In addition, for pediatric care, IM dosing is a particularly poor choice (139), because children often chose to hide their pain rather than risk having to undergo an injection. The end result with intermittent dosing, especially with IM narcotics, is unnecessary undertreatment of pain.

Patient-Controlled Analgesia

Patient-controlled analgesia (PCA) is a sensible approach to the problems inherent with intermittent as-needed dosing of

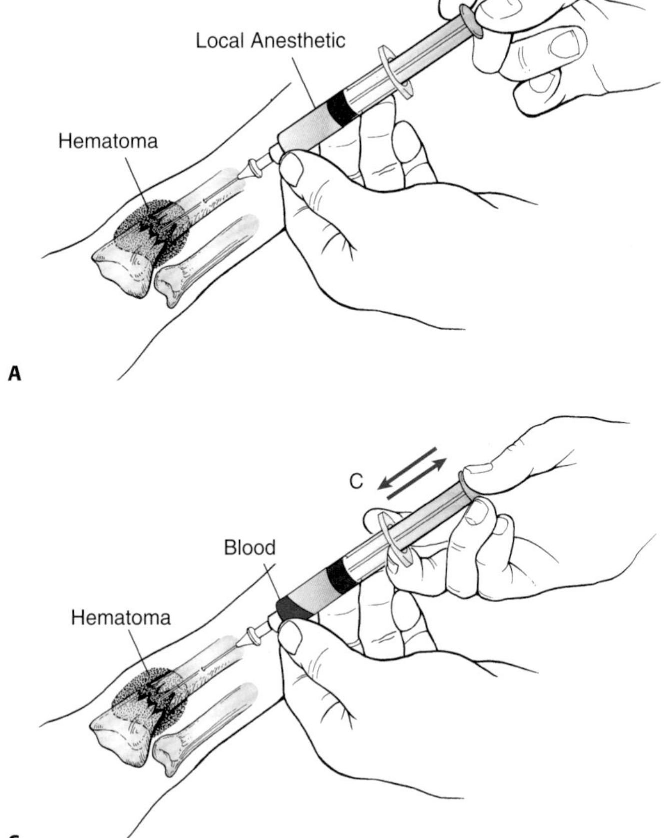

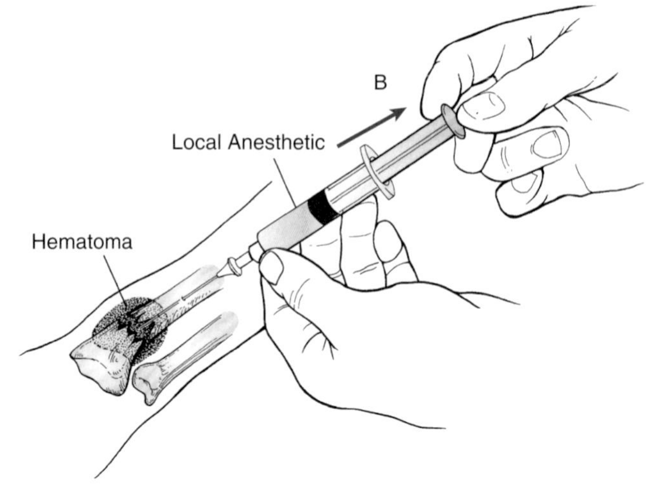

FIGURE 3-11 Barbotage. When performing a hematoma block, the local anesthetic is given by barbotage. **A.** Half the anesthetic is injected in the hematoma. **B.** The blood from the hematoma is withdrawn until the original volume is regained. **C.** This mixed material is repeatedly injected and reaspirated until the anesthetic is dispersed in the hematoma. The final aspirate should contain a volume equal to the original anesthetic; thus, the final volume of fluid in the hematoma has not been increased.

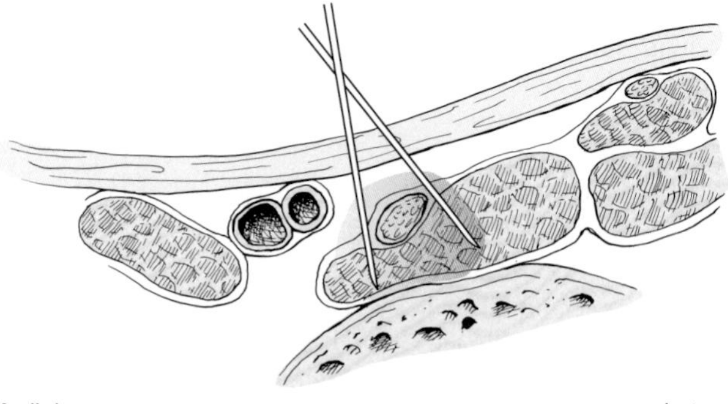

FIGURE 3-12 Section of right thigh immediately below the inguinal ligament, showing femoral nerve under cover of fascia iliaca and its block by a barrage technique. (Berry FR. Analgesia in patients with fractured shaft of femur. *Anesthesia* 1977;32:577; reproduced with permission)

TABLE 3-16 Parenteral Opioid Dosing Schedule for Analgesia in Children*

IM†: Morphine, 0.1–0.15 mg/kg q3–4h; Meperidine, 1.0–1.5 mg/kg q3–4h

IV: Morphine, 0.05–0.1 mg/kg q2h; Meperidine, 0.5–1.0 mg/kg q2h

* Infants < 3 mo old should be dosed in increments of one third to one half because of increased risk of respiratory depression.
† IM dosing should rarely be used.
Adapted from Roger L, Moro M. Acute postoperative and chronic pain in children. In: Rasch DK, Webster DE, eds. *Clinical manual of pediatric anesthesia.* New York: McGraw-Hill, 1994:297; with permission.

opioids (138). With PCA, IV self-titration of small doses of opioids at frequent intervals eliminates the wide variations in plasma drug levels seen with intermittent dosing (138). It also allows patients to gain control over their pain management (140), which may be of psychological importance to the patient's well-being.

PCA was first evaluated in adolescents in 1987, after several years of successful use in adults (140). Since then, this modality has been used for children as young as 6 years of age (141). Depending on the intelligence and cooperative ability of the child, it is conceivable that PCA could be used for younger individuals, although careful assessment of each individual situation is required.

When compared with traditional intermittent dosing, improved pain control and greater patient satisfaction have been demonstrated (141). Further improvement in pain relief may be achieved with the addition of a continuous background infusion of opioids to maintain the plasma concentrations of the analgesic during sleep. However, adding a background infusion may increase the risk of opioid-associated nausea, sedation, and hypoxemia (142,143).

Conceivably, for younger children or for children otherwise unreliably capable of pushing the button on the PCA cord, "parent-controlled analgesia" may be useful. The author has used this approach in a patient as young as 1.5 years of age. In this situation, however, the parents were very motivated and intelligent and had done this before for their child after another surgical procedure. In general, PCA is safest when only the patient is operating the device.

Parameters that must be considered are the loading dose, the maintenance dose, the lockout interval (the period during which no further administration of medication will occur despite attempts to do so by the patient), and the 4-hour maximum dose (Table 3-17). For PCA, morphine is more effective than meperidine (144). Opioids other than morphine should be used only for patients allergic to morphine (145), or in whom morphine produces intolerable side effects. Whenever possible, the persistent use of one medication helps avoid dosing errors (145).

The use of the PCA pump should be explained to patients preoperatively. Effective use of a loading dose will avoid the problem of having to play catch-up with out-of-control levels of pain.

Mishaps have occurred with PCA pumps due to programming errors (146), so ward personnel must be totally familiar with the equipment. Treatment of opioid-related side effects is outlined in Table 3-17.

TABLE 3-17 Patient-Controlled Analgesia in Children

Loading dose: Morphine, 0.025–0.05 mg/kg

Maintenance dose: Morphine, 0.01–0.02 mg/kg

Lockout interval: 6–10 min

4-hr maximum: Morphine, 0.4 mg/kg/4 h

Treatment of Side Effects

Pruritus: Diphenhydramine (0.5 mg/kg IV) OR low-dose naloxone (0.5–1.0 μg/hr)

Nausea/vomiting: Metoclopramide (0.1 mg/kg IV) OR droperidol (10–30 μg/kg IV or IM) OR ondansetron (0.15 mg/kg IV over 15 min) OR low-dose naloxone as for pruritus

Urinary retention (<1 mL/kg/h in the face of adequate fluid intake): Low-dose naloxone infusion as above

Respiratory depression: Specify vital sign parameters that require treatment and method for contracting responsible physician. Stop PCA pump. Give 100% oxygen and maintain the airway. Give naloxone (1–5 μg/kg IV bolus); repeat as needed. Consider naloxone infusion (3–5 μg/kg/h).

Rogers J, Moro M. Acute postoperative and chronic pain in children. In: Rasch DR, Webster DE, eds. *Clinical manual of pediatric anesthesia*. New York: McGraw-Hill, 1994:298; with permission.

Oral Administration of Opioids

Oral dosing of opioids is extremely useful for the continued management of diminishing postoperative pain, once oral analgesics are tolerated. Several oral analgesics are available, and their appropriate use is summarized in Table 3-18. None of these medications is devoid of side effects, including mood changes, nausea, vomiting, constipation, dizziness, and pruritus. The occurrence and degree of side effects vary from patient to patient, so the physician should be prepared to change dosing regimens based on patient response. The use of NSAIDs (see the following section) as part of the analgesic regimen may be helpful in reducing or eliminating troublesome opioid-related side effects.

Other Modes of Opioid Administration

Epidural opioids are being used in children after major surgery with excellent results (147). The author encourages close cooperation between surgeons and anesthesiologists to avail children of this modality of analgesia whenever feasible.

Postoperative Analgesia With NSAIDs

NSAIDs have moderately good analgesic properties (139). Unlike opioids, which produce analgesia by effects on CNS receptors, NSAIDs act peripherally by inhibiting prostaglandin synthesis and decreasing inflammation (148,149). Inflammatory mechanisms play an important part in the pathogenesis of postoperative pain (137); therefore, the use of NSAIDs makes good sense in the postoperative setting. Also, although NSAIDs have

TABLE 3-18 Dosing Schedules and Formulations for Oral Opioids in Children

Agent	Dose	Pediatric Formulations*
Codeine†	0.5–1.0 mg/kg q 4 to 6 h (max. single dose, 60 mg)	15 mg/5 mL oral solution
Codeine with acetaminophen (Tylenol with Codeine, Phenaphen with Codeine, Capital with Codeine)	0.5–1.0 mg/kg codeine q 4 to 6 h + 10–15 mg/kg acetaminophen q 4 to 6 h	12 mg codeine + 120 mg acetaminophen/5 mL solution Tylenol (300 mg) + Codeine tablets #1: 7.5 mg, #2: 15 mg, #3: 30 mg, #4: 60 mg
Hydrocodone with acetaminophen (Lortab, Anexsia, Co-Gesic, DuoCet, Hy-Phen, Vicodin)	Adult dose: hydrocodone 5–10 mg q 4 to 6 h Children (only antitussive dose is published): 0.6 mg/kg day divided in three to four doses/day. <2 yr: Do not exceed 1.25 mg/dose. 2–12 yr: Do not exceed 5 mg/single dose. >12 yr: Do not exceed 10 mg/single dose.	2.5 mg hydrocodone/5 mL + acetaminophen 120 mg/5 mL (Lortab Liquid)
Meperidine (Meperidine HCl, Demerol HCl)†	1.1–1.8 mg/kg q 3 to 4 h Max. single dose 100 mg	50 mg meperidine/5 mL solution
Morphine (morphine sulfate, Raxanol)†	0.2–0.4 mg/kg q 4 h (Adult dose is 10–30 mg q 4 h) Absorption from the GI tract is variable.	10 10 mL/5 mL and 20 mg/5 mL solution
Hydromorphone (Dilaudid, Hydromorphone HCl)†	Optimum pediatric dosage for analgesia not established. Antitussive dose is: 6–12 yr: 0.5 mg q 3–4 h >12 yr: 1 mg q 3–4 h	5 mg hydromorphone/5 mL solution
Oxycodone and Aspirin‡ (Percodan-Demi)†§	6–12 yr: 1/4 tablet q 6 h >12 yr: 1/2 tablet q 6 h	Oxycodone§ + 325 mg aspirin

* This table does not provide an exhaustive list of all available oral opioids and oral opioid/nonsteroidal anti-inflammatory drug combinations. A complete discussion and complete lists of all respective formulations may be found in *AHFS Drug Information '94*.

† Denotes a schedule 1 drug, for which a triplicate prescription is required.

‡ Owing to an association with Reye's syndrome, medications containing aspirin should be expressly avoided in children with flulike symptoms or children with chickenpox.

§ Percodan-Demi contains 2.25 mg oxycodone hydrochloride and 0.19 mg oxycodone terephthalate + 325 mg aspirin.

Adapted from Opiate Agonists. In McEvoy CK, Litvak K, Weish OH, Jr, eds. *AHFS Drug Information '94*. Bethesda, MD American Society of Hospital Pharmacists, 1994; Taketomo CK, Hodding JHJ, Kraus DM. *Pediatric dosage handbook*, 2nd ed. Hudson, OH. Lexi-Comp, 1993; Ragers J, Moro M. *Acute Postoperative and Chronic Pain in Children*. In Rasch DK, Webster DE (eds.). *Clinical Manual of Pediatric Anesthesia*. New York: McGraw-Hill, 1994; with permission.

some troubling side effects of their own, they do not produce respiratory depression, nausea, and vomiting, which are some of the bothersome features of opioids. Thus, using NSAIDs either as an adjunct or as a substitute for opioids when feasible should decrease or eliminate the possibility of drug-induced nausea, vomiting, or respiratory depression in the surgical patient (137).

Potential side effects of this class of drugs include platelet dysfunction, gastritis, and acute renal dysfunction (149,150). A history of sensitivity to aspirin or a history of nasal polyps may be associated with potentially fatal cross-sensitivity to other NSAIDs (148,151). In children with asthma, the prevalence of aspirin sensitivity may be as high as 28% (152). Therefore, asthmatic children should probably receive only those NSAIDs that do not cross-react with aspirin. These medications include acetaminophen, salsalate (Disalcid), and choline magnesium trisalicylate (Trilisate) (see Table 3-18) (153).

In a child with a chronic underlying bleeding disorder, NSAIDs are not necessarily contraindicated. Consultation with the child's hematologist is advised regarding the use of specific medications in this class.

Ketorolac, unlike other NSAIDs, can be administered not only orally but also IV and IM. A loading dose of 1.0 mg/kg may provide similar analgesia as 0.1 mg/kg of morphine (154).

TABLE 3-19 **Dosing Schedules and Formulations for NSAIDs in Children**

Agent	Dose	Formulations*
Ibuprofen (oral)	5–10 mg/kg q 6 h (published dose is for treatment of fever, not specifically for analgesia)	100 mg/5 mL suspension Tablets: 200, 300, 400, 600, 800 mg
Naproxen (oral)	5–7.5 mg/kg q 12 h	125 mg/5 mL suspension Tablets: 250, 375, 500 mg
Ketorolac (IM, IV)	0.5 mg/kg q 6 h	Injectable 30 mg/mL
Choline Magnesium Trisalicylate (Trilisate) (oral)†	50 mg/kg/day Divided into 2 or 3 doses (maximum daily dose, 2.25 g)	500 mg salicylate/5 mL solution Tablets: 500, 750, 1000 mg
Salsalate† (oral) (Disalcid)	Pediatric dose not published; adult maintenance dose is 2–4 g/day.	Tablets: 500, 750 mg
Acetaminophen‡ (oral, rectal)	10–15 mg/kg q 4–6 h	80 mg/0.8 mL drops 80 mg chewable tablets 160 mg/5 mL solution 325, 500 mg tablets 120-, 325-, 650-mg suppositories

* An exhaustive listing of available formulations for NSAIDs may be found in *AHFS Drug Information '94*.

† Although they are salicylates, choline magnesium trisalicylate and salsalate do not crossreact with aspirin and may be used in patients allergic to aspirin. As many as 28% of children with asthma may be in this group of patients. Owing to an association with Reye's syndrome, salicylates should be avoided in children with flu-like symptoms or chickenpox.

‡ Acetaminophen is considered a member of this class of medications, even though it mainly acts centrally and it only very weakly inhibits prostaglandin synthesis. Acetaminophen also does not crossreact with aspirin and may be used in patients allergic to aspirin.

(Adapted from Nonsteroidal Anti-Inflammatory Agents. In McEvoy GK, Litvak K, Welsh OH Jr., eds. *AHFS Drug Information '94*. Bethesda, MD: American Society of Hospital Pharmacists, 1994; Walson PD, Mortensen ME. Pharmacokinetics of common analgesics, anti-inflammatories and antipyretics in children. *Clin Pharmacokinet* 17:116–137, 1989; with permission.

The pharmacology of ketorolac has been extensively reviewed (155), and both its mode of action and adverse reactions are generally typical of NSAIDs. The major controversy with this drug remains its effect on hemostasis and bleeding. Rusy et al (156) found that ketorolac contributed to increased blood loss and more difficulty in achieving surgical hemostasis in pediatric tonsillectomy patients. Caution is advised in administering ketorolac or any other NSAID in a perioperative situation in which bleeding has been or can be significant. Ketorolac has been associated with an increased incidence of nonunion in patients undergoing spine fusion.

Suggested dosing schedules for some of the more common NSAIDs are listed in Table 3-8. Acetaminophen is considered a member of this class of medications, although its mechanism of action is central and its effects on prostaglandin synthesis and the inflammatory response are comparatively very weak (149).

Postoperative Analgesia With Local Anesthetic Agents

Regional anesthesia is an excellent means of providing postoperative analgesia without respiratory depression and with minimal physiologic alterations (157). Both central (epidural) and peripheral (e.g., brachial plexus blocks) nerve blocks may be used for this purpose. The physician must ensure that the pain relief achieved does not mask the signs and symptoms of developing vascular or neurologic compromise (158,159).

TREATMENT OF POSTOPERATIVE NAUSEA

Postoperative nausea is common in children, although not particularly after peripheral orthopaedic procedures (154). The pharmacologic treatment is outlined in Table 3-19. Additional helpful measures include not forcing intake of oral fluids until the child is hungry, and minimizing early postoperative ambulation, especially when opioids have been given (28).

REFERENCES

1. American Academy of Pediatrics Committee on Drugs: Guidelines for monitoring and management of pediatric patients during and after sedation for diagnostic and therapeutic procedures. *Pediatrics* 1992;89:1110–1115.
2. Practice guidelines for sedation and analgesia by non-anesthesiologists. A report by the

American Society of Anesthesiologists Task Force on Sedation and Analgesia by Non-Anesthesiologists. *Anesthesiology* 1996;84:459–471.
3. Maxwell LG, Yaster M. The myth of conscious sedation. *Arch Pediatr Adolesc Med* 1996; 150:665–667.
4. Sacchetti A, Schafermeyer R, Gerardi M, et al. Pediatric analgesia and sedation. *Ann Emerg Med* 1994;23:237–250.
5. Cote CJ, Goldstein EA, Cote MA, et al. A single-blind study of pulse oximetry in children. *Anesthesiology* 1988;68:184–188.
6. Cote CJ. Sedation for the pediatric patient: a review. *Pediatr Clin North Am* 1994;41: 31–51.
7. Brooks TD, Paulus DA, Winkle WE. Infrared heat lamps interfere with pulse oximeters [letter]. *Anesthesiology* 1984;61:630.
8. Barker SJ, Hyatt J, Shah NK, et al. The effect of sensor malpositioning of pulse oximeter accuracy during hypoxemia. *Anesthesiology* 1993;79:248–254.
9. Stoelting RK. Endotracheal intubation. In: Miller RD, ed. *Anesthesiology,* 2nd ed. New York: Churchill-Livingstone, 1986:523–552.
10. Cote CJ, Todres ID. The pediatric airway. In: Ryan JF, Todres ID, Cote CJ, Goudsouzian NG, eds. *A practice of anesthesia for infants and children.* New York: Grune and Stratton, 1986:35–57.
11. Tiret L, Nivoche Y, Hatton F, et al. Complications related to anaesthesia in infants and children. A prospective survey of 40,240 anaesthetics. *Br J Anaesth* 1988;61:263–269.
12. Cote CJ. NPO after midnight for children—a reappraisal. *Anesthesiology* 1990;72: 589–592.
13. Miller M, Wishar HY, Nummo WS. Gastric contents at induction of anaesthesia—is a 4-hour fast necessary? *Br J Anaesth* 1983;55:1185–1187.
14. Schreiner MS, Triebwasser A, Keon TP. Ingestion of liquids compared preoperative fasting in pediatric outpatients. *Anesthesiology* 1990;72:593–597.
15. Splinter WM, Stewart JA, Muir JG. The effect of preoperative apple juice on gastric contents, thirst and hunger in children. *Can J Anaesth* 1989;36:55–58.
16. Ferrari LR, Rooney FM, Rockoff MA. Preoperative fasting practices in pediatrics. *Anesthesiology* 1999;90:978–980.
17. Morris RE, Miller GW. Preoperative management of the patient with a full stomach. *Clin Anesth* 1976;11:25–29.
18. Bricker SRW, McCluckie A, Nightingale DA. Gastric aspirates after trauma in children. *Anaesthesia* 1989;44:721–724.
19. Gibbs PC, Modell JH. Aspiration pneumonitis. In: Miller RD, ed. *Anesthesia,* 2nd ed. New York: Churchill-Livingstone, 1986:2023–2050.
20. Fujigaki T, Fukusaki M, Nakamura H, et al. Quantitative evaluation of gastric contents using ultrasound. *J Clin Anesth* 1993;5:451–455.
21. Striker TW. Anesthesia for trauma in the pediatric patient. In: Gregory GA, ed. *Pediatric anesthesia,* 2nd ed. New York: Churchill-Livingstone, 1989:1273–1288.
22. Webster DE. The pediatric trauma patient. In: Rasch DK, Webster DE, eds. *Clinical manual of pediatric anesthesia.* New York: McGraw-Hill, 1994:189–216.
23. Perkin RM, Levin DL. Shock. In: Levin DL, Morriss FC, eds. *Essentials of pediatric intensive care.* St. Louis: Quality Medical Publishing, 1990:78–79.
24. Wertzel RC. Anesthesia for pediatric trauma. In: Steen JK, Grande CM, eds. *Trauma anesthesia.* Baltimore: Williams & Wilkins, 1991:312–329.
25. Coln D. Trauma in children. In: Levin DL, Morriss FC, eds. *Essentials of pediatric intensive care.* St. Louis: Quality Medical Publishing, 1990:671–676.
26. Magnat D, Orr WC, Smith RO. Sleep apnea, hypersomnolence, and upper airway obstruction secondary to adenotonsillar enlargement. *Arch Otolaryngol Head Neck Surg* 1977;103:383–386.
27. Covino BG. Clinical pharmacology of local anesthetic agents. In: Cousins MJ, Bridenbaugh PO, ed. *Neural blockade in clinical anesthesia and management of pain,* 2nd ed. Philadelphia: JB Lippincott, 1988:111–144.
28. Berry FA. Anesthesia for the child with a difficult airway. In: Berry FA, ed. *Anesthetic management of difficult and routine pediatric patients,* 2nd ed. New York: Churchill-Livingstone, 1990:15–52.
29. Evans JK, Buckley SL, Alexander AH, et al. Analgesia for the reduction of fractures in children: a comparison of nitrous oxide with intramuscular sedation. *J Pediatr Orthop* 1995;15:73–77.
30. Hennrikus WL, Simpson RB, Klingelberger CE, et al. Self-administered nitrous oxide analgesia for pediatric fracture reductions. *J Pediatr Orthop* 1994;14:538–542.
31. Hennrikus WL, Shin AY, Klingelberger CE. Self-administered nitrous oxide and a hematoma block for analgesia in the outpatient reduction of fractures in children. *J Bone Joint Surg [Am]* 1995;77:335–339.
32. Lowe S, Hershey S. Sedation for imaging and invasive procedures. In: Deshpande JK, Tobias JD, ed. *The pediatric pain handbook.* St. Louis: Mosby, 1996:263–317.
33. Corssen G, Miyasaka M, Domino EF. Changing concepts in pain control during surgery: dissociative anesthesia with CI-581, a progress report. *Anesth Analg* 1968;47:746–759.
34. White PF, Way WL, Trever AJ. Ketamine—its pharmacology and therapeutic uses. *Anesthesiology* 1982;56:119–136.
35. Grant IS, Nimmo WS, McNicol LR, et al. Ketamine disposition in children and adults. *Br J Anesth* 1983;55:1107–1111.
36. Stoelting RK. Nonbarbiturate induction drugs. In: *Pharmacology and physiology in anesthetic practice.* Philadelphia: JB Lippincott, 1987:134–147.
37. Saint-Maurice C, Laguenie G, Couturier C, et al. Rectal ketamine in pediatric anesthesia [letter]. *Br J Anesth* 1979;51:573–574.
38. Gutstein HB, Johnson KL, Heard MB, et al. Oral ketamine preanesthetic medication in children. *Anesthesiology* 1992;76:28–33.
39. Tobias JD, Phipps S, Smith B, et al. Oral ketamine premedication to alleviate the distress of invasive procedures in pediatric oncology patients. *Pediatrics* 1992;90:537–541.
40. Weksler N, Ovadia L, Mutai G, et al. Nasal ketamine for paediatric premedication. *Can J Anaesth* 1993;40:119–121.
41. Brown TCK, Fisk GC. *Anaesthesia for children.* Oxford: Blackwell Scientific Publications, 1979:29–31.
42. Lockhart CH, Nelson WL. The relationship of ketamine requirement to age in pediatric patients. *Anesthesiology* 1974;40:507–508.
43. Kohrs R, Durieux ME. Ketamine: teaching an old drug new tricks. *Anesth Analg* 1998; 87:1186–1193.
44. Hollister GR, Burn JMB. Side effects of ketamine in pediatric anesthesia. *Anesth Analg* 1974;53:264–267.
45. Myers EF, Charles P. Prolonged adverse reactions to ketamine in children. *Anesthesiology* 1978;49:39–40.
46. Green SM, Johnson NE. Ketamine sedation for pediatric procedures: part 2, review and implications. *Ann Emerg Med* 1990;19:1033–1046.
47. Tobias JD. Sedation in the pediatric intensive care unit. In: Deshpande JK, Tobias JD, eds. *The pediatric pain handbook.* St. Louis: Mosby, 1996:235–261.
48. Dachs RJ, Ines GM. Intravenous ketamine sedation of pediatric patients in the emergency department. *Ann Emerg Med* 1997;29:146–150.
49. Mitchell RK, Koury SI, Stone CK. Respiratory arrest after intramuscular ketamine in a 2-year-old child. *Am J Emerg Med* 1996;14:580–581.
50. Smith JA, Santer LS. Respiratory arrest following intramuscular ketamine injection in a 4-year-old child. *Ann Emerg Med* 1993;22:613–615.
51. Carson IW, Moore J, Balmer JP, et al. Laryngeal competence with ketamine and other drugs. *Anesthesiology* 1973;38:128–133.
52. Taylor PA, Towey RM. Depression of laryngeal reflexes during ketamine anaesthesia. *Br Med J* 1971;2:688–689.
53. Green SM, Nakamura R, Johnson NE. Ketamine sedation for pediatric procedures: part 1, a prospective series. *Ann Emerg Med* 1990;19:1024–1032.
54. Green SM, Rothrock SG, Lynch EL, et al. Intramuscular ketamine for pediatric sedation in the emergency department: safety profile in 1,022 cases. *Ann Emerg Med* 1998;31: 688–697.
55. Kennedy RM, Porter FL, Miller JP, et al. Comparison of fentanyl/midazolam with ketamine/midazolam for pediatric orthopedic emergencies. *Pediatrics* 1998;102: 956–963.
56. Stoelting RK. Benzodiazepines. In: *Pharmacology and physiology in anesthetic practice.* Philadelphia: JB Lippincott, 1987:117–133.
57. Dretchen K, Ghoneim MM, Long JP. The interaction of diazepam with myoneural blocking agents. *Anesthesiology* 1971;34:463–468.
58. Reeves JG, Fragen RJ, Vinik HR, et al. Midazolam: pharmacology and uses. *Anesthesiology* 62:310–324.
59. Wright SW, Chudnofsky CR, Dronen SC, et al. Comparison of midazolam and diazepam for conscious sedation in the emergency department. *Ann Emerg Med* 1993;22: 201–205.
60. Galletly D, Forrest P, Purdie G. Comparison of the recovery characteristics of diazepam and midazolam. *Br J Anaesth* 1988;60:520–524.
61. Buhrer M, Maitre PO, Crevoisier C, et al. EEG effects of benzodiazepines. II. Pharmacodynamic modeling of the EEG effects of midazolam and diazepam. *Clin Pharmacol Ther* 1990;48:555–567.
62. Forster A, Gardaz JP, Suter PM, et al. Respiratory depression by midazolam and diazepam. *Anesthesiology* 1980;53:494–497.
63. Braunstein MC. Apnea with maintenance of consciousness following intravenous diazepam. *Anesth Analg* 1979;58:52–53.
64. Iber FL, Livak A, Kruss DM. Apnea and cardiopulmonary arrest during and after endoscopy. *J Clin Gastroenterol* 1992;14:109–113.
65. Litman RS. Airway obstruction after oral midazolam [letter]. *Anesthesiology* 1996;85: 1217–1218.
66. Alexander CM, Gross JB. Sedative doses of midazolam depress hypoxic ventilatory responses in humans. *Anesth Analg* 1988;67:377–382.
67. Yaster M, Nichols DG, Deshpande JK, et al. Midazolam–fentanyl intravenous sedation in children: case report of respiratory arrest. *Pediatrics* 1990;86:463–467.
68. Massanari M, Novitsky J, Reinstein LJ. Paradoxical reaction in children associated with midazolam use during endoscopy. *Clin Pediatr* 1997;36:681–684.
69. Peterson MD. Making oral midazolam palatable for children [letter]. *Anesthesiology* 1990;73:1053.
70. Karl HW, Keifer AT, Rosenberger JL, et al. Comparison of the safety and efficacy of intranasal midazolam or sufentanil for preinduction of anesthesia in pediatric patients. *Anesthesiology* 1989;76:209–215.
71. Hennes HM, Wagner V, Bonadio WA, et al. The effect of oral midazolam on anxiety of preschool children during laceration repair. *Ann Emerg Med* 1990;19:1006–1009.
72. Fatovich DM, Jacobs IG. A randomized, controlled trial of oral midazolam and buffered lidocaine for suturing lacerations in children (the SLIC trial). *Ann Emerg Med* 1995; 25:209–214.
73. Feld LH, Negus JB, White PF. Oral midazolam preanesthetic medication in pediatric outpatients. *Anesthesiology* 1990;73:831–834.
74. Sievers TD, Yee JD, Foley ME, et al. Midazolam for conscious sedation during pediatric oncology procedures: safety and recovery parameters. *Pediatrics* 1991;88:1172–1179.
75. Jones RDM, Chan K, Roulson CJ, et al. Pharmacokinetics of flumazenil and midazolam. *Br J Anaesth* 1993;70:286–292.
76. Klotz U, Kanto J. Pharmacokinetics and clinical use of flumazenil (Ro 15-1788). *Clin Pharmacokinet* 1988;14:1–12.
77. Philip BK, Simpson TH, Hauch MA, et al. Flumazenil reverses sedation after midazolam-induced general anesthesia in ambulatory surgery patients. *Anesth Analg* 1990;71: 371–376.

78. Jones RDM, Lawson AD, Andrew LJ, et al. Antagonism of the hypnotic effect of midazolam in children: a randomized double-blind study of placebo and flumazenil administered after midazolam-induced anaesthesia. *Br J Anaesth* 1991;66:660–666.
79. Stoelting RK. Opioid agonists and antagonists. In: *Pharmacology and physiology in anesthetic practice.* Philadelphia: JB Lippincott: 1987:69–101.
80. Bailey PL, Stanley TH. Pharmacology of intravenous narcotic anesthetics. In: Miller RD, ed. *Anesthesia,* 2nd ed. New York: Churchill-Livingstone, 1986:745–797.
81. Gourlay GK, Boas RA. Fatal outcome with use of rectal morphine for postoperative pain control in an infant. *Br Med J* 1992;304:766–767.
82. Stoelting RK. Inhaled anesthetics. In: *Pharmacology and physiology in anesthetic practice.* Philadelphia: JB Lippincott, 1987:2–34.
83. Rita L, Seleny F, Goodarzi M. Comparison of the calming and sedative effects of nalbuphine and pentazocine for paediatric premedication. *Can Anaesth Soc J* 1980;27: 546–549.
84. Hershey LA. Meperidine and central nervous system toxicity [editorial]. *Ann Intern Med* 1983;98:548–549.
85. Kaiko RF, Foley KM, Gabrinski PY, et al. Central nervous system excitatory effects of meperidine in cancer patients. *Ann Neurol* 1983;13:180–185.
86. Schechter NL, Weisman SJ, Rosenblum M, et al. The use of oral transmucosal fentanyl citrate for painful procedures in children. *Pediatrics* 1995;95:335–339.
87. Stoeckel H, Hengstmann JH, Shuttler J. Pharmacokinetics of fentanyl as a possible explanation for recurrent respiratory depression. *Br J Anaesth* 1979;51:741–745.
88. Arandia HY, Patil VU. Glottic closure following large doses of fentanyl [letter]. *Anesthesiology* 1987;66:574–575.
89. Askgaard B, Nilsson T, Ibler M, et al. Muscle tone under fentanyl–nitrous oxide anaesthesia measured with a transducer apparatus in cholecystectomy incisions. *Acta Anaesthesiol Scand* 1977;21:104.
90. Scamman FL. Fentanyl-oxygen-nitrous oxide rigidity and pulmonary compliance. *Anesth Analg* 1983;62:332–334.
91. Sokoll MD, Hoyt JL, Gergis SD. Studies in muscle rigidity, nitrous oxide, and narcotic analgesic agents. *Anesth Analg* 1972;51:16–20.
92. Romagnoli A, Keats AS. Ceiling effect for respiratory depression by nalbuphine. *Clin Pharmacol Therapeut* 1980;27:478–485.
93. Vandam LD. Butorphanol. *N Engl J Med* 1980;302:381–384.
94. Jailon P, Gardin ME, Lecoq B, et al. Pharmacokinetics of nalbuphine in infants, young healthy volunteers, and elderly patients. *Clin Pharmacol Ther* 1989;46:226–233.
95. Deshpande JK, Anand KJS. Basic aspects of acute pediatric pain and sedation. In: Deshpande JK, Tobias JD, eds. *The pediatric pain handbook.* St. Louis: Mosby, 1996: 1–48.
96. Azar I, Turndorf H. Severe hypertension and multiple atrial premature contractions following naloxone administration. *Anesth Anal* 1979;58:524–525.
97. Estilo AE, Cottrell JE. Hemodynamic and catecholamine changes after administration of naloxone. *Anesth Analg* 1965;61:349–353.
98. Emergency drug doses for infants and children and naloxone use in newborns: clarification. *Pediatrics* 1989;83:803.
99. Varela CD, Lorfing KC, Schmidt TL. Intravenous sedation for the closed reduction of fractures in children. *J Bone Joint Surg [Am]* 1995;77:340–345.
100. Proudfoot J, Roberts M. Providing safe and effective sedation and analgesia for pediatric patients. *Emerg Med Reports* 1993;14:207–218.
101. Snodgrass WR, Dodge WF. Lytic/DPT cocktail: time for rational and safe alternatives. *Pediatr Clin North Am* 1989;36:1285–1291.
102. Terndrup TE, Dire DJ, Madden CM, et al. A prospective analysis of intramuscular meperidine, promethazine, and chlorpromazine in pediatric emergency department patients. *Ann Emerg Med* 1991;20:31–35.
103. Bilban P, Baraldi E, Pettenazzo A, et al. Adverse effect of chloral hydrate in two young children with obstructive sleep apnea. *Pediatrics* 1993;92:461–463.
104. Jastak JT, Pallasch T. Death after chloral hydrate sedation: report of a case. *J Am Dent Assoc* 1988;116:345–347.
105. Stoelting RK. Barbiturates. In: *Pharmacology and physiology in anesthetic practice.* Philadelphia: JB Lippincott, 1987:102–116.
106. Kaplan RF. *Sedation and analgesia in pediatric patients for procedures outside the operating room.* #221, American Society of Anesthesiologists Annual Refresher Course Lectures, October 1997.
107. Momota Y, Artu AA, Powers KM, et al. Posttreatment with propofol terminates lidocaine-induced epileptiform electroencephalogram activity in rabbits: effects on cerebrospinal fluid dynamics. *Anesth Analg* 1988;87:900–906.
108. Strichartz GR. Neural physiology and local anesthetic action. In: Cousins MJ, Bridenbaugh PO, eds. *Neural blockade in clinical anesthesia and management of pain,* 2nd ed. Philadelphia: JB Lippincott, 1987:24–45.
109. Tucker GT, Mather LE. Properties, absorption, and disposition of local anesthetic agents. In: Cousins MJ, Bridenbaugh PO, ed. *Neural blockade in clinical anesthesia and management of pain,* 2nd ed. Philadelphia: JB Lippincott, 1988:47–110.
110. Scott DB, Lee A, Fagan D, et al. Acute toxicity of ropivacaine compared with that of bupivacaine. *Anesth Analg* 1989;69:563–569.
111. Eddie R, Deutsch S. Cardiac arrest after interscalene brachial-plexus block. *Anesth Analg* 1977;56:446–447.
112. Moore DC, Crawford RD, Scurlock JE. Severe hypoxia and acidosis following local anesthetic-induced convulsions. *Anesthesiology* 1983;53:1185–1187.
113. Prentiss JE. Cardiac arrest following caudal anesthesia. *Anesthesiology* 1979;50:51–53.
114. Albright GA. Cardiac arrest following regional anesthesia with etidocaine or bupivacaine [editorial]. *Anesthesiology* 1979;51:285–287.
115. Brown DT, Beamish D, Wildsmith JAW. Allergic reaction to an amide local anaesthetic. *Br J Anaesth* 1981;53:435–437.
116. Fisher MM, Graham R. Adverse responses to local anaesthetics. *Anaesthesia Intensive Care* 1984;12:325–327.
117. Chan CYJ. Pediatric pharmacology. In: Rasch DK, Webster DE, eds. *Clinical manual of pediatric anesthesia.* New York: McGraw-Hill, 1994:27–46.
118. Morriss FC. Anaphylaxis. In: Levin DL, Morriss FC, eds. *Essentials of pediatric intensive care.* St. Louis: Quality Medical Publishing, 1990:98–105.
119. Bier A. Uber einen neuen weg lokalansthesie an den gliedmasen zu eruzeugen. *Verhandlungen der Deutschen Gesellschaft fur Chirurgie (Berlin)* 1908;37:204–213.
120. Holmes MC. Intravenous regional analgesia, a useful method of producing analgesia of the limbs. *Lancet* 1963;1:245–247.
121. Barnes CL, Blasier RD, Dodge BM. Intravenous regional anesthesia: a safe and cost-effective outpatient anesthetic for upper extremity fracture treatment in children. *J Pediatr Orthop* 1991;11:717–720.
122. Bolte RG, Stevens PM, Scott SM, et al. Mini-dose Bier block intravenous regional anesthesia in the emergency department treatment of pediatric upper-extremity injuries. *J Pediatr Orthop* 1994;14:534–537.
123. Colizza WA, Said E. Intravenous regional anesthesia in the treatment of forearm and wrist fractures and dislocations in children. *Can J Surg* 1993;36:225–228.
124. Farrell RG, Swanson SL, Walter JR. Safe and effective IV regional anesthesia for use in the emergency department. *Ann Emerg Med* 1985;14:288–292.
125. FitzGerald B. Intravenous regional anesthesia in children. *Br J Anaesth* 1976;48: 485–486.
126. Olney BW, Lugg PC, Turner PL, et al. Outpatient treatment of upper extremity injuries in childhood using intravenous regional anesthesia. *J Pediatr Orthop* 1988;8:576–579.
127. Turner PL, Batten JB, Hjorth D, et al. Intravenous regional anaesthesia for the treatment of upper limb injuries in childhood. *Aust NZ J Surg* 1986;56:153–155.
128. Scott RS, Steinberg RB, Kreitzer JM, et al. Intravenous regional anesthesia using lidocaine and ketorolac. *Anesth Analg* 1995;81:110–113.
129. Holmes MC. Intravenous regional neural blockade. In: Cousins MJ, Bridenbaugh PO, eds. *Neural blockade in clinical anesthesia and management of pain,* 2nd ed. Philadelphia: Lippincott, 1988:443–459.
130. Finegan BA, Bukht MD. Venous pressure in the isolated upper limb during saline injection. *Can Anaesth Soc J* 1984;31:364–367.
131. Case RD. Haematoma block: a safe method of reducing Colles' fractures. *Injury* 1985; 16:469–470.
132. Meinig RP, Quick A, Lobmeyer L. Plasma lidocaine levels following hematoma block for distal radius fractures. *J Orthop Trauma* 1989;3:187–189.
133. Alioto RJ, Furia JP, Marquardt JD. Hematoma block for ankle fractures: a safe and efficacious technique for manipulations. *J Orthop Trauma* 1995;9:113–116.
134. Johnson PQ, Noffsinger MA. Hematoma block of distal forearm fractures. Is it safe? *Orthop Rev* 1991;20:977–979.
135. Younge D. Hematoma block for fractures of the wrist: a cause of compartment syndrome. *J Hand Surg [Br]* 1989;14:194–195.
136. Kongsholm MJ, Olerud C. Neurological complications of dynamic reduction of Colles' fractures without anesthesia compared with traditional manipulation after local infiltration anesthesia. *J Orthop Trauma* 1987;1:43–47.
137. Berry FR. Analgesia in patients with fractured shaft of femur. *Anesthesia* 1977;32: 576–577.
138. Ferrante FM. Patient characteristics influencing effective use of patient-controlled analgesia. In: Ferrante FM, Ostheimer GW, Covino BG, eds. *Patient-controlled analgesia.* Boston: Blackwell Scientific Publications, 1990:51–60.
139. Tyler DC. Pharmacology of pain management. *Pediatr Clin North Am* 1994;41:59–69.
140. Brown RE Jr, Broadman LM. Patient-controlled analgesia for postoperative pain control in adolescents [abstract]. *Anesth Analg* 1987;66:S22.
141. Berde CB, Lehn BM, Yee JD, et al. Patient-controlled analgesia in children and adolescents: a prospective comparison with intramuscular administration of morphine for postoperative analgesia. *J Pediatr* 1991;118:461–466.
142. Doyle E, Robinson D, Morton NS. Comparison of patient-controlled analgesia with and without a background infusion after lower abdominal surgery in children. *Br J Anaesth* 1993;71:670–673.
143. Wu MYC, Purcell GJ. Patient-controlled analgesia—the value of a background infusion [letter]. *Anaesthesia Intensive Care* 1990;18:575–576.
144. Vetter TR. Pediatric patient-controlled analgesia with morphine versus meperidine. *J Pain Symptom Manage* 1992;7:204–208.
145. Broadman LM. Patient-controlled analgesia in children and adolescents. In: Ferrante FM, Ostheimer GW, Covino BG, eds. *Patient-controlled analgesia.* Boston: Blackwell Scientific Publications, 1990:129–138.
146. White PF. Mishaps with patient-controlled analgesia. *Anesthesiology* 1987;66:81–82.
147. Rasmussen GE. Epidural and spinal anesthesia and analgesia. In: Deshpande JK, Tobias JD, eds. *The pediatric pain handbook.* St. Louis: Mosby, 1996:81–112.
148. Stoelting RK. Nonopioid and nonsteroidal analgesic, antipyretic, and anti-inflammatory drugs. In: *Pharmacology and physiology in anesthetic practice.* Philadelphia: JB Lippincott, 1987:240–250.
149. Walson PD, Mortensen ME. Pharmacokinetics of common analgesics, anti-inflammatories and antipyretics in children. *Clin Pharmacokinet* 1989;17(Suppl 1):116–137.
150. McIntire SC, Rubenstein RC, Gartner JC Jr, et al. Acute flank pain and reversible renal dysfunction associated with nonsteroidal anti-inflammatory drug use. *Pediatrics* 1993; 92:459–460.
151. Abrishami MA, Thomas J. Aspirin intolerance: a review. *Annals Allergy Asthma Immunol* 1977;39:28–37.
152. Rachelefsky GS, Coulson A, Siegel SC, et al. Aspirin intolerance in chronic childhood asthma: detected by oral challenge. *Pediatrics* 1975;56:443–448.
153. Stevenson DD, Simon RA. Aspirin sensitivity: respiratory and cutaneous manifestations.

In: Middleton E Jr, Reed CE, Ellis EF, et al., eds. *Allergy principles and practice,* 3rd ed. St. Louis: CV Mosby, 1988:1537–1554.

154. Mason LJ. *Challenges in pediatric anesthesia.* International Anesthesia Research Society Review Course Lectures, 1999:64–70.
155. Litvak KM, McEvoy GK. Ketorolac, an injectable non-narcotic analgesic. *Clin Pharm* 1990;9:921–935.
156. Rusy LM, Houck CS, Sullivan LJ, et al. A double-blind evaluation of ketorolac tromethamine versus acetaminophen in pediatric tonsillectomy patients, effects on analgesia and bleeding. *Anesth Analg* 1995;80:226–229.
157. Yaster M, Maxwell LG. Pediatric regional anesthesia. *Anesthesiology* 1989;70:324–338.
158. Dunwoody JM, Reichert CC, Brown KLB. Compartment syndrome associated with bupivacaine and fentanyl analgesia in pediatric orthopaedics. *J Pediatr Orthop* 1997; 17:285–288.
159. Mubarak SJ, Wilton CTN. Compartment syndromes and epidural anesthesia [editorial]. *J Pediatr Orthop* 1997;17:282–284.

SUGGESTED READINGS

Bassett KE, Anderson JL, Pribble CG, et al. Propofol for procedural sedation in children in the emergency department. *Ann Emerg Med* 2003;42:773–782.

Carre P, Joly A, Cluzel Field B, et al. Axillary block in children: single or multiple injection? *Paediatr Anaesth* 2000;10:35–39.

Davidson AJ, Eyres RL, Cole WG. A comparison of prilocaine and lidocaine for intravenous regional anaesthesia for forearm fracture reduction in children. *Paediatr Anaesth* 2002; 12:146–150.

Dial S, Silver P, Bock K, et al. Pediatric sedation for procedures titrated to a desired degree of immobility results in unpredictable depth of sedation. *Pediatr Emerg Care* 2001;17: 414–420.

Ecoffey C. Local anesthetics in pediatric anesthesia: an update. *Minerva Anesthesiol* 2005;71: 357–360.

Fleischmann E, Marhofer P, Greher M, et al. Brachial plexus anaesthesia in children: lateral infraclavicular vs axillary approach. *Paediatr Anaesth* 2003;13:103–108.

Herrera JA, Wall EJ, Foad SL. Hematoma block reduces narcotic pain medication after femoral elastic nailing in children. *J Pediatr Orthop* 2004;24:254–256.

Hoffman GM, Nowakowski R, Troshynski TJ, et al. Risk reduction in pediatric procedural sedation by application of an American Academy of Pediatrics/American Society of Anesthesiologists process model. *Pediatrics* 2002;109:236–243.

Kennedy RM, Luhmann JD, Luhmann SJ. Emergency department management of pain and anxiety related to orthopedic fracture care: a guide to analgesic techniques and procedural sedation in children. *Paediatr Drugs* 2004;6:11–31.

Marcus RJ, Thompson JP. Anaesthesia for manipulation of forearm fractures in children: a survey of current practice. *Paediatr Anaesth* 2000;10:273–277.

McCarty EC, Mencio GA, Green NE. Anesthesia and analgesia for the ambulatory management of fractures in children. *J Am Acad Orthop Surg* 1999;7:81–91.

MANAGEMENT OF THE MULTIPLY INJURED CHILD

Robert M. Kay and Vernon T. Tolo

INCIDENCE OF INJURIES

Trauma

The most common cause of death in children over the age of 1 year is trauma, not only in the United States but worldwide. Estimates of cost to the American public for the care of pediatric trauma range from over $1 billion (1) to $13.8 billion (2) annually. Although isolated long bone fractures still comprise the bulk of orthopaedic injuries in children, a surprising number of these young patients have multiple system injuries.

Over 1.5 million pediatric injuries have been reported to occur annually in the United States, resulting in more than 500,000 hospitalizations and 15,000 to 20,000 pediatric deaths (3–5). Boys are injured twice as often as girls and may account for even a greater proportion of hospital admissions related to pediatric trauma (6,7). Blunt trauma is the mechanism of injury in most children and preadolescents, whereas penetrating trauma more often is the source of multiple injuries in adults. Although blunt trauma in the youngest children often is due to child abuse, vehicular accidents and falls from a height account for the more severe multiple injuries in the rest of childhood (8). The cause of death from trauma in children generally is severe head injury.

Multiple injuries in teenagers more closely mirror the causes in adults. In the adolescent age group, alcohol abuse now is considered a major factor in over a third of injuries resulting from accidents (9). Orthopaedists treating teenagers involved in vehicular accidents need to be aware of the potential alcohol use in this age group and be prepared to refer adolescents for appropriate counseling to avoid future accidents and injuries (10).

Fractures

Although they are rarely the cause of mortality in a child with multiple injuries, fractures, and other injuries to the musculoskeletal system are commonly a major part of the injuries and associated morbidity (8,11–13). In one series from a pediatric trauma center treating children with polytrauma, femoral shaft fractures accounted for 22% of the fractures and 9% of the fractures were open (8). Although they are less common, fractures of the spine, pelvis, and scapula and clavicle were associated with longer stays in the hospital and in the intensive care unit, in addition to having the highest associated mortality rates.

Knowledge of fracture associations leads to improved diagnostic skill and fracture care. Calcaneal fractures often result from axial loading and most commonly occur after a fall from a height (40%) or from a motor vehicle accident (15%) (14,15). Associated fractures have been reported in approximately one third of children with calcaneal fractures, including spine fractures in 5% (14,15).

Femoral and adjacent pelvic fractures often occur together. If a pedestrian child has been struck by an automobile, there often are fractures in the ipsilateral upper and lower extremity (16). In one study, 58% (87/149) of children with femoral fractures due to motor vehicle accidents were noted to have associated injuries, including 14% with head injuries, 6% with chest injuries, 5% with abdominal injuries, and 4% with genitourinary injuries (17). The coexistence of a femoral fracture and a head injury indicates substantial high-energy trauma and has a more guarded prognosis than does either of these injuries alone.

Child Abuse

Child abuse continues to be a societal problem that crosses all socioeconomic and ethnic groups and is the most common cause of traumatic death in infants and toddlers. Currently, child abuse is estimated to occur in 15 to 42 of every 1,000 children annually, resulting in more than 1,200 deaths annually (18). This diagnosis must be suspected in all cases of multiple injuries in children younger than 2 years of age, if there is no obvious and witnessed plausible explanation of the injuries. Abuse should be considered a possible cause of injury in all young children with multiple long bone fractures in association with head injury. Even a single long bone fracture associated with a head injury or abdominal injury should raise suspicion of child abuse. Although the *corner fracture* usually is thought of as being most characteristic of child abuse, the most common fracture caused by abuse is a single transverse fracture of the femur or humerus, not multiple fractures (19). Although rib fractures occur in only about 5% of children with multiple injuries from trauma of other causes, they are more common in child abuse (13,20). Whereas blunt compressive trauma to the thorax from other causes may result in lateral rib fractures, the rib fractures seen in child abuse are often posterolateral and adjacent to the transverse processes of the thoracic spine (18,21,22).

A skeletal survey is routinely performed in suspected cases of abuse. Some authors have recommended a bone scan in conjunction with the skeletal survey (23), though this recommendation is controversial since the addition of a bone scan requires sedation, elevates radiation exposure, and increases cost (18,24).

COMMON MECHANISMS OF INJURY

Falls

A fall is one of the two primary mechanisms of multiple injuries in children (8,25–28). Occurring more often in younger children, these injuries are due either to the direct impact or to deceleration forces present at the time of landing. Direct impact usually causes fractures, whereas internal injury more often results from the postimpact forces. Falls through a second floor window that may be next to a bed often occur in toddlers and younger children. Although a variety of injuries can result from these falls, the position of the body at impact and the surface on which the child lands are important factors that affect the injury severity (25). Following falls from heights, head injuries have been reported in 39% of children (26), orthopaedic injuries in 34% (26), and mortality in 2% (26,28).

Motor Vehicles

Accidents involving motor vehicles account for most multiple-system injuries in school-age children and preadolescents. These injuries occur when a vehicle strikes a child on foot or riding a bicycle, or when the child is a passenger in a car involved in an accident. In 2002, over 300,000 children age 15 years and younger were injured and over 2,500 were killed in such motor vehicle accidents in the United States (29).

More than 250,000 injuries and 1,700 deaths in this age group in 2002 occurred in passengers in cars and light trucks (29). More than half of the children killed in these accidents were unrestrained at the time of the accident. (29). For childhood passengers injured or killed in car accidents, the risk of death is six times greater for those unrestrained than for those restrained at the time of injury (29).

Noncompliance with car seat use is a major contributor to morbidity and mortality following motor vehicle accidents. Thompson et al reported that only 20% of children treated at a trauma center following motor vehicle accidents were restrained at the time of injury (30). Vaca et al noted that many parents in California with children ages 6 years and younger were unaware of basic safety information regarding child car seats and airbags and that they were also unaware of state laws regarding child seat restraints (31).

Even with appropriate use of car seats, properly restrained children may be injured significantly. Zuckerbraun et al noted a higher incidence of cervical spine injuries in younger children (≤8 years old), thought to be due in part to the suboptimal restraint systems available for these younger children (32). Others have noted the importance of padding in child seats in potentially decreasing the risk of head injury in children restrained in child safety seats (33).

Whereas most states require that infants and toddlers be restrained in car seats when riding in a car, standard adult shoulder and lap belts do not adequately restrain children who are too big for car seats and too small for the standard restraints. Adjustable restraints to better accommodate the size of the car occupant have been proposed to solve this problem. In addition, there is increasing public sentiment to require seat belt use on school buses, a policy that has been in place for physically disabled student transport for some time.

The most important point is that a restraining system which is appropriate for the age and size of the passenger should be used by people of all ages when in a vehicle. Although teaching children better safety while on foot and on bicycles is a laudable and important goal, the safety of automobile travel can be dramatically improved with appropriate parent education regarding child safety seats and airbags and by enforcement of current laws.

ROLE OF THE PEDIATRIC TRAUMA CENTER

After the rapid transport of wounded soldiers to a specialized treatment center proved effective in improving survival in the military setting, trauma centers, using the same principles of rapid transport and immediate care, have been established throughout the United States. These trauma centers are supported by the states on the premise that the first hour after injury is the most critical in influencing the rates of survival from the injuries. Rapid helicopter or ambulance transport to an onsite team of trauma surgeons in the trauma center has led to an improvement in the rates of acute survival after multiple injuries have occurred.

The first trauma centers focused on adult patients, because more adults than children are severely injured. However, pediatric trauma centers have been established at several medical centers across the United States with the idea that the care of pediatric polytrauma patients differs from the care given to adults and that special treatment centers are important for optimal results (34,35). The American College of Surgeons has established specific criteria for pediatric trauma centers, which include the same principles of rapid transport and rapid treatment by an in-house surgical team as in adult trauma centers. A pediatric general surgeon is in the hospital at all times and heads the pediatric trauma team. This surgeon evaluates the child first and the other surgical specialists are immediately available. General x-ray services and computed tomography capability must be available at all times for patient evaluation and an operating room must be immediately available.

Although there is some evidence that survival rates for severely injured children are improved if the children are brought to a pediatric trauma center rather than a community hospital (36), the costs associated with such a center (particularly the on-call costs of personnel) have limited the number of pediatric trauma centers. Given the limited number of pediatric trauma centers, patients frequently are often either (a) stabilized at other hospitals prior to transfer to a pediatric trauma center or (b) treated at an adult trauma center. In one recent study, Larson et al reported that there did not appear to be better outcomes for pediatric trauma patients flown directly to a pediatric trauma center than for those stabilized at nontrauma centers prior to transfer to the same pediatric trauma center (37).

Knudson et al (38) studied the results of pediatric multiple injury care in an adult level I trauma center and concluded that the results were comparable to national standards for pediatric trauma care. Sanchez et al recently reported that adolescent trauma patients admitted to an adult surgical intensive care unit (SICU) had comparable outcomes to comparable patients admitted to a pediatric intensive care unit (PICU) in a single institution (39). However, those admitted to the SICU were more likely to be intubated and to have a Swan-Ganz catheter placed and had longer ICU stays and longer hospital stays (39). The use of a general trauma center for pediatric trauma care may be an acceptable alternative if it is not feasible to fund a separate pediatric trauma center.

INITIAL RESUSCITATION AND EVALUATION

Regardless of the mechanism causing the multiple injuries, the initial medical management focuses on the life-threatening, nonorthopaedic injuries to stabilize the child's condition (2). The responsibility for the initial lifesaving resuscitation is rarely the responsibility of the orthopaedist, though such resuscitative efforts by the orthopaedist may be more commonly required in nontrauma centers and/or those in rural settings.

The Child Is Different

The initial steps in resuscitation of a child are essentially the same as those used for an adult (2,12,40). In severe injuries, the establishment of an adequate airway immediately at the accident site often means the difference between life and death. The cervical spine needs to be stabilized for transport if the child is unconscious or if neck pain is present. A special transport board with a cut-out for the occipital area is recommended for children younger than 6 years of age, because the size of the head at this age is larger in relation to the rest of the body. Because of this larger head size, if a young child is placed on a normal transport board, the cervical spine is flexed, a position that is best avoided if a neck injury is suspected (41).

Fluid Replacement

Once an adequate airway is established, the amount of hemorrhage from the injury, either internally or externally, should be assessed. This blood loss should be replaced initially with intravenous crystalloid solution. In younger children, rapid intravenous access may be difficult. In this situation, the use of intraosseous fluid infusion should be considered for administration of both fluid and medications. Guy et al (42) reported successful intraosseous infusion into the tibias of 15 children between the ages of 3 months and 10 years. In this series, intraosseous needles were placed by prehospital and hospital personnel, and colloid, crystalloid solution, and blood were all given by this route; no complications occurred in the surviving children. Bielski et al (43), in a rabbit tibia model, likewise demonstrated no adverse effects on the histology of bone or the adjacent physis with intraosseous injection of various resuscitation drugs and fluids.

Because death is common if hypovolemic shock is not rapidly reversed, the child's blood pressure must be maintained at an adequate level for organ perfusion. Most multiply injured children have sustained blunt trauma rather than penetrating injuries, and most of the blood loss is internal from visceral injury or from pelvic and femoral fractures. Because of this problem, the blood loss may be easily underestimated at first. The "triad of death," consisting of acidosis, hypothermia, and coagulopathy, has been described to occur in trauma patients as a result of hypovolemia and the systemic response to trauma (44). Peterson et al recently reported that an initial base deficit of ≤ -8 in pediatric trauma patients requiring mechanical ventilation was associated with a 23% mortality rate compared to 6% in those with an initial base deficit >8 (45).

Despite the need to stabilize the child's blood pressure, caution needs to be exercised in children with head injuries so that overhydration is avoided, because cerebral edema is better treated with relative fluid restriction. Excessive fluid replacement also may lead to further internal fluid shifts, which often produce a drop in the arterial oxygenation from interstitial pulmonary edema, especially when there has been direct trauma to the thorax and lungs. In some instances, in order to accurately assess the appropriate amount of fluid replacement, a central venous catheter is inserted during initial resuscitation. A urinary catheter is essential during the resuscitation to monitor urine output as a means of gauging adequate organ perfusion.

EVALUATION AND ASSESSMENT

Trauma Rating Systems

After the initial resuscitation has stabilized the injured child's condition, it is essential to perform a quick but thorough check for other injuries. A number of injury rating systems have been proposed, but the Injury Severity Score (ISS) is a valid, reproducible rating system that can be widely applied in the pediatric polytrauma setting (Table 4-1) (46). Another injury rating system for children that has been shown to be valid and reproducible is the Pediatric Trauma Score (PTS) (Table 4-2) (47). The injury rating system chosen varies among trauma centers, but whether the ISS or PTS is used, these systems allow an objective means to assess mortality risk at the time of initial treatment, as well as allowing some degree of prediction of future disability (7,48,49).

Head injury is most often evaluated and rated by the Glasgow Coma Scale (GCS), which evaluates eye opening (1–4 points), motor function (1–6 points), and verbal function (1–6 points) on a total scale of 3 to 15 points (Table 4-3) (50). There are some limitations in the use of the GCS in children who are preverbal or who are in the early verbal stages of development; but in other children, this rating system has been a useful guide for predicting early mortality and later disability. As a rough guide in verbal children, a GCS score of <8 points means a significantly worse chance of survival for these children than for those with a GCS >8 points. The GCS should be noted on arrival in the trauma center and should be repeated 1 hour after the child arrives at the hospital (Fig. 4-1). Serial changes in the GCS correlate with improvement or worsening of the neurologic injury. Repeated GCS assessments over the initial 72 hours after injury may be of prognostic significance. In addition to the level of oxygenation present at the initial presentation to the hospital, the 72-hour GCS motor response score has been noted to be very predictive of later permanent disability as a sequel to the head injury (51).

Physical Assessment

In a child with multiple injuries, a careful abdominal examination is essential to allow early detection of injuries to the liver, spleen, pancreas, or kidneys. Ecchymosis on the abdominal wall must be noted, because this is often a sign of significant visceral injury or spinal injury (52,53). In one series, 48% (22/46) of children with such ecchymosis required abdominal exploration (52), while in another series 23% (14/61) of children were noted to have spine fractures (53).

Swelling, deformity, or crepitus in any extremity is noted, and appropriate imaging studies are arranged to evaluate potential extremity injuries more fully. If extremity deformity is present, it is important to determine whether the fracture is open or closed. Sites of external bleeding are examined, and pressure dressings are applied if necessary to prevent further blood loss. It has been reported that the presence of a pelvic fracture and one or more other skeletal injuries should serve as a marker for the presence of head and abdominal injuries (54). Major arterial injuries associated with fractures of the extremity usually are diagnosed early by the lack of a peripheral pulse. However, abdominal venous injuries following blunt trauma are less common and are less commonly diagnosed before exploratory lapa-

TABLE 4-1 Injury Severity Score

Abbreviated Injury Scale (AIS)

The AIS classifies injuries as moderate, severe, serious, critical, and fatal for each of the five major body systems. The criteria for each system into the various categories is listed in a series of charts for each level of severity. Each level of severity is given a numerical code (1–5). The criteria for severe level (Code 4) is listed below.

Severity Code	(AIS) Severity Category/Injury Description	Policy Code
4	Severe (Life-Threatening, Survival Probable)	B

General

Severe lacerations and/or avulsions with dangerous hemorrhage.
30%–50% surface second or three degree burns.

Head and Neck

Cerebral injury with or without skull fracture, with unconsciousness >15 min, with definite abnormal neurologic signs; posttraumatic amnesia 3–12 h.
Compound skull fracture.

Chest

Open chest wounds; flail chest; pneumomediastinum; myocardial contusion without circulatory embarrassment; pericardial injuries.

Abdomen

Minor laceration of intra-abdominal contents (ruptured spleen, kidney, and injuries to tail of pancreas)
Intraperitoneal bladder rupture
Avulsion of the genitals
Thoracic and/or lumbar spine fractures with paraplegia

Extremities

Multiple closed long bone fractures
Amputation of limbs

Injury Severity Score (ISS)

The injury severity score (ISS) is a combination of values obtained from the AIS. The ISS is the sum of the squares of the highest AIS grade in each of the three most severely injured areas. For example, a person with a laceration of the aorta (AIS = 5), multiple closed long bone fractures (AIS = 4), and retroperitoneal hemorrhage (AIS = 3) would have an injury severity score of 50 (25 + 16 + 9). The highest possible score for a person with trauma to a single area is 25. The use of the ISS has dramatically increased the correlation between the severity and mortality. The range of severity is from 0 to 75.

Committee on Medical Aspects of Automotive Safety: Rating the severity of tissue damage I. The abbreviated scale. *JAMA* 1971;215: 277–280; Baker SP, O'Neill B, Haddon W Jr, Long WB. The Injury Severity Score: A method for describing patients with multiple injuries and evaluating emergency care. *J Trauma* 1974;14:187–196; with permission.

rotomy. About half of abdominal venous injuries have been reported to be fatal, so the trauma surgeon needs to consider this diagnosis in children who continue to require substantial blood volume support after the initial resuscitation has been completed (55).

Initial splinting of suspected extremity fractures is routinely done by the transporting team members at the scene of the accident. However, once the injured child is in the hospital, the orthopaedist should personally inspect the extremities to determine the urgency with which the extremity injuries need to be definitively treated. Most important are whether a vascular injury has occurred and whether the fracture is open or closed. The back and spine should be carefully examined. If there is not an open fracture and if the peripheral vascular function is normal, there is less urgency in treating the fracture and splinting will suffice until the other organ system injuries are stabilized.

Splinting decreases the child's pain while the child is resuscitated and stabilized and minimizes additional trauma to the soft tissue envelope surrounding the fracture. Splinting also facilitates transport of the child within the hospital while the trauma work-up, including appropriate imaging studies, is completed. If the child is to be transferred to a trauma center, splints prove invaluable for patient comfort and safety during transfer.

Any evident neurologic deficit is noted in order to document the extremity function before any treatment. It is important to remember that a detailed neurologic exam may not be possible since these are often young and/or scared children who are in pain and may have a central nervous system injury. The inability to obtain a reliable exam should also be documented.

Because head injuries and/or extreme pain in certain locations are often present at the time of presentation, it is not uncommon for some injuries to be missed initially. In a series of 149 pediatric polytrauma patients, there were 13 injuries diagnosed an average of 15 days following injury, including five fractures (one involving the spine), four abdominal injuries, two aneurysms, one head injury, and one facial fracture (56). Given this 9% incidence of delayed diagnosis, it is imperative that polytrauma patients be reexamined once they are more comfortable to reassess for potential sites of injury. In addition, children with head injuries need to be reassessed once they awaken enough to cooperate with reexamination. Families and patients need to be informed of the frequency of delayed diagnosis of some injuries in polytrauma patients so that they can partner with the medical team in recognizing such injuries (often evident as previously undetected sites of pain or dysfunction).

Imaging Studies

Radiographs

Imaging studies need to be performed as quickly as possible after the initial resuscitation and physical examination are complete. Any extremity suspected of having a significant injury should be examined on x-ray to assess the degree of injury. If

TABLE 4-2 Pediatric Trauma Score*

	Category		
Component	+2	+1	−1
Size	≥20 kg	10–20 kg	<10 kg
Airway	Normal	Maintainable	Unmaintainable
Systolic BP	≥90 mm Hg	90–50 mm Hg	<50 mm Hg
CNS	Awake	Obtunded/LOC	Coma/decerebrate
Open wound	None	Minor	Major/penetrating
Skeletal	None	Closed fracture	Open/multiple fractures

* This scoring system includes six common determinants of the clinical condition in the injured child. Each of the six determinants is assigned a grade: +2, minimal or no injury; +1, minor or potentially major injury; −1, major, or immediate life-threatening injury. The scoring system is arranged in a manner standard with advanced trauma life-support protocol, and thereby provides a quick assessment scheme. The ranges are from −6 for a severely traumatized child to +12 for a least traumatized child. This system has been confirmed in its reliability as a predictor of injury severity. From Tepas JJ, Mollitt DL, Talbers JL, et al. The Pediatric Trauma Score as a predictor of injury severity in the injured child. *J Pediatr Surg* 1987;22:14–18, with permission.

TABLE 4-3 Glasgow Coma Scale*

Response	Action	Score
Best motor response	Obeys	M6
	Localizes	5
	Withdraws	4
	Abnormal flexion	3
	Extensor response	2
	Nil	1
Verbal response	Oriented	V5
	Confused conversation	4
	Inappropriate words	3
	Incomprehensible sounds	2
	Nil	1
Eye opening	Spontaneous	E4
	To speech	3
	To pain	2
	Nil	1

* This scale is used to measure the level of consciousness using the eye opening, best verbal, and best motor responses. The range of scores is from 3 for the most severe to 15 for the least involved. This is a measure of level and progression of changes in consciousness. From Jeannett E, Teasdale JB, Galbraith S, et al. Severe mood injuries in three countries. *J Neurol Neurosurg Psychiatry* 1977;40:291–298; with permission.

the child has a head injury or if neck pain is noted on the examination, a lateral cervical spine x-ray is obtained. If the lateral cervical spine x-ray is normal, no further views of the cervical spine are needed at this stage. Further work-up with a cervical spine MRI is necessary prior to cervical spine clearance in those who have persistent neck pain and/or tenderness and should be considered in those patients who remain obtunded. (See Magnetic Resonance Imaging section below.)

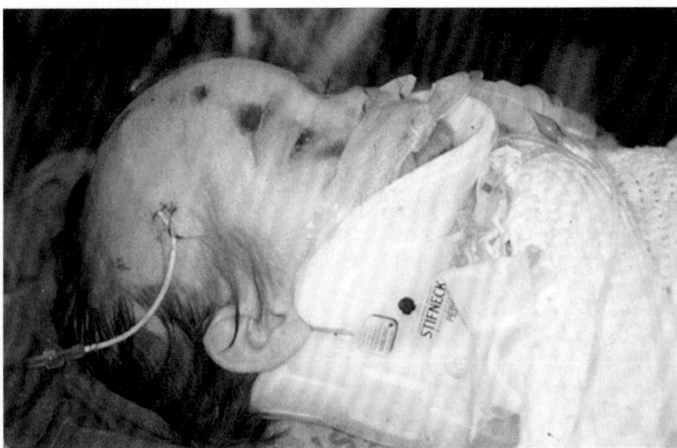

FIGURE 4-1 Temporary cervical spine stabilization is imperative in any child with multi-trauma, especially those who are unconscious or complain of neck pain.

If a cervical spine injury is present, the lateral x-ray of this area almost always will detect it. If there is suspicion of a cervical spine injury on the neutral lateral view, a lateral flexion x-ray of the cervical spine—taken in an awake patient in the presence of the orthopaedist—will help detect any cervical instability. The cervical spine of a young child is much more flexible than the cervical spine in an adult. Under the age of 12 years, the movement of C1 on C2 during flexion of the neck can normally be up to 5 mm, whereas in adults, this movement should be less than 3 mm. Likewise in this young age group, C2 can move up to 3 mm forward on C3 during neck flexion. No forward movement of C2 on C3 should be present in a skeletally mature individual when the neck is flexed. This so-called pseudosubluxation of C2 on C3 in a child should not be diagnosed as instability that requires treatment because this is a normal finding in most young children (57). Because it is difficult to detect a fracture of the thoracic or lumbar spine clinically, x-rays of this area, primarily a lateral view, should be assessed, particularly in a comatose child.

Computed Tomography

Computed tomography (CT) is essential in evaluating a child with multiple injuries. If a head injury is present, the CT of the head will detect skull fractures and intracranial bleeding. With abdominal swelling, pain, or bruising, a CT of the abdomen provides excellent visualization of the liver and spleen and allows quantification of the amount of hemorrhage present. Because most hepatic and splenic lacerations are treated nonoperatively (52,58,59), the CT scan and serial hematocrit levels are used to determine whether surgical treatment of these visceral lacerations is needed.

CT of the pelvis is more sensitive for pelvic fractures than is a screening pelvic x-ray (Fig. 4-2). In one recent study, a screening pelvic x-ray only demonstrated 54% of pelvic fractures identified on CT scan (60). The CT scan also proves invaluable in thoroughly evaluating fracture configuration and appropriate treatment options, both surgical and nonsurgical. If an abdominal CT is being done to evaluate visceral injury, it is simple to request that the abdominal CT be extended distally to include the pelvis. A CT of a fractured vertebra will provide the information needed to classify the fracture as stable or unstable and determine whether operative treatment is needed.

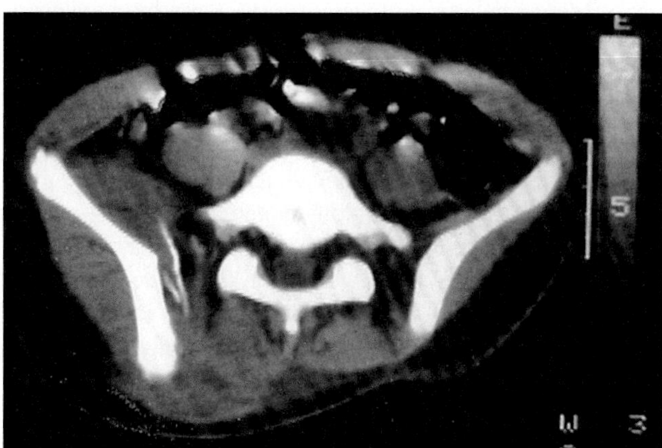

FIGURE 4-2 CT is an excellent addition to x-rays for evaluation of pelvic fractures.

Intravenous Pyelography

There is a strong correlation of urologic injury with anterior pelvic fractures, as well as with liver and spleen injury. Although CT and ultrasonography are used to evaluate renal injuries, the intravenous pyelogram still has a role in helping to diagnose bladder and urethral injuries (61). Regardless of the methods of imaging, the anatomy of the urethral disruption often cannot be accurately demonstrated preoperatively (62).

Radionuclide Scans

Bone scans have a limited role in the acute evaluation of a child with multiple injuries. In conjunction with a skeletal survey, a technetium-99m bone scan is sometimes used in children with suspected child abuse to detect previously undetected new or old fractures (18,23,24).

Heinrich et al (63) reported that bone scans in 48 children with multiple injuries often demonstrated an unsuspected injury. Nineteen previously unrecognized fractures were identified by obtaining x-rays of the areas with increased isotope uptake. In addition, there were 66 false-positive areas of increased uptake in the 48 patients. Of their 48 patients, six had a change in their orthopaedic care as a result of this bone scan, although this treatment was usually simple cast application of a nondisplaced fracture. Nonetheless, the bone scan can be a valuable screening tool in a child with multiple injuries from any cause. In some instances, the bone scan can be useful to differentiate a normal variation in skeletal ossification (normal uptake) from a fracture (increased uptake), particularly in an extremity or a spinal area where pain is present. Areas of increased uptake need to be imaged further to determine whether orthopaedic treatment is required.

Magnetic Resonance Imaging

Magnetic resonance imaging (MRI) is used primarily for the detection of injury to the brain or the spine and the spinal cord. In young children, the bony spine is more elastic than the spinal cord. As a result, a spinal cord injury can occur without an obvious spinal fracture in children with multiple injuries, particularly in automobile accidents (64–66). In the SCIWORA (spinal cord injury without radiographic abnormality) syndrome, MRI is valuable in demonstrating the site and extent of spinal cord injury and in defining the level of injury to the disks or vertebral apophysis. A fracture through the vertebral apophysis is similar to a fracture through the physis of a long bone and may not be obvious on planar x-rays. Recent authors have reported that the use of MRI in obtunded and intubated pediatric trauma patients can lead to a more prompt cervical spine clearance with a resultant decrease in hospital stay and cost (67).

MRI also is very useful in evaluating knee injuries, particularly when a hemarthrosis is present. If blood is present on knee arthrocentesis, MRI can assist in diagnosing an injury to the cruciate ligaments and/or menisci. In addition, a chondral fracture that cannot be seen on routine x-rays may be demonstrated by MRI.

Ultrasonography

Ultrasound evaluation has been shown to be an accurate means of detecting hemoperitoneum following injury. Some trauma centers have replaced peritoneal lavage and laparoscopy with serial ultrasound evaluations to monitor liver, spleen, pancreas, and kidney injury in children with multiple injuries (58,59,68). One problem with ultrasonography is the operator-dependent nature of this imaging study. Another is the fact that, unlike CT scans, ultrasonography cannot be used to rule out the frequently concomitant pelvic fractures. As a result, CT is more often used for assessment and monitoring of visceral injury in children sustaining multiple injuries. Recent comparisons of CT and ultrasonography demonstrated the superiority of CT for diagnosing visceral injury in children with polytrauma (69–72).

NONORTHOPAEDIC CONDITIONS IN THE MULTIPLY INJURED CHILD

Head Injury

Prognosis for Recovery

Head injuries occur in children with multiple injuries even more often than orthopaedic injuries. In a review of 494 pediatric polytrauma patients, Letts et al reported closed head injury in 17%, and skull fracture in 12% (56) while Schalamon et al recently reported injuries to the head and neck region in 87% of pediatric polytrauma patients (6). It has been clearly demonstrated that a child recovers more quickly and more fully from a significant head injury than does an adult (11,73,74). Even children who are in a coma for several hours to several days often recover full motor function. Mild cognitive or learning deficits may persist, however, so educational testing needs to be considered for children who have had head injury and coma. The two factors that have been identified to produce poorer functional recovery and more severe permanent neurologic deficits are a low oxygen saturation level at the time of presentation to the emergency department or trauma center and a low GCS score 72 hours after the head injury.

Despite the fact that excellent motor recovery is expected in most children after a head injury, children are often left with some residual deficits. Many children who sustain traumatic brain injuries (TBI) are unaware of their residual cognitive limitations and tend to overestimate their mental capacities (75). Children who have had a TBI also often have behavioral problems, the presence of which may be predictive of behavioral problems in uninjured siblings as well (76). Greenspan and MacKenzie reported that 55% of children in their series had one or more health problems at 1-year follow-up, many of which were relatively minor (77). Headaches were present in 32% and extremity complaints in 13% of patients. The presence of a lower extremity injury with a head injury led to a higher risk of residual problems.

Because of the more optimistic outlook for children with head injuries than for adults with similar injuries, orthopaedic care must be provided in a timely way, and the orthopaedist must base the orthopaedic care on the assumption that full neurologic recovery will ensue. Waiting for a child to recover from a coma is not appropriate, and comatose children tolerate general anesthesia well. The treatment undertaken for the orthopaedic injury is designed to optimize the orthopaedic outcome from the injury, with the assumption that the child will make a full neurologic recovery. Unless the musculoskeletal injuries are treated with the assumption that full neurologic recovery will take place, long bone fractures may heal in angled or shortened positions. Once neurologic recovery occurs, the primary functional deficit will then be from ill-managed orthopaedic injuries rather than from the neurologic injury.

Intracranial Pressure

After a head injury, intracranial pressure measurements are commonly monitored to prevent excessive intracranial pressure, which may lead to further permanent disability or death. Normally, intracranial pressure does not exceed 15 mm Hg, and all attempts should be made to keep this pressure under 30 mm Hg after a head injury.

This is accomplished by elevating the head of the bed to 30 degrees, lowering the P_{CO_2}, and restricting intravenous fluid administration. Ventilator assistance is used to lower the P_{CO_2}, which, in turn, helps lessen cerebral edema. Fluid restriction is also recommended if peripheral perfusion can be maintained despite the polytrauma. Elevation of serum norepinephrine has been shown to correlate well with the severity of head injury in patients with injury of multiple organ systems (78).

Motion at the site of a long bone fracture will cause an elevation of the intracranial pressure in children with multiple injuries. Because of this problem, long bone fractures must be immobilized to limit fracture motion until definitive fracture care can be provided. Initial immobilization usually is accomplished by splinting or casting of the fractures, or by use of traction for femoral shaft fractures. The use of external or internal fixation of fractures should be strongly considered to help control elevation of intracranial pressure. Fracture stabilization also facilitates dressing changes for the treatment of adjacent soft tissue injury as well as allowing in-hospital transport for imaging studies and other necessary treatments (79,80).

Secondary Orthopaedic Effects of Head Injuries

A head injury can have later impact on the management of musculoskeletal injuries, even after the acute phase has passed. Persistent spasticity, the development of contractures, heterotopic bone formation in soft tissue, and changes in fracture healing rates are all seen in children with sequelae of a head injury.

Spasticity. Spasticity may develop within a few days of head injury. The early effect of this spasticity is to cause shortening at the sites of long bone fractures if traction or splint or cast immobilization is being used. If fracture displacement or shortening occurs in a circumferential cast, the bone ends may cause pressure points between the bone and the cast, leading to skin breakdown at the fracture site, with a higher risk for deep infection. Even with skeletal traction for femoral fractures, fracture shortening and displacement will occur as the spasticity overcomes the traction forces. Once spasticity develops and long bone fractures displace, internal or external fixation is needed to maintain satisfactory reduction. This operative stabilization should be performed as soon as the spasticity becomes a problem for fracture reduction because fracture healing is accelerated by a head injury (79–81).

Contractures. The persistence of spasticity in the extremities often leads to subsequent contractures of the joints spanned by the spastic muscles. Contractures can arise quite quickly, and early preventative stretching or splinting should begin while the child is in the intensive care unit. Nonselective mass action muscle activity associated with brain injury can be used to help prevent these early contractures. If the child lies in bed with the hips and knees extended, there will usually be a strong plantarflexion of the feet at the ankles from the spasticity. If the hip and knee are placed in a flexed position, it will be much easier to dorsiflex the foot at the ankle, so **part-time** positioning in this way will prevent early equinus contractures from developing so quickly. Stretching and splinting can often be effective in preventing contractures; but if these measures are not successful, there should be no hesitation to treat these contractures surgically if they are interfering with subsequent rehabilitation.

Heterotopic Bone Formation. Heterotopic bone may form in the soft tissues of the extremity as early as a few weeks after a head injury with persistent coma (82). Usually, this is in the vicinity of the hip or elbow but may occur elsewhere. There is some evidence that heterotopic bone formation can be stimulated by surgical incisions. In head-injured teenagers who undergo antegrade reamed femoral intramedullary nailing of femoral fractures, heterotopic bone often forms at the nail insertion site that later restricts hip motion (83). Obtaining weekly serum alkaline phosphatase levels on a child with persistent coma may allow early detection of the heterotopic bone, although alkaline phosphatase is also elevated during healing of fractures. A sudden increase of alkaline phosphatase a few weeks after the onset of coma, even with fractures coexisting, may mean that heterotopic bone is starting to form and a more careful examination of the extremities is in order (84). Technetium-99 bone scans show increased isotope uptake in the soft tissue where heterotopic bone forms, and this imaging study should be considered if new swelling is noted in the extremity of a comatose child. Other diagnoses that must be considered in a comatose child with new swelling of the extremity are a new long bone fracture or a deep venous thrombosis (85).

Observation and excision are the two primary approaches taken in managing heterotopic bone formation in an injured child. If the child remains comatose, usually little treatment is administered. There is no conclusive data to support medical treatment if an early diagnosis of heterotopic bone formation is made. However, it may be useful to try to block some of the heterotopic bone formation by use of salicylates or nonsteroidal antiinflammatory medication once an early diagnosis is established. If the child has recovered from the head injury and has heterotopic bone that does not interfere with rehabilitation, no intervention is required. If there is significant restriction of joint motion from the heterotopic bone, this bone should be excised to facilitate rehabilitation. The timing of the heterotopic bone excision is somewhat controversial, but current thinking leans toward resection whenever heterotopic bone significantly interferes with rehabilitation, rather than waiting for 12 to 18 months until the bone is more mature. After surgical excision, it is essential to use prophylaxis to prevent recurrence with local low-dose radiation therapy or medications (salicylates or nonsteroidal antiinflammatory drugs) immediately after the excision to block new heterotopic bone formation at the operative site. Mital et al (84) reported success in preventing recurrence of heterotopic bone after excision by use of salicylates at a dosage of 40 mg/kg/day in divided doses for 6 weeks postoperatively.

Fracture Healing Rates. For reasons that are not entirely clear, long bone fractures heal more quickly in children and adults who have associated head injuries. It has been demonstrated that polytrauma patients in a coma have a much higher serum calcitonin level than do conscious patients with similar long bone fractures, but how or whether this finding influences fracture healing is still unclear (86).

Peripheral Nerve Injuries

Although persistent neurologic deficits in a child who has multiple injuries usually are sequelae of a head injury, peripheral nerve injury should be carefully assessed as the rehabilitation process proceeds. In one clinical review of brain-injured children, 7% had evidence of an associated peripheral nerve injury documented by electrodiagnostic testing (87). The peripheral nerve injury most often is associated with an adjacent fracture or with a stretching injury of the extremity. In most cases, observation is indicated since these injuries often recover spontaneously. However, if the nerve injury is at the level of an open fracture, then exploration of the nerve is indicated. In children being observed following a nerve injury, if function does not return within 2 to 3 months, then electrodiagnostic testing should be undertaken. It is important to recognize these injuries because surgical peripheral nerve repair with nerve grafts offers an excellent chance of nerve function recovery in young patients.

Abdominal Trauma

Abdominal viscera, both solid and hollow, are at high risk of significant injury in children with multiple skeletal injuries. Recent studies have reported abdominal injuries in 8% (56) to 27% (88) of pediatric polytrauma patients. Abdominal swelling, tenderness, or bruising are all signs of injury. CT evaluation has largely replaced peritoneal lavage or laparoscopy as the initial method of evaluation of abdominal injury. Abdominal injury is not unusual if a child in an accident has been wearing a lap seat belt, regardless of whether a contusion is evident (52,89). Bond et al (90) noted that the presence of multiple pelvic fractures strongly correlated (80%) with the presence of abdominal or genitourinary injury, whereas the child's age or mechanism of injury had no such correlation with abdominal injury rates. Though hepatic and splenic injuries are much more common, 22% of pediatric cases of pancreatitis have been reported to result from trauma (91).

The usual practice is to treat hepatic and splenic lacerations nonoperatively, by monitoring the hematocrit, by repeating the abdominal examination frequently, and by serial CT scans or ultrasound examinations (92–97). Once the child's overall condition has stabilized, the presence of abdominal injuries that are being observed should not delay the fracture care as long as the child is stable enough to undergo general anesthesia.

Genitourinary Injuries

Injuries to the genitourinary system are uncommon in the general polytrauma population. Letts reported an incidence of 1% in pediatric polytrauma patients (56). However, injuries to the genitourinary system generally have been reported in 9% (98) to 24% (99) of children with pelvic fractures. Most injuries to the bladder and urethra are associated with fractures of the anterior pelvic ring (Fig. 4-3) (100). Such injuries are more common in males and usually occur at the bulbourethra, but the bladder, prostate, and other portions of the urethra can also be injured (61,100). Though less common following pelvic fracture in girls, such injuries are often associated with severe injuries including those to the vagina and rectum, with long-term concerns regarding continence, stricture formation, and childbearing (101,102). If the iliac wings are displaced or the pelvic ring shape is changed, it may be necessary to reduce these fractures in order to reconstitute the birth canal in female patients. There are increased rates of caesarean section in young women who have had a pelvic fracture compared with those without this injury (103). It is important to inform adolescent females with displaced pelvic fractures of this later potential problem with vaginal delivery. If the injury is severe, kidney injury may also occur, but most urologic injuries that occur with pelvic fractures are distal to the ureters (104).

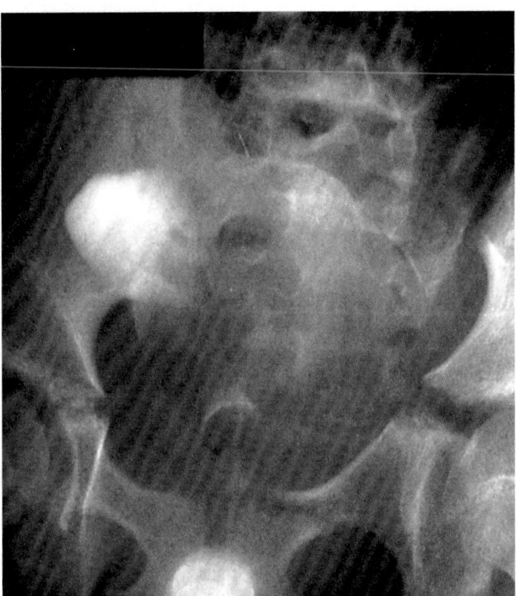

FIGURE 4-3 Most injuries to the bladder and urethra are associated with anterior pelvic ring fractures and should be suspected with these injuries.

Fat Embolism

Although fat embolism and acute respiratory distress syndrome are relatively common in adults with multiple long bone fractures, they are rare in young children (105,106). When they are present, the signs and symptoms are the same as in adults: axillary petechiae, hypoxemia, and x-ray changes of pulmonary infiltrates appearing within several hours of the fractures. It is likely that some degree of hypoxemia develops in some children after multiple fractures, but the full clinical picture of fat embolism seldom develops. If a child with multiple fractures but without a head injury develops a change in sensorium and orientation, hypoxemia is most likely the cause, and arterial blood gases are essential to determine the next step in management. The other primary cause of mental status change after fractures is overmedication with narcotics for pain control.

If fat embolism is diagnosed by low levels of arterial oxygenation, the treatment is the same as in adults. Usually, this management consists of endotracheal intubation, positive pressure ventilation, and hydration with intravenous fluid. The effect of early fracture stabilization, intravenous alcohol, or high-dose corticosteroids on the syndrome of fat embolism has not been studied well in children with multiple injuries.

Nutritional Requirements

Multiple injuries place large caloric demands on the body. If an injured child requires ventilator support for several days, caloric intake via a feeding tube or a central intravenous catheter is necessary to improve healing and help prevent complications from developing. The baseline caloric needs of a child can be determined based on the weight and age of the child. Children on mechanical ventilation in a pediatric intensive care unit have been shown to require 150% of the basal energy or caloric requirements for age and weight (107). The daily nitrogen requirement for a child in the acute injury phase is 250 mg/kg.

ORTHOPAEDIC MANAGEMENT OF THE MULTIPLY INJURED CHILD

Timing

Because fractures are rarely life-threatening in children with multiple system injuries, splinting of the fractures will generally suffice as the initial orthopaedic care needed, while the child's overall condition is stabilized. Loder (108) reported that in 78 children with multiple injuries, early operative stabilization of fractures within the first 2 or 3 days after injury led to a shorter hospital stay, a shorter stay in the intensive care unit, and a shorter time on ventilator assistance. In addition, there were fewer complications in those who underwent surgical treatment of the fractures less than 72 hours after injury. In a more recent study, Loder et al reported a trend toward a higher rate of complications of immobilization (including pulmonary complications) in fractures treated late (after 72 hr), though the difference did not reach statistical significance (109). In this more recent study, age greater than 7 years and MISS (Modified Injury Severity Score) ≥40 were predictive of an increased rate of complications of immobilization. A mixed series of adults and children demonstrated comparable results for early (within 24 hr) and late fixation (after 24 hr) of fractures in the setting of blunt trauma and severe head injuries (110).

Pelvic Fractures

Fractures of the pelvis are common in children and adolescents with multiple injuries, and have been reported in up to 7% of children referred to level I regional trauma centers (111). In one recent series of 166 pelvic fractures, 60% of pelvic fractures involved a pedestrian struck by a motor vehicle, 22% a passenger in a motor vehicle accident, and 13% children who had fallen (98). Though many of these pelvic injuries are stable, a review of 189 pelvic ring fractures reported that unstable patterns were found in 30% of cases (57/189) (112).

Injuries to the axial skeleton have been reported to be associated with the most intense hospital care and higher mortality rates than other injury combinations (8). In their series of 166 consecutive pelvic fractures, Silber et al reported associated "significant" head trauma in 39%, chest trauma in 20% and visceral/abdominal injuries in 19% and a mortality rate of 3.6% (Fig. 4-4) (98). The immediate problem often is control of bleeding, either from the retroperitoneum near the fracture or from the peritoneum from injured viscera (113). However, death of children with pelvic fractures appears to be caused more often by an associated head injury rather than an injury to the adjacent viscera or vessels (114).

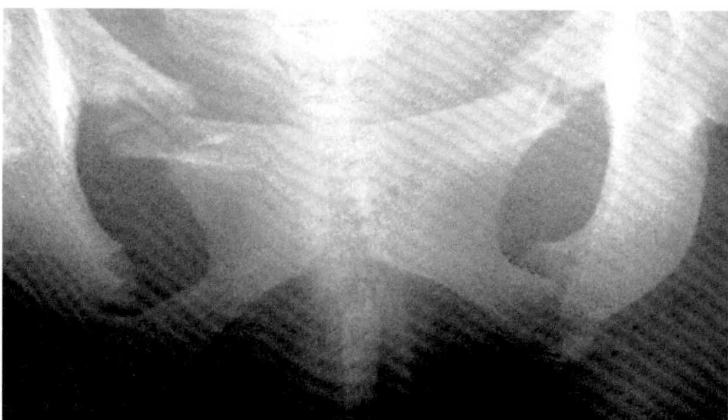

FIGURE 4-4 Bilateral superior and inferior pubic rami fractures. Genitourinary and abdominal injuries must be ruled out with severe pelvic fractures.

The fractures of the anterior pelvic ring are the primary cause of urethral injury (100–102,104), though urethral injuries are reported to occur less frequently in children than in adults (98). Bilateral anterior and posterior pelvic fractures are most likely to cause severe bleeding (115), although death from blood loss in children is uncommon (114,116). Silber et al reported acetabular fractures in 12% (20/166) of pelvic fractures (98). Injury to the sciatic nerve or the lumbosacral nerve roots may result from hemipelvis displacement through a vertical shear fracture. Nonorthopaedic injuries associated with pelvic fractures led to long-term morbidity or mortality in 31% (11/36) of patients in one published review of pediatric pelvic fractures (117).

Most pelvic fractures in children are treated nonoperatively. In a child or preadolescent, an external fixator can be used to close a marked pubic diastasis or to control bleeding by stabilizing the pelvis for transport and other injury care. The external fixator will not reduce a displaced vertical shear fracture, but the stability provided is helpful to control the hemorrhage while the child's condition is stabilized (99,118).

Open Fractures

Background

Most serious open fractures in children result from high-velocity blunt injury involving vehicles. Penetrating injuries are much less common in children than in adults. However, many low-energy blunt injuries can cause puncture wounds in the skin adjacent to fractures, especially displaced radial, ulnar, and tibial fractures. In children with multiple injuries, approximately 10% of the fractures are open (6,8). When open fractures are present, 25% to 50% of patients have additional injuries involving the head, chest, abdomen, and other extremities.

Wound Classification

The classification used to describe the soft tissues adjacent to an open fracture is based primarily on the system described by Gustilo and Anderson and colleagues (119,120). Primary factors that are considered and ranked in this classification system are the size of the wound, the degree of wound contamination, and the presence or absence of an associated vascular injury (Table 4-4).

Type I. Type I fractures usually result from a spike of bone puncturing the skin (inside-out). The wound is less than 1 cm in size, and there is minimal local soft tissue damage or contamination.

Type II. A type II wound is generally larger than 1 cm and is typically associated with a transverse or oblique fracture with minimal comminution. There is adjacent soft tissue injury, including skin flaps or skin avulsion and a moderate crushing component of adjacent soft tissue is usually present. Skin grafts or flaps should not be needed for coverage.

Type III and Subgroups. The most severe open fractures are classified as type III, with associated subgroups A, B, or C, with the letters indicating increasing severity of injury. These fractures typically result from high-velocity trauma and are associated with extensive soft tissue injury, a large open wound, and significant wound contamination. In a type IIIA fracture, there is soft tissue coverage over the bone, which often is a segmental fracture. In a type IIIB fracture, bone is exposed at the fracture site, with treatment typically requiring skin and/or muscle flap coverage of the bone. Type IIIC fractures are defined as those with an injury to a major artery in that segment of the extremity. Though these injuries are commonly associated with extensive soft tissue loss and contamination, a type IIIC injury may, in fact, be associated with even a small wound in some cases.

This classification is widely used and has been shown to correlate in adults with sequelae of the injury, including the potential for infection, delayed union, nonunion, amputation, and residual impairment. The final functional results of type III fractures in children appear to be superior to results after similar fractures in adults, likely due to their better peripheral vascular supply.

TABLE 4-4 Classification of Open Fractures

Type I	An open fracture with a wound <1 cm long and clean
Type II	An open fracture with a laceration >1 cm long without extensive soft-tissue damage, flaps, or avulsions
Type III	Massive soft tissue damage, compromised vascularity, severe wound contamination marked fracture instability
Type IIIA	Adequate soft tissue coverage of a fractured bone despite extensive soft tissue laceration or flaps, or high-energy trauma irrespective of the size of the wound
Type IIIB	Extensive soft-tissue injury loss with periosteal stripping and bone exposure; usually associated with massive contamination
Type IIIC	Open fracture associated with arterial injury requiring repair

Adapted from Gustilo RB, Mendoza RM, Williams DN. Problems in the management of type III (severe) open fractures: a new classification of type III open fractures. *J Trauma* 1984;24:742–746; Gustilo RB, Anderson JT. Prevention of infection in the treatment of 1025 open fractures of long bones, retrospective and prospective analyses. *J Bone Joint Surg Am* 1976;58:453–458; with permission.

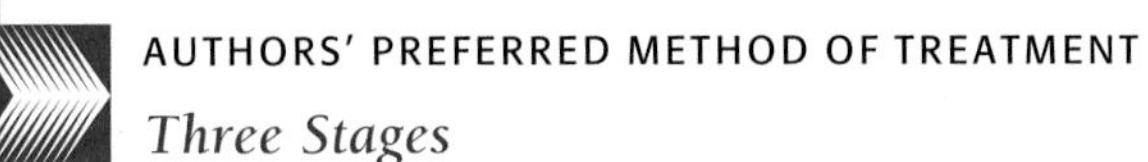

AUTHORS' PREFERRED METHOD OF TREATMENT

Three Stages

We consider the treatment of open fractures in children to be similar to that for open fractures in adults. The primary goals are to prevent infection of the wound and fracture site, while allowing soft tissue healing, fracture union, and eventual return of optimal function. Initial emergency care includes the so-called ABCs of resuscitation, application of a sterile povidone-iodine (Betadine) dressing, and preliminary alignment, and splinting of the fracture for patient transport. If profuse bleeding is present, a compression dressing is applied to limit blood loss. In the emergency room, masks and gloves should be worn as each wound is thoroughly inspected. Tetanus prophylaxis is provided, and the initial dose of intravenous antibiotics is given. The dose of tetanus toxoid is 0.5 mL intramuscularly to be given if the patient's immunization status is unknown, or if it is more than 5 years since the last dose. The second stage of management is the primary surgical treatment, including initial and (if necessary) repeat debridement of the tissues in the area of the open fracture until the entire wound appears viable. The fracture is reduced and stabilized at this time. If the bone ends are not covered with viable soft tissue, muscle or skin flap coverage is considered. Vacuum-assisted closure with the VAC device (Kinetic Concepts, Inc., San Antonio, TX) may be a useful adjunct to facilitate coverage and obviate the need for flaps in some patients (121–123). The third and final stage of this management is bony reconstruction as needed if bone loss has occurred and, ultimately, rehabilitation of the child.

Cultures

Previous studies have demonstrated poor correlation of growth on routine cultures with wound infections (124,125). Lee reported that neither pre- nor postdebridement cultures accurately predicted the risk of infection in open fractures (124). Lee noted that only 20% of wounds (24/119) with positive predebridement cultures and only 28% (9/32) with positive postdebridement cultures became infected. Though postdebridement cultures were more predictive of infection, postdebridement cultures identified the causative organism in only 42% (8/19) of infected wounds. Valenziano et al found that cultures at the time of presentation to the trauma center are also of no value, with only 2 of 28 patients (7%) with positive cultures becoming infected, in comparison to 5 of 89 patients (6%) with negative initial cultures (125). In only 29% (2/7) of cases which became infected were initial cultures positive. Open fractures do not need to be routinely cultured. Cultures should only be obtained only at the time of reoperation in patients with clinical evidence of infection.

Antibiotic Therapy

Antibiotic therapy decreases the risk of infection in children with open fractures. Wilkins and Patzakis (126) reported a 13.9% infection rate in 79 patients who received no antibiotics after open fractures, whereas there was a 5.5% infection rate in 815 patients with similar injuries who had antibiotic prophylaxis. Bacterial contamination has been noted in 70% of open fractures in children, with both gram-positive and gram-negative infections noted, depending on the degree of wound contamination and adjacent soft tissue injury. We limit antibiotic administration generally to 48 to 72 hours after surgical treatment of the open fracture.

For all type I and some type II fractures, we use a first-generation cephalosporin (cefazolin 100 mg/kg/day divided q 8 hr, maximal daily dose 6 g). For more severe type II fractures and for type III fractures, we use a combination of a cephalosporin and aminoglycoside (gentamicin 5–7.5 mg/kg/day divided q 8 hr). For farm injuries or grossly contaminated fractures, penicillin (150,000 units/kg/day divided q 6 hr, maximal daily dose 24 million units) is added to the cephalosporin and aminoglycoside. All antibiotics are given intravenously for 48 to 72 hours. Oral antibiotics are occasionally used if significant soft tissue erythema at the open fracture site remains after the intravenous antibiotics have been completed. Gentamicin levels should be checked after 4 or 5 doses (and doses adjusted as necessary) during therapy to minimize the risk of ototoxicity.

The antibiotic regimen is continued for 48 to 72 hours. An additional 48 to 72 hours course is given around subsequent surgeries such as those for (a) repeat irrigation and debridement, (b) delayed wound closure, (c) open reduction and internal fixation of fractures, and (d) secondary bone reconstruction procedures.

Debridement and Irrigation

We consider debridement and irrigation of the open fracture in the operating room to be the most important step in the primary management of open fractures in children. Some authors have reported that significantly higher infection rates occurred if debridement and irrigation were done more than 6 hours after open fractures in children (127). A recent report, however, demonstrated an overall infection rate of 1% to 2% after open long bone fractures, with no difference in infection rates between groups of patients treated with irrigation and debridement within 6 hours of injury and those treated between 6 and 24 hours following injury (128). One likely reason for the low rate of infection in the aforementioned series is the early administration of intravenous antibiotics in both groups. Though up to a 24-hour delay does not appear to have adverse consequences regarding infection rates, it may be necessary to perform an earlier irrigation and debridement in order to minimize compromise of the soft tissue envelope. The debridement needs to be performed carefully and systematically to remove all foreign and nonviable material from the wound. The order of debridement typically is

1. Excision of the necrotic tissue from the wound edges
2. Extension of the wound to adequately explore the fracture ends
3. Debridement of the wound edges to bleeding tissue
4. Resection of necrotic skin, fat, muscle, and contaminated fascia
5. Fasciotomies as needed
6. Thorough pulsatile irrigation of the fracture ends and wound

Because secondary infection in ischemic muscle can be a major problem in wound management and healing, all ischemic muscle is widely debrided back to muscle which bleeds at the cut edge and contracts when pinched with the forceps.

When debriding and irrigating an open diaphyseal fracture, we always bring the proximal and distal bone ends into the wound to allow visual inspection and thorough irrigation and debridement. This often necessitates extension of the open wound, but is preferable to leaving the fracture site contaminated. We carefully remove devitalized bone fragments and contaminated cortical bone with curettes or a small rongeur. If there is a possibly nonviable bone fragment, judgment is needed as to whether this bone fragment should be removed or left in place. Small fracture fragments without soft tissue attachments are removed, whereas very large ones may be retained if they are not significantly contaminated. Our experience is that reconstruction of a large segmental bone loss has a better outcome in children than in adults, because children have a better potential for bone regeneration and have better vascular supply to their extremities. Nearby major neurovascular structures in the area of the fracture are identified and protected. We consider the debridement complete when all contaminated, dead, and ischemic tissues have been excised; the bones ends are clean with bleeding edges; and only viable tissue lines the wound bed.

We usually use a pulsed lavage system to irrigate the open fracture with sterile normal saline. We routinely use 10 L for the lower extremities, but often use 5 L in the upper extremities due to the smaller compartment size. We previously used bacitracin and polymyxin antibiotics in this irrigation solution, but now irrigate only with normal saline. The antibiotic addition is more costly and does not seem necessary, since the key seems to be local irrigation and debridement to allow the intravenous antibiotics to reach the wound and control the infection. We do not obtain cultures because of the poor correlation of intraoperative cultures with the incidence of infection and with the infecting organisms.

After the debridement and irrigation are complete, we try to use the local soft tissue to cover the neurovascular structures, tendons, and bone ends. If local soft tissue coverage is inadequate, consideration should be given to local muscle flaps or other coverage methods, including vacuum-assisted closure. The area of the wound that has been incised to extend the wound for fracture inspection can be primarily closed with interrupted nylon sutures. The traumatic wound should either be left open to drain or may be closed over one or more drains. Wounds which are left open may be dressed with a moistened Betadine or saline dressing. Grade II and III fractures are routinely reoperated on every 48 to 72 hours thereafter for repeat irrigation and debridement until the wounds appear clean and the tissue viable. This cycle is repeated until the wound can be sutured closed or a split thickness skin graft or local flap is used to cover it. If flap coverage is necessary, this is optimally accomplished within 1 week of injury.

Fracture Stabilization

Fracture stabilization in children with open fractures decreases pain, protects the soft tissue envelope from further injury, decreases the spread of bacteria, allows stability important for early soft tissue coverage, and improves the fracture union rate.

In general terms, our principles for stabilization of open fractures in children include allowing access to the soft tissue wound and the extremity to allow for debridement and dressing changes, allowing weight bearing when appropriate and preserving full motion of the adjacent joints to allow full functional recovery.

Though casts or splints may be used to stabilize type I fractures and occasionally type II fractures with relatively small wounds and minimal soft tissue involvement, difficulties with soft tissue management and loss of alignment as swelling subsides are common with such closed treatment. Most of these injuries involve the radius or ulna in the upper extremity or the tibia in the lower extremity. Splint or cast immobilization generally is not satisfactory for the more unstable type II and most type III injuries.

For diaphyseal forearm fractures, a flexible intramedullary implant in the radius and/or ulna, commonly provides enough stability of the fracture to allow dressing changes through the cast or splint. For intramedullary fixation, we prefer flexible titanium implants of 2 to 4 mm diameter for stabilizing open fractures in the forearm when reduction of either the radial or ulnar fracture is unstable. Since the ulnar canal is straight, the implant chosen is often at least 80% of the narrowest canal diameter, while the implant for the radius is generally 50% to 60% of the narrowest canal diameter. The ulnar implant is inserted antegrade, whereas the radial implant is inserted retrograde just proximal to the distal radial physis. One or both bones can be stabilized, and the implants removed easily after fracture healing.

For distal forearm fractures percutaneous pinning of the radius (and, occasionally, the ulna) is generally appropriate and provides sufficient stability. A short-arm cast is generally sufficient to maintain appropriate alignment following such fixation. The pins are removed in the office at 3 to 4 weeks, though a cast is used for a total of 6 weeks.

We also use flexible intramedullary nails often for open fractures of the femoral shaft. For type III fractures, especially if there is a large or contaminated soft tissue wound present, external fixation may be indicated.

Flexible intramedullary rod fixation has replaced external fixation as our treatment of choice for most open tibial and femoral fractures in children. Both intramedullary rodding and external fixation allow access to the wound for debridement and dressing changes plus any soft tissue reconstruction needed. Such access may be somewhat limited with fixators, especially when there are extensive soft tissue wounds. Intramedullary rods are generally better tolerated by patients and families, do not require daily care, leave more cosmetic scars, and are load-sharing devices. With intramedullary rodding, the child is allowed to weight bear as tolerated following transverse or short oblique fractures, but weight bearing is protected for 4 to 6 weeks following comminuted or spiral fractures.

External fixation is preferable for fractures with segmental bone loss, and ring fixators may even be used in such instances for bone transport. External fixation allows weight bearing relatively soon after the injury. We find that a uniplanar frame is best for most fractures and is relatively easy to apply. For some segmental fractures in the metaphysis and diaphysis, as well as soft tissue injuries, a ring fixator may be a better choice.

We use open reduction and internal fixation for open intraarticular fractures. When feasible, fixation should be parallel to (and avoid) the physis. Cannulated screws are often used in such instances. Screws or threaded pins should never be placed across the physis. If fixation across the physis is necessary, smooth pins are used; they should be removed

3 to 4 weeks postinjury in order to minimize the risk of growth disturbance.

For fractures that involve both the metaphysis and diaphysis, open reduction and internal fixation may be combined with external fixation. For diaphyseal fractures in skeletally immature children, we prefer flexible intramedullary nails to compression plates for internal fixation of type I, type II, and some type III fractures. The role of intramedullary versus external fixation for type IIIB fractures has not been firmly established. For treatment of a *floating joint*, usually the knee or elbow, we almost always stabilize both fractures operatively (129–131).

Wound Management

Serial irrigation and debridement are performed every 2 to 3 days until the wounds are clean and all remaining tissue appears viable. Fracture fixation at the time of initial surgery (as described previously) facilitates wound management. We prefer to provide soft tissue coverage of the open fracture and adjacent soft tissue defect by 5 to 7 days after the injury in order to limit the risk of later infection. Most type I wounds heal with local dressing changes. For some type II and type IIIA fractures, we use delayed wound closure or a split-thickness skin graft over underlying muscle cover.

Large soft tissue loss is most often a problem with types IIIB and IIIC fractures. In the proximal tibia, we often work with the plastic surgeons to provide a gastrocnemius rotational flap, followed by secondary coverage of the muscle with a skin graft. In the middle third of the leg, a soleus flap is used with skin graft coverage, whereas a vascularized free muscle transfer is necessary if local coverage is inadequate. Free flaps may be required for coverage of the distal third of the tibia, especially in teenagers. Vacuum-assisted coverage sometimes can mitigate the need for free tissue transfers.

The flaps and grafts used for reconstructing severe injuries are either muscle flaps or composite grafts. For a massive loss of soft tissue and bone, composite grafts of muscle and bone often are necessary. The younger the child, the better the likelihood that autogenous graft will fill in a bone defect if there is a well-vascularized bed from the muscle flap. Free flaps, especially from the latissimus dorsi, are useful in the midtibial and distal tibial regions to decrease infection rates and improve union rates. Vascularized fibular grafts rarely are used acutely to reconstruct bone defects but may be useful in later reconstruction, after soft tissue wounds are healed.

For the rare case of significant bone defect in a child, we rely on the healing capacity of young periosteum and bone and the vascular supply of a child's extremity. An external fixator is used to hold the bone shortened about 1 to 2 cm to decrease the size of the bone loss. In a growing child, 1 to 2 cm of overgrowth can be expected in the subsequent 2 years after these severe injuries so the final leg length will be satisfactory. Autogenous bone graft can be used early, but if there is surviving periosteum at this site, spontaneous bone formation is often surprisingly robust and may preclude the need for bone grafting. In teenagers with bone loss, once the soft tissue has healed, bone transport using either a uniplanar lengthening device or an Ilizarov device is our preferred method of reconstruction, although use of an allograft or vascularized fibular graft may be considered.

Amputation

In the most severe open fractures, attempts should generally be made to preserve all extremities, even with those type IIIC open fractures that are usually treated with primary amputation in adults. Wounds and fractures that do not heal in adults often heal satisfactorily in children and preservation of limb length and physes are important in young children. Though the Mangled Extremity Severity Score (MESS) correlates very well with the need for amputation in adults, the correlation is less in children (132). In the cited series, the MESS predicted limb amputation or salvage correctly in 86% (31/36) of children, with 93% accuracy in salvaged limbs but only 63% in amputated limbs.

If amputation is absolutely necessary, as much length as possible should be preserved. For example, if the proximal tibial physis is preserved in a child with a below knee amputation at age 7 years, 3 to 4 inches more growth of the tibial stump can be expected by skeletal maturity. Thus, even a very short tibial stump in a skeletally immature child may grow to an appropriate length by skeletal maturity. As a result, even a short below-knee amputation at the time of injury would likely be superior in final function to a knee disarticulation done at the time of injury.

Although amputations performed to treat congenital limb deficits are usually done through the joint to limit bone spike formation (overgrowth) at the end of the stump, we prefer to maintain maximal possible length if amputation becomes necessary as a result of a severe injury.

Management of Other Fractures

When a child with an open fracture is brought to the operating room for irrigation and debridement of the open fracture, the orthopaedist should take advantage of the anesthetic and treat the other fractures as well, whether operative treatment or closed reduction and casting is needed. In order to facilitate patient care and rehabilitation, most long-bone fractures in these children are treated surgically.

STABILIZATION OF FRACTURES

Beneficial Effects

In addition to promoting fracture healing, fracture stabilization also provides a number of nonorthopaedic benefits to a child with multiple injuries. Pulmonary contusions at the time of injury often lead to increasing respiratory problems in the first few days after injury (133). If the lungs have been severely contused, protein leaks into the alveolar spaces, making ventilation more difficult. This may be exacerbated by the systemic inflammatory response syndrome, which is commonly seen following severe trauma (44,106). Surfactant dysfunction follows and is most abnormal in patients with the most severe respiratory failure (134). As the time from the injury increases, pulmonary function deteriorates and general anesthesia becomes more risky. In patients with severe pulmonary contusions and multiple fractures, the use of extracorporeal life support may be the only treatment available to allow patient survival (135).

In adults with multiple injuries, early operative stabilization of fractures decreases pulmonary and other medical complications associated with prolonged bed rest that is a part of nonoperative fracture treatment (136). Most adult trauma centers follow the treatment protocol of early fracture stabilization, even though Poole et al (137) reported that, despite early fracture stabilization simplifying patient care, pulmonary complications in patients with marked chest trauma were not prevented and the course of the head injury was not affected. In children, medical complications are less common so the recommendations that mandate early fracture stabilization are somewhat more difficult to support in the young patients. Nonetheless, bruises on the chest or rib fractures should alert the orthopaedist to potential pulmonary contusions as a part of the injury complex (138). Initial chest x-rays may not clearly demonstrate the degree of pulmonary parenchymal injury, and arterial blood gas determinations are more useful in estimating the anesthetic risk of these patients during operative care of the fractures.

Timing

As noted, splinting is needed at the time of the initial resuscitation. In a child with multiple closed fractures, definitive treatment should proceed expeditiously once the child's condition has been stabilized. Loder (108) reported that operative stabilization of fractures within the first 2 or 3 days after injury led to fewer complications, shorter hospital and intensive care unit stays, and a shorter time on ventilator assistance in children with multiple injuries. A more recent study by Loder et al reported a trend toward a higher rate of complications in fractures treated after 72 hours (109). Although there appear to be other factors besides the timing of surgery that affect the eventual outcomes of polytrauma patients, the timing of surgery is a variable which can be controlled by the surgeon, and it seems prudent to complete fracture stabilization within 2 to 3 days of injury when possible.

Operative Fixation

The type of operative stabilization of closed fractures of long bones in multiply injured children commonly depends, as in other orthopaedic arenas, on the training, experience, and personal preference of the orthopaedist. The most common methods used are intramedullary rod fixation, external fixation, and AO compression plating, though Kirschner wires or Steinmann pins may be used in conjunction with casts.

Intramedullary Rod Fixation

There has been a recent increase in the use of flexible titanium intramedullary rods of 2 to 4 mm diameter for stabilization of long bone fractures of the upper and lower extremities. Intramedullary rodding is most commonly used for unstable closed fractures of the radius and ulna in patients through adolescence, and femoral shaft fractures in patients between the ages of 5 and skeletal maturity (80,139). The tibia may also be fixed in children with an open fracture, polytrauma, a "floating knee" injury, or a high energy, unstable injury (especially during adolescence). A diaphyseal fracture of the humerus may be treated with intramedullary fixation in the presence of a floating shoulder or elbow.

Common indications for intramedullary fixation of forearm fractures include unstable diaphyseal fractures (especially in adolescents) and open fractures (140–143). Forearm fractures generally can be reduced closed, with the intramedullary implant passed across the fracture site under fluoroscopy to stabilize the fracture (141). In one recent study, 23% (10/43) of closed forearm fractures treated with intramedullary rod fixation required open reduction (142). The ulnar implant is placed in antegrade fashion and may be inserted through the lateral proximal metaphyseal area or the tip of the olecranon. The radial implant is inserted retrograde and is contoured to conform to the normal radial bow prior to insertion. The insertion point is proximal to the distal radial physis and may be inserted from the radial aspect of the distal radius or dorsally (slightly ulnar to Lister's tubercle). Stability of both fractures may be achieved by instrumenting only the radius or the ulna in younger children, but both bones are more commonly fixed in adolescents. Intramedullary fixation of open forearm fractures appears to decrease the rate of loss of reduction (140,143). In one recent series, reduction was maintained in all 27 patients treated with rodding of both bones or of only the radius, compared with loss of reduction in 32% (7/22) of patients in whom only the ulna was rodded (142). The high rate of failure may be due to the small diameter pins (1.6 or 2.0 mm) used to fix the ulna in this series (142). A cast is used for further immobilization. The implants are easily removed from the wrist area and the elbow region 6 to 12 months after insertion and after fracture healing has taken place.

Despite the utility of flexible intramedullary implants for stabilizing forearm fractures in children, the radius and ulna in young patients have significant remodeling capacity and not all fractures require anatomic reduction. A closed reduction and cast immobilization often is sufficient treatment. Displaced distal forearm fractures in polytrauma patients often are well treated with closed reduction and percutaneous pinning, thus affording sufficient stability for use of a short-arm cast in these polytrauma patients.

In one reported series of 20 pediatric patients treated with intramedullary rodding of forearm fractures, 50% of patients had complications—including loss of reduction, infection, hardware migration, nerve injury, and delayed union—though 95% (19/20) of patients had excellent or good results on follow-up (144). In another recent series, compartment syndromes occurred in 6 of 80 (7.5%) patients with forearm fractures treated with intramedullary fixation; risk factors in this study were reported to be increased operative time and increased intra-operative use of fluoroscopy (145).

If flexible intramedullary nails are used in the femur, the most common technique is retrograde insertion from the medial and lateral metaphyseal region of the distal femur, 2 to 3 cm proximal to the physis. Two rods are used to cross the fracture site and obtain purchase in the proximal femur, usually with one at the base of the femoral neck and the other at the base of the greater trochanter. Rod diameter is generally 40% of the intramedullary diameter of the femoral isthmus, up to a maximum rod size of 4 mm. A cast is not necessary postoperatively, although a fracture brace can be used to help control rotation at the fracture site and provide some patient comfort during early walking, especially for proximal third fractures or those with significant comminution. The implants are most commonly removed before 1 year from the time of fracture fixation (146,147).

The use of reamed antegrade intramedullary rods to treat femoral shaft fractures in the pediatric population should be reserved, in our view, for those with a closed proximal femoral physis. In younger children, rod insertion at the piriformis fossa may interfere with the vascular supply to the femoral epiphysis, may cause growth arrest of the greater trochanter apophysis with resultant coxa valga, or may interfere with the appositional bone growth at the base of the femoral neck, thereby thinning this region and potentially predisposing the child to a femoral neck fracture (148–152). Some authors have advocated rigid intramedullary rodding using an entrance point at the tip of the greater trochanter (153,154), though there is not sufficient data at this time to confirm the safety and efficacy of such an approach. The specific indications for intramedullary fixation of the femur are discussed in more detail in Chapter 22.

Flexible intramedullary rod fixation is becoming increasingly common for diaphyseal tibial fractures. The most common indications currently are open fractures, "floating knee" injuries, and unstable diaphyseal fractures in adolescents. The rods are inserted in antegrade fashion, with medial and lateral entrance points distal to the physis and avoiding the tibial tubercle. As with femoral fractures, rod diameter is 40% of the narrowest intramedullary diameter, with a maximum rod size of 4 mm. A short-leg walking cast or fracture boot is often used for comfort for the first 4 to 6 weeks postoperatively, though a splint may be used initially to allow access to wounds associated with an open fracture or degloving injury.

Compression Plates

Some have advocated the use of compression plates to stabilize long bone fractures, especially in the femoral shaft, in children with multiple injuries (155,156). Kregor et al (156) reported an average overgrowth of the femur of 9 mm, and all fractures healed in a near anatomic position. Caird et al noted that 3% of patients (2/60) had a limb length discrepancy of greater than 2.5 cm following femoral plating, including a 5 cm discrepancy in one child (155). The disadvantages of compression plating include: the need for more extensive operative exposure at the site of the fracture, the fact that these are not load sharing devices, and the usual need to remove the plate through a relatively long incision once healing is complete. Newer minimally invasive "percutaneous" submuscular plating techniques have eliminated some of the problems associated with traditional plating (Fig. 4-5). Refracture may occur through the screw holes left after plate removal if physical activity is resumed too quickly. Stiffness of adjacent joints is rarely a problem in children unless there has been an associated severe soft tissue injury. As a result, the number of cortices the screws cross on each side of the fracture may be fewer in children than in adults, because a cast or splint is routinely used in young patients.

Although some authors have recommended open reduction and compression plate fixation of displaced radial and ulnar fractures (157), we prefer flexible intramedullary nails, as noted earlier. The use of compression plates in the forearm requires a larger operative incision with the resultant scar, a second extensive procedure for plate removal, and a significant risk of refracture following hardware removal. We do not believe that the healing capability of the young child requires the rigid fixation of compression plating to obtain fracture union.

External Fixation

The most common indications for use of external fixation in a child with multiple injuries have been open fractures with

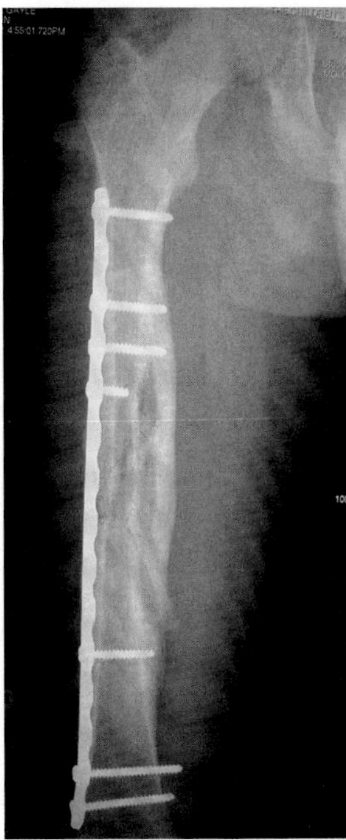

FIGURE 4-5 Stabilization of femoral shaft fractures in children with multi-trauma can be obtained with several methods. Minimally invasive percutaneous submuscular plating techniques can occasionally be used. (Courtesy of Dr. Steven T. Morgan, Denver, CO.)

significant soft tissue injury, fractures in association with a head injury and coma, and so-called floating knee fractures of the femur and tibia (79,129–131,158–163) (Fig. 4-6). With advances in intramedullary rod techniques, external fixation is much less commonly used now than in previous years. The use of an external fixator in these circumstances allows the child to be transported for imaging studies or to the operating room for management of nonorthopaedic injuries. A unilateral fixator generally is sufficient to hold the fracture reduced in this age group.

If external fixation is performed, the pin sites should be predrilled and the pins placed in the operating room under fluoroscopic control. The caliber of the pin should be less than 30% of the diameter of the bone into which it is to be inserted in order to minimize the risk of fracture through a pin site. The distal and proximal pin sites must be inserted at a level to avoid the physis, and we recommend leaving at least 1 to 2 cm between the pin and physis, partly to avoid any adverse effect on the physis should a pin track infection occur. The proximal tibial physis is more distal anteriorly below the tibial tubercle, and this area must be avoided or a recurvatum deformity of the proximal tibia and knee will result.

The external fixator usually is left in place until fracture healing is complete, but it can be removed once the reason for placement has resolved (such as waking from coma or healing of a skin wound) (79,164). If the fixator is removed early, a walking cast is applied. Transverse open fractures reduced out to length take longer to heal than do oblique fractures reduced with slight overlap. Refracture is a well-described risk following fixator removal, though the reported incidence of this complication varies greatly. In a series in which a rigid transfixion type of fixator was used, a 21% refracture rate was noted (81), in contrast to a rate of 1.4% in another series in which a more flexible unilateral frame was used (160). A recent report indicated that if three of the four cortices at the fracture site appear to be healing on anteroposterior and lateral x-rays of the fracture, the refracture rate after frame removal should be small (165).

Laboratory studies have suggested that dynamization of external fixators may stimulate early fracture healing (166,167). Some authors have reported that dynamization decreases the risk of refracture (168), though this has been refuted by others (169). We like to dynamize the fixator early in order to stimulate callus formation.

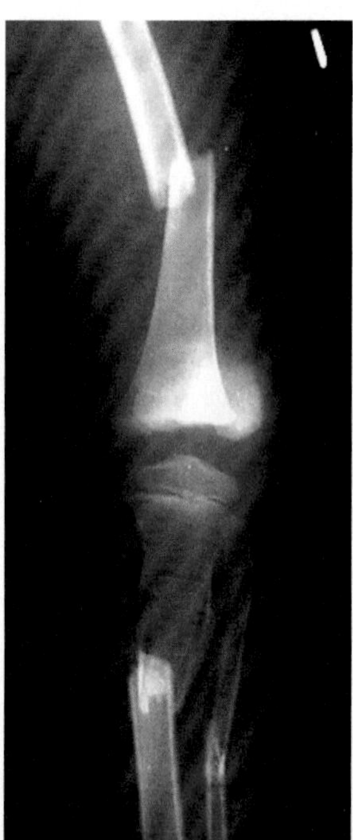

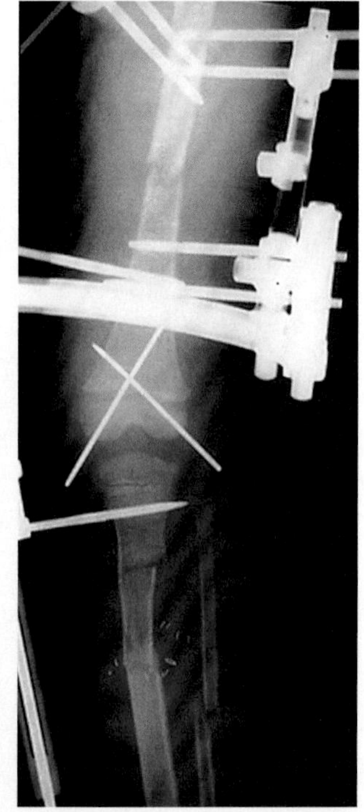

A B

FIGURE 4-6 "Floating knee" injury in a 6-year-old child included **(A)** an open IIIB tibial fracture, an open femoral shaft fracture, and a displaced femoral physeal fracture. **B.** The open fractures were treated with debridement and irrigation and stabilization with external fixation; the femoral physeal fracture was reduced and pinned.

Outcomes of Treatment of the Multiply Injured Child

In one review of 74 children with multiple injuries, 59 (80%) survived, but after 1 year, 22% were disabled, mainly from a brain injury. At 9 years after the injuries, 12% had significant physical disability, whereas 42% had cognitive impairment. In this group, however, the SF-36 or functional outcome survey did not differ from the control population. The best predictor of long-term disability was the Glasgow Outcome Scale from 6 weeks after injury on (170). Letts et al reported that 71.6% of multiply injured children made a full recovery, with a mean of 28 weeks until full recovery (56). Of the 53 residual deficits in 48 patients, the common deficits were neurologic (38%), psychosocial (34%), and musculoskeletal (24%).

Whichever method of fracture treatment—operative or nonoperative—is chosen for a child with multiple injuries, it is important that the orthopaedist be involved in the care of the child from the start. While recognizing the need to care for the other organ system injuries the child has sustained, it is important to advocate for the expeditious and appropriate treatment of the fractures that are present. Failure to do so will leave the multiply injured child with musculoskeletal disability once healing of the other injuries occurs. After multiple injuries, the most common long-term problems relate to either sequelae of the head injury or of the orthopaedic injuries.

REFERENCES

1. MacKenzie EJ, Morris JA Jr, de Lissovoy GV, et al. Acute hospital costs of pediatric trauma in the United States: how much and who pays? *J Pediatr Surg* 1990;25:970–976.
2. Maksoud JG Jr, Moront ML, Eichelberger MR. Resuscitation of the injured child. *Semin Pediatr Surg* 1995;4:93–99.
3. Potoka DA, Schall LC, Gardner MJ, et al. Impact of pediatric trauma centers on mortality in a statewide system. *J Trauma* 2000;49:237–245.
4. Rivara FP. Pediatric injury control in 1999: where do we go from here? *Pediatrics* 1999;103:883–888.
5. Schafermeyer R. Pediatric trauma. *Emerg Med Clin North Am* 1993;11:187–205.
6. Schalamon J, v Bismarck S, Schober PH, et al. Multiple trauma in pediatric patients. *Pediatr Surg Int* 2003;19:417–423.

7. Sullivan T, Haider A, DiRusso SM, et al. Prediction of mortality in pediatric trauma patients: new injury severity score outperforms injury severity score in the severely injured. *J Trauma* 2003;55:1083–1807; discussion 1087–1088.
8. Buckley SL, Gotschall C, Robertson W Jr, et al. The relationships of skeletal injuries with trauma score, injury severity score, length of hospital stay, hospital charges, and mortality in children admitted to a regional pediatric trauma center. *J Pediatr Orthop* 1994;14:449–453.
9. Maio RF, Portnoy J, Blow FC, et al. Injury type, injury severity, and repeat occurrence of alcohol-related trauma in adolescents. *Alcohol Clin Exp Res* 1994;18:261–264.
10. Sindelar HA, Barnett NP, Spirito A. Adolescent alcohol use and injury. A summary and critical review of the literature. *Minerva Pediatr* 2004;56:291–309.
11. Colombani PM, Buck JR, Dudgeon DL, et al. One-year experience in a regional pediatric trauma center. *J Pediatr Surg* 1985;20:8–13.
12. Cramer KE. The pediatric polytrauma patient. *Clin Orthop* 1995;318:125–135.
13. Peclet MH, Newman KD, Eichelberger MR, et al. Patterns of injury in children. *J Pediatr Surg* 1990;25:85–90;discussion 90–91.
14. Schantz K, Rasmussen F. Calcaneus fracture in the child. *Acta Orthop Scand* 1987;58: 507–509.
15. Schmidt TL, Weiner DS. Calcaneal fractures in children. An evaluation of the nature of the injury in 56 children. *Clin Orthop* 1982;171:150–155.
16. Brainard BJ, Slauterbeck J, Benjamin JB. Fracture patterns and mechanisms in pedestrian motor-vehicle trauma: the ipsilateral dyad. *J Orthop Trauma* 1992;6:279–282.
17. Jawadi AH, Letts M. Injuries associated with fracture of the femur secondary to motor vehicle accidents in children. *Am J Orthop* 2003;32:459–462; discussion 462.
18. Kocher MS, Kasser JR. Orthopaedic aspects of child abuse. *J Am Acad Orthop Surg* 2000;8:10–20.
19. King J, Diefendorf D, Apthorp J, et al. Analysis of 429 fractures in 189 battered children. *J Pediatr Orthop* 1988;8:585–589.
20. Garcia VF, Gotschall CS, Eichelberger MR, et al. Rib fractures in children: a marker of severe trauma. *J Trauma* 1990;30:695–700.
21. Barsness KA, Cha ES, Bensard DD, et al. The positive predictive value of rib fractures as an indicator of nonaccidental trauma in children. *J Trauma* 2003;54:1107–1110.
22. Williams RL, Connolly PT. In children undergoing chest radiography what is the specificity of rib fractures for non-accidental injury? *Arch Dis Child* 2004;89:490–492.
23. Mandelstam SA, Cook D, Fitzgerald M, et al. Complementary use of radiological skeletal survey and bone scintigraphy in detection of bony injuries in suspected child abuse. *Arch Dis Child* 2003;88:387–390; discussion 387–390.
24. American Academy of Pediatrics. Diagnostic imaging of child abuse. *Pediatrics* 2000; 105:1345–1348.
25. Greenberg MI. Falls from heights. *JACEP* 1978;7:300–301.
26. Lallier M, Bouchard S, St-Vil D, et al. Falls from heights among children: a retrospective review. *J Pediatr Surg* 1999;34:1060–1063.
27. Rozycki GS, Maull KI. Injuries sustained by falls. *Arch Emerg Med* 1991;8:245–252.
28. Wang MY, Kim KA, Griffith PM, et al. Injuries from falls in the pediatric population: an analysis of 729 cases. *J Pediatr Surg* 2001;36:1528–1534.
29. U.S. Department of Transportation NHTSA. Traffic safety facts 2002. 2004;DOT HS 809 620:1–202.
30. Thompson EC, Perkowski P, Villarreal D, et al. Morbidity and mortality of children following motor vehicle crashes. *Arch Surg* 2003;138:142–145.
31. Vaca F, Anderson CL, Agran P, et al. Child safety seat knowledge among parents utilizing emergency services in a level I trauma center in Southern California. *Pediatrics* 2002;110:e61.
32. Zuckerbraun BS, Morrison K, Gaines B, et al. Effect of age on cervical spine injuries in children after motor vehicle collisions: effectiveness of restraint devices. *J Pediatr Surg* 2004;39:483–486.
33. Kumaresan S, Sances A Jr, Carlin F. Biomechanical analysis of padding in child seats and head injury. *Biomed Sci Instrum* 2002;38:453–458.
34. Haller JA Jr, Shorter N, Miller D, et al. Organization and function of a regional pediatric trauma center: does a system of management improve outcome? *J Trauma* 1983;23: 691–696.
35. Harris BH. Creating pediatric trauma systems. *J Pediatr Surg* 1989;24:149–152.
36. Smith JS Jr, Martin LF, Young WW, et al. Do trauma centers improve outcome over non-trauma centers: the evaluation of regional trauma care using discharge abstract data and patient management categories. *J Trauma* 1990;30:1533–1538.
37. Larson JT, Dietrich AM, Abdessalam SF, et al. Effective use of the air ambulance for pediatric trauma. *J Trauma* 2004;56:89–93.
38. Knudson MM, Shagoury C, Lewis FR. Can adult trauma surgeons care for injured children? *J Trauma* 1992;32:729–737; discussion 737–739.
39. Sanchez JL, Lucas J, Feustel PJ. Outcome of adolescent trauma admitted to an adult surgical intensive care unit versus a pediatric intensive care unit. *J Trauma* 2001;51: 478–480.
40. Armstrong PF. Initial management of the multiply injured child: the ABC's. *Instr Course Lect* 1992;41:347–350.
41. Herzenberg JE, Hensinger RN, Dedrick DK, et al. Emergency transport and positioning of young children who have an injury of the cervical spine. The standard backboard may be hazardous. *J Bone Joint Surg Am* 1989;71:15–22.
42. Guy J, Haley K, Zuspan SJ. Use of intraosseous infusion in the pediatric trauma patient. *J Pediatr Surg* 1993;28:158–161.
43. Bielski RJ, Bassett GS, Fideler B, et al. Intraosseous infusions: effects on the immature physis—an experimental model in rabbits. *J Pediatr Orthop* 1993;13:511–515.
44. Wetzel RC, Burns RC. Multiple trauma in children: critical care overview. *Crit Care Med* 2002;30:S468–477.
45. Peterson DL, Schinco MA, Kerwin AJ, et al. Evaluation of initial base deficit as a prognosticator of outcome in the pediatric trauma population. *Am Surg* 2004;70:326–328.
46. Wesson DE, Spence LJ, Williams JI, et al. Injury scoring systems in children. *Can J Surg* 1987;30:398–400.
47. Tepas JJ 3rd, Mollitt DL, Talbert JL, et al. The pediatric trauma score as a predictor of injury severity in the injured child. *J Pediatr Surg* 1987;22:14–18.
48. Ott R, Kramer R, Martus P, et al. Prognostic value of trauma scores in pediatric patients with multiple injuries. *J Trauma* 2000;49:729–736.
49. Yian EH, Gullahorn LJ, Loder RT. Scoring of pediatric orthopaedic polytrauma: correlations of different injury scoring systems and prognosis for hospital course. *J Pediatr Orthop* 2000;20:203–209.
50. Teasdale G, Jennett B. Assessment of coma and impaired consciousness. A practical scale. *Lancet* 1974;2:81–84.
51. Michaud LJ, Rivara FP, Grady MS, et al. Predictors of survival and severity of disability after severe brain injury in children. *Neurosurgery* 1992;31:254–264.
52. Campbell DJ, Sprouse LR 2nd, Smith LA, et al. Injuries in pediatric patients with seatbelt contusions. *Am Surg* 2003;69:1095–1099.
53. Sivit CJ, Taylor GA, Newman KD, et al. Safety-belt injuries in children with lap-belt ecchymosis: CT findings in 61 patients. *AJR Am J Roentgenol* 1991;157:111–114.
54. Vazquez WD, Garcia VF. Pediatric pelvic fractures combined with an additional skeletal injury is an indicator of significant injury. *Surg Gynecol Obstet* 1993;177:468–472.
55. Payiga YJ, Valentine RJ, Meyers SI, et al. Blunt pediatric vascular trauma: analysis of 41 consecutive patients undergoing operative intervention. *J Vasc Surg* 1994;20: 419–424.
56. Letts M, Davidson D, Lapner P. Multiple trauma in children: predicting outcome and long-term results. *Can J Surg* 2002;45:126–131.
57. Cattell HS, Filtzer DL. Pseudosubluxation and other normal variations in the cervical spine in children. A study of one hundred and sixty children. *J Bone Joint Surg Am* 1965;47:1295–1309.
58. Hoffmann R, Nerlich M, Muggia-Sullam M, et al. Blunt abdominal trauma in cases of multiple trauma evaluated by ultrasonography: a prospective analysis of 291 patients. *J Trauma* 1992;32:452–458.
59. Roche BG, Bugmann P, Le Coultre C. Blunt injuries to liver, spleen, kidney and pancreas in pediatric patients. *Eur J Pediatr Surg* 1992;2:154–156.
60. Guillamondegui OD, Mahboubi S, Stafford PW, et al. The utility of the pelvic radiograph in the assessment of pediatric pelvic fractures. *J Trauma* 2003;55:236–239; discussion 239–240.
61. Onuora VC, Patil MG, al-Jasser AN. Missed urological injuries in children with polytrauma. *Injury* 1993;24:619–621.
62. Andrich DE, O'Malley KJ, Summerton DJ, et al. The type of urethroplasty for a pelvic fracture urethral distraction defect cannot be predicted preoperatively. *J Urol* 2003; 170:464–467.
63. Heinrich SD, Gallagher D, Harris M, et al. Undiagnosed fractures in severely injured children and young adults. Identification with technetium imaging. *J Bone Joint Surg Am* 1994;76:561–572.
64. Aufdermaur M. Spinal injuries in juveniles. Necropsy findings in twelve cases. *J Bone Joint Surg Br* 1974;56B:513–519.
65. Bosch PP, Vogt MT, Ward WT. Pediatric spinal cord injury without radiographic abnormality (SCIWORA): the absence of occult instability and lack of indication for bracing. *Spine* 2002;27:2788–2800.
66. Evans DL, Bethem D. Cervical spine injuries in children. *J Pediatr Orthop* 1989;9: 563–568.
67. Frank JB, Lim CK, Flynn JM, et al. The efficacy of magnetic resonance imaging in pediatric cervical spine clearance. *Spine* 2002;27:1176–1179.
68. Buess E, Illi OE, Soder C, et al. Ruptured spleen in children—15-year evolution in therapeutic concepts. *Eur J Pediatr Surg* 1992;2:157–161.
69. Coley BD, Mutabagani KH, Martin LC, et al. Focused abdominal sonography for trauma (FAST) in children with blunt abdominal trauma. *J Trauma* 2000;48:902–906.
70. Mutabagani KH, Coley BD, Zumberge N, et al. Preliminary experience with focused abdominal sonography for trauma (FAST) in children: is it useful? *J Pediatr Surg* 1999; 34:48–52; discussion 52–54.
71. Richardson MC, Hollman AS, Davis CF. Comparison of computed tomography and ultrasonographic imaging in the assessment of blunt abdominal trauma in children. *Br J Surg* 1997;84:1144–1146.
72. Suthers SE, Albrecht R, Foley D, et al. Surgeon-directed ultrasound for trauma is a predictor of intra-abdominal injury in children. *Am Surg* 2004;70:164–167; discussion 167–168.
73. Levin HS, High WM Jr, Ewing-Cobbs L, et al. Memory functioning during the first year after closed head injury in children and adolescents. *Neurosurgery* 1988;22:1043–1052.
74. Winogron HW, Knights RM, Bawden HN. Neuropsychological deficits following head injury in children. *J Clin Neuropsychol* 1984;6:267–286.
75. Hanten G, Dennis M, Zhang L, et al. Childhood head injury and metacognitive processes in language and memory. *Dev Neuropsychol* 2004;25:85–106.
76. Swift EE, Taylor HG, Kaugars AS, et al. Sibling relationships and behavior after pediatric traumatic brain injury. *J Dev Behav Pediatr* 2003;24:24–31.
77. Greenspan AI, MacKenzie EJ. Functional outcome after pediatric head injury. *Pediatrics* 1994;94:425–432.
78. Woolf PD, McDonald JV, Feliciano DV, et al. The catecholamine response to multisystem trauma. *Arch Surg* 1992;127:899–903.
79. Tolo VT. External fixation in multiply injured children. *Orthop Clin North Am* 1990; 21:393–400.
80. Tolo VT. Orthopaedic treatment of fractures of the long bones and pelvis in children who have multiple injuries. *Instr Course Lect* 2000;49:415–423.
81. Tolo VT. External skeletal fixation in children's fractures. *J Pediatr Orthop* 1983;3: 435–442.

82. Kluger G, Kochs A, Holthausen H. Heterotopic ossification in childhood and adolescence. *J Child Neurol* 2000;15:406–413.
83. Keret D, Harcke HT, Mendez AA, et al. Heterotopic ossification in central nervous system-injured patients following closed nailing of femoral fractures. *Clin Orthop* 1990; 256:254–259.
84. Mital MA, Garber JE, Stinson JT. Ectopic bone formation in children and adolescents with head injuries: its management. *J Pediatr Orthop* 1987;7:83–90.
85. Sobus KM, Sherman N, Alexander MA. Coexistence of deep venous thrombosis and heterotopic ossification in the pediatric patient. *Arch Phys Med Rehabil* 1993;74: 547–551.
86. De Bastiani G, Mosconi F, Spagnol G, et al. High calcitonin levels in unconscious polytrauma patients. *J Bone Joint Surg Br* 1992;74:101–104.
87. Philip PA, Philip M. Peripheral nerve injuries in children with traumatic brain injury. *Brain Inj* 1992;6:53–58.
88. Dereeper E, Ciardelli R, Vincent JL. Fatal outcome after polytrauma: multiple organ failure or cerebral damage? *Resuscitation* 1998;36:15–18.
89. Tso EL, Beaver BL, Haller JA Jr. Abdominal injuries in restrained pediatric passengers. *J Pediatr Surg* 1993;28:915–919.
90. Bond SJ, Gotschall CS, Eichelberger MR. Predictors of abdominal injury in children with pelvic fracture. *J Trauma* 1991;31:1169–1173.
91. Benifla M, Weizman Z. Acute pancreatitis in childhood: analysis of literature data. *J Clin Gastroenterol* 2003;37:169–172.
92. Canarelli JP, Boboyono JM, Ricard J, et al. Management of abdominal contusion in polytraumatized children. *Int Surg* 1991;76:119–121.
93. Cloutier DR, Baird TB, Gormley P, et al. Pediatric splenic injuries with a contrast blush: successful nonoperative management without angiography and embolization. *J Pediatr Surg* 2004;39:969–971.
94. Coburn MC, Pfeifer J, DeLuca FG. Nonoperative management of splenic and hepatic trauma in the multiply injured pediatric and adolescent patient. *Arch Surg* 1995;130: 332–338.
95. Cochran A, Mann NC, Dean JM, et al. Resource utilization and its management in splenic trauma. *Am J Surg* 2004;187:713–719.
96. Leinwand MJ, Atkinson CC, Mooney DP. Application of the APSA evidence-based guidelines for isolated liver or spleen injuries: a single institution experience. *J Pediatr Surg* 2004;39:487–490; discussion 487–490.
97. Uranus S, Pfeifer J. Nonoperative treatment of blunt splenic injury. *World J Surg* 2001; 25:1405–1407.
98. Silber JS, Flynn JM, Koffler KM, et al. Analysis of the cause, classification, and associated injuries of 166 consecutive pediatric pelvic fractures. *J Pediatr Orthop* 2001;21: 446–450.
99. Torode I, Zieg D. Pelvic fractures in children. *J Pediatr Orthop* 1985;5:76–84.
100. Batislam E, Ates Y, Germiyanoglu C, et al. Role of Tile classification in predicting urethral injuries in pediatric pelvic fractures. *J Trauma* 1997;42:285–287.
101. Podesta ML, Jordan GH. Pelvic fracture urethral injuries in girls. *J Urol* 2001;165: 1660–1665.
102. Rourke KF, McCammon KA, Sumfest JM, et al. Open reconstruction of pediatric and adolescent urethral strictures: long-term followup. *J Urol* 2003;169:1818–1821; discussion 1821.
103. Copeland CE, Bosse MJ, McCarthy ML, et al. Effect of trauma and pelvic fracture on female genitourinary, sexual, and reproductive function. *J Orthop Trauma* 1997;11: 73–81.
104. Abou-Jaoude WA, Sugarman JM, Fallat ME, et al. Indicators of genitourinary tract injury or anomaly in cases of pediatric blunt trauma. *J Pediatr Surg* 1996;31:86–89; discussion 90.
105. Limbird TJ, Ruderman RJ. Fat embolism in children. *Clin Orthop* 1978;136:267–269.
106. Robinson CM. Current concepts of respiratory insufficiency syndromes after fracture. *J Bone Joint Surg Br* 2001;83:781–791.
107. Tilden SJ, Watkins S, Tong TK, et al. Measured energy expenditure in pediatric intensive care patients. *Am J Dis Child* 1989;143:490–492.
108. Loder RT. Pediatric polytrauma: orthopaedic care and hospital course. *J Orthop Trauma* 1987;1:48–54.
109. Loder RT, Gullahorn LJ, Yian EH, et al. Factors predictive of immobilization complications in pediatric polytrauma. *J Orthop Trauma* 2001;15:338–341.
110. Velmahos GC, Arroyo H, Ramicone E, et al. Timing of fracture fixation in blunt trauma patients with severe head injuries. *Am J Surg* 1998;176:324–329; discussion 329–330.
111. Smith WR, Oakley M, Morgan SJ. Pediatric pelvic fractures. *J Pediatr Orthop* 2004;24: 130–135.
112. Blasier RD, McAtee J, White R, et al. Disruption of the pelvic ring in pediatric patients. *Clin Orthop* 2000;376:87–95.
113. Ismail N, Bellemare JF, Mollitt DL, et al. Death from pelvic fracture: children are different. *J Pediatr Surg* 1996;31:82–85.
114. Musemeche CA, Fischer RP, Cotler HB, et al. Selective management of pediatric pelvic fractures: a conservative approach. *J Pediatr Surg* 1987;22:538–540.
115. McIntyre RC Jr, Bensard DD, Moore EE, et al. Pelvic fracture geometry predicts risk of life-threatening hemorrhage in children. *J Trauma* 1993;35:423–429.
116. Demetriades D, Karaiskakis M, Velmahos GC, et al. Pelvic fractures in pediatric and adult trauma patients: are they different injuries? *J Trauma* 2003;54:1146–1151; discussion 1151.
117. Garvin KL, McCarthy RE, Barnes CL, et al. Pediatric pelvic ring fractures. *J Pediatr Orthop* 1990;10:577–582.
118. Reff RB. The use of external fixation devices in the management of severe lower-extremity trauma and pelvic injuries in children. *Clin Orthop* 1984;188:21–33.
119. Gustilo RB, Anderson JT. Prevention of infection in the treatment of one thousand and twenty-five open fractures of long bones: retrospective and prospective analyses. *J Bone Joint Surg Am* 1976;58:453–458.
120. Gustilo RB, Mendoza RM, Williams DN. Problems in the management of type III (severe) open fractures: a new classification of type III open fractures. *J Trauma* 1984;24: 742–746.
121. Herscovici D Jr, Sanders RW, Scaduto JM, et al. Vacuum-assisted wound closure (VAC therapy) for the management of patients with high-energy soft tissue injuries. *J Orthop Trauma* 2003;17:683–688.
122. Mooney JF 3rd, Argenta LC, Marks MW, et al. Treatment of soft tissue defects in pediatric patients using the V.A.C. system. *Clin Orthop* 2000;376:26–31.
123. Webb LX. New techniques in wound management: vacuum-assisted wound closure. *J Am Acad Orthop Surg* 2002;10:303–311.
124. Lee J. Efficacy of cultures in the management of open fractures. *Clin Orthop* 1997;339: 71–75.
125. Valenziano CP, Chattar-Cora D, O'Neill A, et al. Efficacy of primary wound cultures in long bone open extremity fractures: are they of any value? *Arch Orthop Trauma Surg* 2002;122:259–261.
126. Wilkins J, Patzakis M. Choice and duration of antibiotics in open fractures. *Orthop Clin North Am* 1991;22:433–437.
127. Kreder HJ, Armstrong P. A review of open tibia fractures in children. *J Pediatr Orthop* 1995;15:482–488.
128. Skaggs DL, Kautz SM, Kay RM, et al. Effect of delay of surgical treatment on rate of infection in open fractures in children. *J Pediatr Orthop* 2000;20:19–22.
129. Bohn WW, Durbin RA. Ipsilateral fractures of the femur and tibia in children and adolescents. *J Bone Joint Surg Am* 1991;73:429–439.
130. Letts M, Vincent N, Gouw G. The "floating knee" in children. *J Bone Joint Surg Br* 1986; 68:442–446.
131. Roposch A, Reis M, Molina M, et al. Supracondylar fractures of the humerus associated with ipsilateral forearm fractures in children: a report of forty-seven cases. *J Pediatr Orthop* 2001;21:307–312.
132. Fagelman MF, Epps HR, Rang M. Mangled extremity severity score in children. *J Pediatr Orthop* 2002;22:182–184.
133. Pfenninger J. Pulmonary problems following multiple trauma in children. *Intensive Care Med* 1989;15(Suppl 1):S50–52.
134. Pison U, Seeger W, Buchhorn R, et al. Surfactant abnormalities in patients with respiratory failure after multiple trauma. *Am Rev Respir Dis* 1989;140:1033–1039.
135. Senunas LE, Goulet JA, Greenfield ML, et al. Extracorporeal life support for patients with significant orthopaedic trauma. *Clin Orthop* 1997;339:32–40.
136. Beckman SB, Scholten DJ, Bonnell BW, et al. Long bone fractures in the polytrauma patient. The role of early operative fixation. *Am Surg* 1989;55:356–358.
137. Poole GV, Miller JD, Agnew SG, et al. Lower extremity fracture fixation in head-injured patients. *J Trauma* 1992;32:654–659.
138. Peclet MH, Newman KD, Eichelberger MR, et al. Thoracic trauma in children: an indicator of increased mortality. *J Pediatr Surg* 1990;25:961–965; discussion 965–966.
139. Verstreken L, Delronge G, Lamoureux J. Orthopaedic treatment of paediatric multiple trauma patients. A new technique. *Int Surg* 1988;73:177–179.
140. Greenbaum B, Zionts LE, Ebramzadeh E. Open fractures of the forearm in children. *J Orthop Trauma* 2001;15:111–118.
141. Lascombes P, Prevot J, Ligier JN, et al. Elastic stable intramedullary nailing in forearm shaft fractures in children: 85 cases. *J Pediatr Orthop* 1990;10:167–171.
142. Lee S, Nicol RO, Stott NS. Intramedullary fixation for pediatric unstable forearm fractures. *Clin Orthop* 2002;402:245–250.
143. Luhmann SJ, Schootman M, Schoenecker PL, et al. Complications and outcomes of open pediatric forearm fractures. *J Pediatr Orthop* 2004;24:1–6.
144. Cullen MC, Roy DR, Giza E, et al. Complications of intramedullary fixation of pediatric forearm fractures. *J Pediatr Orthop* 1998;18:14–21.
145. Yuan PS, Pring ME, Gaynor TP, et al. Compartment syndrome following intramedullary fixation of pediatric forearm fractures. *J Pediatr Orthop* 2004;24:370–375.
146. Heinrich SD, Drvaric DM, Darr K, et al. The operative stabilization of pediatric diaphyseal femur fractures with flexible intramedullary nails: a prospective analysis. *J Pediatr Orthop* 1994;14:501–507.
147. Huber RI, Keller HW, Huber PM, et al. Flexible intramedullary nailing as fracture treatment in children. *J Pediatr Orthop* 1996;16:602–605.
148. Beaty JH, Austin SM, Warner WC, et al. Interlocking intramedullary nailing of femoral-shaft fractures in adolescents: preliminary results and complications. *J Pediatr Orthop* 1994;14:178–183.
149. Canale ST, Tolo VT. Fractures of the femur in children. *Instr Course Lect* 1995;44: 255–273.
150. Letts M, Jarvis J, Lawton L, et al. Complications of rigid intramedullary rodding of femoral shaft fractures in children. *J Trauma* 2002;52:504–516.
151. Mileski RA, Garvin KL, Crosby LA. Avascular necrosis of the femoral head in an adolescent following intramedullary nailing of the femur. A case report. *J Bone Joint Surg Am* 1994;76:1706–1708.
152. O'Malley DE, Mazur JM, Cummings RJ. Femoral head avascular necrosis associated with intramedullary nailing in an adolescent. *J Pediatr Orthop* 1995;15:21–23.
153. Gordon JE, Swenning TA, Burd TA, et al. Proximal femoral radiographic changes after lateral transtrochanteric intramedullary nail placement in children. *J Bone Joint Surg Am* 2003;85-A:1295–1301.
154. Townsend DR, Hoffinger S. Intramedullary nailing of femoral shaft fractures in children via the trochanter tip. *Clin Orthop* 2000;376:113–118.
155. Caird MS, Mueller KA, Puryear A, et al. Compression plating of pediatric femoral shaft fractures. *J Pediatr Orthop* 2003;23:448–452.
156. Kregor PJ, Song KM, Routt ML Jr, et al. Plate fixation of femoral shaft fractures in multiply injured children. *J Bone Joint Surg Am* 1993;75:1774–1780.

157. Wyrsch B, Mencio GA, Green NE. Open reduction and internal fixation of pediatric forearm fractures. *J Pediatr Orthop* 1996;16:644–650.
158. Aronson J, Tursky EA. External fixation of femur fractures in children. *J Pediatr Orthop* 1992;12:157–163.
159. Arslan H, Kapukaya A, Kesemenli C, et al. Floating knee in children. *J Pediatr Orthop* 2003;23:458–463.
160. Blasier RD, Aronson J, Tursky EA. External fixation of pediatric femur fractures. *J Pediatr Orthop* 1997;17:342–346.
161. Kirschenbaum D, Albert MC, Robertson WW Jr, et al. Complex femur fractures in children: treatment with external fixation. *J Pediatr Orthop* 1990;10:588–591.
162. Schranz PJ, Gultekin C, Colton CL. External fixation of fractures in children. *Injury* 1992;23:80–82.
163. Yue JJ, Churchill RS, Cooperman DR, et al. The floating knee in the pediatric patient. Nonoperative versus operative stabilization. *Clin Orthop* 2000;376:124–136.
164. Evanoff M, Strong ML, MacIntosh R. External fixation maintained until fracture consolidation in the skeletally immature. *J Pediatr Orthop* 1993;13:98–101.
165. Skaggs DL, Leet AI, Money MD, et al. Secondary fractures associated with external fixation in pediatric femur fractures. *J Pediatr Orthop* 1999;19:582–586.
166. Claes LE, Wilke HJ, Augat P, et al. Effect of dynamization on gap healing of diaphyseal fractures under external fixation. *Clin Biomech (Bristol, Avon)* 1995;10:227–234.
167. Larsson S, Kim W, Caja VL, et al. Effect of early axial dynamization on tibial bone healing: a study in dogs. *Clin Orthop* 2001;388:240–251.
168. Kesemenli CC, Subasi M, Arslan H, et al. Is external fixation in pediatric femoral fractures a risk factor for refracture? *J Pediatr Orthop* 2004;24:17–20.
169. Domb BG, Sponseller PD, Ain M, et al. Comparison of dynamic versus static external fixation for pediatric femur fractures. *J Pediatr Orthop* 2002;22:428–430.
170. van der Sluis CK, Kingma J, Eisma WH, et al. Pediatric polytrauma: short-term and long-term outcomes. *J Trauma* 1997;43:501–506.

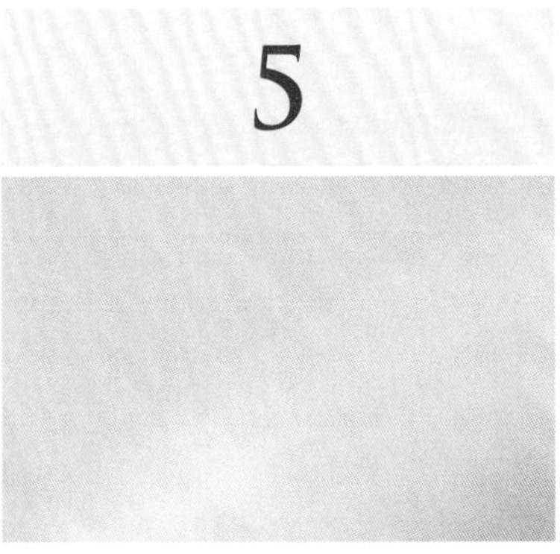

PHYSEAL INJURIES AND GROWTH DISTURBANCES

Karl E. Rathjen and John G. Birch

One of the unique aspects of pediatric orthopedics is the presence of the physis (or growth plate) providing longitudinal growth of children's long bones. Physeal injuries are a common and unique feature of children's bony injuries, in part because the physis is structurally more susceptible to loads that would produce metaphyseal or juxta-articular fractures in adults (1–9). Physeal injury may occur in a variety of ways in addition to trauma (8,10–26). Although physes, similar to the children with them, are resilient to permanent injury, uneventful outcomes are by no means assured (27–42). In this discussion of management of physeal injuries and associated growth disturbances the term *epiphysis* is used to refer to the bulbous end of a long bone incorporating the "growth plate" or "physis" and the secondary ossification center, and the term *physis* is used rather than "growth plate."

PHYSEAL ANATOMY

Normal Physeal Anatomy

Gross

Five regions characterize long bones: the bulbous, articular cartilage-covered ends (epiphyses) tapering to the funnel-shaped metaphyses, with the central diaphysis interposed between the metaphyses. During growth, the epiphyseal and metaphyseal regions are separated by the organized cartilaginous physis, which is the major contributor to longitudinal growth of the bone. The larger long bones (clavicle, humerus, radius, ulna, femur, tibia, and fibula) have physes at both ends, whereas the smaller tubular bones (metacarpals, metatarsals, and phalanges) usually have a physis at one end only.

At birth, with the exception of the distal femur and occasionally the proximal tibia, all of the above-mentioned epiphyses are purely cartilaginous. At various stages of postnatal growth and development, a secondary ossification center forms within the epiphysis. This development helps define the radiolucent zone of the physis, which persists until the physis closes at skeletal maturation. Typical ages for appearance of the major secondary ossification centers and physeal closure are summarized in Figures 5-1 and 5-2.

Microscopic

The microscopic architecture of the physis is highly organized and germane to an understanding of physeal injuries (7). Traditionally, the physis is divided into four zones from the center of the epiphysis to the metaphysis: germinal, proliferative, hypertrophic, and provisional calcification (or enchondral ossification) (Fig. 5-3). The germinal and proliferative zones are the location of cellular proliferation, whereas the hypertrophic and provisional calcification zones are characterized by matrix production, cellular hypertrophy, apoptosis, and matrix calcification. Normal longitudinal growth is dependent on the interaction of many factors, both hormonal and mechanical.

The peripheral margin of the physis comprises two specialized areas important to the mechanical integrity and peripheral growth of the physis (see Fig. 5-3). The zone (or groove) of Ranvier is a triangular microscopic structure at the periphery of the physis, containing fibroblasts, chondroblasts, and osteoblasts. It is responsible for peripheral growth of the physis. The perichondral ring of LaCroix is a fibrous structure overlying the zone of Ranvier, connecting the metaphyseal periosteum and cartilaginous epiphysis, and has the important mechanical function of stabilizing the epiphysis to the metaphysis.

The epiphysis and secondary ossific nucleus must receive blood supply for viability (43). Dale and Harris (44) identified two types of blood supply to the epiphysis (Fig. 5-4). Type A epiphyses (such as the proximal humeral and proximal femoral epiphyses) are nearly completely covered with articular cartilage; therefore, most of the blood supply must enter from the perichondrium. The blood supply to these epiphyses may be easily compromised by epiphyseal separation. Type B epiphyses (such as the proximal and distal tibia and the distal radius) have only a portion of their surface covered with articular cartilage and are theoretically less susceptible to devascularization from epiphyseal separation.

Mechanical Features of the Physis and Patterns of Injury

An understanding of the microscopic characteristics of the physeal zones permits an understanding of the theoretical line of

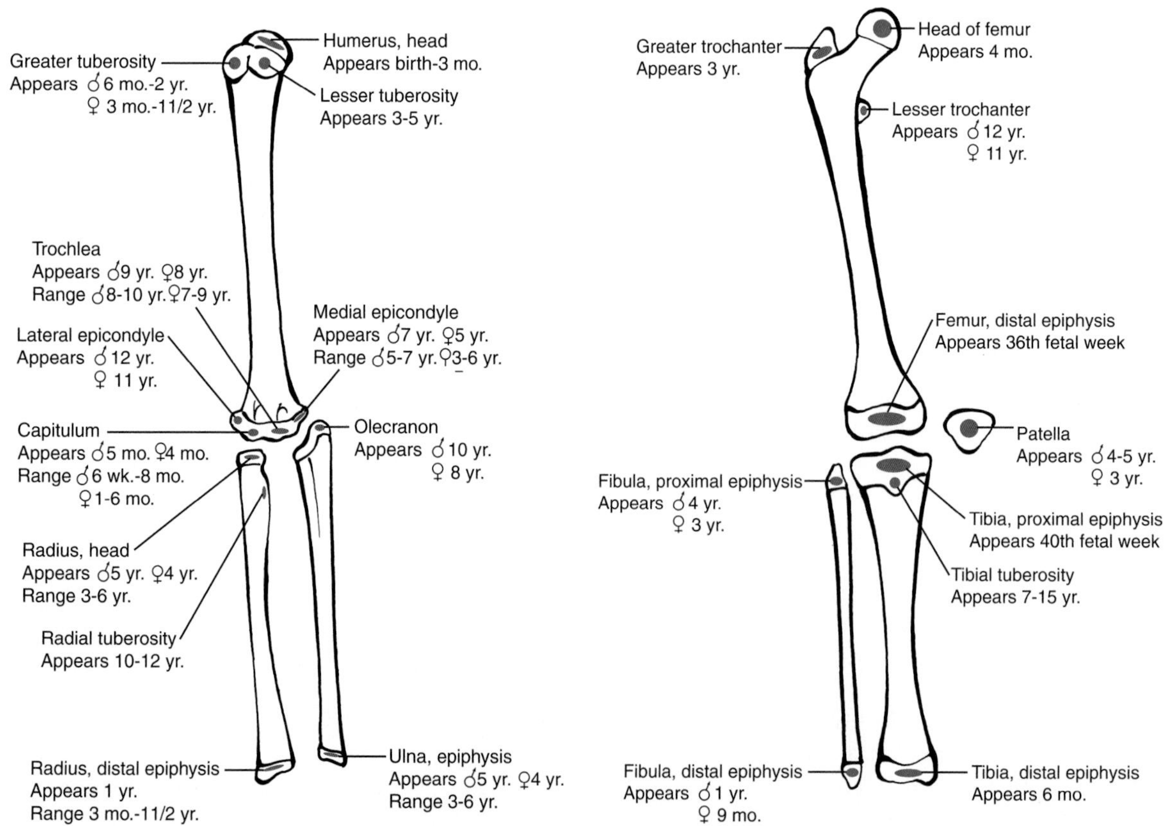

FIGURE 5-1 Typical age (and range) of development of the secondary ossification centers of the epiphyses in the **(A)** upper extremity and **(B)** lower extremity.

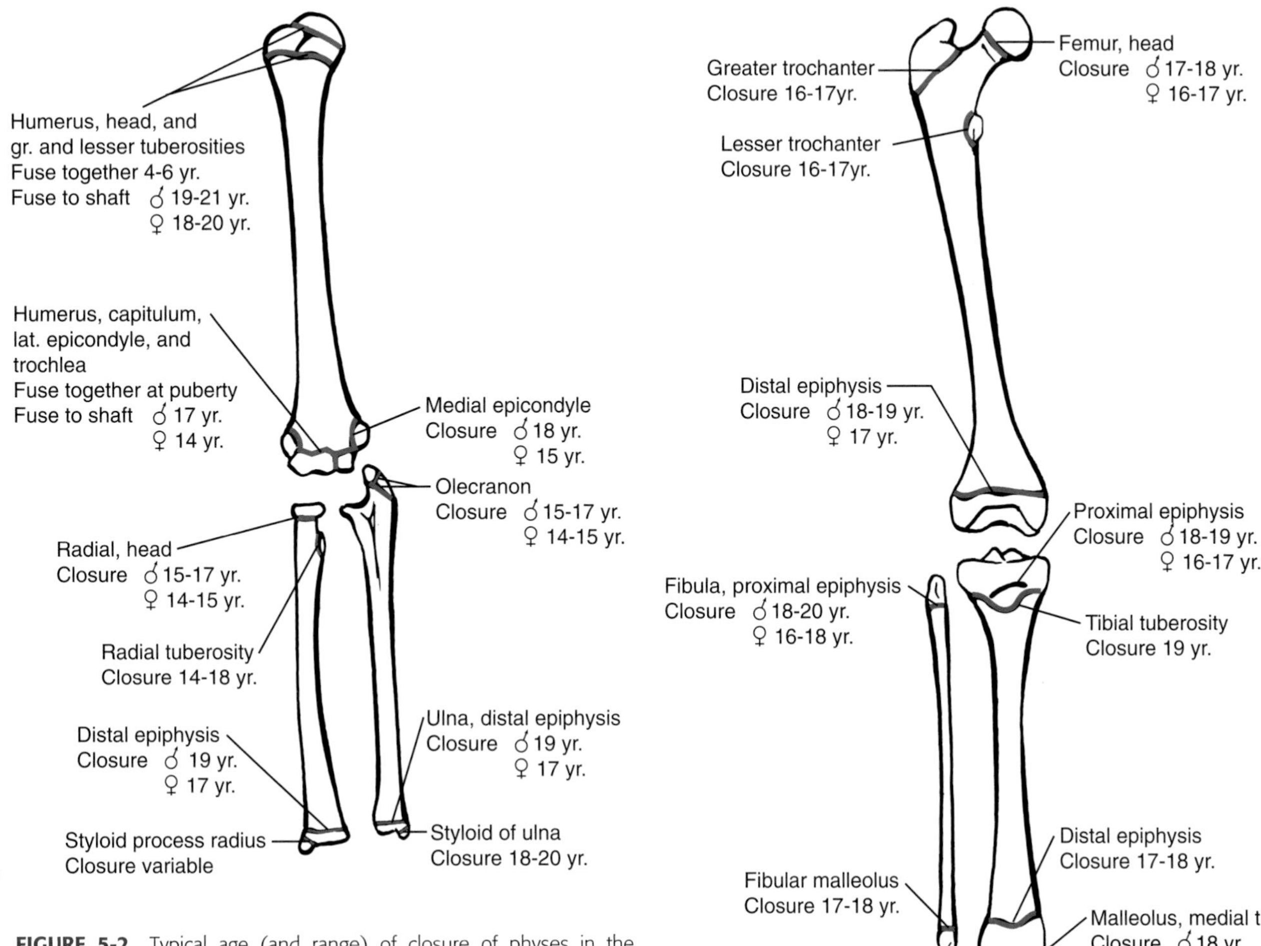

FIGURE 5-2 Typical age (and range) of closure of physes in the **(A)** upper extremity and **(B)** lower extremity.

least resistance (and hence fracture) within the physis. The germinal and proliferative zones are characterized by an abundance of extracellular matrix, whereas the hypertrophic and enchondral ossification zones are primarily apoptotic cells and vascular channels. As a consequence, fracture lines can be predicted to pass through the hypertrophic and enchondral ossification zones, a finding that Salter and Harris reported in their experimental investigation in rats (45). Theoretically, Salter-Harris types I and II fractures should involve these zones only, not affecting the germinal and proliferative zones, and thus should be at lower risk for subsequent growth disturbance. However, types III and IV physeal fractures traverse the entire physis, including the germinal and proliferative zones. In addition, displacement between bone fragments containing portions of the physis may occur. Consequently, growth disturbance is more likely from type III or IV injuries.

Not surprisingly, mechanical and clinical studies of microscopic fracture patterns have demonstrated that fracture lines through the physeal layers are more complex than this simplistic view, and often will undulate through the various zones (2,3,9,46–48). Smith et al (46) reported a Salter-Harris type I fracture of the distal tibia examined microscopically after associated traumatic lower leg amputation. In this high-energy injury, they found that the fracture line involved all four layers of the physis, in part because of the relatively straight plane of fracture and the undulations of the physis. Bright et al (2), in a study of experimentally induced physeal fractures in immature rats, found that not only was the fracture line usually complex, involving all four layers of the physis, but also that the physis contained a number of horizontal "cracks" separate from the fracture itself. They also observed a statistically significant lower force required to produce a physeal fracture in male and prepubescent animals, which might have clinical relevance to the epidemiologic aspects of physeal fractures (see discussion of epidemiology, below). The rate, direction, and magnitude of force are also factors that contribute to the histologic pattern of physeal fractures. Moen and Pelker (3), in an experimental study in calves, found that compression forces produced fractures in the zone of provisional calcification and metaphysis, shear caused fractures in the proliferative and hypertrophic zones, and torque produced fracture lines involving all four layers of the physis. Finally, the energy of injury is a factor in

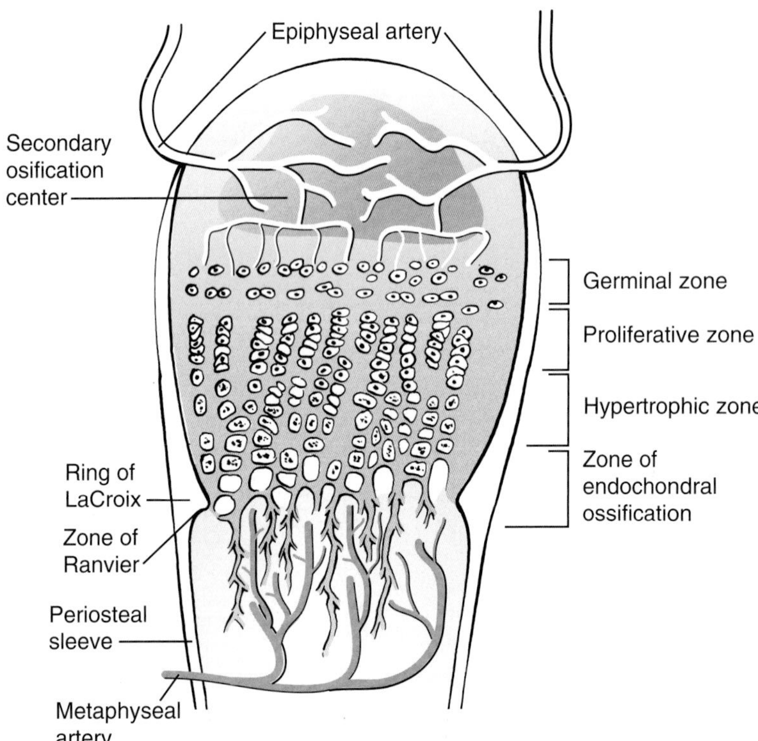

FIGURE 5-3 Schematic diagram of the organization of the physis. Four zones are illustrated: the germinal, proliferative, hypertrophic, and provisional calcification (or enchondral ossification) layers. Note also the groove of Ranvier and the perichondral ring of LaCroix.

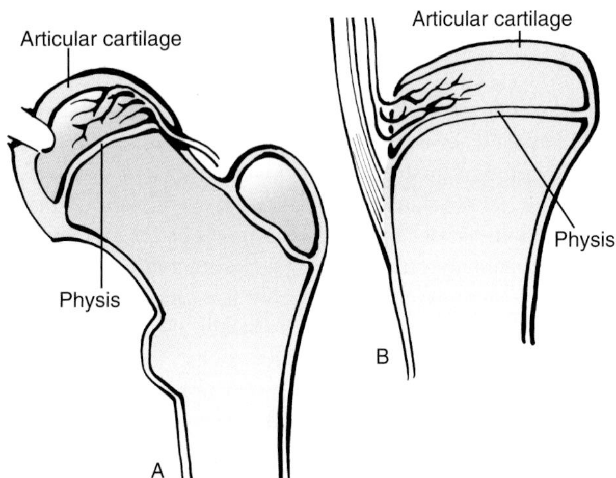

FIGURE 5-4 Classification of epiphyseal blood supply according to Dale and Harris. **A.** Type A epiphyses are nearly completely covered by articular cartilage. Blood supply must enter via the perichondrium. This blood supply is susceptible to disruption by epiphyseal separation. The proximal femur and proximal humerus are examples of type A epiphyses. **B.** Type B epiphyses are only partially covered by articular cartilage. Such epiphyses are more resistant to blood supply impairment by epiphyseal separation. The distal femur, proximal and distal tibia, and distal radius are clinical examples of type B epiphyses.

the extent of physeal injury. Distal femoral physeal fractures are a good example of the overriding significance of the energy of injury in potential for subsequent growth disturbance. High-energy mechanisms of injury are frequent in this region, and the risk of subsequent growth disturbance is high (40,49).

Contributions to Longitudinal Growth and Maturation Characteristics of Selected Physes

Growth of long bones is more complex than simple elongation occurring at their ends. However, as a generality, the physes at the end of long bones contribute known average lengths in percentage of total bone growth and percentage contributions to the total length between two physes at either end of a long bone. This information has come from observations of longitudinal growth by a number of authors (50–55). Knowledge of this information is paramount for the surgeon managing physeal injuries to long bones. Figure 5-5 outlines the generally accepted percentage of longitudinal growth contribution of pairs of physes for each long bone in the upper and lower extremities. Table 5-1 outlines the average amount of growth in millimeters per year of skeletal growth contributed by these same physes. These are estimations only, and growth tables should be consulted when more specific information is required (50–52, 54,55).

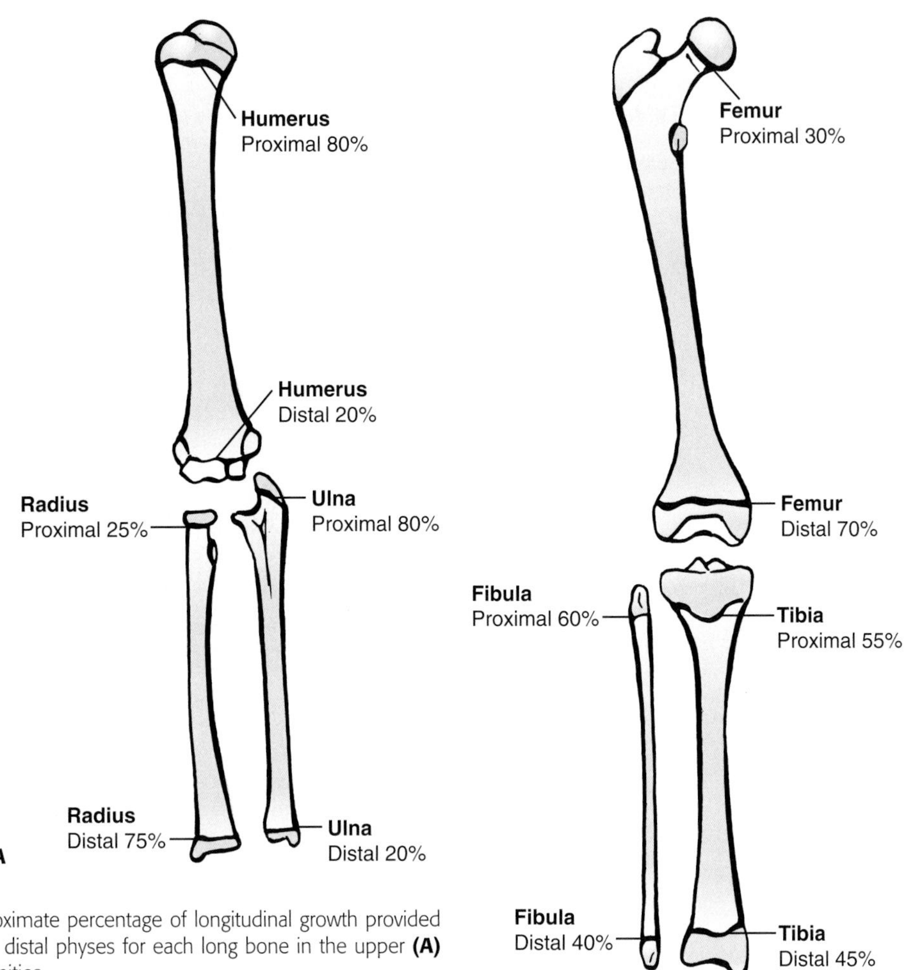

FIGURE 5-5 Approximate percentage of longitudinal growth provided by the proximal and distal physes for each long bone in the upper **(A)** and lower **(B)** extremities.

PHYSEAL INJURIES

Etiology of Physeal Injuries

Physes can be injured in many ways, both obvious and subtle. Obviously, the most frequent mechanism of injury is fracture. Most commonly, fracture injury is direct, with the fracture pattern involving the physis itself. Occasionally, physeal injury from trauma is indirect and associated with a fracture elsewhere in the limb segment, either as a result of ischemia (11) or perhaps compression (27,28,30,33,38,56,57) (see the discussion of Salter-Harris type V physeal fractures, below). Other mechanisms of injuries to the physes include infection (12,13,21,22), disruption by tumor, cysts (10), and tumor-like disorders, vascular insult (11), repetitive stress (20,58–61), irradiation (24,62), and other rare etiologies (18,19,63).

Infection

Long bone osteomyelitis or septic arthritis (particularly of the shoulder, hip, and knee) can cause physeal damage resulting in either physeal growth disturbance or frank growth arrest (12–17,21–23). These septic injuries may be further complicated by joint disruption resulting from associated epiphyseal destruction, articular cartilage damage, and capsular adhesions, particularly in the hip and shoulder.

Multifocal septic arrests can produce significant deformity requiring multiple surgical procedures. The most common causes are fulminant neonatal sepsis, particularly in premature infants or those with neonatal sepsis associated with maternal diabetes, and multiple septic arrests associated with meningococcemia (Fig. 5-6). In the latter case, physeal damage also may result from the cardiovascular collapse and disseminated intravascular coagulation known as purpura fulminans (14–16,23).

Tumor

Both malignant and benign tumors and tumor-like disorders can disrupt normal physeal architecture, resulting in direct physeal destruction. In the case of malignant tumors, the extent of growth lost as the result of local irradiation or limb salvage surgery must be taken into consideration in planning and recommending the therapeutic reconstruction to be undertaken.

Benign tumors and tumor-like conditions can result in de-

TABLE 5-1 Average Growth Per Year (in millimeters) of Specific Physes of the Upper and Lower Extremities*

Location	Average Growth (mm/yr)
Proximal humerus	7
Distal humerus	2
Proximal radius	1.75
Distal radius	5.25
Proximal ulna	5.5
Distal ulna	1.5
Proximal femur	3.5
Distal femur	9
Proximal tibia	6
Distal tibia	5
Proximal fibula	6.5
Distal fibula	4.5

* Estimations only. Gender, skeletal age, percentile height, and epiphyseal growth all influence magnitude of individual bone growth. Growth tables should be consulted when specific calculations are required.

Adapted from growth studies by Anderson et al, Green et al, and Maresh as published in Hensinger (1–9).

struction of all or part of a physis. Examples include enchondromata, either isolated or multiple (Ollier's disease) (Fig. 5-7), and unicameral bone cysts (10). Growth disturbance as a consequence of physeal damage from these disorders generally cannot be corrected by surgical physeal arrest resection (see Physeal Arrest Resection, below), and other treatment strategies must be adopted as clinically indicated.

Vascular Insult

Known vascular insult is a rare cause of physeal injury (11). Partial or complete growth arrests can occur from a pure vascular injury to an extremity (Fig. 5-8). Unrecognized vascular insult may represent the mechanism of subsequent growth disturbance after an injury in an adjacent part of a limb and may represent Salter-Harris type V injuries; the most common location for this is the tibial tubercle after femoral shaft or distal femoral physeal fractures. In addition, ischemia may be the cause of physeal damage associated with purpura fulminans (14–16,23).

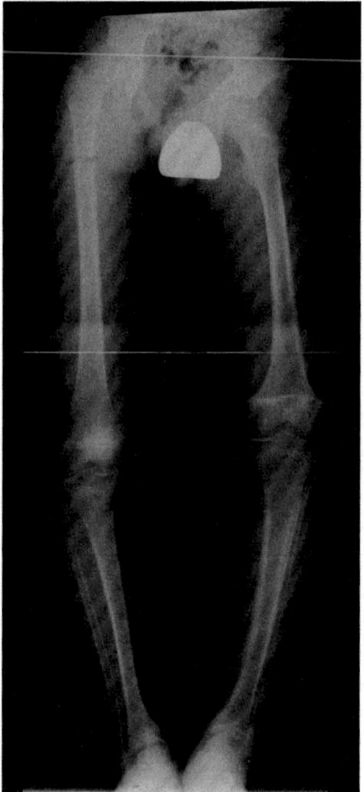

FIGURE 5-6 Standing anteroposterior lower extremity x-ray of a 12-year-old boy with multifocal physeal disturbance from purpura fulminans associated with meningococcemia. X-ray abnormalities are present in the left proximal femur; both distal femoral epiphyses, including partial arrest of the left distal femoral physis; and both distal tibial epiphyses. The patient also has digital amputations and extensive soft-tissue scarring resulting from this septic event.

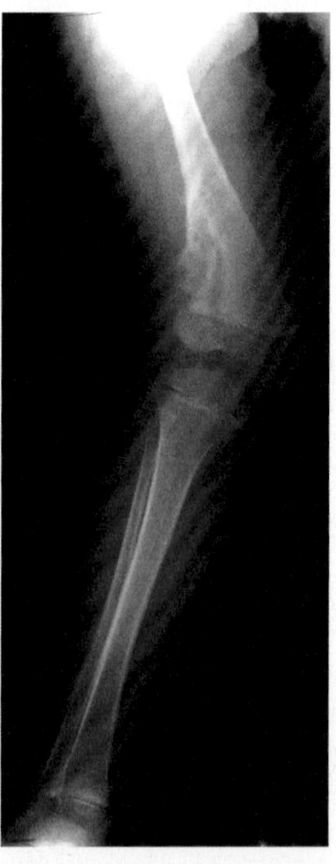

FIGURE 5-7 Valgus deformity of the distal femur associated with the presence of an enchondroma of the distal lateral femur involving the lateral physis.

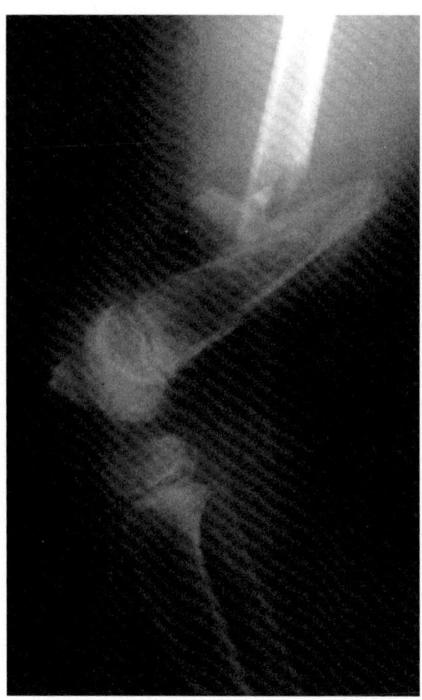

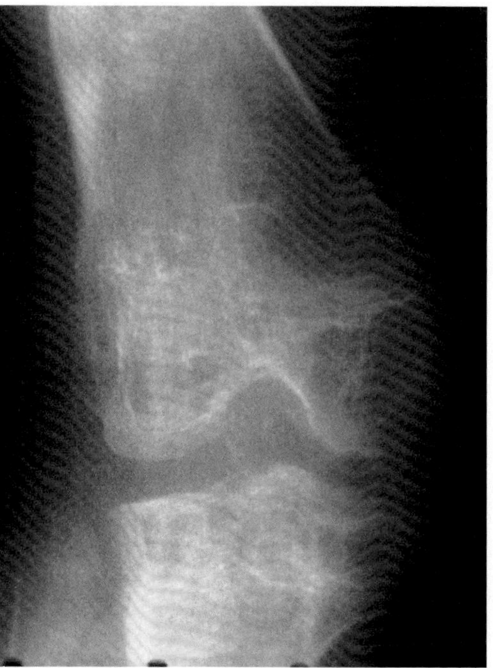

FIGURE 5-8 Physeal injury from presumed vascular insult. **A.** The patient's leg was caught under heavy pipes rolling off a rack, resulting in stripping of the soft tissues from the distal thigh, open comminuted fracture of the distal femur, and popliteal artery injury. **B.** In follow-up, after arterial and soft tissue reconstruction, the patient has physeal growth arrests of the distal femur and proximal tibia. The mechanism of injury to the proximal tibial physis was presumed to be vascular, because of the associated femoral artery injury.

Repetitive Stress

Repetitious physical activities in skeletally immature individuals can result in physeal stress-fracture equivalents (58,59,61). The most common location for such injuries are in the distal radius or ulna, as seen in competitive gymnasts (Fig. 5-9); the proximal tibia, as in running and kicking sports such as soccer (Fig. 5-10); and the proximal humerus, as in baseball pitchers (61). These injuries should be managed by rest, judicious resumption of activities, and longitudinal observation to monitor for potential physeal growth disturbance.

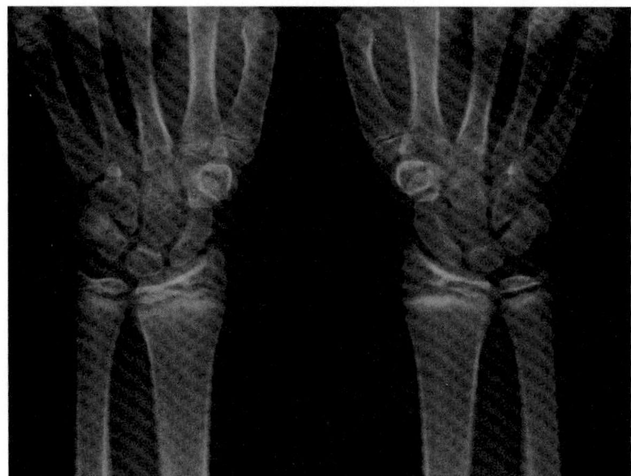

FIGURE 5-9 Stress injury of the distal radius and ulna in both wrists of a competitive gymnast. There was no history of specific injury. The wrists were tender to touch. Note distal radial and ulnar physeal widening and irregularity.

Miscellaneous (Irradiation, Thermal Injury, Electrical, Unrecognized)

Rare causes of physeal injury, usually recognized from consequent growth disturbance, include irradiation (Fig. 5-11) (24,62); thermal injury, especially phalangeal physeal injury from frostbite (Fig. 5-12) (18,19); burns; and electrical injuries. On rare occasions, physeal growth disturbance noted on clinical findings and x-rays has no identifiable cause. Presumably, such events represent unrecognized trauma or infection involving the physis.

Historical Review of Physeal Fractures

Physeal fractures have been recognized as unique since ancient times. Hippocrates is credited with the first written account of this injury. Poland (see Classification, below) reviewed accounts of physeal injuries in his 1898 book, *Traumatic Separation of the Epiphysis* (64). Poland is also credited with the first classification of the patterns of physeal fracture, and the publication of his text closely followed Roentgen's discovery of x-rays in 1895.

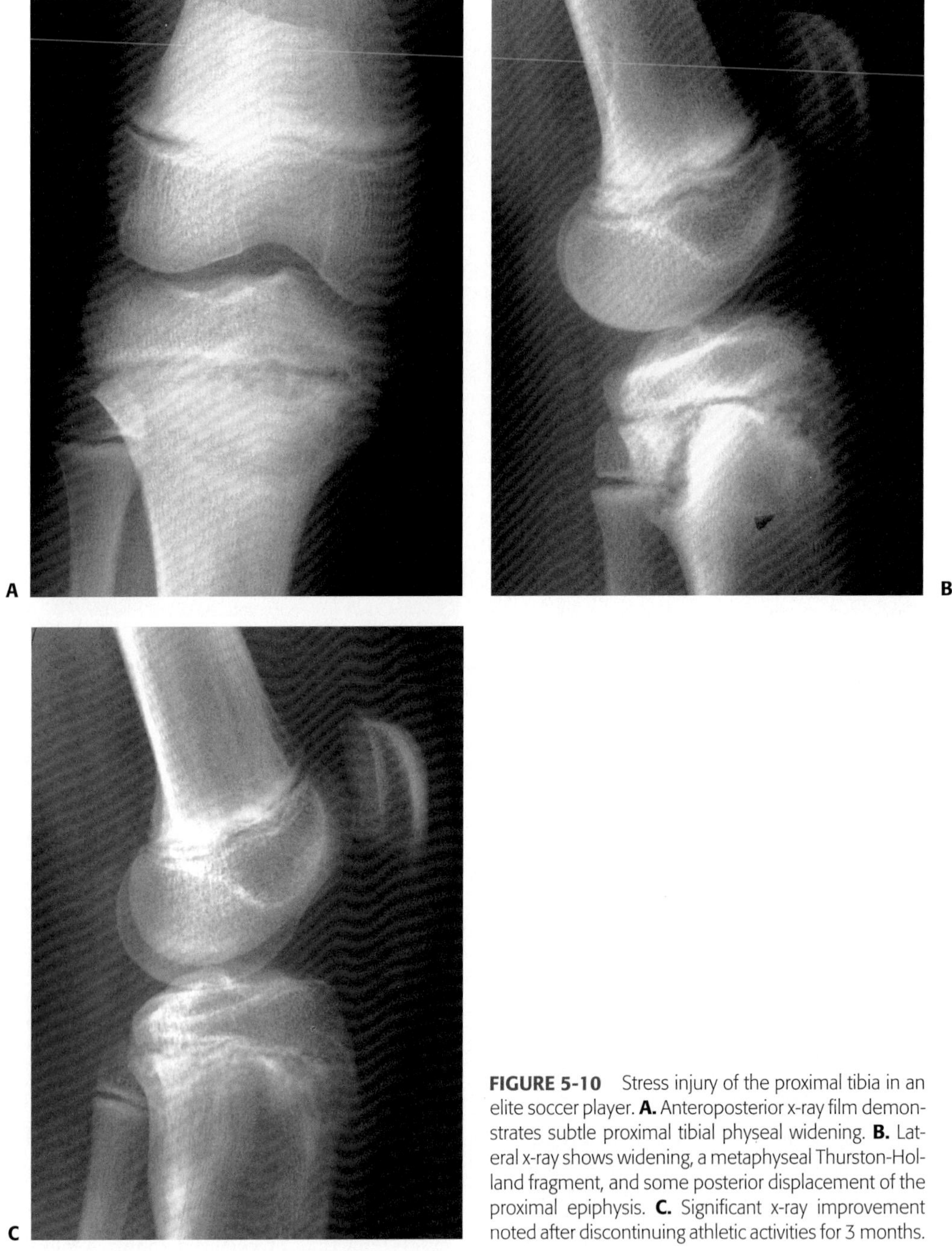

FIGURE 5-10 Stress injury of the proximal tibia in an elite soccer player. **A.** Anteroposterior x-ray film demonstrates subtle proximal tibial physeal widening. **B.** Lateral x-ray shows widening, a metaphyseal Thurston-Holland fragment, and some posterior displacement of the proximal epiphysis. **C.** Significant x-ray improvement noted after discontinuing athletic activities for 3 months.

Classification of Physeal Fractures

Poland (64) proposed the first classification of physeal fractures in 1898. Modifications to Poland's original scheme have been proposed by a number of authors (1,44,45,65–74), including Aitken (65), Salter and Harris (45), Ogden et al (71), and Peterson (72,73). Classifications of physeal fractures are important because they alert the practitioner to potentially subtle x-ray fracture patterns, can be of prognostic significance with respect to growth disturbance potential, and guide general treatment principles based on that risk and associated joint disruption. To some extent, fracture pattern provides some insight into mechanism of injury and the extent of potential physeal microscopic injury (see the sections Normal Physeal Anatomy and Mechanism of Injury).

Currently, the Salter-Harris classification, first published in 1963 (45), is firmly entrenched in the literature and most orthopaedists' minds. Therefore, evolution and specifics of the nature of physeal fractures of the various classification schemes

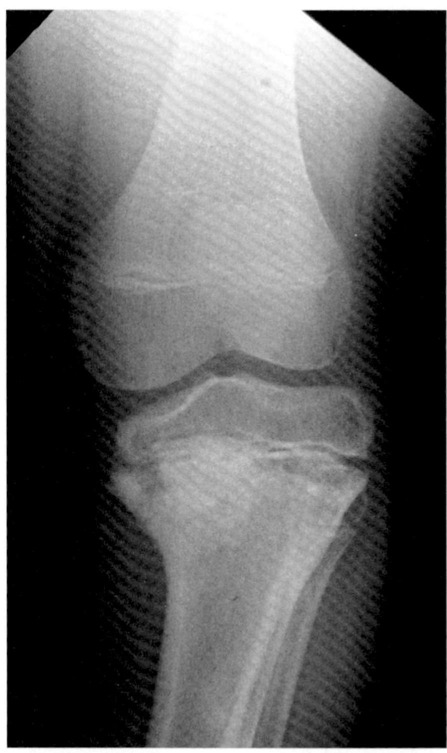

FIGURE 5-11 Proximal tibial physeal growth disturbance with angular deformity after irradiation for Ewing sarcoma.

are discussed relative to the Salter-Harris classification. The reader also should be aware of some deficiencies in that classification, as pointed out by Peterson (72,73,75).

Poland Classification of Physeal Fractures

Poland's classification, published in 1898 (64), consisted of four types of physeal fractures (Fig. 5-13). Types I, II, and III were the foundation of the Salter-Harris classification, as described below. Poland's type IV fracture was effectively a T-condylar fracture of the epiphysis and physis.

Aitken Classification of Physeal Fractures

Aitken in 1936 (65) included three patterns of physeal fracture in his classification (Fig. 5-14). His type I corresponded to Poland and Salter-Harris type II fractures, his type II to Poland and Salter-Harris type III fractures, and his type III was an intra-articular transphyseal metaphyseal-epiphyseal fracture equivalent to a Salter-Harris type IV fracture.

Salter-Harris Classification of Physeal Fractures

Salter and Harris published their commonly used five-part classification of physeal injuries in 1963 (45). The first four types were adopted from Poland (types I, II, and III) and Aitken (Aitken type III became Salter-Harris type IV) (Fig. 5-15). Salter and Harris added a fifth type, which they postulated was an unrecognized compression injury characterized by normal x-rays and late physeal closure. Peterson challenged the existence of true type V injuries (75), but other authors have subsequently

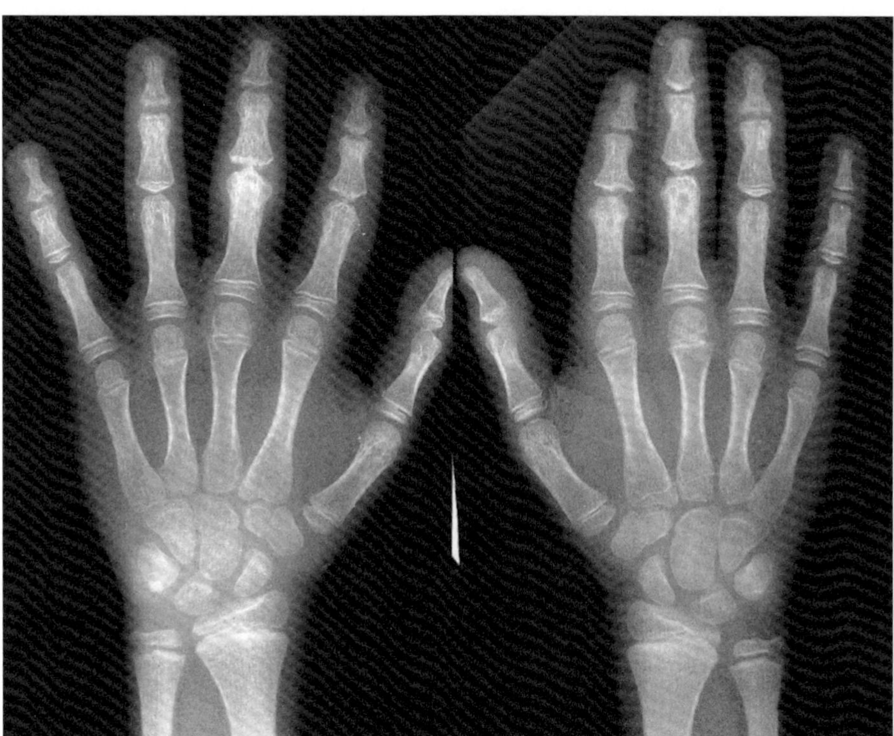

FIGURE 5-12 Premature closure of the distal phalangeal physes after a frostbite injury to the digits.

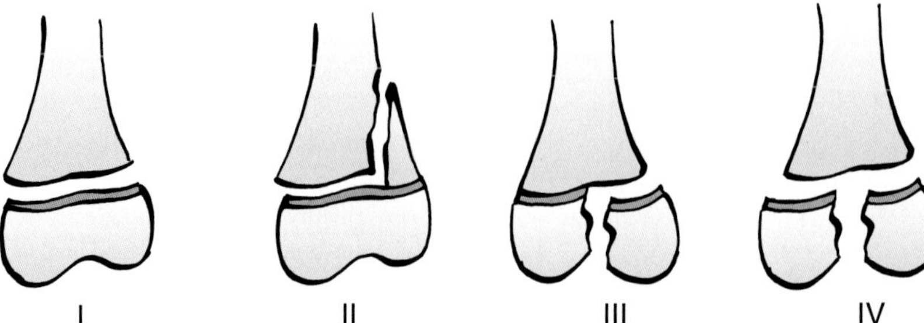

FIGURE 5-13 Poland classification of physeal fractures. Compare to the Salter-Harris classification. Poland type I, epiphyseal separation without metaphyseal fragment, or extension into the epiphysis. Poland type II, physeal fracture line extends into the metaphysis. Poland type III fracture extends from the articular surface to the physis and continues peripherally through the physis. Poland type IV, T-condylar fracture of the epiphysis and physis.

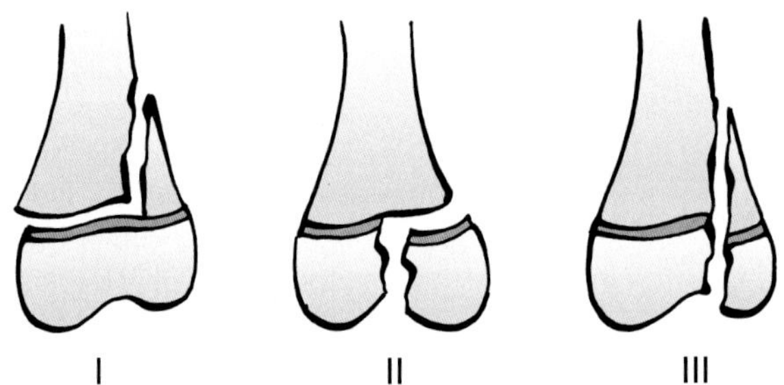

FIGURE 5-14 Aitken classification of physeal fractures: types I, II, and III. Type III is equivalent of Salter-Harris type IV.

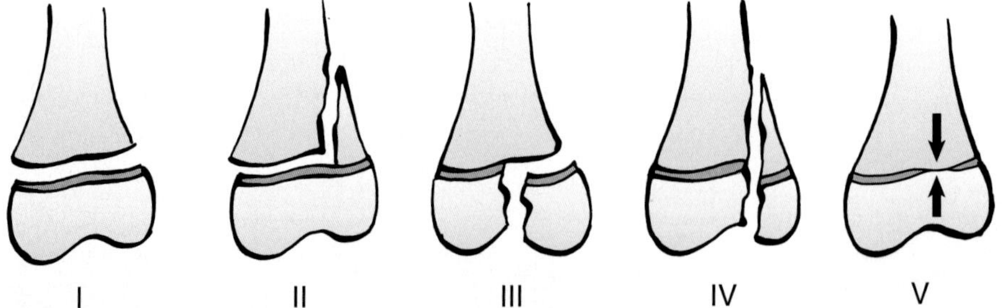

FIGURE 5-15 Salter-Harris classification of physeal fractures. In Salter-Harris type I fractures, the fracture line is entirely within the physis, referred to by Poland as type I. In Salter-Harris type II fractures the fracture line extends from the physis into the metaphysis; describes Poland as type II and Aitken as type I. In Salter-Harris type III fractures the fracture enters the epiphysis from the physis and almost always exits the articular surface. Poland described this injury as type III and Aitken as type II. In Salter-Harris type IV the fracture extends across the physis from the articular surface and epiphysis, to exit in the margin of the metaphysis. Aitken described this as a type III injury in his classification. Salter-Harris type V fractures were described by Salter and Harris as a crush injury to the physis with initially normal x-rays with late identification of premature physeal closure.

documented its existence in some form (27–30,33,57,75–77). Because we believe that delayed physeal closure can occur after some occult injuries, we have chosen to retain this type of injury in our preferred classification scheme.

Type I. Salter-Harris type I injuries are characterized by a transphyseal plane of injury, with no bony fracture line through either the metaphysis or the epiphysis. X-rays of undisplaced type I physeal fractures, therefore, are normal except for associated soft tissue swelling, making careful patient examination particularly important in this injury. In the Olmstead County Survey of physeal fractures (78), type I fractures occurred most frequently in the phalanges, metacarpals, distal tibia, and distal ulna. Epiphyseal separations in infants occur most commonly in the proximal humerus, distal humerus, and proximal femur. If an urgency to make the diagnosis is deemed necessary for patients suspected of having a type I injury, further imaging by ultrasound, magnetic resonance imaging (MRI) (74,79–82), or arthrography may be helpful (83–86). Stress x-rays to document displacement generally are unnecessary and probably unwise. Ultrasound is particularly helpful for assessing epiphyseal separations in infants (especially in the proximal femur and elbow regions) without the need for sedation, anesthetic, or invasive procedure (87–91).

The fracture line of type I injuries usually is in the zone of hypertrophy of the physis, as the path of least resistance during the propagation of the injury (see Normal Physeal Anatomy) (Fig. 5-16). As a consequence, in theory, the essential resting and proliferative zones are relatively spared, and, assuming that there is no vascular insult to these zones as a consequence of the injury, subsequent growth disturbance is relatively uncommon. As discussed above, however, studies have shown this to be a simplistic view of the fracture line through a physis, and that, due to uneven loading and macroscopic undulations in the physis, any zone of the physis can be affected by the fracture line (2,3,5,6,46,48).

Because the articular surface and, at least in theory, the germinal and proliferative layers of the physis are not displaced, the general principles of fracture management are to secure a gentle and adequate reduction of the epiphysis on the metaphysis and stabilize the fragments as needed.

Type II. Type II injuries have physeal and metaphyseal components; the fracture line extends from the physeal margin peripherally across a variable portion of the physis and exits into the metaphysis at the opposite end of the fracture (Fig. 5-17). The epiphyseal fragment thus comprises all of the epiphysis and some portion of the peripheral metaphysis (the Thurston-Holland fragment or sign). The physeal portion of this fracture has microscopic characteristics similar to those of type I injuries, but the fracture line exits the physis to enter the metaphysis (i.e., away from the germinal and proliferative layers) at one margin. Similar to type I injuries, these fractures should have a limited propensity to subsequent growth disturbance as a consequence of direct physeal injury. However, the metaphyseal "spike" of the diaphyseal/metaphyseal fragment may be driven into the physis of the epiphyseal fragment, which can damage the physis (Fig. 5-18). Similar to type I injuries, the articular surface is not affected and the general principles of fracture management are effectively the same.

Type III. Salter-Harris type III fractures begin in the epiphysis (with only rare exception) as a fracture through the articular surface and extend vertically toward the physis. The fracture then courses peripherally through the physis (Fig. 5-19). There are two fracture fragments: a small fragment consisting of a portion of the epiphysis and physis and a large fragment consisting the remaining epiphysis and long bone. This fracture pattern

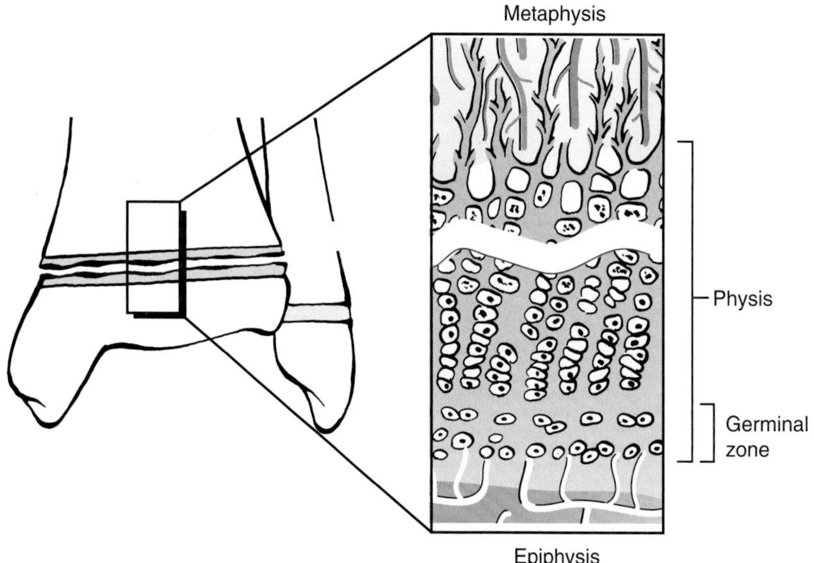

FIGURE 5-16 Scheme of theoretic fracture plane of Salter-Harris type I fractures. Because the hypertrophic zone is the weakest zone structurally, separation should occur at this level. Experimental and clinical studies have confirmed that the fracture plane is more complex than this concept and frequently involves other physeal zones as well.

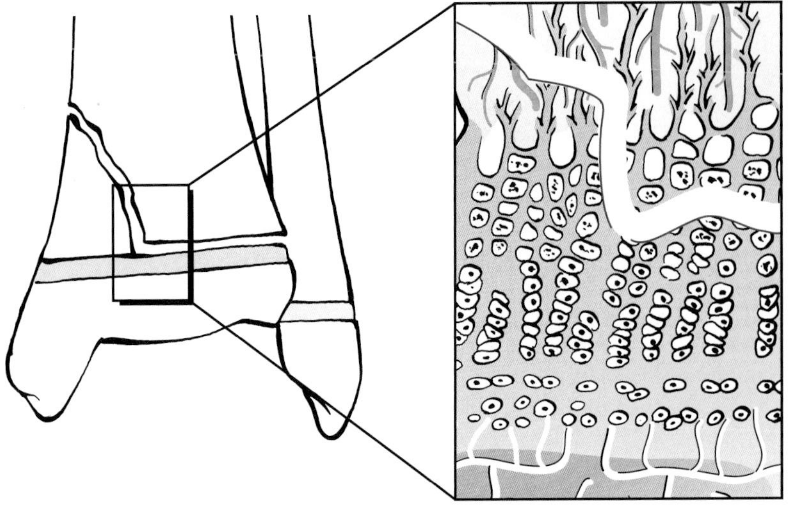

FIGURE 5-17 Fracture plane of Salter-Harris type II fractures. The fracture extends from the physis into the periphery of the metaphysis.

is important for two main reasons: the articular surface is involved (Fig. 5-20) and the fracture line involves the germinal and proliferative layers of the physis. In addition, type III injuries are often associated with high-energy or compression mechanisms of injury, which imply greater potential disruption of the physis and higher risk of subsequent growth disturbance. Anatomic reduction (usually open) and stabilization are required to restore the articular surface and to minimize the potential for growth disturbance.

On occasion, particularly in the distal femur and the distal humerus, high-energy injuries produce either a T-condylar or other complex pattern of injury, with at least three fragments, resulting in a combination of physeal and epiphyseal injuries (Fig. 5-21).

Type IV. Type IV fractures are effectively vertical shear fractures, extending from the articular surface to the metaphysis (Fig. 5-22A). These fractures are important because they disrupt the articular surface, violate all the physeal layers in crossing from the epiphysis to the metaphysis, and, with displacement,

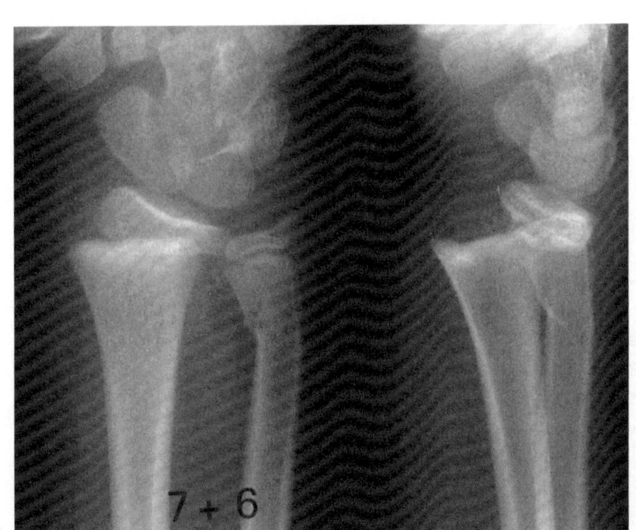

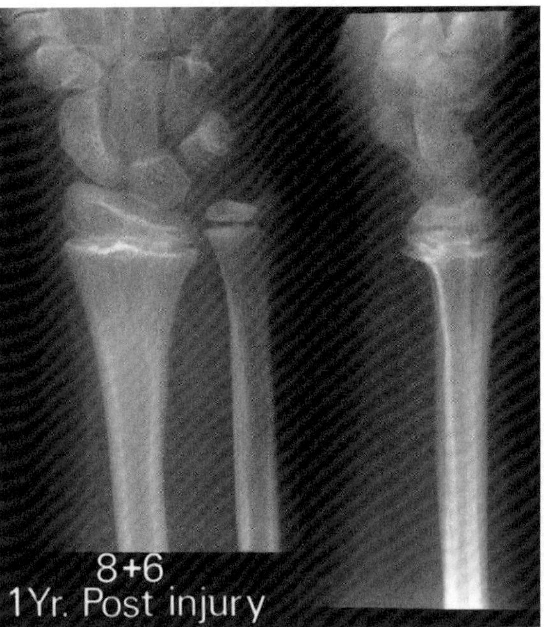

FIGURE 5-18 Potential mechanism of physeal arrest development after Salter-Harris type II fracture of the distal radius. **A.** Dorsally displaced type II fracture of the distal radius. Note the evidence of impaction of the epiphyseal fragment (with the physis) by the dorsal margin of the proximal fragment metaphysis. **B.** One year later, there is x-ray evidence of physeal arrest formation in the distal radial physis.

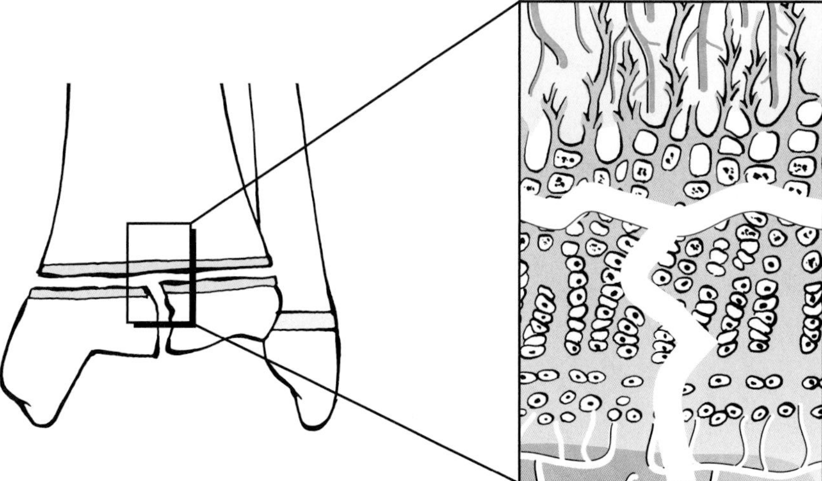

FIGURE 5-19 Scheme of fracture plane in Salter-Harris type III fractures. The fracture plane extends from the physis into the epiphysis and articular surface. "Extra-articular" type III fractures in which the articular surface is intact have been reported but are quite rare.

may result in metaphyseal-epiphyseal cross-union (Fig. 5-22B) (92,93). The latter occurrence almost invariably results in subsequent growth disturbance. This fracture pattern is frequent around the medial malleolus, but may occur in other epiphyses. Lateral condylar fractures of the distal humerus and intra-articular two-part triplane fractures of the distal tibia may be thought of as complex Salter-Harris type IV fractures. Rang (94) described an extra-articular variant (as if a peripheral extra-articular epiphyseal–physeal–metaphyseal fragment were "scooped out" from the rest of the bone) sometimes referred to as a Salter-Harris type VI fracture pattern.

General treatment principles include obtaining anatomic reduction and adequate stabilization to restore the articular surface and prevent metaphyseal-epiphyseal cross union.

Type V. The type V fracture described by Salter and Harris was not described by Poland or Aitken. Salter and Harris postulated that type V fractures represented unrecognized compression injuries with normal initial x-rays that later produced premature physeal closure. The existence of true type V injuries was questioned by Peterson (75) and subsequently became a subject of debate (27–30,33,57,76,77). We believe that delayed physeal closure clearly occurs. The most common example of such an injury is closure of the tibial tubercle, often with the development of recurvatum deformity of the proximal tibia, after

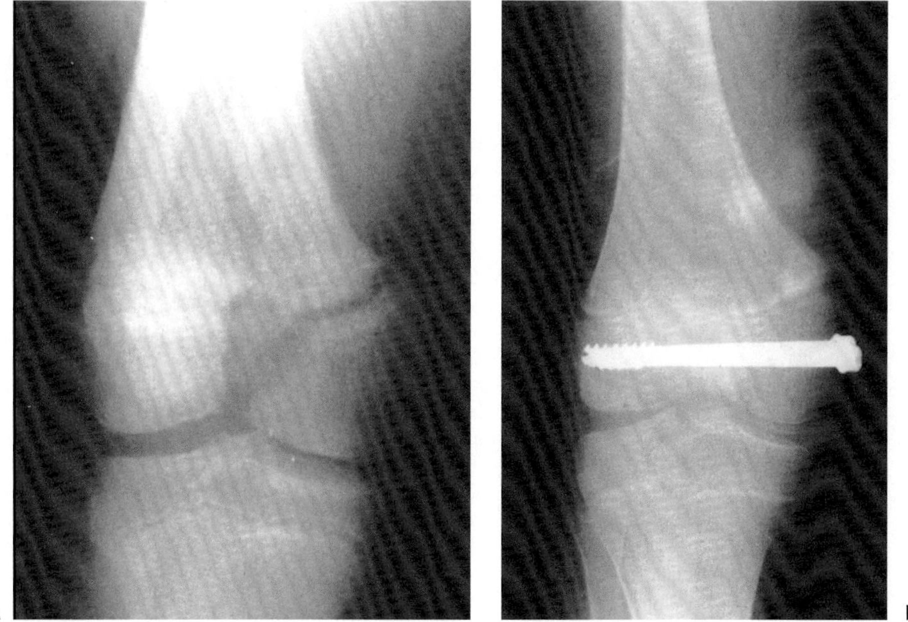

FIGURE 5-20 **A.** Salter-Harris type III fracture of the distal femur. **B.** Fixation with cannulated screws.

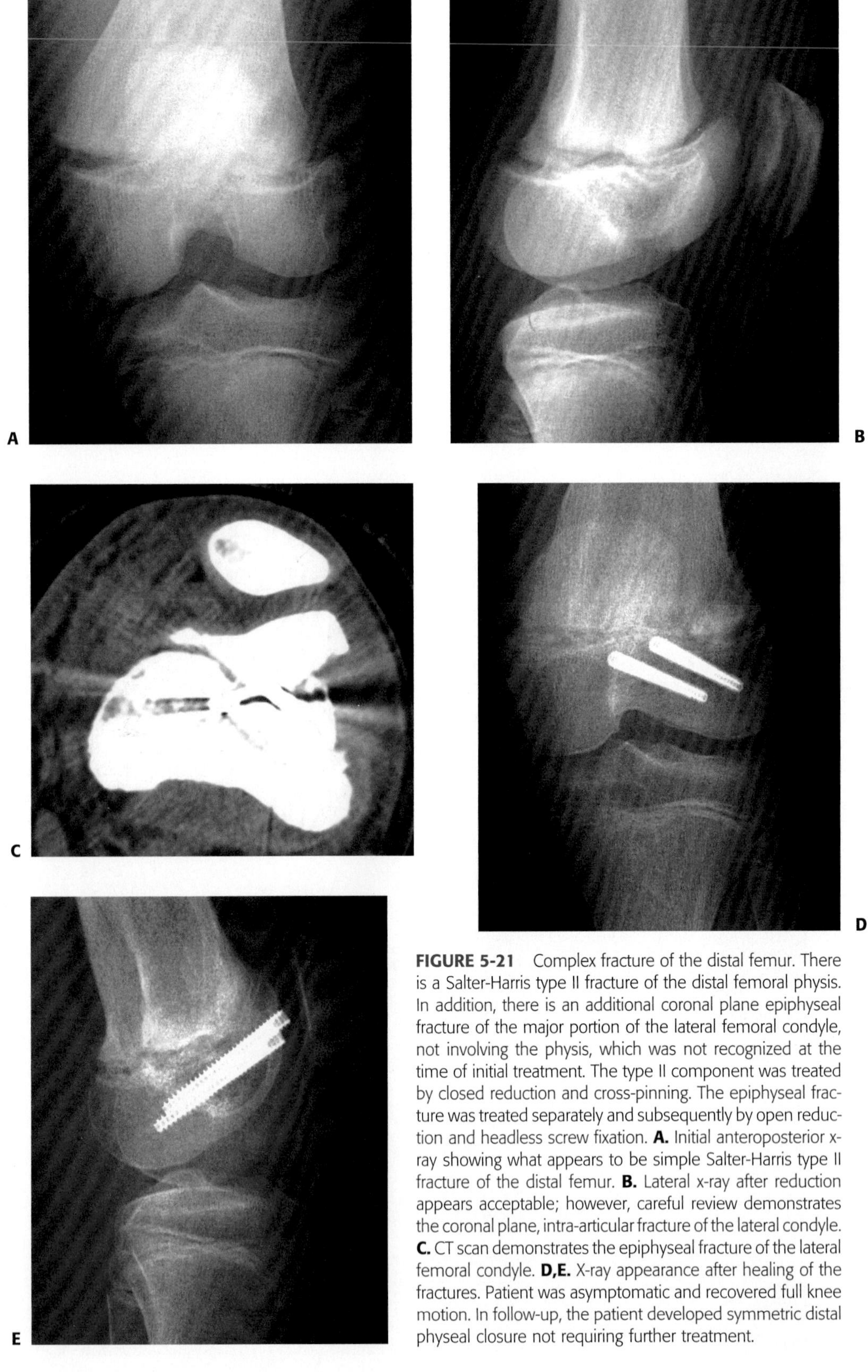

FIGURE 5-21 Complex fracture of the distal femur. There is a Salter-Harris type II fracture of the distal femoral physis. In addition, there is an additional coronal plane epiphyseal fracture of the major portion of the lateral femoral condyle, not involving the physis, which was not recognized at the time of initial treatment. The type II component was treated by closed reduction and cross-pinning. The epiphyseal fracture was treated separately and subsequently by open reduction and headless screw fixation. **A.** Initial anteroposterior x-ray showing what appears to be simple Salter-Harris type II fracture of the distal femur. **B.** Lateral x-ray after reduction appears acceptable; however, careful review demonstrates the coronal plane, intra-articular fracture of the lateral condyle. **C.** CT scan demonstrates the epiphyseal fracture of the lateral femoral condyle. **D,E.** X-ray appearance after healing of the fractures. Patient was asymptomatic and recovered full knee motion. In follow-up, the patient developed symmetric distal physeal closure not requiring further treatment.

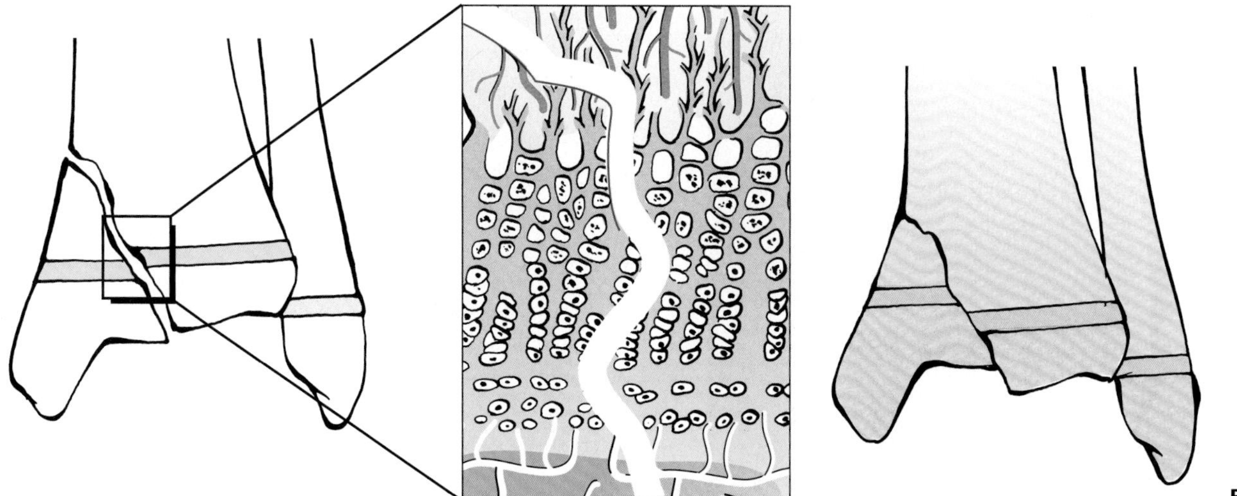

FIGURE 5-22 Scheme of the Salter-Harris type IV fracture. **A.** The fracture line extends across the physis from the epiphysis and articular surface into the peripheral metaphysis. The fracture line extends across the physis. **B.** Displacement of the fragments can lead to horizontal apposition (and cross-union) of the epiphyseal and metaphyseal bone.

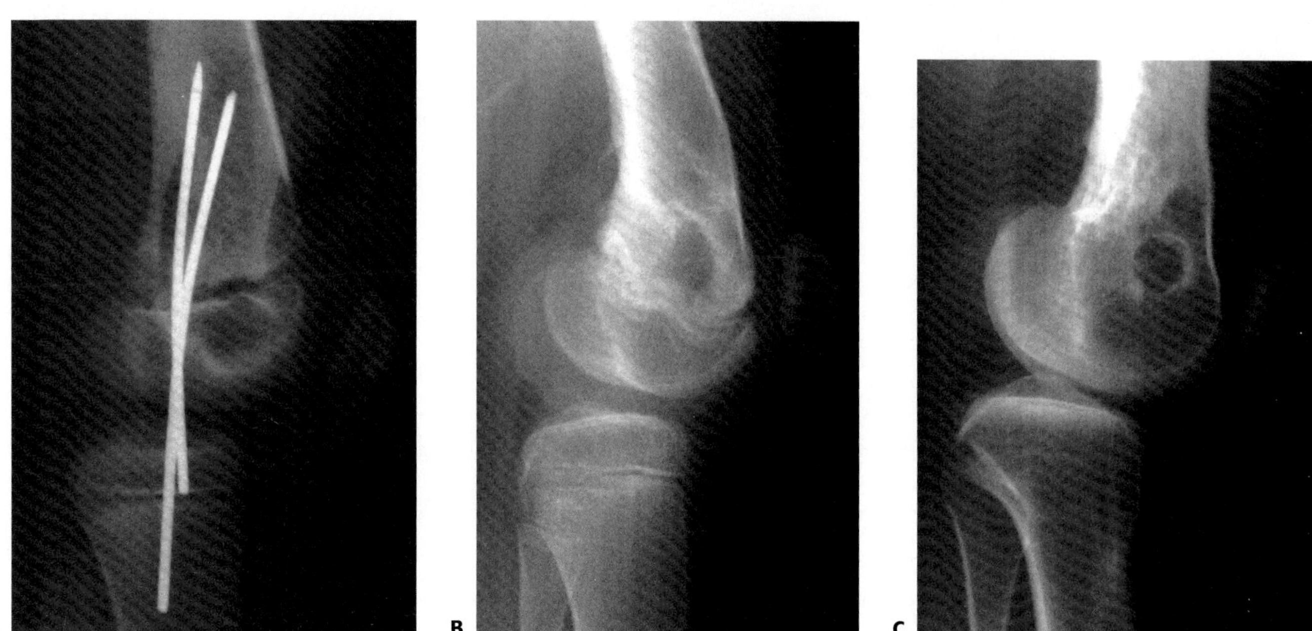

FIGURE 5-23 Post-traumatic closure of the anterior proximal tibial physis after displaced Salter-Harris type II fracture of the distal femoral physis. **A.** Lateral x-rays after reduction. No injury to the proximal tibia was noted at the time of treatment of the distal femoral injury. **B.** At follow-up, distal femoral physeal growth disturbance with flexion deformity is apparent. **C.** At skeletal maturity, proximal tibial extension deformity with sclerosis of the tibial tubercle area is evident, suggestive of arrest in this area. The patient has undergone a distal femoral extension osteotomy.

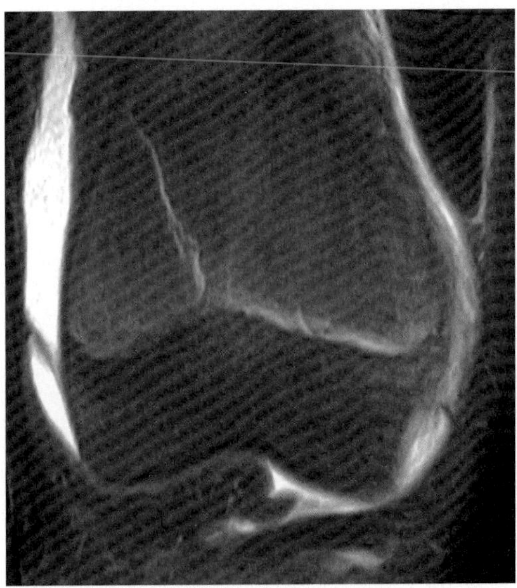

FIGURE 5-24 Magnetic resonance imaging (MRI) of patient after injury with normal x-rays. MRI clearly documents the presence of a Salter-Harris type II fracture of the distal femur.

fractures of the femur or distal femoral epiphysis (Fig. 5-23) (30,76,77). While the mechanism of such injuries may be unclear (perhaps vascular rather than compression trauma), the traditionally held view that such injuries occurred as a result of inadvertent direct injury during the insertion of proximal tibial skeletal traction pins has been unequivocally discounted in some cases (30,76,77). Other locations and case reports of late physeal closure after extremity injury and apparently normal initial x-rays exist in the literature (27–29,33,57,95). By definition, this pattern of injury is unrecognized on initial x-rays. Undoubtedly, more sophisticated imaging of injured extremities (such as with MRI) will identify physeal injuries in the presence of normal plain x-rays (Fig. 5-24). Although the mechanism of injury in type V injuries may be in dispute, in our opinion, the existence of such injuries is not.

Peterson Classification of Physeal Fractures

In an epidemiologic study of physeal injuries, Peterson (78) identified several deficiencies of the Salter-Harris classification and subsequently developed a new classification of physeal fractures (Fig. 5-25). Peterson was not able to identify any Salter-Harris type V injuries caused by compression in this epidemiologic study, challenged their existence, and excluded that type from his classification. His classification retained Salter-Harris types I through IV as Peterson types II, III, IV, and V and added two new types (72,73). It is important to be cognizant of the two new patterns that Peterson described, because they are clinically relevant.

Peterson's type I is a transverse metaphyseal fracture with a longitudinal extension to the physis (Fig. 5-26). He subclassified this pattern of injury into four types, based on the extent of metaphyseal comminution and fracture pattern (73).

Peterson's type VI is a partial physeal loss (Fig. 5-27). Unfortunately, this pattern of injury currently is common, largely as a consequence of lawnmower injuries. Soft tissue loss, neurovascular injury, and partial physeal loss (usually including the epiphysis so that articular impairment also results) further complicate this often-devastating injury.

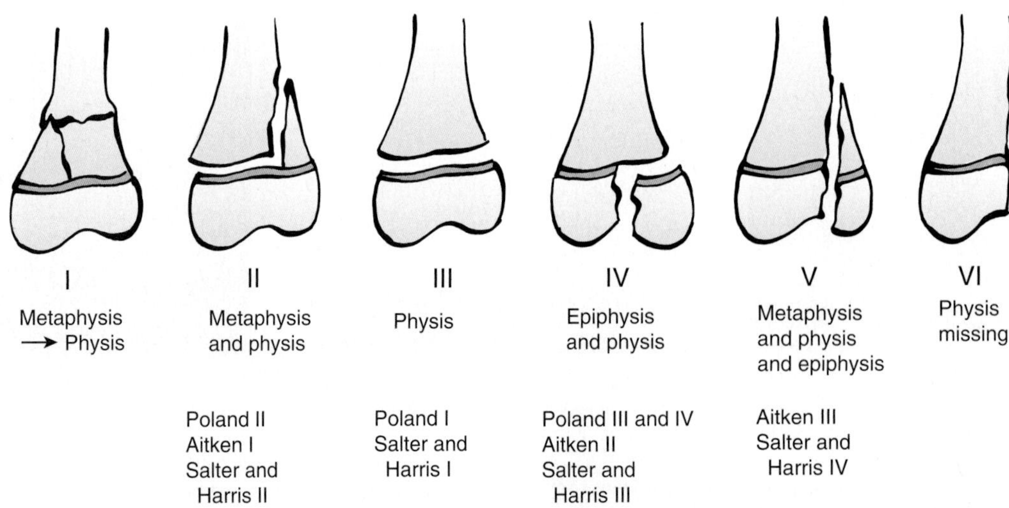

FIGURE 5-25 Peterson classification of physeal fractures. Type I is a fracture of the metaphysis extending to the physis. Types II to V are the equivalents of Salter-Harris types I, II, III, and IV, respectively. Peterson type VI is epiphyseal (and usually articular surface) loss. Lawnmower injuries are a frequent mechanism for type VI injuries. (See text for further discussion.)

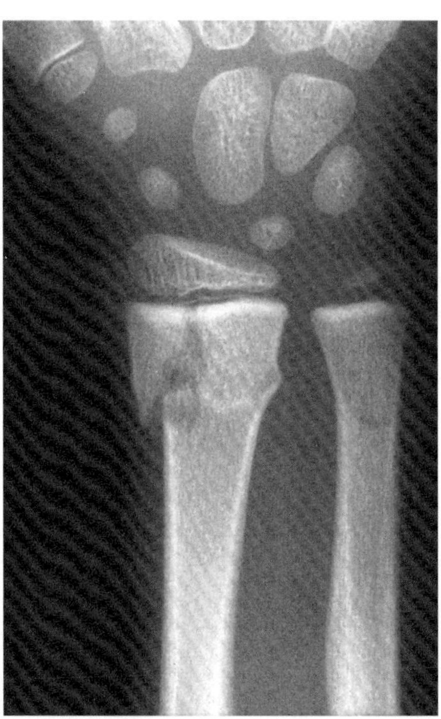

FIGURE 5-26 Peterson type I injury of the distal radius. These injuries typically have a benign course with respect to subsequent growth disturbance.

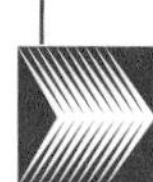

AUTHORS' PREFERRED TREATMENT

We believe that the Salter-Harris classification remains an easily recognized and recalled classification scheme embracing most physeal injuries and continue to use it to describe most physeal fracture patterns. It provides generally useful prognostic and treatment guidelines. We encourage the continued recognition of the Salter-Harris type V physeal injury as a delayed, indirect, or occult injury–induced physeal closure, whose mechanism may be compression, other unrecognized direct injury, or vascular insult. We also believe that Peterson types I and VI physeal fractures are not classifiable by the Salter-Harris scheme and refer to them as Peterson type I and VI fractures, respectively.

Epidemiology of Physeal Fractures

In several population surveys reporting the frequency and distribution of childhood fractures, including physeal injuries (70,78,95,96), 20% to 30% of all childhood fractures were physeal injuries. The phalanges represent the most common location of physeal injuries.

In our opinion, the most useful epidemiologic study of physeal fractures is the Olmstead County Survey (78). This study of the frequency of physeal fractures in a stable population base

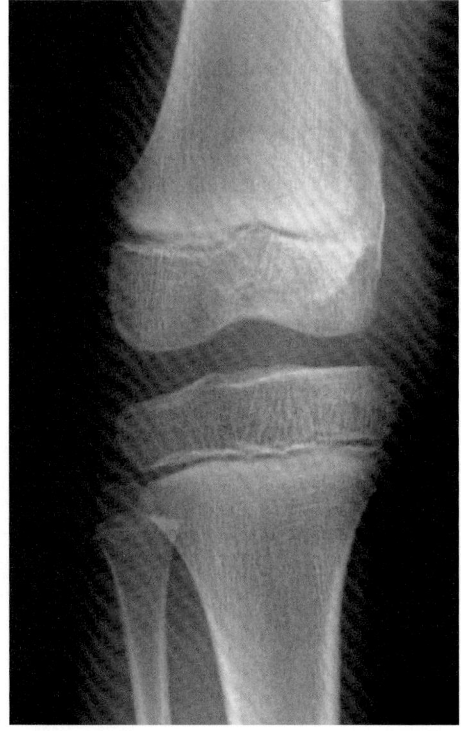

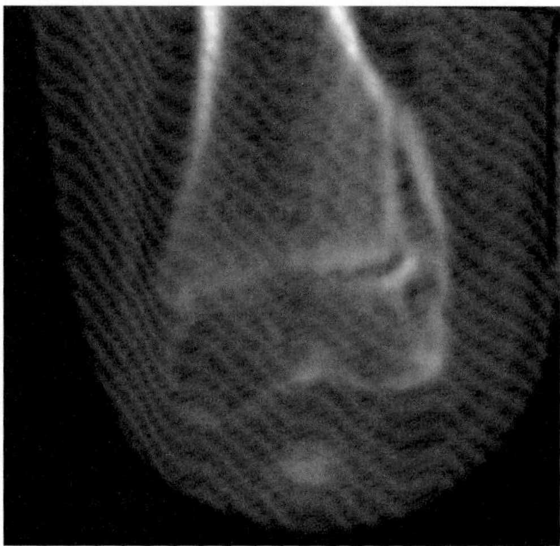

FIGURE 5-27 Sequelae of a Peterson type VI physeal injury. **A.** Anteroposterior x-ray of distal femur of a young girl who suffered a Peterson type VI injury. This particular injury was the result of direct abrasion of the distal femur when the unrestrained child was ejected from a car. **B.** Computed tomography scan 1 year after injury demonstrates the development of a peripheral physeal arrest with valgus deformity.

was performed between 1979 and 1988, in Olmstead County, Minnesota. The most relevant components are summarized in Tables 5-2 and 5-3. During the study period, 951 physeal fractures were identified: 37% of fractures occurred in the finger phalanges, with the next most common site the distal radius; 71% fractures occurred in the upper extremity, 28% in the lower, and 1% in the axial skeleton. Other salient findings of the Olmstead County survey included a 2:1 male to female ratio and age-related incidence by gender (peak incidence at age 14 in boys and 11 to 12 in girls) (Fig. 5-28). The Adelaide, Australia survey by Mizuta et al (95) had similar findings: 30% of physeal fractures were phalangeal, males outnumbered females approximately 2:1, and the prepubertal age-groups had the highest relative frequency of physeal fracture.

TABLE 5-2 Frequency of Physeal Fracture by Location

Skeletal Site	Number	Percent
Phalanges (fingers and toes)	411	43.4
Distal radius	170	17.9
Distal tibia	104	11.0
Distal fibula	68	7.2
Metacarpal	61	6.4
Distal humerus	37	3.9
Distal ulna	27	2.8
Proximal humerus	18	1.9
Distal femur	13	1.4
Metatarsal	13	1.4
Proximal tibia	8	0.8
Proximal radius	6	0.6
Clavicle (medial and lateral)	6	0.6
Proximal ulna	4	0.4
Proximal femur	1	0.1
Proximal fibula	1	0.1

Modified from Peterson HA, Madhok R, Benson JT, et al. Physeal fractures. I. Epidemiology in Olmsted County, Minnesota, 1979–1988. *J Pediatr Orthopedics* 1994;14:423–430.

TABLE 5-3 Distribution of Physeal Fracture Patterns by Salter-Harris and Peterson Types I and VI Classification*

Fracture Type	Number	Percent
Salter-Harris I	126	13.2
Salter-Harris II	510	53.6
Salter-Harris III	104	10.9
Salter-Harris IV	62	6.5
Peterson I	147	15.5
Peterson VI	2	0.2

* See text for description of physeal fracture classification.
Modified from Peterson HA, Madhok R, Benson JT, et al. Physeal fractures. I. Epidemiology in Olmsted County, Minnesota, 1979–1988. *J Pediatr Orthopedics* 1994;14:423–430.

Evaluation of Physeal Fractures

Modalities available for the evaluation of physeal injuries include plain x-rays, CT and MRI scans (48,74,79–82,97), arthrography (83–86,98), and ultrasound (87–91). Plain x-rays remain the preferred initial modality for the assessment of most physeal injuries. X-rays should be taken in true orthogonal views and include the joint both above and below the fracture. If a physeal injury is suspected, dedicated views centered over the suspected physis should be obtained to decrease parallax and increase detail. Oblique views may be of value in assessing minimally displaced injuries.

Although plain x-rays provide adequate detail for the assessment and treatment of most physeal injuries, occasionally greater anatomic detail is necessary. CT scans provide excellent definition of bony anatomy, particularly using reconstructed images. They may be helpful in assessing complex or highly comminuted fractures, as well as the articular congruency of minimally displaced fractures (Fig. 5-29). MRI scans are excellent for demonstrating soft tissue lesions and "minor osseous injuries," which may not be seen using standard radiation techniques.

Both arthrography and ultrasound have been used to assess the congruency of articular surfaces. Arthrography may help define the anatomy in young patients with small or no secondary ossification centers in the epiphyses (83–86,98). Ultrasonography occasionally is useful for diagnostic purposes to identify epiphyseal separation in infants (Fig. 5-30) (87–90,98).

Treatment

The general tenets of physeal fracture management are essentially the same as those for injuries not involving the physis, including

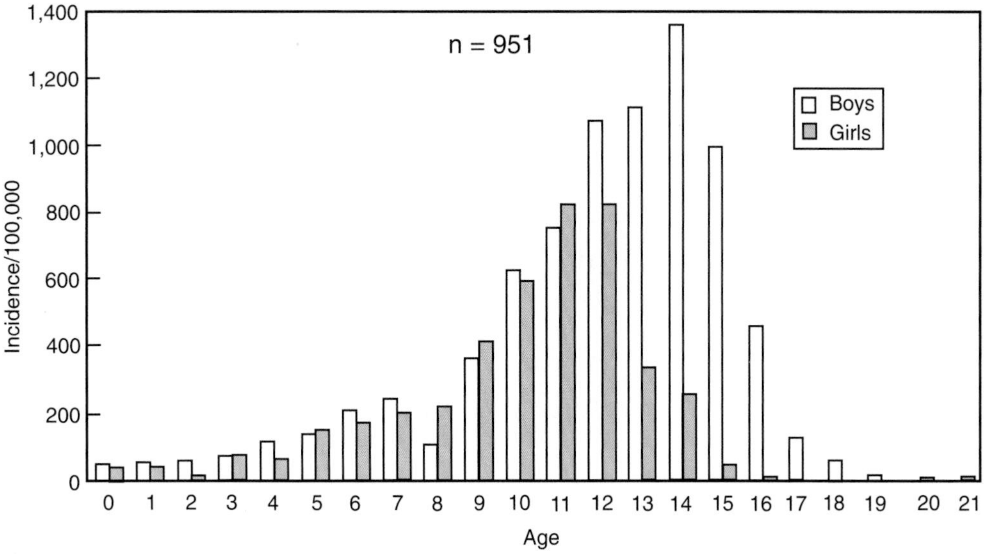

FIGURE 5-28 Relative frequency of physeal fractures by age and sex according to the Olmstead County survey by Peterson et al (78). Peak incidence age 14 in boys, and 11 to 12 in girls.

x-rays of all areas with abnormal physical findings. Once the patient has been stabilized and the initial assessment completed, further studies may be obtained as indicated. Open physeal injuries and those involving neurovascular compromise or impending compartment syndrome should be managed emergently. In most cases, stabilization of the physeal fractures will help facilitate management of the soft tissue injury. All trauma patients should be reassessed as their condition stabilizes to identify occult injuries not identified in the initial assessment.

General Principles of Treatment

In general, fractures in children, including physeal injuries, heal more rapidly than in adults, and they are less likely to experience morbidity or mortality from prolonged immobilization. Additionally, children also are often less compliant with postoperative activity restrictions, making cast immobilization a frequently necessary adjunct to therapy.

Physeal fractures, like all fractures, should be managed in a consistent methodical manner that includes a general assessment and stabilization of the polytraumatized patient, evaluation of the neurovascular and soft tissue status of the traumatized limb, and reduction and stabilization of the fracture. What constitutes an "acceptable" reduction is dictated in part by the fracture pattern and remodeling potential of the fracture. Intra-articular fractures (such as Salter-Harris types III and IV) require

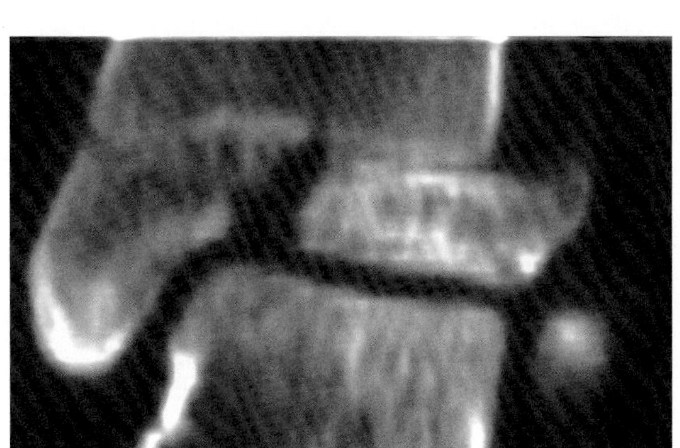

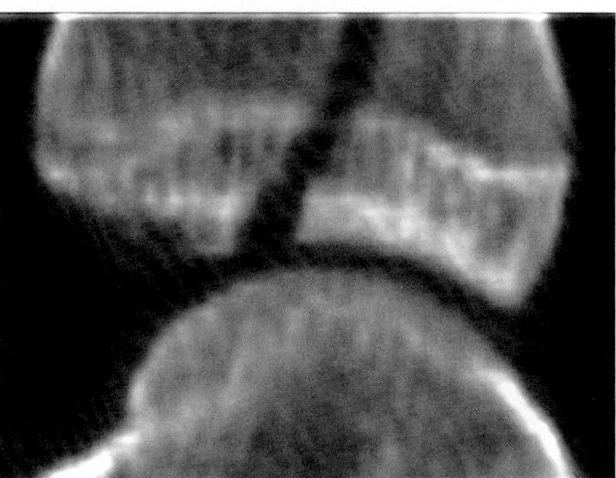

FIGURE 5-29 Computed tomography scans with or without reconstructed images can be helpful in the assessment of physeal fractures. Coronal **(A)** and **(B)** sagittal plane reconstructions of a triplane fracture of the distal tibia.

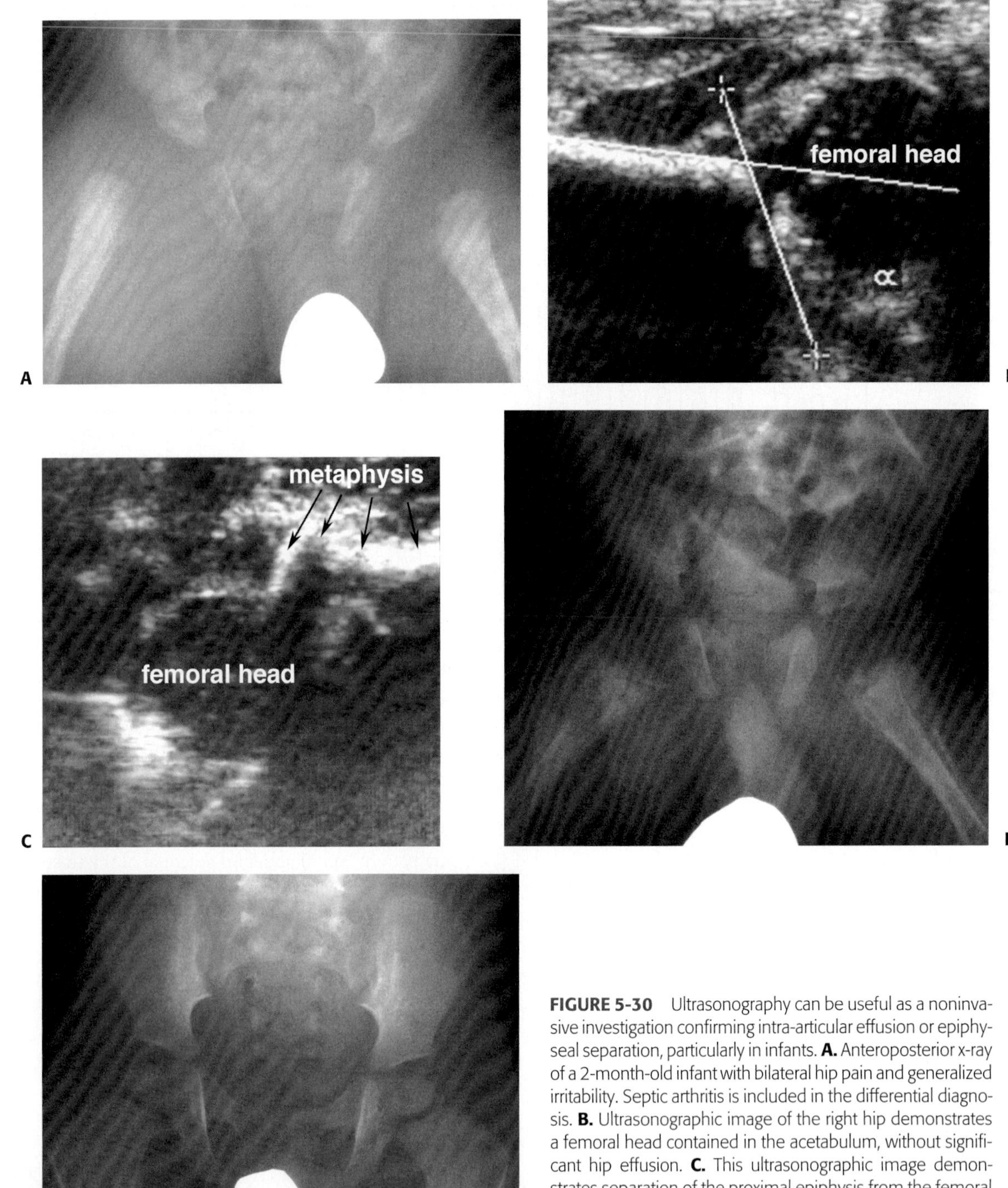

FIGURE 5-30 Ultrasonography can be useful as a noninvasive investigation confirming intra-articular effusion or epiphyseal separation, particularly in infants. **A.** Anteroposterior x-ray of a 2-month-old infant with bilateral hip pain and generalized irritability. Septic arthritis is included in the differential diagnosis. **B.** Ultrasonographic image of the right hip demonstrates a femoral head contained in the acetabulum, without significant hip effusion. **C.** This ultrasonographic image demonstrates separation of the proximal epiphysis from the femoral metaphysis. The diagnosis is non-accidental trauma. **D.** One month later, x-ray demonstrates extensive periosteal reaction bilaterally. **E.** At 18 months of age x-ray demonstrates remarkable remodeling, without evidence of physeal growth disturbance or epiphyseal abnormality.

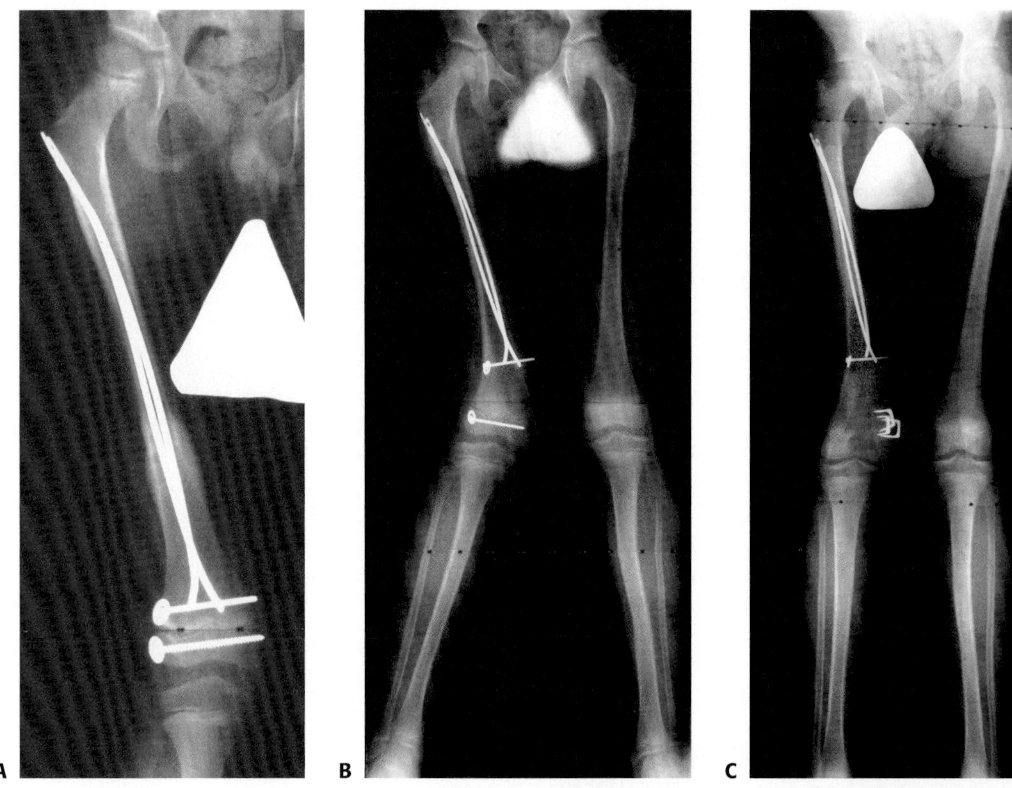

FIGURE 5-31 Growth deceleration in the absence of a true physeal arrest. This patient sustained concurrent ipsilateral femoral shaft and Salter-Harris type IV distal femoral epiphyseal fractures. **A.** Anteroposterior x-ray of the healed femur. Both fractures were treated with internal fixation. **B.** The patient developed valgus deformity of the distal femur due to asymmetric growth of the distal femoral physis. Note that the distance between the screws on either side of the physis has increased asymmetrically, confirming asymmetric growth rather than cessation of growth laterally. **C.** The angular deformity was treated with medial distal femoral epiphyseal stapling.

anatomic reduction to restore the articular surface and prevent epiphyseal–metaphyseal cross-union. Salter-Harris types I and II fractures, particularly those that are the result of low-energy injuries, have minimal risk of growth disturbance (excepting injuries of the distal femur and proximal tibia) and excellent remodeling potential in most patients; in such patients, the surgeon must be cautious not to *create* physeal injury by excessively forceful or invasive reductions.

Complications of Physeal Fractures

Except for the possibility of subsequent growth disturbance, the potential complications of physeal injuries are no different than other traumatic musculoskeletal injuries. Neurovascular compromise and compartment syndrome represent the most serious potential complications (31,39). It is important to remember that, although a high degree of suspicion and diligence may avoid some of these potentially devastating complications, they can occur even with "ideal" management. Infection and soft tissue loss can complicate physeal fracture management, just as they can in other fractures. The one complication unique to physeal injuries is growth disturbance. Most commonly this "disturbance" is the result of a tethering (physeal bar or arrest) that may produce angular deformity or shortening. However, growth disturbance may occur without an obvious tether or bar and growth acceleration also occurs (Fig. 5-31). Finally, growth disturbance may occur without injury to the physis.

PHYSEAL GROWTH DISTURBANCE

An uncommon but important complication of physeal fracture is physeal growth disturbance (36,38,40). The potential consequences of physeal growth disturbance include the development of angular deformity, limb length inequality, epiphyseal distortion, or various combinations of these. Which, if any, of these abnormalities develop depends on the physis affected, location within the affected physis, the duration of time present, and the skeletal maturity of the patient. Frequently, further surgery, often repeated and extensive, is required to correct or prevent deformity caused by an established growth disturbance (99–106).

Etiology

Disturbance of normal physeal growth may result from physical loss of the physis (such as after Peterson type VI injuries), from

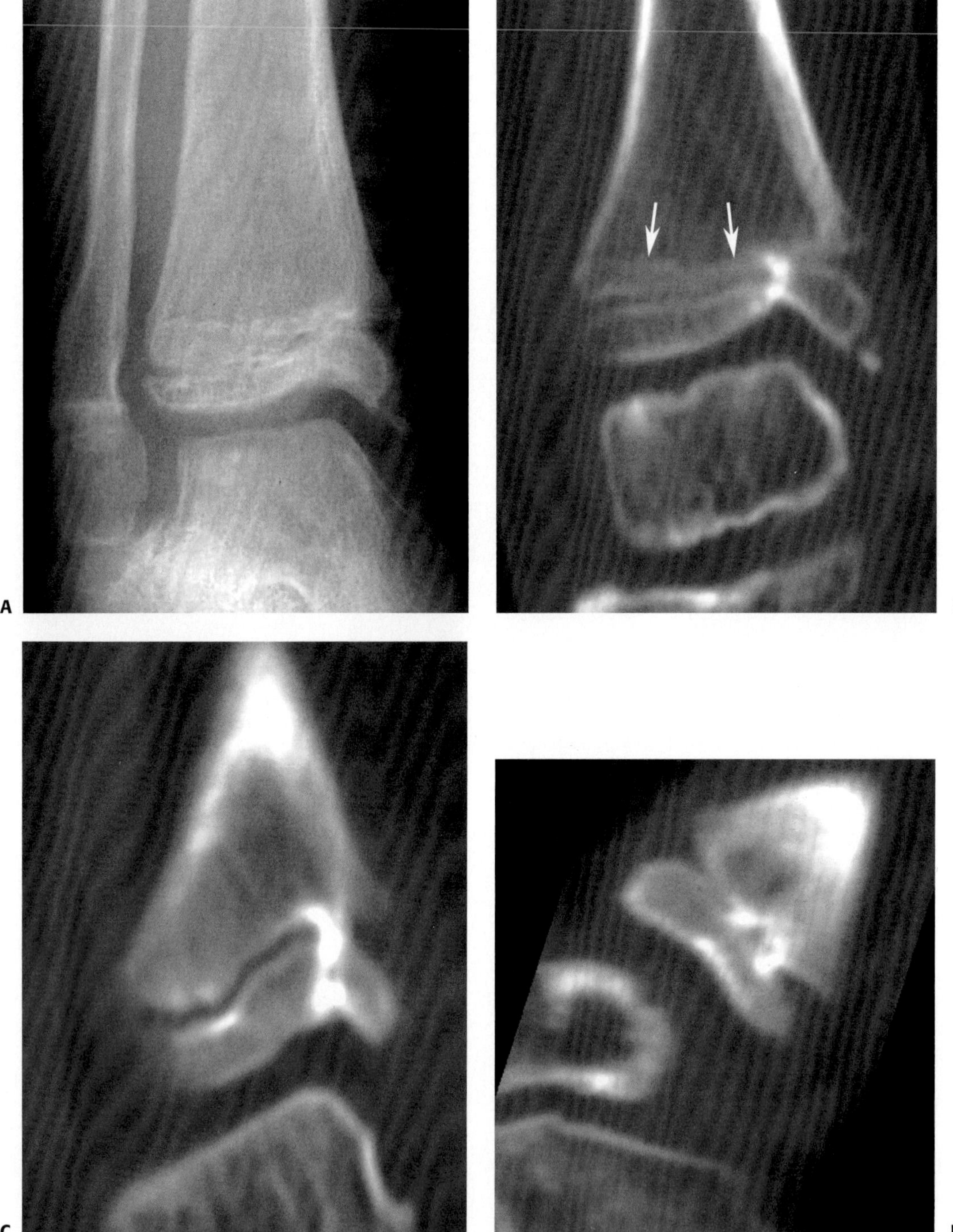

FIGURE 5-32 Harris growth arrest line tapering to the physis at the level of the growth arrest can serve as an excellent x-ray confirmation of the presence of the true growth arrest. Although most commonly noted on plain x-rays, these arrest lines can be seen on computed tomography (CT) scans and magnetic resonance images as well. **A.** Anteroposterior x-ray of the distal tibia after Salter-Harris type IV fracture demonstrates a Harris growth arrest line tapering to the medial distal tibial physis, where a partial physeal arrest has formed. **B.** Harris growth arrest line as noted on CT. CT scans with coronal **(C)** and sagittal **(D)** reconstructions corrected for bone distortion provide excellent images of the location and size of arrest.

disruption of normal physeal architecture and function without actual x-ray loss of the physis, or by the formation of a physeal arrest, also called bony bridges or physeal bars (47). Careful identification of the nature of physeal growth disruption is important, because treatment strategies may differ based on the etiology of growth disturbance and the presence or absence of a true growth arrest.

Growth disturbance as a result of physeal injury may result from direct trauma (physeal fracture) (36,38,40) or associated vascular disruption (11). Infection (21,22), destruction by a space-occupying lesion such as unicameral bone cyst or enchondroma (10), infantile Blount disease (63), other vascular disturbances (such as purpura fulminans) (14–16,23), irradiation (24,29) and other rare causes (18,19,107) also may result in physeal growth disturbance or physeal arrest.

Evaluation

Physeal growth disturbance may present as an x-ray abnormality noted on serial x-rays in a patient known to be at risk after fracture or infection, clinically with established limb deformity (angular deformity, shortening, or both), or occasionally incidentally on x-rays obtained for other reasons. The hallmark of plain x-ray features of physeal growth disturbance is the loss of normal physeal contour and the sharply defined radiolucency between epiphyseal and metaphyseal bone. Frank physeal arrests typically are characterized by sclerosis in the region of the arrest. If asymmetric growth has occurred, there may be tapering of a growth arrest line to the area of arrest (108,109), angular deformity, epiphyseal distortion, or shortening (Fig. 5-32). Physeal growth disturbance without frank arrest typically appears on plain x-rays as a thinner or thicker physeal area with an indistinct metaphyseal border because of alteration in normal enchondral ossification. There may be an asymmetric growth arrest line indicating angular deformity, but the arrest line will not taper to the physis itself (Fig. 5-33) (109). This indicates altered physeal growth (either asymmetric acceleration or deceleration) but not a complete cessation of growth. This distinction is important, because the consequences and treatment are different from those caused by complete growth arrest.

If a growth arrest is suspected on plain x-rays in a skeletally immature child, further evaluation often is warranted. CT scanning with sagittal and coronal reconstructions (orthogonal to the area of interest) may demonstrate clearly an area of bone bridging the physis between the epiphysis and metaphysis (see Fig. 5-32C,D). MRI also is a sensitive method of assessing normal physeal architecture (Fig. 5-34) (79,97). Revealing images of the physis and the region of physeal growth disturbance can be obtained using three-dimensional spoiled recalled gradient echo images with fat saturation or fast spin echo proton density images with fat saturation (Fig. 5-35). MRI has the additional advantage of the opportunity to assess the organization of the residual physis that may indicate its relative "health." This assessment may be helpful in cases of infection, irradiation, or tumor to determine if arrest resection is feasible based on the integrity of the remaining physis. With either CT or MRI, physeal arrests are characterized by an identifiable bridge of bone between the epiphysis and metaphysis, whereas growth disruption without arrest demonstrates some degree of loss of normal physeal contour and architecture without the bony bridge or physeal bar.

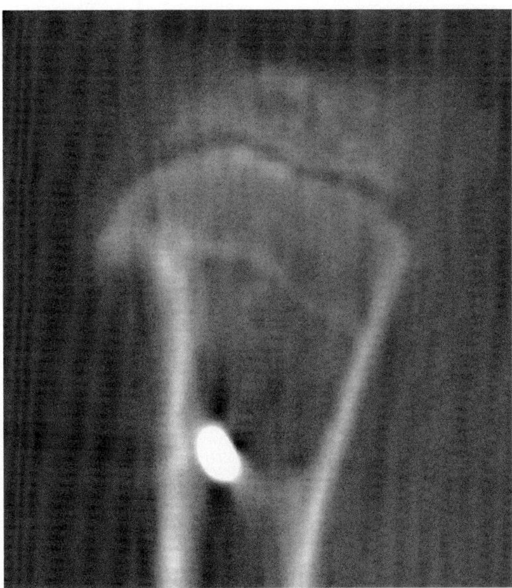

FIGURE 5-33 Asymmetric growth arrest line that does not taper to the physis is a strong indication of the presence of physeal growth disturbance without frank physeal arrest. In this case, the asymmetric growth arrest line is noted in the proximal tibial metaphysis on computed tomography scan.

Although definitive assessment of physeal growth disturbance or arrest usually requires advanced imaging, further eval-

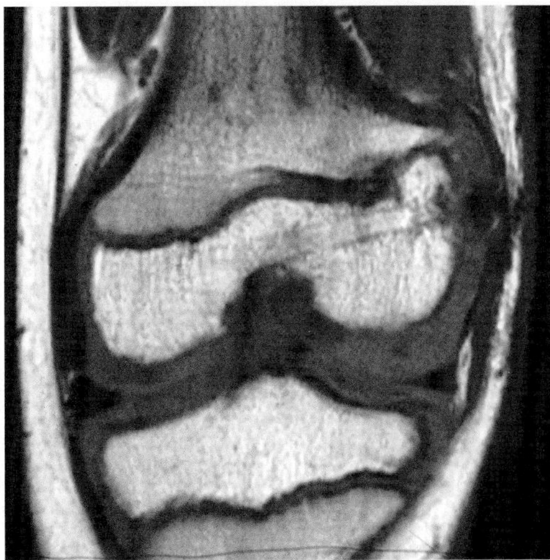

FIGURE 5-34 Magnetic resonance imaging scan of a patient with traumatic lateral distal femoral partial growth arrest. Note Harris arrest line tapering to the site of the arrest.

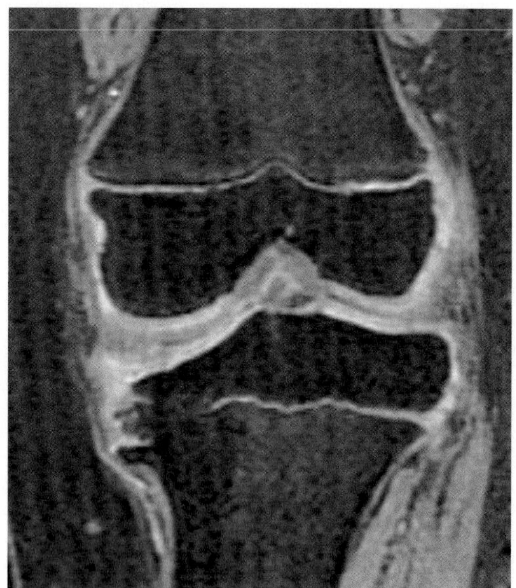

FIGURE 5-35 Magnetic resonance imaging scan (three-dimensional spoiled recalled gradient echo images with fat saturation) provides excellent visualization of the affected area and some sense of the integrity of the residual physis. This patient has infantile Blount disease.

TABLE 5-4 Potential Causes of Physeal Arrest Formation

Potential Causes of Physeal Arrest
Physeal fracture
Traumatic vascular disruption
Transphyseal infection
Vascular collapse associated with infection (purpura fulminans)
Infantile Blount's disease
Irradiation
Unicameral bone cyst
Enchondroma

uation by plain x-rays also is beneficial. X-rays of the entire affected limb should be obtained to document the magnitude of angular deformity. Existing limb length inequality should be assessed by scanogram. An estimation of predicted growth remaining in the contralateral unaffected physis should be made based on a determination of the child's skeletal age and reference to an appropriate growth table (50–55,110).

Physeal Arrests

Whenever a bridge of bone develops across a portion of physis, tethering of the metaphyseal and epiphyseal bone together may result (Table 5-4). These partial physeal arrests can result in angular deformity, joint distortion, limb length inequality, or combinations of these, depending on the location of the arrest, the rate and extent of growth remaining in the physis involved, and the health of the residual affected physis. Although these partial arrests are not common, their presence usually requires preventive or corrective treatment to minimize the long-term sequelae of the disturbance of normal growth they can create (Fig. 5-36).

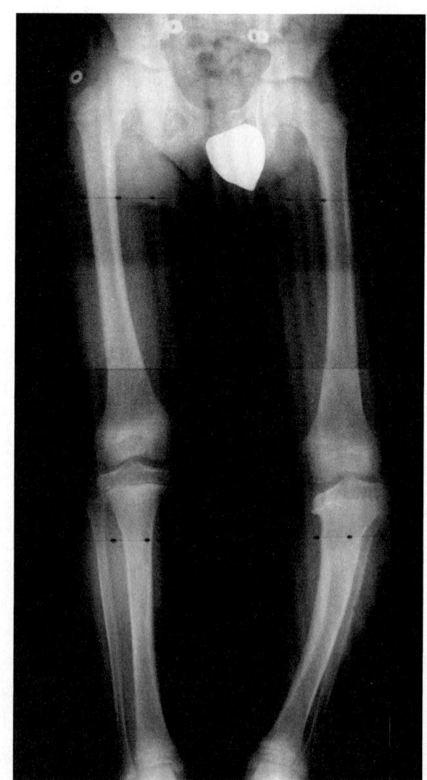

FIGURE 5-36 Physeal arrests create variable amounts of limb shortening, angular deformity, and epiphyseal distortion, depending on the duration of the arrest, the physis affected, and the size of the arrest. A long, standing film of the lower extremities with the hip, knee, and ankle joints included provides an overall assessment of angular deformity and shortening.

Classification

Partial physeal arrests can be classified by etiology and by anatomic pattern. Potential etiologies of physeal arrest are summarized in Table 5-4 and include physeal fracture, Langenskiöld stage VI infantile Blount disease, infection, tumor, and irradiation. Physeal arrests also can be classified based on the anatomic relationship of the arrest to the residual "healthy" physis. Three basic patterns are recognized (Fig. 5-37): central, peripheral,

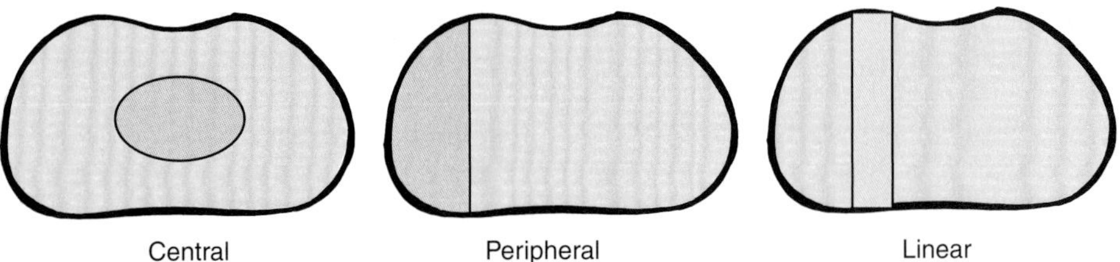

FIGURE 5-37 Anatomic classification of physeal arrests. Central arrests are surrounded by a perimeter of normal physis. Peripheral arrests are located at the perimeter of the physis. Linear arrests are "through-and-through" lesions with normal physis on either side of the arrest area.

and linear. A *central* arrest is surrounded by a perimeter of normal physis, like an island within the remaining physis. Central arrests are most likely to cause tenting of the articular surface, but also may result in angular deformity if eccentrically located and limb length inequality (Fig. 5-38). A *peripheral* arrest is located at the perimeter of the affected physis. This type of arrest primarily causes progressive angular deformity and variable shortening. A *linear* arrest is a "through-and-through" lesion with anatomic characteristics of both a central and peripheral arrest; specifically, the affected area includes the perimeter of the physis, but there is normal physis on either side of the affected area. Linear arrests most commonly develop after Salter-Harris type III or IV physeal fractures of the medial malleolus.

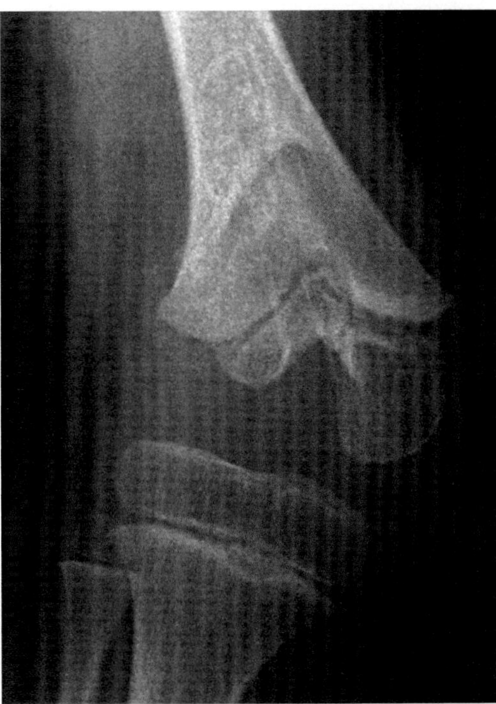

FIGURE 5-38 Central arrests are characterized by tenting of the articular surface. Variable shortening and angular deformity will develop, depending on the size and location of the arrest.

Management

Several management alternatives are available. It is important to be aware of these and to weigh carefully the appropriateness of each for the individual situation.

Prevention of Arrest Formation. Ideally, the surgeon should be proactive in the prevention of physeal arrest formation. Most commonly, this can be accomplished by adhering to the general treatment principles of physeal fractures: gentle, anatomic, and secure reduction of the fracture, especially Salter-Harris types III and IV injuries. Damaged, exposed physes can be protected by immediate fat grafting (111), similar to the principle of interposition material insertion for the resection of established arrests (see following discussion). The most common situation in which this can be considered appropriately is during open reduction of medial malleolar fractures, where comminution or partial physeal damage is identified during reduction.

Some experimental work (112) indicates that nonsteroidal antiinflammatory medications (specifically indomethacin) given for a period of time after physeal injury may prevent formation of physeal arrest. There is, however, no clinical study supporting this experimental study, so the use of nonsteroidal antiinflammatory medications is empiric and not common clinical practice.

Partial Physeal Arrest Resection. Conceptually, surgical resection of a physeal arrest (sometimes referred to as *physiolysis* or *epiphysiolysis*) restoring normal growth of the affected physis is the ideal treatment for this condition (36,93,100–104,106, 113–115). The principle is to remove the bony tether between the metaphysis and physis and fill the physeal defect with a bone reformation retardant, anticipating that the residual healthy physis will resume normal longitudinal growth (100,103,104,113–115). However, this procedure can be technically demanding, and results in our hands are modest. To determine if this procedure is indicated, careful consideration must be given to the location and extent of the arrest and the amount of longitudinal growth to be potentially salvaged.

Physeal Distraction. Physeal arrests have been treated with the application of an external fixator spanning the arrest and gradual distraction until the arrest "separates" (116,117). Angular deformity correction and lengthening can be accomplished after separation as well. However, distraction injury usually results in complete cessation of subsequent normal physeal growth at the distracted level (118). Furthermore, the fixation wires or half-pins may have tenuous fixation of the epiphysis or violate the articular space, risking septic arthritis. Thus, this modality rarely is used in patients near the end of growth.

Repeated Osteotomies During Growth. The simplest method to correct angular deformity associated with physeal arrests is corrective osteotomy in the adjacent metaphysis. Of course, neither significant limb length inequality nor epiphyseal distortion that may result from the arrest is corrected by this strategy. However, in young patients with a great deal of growth remaining in whom previous physeal arrest resection has been unsuccessful or is technically not possible, this treatment may be a reasonable interim alternative until more definitive completion of arrest and management of limb length inequality is feasible.

Completion of Epiphysiodesis and Management of Resulting Limb Length Discrepancy. An alternative strategy for the management of physeal arrests is to complete the epiphysiodesis to prevent recurrent angular deformity or epiphyseal distortion and manage the existing or potential limb length discrepancy appropriately. Management of the latter may be by simultaneous or subsequent lengthening of the affected limb segment or contralateral epiphysiodesis if the existing discrepancy is tolerable and lengthening is not desired. We believe that this course of management is specifically indicated if arrest resection has failed to result in restoration of longitudinal growth and in patients in whom the amount of growth remaining does not warrant an attempt at arrest resection. In our opinion, this treatment should be considered carefully in all patients with a physeal arrest.

Physeal Arrest Resection

Based on our experience with the results of physeal arrest resection, the factors discussed in the following sections should be considered before determining if physeal arrest resection is indicated.

Etiology of the Arrest

Arrests caused by trauma or infantile Blount disease have a relatively good prognosis for resumption of normal growth, whereas those secondary to infection, tumor or tumorlike conditions, or irradiation are less likely to demonstrate growth after resection.

Anatomic Type of the Arrest

Central and linear arrests have been reported to be more likely to demonstrate resumption of growth after resection (101), but our experience has not supported this observation.

Physis Affected

Because proximal humeral and proximal femoral lesions are difficult to expose, a technically adequate resection is less likely in these areas. Distal femoral bars have a poorer prognosis for growth after resection, whereas those of the distal tibia have a more favorable prognosis for the resumption of growth.

Extent of the Arrest

The potential for resumption of longitudinal growth after arrest resection is influenced by the amount of physeal surface area affected (100–102). Arrests affecting more than 25% of the total surface area are unlikely to grow, and, except in patients in whom significant growth potential remains, alternative treatment strategies should be used.

Amount of Growth Remaining in the Physis Affected

Some authors (101–104,115,119) have stated that 2 years of growth remaining based on skeletal age determination is a prerequisite for arrest resection to be considered. Based on our results with this procedure, we find that 2 years of growth remaining is an inadequate indication for physeal arrest resection. We believe that the decision to perform arrest resection should be made on a combination of the calculated amount of growth remaining in the affected physis and the likelihood of resumption of growth. Scanogram and determination of skeletal age (Fig. 5-39) will document the existing discrepancy, and consultation with the growth remaining tables for the affected physis (50–52,54,55,76) will allow calculation of growth remaining in the affected physis.

Preoperative Planning and Surgical Principles

If physeal arrest resection is considered appropriate, some planning is required to maximize the opportunity for resumption of longitudinal growth.

First, the extent and location of the arrest relative to the rest of the physis must be carefully documented. The most cost-effective method to accurately evaluate an arrest is with reconstructed sagittal and coronal CT images to provide views orthogonal to the affected physis. MRI also may be used and, with recent advancements in the capability to identify and quantify physeal arrests, may soon become the imaging study of choice. We currently prefer three-dimensional spoiled recalled gradient echo images with fat saturation or fast spin echo proton density images with fat saturation to visualize the physis. CT images allow precise delineation of bony margins and, at least currently, is cheaper than MRI. An estimation of the affected surface area can be computed with the assistance of the radiologist using a modification of the method of Carlson and Wenger (Fig. 5-40) (120). The procedure should be planned with consideration of the principles discussed in the following section.

Minimize Trauma. The arrest must be resected in a manner that minimizes trauma to the residual physis. Central lesions should be approached through either a metaphyseal window (Fig. 5-41) or through the intramedullary canal after a metaphyseal osteotomy. Peripheral lesions are approached directly, resecting the overlying periosteum to help prevent reformation

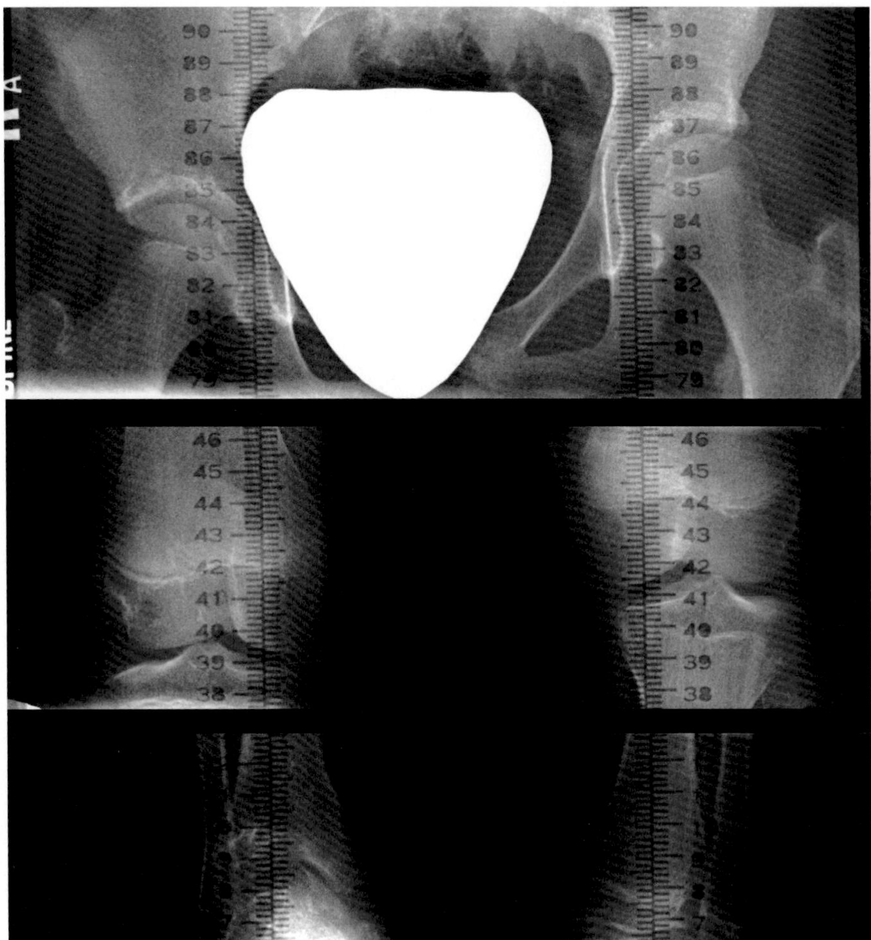

FIGURE 5-39 Scanogram indicates the existing limb length inequality. Bone age determination and growth contribution per year of the affected physis will allow calculation of the extent of limb segment shortening to be expected.

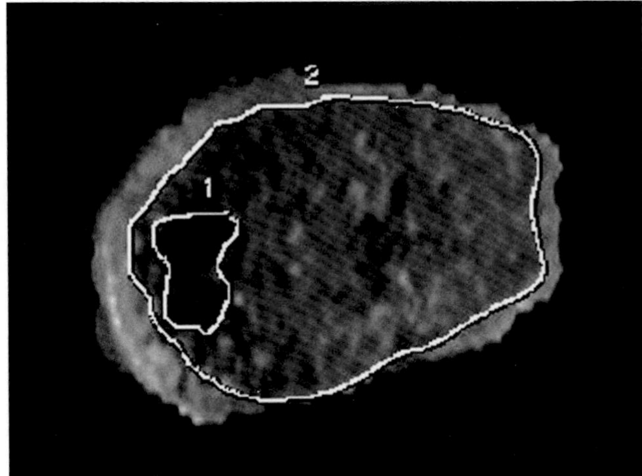

FIGURE 5-40 Reconstructed magnetic resonance images allow estimation of the percentage of surface area of the physis affected by a growth arrest. This workstation reconstruction delineates the perimeter of normal physis (border 2) and that of the physeal arrest (border 1). Surface area affected can be calculated from these reconstructions.

of the arrest. Intraoperative imaging (fluoroscopy) is needed to keep the surgeon oriented properly to the arrest and the residual healthy physis. Care to provide adequate visualization of the surgical cavity is essential, because visualization usually is difficult even under "ideal" circumstances. A brilliant light source, magnification, and a dry surgical field are very helpful. An arthroscope can be inserted into a metaphyseal cavity to permit a circumferential view of the resection area. A high-speed burr worked in a gentle to-and-fro movement perpendicular to the physis usually is the most effective way to gradually remove the bone composing the arrest and expose the residual healthy physis (Fig. 5-42). By the end of the resection, all of the bridging bone between the metaphysis and epiphysis should be removed, leaving a void in the physis where the arrest had been, and the perimeter of the healthy residual physis should be visible circumferentially at the margins of the surgically created cavity (Fig. 5-43).

Prevent Re-forming of Bridge between Metaphysis and Epiphysis. A bone-growth retardant or "spacer" material should be placed in the cavity created by the arrest resection to prevent re-forming of the bony bridge between the metaphysis and epi-

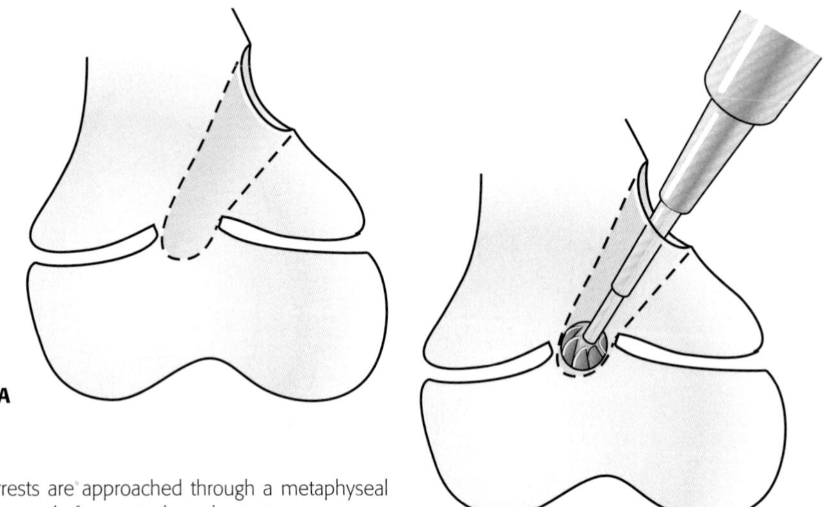

FIGURE 5-41 Central arrests are approached through a metaphyseal "window" or the medullary canal after metaphyseal osteotomy.

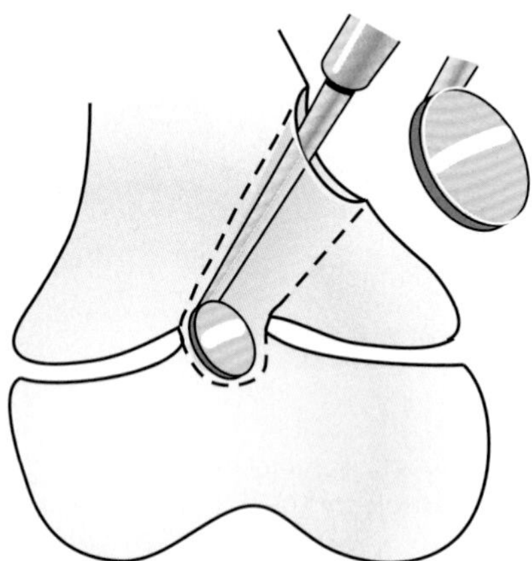

FIGURE 5-42 The arrest is removed, leaving in its place a metaphyseal-epiphyseal cavity with intact physis surrounding the area of resection.

physis. Four compounds have been used for this purpose either clinically or experimentally: autogenous fat (101–104,106,115, 121,122), methylmethacrylate (102,119,123), silicone rubber (100), and autogenous cartilage (63,124–128). Silicone rubber is no longer available and, to our knowledge, autogenous cartilage has been used only experimentally as a press-fit plug or cultured chondroblasts. Currently, only autogenous fat graft, harvested either locally or from the buttock, and methylmethacrylate are used clinically. Autogenous fat has at least a theoretic advantage of the ability to hypertrophy and migrate with longitudinal and interstitial growth (Fig. 5-44) (121,122). Methylmethacrylate is inert, but provides some immediate structural stability (129). This feature may be important with large arrest resections in weight-bearing areas, as in the proximal tibia in association with infantile Blount disease (Fig. 5-45). However, embedded methylmethacrylate, especially products without barium to clearly delineate its location on x-ray, can be extremely difficult to remove and can jeopardize bone fixation if subsequent surgery is required.

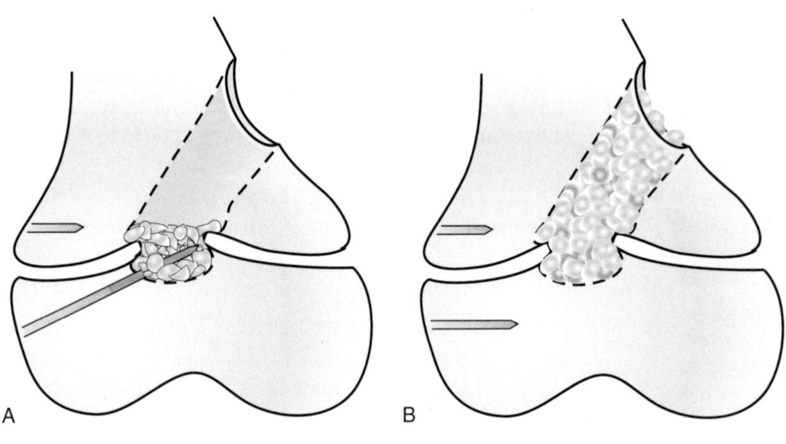

FIGURE 5-43 After complete resection, the healthy physis should be evident circumferentially within the cavity produced by the arrest resection.

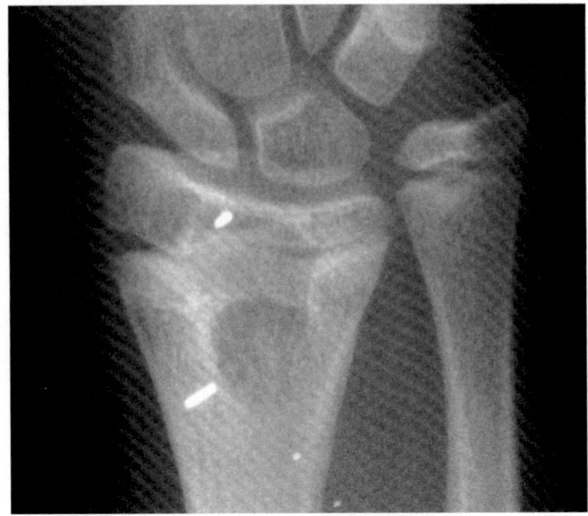

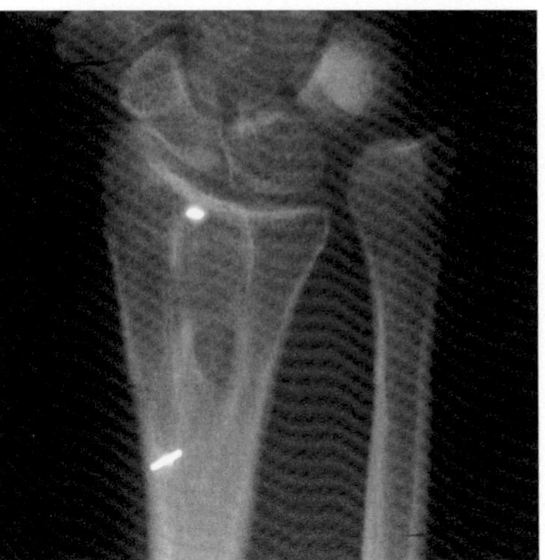

FIGURE 5-44 Fat used as an interposition material in partial physeal arrest resection can persist and hypertrophy during longitudinal growth. **A.** X-ray appearance after traumatic distal radial physeal arrest resection. **B.** Appearance 5 years later. Longitudinal growth between the metallic markers is obvious. The fat-filled cavity created at physeal arrest resection has persisted and elongated with distal radial growth.

Marker Implantation. Metallic markers should implanted in the epiphysis and metaphysis at the time of arrest resection to allow reasonably accurate estimation of the amount of longitudinal growth that occurs across the operated physis, as well as to identify the deceleration or cessation of that growth (Fig. 5-46). We believe that precise monitoring of subsequent longitudinal growth is an important aspect of the management of patients after arrest resection. First, resumption of longitudinal growth may not occur despite technically adequate arrest resection in patients with good clinical indications. Perhaps more importantly, resumption of normal or even accelerated longitudinal growth may be followed by late deceleration or cessation of that growth (105). It is imperative that the treating surgeon be alert to those developments, so that proper intervention can be instituted promptly. Embedded metallic markers serve those purposes admirably.

Authors' Observation. It has been our clinical observation that even patients who have significant resumption of growth following arrest resection will experience premature cessation of

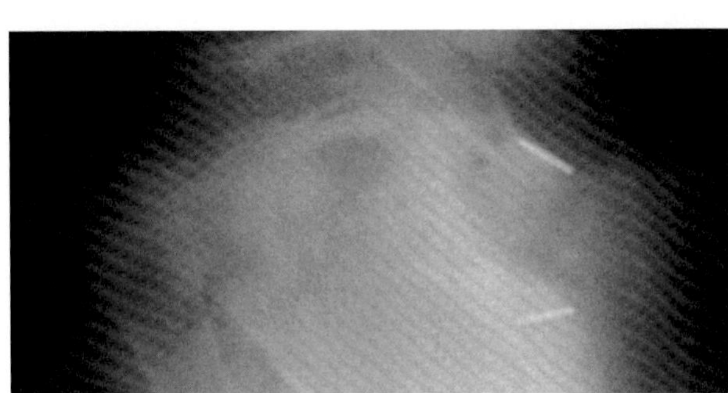

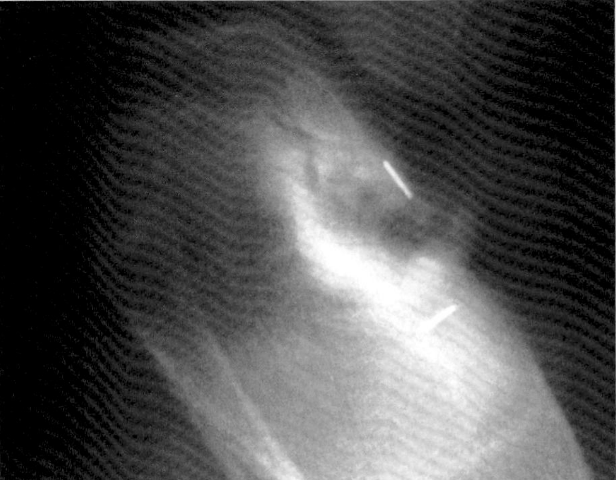

FIGURE 5-45 Resection of substantial physeal arrests in weight-bearing areas may allow subsidence of the articular surface. This is of particular concern in the proximal tibia of patients with infantile Blount disease. **A.** Early postoperative x-ray after partial physeal arrest resection in an obese patient with infantile Blount disease. **B.** One year later, the metallic markers are actually closer together, in addition to demonstrating increased varus. Subsidence of the medial proximal tibial articular surface is the likely explanation of this x-ray finding. Protected weight-bearing or methylmethacrylate as the interposition material may be indicated in such cases.

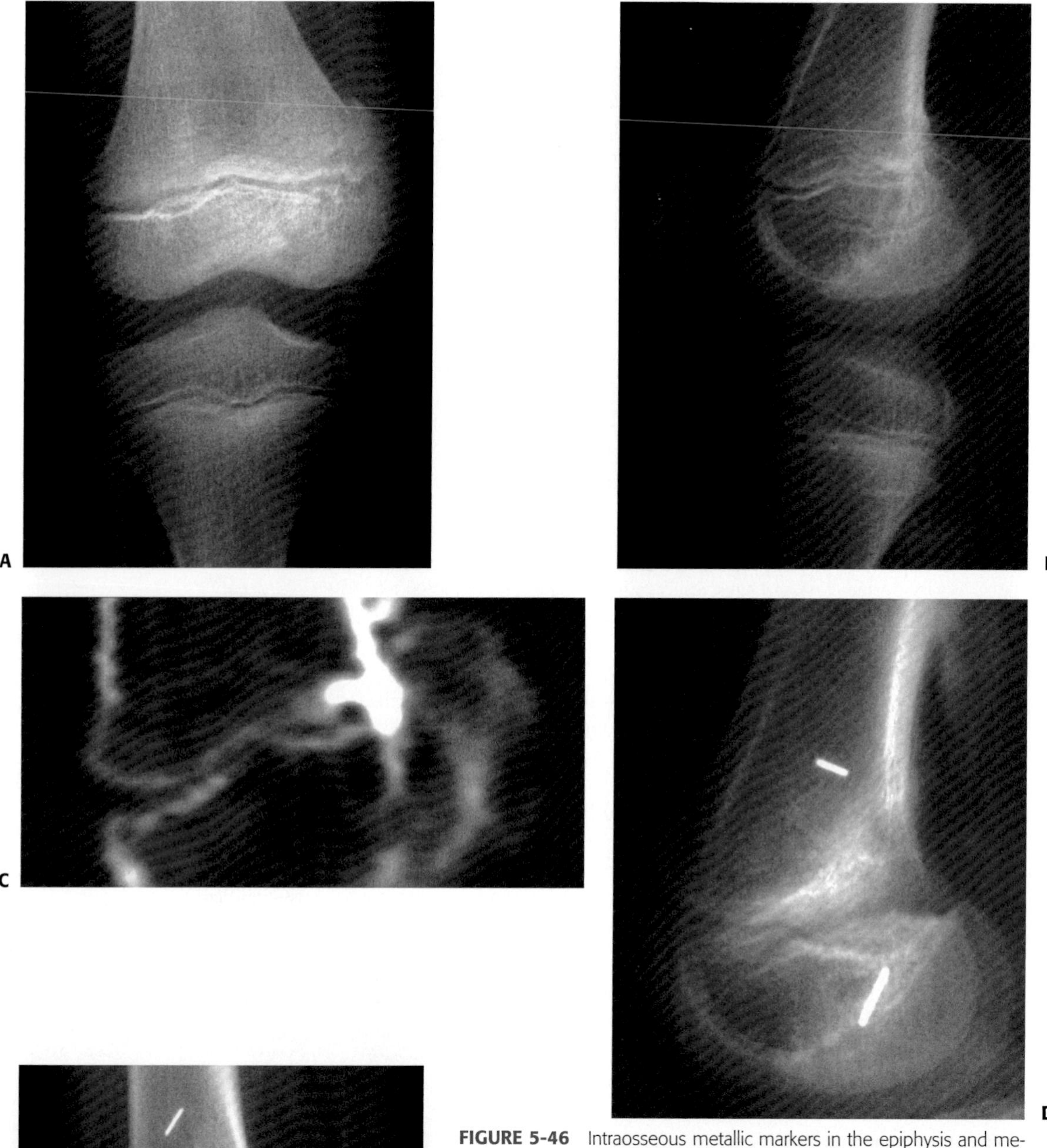

FIGURE 5-46 Intraosseous metallic markers in the epiphysis and metaphysis spanning the area of arrest resection allow sensitive x-ray documentation of the presence and extent of growth after arrest resection and permit early detection of the cessation of restored longitudinal growth. This patient had a small central arrest of the lateral portion of the distal femoral physis after a Salter-Harris type IV fracture. **A.** Injury films show a mildly displaced Salter-Harris type IV fracture of the lateral distal femur. **B.** Several years later, a small central arrest has developed involving a portion of the lateral distal femoral physis. A tapering growth arrest line is faintly visible. **C.** The posterior location of the partial arrest can be seen on the sagittal computed tomography reconstructions. **D.** After arrest resection through a metaphyseal window, a cavity is evident in the region of the original bar. Metallic markers have been placed in the metaphysis and epiphysis. **E.** Three years after arrest resection, substantial growth has occurred, as documented by the increased distance between the markers. However, on x-rays taken at 4 years postoperatively, no further growth was documented. This event was treated by completion of the epiphysiodesis and contralateral distal femoral epiphysiodesis to prevent the development of limb length discrepancy from developing.

longitudinal growth of the affected physis relative to the contralateral uninvolved physis. We believe that even if growth resumes after bar resection, the previously injured physis will cease growing before the contralateral physis. Thus the percent of predicted growth might be expected to decrease over the length of follow-up.

Our experience with physeal arrest resection prompted several conclusions and treatment recommendations:

- On average, approximately 60% of physeal arrests demonstrate clear x-ray evidence of resumption of longitudinal growth of the affected physis after physeal arrest resection.
- There is a correlation between the amount of surface area of the physis affected and the prognosis for subsequent longitudinal growth after arrest resection. Physeal arrests affecting less than 10% of the surface area of the physis have a better prognosis than larger arrests.
- Langenskiöld stage VI infantile Blount disease has results comparable to post-traumatic physeal arrests.
- Etiologies other than post-traumatic and infantile Blount disease have poor prognoses for subsequent growth.
- Central and peripheral arrests have equivalent prognoses with respect to resumption of growth.
- Early growth resumption may be followed by cessation of longitudinal growth before skeletal maturity. As a consequence, patients must be evaluated regularly until skeletal maturity with some reliable method (such as metaphyseal and epiphyseal x-ray markers) to detect such development as promptly as possible.

We believe that physeal bar resection has a role to play in patients with significant longitudinal growth remaining. However, the benefits of such surgery must be weighed against the actual amount of growth remaining, and the etiology, location, and extent of the physeal arrest must be considered. The appropriate time to add a corrective osteotomy to bony bar resection is controversial. Generally, when the angular deformity is more than 10 to 15 degrees from normal, corrective osteotomy should be considered.

Growth Deceleration Without Arrest

Recognition

In contrast to physeal arrest, growth deceleration without frank cessation of growth is characterized by x-ray abnormality of the appearance of an injured physis (usually relative widening of the physis with indistinct metaphyseal boundaries). There may be associated clinical or x-ray deformity if the disturbance is severe and long-standing, but without complete cessation of growth in the affected area. It is important to make a distinction between growth deceleration without complete cessation and true physeal arrest, because management and outcome typically are different in these two disorders. The concept of growth deceleration without arrest is most readily appreciated in patients with adolescent Blount disease and the milder stages of infantile Blount disease. Similar growth deceleration also may occur after infection and physeal fracture. In contrast to physeal arrests, there is no sclerotic area of arrest on plain x-rays (see Fig. 5-33). A growth arrest line, if present, may be asymmetric but will not taper to the physis, thereby suggesting growth asymmetry but not complete arrest. Furthermore, in some cases, deformity will not be relentlessly progressive and can actually improve over time.

Management

The diagnosis of physeal growth disturbance usually is made incidentally by noting physeal abnormality on x-rays during physeal fracture follow-up or after a diagnosis of frank physeal arrest has been excluded during the evaluation of a patient with angular deformity and physeal abnormality on plain x-rays. Once a growth disturbance has been identified in a patient, its full impact should be assessed by determining the presence and extent of limb length inequality and the calculated amount of potential growth remaining for the affected physis.

In some cases, the x-ray abnormality is stable and only longitudinal observation is required. This observation must be regular and careful, because progressive deformity will require treatment. If angular deformity is present or progressive, treatment options include hemiepiphysiodesis (130) or stapling and corrective osteotomy, with or without completion of the epiphysiodesis.

In the absence of frank arrest formation, hemiepiphysiodesis or stapling of the affected physis on the convex side of the deformity may result in gradual correction of the deformity. If correction occurs, options include completion of the epiphysiodesis (with contralateral epiphysiodesis if necessary to prevent the development of significant leg length deformity) or removal of staples with careful longitudinal observation for recurrence or overcorrection of deformity.

Corrective osteotomy is the other option for the management of growth disturbance with established angular deformity. Angular deformity correction in the early stages of infantile and adolescent Blount disease is known to result in resolution of the physeal growth disturbance in some patients, both on x-ray and clinically. We are unaware of confirmation of similar outcome when the etiology of growth disturbance is infection or trauma, although it may occur. Thus, the treating surgeon must decide whether to perform epiphysiodesis of the affected physis (with contralateral epiphysiodesis, if appropriate) to prevent recurrence or to ensure careful longitudinal observation of the growth performance of the affected physis until skeletal maturity.

SUMMARY

Physeal fractures are one of the unique aspects of pediatric orthopedics. These injuries are common and usually have a favorable outcome without long-term sequelae. Physeal fractures must be treated gently and expertly to maximize restoration of normal limb function and longitudinal growth. Depending on the severity and nature of physeal injury, longitudinal follow-up to identify the development of physeal growth disturbance is important.

REFERENCES

1. Ogden JA. Skeletal growth mechanism injury patterns. *J Pediatr Orthop* 1982;2: 371–377.
2. Bright RW, Burstein AH, Elmore SM. Epiphyseal-plate cartilage: a biomechanical and histological analysis of failure modes. *J Bone Joint Surg Am* 1974;56:688–703.
3. Moen CT, Pelker RR. Biomechanical and histological correlations in growth plate failure. *J Pediatr Orthop* 1984;4:180–184.
4. Johnston R. Fractures through human growth plates. *Orthop Trans* 1980;4:295.
5. Shapiro F. Epiphyseal growth plate fracture-separation: a pathophysiologic approach. *Orthopaedics* 1982;5:720–736.
6. Rudicel S, Pelker RR, Lee KE, et al. Shear fractures through the capital femoral physis of the skeletally immature rabbit. *J Pediatr Orthop* 1985;5:27–31.
7. Rivas R, Shapiro F. Structural stages in the development of the long bones and epiphyses: a study in the New Zealand white rabbit. *J Bone Joint Surg Am* 2002;84:85–100.
8. Arriola F, Forriol F, Canadell J. Histomorphometric study of growth plate subjected to different mechanical conditions (compression, tension and neutralization): an experimental study in lambs—mechanical growth plate behavior. *J Pediatr Orthop Br* 2001; 10:334–338.
9. Gomes LS, Volpon JB, Goncalves RP. Traumatic separation of epiphyses: an experimental study in rats. *Clin Orthop Relat Res* 1988;236:286–295.
10. Stanton RP, Abdel-Mota'al MM. Growth arrest resulting from unicameral bone cyst. *J Pediatr Orthop* 1998;18:198–201.
11. Peterson HA. Premature physeal arrest of the distal tibia associated with temporary arterial insufficiency. *J Pediatr Orthop* 1993;13:672–675.
12. Peters W, Irving J, Letts M. Long-term effects of neonatal bone and joint infection on adjacent growth plates. *J Pediatr Orthop* 1992;12:806–810.
13. Langenskiold A. Growth disturbance after osteomyelitis of femoral condyles in infants. *Acta Orthop Scand* 1984;55:1–13.
14. Kruse RW, Tassanawipas A, Bowen JR. Orthopedic sequelae of meningococcemia. *Orthopedics* 1991;14:174–178.
15. Jacobsen ST, Crawford AH. Amputation following meningococcemia: a sequela to purpura fulminans. *Clin Orthop Relat Res* 1984;185:214–219.
16. Grogan DP, Love SM, Ogden JA, et al. Chondro-osseous growth abnormalities after meningococcemia: a clinical and histopathological study. *J Bone Joint Surg Am* 1989; 920–928.
17. Ellefsen BK, Frierson MA, Raney EM, et al. Humerus varus: a complication of neonatal, infantile, and childhood injury and infection. *J Pediatr Orthop* 1994;14:479–486.
18. Carrera GF, Kozin F, Flaherty L, et al. Radiographic changes in the hands following childhood frostbite injury. *Skeletal Radiol* 1981;6:33–37.
19. Brown FE, Spiegel PK, Boyle WE Jr. Digital deformity: an effect of frostbite in children. *Pediatrics* 1983;71:955–959.
20. Boyd KT, Batt ME. Stress fracture of the proximal humeral epiphysis in an elite junior badminton player. *Br J Sports Med* 1997;31:252–253.
21. Bos CF, Mol LJ, Obermann WR, et al. Late sequelae of neonatal septic arthritis of the shoulder. *J Bone Joint Surg Br* 1998;80:645–650.
22. Bergdahl S, Ekengren K, Eriksson M. Neonatal hematogenous osteomyelitis: risk factors for long-term sequelae. *J Pediatr Orthop* 1985;5:564–568.
23. Appel M, Pauleto AC, Cunha LAM. Osteochondral sequelae of meningococcemia: radiographic aspects. *J Pediatr Orthop* 2002;22:511–516.
24. Robertson WW Jr, Butler MS, D'Angio GJ, et al. Leg length discrepancy following irradiation for childhood tumors. *J Pediatr Orthop* 1991;11:284–287.
25. Trueta J, Amato V. The vascular contribution to osteogenesis. III. Changes in the growth cartilage caused by experimentally induced ischaemia. *J Bone Joint Surg Br* 1960;42: 571–587.
26. Trueta J, Trias A. The vascular contribution to osteogenesis. IV. The effect of pressure upon the epiphyseal cartilage of the rabbit. *J Bone Joint Surg Br* 1961;43:800.
27. Abram LJ, Thompson GH. Deformity after premature closure of the distal radial physis following a torus fracture with a physeal compression injury: report of a case. *J Bone Joint Surg Am* 1987;69:1450–1453.
28. Aminian A, Schoenecker PL. Premature closure of the distal radial physis after fracture of the distal radial metaphysis. *J Pediatr Orthop* 1995;15:495–498.
29. Beals RK. Premature closure of the physis following diaphyseal fractures. *J Pediatr Orthop* 1990;10:717–720.
30. Bowler JR, Mubarak SJ, Wenger DR. Tibial physeal closure and genu recurvatum after femoral fracture: occurrence without a tibial traction pin. *J Pediatr Orthop* 1990;10: 653–657.
31. Brogle PJ, Gaffney JT, Denton JR. Acute compartment syndrome complicating a distal tibial physeal fracture in a neonate. *Am J Orthop* 1999;28:587–589.
32. Goldfarb CA, Bassett GS, Sullivan S, et al. Retrosternal displacement after physeal fracture of the medial clavicle in children treatment by open reduction and internal fixation. *J Bone Joint Surg Br* 2001;83:1168–1172.
33. Hunter LY, Hensinger RN. Premature monomelic growth arrest following fracture of the femoral shaft: a case report. *J Bone Joint Surg Am* 1978;60:850–852.
34. Langenskiold A. Traumatic premature closure of the distal tibial epiphyseal plate. *Acta Orthop Scand* 1967;38:520–531.
35. Martin RP, Parsons DL. Avascular necrosis of the proximal humeral epiphysis after physeal fracture: a case report. *J Bone Joint Surg Am* 1997;79:760–762.
36. Mayer V, Marchisello PJ. Traumatic partial arrest of tibial physis. *Clin Orthop Relat Res* 1984;183:99–104.
37. Minami A, Sugawara M. Humeral trochlear hypoplasia secondary to epiphyseal injury as a cause of ulnar nerve palsy. *Clin Orthop Relat Res* 1988;228:227–232.
38. Navascues JA, Gonzalez-Lopez JL, Lopez-Valverde S, et al. Premature physeal closure after tibial diaphyseal fractures in adolescents. *J Pediatr Orthop* 2000;20:193–196.
39. Pape JM, Goulet JA, Hensinger RN. Compartment syndrome complicating tibial tubercle avulsion. *Clin Orthop Relat Res* 1993;295:201–204.
40. Riseborough EJ, Barrett IR, Shapiro F. Growth disturbances following distal femoral physeal fracture-separations. *J Bone Joint Surg Am* 1983;65:885–893.
41. Shelton WR, Canale ST. Fractures of the tibia through the proximal tibial epiphyseal cartilage. *J Bone Joint Surg Am* 1979;61:167–173.
42. Bertin KC, Goble EM. Ligament injuries associated with physeal fractures about the knee. *Clin Orthop Relat Res* 1983;177:188–195.
43. Trueta J, Morgan J. The vascular contribution to osteogenesis. I. Studies by the injection method. *J Bone Joint Surg Br* 1960;42:97–109.
44. Dale G, Harris W. Prognosis of epiphyseal separations: an experimental study. *J Bone Joint Surg Br* 1958;40:116–122.
45. Salter R, Harris W. Injuries involving the epiphyseal plate. *J Bone Joint Surg* 1963;45: 587–622.
46. Smith DG, Geist RW, Cooperman DR. Microscopic examination of a naturally occurring epiphyseal plate fracture. *J Pediatr Orthop* 1985;5:306–308.
47. Wattenbarger JM, Gruber HE, Phieffer LS. Physeal fractures. I. Histologic features of bone, cartilage, and bar formation in a small animal model. *J Pediatr Orthop* 2002;22: 703–709.
48. Jaramillo D, Kammen BF, Shapiro F. Cartilaginous path of physeal fracture-separations: evaluation with MR imaging—an experimental study with histologic correlation in rabbits. *Radiology* 2000;215:504–511.
49. Lombardo S, Harvey J. Fractures of the distal femoral epiphysis: factors influencing prognosis—a review of 34 cases. *J Bone Joint Surg Am* 1977;59:742–751.
50. Anderson M, Green WT. Length of femur and tibia: norms derived from orthoroentgenogram of children from 5 years of age until epiphyseal closure. *Am J Dis Child* 1948; 75:279.
51. Anderson M, Green W, Messner M. Growth and predictions of growth in the lower extremities. *J Bone Joint Surg Am* 1963;45:1–14.
52. Anderson M, Messner M, Green W. Distribution of lengths of the normal femur and tibia in children from one to eighteen years of age. *J Bone Joint Surg* 1964;46: 1197–1202.
53. Green W, Anderson M. Skeletal age and the control of bone growth. *Am Acad Orthop Surg* 1960;17:199–217.
54. Hensinger R. Linear growth of long bones of the lower extremity form infancy to adolescence. In: Hensinger R, ed. *Standards in Pediatric Orthopaedics: Tables, Charts, and Graphs Illustrating Growth.* New York: Raven Press; 1986:232–233.
55. Maresh M. Linear growth of long bones of the extremities from infancy through adolescence. *Am J Dis Child* 1955;89:725–742.
56. Mendez AA, Bartal E, Grillot MB, et al. Compression (Salter-Harris type V) physeal fracture: an experimental model in the rat. *J Pediatr Orthop* 1992;12:29–37.
57. Valverde JA, Albiana J, Certucha JA. Early posttraumatic physeal arrest in distal radius after a compression injury. *J Pediatr Orthop B* 1996;5:57–60.
58. Albanese SA, Palmer AK, Kerr DR, et al. Wrist pain and distal growth plate closure of the radius in gymnasts. *J Pediatr Orthop* 1989;9:23–28.
59. Carter SR, Aldridge MJ. Stress injury of the distal radial growth plate. *J Bone Joint Surg Br* 1988;70:834–836.
60. Liebling MS, Berdon WE, Ruzal-Shapiro C, et al. Gymnast's wrist (pseudorickets growth plate abnormality) in adolescent athletes: findings on plain films and MR imaging. *Am J Roentgenol* 1995;164:157–159.
61. Carson WG Jr, Gasser SI. Little Leaguer's shoulder: a report of 23 cases. *Am J Sports Med* 1998;26:575–580.
62. Butler MS, Robertson WW, Rate WR, et al. Skeletal sequelae of radiation therapy for malignant childhood tumors. *Clin Orthop Relat Res* 1990;251:235–240.
63. Beck CL, Burke SW, Roberts JM, et al. Physeal bridge resection in infantile Blount disease. *J Pediatr Orthop* 1987;7:161–163.
64. Poland J. *Traumatic Separation of the Epiphysis.* Edited. London, Smith, Elder & Company; 1898.
65. Aitken AP. The end result of the fractured distal tibial epiphysis. *J Bone Joint Surg* 1936; 18:685–691.
66. Aitken AP. Fractures involving the distal femoral epiphyseal cartilage. *J Bone Joint Surg Am* 1952;34:96–108.
67. Aitken AP. Fractures of the epiphyses. *Clin Orthop Relat Res* 1965;41:19–23.
68. Aitken AP. Fractures of the proximal tibial epiphysial cartilage. *Clin Orthop Relat Res* 1965;41:92–97.
69. Dias LS, Tachdjian MO. Physeal injuries of the ankle in children: classification. *Clin Orthop Relat Res* 1978;136:230–233.
70. Mann DC, Rajmaira S. Distribution of physeal and nonphyseal fractures in 2,650 long-bone fractures in children aged 0–16 years. *J Pediatr Orthop* 1990;10:713–716.
71. Ogden JA, Ganey T, Light TR, et al. The pathology of acute chondro-osseous injury in the child. *Yale J Biol Med* 1993;66:219–233.

72. Peterson HA. Physeal fractures. II. Two previously unclassified types. *J Pediatr Orthop* 1994;14:431–438.
73. Peterson HA. Physeal fractures. III. Classification. *J Pediatr Orthop* 1994;14:439–448.
74. Petit P, Panuel M, Faure F, et al. Acute fracture of the distal tibial physis: role of gradient-echo MR imaging versus plain film examination. *Am J Roentgenol* 1996;166: 1203–1206.
75. Peterson HA, Burkhart SS. Compression injury of the epiphyseal growth plate: fact or fiction? *J Pediatr Orthop* 1981;1:377–384.
76. Hresko MT, Kasser JR. Physeal arrest about the knee associated with non-physeal fractures in the lower extremity. *J Bone Joint Surg Am* 1989;71:698–703.
77. Keret D, Mendez AA, Harcke HT, et al. Type V physeal injury: a case report. *J Pediatr Orthop* 1990;10:545–548.
78. Peterson HA, Madhok R, Benson JT, et al. Physeal fractures. I. Epidemiology in Olmsted County, Minnesota, 1979–1988. *J Pediatr Orthopedics* 1994;14:423–430.
79. Carey J, Spence L, Blickman H, et al. MRI of pediatric growth plate injury: correlation with plain film radiographs and clinical outcome. *Skeletal Radiol* 1998;27:250–255.
80. Close BJ, Strouse PJ. MR of physeal fractures of the adolescent knee. *Pediatr Radiol* 2000;30:756–762.
81. Jain R, Bielski RJ. Fracture of lower femoral epiphysis in an infant at birth: a rare obstetrical injury. *J Perinatol* 2001;21:550–552.
82. Smith BG, Rand F, Jaramillo D et al. Early MR imaging of lower-extremity physeal fracture-separations: a preliminary report. *J Pediatr Orthop* 1994;14:526–533.
83. Akbarnia BA, Silberstein MJ, Rende RJ, et al. Arthrography in the diagnosis of fractures of the distal end of the humerus in infants. *J Bone Joint Surg Am* 1986;68:599–602.
84. Hansen PE, Barnes DA, Tullos HS. Arthrographic diagnosis of an injury pattern in the distal humerus of an infant. *J Pediatr Orthop* 1982;2:569–572.
85. Marzo JM, d'Amato C, Strong M, et al. Usefulness and accuracy of arthrography in management of lateral humeral condyle fractures in children. *J Pediatr Orthop* 1990; 10:317–321.
86. Yates C, Sullivan JA. Arthrographic diagnosis of elbow injuries in children. *J Pediatr Orthop* 1987;7:54–60.
87. Broker FH, Burbach T. Ultrasonic diagnosis of separation of the proximal humeral epiphysis in the newborn. *J Bone Joint Surg Am* 1990;72:187–191.
88. Dias JJ, Lamont AC, Jones JM. Ultrasonic diagnosis of neonatal separation of the distal humeral epiphysis. *J Bone Joint Surg Br* 1988;70:825–828.
89. Diaz MJ, Hedlund GL. Sonographic diagnosis of traumatic separation of the proximal femoral epiphysis in the neonate. *Pediatr Radiol* 1991;21:238–240.
90. Howard CB, Shinwell E, Nyska M, et al. Ultrasound diagnosis of neonatal fracture separation of the upper humeral epiphysis. *J Bone Joint Surg Br* 1992;74:471–472.
91. Sferopoulos NK. Fracture separation of the medial clavicular epiphysis: ultrasonography findings. *Arch Orthop Trauma Surg* 2003;123:367–369.
92. Gomes LS, Volpon JB. Experimental physeal fracture-separations treated with rigid internal fixation. *J Bone Joint Surg Am* 1993;75:1756–1764.
93. Cass JR, Peterson HA. Salter-Harris type-IV injuries of the distal tibial epiphyseal growth plate, with emphasis on those involving the medial malleolus. *J Bone Joint Surg Am* 1983;65:1059–1070.
94. Rang M. Injuries of the epiphyses, the growth plate, and the perichondral ring. *Children's Fracture.* Philadelphia: JB Lippincott; 1983:10–25.
95. Mizuta T, Benson WM, Foster BK, et al. Statistical analysis of the incidence of physeal injuries. *J Pediatr Orthop* 1987;7:518–523.
96. Worlock P, Stower M. Fracture patterns in Nottingham children. *J Pediatr Orthop* 1986; 6:656–660.
97. Gabel GT, Peterson HA, Berquist TH. Premature partial physeal arrest: diagnosis by magnetic resonance imaging in two cases. *Clin Orthop Relat Res* 1991;272:242–247.
98. Davidson RS, Markowitz RI, Dormans J, et al. Ultrasonographic evaluation of the elbow in infants and young children after suspected trauma. *J Bone Joint Surg Am* 1994;76: 1804–1813.
99. Scheffer MM, Peterson HA. Opening-wedge osteotomy for angular deformities of long bones in children. *J Bone Joint Surg Am* 1994;76:325–334.
100. Bright RW. Operative correction of partial epiphyseal plate closure by osseous-bridge resection and silicone-rubber implant: an experimental study in dogs. *J Bone Joint Surg Am* 1974;56:655–664.
101. Broughton NS, Dickens DR, Cole WG, et al. Epiphysiolysis for partial growth plate arrest: results after four years or at maturity. *J Bone Joint Surg Br* 1989;71:13–16.
102. Kasser JR. Physeal bar resections after growth arrest about the knee. *Clin Orthop Relat Res* 1990;255:68–74.
103. Langenskiold A. Surgical treatment of partial closure of the growth plate. *J Pediatr Orthop* 1981;1:3–11.
104. Langenskiold A. An operation for partial closure of an epiphysial plate in children, and its experimental basis. *J Bone Joint Surg Br* 1975;57:325–330.
105. Hasler CC, Foster BK. Secondary tethers after physeal bar resection: a common source of failure? *Clin Orthop* 2002;405:242–249.
106. Williamson RV, Staheli LT. Partial physeal growth arrest: treatment by bridge resection and fat interposition. *J Pediatr Orthop* 1990;10:769–776.
107. Bigelow DR, Ritchie GW. The effects of frostbite in childhood. *J Bone Joint Surgery Br* 1963;45:122–131.
108. Harris H. Lines of arrested growth in the long bones in childhood: the correlation of histological and radiographic appearance in clinical and experimental conditions. *Br J Radiol* 1931;4:561–588.
109. Ogden JA. Growth slowdown and arrest lines. *J Pediatr Orthop* 1984;4:409–415.
110. Hensinger R. *Standards in Pediatric Orthopaedics: Tables, Charts and Graphs Illustrating Growth.* New York: Raven Press; 1986.
111. Foster BK, John B, Hasler C. Free fat interpositional graft in acute physeal injuries: the anticipatory Langenskiold procedure. *J Pediatr Orthop* 2000;20:282–285.
112. Sudmann E, Husby OS, Bang G. Inhibition of partial closure of epiphyseal plate in rabbits by indomethacin. *Acta Orthop Scand* 1982;53:507–511.
113. Osterman K. Operative elimination of partial premature epiphyseal closure: an experimental study. *Acta Orthop Scand Suppl* 1972;3–79.
114. Freidenberg Z. Reaction of the epiphysis to partial surgical resection. *J Bone Joint Surg,* 1957;39:332–340.
115. Langenskiold A. The possibilities of eliminating premature partial closure of an epiphyseal plate caused by trauma or disease. *Acta Orthop Scand* 1967;38:267–279.
116. Canadell J, de Pablos J. Breaking bony bridges by physeal distraction: a new approach. *Int Orthop* 1985;9:223–229.
117. Connolly JF, Huurman WW, Ray S. Physeal distraction treatment of fracture deformities. *Orthop Trans* 1991;3:231.
118. Fjeld TO, Steen H. Growth retardation after experimental limb lengthening by epiphyseal distraction. *J Pediatr Orthop* 1990;10:463–466.
119. Peterson HA. Partial growth plate arrest and its treatment. *J Pediatr Orthop* 1984;4: 246–258.
120. Carlson WO, Wenger DR. A mapping method to prepare for surgical excision of a partial physeal arrest. *J Pediatr Orthop* 1984;4:232–238.
121. Langenskiold A, Videman T, Nevalainen T. The fate of fat transplants in operations for partial closure of the growth plate: clinical examples and an experimental study. *J Bone Joint Surg Br* 1986;68:234–238.
122. Langenskiold A, Osterman K, Valle M. Growth of fat grafts after operation for partial bone growth arrest: demonstration by computed tomography scanning. *J Pediatr Orthop* 1987;7:389–394.
123. Bollini G, Tallet JM, Jacquemier M, et al. New procedure to remove a centrally located bone bar. *J Pediatr Orthop* 1990;10:662–666.
124. Lennox DW, Goldner RD, Sussman MD. Cartilage as an interposition material to prevent transphyseal bone bridge formation: an experimental model. *J Pediatr Orthop* 1983; 3:207–210.
125. Hansen AL, Foster BK, Gibson GJ, et al. Growth-plate chondrocyte cultures for reimplantation into growth-plate defects in sheep: characterization of cultures. *Clin Orthop Relat Res* 1990;256:286–298.
126. Foster BK, Hansen AL, Gibson GJ, et al. Reimplantation of growth plate chondrocytes into growth plate defects in sheep. *J Orthop Res* 1990;8:555–564.
127. Kawabe N, Ehrlich MG, Mankin HJ. Growth plate reconstruction using chondrocyte allograft transplants. *J Pediatr Orthop* 1987;7:381–388.
128. Barr SJ, Zaleske DJ. Physeal reconstruction with blocks of cartilage of varying developmental time. *J Pediatr Orthop* 1992;11:766–773.
129. Bueche MJ, Phillips WA, Gordon J, et al. Effect of interposition material on mechanical behavior in partial physeal resection: a canine model. *J Pediatr Orthop* 1990;10: 459–462.
130. Ferrick MR, Birch JG, Albright M. Correction of non-Blount's angular knee deformity by permanent hemiepiphysiodesis. *J Pediatr Orthop* 2004;24:397–402.

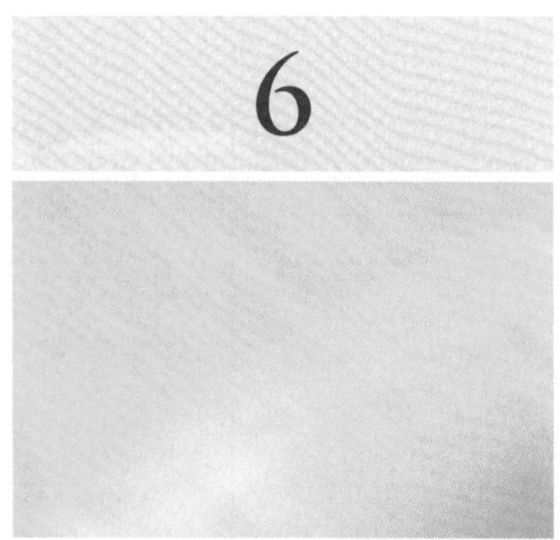

6

PATHOLOGIC FRACTURES ASSOCIATED WITH TUMORS AND UNIQUE CONDITIONS OF THE MUSCULOSKELETAL SYSTEM

John P. Dormans and John M. Flynn

As a child grows, the pattern of injury and the response to injury and treatment change. One of the more difficult situations encountered in caring for children occurs when the diagnosis and treatment of a complex injury are complicated by a preexisting underlying disease process or condition of the skeleton. The diagnosis of both the injury and the underlying condition depends on an accurate understanding of how these conditions alter the presentation of the child, given that evaluation of the traumatic injury may reveal the underlying condition for the first time. This chapter describes the pertinent clinical and radiographic features of the conditions of the pediatric musculoskeletal system that can predispose a child to pathologic fracture, including specific patterns of injury and special concerns of treatment. For most orthopedic surgeons, experience with these conditions is limited, and diligence is needed to avoid pitfalls of treatment. The physician must always be aware of the possibility of a pathologic fracture, especially when a patient presents with a fracture following minimal trauma.

A pathologic fracture is defined as a fracture that occurs through abnormal bone. These fractures occur in bone that lacks normal biomechanical and viscoelastic properties. Pathologic fractures may result from intrinsic or extrinsic processes. Examples of intrinsic processes include the osteopenia of osteogenesis imperfecta or replacement of bone with tumor. With extrinsic processes, the weakness is caused by something that lessens the inherent structural integrity of bone, such as radiation or a hole in bone from biopsy or internal fixation. In addition, pathologic fractures may result from localized (a bone cyst, for example) or generalized processes (such as osteopetrosis), and the fracture may be correctable (rickets) or noncorrectable (metastatic cancer). A fracture similar to a pathologic fracture can occur through anatomically normal bone that is weakened by normal structures, such as vascular foramina (Fig. 6-1).

Pathologic fractures can occur in children with generalized bone conditions and in those with tumors or tumor-like processes of bone. Although the presenting episode of a child with generalized bone disease (osteogenesis imperfecta, osteopetrosis, and rickets) may be a fracture, more commonly, the diagnosis has been made based on clinical findings, such as history, physical examination, x-rays, or laboratory findings. Often, the history is most helpful. For example, pathologic fracture secondary to generalized osteopenia associated with chronic drug therapy (steroids or anticonvulsants) may become evident through the patient's history. Some of the key points in analysis of a pediatric patient with a musculoskeletal tumor or tumor-like lesion are shown in Table 6-1.

TABLE 6-1 Evaluation of a Pediatric Patient with a Musculoskeletal Tumor or Tumor-like Lesion

1. Age of patient (see Table 6-2)
2. Location of lesion (see Table 6-3)
   Epiphysis, metaphysis, diaphysis?
   Central or eccentric?
3. What is the lesion doing to the bone? (Pattern of involvement)
   a. Zone of transition (narrow or wide; can measure)
   b. Geographic versus "moth eaten" versus permeative
4. What is the bone doing to the lesion?
   Periosteal response or "walling off"
   No response?
      Early, immature?
      Late, mature?
5. Is there a characteristic appearance of the lesion, i.e, matrix?
   Lytic, calcified, ossified, "Ground-glass"

Hipp and colleagues proposed a way of quantifying the risk of pathologic fracture in 1995 (1). They defined the *factor of*

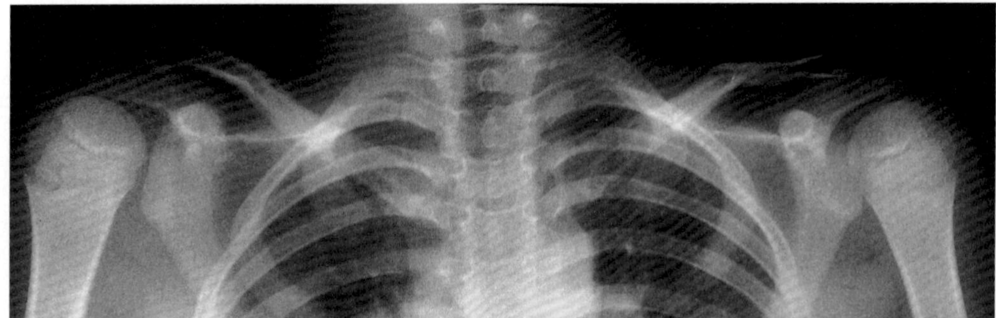

FIGURE 6-1 A fracture through the vascular foramina of this 9-year-old boy's left clavicle. The fracture healed uneventfully.

risk as the load applied to the involved bone divided by the load required for bone failure. Other attempts have been made to measure the risk of pathologic fracture in patients with underlying conditions of bone (2–4). Unfortunately, retrospective studies have failed to find any predictive methods based on radiographic findings that can accurately forecast fracture in most situations. New methods that apply engineering principles to information from computed tomography (CT) scans may provide better noninvasive estimates for the risk of pathologic fracture (1).

With pathologic fractures through a tumor or tumor-like lesion, the age of the patient can also be helpful in making the diagnosis (Table 6-2). Most tumors and tumor-like processes are recognizable by radiographic appearance; the location of the lesion can also be helpful (Table 6-3) (5,6).

Biopsy is sometimes needed to determine the cause of a pathologic fracture, especially with pathologic fractures through tumors or tumor-like processes. In this situation, the surgeon must ensure that biopsy is performed on representative areas of the bony lesion.

Pathologic fractures differ from fractures in normal bone in that the etiology, natural history, and treatment of the underlying abnormality of the bone must be taken into account. Accurate and careful determination of these underlying diagnoses is critical for the appropriate care of these fractures. Fracture management principles often are altered for pathologic fractures because of the abnormal condition responsible for the fracture. The treatment plan must consider both the treatment of the fracture and treatment of the underlying cause of the fracture.

Once a fracture occurs secondary to a previously unrecognized condition, subsequent fractures often can be prevented, usually through patient education. Iatrogenic pathologic fracture often can be prevented by the appropriate use of internal fixation (avoidance of unnecessary cortical penetration with drills and guide pins for example), protection of an extremity with internal fixation by cast or brace when appropriate, and the use of rounded edges of bone biopsy sites (7).

FRACTURES ASSOCIATED WITH CYSTS, TUMORS, OR TUMOR-LIKE PROCESSES

Benign tumors can be classified according to their aggressiveness (Table 6-4). Stage 1, or latent benign lesions, are usually asymptomatic, discovered incidentally, and seldom associated with pathologic fracture. Stage 2 lesions are intermediate in behavior, and stage 3, or aggressive benign lesions, are usually symptomatic, grow rapidly, and may be associated with pathologic fracture.

TABLE 6-2 Peak Age of Common Pediatric Musculoskeletal Conditions (Tumors and Tumor-like Lesions of Bone)

Age (years)	Benign	Malignant
0–5	Langerhans' cell histiocytosis Osteomyelitis	Ewing's sarcoma Leukemia Neuroblastoma (metastasis) Wilms' tumor (metastasis) Neuroblastoma (metastasis)
5–10	Unicameral bone cyst Aneurysmal bone cyst Nonossifying fibroma Fibrous dysplasia Osteoid osteoma Langerhans' cell histiocytosis Osteomyelitis	Ewing's sarcoma Osteosarcoma Rhabdomyosarcoma
10–20	Unicameral bone cyst Aneurysmal bone cyst Osteoid osteoma Fibrous dysplasia Chondroblastoma Osteofibrous dysplasia	Osteosarcoma Ewing's sarcoma (Chondrosarcoma) Rhabdomyosarcoma Synovial cell sarcoma

TABLE 6-3 Location of Tumor and Tumor-like Lesions of Bone

Metaphyeal—Any lesion

Epiphyseal
- Chondroblastoma
- Brodie's abscess of the epiphysis-subacute epiphyseal osteomyelitis
- Giant cell tumor
- Fibrous dysplasia

Diaphyseal
- Fibrous dysplasia
- Osteofibrous dysplasia (child), adamantinoma (adult)
- Langerhans' cell histiocytosis
- Ewing's sarcoma
- Leukemia, lymphoma
- Subacute osteomyelitis
- (Occasionally osteoid osteoma and UBC)

Multiple lesions
- Histiocytosis
- Fibrous dysplasia (Albright's syndrome)
- Leukemia, metastasis
- Enchondroma (Ollier's disease)
- Multiple hereditary exostosis
- Hemangioma of bone

Anterior elements spine
- Eosinophilic granuloma (Langerhans' cell histiocytosis)
- Leukemia
- Hemangioma
- Metastasis
- Infection (end plate, unless tuberculosis)
- Giant cell tumor
- Chondroma (usually adult)

Posterior elements spine
- Aneurysmal bone cyst
- Osteoblastoma
- Osteoid osteoma
- Metastatic (usually adult)

Pelvis
- Ewing's sarcoma
- Osteosarcoma
- Osteochondroma
- Metastasis
- Fibrous dysplasia
- Chondrosarcoma (usually adult)

Rib
- Fibrous dysplasia
- LCH
- Ewing's sarcoma
- Metastatic lesions
- Chondrosarcoma (usually adult)

Benign but locally aggressive tumors:
- Chondroblastoma
- Aneurysmal bone cyst
- Chondromyxoid fibroma
- Giant cell tumor
- Osteoblastoma
- Chordoma
- Adamantamona

TABLE 6-4 Classification of Benign Lesions According to Their Aggressiveness

Stage 1, Latent Benign
- Asymptomatic
- Often discovered incidentally
- Seldom associated with pathologic fracture

Stage 2, Active Benign
- Majority
- Tend to grow steadily
- May be symptomatic

Stage 3, Aggressive Benign
- Generally symptomatic
- Discomfort, usually tender
- May be associated with pathologic fracture
- Growth rapid

Unicameral Bone Cysts

Unicameral bone cysts (UBCs) are radiolucent expansile fluid-filled cystic lesions found most commonly in the metaphyses of long bones. The term *unicameral* suggests a single-chambered cyst, but often, especially after treatment or fracture, the lesions are multiloculated with radiolucent fibrous septa segregating the primary lesion into multiple small chambers (8). The cysts usually contain yellow serous fluid. In order of decreasing frequency, the cysts most commonly occur in the proximal humerus, proximal femur, proximal tibia, distal tibia, distal femur, calcaneus, distal humerus, radius, fibula, ilium, ulna, and rib (4). Approximately 70% of these cysts are found in either the proximal humerus or femur. Some authors have suggested that UBCs evolve from an accumulation of interstitial fluid in the bone because of a defect in venous or lymphatic drainage (9–11).

Approximately 75% of patients who have UBCs present with pathologic fractures (12–17). These cysts usually are diagnosed within the first two decades of life (10,18,19) and the ratio of males to females is about 2:1 (20). Fractures are often incomplete or minimally displaced. Patients with pathologic fractures through UBCs present with mild to moderate pain in the extremity after either mild trauma or no history of injury. In one series (21), 40% of pathologic femoral neck fractures in children were due to UBCs. Pathologic fracture with collapse of the articular surface of the femoral head and joint incongruity also has been reported (22).

Although the fracture commonly heals within 6 weeks of injury, the UBC usually persists, often with further fracture. Only about 10% of cysts heal after fracture. In a 1993 report of 52 pathologic fractures due to UBC, Ahn and Park (23) found that only 8% of cysts healed at an average of 5.5 years after injury.

Radiographic Findings

The classic appearance of a UBC is a centrally located, radiolucent, slightly expansile lesion of the metaphysis (Fig. 6-2) (24). The width of the lesion seldom exceeds that of the adjacent physis [a feature characteristic of the more expansile aneurysmal bone cyst (ABC)]. Occasionally, UBCs are located in the diaphysis when the physis has migrated away from the lesion with growth (Fig. 6-3) (25). The so-called fallen fragment sign, described by Reynolds (24) in 1969, is a fracture fragment seen on plain x-rays at the bottom of a cyst suggesting a hollow cavity in the bone rather than a solid tumor (Fig. 6-4). A cortical fragment also may be tilted into the interior of the lesion. The differential diagnosis of UBC includes ABC, fibrous dysplasia, enchondroma, giant cell tumor, and eosinophilic granuloma.

Natural History—Predicting Fracture

The natural history of UBCs is variable, but typically they gradually improve with growth. Most UBCs persist into adulthood, but some disappear spontaneously at puberty (11). The cysts are traditionally described as active if they are adjacent to the physis (11) or latent if more than 0.5 cm from the physis (Table 6-5) (26). Ahn and Park (23) noted that pathologic fracture occurred when the transverse diameter of the cyst was 85% or more, whereas Nakamura et al (27) reported that the chance of fracture was high if the cyst wall was less than 5 mm in width.

Complications after fracture of the proximal femur include malunion, growth arrest, and osteonecrosis (ON) of the femoral head. Kay and Nason (28) noted growth disturbance in five of their 21 patients (24%) with pathologic proximal humeral fracture before treatment of the UBC. Moed and LaMont (29) reported three patients in whom premature closure of the medial proximal humeral physis resulted in humeral shortening of 2 to 5 cm. Malunion may be a problem in fractures through cysts of the proximal femur (10), and ON of the femoral head has been reported after displaced femoral neck fractures (20) and after an undisplaced femoral neck fracture in an 8-year-old boy (30). Infrequently, the cyst may extend from the metaphysis into the epiphysis (2,12,31) and collapse of the surface of the femoral head has been reported.

Treatment

Pathologic fractures through UBCs invariably heal with simple immobilization; the cyst, however, persists in nearly 85% of patients, and additional fractures are common. Neer et al (4) observed an additional 2.5 fractures per patient during observation periods after the initial injury, and Oppenheim and Galleno (16) emphasized that prolonged observation with inevitable refracture may be stressful to patients and may adversely restrict children from normal childhood activities.

In the upper extremity, minimally displaced, stable pathologic fractures through UBCs are treated with simple immobilization for 4 to 6 weeks to obtain healing. Usually, a sling is adequate treatment for stable fractures of the proximal humerus, and once healed, the options for further treatment are discussed with the patient and family (see later).

With pathologic fracture through UBC in the proximal femur, preliminary traction before surgical intervention may be appropriate (32). Most authors recommend internal fixation if the fracture is unstable or displaced (4,12,20,33). Malunion is common in these fractures (10). Intertrochanteric osteotomies may be necessary later to correct alignment (34).

Operative Treatment

Curettage and Bone Grafting. Many surgical techniques have been developed for the treatment of UBCs, with varying rates of success. Earlier interventions consisted primarily of curettage and bone grafting. Lesions treated with this technique have a recurrence rate varying from 18% to 40% (4,12,15,26,35,36). Delaying the treatment until the cyst converts from an active to a latent stage has been advocated by some physicians, but a 2-year period of observation may be necessary (12). Some data suggest that the response to treatment may be the same for latent as for active cysts (25). After fracture, most authors advocate at least a 6-week delay in treatment to allow the fracture to heal before curettage and bone grafting (10,37). There seems to be no substantial difference in the rate of healing with the use of either autogenous bone graft or allograft.

Open curettage and bone grafting have fallen out of favor for the treatment of upper extremity and smaller lower extremity UBCs due to the invasive nature of the operation and also the still significant persistence and recurrence rates associated with this option. Curettage and bone graft remains a popular method of treatment for larger UBCs of the proximal femur, however; the reported recurrence rates range from 10% to 40% (Fig. 6-5) (12,15,16,35). Although partial persistence or recurrence of the UBC may occur, interim healing usually occurs such that the risk of pathologic fracture and displacement is lessened and subsequent persistence or recurrence can be treated with corticosteroid injections. Follow-up of the treated lesions with periodic x-ray studies is suggested.

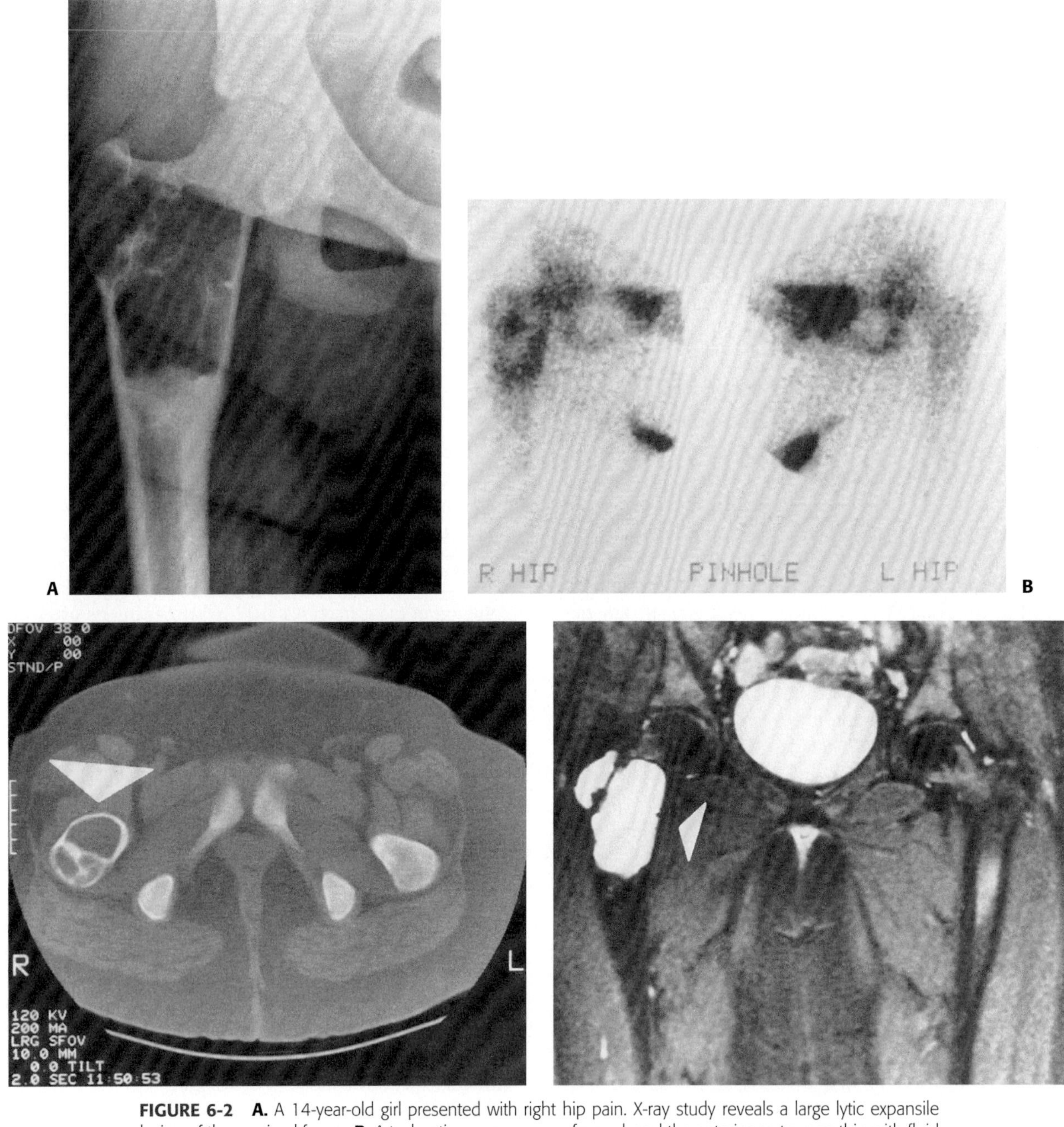

FIGURE 6-2 **A.** A 14-year-old girl presented with right hip pain. X-ray study reveals a large lytic expansile lesion of the proximal femur. **B.** A technetium scan was performed, and the anterior cortex was thin with fluid within the lesion. **C.** MRI was performed, and signal intensity was equal to that within the bladder, and a diagnosis of unicameral bone cyst was made. **D.** It was treated with curettage and bone graft.

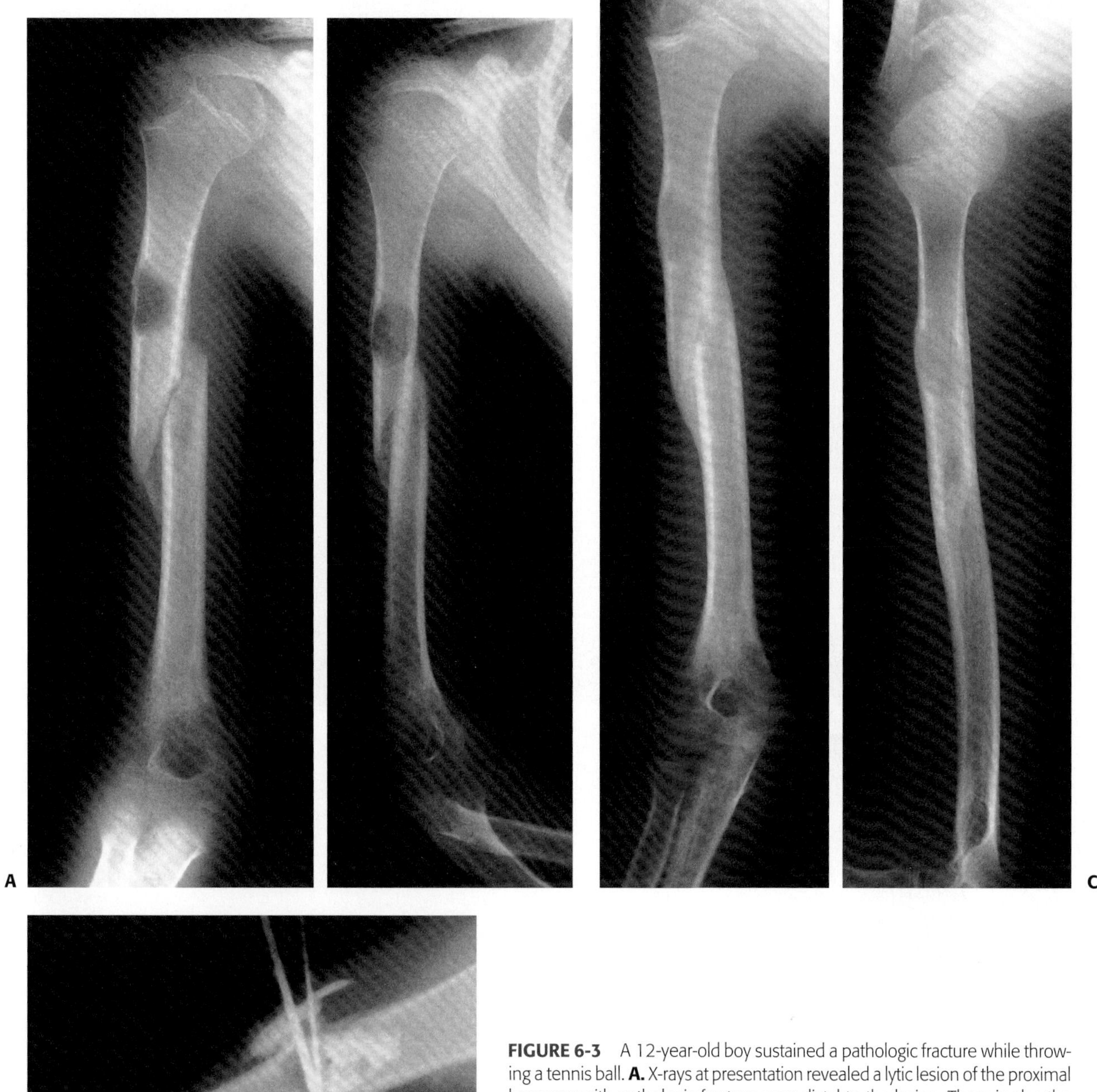

FIGURE 6-3 A 12-year-old boy sustained a pathologic fracture while throwing a tennis ball. **A.** X-rays at presentation revealed a lytic lesion of the proximal humerus with pathologic fracture seen distal to the lesion. There is also the suggestion of a pathologic fracture through the cyst. The lesion was believed to represent a unicameral bone cyst, and the fracture was treated in a hanging arm cast. **B.** At 8-week follow-up, the patient was believed likely to be prone to have a recurrent fracture and was taken to surgery. With the patient under general anesthesia, the lesion was injected with radiopaque dye and was found to be a cystic lesion. Steroid injection was done. **C.** At 12-week follow-up, the patient is asymptomatic, with radiographic improvement of the lesion.

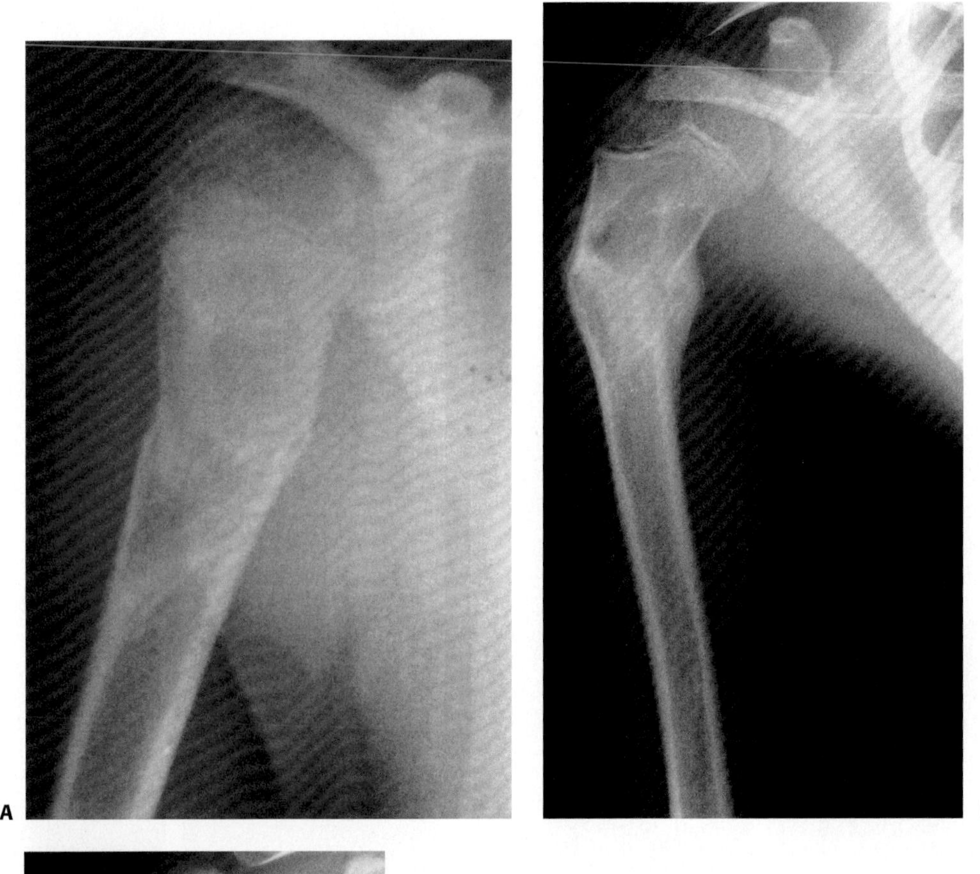

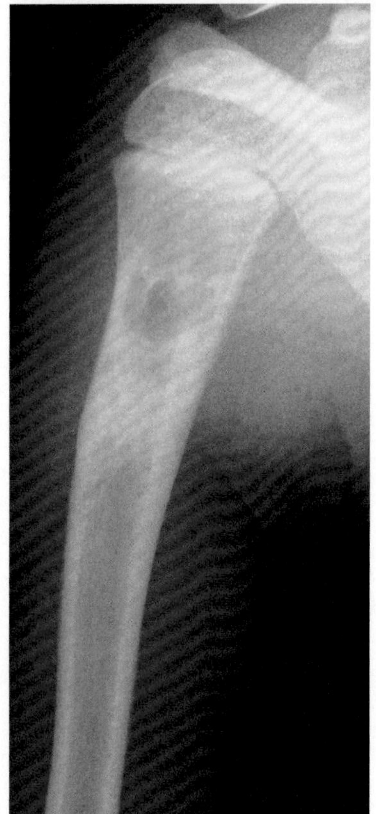

FIGURE 6-4 A 13-year-old boy sustained a pathologic fracture. **A.** X-ray studies at presentation revealed a lytic lesion of the proximal humerus with pathologic fracture. A so-called fallen fragment sign is seen at the bottom of a cyst suggesting a hollow cavity in the bone rather than a solid tumor. The lesion was believed to represent a UBC, and the fracture was treated in a hanging arm cast. **B.** At 8-week follow-up, fracture lines were beginning to obliterate. **C.** At 6-month follow-up, the cyst has partially healed.

TABLE 6-5 Staging of Unicameral Bone Cysts

	Active	Inactive or "Latent"
Age of the patient	≤10–12 years	>12 years
Location	Abutting the physis	Separated from physis by a zone of normal cancellous bone
X-ray appearance	Single cavity	Multiloculated cavity
Intralesional pressure	>30 cm H_2O	6–10 cm H_2O
Pathology	Thin shiny membrane, few osteocytes, little or no hemosiderin, osteoclasts	Thick membrane, frequent giant cells, cholesterol slits, hemosiderin, osteoblasts

The patient with a calcaneal UBC usually presents with pain due to microfracture (38–40). UBCs in this location may not respond as well to injections with methylprednisolone (38,39) and several authors have recommended primary curettage and bone grafting (38,39).

Because of the high rates of recurrence after curettage and bone grafting, a number of approaches were developed, including intentional fracture of the cyst (41), crushing of the lesion with onlay bone grafting (2), and packing of the defect with plaster of Paris pellets (40). Radical excision of the lesion with or without grafting produced recurrence rates of 9% or less (15,19,28) but this procedure is a larger operation with greater risk, can be difficult technically, and requires substantial bone graft.

Aspiration and Injection. In 1974, Scaglietti et al began empiric injection of UBCs with methylprednisolone and in 1979 (42), reported healing rates (mostly radiographic improvement of the cyst) of 96% in 72 patients. Two needles were inserted into each cyst, and the initial corticosteroid dose varied from 40 to 200 mg for large cysts. Complete healing was initially reported in 55% of cysts undergoing this treatment. Local recurrence in 45% of cases was treated with up to five additional injections of 40 to 80 mg of methylprednisolone at 2- to 3-month intervals until healing occurred.

The mechanism for cyst healing after methylprednisolone injection remains unknown. Scaglietti et al (42) suggested that an anti-inflammatory response initiated by the corticosteroids promoted cyst healing. Shindell et al (43) observed elevated levels of prostaglandins in cysts; after serial injections of corticosteroid, levels decreased. Because prostaglandins stimulate osteoclastic activity, these authors suggested that a corticosteroid-induced repression of prostaglandins may indirectly aid in cyst healing. In animal experiments, however, corticosteroids are rapidly cleared from the medullary canal of long bones after injection (44). Others have suggested that cyst healing occurs through decompression of cyst fluid pressure by multiple trephination (18,44,45).

Methylprednisolone injection for UBCs became popular because of its relatively low morbidity and an apparent long-term effectiveness approaching that of more invasive techniques. However, incomplete healing and recurrence are common after the initial injection of corticosteroid, and multiple injections of corticosteroid may be necessary in 50% to 92% of patients (intervals ranging from 2 to 6 months) (8,16).

In those cysts that respond to methylprednisolone treatment, the cortical margins of the lesion usually thicken. By 6 months, the central portion of the cyst assumes a frosted-glass appearance, and by 12 months, the cyst may heal with dense sclerotic bone (13,46).

Aspiration and Injection—Operative Technique. A two-needle injection technique is most commonly used. Some authors (16) recommend the use of two Craig-type needles or Jamshidi biopsy needles so that a biopsy specimen can be obtained at the time of injection. The initial dose of methylprednisolone varies from 40 to 200 mg (8,42,47), and the volume can be adjusted to match radiographic volume of the cyst. The injection can be given under local anesthetic (48), but most prefer general anesthesia. Several authors (16,40,49), have emphasized the importance of outlining the cyst with radiopaque dye injection before placement of the methylprednisolone. With this technique, intracystic fibrous septa were found in 92% of lesions in one series (49) and these may prevent complete filling of the cyst by corticosteroids with later incomplete healing. This cystogram also allows the surgeon to verify that the cyst is indeed fluid filled. If it does not fill with contrast material, other diagnoses, such as fibrous dysplasia or enchondroma, should be considered. Capanna et al (49) recommend vigorous saline irrigation of the cyst through two needles to lyse the fibrous septa, whereas Oppenheim and Galleno (16) simply reinject

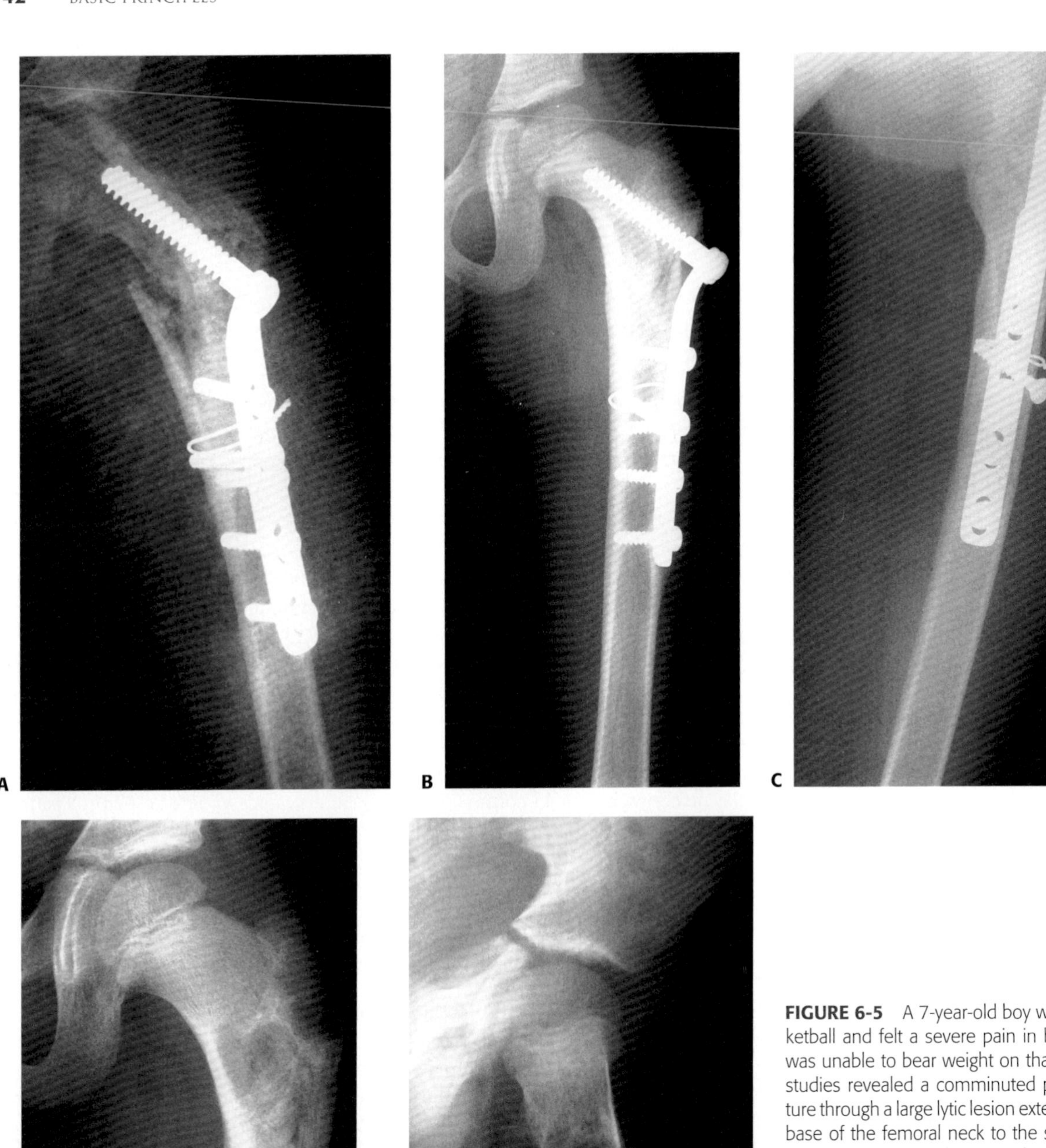

FIGURE 6-5 A 7-year-old boy was playing basketball and felt a severe pain in his left hip and was unable to bear weight on that side. **A.** X-ray studies revealed a comminuted pathologic fracture through a large lytic lesion extending from the base of the femoral neck to the subtrochanteric region (comminuted type IB hip). The appearance of the lesion is believed to be most compatible with a UBC. **B.** The fracture and cyst were approached laterally. Open reduction and internal fixation were performed using a pediatric hip screw and side plate. The cyst contents were consistent with UBC; it was curetted and packed with cancellous bone graft. The patient was placed in a hip spica cast for 6 weeks with healing of the fracture. **C.** At 4-month follow-up, the fracture has healed and the cyst appears to be consolidating. **D.** At 2-year follow-up, x-ray studies show a partial recurrence or persistence of the cyst. The cyst was subsequently grafted again. **E.** At 4-year follow-up, x-ray studies show no evidence of recurrence or persistence of the cyst. The patient has no discomfort and has returned to full activities.

the areas of cyst that are not filled by contrast material in the initial injection.

Aspiration and Injection—The Humerus. With fluoroscopic guidance, the humerus is rotated until an area of thin cortex is identified, and two 20-gauge spinal needles are passed through this area into the cyst so that the needle tips are at opposite ends of the cyst cavity. A more stout, disposable biopsy needle can be used for areas of thicker bone. The presence of serous fluid with removal of the needle stylet is indicative of UBC. A cystogram is then performed by injection of several milliliters of Renografin dye both to confirm the fluid-filled nature of the cyst and to ascertain whether the cyst is indeed unicameral or multiloculated. If the dye does not fill a cyst cavity, the diagnosis of UBC should be questioned. If the cyst is multiloculated, the needles can be used to break up any septations that exist. Methylprednisolone is then injected through one of the needles using a dose ranging from 40 to 200 mg (Fig. 6-6). To guard against recurrent fracture, the arm is protected in a sling for 2 to 6 weeks and x-ray studies are performed every 6 weeks initially to monitor healing. Incomplete healing or persistence of the cyst can be treated with additional injections or with other techniques. Aspiration, cystogram, and steroid injection can also be done for small, stable UBCs of the lower extremity, but if the cyst is potentially unstable and there is a risk of malunion (e.g., varus of the femoral neck), one should consider surgical fixation and bone grafting.

Complications. In addition to recurrence of the cyst, complications that occur with corticosteroid treatment include recurrent pathologic fractures (13,16,31) and osteonecrosis of the femoral head (13,21). Nakamura et al (27) measured the bone mineral content of the corticosteroid injected cyst by densitometer and found that if there was no increase in density 2 months after injection, then the chance of refracture was high. In one series, growth disturbance was a problem in 20% of 141 patients with bone cysts treated by corticosteroid injection (21). Systemic reactions to the corticosteroid injection, such as corticosteroid flush or increased appetite and temporary weight gain, are rare (16,44).

Newer Methods. Some authors believe that relieving the pressure of the interstitial fluid in the lesions can heal the cyst. Chigira et al (18) treated six patients by puncturing the cysts with multiple Kirschner wires, which were then left in place; cysts subsequently recurred in 6 to 8 months in two patients. Santori et al (45) decompressed UBCs with Enders nails or Rush pins without curettage or grafting, and during short-term follow-up, they noted healing in all 11 patients. The effect of the fixation on the adjacent physes awaits long-term follow-up.

New grafting materials also are becoming available. Demineralized bone matrix (DBM) or commercial product paste is composed of demineralized bone particles ranging from 100 to 500 μm in a glycerol base. It has been used in the treatment of delayed unions and nonunion, in some primary bone-healing situations, and more recently, for the treatment of UBCs (3,50,51). Killian et al (3) used DBM in 11 patients with UBCs, and 9 cysts healed (within 4 to 5 months) after a single injection. At 2 years' follow-up, no cysts were deemed active or recurrent (20). Rougraff et al used trephination and injection of allogenic demineralized bone matrix and autogenous bone marrow. Five of 23 patients required a second injection, and at last follow-up, 7 had small, persistent radiolucencies in the area of the cyst (51).

Other materials also have been used. Packing of the defect with plaster of Paris pellets (calcium sulfate) was described by Peltier in 1978 (40). Osteoset pellets bone is composed of medical grade calcium sulfate. This radiopaque product can be used in an open grafting situation or can be injected percutaneously. The biodegradable pellets are resorbed in 30 to 60 days when used according to labeling. This product is not intended to provide structural support during the healing process and therefore is contraindicated when structural support is required.

Adjuvants such as liquid nitrogen have been used for the treatment of UBCs (41), but their efficacy or safety has not been established. Current research includes the use of aspirated bone marrow injected into UBCs.

Internal Fixation of Proximal Femoral Pathologic Fractures. If there is a significant loss of proximal femoral bone because of the UBC, there is a high risk of a coxa vara deformity after treatment without internal fixation. Both the location of the UBC and the amount of bone loss dictate whether fixation can stabilize the fracture after grafting and what type of fixation is appropriate. We have classified pathologic fractures of the femoral neck in children into six types (Fig. 6-7) (52).

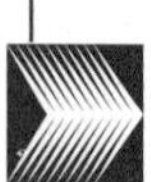

AUTHORS' PREFERRED METHOD OF TREATMENT

Unicameral Bone Cysts

Overall, methylprednisolone injection has a favorable rate of success compared with open surgical treatment; the ease of treatment, relatively low operative morbidity, and the information obtained with aspiration and cystogram make it a favorable initial choice for treatment of UBCs in the upper extremity and smaller cysts in the lower extremity. Because incomplete healing and recurrence are common after the initial injection of corticosteroid, and because multiple injections of corticosteroid are necessary in most patients, new grafting materials are being used more commonly at our institution, especially if the first steroid injection fails. Grafton demineralized bone matrix (Osteotech, Eatontown, NJ) and Osteoset pellets (Wright Medical Technology, Arlington, TN) are the two most often used at present.

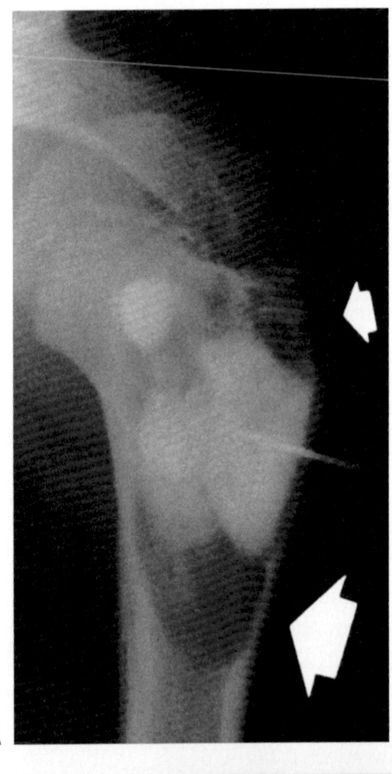

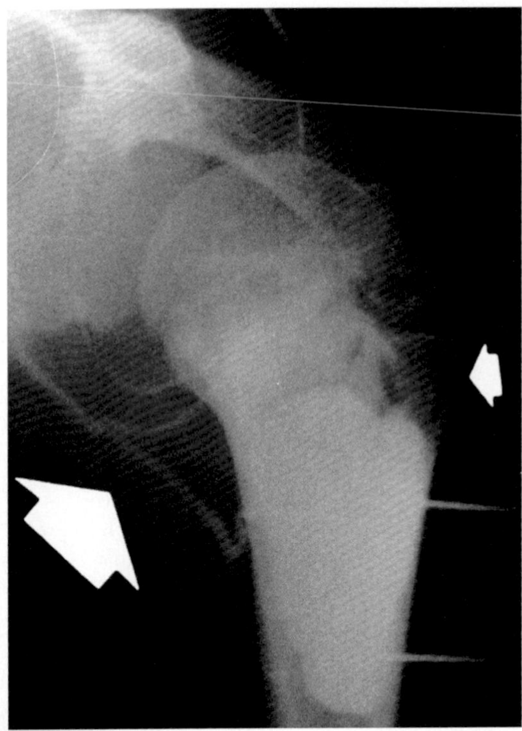

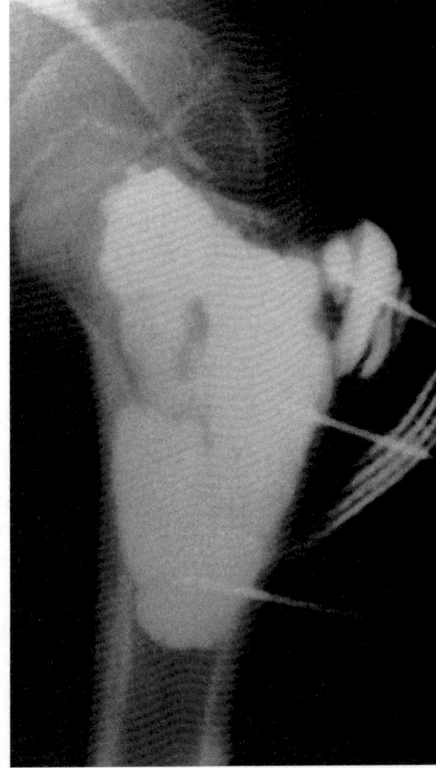

FIGURE 6-6 A. A radiopaque dye injection of a unicameral cyst of the proximal humerus. Note the poor filling of the inferior portion of the cyst (*large arrow*) and the proximal portion (*small arrow*). This suggests that fibrous septa are present in the cyst. **B.** More radiopaque dye was placed in the distal portion of the cyst through a second needle, and a venous drainage of the lesion is now visualized (*large arrow*). The proximal portion of the cyst is still poorly filled (*swag arrow*). **C.** With a third needle superiorly, the proximal portion of the cyst is now filled. The total dose of corticosteroid is divided into equal portions and injected separately through the three needles to ensure complete dispersal throughout the lesion. A single dose through the first needle might not have saturated the entire cyst.

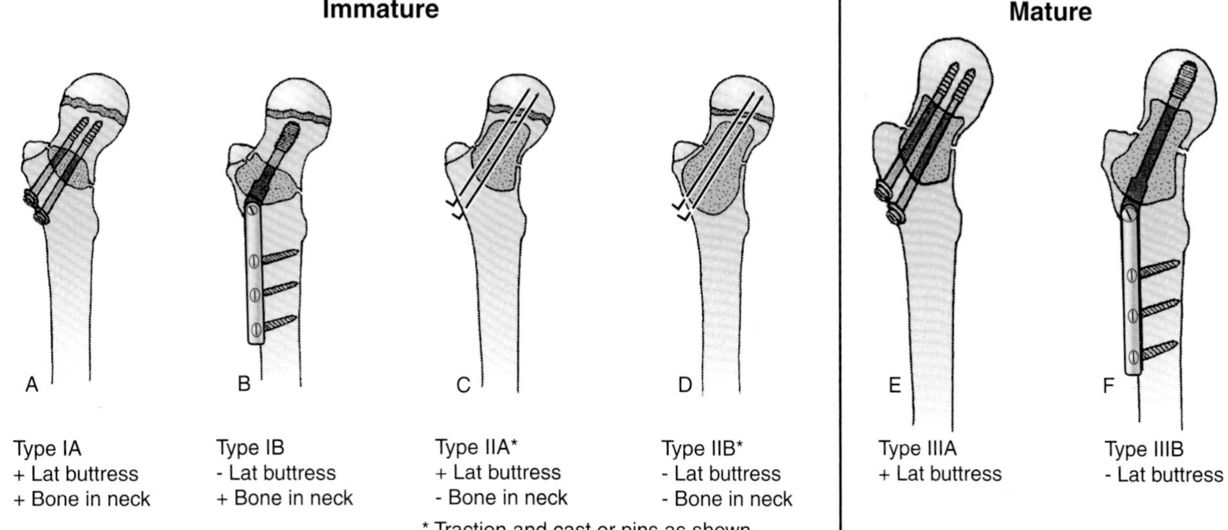

FIGURE 6-7 Our classification system for the treatment of pathologic fractures of the proximal femur associated with bone cysts in children. **A.** In Type IA, a moderately sized cyst is present in the middle of the femoral neck. There is enough bone in the femoral neck and lateral proximal femur (lateral buttress) to allow fixation with cannulated screws after curettage and bone grafting. **B.** In Type IB, a large cyst is present at the base of the femoral neck. Although there is enough bone in the femoral neck, there is loss of lateral buttress, so a pediatric hip screw and a side plate should be considered rather than cannulated screws, after curettage and bone grafting. **C,D.** In Type IIA-B, a large lesion is present in the femoral neck, so there is not enough bone beneath the physis to accept screws. There are two options for treatment of these bone cysts: (a) after curettage and bone grafting, parallel pins across the physis can be used in combination with a spica cast and (b) The patient can be treated in traction until the fracture heals (with subsequent spica cast) followed by curettage and bone grafting. **E,F.** In Type IIIA-B, the physis is closing or closed. The lateral buttress is present in Type IIIA hips, so cannulated screws can be used to stabilize the fracture after curettage and bone grafting. In Type IIIB hips, the loss of lateral buttress makes it necessary to use a pediatric hip screw and a side plate following curettage and bone grafting. In all types, we recommend spica cast immobilization following surgery.

Percutaneous intramedullary decompression and grafting with Osteoset pellets is the authors' preferred method of treatment. Percutaneous intramedullary decompression to allow "streaming in" of local bone marrow, combined with curettage of the cyst lining and grafting using calcium sulfate pellets has shown excellent results in the management of UBCs in children. High healing rates, low rates of recurrence, and low incidence of reoperation are associated with this technique that combines the healing benefits of curettage, grafting, and intramedullary decompression with the low morbidity of a percutaneous procedure. In addition, the use of an effective allograft material such as calcium sulfate pellets avoids the morbidity associated with autograft harvest without sacrificing clinical results. A review of 23 patients with biopsy-confirmed UBCs found complete clinical and radiographic resolution in 91% of patients after treatment with this technique (53).

We recommend simple immobilization for most fractures occurring through UBCs. Spontaneous healing of the cyst can occur, although infrequently. Once the fracture has healed, generally by 6 to 8 weeks, further treatment of the cyst can be rendered, if necessary.

Displaced pathologic fractures of the proximal femur are based on the location of the cyst. The amount of bone loss dictates whether fixation can stabilize the fracture after grafting and what type of fixation would be best to use. We use the classification of pathologic fractures of the proximal femur in children shown in Figure 6-7.

Aneurysmal Bone Cysts

ABCs are eccentric or central, expansile osteolytic lesions usually occurring in the metaphyseal ends of long bones or in the posterior elements of the spine during adolescence. Nearly 75% of ABCs are found in patients younger than 20 years old, and 50% are seen in individuals between 10 and 20 years of age (21,54). Girls are affected slightly more often than boys. ABCs are relatively rare, accounting for approximately 1.5% of all primary bone tumors (54).

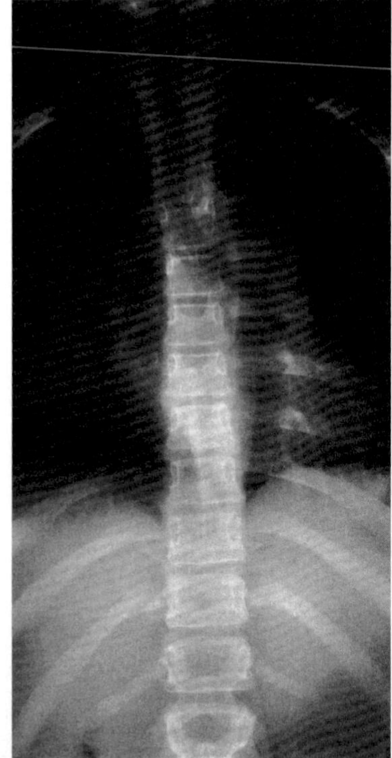

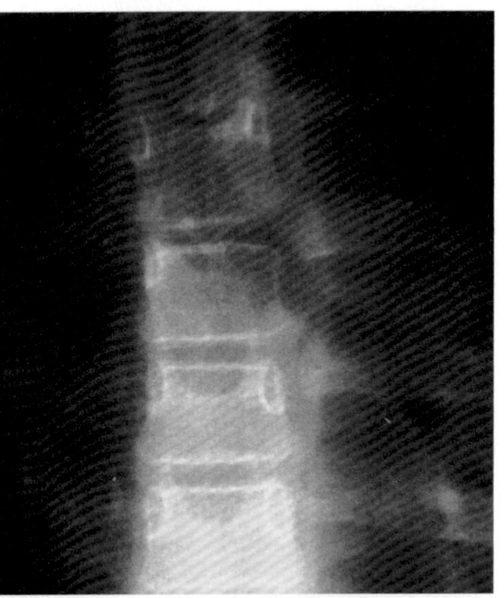

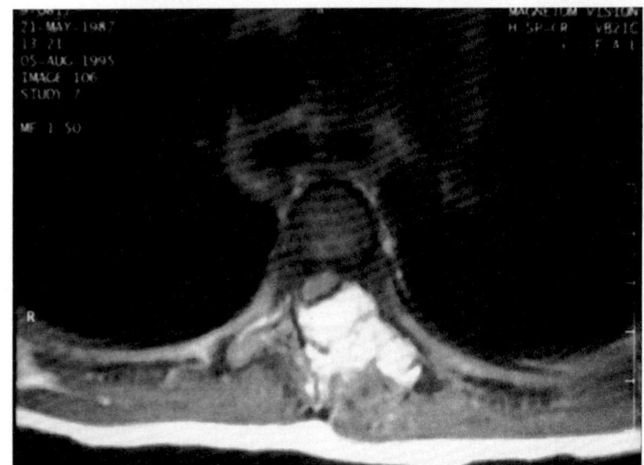

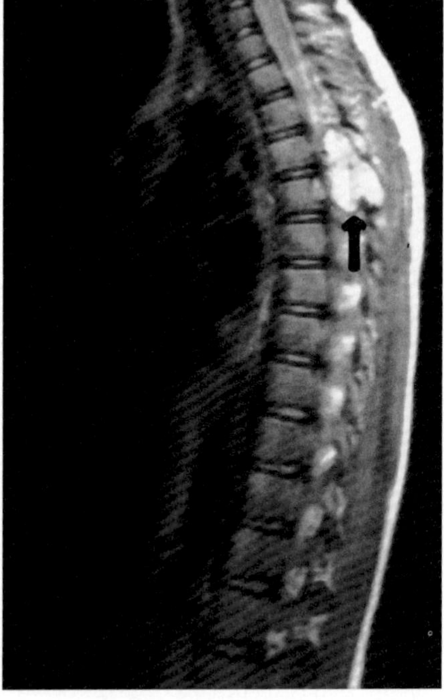

FIGURE 6-8 An 8-year-old girl presented with a 4-week history of back pain. **A.** X-rays show absence of the pedicle of T5 on the left. **B.** Close-up view of the same areas. **C.** The axial T2-weighted image through the body of T5 shows multiple blood-fluid levels within the left sided expansile destructive mass. **D.** Sagittal proton density MRI of the thoracic spine shows a blood fluid level (*arrow*) within an expansile mass. (*continues*)

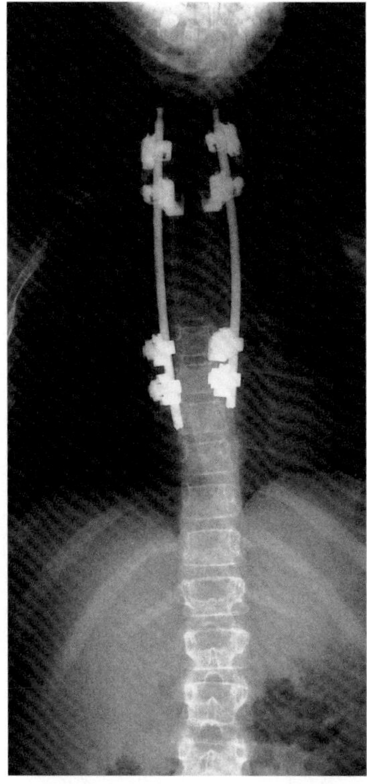

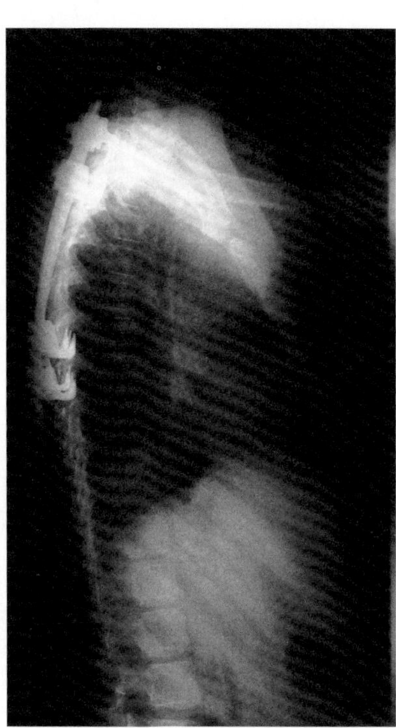

FIGURE 6-8 (*continued*) **E.** Postoperative x-ray studies showing instrumentation and fusion after extended curettage and removal of tumor. The patient is pain free without recurrence or deformity at 4 years after surgery. (From Cohen RB, Dormans JP, Guttenberg ME, et al. Back pain in an 8-year-old girl. *Clin Orthop* 1997;343: 249–252; with permission.)

The long bones are involved in 65% of patients. In order of decreasing frequency, the most commonly involved bones are the distal femur, proximal tibia, proximal humerus, and distal radius. The vertebrae are involved in 12% to 27% of patients (21,55), some of whom have symptoms of radicular pain. The lumbar vertebrae are most commonly affected. The primary site of involvement is the posterior elements of the spine with frequent extension into the vertebral body (56).

The lesions are not true cysts but rather sponge-like collections of interconnected fibrous tissue and blood-filled spaces (55). They tend to be destructive lesions, which replace bone and thin the cortices of the host bone. The elevated viable periosteum usually maintains a thin osseous shell.

The etiology of ABCs is unknown. Some have considered them primary lesions of bone (57), whereas others have noted a secondary association with other lesions such as UBCs, nonossifying fibromas, fibrous dysplasia (58), and osteogenic sarcoma. They also can occur in association with fractures of the long bones (56,59). The most common presenting symptom is localized pain of less than 6 months' duration (21,57). Patients with ABCs are three times more likely to have pain during exercise rather than pain at rest (60).

Radiographic Findings

ABCs are eccentric or central lytic lesions of bone, sometimes with extension beyond the cortex (54,57,58). Septation is common, giving rise to the so-called soap bubble or honeycomb appearance. Lesions in the short tubular bones, such as the metacarpals and metatarsals, are commonly more central. Spinal ABCs usually are located in the posterior elements of the spine but may also occur in the vertebral bodies and can be associated with pathologic fracture and vertebral collapse (Fig. 6-8) (57,61).

The x-ray picture often evolves with time. Initially, there is frank osteolysis of the margins of the bone, and periosteal elevation; with growth of the lesion, there is progressive destruction of bone with poorly demarcated margins. A stabilization phase follows, with formation of a bone shell with septa. Later, with further ossification, a bony mass begins to form (55).

Campanacci et al (21) have classified the ABCs into three groups (Fig. 6-9). An aggressive cyst has signs of reparative osteogenesis with ill-defined margins and no periosteal shell. An active cyst has an incomplete periosteal shell and a defined margin between the lesion and the host bone. An inactive cyst has a complete periosteal shell and a sclerotic margin between the cyst and the long bone.

Angiography may aid diagnosis and treatment; abnormal peripheral vascularization is often present (60). Percutaneous dye injection has been used as an additional diagnostic technique and in evaluation of vertebral lesions (62). Technetium bone scan usually shows an increased uptake of the isotope in the periphery of the lesion, but homogeneous uptake is also seen (63). Magnetic resonance imaging (MRI) often is helpful in demonstrating the characteristic septations and fluid levels, but these findings are not pathognomonic for ABC (Figs. 6-8 and 6-10) (64).

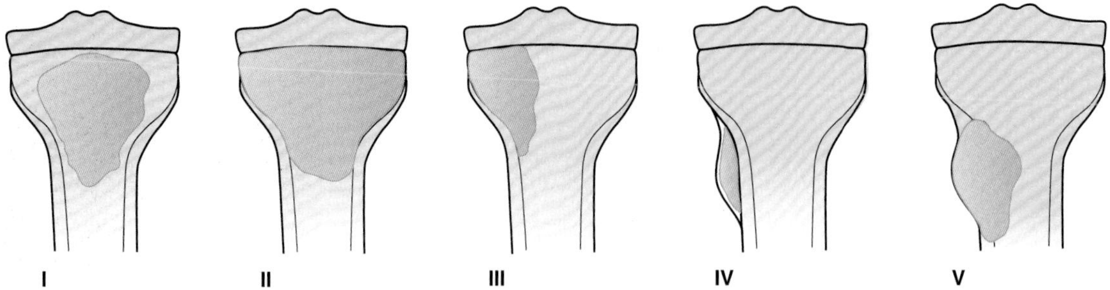

FIGURE 6-9 Classification of morphologic types of ABC. (From Capanna R, Bettelli G, Biagini R, et al. Aneurysmal cysts of long bones. *Ital J Orthop Traumatol* 1985;XI:421–429; with permission.)

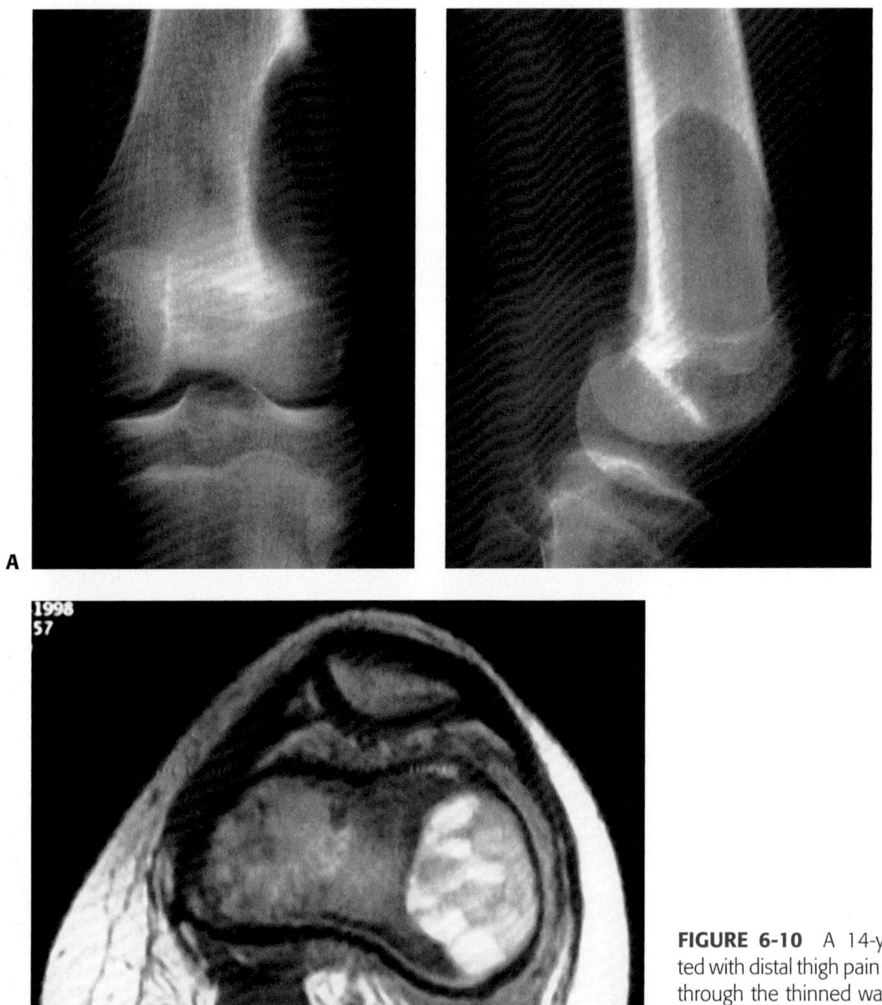

FIGURE 6-10 A 14-year-old-girl presented with distal thigh pain from microfractures through the thinned wall of an aneurysmal bone cyst of the distal femur. **A.** X-ray studies show an eccentric, expansile, lytic lesion of the lateral aspect of the distal femoral metaphysis. There is a narrow zone of transition with a sclerotic border. **B.** MRI shows septation of the lesion with the fluid-fluid levels, which are characteristic of ABC. The patient was treated with extended curettage and bone grafting.

Natural History

ABCs are benign but usually behave in a locally aggressive manner. Pathologic fractures occur in 11% to 35% of patients with ABCs of the long bones (60,65). The humerus and femur are the most commonly fractured long bones (60,66). Other sites of fracture occur, but these are rare. In one series, vertebral body ABC was associated with fracture in 27% of patients (57).

Although rare, epiphyseal involvement by the lesion through metaphyseal extension has been reported (67–69). Capanna et al (49) reported nine patients with invasion of the physis by large metaphyseal ABCs. In five of these patients, growth disturbance of the involved physis subsequently developed.

Conservative treatment with immobilization is inappropriate as a definitive treatment for pathologic fractures of ABCs. Although the pathologic fracture will heal, the ABC will persist and enlarge and a recurrent pathologic fracture will occur.

Treatment

Although ABC healing after simple biopsy has been reported (21), this does not occur often and observation is not recommended because these lesions usually are locally aggressive. Simple curettage and bone grafting have been associated with high recurrence rates (21,55,57,61,67) ranging from 20% to 30% (21,55). In a series of 86 patients with aneurysmal bone cysts, the presence of nodular fasciitis-like fibromyxoid areas and immature osteoid with active osteoblasts was significantly associated with an increased risk of recurrence (70). There appears to be a higher rate of recurrence in patients younger than 15 years of age (57). Freiberg et al (71) treated ABCs with curettage and bone grafting in seven patients younger than 10 years of age and noted recurrence in five of the seven patients at an average of 8 months after the first procedure. Dormans et al (72) reviewed the outcomes of 45 children with primary aneurysmal bone cysts who received surgical treatment, 13 children were 10 years or younger and 32 were older than 10 years. Persistence or recurrence of the lesion requiring additional surgery occurred in 3 children in the younger age group and in 5 children in the older age group. The difference in persistence or recurrence rates based on age was not statistically significant. However, with the author's four-step surgical technique the persistence or recurrence rates are lower than previously reported (82% overall success rate after initial surgery).

Selective arterial embolization is used most commonly in locations where a tourniquet cannot be used and control of bleeding can be difficult (e.g., spine, pelvis, and the proximal portions of the extremities). Green et al (73) reported on eight patients treated with selective arterial embolization. In seven patients, embolization was performed in conjunction with open bone grafting and, in one patient, as definitive treatment. At a follow-up of 3 years, there were no recurrences and no complications related to embolization.

Treatment of ABCs by cryotherapy in conjunction with curettage has a recurrence rate of between 8% and 14% (67,74,75). Dabezies et al (56) obtained healing of ABCs associated with fractures by collapsing the cyst manually after curettage. Polymethylmethacrylate cementation also has been described as an adjuvant to curettage for the treatment of ABCs. Ozaki et al (76) compared curettage and bone grafting in 30 patients with curettage and cementation in 35 patients. At follow-up ranging from 24 to 161 months, the recurrence rate was 37% for curettage and bone grafting compared with 17% for curettage and cementation.

Injection has been used by some physicians (77). Guibaud et al (78) reported on the use of percutaneous embolization with an alcoholic solution of Zein (Ethibloc; Ethnor Laboratories/Ethicon, Norderstedt, Germany) in 18 patients. In two patients, the cystogram showed marked venous drainage and embolization was not attempted. Six patients underwent repeat embolization. At follow-up ranging from 18 months to 4 years, there were no recurrences.

Complete *en bloc* resection is reserved for active or recurrent ABCs (49,53,60,61) and is most feasible in the proximal fibula, distal ulna, ribs, pubic rami, metatarsals (21), and metacarpals (79). Resection of metacarpal lesions with replacement by a fibular autograft often results in soft tissue scarring with reduced joint motion (79). Campanacci et al (21) recommended saucerization of peripheral active and aggressive cysts.

Irradiation should be avoided. Its use has been associated with the development of sarcoma (57). It has been used for lesions that are surgically inaccessible (67), but it is contraindicated in the pelvis, where the reproductive organs may be affected, and in areas of active growth of the long bones (21).

ABCs of the spine can be difficult to treat because of the relative inaccessibility of the lesion, proximity of the lesion to the spinal cord and nerve roots, and the potential for spinal instability (80,81). Papagelopoulos et al (80) reported on 52 consecutive patients with spinal ABCs treated over an 83-year period and recommended preoperative selective arterial embolization, intralesional excisional curettage, bone grafting, and fusion of the affected area if instability is present. Turker et al (81) described three patients with ABCs of the spine and emphasized the need for spinal stabilization and fusion in conjunction with removal of the lesion.

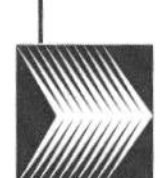

AUTHORS' PREFERRED METHOD OF TREATMENT

Aneurysmal Bone Cysts

The first step in effective treatment of a patient with an ABC is to confirm the diagnosis with open biopsy and frozen section; this biopsy usually is done at the same surgical setting as the definitive surgical procedure. It is important to remember that ABC can be secondary to other tumors, such as nonossifying fibroma, giant cell tumor, and chondroblastoma; telangiectatic osteosarcoma may be difficult to distinguish from ABC with an inadequate biopsy specimen because the aplastic tumor cells are seen only at the periphery of the lesion (82,83).

Once the diagnosis is made, treatment should be initiated as soon as possible because most ABCs are aggressive and often grow and invade rapidly. Preoperative planning is important to ensure adequate exposure, preparation for blood loss, internal fixation, grafting material, and in selected cases, preoperative embolization.

Achieving adequate exposure with a large cortical window for thorough extended curettage is a key component for successful treatment. The use of a high-speed burr allows systematic intralesional excisional curettage. Adjuvants phenol and alcohol, liquid nitrogen, and polymethylmethacrylate (PMMA) usually are reserved for large or recurrent ABCs but may be considered in the initial management. Bone grafting is done for all lesions and can consist of autograft, allograft, bone substitutes, or a combination of these methods, depending on the circumstances. Most patients with fractures through ABCs have microfractures that do not alter treatment. For those with more significant or unstable fractures, internal stabilization is used when appropriate, particularly in the hip, femur, or tibia. The classification and recommendations in Figure 6-7 are applicable for those with proximal femoral fractures associated with ABCs. A walking hip spica cast (i.e., a unilateral hip spica cast with the hip and knee in 20° to 30° of flexion) is sometimes appropriate for young children with stable fractures. Close follow-up is recommended initially because recurrence can be rapid and aggressive.

For ABC of the spine, we recommend preoperative selective arterial embolization, intralesional extended excisional curettage, and bone grafting. Instrumentation and fusion of the affected area should be performed if instability or the potential for instability exists. If instrumentation is used, titanium instrumentation allows follow-up MRI with less metal artifact compared with stainless-steel implants (Fig. 6-11) (84).

Tumors of Bone

Fibrous Cortical Defects and Nonossifying Fibromas

Fibrous cortical defects (FCDs) and a larger variant known as nonossifying fibroma (NOFs) may be associated with pathologic fractures in children. Both lesions contain fibrous tissue, foam cells, and multinucleated giant cells (85). Most pathologic fractures occur in boys (86), and age at presentation varies from 6 to 14 years (87).

FCDs are small metaphyseal lesions ranging from 1 to 2 cm in diameter and most commonly occur in the distal femur, proximal tibia, and fibula. They are eccentric and usually are surrounded by the thinned cortex, with the medullary wall of the lesion tending to be sclerotic. FCDs are common and can be seen on x-ray studies of the lower extremity in approximately 25% of pediatric patients (88). In view of their usually asymptomatic nature, it is difficult to estimate the true incidence. They usually require no treatment other than observation.

Radiographic Findings. NOFs also are eccentric lesions of the metaphysis, but they may achieve a length of 5 cm (89) or more and can extend across a substantial portion of the width of the long bone. They present at a similar age as FCDs, and follow a similar distribution of bone involvement, and multiple lesions are present in approximately one third of patients (86,90). On x-ray study, the lesions are usually eccentric, radiolucent cyst-like areas that can be either uniloculated or multiloculated; in small bones such as the fibula, they may occupy the entire width of the shaft (85). Sclerotic scalloping is often present along the endosteal margin (91). Usually, NOFs are asymptomatic unless a pathologic fracture is present (85). They become clinically significant when they present with or predispose to pathologic fracture.

Natural History. Arata et al (92) found that 43% of pathologic fractures through NOFs were in the distal tibia. Several previous reports suggested that these lesions regress spontaneously (85,86,89,90,93,94). Ritschl et al (94) described the radiomorphic course of NOFs, demonstrating that the defects become sclerotic and resolve. Typically, this tumor remains asymptomatic and is commonly an incidental radiographic finding. However, lesions with extensive cortical involvement can cause pathologic fractures.

Previous reports suggest that the absolute size of the lesion correlates directly with the risk of pathologic fracture (92). Based on this factor, prophylactic curettage and bone grafting of larger NOFs have been recommended. Arata et al (92) noted that all pathologic fractures associated with NOFs in the lower extremity occurred through lesions involving *more than 50% of the transverse cortical diameter*. These large lesions were defined as exhibiting more than 50% cortical involvement on anteroposterior (AP) and lateral x-ray studies and a height measurement of more than 33 mm (92). Although the authors recommended careful observation of these large NOFs, they suggested that "prophylactic curettage and bone grafting be considered if there is a reasonable chance of fracture." Their series does not include any large lesions meeting their size criteria that did not fracture, and their hypothesis has never been tested in any published series. Drennan et al (90) suggested that large NOFs causing pain may predispose to fracture and recommended prophylactic curettage and bone grafting for selected larger lesions.

Fractures through NOFs exhibit excellent healing potential (85,90,92), but the lesion usually persists after healing of the fracture (Figs. 6-12 and 6-13). Recurrent fractures have been reported, but the incidence of documented refracture is low (90,92). Fracture union takes place normally, but often multiple radiolucencies remain (85). Overall, fracture healing does not usually obliterate the lesions so recurrent fracture can occur (91,92).

Large lesions, defined as having a diameter more than 50% of the width of a long bone on both AP and lateral x-rays, are believed to be prone to pathologic fracture; most authors have recommended curettage and bone grafting for these large lesions (85–87,90,91,95).

Easley and Kneisl et al (96) reported that although absolute size parameters were helpful in predicting pathologic fracture,

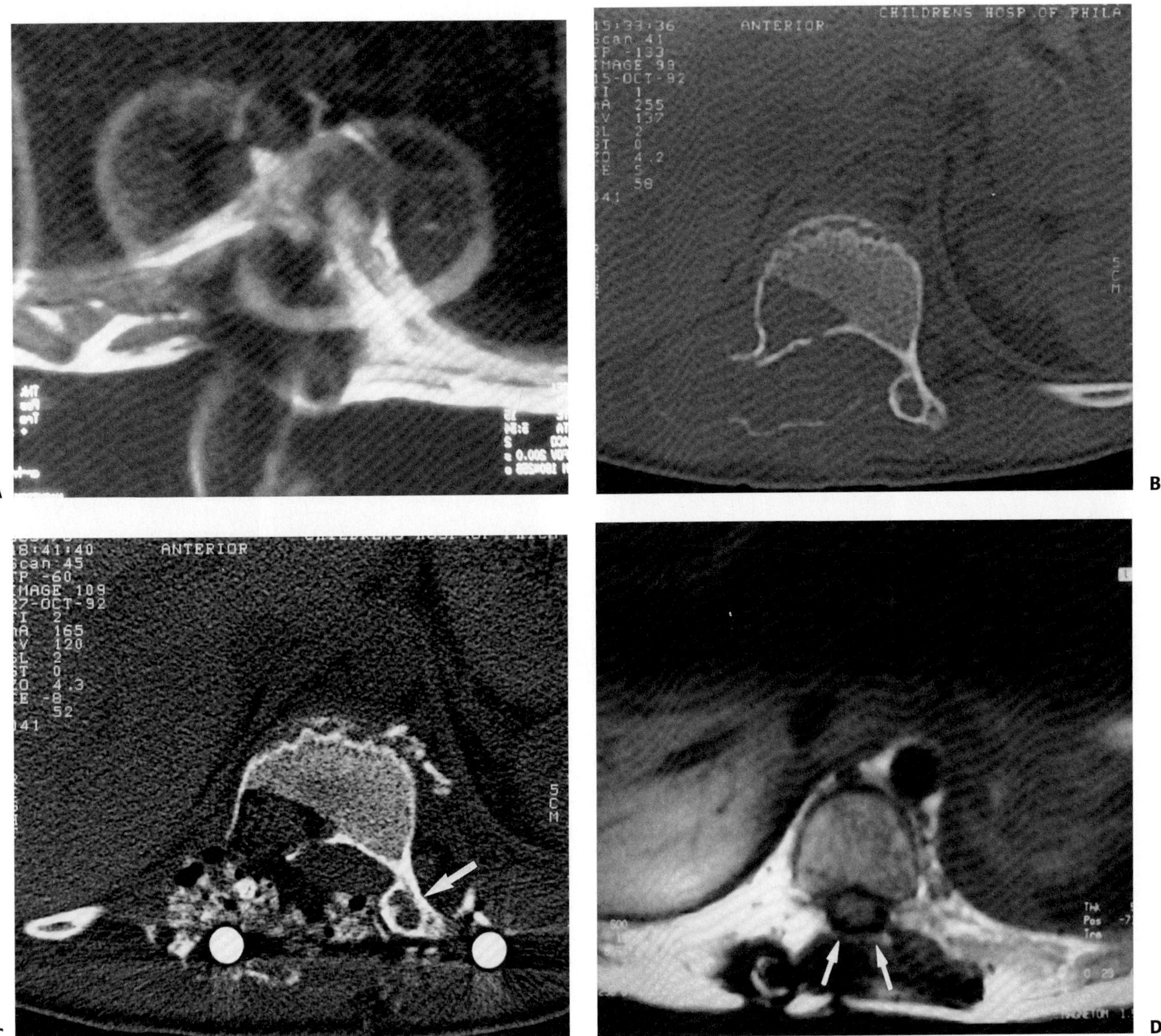

FIGURE 6-11 When dealing with pathologic fractures secondary to tumors or tumor-like processes of the spine, if instrumentation is needed, titanium instrumentation allows much better postoperative visualization with both CT and MRI for the detection of tumor recurrence as compared with standard stainless-steel instrumentation. **A.** Postoperative MRI of the spine with standard stainless-steel instrumentation showing a large degree of artifact that makes interpretation difficult. **B.** Preoperative CT scan of a patient with an ABC of the spine. **C.** Postoperative CT scan of the same patient showing an adequate view of the surgical area. **D.** Postoperative MRI of a patient with a previous spinal tumor again adequately showing the surgical site to monitor for recurrence or persistent tumor.

they did not imply a requirement for prophylactic curettage and bone grafting. In their series, 13 (59%) large NOFs had not had pathologic fracture despite exceeding the previously established size threshold. In the nine (41%) patients in whom pathologic fracture occurred, healing was uneventful after closed reduction and cast immobilization, and no refractures occurred. They suggested that most patients with large NOFs can be monitored without intervention, because previous studies support spontaneous resolution of most of these lesions (85,90,92). All fractured NOFs in their series healed with closed reduction and immobilization. It may be reasonable to restrict the activity of patients with large NOFs based on the nine patients in their study with pathologic fractures caused by trauma.

Fractures usually are treated with immobilization until healing is obtained (86,95). Surgery is necessary only if the residual lesion is of significant size to predispose the patient to further

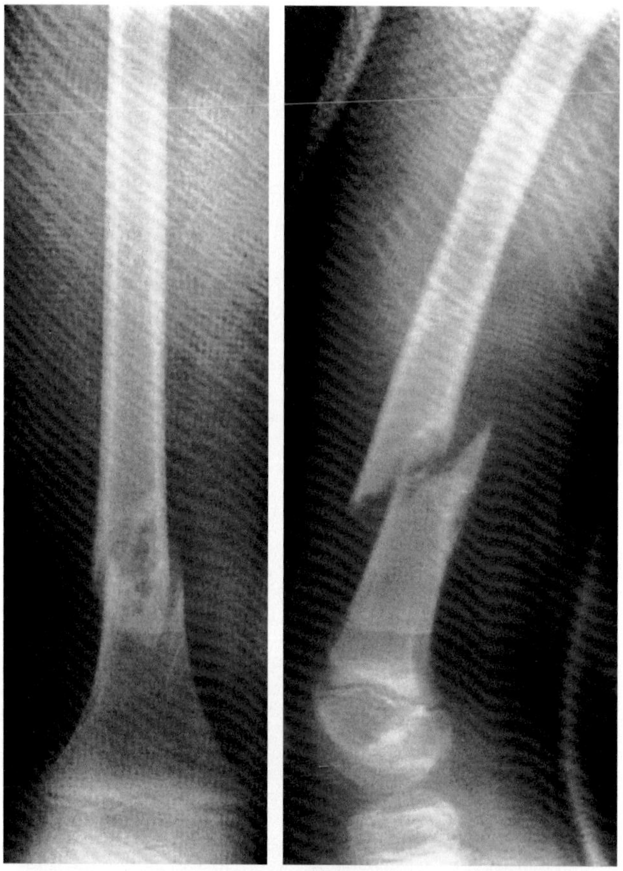

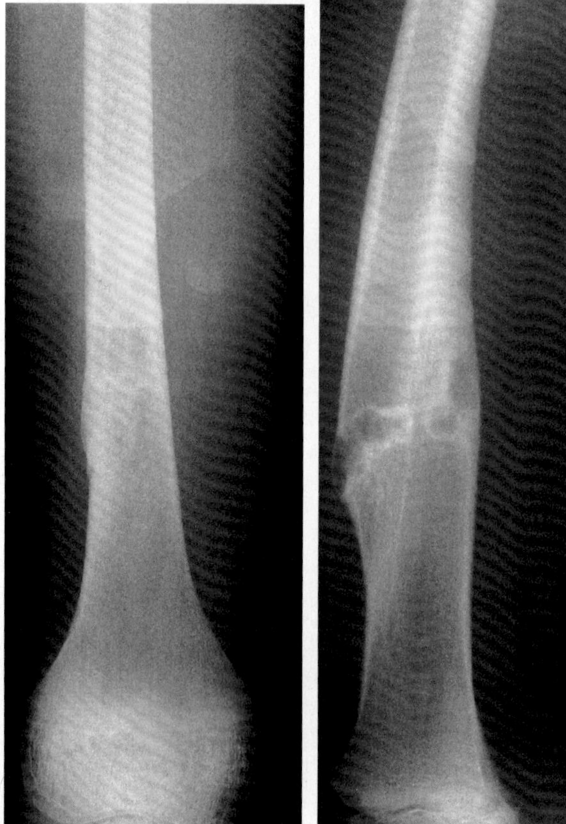

FIGURE 6-12 **A.** An 8-year-old boy was referred after being casted at another institution for a pathologic fracture of the right femur. The x-ray studies in the cast show a pathologic fracture of the right distal femur through an NOF. **B.** At 14 weeks after the injury, the fracture has united with some posterior displacement of the distal fragment. **C.** At 7 months after fracture, there has been good remodeling at the fracture site with persistence of the NOF. The patient returned to full activities and has had no further problems at 7-year follow-up.

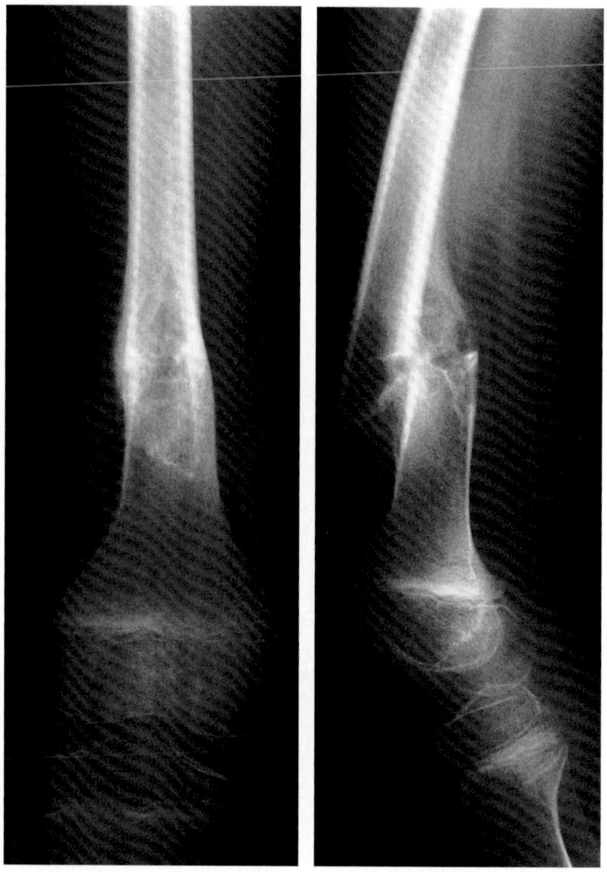

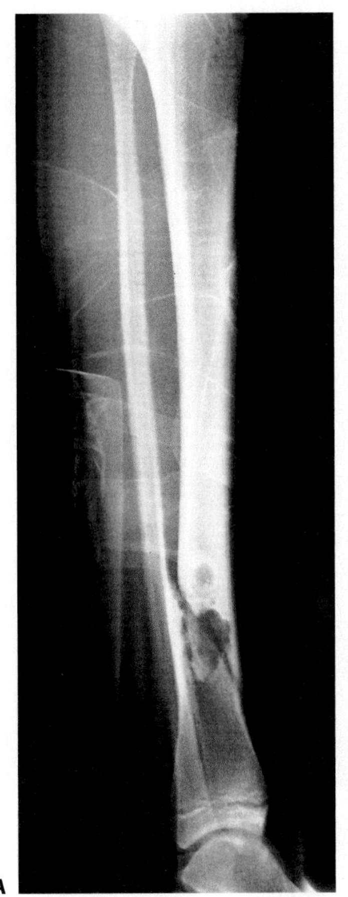
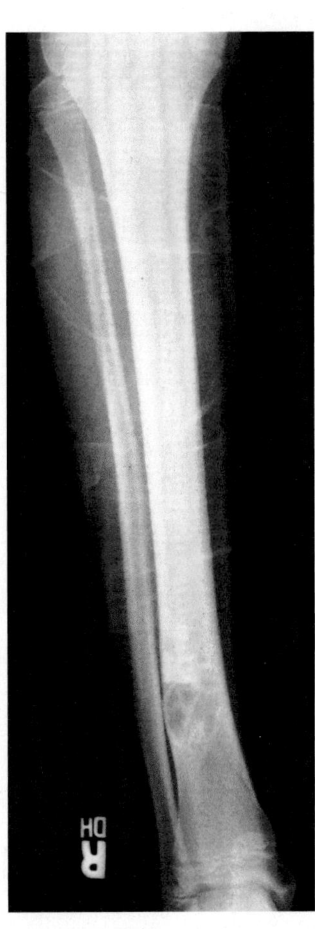

FIGURE 6-13 A 13-year-old athlete presented with a pathologic fracture through the distal tibia after a fall on the ice. **A.** The patient was treated with a long leg cast immobilization. After the fracture had healed, the patient underwent open curettage and bone grafting of the lesion. **B.** Follow-up x-ray studies show healing of both the fracture and the lesion, and the patient has returned to full activities.

pathologic fractures or there is doubt about the identity of the lesion (85). Displaced pathologic supracondylar fractures of the distal femur may require open reduction, bone grafting, and intramedullary fixation (90). Subperiosteal resection of a pathologic humeral shaft fracture followed by bone grafting has resulted in pseudoarthrosis (91).

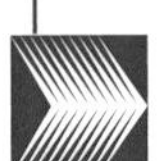

AUTHORS' PREFERRED METHOD OF TREATMENT

Fibrous Cortical Defects and Nonossifying Fibromas

Treatment is based on the size and location of the lesion and the type of pathologic fracture. Small lesions without fracture can be observed and may require 1 to 3 years to spontaneously resolve (86). Substantial lesions of the lower extremity in active children, even if they are asymptomatic, should either be followed carefully with serial x-ray studies or should undergo curettage and bone grafting to avoid pathologic fracture. Although absolute size parameters may be useful in predicting pathologic fracture, they do not imply a requirement for prophylactic curettage and bone grafting. Most patients with large NOFs can be monitored without surgical intervention, and fractures can be successfully managed with nonoperative treatment. Our experience is that a considerable number of incidentally discovered large NOFs do not fracture. Although we cannot readily identify an accurate denominator, we infer that many large NOFs remain unidentified and nonproblematic. Patient and family wishes and the individual's activity demands also obviously influence the decision. Given the historic evidence for spontaneous resolution and favorable healing characteristics of NOFs, patients with lesions larger than 50% of the width of the bone should be approached individually. Dormans et al recently reported a comparison of 15 patients (15 NOFs) treated with open curettage, with or without bone grafting, versus 15 patients (20 NOFs) treated with a minimally invasive percutaneous curettage, intramedullary decompression, and grafting with calcium sulfate pellets. Complete resolution of pain and return to activity was noted at the last follow-up visit for all patients in both groups; the group receiving percutaneous treatment demonstrated statistically significant accelerated rates of healing and resolution of clinical symptoms (97).

Giant Cell Tumors of Bone

Giant cell tumors of bone are rare in the pediatric population; most occur in skeletally mature individuals. In a series of 221

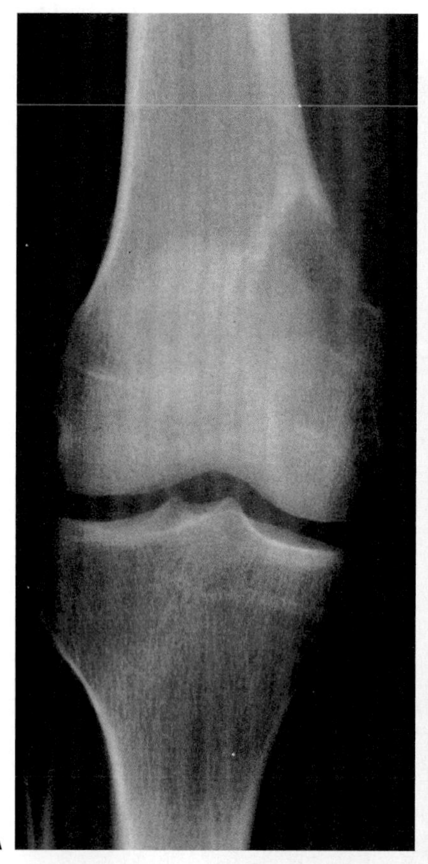
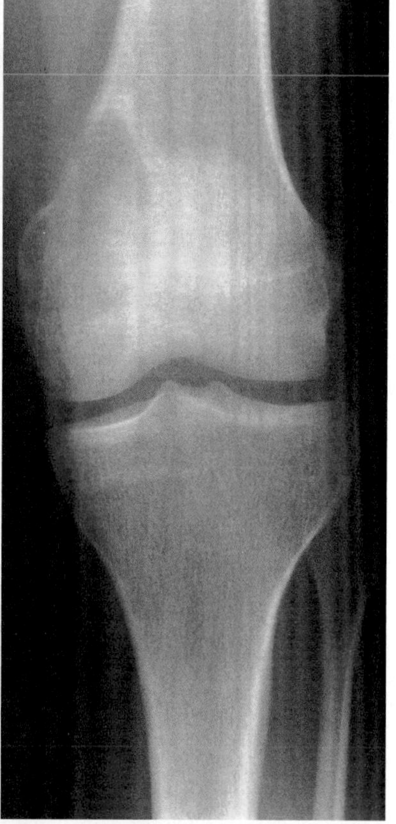
A

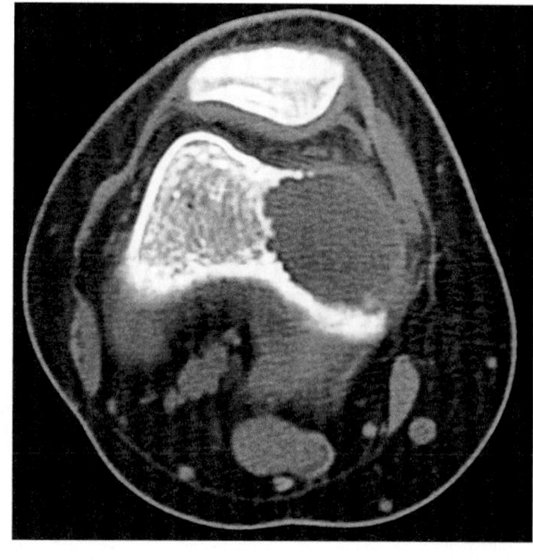
B

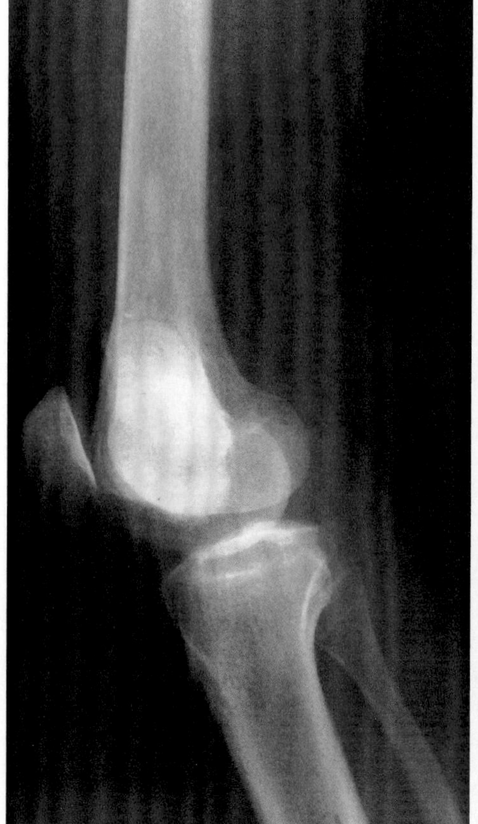
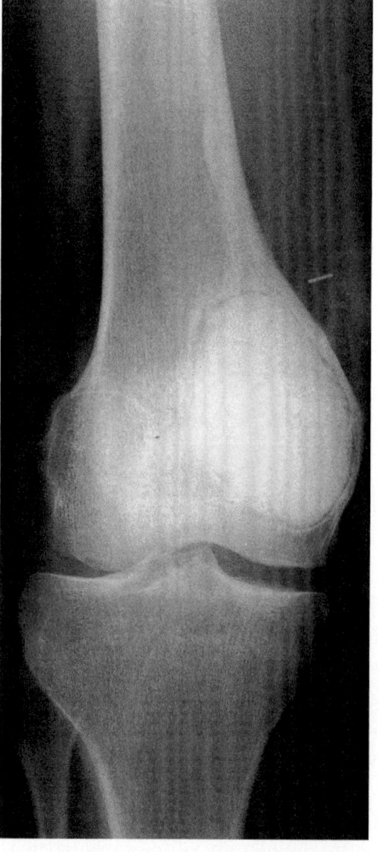
C

FIGURE 6-14 An 18-year-old girl presented with left medial knee pain. **A.** X-ray studies showed an eccentric, lytic, destructive lesion involving the distal portion of the medial metaphysis with extension into the epiphysis. **B.** CT scan showed the destructive lesion with thinning of the cortex and no external soft tissue mass. Open biopsy and frozen sections were consistent with giant cell tumor of the distal femur. An extended curettage was then performed with phenol as an adjuvant and subsequent cementation using methylmethacrylate bone cement. **C.** Follow-up x-ray studies at 2 years after surgery showing no evidence of recurrence. The patient is asymptomatic and has full range of motion and function of the knee.

patients with giant cell tumors of bone (98), only 20% of patients were younger than 20 years of age. In order of decreasing frequency, these tumors most commonly occur in the distal femur, proximal tibia, proximal humerus, and distal radius. The incidence of pathologic fractures with these lesions is approximately 16% (98–102).

Radiographically, they are osteolytic, metaphyseal lesions that can extend into the epiphysis, usually after physeal closure (Fig. 6-14). They can be eccentric, but larger lesions can involve the full width of the bone. Little or no sclerosis usually is present around the margin of the tumor. Although heavy trabeculation may be present, new periosteal bone formation is uncommon.

Giant cell tumors usually are treated by extended curettage in combination with adjuvants, such as phenol or liquid nitrogen, and filling with material such as PMMA (Fig. 6-14) (98–100). *En bloc* or wide resection is a more aggressive option. Simple curettage and bone grafting are associated with a high recurrence rate. In one series (98), simple curettage and bone grafting had a 34% recurrence rate, whereas wide resection of the lesion resulted in only a 7% recurrence rate. Wide resection is most appropriate for giant cell tumors involving expendable bones and for aggressive lesions with significant involvement of the articular surface. The location and extent of the lesion and the proximity of the tumor to articular cartilage and physis influence the treatment of giant cell tumors in children.

TABLE 6-6 Treatment of Giant Cell Tumors

Scenario	Treatment
1. Fracture undisplaced, structurally insignificant, non-articular	No change in treatment plan (Usually extended curettage and cementation with adjuvant such as phenol)
2. Fracture simple, but displaced a. Fracture can be reduced closed b. Fracture cannot be reduced closed	Joint preserving options: a. closed reduction and delayed extended curettage[a] b. Open reduction, extended curettage, simultaneous internal fixation and cementation[b]
3. Fracture displaced, intraarticular; Open reduction, extended curettage and internal fixation cannot be achieved satisfactorily (uncommon in children)	Resection or partial resection of the joint

[a] If a fracture can be reduced and held by closed methods, it may be preferable to delay the definitive surgery until initial fracture healing has occurred. Fracture healing is biologically faster than the growth of the tumor: a delay of 4 to 6 weeks will have a minimal effect on tumor progression.

[b] A technically demanding and difficult procedure: i.e., mechanically removing all tumor (with curets and high-speed bur), use of adjuvant such as phenol, reduction and fixation of thin "shell" of bone and cementation around the internal fixation device.

Pathologic Fractures Associated with Giant Cell Tumors of Bone. Pathologic fractures are associated with giant cell tumors in 6% to 30% of patients. The complexity of treatment is markedly increased if a pathologic fracture is present. Management depends on the type of fracture and fracture displacement (Table 6-6).

A biopsy may be needed before fracture treatment if the diagnosis is not certain. Most pathologic fractures are undisplaced, structurally insignificant, or nonarticular, and require no change in the treatment plan. For more significant fractures, an attempt at preserving the joint should be made. Overall, the presence of a pathologic fracture itself does not seem to directly influence the recurrence rate of giant cell tumor; it may influence the reconstruction options and the overall functional result.

Enchondroma

Solitary enchondroma is a rare lesion in children. In one series of enchondromas (103), 57% of patients were between 11 and 30 years of age. The common presenting symptom is pain, usually associated with a pathologic fracture. Most common sites of involvement in decreasing order of frequency are the phalanges, metacarpals, metatarsals, humerus, and femur. Pathologic fracture is commonly the presenting symptom for enchondromas located in the phalanges of the hands or feet, but is rare for enchondromas in other locations.

On x-ray studies, the lesions can be central or eccentric and a stippled calcification of the cartilage tumor matrix may be seen. In the long bones, lesions tend to be central with only slight bulging of the cortex. The short tubular bones with enchondromas show a cloudy radiolucency with bulging and thinning of the cortex (Fig. 6-15) (103).

Children can also have multiple enchondromas or enchondromatosis (Ollier's disease), which is commonly seen between 2 and 10 years of age (Fig. 6-16). X-ray studies show lesions similar to solitary enchondroma, but usually with deformity and shortening of the extremity due to growth disturbance. A unique x-ray finding that is believed to be pathognomonic for enchondromatosis is the presence of linear radiolucencies extending from the metaphysis down the shaft of the long bone.

When these lesions are associated with multiple hemangiomas, the general condition is known as Maffucci's syndrome (104,105). In this syndrome, 30% of patients have one or more pathologic fractures (105). Approximately half of these fractures

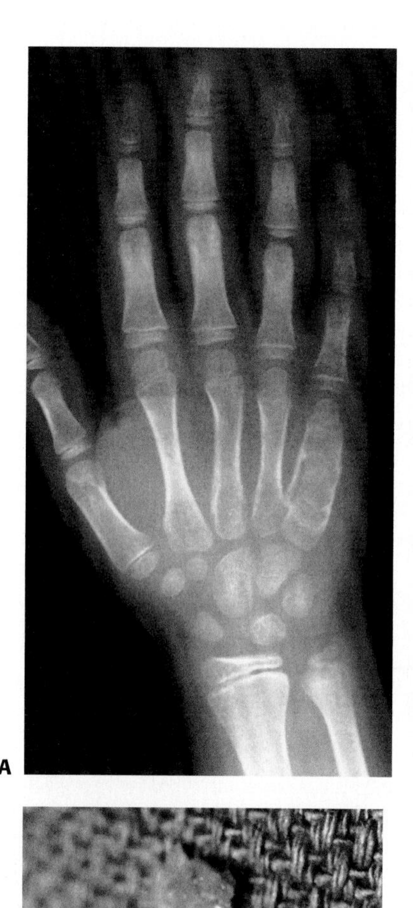

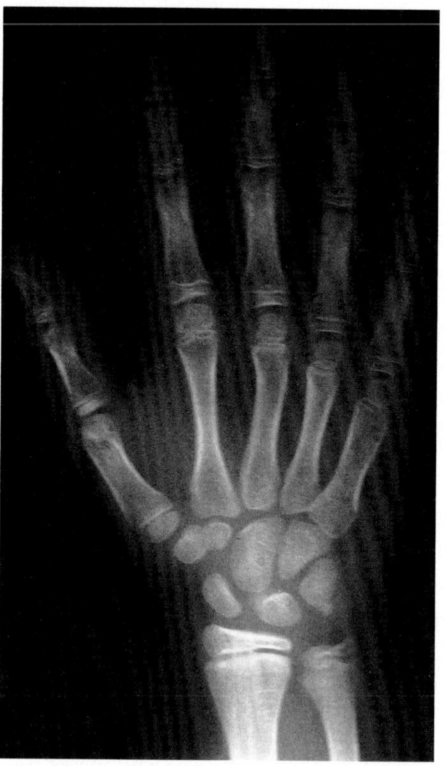

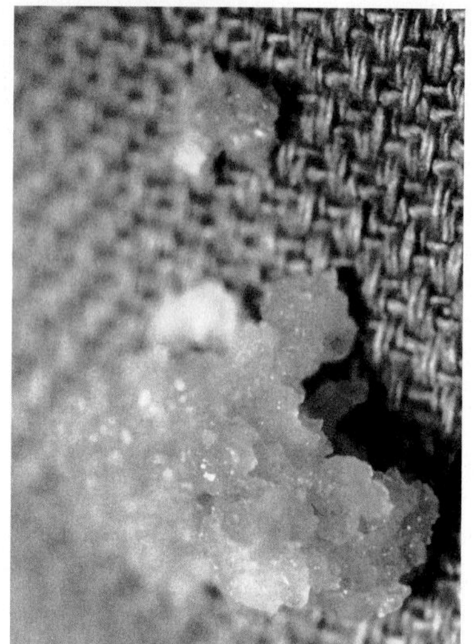

FIGURE 6-15 An 8-year-old boy presents with pain and swelling of the ulnar border of his right hand. **A.** X-ray studies showed an expansile, lucent lesion of the diaphysis of the patient's right fifth metacarpal with microfractures. The patient had an open incisional biopsy with frozen section, which was consistent with enchondroma with subsequent curettage and bone grafting. **B.** Gross appearance of material removed at the time of surgery, which is consistent with enchondroma. **C.** At 6-month follow-up, the fracture is well healed, and there is no sign of recurrent tumor.

go on to delayed union or nonunion. Unilateral skeletal involvement occurred in 48% of patients, with involvement in the order of frequency of the hand, foot, tibia, femur radius and ulna, humerus, and ribs. Skeletal deformities tend to stabilize at maturity. Sarcomatous degeneration has been reported in approximately 15% of patients.

Asymptomatic lesions can be observed. Biopsy may be necessary when the identity of the lesion is uncertain. Symptomatic lesions respond well to curettage and bone grafting (104,106). Treatment is individualized for displaced fractures (Fig. 6-15).

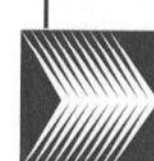

AUTHORS' PREFERRED METHOD OF TREATMENT

Enchondroma

Solitary enchondromas often require biopsy to establish the diagnosis. For asymptomatic patients with small lesions with classic x-ray findings, biopsy usually is not necessary. A recent comparison of immediate and delayed treatment of fractures and tumors in pathological fractures through enchondromas noted a higher complication rate for the group receiving immediate treatment: 67% versus 10% (107). Cau-

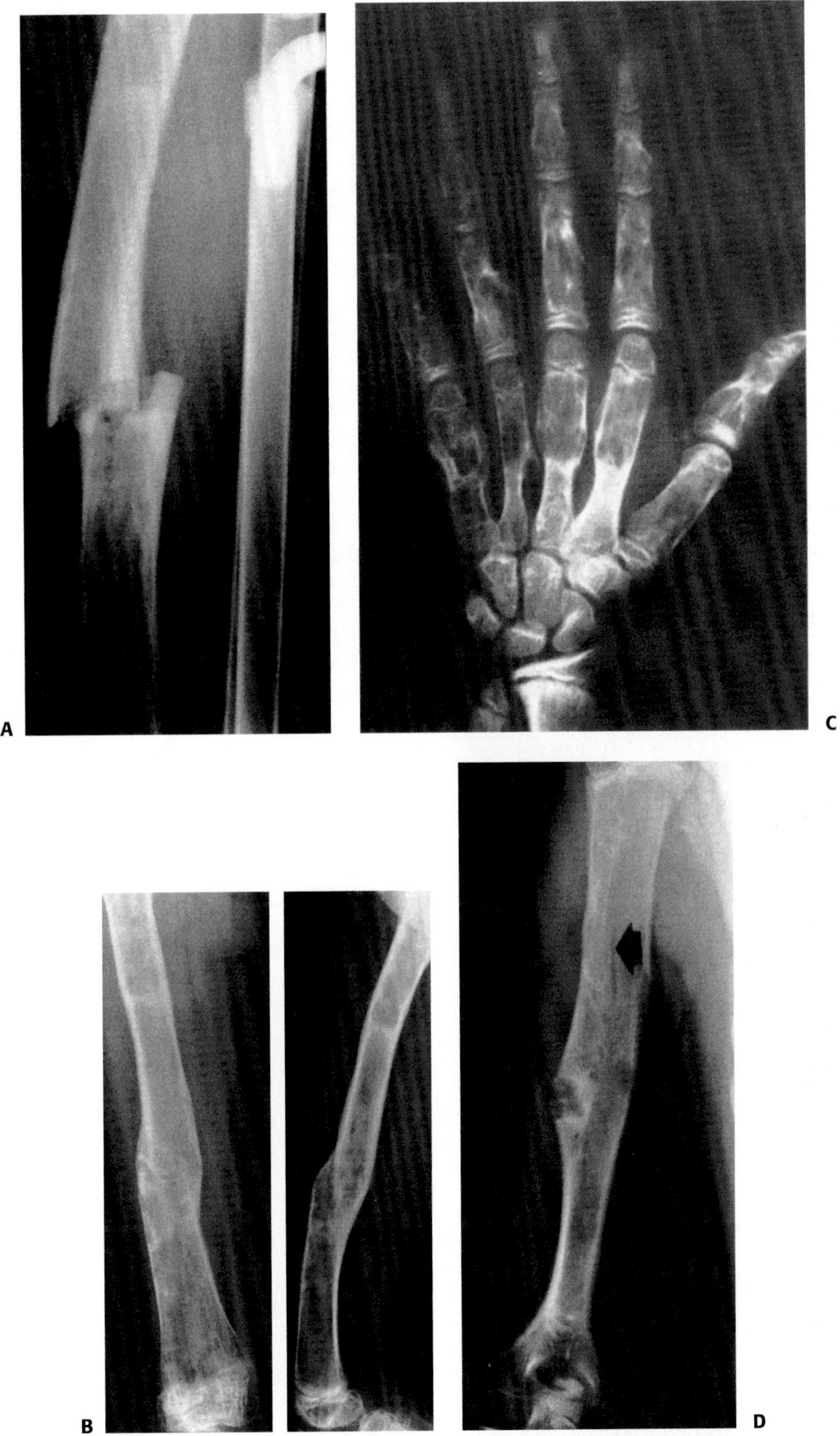

FIGURE 6-16 Multiple enchondromatosis. **A.** A 10-year-old girl with multiple enchondromas sustained a spontaneous pathologic fracture of the femur while running. The lateral x-ray study shows overriding of the fracture. **B.** At 3-year follow-up, the fracture is well healed. **C.** The anteroposterior x-ray study of the hand in this patient demonstrated multiple expansile enchondromas of the small bones. **D.** An x-ray study of the humerus shows the streaked-mud appearance of the lateral humerus (*arrow*).

tion is advised when considering immediate treatment of pathologic fractures associated with enchondromas. Curettage and bone grafting is necessary for those lesions with acute or impending pathologic fracture. Fixation is not necessary for those lesions of the short tubular bones but may be necessary for lesions of the proximal femur or long bone of the lower extremity. Standard fracture care is adequate to treat most injuries.

Osteochondromas

Osteochondromas are one of the most common tumors of bone in children, and clinical symptoms usually are related to irritation of the surrounding soft-tissue structures. Peroneal nerve palsy may occur in association with osteochondroma of the proximal fibula (108). Radiation induced osteochondromas also can occur (109).

Although they are rare, fractures may occur through the base or stalk of a pedunculated osteochondroma (110); conservative treatment is adequate (Fig. 6-17). Fractures through solitary osteochondromas should be observed, and excision should be reserved for those patients with persistent symptoms after healing.

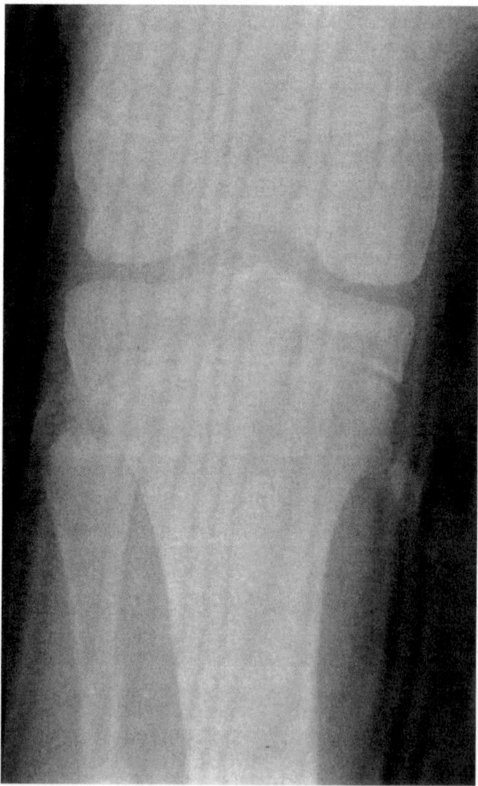

FIGURE 6-17 A 10-year-old-boy with pain over the right medial tibia after a direct blow. An exostosis is present, and the transverse radiolucency at its base may represent a fracture. The patient continued to have symptoms after healing of the fracture and the osteochondroma was excised.

Eosinophilic Granuloma (Langerhans' Cell Histiocytosis)

Eosinophilic granuloma of bone is a benign condition with either solitary or multiple lytic bone lesions. It is considered part of a general family of diseases collectively known as Langerhans' cell histiocytosis (LCH) or histiocytosis X, which also includes Hand-Schüller-Christian and Letterer-Siwe diseases (111,112). Bone lesions contain large coffee bean–shaped histiocytes, eosinophils, and multinucleated giant cells (113).

Nearly 75% of patients with eosinophilic granuloma of bone are younger than 20 years old, and 34% are younger than 4 years old. The ratio of male to female is approximately 3:2 (113). Nearly 50% of patients present with localized pain and tenderness (113,114); the duration of symptoms ranges from 2 weeks to 2 months, with occasional associated trauma. Swelling may be present over superficial bones, such as the skull, clavicle, and tibia (114). In order of decreasing frequency, the sites of involvement are the skull, femur, pelvis, ribs, humerus, spine, clavicle, mandible, tibia, radius, scapula, and fibula. In one series (115), 14% of patients with solitary eosinophilic granuloma of bone had additional lesions within 2 years of diagnosis, whereas 85% of patients with multiple lesions at the time of initial diagnosis had additional bone involvement. Patients with solitary or multiple bone involvement have a high potential for spontaneous remission, whereas patients with multiple system involvement have a worse prognosis and are best managed by a hematologist (116). The incidence of pathologic fracture in patients with LCH is approximately 14% (113,114). Laboratory tests usually are not very helpful; eosinophilia is infrequent (113). Glotzbecker et al (117) recently demonstrated an association between HHV-6 and LCH, suggesting a role for the HHV-6B in the etiology of this disease. The authors analyzed tissue from 35 children diagnosed with LCH for the presence of viral proteins and DNA and found that the difference in the prevalence of HHV-6 in LCH-positive tissues (25/35), when compared with control tissues from patients without LCH involvement (5/18), was statistically significant.

Patients with vertebral body involvement present with back pain and may have neurologic signs or symptoms. Although it has been reported that the thoracic spine is the most commonly involved part of the spine (115), a more recent case series of LCH of the spine reported a high incidence of cervical spine involvement (118). A meta-analysis based on 53 cases of cervical eosinophilic granuloma reported that immobilization is usually adequate therapy (119).

Radiographic Findings. In children, long bone lesions may occur in both the diaphysis and metaphysis, with destructive osteolysis that erodes the cortex and overlying expansion by periosteal layering (114,115,120). Epiphyseal involvement is rare. Defects in bone may be lobulated, and aggressive subperiosteal bone formation may suggest malignancy. The size of the lytic area may vary from 1 to 4 cm (113).

Classic vertebral plana is uncommon with eosinophilic granuloma of the spine in a child. When present, however, usually only one vertebra is involved, and it assumes a coin-on-end appearance with intact adjacent disk spaces. X-ray studies of patients with skull involvement show characteristic punched-out round lytic lesions that are beveled on tangential views.

The lesion may mimic osteomyelitis, Ewing's sarcoma, Brodie's abscess, metastatic disease, and osteogenic sarcoma (114). Bone scans tend to be unpredictable, with the incidence of false-negative scans ranging from 28% to 35% (121). In one series (121), the increased uptake of isotope was seen in 60% of patients, and there was an 11% incidence of cold lesions found only in the vertebral column and the ribs. Although bone scans may be useful in identifying recurrent lesions (121), the skeletal survey is most valuable in identifying the lesions. A bone scan should be used only when the x-ray studies are normal or equivocal.

Treatment. Biopsy usually is needed for diagnosis because of the lesion's tendency to mimic more serious conditions. Once the diagnosis is established, treatment options may include curettage, curettage and bone grafting, irradiation, chemotherapy (113, 114) and corticosteroid injection (112). All of these forms of treatment result in healing of the lesions (114). For small lesions and an established diagnosis, observation may be the best option; marginal sclerosis about the lytic area suggests healing.

Sbarbaro and Francis (113) reported an average healing time of 16 months after curettage without grafting. McCollough (115) noted that if a lesion increased in size after surgery, then additional bone or soft-tissue lesions usually appeared. Yasko et al (122) described a percutaneous needle biopsy technique for diagnosis with subsequent methylprednisolone injection for patients with localized LCH; 34 of 35 lesions injected with methylprednisolone healed, and there were no complications. Other investigators (123) have had similar results. Radiation therapy has been recommended for some inaccessible lesions (114), but one series suggested an association of this treatment with subsequent lymphosarcoma (114). Chemotherapy, usually consisting of oral methotrexate and prednisone, is used in patients with severe, painful, or progressive lesions or visceral involvement (112).

Fracture bracing is useful for both acute fractures and prophylactic use for impending fracture or after biopsy of lower extremity lesions (124). Surgery may be necessary for unstable fractures (Fig. 6-18). The diagnosis of vertebral lesions usually is best established by biopsy, especially if there are any atypical radiographic feature of a lesion, such as a soft-tissue mass. After diagnosis, they usually are treated with activity modification and a spinal orthosis (Fig. 6-19) (125,126). Seimon (127) recommended biopsy "only if there is any uncertainty in diagnosis," and irradiation only for progressive disease. Surgery may be necessary when there are associated neurologic deficits (115). Remodeling is seen with some spinal lesions but does not seem to correlate with patient age (125,126,128).

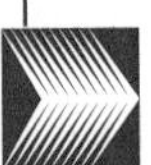

AUTHORS' PREFERRED METHOD OF TREATMENT

Eosinophilic Granuloma (Langerhans' Cell Histiocytosis)

Pathologic fracture is uncommon in patients with LCH. The correct diagnosis should be established with biopsy for most lesions, and the use of newer diagnostic methods such as immunohistochemistries (such as CD1A) can be helpful in confirming the diagnosis of these lesions. The natural history is one of gradual regression and healing. Standard fracture care is usually sufficient for pathologic fractures.

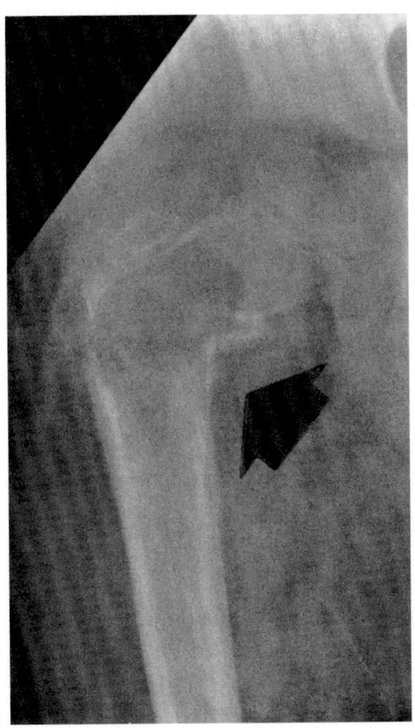

A

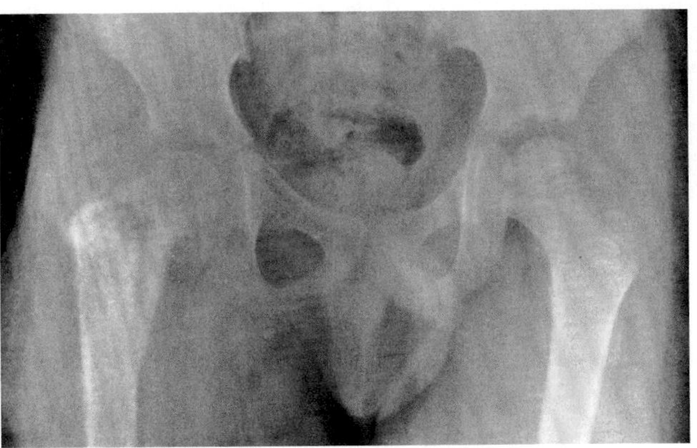

B

FIGURE 6-18 Eosinophilic granuloma. **A.** A 4-year-old boy with a pathologic fracture of the right femoral neck secondary to eosinophilic granuloma (*arrow*). **B.** The pins were removed, and at 3-month follow-up, the fracture was healed with acceptable alignment.

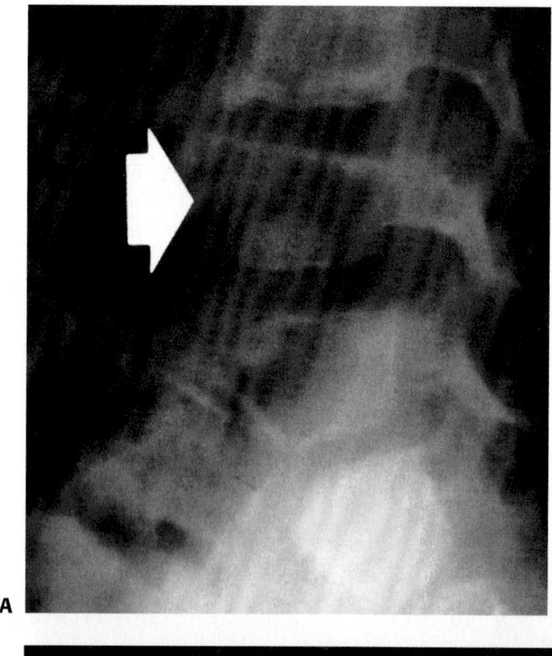
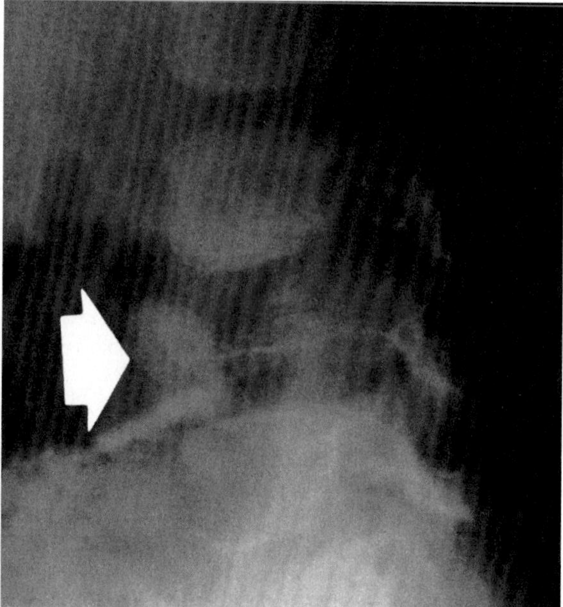
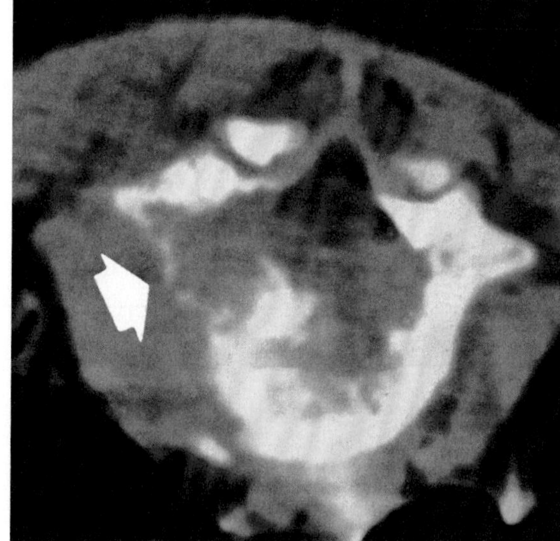

FIGURE 6-19 Eosinophilic granuloma. **A.** A 5-year-old boy presented with mild back pain and normal results of physical examination. A lateral x-ray study showed equivocal posterior wedging of L4 (*arrow*). Bone scan was read as normal. **B.** Nineteen days later on follow-up, he had marked spasm of the lower back. The lateral x-ray study now shows vertebral plana of L4 (*arrow*). **C.** CT scan shows marked expansion and erosion of the pedicle (*arrow*) and vertebral body. (*continues*)

Malignant Bone Tumors and Metastasis

The two most common primary sarcomas of the long bones in children are Ewing's sarcoma and osteosarcoma. Destructive lesions also can be caused by metastatic cancer to bone.

Careful staging (129,130) and subsequent biopsy (131–134) are critical in the evaluation of children with malignant bone tumors. To avoid pathologic fracture from biopsy of bone, an oval hole with smooth edges should be used and should be filled with PMMA (130). Many malignant tumors have a large soft-tissue mass that can be biopsied, obviating the need to make a hole in the bone. There has been a great deal of progress in the understanding of the molecular biology and genetics of cancer (135–138). These advances have already led to better diagnostic analysis of these tumors. Immunohistochemical, molecular genetic, and cytogenetic tests often are critical in establishing the correct diagnosis, especially small round blue cell tumors. The evaluation and biopsy of these children should preferably be done at a center where these techniques are known and available (131–133,139).

One of the major advances in the care of children with isolated extremity sarcoma has been the development of limb-sparing surgical techniques for local control of the tumors. Pathologic fracture has been cited as a contraindication to this procedure because of concerns about tumor dissemination by fracture hematoma (Fig. 6-20). Until recently, there has been little clinical data in the literature on which to base the treatment of these patients. A number of recent studies, however, have shown that pathologic fractures heal with neoadjuvant chemo-

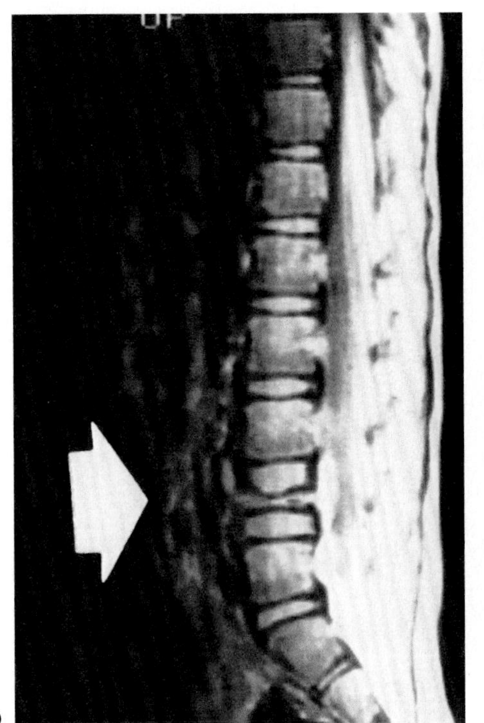
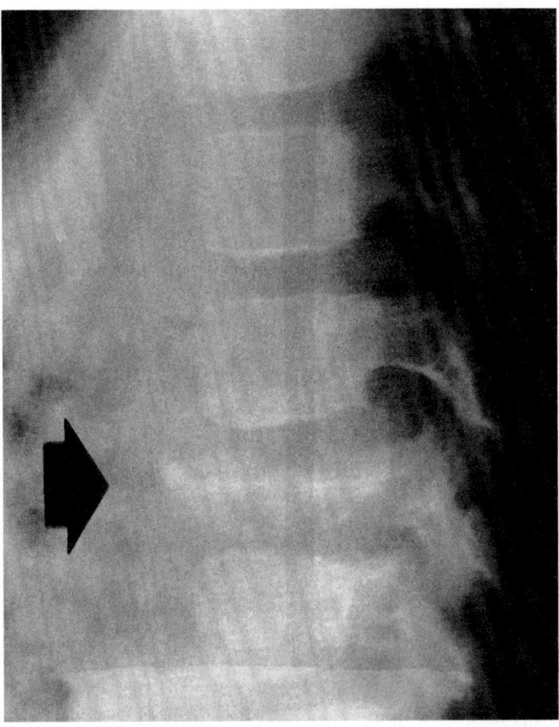

D E

FIGURE 6-19 *(continued)* **D.** MRI shows marked collapse of L4 with thickening of the adjacent intervertebral disks. Soft-tissue mass is also seen adjacent to L4 (*arrow*). Eosinophilic granuloma was diagnosed by Craig needle biopsy guided by CT scan, and the patient was treated with a spinal orthosis. Radiation treatment was also recommended, and a total of 600 rads was given in three divided doses. **E.** At 2-month follow-up, the compressed vertebra was beginning to regain density (*arrow*). The patient was asymptomatic. Bracing was continued for a total of 6 months.

therapy and do not affect survival rates (140–142). Abudu et al (143) reviewed the surgical treatment and outcome of pathologic fractures in 40 patients with localized osteosarcomas and found that limb-sparing surgery with adequate margins of excision could be achieved in many patients without compromising survival, but that 19% of those treated with limb-sparing surgery had local recurrences. Scully et al (135) reviewed the surgical treatment of 18 patients with osteosarcomas pathologic fractures. Of the 10 patients who had limb-sparing surgery, three had local recurrences and six had distant recurrences. Although the distant recurrence rate for patients undergoing amputation was no different from the rate for those undergoing limb salvage, the difference in local tumor control approached statistical significance. All patients who developed local recurrence died. The authors stated that surgical treatment should be individualized (135). Limb-sparing surgery is possible and appropriate in carefully selected patients as long as wide margins can be safely achieved and the function of the child will be better than that achieved with an amputation and a well-fitting prosthesis.

Pathologic fracture after limb-sparing surgery is a major complication, occurring most commonly after allograft reconstruction (144,145). Berrey et al (144) reviewed 43 patients in whom allografts used in reconstruction after resection of tumors had subsequently fractured. Four fractures healed with immobilization alone, and the remainder of patients attained satisfactory results with open reduction and grafting, replacement of the internal fixation device, or total joint replacement (144). San-Julian and Canadell (145) reported on 12 patients with 14 fractures (10.2% of 137 patients with allografts for limb-sparing surgery in their series). They recommended intramedullary fixation whenever possible to reduce the incidence of allograft fracture.

Pathologic fractures also can occur in children with metastatic disease but are less common in children than in adults. Most are microfractures and can be managed with conservative fracture management techniques.

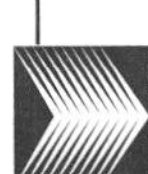

AUTHORS' PREFERRED METHOD OF TREATMENT

Malignant Bone Tumors and Metastasis

In all suspicious lesions, careful staging and biopsy are the appropriate treatments by individuals who have experience in the management of children with musculoskeletal sarcomas. Furthermore, access to special diagnostic modalities, such as immunohistochemistry and cytogenetics, will lessen the chances of misdiagnosis. The decision for or against limb-sparing surgery in patients with pathologic fractures should

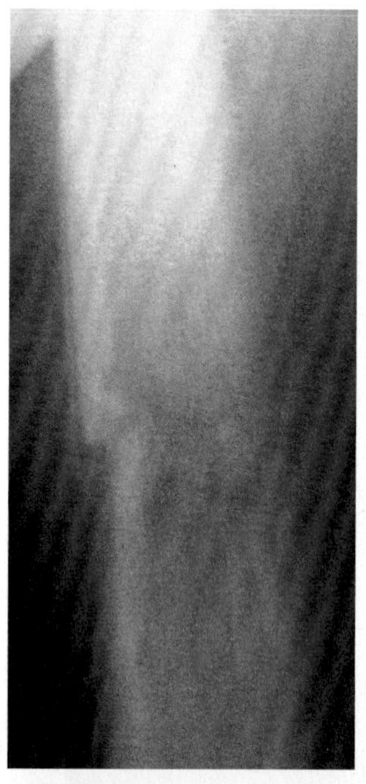

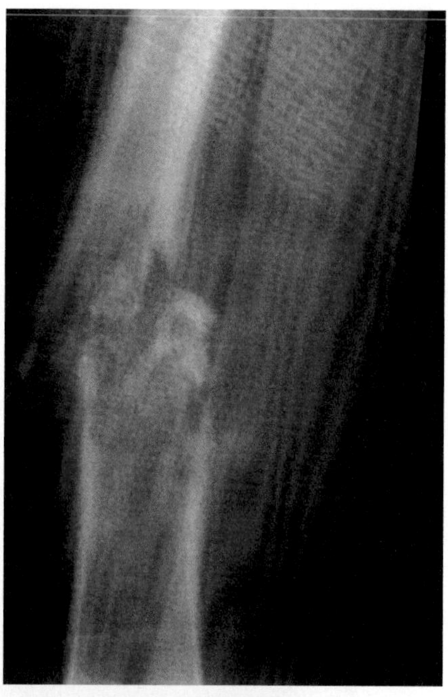

A

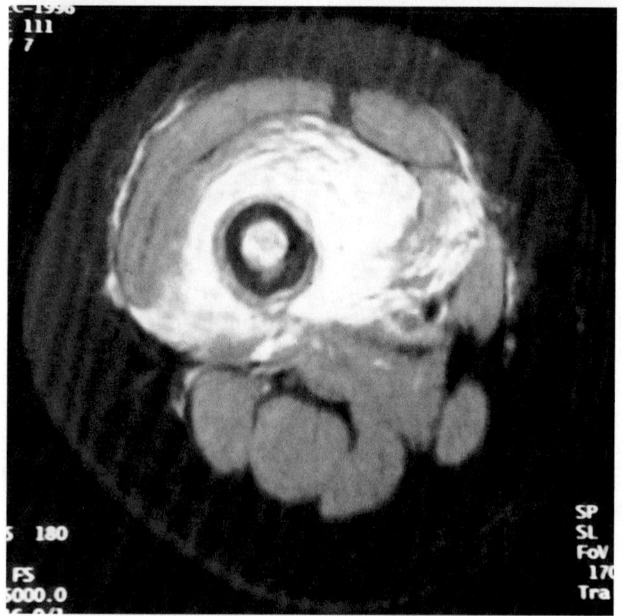

B

FIGURE 6-20 A 15-year-old girl was referred with a pathologic fracture of the femoral shaft after a fall while going down stairs. On close questioning, she stated that she had had pain in her thigh for several weeks before the fall and that the fall occurred after her leg gave way while going down the stairs. As an infant, she had already been treated with a cast for 2 months. **A.** The patient had been casted at another hospital, and x-ray studies in the cast show a transverse fracture of the mid-femoral shaft with destructive changes and worrisome periosteal elevation. **B.** MRI showed destructive changes of the mid-shaft of the femur with a soft tissue mass and bleeding from the fracture. An open biopsy established the diagnosis of Ewing's sarcoma of the femur, which was treated with neoadjuvant chemotherapy.

be individualized based on factors such as the fracture displacement, fracture stability, histologic and radiologic response to chemotherapy, and most important, the ability to achieve wide margins for local tumor control. Pathologic fractures that occur after reconstruction through allograft or endoprosthetic reconstruction often can be successfully treated with bone grafting or exchange of allograft or endoprosthesis.

Bone and Fibrous Tissue Diseases

Fibrous Dysplasia

Fibrous dysplasia, a developmental abnormality of bone presenting as expansile fibrous lesions, can result in pathologic fracture and deformity. Three forms exist: monostotic fibrous dysplasia, polyostotic fibrous dysplasia, and McCune-Albright syndrome (MAS). In 1937, McCune and Bruch (146) and Albright et al (147) described patients with these osseous lesions in association with cutaneous pigmentation and endocrine dysfunction. Later, Lichtenstein and Jaffe (148,149) coined the term fibrous dysplasia and further divided the entity into monostotic and polyostotic forms without endocrine disorder. The common factor is expansile fibrous tissue lesions of the bone, which contain woven bone formed by metaplasia with poorly oriented bone trabeculae.

Studies have demonstrated that MAS is caused by activating mutations in the gene for the alpha subunit of the heterotrimeric stimulatory G protein of adenylate cyclase (*GNAS1* gene), located on the long arm of chromosome 20 at locus 20q13.2-q13.3 (150,151). The mutation in this gene likely occurs in embryonic development and is expressed in a mosaic pattern, resulting in the often lateralized pattern of skin and bone involvement in patients with MAS. This mutation is not present in tissue from patients with aggressive fibromatosis involving bone or osteofibrous dysplasia (150).

Monostotic Fibrous Dysplasia

Clinical Presentation. The diagnosis usually is made between the ages of 10 and 15 years of age, although neonatal fibrous dysplasia has been reported (151). The lesions usually are asymptomatic until a fracture occurs, then patients may have pain and swelling (152). Incomplete fractures are most common. The sites of fracture in order of decreasing frequency are the proximal femur, tibia, ribs, and bones of the face (152). Cutaneous lesions usually are not present in monostotic fibrous dysplasia. Although pregnancy may stimulate the lesions (153), overall progression is rare after initial presentation. Sarcomatous degeneration has an incidence of approximately 0.5% and generally occurs approximately 15 years after initial diagnosis.

The central dilemma in monostotic fibrous dysplasia is distinguishing the lesion from other benign disorders. The differential diagnosis usually includes eosinophilic granuloma, UBC, giant cell tumor, enchondroma, solitary fibroma, and osteomyelitis. MRI can be helpful in evaluating these lesions, but biopsy is sometimes necessary to establish the correct diagnosis. Recent work has also suggested that analysis of FD-associated GNAS1 mutations may prove to be helpful in confirming the diagnosis of monostotic fibrous dysplasia (154).

Radiographic Findings. Radiographically, lesions of monostotic fibrous dysplasia usually are elliptical, central lesions in the mid-diaphysis. The borders of the lesion are commonly sclerotic; trabeculation is more common than a ground-glass appearance. There often is a slight bowing of the tibia, but bowing of the femur is uncommon.

With evaluation by CT scan, the extent of cortical thinning can be studied and relative central densities measured. Eosinophilic granuloma, neoplasm, and osteomyelitis have a density on CT scan ranging from 20 to 40 Hounsfield units, whereas fibrous dysplasia has a higher density, ranging from 70 to 130 Hounsfield units. MRI may be useful to differentiate fibrous dysplasia from other lesions, especially UBC.

Injury. Pathologic fractures occur in nearly 45% of patients. Fractures of the long bones are generally not displaced; many are microfractures. Although the fractures heal rapidly, endosteal callus is poorly formed and periosteal callus is normal (155). With mild deformity, the cortex thickens on the concave side of the long bone. Nonunion is rare.

Treatment. Conservative treatment with immobilization is indicated for most fractures that occur in conjunction with monostotic fibrous dysplasia. Traction with subsequent casting can be used for femoral shaft fractures in young children; casts or cast-bracing for upper and other lower extremity fractures is often appropriate (152).

Operative intervention is indicated for fractures of severely deformed long bones and those through large cystic areas. Bone graft can be resorbed, but total obliteration of the lesion often can be accomplished with grafting. Deformity can occur, and internal fixation may be required for stabilization. Complete *en bloc* extraperiosteal excision with grafting has been shown to be successful for severe lesions but is seldom needed. Both painful lesions without fracture and impending pathologic fractures can be treated with bone grafting.

Proximal femoral lesions with pathologic fracture are especially troublesome because of the propensity for malunion with coxa vara. For fractures through small lesions, either cast immobilization or curettage with grafting can be used; osteotomy can be done for residual deformity (156). For larger lesions, internal fixation is necessary. Proximal femoral pathologic fractures have been stabilized with lag screws, blade plates (152), intramedullary nails, and Enders nails. Cast immobilization and protected weight-bearing are necessary after these procedures to protect the reduction. Spine fractures are rare but can be treated with bed rest followed by immobilization with an orthosis (152).

Polyostotic Fibrous Dysplasia

Clinical Presentation. Most patients with polyostotic fibrous dysplasia present before age 10 years with pain, limp, deformity, or pathologic fracture (148,151). The bones most commonly affected are the femur, tibia, humerus, radius, facial bones, pelvis, ribs, and phalanges (148). Involvement is often unilateral, usually affecting a single extremity. In one series, 50% of patients had facial involvement (151). Spine involvement occurs with polyostotic fibrous dysplasia, and limb-length discrepancy is common (151,155). Although most laboratory studies are normal, serum alkaline phosphatase levels may be elevated (155). Some authors believe that polyostotic fibrous dysplasia does not usually progress significantly after adulthood (151,157), but others (155) believe that puberty does not affect the bone lesions.

Both intramuscular myxoma and myositis ossificans progressiva have been associated with polyostotic fibrous dysplasia. When it occurs, sarcomatous degeneration of the lesions occurs 10 to 12 years after the initial diagnosis of fibrous dysplasia; osteogenic sarcomas, chondrosarcomas, and giant cell sarcomas also have been reported. The warning signs for sarcoma in existing lesions of fibrous dysplasia are pain and rapid enlargement of the lesion.

Radiographic Findings. Polyostotic fibrous dysplasia appears as multiple expansile lesions with cortical erosion. Most have a multilocular appearance associated with a scalloped pattern of endosteal erosion (158). A ground-glass appearance on x-ray study is caused by the metaplastic woven bone comprising the lesion. A radiolucent cystic appearance also is common. Cartilage may be present in approximately 10% of lesions, and radiographic stippling may be seen (147). In contrast to those in monostotic fibrous dysplasia, the lesions in the polyostotic form have little increased peripheral density, and they usually form a characteristic fusiform expansion of the bone (Fig. 6-21). Bowing of the long bones is common, and normal tubulation may not occur with growth (155).

Distinguishing polyostotic from monostotic fibrous dysplasia may be difficult. Plain x-ray skeletal surveys usually are done; technetium bone scans are helpful in identifying multiple lesions that may not be present on plain x-ray studies (14,159). Harris et al (155) suggested that the hallmarks of polyostotic fibrous dysplasia is the characteristic long bone lesions with extension from epiphysis to epiphysis and increased density at the base of the skull. They suggest that a survey of the pelvis and femurs is most helpful in noting multiple lesions. Epiphyseal lesions can also occur (155).

Injury. In one series of 37 patients with polyostotic fibrous dysplasia, nearly 85% had at least one fracture and 40% had an average of three fractures (155). Fractures are most common in the femur, humerus, radius, and wrist (148,149). Like fractures in monostotic fibrous dysplasia, fractures in the polyostotic form generally are not displaced and healing is not delayed; nonunion can occur, however (155). Rib fractures are rare, and generally rib lesions are asymptomatic. A shepherd's crook deformity of the humerus associated with polyostotic fibrous dysplasia has been reported (14,160). Compression of the spinal cord by fibrous tissue also has been reported.

Treatment. The fractures of polyostotic fibrous dysplasia usually occur through very diseased bone and are associated with marked deformity. They often require more aggressive treatment than fractures seen in the monostotic form. Conservative immobilization techniques usually are appropriate for most

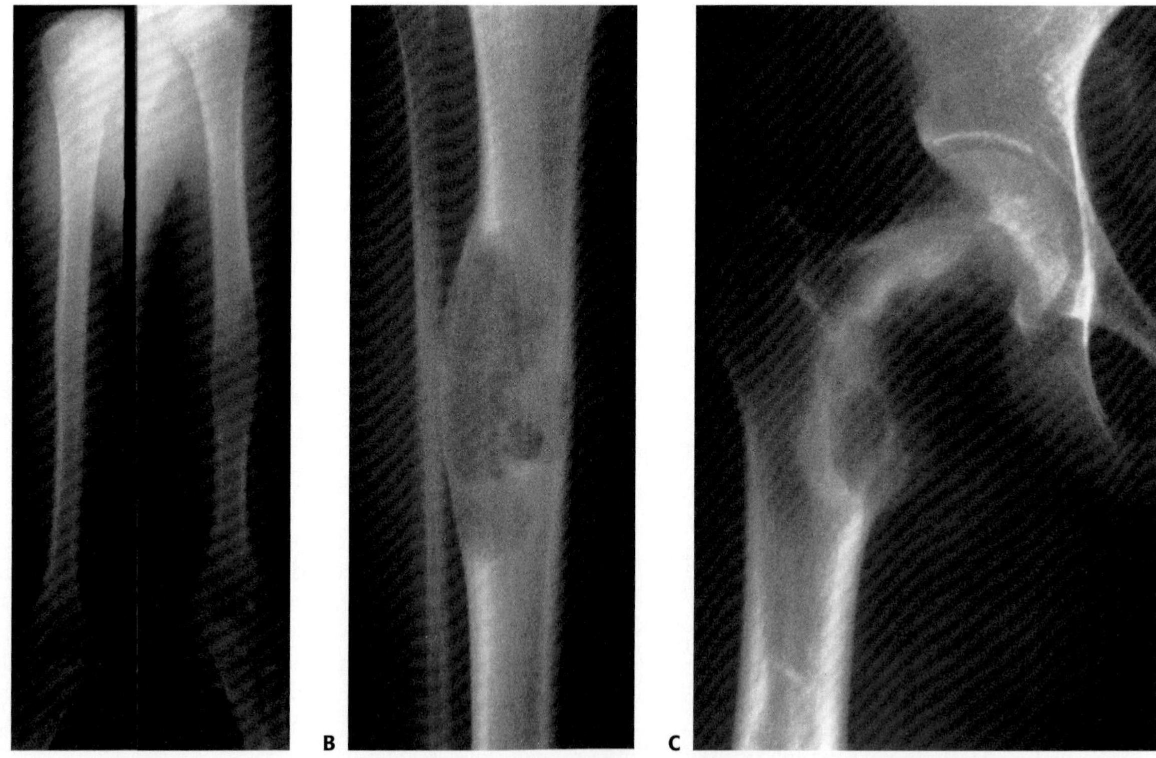

FIGURE 6-21 Polyostotic fibrous dysplasia in a 10-year-old girl. **A.** A fusiform expansile lesion is present in the mid-shaft of the humerus. **B.** A more eccentric expansile lesion is seen in the tibial shaft. There is scalloping due to endosteal erosion with a central ground-glass appearance. The lesion was painful and was treated with curettage and bone graft. (Courtesy of Jack Henry, M.D., San Antonio, Texas.) **C.** Polyostotic fibrous dysplasia in a 26-year-old woman. A large erosive lesion is present in the inferior neck of the femur. This lesion was treated by curettage with both fibula and iliac crest bone graft. (Courtesy of Gregorio Canales, MD, San Antonio, Texas.)

shaft fractures in children before puberty. Fractures of the femur can be treated with traction and subsequent casting in young patients. After adolescence, however, the recurrence of deformity after surgery is less, and curettage and grafting should be considered for fractures, especially for large lesions with associated deformity (149,155). Stephenson et al (160) found that in patients younger than 18 years of age, closed treatment or curettage and bone grafting of lower extremity fractures gave unsatisfactory results, but internal fixation produced more satisfactory outcomes. A Sofield procedure (osteotomy and intramedullary nailing) can be used for tibial deformity.

The greatest challenge in polyostotic fibrous dysplasia is treatment of fractures of the proximal femur. With recurrent fracture and deformity, a severe coxa vara resembling a shepherd's crook develops. Curettage of the lesion with abundant bone grafting has been recommended for mild deformities (149,159), and fixation usually is needed for large lesions. Femoral neck fracture or osteotomy for deformity can be stabilized with internal fixation. For severe shepherd's crook deformity, medial displacement valgus osteotomies with plate fixations are needed to restore the biomechanical stability of the hip (161). For severe lesions, Funk and Wells (158) recommended complete excision of the intertrochanteric area and advancement of the psoas and gluteus medius tendons. Breck (162) recommended securing the side plate of the femoral nail with bolts and washers rather than with screws to obtain better stability. Massive autogenous bone grafting is believed to be superior to donor bone graft (155), but it may be impractical because the iliac crests of a young child may be small and the pelvis may have coexisting disease.

The use of bisphosphonates may offer hope for a medical treatment for patients with severe fibrous dysplasia. Radiation therapy is not recommended (148).

McCune-Albright Syndrome

Clinical Presentation. McCune-Albright syndrome is a rare variant of fibrous dysplasia associated with endocrine dysfunction (such as precocious puberty in females), characteristic bone lesions (osteitis fibrosa disseminata), and areas of cutaneous pigmentation (144,147). It affects both women and men and has been associated with pituitary adenoma, gigantism, hyperthyroidism, and Cushing's syndrome (163). The skin lesions generally are flat, multiple melanotic areas that stop at the midline and parallel the distribution of bone lesions (151). The irregular margins have been compared to the coast of Maine in contrast to the smoother lesions found in neurofibromatosis, which are likened to the coast of California. Skin lesions may also be absent.

On x-ray studies, a polyostotic presentation is seen. With precocious sexual development, there is rapid bone maturation with early physeal closure and short stature (151). Pathologic fractures in childhood occur with a pattern and appearance similar to those in polyostotic fibrous dysplasia.

Treatment. The literature is limited regarding specific treatment of McCune-Albright syndrome, but both conservative treatment and aggressive surgical intervention have been used with apparent success. Internal fixation may be necessary in severe cases (Fig. 6-22). Ippolito et al found that conservative treatment, curettage and bone grafting, and fixation with screws and plates were not as successful as internal fixation with intramedullary nails for treating cases in which the femur or other limb long bones were extensively involved. Intramedullary nails provided effective stabilization and successfully prevented further fractures and major deformities (151). With the recent progress in understanding the genetic basis of this disorder, newer treatment alternatives may become available.

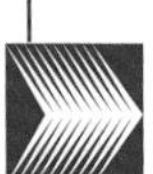

AUTHORS' PREFERRED METHOD OF TREATMENT

Fibrous Dysplasia

Conservative treatment with immobilization is indicated for most fractures in children with monostotic fibrous dysplasia. In younger children, immediate casting, or traction and subsequent casting are used for most femoral shaft fractures. Because fractures in patients with polyostotic fibrous dysplasia usually occur through very abnormal bone and can result in marked deformity, they often require more aggressive treatment (e.g., internal fixation).

After adolescence, the occurrence of deformity after surgery is less frequent. Nonoperative treatment of fractures and curettage and cancellous bone grafting do not generally produce satisfactory results in children with fibrous dysplasia of the lower extremity. Curettage and grafting are indicated for fractures of severely deformed long bones and those through large cystic areas, with internal fixation appropriate for the location and age. Bone graft can be resorbed after placement in extensive lesions, and proximal deformity can occur after corrective osteotomy.

Proximal Femoral Lesions. One of the most common sites of fracture and deformity is the proximal femur. Proximal femoral lesions with pathologic fracture are especially difficult because of the tendency for varus deformity and repeated fracture. Stable fractures through small lesions can be treated with cast immobilization, but one must be vigilant and ready to intervene at any sign of varus displacement.

Femoral neck fractures can be stabilized *in situ* with a cannulated screw, or compression screw and side plate, depending on the extent of involvement and the nature and location of the fracture. Fixation can be combined with valgus osteotomy if there is preexisting deformity or with curettage and grafting if there is a large area of bone loss. Postoperative cast immobilization and protected weight-bearing usually are necessary. Varus deformity is best treated with valgus osteotomy of the subtrochanteric region and internal fixation early in the course of the disease to restore the normal neck shaft angle and mechanical axis. Intramedullary load-sharing fixation (such as flexible intramedullary nails) can be used for juvenile patients with femoral shaft fractures.

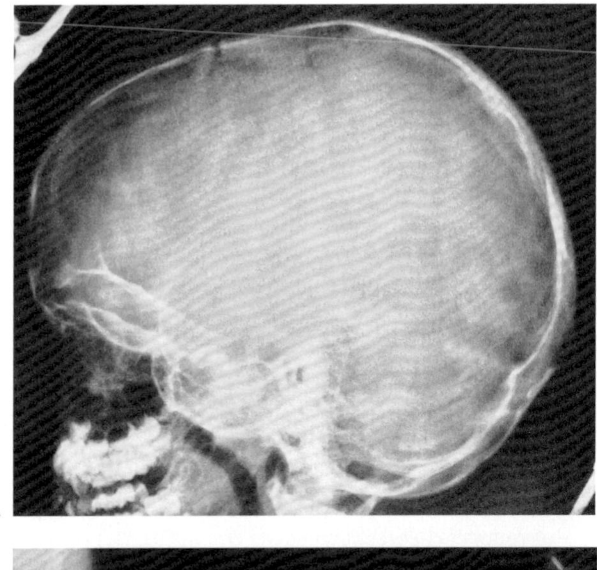

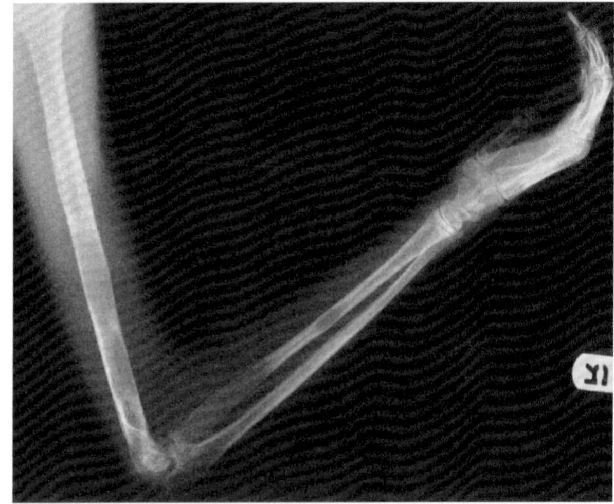

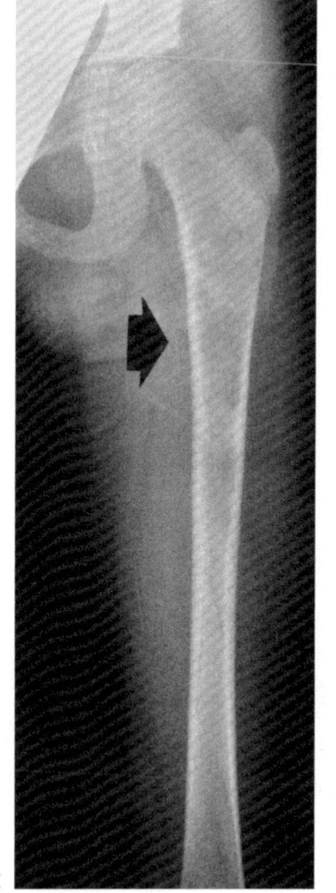

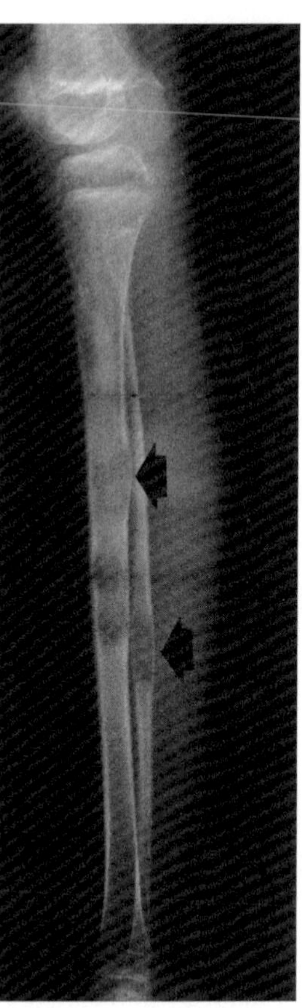

FIGURE 6-22 **A.** A 7-year-old girl presented with McCune-Albright syndrome. Skull x-rays show multiple lesions consistent with this condition. **B.** Expansile rarefied lesions are present throughout the humerus and the radius. **C.** Both proximal femurs have areas of rarefaction with expansile lesions (*arrows*). **D.** Both tibiae and fibulae show areas of expansile fibrous dysplasia (*arrows*).

For larger lesions with more severe deformity, and in older patients, rigid fixation often is necessary. Depending on the situation, intramedullary load-sharing fixation devices that support not only the femoral neck but also the shaft of the femur (such as *custom intramedullary reconstruction nails*) are better and should be used when possible. For severe shepherd's crook deformity, medial displacement osteotomies are needed to restore the biomechanical stability of the hip.

Patients with McCune-Albright syndrome should have careful preoperative evaluation in preparation for anesthesia and surgery. The reader is referred to an excellent review by Langer et al (164) for further information.

Osteofibrous Dysplasia of the Tibia and Fibula

Clinical Presentation. The term osteofibrous dysplasia of the tibia and fibula is advocated to describe specific, uncommon fibrous lesions of the tibia and fibula in young children (165). These lesions superficially resemble monostotic fibrous dysplasia but exhibit unique natural history, response to treatment, and specific histology.

Most patients present before the age of 5 years, but the range varies from 5 weeks to 15 years of age (165,166). There usually is painless enlargement of the tibia with slight to moderate anterior or anterolateral bowing. The disease process is almost always confined to one tibia, but the ipsilateral fibula can also be involved. Solitary involvement of the fibula is infrequent, and bilateral involvement of both tibias is rare. Both distal and proximal lesions can occur, and with fibular involvement, the lesion is located distally.

Biopsy specimens distinguish this entity from fibrous dysplasia or adamantinoma. The fibrous tissue present is less cellular than in fibrous dysplasia. Woven bone is at the center of the lesion, with newly formed bone trabeculae bordered by active osteoblasts and lamellar structure near the periphery of the lesion. This pattern is unusual in fibrous dysplasia. A particular zonal architecture is present in large biopsy specimens and shows increasing size and maturity of the bone trabeculae toward the edge of the lesion. Some authors believe that osteofibrous dysplasia may be related to adamantinoma (167,168).

Radiographic Findings. An eccentric intracortical lesion of osteolysis usually is present in the middle third of the tibia, with extension proximally or distally (Fig. 6-23) (166). The cortex overlying the lesion is expanded and thinned, and in the medullary canal, a dense band of sclerosis borders the lesion with narrowing of the medullary canal. A single area of radiolucency may be present and has a ground-glass appearance, but often there are several areas of involvement with a bubble-like appearance.

The differential diagnosis usually includes both monostotic fibrous dysplasia and adamantinoma, but some authors (165) believe that the characteristic x-ray appearance and the early onset of the disease effectively exclude these two disorders and that biopsy is not necessary. Others support the need for biopsy to establish diagnosis. Bracing with orthotics is advisable after open biopsy for diagnostic purposes.

Injury. Pathologic fractures are present in nearly one third of patients (165). These fractures are either incomplete or minimally displaced and heal well with both closed and open methods (165), although delayed union may be a problem. Pseudarthrosis is rare.

Treatment. The natural history of this disorder in untreated patients is variable. Most lesions show slight or moderate progres-

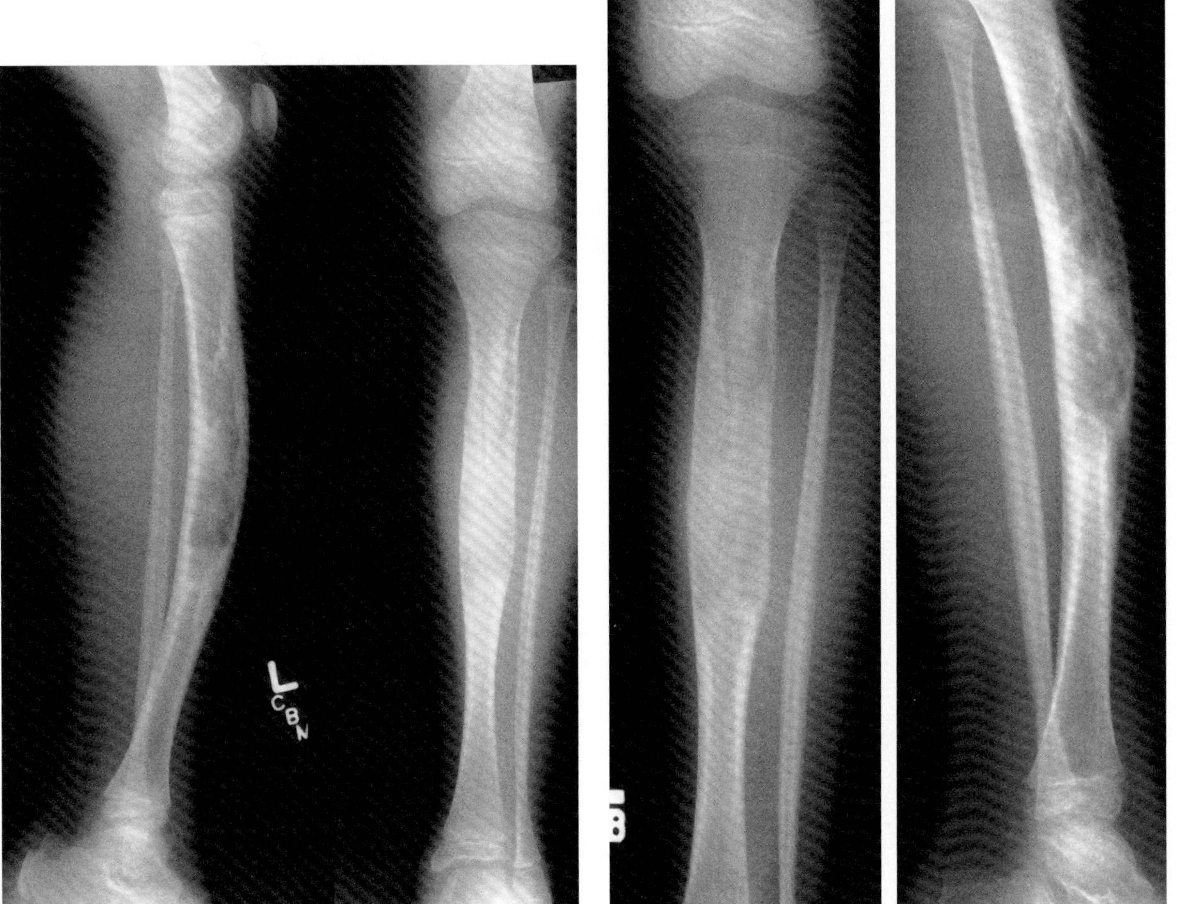

FIGURE 6-23 Osteofibrous dysplasia of the tibia. **A.** An 8-year-old girl presented with slight bowing of the left leg. X-ray study showed a circumscribed sclerotic and lytic lesion of the diaphysis of the tibia. Lateral x-rays show bowing of the tibia with a diaphyseal intracortical lesion. The patient was thought to have osteofibrous dysplasia, and was braced and followed yearly. **B.** Eight years later, the lesion has become slightly more extensive and is associated with slight progression of anterior bowing of the tibia. The patient underwent open biopsy, and pathologic diagnosis was consistent with adamantinoma. Chest CT showed no sign of lung involvement. The patient was treated with wide excision of the entire lesion and free vascular fibula bone graft reconstruction.

sion in late childhood, but others may show aggressive expansion with bowing of the tibia in patients up to 15 years of age. Rarely, the lesions may even regress or remain stationary over 3 to 4 years. Most lesions stop expanding after completion of skeletal growth. What appears to be osteofibrous dysplasia may actually be early adamantinoma (167). MRI showing a soft-tissue extension is indicative of adamantinoma. Open biopsy also may be needed to establish the biphasic histology of adamantinoma.

Curettage and grafting were associated with a local recurrence rate of up to 64% in children 14 years old or younger in one series (165). Others reported a lower local recurrence rate. Ozaki et al (169) showed the course of six tibial lesions in five patients with osteofibrous dysplasia who were followed longer than 10 years (average: 16.8 years). Curettage and autogenic bone grafting were performed on two lesions, which then healed. Of four lesions on which curettage and autogeneic bone grafts were performed, three healed and one recurred. The recurrent lesion healed after curettage and xenogeneic bone grafting. Three lesions healed without surgical treatment. During long-term follow-up, this disease showed a clear tendency for healing (169). Wide extraperiosteal resection can be performed, but graft resorption can still occur (165). Some authors (170,171) believe that bracing until skeletal maturity is preferable to surgery.

Pathologic fractures in this disorder should heal with cast immobilization in plaster casts. If fractures recur, or if the lesion is rapidly progressive, wide extraperiosteal resection with grafting is necessary (165). Open reduction with bone grafting and internal fixation is recommended for fractures with angular deformity. Early osteotomy is recommended for severe bowing deformity.

Neurofibromatosis

Neurofibromatosis, also known as von Recklinghausen's disease, is an autosomal dominant condition with variable penetrance that occurs in 1 in 2,500 to 3,000 live births (172). It affects neural tissue, vascular structures, skin, and the skeleton. The diagnosis of neurofibromatosis can be based on the presence of two of the four following criteria, according to Crawford and Bagamery (172):

1. Multiple café-au-lait spots
2. Positive family history for neurofibromatosis
3. Diagnostic biopsy of a neurofibroma
4. Presence of pseudarthrosis of the tibia, hemihypertrophy, or a short, angular scoliosis

Crowe and Schull (173) pointed out that adult patients with neurofibromatosis usually had more than five café-au-lait spots with a diameter of more than 1.5 cm. The presence of café-au-lait spots, however, is not pathognomonic for neurofibromatosis. Whitehouse (174) noted that 23% of normal children have one or two café-au-lait spots with a diameter of more than 0.5 cm, and the presence of five or more café-au-lait spots is needed to suggest the diagnosis of neurofibromatosis. Although café-au-lait spots may be present at birth, usually they are not seen until the patient is 5 or 6 years old (172). Generalized soft-tissue hypertrophy of the limbs is present in 37% of adults with neurofibromatosis (175), whereas children have an 11% incidence of limb-length discrepancy and only a 3% incidence of soft-tissue enlargement of the extremities (172).

A diagnostic biopsy of a dermal neurofibroma is considered a valuable criterion for the diagnosis of neurofibromatosis. These tumors, however, tend not to be clinically apparent until the child is older than 12 years of age (172). Plain x-ray studies are not helpful in identifying these soft-tissue tumors. MRI can be helpful in identifying the soft-tissue masses. Technetium 99m–labeled diethylenetriaminepentaacetic acid (DTPA) accumulates in the soft-tissue tumors of neurofibromatosis (176,177). Routine isotopic imaging with this technique can identify lesions as small as 1.5 cm. Lesions as small as 0.8 cm were seen through a more advanced technique known as single proton emission computed tomography. Such techniques may be useful in identifying occult neurofibromatosis and pseudarthrosis of the long bones.

Injury. Pseudarthrosis of the long bones in patients with neurofibromatosis can be a therapeutic dilemma. The appearance of pseudarthroses and their resistance to treatment has been postulated to be due to a deficiency of bone formation secondary to mesodermal dysplasia. More recently, the abnormal soft tissue associated with these pseudarthroses has been postulated to be the major associated factor in causing pseudarthrosis (178). Wright et al (178) developed a rabbit tibia congenital pseudarthrosis model and suggested that a possible underlying abnormality in congenital pseudarthrosis might actually be the abnormal soft tissue surrounding the bone rather than the bone itself (178).

Approximately 5% of patients with neurofibromatosis are thought eventually to have pseudarthrosis of the long bones. The tibia is the bone most often affected, but only 55% of the cases of congenital pseudarthroses of the tibia are thought to be associated with neurofibromatosis (153).

The term congenital pseudarthrosis in neurofibromatosis is misleading because a substantial number of patients do not have a pseudarthrosis at birth but rather develop it later after a pathologic fracture (179). Brown et al (158) found that in six children with neurofibromatosis, anterior bowing of the leg developed at an average age of 8 months and then went on to fracture and pseudarthrosis an average of 4.5 months after the initial clinical observation of deformity.

The focus of the recent orthopaedic literature has been treatment of congenital pseudarthrosis of the tibia (179), but pseudarthroses in other locations in children with neurofibromatosis also occur and can be a challenge. Pseudarthroses have been reported in the radius (158,176,177,180–190) ulna (180,186,191–195) both the radius and the ulna (188,190,192,193,196,197) femur, clavicle, and humerus. Most patients had associated neurofibromatosis, but some with pseudarthroses in each of the above-mentioned locations did not.

Radiographic Findings. Anterolateral bowing of the tibia with loss of the medullary canal usually is present before fracture (Fig. 6-24) (158). Another x-ray characteristic is a prefracture cystic lesion of the tibia with anterolateral bowing (153). Biopsy specimens of these pseudarthroses invariably reveal fibrous tissue, but there are reports of (189,192) found evidence of neural tissue in biopsy specimens. None of these findings, however, has been confirmed by electron microscopy to document the presence of Schwann cells. X-ray findings in patients with estab-

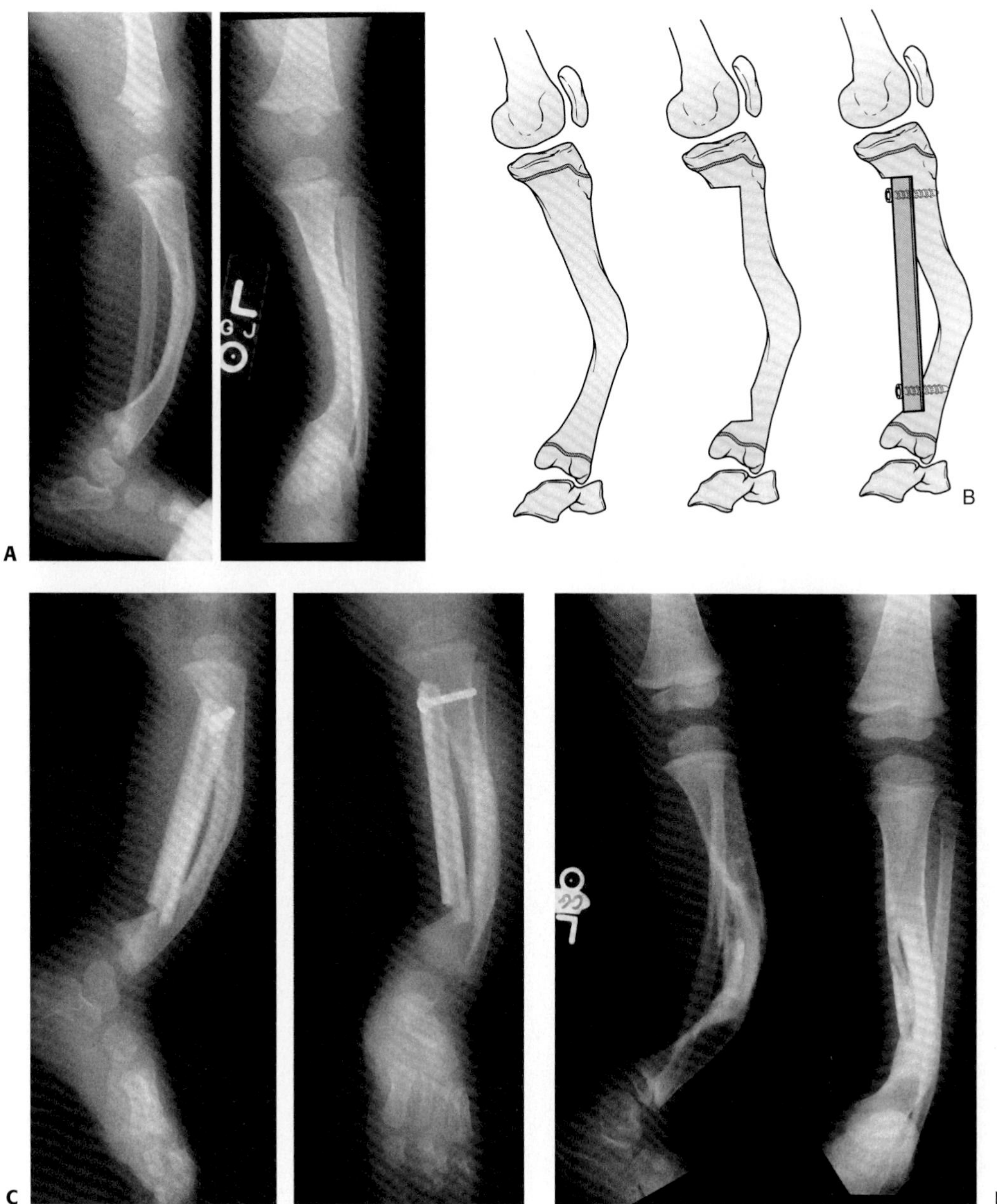

FIGURE 6-24 **A.** A 2-year-old boy with neurofibromatosis presented with anterolateral bowing, sclerosis, and partial obliteration of the medullary canal of the tibia without fracture. **B.** A modified McFarland technique for prophylactic bypass grafting was performed as shown. **C.** Immediate postsurgical x-ray studies of the tibia after prophylactic bypass grafting. **D.** Three years later, x-ray studies show continued growth of the tibia without fracture but some absorption of the allograft and relative loss of structural support by the allograft related to continued growth. (From Dormans JP. Modified sequential McFarland bypass procedure for prepseudarthrosis of the tibia. *J Orthop Tech* 1995;3:176–180, with permission.)

lished pseudarthroses of the tibia include narrowing or obliteration of the medullary canal at the pseudarthrosis site, with sclerosis and anterolateral angulation (Fig. 6-25). Pseudarthrosis of the fibula is associated with valgus deformity of the ankle.

In upper extremity pseudarthroses of neurofibromatosis, the x-ray signs of the bone at risk are narrowing of the diaphysis (195), sclerosis and hypoplasia with associated absent medullary canal (188), and the presence of a cystic lesion in the bone. Once a fracture has occurred, a pseudarthrosis is likely when the fracture line persists for more than 7 weeks after injury (189). The ends of the fracture gradually become tapered, there is little callus, and the cortex of the healing bone thickens with a decreased diameter of the medullary canal. The cause of these radiographic changes is unclear. Biopsy specimens from upper extremity pseudarthrosis have consistently shown the presence of dense fibrous tissue without evidence of neurofibroma. Pseudarthroses have developed in children with neurofibromatosis after fracture through normal-appearing forearm bones (182,183).

Treatment. A tibia with an anterolateral bow in an infant or child will eventually fracture; corrective osteotomy to correct angular deformity will only accelerate the progression to pseudarthrosis and should not be done. Once the fracture occurs, there is no indication for closed treatment. In conjunction with excision of the hypotrophic bone ends, methods of treatment of this congenital pseudarthrosis include intramedullary fixation with iliac bone graft, fixation with vascularized fibular graft, and Ilizarov's compression of the pseudarthrosis with callotastic lengthening of the proximal tibia. All of these methods may be complicated by further pathologic fracture.

In contrast to pseudarthrosis of the upper extremity, there is substantial experience with treatment of pseudarthrosis of the tibia, but results are also disappointing. Bracing has proved ineffectual in the treatment of an established pseudarthrosis. Surgical procedures have included bypass grafts (198), onlay grafts (199), grafting with small bone chips, intramedullary nailing procedures (200,201), and intramedullary rod fixation after segmental osteotomies (202). The rate of union with these procedures ranges from 7% to 90%, and eventual amputation has been common. Electrical stimulation has been used with some success, but most series reporting its use have short patient follow-up and the electrical stimulation was used in combination with other surgical techniques. In one series, a 20% success

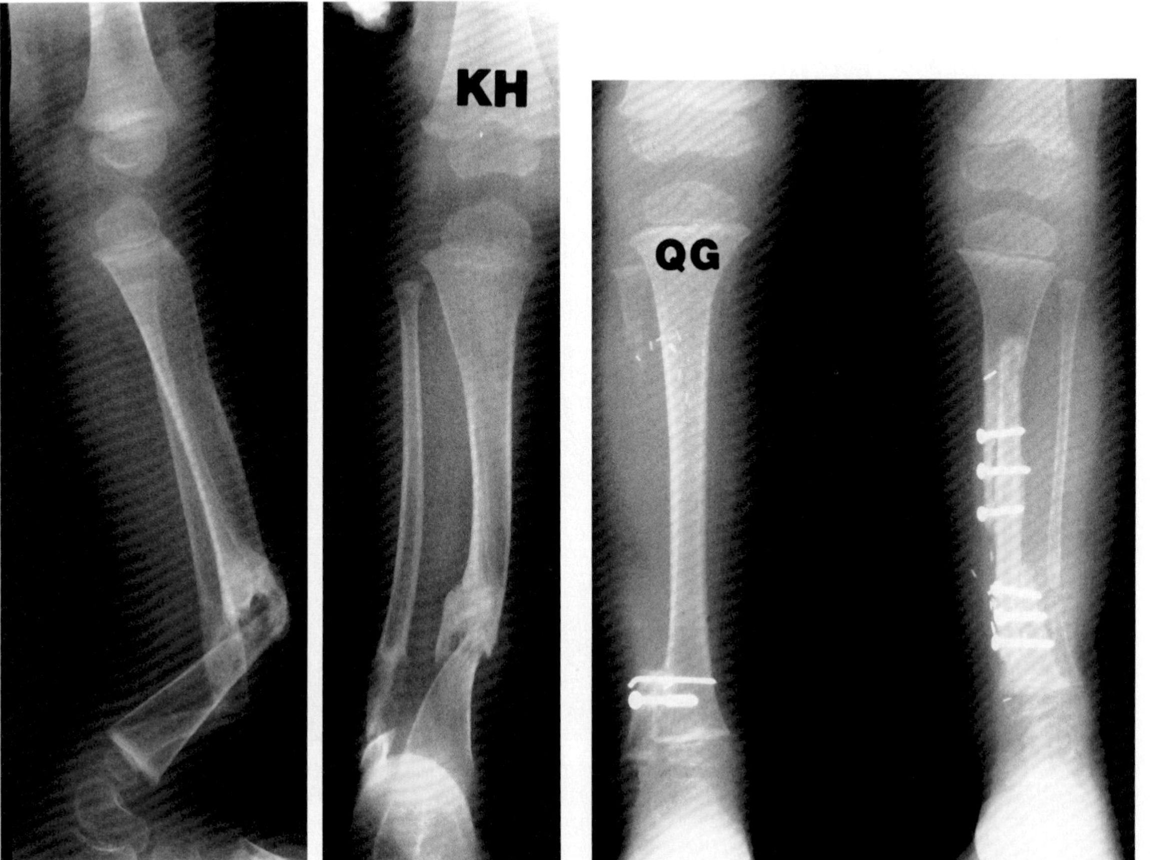

FIGURE 6-25 A. Untreated congenital pseudarthrosis of the tibia in children with neurofibromatosis. **B.** After resection and reconstruction with a vascularized free fibula interposition.

rate was achieved using direct-current stimulation (203). In another series, union was achieved in 10 of 12 patients with pseudarthrosis of the tibia through rigid intramedullary rod fixation and electrical stimulation through implanted electrodes (204). The Farmer procedure, a skin and bone pedicle from the contralateral leg, has a reported union rate approaching 53% (205). Free vascularized fibular grafts also have been used for reconstruction after excision of the involved tibia (205). In one series, 11 of 12 patients with neurofibromatosis and pseudarthrosis of the tibia were successfully treated with free vascularized fibular grafts. Union of the pseudarthrosis occurred between 3 to 8 months after surgery (206–208). A free vascularized iliac graft has been used in one patient with neurofibromatosis, resulting in union within 10 weeks (185). Fabry et al (209) obtained union of pseudarthrosis of the tibia in two patients with compression through an Ilizarov fixator. In another series (210), the fractures in three of five patients healed in 4.5 months. The other two patients needed supplementary iliac grafts, and eventually, the bone united. It is important to stress that treatment cannot be considered successful until skeletal maturity has been reached; many of these series included patients with short follow-up, and few included follow-up to skeletal maturity.

A prophylactic bypass grafting of the prepseudarthrotic tibia in neurofibromatosis has been performed with some success. This modification of the original McFarland bypass procedure, which was originally done for established pseudarthrosis, was successful in a series of patients from several centers reviewed by Strong and Wong-Chung (211). A modified sequential McFarland bypass procedure for prepseudarthrosis of the tibia also has been described (Fig. 6-24) (212).

Amputation should be considered and discussed with the family early when previous operative interventions have been unsuccessful. Amputation usually is at the Syme level, with prosthetic fitting around the pseudarthrosis. In a gait analysis study, Karol et al (184) compared 12 patients with previously operated and healed congenital pseudarthroses of the tibia with four children with amputations for final treatment of congenital pseudarthroses of the tibia. They found marked disturbance of gait and muscle strength in patients with healed congenital pseudarthroses of the tibia. They concluded that patients with early onset of disease, early surgery, and transankle fixation had more inefficient gaits than amputees. Patients with forearm pseudarthroses can be pain free and function may be satisfactory with observation or splinting. However, persistence of an ulnar pseudarthrosis in a growing child often leads to bowing of the radius and posterior lateral subluxation or dislocation of the radial head (185,191,192,195). Healing after 6 months of casting has been reported in a 2-month-old infant with a congenital pseudarthrosis of the radius. There was no clinical evidence of neurofibromatosis at the time of treatment of this patient (213). Union after conventional bone grafting and fixation has been reported in only a small number of patients with congenital pseudarthrosis of the forearm (180,182,183,188,193,214). Many of these patients require multiple conventional bone grafting procedures and often years of immobilization. There are more reports of patients (and probably many more patients) with pseudarthroses of the forearm bones who did not respond to multiple grafting procedures (158,180,189,191,195). The results of treatment of congenital pseudarthrosis of the forearm in neurofibromatosis by free vascularized fibular grafts are encouraging. Allieu et al (192) treated one patient with radial and ulnar pseudarthroses and another with ulnar pseudarthrosis with free vascularized fibular grafts. They obtained union in the patient with radial and ulnar pseudarthroses in 6 weeks and in the patient with ulnar pseudarthroses in 3 months. Earlier conventional grafting techniques had failed in both. Two additional patients with pseudarthroses of the radius without evidence of neurofibromatosis were treated with free vascularized fibular grafts, resulting union within 6 weeks (178,197). Mathlin et al (190) reported six pseudarthroses of the forearm bones treated with vascularized fibular grafting with union in five ranging from 6 to 18 months after surgery. Other surgical options include excision of the ulnar pseudarthrosis to avoid a later tethering effect on the growing radius (191) and fusion of the distal radius and ulnar joint (195). Creation of a one-bone forearm is often technically successful, but both length and rotation of the forearm are sacrificed with this procedure (186,195).

Extreme care should be taken in surgical treatment of children with neurofibromatosis, in whom the periosteum of the long bones is believed to be less adherent to the bone than normal periosteum.

Complications. Extensive subperiosteal hemorrhage with subsequent ossification was reported in a 9-year-old patient who underwent surgical epiphysiodesis of the proximal tibia and fibula (215). Massive subperiosteal hemorrhage due to minor trauma in children with neurofibromatosis occurred in the tibia and femur (215). The amount of blood loss in subperiosteal hemorrhages can be life-threatening. Yaghmai and Tafazoli (215) evacuated a subperiosteal hemorrhage of a femur in an 11-year-old boy with neurofibromatosis who presented with a rapidly growing mass of the thigh after a minor fall. An eggshell calcification was visible around the femur within weeks of the trauma. The cyst held 2,100 mL of serous fluid and went on to complete ossification within 12 weeks of surgery with marked thickening and distortion of the involved femur.

It is important preoperatively to rule out hypertension in children with neurofibromatosis because 16% of children with neurofibromatosis had hypertension in one series (216).

Injuries of the Spine in Neurofibromatosis. Spinal deformity is the most common musculoskeletal abnormality seen in individuals with neurofibromatosis. Although scoliosis was present in 64% of patients with neurofibromatosis in one series (172), kyphoscoliosis may be the primary contributor to the development of paraplegia (217). Patients younger than 19 years of age may have paraplegia secondary to vertebral deformity, whereas those patients older than 19 are more likely to have neurologic deficits secondary to a neurofibroma. Complete dislocation of the spine with neurologic defect has been reported in two patients with neurofibromatosis (218). Rib penetration of the enlarged neural foramen with spinal cord compression in neurofibromatosis has also been reported in four patients (187,219). CT scan and MRI are useful for evaluating these patients. Resection through either an anterior or a posterior approach seems satisfactory (187).

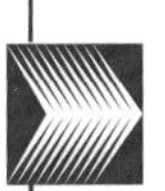

AUTHORS' PREFERRED METHOD OF TREATMENT

Neurofibromatosis

The treatment of congenital pseudarthrosis of the tibia remains controversial. When a child presents with prepseudarthrosis (angulation without fracture), either bypass grafting with fibular allograft or bracing are reasonable options. Once pseudarthrosis has developed, our preference is inserting an intramedullary rod and bone grafting of both the tibia and fibula when possible. If these procedures fail, free vascularized fibula transfer or resection and bone transport with circular frame techniques can be considered. Amputation and prosthetic fitting should be considered early in patients with failure of the above-mentioned techniques and severe shortening and a stiff ankle and foot. Conservative options, such as bracing or observation, for upper extremity pseudarthroses may be justified in a patient with a nonprogressive deformity and a satisfactory functional use of the extremity. Conventional bone grafting and fixation procedures for treatment of pseudarthrosis of the upper extremity have very limited success, and other approaches should be considered. Free vascularized fibular grafts seem the treatment of choice for upper extremity pseudarthrosis associated with neurofibromatosis.

CONGENITAL INSENSITIVITY TO PAIN

Congenital insensitivity to pain is a rare disorder characterized by the absence of normal subjective and objective responses to noxious stimuli in patients with intact central and peripheral nervous systems. The cause is unknown, but sporadic reports have appeared in the orthopaedic literature (220–223).

Orthopaedic manifestations of congenital insensitivity to pain include recurrent fractures, osteomyelitis, and neuropathic joints (Fig. 6-26). Limb-length discrepancy may occur from physeal damage. Lack of pain perception is associated with the development of Charcot's joints, which may lead to later neuropathic arthropathy. The weight-bearing joints usually are affected, especially the knees and ankles.

The differential diagnosis includes a spectrum of closely related sensory disorders including congenital sensory neuropathy, hereditary sensory radicular neuropathy, familial sensory neuropathy with anhidrosis, and familial dysautonomia (Riley-Day syndrome). Acquired conditions with pain insensitivity include syringomyelia, diabetes mellitus, tabes dorsalis, alcoholism, and leprosy. Loss of protective sensation promotes self-mutilation, burns, bruises, and fractures. The disease comes to light when the child develops teeth and then bites his or her tongue, lips, and fingers.

Management should aim at education and prevention of injury. Prevention of joint disease is the best early option (220,223). Joint injury should be recognized and treated early to prevent progression to gross arthropathy. Early diagnosis of injury is important, with signs of instability, swelling, and local warmth prompting early investigation and treatment. Most fractures are treated nonoperatively, when appropriate. Immobilization, bed rest, or appropriate bracing usually is indicated (220,222).

In a severely unstable, degenerated joint, arthrodesis may eventually be appropriate; however, poor healing, nonunion, and pseudarthrosis are common in neuropathic joints. The condition appears to improve with time with the gradual recovery of pain sensation.

MARROW DISEASE OF BONE

Gaucher's Disease

Gaucher's disease is a hereditary disorder of lipid metabolism. A deficiency of the lysosomal enzyme glucocerebrosidase results in an abnormal accumulation of glucocerebroside (glucosylceramide) in macrophages of the reticuloendothelial system. The most common sphingolipidosis, it is inherited as an autosomal recessive trait (224), with most cases noted in Ashkenazic Jews of eastern European origin (225). There are three types. Type I is a chronic nonneuropathic form with visceral (spleen and liver) and osseous involvement. More than 90% of children with Gaucher's have type I, so it is the most common type seen by orthopaedic surgeons. Type I is also known as the adult form, although, patients present during childhood (226). Type II is an acute, neuropathic type with central nervous system involvement and early infantile death. Type III is a subacute nonneuropathic type with chronic central nervous system involvement. These later two types, characterized as either infantile or juvenile, are notable for severe progressive neurologic disease and usually are fatal.

Lipid-laden histiocytes, known as Gaucher's cells, provoke clinical symptoms by accumulating in the liver, spleen, and bone marrow. Osseous lesions result from marrow accumulation and include Erlenmeyer's flask appearance, osteonecrosis (particularly of the femoral head), and pathologic fractures, especially of the spine and femoral neck.

Clinical Presentation

Most patients with Gaucher's disease are diagnosed before age 10 years (227). Common clinical findings include hepatosplenomegaly, yellowish pigmentation of the skin, pingueculae of the eyes (228,229), and bone lesions in 50% to 75% of patients (228). Bone pain, presenting as a dull extremity ache, is present

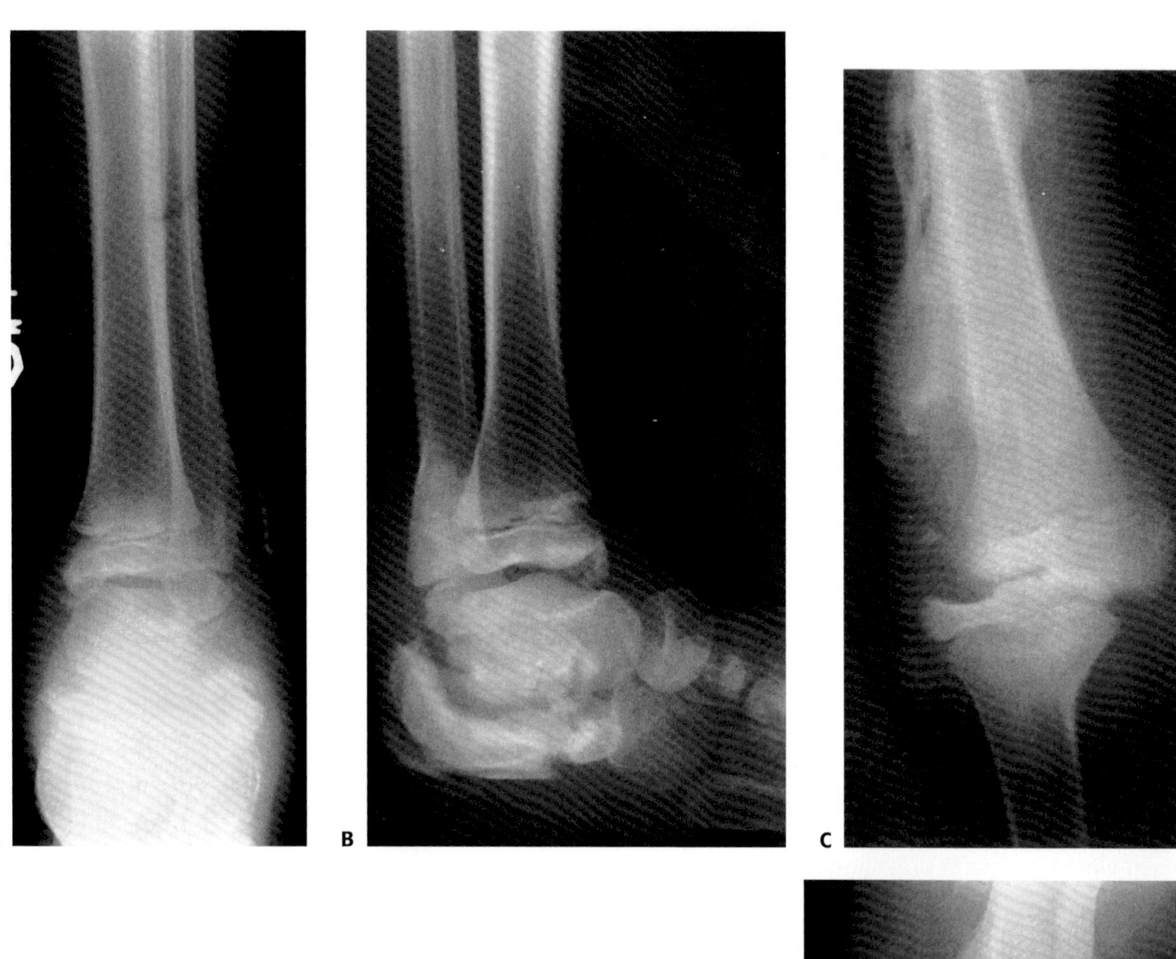

FIGURE 6-26 **A.** This 6-year-old child with anhidrosis, congenital insensitivity to pain, and attention deficit disorder presented with a history of swollen ankles and knees. This AP x-ray and **B.** this lateral x-ray shows Charcot changes in the subtalar joint with calcaneus and distal fibula fracture. **C.** This AP x-ray of the right knee and **D.** this lateral x-ray of the right knee show large, loose osteochondral fragments, medial subluxation of the femur on the tibia and extensive periosteal new bone formation in the distal femur. Soft-tissue shadows are consistent with her huge knee hemarthrosis. More than 100 mL of sterile serosanguineous fluid was aspirated from the knee at her initial visit. The effusion quickly returned in the days following the aspiration. Because management with casts at another hospital resulted in significant skin breakdown, we stabilized the knees with removable hinged braces. The effusions improved but did not resolve.

in most patients, and joint pain is equally common (225). Hemolytic anemia, leukopenia, and thrombocytopenia result from both hypersplenism and marrow replacement. These factors, along with abnormal liver function, tend to make these patients susceptible to infection and abnormal bleeding (225,230–233). Patients often have an increased serum acid phosphatase level and may have a decreased level of activity of glucocerebrosidase enzyme in white cells.

Bone lesions are most common in the femur, but they also occur in the pelvis, vertebra, humerus, and other locations (228). Infiltration of bone by Gaucher's cells leads to vessel thrombosis; compromise of the medullary vascular supply leads to localized osteonecrosis of the long bones (229), osteonecrosis of the femoral head occurs in most patients in whom the disease is diagnosed in childhood (225).

Bone crisis and osteomyelitis in patients with Gaucher's disease presents with similar symptoms. Nearly half of patients with Gaucher's disease have episodes of bone crisis, also known as pseudo-osteomyelitis, in which they present with acute sharp pains of the extremity with associated local warmth, redness, and tenderness (234). Distinguishing this problem from osteomyelitis can be difficult. With bone crisis, a patient may have severe pain in the back or extremities, rubor, fever, and an elevated white blood cell count (234). X-rays may show periosteal reaction or lytic lesions that are difficult to differentiate from osteomyelitis. Blood cultures are sterile, and aspiration of the affected bone is often necessary to provide correct diagnosis (230).

Osteomyelitis is present in a significant number of patients with Gaucher's disease. Hematogenous osteomyelitis was found in 10% of 49 patients in one series (230). Acute osteomyelitis is best managed conservatively when possible. Open irrigation and debridement of the bone may result in chronic osteomyelitis.

Plain x-ray studies usually are not helpful in differentiating crisis from infection (230). Technetium 99 bone scanning often demonstrates no increased uptake with a crisis (230) and shows decreased uptake in the area of osteonecrosis secondary to bone crisis, usually within 1 to 3 days after onset (231). Gallium 67 scintigraphy may be useful in differentiating crisis from infection by showing a lack of uptake in osteonecrosis and bone crisis, which may prove useful in excluding the presence of osteomyelitis (227). Bell et al recommended the use of CT scans to document the presence of purulent exudate in osteomyelitis in patients with Gaucher's disease (230). Some authors have found MRI useful for excluding osteomyelitis in patients with Gaucher's disease (229), but others (231) believe that MRI cannot distinguish between osteomyelitis and pseudo-osteomyelitis of bone crisis.

Radiographic Findings

Radiographically, three patterns of bone involvement have been described:

1. Generalized infiltration of the bone marrow of long bones by Gaucher cells causes a decreased density and cortical thinning. There is a general tendency for failure of tubulation (235), and this problem is most pronounced in the distal femur, where it produces an Erlenmeyer's flask appearance (Fig. 6-27).
2. The bone is moth-eaten with occasional osteosclerosis, and a centrally located curvilinear or vertical radiolucent streak is seen in the distal femur.
3. Dense collections of Gaucher cells form localized bubbly expansile lytic lesions in the bone, and associated areas of aseptic necrosis with medullary infarction form diaphyseal lytic lesions with reparative periosteal reaction surrounding them (235).

Osteonecrosis of the femoral head is similar to that seen in Legg-Calvé-Perthes disease, and vertebral plana may be present with lesions of the spine (235). MRI is more sensitive than x-rays or CT in demonstrating marrow involvement.

Injury

Pathologic fractures, especially of the femoral neck or shaft after biopsy, and of the spine, usually are best managed conservatively. Katz et al reported 23 pathologic fractures in 9 children with

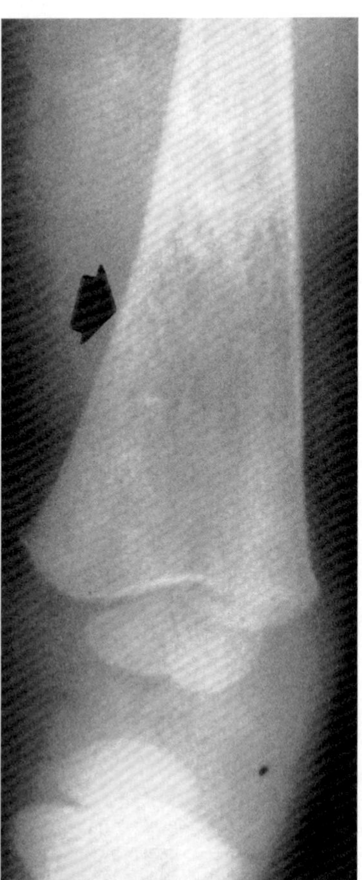

FIGURE 6-27 A 2-year-old child with Gaucher's disease. Early flaring of the distal femur is already present and will likely develop into a classic Erlenmeyer's flask deformity. Note the moth-eaten appearance of the metaphysis (*arrow*).

Gaucher's disease; 7 had multiple fractures (224). In decreasing order of frequency, the site of involvement included the distal femur, basilar neck of the femur, spine, and proximal tibia. Fractures also occurred infrequently in the distal tibia, proximal humerus, rib, and acetabulum. Fractures of the long bones were transverse and usually in the metaphysis. Fractures of the spine were either wedge shaped or centrally depressed at the end plate. The factors predisposing these children to fracture included significant medullary space infiltration, cortical bone erosion, osteonecrosis, and associated disuse osteoporosis (224).

In another report of 53 patients with Gaucher's disease aged 9 to 18 years (236), 11 children had vertebral fractures, usually at two or three sites in each patient, with either anterior wedging, central vertebral collapse, or total rectangular collapse. Most patients had relief of their pain after 1 to 4 months of conservative treatment; two required decompression laminectomies, and one had a posterior lateral fusion to stabilize the spine.

Katz et al (237) found that fractures of the upper extremities in Gaucher's disease were prone to occur in areas of prior crisis. Although external callus formed in 6 to 8 weeks in most patients, complete healing with internal callus took almost 2 years in some. Other authors have found fracture union to be rapid (235). Both delayed union and nonunion (229) have been reported in older patients with Gaucher's disease.

Pathologic femoral neck fractures with minimal associated trauma in children with Gaucher's disease often heal with a varus malunion and minimal subsequent remodeling; osteonecrosis of the femoral head also can be associated with femoral neck fractures (228,235). Goldman and Jacobs stated that the presence of a mixed density of bone of the femoral neck on x-ray with narrowing of the medial cortex was a risk factor for fracture (235).

Treatment

In the past, there was no specific treatment for Gaucher's disease. Splenectomy was often performed to help correct thrombocytopenia, but some authors believed that splenectomy worsened the orthopaedic complications of Gaucher's disease and recommended that it should be delayed as long as possible (235). Enzyme replacement therapy for the deficit found in Gaucher's disease has been developed (238). Alglucerase (Ceredase) is given in intravenous infusions every 2 weeks, resulting in a decrease in the size of the liver and spleen in most patients, and improvement in their anemia. With the recommended dosage of 60 units of alglucerase per kilogram, a 30-kg child requires a yearly amount of enzyme costing $163,800 (233). Low-dose imiglucerase (Cerezyme, Genxyme), a placental recombinant human-derived beta-glucocerebrosidase enzyme replacement, is also being used to treat patients with type I Gaucher's disease (239). Studies have shown that either a reduced dose or a low-dose–high-frequency regimen can achieve similar clinical effects with less cost (233,240). Less costly home intravenous enzyme replacement treatment is possible (241). After 1 year of treatment with replacement enzyme, patients with Gaucher's disease seem to have a decreased tendency for infection (240). The effects of the enzyme on the bone disease are unclear. Zirman et al (241) found no change in bone appearance after 1 year of replacement therapy, whereas Hill et al (242) noted improved appearance of the long bones and involved spine after 16 months of enzyme replacement therapy. Bembi et al suggest that enzyme replacement therapy with alglucerase and imiglucerase may reduce the risk of pathological fracture and may also be an effective treatment for osteopenia. Enzyme replacement therapy may maintain bone mineral density and decrease the risk of developing osteopenia (243). Bone marrow transplantation also has been shown to be helpful in reversing the medical effects of Gaucher's disease (244), but the mortality rate of patients undergoing allogenic marrow transplantation is greater than 15% (233).

Fracture Management

Pathologic fractures of the upper extremities and the spine respond well to conservative immobilization techniques. For fractures of the lower extremity, prolonged bed rest is to be avoided because of the additional complication of disuse osteoporosis. Early mobilization with non–weight-bearing casts is necessary to avoid angulation of the fractures. Complete healing, as defined by the appearance of internal callus may require, from 10 to 32 weeks of immobilization. Corrective osteotomy may be necessary for residual angulation. Some authors have recommended conservative treatment with non–weight-bearing for minimally angulated femoral neck fractures (224,225), with internal fixation reserved for unstable femoral fractures with progressive or marked displacement (223,228).

All patients with Gaucher's disease considered for a surgical procedure should undergo extensive preoperative evaluation of their abnormal clotting function. Excessive bleeding may even occur when clotting tests are normal (230). It is important for the anesthesiologist to recognize that patients with Gaucher's disease may be prone to upper airway obstruction because of infiltration of the upper airway with glycolipids and commonly may have an airway up to 50% smaller than predicted for age (245). These patients are prone to infection, likely due to abnormal neutrophil chemotaxis (245), and needle biopsy under operating room conditions is preferable to open biopsy (229).

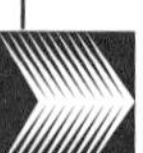

AUTHORS' PREFERRED METHOD OF TREATMENT

Gaucher's Disease

Conservative immobilization with non–weight-bearing is suggested for long bone fractures when appropriate. Stable fractures of the femoral neck should be treated by immobilization with frequent follow-up x-rays. Internal fixation should be used in unstable femoral neck fractures. Preoperative planning is important, with careful evaluation of clotting function and preoperative consultation by the anesthesiologist. Femoral head osteonecrosis is managed symptomatically, at first with osteotomy or joint replacement later when necessary.

Sickle Cell Disease

The term sickle cell disease (SCD) characterizes conditions caused by the presence of sickle cell hemoglobin (HbS). The most common type of SCD, HbS-S, is a homozygous recessive condition in which individuals inherit the β-S globin gene from each parent. SCD has systemic effects particularly on splenic function and on the central nervous, renal, hepatic, and musculoskeletal systems. SCD affects approximately 1 in 400 African-Americans. Sickle cell trait affects 8% to 10% of the African-American population and other groups less frequently (247). With sickle cell trait, each individual has inherited a beta-S globin gene and a beta-A globin gene. Clinical manifestations of sickle cell trait usually are not apparent. The presence of these abnormal hemoglobins in red blood cells causes them to be mechanically fragile, and when they are deoxygenated, the cells assume a sickle shape, which makes them prone to clumping with blockage of the small vessels of the spleen, kidneys, and bones (248,249). Chronic hemolytic anemia is present in most severely affected patients, and marrow hyperplasia is found in both the long bones and the short tubular bones. These disorders are diagnosed by hemoglobin electrophoresis (250).

Clinical Presentation

Musculoskeletal involvement results from small vessel occlusion by clumped sickle cells with bone infarction, osteonecrosis, and increased susceptibility to infection. These problems are most commonly seen in sickle cell anemia and sickle cell disease. Bone infarction is caused by blockage of marrow vascular channels by sickled erythrocytes. It is seen in patients as young as 6 to 12 months of age. Ultimate infarction occurs in as many as 74% of patients. Patients with acute long bone infarctions present with pain and swelling of the affected extremity and a low-grade fever. The long bone usually is tender, and infrequently, both erythema and warmth also are present (251). Acute symptoms usually resolve within a week. Sickle cell dactylitis, or infarction of the small bones of the hands and feet, may resemble infection and is common in infancy and childhood (252). Infarct can occur when young children get their feet wet or walking in the snow (253). Pain and swelling may last for 1 to 2 weeks. X-ray studies may show osteolysis and periosteal new bone formation.

Acute bone infarct in patients with SCD may be difficult to distinguish from osteomyelitis. Osteomyelitis occurs in fewer than 1% of affected patients. Acute long bone infarctions are 50 times more common than bacterial osteomyelitis in patients with sickle cell disease (251), but in Africa, osteomyelitis is 200 times more common in patients with SCD than in normal individuals (254). Osteoarticular bacterial infection was diagnosed in 1.6% of 247 admissions in one series of children with sickle cell disease admitted to the hospital for musculoskeletal complaints (255). These authors recommended aspiration as the diagnostic procedure of choice for infection. Clinical and x-ray presentations in both of these conditions are quite similar, except that high fevers are more common in osteomyelitis. Patients present with a warm, swollen, painful extremity. Multifocal bone involvement was reported in 73% of patients with osteomyelitis in one series (256), and the most common site in decreasing order of frequency was the humerus, metatarsal, tibia, femur, radius, metacarpal, and ulna. Routine evaluation should include blood cultures and needle aspiration of the affected area. Typical causative organisms in osteomyelitis include *Staphylococcus aureus, Salmonella,* and *Streptococcus pneumoniae.* Bennett et al (257) reviewed bone and joint manifestations in 57 patients with sickle cell anemia and found that osteomyelitis occurred in 61% and that *Salmonella* was the causative organism in 71% of these patients. Others have also found that *Salmonella* is a common organism seen in osteomyelitis in SCD (254,256), but Epps and co-workers (258) found that *Staphylococcus* was the most common organism in their patients with SCD osteomyelitis. Al-Salem (259) also found that *Staphylococcus* was the most common organism in osteomyelitis in those patients with sickle cell trait. Both the metaphysis and diaphysis are common locations of infection (256,260). Septic arthritis is rare in patients with SCD. Surgical drainage of septic joints, osteomyelitis, and subperiosteal abscesses is indicated.

Other common problems in SCD include osteonecrosis of both the femoral head and proximal humerus. Wedging or flattening of the vertebral bodies is also seen in older patients (253). Fat emboli, secondary to marrow infarcts, can occur in patients with less severe SCD (HbS-C) and less frequently in patients with sickle cell anemia. Pneumococcal sepsis is the leading cause of death in young children with SCD.

Radiographic Findings

In young patients, marrow hyperplasia results in a generalized osteoporosis with widening of the medullary canal and thinning of the cortex. As the patients become older, endosteal bone apposition causes sclerosis (Fig. 6-28) and the medullary canal may actually become narrowed with thickening of the cortex. Large bone infarctions may not be visible on plain x-ray studies because of limited circulation, but commonly within 2 weeks of onset of symptoms, areas of involvement appear moth-eaten, with irregularly distributed translucent areas commonly bound by elevated periosteum with new bone formation (250). Widespread involvement may form a "bone within a bone" appearance (253). Nearly 85% of long bone infarcts are found at the junction between the metaphysis and diaphysis, and 10% are centrally located (261). Plain x-ray studies cannot distinguish between osteomyelitis and bone infarction in these patients. Although Keeley and Buchanan (251) believe that bone scans are not helpful in the diagnosis of bone infarction, Koren et al (262) noted that in the first 48 hours of symptoms, there was decreased uptake in the affected area of bone infarct by technetium bone scan. Normal isotope uptake developed approximately 1 week later. They found that increased isotope uptake was common 2 to 4 weeks after the onset of symptoms. Gallium bone scan was thought to be a helpful adjunct to this technique when osteomyelitis was suspected. Skaggs et al (263) suggest

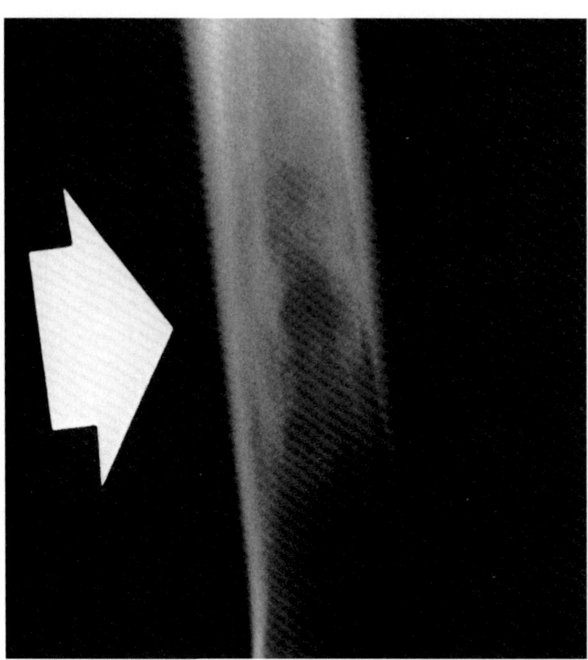

FIGURE 6-28 A young man with sickle cell disease. The lateral x-ray of the femur shows evidence of past osteonecrosis, and scalloping and radiolucencies of the shaft with sclerosis are seen posteriorly (*arrow*). This x-ray appearance can mimic osteomyelitis.

that osteomyelitis can be differentiated from bone infarction in these patients by a combination of sequential bone-marrow and bone scintigraphy. Bone infarction led to decreased activity of the radionuclide on bone-marrow scans and analogous abnormal activity on bone scans. In contrast, osteomyelitis resulted in normal activity on bone-marrow scans and abnormal activity on bone scans. These findings indicate that the combination of sequential bone marrow and bone scans within a 24-hour period is useful for early differentiation between osteomyelitis and bone infarction. MRI has not been found useful in distinguishing osteomyelitis from acute infarcts (264), but contrast material–enhanced CT scan can aid in diagnosis of osteomyelitis in these patients by its ability to visualize subperiosteal abscess (265). Differentiation of infection from infarction can be aided by aspiration and by comparing the results of technetium 99 scans with those of a bone marrow scan. Both partial and full femoral head involvement can occur in ON of the capital femoral epiphysis in SCD (253), and coxa vara also has been reported (252).

Injury

Pathologic fractures of the long bones in SCD frequently may be the first symptom of the disorder (248), and many authors report pathologic fractures in their series (250,252,257,260,266,267). In a series of 81 patients with 198 long bone infarcts with occasional concurrent osteomyelitis, Bohrer (261) found evidence of fracture in 25% of femoral lesions, 20% of humeral lesions, and a significant percentage also in tibial bone infarcts. Ebong (266) reported pathologic fractures in 20% of patients with SCD and osteomyelitis. The most common site of fracture was the femur. The fractures are transverse and commonly located in the shaft of the long bone (253), and although minimal trauma is needed to cause them (252), they often have significant displacement (261,268). The exact mechanism for pathologic fracture in these patients is unclear; although it is often associated with bone infarct, the fracture itself is seldom through the area of infarction (252). Marrow hyperplasia may be a major contributing factor; not only does the hypercellular bone marrow expand the medullary canal with thinning of both trabecular and cortical bone, but it also extends into widened haversian and Volkmann canals (253). This process probably weakens the bone sufficiently so that fractures occur. The healing process seems unaffected, and union usually occurs normally (248).

Treatment

Vaso-occlusive episodes are managed with nonsteroidal anti-inflammatory medications, oxygen, and hydration. Symptomatic bone infarction should be treated with bed rest, analgesics, and intravenous or oral administration of fluids (251). If osteomyelitis is suspected, identification of the organism should be attempted by both blood cultures and aspiration of subperiosteal fluid (256). The choice of antibiotics is based on Gram's stain. Changes in antibiotics are based on later culture results and sensitivities. The patient is monitored by C-reactive protein or sedimentation rate, and intravenous antibiotics usually are continued for at least 6 weeks. Operative management of fractures or infections in patients with SCD is potentially hazardous. Extreme care must be taken to oxygenate the patient's tissues adequately during the procedure, and ideally, elective procedures should be preceded by multiple transfusions to reduce hemoglobin (S) to less than 30% of total hemoglobin levels. A randomized multicenter study found that a simple conservative transfusion regimen to raise Hb levels to 10 g/dL was as effective as an aggressive exchange transfusion regimen (to reduce HgS to less than 30%) in preventing perioperative complications. The conservative approach resulted in only half as many transfusion-associated complications (269). Intravenous hydration also is important, with one and a half to two times the daily fluid requirements needed in addition to routine replacement of fluid losses. The use of a tourniquet in surgery for patients with SCD is somewhat controversial. Some authors believe that it is not indicated because it is potentially dangerous (253,258); others found no increased risks associated with its use in these patients (252,247). Koc et al recently found that the use of hydroxyurea lowers circulating levels of coagulation factors and increases levels of coagulation inhibitors; however, more research must be done to determine the impact of this finding on the pathogenesis and treatment of occlusive problems in SCD (270). Hydroxyurea treatment raises concerns regarding its carcinogenic potential and effect on growth of children. A recent study found 49 patients with 52 malignancies, out of 16,613 patients with SCD (271). Only three of the patients with malignancies had received hydroxyurea treatment. Results of a Phase I-II trial of hydroxyurea in children, which demonstrated no effect on height or weight, have addressed concerns regarding the potential adverse effects of hydroxyurea on growth (272).

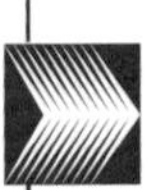

AUTHORS' PREFERRED METHOD OF TREATMENT

Sickle Cell Disease

Pathologic fractures in patients with SCD usually heal well with conservative immobilization techniques (253). Customary precautions should be followed in those patients who require open surgical procedures for displaced or unstable fractures. Osteonecrosis of the femoral head is an especially difficult problem in patients with SCD. Treatment options include conservative measures and core decompression (a multicenter trial is under way). Patients with total head involvement may require femoral or pelvic osteotomies. Athanassiou-Metaxa et al show that out of 9 children treated with subtrochanteric varus femoral osteotomy for femoral head osteonecrosis, 8 children experienced improvements in pain, joint motion, and walking (273). Total joint replacement is occasionally indicated in young adults. Before general anesthesia, the patient's hematocrit should be raised to more than 30 Hb to more than 10 g/dL.

Leukemias

Leukemia accounts for over 30% of cases of childhood cancer. Acute lymphocytic leukemia (ALL) is one of the most common malignant diseases in childhood and accounts for 80% of pediatric leukemias. There is an increased occurrence of lymphoid leukemias in patients with Down syndrome, immunodeficiencies, and ataxic telangiectasia. The peak incidence occurs at 4 years of age.

Leukemic involvement of bones and joints is common. Skeletal lesions occur more frequently in leukemic children than in adults because a child's small marrow reserve can be replaced quickly by leukemic cells. Approximately 50% to 75% of children with acute leukemia develop radiographic skeletal manifestations during the course of their disease (274,275). Rogalsky et al (276) reported a 12% incidence of fracture associated with acute leukemic lesions.

Clinical Presentation

Patients present with fatigue, pallor, purpura, fever, hepatosplenomegaly, or bone and joint pain; 20% to 60% of patients present with musculoskeletal signs or symptoms (277). In one series, bone pain was a presenting symptom in 59% of patients (278,279). Rogalsky et al (276) reported a 20.6% incidence of reports of problems with the skeletal system at initial presentation. Migratory arthritis may be present in some patients; point pain is believed to be secondary to leukemic cell infiltrate of the metaphyseal periosteum (279). Leukemia may mimic osteomyelitis, rheumatic fever, septic arthritis, and tuberculosis (280). Either leukocytosis or leukopenia is present, and the presence of immature leukocytes in the peripheral blood smear should suggest a diagnosis of leukemia. In the early phase of the disease, anemia, neutropenia, and thrombocytopenia occur in 80% of patients; 10% of children have normal peripheral blood counts. Bone marrow aspirate usually is diagnostic.

Radiographic Findings

No pathognomonic osseous manifestations occur in acute leukemia. Skeletal involvement occurs in approximately 50% of patients, and diffuse osteopenia is the most frequent manifestation. Lucencies and periostitis may mimic osteomyelitis.

Nonspecific juxtaepiphyseal lucent lines are a result of generalized metabolic dysfunction. Sclerotic bands of bone trabeculae are more typical in older children. A characteristic lesion seen within a month of onset of symptoms is a radiolucent metaphyseal band adjacent to the physis. These are usually bilateral and vary from 2 to 15 mm in width (279). Similar radiolucent bands are seen both in infants with scurvy and in older children with neuroblastoma.

Osteolytic lesions with punctate areas of radiolucency are found in the metaphyses and can either appear moth-eaten or as a confluent radiolucency. Similar lesions can be present in the diaphysis (281), the skull, pelvis, ribs, and bones of the hands and feet. Large geographic lesions also may be seen. Periosteal reaction often is present with osteolytic lesions and is most common in the posterior cortex of the distal femoral metaphysis, the medial neck of the femur, and the diaphyses of the tibia and fibula (282).

With medical management, remission rates are now up to 98%, with cure rates approaching 80% (283). The complication seen most commonly by orthopaedic surgeons is osteonecrosis (ON) of the femoral head (284,285). This may occur after chemotherapy, after chemotherapy and allogenic bone marrow transplantation (BMT), or after graft-versus-host disease (GVH) related to BMT (286). Although most ON is attributed to glucocorticoid therapy, L-asparaginase can contribute to thrombophilia and has been implicated in the production of ON. The risk of ON is especially high after BMT in boys older than 16 years who are treated for GVH with steroids or irradiation. MRI is best for the early detection of ON. Treatment modalities include weight relief, symptomatic treatment, core decompression, and total hip replacement. Bizot et al (287) described the results in 27 patients treated with total hip arthroplasty for ON after allogenic BMT.

Most bone lesions in leukemia improve during remission after treatment and tend to progress with worsening of the disease. The radiolucent metaphyseal bands usually are not affected by treatment, however, and further demineralization of the skeleton may occur with both corticosteroid use and methotrexate therapy. Diffuse demineralization of the skeleton occurs in almost all patients with widening of the medullary canal and thinning of the cortex (279). Although increased uptake of isotope is seen on technetium bone scan in 80% of patients, positive areas of isotope uptake correlate poorly with both sites of clinical bone pain and the presence of lesions on x-ray study (288).

Several authors (274,289–291) have attempted to evaluate

the prognostic significance of the extent of bone involvement in childhood leukemia. Hughes et al (284) reported that major skeletal involvement, in fact, may correlate with a better overall outcome in childhood leukemia. Heinrich et al (274) concluded that children without radiographic skeletal abnormalities have an aggressive form of acute leukemia that results in a worse prognosis.

Injury

Pathologic lesions predisposing children to a fracture usually resolve during treatment. Fracture is most commonly associated with osteoporosis of the spine, resulting in vertebrae plana. Fractures occasionally occur at other locations and usually after minor trauma (Fig. 6-20).

Vertebral compression fractures are the most commonly reported fractures associated with leukemia. The thoracic vertebrae are the most commonly involved; uniform spinal osteoporosis often is present (284,292). A bone scan may aid in identifying clinically silent areas but may not correlate with areas of obvious destruction on x-rays. Spastic paraparesis has been reported in one patient with vertebral fracture due to leukemia (284).

Treatment

Most fractures are treated using standard methods (Fig. 6-29). Newman and Melhorn (292) noted a prompt decrease in pain in four patients with vertebral fractures due to leukemia once chemotherapy was initiated. No bracing was used in these patients, and full activity was encouraged. In one of their patients observed for more than 5 years, there was no evidence of healing of the fractured vertebra on x-ray study. There are no specific treatment recommendations for any other associated pathologic fractures of leukemia in the literature.

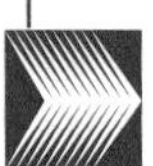

AUTHORS' PREFERRED METHOD OF TREATMENT

Leukemias

Prompt diagnosis and initiation of chemotherapy is the first step in the treatment of pathologic fractures associated with leukemia. Most fractures are stable microfractures and can be treated with conservative immobilization techniques with emphasis on early ambulation to avoid further problems with disuse osteoporosis. Most vertebral fractures can be treated nonoperatively with close observation.

Hemophilia

Hemophilia is a sex-linked recessive disorder of the clotting mechanism that presents most commonly as a functional defi-

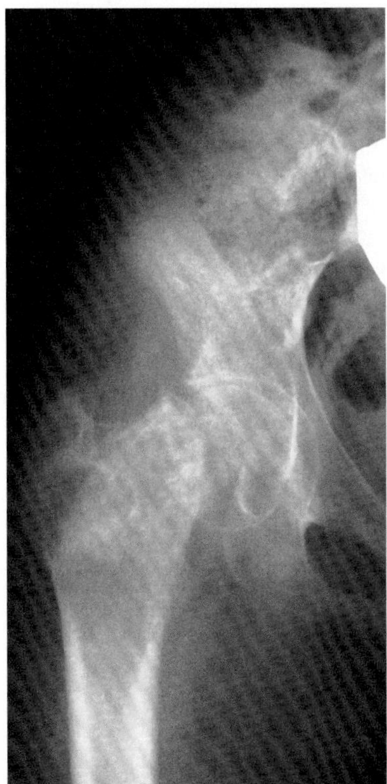

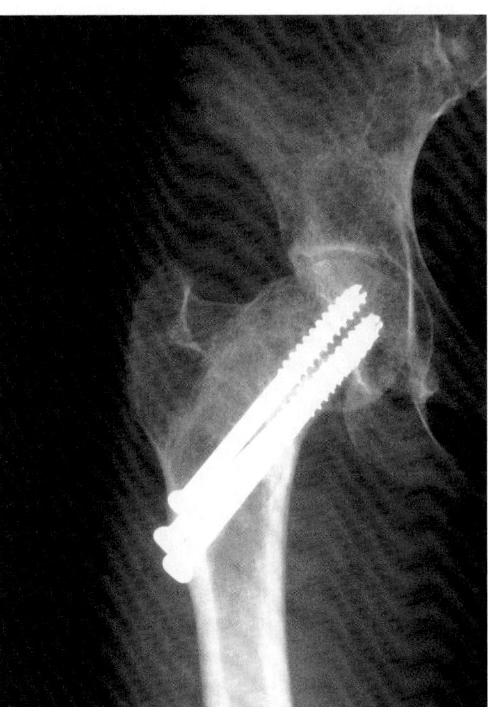

A B

FIGURE 6-29 **A.** A 13-year-old girl with acute lymphocytic leukemia presented with a pathologic fracture of the right hip. Note the destructive changes associated with the displaced femoral neck fracture. **B.** Follow-up x-ray studies 1 year after surgery show healing with slight varus and without evidence of osteonecrosis. At present, the patient is alive and well, has no hip pain and walks with a very slight Trendelenburg gait.

ciency of either factor VIII (hemophilia A) or factor IX (hemophilia B). Classic hemophilia, or hemophilia A (factor VIII deficiency), is an inherited sex-linked recessive disorder. The incidence is 1 per 10,000 live male births in the United States (293). Christmas disease, or hemophilia B, is a sex-linked recessive factor IX deficiency and occurs in 1 per 40,000 live births.

When hemophilia is suspected, screening tests should be performed, including platelet count, bleeding time, prothrombin time, and partial thromboplastin time. Deficiency of factor VII, the most common form of hemophilia, causes a marked prolongation in the partial thromboplastin time (294). Once the disease is suspected, specific factor assays can document the type of hemophilia.

Musculoskeletal complications in a child with hemophilia include acute hemarthroses (knee, elbow, and ankle, in decreasing order of frequency), soft tissue and muscle bleeds, acute compartment syndrome, carpal tunnel syndrome, and femoral nerve neuropraxia. The severity of the deficiency often is correlated with circulating levels of factor VIII or IX (Table 6-7). The disease is classified as severe when clotting activity is less than 1%, moderate when clotting activity is 1% to 5%, and mild when clotting activity is more than 5%. By definition, each milliliter of normal human plasma contains one unit of factor activity, and the clinical severity of hemophilia correlates with the patient's percentage of normal levels of plasma factor activity (Table 6-7). Early diagnosis and aggressive management are the keys to lessening complications.

Treatment—Bleeding Episodes

During bleeding episodes, the primary therapy is intravenous replacement of the deficient factor. Several different treatment plans exist. In on-demand therapy, the traditional method of hemophilia management, factor replacement is given at the first sign of a bleeding episode. Primary prophylaxis involves initiation of regular factor replacement therapy soon after the diagnosis of severe hemophilia (usually when the child is 1 to 2 years of age) with the intention of preventing joint bleeds. Secondary prophylaxis is used after a child has established a pattern of frequent bleeding but before frequent joint bleeds occur.

Empirically, one unit of factor VIII per kilogram of body weight will raise plasma activity by 2%, and a similar dose of factor IX will elevate the plasma level of that factor by 1.5% (293). The usual half-life of factor VIII varies from 6 to 12 hours and that of factor IX varies from 8 to 18 hours. Routinely in the nonbleeding patient, factor VIII must be given every 8 hours and factor IX must be given every 12 hours to maintain a stable factor level. Higher than usual dosages given more frequently are necessary in patients with active bleeding. In the past, factor replacement was accomplished through plasma transfusion, but the quantities necessary for adequate factor levels may result in circulatory overload and pulmonary edema (295). This problem was eventually solved through the use of cryoprecipitate, protein prepared from plasma that is rich in factor VIII and fibrinogen. More concentrated forms of both factor VIII and factor IX (Konyne 80) have become available. The reader is referred to an excellent review by Connelly and Kaleko (296) for a summary of gene therapy for patients with hemophilia A.

TABLE 6-7 Severity of Hemophilia Correlated with Plasma Factor Activity Levels

Degree of Hemophilia	Percentage of Factor	Clinical Characteristics
Mild	20%–60%	Usually clinically occult, excessive bleeding after major trauma or surgery
Moderate	5%–20%	Excessive bleeding during surgery and after minor trauma
Moderately severe	1%–5%	Excessive bleeding with mild injury and infrequent spontaneous hemarthrosis
Severe	Less than 1%	Frequent excessive bleeding with trauma and spontaneous bleeding into the soft tissue and joints

Surgery in Hemophilia

Should a child with hemophilia require operative management of a fracture, the orthopedist and the hematologist should work closely together. Preoperatively, the patient should be tested for the presence of inhibitor and a test dose of factor replacement should be given to determine the biologic half-life of that factor for that particular patient (293). Elective surgery usually is contraindicated in the presence of inhibitor. Most authors recommend a level of factor activity during surgery ranging from 70% to 100% (293,295,297), although others believe that approximately 50% is adequate (298,299). Tourniquets are recommended for extremity surgery. The use of routine drains is not advised, but 24 hours of suction drainage is favored by some (293,295,297). Factor levels are checked immediately after surgery and then at least daily. Factor VIII is given every 6 hours, and factor IX is given every 8 hours. It is useful to check a trough level factor activity immediately before the next dose of factor supplementation. In the immediate postoperative period, factor levels are maintained at 30% to 40% (293,297), and these levels should be maintained until sutures are removed. During the rehabilitative period, maintenance levels of factor ranging from 20% to 50% immediately before sessions of physical therapy should be maintained (293,295,298,300). Intramuscular injections of analgesics should obviously be avoided, as should aspirin compounds and nonsteroidal antiinflammatory medications that affect platelet function. Both acetaminophen (Tylenol) and codeine medications are safe oral analgesics (301). In the past, hemophiliac patients had an increased risk of operative infections and delayed wound healing, but aggressive replacement therapy has minimized those problems (295).

Injury

Fractures and Dislocations

Clinical Presentation. Fractures in patients with hemophilia do not appear to happen more or less frequently than in nonhemophilic patients (302). Most authors have noted that healing of fractures proceeds primarily with endosteal callus and very little periosteal callus (303–305), but Lancourt et al (300) observed significant periosteal calcification in these fractures with a normal rate of healing. Fractures occur in both the upper and lower extremities (303,304,306–308). Joint dislocations are rare in hemophiliac patients. Floman and Niska (309) reported on a 6-year-old boy who sustained a posterior dislocation of the hip with mild trauma that required a closed reduction under general anesthesia and immobilization in a hip spica cast. The joint was found to be ankylosed at 6-year follow-up. Ackroyd and Dinley (310) reported on two patients who had their patellas locked into the intercondylar notch of the distal femur after sustaining hyperflexion injuries of the knees, which had limited range of motion owing to arthropathy. These injuries were treated by flexion of the knee under general anesthesia, depression of the inferior pole of the patella to unlock it, and then extension of the knee followed by splinting.

Treatment. Most fractures in hemophiliac patients are treated conservatively with immobilization. Factor replacement is important for about the first week after the fracture, and levels of factor activity recommended vary from 20% to 50% (293,300,303,306,307,311). Circumferential plaster casts are extremely hazardous in the treatment of these fractures because of the risk of swelling from bleeding as well as subsequent compartment syndrome and skin necrosis (312). A Robert Jones dressing may be preferable for fracture immobilization immediately after injury, and a cast should be applied once active swelling has stopped (311). All casts applied should be well padded and split, and the patient should be monitored carefully for swelling. Fractures of the femur can be treated with traction and subsequent spica casting (307). Some authors consider skeletal traction to be hazardous because of the risk of infection or bleeding (293,311), but Boardman and English (307) believe that with proper replacement therapy, skeletal pins can be used in the hemophiliac. Replacement therapy is advisable while fractures are manipulated and casts are changed. Most authors think that open reduction and internal fixation should be performed in hemophiliac patients for fractures that would customarily be treated with such methods (293,300,307). External fixators are not commonly used for patients with hemophilia, however, in a recent study, Lee et al describes the use of external fixators (Ilizarov, AO-uni- and bi-planar fixators and Charnley clamp) in nine patients with hemophilia for arthrodesis of infected joints, treatment of open fractures and osteoclasis. One major complication related to external fixators occurred, in a patient who developed inhibitors. They conclude that external fixators can be used safely in hemophilic patients without inhibitors and does not require prolonged factor replacement (313).

Muscle Hematoma

Clinical Presentation. Hematomas of the soft tissues in hemophiliacs occur in superficial tissues but are more of a clinical problem when they develop in muscle (300). Although most are spontaneous, a history of trauma was noted in 24% of 178 episodes of muscle hematoma in one series (314). In order of frequency, the most common sites of involvement in that series were the quadriceps, calf, anterior compartment of the leg, thigh adductors, hamstrings, and sartorius muscle. The first clinical symptoms are tenderness, stiffness, and swelling of the involved muscle group with pain on motion (314). A hematoma in the iliacus muscle can present as severe groin pain, flexion deformity of the hip, and a tender mass palpable along the iliac crest. Passive extension of the hip increases pain, and significant swelling of the muscle can cause compression of the femoral nerve by the inguinal ligament superiorly and the iliopectineal ligament medially (with subsequent femoral nerve palsy and quadriceps muscle paralysis). Ultrasound (315), CT scan (316), and MRI are useful in documenting the presence of muscle hematoma. Wilson et al (317) noted that in early hemorrhage of the muscle, the ultrasound shows increased echogenicity, but in established muscle hematoma, the echogenicity is decreased. This may be helpful in recurrence, because fresh hemorrhage into an organizing hematoma can be distinguished by this technique. One should not assume that all groin pain in hemophilia is due to an iliacus muscle hematoma. Although rare, hip hemarthrosis can occur, and septic arthritis of the hip has also been reported in hemophiliac patients. In this clinical situation, a hip ultrasound and aspiration can help make the correct diagnosis (317).

Treatment. The most important consideration in the treatment of a patient with muscle hematoma is early initiation of replacement therapy. Aronstam et al (318) found that if replacement therapy was initiated within 2 hours of onset of symptoms, then excellent recovery ensued. The only exception to this finding was hematomas of the calf muscles, which responded equally well to replacement therapy if it was treated within 3 hours of the onset of symptoms. Most authors recommend raising factor levels to between 20% and 50% (293,311,314,319,320) and continuing treatment for 24 hours (314) to 5 days (300). The patient should not bear weight on the extremity (314), and the affected joints should be placed in a position of comfort, with a compression dressing and ice packs applied to the swollen muscle (311,314). Quadriceps muscle function usually returns with recovery from quadriceps hematoma. Infrequently, ectopic bone may form in the soft tissues after hematoma (321). In severe cases of muscle hemorrhage that do not respond to conservative treatment, fasciotomy and neurolysis (with proper replacement therapy) may be necessary (300).

Neurapraxia. In addition to the compression of the femoral nerve seen in iliacus hematoma, neurapraxia in hemophiliacs can occur in the peroneal, sciatic, median, and ulnar nerves (293). Carpal tunnel syndrome due to hemorrhagic compression of the median nerve has been reported (303,322). Factor levels for these patients should be raised to 80% to 100% of normal for 2 days and then maintained at 40% of factor levels for another 7 days with splinting of the extremity (293). Another neurologic complication in patients with hemophilia is significant intracranial bleeding from minor head trauma. This has been reported in 2% to 13% of children who have hemophilia and von Willebrand's disease (323).

Pseudotumor of Hemophilia

Clinical Presentation. The pseudotumor of hemophilia is a cystic swelling of the muscle due to hematoma. Adjacent bone erosion is often evident on plain x-ray study and is seen most frequently in the ilium and femur (324). In children, a pathologic fracture can occur after a destructive pseudotumor of the femoral shaft. Pseudotumors can also evolve after fracture of the femur (325). These lesions may develop through subperiosteal hemorrhage, which causes pressure necrosis of the overlying muscle and underlying bone (305). Progressive enlargement can compress surrounding vital soft-tissue structures, and extreme enlargement may eventually result in skin perforation, with infection and possible death (325). In children, the peripheral skeleton is most commonly affected by pseudotumor (311), and the small bones in the hands and feet are the most common sites; the prognosis is better with these sites than with more centrally located pseudotumors (306). Large pseudotumors may develop calcific deposits that are visible on plain x-ray studies. An established cyst may be associated with semilunar struts of bone projecting from the adjacent bone at the proximal and distal ends of the pseudocyst (325). With involvement of the small bones of hands and feet, interosseous expansile lesions with surrounding periosteal elevation are seen (300). The CT scan is useful in delineating the extent of pseudotumor (326).

Treatment. Aspiration is contraindicated in treatment of pseudocysts—the needle track may fail to heal, the hematoma soon recurs, with the possibility of infection and bleeding from the needle wound (293,305,320,325). Very early treatment of small pseudotumors with replacement therapy, compression dressings, and prolonged immobilization may arrest their development (200,306,311,327). Factor levels of 50% were used in one series (306). Surgical excision of the pseudotumor may be necessary if the diagnosis is in question or if the lesion is enlarging with danger of skin perforation (293,328).

Hemarthrosis

Clinical Presentation. Patients with severe hemophilia have a high rate of hemarthrosis. The joints most commonly involved in decreasing order of frequency include the knees, elbows, ankles, hips, and shoulders (293). There usually is a prodrome of stiffness and pain before clinical swelling, and trauma usually is absent. The joint is held in a position of flexion that is most comfortable, and eventually, the joint becomes tense and swollen with decreased range of motion. A subacute hemarthrosis of the knee is said to be present when two or more episodes of acute hemarthrosis have preceded it. On clinical examination, the synovium is very thick and boggy with decreased range of motion of the joint. Pain is uncommon. In chronic hemarthrosis, generally a subacute arthrosis has been present for at least 6 months, and destructive changes are present on the x-ray studies of the knee with osteoporosis, overgrowth of the epiphysis with subchondral cysts, and eventual narrowing of the joint space (Fig. 6-30) (293). MRI was found to be useful in examining both the hypertrophied synovium in hemophilia arthropathy as well as subchondral cysts (329,330). Various systems of classification of joint arthropathy of the knee in hemophilia have been proposed (293,331). The chronic phase of articular involvement for patients with hemophilia can lead to articular cartilage degeneration from recurrent bleeds and effusions. Initially, synovial hypertrophy and chronic hyperemia occur, followed by epiphyseal overgrowth. Articular involvement may be graded as shown in Table 6-8.

Treatment. The first step in the treatment of joint hemarthrosis is prompt factor replacement with levels ranging from 30% to 50% (293,294,332,333), maintaining levels for up to 4 days for severe cases (332). Home care factor replacement provides a means of rapid initiation of therapy (293). With effective treatment, usually prompt pain relief is achieved in minutes after initiation of replacement therapy, and the extremity should be splinted and ice should be applied to the joint (293). In acute hemarthrosis of the knee with a very tense, swollen joint that is not responding well to replacement therapy, early aspiration may be of some value. For aspiration to be successful, a large

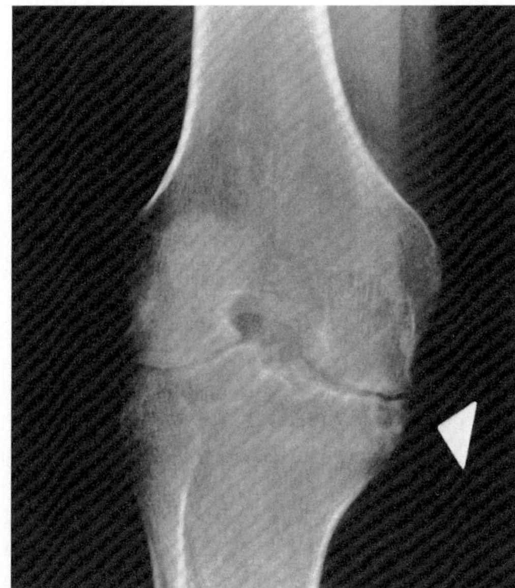

FIGURE 6-30 A 22-year-old man with hemophilia had frequent hemarthrosis of the knee. Moderately severe arthropathy is present, with joint space narrowing, spurring, and subchondral cyst (*arrow*).

TABLE 6-8 Grades of Articular Involvement

Grade 1	Transitory synovitis; no bleeding sequelae, and with no more than three episodes in 3 months
Grade 2	Permanent synovitis with increased joint size, synovial thickening, and limitation of movement
Grade 3	Chronic arthropathy with axial deformity and muscular atrophy
Grade 4	Ankylosis

needle, such as a 16-gauge needle, must be used (300), and aspiration must be accomplished within 24 hours of the onset of swelling because the clot begins to loculate after that time (311). Factor replacement must not be given before the aspiration because this will promote clotting of the hemarthrosis fluid and prevent removal; ideally, therapy is initiated at the same time as aspiration (319). The value of aspiration is uncertain because there was no difference in the range of motion between aspirated and unaspirated knees at 5-day follow-up in one controlled trial (334). In addition to factor replacement, splinting, ice packs, and compression bandages are helpful (300).

Nonsteroidal antiinflammatory drugs (NSAIDs) and intraarticular dexamethasone are used by some. A short course of corticosteroids seems to reduce the need for long-term replacement therapy (335). In subacute hemarthrosis, aspiration is not necessary, and factor replacement with levels from 20% to 30% is used three times weekly to protect the patient from further bleeding during physical therapy sessions (336). Mobilization should continue for 3 to 4 weeks, and if there is no response to therapy, synovectomy may be indicated (300). A target joint is defined as one with four bleeding episodes in a 6-month period. Treatment involves regular replacement therapy for at least 6 to 12 weeks to interrupt bleeding cycles. Replacement therapy can include recombinant or plasma-derived factor; most patients use recombinant factor. In general, 1 unit per kg of body weight of factor VIII concentrate provides a 2% increase in the factor VIII plasma activity. Today, acute joint bleeds are treated with a more intensive therapy than was used previously (294,333).

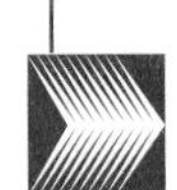

AUTHORS' PREFERRED METHOD OF TREATMENT

Hemophilia

Collaboration between the orthopedist and the hematologist is important in providing care for children with hemophilia. Most fractures in children with hemophilia can be treated with either traction or cast techniques. Care must be taken to avoid complications related to compression in these patients, and a monovalved, well-padded plaster cast provides a safe means of treatment. A fiberglass cast is not as desirable because a simple monovalve will fail to expand the cast completely. Operative treatment should be reserved for fractures that normally require surgery, and the usual precautions for hemophiliac patients for surgery are observed. Muscle hematomas are treated with a combination of replacement therapy, ice packs, bed rest, and a particular emphasis on rehabilitation. CT scans are extremely helpful in following the course of an iliopsoas muscle hematoma. Pseudotumors of the small bones of the hands and feet can be treated with excision and bone grafting. Hemarthrosis of the knee responds well to prompt factor replacement therapy and immobilization; aspiration is seldom needed. The orthopaedic surgeon caring for patients with hemophilia must be ever mindful of the possible presence of both hepatitis and HIV, and the utmost care should be used in any sort of invasive procedure with these patients.

OSTEOMYELITIS

The character of pediatric acute hematogenous osteomyelitis in North America has changed during the past several decades. Although the typical clinical picture of acute osteomyelitis in children is still seen, subtle presentations have become more frequent. There are several reasons for this change, including modification of the clinical course by antibiotics given before admission (337) and, possibly, increased awareness and an earlier presentation to a medical facility resulting in earlier diagnosis. Children often present with subacute osteomyelitis (Fig. 6-31 and Table 6-9). Less common variants include Brodie's abscess, subacute epiphyseal osteomyelitis, viral osteomyelitis (338), and chronic recurrent multifocal osteomyelitis (339). Some patients present with a bone lesion that may be confused with other disease entities, including neoplasm (340). All can masquerade as osteomyelitis with fever and tenderness over areas of focal leukemic bone destruction (341). Biopsy often is needed to clarify the diagnosis. Even with appropriate antibiotic therapy, some patients have recurrent infection, growth disturbance, or pathologic fractures.

Definitions

Acute hematogenous osteomyelitis can be classified by age (neonatal, childhood, and adult osteomyelitis), organism (pyogenic and granulomatous infections), onset (acute, subacute, and chronic osteomyelitis), and routes of infection (hematogenous and direct inoculation). Chronic osteomyelitis is defined by most authors as osteomyelitis with symptoms that have been present for longer than 1 month.

Clinical Presentation

Most patients with acute hematogenous osteomyelitis present with fever, pain, and localized tenderness at the site of infection.

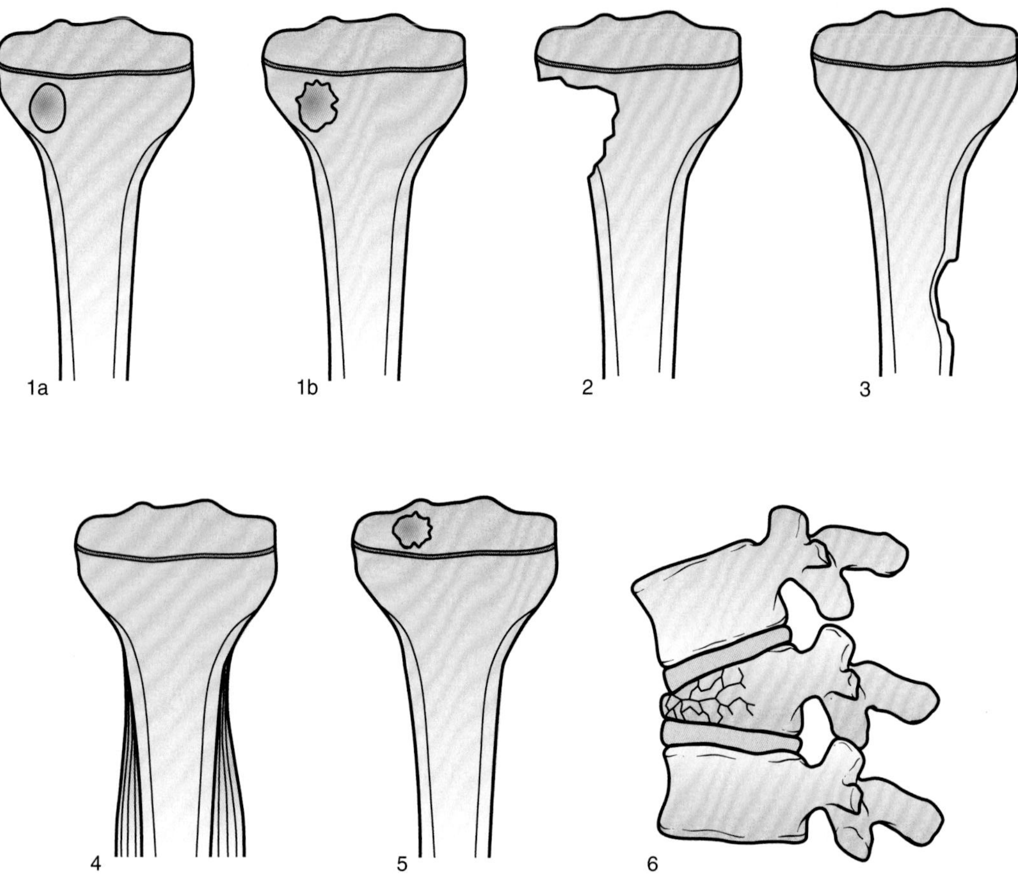

FIGURE 6-31 Classification of subacute osteomyelitis. (From Dormans JP, Drummond DS. Pediatric hematogenous osteomyelitis: new trends in presentation, diagnosis, and treatment. Redrawn from *J Am Acad Orthop Surg* 1994;2:333–341; with permission.)

In order of decreasing frequency, the most commonly involved bones include the femur, tibia, humerus, fibula, radius, phalanges, calcaneus, ulna, ischium, metatarsals, and vertebral bodies. Although the erythrocyte sedimentation rate is commonly elevated in osteomyelitis, the white blood count is normal in 40% to 75% of patients (342). Blood cultures are positive for the infecting organism in 40% to 50% of patients (343), and direct cultures of the site of infection are positive in no more than 70% (342). The most common organism in hematogenous osteomyelitis is *Staphylococcus aureus.* In very young children, *Streptococcus pneumoniae* has a significant prevalence (342), and *Haemophilus influenzae* has virtually been eliminated as a musculoskeletal pathogen by immunization. Table 6-10 shows the most common organisms affective individuals by age.

Radiographic Evaluation

Only 20% of patients have plain x-ray findings of osteomyelitis within 10 to 14 days after onset of symptoms; the earliest finding is loss of defined deep soft-tissue planes (342). Because of this early insensitivity of plain x-ray studies, isotope scanning techniques have been used to aid in diagnosis with varying rates of success. In proven osteomyelitis, abnormal technetium scans are seen in 63% to 90% of patients (344). In neonates with osteomyelitis, only 31.5% had abnormal technetium bone scans in one series (345). After plain x-ray studies, MRI is the study of choice for defining the stage and extent of osteomyelitis (346). Bone infection can be identified by soft-tissue changes through MRI techniques in 92% of patients, but the presence of previous surgery or coexisting fractures affects the accuracy of this study (347).

Injury

In 1932, Capener and Pierce (348) reviewed 1,068 patients with osteomyelitis and found only 18 pathologic fractures, 13 of which occurred in the femur. They thought these fractures were due to delayed recognition of the infection or inadequate treatment. Other factors were disuse osteopenia, presence of a weak involucrum, and excessive surgical removal of involved bone. In that pre-antibiotic era, most of the fractures were sustained after surgical treatment of the osteomyelitis, and the au-

TABLE 6-9 Comparison of Acute to Subacute Osteomyelitis

Presentation	Subacute	Acute
Pain	Mild	Severe
Fever	Few patients	Majority
Loss of function	Minimal	Marked
Prior antibiotics	Often (30%–40%)	Occasional
Elevated WBC	Few	Majority
ESR	Majority	Majority
Blood cultures	Few positive	50% positive
Bone cultures	60% positive	85% positive
Initial x-ray study	Frequently abnormal	Often normal
Site	Any location (may cross physis)	Usually metaphysis

From Dormans JP, Drummond DS. Pediatric hematogenous osteomyelitis: new trends in presentation, diagnosis, and treatment. *J Am Acad Ortho Surg* 1994;2:333–341.

TABLE 6-10 Initial Antibiotic Therapy for Osteomyelitis

Patient Type	Probable Organism	Initial Antibiotic
Neonate	Grp. B Strep, *S. aureus*, gram-negative rods (*H. influenza*)	Cefotaxime (100–120 mg/kg/24 h) or oxacillin and gentamicin (5–7.5 mg/kg/24 h)
Infants and children	*S. aureus* (90%) if allergic to penicillin[a] if allergic to penicillin and cephalosporins[a]	Oxacillin (150 mg/kg/24 h) Cefazolin (100 mg/kg/24 h) Clindamycin (25–40 mg/kg/24 h) or Vancomycin (40 mg/kg/24 h)
Sickle cell disease	*S. aureus* or Salmonella	Oxacillin and ampicillin or chloramphenicol or cefotaxime (100–120 mg/kg/24 h)

[a] Overall 80% due to *S. aureus.*

thors believed that conservation of the involucrum and proper immobilization could have prevented these injuries. White and Dennison (349) noted that before antibiotics, pathologic fractures of osteomyelitis were common, but union occurred with certainty in the presence of dense involucrum. Daoud and Saighi-Bouaouina (350) reported on 34 patients with hematogenous osteomyelitis complicated by pathologic fracture, pseudarthrosis, or significant segmental bone loss. The tibia was affected in 24 cases, the femur was affected in 8 cases, and the humerus was affected in 2 cases. A pathologic proximal femoral fracture has been reported in neonatal osteomyelitis (345). Although the condition is rare, hematogenous osteomyelitis can also develop at the site of a closed fracture from 1 to 6 weeks after injury (351–353). Canale et al (351) reported three children with osteomyelitis after closed fracture. They pointed out that progressive pain and swelling at a fracture site during healing are suggestive of possible osteomyelitis. Daoud et al (354) reported 35 children with upper femoral osteomyelitis with associated septic arthritis. The incidence of ON of the femoral head was approximately 50% both in the group that was treated with arthrotomy and in the group in which no surgery had been done. They postulated that ON of the femoral head may be due to compression by abscess of the vessels lying on the posterior superior femoral neck. The complications of fracture, dislocation, and displacement of the capital femoral epiphysis occurred in two thirds of their patients, and these usually were patients who presented long after an acute phase of the disease. They recommended surgical drainage of septic hips, and reduction and stabilization of hips with ON using skin traction and plaster immobilization for 40 to 60 days. Lewallen and Peterson (353) documented osteomyelitis in 40% of 20 nonunions of diaphyseal open fractures in children. They believed that the presence of infection was a significant factor in their failure to heal. Long bone lesions also may be present in congenital rubella (356), and pathologic fractures have been reported in congenital cytomegalic inclusion disease (357).

Treatment

Once osteomyelitis is clinically suspected, needle aspiration of the area of maximal tenderness of the long bone is recommended to obtain the causative organism either from subperiosteal fluid or from the metaphysis directly. If gross purulent material is obtained, surgical drainage should follow (341). Ultrasound or MRI may be helpful in evaluating equivocal cases. Decreasing the duration of intravenous antibiotic treatment of osteomyelitis appears to be appropriate as long as certain criteria are met. If oral antibiotics are inappropriate or the organism is not isolated by culture, then longer-term parenteral antibiotics must be considered. Total length of therapy is based on the type of organism isolated and the patient's response to treatment. Unkila-Kallio et al (358) found that in acute hematogenous osteomyelitis in children, the serum C-reactive protein correlated more closely than erythrocyte sedimentation rate to the clinical course of osteomyelitis, with rapid elevation at the onset of disease and a significantly faster decline with effective treatment than the erythrocyte sedimentation rate.

Fracture Management

Fractures associated with osteomyelitis may be difficult to treat and may be associated with complications such as malunion and growth disturbance (359). Pathologic fractures associated with osteomyelitis are rare in North America and usually are associated with neglected or chronic osteomyelitis, neonatal osteomyelitis, or septic arthritis (Fig. 6-32). In children with chronic osteomyelitis, the purulent material elevates the periosteum and a supportive involucrum develops. Sequestrectomy of a portion of the necrotic diaphysis while leaving the supportive involucrum is often needed to bring the infection under control, but the timing of this procedure is controversial. Langenskiold (360) delayed sequestrectomy of a necrotic femoral shaft for 10 months in a 6-year-old patient to allow the involucrum to develop, but Daoud and Saighi-Bouaouina (350) recommended much earlier debridement. In patients with active infection, they performed sequestrectomy with debridement, followed by antibiotic therapy for up to 6 months. Prolonged cast immobilization was necessary. They obtained healing in 33 of 34 patients with pathologic fractures or pseudarthroses due to osteomyelitis. The mean healing time of fractures was 5 months in patients with involucrum. Patients with active infection without involucrum required debridement, antibiotics, and subsequent treatment with corticocancellous iliac graft. The mean healing time was 8.7 months. Their patients without active infection and no involucrum were treated with prolonged immobilization and cancellous bone graft supplemented by fixation. Angular deformities were treated with cast manipulation. Tudisco et al (361) reported on 26 patients with chronic osteomyelitis with average follow-up of 23 years. Approximately 15% had shortening and angular deformity of the affected limb. Newer techniques for difficult cases have also been developed.

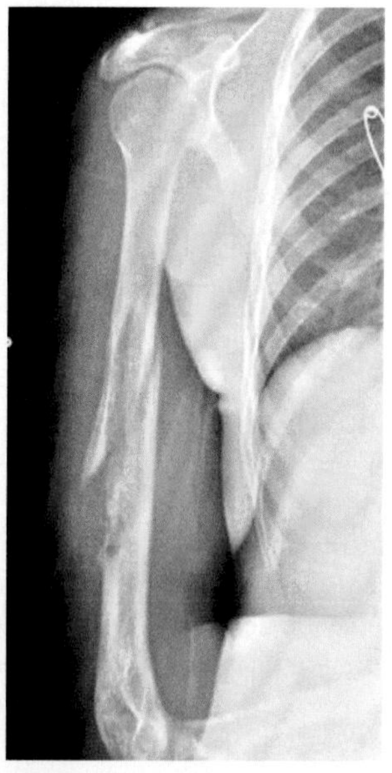

FIGURE 6-32 This lateral x-ray of the humeral shaft of a 17-year-old boy shows a pathologic fracture through chronic osteomyelitis of the humerus. (Case courtesy of B. David Horn, MD.)

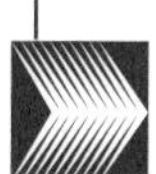

AUTHORS' PREFERRED METHOD OF TREATMENT

Osteomyelitis

With early recognition and appropriate treatment, osteomyelitis leading to pathologic fracture is uncommon. When osteomyelitis is associated with pathologic fracture, it usually is neglected chronic osteomyelitis, or rarely, neonatal osteomyelitis or septic arthritis. The most important step in the treatment of fracture associated with osteomyelitis is to control the underlying infection. At a minimum, this requires drainage and debridement of the infection with immobilization in association with antibiotic therapy. In advanced infections, sequestrectomy may be necessary. MRI is useful in identifying the sequestrum; an attempt should be made to leave as much supporting involucrum as possible at the time of sequestrectomy. Bone transport and lengthening may be valuable in certain cases. Prolonged immobilization with either plaster casts or external fixation devices may be needed, and segmental bone loss can be treated with bone transport or grafting.

PATHOLOGIC FRACTURES AFTER LIMB LENGTHENING

Limb lengthening has evolved dramatically over the past several decades. Surgeons experienced with lengthening techniques can now correct problems that previously had no satisfactory solution. The very high complication rate that has come with these advances has decreased with newer techniques and more extensive surgical experience. Complications with the Wagner method, popular 20 to 30 years ago, were as high as 92% (362,363). Newer techniques, using gradual lengthening with either monolateral fixators or fine wire fixators, such as the Ilizarov fixator, have decreased the complication rate.

Fractures that occur in association with limb lengthening fall into three general categories: (a) fractures through pin tracks, (b) fractures through regenerate bone, or (c) fractures through bone weakened by disuse osteoporosis. Fractures that occur through holes left after removal of screws or fine wires generally occur a few weeks after device removal. The incidence of these fractures can be minimized by protective weight-bearing after removal of the device and using the smallest possible screw diameter that is appropriate for the fixation device needed.

Fractures through regenerate bone are true pathologic fractures. The bone that is formed by distraction callotasis must be subjected to normal weight-bearing forces over a period of time before normal bony architecture is established. Fractures that occur through the lengthening gap can occur either soon after removal of the fixator, or years later. Various reports describe fractures through regenerative bone occurring as late as 2 to 8 years after lengthening (363–365). The incidence of fractures has been reported to be as high as 18% for Wagner lengthenings but only 3% for newer techniques (362,365–369). At present, most lengthenings are performed through the metaphysis, which has a larger bone diameter and better blood supply than the diaphysis (where Wagner lengthening was done) (370). When fractures occur in regenerate bone, they can be treated with simple cast immobilization. However, because this method further promotes osteopenia, many surgeons reapply a fixator, correct any malalignment caused by the fracture, and compress at the fracture site until healing. To ensure that the regenerate bone can bear the forces of normal activity, a variety of imaging methods have been used (364,371). When the regenerate bone attains the density and ultrastructural appearance (development of the cortex and the medullary canal) of the adjacent bone, fixator removal is generally safe.

Pathologic fracture also can be caused by the osteopenia and joint contractures that can occur after months in an external fixation device. Some children, because of pain or anxiety, are reluctant to bear sufficient weight on their fixator devices, putting them at risk for disuse osteoporosis. Joint contractures can be related to either the lengthening itself or insufficient rehabilitation during and after lengthening. Many of the fractures due to these causes are avoidable; when they do occur, appropriate immobilization or internal fixation is used.

FRACTURES IN CONDITIONS THAT WEAKEN BONE

Osteogenesis Imperfecta

Osteogenesis imperfecta (OI) is a heterogenous group of inherited disorders in which the structure and function of type I collagen is altered. The fragile bone is susceptible to frequent fractures and progressive deformity (372, 373). OI is identifiable in 1 in 20,000 total births, with an overall prevalence of approximately 16 cases per million index patients (373,374). The wide spectrum of clinical severity—from perinatal lethal forms to clinically silent forms—reflects the tremendous genotypic heterogeneity (more than 150 different mutations of the type 1 procollagen genes *COL1A1* and *COL1A2* have been described). As the molecular basis of this continuum of severity is further elucidated, the phenotypic groupings of the various classifications and subclassifications may seem arbitrary. However, these classifications facilitate communication, predict natural history, and help the clinician plan management strategies (373). From a practical viewpoint of orthopaedic care, patients with OI can be divided into two groups. One group of patients with severe disease develops long-bone deformity through repetitive fractures, eventually requiring open treatment with intramedullary fixation. Another group of patients has mild disease with frequent fractures, but most of their injuries respond well to closed methods of treatment and there is less residual deformity.

Clinical Presentation

Children with severe OI may present with a short trunk, marked deformity of the weight-bearing lower extremities, prominence of the sternum, triangular facies, thin skin, muscle atrophy, and ligamentous laxity; some develop kyphoscoliosis (375–377), basilar impression (378,379), and deafness (due to otosclerosis) (380). Despite this multitude of physical problems, children with OI usually have normal intelligence. Blue sclera, a classic finding in certain forms of OI, can also be present in normal infants, as well as in children with hypophosphatasia, osteopetrosis, Marfan's syndrome, and Ehlers-Danlos syndrome (381). Osseous histologic findings in severe cases reveal a predominance of woven bone, an absence of lamellar bone, and thinning of the cortical bone with osteopenia.

Patients with OI may present with swelling of the extremity, pain, and low-grade fever and an x-ray showing exuberant, hyperplastic, callus formation (Fig. 6-33). The callus may occur without fracture and can have a distinct butterfly shape (381), as opposed to the usual fusiform callus of most healing fractures. The femur is most commonly involved, but cases noting involvement of the tibia and humerus have been reported (382). The sedimentation rate and serum alkaline phosphatase may be elevated. Because osteosarcoma has been associated with OI (383,384), aggressive-appearing lesions may occasionally require biopsy to confirm their benign nature.

Radiographic Findings

Radiographic findings vary. In severe involvement, there is marked osteoporosis, thin cortical bone, and evidence of past fracture with angular malunion (Fig. 6-34). Both anterior and lateral bowing of the femur and anterior bowing of the tibia are common. The long bones may be gracile with multiple cystic areas. Spinal x-rays may show compression of the vertebrae between the cartilaginous disc spaces (so-called codfish vertebra). The presence of wormian bones on a skull x-ray is relatively specific for OI. Subsequent development of multiple pathologic fractures with callus and deformity firmly establishes the diagnosis (Fig. 6-35).

The diagnosis of OI is based on clinical and radiographic findings. There is no specific laboratory diagnostic test, although fibroblast cell culture can detect the collagen abnormality in 85% of OI patients (385). In the absence of multiple fractures, the initial radiographic diagnosis can be difficult. It is crucial, but often difficult, to distinguish OI from nonaccidental injury (386,387). Unexplained fractures in mild, undiagnosed OI can drag a family through unnecessary legal proceedings; conversely, a child with OI may be abused but not exhibit classic fracture patterns (e.g., corner fractures) owing to the fragility

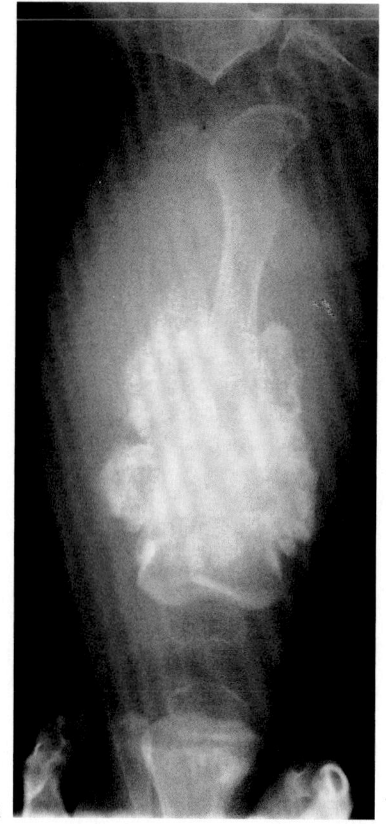

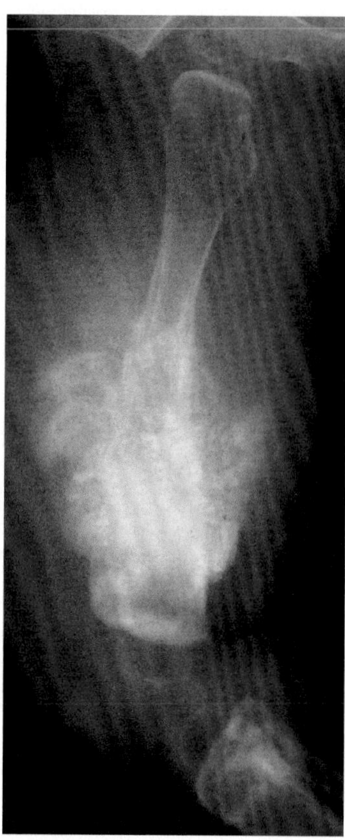

FIGURE 6-33 **A.** This 10-month-old boy with a history of osteogenesis imperfecta presented with a right thigh pain and swelling and refusal to bear weight. This AP x-ray and **(B)** this lateral x-ray of the right femur show the extraordinarily abundant, hyperplastic callus—with the characteristic butterfly shape—that can occur in osteogenesis imperfecta. This appearance may be mistaken for an infection or a neoplastic process.

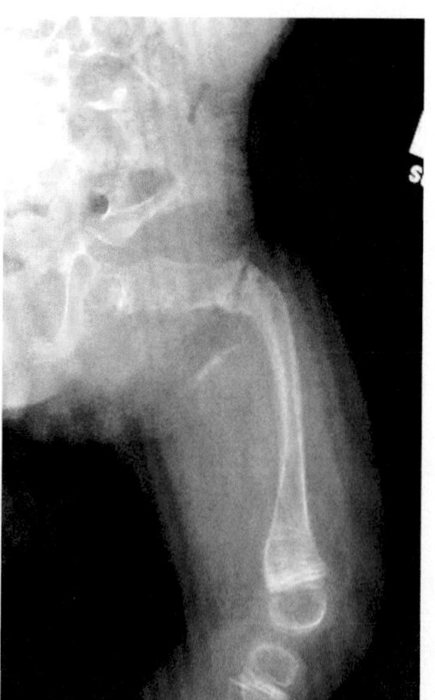

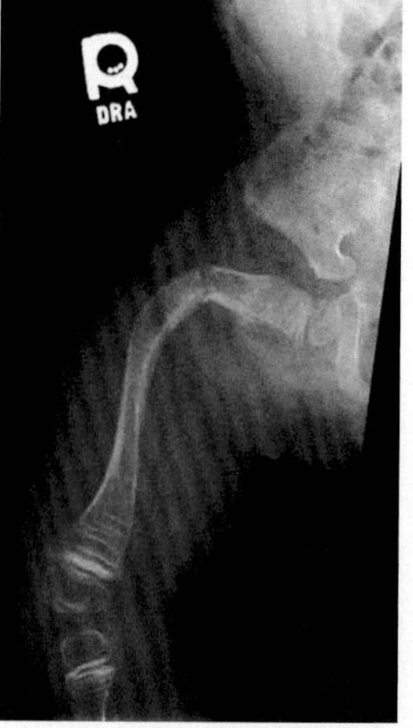

FIGURE 6-34 Fractures and deformity of the proximal femur in osteogenesis imperfecta. **A,B.** X-rays of the left and right femora in a 3-year-old boy with severe osteogenesis imperfecta and recurrent fractures of the proximal femur.

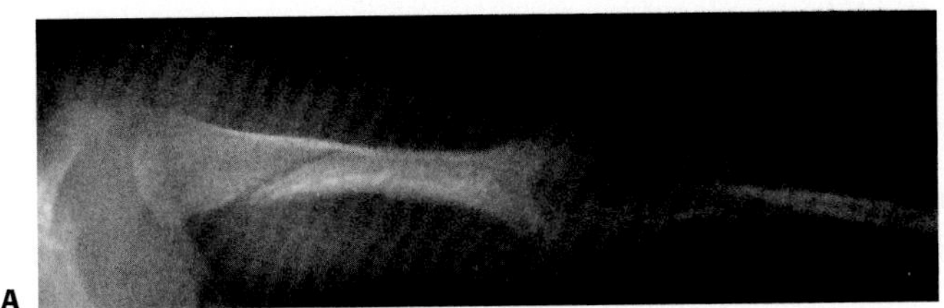

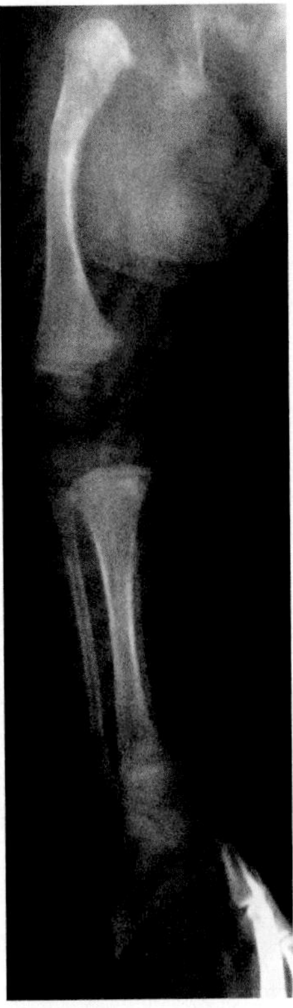

FIGURE 6-35 **A.** This 6-week-old girl presented with multiple fractures in different stages of healing. She was evaluated for osteogenesis imperfecta and nonaccidental injury. She had a strong family history of osteogenesis imperfecta. An AP x-ray of the left upper extremity shows marked osteopenia and a nondisplaced spiral fracture of the left proximal humerus. **B.** An AP x-ray of the right lower extremity showing osteopenia and healing fractures of both the femur and the tibia. There is already some varus angulation and bowing to the mid-shaft of the right femur.

of their bones. Although no test or finding is specific, skin biopsy plays an important role (388,389).

Treatment

Multiple fractures in OI usually are transverse, diaphyseal, and seldom displaced, and they usually heal at a relatively normal rate in most patients (379,381). Most fractures in patients with OI occur before skeletal maturity. In a series of 31 patients, Moorefield and Miller (377) noted 951 fractures, 91% of which occurred before skeletal maturity. Fractures of the femur and tibia predominate. The humerus is the most commonly fractured bone in the upper extremity. Multiple long bone fractures may result in coxa vara, genu valgum, and leg-length discrepancy. Lateral dislocation of the radial head has been noted in some patients (381). Olecranon fractures, which are rare in unaffected children, are more common in patients with OI, especially the tarda form (390,391). Zionts and Moon reviewed 17 fractures of the olecranon apophysis in 10 children with mild OI; 15 of these fractures were treated operatively. The same injury presented in the opposite extremity 1 to 70 months after the initial fracture in 7 of the 10 patients. All fractures had healed by the time of cast removal; however, two refractured. The authors concluded that with careful follow-up, cast immobilization may be used for minimally displaced fractures, but operative management is suggested for displaced fractures. The high rate of bilateral injury (70%) suggests that children with OI who sustain this fracture be counseled about the possible risks of injury to the opposite extremity (392).

Nonunion is more common in OI than in similar fractures in unaffected children. Although nonunion was mentioned in several series (377), Gamble et al (393) emphasized the problem with a report of 12 nonunions in 10 patients. Almost all had type III OI (394) and presented with nonpainful clinical deformity and decreased functional ability. A history of inadequate treatment of the initial fracture was seen in 50% of these nonunions. One patient eventually required an amputation for a painful nonunion of a distal femoral supracondylar fracture.

Prevention

The role of medical therapy to limit the fracture frequency in OI is still investigational but promising. The tremendous genotypic and phenotypic variations in OI must be considered as the results of these trials are analyzed: A drug that works well for children with certain forms of OI may be ineffective for others. Sodium fluoride, growth hormones, and anabolic steroids have all been shown to be ineffective. Calcitonin, which limits osteoclasts, has had variable success. Nishi et al (395) reported that the fracture rate decreased in 10 patients with OI treated with either calcitonin injection or nasal spray.

At present the most promising agents are the bisphosphonates (396–399). Pamidronate, like other bisphosphonates, is a potent inhibitor of bone resorption. In a trial of 30 children with severe OI, Glorieux et al (397) showed that cyclic intravenous administration of pamidronate every 4 to 6 months resulted in a 41.9% increase per year in bone mineral density, an increase in metacarpal cortical width, and a decrease in fracture incidence of 1.7 fractures per year. Mobility improved in 16 of the 30 children, and all reported substantial relief of chronic pain. The results of a recent study performed by Falk et al supports the findings of Glorieux et al. However, they have concluded that long-term follow-up will be required to determine whether bisphosphonate therapy will decrease fracture rates and increase mobility in children with moderate to severe OI (398). Sakkers et al report a reduction of fracture risk of long bones in children with OI using oral treatment with olpadronate at a daily dose of 10 mg. However, the issue of whether bisphosphonates will alter the natural course of OI remains unresolved (399). Recently, Zeitlin et al have also shown that administering cyclical intravenous pamidronate to children with OI reduces bone pain and fracture incidence, and increases bone density and level of ambulation, with minimal side effects. Effects on bone include an increase in the size of vertebral bodies as well as thickening of cortical bone; therefore allowing for more effective corrective surgery using intramedullary rodding of the long bones and spinal instrumentation. Specific occupational and physiotherapy programs are important parts of the treatment procedure. This multidisciplinary approach will prevail until strategies aiming at the correction of the basic defect(s) are found (400).

Closed Methods

The orthopedist caring for children with OI must balance good, standard fracture care (satisfactory reduction and casting) with the goal of minimizing immobilization to avoid a vicious circle: immobilization, weakness and osteopenia, then refracture (373,377,401). Plaster splints and casts, braces, and air splints have all been used (377,379,402–404).

Protected weight-bearing is thought to reduce the incidence of lower extremity fractures (405). Customized splints and braces can add support to limbs weakened by fragile and deformed bone. Letts et al (406) encouraged weight-bearing in patients by protecting them with vacuum pants. The splinting system is a two-layer set of pants with Styrofoam beads between the layers. By evacuating the interval between the layers, a form-fitting orthosis results, much like the bean bag seating systems. Both decreased frequency of fracture and increased bone density were reported after use of this support system.

Operative Treatment

Load-sharing devices (such as intramedullary rods) are used for internal fixation of long bone fractures or osteotomies in children with OI. Plates and screws should be avoided. In patients with OI, most internal fixation is used for stabilization after corrective osteotomies. The goals of these osteotomies are to improve function and reduce fractures in weight-bearing bones by correcting angulation. Porat et al (407) found that the percentage of ambulatory patients in their series went from 45% to 75% after intramedullary rodding. The amount of bowing that requires osteotomy has not been defined. In one series (408), the average preoperative bowing was 71 degrees for the femur and 40 degrees for the tibia, but many patients had much less angulation.

Traditionally, multiple osteotomy and rodding procedures (Sofield technique) involved extensive incisions with significant soft-tissue stripping and blood loss. Sijbrandij (409) reported a percutaneous technique in which the deformity is straightened by closed osteoclasis and Rush pins are inserted along the proximal axis of the long bones, partially transfixing them to stabilize them in a new alignment. Most centers now use limited incisions, thus minimizing blood loss and periosteal stripping, while ensuring optimally placed osteotomies and efficient, controlled instrumentation. The choice of fixation device should be based on the age of the patient and the width of the medullary canal of the bone. Both fixed-length rods (202,381,407) and extensible Bailey-Dubow rods (393,407,408,410–414), are used. Skeletally mature patients and patients with very small medullary canals are best treated with nonelongating rods, whereas skeletally immature patients with adequate width of the medullary canal are best treated with extensible rods (393). Luhmann et al (415) reported a 20-year experience with extensible nails: both overlapping Rush rods and Bailey-Dubow rods. They first implanted the rods at an average age of 7 years and averaged more than 5 years before the first revision. They recommended a posterior position in the canal and using the stronger overlapping Rush rods technique in the femur whenever the canal diameter permitted; they advised against using overlapping Rush rods in the tibia. Malpuri and Joseph reported the results of intramedullary rodding of long bones in 16 children with OI, over a 10-year period. Sheffield elongating rods or nonelongating rods were used. The rate of fractures reduced drastically after insertion of either type of rod, and the ambulatory status improved in all patients. With regard to the frequency of complications requiring re-operations and the longevity of the rods, Mulpuri and Joseph determined results were notably superior after Sheffield rodding (416).

Displaced fractures of the apophysis of the olecranon in patients with OI can be treated with open reduction and internal fixation using two Kirschner wires and tension band technique by figure-of-eight absorbable suture in older children (Fig. 6-36) (391). Tibial tubercle avulsion injuries should be treated by surgical stabilization if displaced.

Complications

Complication rates are high after osteotomies and intramedullary fixation in OI (Fig. 6-37). Problems include fracture at the rod tip, migration of the fixation device, joint penetration, loosening of components of extensible rods, and fractures through the area of uncoupled rods. Harrison and Rankin (417) compared the complications of 23 extensible rods with those of 27 fixed-length rods. They found that the refracture rate was higher in the fixed-length rods and fewer surgical interventions were necessary when extensible rods were used. Gamble et al (413) reported that, although the complication rate approached 69% for Bailey-Dubow rods (mostly due to loosening of the T-piece), the fixed-length rods had a complication rate of 55%; however, the replacement rate for nonelongating rods was 24% but only 12% for the Bailey-Dubow rods. They recommended

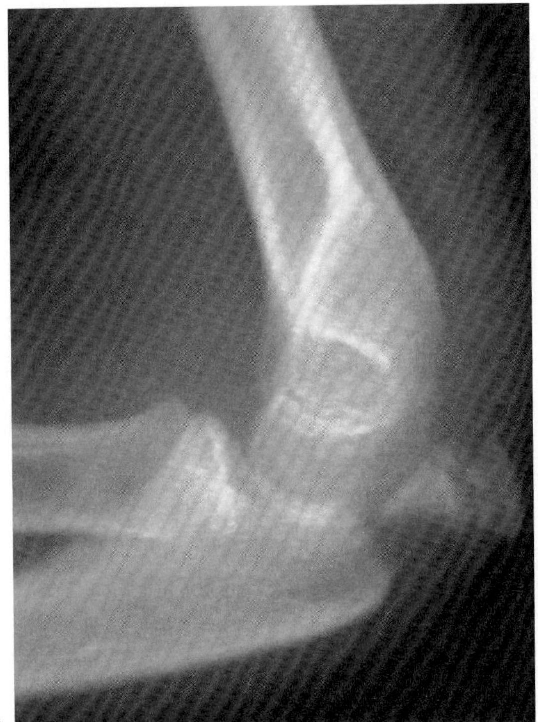

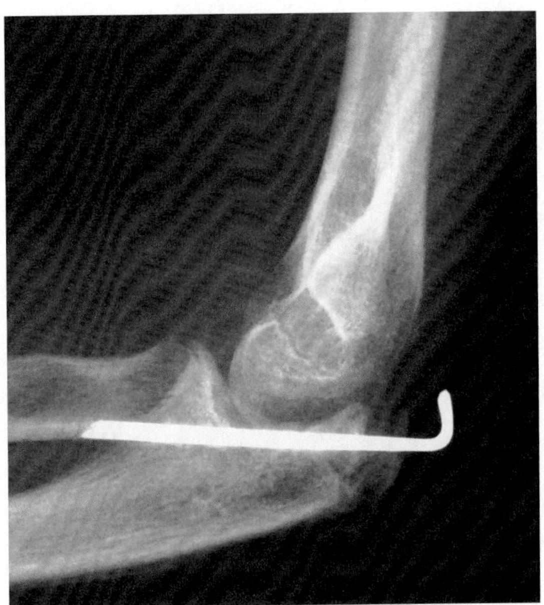

FIGURE 6-36 This 10-year-old girl with osteogenesis imperfecta presented with a displaced olecranon sleeve fracture of the left elbow. This was her first fracture. **A.** This lateral x-ray shows a widely displaced fracture involving the posterior portion of the articular surface. **B.** She was treated with open reduction and internal fixation with two K-wires and tension band construct using no. 2 Vicryl suture. She was maintained in a cast for 3 weeks and then started on range-of-motion exercises.

crimping the T-piece to the sleeve and burying it slightly under the bone of the greater trochanter to prevent displacement. Jerosch (418) found a similar 63.5% complication rate for Bailey-Dubow rods but also thought that they were the best device available. Porat et al (407) found that the complication rate was 75% for Bailey-Dubow rods and 50% for nonelongating rods, with a similar percentage requiring reoperation for both types of nails. Zionts et al (419) reported 40 complications in 40 extensible nailings of 15 children, finding a much higher complication rate when insertion of the rods was initiated before 5 years of age. Complications were also higher for tibial nailings.

Postoperative bracing is suggested for lower extremity fractures (408). Upper extremity fractures should also undergo prolonged splinting after removal of fracture fixation. Immobilization also may be adequate to treat stable, minimally displaced fractures just distal or proximal to the intramedullary rods (393).

Nonunions, after fracture or surgical intervention, may cause difficulty in both ambulation and transfer. In one series of nonunions (393), the average age at diagnosis was close to 10 years and most patients responded to treatment with intramedullary rods and bone grafting, with healing in approximately 9 weeks. Nonunion can occur after insertion of rods for upper extremity fractures. Growth arrest also can follow the use of intramedullary rods in the lower extremities.

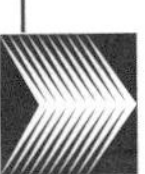

AUTHORS' PREFERRED METHOD OF TREATMENT

Osteogenesis Imperfecta

Protected weight-bearing is the goal for patients with severe OI. Close follow-up is necessary in the first few years of life, with protective posterior plaster splinting for fractures. Orthoses are constructed for bracing of the lower extremities to aid in both standing and ambulation. Standing frames also are used. Once ambulatory, the child is advanced to the use of a walker or independent ambulation.

Severe bowing of the extremities after recurrent fractures is an indication for osteotomy and intramedullary rodding. Whenever possible, surgery is delayed until 6 or 7 years of age. We recommend extensible rods in skeletally immature patients and nonelongating rods both in older patients and in younger patients whose canal is not wide enough for insertion of Bailey-Dubow rods. When possible, we use limited incisions for insertion of Bailey-Dubow rods to minimize blood loss and to avoid devascularization of the long bones, which occurs commonly in the so-called open shish-kabob technique.

Operative Technique—Bailey-Dubow Rod. Multiple small skin incisions are made at the point of maximal deformity of the

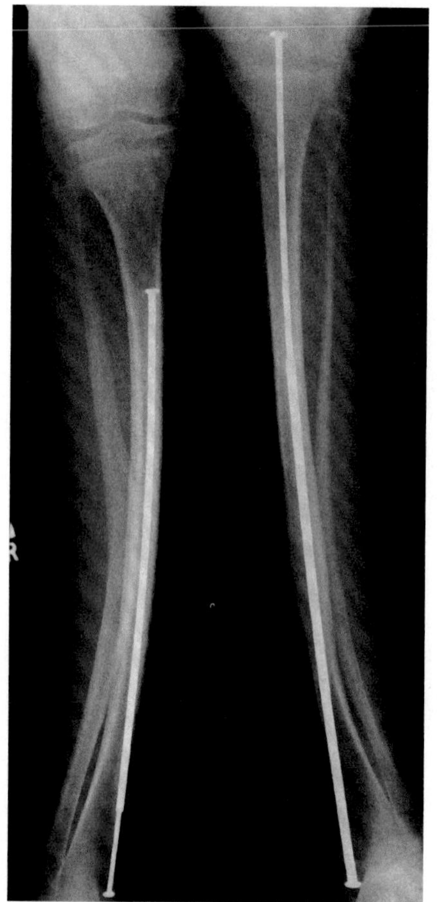

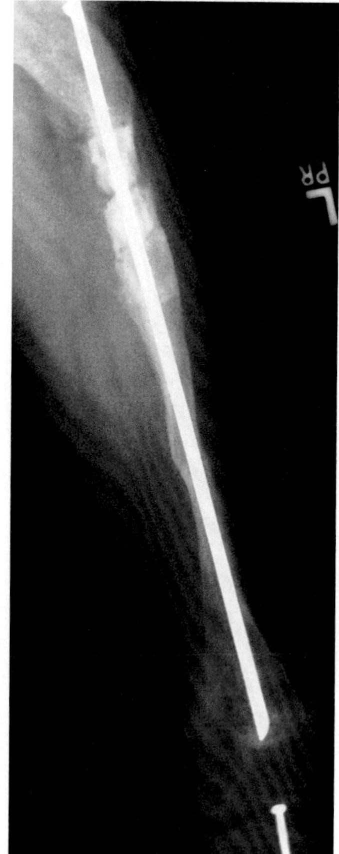

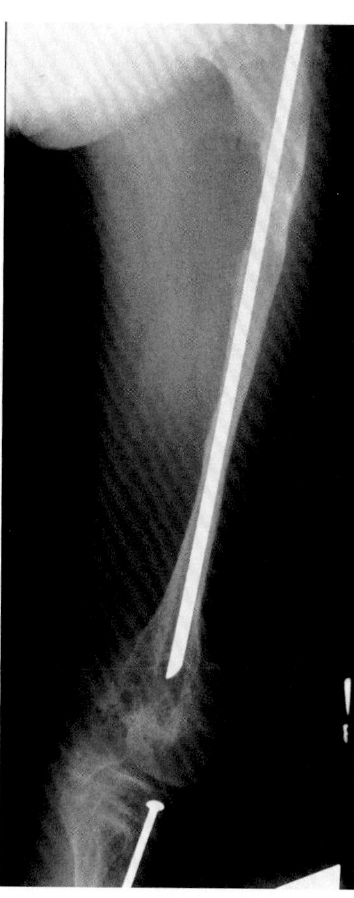

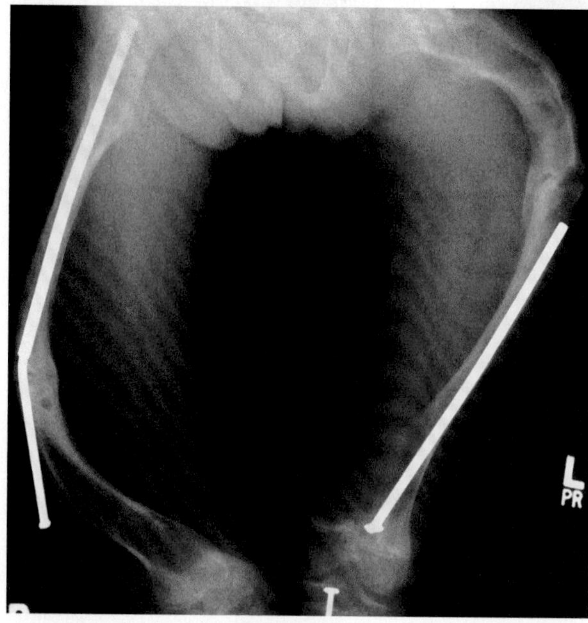

FIGURE 6-37 **A.** The lower extremity deformities of this 14-year-old girl with severe osteogenesis imperfecta were managed throughout childhood with Bailey-Dubow rods. This AP x-ray of both legs shows successful lengthening and maintenance of alignment of the left tibia but failure of rod lengthening with valgus angulation of the right tibia. **B.** The AP x-ray of both femurs, also taken at age 14, shows signs of several of the problems in the management of the femoral deformities throughout childhood. The right Bailey-Dubow rod protrudes into the soft tissues distally. There is femoral bowing with a fracture and bending of the Bailey-Dubow rod at the junction of the male and female ends. In the left femur, part of the Bailey-Dubow rod has been removed because it was protruding into the soft tissues. There is a pathologic fracture through the bowing of the proximal femur. **C.** Deformities of both femurs were treated by osteotomy and exchange of the Bailey-Dubow rods for a Rush nail. **D.** One year after the exchange, the osteotomy has healed. The femoral alignment is good, but the proximal portion of the Rush rod is prominent in the soft tissues.

long bones, and a small periosteal incision is made to permit introduction of a drill bit. After the cortex is drilled repeatedly, manual osteoclasis completes the osteotomy and the long bone is straightened. A guide pin is drilled in to the medial edge of the tip of the greater trochanter, and down into the intertrochanteric femur, and then is tapped distally through the intramedullary canal through the knee. If callus from old fracture halts progress, the guide pin can be drilled through the obstruction and then tapped farther distally into the middle of the distal flexed knee joint. Next, the reamer is advanced over the guide pin and the female portion of the Bailey-Dubow rod is threaded over the guide pin and driven down the canal. The guide pin is pulled out of the knee joint through a small arthrotomy incision, and the T-piece is attached to the Bailey-Dubow sleeve. The T-piece is tapped down into the greater trochanter. The male portion is then slid into the sleeve to complete assembly of the expandable rod.

The patient is immobilized for approximately 4 weeks in a hip spica cast and then in a brace for 3 to 6 months. When there are fractures associated with intramedullary rods, these are treated with either rod revision or immobilization. Every effort should be made to keep patients ambulatory early after fractures occur to minimize disuse osteoporosis.

Osteopetrosis

Osteopetrosis, also known as Albers-Schönberg disease, is a condition in which excessive density of bone occurs as a result of abnormal function of osteoclasts (420,421). The resultant bone of these children is dense, brittle, and highly susceptible to pathologic fracture. The incidence of osteopetrosis is approximately 1 per 200,000 births. The inherent problem is a failure of bone resorption with continuing bone formation and persistent primary spongiosa. The disorder classically has been divided into a severe infantile type and a milder form that presents later in life. Intermediate forms have been identified in which osteopetrosis presents as renal tubular acidosis (422). Although the number of osteoclasts present in the affected bone is variable (378,423), in the severe form of this disease, the osteoclasts may be increased but function poorly (424).

Radiographically, the bones have a dense, chalklike appearance (Fig. 6-38). The spinal column may have a sandwich or rugger jersey appearance because of dense, sclerotic bone at each end plate of the vertebrae and less involvement of the central portion. The long bones tend to have a dense, marblelike appearance and may have an Erlenmeyer's flask shape at their ends owing to deficient cutback remodeling. Radiolucent transverse bands may be present in the metaphysis of the long bones, and these may represent a variable improvement in the resorption defect during growth of the child (425). There may be bowing of the bones due to multiple fractures (426), spondylolysis (427), or coxa vara (421). The small bones of the hands and feet may show a bone-within-bone appearance with increased density around the periphery. The unusual radiographic appearance may initially obscure occult, nondisplaced fractures.

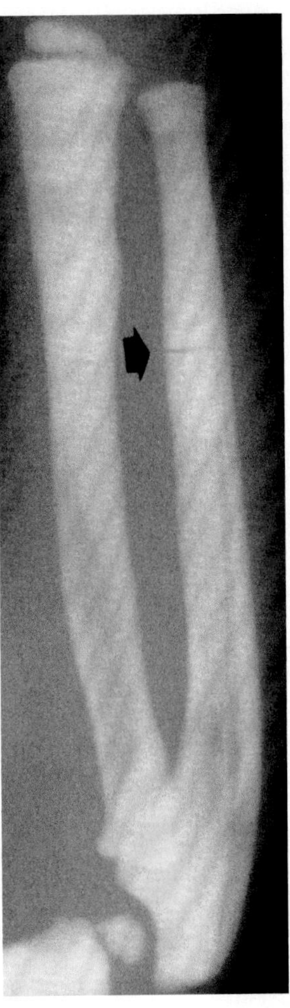

FIGURE 6-38 This 2-year-old with osteopetrosis presented with forearm pain. An AP x-ray shows the characteristic increased bone density and absence of a medullary canal, especially in the distal radius and ulna. There is a typical transverse, nondisplaced fracture (*arrow*) in the distal ulnar diaphysis.

Treatment

Pathologic fractures are quite common in patients with osteopetrosis (378,421,426,428–431). Patients with a severe form of the disease have more fractures than those with presentation later in childhood. Concurrent blindness can make patients more susceptible to accidental trauma. Patients with autosomal dominant osteopetrosis with rugger jersey spine and endobones of the pelvis (type II) are six times more likely to have fractures than patients with only sclerosis of the cranial vault (type I) (428).

Patients with the severe, congenital disease have transverse or short oblique fractures of the diaphysis, particularly the femur (Fig. 6-39). Distal physeal fractures with exuberant callus may be confused with osteomyelitis (425). Common locations for fractures include the inferior neck of the femur, the proximal third of the femoral shaft, and the proximal tibia (420,425). Although most fractures involve the long bones of the lower

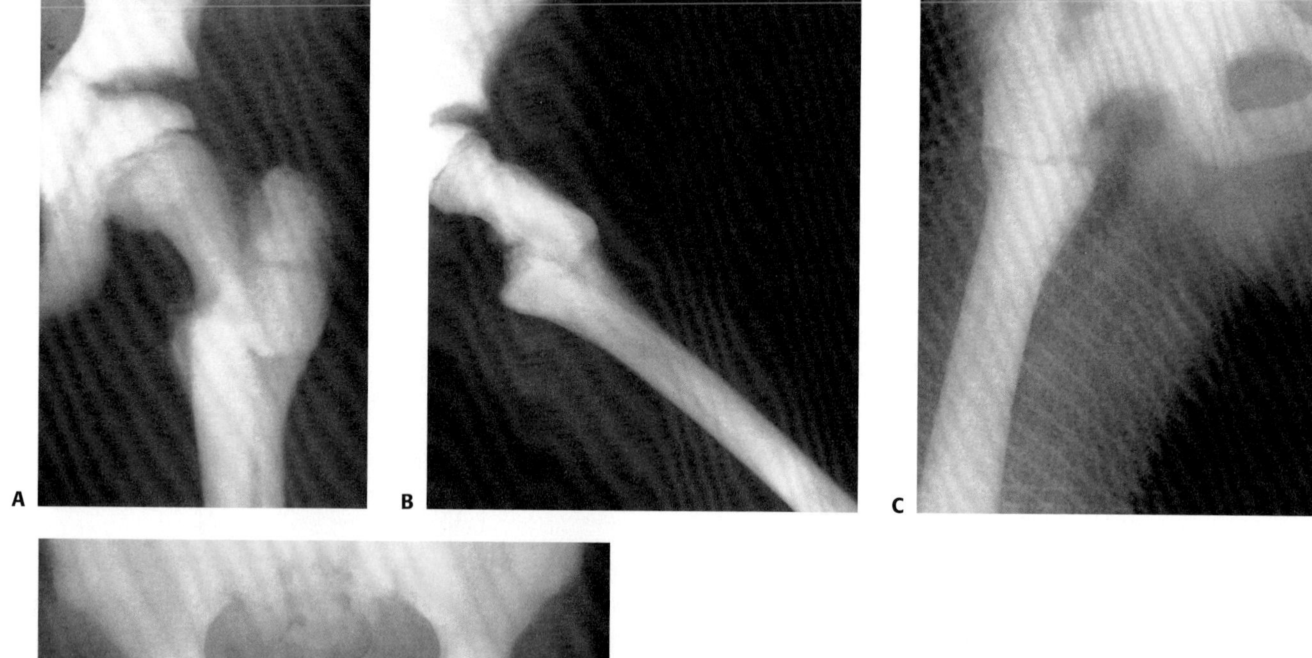

FIGURE 6-39 **A.** This 9-year-old with osteopetrosis sustained similar bilateral subtrochanteric fractures of the femur over a 2-year period. This AP femoral x-ray and **B.** this lateral femoral x-ray shows a healing transverse subtrochanteric fracture of the left femur. **C.** One year later, at age 10, she sustained a similar right transverse minimally displaced subtrochanteric femur fracture, which was treated with reduction and a spica cast. **D.** This AP x-ray taken at age 14 years shows that both proximal femur fractures have healed and there is mild residual coxa vara, especially on the right side.

extremities, upper extremity fractures also occur frequently (420,426). The onset of callus formation after fracture in osteopetrosis is variable (420,423,426). Although many studies state that fractures in osteopetrosis heal at a normal rate (421,423), others report delayed union and nonunion (420). In a rat model of osteopetrosis, Marks and Schmidt (432) found delayed fracture healing and remodeling. Hasenhuttl (426) observed that in one patient with recurrent fractures of the forearm, each succeeding fracture took longer to heal, with the last fracture taking nearly 5 months to unite.

The orthopedist treating fractures in children with osteopetrosis should follow the principles of standard pediatric fracture care, with additional vigilance for possible delayed union and associated rickets (426,431). Immobilization is prolonged when delayed union is recognized. Armstrong et al (420) surveyed the membership of the Pediatric Orthopaedic Society of North America and compiled the combined experience of 58 pediatric orthopaedic surgeons with experience treating pathologic fractures in osteopetrosis. In this comprehensive review, they concluded that nonoperative treatment should be strongly considered for most diaphyseal fractures of the upper and lower limbs in children, but surgical management is recommended for femoral neck fractures and coxa vara.

Open treatment of these fractures with fixation is technically difficult. One author (433) described insertion of fixation into this bone like "drilling into a rock." In intramedullary fixation of femoral fractures, extensive reaming may be required because the intramedullary canal can be completely obliterated by sclerotic bone (434). Other authors have found fixation of hip fractures with fixation to be a formidable task (420,425), with damage occurring to the fixation devices on insertion. The bone is hard enough to break the edges off both chisels and drill bits. Armstrong et al (420) cautioned, "the surgeon should expect to use several drill bits and possibly more than one power driver."

In addition to these technical difficulties, patients with osteopetrosis are at risk for excessive bleeding and infection, probably related to the hematopoietic dysfunction caused by obliteration of the marrow cavity (431). Procedures should not be performed unless the platelet count is greater than 50,000 mm^3; preoperative platelet transfusions may be necessary (431). Prophylactic antibiotic coverage is advised. Minor procedures should be performed percutaneously whenever possible (431).

In the past, primary medical treatment for osteopetrosis included transfusions, splenectomy, calcitriol, and adrenal corticosteroids, but these techniques have proved ineffectual

(435,436). Bone marrow transplantation for severe infantile osteopetrosis has proved to be an effective means of treatment for some patients, but it is not possible in all patients, it does not guarantee survival, and it may be complicated by hypercalcemia (420,437–439).

Pyknodysostosis

Pyknodysostosis is a rare syndrome of short stature and generalized sclerosis of the entire skeleton. The dense brittle bones of affected children are highly susceptible to pathologic fractures. Henri Toulouse-Lautrec was thought to be afflicted by this disorder (440). Pyknodysostosis is inherited as an autosomal recessive trait, with an incidence estimated as 1.7 per 1 million births. The long bones are sclerotic, with poorly formed medullary canals; histologic section show attenuated haversian canal systems.

Patients with pyknodysostosis have short stature, a hypoplastic face, a nose with a parrot-like appearance, and both frontal and occipital bossing. Bulbous distal phalanges of the fingers and toes with spooning of the nails are common. Coxa vara, coxa valgum, genu valgum, kyphosis, and scoliosis may be present. Failure of segmentation of the lower lumbar spine has been reported. (441) Results of laboratory studies usually are normal.

X-rays show a sclerotic pattern very similar to that of osteopetrosis. In pyknodysostosis, however, the medullary canals, although poorly formed, are present and a faint trabecular pattern is seen. Such sclerotic bone is also seen in Engelmann's disease, but clinically those patients are tall and eventually develop muscle weakness. The distal femur in a patient with pyknodysostosis usually has an Erlenmeyer's flask deformity similar to that found in patients with Gaucher's disease (442).

Treatment

Although pathologic fractures are thought to be less common in pyknodysostosis than in OI, almost all patients with pyknodysostosis reported in the literature have had pathologic fractures (443). By age 22 years, one patient had sustained more than 100 fractures (444). The fractures are usually transverse and diaphyseal, and heal with scanty callus (445). The fracture line can persist for nearly 3 years after clinical union, with an appearance similar to a Looser line. Lower extremity fractures are the most common (444), and clinical deformity of both the femur and tibia is frequent.

Fracture healing has been described as both normal (446) and delayed (444). Nonunion is reported in the ulna, clavicle, and tibia (445). One series (445) with long-term follow-up suggests that fractures tend to heal readily in childhood, but nonunion can be a problem in adulthood. Edelson et al (447) reported 14 new cases of pyknodysostosis from a small Arab village. They described a Hangman's fracture of C2 in a 2-year-old child that went on to asymptomatic nonunion. There was 100% incidence of spondylolysis in their patients aged 9 years or older, with most located at L4–L5. None of the spondylolytic lesions showed uptake on technetium 99m bone scan. Treatment was conservative, with one patient with symptomatic spondylolysis responding to bed rest.

Cast immobilization is successful in the treatment of most of these fractures. Taylor et al (448) treated a femoral fracture in an 11-year-old boy with skin traction and a one-and-a-half hip spica cast. At 6-month follow-up, clinical union with persistent fracture line was seen. In adults, both plates and screws and hip screws have been used for proximal femoral fractures (449). Delayed union of tibial fractures has been treated with both compression plating and bone grafting (445) and intramedullary nailing with cast immobilization. Roth (449) noted that treatment of a hip fracture with fixation was technically difficult. Cervical immobilization through a Minerva cast and soft cervical collar has been used for a C2 fracture in a child, and the patient did well, although immobilization was prematurely discontinued (444).

Rickets

Rickets is a disease of growing children caused by either a deficiency of vitamin D or an abnormality of its metabolism. The osteoid of the bone is not mineralized, and broad unossified osteoid seams form on the trabeculae. With failure of physeal mineralization, the zone of provisional calcification widens and the ingrowth of blood vessels into the zone is disrupted. In the rickets of renal failure, the effects of secondary hyperparathyroidism (bone erosion and cyst formation) are also present. Before widespread fortification of common foods, vitamin D deficiency was a common cause of rickets, but other diseases affecting the metabolism of vitamin D have become a more common cause. Regardless of the underlying cause, the various types of rickets share similar clinical and radiographic features. Although many of the metabolic findings are the same, there are some differences (Table 6-11).

Both pathologic fractures (423,450–453) and epiphyseal displacement (454,455) can occur in rickets with associated renal disease. The treatment of rickets with associated pathologic fractures depends on identification of the underlying cause. In addition to nutritional rickets, many diseases of the various organ systems can affect vitamin D metabolism, and their treatment is necessary before the clinical rickets can be resolved.

Nutritional Rickets

Inadequate dietary vitamin D and lack of exposure to sunlight can lead to a vitamin D deficiency (Fig. 6-40). Pathologic fractures from vitamin D deficiency rickets also occur in children on certain diets: unsupplemented breast milk (456), diets restricted by religious beliefs (450), and fad diets (457).

Fractures are treated with both cast immobilization and correction of the vitamin deficiency by oral vitamin D supplementation. Oral calcium supplements also may be necessary, and patients should consume a vitamin D–fortified milk source (450).

TABLE 6-11 Rickets: Metabolic Abnormalities

Disorder	Cause	1,25 $(OH)_2$ Vitamin D	PTH	Ca^{2+}	P	Alk Phos
Vitamin D deficiency rickets	Lack of vitamin D in the diet	↓	↑	↓ or →	↓	↑
Gastrointestinal rickets	Decreased gastrointestinal absorption of vitamin D or Ca^{2+}	↓ or →	↑	↓	↓	↑
Vitamin D–dependent rickets	Reduced 1,25$(OH)_2$ vitamin D production	↓↓	↑	↓	↓	↑
Vitamin D–resistant rickets—end-organ insensitivity	Intestinal cell insensitivity to vitamin D causing decreased Ca^{2+} absorption	↑ or →	↑	↓	↓	↑
Renal osteodystrophy	Renal failure causing decreased vitamin D synthesis, phosphate retention, hypocalcemia and secondary hyperparathyroidism	↓↓	↑↑	↓	↑	↑

Rickets in Malabsorption Diseases

Celiac disease caused by gluten-sensitive enteropathy affects intestinal absorption of fat-soluble vitamins (such as vitamin D), resulting in rickets. Biopsy of the small intestine shows characteristic atrophy of the villi. Treatment is oral vitamin D and a gluten-free diet. Infants with short gut syndrome may have vitamin D–deficiency rickets. This syndrome may develop after intestinal resection in infancy for volvulus or necrotizing enterocolitis, in intestinal atresia, or after resection of the terminal ileum and the ileocecal valve (458). Pathologic fractures have been reported, and treatment is immobilization and administration of vitamin D_2 with supplemental calcium gluconate.

Hepatobiliary disease also is associated with rickets (Fig. 6-41) (459,460). With congenital biliary atresia, the bile acids, essential for the intestinal absorption of vitamin D, are inadequate. By age 3 months, nearly 60% of patients with biliary atresia may have rickets (461). Intravenous vitamin D often is needed for effective treatment of these patients. After appropriate surgical correction of the hepatic syndrome, the bone disease gradually improves. The pathologic fractures that develop in these disorders (459) can be treated with immobilization.

Anticonvulsant therapy can interfere with the hepatic metabolism of vitamin D and result in rickets and pathologic fractures. Fewer fractures occur in institutionalized patients receiving vitamin D prophylaxis (462). In a study of 20 children with epilepsy, there was no difference in the bone mineral density of the femoral neck in patients on either phenobarbital or phenytoin compared with control subjects (463).

Ifosfamide, a chemotherapeutic agent used for treatment of Ewing's sarcoma, can cause hypophosphatemic rickets in children. The onset of rickets may occur anywhere from 2 to 14 months after chemotherapy and can be corrected with the administration of oral phosphates (464). Other mineral deficiencies such as magnesium (a cofactor for parathyroid hormone) can cause rare forms of rickets.

Rickets and Very-Low-Birth-Weight Infants

Very-low-birth-weight infants (1,500 g or less) can have pathologic fractures. In one study of 12 very-low-birth-weight infants, the incidence of pathologic fracture was 2.1%, nearly twice the rate of other premature infants with a birth weight of more than 1,500 g (465). The fractures are likely caused by a nutritional osteomalacia that may evolve into frank rickets in nearly 30% of very-low-birth-weight infants (Fig. 6-42) (465–468). During the last trimester of pregnancy, the intrauterine growth rate is exponential—almost two thirds of the birth weight is gained at that time (469). Eighty percent of both calcium and phosphorus is acquired then (470). Bone loss can be graded by either loss of cortical bone of the humerus (471) or loss of bone of the distal radius (467). Other than craniotabes (thinning and softening of the skull bone, with widening of the sutures and fontanelles), the clinical signs of rickets are generally lacking in these patients (466). The risk factors predisposing these patients to both rickets and fractures include hepatobiliary disease (460,461,464), prolonged total parenteral nutrition (464), chronic lung disease (465), necrotizing enterocolitis (458), patent ductus arteriosus (472), and physical therapy with passive range-of-motion exercises (466,468). In a prospective study of 78 low-birth-weight infants, Koo et al (468) observed a 73% incidence of rickets with associated pathologic fractures in patients with a birth weight of 800 g or less and only a 15% incidence of rickets with fractures in patients with a birth weight ranging from 1,000 to 1,500 g.

Treatment. In most cases, pathologic fractures in very-low-birth-weight infants are found incidentally on chest x-ray or gastrointestinal studies. The fractures may be suspected when physical examination reveals swelling and decreased movement of an extremity. The differential diagnosis of these fractures is limited but important: OI, copper deficiency syndrome, child

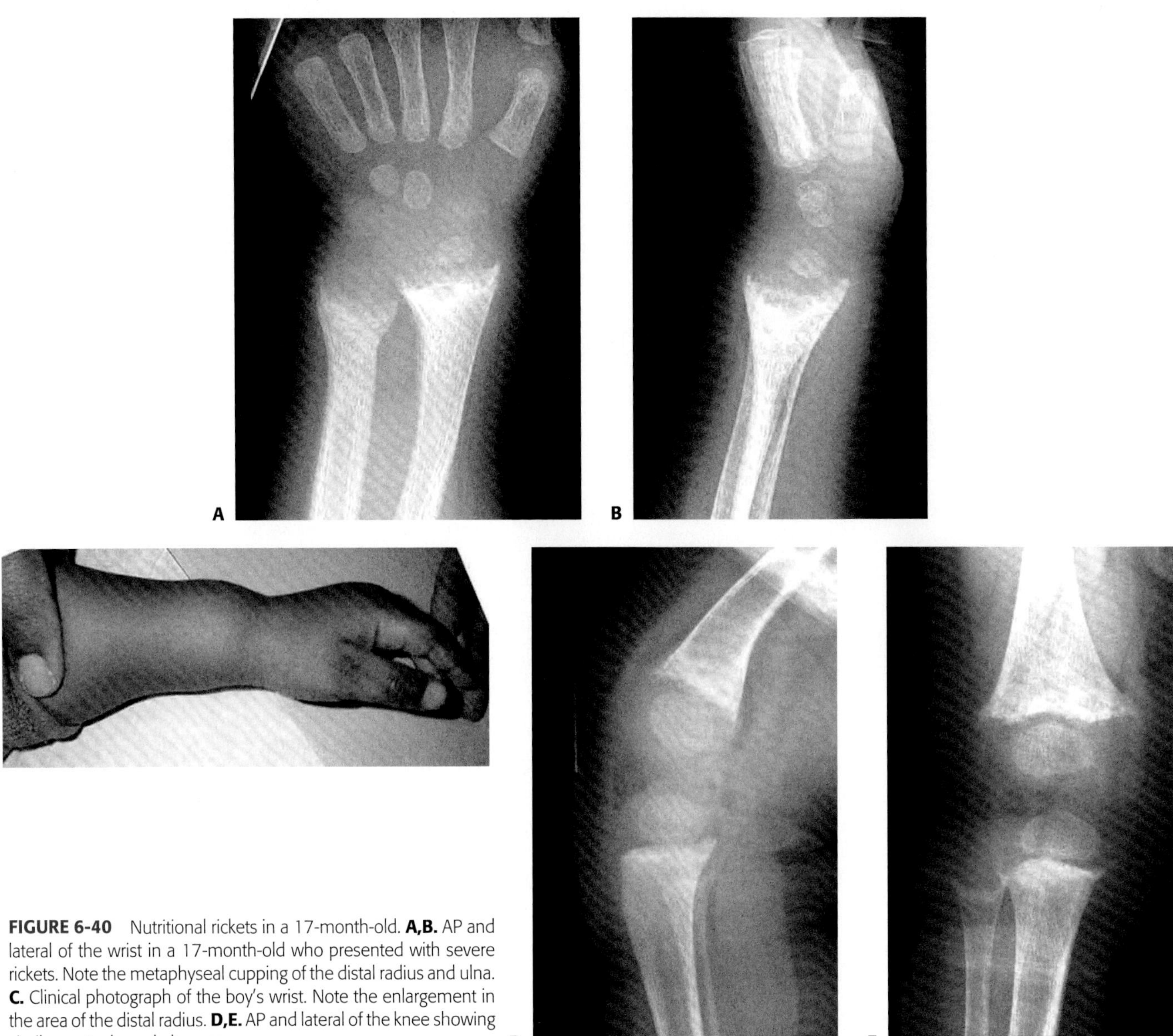

FIGURE 6-40 Nutritional rickets in a 17-month-old. **A,B.** AP and lateral of the wrist in a 17-month-old who presented with severe rickets. Note the metaphyseal cupping of the distal radius and ulna. **C.** Clinical photograph of the boy's wrist. Note the enlargement in the area of the distal radius. **D,E.** AP and lateral of the knee showing similar metaphyseal changes.

abuse, and pathologic fracture from overzealous physical therapy (466). Recurrent fractures, physical findings, and a positive family history are the hallmarks of OI; serum copper levels are useful in establishing copper deficiency syndrome. Neonatal osteomyelitis may also present a similar x-ray appearance. If risk factors for infection are present, the bone lesion should be aspirated and cultured (465).

In the series reported by Amir et al (465), 12 (1.2%) of 973 preterm infants had fractures; 11 of 12 had more than 1 fracture. Radiographically, osteopenia is first seen at the fourth week of life. Typically, rib fractures are next seen at 6 to 8 weeks of life, then fractures of the long bones at 11 to 12 weeks (469). In one study, 54% of fractures were in the upper extremities, 18% in the lower extremities, 22% in the ribs, and approximately 6% in either the scapula or the clavicle (468). Most long bone fractures are metaphyseal and may be transverse or greenstick with either angulation or complete displacement (465). Callus is seen at the fracture site in less than a week, and complete remodeling occurs in 6 to 12 months (465,468). Passive range-of-motion exercises for these infants, by both physical therapists and parents, should be avoided unless it is absolutely necessary (466). Rib fractures have been associated with vigorous chest physiotherapy (468). Care also should be taken even with routine manipulation of the extremities during nursing care, and special care should be taken in restraining the extremities during surgical procedures (468).

Splinting is the treatment of choice for pathologic fractures of the long bones in very-low-birth-weight infants (Fig. 6-43).

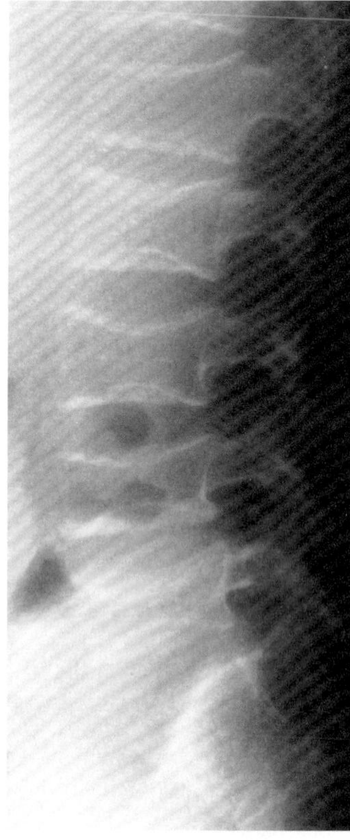

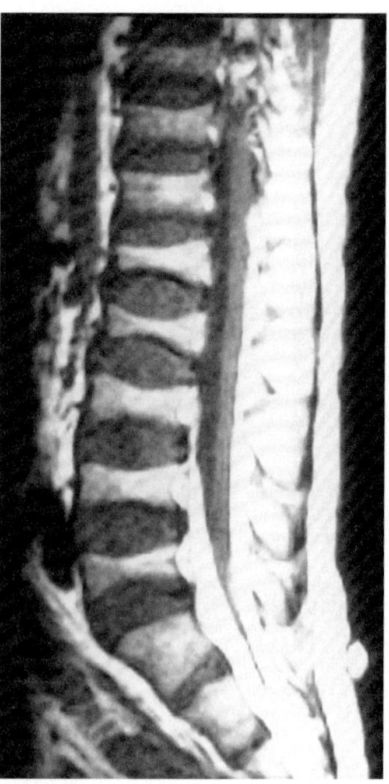

FIGURE 6-41 **A.** This 18-year-old boy with sclerosing cholangitis and a history of steroid use presented with several months of worsening low back pain. This lateral x-ray of his lumbar spine shows marked osteopenia, collapsed codfish vertebra with sclerotic end plates and widened disc spaces and Schmorl's nodes. **B.** This MRI shows flattened concave vertebra that are smaller in most locations than the adjacent intervertebral disc. He was successfully treated with 3 months in a thoraco-lumbar-sacral-orthosis (TLSO) brace, followed by weaning from the brace and conditioning exercises.

Hip spica casts are contraindicated because they may compromise cardiopulmonary support and hamper nursing care (468). Regardless of the means of immobilization, the prognosis is excellent for most of these fractures because they go on to complete remodeling within 12 months; prolonged follow-up is advised. Preventive measures are important to minimize the risk of fracture in low-birth-weight infants. Their nutritional need for high levels of calcium, phosphorus, and vitamin D should be recognized. Alternating high levels of calcium with low levels of phosphorus in hyperalimentation solutions can help meet

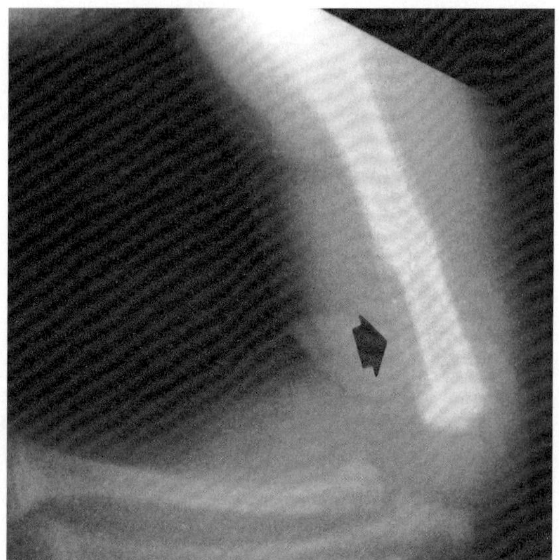

FIGURE 6-42 A 4-month-old premature infant of low birth weight with healing rickets. New periosteal bone is cloaking the humerus (*arrow*).

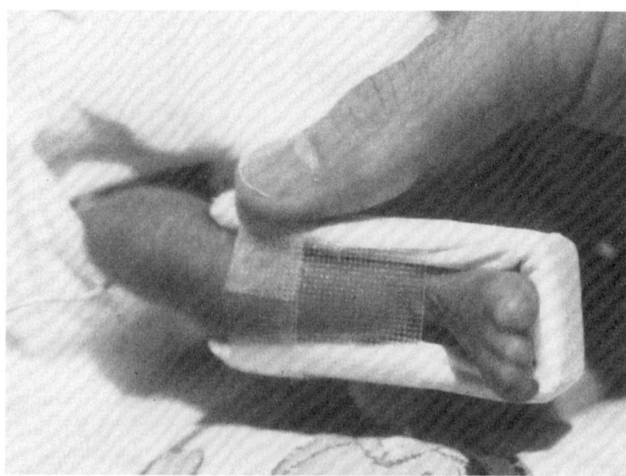

FIGURE 6-43 A tibia splint has been constructed for this premature infant by wrapping a tongue blade in a heavy layer of Webril and then fracturing the tongue depressor so that it assumes a sugar tong appearance. Tape is gently wound around the splint to hold it in place.

these needs. Because growth arrest is possible after fractures, follow-up over the first 2 to 3 years of life is advised.

Rickets and Renal Osteodystrophy

Renal osteodystrophy is common in patients with end-stage renal failure (473). Typically developing about 1.4 years after diagnosis of the kidney disease (473), the clinical syndrome is a combination of rickets and secondary hyperparathyroidism with marked osteoporosis. Affected children present with short stature, bone pain, muscle weakness, delayed sexual development, and bowing of the long bones (474). The underlying renal disease may be chronic nephritis, pyelonephritis, congenitally small kidneys, or cystinosis (453). Identification of the renal disorder is important because patients presenting with rickets due to obstructive uropathy may respond to surgical treatment of the renal disease.

Specific clinical deformities include genu valgum (most common), genu varum, coxa vara, and varus deformities of the ankle (474–476). These deformities are most common in patients diagnosed before 3 years of age. Davids et al (476) showed that periods of metabolic instability, characterized as an alkaline phosphatase of 500 U for at least 10 months, were associated with progression of deformity. With the adolescent growth spurt, osseous deformities can accelerate rapidly over a matter of weeks (476).

X-rays show rickets and osteopenia with osteitis fibrosa cystica (475). Osteoclastic cysts (brown tumors) may form. Metaphyseal cortical erosions occur in the lateral clavicle, distal ulna and radius, neck of the humerus, medial femoral neck, medial proximal tibia, and middle phalanges of the second and third fingers (473). The proximal femur may become so eroded with tapering and thinning that it has been likened to a rotting fence post (477). In renal osteodystrophy, the Looser zone may represent a true stress fracture and, with minor trauma, may extend across the full thickness of the bone with development of a true fracture. Callus may be scanty in patients with fractures who have untreated renal disease, but in patients on hemodialysis, abundant callus may form at the fracture site (452). Phalangeal quantitative ultrasound may be a useful method to assess bone quality and fracture risk in children and adolescents with bone and mineral disorders (478).

Treatment.

In renal osteodystrophy, pathologic fractures of the long bones, as rib fractures, vertebral compression fractures, and epiphyseal displacement of the epiphyses occur frequently. Fractures occur in areas of metaphyseal erosion or through cysts. Immobilization is used to treat pathologic fractures through both generalized weakened bone and brown tumors.

Once the underlying bone disease is under control, open procedures such as curettage of cysts with bone grafting and open reduction of fractures may be considered when appropriate (452). Internal fixation is preferable to external fixation (479). Preoperative tests needed for these patients before surgery include electrolytes, calcium, phosphorus, and alkaline phosphatase. Before surgery, these patients may need dialysis, phosphate adjustment, either medical or surgical correction of hyperparathyroidism, or chelation therapy for aluminum toxification. Supplemental vitamin D should be discontinued or the dose halved 2 to 4 weeks before any procedure that may require immobilization (474). It is important to rule out dental abscess, which may be present in as many as 25% of patients with vitamin D–resistant rickets (480). Postoperative infection may be more common in patients who are on corticosteroid therapy after renal transplantation (481). Prophylactic antibiotics are highly recommended for surgery of all patients with renal osteodystrophy (482).

Osteonecrosis may occur in weight-bearing bones, with the femoral head most often symptomatic (483). Other sites of involvement include the distal femoral condyles and the talus (475,484). Osteonecrosis may result from the use of immunosuppressive corticosteroids, because there is less osteonecrosis when the corticosteroid dose is decreased (485). Ferris et al (482) described osteochondritis dissecans lesions of the medial femoral condyles in young adults with hypophosphatemic rickets. Both loose bodies and so-called trap-door lesions were seen in these patients. Older patients developed calcification of the ligaments about the hip, knees, and spine. Lesions of bilateral osteochondritis dissecans may require repeated arthroscopic irrigations and removal of loose bodies (486). Joint stiffness in older patients due to ligamentous calcification about the knees, hips, and spine can be minimized if early corrective osteotomies of the lower extremities are performed to place them in the optimal position for function. Osteonecrosis in renal osteodystrophy can be treated with repeated joint aspiration, crutch ambulation, and physical therapy (476).

Rickets and Renal Osteodystrophy—Slipped Capital Femoral Epiphysis

The incidence of epiphyseal displacement in children with renal osteodystrophy ranges from 20% to 30% (455,487). Sites of involvement include the distal femur, proximal femur, and proximal humerus, the heads of both the metatarsals and metacarpals, and the distal radial and ulnar epiphyses, which tend to displace in an ulnar direction (487). In the proximal femur, both femoral neck fractures (454) and slipped capital femoral epiphysis occur (Fig. 6-44).

Possible explanations for displacement of the proximal femoral epiphysis include metaphyseal erosion with subsequent fracture (454,487), and a layer of fibrous tissue that forms between the physis and the metaphysis because of the destructive effects of the renal osteodystrophy (488). The warning signs and risk factors for slipped capital femoral epiphysis in renal osteodystrophy include subperiosteal erosion of the medial femoral neck, increasing width of the physis, bilateral coxa vara, male gender, and an age between 10 and 20 years (454). With erosion of the cortex of the inferior medial femoral neck, the femoral head collapses, decreasing the neck shaft angle, and subjecting the physis to shear forces as it assumes a vertical orientation.

The aggressive medical treatment of renal osteodystrophy, including administration of vitamin D (489), calcitriol, hemodi-

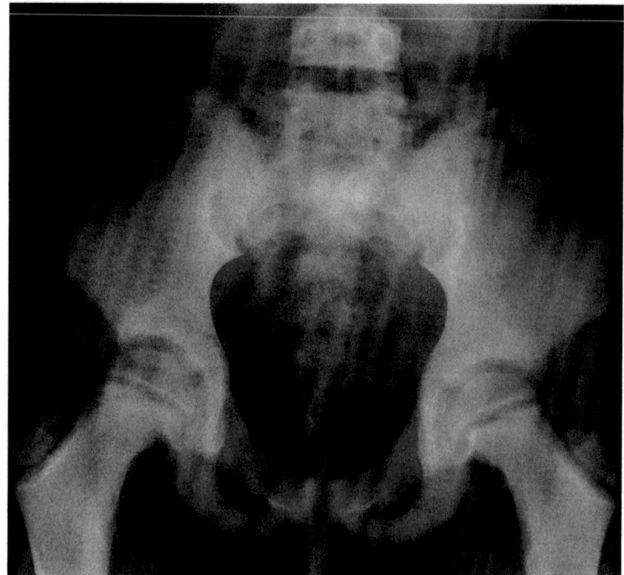

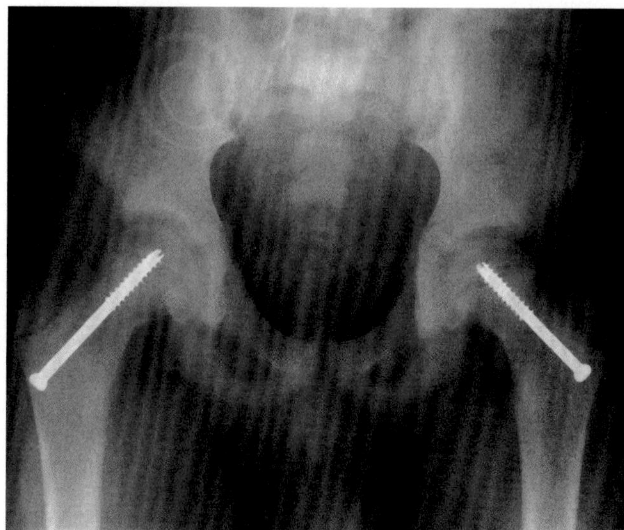

FIGURE 6-44 **A.** This 13-year-old boy with renal osteodystrophy presented with bilateral hip and thigh pain. This AP pelvis x-ray shows widening of the proximal femoral physes with sclerosis. Slipped capital femoral epiphyses were diagnosed. **B.** This AP pelvis x-ray taken 9 months after surgery shows narrowing of the physis and no evidence of further displacement of the capital femoral epiphyses.

alysis, renal transplantation, and parathyroidectomy, has improved the long-term survival and quality of life for these patients. Temporary limitation of weight bearing is recommended if there is little metaphyseal erosion, minimal coxa vara, and fusion of the physis is expected within 1 to 2 years (452). Goldman et al (454) recommended prophylactic hip pinning or close follow-up if risk factors are present for slipped capital femoral epiphysis in patients with renal osteodystrophy. With continuing slippage after medical treatment, most authors recommend in situ fixation (454,474,490). Continuing displacement of the proximal femoral epiphysis may occur even after pinning. Fixation holds poorly, possibly because the wide radiolucent zone of the femoral neck in this disorder is not true physis, but rather poorly mineralized woven bone and fibrous tissue (455). In a very young child, threaded pin fixation of the proximal femoral epiphysis may result in growth abnormality with trochanteric overgrowth.

Smooth pins can be used to stabilize the epiphysis temporarily until medical treatment resolves the underlying bone disease. For patients younger than 5 years, Hartjen and Koman (491) recommended treatment of slipped capital femoral epiphysis with reduction through Buck's traction and fixation with a single specially fabricated 4.5-mm cortical screw. The distal threads of the screw were machined off so that only the smooth shank of the screw extended across the physis. Subtrochanteric osteotomy with fixation or total hip arthroplasty may be necessary in older patients with severe coxa vara after slipped capital femoral epiphysis (454,474). Medical management of the underlying renal disease and of hyperparathyroidism is mandatory. Pinning of the proximal femur may not be necessary.

Renal Osteodystrophy Complicated by Aluminum Toxicity

Oppenheim et al (492) noted the contribution of aluminum toxicity to the development of fractures in renal osteodystrophy. Because phosphorus restriction is important in children with renal disease, aluminum hydroxide has been commonly used as a phosphate binder (493). Aluminum intoxication causes defective mineralization. Multiple pathologic fractures may occur with poor healing. Serum aluminum levels are not diagnostic, but the use of deferoxamine, a chelation agent, in an infusion test may provide the diagnosis (494). A bone biopsy often is necessary.

After treatment of the renal disease with correction of the aluminum toxicity by chelation agents, acute fractures will heal. Severe bowing of the long bones due to fractures can be treated with multiple osteotomies with intramedullary Rush rod or plate fixation (492). Recurrence of the syndrome is prevented by use of aluminum-free phosphate-binding agents such as calcium carbonate (495).

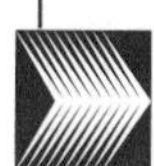

AUTHORS' PREFERRED METHOD OF TREATMENT

Rickets

Recognition of the underlying metabolic abnormalities is the most important aspect in the care of all of these injuries. Slipped capital femoral epiphysis may be the first presenting sign of renal failure (454). A slipped capital femoral epiphysis should be stabilized with in situ screw fixation in older children if progression is noted despite medical treatment. Multiple screws should be considered because the underlying metaphyseal bone is quite soft. For treatment of progressive slipped capital femoral epiphysis in very young children, some form of unthreaded fixation seems most logical.

Most fractures of the long bones respond readily to cast or splint immobilization, with concurrent aggressive medical treatment of the underlying metabolic disease. Femoral neck fractures are treated with anatomic reduction and internal fixation. The underlying bone disease should be medically treated to ensure success of open procedures. Significant cysts should be treated with curettage and bone grafting. Angular deformities of the long bones should be corrected when the patient is close to maturity.

Idiopathic Osteoporosis

Osteoporosis in a child generally is associated with either congenital disease such as osteogenesis imperfecta or metabolic disorders such as Cushing's syndrome. Rarely, children develop idiopathic osteoporosis with pathologic fractures (Fig. 6-45). Idiopathic osteoporosis is characteristically seen 2 years before puberty, but age at presentation may range from 4 to 16 years (496). Unique metaphyseal impaction fractures are a hallmark of this disorder (497). Biopsy specimens show a quantitative decrease in the amount of bone that has been linked to both increased resorption (498) and primary failure bone formation (496). Osteoblasts in this disorder seem to function normally when stimulated by oral 1,25-hydroxyvitamin D_3 (499). Symptoms can persist for 1 to 4 years after diagnosis, with spontaneous resolution in most patients after the onset of puberty. The only consistent metabolic abnormality is a negative calcium balance with high rates of fecal excretion of calcium (497). This finding supports the hypothesis that idiopathic juvenile osteoporosis results from intestinal malabsorption of calcium (500).

Although many children present with back pain as the only complaint, the most severely affected present with generalized skeletal pain (496,498,501,502). Patients have difficulty walking, and their symptoms may be initiated by mild trauma. In a review of 40 patients with idiopathic osteoporosis, Smith (496) observed that 87% had vertebral fractures and 42% had metaphyseal fractures. Symptoms of back or extremity pain can predate fractures by 6 months (501). Generally, 30% of bone mass must be absent before osteoporosis is detected on x-rays (503). Serum calcium, phosphorus, and alkaline phosphatase levels are usually normal (497). Low plasma calcitriol, a vitamin D metabolite that aids calcium absorption in the gut, has been observed in juvenile osteoporosis (504).

X-ray of the spine show decreased density in the central areas of the vertebral bodies, and clarity of the dense vertebral end plates is increased. The long bones lose trabecular anatomy and show thinning of the cortex (497,505). Once symptoms begin, a mildly lucent area of newly formed bone, a so-called neo-osseous porosis, is observable in the metaphysis. This is considered weaker than the surrounding bone, which formed before onset of the disease (496).

Treatment

Lower extremity and vertebral fractures (506) are common, although fractures of the proximal humerus, radius, ulna, and ribs are frequent (497). Nonunions of the tibia, radius, and ulna have been reported (497,500). Spinal cord compression has also been reported with vertebral fractures of osteoporosis in a child (507). Metaphyseal fractures can start as hairline cracks that gradually extend across the width of the shaft, and with further collapse in the femoral shaft, the cracks may telescope into the distal femur, with later distortion of the femoral condyles (497). Tibia and femoral shaft fractures may heal with bowing. Long bone shaft fractures are either transverse or oblique (497), and the callus formed seems to be normal (497,504). A technetium bone scan may be useful in showing healing fractures that are not obvious on plain x-ray studies (504). No clear-cut effective medical treatment has been found for idiopathic juvenile osteoporosis (497,498,508). Many patients have been treated by both vitamin D and calcium supplements with equivocal benefit, and usually mineralization of the skeleton does not improve until puberty, when the disease spontaneously resolves. Low does pamidronate appears promising in the treatment of childhood osteoporosis (509).

Dent and Friedman (500) summarized the treatment of fractures in juvenile osteoporosis when they stated that these fractures should undergo anatomic reduction with immobilization "as little as practical." They noted both severe deformity of the long bones and pseudarthrosis when the fractures could not be immobilized. The bones usually are so soft that they are thought to be unsuitable for the usual forms of fixation, but femoral neck fractures in this disorder have been treated with internal fixation (497).

Iatrogenic Osteoporosis

Osteoporosis of Chemotherapy

Osteoporosis is common in association with chemotherapeutic agents. Methotrexate, for example, is believed to inhibit osteogenesis, causing both delayed union and nonunion of fractures (510). The incidence of pathologic fractures after methotrexate use ranges from 19% to 57% (510–512). Generalized demineralization of the skeleton is seen with marked radiolucency of the metaphyseal regions of the long bones. Radiographic changes in the metaphysis and epiphysis resemble those seen in scurvy (510). Minimally displaced transverse fractures occur in the long bones of both the upper and lower extremities, and the small bones of the feet (510,512). Schwartz and Leonidas (513) caution that stress fractures of the long bones that can occur after methotrexate therapy can be mistaken for recurrence of leukemia. If feasible from an oncologic viewpoint, methotrexate should be discontinued to allow these fractures to heal in a cast. The cast immobilization itself may result in additional osteopenia and fractures even though methotrexate

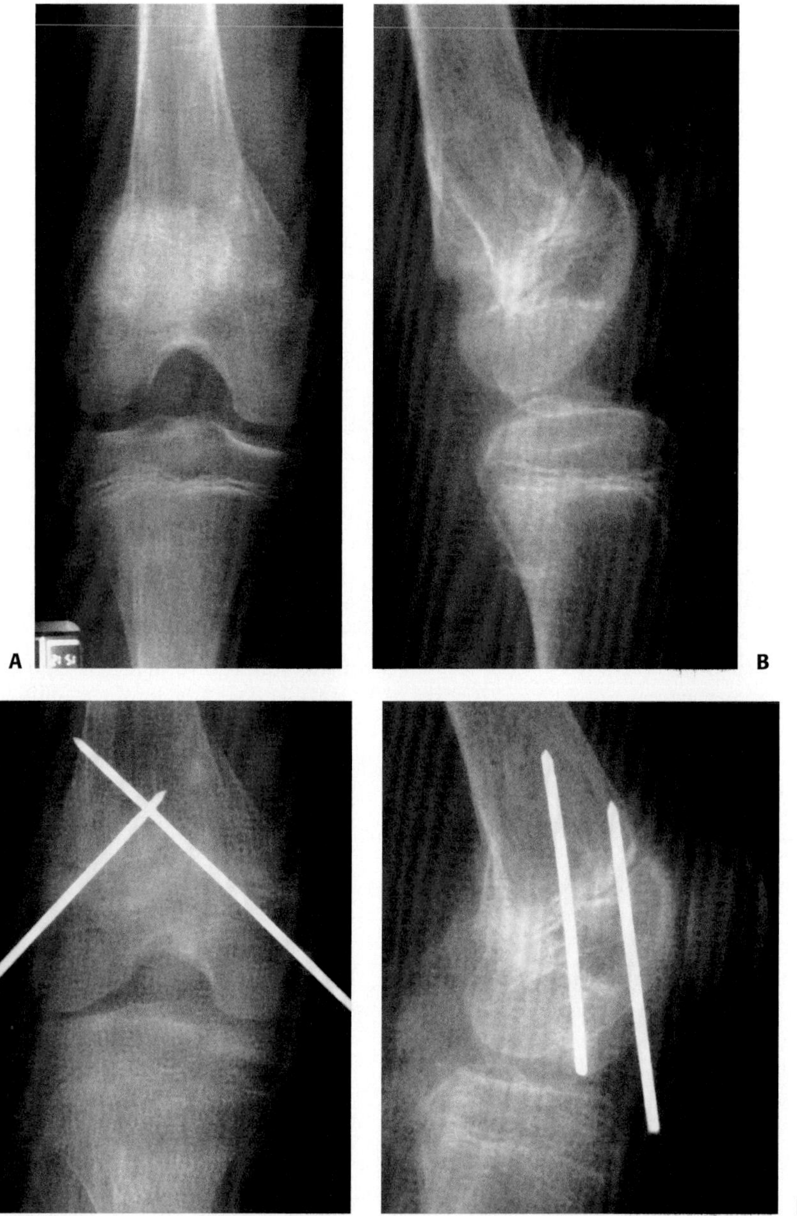

FIGURE 6-45 **A.** This case demonstrates multiple pathologic fractures in a previously healthy teenage boy who developed idiopathic osteoporosis. This AP x-ray of the right knee and this lateral x-ray **(B)** demonstrates a displaced distal femoral metaphyseal fracture with apex posterior angulation. **C.** This was treated with closed reduction and percutaneous pinning and application of a cast. **D.** This lateral x-ray shows satisfactory alignment with the pins in place. *(continues)*

is discontinued (513). Persistent nonunions require open reduction and internal fixation with bone graft (512). Patients with severe osteoporosis and bone pain without fracture also respond to a halt in methotrexate therapy (510).

Immobilization Osteoporosis

Immobilization of an extremity for fracture treatment can result in loss of as much as a 44% of mineralization of trabecular bone. In some patients, osteoporosis may persist for 6 months after injury (514). Immobilization leads to bone resorption, especially in unstressed areas (511). In one study (514), bone density of the distal radius returned to normal in all patients at l-year follow-up. Nilsson and Westlin (515) found a residual decrease in bone mineralization of the distal femur of 7% at nearly 11 years of follow-up in a study of 30 patients. Persistent osteoporosis after cast immobilization for fracture can contribute to refracture.

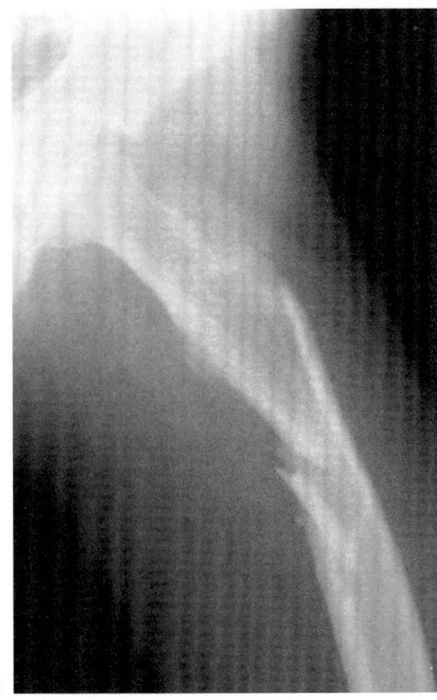
E

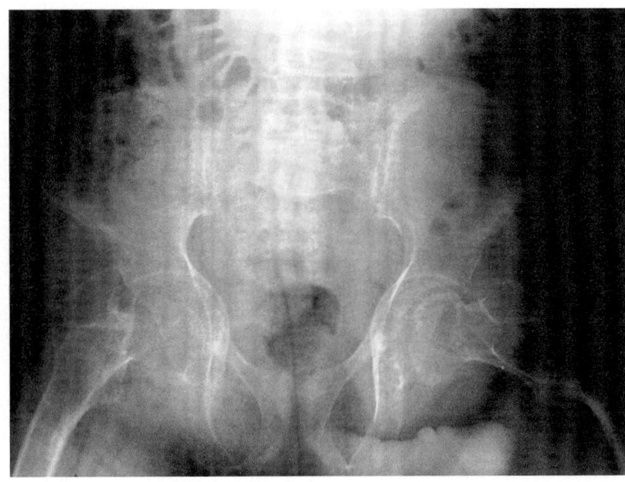
F

FIGURE 6-45 *(continued)* **E.** A few months later, he sustained a left proximal femur fracture, which was treated with a spica cast. **F.** This AP pelvis x-ray taken 3 years later shows healed proximal femoral fractures with varus angulation, and severe osteopenia of the pelvis and femora with profusion of both acetabuli.

Hyperparathyroidism

Primary hyperparathyroidism in childhood results from either hyperplasia of the parathyroid gland in very young children or parathyroid adenoma in older children (516). Increased parathyroid hormone increases osteoclastic activity, leading to general demineralization of the skeleton. In severely affected patients, osteitis fibrosa cystica may develop with fibrous tissue replacement of bone and formation of cysts (517). Hypercalcemia is common.

A particularly severe form of primary hyperparathyroidism seen in infants is congenital primary hyperparathyroidism, which results from an autosomal recessive trait (518) and is lethal without parathyroidectomy. These patients present with respiratory difficulty, hypotonia, poor feeding with constipation, and failure to thrive (519). Serum calcium is markedly increased in most patients, but a gradual rise above normal serum levels may occur in some infants with serial measurements (520). X-rays reveal demineralization of the skeleton. Marked resorption is present in the femoral necks and distal tibiae, with decreased trabeculae and poorly defined cortices (518). Periosteal elevation is common, and when it is severe, the long bones may actually look cloaked with new bone (Fig. 6-46). Periosteal resorption of the bone of the middle phalanges is believed to be characteristic of this disease. Brown tumors are rare in infancy.

In older children and adolescents, the clinical presentation is more subtle. Weakness, anorexia, and irritability are present in 50% of patients, and constipation is present in 28% (516). Renal calculi also are present in 25% of patients, and polyuria, excessive thirst, bone pain, abdominal distention, pancreatitis, and swelling of the knees are occasionally present (516,521,522). Approximately 50% of older patients have osteopenia and other osseous signs of hyperparathyroidism (516). The serum calcium is only moderately elevated in many patients, but 24-hour urine calcium excretion is abnormally high (516,523). If the diagnosis is uncertain, selective venous catheterization for parathyroid hormone can be done, localizing the gland by either ultrasound, CT scan, or MRI (524).

Treatment

Pathologic fractures of the long bones are common in patients with hyperparathyroidism (523,525), especially in infancy. Vertebral fractures, which occur in 4.4% of adult patients (526), are rare in infancy. Increased levels of parathyroid hormone results in decreased function and numbers of osteoblasts, and hence delayed union of pathologic fractures (297), but this problem has only been reported in adults; healing occurred after parathyroidectomy (423).

Most fractures are successfully treated with simple immobilization. Occasionally, a fracture through a cyst requires curettage and bone grafting after a period of initial healing (527). Partial or total parathyroidectomy is the primary treatment for hyperparathyroidism (524,528). Solitary bone cysts often heal after parathyroidectomy.

Cushing's Syndrome

Cushing's syndrome results from excessive production of cortisol and its related compounds. If the hyperactivity of the adrenal cortex is due to pituitary gland stimulation, the syndrome is most precisely known as Cushing's disease (529). In children, hypercortisolism is most often caused by carcinoma, adenoma, hyperplasia of the adrenal cortex (530), Ewing's sarcoma (531),

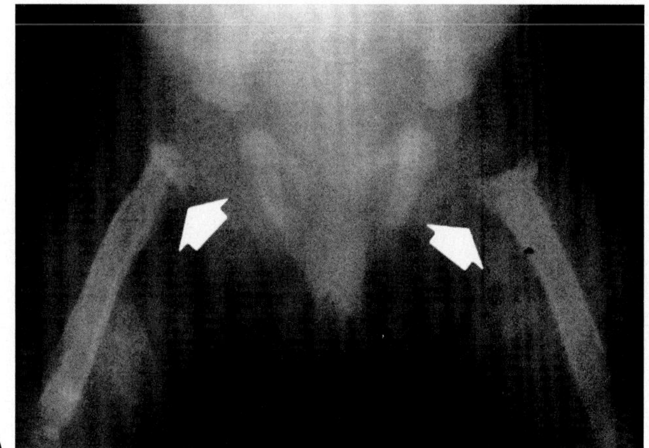
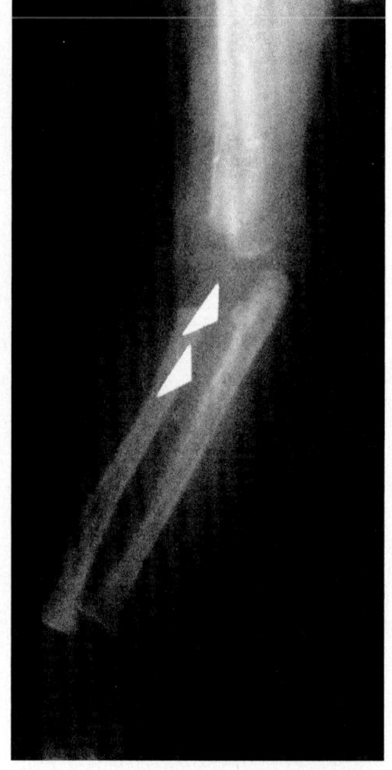

FIGURE 6-46 **A.** Newborn with hyperparathyroidism. There is marked demineralization of bone, and marked resorption is present in the proximal femora (*arrows*). **B.** Periosteal elevation is present along the ulna (*arrows*). (Courtesy of Bruce Mewborne, MD, San Antonio, Texas.)

or exogenous corticosteroid therapy. The elevated adrenal corticosteroids inhibit the formation of osteoblasts (532), resulting in increased resorption of the bone matrix and decreased bone formation (533).

In infancy, carcinoma and adenoma are the primary causes of Cushing's syndrome; the remaining cases are secondary to hyperplasia of the adrenal cortex. Presenting symptoms include failure to thrive, short stature with excessive weight gain, moon facies, presence of a buffalo hump, hirsutism, weakness, and hypertension (530). Cutaneous striae are rare, and the genitalia are of normal size. Mortality is well over 50% (530). In older children, the clinical picture is somewhat different: truncal obesity, short stature, a lowered hairline, acne, weakness, emotional lability, hirsutism, cutaneous striae, hypertension, and ecchymosis. Radiographic findings may include severe osteopenia and a retarded bone age. Fractures of the ribs, vertebrae, and long bones have been reported in children with Cushing's syndrome (534,535).

Treatment

The primary treatment of Cushing's syndrome of childhood is total adrenalectomy (535). The associated fractures usually can be treated with standard immobilization techniques, but care should be taken not to increase the extent of osteopenia through excessive immobilization. In patients on corticosteroid therapy, the dose should be reduced, converted to an alternate-day schedule, or discontinued, if possible (531).

Scurvy

The rarity of scurvy makes its diagnosis difficult. In children, scurvy may follow 6 to 12 months of a vitamin C–deficient diet (536). Because vitamin C is essential for normal collagen formation, deficiency of the vitamin results in defective osteogenesis, vascular breakdown, delayed healing, and wound dehiscence (537). With abnormal crosslinking, the defective collagen formed inhibits formation of osteoid matrix. Meanwhile, the chondroid tissue continues to be mineralized and can become completely calcified (538). Increased resorption and decreased formation of bone lead to generalized skeletal demineralization. The ends of the long bones resorb, leaving only a cuff of thickened periosteum to stabilize the epiphysis (539). Although scurvy is often due to a dietary deficiency of vitamin C (537,538,540), both aspirin and phenytoin are associated with decreased plasma levels of ascorbic acid. Vitamin C deficiency also is present in patients with myelomeningocele (541), although its contribution to fracture in that population is unclear.

Infants with scurvy present with irritability, tenderness of the lower extremities, weakness, pseudoparalysis, and possibly bleeding gums (if teeth have erupted). Subperiosteal hemorrhages may exist as well as hemorrhage into the subcutaneous tissues, muscles, urinary system, and gastrointestinal tract (542). Anemia is also a common finding. In older children, tenderness and swelling of the extremities are the most common findings. Fever was noted at the time of presentation in 70% of 52 patients in one series (543). Therefore, both osteomyelitis and septic arthritis must be initially considered in the differential diagnosis. In developing countries, older children with scurvy presenting with inability to walk may be misdiagnosed as having poliomyelitis (544).

X-rays show profound demineralization. In advanced disease, the long bones become almost transparent with a ground-glass appearance and extreme thinning of the cortex. Calcium accumulates in the zone of provisional calcification adjacent to the physis and becomes densely white (Fränkel's line). Fractures generally occur in the scurvy line (Trummerfeld zone)—the radiolucent juxtaepiphyseal area above Frankel's line where the matrix is not converted to bone. Dense lateral spurs, known as Pelken's sign, may be seen (537). A characteristic finding of scurvy is the corner sign, in which a peripheral metaphyseal defect exists where fibrous tissue replaces absorbed cortex and cartilage (539). Cupping of the metaphysis is common in both scurvy and rickets; in rickets, the metaphysis is ragged, whereas in scurvy, the metaphysis is sharply outlined (537). The epiphysis becomes ringed with a thin, dense line (Wimberger's sign). The periosteal elevation caused by hemorrhage calcifies within 10 days of treatment with vitamin C (Fig. 6-47).

Treatment

Fractures and epiphyseal displacement occur in both infants and older children with scurvy (536,539,543,545,546). The most common sites of fracture, in order of frequency, are the distal femur, proximal humerus, costochondral junction of the

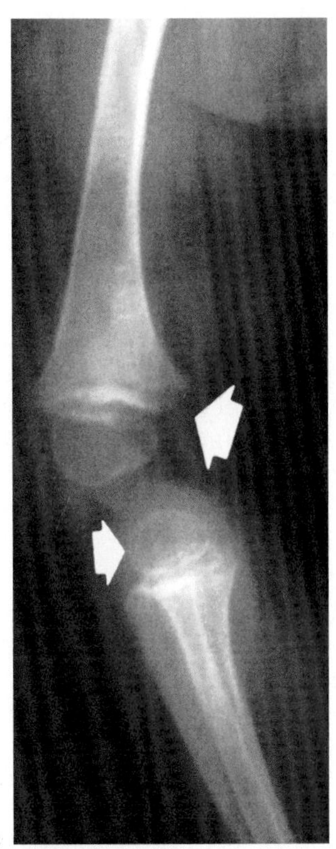

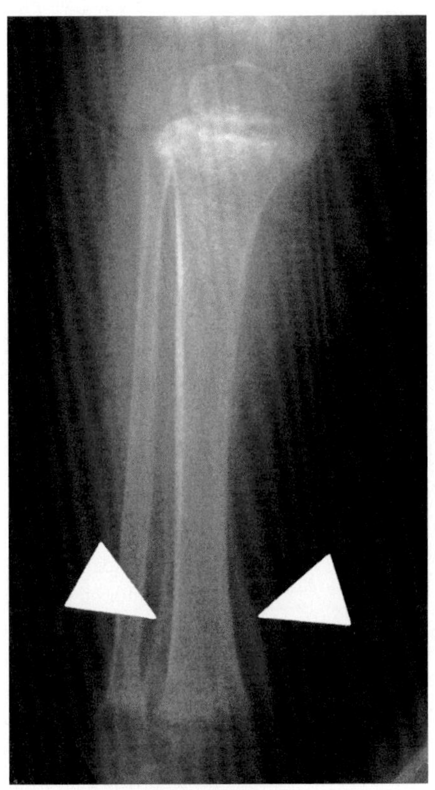

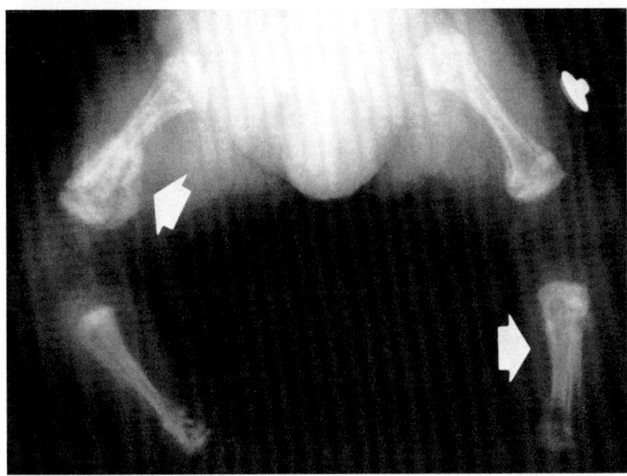

FIGURE 6-47 Scurvy. **A.** A 10-month-old boy presented with a 2-week history of refusal to walk with tenderness of the lower extremities. He had a history of milk and cereal intake only. There are signs of scurvy in the metaphysis (*large arrow*). The dense white line in the zone of the provisional calcification of the distal femur is known as Fränkel's line. The radiolucent juxtaepiphyseal line above the white line is known as the scurvy line. The peripheral metaphyseal defect, where fibrous tissue replaces absorbed cortex in cartilage, is known as the corner sign. Wimberger's sign is a thin, dense line surrounding the epiphysis (*small arrow*). **B.** This is a child with healing scurvy. There is marked periosteal calcification around the distal tibia (*arrows*). **C.** A newborn with scurvy. Periosteal hemorrhage has become calcified in the bones of the lower extremity (*arrows*). (Courtesy of Bruce Mewborne, MD, San Antonio, Texas.)

ribs, and distal tibia (537). Fractures of the long bones generally are nondisplaced metaphyseal buckle fractures with mild angulation. In contrast, marked epiphyseal displacement occurs with a moderate amount of callus present even in untreated patients. Exuberant callus forms once vitamin C is administered. Standard immobilization, with administration of vitamin C, is adequate for most fractures. Remodeling potential is high in these patients (545). Even healed fractures that appear to have undergone growth arrest should just be observed, because the potential for continued growth with medical treatment of the vitamin C deficiency can be nearly normal (547). For infants who are older than 12 months of age and have begun weight-bearing, spine films are recommended to rule out vertebral fractures (536).

The literature of fracture treatment in scurvy consists primarily of case reports. Hoeffel et al (548) reported on a 14-month-old girl with scurvy with bilateral distal femoral epiphysis displacement. This condition resolved after treatment with vitamin C, but limb-length discrepancy developed on one side (549). In two patients with distal femoral fractures, healing went on to cupping of the metaphysis with an appearance similar to that in central growth arrest (543,546).

Copper Deficiency and Scurvy-like Syndrome

Copper is a vital trace element needed in the production of collagen. Copper deficiency results in a decreased number of collagen crosslinks, with adverse effects on both bone and blood vessels (550). Copper deficiency can occur by 3 months in low-birth-weight infants (551) and after prolonged total parenteral nutrition. Copper deficiency can also develop as a result of excessive supplemental zinc ingestion (552).

Infants at risk for this syndrome are those who are primarily milk fed and are on semistarvation diets with concurrent vomiting and diarrhea (553). Both rib and wrist enlargement are frequent (550), and neutropenia is common (551). The diagnosis is commonly based on clinical presentation and decreased levels of serum copper.

Radiographic findings in copper deficiency syndrome are very similar to those in rickets, including metaphyseal cupping, flaring, demineralization of the skeleton, and subperiosteal elevation with calcification (483). There are some radiographic differences between scurvy and copper deficiency syndrome (550). The corner sign is frequently absent in copper deficiency, the metaphyseal spurs are not strictly lateral but sickle shaped, and radiolucent bands of the metaphysis are absent. Bone age also is frequently retarded.

Pathologic fractures have been reported in copper deficiency syndrome. Cordano et al (553) noted prompt healing of a distal femoral fracture in an infant, but the fracture recurred before treatment of the copper deficiency. Such injuries could be treated like those in scurvy, with simple immobilization and concurrent correction of the copper deficiency.

FRACTURES IN NEUROMUSCULAR DISEASE

Cerebral Palsy

The management of fractures in patients with severe cerebral palsy can prove challenging. Low bone mineral density (BMD) is common in children with moderate to severe cerebral palsy (CP) and is associated with significant fracture risk. The underlying pathophysiology is complex, with several factors contributing to the problem and significant variation between different regions of the body (554). In a review of 1,232 institutionalized patients with cerebral palsy, McIvor and Samilson (555) documented 134 extremity fractures, primarily in quadriplegics. When the mechanism of injury was known, most of these fractures were the consequence of a fall, often associated with seizure activity. Approximately 46% of these fractures involved the femoral shaft, 6% were fractures of the head or neck of the femur, 15% involved the tibia and fibula, and 13% were humeral fractures. These authors believed that contracture or paralytic dislocation of the hip joint predisposed these patients to femoral fractures (Fig. 6-48).

Miller and Glazer (556) emphasized that spontaneous fractures can occur in patients with cerebral palsy without episodes of trauma, and factors such as disuse atrophy, nutritional deficiencies, and preexisting joint contractures contributed to these injuries. Nearly 50% of the full-time bedridden patients they studied developed spontaneous fractures. The diagnosis usually was delayed because the patients were noncommunicative. Anticonvulsant therapy may contribute to osteoporosis in patients with multiple fractures—low levels of serum vitamin D were seen in 42% of patients in one series (557). One study concluded that unless sunlight exposure can be guaranteed, vitamin D supplementation should be considered for children and adults in residential care, especially if they are on anticonvulsant therapy, even in areas with year-round sunshine (558). Fractures through osteoporotic bone can occur both above and below fixation devices.

Although long bone fractures in patients with cerebral palsy heal quickly with abundant callus (556), their treatment through either closed or open methods can be quite difficult. In a large series of patients, McIvor and Samilson (555) recommended closed treatment through skeletal traction, hip spica cast, or long-leg cast. Approximately 65% of the femoral shaft fractures and 86% of distal femoral fractures went on to malunion. Despite malunion, most patients regained their prefracture function. Nearly 21% of their patients had refractures, and the authors believed that this was due to disuse osteopenia, inadequate reduction, or joint contractures. Closed treatment of these fractures can be complicated by the development of decubitus ulcers. Closed fractures, especially those of the femur, can become open injuries during treatment, owing to spasticity or inadequate immobilization (555,556). Hip spica casts are difficult to use in patients with severe flexion contractures or dislocation of the hip. The healing time of femoral fractures

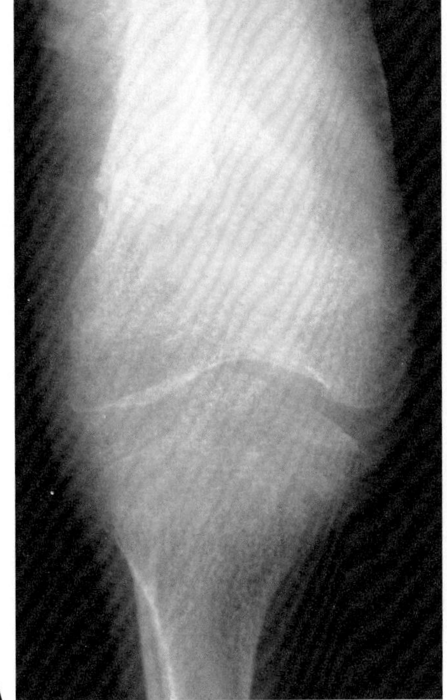

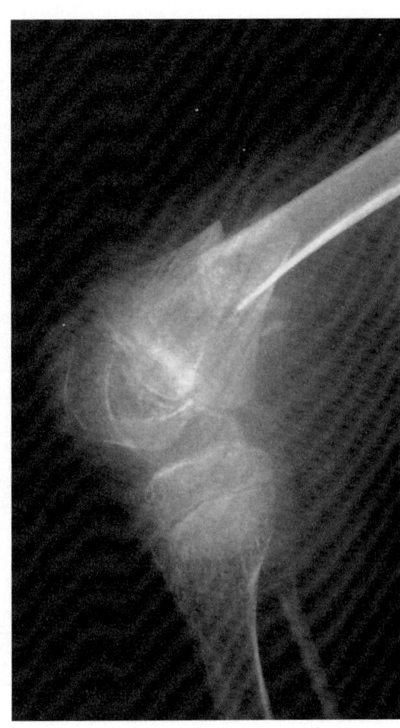

FIGURE 6-48 **A.** This 11-year-old boy with quadriplegic cerebral palsy had a varus derotation osteotomy followed by spica casting. Two weeks after cast removal, he sustained this distal femoral fracture during physical therapy. An AP x-ray of the right knee and **(B)** a lateral x-ray of the right knee show a distal femoral metaphyseal fracture in a location typical for insufficiency fractures in children with neuromuscular disease. The fracture was minimally displaced and was treated with closed reduction and a carefully applied, well-padded spica cast. Note the osteopenia and the typical changes around the knee associated with long-standing knee flexion contracture.

treated through immobilization varies from 1 to 3.5 months (555,556). Fractures of the humerus have been treated with light hanging-arm casts or sling-and-swath bandages (556). Hip nails with side plates, compression plates, and intramedullary fixation also have been used for femoral shaft fractures in patients with cerebral palsy. The mean healing time has been 5.3 months (555).

Numerous reports note success in treating fractures of neurologically impaired children with internal or external fixation (559,560). Heinrich et al (560) treated four femoral fractures in young patients with cerebral palsy with flexible intramedullary nails with good outcomes. Femoral neck fractures may require in situ pinning, but observation may be adequate in asymptomatic bedridden patients. Although he advocated open fixation of some lower extremity fractures in patients with mental retardation, Sherk (561) cautioned that some patients may have inadequate motivation to resume ambulation even with successful healing of their injuries. Medical management of these patients must also be emphasized. In patients with cerebral palsy and multiple fractures, Lee and Lyne (557) recommended metabolic supplementation, along with traditional fracture care.

Fractures of the distal pole of the patella have been reported in children with cerebral palsy due to spasticity of the extensor mechanism of the knee in the presence of established knee flexion contracture (562–564). Lloyd-Roberts et al (563) reported on eight patients with this injury who presented with deterioration in walking and decreased endurance. All had knee flexion contractures. Seven of the eight patients complained of pain and local tenderness at the distal pole of the patella. In a series of 88 patients, fragmentation was seen in only 8% (564). Patella alta and elongation of the patella are frequent in affected patients (Fig. 6-49) (562,564). Children predisposed to distal pole patellar fractures are spastic ambulators with flexion contractures of the knees, patella alta, and a history of falls (562). Extension casting may be helpful in symptomatic patients (564). If conservative treatment is unsatisfactory, then hamstring lengthening with correction of the knee flexion contracture can result in both healing of the fracture and relief of symptoms (563,564). Some authors (562,563) also have excised the avulsed distal pole of the patella to relieve chronic symptoms.

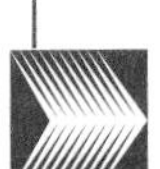

AUTHORS' PREFERRED METHOD OF TREATMENT

Cerebral Palsy

The goal of fracture treatment in cerebral palsy is to restore the child to his or her prefracture level of function. If the patient is ambulatory, conventional forms of fracture treatment should be used. In nonambulatory children with cerebral palsy, a goal of fracture care should be to preserve the ability to transfer. Special precautions should be used in closed treatment of fractures in these patients. The patients' spasticity and inability to communicate make them prone to skin problems, so casts should be properly applied and well padded, usually with felt and polyurethane foam. Extra

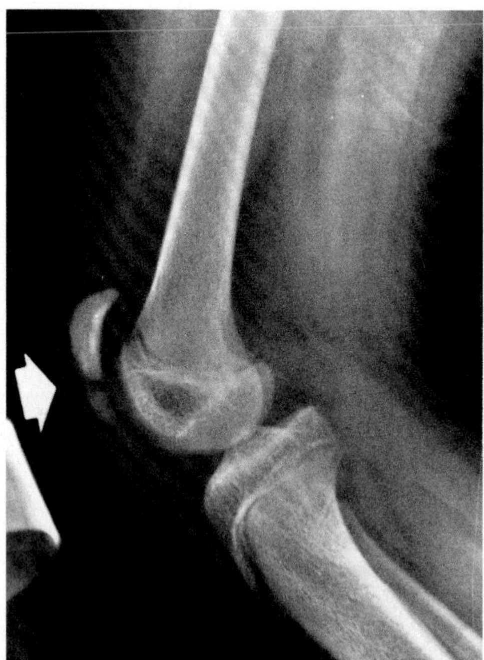

FIGURE 6-49 A 10-year-old girl with cerebral palsy had a healing stress fracture of an elongated patella (*arrow*). Patella alta is also present. The injury responded to conservative treatment.

padding should be placed over the patella, anterior ankle, and heel, and a snug cast mold should be placed above the calcaneus to prevent proximal migration of the heel (Fig. 6-50). When indicated, operative fracture fixation should be used in ambulatory patients. Elastic intramedullary nails can be a very effective way to treat femoral fractures in children with spasticity.

Prevention should be an important part of managing fractures in children with cerebral palsy. Traditionally, long-leg casts or spica casts were used after multiple muscle lengthenings or hip osteotomies, then after several weeks, the cast was removed and therapy begun. After cast treatment, however, the osteopenia was worse, the joints were stiff, and fractures—especially in the distal femoral metaphysis—occurred during therapy or transfers. We and others (565,566) use foam abduction pillows and knee immobilizers and an intensive therapy program in the immediate postoperative period to avoid the deconditioning, osteopenia, and joint stiffness that develop after prolonged cast immobilization. In ambulatory children who need hip osteotomies, use of rigid internal fixation allows standing and gait training within 2 weeks, preventing not only osteopenia but also the risk that the child may never regain the full level of preoperative function after a prolonged period of cast immobilization.

In nonambulatory children with severe cerebral palsy, some degree of both malunion and shortening may be accepted. Well-padded splints or casts are adequate treatment for many displaced fractures. Acute femoral shaft fractures can be treated with a heavily padded hip spica cast and distal fractures of the femur by a long-leg cast. Distal femoral buckle fractures in nonambulatory children are safely treated with a knee immobilizer. If a long-leg cast is used for a fracture of the lower extremity and the joint of the involved side is dislocated, the rigid cast may function as a lever arm, with the posterior fracture of the proximal femur beyond the cast.

Myelomeningocele

Insufficiency Fractures

Children with myelomeningocele sustain fractures of the lower extremities through bone weakened by either disuse or immobilization after reconstructive surgical procedures. The incidence of fractures in children with myelomeningocele ranges from 12% to 31% (564–571). The locations of these fractures, in order of decreasing frequency, are mid-shaft of the femur, distal femur, mid-shaft of the tibia, proximal femur, femoral neck, distal femoral physis, and proximal tibia (567). Fractures of the distal tibia also have been reported in numerous series (570–574). Both metaphyseal and diaphyseal fractures, usually resulting from minor trauma, are often either incomplete or impacted with intact periosteum (575). They tend to heal rapidly—nonunion is rare (567). Physeal fractures, however, may take 3 to 33 months to heal (571).

Numerous factors predispose these patients to fracture. Children with flail limbs tend to pick up one leg and drop it out of the way when they roll over in bed or twist around while in a sitting position, and this may be enough force to cause a fracture (570). Because protective sensation is absent, the child can neither anticipate impending injury nor be aware of injury once it has occurred. The level of neurologic involvement also affects the incidence of fractures. In a series of 76 fractures, Lock and Aronson (575) found that 41% occurred with neurologic deficit at the thoracic level, 36% occurred with deficit at the upper lumbar level, and only 13% occurred in patients with lower lumbar or sacral deficits. Nearly 86% of these fractures occurred before 9 years of age, and 76% were associated with cast immobilization. Most fractures after immobilization occur within 4 weeks of cast removal (568), and in one series (575), 30% of patients with casts had multiple cluster fractures of either the casted extremity or the partially casted contralateral extremity. In addition to the inherent disuse osteoporosis from immobilization, casting causes stiffness of joints, with concentration of force on the osteoporotic bone adjacent to the joints (575). Boytim et al (576) reported neonatal fractures in 6 infants with myelomeningocele and concluded that the risk of fracture was 17% for patients with thoracic or high lumbar level deficits with significant contracture of the lower extremities. The authors cautioned that particular care must be used to avoid fractures in these patients during physical therapy, x-ray positioning, or surgical procedures.

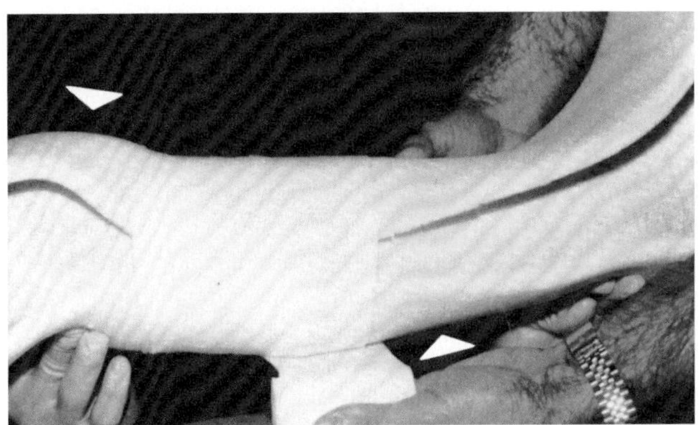

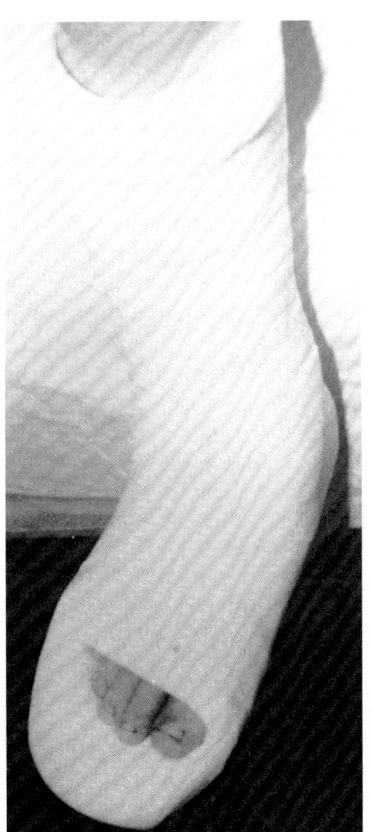

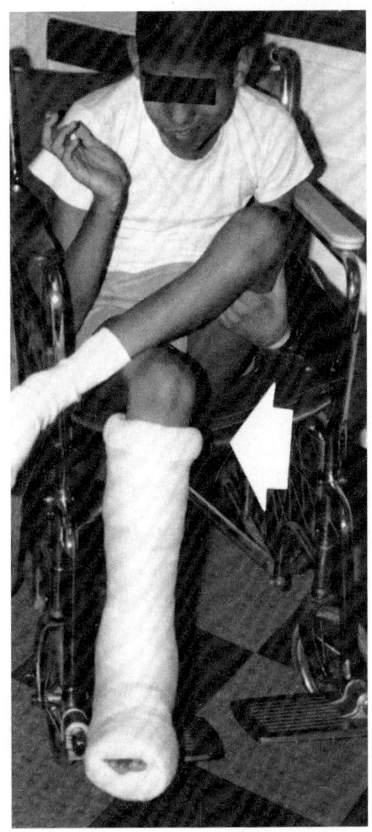

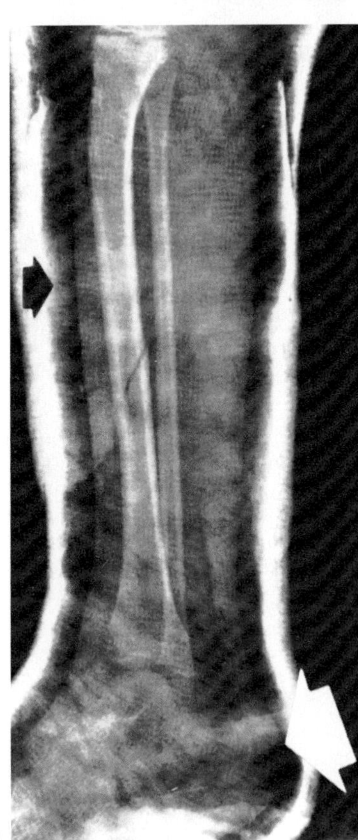

FIGURE 6-50 Casting in neuromuscular fractures. **A.** A polyurethane foam short-leg cast is being placed on a patient. Two long rectangular sheets of foam (*arrows*) are placed anteriorly and posteriorly over the stockinette, and Webril padding is wrapped around the foam. **B.** A long toe plate is needed to prevent injury to the foot of the patient. **C.** A thick, protective cuff of foam is formed by folding the polyurethane toward the center of the cast with the stockinette (*arrow*). **D.** The Webril must be wrapped quite snugly to compress the foam against the underlying extremity evenly (*black arrow*). Extra foam is placed over the anterior ankle and over the Achilles tendon to prevent proximal migration of the foot in the cast. A plaster cast is usually applied and covered with a layer of fiberglass for strength. A lateral x-ray verifies the position of the heel in the cast (*white arrow*).

Stable fractures of the long bones may not require complete immobilization (568). Femoral shaft fractures have been treated with padding and sandbags (577). Skin traction of anesthetic limbs may cause massive skin necrosis (567,577). Skeletal traction usually is inadvisable because of problems with decubitus ulcers and poor fixation in atrophic bone (567,577). However, Drummond et al (578) treated 9 of 18 patients with skeletal traction without mention of failure or fixation.

Preventive measures include limiting cast immobilization after reconstructive surgery (568,578). Solid side cushions may prevent fractures that occur when patients catch their lower extremities in bed rails (579). The most important consideration was noted by Norton and Foley (580) in 1959, when they stated "the quality of bone developed by activity appears to be the best protection against pathologic fractures," and the orthopedist should assist these patients in maintaining the highest activity level possible.

Physeal Fractures

Fractures of the physes in patients with myelomeningocele are relatively uncommon, but for the unwary, the diagnosis can be difficult (581). The clinical presentation may mimic infection, with elevated temperature and swelling, redness, and local warmth at the fracture site (574,582). Fractures of the proximal tibia may be confused with septic arthritis of the knee, with swelling up to the mid-thigh and limited knee flexion. Both the white blood cell count and erythrocyte sedimentation rate are often elevated. Immobilization of these injuries usually results in a dramatic decrease in swelling and redness of the extremity within 2 to 3 days of casting. With healing, the x-ray picture can be alarming, with epiphyseal plate widening, metaphyseal fracture, and periosteal elevation (583). The radiographic differential diagnosis should include osteomyelitis, sarcoma, leukemia, and Charcot's joint (571,574,582).

Recurrent trauma to the physis, from either continued walking or passive joint motion after injury, results in an exuberant healing reaction (Fig. 6-51) (572). Repetitive trauma delays resumption of normal endochondral ossification, resulting in abnormal thickening of the cartilage in the zone of hypertrophy and the physeal widening seen on x-rays (Fig. 6-52) (571). In a study of 19 chronic physeal fractures, Rodgers et al (572) compared MRI with histology and found that adjacent to this thickened, disorganized zone of hypertrophy is juxtametaphyseal fibrovascular tissue that enhances gadolinium on MRI. Delayed union is common, and premature growth arrest occurs in 29% to 55% of patients (571,575). Anschuetz et al (584) reported a unique syndrome in three patients with myelomeningocele and fracture. These children sustained fractures of the lower extremities during long-term immobilization and with cast removal went on to dramatic cardiopulmonary distress with increased pulse rate, hypotension, and increased respiratory rate. Fever also developed with decreased hematocrit levels. They suggested that the etiology of this problem was loss of intravascular volume into the fracture sites and recommended intravenous replacement of fluid losses, along with careful splinting of associated fractures.

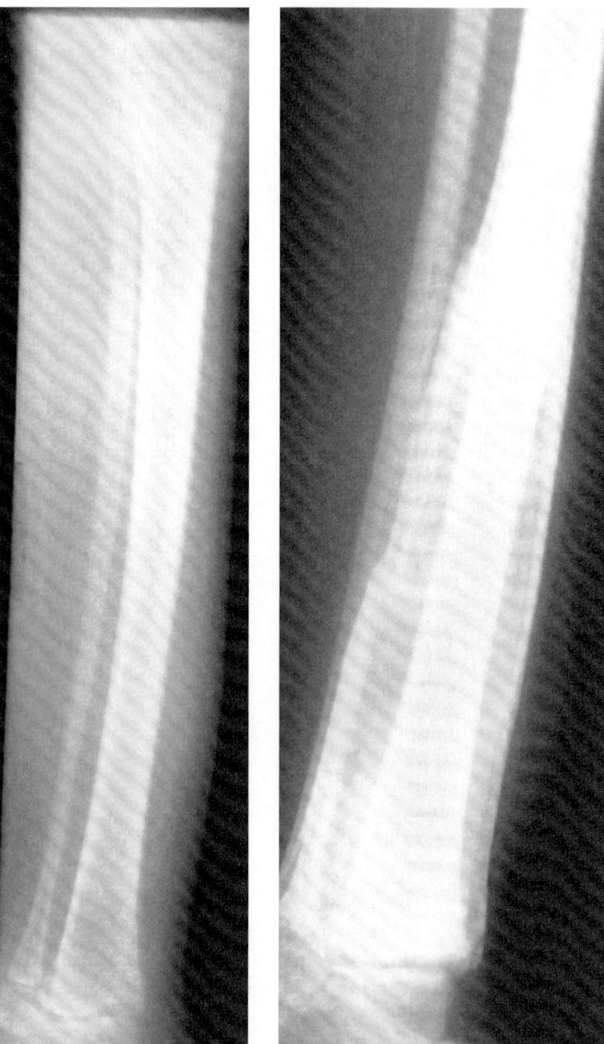

FIGURE 6-51 **A.** This 7-year-old boy with spina bifida presented with increasing swelling of the distal tibia. This lateral x-ray of the entire tibia shows slight widening of the distal tibial physis with subtle signs of posterior displacement of the distal tibial physis. There was a high suspicion of a fracture, so the leg was treated with a well-padded cast. **B.** This lateral x-ray, taken 2 months later, shows slight physeal widening with extraordinary periosteal new bone formation.

Physeal injuries in patients with myelomeningocele are more difficult to treat than metaphyseal or diaphyseal long bone fractures and require lengthy immobilization with strict avoidance of weight-bearing to avoid destructive repetitive trauma to the physis (572). Either a plaster cast or a snug-fitting total-contact orthosis is suggested for immobilization, and union can be determined by return of the physis to normal width on x-ray study (571). Kumar et al (573) emphasized that application of a long leg cast for 8 to 12 weeks is necessary to obtain satisfactory healing of physeal fractures of the tibia, and weight-bearing is to be avoided until union occurs.

Cast Technique

Immediate casting (570) and bivalved casting (577) have been used for long-bone fractures in children with myelomeningo-

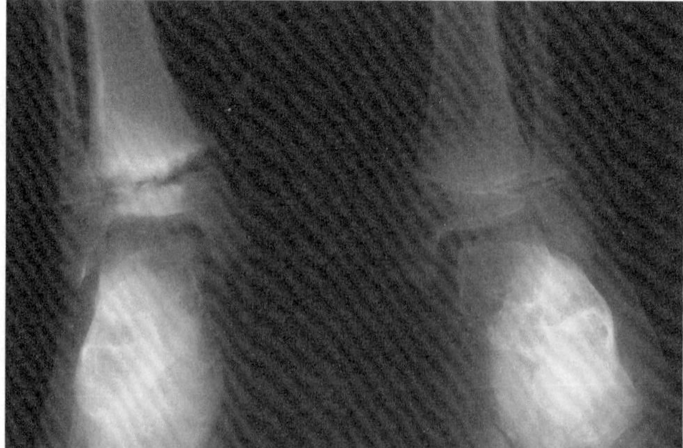

FIGURE 6-52 This 11-year-old boy with L4 myelomeningocele presented with a warm, swollen right ankle and no clear history of trauma. This AP x-ray of both ankles shows right distal tibial physeal widening with adjacent sclerosis, consistent with a chronic physeal injury. The child was treated in a well-padded, non–weight-bearing short leg cast. He had complete resolution of symptoms when the cast was removed 6 weeks later.

cele. A bilateral hip spica cast is suggested for supracondylar fractures of the femur, because use of a one-and-a-half hip spica cast may predispose the uninjured side to fracture (567). A bulky Webril dressing approximately 1.5 cm thick wrapped with an elastic bandage can be used instead of a plaster or fiberglass cast. Lock and Aronson (575) used Webril immobilization for an average of 1 to 3 weeks in their patients with fractures and discontinued immobilization when callus was visible. They found similar outcomes in patients treated with Webril dressings and those treated with casts; however, there was much less difficulty with pressure sores in the group treated with Webril dressings. Kumar et al (573) used a polyurethane padded long leg posterior plaster splint for metaphyseal and diaphyseal fractures for 3 weeks, followed by bracing.

Drennan and Freehafer (567) recommend a well-padded cast for 2 to 3 weeks for infants with fracture and braces or Webril immobilization for incomplete fractures that followed surgery. Injuries with deformity were placed in a cast. Mobilization was begun as soon as practical to prevent further osteopenia—patients with shaft fractures began ambulation 2 weeks after injury. Shortening was not a problem in their series. Lock and Aronson (575) cautioned that brace treatment of acute fractures may cause pressure sores. Drummond et al (568) reported on 18 fractures treated by closed techniques that resulted in three malunions, two shortenings, and two episodes of pressure sores; one patient had four refractures. Drabu and Walker (585) noted a mean loss of knee movement of 58° in 67% of fractures about the knee. The stiffness began 2 months after fracture and was well established by 6 months but resolved almost completely in all patients 3 years after injury. They suggested that aggressive physical therapy to restore knee motion is probably not necessary in these injuries.

Operative Treatment

Operative fixation of fractures in children with myelomeningocele is associated with a high rate of infection (577). Wenger et al (571) reported that most patients with proximal femoral epiphyseal displacement can be treated with hip spica casts. Reduction and pinning with subtrochanteric osteotomy may be necessary in certain patients. Bailey-Dubow rods may be valuable in multiple recurrent pathologic fractures of the femoral or tibial shaft (586). If operative treatment is necessary, it should be noted that the incidence of malignant hyperthermia is higher in patients with myelomeningocele than in other children (587).

Latex Allergy

Life-threatening anaphylactic reactions due to latex allergy in children with myelomeningocele have been reported with increasing frequency (575,588). Minor allergic reactions, such as rash, edema, hives, and respiratory symptoms are common when children with myelodysplasia are exposed to latex products such as gloves, catheters, and balloons. Between 18% and 40% of children with myelodysplasia are allergic to latex (589). Meeropol et al (590) emphasized that every child with myelomeningocele should be screened for latex allergy, and those with a positive history should be evaluated individually by the anesthesiologist for preoperative prophylaxis. Current preoperative prophylaxis begins 24 hours before surgery and is continued for 24 hours after surgery. Medications used include diphenhydramine, 1 mg/kg every 6 hours (maximum 50 mg); methylprednisolone, 1 mg/kg every 6 hours (maximum 125 mg); and cimetidine, 5 mg/kg every 6 hours (maximum 300 mg). A latex-free environment must also be provided throughout the hospitalization.

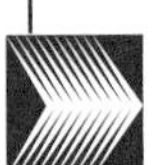

AUTHORS' PREFERRED METHOD OF TREATMENT

Myelomeningocele

In nonambulatory patients, mild malunion and shortening can be tolerated, and stable or minimally angulated fractures can be treated with either polyurethane splints or Webril dressings. Fractures with significant deformity may require reduction and immobilization in a cast heavily padded with polyurethane foam. In children who walk, fractures should be carefully aligned with heavily padded casts that allow continued protective weight-bearing, if possible. Hip spica casts may be necessary for femoral shaft fractures. Fractures of the proximal femur should be treated by immobilization and any later deformity corrected by osteotomy. Any patient considered for operative intervention should be screened for latex allergy, and if needed, given appropriate prophylaxis. Physeal fractures are treated with padded long leg casts and non–weight-bearing. Long-term follow-up is encouraged for physeal injuries because of the risk of growth arrest. Significant discrepancies can be addressed through contralateral epiphysiodesis or bridge resection.

Muscular Dystrophy

Fractures of the lower extremity in children with Duchenne muscular dystrophy must be managed so as not to cause premature loss of the ability to walk (591,592) or transfer (593). In patients 9 to 10 years old, increasing muscle weakness and joint contractures contribute to falls, and a loss of normal muscle bulk and fat limit the cushioning on impact (594). Patients in lower extremity braces seem to sustain few fractures in falls (591), probably because the overlying orthoses provide some protection (594). Patients confined to a wheelchair can fall because they have poor sitting balance, and fractures are frequent because these patients are more osteoporotic than ambulatory individuals (594).

Concentric "osseous atrophy" occurs in the long bones of patients with Duchenne muscular dystrophy; osteoporosis is also common (595,596). Osteoporosis is most profound in the lower extremities, and begins to develop early while still ambulating. Consequently, frequent fractures may result in loss of ambulation (597). Larson and Henderson reported that bone density in the proximal femur was profoundly diminished even when gait was minimally affected, and then progressively decreased to nearly 4 standard deviations below age-matched normals (597). Fractures are seldom displaced and are frequently minimally painful because there is minimal muscle spasm (594). Fractures tend to heal rapidly. The most commonly fractured bone is the femur (Fig. 6-53) (593,594,598) followed by the proximal humerus (594).

Corticosteroid therapy given to children with Duchenne muscular dystrophy to prolong mobility has been shown to increase the rate of osteoporosis and consequently, increase the risk of fracture. A study of 33 boys with Duchenne muscular dystrophy demonstrated the incidence of vertebral fractures in these patients after the initiation of corticosteroid treatment; 40 months after commencement of steroids the first vertebral fracture emerged. By 100 months of treatment, approximately 75% of patients had sustained a vertebral fracture (599).

There are two goals of fracture care in children with muscular dystrophy: limb stability and maintenance of maximal function during fracture healing. In ambulatory patients, treatment methods should allow children to maintain the ability to walk as the fracture heals. When ambulatory ability is tenuous, even minor bruises or ankle sprains (591) may end walking ability. As little as 1 week in a wheelchair can prematurely end ambulation (591); patients at bed rest for more than 2 weeks will likely lose the ability to ambulate (592). Hsu (598) reported that 25% of ambulatory patients with muscular dystrophy lost the ability to walk after sustaining fractures. In one of these patients, the ankle was casted in 20 degrees of plantar flexion, and the resulting contracture prevented ambulation at the end of treatment.

Treatment of specific fractures should be individualized. Upper extremity fractures can be treated with lightweight slings (594). Lower extremity fractures can be treated with either light walking casts or long leg double upright braces (591,594). Splints also can be used until the patients are pain free. Routine activities are begun as soon as possible (598). Protected standing and ambulation with physical therapy are crucial in maintaining independent ambulation (591).

Hsu and Garcia-Ariz (593) reported on 20 femoral fractures in 16 patients with muscular dystrophy. Six of the seven ambulatory patients were able to walk after treatment. In the nonambulatory patients in this series, most had supracondylar femoral fractures, which were splinted for 2 to 3 weeks, with emphasis on physical therapy to maintain functional abilities. Although union was achieved rapidly, hip and knee flexion contractures often increased in these patients, and up to 20 degrees of angulation of the fracture was routinely accepted. One patient with slipped capital femoral epiphysis was treated successfully with pinning in situ.

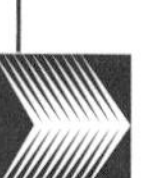

AUTHORS' PREFERRED METHOD OF TREATMENT

Muscular Dystrophy

The first goal of fracture treatment in children with muscular dystrophy is to avoid making matters worse. The patient should be mobilized as soon as possible in a lightweight cast or orthosis. Aggressive physical therapy should be used to maintain functional status. In a very young child, mid-shaft femoral fractures can be treated by traction and hip spica techniques, but in an older patient, ambulatory cast bracing might be a better choice.

Arthrogryposis and Poliomyelitis

Arthrogryposis is a rare disorder with an incidence of 3 in 10,000 live births (600). In this disease, muscle fiber is lost in utero, joint motion is limited during development, and taut ligaments and capsular tightness result in joint stiffness. Dislocations can occur with severe shortening of the involved muscles.

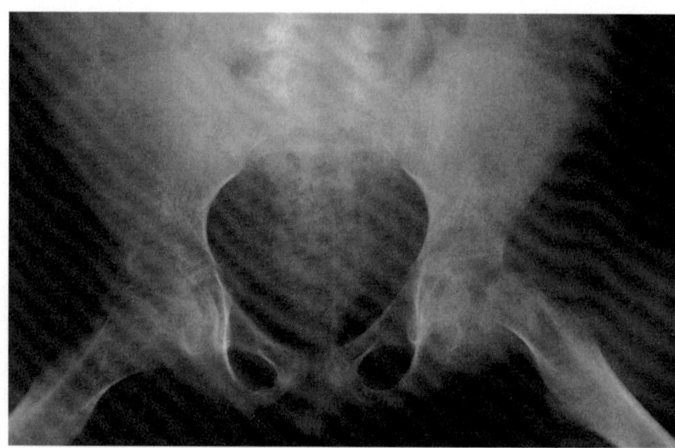

A

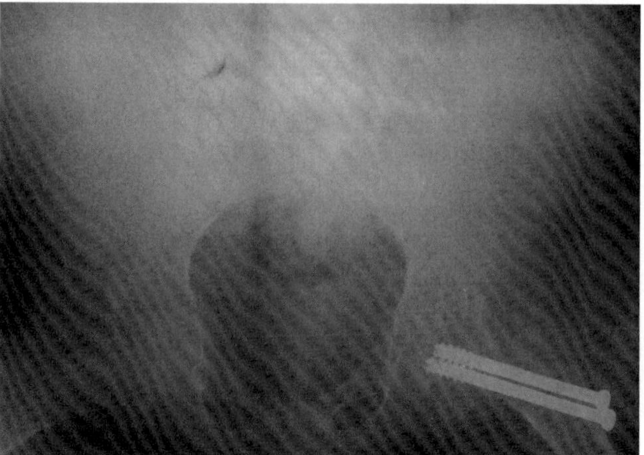

B

FIGURE 6-53 A. This 14-year-old nonambulatory boy with Duchenne muscular dystrophy crashed his wheelchair into the bumper of a stationary car, sustaining a displaced subcapital femoral fracture. This AP pelvis x-ray at the time of injury shows a displaced fracture and marked osteopenia of the pelvis and proximal femur. **B.** The fracture was treated by reduction and internal fixation with two cannulated screws.

Fractures may occur in 25% of infants with arthrogryposis multiplex congenita (601). A difficult delivery or forceful manipulation of the extremities can lead to fracture (601). Diamond and Alegado (601) reported on 16 fractures in 9 infants with arthrogryposis; an ipsilateral dislocated hip was present in 35% of patients. Most fractures involved the femur, with the remainder mostly tibial fractures, one humeral fracture, and one clavicular fracture. Epiphyseal separations occurred in the proximal tibia, distal femur, and proximal humerus. Clinical symptoms included poor feeding, irritability, and fussiness when handled. The involved extremity was thickened, and there was often an increased white blood cell count. Plain x-rays after acute injury, especially with epiphyseal separations, were not helpful, and arthrography was used in one patient to evaluate a distal femoral epiphyseal separation. With healing, these fractures develop exuberant callus with rapid union, and ready remodeling of angulated mid-shaft fractures.

Short-term immobilization is adequate to treat undisplaced fractures in these patients. Heavy plaster splints are not necessary (602). Some authors (603) recommend closed reduction of acutely displaced epiphyseal fractures and fractures with rotatory malalignment. Postnatal fractures are most common in patients with either knee contracture or dislocation of the hip, and postnatal injury could possibly be reduced by avoidance of forceful manipulation of these extremities. Older patients with lower extremity contractures do not seem to have difficulty with pathologic fractures (604).

Acute poliomyelitis has become a relatively rare disease in most Western countries but occasionally occurs in children who live in less developed countries. There are few reports in the literature concerning fractures in patients with poliomyelitis. Robin (602) reported 62 fractures in patients with poliomyelitis. More than half were fractures of the femur, and 90% of those injuries were supracondylar fractures. More than half of the fractures occurred after cast immobilization, and joint stiffness also was associated with a significant number of fractures. There were no epiphyseal injuries in this series.

Treatment of these fractures is simple immobilization. Because most fractures have very little displacement, reduction is seldom necessary; if there is preexisting deformity, manual osteoclasis through the fracture site can be used to correct deformities. Robin (602) stressed that joint mobility must be obtained before general mobilization of the patient to reduce the incidence of fracture after plaster immobilization. He also emphasized that fractures in these patients heal rapidly, and immobilization times should be reduced accordingly, with walking or standing in casts to decrease osteoporosis.

Spinal Cord Injury

Fortunately, childhood spinal cord injury is rare, and reports of pathologic fractures usually are included in larger series of patients with fractures and myelomeningocele because of the clinical similarities in presentation (605,606). Fractures of the femur, especially supracondylar fractures, are most common (607), but tibial fractures also are common (607). In most patients, these are pathologic fractures through osteoporotic bone. Children may be much more susceptible to these fractures than adults. Although fractures in paraplegics appear to heal rapidly with abundant callus (607), animal experiments suggest that in denervated limbs, the quality of the callus in fractures is compromised (608). Children with traumatic peripheral nerve lesions may have distal tibial physeal lesions similar to those in patients with myelomeningocele, neuropathic arthropathy of the small joints of the foot, and soft tissue ulcers (609).

Conservative treatment of fractures in patients with spinal cord injury is most commonly recommended. Skin traction is contraindicated because of the possibility of skin necrosis (577). Comarr et al (610) also use pillow sandbag splints and, for certain fractures, treat patients with a turning frame. Open reduction and internal fixation of these fractures is controversial. The conservative techniques used for the treatment of similar fractures in children with myelomeningocele might best be applied to fractures in children with traumatic paraplegia (567,605,606).

Although crutch and brace ambulation in paraplegics reportedly restores bone integrity (611), fractures continue to occur through osteoporotic bone in children actively ambulating with brace support (605). Some authors advocate light protective braces (610), but Katz (605) suggested that continuous splinting will worsen the disuse osteoporosis. He recommended careful manipulation of the lower extremities when they are out of ambulatory braces to reduce the incidence of fracture. Robin (606) emphasized that immobilization should be discontinued as soon as possible after fracture healing. Patient activity should be limited until knee motion is restored.

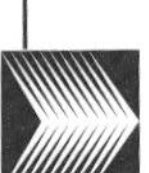

AUTHORS' PREFERRED METHOD OF TREATMENT

Spinal Cord Injury

Heavily padded casts or splints are recommended for most lower extremity fractures in children with traumatic paraplegia. Returning to ambulation with protection by walking braces is permitted once callus and joint motion are adequate. Every effort should be made to restore the child's prefracture function. Moderate malunion and shortening are acceptable in patients who are nonambulatory. Operative treatment of such fractures should be reserved for selected patients whose function would be significantly compromised by less than anatomic reduction.

REFERENCES

1. Hipp JA, Springfield DS, Hayes WC. Predicting pathologic fracture risk in the management of metastatic bone defects. *Clin Orthop* 1995;312:120–135.
2. Badgley C. Unicameral cyst of the long bones: treatment by crushing cystic walls and onlay grafts. *J Bone Joint Surg Am* 1957;39A:1429–1430.
3. Killian JT, Wilkinson L, White S, et al. Treatment of unicameral bone cyst with demineralized bone matrix. *J Pediatr Orthop* 1998;18(5):621–624.

4. Neer CS, Francis KC, Johnson AD, et al. Current concepts on the treatment of solitary unicameral bone cyst. *Clin Orthop* 1973;97:40–51.
5. Copley L, Dormans JP. Benign pediatric bone tumors. Evaluation and treatment. *Pediatr Clin North Am* 1996;43(4):949–966.
6. Dormans JP, Pill SG. Fractures through bone cysts: unicameral bone cysts, aneurysmal bone cysts, fibrous cortical defects, and nonossifying fibromas. *Instr Course Lect* 2002; 51:457–467.
7. Clark CR, Morgan C, Sonstegard DA, et al. The effect of biopsy-hole shape and size on bone strength. *J Bone Joint Surg Am* 1977;59(2):213–217.
8. Capanna R, Albisinni U, Picci P, et al. Aneurysmal bone cyst of the spine. *J Bone Joint Surg Am* 1985;67(4):527–531.
9. Cohen J. Simple bone cysts. Studies of cyst fluid in six cases with a theory of pathogenesis. *Am J Orthop* 1960;42-A:609–616.
10. Cohen J. Unicameral bone cysts. a current synthesis of reported cases. *Orthop Clin North Am* 1977;8(4):715–736.
11. Jaffe H. *Tumors and tumorous conditions of bone and joints*. Philadelphia: Lea & Febiger, 1958.
12. Boseker EH, Bickel WH, Dahlin DC. A clinicopathologic study of simple unicameral bone cysts. *Surg Gynecol Obstet* 1968;127(3):550–560.
13. Capanna R, Dal Monte A, Gitelis S, et al. The natural history of unicameral bone cyst after steroid injection. *Clin Orthop* 1982;166:204–211.
14. DePalma AF, Ahmad I. Fibrous dysplasia associated with Shepherd's Crook deformity of the humerus. *Clin Orthop* 1973;97:38–39.
15. Fahey JJ, O'Brien ET. Subtotal resection and grafting in selected cases of solitary unicameral bone cyst. *J Bone Joint Surg Am* 1973;55(1):59–68.
16. Oppenheim WL, Galleno H. Operative treatment versus steroid injection in the management of unicameral bone cysts. *J Pediatr Orthop* 1984;4(1):1–7.
17. Schreuder HW, Conrad EU 3rd, Bruckner JD, et al. Treatment of simple bone cysts in children with curettage and cryosurgery. *J Pediatr Orthop* 1997;17(6):814–820.
18. Chigira M, Maehara S, Arita S, et al. The aetiology and treatment of simple bone cysts. *J Bone Joint Surg Br* 1983;65(5):633–667.
19. Gartland JJ, Cole FL. Modern concepts in the treatment of unicameral bone cysts of the proximal humerus. *Orthop Clin North Am* 1975;6(2):487–498.
20. Khermosh O, Weissman SL. Coxa vara, avascular necrosis and osteochondritis dissecans complicating solitary bone cysts of the proximal femur. *Clin Orthop* 1977;126: 143–146.
21. Campanacci M, Capanna R, Picci P. Unicameral and aneurysmal bone cysts. *Clin Orthop* 1986;204:25–36.
22. Czitrom AA, Pritzker KP. Simple bone cyst causing collapse of the articular surface of the femoral head and incongruity of the hip joint. A case report. *J Bone Joint Surg Am* 1980;62(5):842–845.
23. Ahn JI, Park J. Pathological fractures secondary to unicameral bone cysts. *Int Orthop* 1994;18(1):20–22.
24. Reynolds J. The fallen fragment sign in the diagnosis of unicameral bone cysts. *Radiology* 1969;92(5):949–953 passim.
25. Harrer MD, Stanton JP, Davidson RS. Diaphyseal unicameral bone cysts in children. *Orthop Trans* 1997–1998;21:1187–1188.
26. Neer CS 2nd, Francis KC, Marcove RC, et al. Treatment of unicameral bone cyst: a follow-up study of one hundred seventy-five cases. *J Bone Joint Surg Am* 1966;48: 731–745.
27. Nakamura T, Takagi K, Kitagawa T, et al. Microdensity of solitary bone cyst after steroid injection. *J Pediatr Orthop* 1988;8(5):566–568.
28. McKay DW, Nason SS. Treatment of unicameral bone cysts by subtotal resection without grafts. *J Bone Joint Surg Am* 1977;59(4):515–519.
29. Moed BR, LaMont RL. Unicameral bone cyst complicated by growth retardation. *J Bone Joint Surg Am* 1982;64(9):1379–1381.
30. Taneda H, Azuma H. Avascular necrosis of the femoral epiphysis complicating a minimally displaced fracture of solitary bone cyst of the neck of the femur in a child. A case report. *Clin Orthop* 1994;304:172–175.
31. Fernbach SK, Blumenthal DH, Poznanski AK, et al. Radiographic changes in unicameral bone cysts following direct injection of steroids: a report on 14 cases. *Radiology* 1981; 140(3):689–695.
32. Weisel A, Hecht HL. Development of a unicameral bone cyst. Case report. *J Bone Joint Surg Am* 1980;62(4):664–666.
33. Malkawi H, Shannak A, Amr S. Surgical treatment of pathological subtrochanteric fractures due to benign lesions in children and adolescents. *J Pediatr Orthop* 1984;4(1): 63–69.
34. Kaelin AJ, MacEwen GD. Unicameral bone cysts. Natural history and the risk of fracture. *Int Orthop* 1989;13(4):275–282.
35. Baker DM. Benign unicameral bone cyst. A study of forty-five cases with long-term follow up. *Clin Orthop* 1970;71:140–151.
36. Spence KF, Sell KW, Brown RH. Solitary bone cyst: treatment with freeze-dried cancellous bone allograft. A study of one hundred seventy-seven cases. *J Bone Joint Surg Am* 1969;51(1):87–96.
37. Robins PR, Peterson HA. Management of pathologic fractures through unicameral bone cysts. JAMA 1972;222(1):80–81.
38. Glaser DL, Dormans JP, Stanton RP, et al. Surgical management of calcaneal unicameral bone cysts. *Clin Orthop* 1999;360:231–237.
39. Moreau G, Letts M. Unicameral bone cyst of the calcaneus in children. *J Pediatr Orthop* 1994;14(1):101–104.
40. Peltier LF, Jones RH. Treatment of unicameral bone cysts by curettage and packing with plaster-of-Paris pellets. *J Bone Joint Surg Am* 1978;60(6):820–822.
41. Siegel IM. Brisement force with controlled collapse in treatment of solitary unicameral bone cyst. *Arch Surg* 1966;92(1):109–114.
42. Scaglietti O, Marchetti PG, Bartolozzi P. The effects of methylprednisolone acetate in the treatment of bone cysts. Results of three years follow-up. *J Bone Joint Surg Br* 1979; 61-B(2):200–204.
43. Shindell R, Huurman WW, Lippiello L, et al. Prostaglandin levels in unicameral bone cysts treated by intralesional steroid injection. *J Pediatr Orthop* 1989;9(5):516–519.
44. Colville MR, Aronson DD, Prcevski P, et al. The systemic and local effects of an intramedullary injection of methylprednisolone acetate in growing rabbits. *J Pediatr Orthop* 1987;7(4):412–414.
45. Santori F, Ghera S, Gallucci M. Treatment of solitary bone cysts with intramedullary nailing. *Orthopedics* 1988;11(6):873–878.
46. Rosenborg M, Mortensson W, Hirsch G, et al. Considerations in the corticosteroid treatment of bone cysts. *J Pediatr Orthop* 1989;9(2):240–243.
47. de Palma L, Santucci A. Treatment of bone cysts with methylprednisolone acetate. A 9 to 11 year follow-up. *Int Orthop* 1987;11(1):23–28.
48. Campos OP. Treatment of bone cysts by intracavity injection of methylprednisolone acetate: a message to orthopedic surgeons. *Clin Orthop* 1982;165:43–48.
49. Capanna R, Springfield DS, Biagini R, et al. Juxtaepiphyseal aneurysmal bone cyst. *Skeletal Radiol* 1985;13(1):21–25.
50. Kresler TK, Kling TF, Rougraff BT. Unicameral bone cysts. *Curr Opin Orthop* 1994;5: 75–81.
51. Rougraff BT, Kling TJ. Treatment of active unicameral bone cysts with percutaneous injection of demineralized bone matrix and autogenous bone marrow. *J Bone Joint Surg Am* 2002;84-A(6):921–929.
52. Campbell RJ. Problem injuries in unique conditions of the musculoskeletal system. In: Rockwood CJW, Beaty KE, eds. *Fractures in children*. Philadelphia: Lippincott–Raven, 1996:167–320.
53. Dormans JP, Dormans NJ. Use of percutaneous intramedullary decompression and medical-grade calcium sulfate pellets for treatment of unicameral bone cysts of the calcaneus in children. Orthopedics 2004:27:S137–S139.
54. Besse BE Jr, Dahlin DC, Ghormley RK, et al. Aneurysmal bone cysts: additional considerations. *Clin Orthop* 1956;38(7):93–102.
55. Dabska M, Buraczewski J. Aneurysmal bone cyst. Pathology, clinical course and radiologic appearances. *Cancer* 1969;23(2):371–389.
56. Dabezies EJ, D'Ambrosia RD, Chuinard RG, et al. Aneurysmal bone cyst after fracture. A report of three cases. *J Bone Joint Surg Am* 1982;64(4):617–621.
57. Tillman BP, Dahlin DC, Lipscomb PR, et al. Aneurysmal bone cyst: an analysis of ninety-five cases. *Mayo Clin Proc* 1968;43(7):478–495.
58. Bonakdarpour A, Levy WM, Aegerter E. Primary and secondary aneurysmal bone cyst: a radiological study of 75 cases. *Radiology* 1978;126(1):75–83.
59. Ginsburg LD. Congenital aneurysmal bone cyst. Case report with comments on the role of trauma in the pathogenesis. *Radiology* 1974;110(1):175–176.
60. Koskinen EV, Visuri TI, Holmstrom T, et al. Aneurysmal bone cyst: evaluation of resection and of curettage in 20 cases. *Clin Orthop* 1976;118:136–146.
61. Hay MC, Paterson D, Taylor TK. Aneurysmal bone cysts of the spine. *J Bone Joint Surg Br* 1978;60-B(3):406–411.
62. Macpherson RI. Aneurysmal bone cyst of spine diagnosed by percutaneous opacification. *J Can Assoc Radiol* 1980;31(3):210–212.
63. Hudson TM. Scintigraphy of aneurysmal bone cysts. *AJR Am J Roentgenol* 1984;142(4): 761–765.
64. Sullivan RJ, Meyer JS, Dormans JP, et al. Diagnosing aneurysmal and unicameral bone cysts with magnetic resonance imaging. *Clin Orthop* 1999;366:186–190.
65. Hooper JC. Aneurysmal bone cysts penetrating the tibial epiphysis after curettage. *Med J Aust* 1971;1(4):200–201.
66. Clough JR, Price CH. Aneurysmal bone cyst: pathogenesis and long term results of treatment. *Clin Orthop* 1973;97:52–63.
67. Biesecker JL, Marcove RC, Huvos AG, et al. Aneurysmal bone cysts. A clinicopathologic study of 66 cases. *Cancer* 1970;26(3):615–625.
68. Dyer R, Stelling CB, Fechner RE. Epiphyseal extension of an aneurysmal bone cyst. *AJR Am J Roentgenol* 1981;137(1):172–173.
69. Jaffe KA, Dunham WK. Treatment of benign lesions of the femoral head and neck. *Clin Orthop* 1990;257:134–137.
70. de Silva MV, Raby N, Reid R. Fibromyxoid areas and immature osteoid are associated with recurrence of primary aneurysmal bone cysts. *Histopathology* 2003;43(2): 180–188.
71. Freiberg AA, Loder RT, Heidelberger KP, et al. Aneurysmal bone cysts in young children. *J Pediatr Orthop* 1994;14(1):86–91.
72. Dormans JP, Hanna BG, Johnston DR, et al. Surgical treatment and recurrence rate of aneurysmal bone cysts in children. *Clin Orthop* 2004;421:205–211.
73. Green JA, Bellemore MC, Marsden FW. Embolization in the treatment of aneurysmal bone cysts. *J Pediatr Orthop* 1997;17(4):440–443.
74. Marcove RC, Sheth DS, Brien EW, et al. The treatment of aneurysmal bone cyst. *Clin Orthop* 1995;311:157–163.
75. Schreuder HW, Veth RP, Pruszczynski M, et al. Aneurysmal bone cysts treated by curettage, cryotherapy and bone grafting. *J Bone Joint Surg Br* 1997;79(1):20–25.
76. Ozaki T, Hillmann A, Lindner N, et al. Cementation of primary aneurysmal bone cysts. *Clin Orthop* 1997;(337):240–248.
77. Fraser RK, Coates CJ, Cole WG. An angiostatic agent in treatment of a recurrent aneurysmal bone cyst. *J Pediatr Orthop* 1993;13(5):668–671.
78. Guibaud L, Herbreteau D, Dubois J, et al. Aneurysmal bone cysts: percutaneous embolization with an alcoholic solution of zein—series of 18 cases. *Radiology* 1998;208(2): 369–373.
79. Burkhalter WE, Schroeder FC, Eversmann WW Jr. Aneurysmal bone cysts occurring in the metacarpals: a report of three cases. *J Hand Surg Am* 1978;3(6):579–584.

80. Papagelopoulos PJ, Currier BL, Shaughnessy WJ, et al. Aneurysmal bone cyst of the spine. Management and outcome. *Spine* 1998;23(5):621–628.
81. Turker RJ, Mardjetko S, Lubicky J. Aneurysmal bone cysts of the spine: excision and stabilization. *J Pediatr Orthop* 1998;18(2): 209–213.
82. Kaufman RA, Towbin RB. Telangiectatic osteosarcoma simulating the appearance of an aneurysmal bone cyst. *Pediatr Radiol* 1981;11(2):102–104.
83. Reed RJ, Rothenberg M. Lesions of bone that may be confused with aneurysmal bone cyst. *Clin Orthop* 1964;35:150–162.
84. Torpey BM, Dormans JP, Drummond DS. The use of MRI-compatible titanium segmental spinal instrumentation in pediatric patients with intraspinal tumor. *J Spinal Disord* 1995;8(1):76–81.
85. Cunningham JB, Ackerman LV. Metaphyseal fibrous defects. *J Bone Joint Surg Am* 1956; 38-A(4):797–808.
86. Campbell CJ, Harkess J. Fibrous metaphyseal defect of bone. *Surg Gynecol Obstet* 1957; 104(3):329–336.
87. Phelan JT. Fibrous cortical defect and nonosseous fibroma of bone. *Surg Gynecol Obstet* 1964;119:807–810.
88. Selby S. Metaphyseal cortical defects in the tubular bones of growing children. *J Bone Joint Surg Am* 1961;43:395–400.
89. Hatcher C. The pathogenesis of localized fibrous lesions in the metaphyses of long bones. *Ann Surg* 1945;122:1016–1030.
90. Drennan DB, Maylahn DJ, Fahey JJ. Fractures through large non-ossifying fibromas. *Clin Orthop* 1974;103:82–88.
91. Evans GA, Park WM. Familial multiple non-osteogenic fibromata. *J Bone Joint Surg Br* 1978;60-B(3):416–419.
92. Arata MA, Peterson HA, Dahlin DC. Pathological fractures through non-ossifying fibromas. Review of the Mayo Clinic experience. *J Bone Joint Surg Am* 1981;63(6):980–988.
93. Dahlin DC. *Bone tumors: general aspects and data on 6,221 cases*. Springfield, IL: Charles C. Thomas, 1978.
94. Ritschl P, Karnel F, Hajek P. Fibrous metaphyseal defects—determination of their origin and natural history using a radiomorphological study. *Skeletal Radiol* 1988;17(1): 8–15.
95. Devlin JA, Bowman HE, Mitchell CL. Non-osteogenic fibroma of bone; a review of the literature with the addition of six cases. *J Bone Joint Surg Am* 1955;37-A(3):472–486.
96. Easley ME, Kneisl JS. Pathologic fractures through nonossifying fibromas: is prophylactic treatment warranted? *J Pediatr Orthop* 1997;17(6):808–813.
97. Dormans JP, Landa J, Mahlberg M. Use of a new minimally invasive percutaneous technique for the treatment of non-ossifying fibromas. Podium presentation, Pediatric Orthopaedic Society of North America, April 29, 2004.
98. McDonald DJ, Sim FH, McLeod RA, et al. Giant-cell tumor of bone. *J Bone Joint Surg Am* 1986;68(2):235–242.
99. Campanacci M, Baldini N, Boriani S, et al. Giant-cell tumor of bone. *J Bone Joint Surg Am* 1987;69(1):106–114.
100. Dahlin DC, Cupps RE, Johnson EW Jr. Giant-cell tumor: a study of 195 cases. *Cancer* 1970;25(5):1061–1070.
101. Muscolo DL, Ayerza MA, Calabrese ME, et al. The use of a bone allograft for reconstruction after resection of giant-cell tumor close to the knee. *J Bone Joint Surg Am* 1993; 75(11):1656–1662.
102. Sung HW, Kuo DP, Shu WP, et al. Giant-cell tumor of bone: analysis of two hundred and eight cases in Chinese patients. *J Bone Joint Surg Am* 1982;64(5):755–761.
103. Jaffe H. Solitary benign enchondroma of bone. *Arch Surg* 1943;46:480–493.
104. Bean WB. Dyschondroplasia and hemangiomata (Maffucci's syndrome). II. *AMA Arch Intern Med* 1958;102(4):544–550.
105. Lewis RJ, Ketcham AS. Maffucci's syndrome: functional and neoplastic significance. Case report and review of the literature. *J Bone Joint Surg Am* 1973;55(7):1465–1479.
106. Bauer RD, Lewis MM, Posner MA. Treatment of enchondromas of the hand with allograft bone. *J Hand Surg Am* 1988;13(6): 908–916.
107. Ablove RH, Moy OJ, Peimer CA, et al. Early versus delayed treatment of enchondroma. *Am J Orthop* 2000;29(10):771–772.
108. Cardelia JM, Dormans JP, Drummond DS, et al. Proximal fibular osteochondroma with associated peroneal nerve palsy: a review of six cases. *J Pediatr Orthop* 1995;15(5): 574–577.
109. Mahboubi S, Dormans JP, D'Angio G. Malignant degeneration of radiation-induced osteochondroma. *Skeletal Radiol* 1997;26(3):195–198.
110. Theodorou SD, Karamitsos S, Tsouparopoulos D, et al. Rare complications of exostosis. Fractures and injury to the common peroneal nerve. *Acta Orthop Belg* 1978;44(4): 496–505.
111. Lieberman PH, Jones CR, Stinman RM, et al. Langerhans cell (eosinophilic) granulomatosis. A clinicopathologic study encompassing 50 years. *Am J Surg Pathol* 1996;20(5): 519–552.
112. Osenbach RK, Youngblood LA, Menezes AH. Atlanto-axial instability secondary to solitary eosinophilic granuloma of C2 in a 12-year-old girl. *J Spinal Disord* 1990;3(4): 408–412.
113. Sbarbaro JL Jr, Francis KC. Eosinophilic granuloma of bone. JAMA 1961;178:706–710.
114. Fowles JV, Bobechko WP. Solitary eosinophilic granuloma in bone. *J Bone Joint Surg Br* 1970;52(2):238–243.
115. McCullough CJ. Eosinophilic granuloma of bone. *Acta Orthop Scand* 1980;51(3): 389–398.
116. Ghanem I, Tolo VT, D'Ambra P, Malogalowkin MH. Langerhans cell histiocytosis of bone in children and adolescents. *J Pediatr Orthop* 2003;23(1):124–130.
117. Glotzbecker MP, Carpentieri DF, Dormans JP. Langerhans cell histiocytosis: a primary viral infection of bone? Human herpes virus 6 latent protein detected in lymphocytes from tissue of children. *J Pediatr Orthop* 2004;24(1):123–129.
118. Garg S, Mehta S, Dormans JP. Langerhans cell histiocytosis of the spine in children. Long-term follow-up. J Bone Joint Surg Am 2004 Aug;86:1740–1750.
119. Bertram C, Madert J, Eggers C. Eosinophilic granuloma of the cervical spine. *Spine* 2002;27(13):1408–1413.
120. Meyer JS, Harty MP, Mahboubi S, et al. Langerhans cell histiocytosis: presentation and evolution of radiologic findings with clinical correlation. *Radiographics* 1995;15(5): 1135–1146.
121. Crone-Munzebrock W, Brassow F. A comparison of radiographic and bone scan findings in histiocytosis X. *Skeletal Radiol* 1983;9(3):170–173.
122. Yasko AW, Fanning CV, Ayala AG, et al. Percutaneous techniques for the diagnosis and treatment of localized Langerhans-cell histiocytosis (eosinophilic granuloma of bone). *J Bone Joint Surg Am* 1998;80(2):219–228.
123. Egeler RM, Thompson RC Jr, Voute PA, et al. Intralesional infiltration of corticosteroids in localized Langerhans' cell histiocytosis. *J Pediatr Orthop* 1992;12(6):811–814.
124. Greis PE, Hankin FM. Eosinophilic granuloma. The management of solitary lesions of bone. *Clin Orthop* 1990;(257):204–211.
125. Levine SE, Dormans JP, Meyer JS, et al. Langerhans' cell histiocytosis of the spine in children. *Clin Orthop* 1996;(323):288–293.
126. Mammano S, Candiotto S, Balsano M, et al. Cast and brace treatment of eosinophilic granuloma of the spine: long-term follow-up. *J Pediatr Orthop* 1997;17(6):821–827.
127. Seimon LP. Eosinophil granuloma of the spine. *J Pediatr Orthop* 1981;1(4):371–376.
128. Raab P, Hohmann F, Kuhl J, et al. Vertebral remodeling in eosinophilic granuloma of the spine. A long-term follow-up. *Spine* 1998;23(12):1351–1354.
129. Enneking WF. A system of staging musculoskeletal neoplasms. *Instr Course Lect* 1988; 37:3–10.
130. Massengill AD, Seeger LL, Eckardt JJ. The role of plain radiography, computed tomography, and magnetic resonance imaging in sarcoma evaluation. *Hematol Oncol Clin North Am* 1995;9(3):571–604.
131. Ayala AG, Ro JY, Fanning CV, et al. Core needle biopsy and fine-needle aspiration in the diagnosis of bone and soft-tissue lesions. *Hematol Oncol Clin North Am* 1995;9(3): 633–651.
132. Mankin HJ, Lange TA, Spanier SS. The hazards of biopsy in patients with malignant primary bone and soft-tissue tumors. *J Bone Joint Surg Am* 1982;64(8):1121–1127.
133. Peabody TD, Simon MA. Making the diagnosis: keys to a successful biopsy in children with bone and soft-tissue tumors. *Orthop Clin North Am* 1996;27(3):453–459.
134. Simon MA. Biopsy of musculoskeletal tumors. *J Bone Joint Surg Am* 1982;64(8): 1253–1257.
135. Scully SP, Temple HT, O'Keefe RJ, et al. The surgical treatment of patients with osteosarcoma who sustain a pathologic fracture. *Clin Orthop* 1996;(324):227–232.
136. Hahn M, Dormans JP. Primary bone malignancies in children. *Curr Opin Pediatr* 1996; 8(1):71–74.
137. Himelstein BP, Dormans JP. Malignant bone tumors of childhood. *Pediatr Clin North Am* 1996;43(4):967–984.
138. Kruzelock RP, Hansen MF. Molecular genetics and cytogenetics of sarcomas. *Hematol Oncol Clin North Am* 1995;9(3):513–540.
139. Letson GD, Greenfield GB, Heinrich SD. Evaluation of the child with a bone or soft-tissue neoplasm. *Orthop Clin North Am* 1996;27(3):431–451.
140. Ehara S, Kattapuram SV, Egglin TK. Ewing's sarcoma. Radiographic pattern of healing and bony complications in patients with long-term survival. *Cancer* 1991;68(7): 1531–1535.
141. Pochanugool L, Subhadharaphandou T, Dhanachai M, et al. Prognostic factors among 130 patients with osteosarcoma. *Clin Orthop* 1997;(345):206–214.
142. Wunder JS, Paulian G, Huvos AG, et al. The histological response to chemotherapy as a predictor of the oncological outcome of operative treatment of Ewing sarcoma. *J Bone Joint Surg Am* 1998;80(7):1020–1033.
143. Abudu A, Sferopoulos NK, Tillman RM, et al. The surgical treatment and outcome of pathological fractures in localised osteosarcoma. *J Bone Joint Surg Br* 1996;78(5): 694–698.
144. Berrey BH Jr, Lord CF, Gebhardt MC, et al. Fractures of allografts. Frequency, treatment, and end-results. *J Bone Joint Surg Am* 1990;72(6):825–833.
145. San-Julian M, Canadell J. Fractures of allografts used in limb preserving operations. *Int Orthop* 1998;22(1):32–36.
146. McCune DB, Bruch H. Osteodystrophia fibrosa, report of a case in which condition was combined with precocious puberty, pathologic pigmentation of the skin and hyperthyroidism, with review of the literature. *Am J Dis Child* 1937;54:806–848.
147. Albright FB, Butler AM, Hampton AO, et al. Syndrome characterized by osteitis fibrosa disseminata, areas of pigmentation and endocrine dysfunction, with precocious puberty in females: a report of five cases. *N Engl J Med* 1937;216:727–746.
148. Lichtenstein L. Polystotic fibrous dysplasia. *Arch Surg* 1938;36:874–898.
149. Lichtenstein L, Jaffee HL. Fibrous dysplasia of bone: a condition affecting one, several or many bones, the graver cases of which may present abnormal pigmentation of skin, premature sexual development, hyperthyroidism or still other extra skeletal abnormalities. *Arch Pathol* 1942;33:777–815.
150. Alman BA, Greel DA, Wolfe HJ. Activating mutations of Gs protein in monostotic fibrous lesions of bone. *J Orthop Res* 1996;14(2):311–315.
151. Hindman BW, Bell S, Russo T, et al. Neonatal osteofibrons dysplasia; a case report. *Pediatr Radiol* 1996;26:303–306.
152. Grabias SL, Campbell CJ. Fibrous dysplasia. *Orthop Clin North Am* 1977;8(4):771–783.
153. Crawford AH. Neurofibromatosis in the pediatric patient. *Orthop Clin North Am* 1978; 9(1):11–23.
154. Ippolito E, Bray EW, Corsi A, et al. Natural history and treatment of fibrous dysplasia of bone: a multicenter clinicopathologic study promoted by the European Pediatric Orthopaedic Society. *J Pediatr Orthop* 2003;B-12(3):155–177.

155. Harris WH, Dudley HR Jr, Barry RJ. The natural history of fibrous dysplasia. An orthopaedic, pathological, and roentgenographic study. *Am J Orthop* 1962;44-A:207–233.
156. Funk FJ Jr, Wells RE. Hip problems in fibrous dysplasia. *Clin Orthop* 1973;90:77–82.
157. Warric C. Polystotic fibrous dysplasia—Albright's syndrome. A review of the literature and report of four male cases, two of which were associated with precocious puberty. *J Bone Joint Surg Am* 1949;31:175–183.
158. Brown GA, Osebold WR, Ponseti IV. Congenital pseudarthrosis of long bones: a clinical, radiographic, histologic and ultrastructural study. *Clin Orthop* 1977;(128):228–242.
159. Higashi T, Iguchi M, Shimura A, et al. Computed tomography and bone scintigraphy is polyostotic fibrous dysplasia. Report of a case. *Oral Surg Oral Med Oral Pathol* 1980; 50(6):580–583.
160. Stephenson RB, London MD, Hankin FM, et al. Fibrous dysplasia. An analysis of options for treatment. *J Bone Joint Surg Am* 1987;69(3):400–409.
161. Kensinger DR, Guille JT, Horn BD, et al. The stubbed great toe: importance of early recognition and treatment of open fractures of the distal phalanx. *J Pediatr Orthop* 2001; 21(1):31–34.
162. Breck LW. Treatment of fibrous dysplasia of bone by total femoral plating and hip nailing. A case report. *Clin Orthop* 1972;82:82–83.
163. Kupcha PC, Guille JT, Tassanaipas A, et al. (1991). Polyostotic fibrous dysplasia and acromegaly. *J Pediatr Orthop* 1991;11(1):95–99.
164. Langer, RA, Yook I, Capan LM. Anesthetic considerations in McCune-Albright syndrome: case report with literature review. *Anesth Analg* 1995;80(6):1236–1239.
165. Campanacci M, Laus M. Osteofibrous dysplasia of the tibia and fibula. *J Bone Joint Surg Am* 1981;63(3):367–375.
166. Park YK, Unni KK, McLeod RA, et al. Osteofibrous dysplasia: clinicopathologic study of 80 cases. *Hum Pathol* 1993;24(12):1339–1347.
167. Springfield DS, Rosenberg AE, Mankin HJ, et al. Relationship between osteofibrous dysplasia and adamantinoma. *Clin Orthop* 1994;(309):234–244.
168. Sweet DE, Vinh TN, Devaney K. Cortical osteofibrous dysplasia of long bone and its relationship to adamantinoma. A clinicopathologic study of 30 cases. *Am J Surg Pathol* 1992;16(3):282–290.
169. Ozaki T, Hamada M, Sugihara S, et al. Treatment outcome of osteofibrous dysplasia. *J Pediatr Orthop* 1998;B-7(3):199–202.
170. Akamatsu N, Hamada Y, Kohno H, et al. Osteofibrous dysplasia of the tibia treated by bracing. *Int Orthop* 1992;16(2):180–184.
171. Komiya S, Inoue A. Aggressive bone tumorous lesion in infancy: osteofibrous dysplasia of the tibia and fibula. *J Pediatr Orthop* 1993;13(5):577–581.
172. Crawford AH Jr, Bagamery N. Osseous manifestations of neurofibromatosis in childhood. *J Pediatr Orthop* 1986;6(1):72–88.
173. Crowe FW, Schull WJ. Diagnostic importance of cafe-au-lait spot in neurofibromatosis. *AMA Arch Intern Med* 1953;91(6):758–766.
174. Whitehouse D. Diagnostic value of the cafe-au-lait spot in children. *Arch Dis Child* 1966;41(217):316–319.
175. McCarroll H. Clinical manifestations of congenital neurofibromatosis. *J Bone Joint Surg Am* 1950;32(A):601–617.
176. Mandell GA, Harcke HT, Harkey C, et al. SPECT imaging of para-axial neurofibromatosis with technetium-99m DTPA. *J Nucl Med* 1987;28(11):1688–1694.
177. Mandell GA, Herrick WC, Harcke HT, et al. Neurofibromas: location by scanning with Tc-99m DTPA. Work in progress. *Radiology* 1985;157(3): 803–806.
178. Wright J, Dormans J, Rang M. Pseudarthrosis of the rabbit tibia: a model for congenital pseudarthrosis? *J Pediatr Orthop* 1991;11(3):277–283.
179. Morrissy RT, Riseborough EJ, Hall JE. Congenital pseudarthrosis of the tibia. *J Bone Joint Surg Br* 1981;63-B(3):367–375.
180. Bell DF. Congenital forearm pseudarthrosis: report of six cases and review of the literature. *J Pediatr Orthop* 1989;9(4):438–443.
181. Gregg PJ, Price BA, Ellis HA, et al. Pseudarthrosis of the radius associated with neurofibromatosis. A case report. *Clin Orthop* 1982;(171):175–179.
182. Kaempffe FA, Gillespie R. Pseudarthrosis of the radius after fracture through normal bone in a child who had neurofibromatosis. A case report. *J Bone Joint Surg Am* 1989; 71(9):1419–1421.
183. Kameyama O, Ogawa R. Pseudarthrosis of the radius associated with neurofibromatosis: report of a case and review of the literature. *J Pediatr Orthop* 1990;10(1):128–131.
184. Karol LA, Haideri NF, Halliday SE, et al. Gait analysis and muscle strength in children with congenital pseudarthrosis of the tibia: the effect of treatment. *J Pediatr Orthop* 1998;18(3):381–386.
185. Leung PC. Congenital pseudarthrosis of the tibia. Three cases treated by free vascularized iliac crest graft. *Clin Orthop* 1983;(175):45–50.
186. Lloyd-Roberts GC. Treatment of defects of the ulna in children by establishing cross-union with the radius. *J Bone Joint Surg Br* 1973;55(2):327–330.
187. Major MR, Huizenga BA. Spinal cord compression by displaced ribs in neurofibromatosis. A report of three cases. *J Bone Joint Surg Am* 1988;70(7):1100–1102.
188. Manske PR. Forearm pseudarthrosis—neurofibromatosis: case report. *Clin Orthop* 1979;(139):125–127.
189. Masihuz Z. Pseudarthrosis of the radius associated with neurofibromatosis. A case report. *J Bone Joint Surg Am* 1977;59(7):977–978.
190. Mathoulin C, Gilbert A, Azze RG. Congenital pseudarthrosis of the forearm: treatment of six cases with vascularized fibular graft and a review of the literature. *Microsurgery* 1993;14(4):252–259.
191. Ali MS, Hooper G. Congenital pseudarthrosis of the ulna due to neurofibromatosis. *J Bone Joint Surg Br* 1982;64(5):600–602.
192. Allieu Y, Gomis R, Yoshimura M, et al. Congenital pseudarthrosis of the forearm-two cases treated by free vascularized fibular graft. *J Hand Surg Am* 1981;6(5):475–481.
193. Bayne LG. Congenital pseudarthrosis of the forearm. *Hand Clin* 1985;1(3):457–465.
194. Murray HH, Lovell WW. Congenital pseudarthrosis of the tibia. A long-term follow-up study. *Clin Orthop* 1982;(166):14–20.
195. Ostrowski DM, Eilert RE, Waldstein G. Congenital pseudarthrosis of the ulna: a report of two cases and a review of the literature. *J Pediatr Orthop* 1985;5(4):463–467.
196. Richin PF, Kranik A, Van Herpe L, et al. Congenital pseudarthrosis of both bones of the forearm. A case report. *J Bone Joint Surg Am* 1976;58(7):1032–1023.
197. Sellers DS, Sowa DT, Moore JR, et al. Congenital pseudarthrosis of the forearm. *J Hand Surg Am* 1988;13(1):89–93.
198. McFarland B. Pseudarthrosis of the tibia in childhood. *J Bone Joint Surg Br* 1951;33-B(1):36–46.
199. Boyd HB, Sage FP. Congenital pseudarthrosis of the tibia. *J Bone Joint Surg Am* 1958; 40-A(6):1245–1270.
200. Anderson DJ, Schoenecker PL, Sheridan JJ, et al. Use of an intramedullary rod for the treatment of congenital pseudarthrosis of the tibia. *J Bone Joint Surg Am* 1992;74(2): 161–168.
201. Baker JK, Cain TE, Tullos HS. Intramedullary fixation for congenital pseudarthrosis of the tibia. *J Bone Joint Surg Am* 1992;74(2):169–178.
202. Sofield H, Millar EA. Fragmentation, realignment, and intramedullary rod fixation of deformities of the long bones in children. *J Bone Joint Surg Am* 1959;41:1371–1391.
203. Brighton CT, Friedenberg ZB, Zemsky LM, et al. Direct-current stimulation of non-union and congenital pseudarthrosis. Exploration of its clinical application. *J Bone Joint Surg Am* 1975;57(3):368–377.
204. Paterson DC, Simonis RB. Electrical stimulation in the treatment of congenital pseudarthrosis of the tibia. *J Bone Joint Surg Br* 1985;67(3):454–462.
205. Morrissy RT. Congenital pseudarthrosis of the tibia. Factors that affect results. *Clin Orthop* 1982;(166):21–27.
206. de Boer HH, Verbout AJ, Nielsen HK, et al. Free vascularized fibular graft for tibial pseudarthrosis in neurofibromatosis. *Acta Orthop Scand* 1988;59(4):425–429.
207. Dormans JP, Krajbich JI, Zuker R, et al. Congenital pseudarthrosis of the tibia: treatment with free vascularized fibular grafts. *J Pediatr Orthop* 1990;10(5):623–628.
208. Weiland AJ, Daniel RK. Congenital pseudarthrosis of the tibia: treatment with vascularized autogenous fibular grafts. A preliminary report. *Johns Hopkins Med J* 1980; 147(3): 89–95.
209. Fabry G, Lammens J, Van Melkebeek, et al. Treatment of congenital pseudarthrosis with the Ilizarov technique. *J Pediatr Orthop* 1988;8(1):67–70.
210. Rathgeb JM, Ramsey PL, Cowell HR. Congenital kyphoscoliosis of the tibia. *Clin Orthop* 1974;0(103):178–190.
211. Strong ML, Wong-Chung J. Prophylactic bypass grafting of the prepseudarthrotic tibia in neurofibromatosis. *J Pediatr Orthop* 1991;11(6):757–764.
212. Dormans JP. Modified sequential McFarland bypass procedure for pre-pseudarthrosis of the tibia. *J Orthop Tech* 1995;3:176–180.
213. Greenberg LA, Schwartz A. Congenital pseudarthrosis of the distal radius. *South Med J* 1975;68(8):1053–1054.
214. Shertzer JH, Bickel WH, Stubbins SG. Congenital pseudarthrosis of the ulna. Report of two cases. *Minn Med* 1969;52(7):1061–1066.
215. Yaghmai I, Tafazoli M. Massive subperiosteal hemorrhage in neurofibromatosis. *Radiology* 1977;122(2):439–441.
216. Virdis R, Balestrazzi P, Zampolli M, et al. Hypertension in children with neurofibromatosis. *J Hum Hypertens* 1994;8(5):395–397.
217. Winter RB, Moe JH, Bradford DS, et al. Spine deformity in neurofibromatosis. A review of one hundred and two patients. *J Bone Joint Surg Am* 1979;61(5):677–694.
218. Rockower S, McKay D, Nason S. Dislocation of the spine in neurofibromatosis. A report of two cases. *J Bone Joint Surg Am* 1982;64(8):1240–1242.
219. Flood BM, Butt WP, Dickson RA. Rib penetration of the intervertebral foraminae in neurofibromatosis. *Spine* 1986;11(2):172–174.
220. Guidera KJ, Multhopp H, Ganey T, et al. Orthopaedic manifestations in congenitally insensate patients. J Pediatr Orthop 1990;10(4): 514–521.
221. Guille JT, Forlin E, Bowen JR. Charcot joint disease of the shoulders in a patient who had familial sensory neuropathy with anhidrosis. A case report. *J Bone Joint Surg Am* 1992;74(9):1415–1417.
222. Kuo RS, Macnicol MF. Congenital insensitivity to pain: orthopaedic implications. *J Pediatr Orthop* 1996;B-5(4):292–295.
223. Okuno T, Inoue A, Izumo S. Congenital insensitivity to pain with anhidrosis. A case report. *J Bone Joint Surg Am* 1990;72(2):279–282.
224. Katz K, Cohen IJ, Ziv N, et al. Fractures in children who have Gaucher disease. *J Bone Joint Surg Am* 1987;69(9):1361–1370.
225. Goldblatt J, Sacks S, Beighton P. The orthopedic aspects of Gaucher disease. *Clin Orthop* 1978;(137):208–214.
226. Schein AJ, Arkin AM. The classic: hip-joint involvement in Gaucher's disease. *Clin Orthop* 1973;90:4–10.
227. Miller JH, Ortega JA, Heisel MA. Juvenile Gaucher disease simulating osteomyelitis. *AJR Am J Roentgenol* 1981;137(4): 880–882.
228. Lachiewicz PF. Gaucher's disease. *Orthop Clin North Am* 1984;15(4):765–774.
229. Rosenthal DI, Scott JA, Barranger J, et al. Evaluation of Gaucher disease using magnetic resonance imaging. *J Bone Joint Surg Am* 1986;68(6):802–808.
230. Bell RS, Mankin HJ, Doppelt SH. Osteomyelitis in Gaucher disease. *J Bone Joint Surg Am* 1986;68(9):1380–1388.
231. Bilchik TR, Heyman S. Skeletal scintigraphy of pseudo-osteomyelitis in Gaucher's disease. Two case reports and a review of the literature. *Clin Nucl Med* 1992;17(4): 279–282.
232. Cremin BJ, Davey H, Goldblatt J. Skeletal complications of type I Gaucher disease: the magnetic resonance features. *Clin Radiol* 1990;41(4):244–247.

233. Figueroa ML, Rosenbloom BE, Kay AC, et al. A less costly regimen of alglucerase to treat Gaucher's disease. *N Engl J Med* 1992;327(23):1632–1636.
234. Schubiner H, Letourneau M, Murray DL. Pyogenic osteomyelitis versus pseudo-osteomyelitis in Gaucher's disease. Report of a case and review of the literature. *Clin Pediatr* (Phila) 1981;20(10):667–669.
235. Goldman AB, Jacobs B. Femoral neck fractures complicating Gaucher disease in children. *Skeletal Radiol* 1984;12(3):162–168.
236. Katz K, Sabato S, Horev G, et al. Spinal involvement in children and adolescents with Gaucher disease. *Spine* 1993;18(3):332–335.
237. Katz K, Horev G, Rivlin E, et al. Upper limb involvement in patients with Gaucher's disease. *J Hand Surg Am* 1993;18(5):871–875.
238. Hermann G, Pastores GM, Abdelwahab IF, et al. Gaucher disease: assessment of skeletal involvement and therapeutic responses to enzyme replacement. *Skeletal Radiol* 1997; 26(12):687–696.
239. Zimran A, Elstein D, Levy-Lahad E, et al. Replacement therapy with imiglucerase for type 1 Gaucher's disease. *Lancet* 1995;345:1479–1480.
240. Zimran A, Elstein D, Kannai R, et al. Low-dose enzyme replacement therapy for Gaucher's disease: effects of age, sex, genotype, and clinical features on response to treatment. *Am J Med* 1994;97(1):3–13.
241. Zimran A, Hollak CE, Abrahamov A, et al. Home treatment with intravenous enzyme replacement therapy for Gaucher disease: an international collaborative study of 33 patients. *Blood* 1993;82(4):1107–1109.
242. Hill SC, Parker CC, Brady RO, et al. MRI of multiple platyspondyly in Gaucher disease: response to enzyme replacement therapy. *J Comput Assist Tomogr* 1993;17(5):806–809.
243. Bembi B, Ciana G, Mengel E, et al. Bone complications in children with Gaucher disease. *Br J Radiol* 2002;75[Suppl 1]:A37–A44.
244. Tsai P, Lipton JM, Sahdev I, et al. Allogenic bone marrow transplantation in severe Gaucher disease. *Pediatr Res* 1992;31(5):503–507.
245. Tobias JD, Atwood R, Lowe S, et al. Anesthetic considerations in the child with Gaucher disease. *J Clin Anesth* 1993;5(2):150–153.
246. Aker M, Zimran A, Abrahamov A, et al. Abnormal neutrophil chemotaxis in Gaucher disease. *Br J Haematol* 1993;83(2):187–191.
247. Stein RE, Urbaniak J. Use of the tourniquet during surgery in patients with sickle cell hemoglobinopathies. *Clin Orthop* 1980;(151):231–233.
248. Piehl FC, Davis RJ, Prugh SI. Osteomyelitis in sickle cell disease. *J Pediatr Orthop* 1993; 13(2):225–227.
249. Sennara H, Gorry F. Orthopedic aspects of sickle cell anemia and allied hemoglobinopathies. *Clin Orthop* 1978;(130):154–157.
250. Chung SM, Alavi A, Russell MO. Management of osteonecrosis in sickle-cell anemia and its genetic variants. *Clin Orthop* 1978;(130):158–174.
251. Keeley K, Buchanan GR. Acute infarction of long bones in children with sickle cell anemia. *J Pediatr* 1982;101(2):170–175.
252. Middlemiss JH, Raper AB. Skeletal changes in the haemoglobinopathies. *J Bone Joint Surg Br* 1966;48(4):693–702.
253. Diggs LW. Bone and joint lesions in sickle-cell disease. *Clin Orthop* 1967;52:119–143.
254. Golding JS, Maciver JE, Went LN. The bone changes in sickle cell anaemia and its genetic variants. *J Bone Joint Surg Br* 1959;41-B:711–718.
255. Dalton GP, Drummond DS, Davidson RS, et al. Bone infarction versus infection in sickle cell disease in children. *J Pediatr Orthop* 1996;16(4):540–544.
256. Specht EE. Hemoglobinopathic salmonella osteomyelitis. Orthopedic aspects. *Clin Orthop* 1971;79:110–118.
257. Bennett OM, Namnyak SS. Bone and joint manifestations of sickle cell anaemia. *J Bone Joint Surg Br* 1990;72(3):494–499.
258. Epps CH, Bryant DD Jr, Coles MJ 3rd, et al. Osteomyelitis in patients who have sickle-cell disease. Diagnosis and management. *J Bone Joint Surg Am* 1991;73(9):1281–1294.
259. al-Salem AH, Ahmed HA, Qaisruddin S, et al. Osteomyelitis and septic arthritis in sickle cell disease in the eastern province of Saudi Arabia. *Int Orthop* 1992;16(4): 398–402.
260. Bohrer SP. Growth disturbances of the distal femur following sickle cell bone infarcts and-or osteomyelitis. *Clin Radiol* 1974;25(2):221–235.
261. Bohrer SP. Acute long bone diaphyseal infarcts in sickle cell disease. *Br J Radiol* 1970; 43(514):685–697.
262. Koren A, Garty I, Katzuni E. Bone infarction in children with sickle cell disease: early diagnosis and differentiation from osteomyelitis. *Eur J Pediatr* 1984;142(2):93–97.
263. Skaggs DL, Kim SK, Greene NW, et al. Differentiation between bone infarction and acute osteomyelitis in children with sickle-cell disease with use of sequential radionuclide bone-marrow and bone scans. *J Bone Joint Surg Am* 2001;83-A(12):1810–1813.
264. Bonnerot V, Sebag G, de Montalembert M, et al. Gadolinium-DOTA enhanced MRI of painful osseous crises in children with sickle cell anemia. *Pediatr Radiol* 1994;24(2): 92–95.
265. Stark JE, Glasier CM, Blaisier RD, et al. Osteomyelitis in children with sickle cell disease: early diagnosis with contrast-enhanced CT. *Radiology* 1991;179(3):731–733.
266. Ebong WW. Pathological fracture complicating long bone osteomyelitis in patients with sickle cell disease. *J Pediatr Orthop* 1986;6(2):177–181.
267. Smith JA. Bone disorders in sickle cell disease. *Hematol Oncol Clin North Am* 1996; 10(6):1345–1356.
268. Bohrer SP. Fracture complicating bone infarcts and-or osteomyelitis in sickle-cell disease. *Clin Radiol* 1971;22(1):83–88.
269. Vichinsky EP, Haberkern CM, Neumayr L, et al. A comparison of conservative and aggressive transfusion regimens in the perioperative management of sickle cell disease. The Preoperative Transfusion in Sickle Cell Disease Study Group. *N Engl J Med* 1995; 333(4):206–213.
270. Koc A, Gumruk F, Gurgey A. The effect of hydroxyurea on the coagulation system in sickle cell anemia and beta-thalassemia intermedia patients: a preliminary study. *Pediatr Hematol Oncol* 2003;20(6):429–434.
271. Schultz WH, Ware RE. Malignancy in patients with sickle cell disease. *Am J Hematol* 2003;74(4):249–253.
272. Wang WC, Helms RW, Lynn HS, et al. Effect of hydroxyurea on growth in children with sickle cell anemia: results of the HUG-KIDS Study. *J Pediatr* 2002;140(2):225–229.
273. Athanassiou-Metaxa M, Kirkos J, Koussi A, et al. Avascular necrosis of the femoral head among children and adolescents with sickle cell disease in Greece. *Haematologica* 2002;87(7):771–772.
274. Heinrich SD, Gallagher D, Warrior R, et al. The prognostic significance of the skeletal manifestations of acute lymphoblastic leukemia of childhood. *J Pediatr Orthop* 1994; 14(1):105–111.
275. Meehan PL, Viroslav S, Schmitt EW Jr. Vertebral collapse in childhood leukemia. *J Pediatr Orthop* 1995;15(5):592–595.
276. Rogalsky RJ, Black GB, Reed MH. Orthopaedic manifestations of leukemia in children. *J Bone Joint Surg Am* 1986;68(4):494–501.
277. Gallagher DJ, Phillips DJ, Heinrich SD. Orthopedic manifestations of acute pediatric leukemia. *Orthop Clin North Am* 1996;27(3):635–644.
278. Silverstein MN, Kelly PJ. Leukemia with osteoarticular symptoms and signs. *Ann Intern Med* 1963;59:637–645.
279. Thomas LB, Forkner CE Jr, Frei E 3rd, et al. The skeletal lesions of acute leukemia. *Cancer* 1961;14:608–621.
280. Samuda GM, Cheng MY, Yeung CY. Back pain and vertebral compression: an uncommon presentation of childhood acute lymphoblastic leukemia. *J Pediatr Orthop* 1987; 7(2):175–178.
281. Bos GD, Simon MA, Spiegel PG, et al. Childhood leukemia presenting as a diaphyseal radiolucency. *Clin Orthop* 1978;(135):66–68.
282. Van Slyck EJ. The bony changes in malignant hematologic disease. *Orthop Clin North Am* 1972;3(3):733–734.
283. Bleyer WA. Acute lymphoblastic leukemia in children. Advances and prospectus. *Cancer* 1990;65[Suppl 3]:689–695.
284. Hughes RG, Kay HE. Major bone lesions in acute lymphoblastic leukaemia. *Med Pediatr Oncol* 1982;10(1):67–70.
285. Wei SY, Esmail AN, Bunin N, et al. Avascular necrosis in children with acute lymphoblastic leukemia. *J Pediatr Orthop* 2000;20(3):331–335.
286. Beredjiklian PK, Drummond DS, Dormans J, et al. Orthopaedic manifestations of chronic graft-versus-host disease. *J Pediatr Orthop* 1998;18(5):572–575.
287. Bizot P, Witvoet J, Sedel L. Avascular necrosis of the femoral head after allogenic bone-marrow transplantation. A retrospective study of 27 consecutive THAs with a minimal two-year follow-up. *J Bone Joint Surg Br* 1996;78(6):878–883.
288. Clausen N, Gotze H, Pedersen A, et al. Skeletal scintigraphy and radiography at onset of acute lymphocytic leukemia in children. *Med Pediatr Oncol* 1983;11(4):291–296.
289. Aur RJ, Westbrook HW, Riggs W Jr. Childhood acute lymphocytic leukemia. Initial radiological bone involvement and prognosis. *Am J Dis Child* 1972;124(5):653–654.
290. Hann IM, Gupta S, Palmer MK, et al. The prognostic significance of radiological and symptomatic bone involvement in childhood acute lymphoblastic leukaemia. *Med Pediatr Oncol* 1979;6(1):51–55.
291. Masera G, Carnelli V, Ferrari M, et al. Prognostic significance of radiological bone involvement in childhood acute lymphoblastic leukaemia. *Arch Dis Child* 1977;52(7): 530–533.
292. Newman AJ, Melhorn DK. Vertebral compression in childhood leukemia. *Am J Dis Child* 1973;125(6):863–865.
293. Ahlberg A, Nilsson IM. Fractures in haemophiliacs with special reference to complications and treatment. *Acta Chir Scand* 1967;133(4):293–302.
294. Shopnick RI, Brettler DB. Hemostasis: a practical review of conservative and operative care. *Clin Orthop* 1996(328):34–38.
295. Post M, Telfer MC. Surgery in hemophilic patients. *J Bone Joint Surg Am* 1975;57(8): 1136–1145.
296. Connelly S, Kaleko M. Gene therapy for hemophilia A. *Thromb Haemost* 1997;78(1): 31–36.
297. Lancourt JE, Hochberg F. Delayed fracture healing in primary hyperparathyroidism. *Clin Orthop* 1977;(124):214–218.
298. Patel MR, Pearlman HS, Lavine LS. Arthrodesis in hemophilia. *Clin Orthop* 1972;86: 168–174.
299. Pietrogrande V, Dioguardi N, Mannucci PM. Short-term evaluation of synovectomy in haemophilia. *Br Med J* 1972;2(810):378–381.
300. Lancourt JE, Gilbert MS, Posner MA. Management of bleeding and associated complications of hemophilia in the hand and forearm. *J Bone Joint Surg Am* 1977;59(4):451–460.
301. Kasper CK, Rapaport SI. Bleeding times and platelet aggregation after analgesics in hemophilia. *Ann Intern Med* 1972;77(2):189–193.
302. Rodriguez-Merchan E. Bone fracture in the haemophilic patient. *Haemophilia* 2002;8: 104.
303. Feil E, Bentley G, Rizza CR. Fracture management in patients with haemophilia. *J Bone Joint Surg Br* 1974;56-B(4):643–649.
304. Kemp HS, Matthews JM. The management of fractures in haemophilia and Christmas disease. *J Bone Joint Surg Br* 1968;50(2):351–358.
305. Fernandez V, Spain M, Matthews JM. The Haemophilic pseudotumour or haemophilic subperiosteal haematoma. *J Bone Joint Surg Br* 1965;47:256–265.
306. Ahlberg AK. On the natural history of hemophilic pseudotumor. *J Bone Joint Surg Am* 1975;57(8):1133–1136.
307. Boardman KP, English P. Fractures and dislocations in hemophilia. *Clin Orthop* 1980; (148):221–232.
308. Robins RH, Murrell JS. Traumatic ischaemia in a haemophiliac. Report of a case of

prolonged haemostasis with cryoprecipitate during decompression and skin grafting. *J Bone Joint Surg Br* 1971;53(1):113–117.
309. Floman Y, Niska M. Dislocation of the hip joint complicating repeated hemarthrosis in hemophilia. *J Pediatr Orthop* 1983;3(1):99–100.
310. Ackroyd CE, Dinley RJ. The locked patella. An unusual complication of haemophilia. *J Bone Joint Surg Br* 1976;58-B(4):511–512.
311. Houghton GR, Duthie RB. Orthopedic problems in hemophilia. *Clin Orthop* 1979;(138):197–216.
312. Stein H, Dickson RA. Reversed dynamic slings for knee-flexion contractures in the hemophiliac. *J Bone Joint Surg Am* 1975;57(2):282–283.
313. Lee V, Srivastava A, PalaniKumar C, et al. External fixators in haemophilia. *Haemophilia* 2004;10(1):52–57.
314. Arnold WD, Hilgartner MW. Hemophilic arthropathy. Current concepts of pathogenesis and management. *J Bone Joint Surg Am* 1977;59(3):287–305.
315. Kumari S, Fulco JD, Karayalcin G, et al. Gray scale ultrasound: evaluation of iliopsoas hematomas in hemophiliacs. *AJR Am J Roentgenol* 1979;133(1):103–105.
316. Shirkhoda A, Mauro MA, Staab EV, et al. Soft-tissue hemorrhage in hemophiliac patients. Computed tomography and ultrasound study. *Radiology* 1983;147(3):811–814.
317. Wilson DJ, Green DJ, MacLamon JC. Arthrosonography of the painful hip. *Clin Radiol* 1984;35(1):17–19.
318. Aronstam A, Browne RS, Wassef M, et al. The clinical features of early bleeding into the muscles of the lower limb in severe haemophiliacs. *J Bone Joint Surg Br* 1983;65(1):19–23.
319. Lurie A, Bailey BP. The management of acute haemophilic haemarthroses and muscle haematomata. *S Afr Med J* 1972;46(21):656–659.
320. Miller EH, Flessa HC, Glueck HI. The management of deep soft tissue bleeding and hemarthrosis in hemophilia. *Clin Orthop* 1972;82:92–107.
321. Hutcheson J. Peripelvic new bone formation in hemophilia. Report of three cases. *Radiology* 1973;109(3):529–530.
322. Moneim MS, Gribble TJ. Carpal tunnel syndrome in hemophilia. *J Hand Surg Am* 1984;9(4):580–583.
323. Dietrich AM, James CD, King DR, et al. Head trauma in children with congenital coagulation disorders. *J Pediatr Surg* 1994;29(1):28–32.
324. Rosenthal RL, Graham JJ, Selirio E. Excision of pseudotumor with repair by bone graft of pathological fracture of femur in hemophilia. *J Bone Joint Surg Am* 1973;55(4):827–832.
325. Brant EE, Jordan HH. Radiologic aspects of hemophilic pseudotumors in bone. *Am J Roentgenol Radium Ther Nucl Med* 1972;115(3):525–539.
326. Pettersson H, Ahlberg A. Computed tomography in hemophilic pseudotumor. *Acta Radiol Diagn (Stockh)* 1982;23(5):453–457.
327. Krill CE Jr, Mauer AM. Pseudotumor of calcaneus in Christmas disease. *J Pediatr* 1970;77(5):848–855.
328. Castaneda VL, Parmley RT, Bozzini M, et al. Radiotherapy of pseudotumors of bone in hemophiliacs with circulating inhibitors to factor VIII. *Am J Hematol* 1991;36(1):55–59.
329. Idy-Peretti I, Le Balc'h T, Yvart J, et al. MR imaging of hemophilic arthropathy of the knee: classification and evolution of the subchondral cysts. *Magn Reson Imaging* 1992;10(1):67–75.
330. Nuss R, Kilcoyne RF, Geraghty S, et al. Utility of magnetic resonance imaging for management of hemophilic arthropathy in children. *J Pediatr* 1993;123(3):388–392.
331. Greene WB, Yankaskas BC, Guilford WB. Roentgenographic classifications of hemophilic arthropathy. Comparison of three systems and correlation with clinical parameters. *J Bone Joint Surg Am* 1989;71(2):237–244.
332. Gregosiewicz A, Wosko I, Kandzierski G. Intraarticular bleeding in children with hemophilia: the prevention of arthropathy. *J Pediatr Orthop* 1989;9(2):182–185.
333. Rodriguez-Merchan EC. Pathogenesis, early diagnosis, and prophylaxis for chronic hemophilic synovitis. *Clin Orthop* 1997;(343):6–11.
334. Ingram GI, Mathews JA, Bennett AE. Controlled trial of joint aspiration in acute haemophilic haemarthrosis. *Ann Rheum Dis* 1972;31(5):423.
335. Kisker CT, Burke C. Double-blind studies on the use of steroids in the treatment of acute hemarthrosis in patients with hemophilia. *N Engl J Med* 1970;282(12):639–642.
336. Erken EH. Radiocolloids in the management of hemophilic arthropathy in children and adolescents. *Clin Orthop* 1991;(264):129–135.
337. Ferguson AB Jr. Osteomyelitis in children. *Clin Orthop* 1973;96:51–56.
338. Silverman FN. Virus diseases of bone. Do they exist? The Neuhauser Lecture. *Am J Roentgenol* 1976;126(4):677–703.
339. Jurik AG, Helmig O, Ternowitz T, et al. Chronic recurrent multifocal osteomyelitis: a follow-up study. *J Pediatr Orthop* 1988;8(1):49–58.
340. Cabanela ME, Sim FH, Beabout JW, et al. Osteomyelitis appearing as neoplasms. A diagnostic problem. *Arch Surg* 1974109(1):68–72.
341. Sitarz AL, Berdon WE, Wolff JA, et al. Acute lymphocytic leukemia masquerading as acute osteomyelitis. A report of two cases. *Pediatr Radiol* 1980;9(1):33–35.
342. Jackson MA, Nelson JD. Etiology and medical management of acute suppurative bone and joint infections in pediatric patients. *J Pediatr Orthop* 1982;2(3):313–323.
343. Septimus EJ, Musher DM. Osteomyelitis: recent clinical and laboratory aspects. *Orthop Clin North Am* 1979;10(2):347–359.
344. Howie DW, Savage JP, Wilson TG, et al. The technetium phosphate bone scan in the diagnosis of osteomyelitis in childhood. *J Bone Joint Surg Am* 1983;65(4):431–437.
345. Ash JM, Gilday DL. The futility of bone scanning in neonatal osteomyelitis: concise communication. *J Nucl Med* 1980;21(5):417–420.
346. Dormans JP, Drummond DS. Pediatric hematogenous osteomyelitis: new trends in presentation, diagnosis, and treatment. *J Am Acad Orthop Surg* 1994;2(6):333–341.
347. Berquist TH, Brown ML, Fitzgerald RH Jr, et al. Magnetic resonance imaging: application in musculoskeletal infection. *Magn Reson Imaging* 1985;3(3):219–230.
348. Capener MP. Pathological fractures in osteomyelitis. *J Bone Joint Surg Am* 1932;14:501–510.
349. White M, Dennison WM. Acute haematogenous osteitis in childhood. *J Bone Joint Surg Br* 1952;34-B(4):608–623.
350. Daoud A, Saighi-Bouaouina A. Treatment of sequestra, pseudarthroses, and defects in the long bones of children who have chronic hematogenous osteomyelitis. *J Bone Joint Surg Am* 1989;71(10):1448–1468.
351. Canale ST, Puhl J, Watson FM, et al. Acute osteomyelitis following closed fractures. Report of three cases. *J Bone Joint Surg Am* 1975;57(3):415–418.
352. Kavanaugh JH. Occult infected fracture of the femur: report of two cases with long-term followup. *J Trauma* 1978;18(12):813–815.
353. Seftion G. Osteomyelitis after closed femoral fracture in a child. *J R Coll Surg Edinb* 1982;27:113.
354. Daoud AS-B, Descamps L, Maestro M. Hematogenous osteomyelitis of the femoral neck in children. *J Pediatr Orthop B* 1993;(2):83–95.
355. Lewallen RP, Peterson HA. Nonunion of long bone fractures in children: a review of 30 cases. *J Pediatr Orthop* 1985;5(2):135–42.
356. Sacks R, Habermann ET. Pathological fracture in congenital rubella. A case report. *J Bone Joint Surg Am* 1977;59(4):557–559.
357. Smith RK, Specht EE. Osseous lesions and pathologic fractures in congenital cytomegalic inclusion disease: report of a case. *Clin Orthop* 1979;(144):280–283.
358. Unkila-Kallio L, Kallio MJ, Eskola J, et al. Serum C-reactive protein, erythrocyte sedimentation rate, and white blood cell count in acute hematogenous osteomyelitis of children. *Pediatrics* 1994;93(1):59–62.
359. Morrey BF, Peterson HA. Hematogenous pyogenic osteomyelitis in children. *Orthop Clin North Am* 1975;6(4):935–951.
360. Langenskiold A. Femur remodelled during growth after osteomyelitis causing coxa vara and shaft necrosis. *J Pediatr Orthop* 1982;2(3):289–294.
361. Tudisco C, Farsetti P, Gatti S, et al. Influence of chronic osteomyelitis on skeletal growth: analysis at maturity of 26 cases affected during childhood. *J Pediatr Orthop* 1991;11(3):358–363.
362. Hood RW, Riseborough EJ. Lengthening of the lower extremity by the Wagner method. A review of the Boston Children's Hospital Experience. *J Bone Joint Surg Am* 1981;63(7):1122–1131.
363. Malhis TM, Bowen JR. Tibial and femoral lengthening: a report of 54 cases. *J Pediatr Orthop* 1982;2(5):487–491.
364. Maffulli N, Hughes T, Fixsen JA. Ultrasonographic monitoring of limb lengthening. *J Bone Joint Surg Br* 1992;74(1):130–132.
365. Mosca VM, Moseley C. Complications of Wagner leg lengthening and their avoidance. *Orthop Trans* 1986;10:462.
366. Eldridge JC, Bell DF. Problems with substantial limb lengthening. *Orthop Clin North Am* 1991;22(4):625–631.
367. Epps CH, Bowen JR, Bowen JR, eds. *Complications in pediatric orthopaedic surgery*. Philadelphia: JB Lippincott, 1995:747.
368. Osterman K, Merikanto J. Diaphyseal bone lengthening in children using Wagner device: long-term results. *J Pediatr Orthop* 1991;11(4):449–451.
369. Price CT, Cole JD. Limb lengthening by callotasis for children and adolescents. Early experience. *Clin Orthop* 1990;(250):105–111.
370. Paley D. Problems, obstacles, and complications of limb lengthening by the Ilizarov technique. *Clin Orthop* 1990;(250):81–104.
371. Blane CE, Herzenberg JE, DiPietro MA. Radiographic imaging for Ilizarov limb lengthening in children. *Pediatr Radiol* 1991;21(2):117–120.
372. Cole WG. The Nicholas Andry Award-1996. The molecular pathology of osteogenesis imperfecta. *Clin Orthop* 1997;(343):235–248.
373. Kocher MS, Shapiro F. Osteogenesis imperfecta. *J Am Acad Orthop Surg* 1998;6(4):225–236.
374. Wynne-Davies RH, Apley CM, eds. *Atlas of skeletal dysplasias*. New York: Churchill Livingstone, 1985.
375. Benson DR, Newman DC. The spine and surgical treatment in osteogenesis imperfecta. *Clin Orthop* 1981;(159):147–153.
376. Hanscom DA, Winter RB, Lutter L, et al. Osteogenesis imperfecta. Radiographic classification, natural history, and treatment of spinal deformities. *J Bone Joint Surg Am* 1992;74(4):598–616.
377. Moorefield WG Jr, Miller GR. Aftermath of osteogenesis imperfecta: the disease in adulthood. *J Bone Joint Surg Am* 1980;62(1):113–119.
378. McKusick V. *Heritable disorders of connective tissue*, 3rd ed. St. Louis: CV Mosby, 1972.
379. Shoenfeld, Y. Osteogenesis imperfecta. Review of the literature with presentation of 29 cases. *Am J Dis Child* 1975;129(6):679–687.
380. Harkey HL, Crockard HA, Stevens JM, et al. The operative management of basilar impression in osteogenesis imperfecta. *Neurosurgery* 1990;27(5):782–786; discussion 786.
381. King JB, Bobenchko WP. Osteogenesis imperfecta: an orthopaedic discussion and surgical review. *J Bone Joint Surg Br* 1971;53:72–89.
382. Roberts JB. Bilateral hyperplastic callus formation in osteogenesis imperfecta. *J Bone Joint Surg Am* 1976;58(8):1164–1166.
383. Jewell FL. Osteogenetic sarcoma occurring in fragilitas ossium: a case report. *Radiology* 1940;34:741–743.
384. Klenerman L, Ockenden BG, Townsend AC. Osteosarcoma occurring in osteogenesis imperfecta. Report of two cases. *J Bone Joint Surg Br* 1967;49(2):314–323.
385. Cohn DH, Byers PH. Clinical screening for collagen defects in connective tissue diseases. *Clin Perinatol* 1990;17(4):793–809.

386. Knight DJ, Bennet GC. Nonaccidental injury in osteogenesis imperfecta: a case report. *J Pediatr Orthop* 1990;10(4):542–544.
387. Minch CM, Kruse RW. Osteogenesis imperfecta: a review of basic science and diagnosis. *Orthopedics* 1998;21(5):558–567; quiz 568–569.
388. Paterson CR, Burns J, McAllion SJ. Osteogenesis imperfecta: the distinction from child abuse and the recognition of a variant form. *Am J Med Genet* 1993;45(2):187–192.
389. Steiner RD, Pepin M, Byers PH. Studies of collagen synthesis and structure in the differentiation of child abuse from osteogenesis imperfecta. *J Pediatr* 1996;128(4): 542–547.
390. DiCesare PE, Sew-Hoy A, Krom W. Bilateral isolated olecranon fractures in an infant as presentation of osteogenesis imperfecta. *Orthopedics* 1992;15(6):741–743.
391. Stott NS, Zionts LE. Displaced fractures of the apophysis of the olecranon in children who have osteogenesis imperfecta. *J Bone Joint Surg Am* 1993;75(7):1026–1033.
392. Zionts LE, Moon CN. Olecranon apophysis fractures in children with osteogenesis imperfecta revisited. *J Pediatr Orthop* 2002;22(6):745–750.
393. Gamble JG, Strudwick WJ, Rinsky LA, et al. Complications of intramedullary rods in osteogenesis imperfecta: Bailey-Dubow rods versus nonelongating rods. *J Pediatr Orthop* 1988;8(6):645–649.
394. Sillence D. Osteogenesis imperfecta: an expanding panorama of variants. *Clin Orthop* 1981;(159):11–25.
395. Nishi Y, Hamamoto K, Kajiyama M, et al. Effect of long-term calcitonin therapy by injection and nasal spray on the incidence of fractures in osteogenesis imperfecta. *J Pediatr* 1992;121(3):477–480.
396. Bembi B, Parma A, Bottega M, et al. Intravenous pamidronate treatment in osteogenesis imperfecta. *J Pediatr* 1997;131(4):622–625.
397. Glorieux FH, Bishop NJ, Plotkin H, et al. Cyclic administration of pamidronate in children with severe osteogenesis imperfecta. *N Engl J Med* 1998;339(14):947–952.
398. Falk MJ, Heeger S, Lynch KA, et al. Intravenous bisphosphonate therapy in children with osteogenesis imperfecta. *Pediatrics* 2003;111(3):573–578.
399. Sakkers R, Kok D, Engelbert R, et al. Skeletal effects and functional outcome with olpadronate in children with osteogenesis imperfecta: a 2-year randomised placebo-controlled study. *Lancet* 2004;363(9419):1427–1431.
400. Zeitlin L, Fassier F, Glorieux FH. Modern approach to children with osteogenesis imperfecta. *J Pediatr Orthop B* 2003;12(2):77–87.
401. Alman B, Frasca P. Fracture failure mechanisms in patients with osteogenesis imperfecta. *J Orthop Res* 1987;5(1):139–143.
402. Bleck EE. Nonoperative treatment of osteogenesis imperfecta: orthotic and mobility management. *Clin Orthop* 1981;(59):111–122.
403. Byers PH, Bonadio JF, Steinmann B. Osteogenesis imperfecta: update and perspective. *Am J Med Genet* 1984;17(2):429–435.
404. Furey JG, McNamee DC. Air splints for long-term management of osteogenesis imperfecta. *J Bone Joint Surg Am* 1973;55(3):645–649.
405. Gerber LH, Binder H, Weintrob J, et al. Rehabilitation of children and infants with osteogenesis imperfecta. A program for ambulation. *Clin Orthop* 1990;(51):254–262.
406. Letts M, Monson R, Weber K. The prevention of recurrent fractures of the lower extremities in severe osteogenesis imperfecta using vacuum pants: a preliminary report in four patients. *J Pediatr Orthop* 1988;8(4):454–457.
407. Porat S, Heller E, Seidman DS, Meyer S. Functional results of operation in osteogenesis imperfecta: elongating and nonelongating rods. *J Pediatr Orthop* 1991;11(2): 200–3.
408. Nicholas RW, James P. Telescoping intramedullary stabilization of the lower extremities for severe osteogenesis imperfecta. *J Pediatr Orthop* 1990;10(2):219–223.
409. Sijbrandij S. Percutaneous nailing in the management of osteogenesis imperfecta. *Int Orthop* 1990;14(2):195–197.
410. Bailey RW, Dubow HI. Evolution of the concept of an extensible nail accommodating to normal longitudinal bone growth: clinical considerations and implications. *Clin Orthop* 1981;(59):157–170.
411. Bailey RW, Dubow HI. Studies of longitudinal bone growth resulting in an extensible nail. *Surg Forum* 1963;14:455–458.
412. Bailey RW. Further clinical experience with the extensible nail. *Clin Orthop* 1981;(59): 171–176.
413. Gamble JG, Rinsky LA, Strudwick J, et al. Non-union of fractures in children who have osteogenesis imperfecta. *J Bone Joint Surg Am* 1988;70(3):439–443.
414. Niemann KM. Surgical treatment of the tibia in osteogenesis imperfecta. *Clin Orthop* 1981;(59):134–140.
415. Luhmann SJ, Sheridan JJ, Capelli AM, et al. Management of lower-extremity deformities in osteogenesis imperfecta with extensible intramedullary rod technique: a 20-year experience. *J Pediatr Orthop* 1998;18(1):88–94.
416. Mulpuri K, Joseph B. Intramedullary rodding in osteogenesis imperfecta. *J Pediatr Orthop* 2000;20(2):267–273.
417. Harrison WJ, Rankin KC. Osteogenesis imperfecta in Zimbabwe: a comparison between treatment with intramedullary rods of fixed-length and self-expanding rods. *J R Coll Surg Edinb* 1998;43(5):328–332.
418. Jerosch J, Mazzotti I, Tomasevic M. Complications after treatment of patients with osteogenesis imperfecta with a Bailey-Dubow rod. *Arch Orthop Trauma Surg* 1998; 117(4–5):240–245.
419. Zionts LE, Ebramzadeh E, Stott NS. Complications in the use of the Bailey-Dubow extensible nail. *Clin Orthop* 1998;(48):186–195.
420. Armstrong DG, Newfield JT, Gillespie R. Orthopedic management of osteopetrosis: results of a survey and review of the literature. *J Pediatr Orthop* 1999;19(1):122–132.
421. Popoff SN, Marks SC Jr. The heterogeneity of the osteopetroses reflects the diversity of cellular influences during skeletal development. *Bone* 1995;17(5):437–445.
422. Whyte MP. Carbonic anhydrase II deficiency. *Clin Orthop* 1993;(94):52–63.
423. Jaffe H. *Metabolic, degenerative, and inflammatory diseases of bone and joints*. Philadelphia: Lea & Febiger, 1972.
424. Shapiro F, Glimcher MJ, Holtrop ME, et al. Human osteopetrosis: a histological, ultrastructural, and biochemical study. *J Bone Joint Surg Am* 1980;62(3):384–399.
425. Milgram JW, Jasty M. Osteopetrosis. A morphological study of twenty-one cases. *J Bone Joint Surg Am* 1982;64(6):912–929.
426. Hasenhuttl K. Osteopetrosis. Review of the literature and comparative studies on a case with a twenty-four-year follow-up. *Am J Orthop* 1962;44-A:359–370.
427. Martin RP, Deane RH, Collett V. Spondylolysis in children who have osteopetrosis. *J Bone Joint Surg Am* 1997;79(11):1685–1689.
428. Bollerslev J, Andersen PE Jr. Fracture patterns in two types of autosomal-dominant osteopetrosis. *Acta Orthop Scand* 1989;60(1):110–112.
429. Kaplan FS, August CS, Fallon MD, et al. Osteopetrorickets. The paradox of plenty. Pathophysiology and treatment. *Clin Orthop* 1993;(94):64–78.
430. Manusov EG, Douville DR, Page LV, et al. Osteopetrosis ('marble bone' disease). *Am Fam Physician* 1993;47(1):175–180.
431. Shapiro F. Osteopetrosis. current clinical considerations. *Clin Orthop* 1993;(94):34–44.
432. Marks SC Jr, Schmidt CJ. Bone remodeling as an expression of altered phenotype: studies of fracture healing in untreated and cured osteopetrotic rats. *Clin Orthop* 1978; (37):259–264.
433. Greene WB, Torre BA. Femoral neck fracture in a child with autosomal dominant osteopetrosis. *J Pediatr Orthop* 1985;5(4):483–485.
434. Cameron HU, Dewar FP. Degenerative osteoarthritis associated with osteopetrosis. *Clin Orthop* 1977;(27):148–149.
435. Reeves JD, Huffer WE, August CS, et al. The hematopoietic effects of prednisone therapy in four infants with osteopetrosis. *J Pediatr* 1979;94(2):210–214.
436. van Lie Peters EM, Aronson DC, Everts V, et al. Failure of calcitriol treatment in a patient with malignant osteopetrosis. *Eur J Pediatr* 1993;152(10): 818–821.
437. Coccia PF, Krivit W, Cervenka J, et al. Successful bone-marrow transplantation for infantile malignant osteopetrosis. *N Engl J Med* 1980;302(13):701–708.
438. Gerritsen EJ, Vossen JM, van Loo IH, et al. Autosomal recessive osteopetrosis: variability of findings at diagnosis and during the natural course. *Pediatrics* 1994;93(2):247–253.
439. Rawlinson PG, Green RH, Coggins AM, et al. Malignant osteoporosis: hypercalcaemia after bone marrow transplantation. *Arch Dis Child* 1995;66:638–639.
440. Maroteaux P, Lamy M. The Malady of Toulouse-Lautrec. *JAMA* 1965;191:715–717.
441. Riseborough EJ, Herndon JH. Scoliosis of other deformities of the axial skeleton. Boston: Little, Brown, and Company; 1975:242.
442. Benz G, Schmid-Ruter E. Pycnodysostosis with Heterozygous beta-thalassemia. *Pediatr Radiol* 1977;5(3):164–171.
443. Bathi RJ, Masur VN. Pyknodysostosis—a report of two cases with a brief review of the literature. *Int J Oral Maxillofac Surg* 2000;29(6):439–442.
444. Dusenberry JF Jr, Kane JJ. Pycnodysostosis. Report of three new cases. *Am J Roentgenol Radium Ther Nucl Med* 1967;99(3): 717–723.
445. Meredith SC, Simon MA, Laros GS, et al. Pycnodysostosis. A clinical, pathological, and ultramicroscopic study of a case. *J Bone Joint Surg Am* 1978;60(8):1122–1127.
446. Tachdjian M. *Pediatric orthopaedics*, 2nd ed. Philadelphia: WB Saunders, 1989.
447. Edelson JG, Obad S, Geiger R, et al. Pycnodysostosis. Orthopedic aspects with a description of 14 new cases. *Clin Orthop* 1992;(80):263–276.
448. Taylor MM, Moore TM, Harvey JP Jr. Pycnodysostosis. A case report. *J Bone Joint Surg Am* 1978;60(8):1128–1130.
449. Roth VG. Pycnodysostosis presenting with bilateral subtrochanteric fractures: case report. *Clin Orthop* 1976;(17):247–253.
450. Bachrach S, Fisher J, Parks JS. An outbreak of vitamin D deficiency rickets in a susceptible population. *Pediatrics* 1979;64(6):871–877.
451. Mankin HJ. Rickets, osteomalacia, and renal osteodystrophy. Part II. *J Bone Joint Surg Am* 1974;56(2):352–386.
452. Parfitt AM. Renal osteodystrophy. *Orthop Clin North Am* 1972;3(3):681–698.
453. Smith R. The pathophysiology and management of rickets. *Orthop Clin North Am* 1972; 3(3):601–621.
454. Goldman AB, Lane JM, Salvati E. Slipped capital femoral epiphyses complicating renal osteodystrophy: a report of three cases. *Radiology* 1978;126(2):333–339.
455. Mehls O, Ritz E, Krempien B, et al. Slipped epiphyses in renal osteodystrophy. *Arch Dis Child* 1975;50:545–554.
456. Lebrun JB, Moffatt ME, Mundy RJ, et al. Vitamin D deficiency in a Manitoba community. *Can J Public Health* 1993;84(6):394–396.
457. Edidin DV, Levitsky LL, Schey W, et al. Resurgence of nutritional rickets associated with breast-feeding and special dietary practices. *Pediatrics* 1980;65(2):232–235.
458. Touloukian RJ, Gertner JM. Vitamin D deficiency rickets as a late complication of the short gut syndrome during infancy. *J Pediatr Surg* 1981;16(3):230–235.
459. Holda ME, Ryan JR. Hepatobiliary rickets. *J Pediatr Orthop* 1982;2(3):285–287.
460. Kooh SW, Jones G, Reilly BJ, et al. Pathogenesis of rickets in chronic hepatobiliary disease in children. *J Pediatr* 1979;94(6):870–874.
461. Kobayashi A, Kawai S, Utsunomiya T, et al. Bone disease in infants and children with hepatobiliary disease. *Arch Dis Child* 1974;49(8):641–646.
462. Sherk HH, Cruz M, Stambaugh J. Vitamin D prophylaxis and the lowered incidence of fractures in anticonvulsant rickets and osteomalacia. *Clin Orthop* 1977;(29):251–257.
463. Timperlake RW, Cook SD, Thomas KA, et al. Effects of anticonvulsant drug therapy on bone mineral density in a pediatric population. *J Pediatr Orthop* 1988;8(4):467–470.
464. Sweeney LE. Hypophosphataemic rickets after ifosfamide treatment in children. *Clin Radiol* 1993;47(5):345–347.
465. Amir J, Katz K, Grunebaum M, et al. Fractures in premature infants. *J Pediatr Orthop* 1988;8(1):41–44.
466. Helfer RE, Scheurer SL, Alexander R, et al. Trauma to the bones of small infants from passive exercise: a factor in the etiology of child abuse. *J Pediatr* 1984;104(1):47–50.
467. Koo WW, Gupta JM, Nayanar VV, et al. Skeletal changes in preterm infants. *Arch Dis Child* 1982;57(6):447–452.
468. Koo WW, Oestreich AE, Sherman R, et al. Radiological case of the month. Osteopenia, rickets, and fractures in preterm infants. *Am J Dis Child* 1985;139(10):1045–1046.

469. Roberts WA, Badger VM. Osteomalacia of very-low-birth-weight infants. *J Pediatr Orthop* 1984;4(5):593–598.
470. Kelly HJ, Sloan RE, Hoffman W, et al. Accumulation of nitrogen and six minerals in the human fetus during gestation. *Hum Biol* 1951;23(1):61–74.
471. Poznanski AK, Kuhns LR, Guire KE. New standards of cortical mass in the humerus of neonates: a means of evaluating bone loss in the premature infant. *Radiology* 1980; 134(3):639–644.
472. Bosley AR, Verrier-Jones ER, Campbell MJ. Aetiological factors in rickets of prematurity. *Arch Dis Child* 1980;55(9):683–686.
473. Hsu AC, Kooh SW, Fraser D, et al. Renal osteodystrophy in children with chronic renal failure: an unexpectedly common and incapacitating complication. *Pediatrics* 1982;70(5):742–750.
474. Cattell H S, Levin S, Kopits S, et al. Reconstructive surgery in children with azotemic osteodystrophy. *J Bone Joint Surg Am* 1971;53(2):216–228.
475. Apel DM, Millar EA, Moel DI. Skeletal disorders in a pediatric renal transplant population. *J Pediatr Orthop* 1989;9(5):505–511.
476. Davids JR, Fisher R, Lum G, et al. Angular deformity of the lower extremity in children with renal osteodystrophy. *J Pediatr Orthop* 1992;12(3):291–299.
477. Teall C. A radiological study of the bone changes in renal infantilism. *Br J Radiol* 1928; 1:49–58.
478. Baroncelli GI, Federico G, Bertelloni S, et al. Assessment of bone quality by quantitative ultrasound of proximal phalanges of the hand and fracture rate in children and adolescents with bone and mineral disorders. *Pediatr Res* 2003;54(1):125–136.
479. Chalmers J. Subtrochanteric fractures in osteomalacia. *J Bone Joint Surg Br* 1970;52(3): 509–513.
480. McWhorter AG, Seale NS. Prevalence of dental abscess in a population of children with vitamin D-resistant rickets. *Pediatr Dent* 1991;13(2):91–96.
481. Nelson CL, Evarts CM, Popowniak K. Musculoskeletal complications of renal transplantation. *Surg Clin North Am* 1971;51(5):1205–1209.
482. Eyres KS, Brown J, Douglas DL. Osteotomy and intramedullary nailing for the correction of progressive deformity in vitamin D-resistant hypophosphataemic rickets. *J R Coll Surg Edinb* 1993;38(1):50–54.
483. Stern PJ, Watts HG. Osteonecrosis after renal transplantation in children. *J Bone Joint Surg Am* 1979;61(6A):851–856.
484. Ruderman RJ, Poehling GG, Gray R, et al. Orthopedic complications of renal transplantation in children. *Transplant Proc* 1979;11(1):104–106.
485. Davidson JK, Tsakiris D, Briggs JD, et al. Osteonecrosis and fractures following renal transplantation. *Clin Radiol* 1985;36(1):27–35.
486. Ferris B, Walker C, Jackson A, et al. The orthopaedic management of hypophosphataemic rickets. *J Pediatr Orthop* 1991;11(3):367–373.
487. Kirkwood JR, Ozonoff MB, Steinbach HL. Epiphyseal displacement after metaphyseal fracture in renal osteodystrophy. *Am J Roentgenol Radium Ther Nucl Med* 1972;115(3): 547–554.
488. Krempien B, Mehls O, Ritz E. Morphological studies on pathogenesis of epiphyseal slipping in uremic children. *Virchows Arch A Pathol Anat Histol* 1974;362(2):129–143.
489. Llach F, Nikakhtar B. Current advances in the therapy of secondary hyperparathyroidism and osteitis fibrosa. *Miner Electrolyte Metab* 1991;17(4):250–255.
490. Nixon JR, Douglas JF. Bilateral slipping of the upper femoral epiphysis in end-stage renal failure. A report of two cases. *J Bone Joint Surg Br* 1980;62-B(1):18–21.
491. Hartjen CA, Koman LA. Treatment of slipped capital femoral epiphysis resulting from juvenile renal osteodystrophy. *J Pediatr Orthop* 1990;10(4):551–554.
492. Oppenheim WL, Namba R, Goodman WG, et al. Aluminum toxicity complicating renal osteodystrophy. A case report. *J Bone Joint Surg Am* 1989;71(3):446–452.
493. Andreoli SP, Bergstein JM, Sherrard DJ. Aluminum intoxication from aluminum-containing phosphate binders in children with azotemia not undergoing dialysis. *N Engl J Med* 1984;310(17):1079–1084.
494. Milliner DS, Nebeker HG, Ott SM, et al. Use of the deferoxamine infusion test in the diagnosis of aluminum-related osteodystrophy. *Ann Intern Med* 1984;101(6):775–779.
495. Salusky IB, Coburn JW, Foley J, et al. Effects of oral calcium carbonate on control of serum phosphorus and changes in plasma aluminum levels after discontinuation of aluminum-containing gels in children receiving dialysis. *J Pediatr* 1986;108(5 Pt 1): 767–770.
496. Smith R. Idiopathic osteoporosis in the young. *J Bone Joint Surg Br* 1980;62-B(4): 417–427.
497. Houang MTW, Brenton DP, Renton P, et al. Idiopathic juvenile osteoporosis. *Skeletal Radiol* 1978;3:17–23.
498. Jowsey J, Johnson KA. Juvenile osteoporosis: bone findings in seven patients. *J Pediatr* 1972;81(3):511–517.
499. Bertelloni S, Baroncelli GI, Di Nero G, et al. Idiopathic juvenile osteoporosis: evidence of normal osteoblast function by 1,25-dihydroxyvitamin D3 stimulation test. *Calcif Tissue Int* 1992;51(1):20–23.
500. Dent CE, Friedman M. Idiopathic juvenile osteoporosis. *Q J Med* 1965;34:177–210.
501. Berglund GL. Osteopenia in adolescents. *Clin Orthop* 1960;17:259–264.
502. Dent CE. Osteoporosis in childhood. *Postgrad Med J* 1977;5:3(622):450–457.
503. Lane JM, Vigorita VJ. Osteoporosis. *J Bone Joint Surg Am* 1983;65(2):274–278.
504. Marder HK, Tsang RC, Hug G, et al. Calcitriol deficiency in idiopathic juvenile osteoporosis. *Am J Dis Child* 1982;136(10):914–917.
505. Singh M, Nagrath AR, Maini PS. Changes in trabecular pattern of the upper end of the femur as an index of osteoporosis. *J Bone Joint Surg Am* 1970;52(3):457–467.
506. Marhaug G. Idiopathic juvenile osteoporosis. *Scand J Rheumatol* 1993;22(1):45–47.
507. Cloutier MD, Hayles AB, Riggs BL, et al. Juvenile osteoporosis: report of a case including a description of some metabolic and microradiographic studies. *Pediatrics* 1967;40(4): 649–655.
508. Gooding CA, Ball JH. Idiopathic juvenile osteoporosis. *Radiology* 1969;93(6): 1349–1350.
509. Gandrud LM, Cheung JC, Daniels MW, et al. Low-dose intravenous pamidronate reduces fractures in childhood osteoporosis. *J Pediatr Endocrinol Metab* 2003;16(6): 887–892.
510. Ragab AH, Frech RS, Vietti TJ. Osteoporotic fractures secondary to methotrexate therapy of acute leukemia in remission. *Cancer* 1970;25(3):580–585.
511. Lane MN, Hall TC. Chemotherapy: discussion. *Cancer* 1976;37[Suppl]:1055–1057.
512. Stanisavljevic S, Babcock AL. Fractures in children treated with methotrexate for leukemia. *Clin Orthop* 1977;(25):139–144.
513. Schwartz AM, Leonidas JC. Methotrexate osteopathy. *Skeletal Radiol* 1984;11(1):13–16.
514. Elsasser U, Ruegsegger P, Anliker M, et al. Loss and recovery of trabecular bone in the distal radius following fracture—immobilization of the upper limb in children. *Klin Wochenschr* 1979;57(15):763–767.
515. Nilsson BE, Westlin NE. Restoration of bone mass after fracture of the lower limb in children. *Acta Orthop Scand* 1971;42(1):78–81.
516. Bjernulf A, Hall K, Sjogren L, et al. Primary hyperparathyroidism in children. Brief review of the literature and a case report. *Acta Paediatr Scand* 1970;59(3):249–258.
517. Jackson CE, Frame B. Diagnosis and management of parathyroid disorders. *Orthop Clin North Am* 1972;3(3):699–712.
518. Eaton DG, Hewitt CA. Renal function in hyperparathyroidism with complicating nephrocalcinosis. *Acta Paediatr* 1993;82(1):111–112.
519. Randall C, Lauchlan SC. Parathyroid hyperplasia in an infant. *Am J Dis Child* 1963; 105:364–367.
520. Rajasuriya K, Peiris OA, Ratnaike VT, et al. Parathyroid adenomas in childhood. *Am J Dis Child* 1964;107:442–449.
521. Anspach WC. Hyperparathyrodism in children: a report of two cases. *Am J Dis Child* 1939;58:540–557.
522. Dauphine RT, Riggs BL, Scholz DA. Back pain and vertebral crush fractures: an unemphasized mode of presentation for primary hyperparathyroidism. *Ann Intern Med* 1975; 83(3):365–367.
523. Parfitt AM. The actions of parathyroid hormone on bone: relation to bone remodeling and turnover, calcium homeostasis, and metabolic bone disease. Part III of IV parts; PTH and osteoblasts, the relationship between bone turnover and bone loss, and the state of the bones in primary hyperparathyroidism. *Metabolism* 1976;25(9):1033–1069.
524. Bleck EK. Special injuries of the musculoskeletal system. In: CA Rockwood, Wilkins KE, King RE, eds. *Fractures in children*. Philadelphia: JB Lippincott, 1984:173–228.
525. Adam A, Ritchie D. Hyperparathyroidism with increased bone density in the areas of growth. *J Bone Joint Surg Br* 1954;36-B(2):257–260.
526. Clark OH, Duh QY. Primary hyperparathyroidism. A surgical perspective. *Endocrinol Metab Clin North Am* 1989;18(3):701–714.
527. Wilkinson H, James J. Self limiting neonatal primary hyperparathyroidism associated with familial hypocalciuric hypercalcaemia. *Arch Dis Child* 1993;69(3 Spec No): 319–321.
528. Grantmyre EB. Roentgenographic features of primary hyperparathyroidism in infancy. *J Can Assoc Radiol* 1973;24(3):257–260.
529. Cushing H. The basophil adenomas of the pituitary body and their clinical manifestations. *Bull Johns Hopkins Hosp* 1932;50:137–195.
530. McArthur RG, Bahn RC, Hayles AB. Primary adrenocortical nodular dysplasia as a cause of Cushing's syndrome in infants and children. *Mayo Clin Proc* 1982;57(1):58–63.
531. Preeyasombat C, Sirikulchayanonta V, Mahachokelertwattana P, et al. Cushing's syndrome caused by Ewing's sarcoma secreting corticotropin releasing factor-like peptide. *Am J Dis Child* 1992;146(9):1103–1105.
532. Harris WH, Heaney RP. Skeletal renewal and metabolic bone disease. *N Engl J Med* 1969;280(6):303–311.
533. Jowsey J, Riggs BL. Bone formation in hypercortisonism. *Acta Endocrinol (Copenh)* 1970; 63(1):21–28.
534. Iannaccone A, Babrilove JL, Brahms SA, et al. Osteoporosis in Cushing's syndrome. *Ann Intern Med* 1960;52:570–586.
535. McArthur RG, Cloutier MD, Hayes AB, et al. Cushing's disease in children. Findings in 13 cases. *Mayo Clin Proc* 1972;47(5):318–326.
536. Maclean AD. Spinal changes in a case of infantile scurvy. *Br J Radiol* 1968;41(485): 385–387.
537. Grewar D. Infantile scurvy. *Clin Pediatr (Phila)* 1965;35:82–89.
538. Nerubay J, Pilderwasser D. Spontaneous bilateral distal femoral physiolysis due to scurvy. *Acta Orthop Scand* 1984;55(1):18–20.
539. Banks S. Bone changes in acute and chronic scurvy: an experimental study. *J Bone Joint Surg Am* 1943;15:553–565.
540. Ossofsky HJ. Infantile scurvy. *Am J Dis Child* 1965;109:173–176.
541. McKibbin B, Porter RW. The incidence of vitamin-C deficiency in meningomyelocele. Dev *Med Child Neurol* 1967;9(3):338–344.
542. Lee RV. Scurvy: a contemporary historical perspective (3). *Conn Med* 1984;48(1): 33–35.
543. McLean SM. Healing in infantile scurvy as shown by x-ray. *Am J Dis Child* 1928;36: 875–930.
544. Ramar S, Sivaramakrishnan V, Manoharan K. Scurvy—a forgotten disease. *Arch Phys Med Rehabil* 1993;74(1):92–95.
545. Scott W. Epiphyseal dislocations in scurvy. *J Bone Joint Surg Am* 1941;23:314–322.
546. Silverman FN. Recovery from epiphyseal invagination: sequel to an unusual complication of scurvy. *J Bone Joint Surg Am* 1970;52(2):384–390.
547. Silverman FN. An unusual osseous sequel to infantile scurvy. *J Bone Joint Surg Am* 1953;35-A(1):215–220.
548. Hoeffel JC, Lascombes P, Mainard L, et al. Cone epiphysis of the knee and scurvy. *Eur J Pediatr Surg* 1993;3(3):186–189.

549. Quiles M, Sanz TA. Epiphyseal separation in scurvy. *J Pediatr Orthop* 1988;8(2): 223–225.
550. Grunebaum M, Horodniceanu C, Steinherz R. The radiographic manifestations of bone changes in copper deficiency. *Pediatr Radiol* 1980;9(2):101–104.
551. Heller RM, Kirchner SG, O'Neill JA Jr, et al. Skeletal changes of copper deficiency in infants receiving prolonged total parenteral nutrition. *J Pediatr* 1978;92(6):947–949.
552. Botash AS, Nasca J, Dubowy R, et al. Zinc-induced copper deficiency in an infant. *Am J Dis Child* 1992;146(6):709–711.
553. Cordano A, Baertl JM, Graham GG. Copper deficiency in infancy. *Pediatrics* 1964;34: 324–336.
554. Henderson RC, Lark RK, Gurka MJ, et al. Bone density and metabolism in children and adolescents with moderate to severe cerebral palsy. *Pediatrics* 2002;110(1 Pt 1): e5.
555. McIvor WC, Samilson RL. Fractures in patients with cerebral palsy. *J Bone Joint Surg Am* 1966;48(5):858–866.
556. Miller PR, Glazer DA. Spontaneous fractures in the brain-crippled, bedridden patient. *Clin Orthop* 1976;(120):134–137.
557. Lee JJ, Lyne ED. Pathologic fractures in severely handicapped children and young adults. *J Pediatr Orthop* 1990;10(4):497–500.
558. Bischof F, Basu D, Pettifor JM. Pathological long-bone fractures in residents with cerebral palsy in a long-term care facility in South Africa. *Dev Med Child Neurol* 2002; 44(2):119–122.
559. Fry K, Hoffer MM, Brink J. Femoral shaft fractures in brain-injured children. *J Trauma* 1976;16(5):371–373.
560. Heinrich SD, Drvaric DM, Darr K, et al. The operative stabilization of pediatric diaphyseal femur fractures with flexible intramedullary nails: a prospective analysis. *J Pediatr Orthop* 1994;14(4):501–507.
561. Sherk HH. Indications for orthopedic surgery in the mentally retarded patient. *Clin Orthop* 1973;90:174–177.
562. Kaye JJ, Freiberger RH. Fragmentation of the lower pole of the patella in spastic lower extremities. *Radiology* 1971;101(1):97–100.
563. Lloyd-Roberts GC, Jackson AM, Albert JS. Avulsion of the distal pole of the patella in cerebral palsy. A cause of deteriorating gait. *J Bone Joint Surg Br* 1985;67(2):252–254.
564. Rosenthal RK, Levine DB. Fragmentation of the distal pole of the patella in spastic cerebral palsy. *J Bone Joint Surg Am* 1977;59(7):934–939.
565. Miller F, Cardoso Dias R, Dabney KW, et al. Soft-tissue release for spastic hip subluxation in cerebral palsy. *J Pediatr Orthop* 1997;17(5):571–584.
566. Miller F, Girardi H, Lipton G, et al. Reconstruction of the dysplastic spastic hip with peri-ilial pelvic and femoral osteotomy followed by immediate mobilization. *J Pediatr Orthop* 1997;17(5):592–602.
567. Drennan JC, Freehafer AA. Fractures of the lower extremities in paraplegic children. *Clin Orthop* 1971;77:211–217.
568. Drummond DS, Moreau M, Cruess RL. Post-operative neuropathic fractures in patients with myelomeningocele. *Dev Med Child Neurol* 1981;23(2):147–150.
569. Feiwell E, Sakai D, Blatt T. The effect of hip reduction on function in patients with myelomeningocele. Potential gains and hazards of surgical treatment. *J Bone Joint Surg Am* 1978;60(2):169–173.
570. James CC. Fractures of the lower limbs in spina bifida cystica: a survey of 44 fractures fin 122 children. *Dev Med Child Neurol* 1970;[Suppl 22]:88.
571. Wenger DR, Jeffcoat BT, Herring JA. The guarded prognosis of physeal injury in paraplegic children. *J Bone Joint Surg Am* 1980;62(2):241–246.
572. Edvardsen P. Physeo-epiphyseal injuries of lower extremities in myelomeningocele. *Acta Orthop Scand* 1972;43(6):550–557.
573. Kumar SJ, Cowell HR, Townsend P. Physeal, metaphyseal, and diaphyseal injuries of the lower extremities in children with myelomeningocele. *J Pediatr Orthop* 1984;4(1): 25–27.
574. Townsend PF, Cowell HR, Steg NL. Lower extremity fractures simulating infection in myelomeningocele. *Clin Orthop* 1979;(44):255–259.
575. Lock TR, Aronson DD. Fractures in patients who have myelomeningocele. *J Bone Joint Surg Am* 1989;71(8):1153–1157.
576. Boytim MJ, Davidson RS, Charney E, et al. Neonatal fractures in myelomeningocele patients. *J Pediatr Orthop* 1991;11(1):28–30.
577. Eichenholtz S. Management of long-bone fractures in paraplegic patients. *J Bone Joint Surg Am* 1963;45:299–310.
578. Drummond DS, Moreau M, Cruess RL. The results and complications of surgery for the paralytic hip and spine in myelomeningocele. *J Bone Joint Surg Br* 1980;62-B(1): 49–53.
579. Quilis AN. Fractures in children with myelomeningocele. *Acta Orthop Scand* 1974; 45(6): 883–897.
580. Norton, PL, Foley JJ. Paraplegia in children. *Am J Orthop* 1959;41-A:1291–1309.
581. Khoury JG, Morcuende JA. Dramatic subperiosteal bone formation following physeal injury in patients with myelomeningocele. *Iowa Orthop J* 2002;22:94–98.
582. Rodgers WB, Schwend RM, Jaramillo D, et al. Chronic physeal fractures in myelodysplasia: magnetic resonance analysis, histologic description, treatment, and outcome. *J Pediatr Orthop* 1997;17(5):615–621.
583. Gyepes MT, Newbern DH, Neuhauser EB. Metaphyseal and physeal injuries in children with spina bifida and meningomyeloceles. *Am J Roentgenol Radium Ther Nucl Med* 1965; 95:168–177.
584. Anschuetz RH, Freehafer AA, Shaffer JW, et al. Severe fracture complications in myelodysplasia. *J Pediatr Orthop* 1984;4(1):22–24.
585. Drabu KJ, Walker G. Stiffness after fractures around the knee in spina bifida. *J Bone Joint Surg Br* 1985;67(2):266–267.
586. Laidlaw AT, Loder RT, Hensinger R. Telescoping intramedullary rodding with Bailey-Dubow nails for recurrent pathologic fractures in children without osteogenesis imperfecta. *J Pediatr Orthop* 1998;18(1):4–8.
587. Anderson TE, Drummond DS, Breed AL, et al. Malignant hyperthermia in myelomeningocele: a previously unreported association. *J Pediatr Orthop* 1981;1(4):401–403.
588. Dormans JP, Templeton J, Schreiner MS, et al. Intraoperative latex anaphylaxis in children: classification and prophylaxis of patients at risk. *J Pediatr Orthop* 1997;17(5): 622–625.
589. FDA Allergic Reactions to Latex Containing Medical Devices: FDA Medical Alert. DHHS (NIOSH) 1997;No. 97-135.
590. Meeropol E, Frost J, Pugh L, et al. Latex allergy in children with myelodysplasia: a survey of Shriners hospitals. *J Pediatr Orthop* 1993;13(1):1–4.
591. Vignos PJ Jr, Archibald KC. Maintenance of ambulation in childhood muscular dystrophy. *J Chronic Dis* 1960;12:273–290.
592. McDonald DG, Kinali M, Gallagher AC, et al. Fracture prevalence in Duchenne muscular dystrophy. *Dev Med Child Neurol* 2002;44(10):695–698.
593. Hsu JD, Garcia-Ariz M. Fracture of the femur in the Duchenne muscular dystrophy patient. *J Pediatr Orthop* 1981;1(2):203–207.
594. Siegel IM. Fractures of long bones in Duchenne muscular dystrophy. *J Trauma* 1977; 17(3):219–222.
595. Epstein BA. Roentgenological changes in the bones in cases of pseudohypertrophic muscular dystrophy. *Arch Neurol Psychiatry* 1941;46:868–876.
596. Maybarduk PL. Osseous atrophy associated with progressive muscular dystrophy. *Am J Dis Child* 1941;61:565–576.
597. Larson CM, Henderson RC. Bone mineral density and fractures in boys with Duchenne muscular dystrophy. *J Pediatr Orthop* 2000;20(1):71–74.
598. Hsu JD. Extremity fractures in children with neuromuscular disease. *Johns Hopkins Med J* 1979;145(3):89–93.
599. Bothwell JE, Gordon KE, Doley JM, et al. Vertebral fractures in boys with Duchenne muscular dystrophy. *Clin Pediatr (Phila)* 2003;42(4):353–356.
600. Williams P. The management of arthrogryposis. *Orthop Clin North Am* 1978;9(1): 67–88.
601. Diamond LS, Alegado R. Perinatal fractures in arthrogryposis multiplex congenita. *J Pediatr Orthop* 1981;1(2):189–192.
602. Robin GC. Fractures in poliomyelitis in children. *J Bone Joint Surg Am* 1966;48(6): 1048–1054.
603. Neuhauser EB. Arthrogryposis multiplex congenita. Susceptibility to injury. *Postgrad Med* 1969;46(4):61–63.
604. Sodergard J, Ryoppy S. The knee in arthrogryposis multiplex congenita. *J Pediatr Orthop* 1990;10(2):177–182.
605. Katz JF. Spontaneous fractures in paraplegic children. *J Bone Joint Surg Am* 1953;35-A(1):220–226.
606. Robin GC. Fracture in childhood paraplegia. *Paraplegia* 1965;3(3):165–170.
607. Freehafer AA, Mast WA. Lower extremity fractures in patients with spinal-cord injury. *J Bone Joint Surg Am* 1965;47:683–694.
608. Hulth A, Olerud S. The healing of fractures in denervated limbs. An experimental study using sensory and motor rhizotomy and peripheral denervation. *J Trauma* 1965;5(5): 571–579.
609. Schneider R, Goldman AB, Bohne WH. Neuropathic injuries to the lower extremities in children. *Radiology* 1978;128(3):713–718.
610. Comarr AE, Hutchinson RH, Bors E. Extremity fractures of patients with spinal cord injuries. *Am J Surg* 1962;103:732–739.
611. Abramson A. Bone disturbances in injuries to the spinal cord and cauda equina (paraplegia): their prevention by ambulation. J Bone Joint Surg Am 1948;30:982–987.

7

CHILD ABUSE

Robert M. Campbell, Jr and Timothy Schrader

THE ORTHOPAEDIC RECOGNITION OF CHILD ABUSE

Epidemiology

Child abuse is maltreatment of a child by either parents or caretakers, and includes physical, sexual, and emotional abuse, as well as emotional and physical neglect (1). The incidence of physical abuse nationally is estimated to be 4.9 children per 1,000, and 1 of every 1,000 abused children die (2). The epidemic of child abuse continues to worsen in the United States, with approximately 2.9 million reports now filed annually compared with 1.2 million in 1982 (3). In the United States 3 children a day die of abuse or neglect (4). In Texas alone, 50,746 children were confirmed victims of child abuse or neglect in fiscal year 1995, with 101 deaths recorded (5). The types of abuse these children were subjected to included physical abuse in 31.5%, sexual abuse in 15.6%, emotional abuse in 6.8%, abandonment in 2%, medical neglect in 4.7%, physical neglect in 15.4%, and neglectful supervision in 40.3%. The minimal annual cost of child abuse in the United States is estimated to be 9 billion dollars (3), but additional costs, both direct and indirect, exist. The estimated national cost of child abuse for the child welfare system is 14 billion dollars, law enforcement 24 million, and the court system 341 million (4). The median cost of hospital admission for child maltreatment in Pennsylvania in 1995 was $15,587 (6). The long-term social costs of child abuse are impossible to estimate: one third of the victims of child abuse grow up to be seriously inept, neglectful, or abusive parents; one third are at high risk for eventually becoming abusive parents; and only one third do not repeat the destructive patterns they were exposed to as children (7). Indirect estimated national costs of child abuse, including special education for learning disorders of abused children, maternal mental and health care, legal costs of juvenile delinquency, lost productivity to society of abused children as unemployed adults, and later adult criminality of abused children are 94 billion dollars (4). The orthopaedist becomes involved in the care of 30% to 50% of abused children (8). Early recognition of these abused patients by the orthopaedist is critical, because the children who are returned to their homes after an unrecognized episode of child abuse have a 25% risk of serious reinjury and a 5% risk of death (9).

Overview

In 1946, Caffey (10) described six infants with long-bone fractures, chronic subdural hematomas, and intraocular bleeding without a history of trauma to explain the injuries. Although his work is often cited as the first report in the English literature of child abuse, Caffey did not speculate about the etiology of the children's injuries. In 1953, Silverman (11) characterized the unique metaphyseal fractures found in abused children in the pediatric literature and clearly emphasized that these were due to nonaccidental trauma. Altman and Smith (12) in 1960 published the first series in the orthopaedic literature of injuries caused by child abuse. General public awareness of child abuse increased with the 1962 publication of a report by Kempe et al (13) characterizing the problems as the *battered child syndrome*. In 1974, Caffey introduced the term *whiplash-shaken infant syndrome* to the literature to emphasize the etiology of subdural hematomas in infants caused by shaking episodes (14). In 1974, Congress acknowledged the national importance of the prevention of child abuse by the passage of the Child Abuse Prevention and Treatment Act.

THE RISK FACTORS FOR CHILD ABUSE

The Home at Risk

In assessing where abuse of children may occur, households in turmoil from marital separation, job loss, divorce, family death, housing difficulties, or money problems are more likely to have abusive episodes (15). Families with two unplanned births are 2.8 times more likely to have an episode of child abuse than families with no unplanned births (16). In these homes at risk, stepparents, babysitters, boyfriends, relatives, and even larger siblings frequently are abusers (17–19). The parents of battered children may themselves have been abused when they were children (20). High levels of parental stress and high belief in the worth of corporal punishment are predictors of child abuse (21). Parental substance abuse, whether alcohol or other drugs, makes child abuse more likely (22). The risk of physical abuse is fivefold more likely with maternal cocaine use (23). Young, unmarried mothers are more likely to have their infants die from intentional injury, with a peak incidence of 10.5 intentional deaths per 10,000 live births in one study (24). Violence in the home is not directed solely toward the child; in one study (25) of families with substantiated child abuse, 30% of the mothers had been battered. Although the youngest, poorest, most socially isolated and economically frustrated caretakers are the most likely to act violently toward their children (26), any adult from any social or economic level may be guilty of abusing a child (17). Primary parental predictors of child abuse are listed in Table 7-1 (27).

The Child at Risk

Certain children of all ages are more likely to experience abuse, and younger children are particularly at risk. Most reported

TABLE 7-1 Parental Predictors of Child Abuse

Mother
- Age <20 years
- Lower educational achievement
- History of sexual abuse
- Child guidance issues
- Absent father during childhood
- History of psychiatric illness

Father
- Age <20 years
- Lower educational achievement
- Child guidance issues
- History of psychiatric illness

General
- Parent history of child abuse
- Divorce or separation of mother's parents
- Maternal history of being separated from mother, parental alcohol or drug abuse
- Maternal history of depression

From Sidebotham P, Golding J. The ALSPAC Study Team: child maltreatment in the "Children of the Nineties"—a longitudinal study of parental risk factors. *Child Abuse Negl* 2001;25:1177–1200; with permission.

cases of child abuse involve children younger than 3 years of age (28). In one report of child abuse (29), 78% of all fractures reported were in children younger than 3 years of age and 50% of all fractures occurred in children younger than 1 year of age. Infants younger than 1 year are especially at risk for the most severe form of child abuse: infant homicide (30,31). With severe shaking injuries by caretakers, 30% of infants are disabled and another 30% die (32). The problem probably is more widespread than suspected. There is evidence that suggests that in the United Kingdom, 10% to 20% of children diagnosed as having sudden infant death syndrome may be intentional infant homicide (33). In one report (34), covert video recordings of adults attending their children who were hospitalized for suspicious illness documented 14 separate instances of caretaker attempts at upper airway obstruction. First-born children (29), premature infants, stepchildren, and handicapped children are at a greater risk for child abuse (8). Benedict et al (35), in a longitudinal study of 500 handicapped children followed from birth to age 10 years, documented a 4.6% incidence of physical abuse. Surprisingly, they found that the most severely involved children were less likely to be abused, whereas the marginally functioning children were at greater risk, with parental frustration possibly being a factor.

The Risk for Munchausen Syndrome by Proxy

Children who are persistently presented by parents for medical assessment of vague illness, and have a history of multiple diagnostic or therapeutic procedures with unclear outcome, are at risk for having a form of child abuse known as Munchausen syndrome by proxy (36,37). Munchausen syndrome is named for Baron von Munchausen, an 18th-century mercenary whose exaggerated tales of adventure were viewed with great suspicion. Asher (36), in 1951, described Munchausen syndrome in adults who presented with apparent acute illness accompanied by dramatic, untruthful medical histories to gain attention. In Munchausen syndrome by proxy, children become the victims of this adult behavior when parents with a misguided sense of purpose fabricate a wide range of childhood illnesses for their children, often subjecting them to needless diagnostic workups and treatment (37). Symptoms of the child's "illness" are based on an imaginary medical history given by the parent, with signs of the illness either simulated or induced by the parent. For example, a child may be brought into the emergency room by a parent with a complaint of vomiting. In Munchausen syndrome by proxy, this complaint may either be a total fabrication by the parent or the parent may simulate the complaint by producing "vomitus" from some source as proof of illness. In one report, bloodstained material has been presented by a caretaker as proof of a child's "gastrointestinal bleeding," but DNA testing revealed that the source was actually the caretaker (38). Conjunctivitis from a caustic agent placed on an infant by a caretaker has been reported (39). Children have been given clozapine and clonidine by caretakers to simulate illness (40). A parent has caused vomiting in a child by the administration of salt (41) or ipecac. In the most extreme situations, a rodenticide-induced coagulopathy was induced in a 2-year-old child (42), a deliberate self-induced preterm labor was caused by a parent (43), and another gave chronic illicit insulin to a 1-year-old child (37). Over half of reported cases of Munchausen syndrome by proxy involve induced symptoms, whereas another 25% involve a combination of both simulation and induction of symptoms (44).

The biologic mother is almost always the perpetrator of this pattern of abuse (45), but men, especially those with a history of Munchausen syndrome themselves, also can be responsible for this form of child abuse (46). Caretakers in Munchausen syndrome by proxy almost all have a medical background: 35% to 45% are nurses, 5% are medical office workers, 3% are social workers, and 1% are orderlies (45). The perpetrator of the child's illness denies the knowledge of its etiology, but the acute signs and symptoms of the child's illness in Munchausen syndrome by proxy will resolve if the syndrome is recognized and the child is separated from the parent (45). Follow-up of families with this disorder is crucial. Davis et al (47) reported a reoccurrence of abuse rate of Munchausen by proxy of 17%, new sibling abuse in 50% of families with a suffocated child, and 40% of families involved with nonaccidental poisoning. Failure to diagnose this condition places a child at risk for either serious long-term sequelae or death in approximately 9% of cases.

The diagnosis of Munchausen syndrome by proxy remains difficult. Covert in-hospital video surveillance (CVS) of caretakers with their children may be a valuable means to substantiate or disprove this diagnosis. Hall et al (48) reported that CVS with audio surveillance added allowed diagnosis of Munchausen syndrome by proxy in 56% of patients monitored and was supportive of the diagnosis in another 22% of children. Both suffocation and injection of bodily fluids were documented by this approach. Privacy concerns were addressed by routine consent of the caretakers on the admission form that "closed-circuit monitoring of patient care may be used for educational or clinical purposes," and a multispecialty team approved the 24-hour use of security officers to monitor selected patients and make log entries on at least an hourly basis. The approach, though, is expensive and cannot be covered by third party payers. The diagnosis of Munchausen syndrome by proxy depends on health care workers maintaining a high degree of suspicion when children present with repetitive illness with no physiologic explanation.

The Risk for Sexual Abuse

Although the orthopaedist usually considers child abuse in the context of fractures and other obvious injuries, an increasingly important aspect of child abuse to recognize is sexual abuse. It is estimated that 25% of abused or neglected children have been sexually abused (49). Physically abused children have a 1 in 6 chance of being sexually abused, whereas sexually abused children have a 1 in 7 risk of being physically abused (50). Children living with nonbiologic parents or with caretakers who are substance abusers are most at risk. The child usually discloses sexual abuse under three types of circumstances. The child may have just experienced an argument with the abuser and may "accidentally" reveal the existence of the abusive relationship, the child is permanently separated from the abuser, or the abusive adult is shifting attention to a younger sibling (51). The incidence of sexual abuse of handicapped patients has been estimated as ranging from 25% to 83%, with handicapped males being more likely to be sexually abused than nonhandicapped males in the general population (52). Both sexual and physical abuse may be associated with cults, which may be identified by their symbols. Satanic cults may use a pentagram (an encircled five-pointed star with an inverted apex), the eye of Horus (an eye within a triangle), or various symbols that modify a cross, and the middle or little finger of the left hand may be painted black (2). Sadistic ritual abuse has been reported in preschool and elementary school children (53).

The Risk for Atypical Child Abuse

Bizarre forms of child abuse may cause a confusing illness or injury. There are reports of young children forced to aspirate pepper, of intentional burns of infants by placing them in microwave ovens (54), of children denied water who developed hypernatremic dehydration, and of infants poisoned with cocaine given to them by caretakers (55). In one case of abuse an infant presented with bloody stools and persistent acidosis due to intentional iron poisoning (56). A high index of suspicion is needed to avoid missing the diagnosis of nonaccidental trauma in these situations.

OBTAINING THE HISTORY

The history is critical in the diagnosis of child abuse. It usually is taken in the chaotic environment of a busy emergency room, so it is important to find a quiet area for the interview where tempers can cool and distractions can be minimized. In addition to taking a thorough history with regard to the mechanism of injury, the orthopaedist must question the patient and the family in an investigative fashion to establish accurately the circumstances of the injury and the environment in which the child lives. These skills rarely are taught in residency training. In a survey of pediatric residents (57), 42% of them had 1 hour or less in training for detection of child abuse, and most orthopaedic residents likely have even less training in this area. Unfortunately, little progress has been made. In a study comparing the documentation of physical abuse between 1980 and 1995 in a teaching hospital, very little improvement was noted (58). It has been found that use of a structured clinical form increased the information collected to support the diagnosis of child abuse (59). Precise documentation in child abuse is vital for reasons beyond medical care. Although most subpoenas for testimony by physicians in child abuse cases do not result in courtroom appearances (60), it must be clear that all documentation in child abuse cases is clearly at risk for becoming evidence in courtroom proceedings and clear, detailed records are the best defended in courtroom testimony by physicians (61).

The Investigative Interview

The extensive history needed to detect child abuse is termed the investigative interview. It begins with documenting the history (or the lack of history) of the injury and, more importantly, goes on to uncover enough details about the child's life so that plausible scenarios can be created to explain the injury. A full physical examination and skeletal survey should precede this interview to search for any possible evidence of additional undocumented child abuse. The orthopaedist must become social worker and detective, calmly and methodically establishing how the injured child lives; finding out which family members, friends, or other caretakers have access to the child; and how likely it is that they might have contributed to the child's injuries. A detailed history of injury is obtained individually from each adult family member in a private setting. If the patient and siblings can communicate, they should be interviewed separately from the parents and other members of the family.

Once full injury physical and x-ray assessments of the child are complete, the investigative interview is begun by asking the primary caregiver in a nonjudgmental way how the child was acutely injured. To avoid provoking emotions, any additional soft tissue or skeletal trauma discovered should be brought up at the end of the interview for explanation once the presentation injury has been thoroughly discussed. Each investigative interview should follow a systematic review of symptoms: what happened, who was there, when was the injury recognized, and how long before medical treatment was sought. Inconsistencies are not challenged. Leading questions are avoided in favor of open-end questions. Medical terms should be explained in plain English, with care taken to avoid medical jargon. More plausible explanations for the injury are not volunteered. The place where the injury occurred and which individuals were actually present are determined. Open prompts can enhance the interview (62). Never ask who caused the injury, but rather ask what they saw or what they think happened. Exactly who discovered the injury and how soon the child received medical care after onset of symptoms should be established. Delays in seeking medical care for an injured child are very suggestive of child abuse (15). The crucial questions to be answered are not only whether the given history of trauma is sufficient to explain the severity of injury but what other possible scenarios could explain the injury if the volunteered explanation is not plausible. This requires acquiring a working knowledge of the child's environment, which can be obtained by asking specific, detailed questions (Table 7-2).

When interviewing injured children, it is essential to be as gentle as possible, asking how they got hurt rather than who hurt them. Any question asked should be appropriate for the child's age. The child's account of what he or she was doing at time of injury should be compared with the accounts of the adult witnesses. If possible, the siblings of the injured child

TABLE 7-2 Child Abuse: Investigative Interview

Environmental Issues

Primary caretakers
- Unsupervised
- Responsible for feeding, discipline, toilet training
- Easy or difficult child

Home environment
- Place of residence
- Living conditions
- Adults employed or unemployed
- Sleeping arrangements
- Marital status of parents
- Boyfriend or girlfriend of single parent
- Substance abuse

Home stress level
- Recent job loss
- Marital problems (separation or divorce)
- Death in the family
- Housing problems
- Inadequate funds for food

Parental or Caregiver Responses and Attitudes
- Evasive, not readily responsive to questions
- Irritated by questioning
- Contradictory in responses
- Hostile and critical toward child
- Fearful of losing child or criminal prosecution, or both
- Unconcerned about child's injuries
- Disinterested in treatment and prognosis
- Intermittently unavailable for interview (without valid reason)
- Unwilling to give medical information
- Unwilling to give consent for tests
- Indifferent to child's suffering (seldom touches or looks at child)

Selected data from Akbarnia BA. The role of the orthopaedic surgeon in child abuse. In: Morrissy RP, ed. *Lowell and Winter's pediatric orthopaedic.* Philadelphia: JB Lippincott; 1990; and Green FC. Child abuse and neglect: a priority problem for the private physician. *Pediatr Clin North Am* 1975;22:329–339; with permission.

should be interviewed because they also are at risk for child abuse. Nonvisual clues during the interview also may be helpful (Table 7-2).

To make the diagnosis of child abuse, the orthopaedist must make one crucial decision: Is the history of trauma adequate to explain the severity of injury? That decision should be based on experience in the care of fractures with knowledge of their mechanisms of injury and special insight into the types of trauma most likely to cause significant injury. In addition, it is also extremely important to have knowledge of the developmental abilities of a child when a caretaker states the child's injuries are self-inflicted (2). It is patently absurd for the parents to explain that an infant's femoral fracture occurred in a fall while the infant was standing alone when the infant is too young to even roll over. Details of the accident given as the reason of the injury should be carefully considered. Although it is not unusual for a young child to sustain an accidental fall, it is unusual to sustain a serious injury from that fall alone. Infants fall from a bed or a raised surface during a diaper change fairly frequently. In a study of 536 normal infants (63), nearly 50% of them had fallen accidentally from an elevated surface, usually after the first 5 months of life, when the children were able to roll over and pull themselves up. Significant injury in such falls is, however, extremely rare. Combining two studies (64,65) of 782 children younger than 5 years of age who accidentally fell off an elevated surface, such as bed or sofa, injuries were limited to three clavicular fractures, six skull fractures, one humeral fracture, and one subdural hematoma. In another report a much higher rate of fracture was seen in falls from furniture with 98% having fractures, most in the upper extremity (66). More, injuries occur in falls from greater heights. In a report of 363 stairway injuries (13), 10 were in infants who fell with their caretaker while being carried on stairways and four of those sustained skull fractures. In patients aged 6 months to 1 year, 60% were using walkers at the time of injury. Only 4% of patients had extremity fractures, and 1% had skull fractures. Abrasions and contusions were present in 55% of patients, whereas 26% had lacerations. In another study (67) of 76 children who had fallen from a bed, a crib, or a chair (estimated height 1 to 3 feet), while in the hospital for other illness, 18% had scalp or facial hematomas and 12% had lacerations about the head. There was only one nondisplaced skull fracture and one long-bone fracture in a patient with osteogenesis imperfecta.

Additional important information about the child and the family may be obtained by a review of past medical records or by contacting social workers who may have been involved with the family. Conferring with the family's primary health care provider also may be extremely helpful. A medical release from the family is necessary before these sources of information can be explored (15). The physician or social worker should be asked if there has been a suspicious pattern of injury, illness, ingestion of objects or medications, or noncompliance with health care recommendations; whether the family is receiving counseling or other support from any community groups; and whether the family has any previous involvement with child protective services or the police (15).

Documentation Requirements

Careful documentation is critical. Chart notes may later be needed in court as evidence for either custodial hearings or criminal trial (58), and defending inaccurate or partial chart notes in court can be extremely embarrassing. Each account should be recorded in as much detail as possible, using quotation marks for exact quotes and specifying who is giving the history. Particularly with crucial answers, the exact question preceding the response should be documented. In addition, the general emotional state of the individual providing the account,

TABLE 7-3 Documentation of Child Abuse

- Mechanism of injury
- Family social history
- Past medical history
- Family history of diseases such as osteogenesis imperfecta or other metabolic disease
- Physical examination findings (positive and negative)
- X-ray findings
- Laboratory results
- Photographs of soft tissue injuries
- Results of consultations
- Diagnosis of child abuse
- Treatment recommendations
- Acute injuries
- Investigation by child protective services

as well as the individual's reactions to emotionally charged questions should be documented to assist in later evaluation of the credibility of the account. If the family wishes to change their story after the initial account, no changes should be made to the earlier record, but an addendum should be placed detailing the new account. The completed record should include several specific items (Table 7-3). If child protective services recommends emergency transfer of custody of the child to a foster home or a shelter, then the orthopaedist should summarize chart documentation in a separate notarized narrative, which is preferred by most courts.

PHYSICAL EXAMINATION

After the initial musculoskeletal evaluation for acute fracture assessment, an extremely thorough physical examination of the entire patient should follow, systematically going from the head to the toes, to detect any signs of additional acute or chronic injury. Additional acute and subacute fractures may cause local tenderness and swelling, whereas chronic fractures may produce swelling from the presence of callus and clinical deformity from malunion. Specific x-rays should be used to confirm clinically suspected fractures, with the skeletal surveys being used to show most occult fractures not detectable by clinical examination. The thorough review should focus specifically on the other body areas commonly involved in child abuse including the skin, the central nervous system, the abdomen, and the genitalia. These areas should be carefully evaluated for signs of acute and especially chronic injury, because 50% of verified abuse cases show evidence of prior abuse (20).

Soft Tissue Injuries

In addition to examination of the soft tissue around the acute fracture site for swelling and bruising, the patient's entire body should be carefully and systematically evaluated to detect acute and chronic soft tissue trauma. Deliberate soft tissue injuries are present in 81% to 92% of abused patients (28,68) making these the most common physical examination findings in abused children. The types of skin lesions commonly encountered include ecchymosis, welts, abrasions, lacerations, scars, and burns.

The typical toddler often has multiple accidental bruises over bony prominences such as the chin, the brow, the knees, and the shins (9,17,69). Babies who are not yet mobile have a much lower prevalence of accidental bruising compared to mobile toddlers, and accidental bruises in babies are also typically noted over bony prominences on the front of the body (70). Bruises on the back of the head, neck (17), arms and legs, on the buttocks, abdomen, cheeks, or genitalia may be suspicious for abuse, although accidental bruises can also occur in all these locations (9). Accidental bruising of the face, though, is much less common and should be carefully evaluated. Although nonaccidental bruises often are concentrated on the trunk and buttocks, they are also commonly present on the head and proximal extremities. In a study of 400 nonabused children, Robertson and Barbor (71) found an overall incidence of just 7% for accidental soft tissue injuries of the face and head, with the peak incidence of 17% seen in toddlers. Soft tissue injuries were present on the lower extremities and buttocks in only 31% of children and on the upper extremities of only 9%. In a study of 1,467 patients seen for reasons other than trauma at a medical center over a 1-year period, 76.6% had at least one recent skin lesion, 17% had at least five injuries, 4% had at least 10 injuries, and fewer than 1% had more than 15 injuries. In children over 9 months of age, skin lesions were rare (11.4%) and they were concentrated on the head and face. In children over 9 months of age, the skin lesions were mostly on the lower extremities, with fewer than 1% on the chin, ears, or neck (72). It is clear that there is no threshold number of bruises that are consistent with abuse; some children will only have one bruise from abuse, whereas others may have 20 accidental bruises. What is crucial is the location and configuration of the bruises and the mobility of the child, taken together with the rest of the medical and social history.

The configuration of the bruise resulting from abuse may resemble the implement used to inflict the injury (Fig. 7-1). One study, however, determined that the soft tissue injuries of abuse are weapon specific in fewer than 10% of patients (68). The weapons used to abuse children can be almost any common

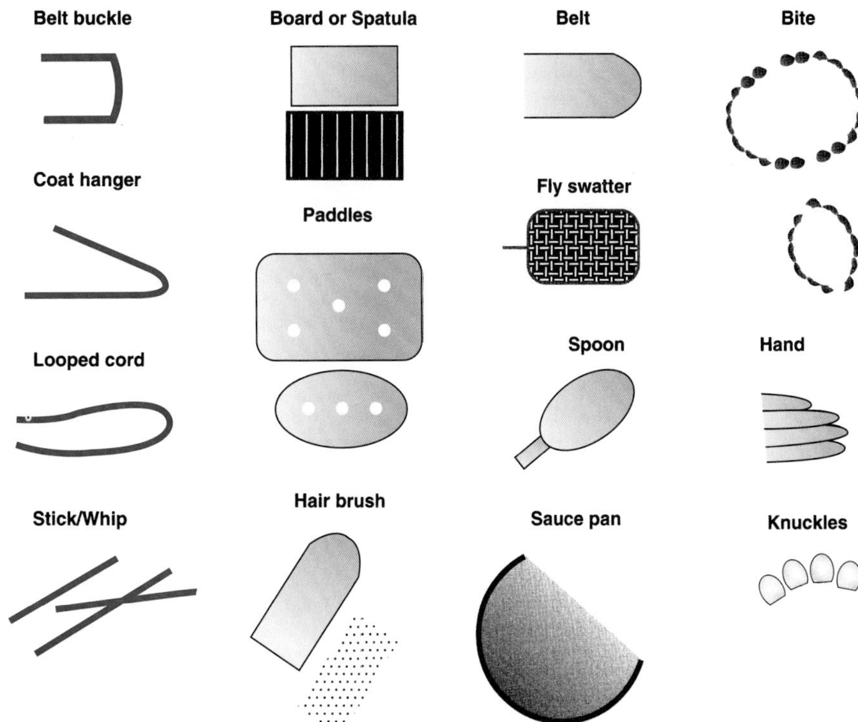

FIGURE 7-1 Healing soft tissue injuries may resemble the instrument used to inflict the lesion.

object, but they often include belt buckles, staplers, ropes, switches, coat hangers, ironing cords, and the open or closed human hand (73,74). Bruises inflicted by an open hand may appear on the face or a flat area of skin, and grasp marks may appear as ovoid lesions when the fingertips are deeply embedded in the extremities or the shoulders of the child during extreme shaking (75). The injury pattern and the severity of the ecchymosis depend on the amount of force used, how directly the instrument made contact, and the specific type of implement used to strike the child (75). Welts are more complex skin lesions in which swelling accompanies bruising from injury through lashing or whipping.

The type of soft tissue injuries seen in child abuse may depend on the age of the child (Table 7-4). In the pediatric dentistry literature, in a series of 266 children suspected of being abused, Jessee and Rieger (76) also found that bruises were the most common soft tissue injury, with the most common facial injury being ecchymosis of the cheek, forehead, periorbital area, or the lip.

The age of a cutaneous contusion reportedly can be estimated by a change in its color over the 2 to 4 weeks following injury, with fading of the lesions beginning at the periphery. An acute contusion is blue or reddish purple; it gradually changes to green, then to yellow, with final resolution as a brownish stain

TABLE 7-4 **Distribution of Soft Tissue Injuries in 371 Abused Children**

Age	Bruises/Abrasions	Lacerations	Scars	Burns	Head/Neck	Injury
≤9 mo	71%	8%	–	–	16%	50%
10–35 mo	64%	13%	6%	6%	12%	38%
≥36 mo	61%	21%	4%	11%	3%	24%

Data from McMahon P, Grossman W, Gaffney M, et al. Soft tissue injury as an indication of child abuse. *J Bone Joint Surgery Am* 1995;77:1179–1183; with permission.

as the hemoglobin is finally broken down (77). Langlois and Gresham (78) noted that a yellowish bruise must be older than 18 hours; a red, purple, blue, or black coloration of the bruise may be present from 1 hour after injury to resolution; red is always present in bruises regardless of the age; and bruises of identical age and etiology on the same person may be of different appearances and may change at different rates. Although the age of a superficial contusion may be approximately dated by its appearance, a deep contusion may take some time to rise to the skin surface because of fascial planes and thus delay visible ecchymosis. Even though the color of a bruise can aid in determining the length of time it has been present, the clinical precision of this practice has been questioned (79).

Natural skin lesions should not be mistaken for bruises. Mongolian spots are naturally occurring deep-blue pigmented areas that are present on the lower back at birth, usually just proximal to the buttocks. They occur more commonly in black and Asian infants than in white infants (80). Unlike traumatic bruises, they do not change in color but gradually resolve as the child matures (75). Cultural differences should always be considered when unusual skin lesions are noted. Vietnamese children may be subjected to a folklore medical practice known as *cao-gio,* which causes suspicious scratches and bruises on the back and may be mistaken for child abuse (81).

Acute lacerations in various stages of healing and chronic scarring may be present in an abused child. Like bruises, the configuration of the injury can resemble the weapon used to inflict the injury on the child. Although minor lacerations around the eye are fairly common, multiple scars resulting from either lacerations or burns (82,83) are suspicious for abuse.

Burns

Burns are found in approximately 20% of abused patients (28) and are most likely to be found in patients younger than 3 years of age (68). Burn evaluation should include configuration, approximate percentage of body surface area, location, distribution, uniformity, length of time the child was in contact with the burning agent, temperature of the burning agent, and presence or absence of splash marks when hot liquids are involved (75). Most self-inflicted accidental pour or spill burns occur anteriorly on the child, but accidental burns can also occur on the back. In accidental burns, the injury usually has an arrowhead configuration in which the burn becomes shallower and more narrow as it moves downward, and there may be splash marks surrounding the lesion (75). The burn pattern in accidental burns may also be indicative of flowing water (84). Abuse should be suspected when deep second- or third-degree burns are seen well demarcated with circumferential definition. In accidental hot water immersion, an indistinct stocking or glove configuration may be seen with varying burn depths and indistinct margins. In deliberate immersion burns, the burn demarcation shows uniform depth and a well-demarcated water line (75). Particularly severe burns occur when a child's buttocks are immersed in hot tap water as abusive punishment. The central aspect of the buttocks may be spared, giving a doughnut-like appearance to the burn. Galleno and Oppenheim (28) noted that in accidental hot water immersion, the child is uniformly scalded about the lower extremities as the legs are quickly extended by the child to climb out of the water, but in deliberate, abusive immersion the children are lowered into the water, so they instinctively pull up their legs to avoid the scalding hot water, and knee flexion may protect the popliteal areas from burn (Fig. 7-2). The average child abused by scalding burns is an undernourished 2-year-old child with burns involving 15% to 20% of the body, usually the buttocks; these children have a 10% to 15% mortality rate from burns owing to sepsis (84).

Burns also can be inflicted by many objects commonly found in the household. Sometimes the object can be identified by the configuration of the burn. Intentional burns by cigarettes are circular, deeply excavated, and sometimes repetitive, usually about 8 mm in diameter (75). Isolated cigarette burns may be accidental, and in such cases they are usually superficial, pointing downward, and often appearing triangular. Lesions of impetigo resemble those of cigarette burns, but they are much more superficial. Severe eczema may mimic burns suspicious for child abuse (85).

Contact with heated objects may cause burns of unique shape that allow identification of their etiology (Fig. 7-3). Children accidentally grasping curling irons sustain burns of the palms, whereas burns on the dorsum of the hands are more suspicious for abuse (2). Hair dryers can be used to inflict burns on children, and full-thickness skin burns can result from contact with the grill of a dryer up to 2 minutes after it has been turned off (86). Such burns can resemble those caused by hot water or could have a grill pattern caused by direct contact with the dryer. Abuse burns have also been inflicted by stun guns (87). These devices deliver a high-voltage impulse of up to 100,000 volts at 3 to 4 mA, incapacitating the individual and leaving hypopigmented burn scars on the skin 0.5 cm apart. Rope burns, sustained when children are restrained about the wrists for beatings, may be seen as circular scars about the wrists (2). Full-thickness skin burns have been reported in small children who were placed in microwave ovens (54).

Certain folklore practices may cause lesions simulating abusive burns. Round burns on the abdomen, buttock, or between the thumb and forefinger of Southeast Asian children may be due to a variant on the Chinese medical practice of moxibustion. Folk medical practitioners burn balls of the moxa herb on the surface of the skin for therapeutic purposes, and both cigarettes and yarn have been similarly used in refugee camps. The knowledge of these practices may help to avoid inappropriate accusations of child abuse (88). Infants may sustain second-degree burns when they accidentally come in contact with the hot vinyl upholstery of a car (89).

It is critical that the orthopaedist examine and carefully document all soft tissue injuries that are present before treating the acute fractures. The cast applied in the treatment of the fracture, especially a spica cast, may cover up potentially incriminating

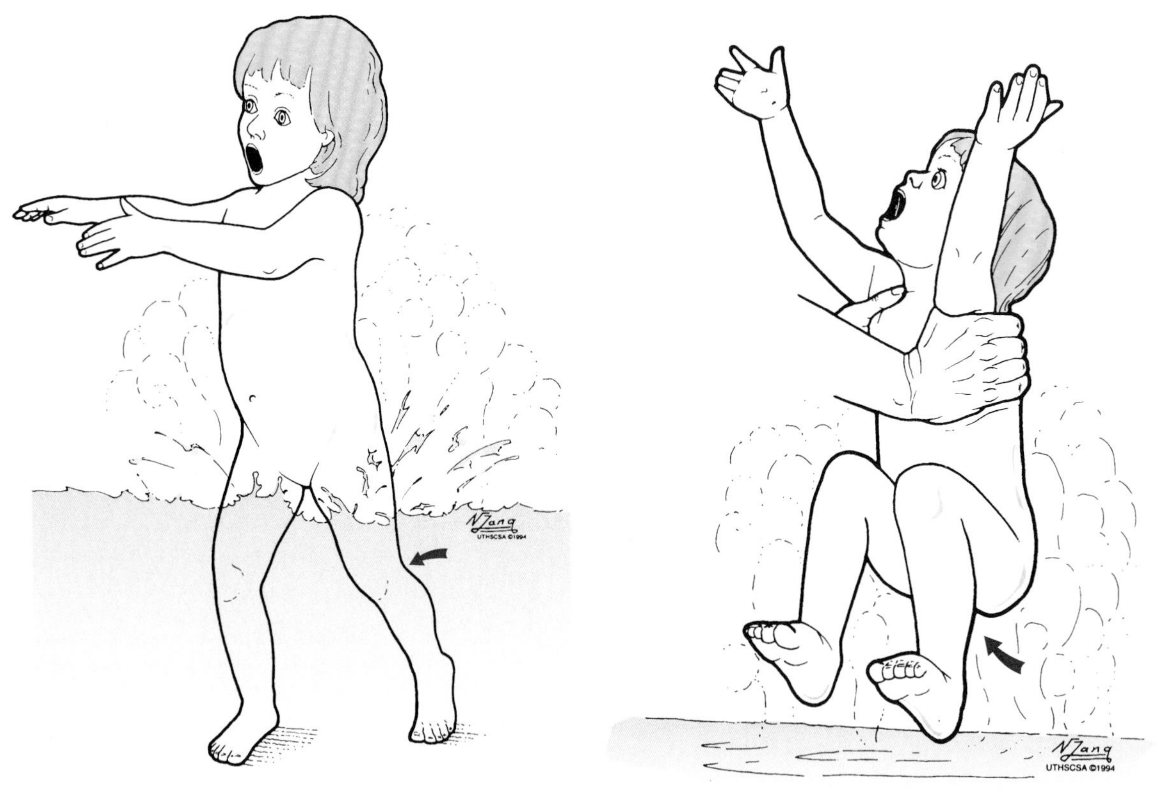

FIGURE 7-2 **A.** In accidental hot water immersion, the child is uniformly scalded about the lower extremities as the legs are extended quickly by the child to climb out of the water, with burns occurring behind the knee (*curved arrow*). **B.** In nonaccidental immersion, the child instinctively pulls up the legs to avoid the hot water, and knee flexion may protect the popliteal areas from burn (*curved arrow*).

skin lesions and will preclude other members of the child advocacy team from being able to identify or document them. Photographs can be used to document lesions before cast placement.

Head Trauma and Spinal Fracture

In physical abuse the most common cause of death is head trauma (90). An excellent review on fatal abusive head injury was published by the National Association of Medical Examiners Ad Hoc Committee on shaken baby syndrome (91). A complete neurologic examination is required in any child suspected of being abused. This should include assessment of the child's mental status, motor function and sensation, reflexes, and gait, if possible. Any abnormal findings warrant further investigation. Skull x-rays, a head computed tomography (CT) scan and spinal x-rays should be considered in the work up of such patients. Also included should be an ophthalmologic evaluation looking for retinal hemorrhages.

According to the American Academy of Pediatrics Section on Radiology (92), anteroposterior (AP) and lateral skull x-rays are mandatory in head trauma of children. CT scans alone may miss skull fractures. All children with suspected intracranial injury should also undergo either cranial CT scan or magnetic resonance imaging (MRI), or both, to document soft tissue brain injury. Unenhanced CT scans are readily available and can diagnose acute parenchymal, subarachnoid, subdural, and epidural hemorrhage better than MRI. Even in abused children without neurologic findings or retinal hemorrhages, occult head injury should be suspected. One study using both CT scans and skeletal surveys to evaluate 51 neurologically intact abused children identified skull fractures in 74% and intracranial injury in 53% in high-risk groups of those with rib fractures, multiple fractures, facial injury, or those younger than 6 months (93). These high-risk patients without neurologic findings should be screened by CT scan or, if inconclusive, also with MRI. The MRI can be a sensitive means of diagnosing small extra-axial cranial hemorrhage (94). If routine MRI is inconclusive, diffusion-weighted MRI can show subtle hypoxic-ischemic brain injury (95,96). Jaspan et al (96a) noted that cerebral contusion tears could be noted by sonography, and in another study Jaspan et al suggested a detailed protocol for imaging work-up of head injury in child abuse (97).

When an infant with musculoskeletal injury presents with altered mental status, whiplash-shaken infant syndrome should be suspected. Violent shaking of a small child whiplashes the relatively large head back and forth over the thorax, with possi-

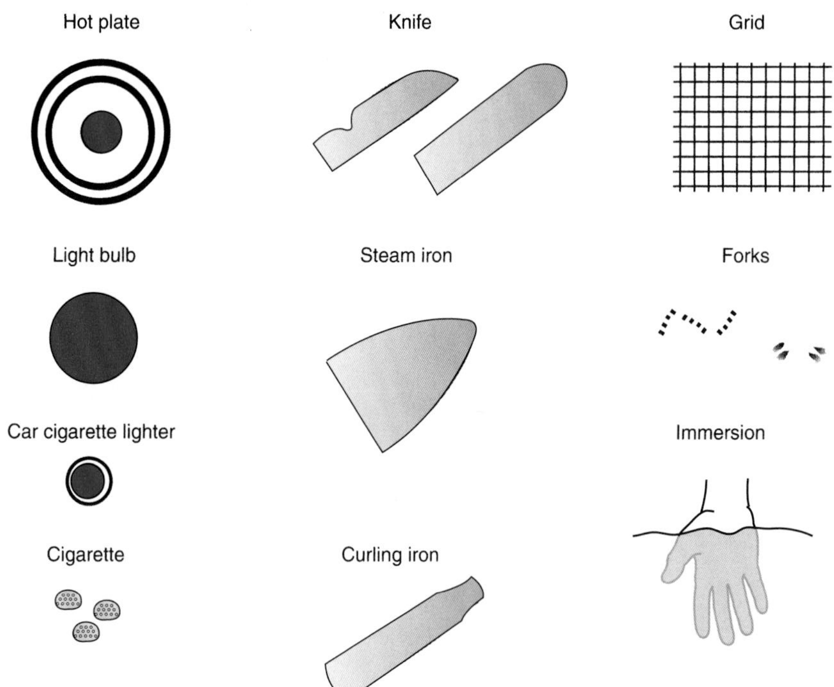

FIGURE 7-3 Contact burns by heated objects may cause burns of unique shape that allow identification of their cause.

ble development of subdural hematomas (Fig. 7-4). Some authors (94) believe these head injuries actually occur when the child's head is slammed onto a soft surface such as a mattress. On impact, deceleration forces approaching 400 G's may be seen, tearing the bridging vessels between the skull and the brain and producing intracranial hemorrhage and cerebral edema. Skull fractures, though, are rare unless the child is thrown onto a hard object. Simple linear skull fractures usually are due to a fall of less that 4 feet and may be accidental, but complex skull fractures without a history of significant trauma, including comminuted, diastatic (separated sutures), displaced fractures, and fractures crossing suture lines, are suspicious for abuse (44). Children with head injuries caused by direct impact trauma are described as having shaken impact syndrome (94). Children with head injuries have fevers, bulging fontanelles, and sometimes enlargement of the head. A pattern of paresis may be present, and reflexes may be increased (14). Skull fractures generally are uncommon, and either ultrasound or CT scans are commonly used to diagnose subdural hematomas. Cerebral edema may be lethal (98), and emergency neurosurgical consultation is needed. Funduscopic examination by an ophthalmologist is indicated because of concurrent retinal hemorrhage (14). The examiner should be aware, however, that retinal hemorrhages resulting from normal vaginal birth are present in 40% of newborns, but these injuries resolve by 3 to 4 weeks of age (99). Shaken baby syndrome has a high mortality rate: 30% of infants die of their injuries (32).

Fatal cerebral injury also occurs in the abusive tin ear syndrome: a clinical triad of unilateral ear bruising, CT scan evi-

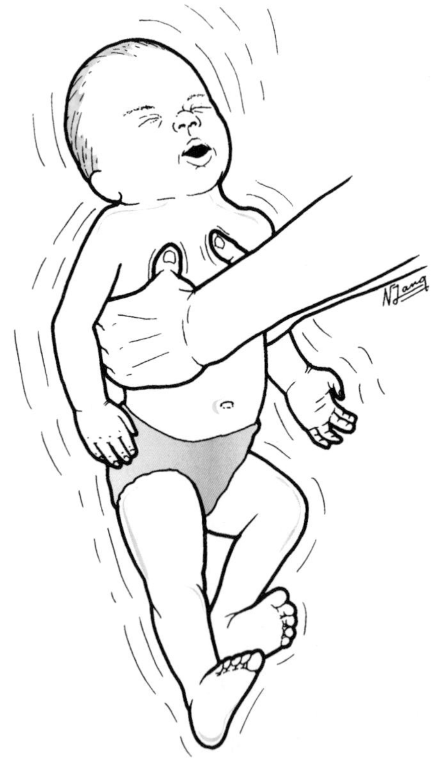

FIGURE 7-4 Violent shaking of a small child held by the chest whiplashes the head back and forth over the thorax, with the possible development of subdural hematomas as well as rib fractures. Infants held by the extremities are also at risk for long-bone fracture.

dence of ipsilateral cerebral edema, and hemorrhagic retinopathy, with a 100% mortality rate in one series (100).

Pediatric spinal fractures and spinal cord injuries are rare with nonaccidental trauma.

An excellent review of pediatric spinal fractures in general was published by Akbarnia (101). These injuries often can be subtle, and a high index of suspicion is necessary. The actual incidence of these injuries may be underreported (102). Spinal fractures may occur in child abuse when a child is forcibly slammed onto a countertop with hyperflexion of the spine (17). Although neurologic deficit with this type of injury is uncommon (103), children should be carefully evaluated for signs of spinal cord injury secondary to spinal fracture when abuse is suspected.

Abdominal Injuries

Trauma to the abdomen is the second most common reason for death from child abuse (44). Careful evaluation is needed to rule out occult abdominal injury in an abused child, and often abdominal trauma is the presenting complaint in abused children. In a review of the National Pediatric Trauma Registry, 16% of all blunt abdominal trauma in a group of children 0 to 4 years of age was attributable to child abuse (104). These are injuries due to beatings with the hand or fist and also can occur when the child is thrown into a fixed object. External abdominal bruising is present in only 12% to 15% of cases of major abdominal injuries (75). Patients with abdominal injury resulting from child abuse may have fever, vomiting, and anemia, with abdominal distention, localized involuntary spasm, and absent bowel sounds (19). One of the most common abdominal injuries is a ruptured liver or spleen, and the hypovolemic shock from blood loss can be fatal (105). Blunt trauma to the abdomen also may cause intestinal perforation, usually involving the large intestine, and the physical examination suggests peritonitis with free air seen on abdominal x-ray. Intramural duodenal hematoma may cause obstruction and projectile vomiting (75). More severe trauma may cause duodenal avulsion or transection with nausea, vomiting, and clinical acute abdomen (106). Severe blunt trauma to the abdomen or a blow to the back may cause renal or bladder contusion with hematuria. Blunt trauma to the abdomen also may result in shearing of the mesenteric vessels, leading to hypovolemic shock due to blood loss. Pancreatic transection can occur where the pancreas overlies the vertebral column, and a pseudocyst may form (75).

Liver function tests are useful in detecting abdominal injury resulting from occult liver injury in child abuse. In one study (107), elevated aspartate aminotransferase, alanine aminotransferase, and lactic dehydrogenase enzyme levels were useful markers for occult liver lacerations in abused children who had false-negative abdominal examinations.

The American Academy of Pediatrics Section on Radiology (92) recommends CT scans with nonionic intravenous contrast to define injury to abdominal organs. Contrast should not be used if there is a history of iodine allergy, severe shock, or renal failure. The use of oral contrast is debatable with CT scans and may place the patient at risk of aspiration. If CT scan is not possible, peritoneal lavage may be considered in rare cases. Acute abdominal sonography is controversial and may not add useful information after CT scan, but may have worth in follow-up evaluations. An upper GI series is sometimes used to evaluate duodenal hematoma. If a bone scan is obtained to diagnose occult fracture, there may be abnormal patterns of isotope uptake in the abdomen as a result of intestinal injury, renal contusion, or muscle trauma of the abdominal wall (108).

When abdominal injury is suspected in an abused child, the hematocrit and hemoglobin levels are checked, the child is typed and cross-matched for blood, and an intravenous line is placed to provide replacement fluids. Emergency general surgery consultation should be obtained. The overall mortality rate associated with visceral injury in child abuse is 40% to 50% (107). In fatal cases with liver injury, hepatic glycogen staining may be helpful in establishing time of death for legal reasons (109).

Genital Injuries

Sexual abuse should always be considered when evaluating a physically abused child. Children who have been sexually abused can have symptoms of bed wetting, fecal incontinence, painful defecation, pelvic pain, abdominal pain, vaginal itching and bleeding, sexually transmitted diseases, and pregnancy in postmenarchal women. Types of sexually transmitted diseases found in abused children include gonorrhea, syphilis, chlamydiosis, trichomoniasis, and lymphogranuloma venereum. Although the percentage of sexually assaulted children with obvious physical trauma to the genitalia is low, failure to document such findings is a serious matter because sexual abuse is always a criminal offense and must be reported to legal authorities.

The genitalia should always be examined in a chaperoned setting. Infant and toddler girls are placed in a supine frog-leg position, and boys are placed in either a prone knee-chest position or in a lateral decubitus position (110). Patterns of injury that suggest sexually motivated assault include bruises, scratches, and burns around the lower trunk, genitalia, thighs, buttocks, and upper legs, including the knees. Pinch or grip marks may be found where the child was held. Attempted or achieved penetration may involve the mouth, vagina, or anus (50). Sexually abused boys may have poor rectal sphincter tone, perianal scarring, or urethral discharge. Female genital examination findings that are consistent with, but not diagnostic of, sexual abuse include chafing, abrasion, or bruising of the inner thighs or genitalia; distortion of the hymen; decreased or absent hymen; scarring of the external genitalia; and enlargement of the hymenal opening (111). The size of the transverse hymenal orifice does not correlate as a marker of child abuse (112). The examination of the female genitalia can be normal even when there has been penetration, because hymenal tissue is elastic and there can be rapid healing. In a study of 36 adolescent pregnant girls evaluated for sexual abuse evaluation only two of 36 had genital changes diagnostic of penetrating trauma, suggesting injuries either may not occur or may heal completely (113). There also is a wide variability of appearance of normal female genitalia (98,114), but posterior hymen disruption is rare and should raise suspicion for abuse (115). If the sexual assault occurred within 72 hours of evaluation, then a rape kit must be used by the evaluating physician or nurse examiner to provide medical evidence of the attack (49).

The physical signs of sexual abuse, including genital trauma, sexually transmitted diseases, or presence of sperm are present in only 3% to 16% of verified sexual assaults (110,116), but even this minority of patients will be undiagnosed if sexual abuse is not considered when a child presents with musculoskeletal injury resulting from abuse. The orthopaedist or a consultant such as a pediatrician or a gynecologist must perform and document the genital examination in children with physical abuse.

FRACTURES IN CHILD ABUSE

Overview

Fractures documented on plain x-ray studies are present in 11% to 55% of abused children and are most common in children younger than 3 years of age (17,20,117). Fractures resulting from abuse should be suspected in a young child if the caretaker brings in the child for evaluation, reporting no accident, but does report a change in the child such as extremity swelling or decreased movement of the limb (118). Unexplained systemic hypertension in infants may be due to the pain of occult long-bone fractures (119). Femoral fractures are especially suspicious for child abuse in younger children. One study (120) found that 79% of patients younger than 2 years of age with femoral fractures were battered, and, of those, two thirds had femoral fractures as their only sign of abuse. Accidental femoral fractures can occur in children old enough to stand or run who fall with a twisting injury to the lower extremities, but femoral fractures in children younger than 1 year of age are most likely due to abuse (121). Fractures of both the lateral clavicle and the scapula are suggestive of abuse in young children (122). Infants may normally have a separate ossification center adjacent to the tip of the acromion, simulating a fracture (123), but a true fracture has sharp, demarcated edges, may be positive on bone scan, and will show callus on healing (Fig. 7-5). Although fractures of the sternum are believed to be specific for child abuse by Kleinmann (124), accidental midsternal fractures in children have been reported (125).

Fractures of the hands and feet are most commonly due to accidental trauma in older children (126) but are suspicious for abuse in infants. Nimkin et al (127) reviewed 11 hand and foot fractures in abused children younger than 10 months of age and found mostly torus fractures either of the metacarpals or the proximal phalanges of the hand and similar fractures of the first metatarsals of the feet. Clinical signs of fracture were present in only one patient, and bones scans were insensitive to the presence of the fractures in all patients.

All types of fractures have been reported in the child abuse literature. In one of the largest series, King et al (128) reported 429 fractures in 189 abused children. Fifty percent of these patients had a single fracture, and 17% had more than three fractures. Approximately 60% of fractures were found in roughly equal numbers in the humerus, femur, and tibia. Fractures also occurred in the radius, skull, spine, ribs, ulna, and fibula, in order of decreasing frequency. Another study (19) found a similar incidence of fractures of the humerus, femur, and tibia in abused children, with skull fractures seen in 14% of patients (Fig. 7-6). In contrast, Akbarnia et al (129) found that rib fractures in abused patients were twice as prevalent as fractures of any one long bone; the next most frequently fractured bone was the humerus, followed by the femur and the tibia. Nearly a third of their patients had skull fractures. Loder and Bookout (130) found the tibia to be the bone most commonly fractured in their series of abused children, followed by the humerus, the femur, the radius, and the ulna.

New Developments: Biomechanical Evaluation of Abuse Fractures and Computer Models of Childhood Injury

The past literature of child abuse orthopedic injury is based solely on clinical series and pathology specimens from autopsy specimens. For example, injury from falls from furniture by children are almost always accidental (64), except in infants (66), but little is known about the biomechanics of these injuries. Recently there have been attempts to study the biomechanics of the injuries of children in an abuse scenario using a test dummy and computer models of injury (131). Bertocci et al (132) conducted feet-first free-fall experiments using an instrumented Hybrid II simulated 3-year-old test dummy using varying heights and impact surfaces. They found that in falls on playground foam, increasing fall heights increased femoral compression loads and compression moments. Falls from short distances of 27 inches were associated with a low risk of contact-type head injury, but they also found that head acceleration was less for playground foam falls compared with falls on wood, linoleum, or padded carpet. In another study (133), the same authors examined the biomechanics of the same test dummy falling 0.68 meters, an estimation of typical bed height, through a roll onto different surfaces. They found that either the pelvis or the legs made first contact, and head deceleration, femoral loading, and pelvis deceleration were below known head injury criteria and lower extremity thresholds for injury. In 2001 they reported a computer simulation of pediatric stair falls (134) and in 2005 reported an "injury plausible" biomechanical model to assess femoral fractures in 29 children who fell down stairs. They found that with scoring for detail of history, biomechanical compatibility of fracture pattern, time to seeking care, and presence of other injuries, their model allowed them to distinguish between two groups of either plausible injury or suspicious

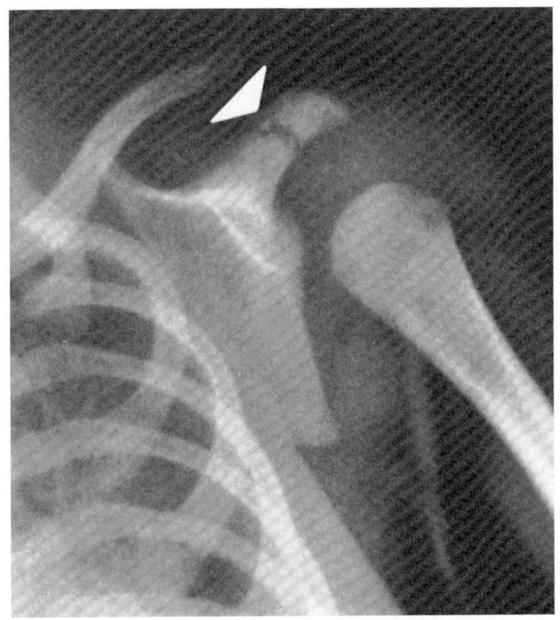

A

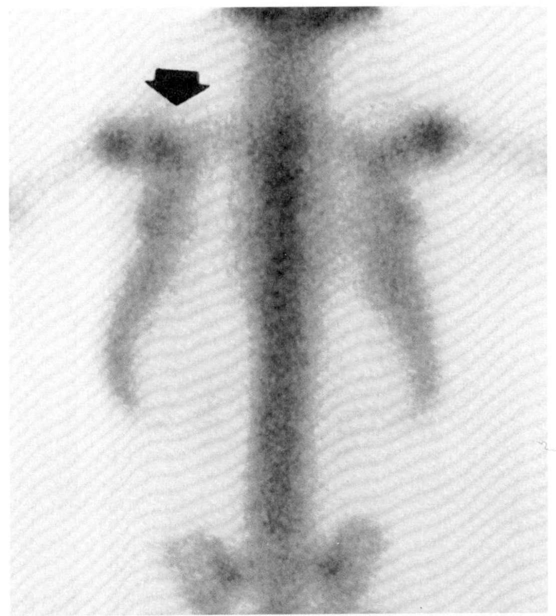

B

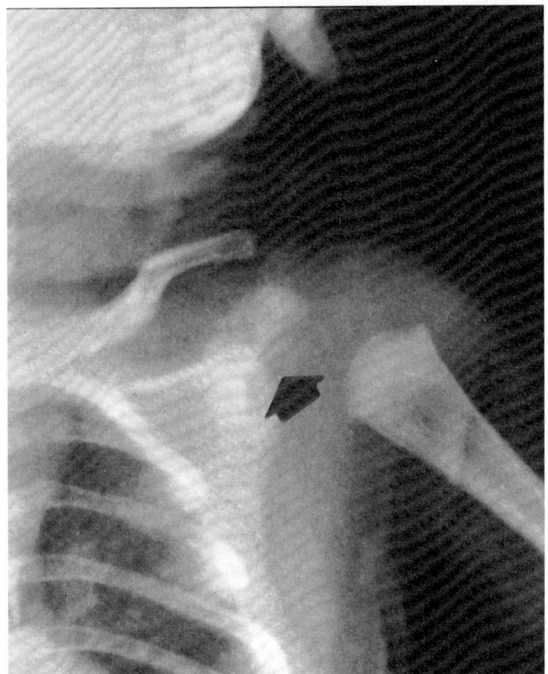

C

FIGURE 7-5 **A.** A 7-week-old girl was seen in the emergency department with swelling of the left shoulder. History revealed her being roughly grabbed by the shoulder by one of her parents. The anteroposterior x-ray study shows a transverse lucency of the acromion, which was thought to represent either a congenital lesion or a traumatic fracture (*arrow*). **B.** A technetium bone scan was obtained. Although the delayed anterior image was normal, the posterior view showed increased uptake in the left shoulder in the area of the acromion (*arrow*) and a fracture was diagnosed. The incident was investigated. **C.** A follow-up x-ray 9 days later showed callus bridging the fracture site of the acromion (*arrow*).

injury. In the plausible group a transverse femoral fracture had a 10-fold greater linear momentum compared to spiral or buckle fractures (135). Much more research is needed in this area.

Skull Fractures

Infants in the first year of life with fractures of the skull or the extremities have an equal risk of the etiology being either accident or abuse (136). Skull fractures were the most commonly reported fracture in one series (68), but only 10% of their patients underwent x-ray evaluation. Skeletal surveys missed 26% of skull fractures confirmed on CT scan in one study (93).

Extremity Fractures

There is no predominant pattern of diaphyseal fracture in child abuse. Traditionally, a midshaft spiral fracture is believed to be caused by a violent twisting injury to the extremity of the child. In a study of 23 long-bone fractures in battered children, Herndon (18) found spiral fractures in 78%. He suggested that in

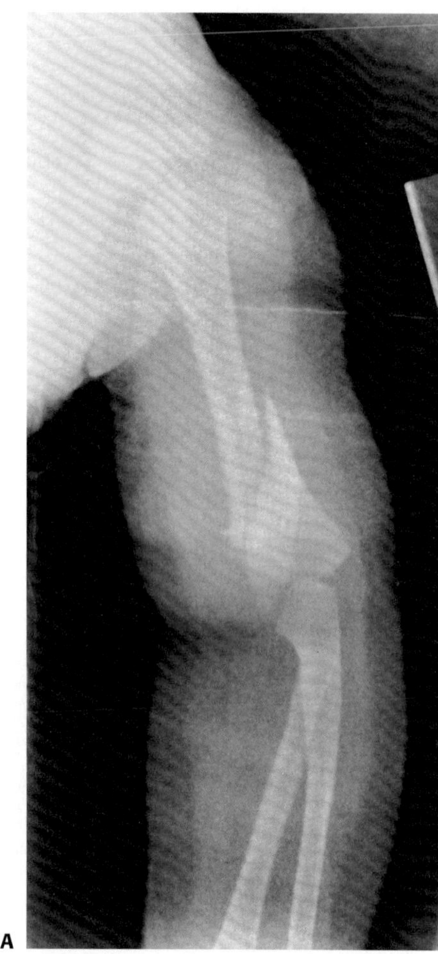

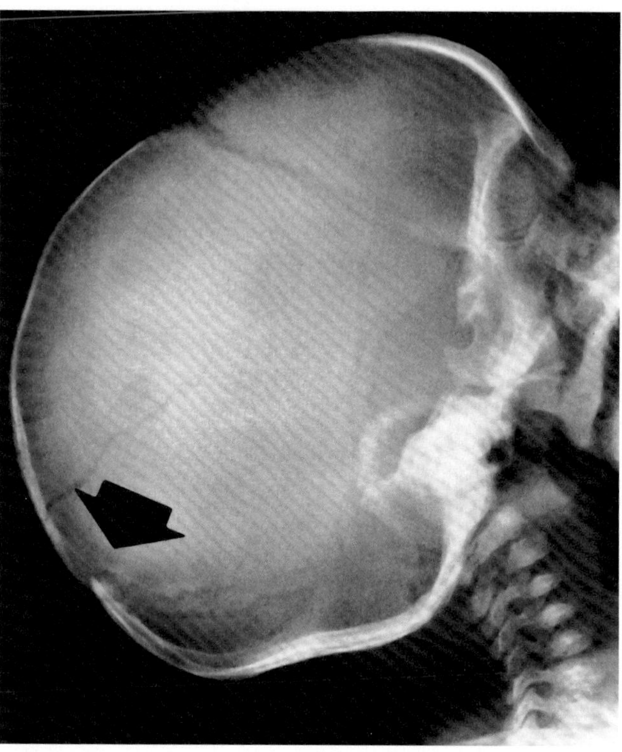

FIGURE 7-6 **A.** A 4-month-old male without history of trauma was brought into the emergency department by his parents with a history of decreased use of the arm. This distal humeral shaft fracture was seen on x-ray. **B.** Skeletal survey disclosed a posterior skull fracture (*arrow*), and the injuries were investigated.

children younger than 3 years of age, a spiral fracture of a long bone is highly suggestive of child abuse. Other authors (28), however, found that 71% of diaphyseal fractures were transverse in abused children. In another study of 34 patients in the first year of life, there was no difference in fracture patterns between those injured by accidental trauma and those injured by abuse. Loder and Bookout (130) reviewed 69 long-bone fractures in abused children and found that 56% were transverse, 36% oblique, and only 8% spiral. In another study of 429 fractures (88), 48% of fractures were transverse and 26% were spiral. Most of these long-bone fractures were in either the middle or distal third of the shaft. Transverse fractures are most commonly associated with either violent bending force or a direct blow to the extremities, whereas spiral or oblique fractures of the long bones are due to twisting injuries or a fall. Significant rotational force is required, however, to produce a spiral fracture with a fall (17). Humeral shaft fractures in children under age 3 years have a 18% risk of being due to probable abuse (137). In delayed follow-up, long-bone fractures may show exuberant callus because of a lack of immobilization, and multiple fractures may be present in different stages of healing (8). Juxtacortical calcification may be seen without fracture when there is diaphyseal periosteal separation resulting from tractional or torsional force when the limb is grasped or pulled along the shaft of the bone (138).

Femoral fractures are especially suspicious for abuse when seen in infants; whereas children old enough to run can fall and accidentally fracture their femurs if there is a significant twisting motion at the time of injury (121). Comparing accidental femoral fractures to those of child abuse, there was no difference in site or pattern of fractures between groups in one study, but 93% of femoral fractures in those younger than 1 year were due to abuse (139). In one report (140) there was equal risk of having a spiral or transverse femoral fracture as a result of abuse. Gross and Stanger (140a) found that 65% of femoral shaft fractures were due to abuse in children younger than 1 year. Schwend et al (141) reported that 42% of femoral fractures in infants not walking were due to abuse while only 2.6% of femoral fractures in ambulatory toddlers were due to abuse. Blakemore et al (142) noted that only 2% of femoral fractures from age 1 to 5 years were due to abuse. It appears the most important predictor of abuse in childhood femoral fractures is an age under 1 year.

Metaphyseal and epiphyseal fractures of the long bones are

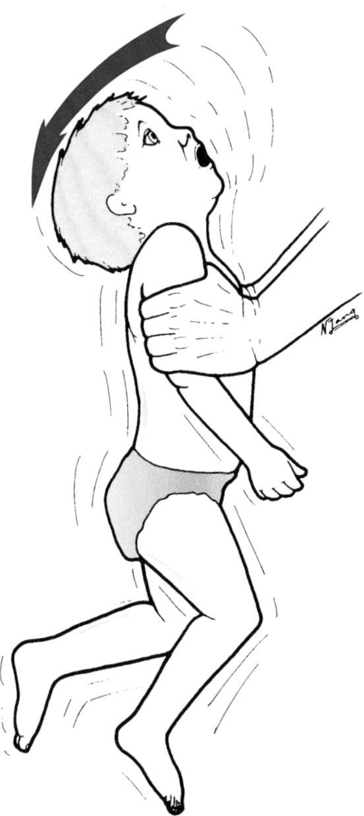

FIGURE 7-7 When a toddler is violently shaken by the extremities, long-bone fractures can occur through either direct violent traction or rotation of the extremity. These children are also at risk for closed-head injury because of violent motion of the head during the shaking episode (*arrow*).

TABLE 7-5 Specificity of Skeletal Trauma for Abuse

High specificity
- Any metaphyseal lesion
- Posterior rib fracture
- Scapular fracture
- Spinous process fracture
- Sternal fracture

Moderate specificity
- Multiple fractures, especially bilateral
- Fractures of different ages
- Epiphyseal separation
- Vertebral body fracture or subluxation
- Digital fracture
- Complex skull fracture

Low specificity
- Clavicular fracture
- Long-bone shaft fracture
- Linear skull fracture

Data from Kleinman PK, ed. *Diagnostic Imaging of Child Abuse*. Baltimore: Williams & Wilkins, 1987; with permission.

classically associated with child abuse (10,11). In toddlers, these fractures can occur when the child is violently shaken by the extremities (Fig. 7-7) with direct violent traction on or rotation of the extremity (126). Metaphyseal fractures may be characterized by impaction into the epiphysis, with profound production of new periosteal bone. Buckle fractures may be present in multiple sites, and these injuries seldom produce exuberant callus. Repeated injury causes irregular metaphyseal deformities. Periosteal avulsion produces new bone formation within 2 to 3 weeks of injury and can be confused with osteomyelitis (8). New bone formation may be delayed, however, in children with malnutrition. Metaphyseal fractures constituted 4% of fractures in one series (28) but fewer than 15% in another (65).

Kleinman (124) ranked the specificity of skeletal trauma for abuse (Table 7-5). Distinguishing between an accident and child abuse is based on both location and type of fracture. He cautioned that both moderate- and low-specificity x-ray findings of child abuse become more highly specific when there is an inadequate explanation for the injury.

Corner Fracture of Child Abuse

The so-called pathognomonic fracture of child abuse is the corner or bucket-handle fracture of the metaphysis (8,17). On x-ray study, there is no gross displacement of the epiphysis, but a corner or chip fracture is seen at the edge of the involved metaphysis (Fig. 7-8). If a significant portion of the metaphyseal rim is involved, a bucket-handle fracture pattern is produced. Another fracture pattern that may be seen is a faint metaphyseal lucency just adjacent to the physis. Classically, these fractures have been believed to result from avulsion of metaphyseal fragments through the periosteal attachment of the epiphysis (10,143). Kleinman et al (144,145) challenged this view based on their histopathologic study at autopsy of metaphyseal fractures in abused infants. They found that in bucket-handle or corner fractures, there was actually a full-thickness metaphyseal fracture extending through the primary spongiosa of bone just above the zone of provisional calcification. This fracture corresponded to the zone of metaphyseal lucency occasionally seen on x-ray. Centrally, the amount of metaphysis remaining attached to the physis was thin, but peripherally the fracture line curved away from the physis so that a substantial metaphyseal rim remained attached to the physis. On x-ray study, this metaphyseal rim formed the basis for both corner and bucket-handle fractures (Fig. 7-9). In healing fractures, biopsy specimens showed metaphyseal extension of hypertrophied chondrocytes (146,147). These fractures are most likely caused by either violent shaking or traction injuries to the extremity and are specifically suggestive of child abuse (17) (see Fig. 7-8); however, they are not the most common fractures in abused children, with their incidence in large series ranging from 15% to 32% (28,65,128,130). Subepiphyseal-metaphyseal lucency

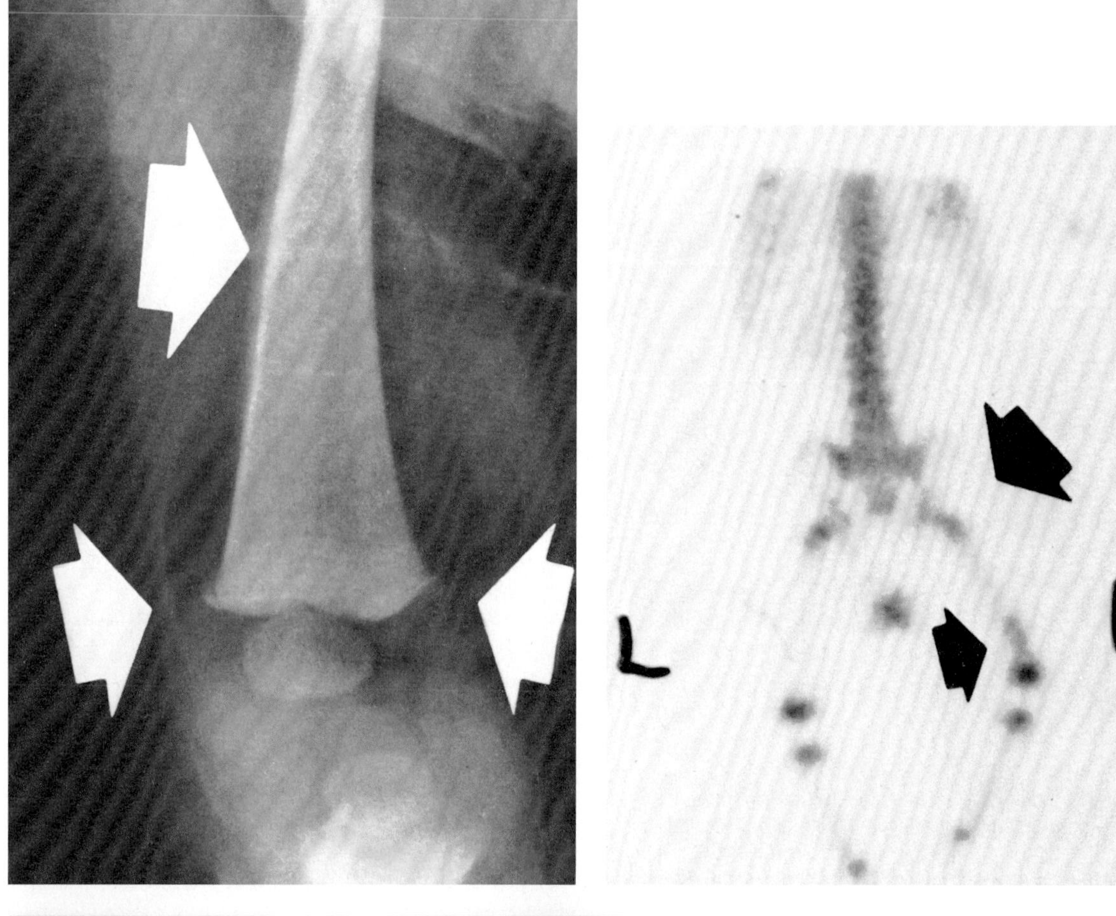

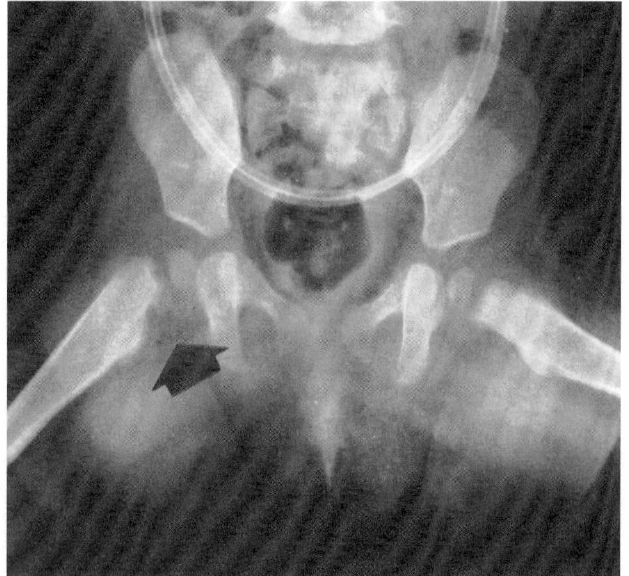

FIGURE 7-8 **A.** An 11-month-old girl with a history of right thigh swelling was seen. X-rays of the right femur show corner or "chip" fractures of the distal femur (*bottom arrows*). Faint periosteal calcification is also visible along the lateral cortex (*top arrow*). Such fractures raise suspicion for child abuse. **B.** A technetium bone scan showed increased uptake of isotope in the distal and proximal femur (*arrows*). **C.** A healing physeal fracture of the proximal femur is seen (*arrow*).

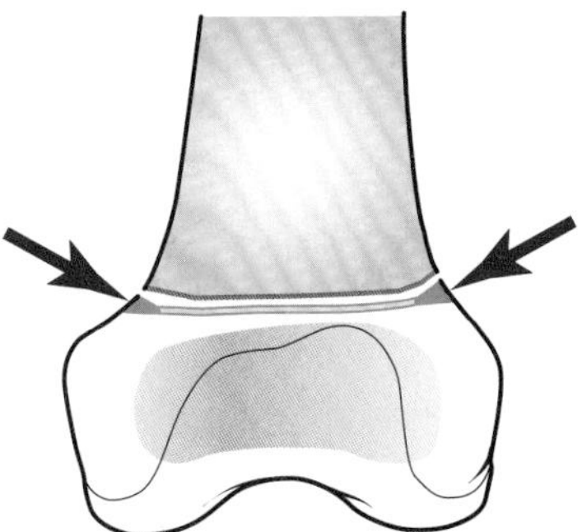

FIGURE 7-9 In the corner or bucket-handle fracture, a full-thickness metaphyseal fracture extends through the primary spongiosa just above the zone of provisional calcification. Centrally, the amount of metaphysis remaining attached to the physis is thin, but peripherally the fracture line curves away from the physis so a substantial metaphyseal rim remains attached to the physis (*arrows*). On x-ray study, this metaphyseal rim (*dark shaded area*) forms the basis for both the corner and bucket-handle fractures.

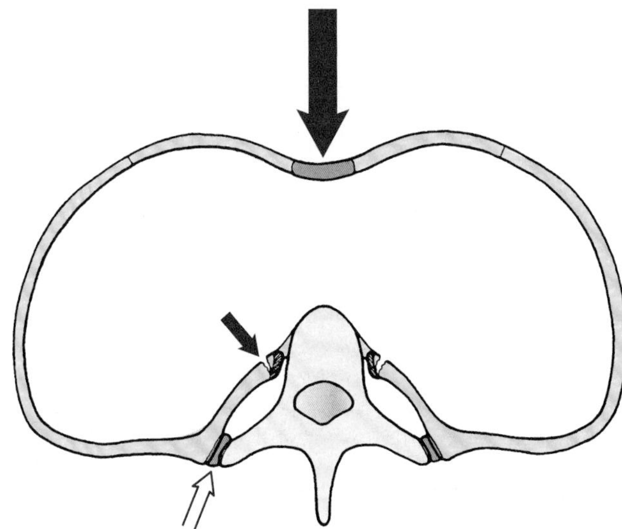

FIGURE 7-10 With anterior compression of the chest, the posterior rib is levered over the transverse process of the vertebral body (*open arrow*), causing fractures of the rib head adjacent to the vertebra (*shaded arrow*) as well as avulsion fractures of the rib at the transverse process.

also can be caused by systematic disease such as rickets and leukemia. "Corner fractures" of the distal radius, ulna, tibia, and proximal humerus also have been reported with developmental coxa vara associated with spondylometaphyseal dysplasia (148).

Rib Fractures

Rib fractures are uncommon in childhood accidents, so their presence is very suspicious for child abuse, especially when other long-bone fractures are present (149). Abusive rib fractures may be caused by squeezing of the chest by a caretaker (14), hitting the child from behind, or stepping on the chest (150,151). Kleinman et al (152) postulated that severe shaking of an infant (see Fig. 7-1) can cause front-to-back chest compression, which levers the posterior rib over the transverse process of the vertebral body, causing fractures of the posterior rib shaft at the transverse process and of the rib head adjacent to the vertebra (Fig. 7-10). These posterior rib fractures are difficult to diagnose acutely because of a lack displacement. Even with healing, the callus on x-ray study may be obscured by the overlying transverse process (31), and a bone scan may be needed to make the diagnosis (Fig. 7-11). Posterior rib fractures are believed to be most common in child abuse, but fractures may occur anywhere along the arc of the rib, including disruption of the anterior costochondral junction (Fig. 7-12). Posterior paraspinal rib fractures tend to occur between T4 and T9, rib fractures in the axillary line occur mostly in the lower rib cage, and disruption of the anterior costochondral junction usually occurs from the second to the ninth ribs (153).

Lateral rib fractures, both acute and chronic, may be difficult to see on standard AP x-rays, so oblique views may be necessary. Healing fractures show early callus, but healed fractures may be subtle, with only a fusiform thickening of the rib (see Fig. 7-12). Old fractures of the ribs in child abuse may form lytic, expansile lesions that mimic a tumor (154). Fractures along the lateral arc of the rib are likely due to AP compression of the chest (Fig. 7-13), while lateral compression of the chest likely causes fractures of the rib along its posterior arc lateral to the transverse process as well as disruptions of the costochondral junction (Fig. 7-13B). Acute anterior costochondral separations of the ribs may be difficult to see on x-rays, but ultrasound can show costochondral dislocation (155), and, with healing, the anterior end of the osseous rib becomes widened and clubbed on x-rays (19,65). They are commonly associated with abdominal injury and can be detected on CT scan, resembling bucket-handle metaphyseal fractures (156).

In the rare instances when rib fractures are discovered in abused infants undergoing resuscitation for cardiac arrest, there may be confusion about the etiology of the fractures (157), but the elasticity of the infant chest seems to enable it to tolerate compressions, with only 2% of 94 nonabused infants resuscitated having rib fractures in one series (158). Death from cardiac arhythmia from a blow to the chest has been reported in a 7-week-old abused infant whose rib fractures at autopsy were initially thought to be due to resuscitation efforts (159). In addition to rib fractures, abused infants can sustain severe lung contusion and respiratory distress from chest wall trauma (160), with fatal fat embolus reported (161). Necklace calcifications may be present in strangulation cases (162).

In the case of infant fatalities of suspicious origin, postmortem high-detailed skeletal surveys and specimen x-rays can be helpful in diagnosing child abuse (163). In a postmortem study of 31 infants who died of inflicted skeletal injury, Kleinman et al (164) found a total of 165 fractures (51% rib fractures, 39% metaphyseal long bone fractures, 5% long-bone shaft fractures, 4% fractures of the hands and feet, 1% clavicular fractures, and less than 1% spinal fractures). It is important to obtain skeletal

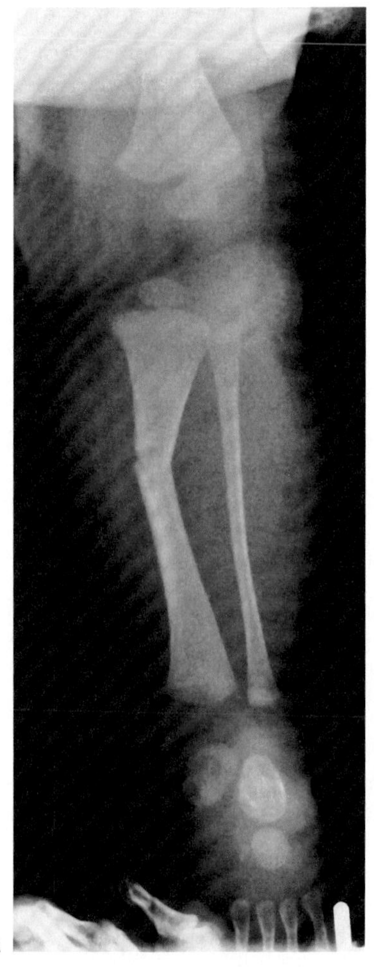

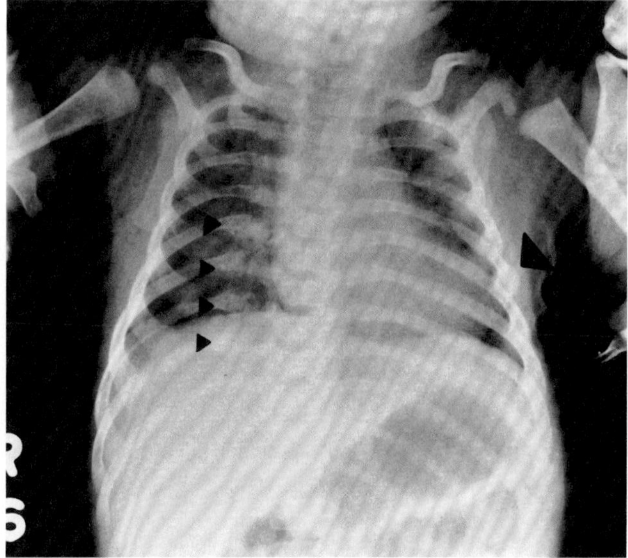

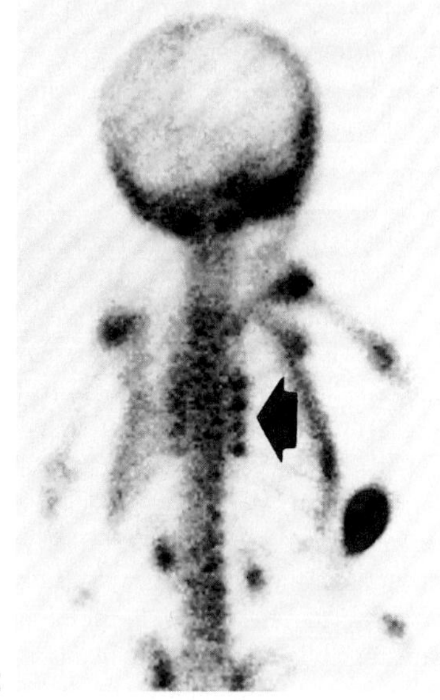

FIGURE 7-11 **A.** This 5-week-old infant was presented by her parents with a complaint of irritability when her left leg was handled. Her mother stated the infant's 18-month-old sibling may have "kicked" her in the leg. X-rays showed an acute fracture of the proximal tibia. **B.** Skeletal survey showed a healing fracture of the left distal clavicle (*arrow*), a healed fracture of the anterior left 5th rib (*arrow*), and probable healing of the posterior right 6th, 7th, 8th, and 9th ribs (*arrows*). **C.** The posterior image of the delayed phase of the bone scan confirmed the presence of healing posterior rib fractures (*arrows*).

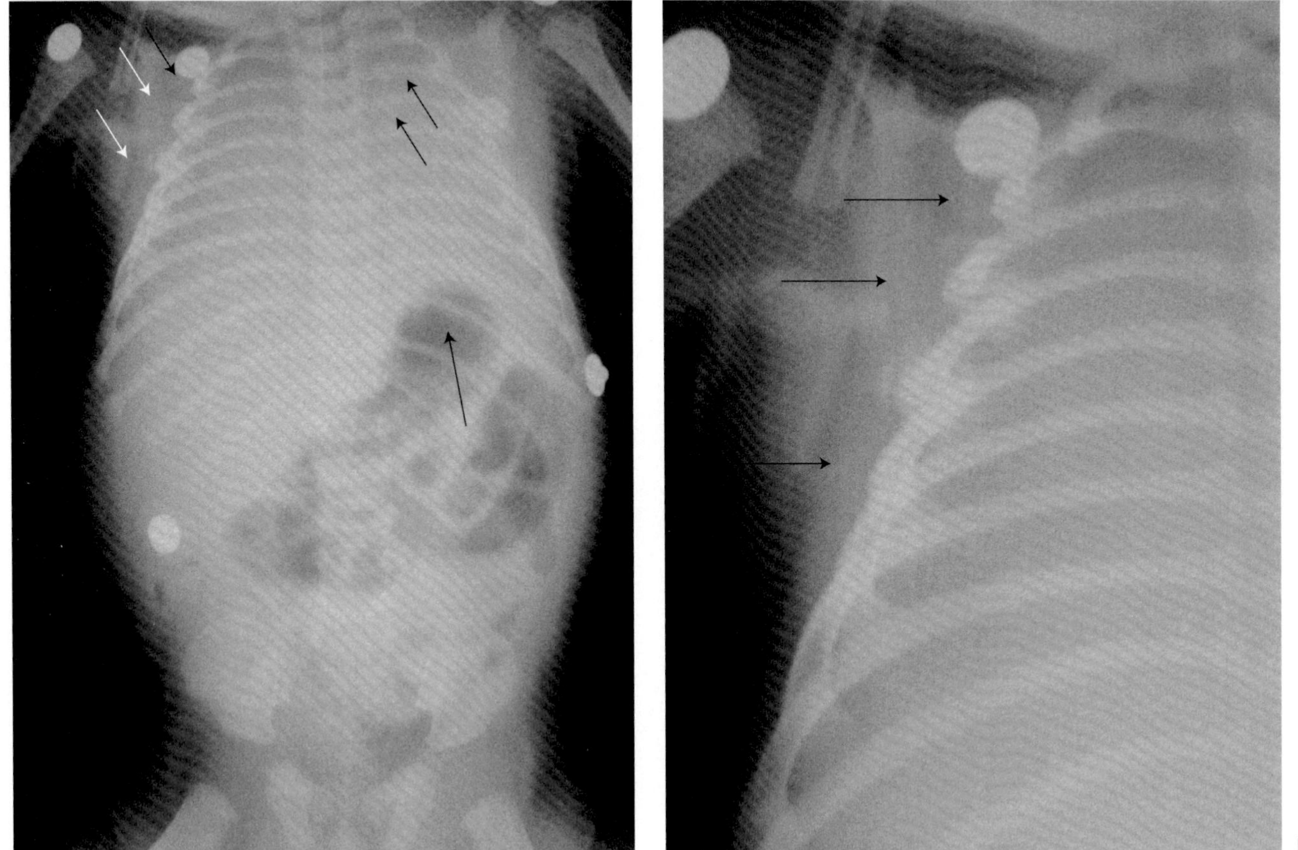

FIGURE 7-12 A. An anteroposterior "baby-gram" x-ray of an infant who died without clear-cut reason. Note the "halo" calcifications around the anterior rib costochondral junctions, equivocal at the second rib (*black arrows*), definitive at the 3rd and 4th ribs of the right hemithorax (*white arrows*) suggestive of anterior costochondral junction rib fracture. On the patient's left side, note the fusiform swelling of the 3rd and 4th ribs posteriorly (*black arrows*), which suggests nondisplaced posterior rib fractures, and a minimally displaced fracture of the 10th rib posteriorly (*large black arrow*). **B.** A close-up view of the right hemithorax. Note the subtle calcification around the 2nd rib costochondral junction, suggesting fractures from the 2nd to the 4th rib.

x-rays before autopsy to avoid artifact (P. Kleinman, Personal communication, 1998).

Spinal Fractures

Spinal fractures in child abuse are rare but can occur when a child is forcibly slammed onto a flat surface, with hyperflexion of the spine (17,101). Based on autopsy findings (165), spinal fractures of fatally abused children generally involved 25% or less compression of the vertebrae. Half of the fractures involved the anterosuperior end plate associated with a compression deformity, 30% had pure compression fractures, and 20% had fractures of the superior end plate without significant compression. In another study of fractures of the cervical spine, prevertebral soft tissue edema on x-ray was the only sign of cervical injury, because spontaneous reduction of the cervical vertebrae after dislocation was common (166). In a report of 103 children with cervical spine injury, only three patients had injury due to abuse and all had spinal cord injury without radiographic abnormality (SCIWORA) (167). Thomas et al (168) reported a 9-week-old boy with spinal cord injury resulting from cervical spine fracture who presented as a floppy infant. Although routine cervical x-rays were normal, MRI studies showed retropulsion of a fragment of the primarily cartilaginous C3 vertebrae into the spinal canal. Kleinman and Shelton (169) reported a hangman's fracture in a 6-month-old infant with multiple rib fractures that went on to nonunion and required fusion. This must be distinguished from C-2 primary spondylolysis which may be associated with pyknodysostosis (170). Ravandrin et al (171) reported a 23-month-old child with a hangman's fracture resulting from abuse that healed with immobilization. The CT scan was helpful in showing the fracture, but a bone scan was nondiagnostic. Rooks et al (172) reported a compression fracture of C-5 with anterior subluxation of C-4 on C-5 in a 3-month-old premature twin requiring decompression and cer-

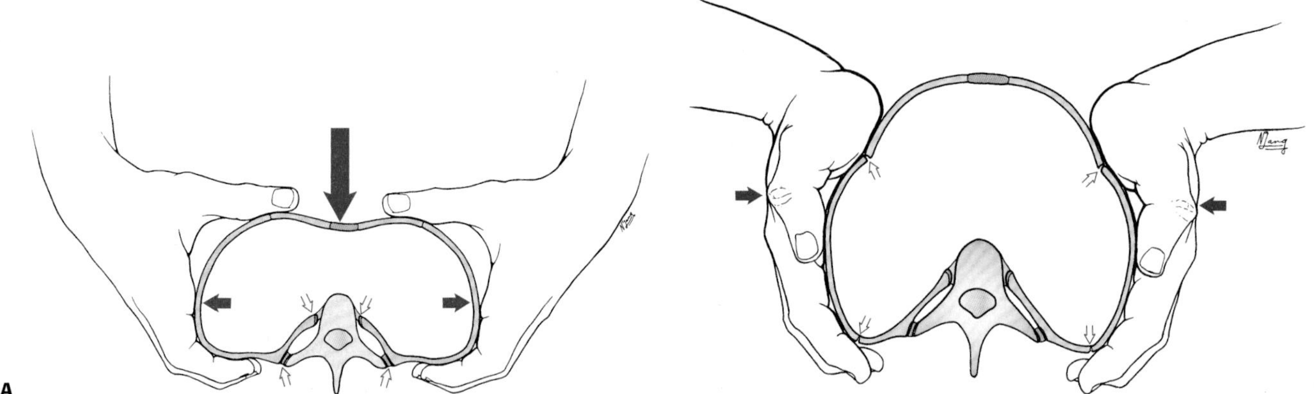

FIGURE 7-13 **A.** Anteroposterior compression of the infant chest causes fractures both at the rib head and adjacent to the transverse processes (*open arrow*), but fractures along the lateral arc of the rib are also possible because of the acute bending of the ribs at this point by compression (*shaded arrow*). **B.** Lateral compression of the chest likely causes fractures of the rib along its posterior arc lateral to the transverse process, as well as possible disruption of the costochondral junction (*open arrows*).

vical fusion. The other twin had a C-5 on C-6 fracture-subluxation treated with casting but later required surgery to reduce and fuse the subluxation. MRI was very helpful in showing cord compression in both cases. Carrion et al (173) reported circumferential physeal fractures of the spine associated with child abuse that required open reduction. Positioning premature infants in extreme flexion for lumbar puncture may cause iatrogenic lumbar spine fracture (173a). Bone scans using single photon emission computed tomography can be helpful for diagnosing occult compression fractures of the thoracic spine (153). Although neurologic injury in spinal fractures resulting from child abuse is uncommon (103), any patient with abusive spinal injury should undergo complete neurologic examination.

The Skeletal Survey

In addition to standard x-ray studies of the acute injury, a skeletal survey is used to detect the presence of additional fractures in battered children (143). The standard skeletal survey recommended by the American College of Radiology (174) includes the following:

- AP of the humeri
- AP of the forearms
- Oblique and AP of the hands
- AP of the femurs
- AP of the lower legs
- AP of the feet
- AP and lateral of the chest
- AP of the pelvis, including mid and lower lumbar spine
- Lateral of lumbar spine
- Lateral of cervical spine
- AP and lateral of skull

The technique should have high resolution, high contrast, screen/film speed of no more than 200, low kVp (bone technique), and single emulsion or special film-screen combination.

An oblique view of the thorax can be helpful in diagnosis of subtle rib fractures and should be added to the skeletal survey when indicated. Oblique x-ray studies of the hand are recommended to detect subtle torus fractures of the metacarpals and the phalanges (127). The indications for skeletal survey are not completely clear. Merten and Carpenter (138) recommended skeletal survey in infants 1 year of age or younger when there is evidence of neglect and in children age 2 years or younger when clinical abuse is evident. The American Academy of Pediatrics Section on Radiology (92) considered a "baby gram" to have no value in diagnosing the fractures of child abuse because the obliquity of the angle at which the x-ray transverses the skeleton may obscure subtle fractures (153). Imaging systems should have a spatial resolution of at least 10 line pairs per millimeter and should be used without a grid (174).

A skeletal survey is mandatory in all cases of suspected physical abuse in children younger than 2 years of age (92), but the sensitivity of skeletal surveys is unclear in older patients. The cost-effectiveness of such skeletal surveys appears to be low because in one study of 331 children, only eight patients without overt physical signs of child abuse had occult fractures revealed by the survey (175), but the use of the skeletal survey in these eight patients possibly prevented both reinjury and death. Perhaps when the death of a child is the ultimate risk of the misdiagnosis of child abuse, we should not play the odds but use very best medical test at our disposal to identify the child at risk for abuse so we can try to protect him or her from further possible fatal abuse.

Sty and Starshak (176) reported a false-negative rate of 12.3% in skeletal surveys of abused children and suggested that a technetium bone scan is the best screening test for occult fractures. Technetium bone scans, however, may fail to diagnose either epiphyseal or metaphyseal fractures and often fail to show skull fractures (126,176). Although CT scans may miss skull fractures, they may conversely show skull fractures even when skeletal surveys are negative (93). Jaudes (177) found that when results of either a bone scan or a skeletal survey were normal in an abused child, the use of both tests often revealed additional occult fractures. Technetium bone scans are especially useful in the diagnosis of occult rib fractures (151,153), but consistent interpretation is difficult in children younger than 18 months of age. Technetium scans are not useful for dating fractures, because increased isotope uptake may occur at a fracture as early as 24 hours after injury and scan abnormalities may persist for years (178). Kleinman et al (150) reported that a follow-up skeletal survey 2 weeks after the initial series detected 27% more fractures and provided assistance in dating 20% of previously detected fractures.

Digital radiography through the picture archiving and communication system (PACS) is gradually replacing standard film-screen imaging in many hospitals, and its role in the detection of the subtle fractures of child abuse is becoming controversial. Youmans et al noted that child abuse fractures can be missed by digitalized images (179). Kleinman et al (180) noted that digital imaging of child abuse fractures had a spatial resolution lower than film-screen imaging, but the difference was not appreciable in detecting rib fractures in a postmortem evaluation.

Additional Imaging Studies

Other imaging techniques may be useful in investigating suspicious x-ray or bone scan findings. Markowitz et al (181) found that sagittal and coronal sonograms of injured knees in abused children were helpful in diagnosing epiphyseal fractures when compared with the normal side. They cautioned that epiphyseal fractures resulting from rickets in neonates can be confused with child abuse on ultrasound evaluation. Rogers and Poznanski (182) pointed out that acute interruption of the physis in trauma of any etiology can be seen on MRI. They recommended multiplanar gradient-echo imaging with a repetition time of 50 to 700 ms, an echo time of 200 ms, and a flip angle of 20 degrees for optimal imaging of the physis.

Dating Fractures

X-ray proof of unexplained fractures in various stages of healing is believed to be strong evidence of child abuse (Fig. 7-14) (129). The orthopaedist often is asked to estimate the age of

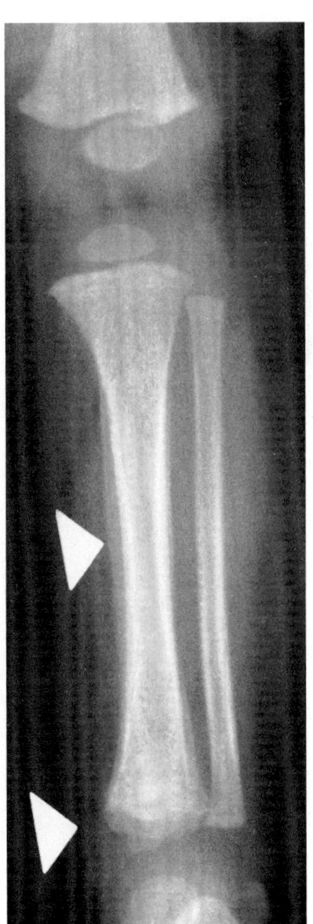

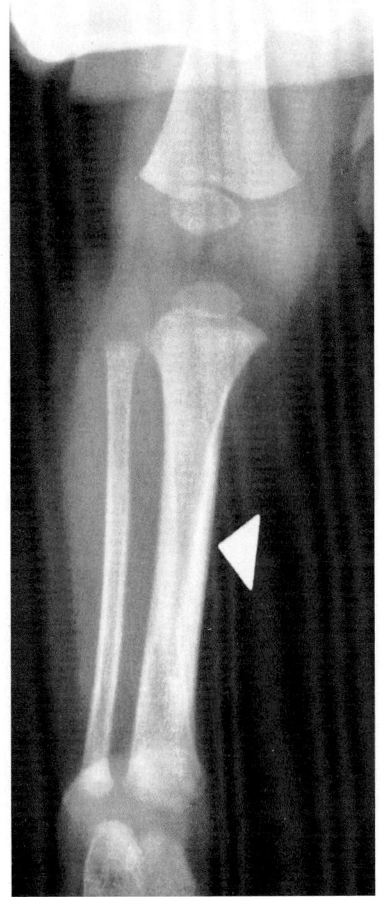

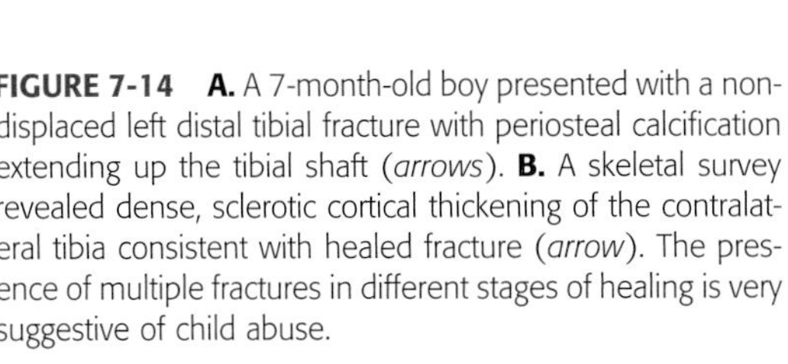
FIGURE 7-14 **A.** A 7-month-old boy presented with a nondisplaced left distal tibial fracture with periosteal calcification extending up the tibial shaft (*arrows*). **B.** A skeletal survey revealed dense, sclerotic cortical thickening of the contralateral tibia consistent with healed fracture (*arrow*). The presence of multiple fractures in different stages of healing is very suggestive of child abuse.

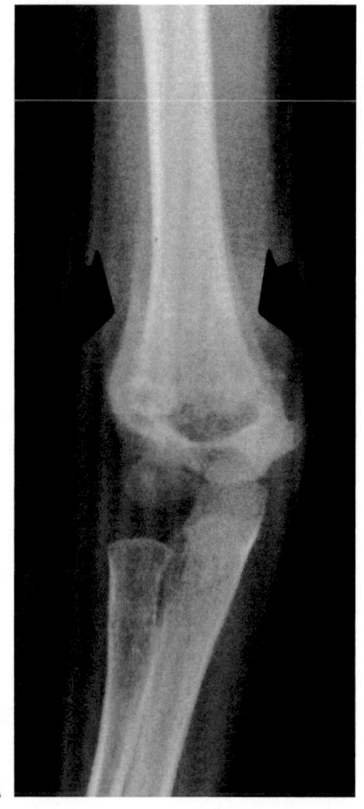

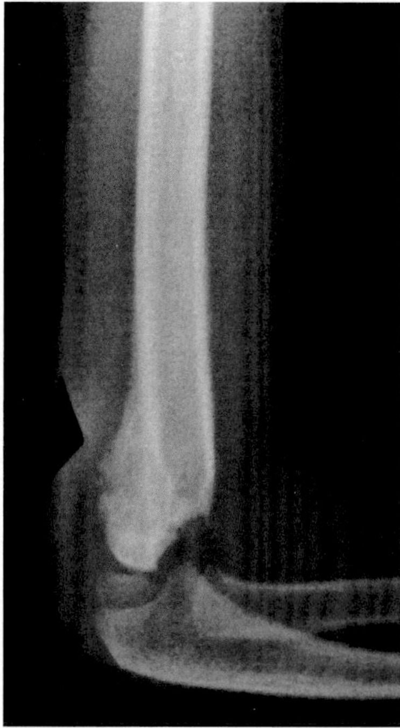

FIGURE 7-15 A 3-year-old female was brought to the clinic with a swollen elbow. The mother stated that the child had fallen only a week ago, but x-rays of the elbow showed a healing supracondylar fracture of the distal humerus that was likely 2 to 3 weeks old based on presence of soft callus (*arrows*). Child protective services was contacted, and a full examination including skeletal survey was performed. No other signs or risk factors for child abuse were detected. The mother then admitted that the child had indeed fallen 3 weeks ago. She was allowed to take her child home after treatment and was counseled about the need for prompt medical care when her children were injured.

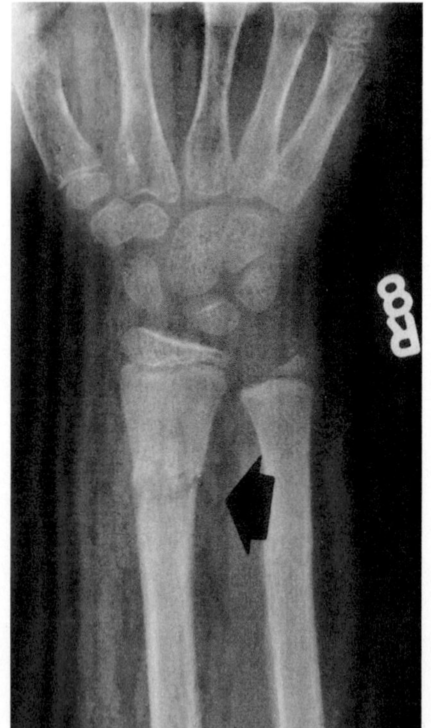

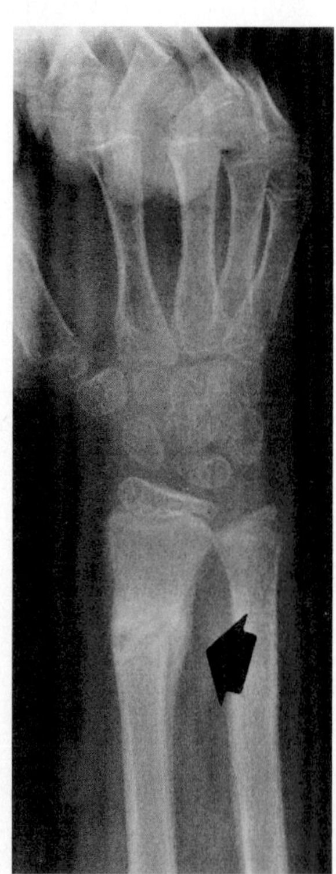

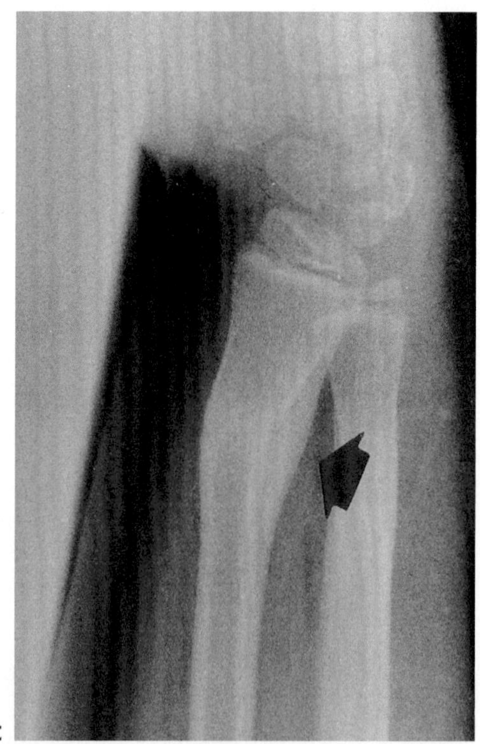

FIGURE 7-16 **A.** A 6-year-old patient presented with a nondisplaced transverse fracture of the distal radius (*arrow*). **B.** At 4-week follow-up, soft callus is seen enveloping the fracture site (*arrow*). **C.** At 6-week follow-up, hard callus is seen and early remodeling is occurring at the fracture site.

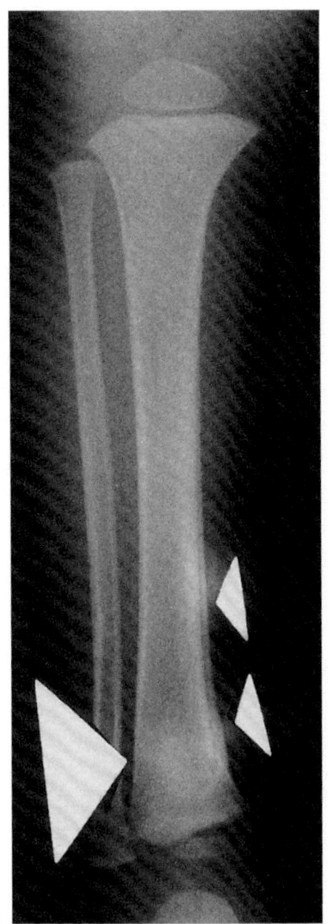

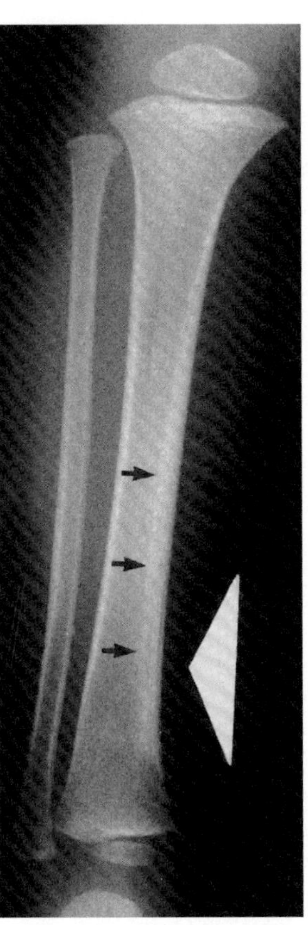

FIGURE 7-17 **A.** An 18-month-old child presented with a 1-month-old nondisplaced fracture of the distal tibia (*large arrow*). The fracture line is beginning to fade, but periosteal calcification is seen medially (*small arrows*). **B.** At 5 months after injury, the fracture shows almost complete remodeling (*large arrow*) with the only sign of past injury a thickened medial cortex of the tibia (*small black arrows*). Subtle signs of past fracture are best noted by comparing the x-rays of the injured side to the contralateral uninjured side.

fractures with some certainty to corroborate a history of injury given by caretakers (Fig. 7-15). Whereas most experienced orthopaedists can roughly estimate the age of fractures based on x-ray appearance, specific guidelines have been established for estimating the age of fractures in children (183). Growth lines present on x-rays may be helpful in dating fractures (184). In general, fractures on x-rays are acute until callus appears, then their age is based on the presence of either soft or hard callus some weeks later (Fig. 7-16). The most difficult fractures to date are those that are completely healed, with substantial remodeling, and often the only sign of fracturing is a thickened cortex (Fig. 7-17).

LABORATORY STUDIES

An abused child should have a complete blood cell count with sedimentation rate, liver function studies, and urinalysis. Clotting studies should be performed routinely, especially in patients with ecchymosis, to rule out a blood disorder as a cause for the bruises. If there is any suspicion of substance abuse by any family member, a toxicology screen should also be performed on the patient (28).

SPECIALTY CONSULTATIONS

Any significant nonorthopaedic injury should prompt appropriate consultations by neurosurgery, general surgery, plastic surgery, or ophthalmology specialists (8). Any female patients who require pelvic examination to rule out sexual abuse should have a gynecologic consultation.

THE DIFFERENTIAL DIAGNOSIS

Although it is extremely important not to miss the diagnosis of child abuse, it is equally important not to make the diagnosis in error. Kaplan (185) pointed out that overdiagnosing battered child syndrome can be harmful to the family, with the parents being placed at risk of losing custody of their child and also facing criminal charges. Even direct allegations of child abuse may turn out to be false. Bernet (186) pointed out that patients or family friends may make false statements about an abuse situation through misinterpretation, confabulation, fantasy, delusions, and other situations. The American Academy of Child and Adolescent Psychiatry (187) has published guidelines for the evaluation of abuse that state that the possibility of false allegations needs to be considered, particularly if allegations are coming from the parent rather than the child, the parents are engaged in a dispute over custody or visitation, or the child is a preschooler.

Normal metaphyseal x-ray appearance should not be confused with child abuse. The x-ray metaphyseal variants include acute angulation of the ossified peripheral tip of the metaphysis adjacent to the physis (most commonly seen in the proximal tibia, distal femur, proximal fibula, distal radius, and distal ulna), which is bilateral in 41% of individuals. A bony beak may be seen medially in the proximal humerus and tibia in rare cases and is bilateral in 77% of individuals. Cortical irregularity in the medial proximal tibia may be seen in 4% of individuals and is bilateral in 25%. Spurs may extend beyond the metaphyseal margins in both the distal radius and lateral aspect of the distal femur, with bilateral variants in 25% of individuals (188).

The signs of child abuse found on x-ray study also can be mimicked by systemic diseases such as scurvy, osteogenesis imperfecta, Caffey disease, osteomyelitis, septic arthritis, fatigue fracture, osteoid osteoma and other tumors, rickets, leukemia, hypophosphatasia, neuromuscular disease, metastatic neuroblastoma, congenital indifference to pain, osteopetrosis, kinky hair syndrome, and prostaglandin therapy (8,44). Fractures resulting from both vitamin D deficiency rickets and drug-induced rickets have been mistaken for child abuse (189). Children with biliary atresia may present with osteopenia and fractures without history of significant injury and should not be mistaken for child abuse (190). Rib fractures are commonly seen in rickets of prematurity as well as rickets of low birth weight and also have been reported after chest physiotherapy (191). There has been an increase in the incidence of syphilis in females of childbearing age, and congenital syphilis can mimic fractures of child abuse with diaphysitis, metaphysitis, and multiple pathologic fractures in different stages of healing (192). Physiologic periostitis (Fig. 7-18), in contrast to lesions from child abuse, is usually bilateral with no excessive uptake of isotope on bone scan (153). The presence of metabolic disease and pathologic fractures does not exclude the possibility of child abuse. Duncan and Chandry (193) reported a 3-month-old girl with multiple fractures associated with rickets who died suddenly at 5 months of age. Child abuse was suspected but not proven. Three years later, evidence of child abuse was found in a subsequent sibling in the same family. Several diseases are commonly brought up in custodial hearings as alternative possibilities to child abuse to explain trauma findings, and these diseases should be carefully explored in the differential diagnosis.

Line lucencies of the proximal tibia resulting from intraosseous vascular access needles may mimic fracture (194). Metaphyseal corner fractures of the distal tibia and fibula were seen in eight children treated with serial casting for clubfoot, with only one thought to be associated with abuse (195). The senior author (RMC) has seen bilateral fractures of the distal tibia and fibula in an infant undergoing serial casting for clubfoot whose father forcedly pulled off the casts.

McClain et al (196) reported a 2-year-old child who died of undiagnosed acute lymphoblastic leukemia. The child had been reported as a possible victim of child abuse because of ecchymosis on the back and extremities. They emphasized that the clinical signs of leukemia, including fever, pallor, petechia, purpura, adenopathy, hepatosplenomegaly, and bone pain, should be sought in children with bruising of unknown origin. Factor XIII deficiency may cause unexplained bleeding from minor trauma and be mistaken for child abuse because the standard coagulation profile may be negative and factor-specific tests may be negative if performed post-transfusion (197).

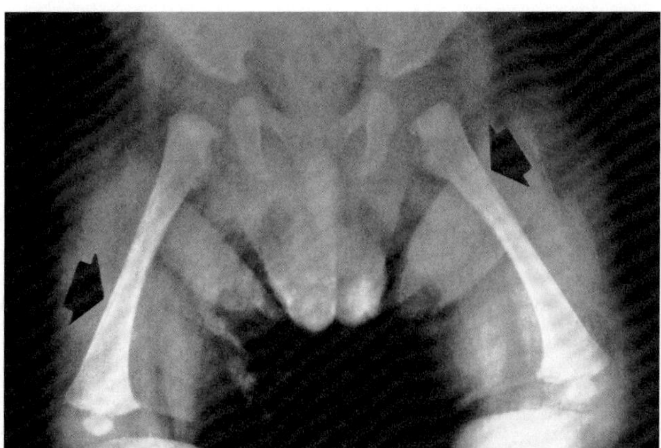

FIGURE 7-18 A 10-month-old infant with physiologic periostitis of the femurs (*arrows*). This type of x-ray appearance may be confused with fractures of child abuse, but this periostitis tends to be bilateral with a uniform appearance in contrast to multiple fractures in different stages of healing seen in battered children.

Osteogenesis Imperfecta

Undiagnosed osteogenesis imperfecta should always be considered when a child presents with multiple fractures of unknown etiology, but it may be a very difficult diagnosis clinically. Osteogenesis imperfecta caused by spontaneous mutation can occur without a family history (198). The so-called hallmark of osteogenesis imperfecta is an intensely blue sclerae, but this feature is consistently present only in type I (199) and may be completely absent in patients with type IV osteogenesis imperfecta (198). Sillence and Butler (200) noted that patients with either type II or III osteogenesis imperfecta may have blue sclerae at birth but the sclerae can become normal by adolescence. The rare type II osteogenesis imperfecta has normal sclerae, but bone abnormalities and osteopenia are severe and early death is likely (198). Blue sclerae may be present in normal young children and can be misleading as a sign of pathologic bone fragility. The presence of abnormal teeth, known as dentinogenesis imperfecta, may be helpful in a diagnosis of osteogenesis imperfecta if the child is old enough for teeth to have erupted. Plain x-ray studies, however, may show long bones of normal density in both types I and IV osteogenesis imperfecta. Another x-ray sign of osteogenesis imperfecta, wormian bones of the skull, is consistently present only in type III and is often absent in types I and IV (198). Some authors believe that the presence of metaphyseal fracture is pathognomonic for child abuse and, therefore, helpful to distinguish abuse from osteogenesis imperfecta (201), but other authors (198,202) believe that there is no particular fracture pattern that renders the diagnosis of osteogenesis imperfecta likely. Patients with osteogenesis imperfecta tend to bruise to excess, which simulates lesions of child abuse (203), and sudden infant death has also been recorded in patients with undiagnosed osteogenesis imperfecta (204).

Sometimes, when the diagnosis of osteogenesis imperfecta cannot be made on clinical grounds, the diagnosis can be made by biochemical assay. Gahagan and Rimsza (205) stated that 87% of patients with osteogenesis imperfecta have abnormal procollagen that can be detected by current techniques. A skin biopsy is performed for fibroblast culture, and fibroblasts are assayed for both abnormally low levels of procollagen and primary abnormal procollagen (206). Steiner et al (207) reported that over a 4-year period, 48 patients were referred to them for collagen analysis to rule out the presence of osteogenesis imperfecta in cases of suspected child abuse. Only six of these children had abnormal collagen test results, and in five of those six patients, the diagnosis of osteogenesis imperfecta could have been made on clinical and x-ray grounds. They concluded that routine collagen biochemical testing for osteogenesis imperfecta is unwarranted in these children, and collagen analysis should be reserved for the rare instances when diagnostic uncertainty persists in cases of suspected child abuse.

Even when a child has osteogenesis imperfecta, fractures may be due to abuse. Knight and Bennett (208) reported on a young child with osteogenesis imperfecta whose abuse could not be proved until linear bruising of the face suggestive of slapping was documented.

Temporary Brittle Bone Disease

In 1993, Patterson et al (198) described 39 patients with a variant of osteogenesis imperfecta that they described as a temporary brittle bone disease in which fractures were limited to the first year of life and then there was spontaneous improvement. These patients presented with vomiting, followed by diarrhea, anemia, hepatomegaly, episodes of apnea, neutropenia, and edema. The most common x-ray findings were metaphyseal corner fractures, rib fractures, diaphyseal fractures, periosteal reaction of long bones, expanded costochondral junctions, and delayed bone age. Only 31% of patients had osteopenia on x-ray study. They suggested that a self-limiting period of copper deficiency was the cause of this problem, but limited serum copper assays were inconclusive. Other authors (209–211) doubt the existence of "temporary" brittle bone disease because of the rarity of fractures associated with proven copper deficiency syndrome, but another author (212–215) supports the existence with indirect evidence. Judicial authorities (51,216, 217) have commented that although one patient in the series of Patterson et al had injuries resulting from child abuse, this fact was not included in the report, and they had concerns that assumptions proposed by medical experts that injuries may be considered solely the result of disease may inhibit full investigation of such injuries by civil authorities and place children at risk for further abuse.

Sudden Infant Death Syndrome

In sudden infant death syndrome (SIDS), there is a distinct possibility of child abuse (33), with one study noting 50% of 81 infants dying from child abuse had an initial diagnosis of SIDS before the correct diagnosis was made (218), but other causes of sudden death must be excluded. Byard et al (219) reported a 5-month-old girl who died suddenly because of spontaneous subarachnoid hemorrhage from undiagnosed Ehlers-Danlos syndrome. They recommended collagen analysis in patients with unexplained multifocal spontaneous hemorrhages to exclude this rare syndrome. Sperry and Pfalzgraf (220) reported a 9-month-old infant whose diagnosis of sudden infant death syndrome became uncertain when postmortem x-rays showed healing symmetric clavicular fractures and a healing left medial humeral epicondylar fracture. Subsequent investigation showed that the child had undergone "chiropractic" manipulation 4 weeks before death by an unlicensed therapist to correct "shoulder dislocations," and the parents were exonerated of abuse charges.

Accidental Trauma

In considering the differential diagnosis of child abuse, accidental trauma should always be considered. The orthopaedist, however, should be comfortable with the diagnosis of accidental trauma only when the acute injury is brought promptly to medical attention and has a plausible mechanism of injury and there are no risk factors for child abuse.

POST-EMERGENCY ROOM TREATMENT AND LEGAL REPORTING REQUIREMENTS

Once child abuse is recognized, the first step in treatment is hospital admission. This is therapeutic in that it places the child in a safe, protected environment and provides the opportunity for additional diagnostic workup and, more importantly, investigation of the family's social situation by appropriate personnel. In university settings, multidisciplinary teams often are available to evaluate and treat such children, but in other circumstances, the orthopaedist may be primarily responsible for coordinating both evaluation and treatment. Court custody may be required for children of uncooperative families who refuse admission, and hospitalization should be continued until a full investigation is completed by the appropriate child protective services. In the United States, the physician is required by law to report all suspected child abuse to appropriate child protective services or legal authorities. When the reporting is done in good faith, the physician has immunity against criminal or civil liability for these actions, but in only three states—Ohio, California, and Alabama—is this protection extended to include absolute immunity (221). The distinction is critical. Absolute immunity means that the physician who reports suspected child abuse cannot ever be held for damages sought by families for allegedly inappropriate reports of child abuse or neglect. The granting of absolute immunity, even for physicians, is not encouraged by the American legal system because in theory it would protect individuals who make false reports of child abuse in order to harass families and would deprive the injured parties their legal right to seek damages for harmful actions. In contrast, physician immunity based on good faith reporting of suspected child abuse is contingent on the physician having a reasonable belief that abuse or neglect has occurred. Although in theory this protection seems to be quite adequate, recently there has been a dramatic rise in the number of lawsuits filed by families seeking damages for alleged, unfounded reports of child abuse and neglect. Although it is true that by the time these lawsuits are eventually resolved, physicians have almost never been held liable for good faith reports of child abuse, in a substantial number of these cases, the physicians first lost at trial level before eventually prevailing at appeal. Considerable expense, frustration, and loss of time can be experienced by the physician in defending against such allegations as the families and their attorneys pursue multiple forms of legal theories in court an attempt to evade the immunity provisions (221). On the other hand, failure to report suspected child abuse may expose the physician to charges of malpractice (17). All states require physicians to report not only cases of definitive child abuse or neglect but also cases when abuse is just suspected or is considered a possibility. Physicians have been held liable for damages for their negligence in failing to diagnose child abuse when the child subsequently was reinjured by more abuse, and, ironically, the parents also may be able to collect additional compensation for losses resulting from medical expenses. For families to be successful in these lawsuits, they must be able to prove that the failure to make the diagnosis of child abuse was negligent and that, had the diagnosis been made, steps would have been taken to protect the child from additional abuse. Although the probability of a physician being held liable under such circumstances is low, the amount of damages can be high if the family does prevail when the child has suffered permanent sequelae (221). Researchers of child abuse have no legal requirement to report suspected child maltreatment, so they may be exposed to both civil and criminal liability for even "good faith" reports that may turn out to be false and injurious (222).

After admission, the orthopaedist proceeds with care of the child's musculoskeletal injuries and coordinates various medical consultations. There should be frequent communications with child protective services to stay current with the results of their investigations. Recommendations for disposition of the child after completion of medical treatment may be a group decision through a multidisciplinary team or, more often, the decision of the primary physician, who may be the orthopaedist. Final disposition choices may include return to the family, return to a family member who does not live in the child's home, or placement in a shelter or a foster home setting. The risk of reinjury and death is significant if the abused child is returned to the unsafe home, so the orthopaedist must strongly support child protective services in custodial actions when it is believed that a child's injury truly occurred from abuse at home. Not only must the definitive diagnosis of child abuse be documented in the chart but a separate notarized affidavit may be necessary. Commonly, custodial actions by child protective services are reviewed in a court hearing in a matter of weeks, and the physician is likely to be called to testify in the hearing. Criminal charges also may be brought against the perpetrator of the child abuse, and the physician likely also serves as a witness in these proceedings.

The Orthopaedic Legal Complications of Child Abuse

The orthopaedist fills a dual role in the courtroom in child abuse proceedings. First, he or she serves as a material witness whose testimony is confined to the physician's personal involvement in the legal matter. The testimony may include clarification to the court of information contained in progress notes in the chart or of other past documentation. As a material witness, the physician, like the layman, cannot render opinions about the facts as stated during his or her testimony. In addition, however, the physician may also be sworn in as an expert witness (223). This is an individual considered by the court to have special knowledge and experience that qualifies him or her to render opinions about certain facts presented in the courtroom. The limits of the physician's expertise usually are defined by the attorneys in court before the testimony of the expert witness.

Physicians usually are reluctant to testify in court for many reasons. The courtroom is an unfamiliar setting for almost all physicians, and the adversarial nature of the American law system makes it a hostile environment. In the courtroom, the perception of truth is just as important as the truth itself, and opposing attorneys will search for inconsistencies in the testimony or unfamiliarity with the record to discredit the physician witness. To avoid being a poor witness, the orthopaedist must meticulously prepare to give testimony.

The orthopaedist preparing to testify in a child abuse case should begin with a thorough review of the child's medical records and a review of recent medical literature on the subject of child abuse (223). Often, there is a pretestimony discussion with child protective services counsel in family court cases or the district attorney's office in criminal cases. Such meetings should preferably be in person, and the orthopaedist's professional training and expertise are examined to determine whether he or she may serve as a material witness, an expert witness, or both. The attorney should be provided the orthopaedist's curriculum vitae, and another copy should be made available to the court. If the orthopaedist is to serve as a material witness, the factual information of the case as well as the limitations of the physician's knowledge are discussed, as are questions that may be posed during testimony. Orthopaedists functioning as expert witnesses should indicate relevant information that should be provided through questioning during testimony. In addition, anticipated testimony from any opposing expert witness and cross-examination questions from the opposing attorney should be discussed. The opposing attorney also may request an informal pretestimony meeting. The orthopaedist should request a list of questions that will be asked in this session ahead of time and request that both the prosecution attorney and the opposing attorney be present during the session, which often is recorded. The next step may be a deposition in which both attorneys question the witness under oath to "discover" the testimony that the witness will provide in court. The primary purpose for a deposition in the discovery process is to keep attorneys from later being surprised in court by testimony of witnesses (224). Preparations for depositions should be meticulous. Any testimony the physician gives during the deposition will be recorded, and later in court any inconsistencies between testimony and prior depositions will be vigorously attacked by attorneys in cross-examination. Depositions rarely are used in criminal prosecutions (223).

A subpoena is issued requiring a physician witness to appear at the courtroom at a certain time, but often there may be hours of delay before the testimony actually begins. Through prior arrangements with the attorneys, the orthopaedist may be placed "on call" if he or she works within a reasonable distance of the courtroom and can be available a short time before the actual testimony is needed. The physician has no legal right to such treatment and must be prepared to honor the exact conditions of the subpoena if alternative arrangements cannot be made. If significant delays are encountered to giving testimony and the attorneys are not responsive to physician hardship, then the orthopaedist should contact the judge directly to remedy the situation (224). In the courtroom, the orthopaedist should be conservatively dressed and appear attentive, competent, poised, and at ease (223,224).

Once called to the stand, the orthopaedist is sworn in and identified. Next follows qualification, direct examination, and then cross-examination. In the qualification process, the attorney asks the physician fairly detailed questions about the orthopaedist's training and background to establish whether he or she is a credible witness (223). The attorney wishes to impress the judge or jury with the orthopaedist's qualifications as a witness, whereas the opposing attorney may challenge the witness with questions to cast doubt on his or her expertise (224). During this phase, the attorneys also may establish the limits of the physician's expertise as an expert medical witness. Next, the attorney will proceed with direct examination. A series of questions are asked that aim at developing a logical and progressive line of thought leading to a conclusion (224). In child abuse cases, in particular, the testimony will lead to the fact that the abuse has occurred and that it has been appropriately diagnosed. In addition, the physician expert witness may be asked to give an opinion of the risk for subsequent abuse if the child returns to the home where the alleged abuse occurred. Almost never will the physician witness be asked about the guilt or innocence of the caretaker accused of abuse, but the orthopaedist in certain circumstances will come close to answering the "ultimate question" (224), by testifying about a child's statement of history if it identifies the abuser. Some states, however, restrict such testimony. In Maryland, a physician may not testify regarding any disclosures made by a child abuse victim unless the disclosure is admissible under a recognized exception to the rule prohibiting hearsay evidence (69). The orthopaedist should ask about any possible restrictions on his or her testimony with the attorney in pretrial discussion. In testimony, the orthopaedist will want to use the courtroom setting to advocate for the safety and well-being of the child (223). Questions regarding medical findings often will be prefaced in the courtroom by the words "reasonable medical certainty," a term that is poorly understood by most physicians. Chadwick (224) offered a definition of reasonable medical certainty as "certain as a physician should be in order to recommend and carry out treatment for a given medical condition." He offered an example that the certainty for the diagnosis and treatment of leukemia must be much higher than that for diagnosis and treatment of a viral upper respiratory tract infection.

During testimony, the orthopaedist's words should be carefully chosen and should be understandable by a lay jury. Testimony should be objective, honest, and thorough (223). Attorneys may frame questions in ways that are difficult to understand, and the orthopaedist should not hesitate to ask the attorney to clarify a question (224). Answers should be brief, without volunteering extra information, but the perception listeners will have of the answers should be carefully considered by the orthopaedist. In particular, attorneys may phrase yes or no questions that could place misleading words in the mouth of the orthopaedist. In such situations, when neither response is appropriate, the orthopaedist should answer in a sentence that provides an accurate answer (223). Language should be straightforward, and visual aids may be used in providing clear testimony. The expert should use testimony as an educational process for the court, in which the common experience and knowledge of the jury is used to build understanding with common sense explanations of medical findings (224).

Cross-examination by the opposing attorney follows direct examination. The opposing attorney's role is to challenge the material presented by the physician witness to protect the defendant (223). This may involve an attempt to bring into question the physician's credibility, the medical record, the physician's training or expertise, or the physician's objectivity or composure and clarity of thought before the jury (223). Attorneys may accomplish this by finding inconsistencies with prior statements, asking leading questions as well as questions that allow only certain desired answers, and minimizing physician qualifications (224). The attorney may frame a question that contains certain elements that the physician agrees with and others that are misleading, and often the question will end with "Isn't that so, doctor?" The physician witness should be firm in answering such questions, clearly stating what in the question he or she agrees with and what he or she does not. It is also common to encounter questions from attorneys based on hypotheses that are extremely unlikely, and the physician needs to point out that unlikelihood (224). Part of the strategy of aggressive cross-examination is to provoke the physician into arguments or unprofessional behavior that could discredit the physician or his or her testimony before the court. In particular, juries will allow aggression on the part of an attorney, but they expect physician witnesses to respond professionally, even under extreme duress (117). Inexperienced potential physician witnesses can prepare themselves by either watching trials or participating in mock trials (224). Brent (226) assembled an excellent series of vignettes of expert medical witness case studies in court and provided detailed instructions with regard to the responsibilities of such experts. Both redirect examination and recross-examination may follow cross-examination at the discretion of attorneys, but usually these procedures are very short (224).

Disposition Following Custody Hearings

After a hearing or trial, the child historically either remained in the protective custody of the state or was returned to the home, but the danger of further abuse exists in both situations. In a study of recurrent maltreatment in 10 states based on the National Child Abuse and Neglect Data System, Fluke et al (227) found that the recurrence rate was 13% by 6 months after the first episode of reported abuse, increasing to 17% by 12 months. In a report of 206 care and protection petitions brought to the Boston juvenile courts (228), 31 were dismissed with return of the child to the parents. During a 2-year follow-up of these dismissed cases, 29 had reports of further mistreatment and 16 were returned to court under another care and protection petition. One risk factor identified by the study was a previous appearance in court. Half of dismissed cases with this risk factor returned to court again. Of the children ordered permanently removed from parental custody by the court, six returned to court with evidence of further abuse by another caretaker. Another alternative pathway of custody is gaining popularity with the court systems in which the abused child is released to the custody of a relative of the family with consideration given to the wishes of the parents or other prior custodians of the child. Although in theory this approach may help preserve the integrity of the family unit, the child may still be in danger in this sort of arrangement. Handy et al (229) of the Pediatric Forensic Medicine Program of the Kentucky State Medical Examiner's Office noted evidence of recurrent abuse 2 to 9 months after the original injury in six patients out of 316 referrals to the program. They emphasized that in two of these cases, the child was in protective custody of a family relative when the original perpetrator was allowed unsupervised access to the child in violation of court order. One 6-month-old infant placed in the custody of a grandmother was bent backward by the original perpetrator until his head touched his feet, sustaining a thoracic spinal fracture with fatal outcome. Another 4-year-old was in the custody of her grandmother when the child's mother gained unauthorized access to her and the child was reinjured with a burn on the face with an iron. It is possible that such reinjuries occur because either the close relatives of the child abuser may not believe that the caretaker committed the original abuse or the relatives are under emotional pressure to allow the caretaker to have access to the child in spite of court order. It is hoped that the court systems can strike a balance between the need to preserve the family unit and the need to protect the child from further abuse.

PREVENTION OF CHILD ABUSE

Prevention of child abuse lies in early intervention. Home visitor programs can contact a mother immediately after the birth of her child and arrange for a visit in which the mother's parenting strengths are assessed. Parents requiring additional support are linked to community agencies and family resources (122,230). Such support seems to enhance parent and child interactions, and mothers report a diminished need to punish or restrict their children. Anti-victimization programs teach children certain concepts believed to facilitate self-protection, such as identification of strangers, types of touching, saying "no" to inappropriate advances, and telling someone about inappropriate behavior.

Parenting education offers instruction in specific parenting skills such as discipline methods, basic child care, infant stimulation, child development, education, and familiarity with local support services and introduction to other new parents in the community (105). Continuing abuse can be prevented by the orthopaedist's prompt recognition of child abuse in the emergency department and appropriate intervention. The most important issue in dealing with child abuse is to help both the child and the family through early recognition of the problem and appropriate therapeutic measures by all health personnel. The failure to diagnose child abuse may result in serious injury to or death of the child.

ACKNOWLEDGMENTS

Special thanks is given to Hope Trevino and Randy Llamas for technical assistance.

REFERENCES

1. Kocher MS, Kasser JR. Orthopaedic aspects of child abuse. *J Am Acad Orthop Surg* 2000;8:10–20.
2. Johnson CF. Inflicted injury versus accidental injury. *Pediatr Clin North Am* 1990;37:791–814.
3. Texas Department of Health. *Children's Health and Safety Initiative: Building Blocks for Healthy Children*. Texas Department of Health 1996:24.
4. Prevent child abuse America: http://www.preventchildabuse.org/learn_more/research_docs/cost_analysis.pdf. Accessed August, 2005.
5. Texas Medical Association Foundation. *A Report by the Blue Ribbon Panel on Family Violence*. Texas Medical Association Foundation.
6. Forjuoh SN. Child maltreatment related injuries: incidence, hospital charges, and correlates of hospitalization. *Child Abuse Negl* 2000;24:1019–1025.
7. Oliver JE. Intergenerational transmission of child abuse: rates, research, and clinical implications. *Am J Psychiatry* 1993;150:1315–1324.
8. Akbarnia BA, Akbarnia NO. The role of the orthopedist in child abuse and neglect. *Orthop Clin North Am* 1976;7:733–742.
9. Schmitt BD. Child abuse. In: Green M, Haggerty RJ, eds. *Pediatrics*. Philadelphia: WB Saunders; 1984:111.
10. Caffey J. Multiple fractures in long bones of infants suffering from chronic subdural hematoma. *Am J Roentgenol* 1946;56:163–173.
11. Silverman FN. The roentgen manifestations of unrecognized skeletal trauma in infants. *Am J Roentgenol* 1953;69:413–427.
12. Altman DH, Smith RL. Unrecognized trauma in infants and children. *J Bone Joint Surg Am* 1960;42:407–413.
13. Kempe CH, Silberman FN, Steele BF, et al. The battered-child syndrome. *JAMA* 1962;181:105–112.
14. Caffey J. The whiplash shaken infant syndrome: manual shaking by the extremities with whiplash-induced intracranial and intraocular bleedings, linked with residual permanent brain damage and mental retardation. *Pediatrics* 1974;54:396–403.
15. Dubowitz H, Bross DC. The pediatrician's documentation of child maltreatment. *Am J Dis Child* 1992;146:596–599.
16. Zuravin SJ. Unplanned childbearing and family size: their relationship to child neglect and abuse. *Fam Planning Perspect* 1991;23:155–161.
17. Akbarnia BA. The role of the orthopaedic surgeon in child abuse. In: Morrissy RM, ed. *Lovell and Winter's pediatric Orthopaedics*. Philadelphia: JB Lippincott; 1996:1315.
18. Herndon WA. Child abuse in a military population. *J Pediatr Orthop* 1983;3:73–76.
19. O'Neill JA Jr, Meacham WF, Griffin PP, et al. Patterns in injury in battered child syndrome. *J Trauma* 1973;13:332–339.
20. Green FC. Child abuse and neglect: a priority problem for the private physician. *Pediatr Clin North Am* 1975;22:329–339.
21. Crouch JL, Behl LE. Relationships among parental beliefs in corporal punishment, reported stress, and physical child abuse potential. *Child Abuse Negl* 2001;25:413–419.
22. Helfer RE. The epidemiology of child abuse and neglect. *Pediatr Ann* 1984;13:745–751.
23. Wasserman DR, Leventhal JM. Maltreatment of children born to cocaine-dependent mothers. *Am J Dis Child* 1993;147:1324–1328.
24. Siegel CD, Graves P, Maloney K, et al. Mortality from intentional and unintentional injury among infants of young mothers in Colorado, 1986 to 1992. *Arch Pediatr Adolesc Med* 1996;150:1077–1083.
25. Campbell JC. Child abuse and wife abuse. *Md Med J* 1994;43:349–350.
26. Wolfner GD, Gelles RJ. A profile of violence toward children: a national study. *Child Abuse Negl* 1993;17:197–212.
27. Sidebotham P, Golding J. The ALSPAC Study Team: child maltreatment in the "Children of the Nineties"—a longitudinal study of parental risk factors. *Child Abuse Negl* 2001;25:1177–1200.

28. Galleno H, Oppenheim WL. The battered child syndrome revisited. *Clin Orthop* 1982; 62:11–19.
29. Beals RK, Tufts E. Fractured femur in infancy: the role of child abuse. *J Pediatr Orthop* 1983;3:583–586.
30. Desilva S, Oates RK. Child homicide: the extreme of child abuse. *Med J Aust* 1993; 158:300–301.
31. Kleinman PK, Marks SC, Adams VI, et al. Factors affecting visualization of posterior rib fractures in abused infants. *Am J Roentgenol* 1988;150:635–638.
32. Bruce DA, Schut L, Bruno LA, et al. Outcome following severe head injuries in children. *J Neurosurg* 1978;48:679–688.
33. Emery JL. Child abuse, sudden infant death syndrome, and unexpected infant death. *Am J Dis Child* 1993;147:1097–1100.
34. Samuels MP, McClaughlin W, Jacobson RR, et al. Fourteen cases of imposed upper airway obstruction. *Arch Dis Child* 1992;67:162–170.
35. Benedict RB, Wulff LM, Hall BJ. Reported maltreatment in children with multiple disabilities. *Child Abuse Negl* 1990;14:207–217.
36. Asher R. Munchausen syndrome. *Lancet* 1951;1:339.
37. Mehl AL, Coble L, Johnson S. Munchausen syndrome by proxy: a family affair. *Child Abuse Negl* 1990;14:577–585.
38. Wenk, RE. Molecular evidence of Munchausen syndrome by proxy. *Arch Pathol Lab Med* 2003;127:e36–e37.
39. Baskin DE, Stein F, Coats DK, et al. Recurrent conjunctivitis as a presentation of Munchausen syndrome by proxy. *Ophthalmology* 2003;110:1582–1584.
40. Bartsh C, Risse M, Schutz H, et al. Munchausen syndrome by proxy (MSBP): an extreme form of child abuse with a special forensic challenge. *Forensic Sci Int* 2003;137: 147–151.
41. Meadow SR. Non-accidental salt poisoning. *Arch Dis Child* 1993;68:448–452.
42. Babcock J, Hartman K, Pedersen A, et al. Rodenticide-induced coagulopathy in a young child: a case of Munchausen syndrome by proxy. *Am J Pediatr Hematol Oncol* 1993; 15:126–130.
43. Goss PW, McDougall PN. Munchausen syndrome by proxy: a cause of preterm delivery. *Med J Aust* 1992;157:814–817.
44. Berkowitz CD. Pediatric abuse: new patterns of injury. *Emerg Med Clin North Am* 1995; 13:321–341.
45. Rosenberg DA. Web of deceit: a literature review of Munchausen syndrome by proxy. *Child Abuse Negl* 1987;11:547–563.
46. Meadow R. Munchausen syndrome by proxy abuse perpetuated by men. *Arch Dis Child* 1998;78:210–216.
47. Davis P, McClure RJ, Rolfe K, et al. Procedures, placement, and risks of further abuse after Munchausen's by proxy, non-accidental poisoning, and non-accidental suffocation. *Arch Dis Child* 1998;78:217–221.
48. Hall DE, Eubanks L, Swarnalatha M, et al. Evaluation of covert surveillance in the diagnosis of Munchausen syndrome by proxy: lessons from 41 cases. *Pediatrics* 2000; 105:1305–1312.
49. Krugman RD. Recognition of sexual abuse in children. *Pediatr Rev* 1986;8:25–30.
50. Hobbs CJ, Wynne JM. The sexually abused battered child. *Arch Dis Child* 1990;65: 423–427.
51. Wissow LS. Child abuse and neglect. *N Engl J Med* 1995;332:1425–1431.
52. Sullivan PM, Brookhouser PE, Scanlan JM, et al. Patterns of physical and sexual abuse of communicatively handicapped children. *Ann Otol Rhinol Laryngol* 1991;100:188–427.
53. Young WC. Sadistic ritual abuse: an overview in detection and management. *Primary Care* 1993;20:447–458.
54. Alexander RC, Surrell JA, Cohle SD. Microwave oven burns to children: an unusual manifestation of child abuse. *Pediatrics* 1987;79:255–260.
55. Reece RM. Unusual manifestations of child abuse. *Pediatr Clin North Am* 1990;37: 905–912.
56. Black J, Zenel JA. Child abuse by intentional iron poisoning presenting as shock and persistent acidosis. *Pediatrics* 2003;111:197–199.
57. Dubowitz H, Black M. Teaching pediatric residents about child maltreatment. *Dev Behav Pediatr* 1991;12:305–307.
58. Limbos MAP. Documentation of child abuse: how far have we come? *Pediatrics* 1998; 102:53–58.
59. Bar-on ME, Zanga JR. Child abuse: a model for use of structured clinical forms. *Pediatrics* 1996;81:17–24.
60. Palusci VJ, Hicks RA, Vandervort FE. "You are hereby commanded to appear": pediatrician subpoena and court appearance in child maltreatment. *Pediatrics* 2001;107: 1427–1431.
61. Hanes M, Mc Aufliff T. Preparation for child abuse litigation: perspectives of the prosecutor and the pediatrician. *Pediatr Ann* 1977;26:288–295.
62. Orebach Y, Lamb ME. Enhancing children's narratives in investigative interviews. *Child Abuse Negl* 2000;24:1631–1648.
63. Kravitz H, Driessen G, Gomberg R, et al. Accidental falls from elevated surfaces in infants from birth to one year of age. *Pediatrics* 1969;44:869–876.
64. Helfer RE, Slovis TL, Black M. Injuries resulting when small children fall out of bed. *Pediatrics* 1977;60:533–535.
65. Kogutt MS, Swischuk LE, Fagan CJ. Patterns of injury and significance of uncommon fractures in the battered child syndrome. *Radiology* 1974;121:143–149.
66. Hennrikus WL, Shaw BA, Gerardi JA. Injuries when children reportedly fall from a bed or a couch. *Clin Orthop Rel Res* 2003;407:148–151.
67. O'Connor JF, Cohen J. Dating fractures. In: Kleinman PK, ed. *Diagnostic Imaging of Child Abuse*. Baltimore: Williams & Wilkins; 1987:103.
68. McMahon P, Grossman W, Gaffney M, et al. Soft-tissue injury as an indication of child abuse. *J Bone Joint Surg Am* 1995;77:1179–1183.
69. Sugar NF, Taylor JA, Feldman KW. Bruises in infants and toddlers: those who don't cruise rarely bruise. Puget Sound Pediatric Research Network. *Arch Pediatr Adolesc Med* 1999;153:399–403.
70. Carpenter RF, The prevalence and distribution of bruising in babies. *Arch Dis Child* 1999;80:363–366.
71. Robertson DM, Barbor P. Unusual injury? Recent injury in normal children and children with suspected non-accidental trauma. *Br Med J* 1982;285:1399–1401.
72. Labbe J, Caouette G. Recent skin injuries in normal children. *Pediatrics* 2001;108: 271–276.
73. Johnson CF, Kaufman KL. The hand as a target organ in child abuse. *Clin Pediatr* 1990; 29:66–72.
74. Sussman SJ. Skin manifestations of the battered-child syndrome. *J Pediatr* 1968;72: 99–101.
75. Hyden PW, Gallagher TA. Child abuse intervention in the emergency room. *Pediatr Clin North Am* 1992;39:1053–1081.
76. Jessee SA, Rieger M. Physical abuse: a study of age-related variables among physically abused children. *J Dent Child* 1996;14:275–280.
77. Wilson FF. Estimation of age of continuous contusions in child abuse. *Pediatrics* 1977; 60:750–752.
78. Langlois NEI, Gresham GA. The age of bruises: a review and study of the color changes with time. *Forensic Sci Int* 1991;50:227–238.
79. Stephenson T, Bialas Y. Estimation of the age of bruising, *Arch Dis Child* 1996;74: 53–55.
80. Asnes RS. Buttock bruises = mongolian spot [Letter]. *Pediatrics* 1984;74:321.
81. Anh NT. "Pseudo-battered child" syndrome. *JAMA* 1976;236:2288.
82. Purdue GF, Hunt JL, Prescott PR. Child abuse by burning: an index of suspicion. *J Trauma* 1988;28:221–224.
83. Titus MO, Baxter AL, Starling SP. Accidental scald burn in sinks. *Pediatrics* 2003;111: E191–E194.
84. Renz BM, Sherman R. Abusive scald burns in infants and children: a prospective study. *Am Surgeon* 1993;59:329–334.
85. Heider TR, Priolo D, Hultman CS, et al. Eczema mimicking child abuse: a case of mistaken identity. *J Burn Care Rehabil* 2002;23:357–359.
86. Prescott PR. Hair dryer burns in children. *Pediatrics* 1990;86:692–697.
87. Frechette A, Rimsza ME. Stun gun injury: a new presentation of the battered child syndrome. *Pediatrics* 1992;89:898–901.
88. Feldman KW. Pseudoabusive burns in Asian refugees. *Am J Dis Child* 1984;138: 768–769.
89. Schmitt BD, Gray JD, Britton HL. Car seat burns in infants: avoiding confusion with inflicted burns. *Pediatrics* 1978;62:607–609.
90. Reece RM, Sege R. Childhood head injuries: accidental or inflicted? *Arch Pediatr Adolesc Med* 2000;154:11–15.
91. Case ME, Graham MA, Handy TC, et al. Position paper on fatal abusive head injuries in infants and young children. *Am J Forensic Med Pathol* 2001;22:112–122.
92. American Academy of Pediatrics Section on Radiology. Diagnostic imaging of child abuse. *Pediatrics* 2000;105:1345–1348.
93. Rubin DM, Christian CW, Bilaniuk LT, et al. Occult head injury in high-risk abused children. *Pediatrics* 2003;111:1382–1386.
94. Duhaime AC, Gennarelli TA, Thibault LE, et al. The shaken baby syndrome: a clinical, pathological, and biomechanical study. *J Neurosurg* 1987;66:409–415.
95. Pariziel PM, Ceulemans B, Laridon A, et al. Cortical hypoxic-ischemic brain damage in shake-baby (shaken impact) syndrome: value of diffusion-weighted MRI. *Pediatr Radiol* 2003;33:868–871.
96. Suh DY, Davis PC, Hopkins KL. Nonaccidental pediatric head injury: diffusion-weighted imaging findings. *Neurosurgery* 2001;49:309–320.
96a. Jaspan T, Narborough G, Punt JAG, et al. Cerebral contusion tears as a marker of child abuse: detection by cranial sonography. *Pediatr Radiol* 1992;22:237–245.
97. Jaspan T, Griffiths PD, McConachie NS, et al. Neuroimaging for non-accidental head injury in childhood: a proposed protocol. *Clin Radiol* 2003;58:44–53.
98. Cho D-R, Wang Y-C, Chi C-S. Decompression craniotomy for acute shaken/impact baby syndrome. *Pediatr Neurosurg* 1995;23:192–198.
99. Eller AW, Brown GC. Retinal disorders of childhood. *Pediatr Clin North Am* 1983;301: 87–101.
100. Hanigan WC, Peterson RA, Njus G. Tin ear syndrome: rotational acceleration in pediatric head injuries. *Pediatrics* 1987;80:618–622.
101. Akbarnia BA. Pediatric spine fractures. *Orthop Clin North Am* 1999;30:521–536.
102. Ghatan S, Ellenbogen RG. Pediatric spine and spinal cord injury after inflicted trauma. *Neurosurg Clin North Am* 2002;13:227–233.
103. Cullen JC. Spinal lesions in battered babies. *J Bone Joint Surg Br* 1975;57:364–366.
104. Trokel M, DiScala C, Terrin NC, et al. Blunt abdominal injury in the young pediatric patient: child abuse and patient outcomes. *Child Maltreat* 2004;9:111–117.
105. Touloukian RJ. Abdominal visceral injuries in battered children. *Pediatrics* 1968;42: 642–646.
106. Tracy T Jr, O'Connor TP, Weber TR: Battered children with duodenal avulsion and transection. *Am Surgeon* 1993;59:342–345.
107. Coant PN, Kornberg AE, Brody AS, et al. Markers for occult liver injury in cases of physical abuse in children. *Pediatrics* 1992;89:274–278.
108. Howard JL, Barron BJ, Smith GG. Bone scintigraphy in the evaluation of extraskeletal injuries from child abuse. *Radiographics* 1990;10:67–81.
109. Thogmartin JR, England D, Siebert Jr CF. Hepatic glycogen staining: applications in injury survival time and child abuse. *Am J Forensic Med Pathol* 2001;22:313–318.
110. Sinal SH. Sexual abuse of children and adolescents. *South Med J* 1994;87:1242–1258.
111. American Academy of Pediatrics. Guidelines for the evaluation of sexual abuse of children. *Pediatrics* 1991;87:254–260.
112. Ingram DM, Everett VD, Ingram DL. The relationship between the transverse hymenal orifice diameter by the separation technique and other possible markers of sexual abuse. *Child Abuse and Negl* 2001;25:1109–1120.

113. Kellog ND, Menard SW, Santos A. Genital anatomy in pregnant adolescents: "normal" does not mean "nothing happened." *Pediatrics* 2004;113:e67–e69.
114. Cantwell HB. Vaginal inspection as it relates to child sexual abuse in girls under thirteen. *Child Abuse Negl* 1983;7:171–176.
115. Berenson AB, Heger AH, Hayes JM, et al. Appearance of the hymen in prepubescent girls. *Pediatrics* 1992;89:387–394.
116. Bays J, Chadwick D. Medical diagnosis of the sexually abused child. *Child Abuse Negl* 1993;17:91–110.
117. Dalton HJ, Slovis T, Helfer RE, et al. Undiagnosed abuse in children younger than 3 years with femoral fracture. *Am J Dis Child* 1990;140:875–878.
118. Leventhal JM, Thomas SA, Rosenfield NS, et al. Fractures in young children: distinguishing child abuse from unintentional injuries. *Am J Dis Child* 1993;147:87–92.
119. Adelman, RD, Fink RA, Rohn RD et al. Child abuse in an infant presenting as unexplained acute systemic hypertension. *Pediatr Nephr* 200;14:811–812.
120. Ander WA. The significance of femoral fractures in children. *Ann Emerg Med* 1982; 11:174–177.
121. Thomas SA, Rosenfield NS, Leventhal JM, et al. Long-bone fractures in young children: distinguishing accidental injuries from child abuse. *Pediatrics* 1991;88:1–476.
122. American Academy of Pediatrics: Section on Child Abuse and Neglect. *A Guide to References and Resources in Child Abuse and Neglect*. Elk Grove Village, IL: American Academy of Pediatrics; 1994:107–190.
123. Kleinman PK, Spevak MR. Variations in acromial ossification simulating infant abuse in victims of sudden infant death syndrome. *Radiology* 1991;180:185–187.
124. Kleinman PK. *Diagnostic Imaging of Child Abuse*, 2nd ed. St. Louis: Mosby; 1998.
125. Hechter S, Huyer D, Manson D. Sternal fractures as a manifestation of abusive injury in children. *Pediatr Radiol* 2002;32:902–906.
126. Merter LDF, Radkowski MA, Leonidas JC. The abused child: a radiological reappraisal. *Radiology* 1983;146:377–381.
127. Nimkin K, Spevak MR, Kleinman PK. Fractures of the hands and feet in child abuse: imaging and pathological features. *Radiology* 1997;203:233–236.
128. King J, Diefendorf D, Apthorp J, et al. Analysis of 429 fractures in 189 battered children. *J Pediatr Orthop* 1988;8:585–589.
129. Akbarnia B, Torg JS, Kirkpatrick J et al: Manifestations of battered-child syndrome. *J Bone Joint Surg Am* 1974;56:1159–1166.
130. Loder RT, Bookout C. Fracture patterns in battered children. *J Orthop Trauma* 1991; 5:428–433.
131. Pierce MC, Bertocci GE, Vogeley E, et al. Evaluating long bone fractures in children: a biomechanical approach with illustrative cases. *Child Abuse Negl* 2004;28:505–524.
132. Bertocci GE, Pierce MC, Deemer E, et al. Influence of fall height and impact surface on biomechanics of feet-first free falls in children. *Injury* 2004;35:417–424.
133. Bertocci GE, Pierce MC, Deemer E, et al. Using test dummy experiments to investigate pediatric injury risk in simulated short-distance falls. *Arch Pediatr Adolesc Med* 2003; 157:480–486.
134. Bertocci GE, Pierce MC, Deemer E, et al. Computer simulation of stair falls to investigate scenarios in child abuse. *Arch Pediatr Adolesc Med* 2001;155:1008–1014.
135. Pierce MC, Bertocci GE, Janosky JE, et al. Femur fractures resulting from stair falls among children: an injury implausibility model. *Pediatrics* 2005;115:1712–1722.
136. McClelland CQ, Heiple KG. Fractures in the first year of life: a diagnostical dilemma? *Am J Dis Child* 1982;136:26–29.
137. Shaw BA, Murphy KM, Shaw A, et al. Humerus shaft fractures in young children: accident or abuse? *J Pediatr Orthop* 1997;17:293–297.
138. Merten DF, Carpenter BLM. Radiologic imaging of inflicted injury in the child abuse syndrome. *Pediatr Clin North Am* 1990;37:815–837.
139. Rex C, Kay PR. Features of femoral fractures in nonaccidental injury. *J Pediatr Orthop* 2000;20:411–413.
140. Scherl SA, Miller L, Lively N, et al. Accidental and nonaccidental femur fractures in children. *Clin Orthop Relat Res* 2000;376:96–105.
140a. Gross RH, Stanger M. Causative factors responsible for femoral shaft fractures in infants and young children. *J Pediatr Orthop* 1983;3:341–343.
141. Schwend RM, Werth C, Johnston A. Femur fractures in toddlers and young children: rarely from child abuse. *J Pediatr Orthop* 2000;20:475–481.
142. Blakemore LC, Loder RT, Hensinger RN. Role of intentional abuse in children one to five years old with isolated femoral shaft fractures. *J Pediatr Orthop* 1996;16:585–588.
143. Leonidas JC. Skeletal trauma in the child abuse syndrome. *Pediatr Ann* 1983;12: 875–881.
144. Kleinman PK, Marks SC. Relationship of the subperiosteal bone collar to metaphyseal lesions in abused infants. *J Bone Joint Surg Am* 1995;77:1471–1476.
145. Kleinman PK, Marks SC, Blackbourne B. The metaphyseal lesion in abused infants: a radiologic-histopathologic study. *Am J Roentgenol* 1986;146:895–905.
146. Kleinman PK, Marks SC Jr, Spevak MR, et al. Extension of growth-plate cartilage into the metaphysis: a sign of healing fracture in abused infants. *Am J Roentgenol* 1991;156: 775–779.
147. Osier LK, Marks SC Jr, Kleinman PK. Metaphyseal extensions of hypertrophied chondrocytes in abused infants indicate healing fractures. *J Pediatr Orthop* 1993;13: 249–254.
148. Currarino G, Birch J G, Herring, JA. Developmental coax vara associated with spondylometaphyseal dysplasia (DCV/SMD): " SMD-Corner fracture type" DCV/SMD-CF) demonstrated inmost cases. *Pediatr Radiol* 2000;30:14–24.
149. Strouse PJ, Owings CL. Fractures of the first rib in child abuse. *Radiology* 1995;197: 763–765.
150. Kleinman PK, Nimkin K, Spevak MR, et al. Follow-up skeletal surveys in suspected child abuse. *Am J Roentgenol* 1996;167:893–896.
151. Smith FW, Gilday DL, Ash JM, et al. Unsuspected costo-vertebral fractures demonstrated by bone scanning in the child abuse syndrome. *Pediatr Radiol* 1980;10:103–106.
152. Kleinman PK, Marks SC Jr, Spevak MR, et al. Fractures of the rib head in abused infants. *Radiology* 1992;185:119–123.
153. Conway JJ, Collins M, Tanz RR, et al. The role of bone scintigraphy in detecting child abuse. *Semin Nucl Med* 1993;23:321–333.
154. Magid N, Glass T. A "hole in a rib" as a sign of child abuse. *Pediatr Radiol* 1990;20: 334–336.
155. Smeets AJ, Robben SGF, Meradji M. Sonographically detected costo-chondral dislocation in an abused child. *Pediatr Radiol* 1990;20:566–567.
156. Ng SC, Hall CM. Costochondral junction fractures and intra-abdominal trauma in non-accidental injury (child abuse). *Pediatr Radiol* 1998;28:671–676.
157. Cumming WA. Neonatal skeletal fractures: birth trauma or child abuse? *J Can Assoc Radiol* 1979;30:30–33.
158. Betz P, Liebhardt E. Rib fractures in children: resuscitation or child abuse? *Int J Legal Med* 1994;106:215–218.
159. Baker AM, Craig BR, Lonnergan GJ. Homicidal commotion cordis: the final blow in a battered infant. *Child Abuse Neglect* 2003;27:125–130.
160. McEniery J, Hanson R, Grigor W, et al. Lung injury resulting from a nonaccidental crush injury to the chest. *Pediatr Emerg Care* 1991;7:166–168.
161. Nichols GR II, Corey TS, Davis GJ. Case report: non-fracture-associated fatal fat embolism in a case of child abuse. *J Forensic Sci* 1990;35:493–499.
162. Carty H. Case report: child abuse—necklace calcification—of strangulation. *Br J Radiol* 1993;66:1186–1188.
163. Kleinman PK, Blackbourne BD, Marks SC, et al. Radiologic contributions to the investigation and prosecution of cases of fatal infant abuse. *N Engl J Med* 1989;320:507–511.
164. Kleinman PK, Marks SC, Richmond JM, et al. Inflicted skeletal injury: a postmortem radiologic–histopathologic study in 31 infants. *Am J Roentgenol* 1995;165:647–650.
165. Kleinman PK, Marks SC. Vertebral body fractures in child abuse: radiologic–histopathologic correlates. *Invest Radiol* 1992;27:715–722.
166. Swischuk LE. Spine and spinal cord trauma in the battered child syndrome. *Radiology* 1969;932:733–738.
167. Brown R, Brunn MA, Garcia VF. Cervical spine injuries in children: a review of 103 patients treated conservatively at a level 1 pediatric trauma center. *J Pediatr Surg* 2001; 36:1107–1114.
168. Thomas NH, Robinson L, Evans A, et al. The floppy infant: a new manifestation of nonacccidental injury. *Pediatr Neurosurg* 1995;23:188–191.
169. Kleinman PK, Shelton YA. Hangman's fracture in an abused infant: imaging features. *Pediatr Radiol* 1997;27:776–777.
170. Currarino G. Primary spondylolysis of the axis vertebrae (C-2) in three children, including one with pyknodysostosis. *Pediatr Radiol* 1989;19:535–538.
171. Ravindran RK, Mullett JH, Burke TE. Hangman's fracture caused by suspected child abuse: a case report. *J Pediatr Orthop B* 2002;11:329–332.
172. Rooks VJ, Sisler C, Burton B. Cervical spine injury in child abuse: a report of two cases. *Pediatr Radiol* 1998;28:193–195.
173. Carrion WV, Dormans JP, Drummond DS, et al. Circumferential growth plate fracture of the thoracolumbar spine from child abuse. *J Pediatr Orthop* 1996;16:210–214.
173a. Habert J, Haller JO. Iatrogenic vertebral body compression fracture in a premature infant caused by extreme flexion during positioning for a lumbar puncture. *Pediatr Radiol* 2000;30:410–411.
174. American College of Radiology. Imaging of the child with suspected child abuse. In: *American College of Radiology Standards for Skeletal Surveys in Children. Resolution 22*. Reston, VA: American College of Radiology; 1997;23.
175. Ellerstein NS, Norris KJ. Value of radiologic skeletal survey in assessment of abused children. *Pediatrics* 1984;74:1075–1078.
176. Sly JR, Starshak RJ. The role of bone scintigraphy in the evaluation of the suspected abused child. *Radiology* 1983;146:369–375.
177. Jaudes PK. Comparison of radiography and radionuclide bone scanning and the detection of child abuse. *Pediatrics* 1984;73:166–168.
178. Fordham EW, Ramachandran PC. Radionuclide imaging of osseous trauma. *Semin Nucl Med* 1974;4:411–429.
179. Youmans DC, Don S, Hidebolt C, et al. Skeletal surveys for child abuse: comparison of interpretation using digitized images and screen-film radiographs *Am J Roentgenol* 1998;171:1415–1419.
180. Kleinman PK, O'Connor B, Nimkin K, et al. Detection of rib fractures in an abused infant using digital radiography: a laboratory study. *Pediatr Radiol* 2002;32:896–901.
181. Markowitz RI, Hubbard AM, Harty MP, et al. Sonography of the knee in normal and abused infants. *Pediatr Radiol* 1993;23:264–267.
182. Rogers LF, Poznanski AK. Imaging of epiphyseal injuries. *Radiology* 1994;191:297–308.
183. Dreizen S, Spirakis CN, Stone RE. The influence of age and nutrition on "bone scar" formation in the distal end of the growing femur. *Am J Phys Anthropol* 1964;22: 295–306.
184. Edwards DK. Skeletal growth lines seen on radiographs of newborn infants: prevalence and possible association with obstetric abnormalities. *Am J Roentgenol* 1993;161: 141–145.
185. Kaplan JM. Pseudoabuse: the misdiagnosis of child abuse. *J Forensic Sci* 1986;31: 1420–1428.
186. Bernet W. False statements and the differential diagnosis of abuse allegations. *J Am Acad Child Adolesc Psychiatry* 1993;32:903–910.
187. American Academy of Child and Adolescent Psychiatry. *Policy Statement: Guidelines for the Clinical Evaluation of Child and Adolescent Sexual Abuse*. Washington, DC: American Academy of Child and Adolescent Psychiatry; 1990.
188. Kleinman PK, Belanger PL, Karellas A, et al. Normal metaphyseal radiologic variants not to be confused with findings of infant abuse. *Am J Roentgenol* 1991;156:781–783.
189. Zeiss J, Wycliffe ND, Cullen BJ, et al. Radiological case of the month. *Am J Dis Child* 1988;142:1367–1368.
190. DeRusso PA, Spevak MR, Schwarz KB. Fractures in biliary atresia misinterpreted as child abuse. *Pediatrics* 2003;112:185–188.

191. Chalumeau M, Fox-l'Helias L, Scheinmann P, et al. Rib fractures after chest physiotherapy for bronchiolitis or pneumonia in infants. *Pediatr Radiol* 2002;32:644–647.
192. Lim HK, Smith WL, Sato Y, et al. Congenital syphilis mimicking child abuse. *Pediatr Radiol* 1995;25:560–561.
193. Duncan AA, Chandry J. Case report: multiple neonatal fractures—dietary or deliberate? *Clin Radiol* 1993;48:137–139.
194. Harty MP, Kao SC. Intraosseous vascular access defect: fracture mimic in the skeletal survey for child abuse. *Pediatr Radiol* 2002;32:188–190.
195. Grayev AM, Boal DKB, Wallach DM, et al. Metaphyseal fractures mimicking abuse during treatment for clubfoot. *Pediatr Radiol* 2001;31:559–563.
196. McClain JL, Clark MA, Sandusky GE. Undiagnosed, untreated acute lymphoblastic leukemia presenting as suspected child abuse. *J Forensic Sci* 1990;35:735–739.
197. Newman RS, Jalili M, Kolls BJ, et al. Factor XIII deficiency mistaken for battered child syndrome: case of a commonly accepted qualitative test with limited negative predictive value. *Am J Hematol* 2002;71:328–330.
198. Patterson CR, Burns J, McAltion SJ. Osteogenesis imperfecta: the distinction from child abuse and the recognition of a variant form. *Am J Med Genet* 1993;45:187–192.
199. Sillence D. Osteogenesis imperfecta: an expanding panorama of variants. *Clin Orthop* 1981;159:11–25.
200. Sillence D, Butler B, Latham M, et al. Natural history of blue sclerae in osteogenesis imperfecta. *Am J Med Genet* 1993;45:183–186.
201. Albin DS, Greenspan A, Reinhart M et al. Differentiation of child abuse from osteogenesis imperfecta. *Am J Roentgenol* 1990;154:1035–1046.
202. Dent JA, Patterson CR. Fractures in early childhood: osteogenesis imperfecta or child abuse? *J Pediatr Orthop* 1991;11:184–186.
203. Shoenfeld Y, Fried A, Ehrenfeld NE. Osteogenesis imperfecta: review of the literature with presentation of 29 cases. *Am J Dis Child* 1975;129:679–687.
204. Ojima K, Matsumoto H, Hayase T, et al. An autopsy case of osteogenesis imperfecta initially suspected as child abuse. *Forensic Sci Int* 1994;65:97–104.
205. Gahagan S, Rimsza ME. Child abuse or osteogenesis imperfecta: how can we tell? *Pediatrics* 1991;88:987–991.
206. Byers PH. Disorders of collagen biosynthesis and structure. In: Scriver CR, Beaudet AL, Sly WS, et al, eds. *The Metabolic Basis of Inherited Disease*. New York: McGraw-Hill; 1989:2814–2824.
207. Steiner RD, Pepin M, Beyers PH. Studies of collagen synthesis and structure in the differentiation of child abuse from osteogenesis imperfecta. *J Pediatr* 1996;128:542–547.
208. Knight DJ, Bennet GC. Nonaccidental injury in osteogenesis imperfecta: a case report. *J Pediatr Orthop* 1990;10:542–544.
209. Albin D. Osteogenesis imperfecta: a review. *Can Assoc Radiol J* 1998;49:110–123.
210. Ablin DS, Sane SM. Non-accidental injury: confusion with temporary brittle bone disease and mild osteogenesis imperfecta. *Pediatr Radiol* 1997;27:111–113.
211. Chapman S, Hall CM. Non-accidental injury, or brittle bones. *Pediatr Radiol* 1997;27:106–110.
212. Miller M. Fractures during physical therapy [Letter]. *Pediatr Radiol* 2002;32:536–537.
213. Miller ME, Hangartner TN. Temporary brittle bone disease: association with decreased fetal movement and osteopenia. *Calcif Tissue Int* 1999;64:137–143.
214. Miller ME. Temporary brittle bone disease: a real entity? *Semin Perinatol* 1999;23:174–182.
215. Miller ME. Another perspective as to the cause of bone fractures in potential child abuse. *Pediatr Radiol* 2000;30:495–496.
216. Cazalet J. Note Re R (A Minor). Expert Evidence. [1991] 1 FLR 291.
217. Lynch MA. A judicial comment on temporary brittle bone disease [Letter]. *Arch Dis Child* 1995;73:379.
218. Meadow R. Unnatural sudden infant death. *Arch Dis Child* 1999;80:7–14.
219. Byard RW, Keeley FW, Smith CR. Type IV Ehlers-Danlos syndrome presenting as sudden infant death. *Am J Clin Pathol* 1990;93:579–582.
220. Sperry K, Pfalzgraf R. Inadvertent clavicular fractures caused by "chiropractic" manipulations in an infant: an unusual form of pseudoabuse. *J Forensic Sci* 1995;35:1211–1216.
221. Clayton EW. Potential liability in cases of child abuse and neglect. *Pediatr Ann* 1997;26:173–177.
222. Steinberg AM, Pynoos RS, Goenjian AK, et al. Are researchers bound by child abuse reporting laws? *Child Abuse Negl* 1999;8:771–777.
223. Halverson KC, Elliott BA, Rubin MS, et al. Legal considerations in cases of child abuse. *Primary Care* 1993;20:407–415.
224. Chadwick DL. Preparation for court testimony in child abuse cases. *Pediatr Clin North Am* 1990;37:955–970.
225. Drake JA. Physicians and attorneys: a partnership on behalf of the youngest victims of family violence. *Md Med J* 1994;43:365–367.
226. Brent RL. The irresponsible expert witness: a failure of biomedical graduate education and professional accountability. *Pediatrics* 1982;7:754–762.
227. Fluke JD, Yuan Y-Y, Edwards M. Recurrence of maltreatment: an application of the National Child Abuse and Neglect Data System (NCANDS). *Child Abuse Negl* 1999;23:633–650.
228. Murphy JM, Bishop SJ, Jellinek MS, et al. What happens after the care and protection petition? Reabuse in a court sample. *Child Abuse Negl* 1992;16:485–493.
229. Handy TC, Nichols GR II, Smock WS. Repeat visitors to a pediatric forensic medicine program. *J Forensic Sci* 1996;41:841–844.
230. Smith PB, Poertner J, Fields JD. Preventing child abuse and neglect in Texas. *Texas Med* 1990;86:44–45.

RECOMMENDED READING

Two references invaluable for preparation for testimony in the courtroom about child abuse:

Chadwick DL. Preparation for court testimony in child abuse cases. *Pediatr Clin North Am* 1990;37:955–970.

Halverson KC, Elliott BA, Rubin MS, et al. Legal considerations in cases of child abuse. *Primary Care* 1993;20:407–415.

The bible of child abuse radiology:

Kleinman PK. Diagnostic imaging of child abuse, 2nd ed. St. Louis: Mosby; 1998.

A current, concise review of the orthopaedic detection of child abuse:

Kocher MS, Kasser JR. Orthopaedic aspects of child abuse. *J Am Acad Orthop Surg* 2000;8:10–20.

A handy reference for courtroom testimony involving dating fractures:

O'Connor JF, Cohen J. Dating fractures. In: Kleinman PK, ed. *Diagnostic Imaging of Child Abuse*. Baltimore: Williams & Wilkins, 1987.

SECTION

TWO

UPPER EXTREMITY

FRACTURES AND DISLOCATIONS OF THE HAND AND CARPUS IN CHILDREN

Scott H. Kozin and Peter M. Waters

PEDIATRIC HAND INJURIES

Epidemiology

Incidence

The pediatric hand is vulnerable to injury for several reasons. Usage pattern of the exposed hand and the child's curiosity about the surrounding world are prime factors. Youngsters often are unaware of dangers and place their hands in vulnerable situations (1–5). Hand and wrist injuries account for up to 25% of pediatric fractures (Table 8-1) (2,6,7). The annual incidence is approximately 26.4 fractures per 10,000 children (4).

Biphasic Distribution

Pediatric hand fractures occur primarily in two distinct age groups, the toddler and the adolescent. In the toddler age group, the injury usually is secondary to a crush (2–4,8–10), often involving a finger caught in a closing door. In the adolescent age group, the injury is most commonly from participation in sports (2,11–17). Football and skiing are prime examples of sports prone to athletic hand injuries (12,18,19). Hand fractures in children peak around age 13, which coincides with active participation in organized contact sports (Fig. 8-1).

TABLE 8-1 Incidence of Pediatric Hand Injuries

Peak age: 13 years
Annual incidence: 26.4 per 10,000 children
Percentage of all pediatric emergency patients: 1.7%
Right side incidence equals left
Male incidence is greater than female incidence
Most common areas Nonphyseal: distal phalanx (crush) Physeal: proximal phalanx
Index and small fingers most commonly injured

Incidence of Specific Fractures

The most common fractures are distal phalangeal crush injuries and Salter-Harris (S-H) II fractures of the proximal phalangeal base (2–4,7,20,21). The border digits (index and small fingers) are the most commonly injured rays (1–4,20,21). Although dislocations of the pediatric hand are relatively uncommon injuries, the metacarpal-phalangeal (MCP) joint is the most commonly dislocated joint in the immature hand (22–25) and the proximal interphalangeal (PIP) joint most commonly injured joint from volar plate tears.

Incidence of Physeal Fractures

Fracture forces often are transmitted through the physis in a child's hand because this course is the path of least resistance (2–4,8,14,26). A S-H II fractures is the predominate type of phalangeal fracture and the proximal phalanx is the most commonly injured bone.

Anatomy of the Immature Hand

Adults and children have disparate patterns of hand injury because of different usage patterns and differences in underlying skeleton and soft-tissue composition. Knowledge of the architecture of the physis, the soft tissue origins and insertions, and the surrounding periosteum is useful for recognition and treatment of children's hand fractures.

Osseous Anatomy

There are potential epiphyses at both the proximal and distal ends of all the tubular hand bones. Secondary ossification centers, however, develop only at the distal ends of the metacarpals of the index, long, ring, and small rays, and at the proximal end of the thumb. Conversely, the secondary centers of ossification are present only at the proximal ends of the phalanges in all digits (27,28).

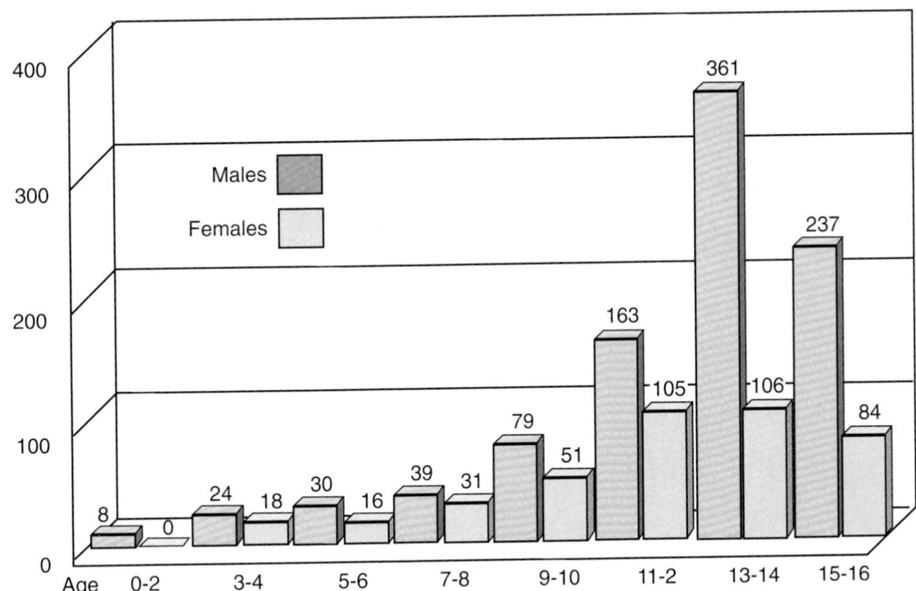

FIGURE 8-1 Total number of fractures of the hand, 1970–1975, Malmo, Sweden. (Reprinted from Landin LA. Fracture patterns in children. *Acta Orthop Scand Suppl* 1983;202:54, with permission.)

Secondary Ossification Centers

In boys, the secondary ossification centers within the proximal phalanges appear at 15 to 24 months and fuse at bone age of 16 years (Fig. 8-2) (27,28). In girls, the appearance and fusion occur earlier, at 10 to 15 months and bone age of 14 years, respectively. The appearance of the secondary ossification centers of the middle and distal phalanges is later than the proximal phalanx, usually by 6 to 8 months. Fusion of the secondary ossification centers, however, occurs from distal to proximal.

Within the metacarpal, the secondary ossification centers appear at 18 to 27 months in boys and at 12 to 17 months in girls. The proximal thumb metacarpal secondary ossification center appears 6 to 12 months after the fingers. The secondary centers within the metacarpals fuse between 14 to 16 years of age in girls and boys.

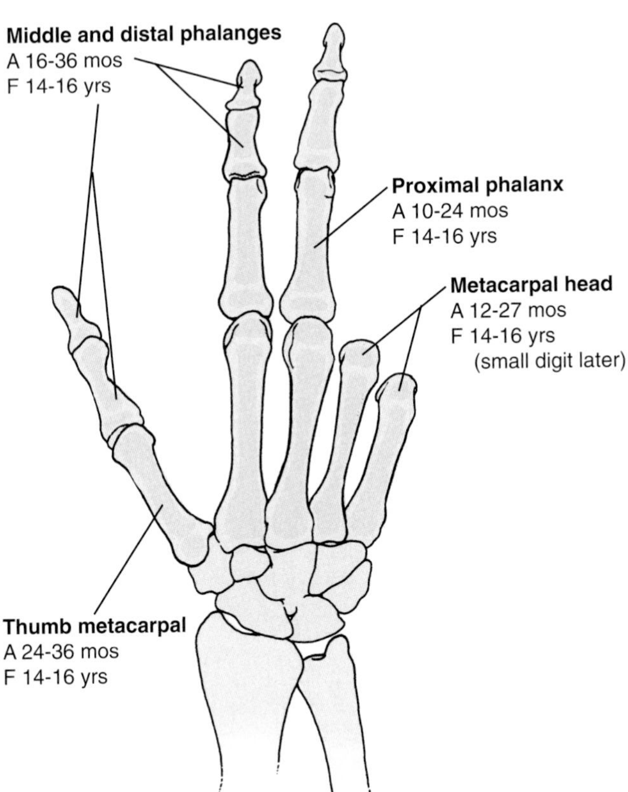

FIGURE 8-2 Appearance of secondary ossification centers (*A*). Fusion of secondary centers to the primary centers (*F*).

Physeal Anatomy

The anatomy of the physis has direct impact on fracture geometry (29). The zone of chondrocyte hypertrophy (zone III) is the least resistant to mechanical stresses. This zone is devoid of the collagen that provides inherent stabilizing properties. The collagen is present in zones I and II, and the calcium present in zone IV provides similar structural strength (7,30). Therefore, the fracture often propagates through the zone of chondrocyte hypertrophy (zone III) as the path of least resistance.

The irregularity of the physeal zones increases near skeletal maturity (29). Thus, a fracture line may be transmitted through several zones. This variable path through irregular topography may contribute to partial growth arrest after adolescent fractures that involve the physis. This change in irregularity also explains the differing patterns of physeal injuries dependent on age: S-H I and II fractures tend to occur in younger patients compared to S-H III or IV fractures, which are more prevalent in children close to skeletal maturity (6,31).

Pseudoepiphyses and Double Epiphyses

A persistent expression of the distal epiphysis of the thumb metacarpal is called a pseudoepiphysis (32). The pseudoepi-

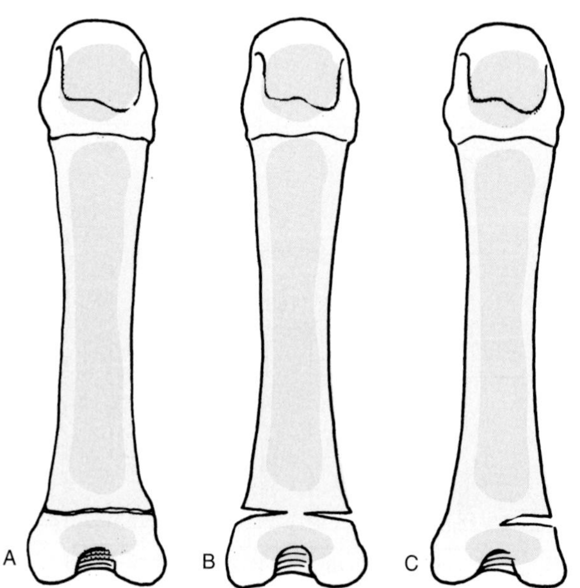

FIGURE 8-3 Abnormal epiphyseal appearance. **A.** Double epiphysis. **B.** Pseudoepiphysis. **C.** Notched epiphysis.

physis appears earlier than the proximal epiphysis and fuses rapidly. By the sixth or seventh year, the pseudoepiphysis is incorporated within the metacarpal and is inconspicuous. Pseudoepiphyses also have been noted at the proximal ends of the finger metacarpals, usually of the index ray. The only clinical significance is differentiation from an acute fracture (Fig. 8-3).

Double epiphyses can be present in any bone of the hand, but these anomalies are more common in the metacarpals of the index finger and thumb. There are variable expressions of double epiphyses, but the true entity is considered only when a fully developed growth mechanism is present on both ends of a tubular bone. Double epiphyses usually are seen in children with other congenital anomalies, but their presence does not appear to influence overall bone growth. When fractures occur in bones with double epiphyses, growth of the involved bone appears to be accelerated (33).

Double epiphyses must be delineated from a pseudoepiphysis or metaphyseal "notching" (32–35). Periphyseal notching can be confused with trauma or double epiphyses. The location of the notches can coincide with the physis or may be slightly more distant from the epiphysis. Notching is a benign condition that does not influence the structural properties of the bone (33).

Soft-Tissue Anatomy

The tensile strength of a child's soft tissues usually exceeds that of the adjacent physis and epiphysis (36). For this reason, ligament ruptures and tendon avulsions are uncommon compared to physeal or epiphyseal fractures (37,38).

Tendons

The extensor tendons insert onto the epiphyses. The terminal tendon of the digital extensor mechanism and the extensor pollicis longus insert on the epiphyses of the distal phalanx. The

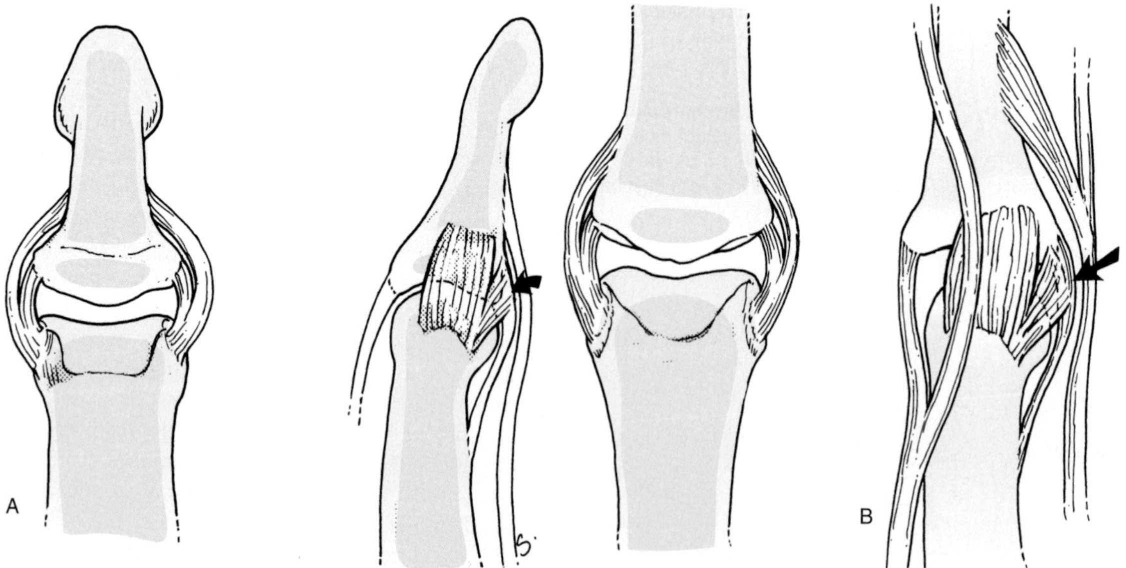

FIGURE 8-4 Anatomy of the collateral ligaments at the distal **(A)** and proximal **(B)** interphalangeal joints. The collateral ligaments at the interphalangeal joints originate in the collateral recesses and insert into both the metaphyses and epiphyses of their respective middle and distal phalanges. Additional insertion into the volar plane (*arrows*) is seen at the the interphalangeal joints.

central slip of the extensor mechanism inserts onto the epiphysis of the middle phalanx. The extensor pollicis brevis inserts onto the epiphysis of the proximal phalanx. The abductor pollicis longus has a broad-based insertion onto both the epiphysis and metaphysis of the thumb metacarpal. The extensor digitorum communis inserts onto the sagittal band at the MCP joint, which in turn lifts the proximal phalanx into extension by its insertion volarly.

The flexor tendons do not insert onto the epiphyses. The long digital flexor tendons (the flexor digitorum profundus and the flexor pollicis longus) insert into the metadiaphyseal region of their respective terminal phalanges (39). The flexor digitorum superficialis inserts onto the central three fifths of the middle phalanx.

Collateral Ligaments

The collateral ligaments about the interphalangeal joint originate from the collateral recesses of the phalangeal head, span the physis, and insert onto both the metaphysis and epiphysis of the middle and distal phalanges (Fig. 8-4). The collaterals also insert onto the volar plate to create a three-sided box that protects the physes and epiphyses of the interphalangeal joints from laterally directed forces (22). This configuration explains the rarity of S-H III injuries at the interphalangeal joints.

The collateral ligaments about the MCP joints originate from the metacarpal epiphysis and insert almost exclusively onto the epiphysis of the proximal phalanx (Fig. 8-5). This anatomic arrangement accounts for the frequency of S-H III injuries at the MCP joint level. Some fibers may originate from the distal metaphysis of the metacarpal, but this represents only a minor component of the ligament. The ligamentous anatomy about the thumb MCP joint more closely resembles that of the interphalangeal joints, which mirrors the arrangement of the adjacent physes.

Volar Plate

The volar plate is a stout stabilizer of the interphalangeal joint and MCP joints and resists hyperextension forces. The volar plate originates from the metaphysis of the respective proximal digital segment and inserts onto the epiphysis of the distal segment (Fig. 8-4B). The plate receives insertional fibers from the accessory collateral ligaments to create a three-sided box that protects the joint.

Periosteum

The periosteum is robust in a child's hand and can act as a considerable asset or liability in fracture management. The periosteal sleeve can minimize fracture displacement, aid in fracture reduction, or interpose between displaced fracture fragments and prevent reduction.

Remodeling

Children's ability to remodel must be considered during fracture management. Factors that influence remodeling are the patient's age, the proximity of the fracture to the physis, and the plane of motion of the adjacent joint and the plane of malalignment (40). The remodeling capacity is greater in younger children, fractures near a physis, and deformity in the plane of motion (7,31,41,42). Several clinicians have observed remodeling between 20 to 30 degrees in the sagittal plane in children under 10 years of age and about 10 to 20 degrees in older children (26,43). Remodeling in the coronal or adduction-abduction plane is considerably reduced compared to the sagittal plane. The amount is rarely quantified but is probably 50% or less than remodeling in the sagittal plane. Rotational remodeling does not occur.

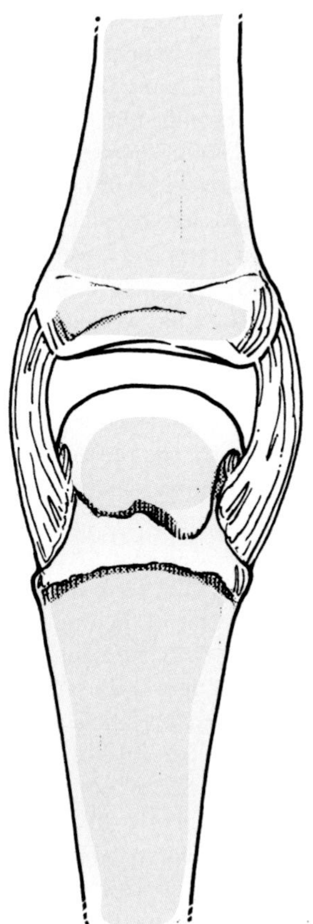

FIGURE 8-5 The collateral ligaments at the metacarpophalangeal joint both originate and insert almost exclusively on the epiphyseal regions of the metacarpal and the proximal phalanx.

EVALUATION OF PEDIATRIC HAND INJURIES

Clinical Examination

The evaluation of a child is more difficult than an adult, especially infants and toddlers. The child frequently is noncompliant, unable to understand instructions, and fearful of the physician. The physician must be patient and engage the child.

Observation and play are the mainstays of the examination. The child's hand posture and movements provide clues about the location and severity of the injury as the child interacts with toys, parents, and the environment in the examining area. Fracture is diagnosed by swelling, ecchymosis, deformity, or limited movement. Fracture rotation is noted by digital scissoring during active grasp or passive tenodesis. Tendon integrity is observed by digital posture at rest and during active grasp around objects of varying size. Comparison to the noninjured hand is invaluable. In a frightened child with an acute injury, passive wrist motion to assess tenodesis for digital alignment and cascade is critical to an accurate diagnosis. A hurried exam or frightened child can lead to a missed malrotated fracture.

After the child is relaxed, the physician may palpate areas of tenderness and move injured joints to assess their integrity. Stress testing should be gentle, and joint stability should be recorded in the anteroposterior and lateral directions. Neurologic injuries are especially difficult to detect in a young child. Excessive bleeding at the time of the original injury or during evaluation in the emergency department are clues to a nerve injury. The proper digital artery is dorsal to the proper digital nerve within the finger. Therefore, there is a high concordance between pulsatile bleeding indicative of a digital artery injury and laceration of the digital nerve.

Sensory function is particularly difficult to determine in a young child. Normal discriminatory sensibility developmentally has not occurred at ages 5 to 7 years. Therefore, meaningful objective data is not obtainable and gross observations, such as withdrawal to stimuli, are inadequate grounds on which to base therapeutic decisions. A helpful examination maneuver to assess nerve integrity is the wrinkle test. Immersion of an innervated digit in warm water for 5 minutes or more usually results in corrugation or wrinkling of the volar skin of the tuft. Wrinkling often is absent in a denervated digit. True objective sensibility testing requires patient cooperation and maturity. Repeat testing of multiple uninjured digits is necessary to ensure the validity of two-point discrimination. If there is doubt, operative exploration is appropriate.

Radiographic Examination

A careful clinical evaluation is a prerequisite for conducting a proper radiographic examination. Localization of areas of tenderness or deformity directs a thorough radiographic assessment. Several pediatric imaging factors complicate interpretation of plain x-rays, including lack of bony detail and normal variations. The normal ossification pattern of the immature hand creates problems with the detection of fractures and also promotes false interpretation of ligamentous injuries. Uncertain interpretation requires comparison to the noninjured hand or consultation with a pediatric atlas of child development and normal radiographic variants (27,28).

Anteroposterior, lateral, and oblique views are needed for complete evaluation of the injured hand or digit. The phalangeal line test is useful in recognizing displaced fractures and joint malalignment. If a line is drawn from the center of the phalangeal neck through the center of the phalangeal metaphysis at the level of the physis, it should pass through the exact center of the metacarpal or phalangeal head in a normal finger, regardless of joint flexion (Fig. 8-6) (44). Oblique views are particularly useful for assessing displacement and intra-articular extension. A common x-ray pitfall is failure to obtain a true lateral x-ray of the injured digit. Isolation of the affected digit on the film or splaying of the fingers projects a true lateral view. Stress views are rarely used for fracture evaluation. Mini-fluoroscopy units are invaluable and allow a real-time assessment of articular congruity and joint stability. These units have considerable advantages, including the ability to obtain multiple views, and stress views with low-radiation exposure for the patient and physician.

Differential Diagnosis

The differential diagnosis includes nontraumatic entities that may be interpreted as acute injuries. These diagnoses are uncommon but may cause swelling, deformity, or decreased motion.

Congenital

A Kirner deformity is a palmar and radial curving of the terminal phalanx of the small digit distal phalanx. This deformity occurs spontaneously between the ages of 8 and 14 years and may be confused with an acute fracture or epiphyseal separation (Fig. 8-7) (45). A Kirner deformity, however, usually is bilateral and not associated with trauma (46). A trigger thumb in a young child sometimes is mistaken for an interphalangeal joint dislocation because of the fixed flexion posture. The key diagnostic feature of a trigger thumb is the palpable nodule over the A1 pulley.

Thermal Injury

Thermal injury to the growing hand (e.g., frostbite, burns from flame or radiation) may cause bizarre deformities from altered appositional and interstitial bone growth. An ischemic necrosis of the physes and epiphyses may result (Fig. 8-8). The clinical result may yield altered bone width, length, or angulation secondary to the unpredictable effect on the growing elements that make interpretation of subsequent trauma difficult (47,48).

Osteochondrosis (Thiemann Disease)

Osteochondrosis of the phalangeal epiphyses may cause epiphyseal narrowing and fragmentation, which are characteristic of Thiemann disease. This hereditary entity usually involves the middle and distal phalanges and typically resolves without treatment, although some permanent joint deformity has been reported (49,50).

Tumors

A tumor may be discovered after fracture of the weakened bone or confused with fracture secondary to swelling and pain. An

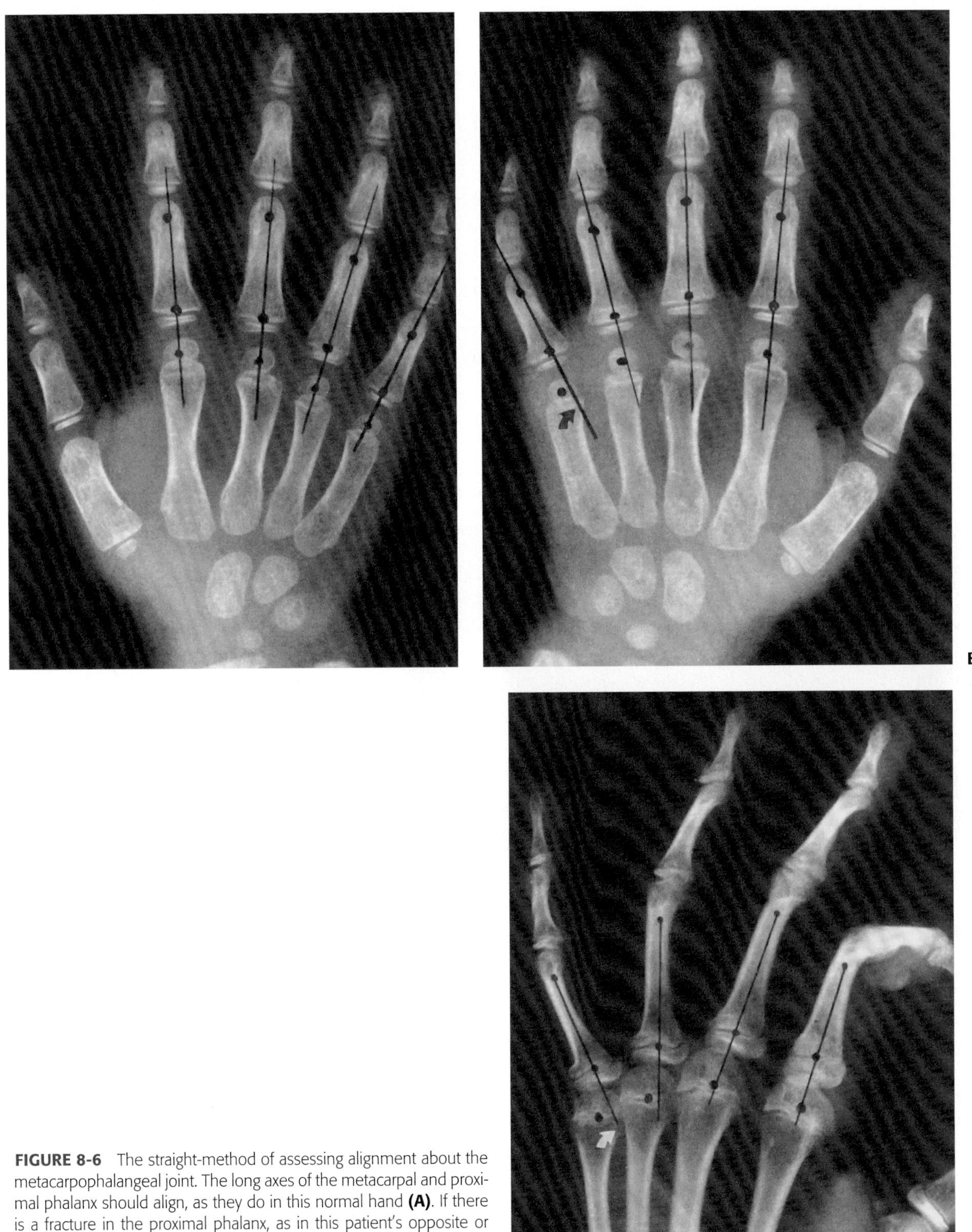

FIGURE 8-6 The straight-method of assessing alignment about the metacarpophalangeal joint. The long axes of the metacarpal and proximal phalanx should align, as they do in this normal hand **(A)**. If there is a fracture in the proximal phalanx, as in this patient's opposite or injured hand **(B,C)**, the axes will not be colinear (*arrows*). (Courtesy of Robert M. Campbell, Jr., MD.)

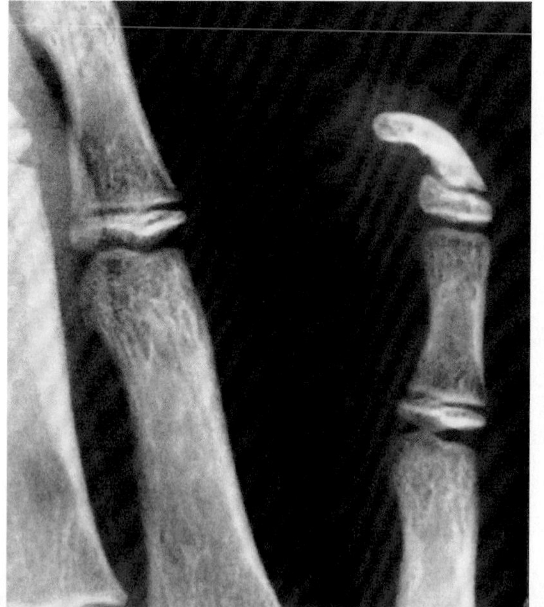

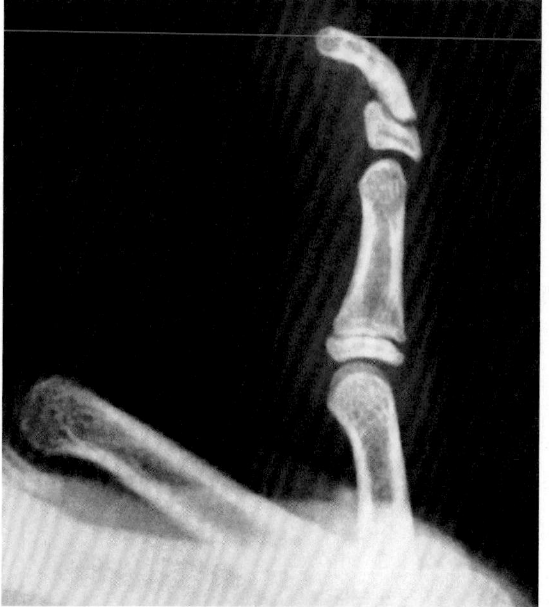

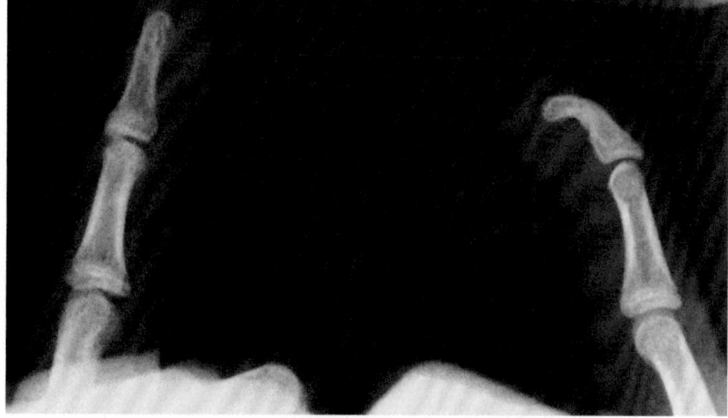

FIGURE 8-7 A,B. A 12-year-old boy with incurving of the tip of the right small finger. The anteroposterior and lateral x-rays show radial and palmar incurving of the distal phalanx, characteristic of Kirner's deformity. **C.** Two years later, healing has occurred, but the deformity has persisted.

enchondroma of the proximal phalanx is the classic benign tumor that may fracture after trivial trauma. The malignant bone, cartilage, or muscle tumors are rare. X-rays reveal intrinsic destructive bony changes in an osteogenic sarcoma or extrinsic compression with adjacent periosteal reaction secondary to an adjacent rhabdomyosarcoma.

Inflammatory and Infectious Processes

Dactylitis from sickle cell anemia can masquerade as a traumatic injury. The affected digit(s) presents with fusiform swelling and decreased motion. The medical history usually is positive for sickle cell disease. The inflammatory arthropathies (e.g., juvenile rheumatoid arthritis, psoariatic arthritis, scleroderma, systemic lupus) may be confused with trauma. A joint effusion and tenosynovitis are common findings that require further diagnostic evaluation. Aside from standard laboratory testing, magnetic resonance imaging is important for diagnosis of an inflammatory synovitis or tenosynovitis. An infectious process often can be mistaken for injury, although local and systemic evaluation usually ascertains this diagnosis.

GENERAL PRINCIPLES OF TREATMENT

Nonoperative Management

Most children's hand fractures can be treated without surgery. Children have a remarkable ability to remodel moderate fracture malalignment in the coronal and sagittal planes. In contrast, children cannot remodel malrotation, which requires reduction and stabilization to prevent digital scissoring. It is essential that the clinician properly diagnose and adequately treat the problematic fractures. Anesthesia is required for fracture reduction. Conscious sedation, regional anesthesia, and general anesthesia are alternatives. A digital block may be used for finger fracture reduction in adolescents. Rapid fracture manipulation without anesthesia should be avoided. Immobilization is best applied

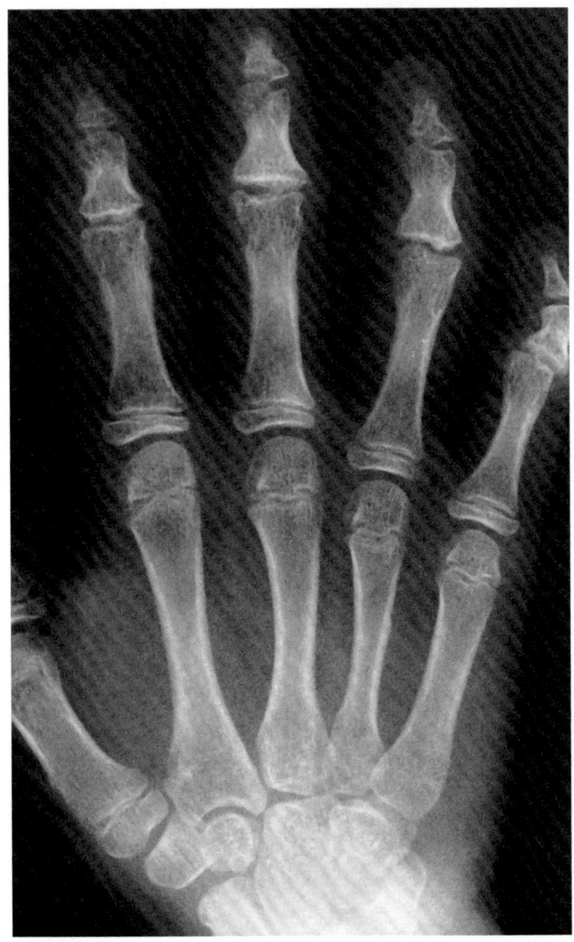

FIGURE 8-8 An 11-year-old girl sustained a frostbite injury to the right hand. X-ray reveals premature fusion of the physis of the distal and proximal phalanges with irregularity of the bases of the shortened phalanges.

immediately after reduction. The choice of splint or a cast depends on the degree of swelling, the difficulty of reduction, and the age of the patient. The amount of padding is an important consideration during cast application. Too much padding renders the cast ineffective in maintaining the reduction. In contrast, too little padding may cause skin compromise from thermal injury or direct pressure. The use of rigid materials other than accepted casting materials (e.g., tongue blades, arm boards, metal rods) should be discouraged. Immobilization of a solitary digit in a child should be avoided because it is ineffective.

Fractures of the phalanges and metacarpals require immobilization of the injured digit with at least one of the adjacent digits. Similar to the adult hand, the child's hand is best immobilized in the "safe position" with the MCP joints in flexion and the interphalangeal joints in extension. Short-arm immobilization usually is adequate for hand fractures, provided cooperation is reasonable. Fractures in infants and toddlers require long-arm immobilization to encircle the elbow and decrease the chances of escaping from the cast.

Fractures that are truly nondisplaced are treated with immobilization and reevaluation in 3 to 4 weeks for cast or splint removal. Fractures that required reduction necessitate weekly evaluation to ensure maintenance of alignment. The first evaluation should be within a week to allow detection of recurrent displacement and provide ample time to perform repeat reduction before the rapid healing that occurs in children. To assess for maloration, it is necessary to remove the immobilization and check alignment by tenodesis and active motion because x-rays can be misleading regarding rotational alignment. An unstable malaligned fracture should be treated aggressively with pin fixation to avoid malunion.

Children's fractures possess a remarkable propensity to heal. Therefore, delayed union and nonunion are uncommon problems except after open fractures or open surgery that disrupts the inherent blood supply. A frequent concern is growth arrest following a physeal injury. The arrest usually is secondary to the initial injury, although repeated manipulations impart additional trauma to the damaged physis and should be avoided. Growth arrests are very rare and usually associated with a dysvascular or infectious situation related to the trauma.

Surgical Management

Surgery in children is different than that in adults. There are inherent differences in anatomy that require special consideration. The periosteum is thick and periosteal flaps can be created and later approximated to enhance healing and remodeling. The periosteal layer also provides an excellent cover for implants and a good sliding surface for tendons.

The physis requires meticulous respect. Surgical dissection around the physis should be minimized to avoid injury. Fixation across a physis requires thoughtful consideration concerning growth arrest. When fixation is necessary, the smallest diameter nonthreaded wire that effectively holds the fracture fragments should be used. Implants, such as plates, should also avoid the physis.

Rehabilitation

Following fracture union, formalized therapy rarely is necessary. Simple liberation from immobilization and instructions to the patient and parents regarding range of motion, strengthening, and activity return usually are sufficient. In uncommon circumstances (e.g., complicated fractures or multiple trauma), formal hand therapy is indicated.

Complications

Complications from pediatric hand fractures are relatively uncommon. However, the physician should avoid being nonchalant in thinking that the pediatric hand is forgiving in its ability to remodel and regain motion. Recognition of the potential pitfalls is important, as is the development of a systematic plan for rectifying complications.

The most common complication of pediatric hand fractures is failure to diagnose the fracture or an under appreciation of the extent of injury. Anteroposterior, lateral, and oblique x-rays are needed for complete evaluation of the injured hand or digit. Imaging of the contralateral hand for comparison and consultation with a pediatric atlas of child development and normal radiographic variants (27,28) should be done whenever the diagnosis is in question.

Once the fracture is recognized, the appropriate treatment is instituted to ensure anatomic healing and return of normal function. Displacement or rotation at the fracture site may be subtle on x-rays. Inspection of the x-rays and a meticulous examination are necessary. Finger fractures must be scrutinized for evidence of malrotation by evaluating the plane of the fingernails with the fingers semi-flexed by tenodesis or active motion. A malrotated or markedly displaced fracture requires reduction under anesthesia to regain bony alignment. The degree of reduction required depends on the configuration, location, and extent of the fracture as well as the age of the child. Although sagittal and coronal remodeling can occur in the immature skeleton, roational malalignment will not remodel (51).

SPECIFIC FRACTURES OF THE PEDIATRIC HAND

Fractures of the Distal Phalanx

Relevant Anatomy

The skin, nail elements, soft tissues, and bone of the distal digit are closely related (Fig. 8-9). The dorsal periosteum of the distal phalanx is the underlying nutritional and structural support for the sterile matrix and nail bed. The germinal matrix is responsible for generating the nail plate. The volar aspect of the distal phalanx anchors the pulp through tough, fibrous septae that stabilize the skin against shear forces. The terminal extensor tendon inserts onto the epiphysis of the distal phalanx. The flexor digitorum profundus bypasses the physis to insert onto the metadiaphysis of the distal phalanx.

Mechanism of Injury

The primary mechanisms of injury are crush, hyperflexion, and hyperextension. A crush injury creates a spectrum of injury from minor tissue disruption with little need for intervention to severe tissue trauma that requires bony fixation, meticulous nail bed repair, and skin coverage (Fig. 8-10). A flexion force applied to the extended tip of the finger results in a mallet injury. The distal interphalangeal (DIP) joint rests in flexion and active extension is impossible. A hyperextension force can produce a bony avulsion injury of the flexor digitorum profundus tendon (pediatric jersey finger).

Fracture Patterns

Fractures of the distal phalanx can be divided into extraphyseal and physeal injuries (Table 8-2). Extraphyseal fractures are common and range from a simple distal tuft fracture to an unstable diaphyseal fracture underlying a nail bed laceration. The fracture pattern can be divided into three types (Fig. 8-11). A transverse fracture (Fig. 8-11A) may occur either at the distal extent of the terminal phalanx or through the diaphysis. Displaced transverse fractures through the diaphysis are almost

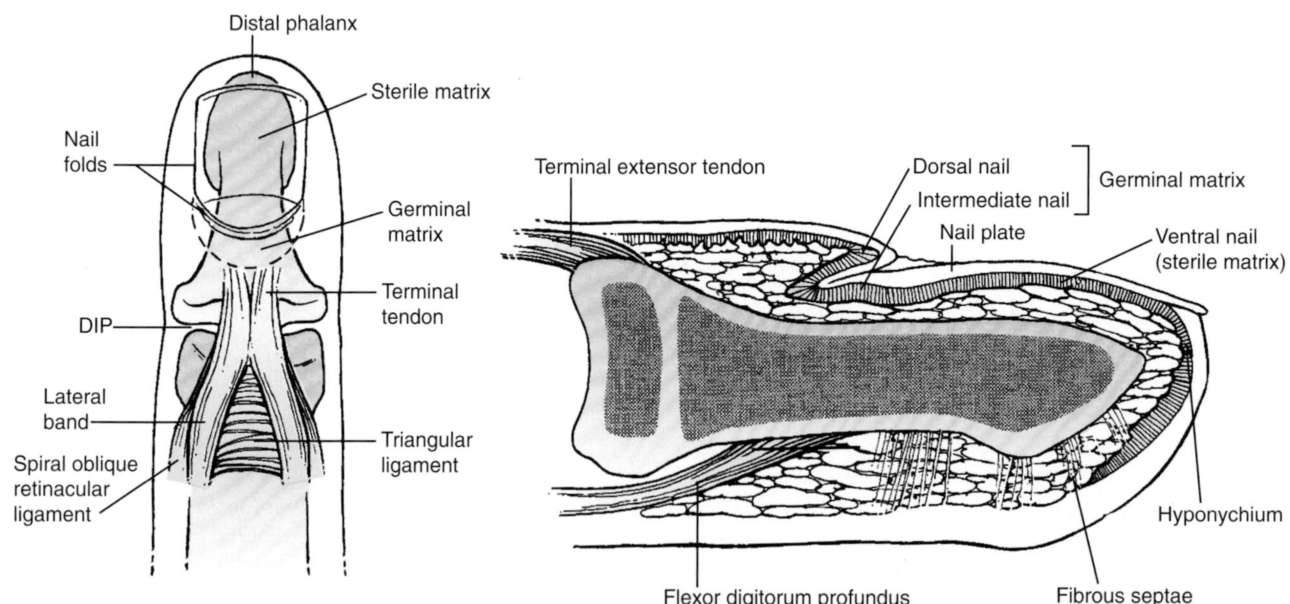

FIGURE 8-9 Anatomy about the distal phalanx. **A.** The skin, nail, and extensor apparatus share a close relationship with the bone of the distal phalanx. Specific anatomic structures at the terminal aspect of the digit are labeled. **B.** This lateral view of the nail demonstrates the tendon insertions and the anatomy of the specialized nail tissues.

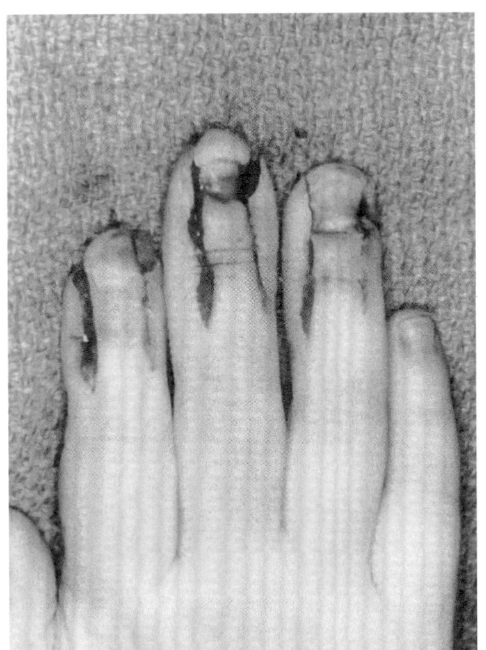

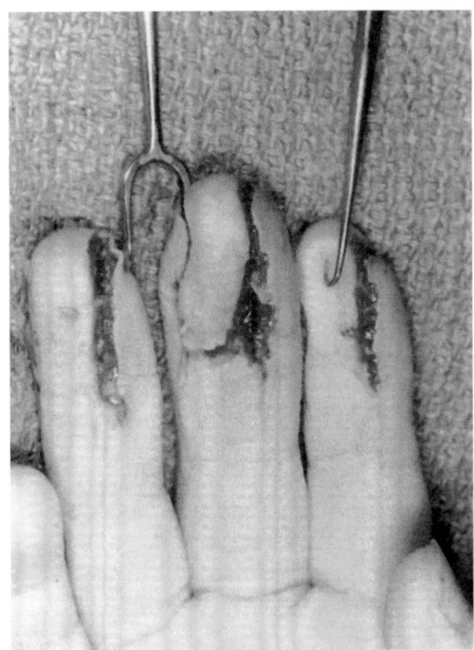

FIGURE 8-10 A,B. Crush injury to the fingers of a 4-year-old with nail bed laceration requiring meticulous repair with absorbable suture.

always associated with a considerable nail bed injury that requires repair. A longitudinal splitting type fracture is much less common (Fig. 8-11B). This pattern is the result of excessive hoop stress within the tubular distal phalanx at the time of a crush injury. The "cloven-hoof" appearance of the fracture is characteristic (Fig. 8-12). The fracture may be contained within the shaft or can propagate through the physis and even into the joint (10). A comminuted fracture of the distal diaphysis also can occur and usually is accompanied by extensive soft-tissue injury (Figs. 8-11C and 8-13).

A less common etiology of extraphyseal fracture is forced extension of the flexed DIP joint. This mechanism can result in either a bony avulsion injury or a soft-tissue disruption of the flexor digitorum profundus (Fig. 8-14) (52,53). An avulsion fracture often limits flexor digitorum profundus retraction in the pulley system by tethering of the bone fragment on the A5 or A4 pulley. The radiographic location of the bony fragment identifies the level of tendon retraction. In contrast, soft-tissue disruption of the flexor digitorum profundus frequently retracts into the palm. Diagnosis of this situation often is missed acutely.

TABLE 8-2 Classification of Distal Phalanx Fractures

Extraphyseal (see Fig. 8-10)
- Transverse diaphysis
- Longitudinal splitting
- Comminuted separations
- Avulsion of flexor with bone (jersey finger) (see Fig. 8-14)

Physeal

Dorsal mallet injuries (see Fig. 8-13)
- Salter-Harris I or II
- Salter-Harris III or IV
- Salter-Harris I or II joint dislocation
- Avulsion of extensor + Salter-Harris fracture

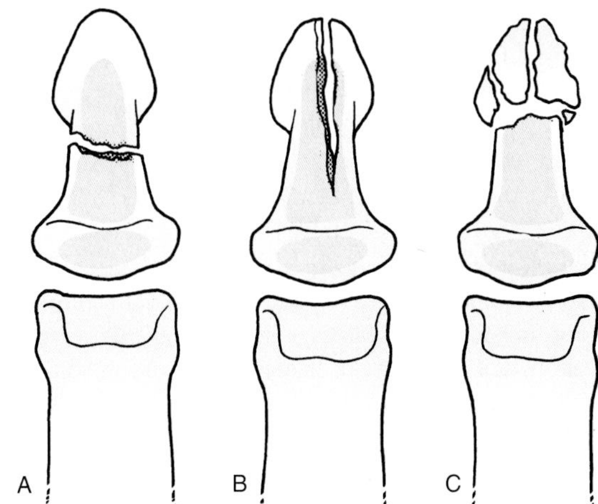

FIGURE 8-11 Three types of extraepiphyseal fractures of the distal phalanx. **A.** Transverse diaphyseal fracture. **B.** Cloven-hoof longitudinal splitting fracture. **C.** Comminuted distal tuft fracture with radial fracture lines.

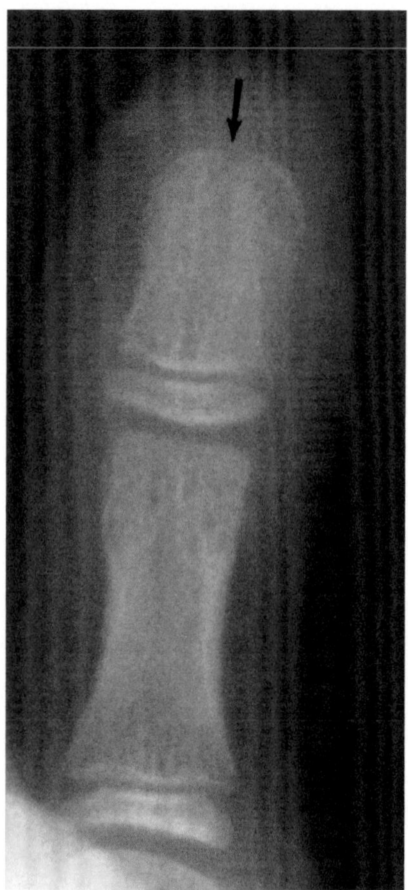

FIGURE 8-12 Extraepiphyseal fracture of the distal phalanx, the cloven-hoof longitudinal splitting fracture. In this patient, the fracture line (*arrow*) does not appear to extend across the physis.

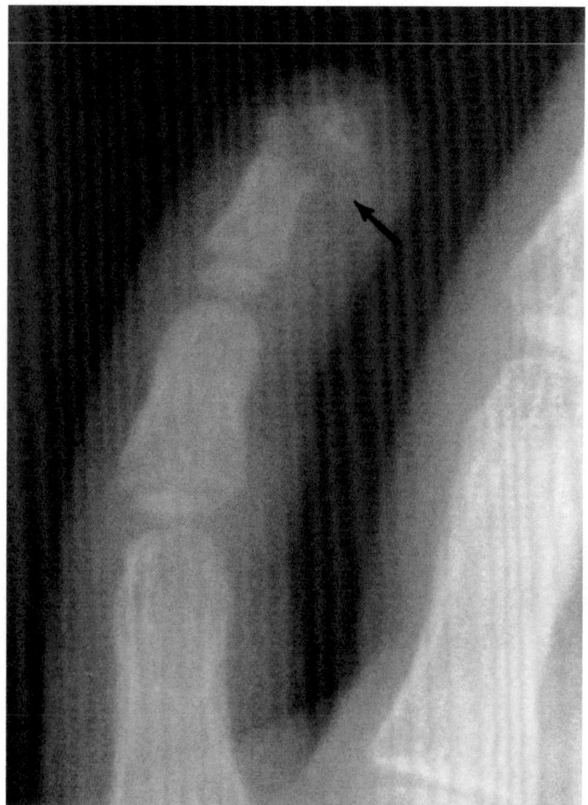

FIGURE 8-13 Extraepiphyseal distal phalangeal fracture. The fracture line is distal to the insertion of the flexor digitorum profundus tendon. The accompanying soft-tissue disruption (*arrow*) can be seen.

Physeal fractures clinically resemble a mallet finger. There are four basic fracture patterns and all result in a flexed posture of the DIP joint (Fig. 8-15). A S-H I or II fracture with flexion of the distal fragment occurs predominantly in young patients less than 12 years of age. The unopposed flexor digitorum profundus flexes the distal fragment. The injury often is open and associated with a nail bed injury. There is a high risk for incarceration of the germinal or sterile matrix in the fracture site, known as a Seymour fracture (54). Closed reduction may be blocked by interposition of the nail bed in the dorsal physis deep to the nail plate. Rarely, a S-H I or II fracture causes extrusion of the epiphyseal fragment (5,55). This "epiphyseal dislocation" is challenging to diagnose with an unossified epiphysis because the remaining distal phalanx remains colinear with the axis of the digit, whereas the displaced unossified epiphysis is dorsally dislocated by traction produced by the extensor tendon. A dorsal Salter-Harris III fracture of the distal phalanx occurs in teenagers and results in an extension lag at the DIP joint. Rarely, the epiphysis also may separate from the terminal extensor tendon (56).

Diagnosis

Signs and Symptoms

The diagnosis usually is straightforward. The history and physical examination are consistent with a distal phalanx fracture. A nail bed injury or a subungual hematoma greater than 50% creates a high index of suspicion for bony injury (Fig. 8-16) (57). X-rays are confirmatory and detail the fracture pattern. Anteroposterior and lateral views of the distal phalanx are necessary to ascertain fracture configuration.

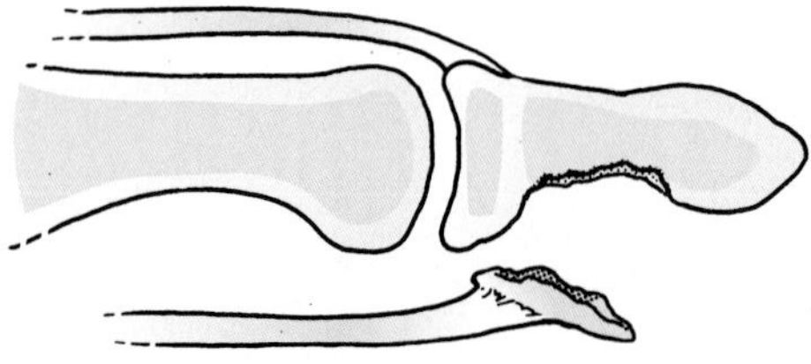

FIGURE 8-14 Flexor digitorum profundus avulsion fracture of the distal phalanx (jersey finger). This bony avulsion is apparent on x-rays, indicating the extent of proximal migration.

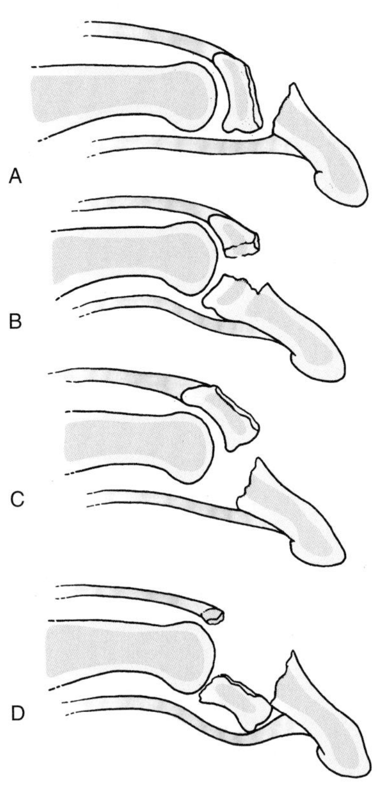

FIGURE 8-15 **A–D.** Mallet-equivalent fracture types.

Treatment Options

Fractures associated with nail bed lacerations require attention to the soft-tissue and bony injuries. The soft-tissue repair is as critical to outcome as the bony treatment. Any substantial nail bed laceration requires repair. The distal phalangeal fracture is assessed for alignment and stability. An unstable fracture that cannot support the nail bed necessitates stabilization.

Nonoperative Management

Most distal phalangeal fractures can be treated with nonoperative measures using a splint or cast. Mild and moderate displacement of extraphyseal fractures will heal without difficulty. Even physeal injuries with mild displacement of the dorsal epiphyseal fragment have favorable results with splinting.

Hematoma Evacuation

Indications for a hematoma evacuation include subungual hematoma involving more than 50% of the nail plate or painful pressure under the nail (58). Decompression can be done with a hypodermic needle that penetrates the nail plate. A heated paper clip or cautery tip may also be used, but the heat can cause further nail bed injury if penetration is too deep.

Nail Bed Repair

Nail bed repair is required for obvious nail bed lacerations and potentially for subungual hematomas that involve more than 50% of the nail plate. A blunt Freer elevator is used to remove the nail plate to avoid additional nail bed injury. Partial nail removal rarely is indicated for nail bed repair in children. Proximal exposure of the germinal matrix requires incisions along the eponych-

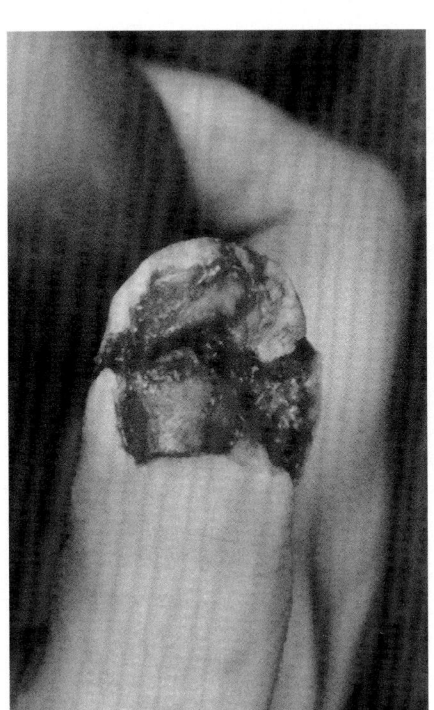

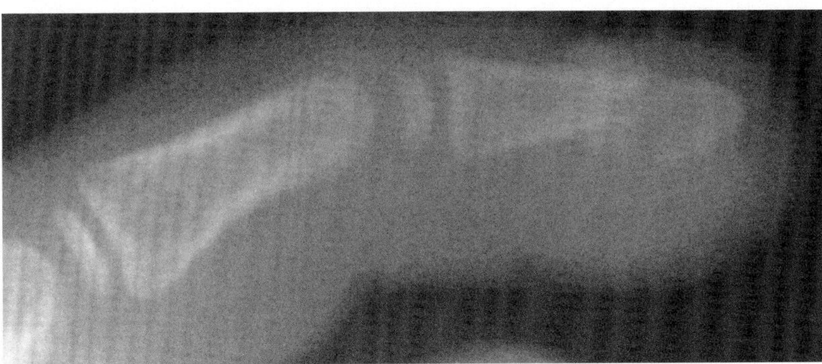

FIGURE 8-16 **A.** A crush injury to the thumb of a 4-year-old with a stellate nail bed laceration and fracture of the tuft. **B.** Radiograph reveals a comminuted tuft fracture.

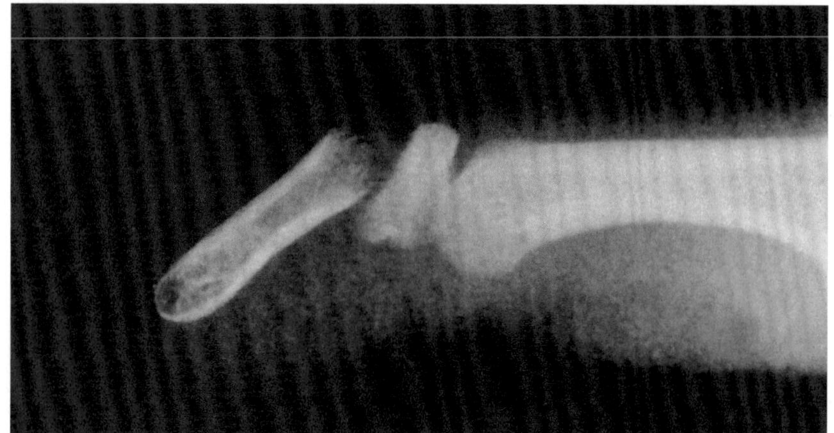

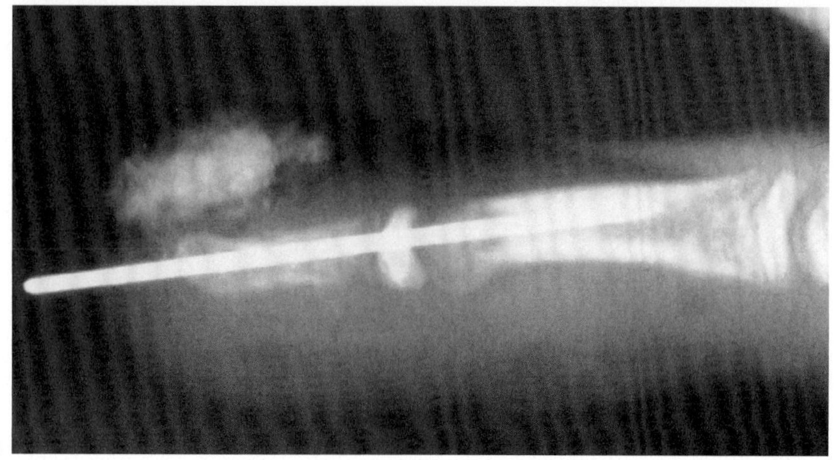

FIGURE 8-17 **A.** An irreducible distal phalangeal fracture that required extrication of the nail bed from within the fracture site. **B.** Stabilization of the fracture fragments with a longitudinal Kirschner wire across the distal interphalangeal joint.

ial folds. The nail bed is repaired with interrupted 6-0 or 7-0 absorbable sutures under loupe magnification. Following repair, the nail bed is supported using the nail plate or using other substitutes, such as the foil from the suture pack (57,59–61).

Operative Management

Extremely unstable extraphyseal fractures with wide displacement may require stabilization. Usually a smooth Kirschner wire can be inserted across the fracture through the tip of the finger. A hypodermic needle can be used as a substitute for the smooth wires (62). Physeal fractures with a dorsal fragment larger than 50% of the epiphysis or considerable DIP joint subluxation may require operative intervention (22,26). Closed manipulation and percutaneous Kirschner wire fixation usually are sufficient.

Open unstable injuries with severe displacement or irreducible fractures require stabilization (Fig. 8-17) (44,63). The Sey-

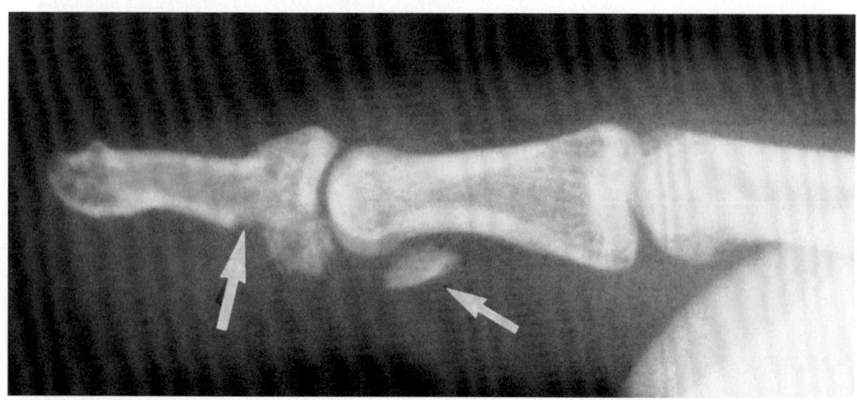

FIGURE 8-18 A 17-year-old athlete with an avulsion fracture from the flexor digitorum profundus tendon. The fracture extends through the epiphysis and into the joint (*large arrow*). The flexor digitorum profundus tendon with its attached bony fragment has retracted to the level of the A4 pulley (*small arrow*).

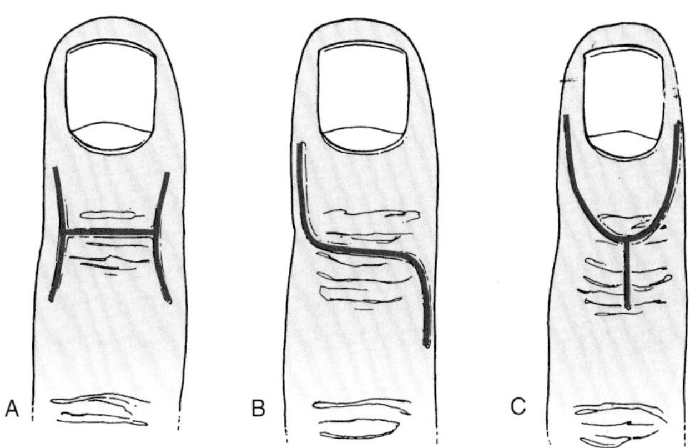

FIGURE 8-19 Exposures to the distal interphalangeal joint. **A.** H-type flap with the transverse limb over the distal interphalangeal joint. **B.** S-shaped exposure of the distal interphalangeal joint. **C.** An extended exposure of the DIP joint. All exposures must avoid injury to the germinal matrix, which is located just proximal to the nail fold.

mour fracture represents an irreducible fracture that requires open reduction. The sterile matrix must be extricated from the fracture site and repaired beneath the epinychium. Epiphyseal dislocations also require operative intervention to both restore joint congruity and reestablish extensor tendon continuity.

An avulsion of the flexor digitorum profundus is an indication for open reduction. Surgery should be done as soon as possible to limit tendon ischemia and shortening. The profundus tendon is identified at the level of retraction and repaired to the distal phalanx (Fig. 8-18). Too often this diagnosis is made late.

Surgical Approach

A dorsal approach is used for most extraphyseal and physeal fractures that require open reduction (Fig. 8-19) (64,65). The doral fragment is isolated and reduced (Fig. 8-20). A small portion of the collateral ligaments may be recessed to enhance exposure; however, soft-tissue dissection should be limited to prevent osteonecrosis of small bony fragments. Fracture fixation can be accomplished with a smooth wire, pullout wire, tension band, or heavy suture (2,7,41,51,66–68). Fixation across the DIP joint usually is necessary to maintain joint and physeal

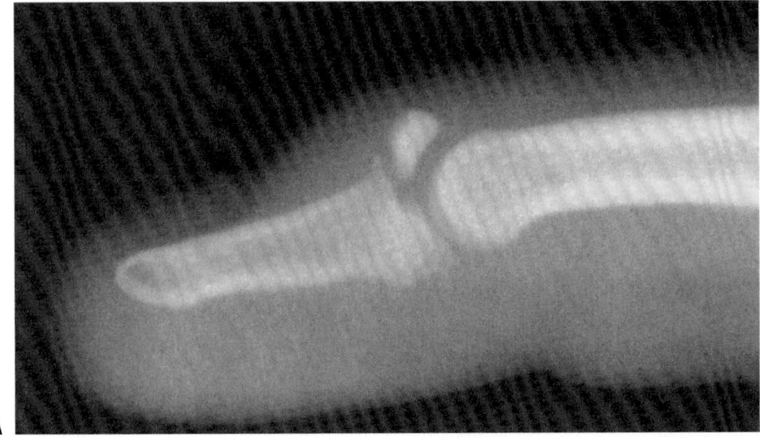
A

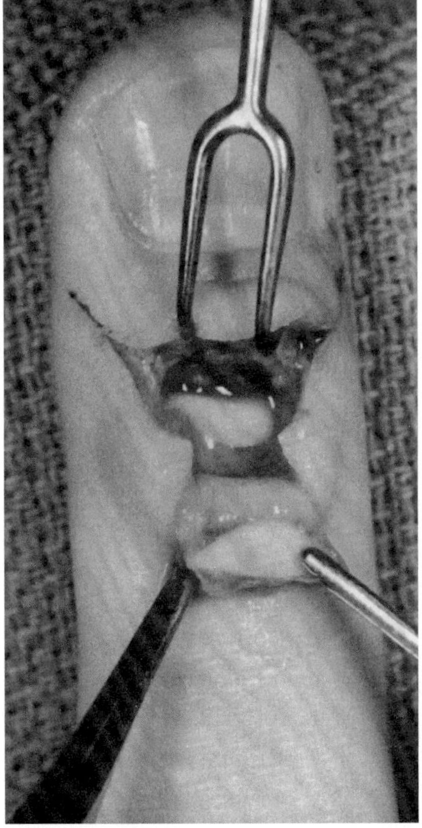
B

FIGURE 8-20 **A.** Displaced mallet fracture with considerable articular involvement and dorsal prominence. **B.** Open reduction through a dorsal approach reveals the articular fragment attached to the terminal tendon.

congruity. A volar approach is used for avulsion of the flexor digitorum profundus tendon.

Amputations

Amputations of the fingertip often are open distal phalangeal fractures. The injury may involve skin, nail tissue, and bone. Support for nail growth is a primary consideration. Minimal loss of tissue can be treated with local wound care and healing through secondary intention. A small amount of exposed bone does not preclude spontaneous healing in children. The likelihood of nail deformity (hooked or "parrot"s beak") is high for amputations that involve more than 50% of the distal phalanx.

Soft-Tissue Coverage of Amputations

Soft-tissue coverage varies depending on the degree of tissue loss and direction of injury (39,69,70). Simple healing by primary closure is preferred for most volar oblique fingertip amputations. Dorsal oblique amputations are complicated by nail bed injury and are more difficult to cover. Composite grafts of skin and subcutaneous tissue from the amputated part have been used in young children with variable results. Local flaps are another option for coverage of large volar or dorsal oblique amputations. Options include a variety of flaps, such as a V-Y volar advancement, a thenar flap, a cross-finger flap, a pedicled flap, and a neurovascular island flap (Figs. 8-21 and 8-22) (71–73). Fortunately coverage issues are rare in children. An amputation of the distal thumb also can be covered with a bipedicle (Moberg volar ad-

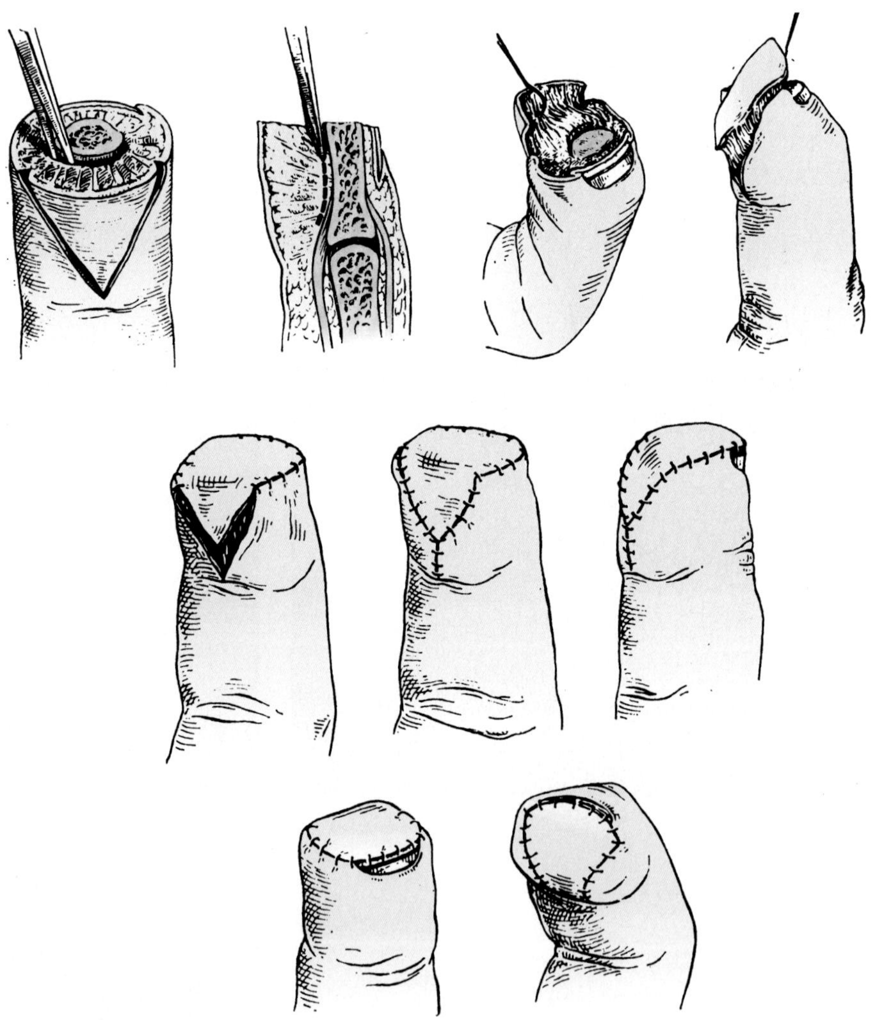

FIGURE 8-21 The reversed cross-finger subcutaneous flap. A full-thickness skin flap is elevated from the donor digit based on the side opposite the injured digit. The subcutaneous tissues are then elevated from the epitenon, based on the side of the injured digit. The subcutaneous tissues are reflected in a reversed fashion into the defect, and a thin full-thickness skin graft is applied to the recipient. The full-thickness skin flap from the donor is then replaced over the vascular epitenon. The flap can be divided at 2 weeks. (Reprinted from Atasoy E. Reversed cross-finger subcutaneous flap. *J Hand Surg [Am]* 1982;7:481–483; with permission.)

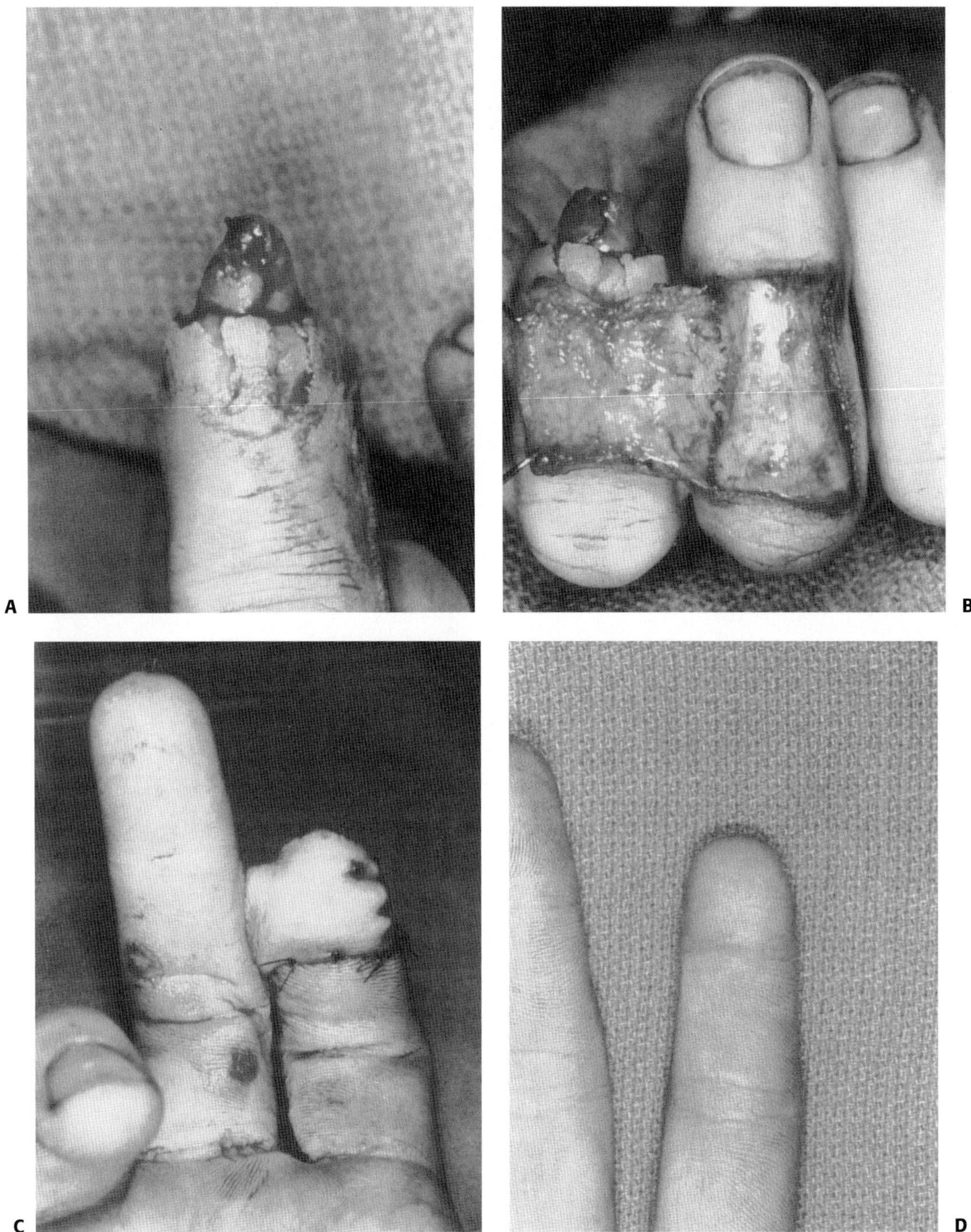

FIGURE 8-22 Cross-finger flap in a 17-year-old male with open distal phalangeal injury and tissue loss. **A.** Extensive volar and distal soft-tissue loss with preservation of the bone and nail bed. **B.** A cross-finger flap of skin and subcutaneous tissue is elevated from the dorsal aspect of the adjacent donor digit based on the side of the index finger. **C.** The vascular epitenon is preserved on the donor digit to support a skin graft. The flap is transferred to the volar aspect of the index finger to recreate the tuft. **D.** Satisfactory coverage and functional and result.

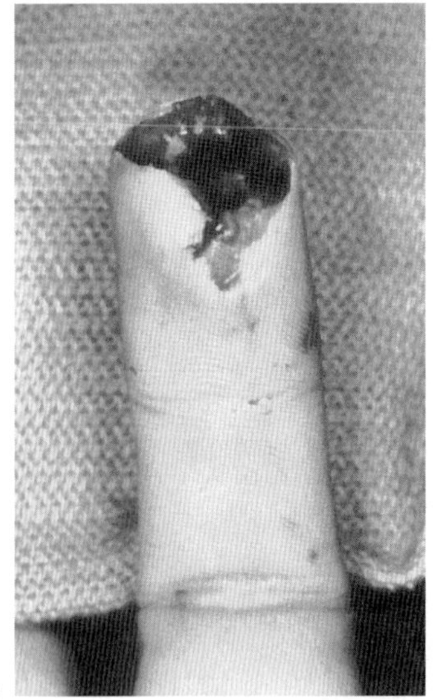
A

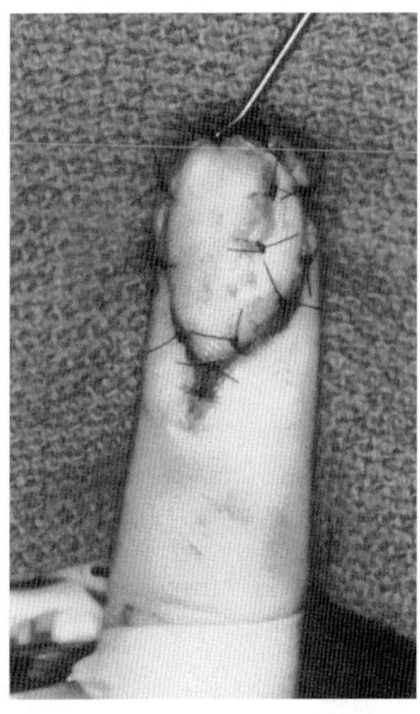
B

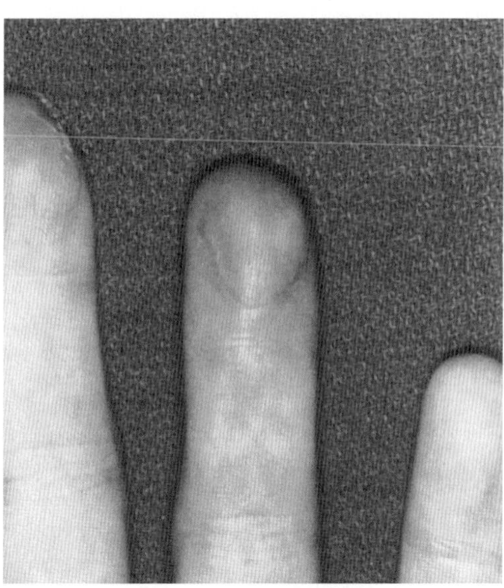
C

FIGURE 8-23 Volar V-Y advancement flap for coverage. **A.** A volar oblique tissue loss of the ring finger with intact nail bed. **B.** Flap designed with apex at the distal interphalangeal joint and mobilized to cover the fingertip. The defect is closed proximal to the flap creating the Y. **C.** Satisfactory result with good durability and sensibility.

vancement flap) or unipedicle neurovascular flap (Fig. 8-23) (74). The choice of coverage depends on the degree and direction of soft tissue loss, age of the patient, and preference of the surgeon.

Postoperative Care and Rehabilitation

Children younger than 4 or 5 years are immobilized with long-arm mitten casts. As the child ages, the degree of immobilization is decreased. An adolescent with a simple distal phalangeal fracture or nail bed repair usually can be treated similar to an adult with only DIP joint immobilization. Percutaneous fixation is removed in the office 4 to 6 weeks after surgery. Formal hand therapy usually is not required, although an instructed home program with emphasis on DIP joint motion is useful. DIP blocking exercises are particularly helpful to regain full joint movement. Formal therapy is reserved for patients who fail to regain motion and strength after 3 to 4 weeks on a home program.

Prognosis

The overall results following distal phalangeal fractures are favorable. A small loss of motion has little functional impact. A small extensor lag or minor longitudinal nail ridge is well tolerated by most patients. Considerable nail irregularity or deformity is a frequent source of dissatisfaction.

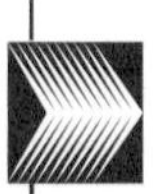

AUTHORS' PREFERRED TREATMENT

Extraphyseal Fractures

Most simple closed fractures are treated with immobilization. Immobilization for 3 to 4 weeks allows clinical union, which proceeds complete radiographic healing by about 1 month. Uncommonly, an unstable distal phalangeal fracture requires percutaneous pinning with a small Concept or Kirschner wire. The DIP joint usually is transfixed to provide additional stability. The pin is removed approximately 4 weeks after injury.

Fractures with a nail bed laceration require adequate anesthesia, removal of the nail plate, and nail bed repair. The parents and patient are told that it takes several cycles of nail growth (3 to 6 months) before the final morphology of the nail is known. Fortunately in properly treated nail bed injuries, chronic deformity is rare.

Physeal Fractures

Most closed pediatric physeal fractures are treated by reduction and splinting. Placement of the DIP joint into extension reduces most fractures. A splint is applied and x-rays are taken to assess the degree of reduction (Fig. 8-24). Adequate alignment requires full-time splinting for 4 to 6 weeks depending on the age of the child, size of the fracture fragment, and amount of bony apposition. The DIP joint is positioned in neutral to 15 degrees of extension. Extreme hyperextension is contraindicated because dorsal skin hypoperfusion and necrosis may result (75). The patient and parent should check the skin daily to avoid skin necrosis from splint pressure. X-rays are taken weekly for the first 2 weeks, then every 2 weeks to monitor for loss of reduction or volar joint subluxation (76).

Surgery is indicated for fractures that are open, grossly unstable or irreducible, or have unacceptable alignment. Closed reduction and percutaneous fixation are preferred unless the fracture is irreducible. Additional fixation of the

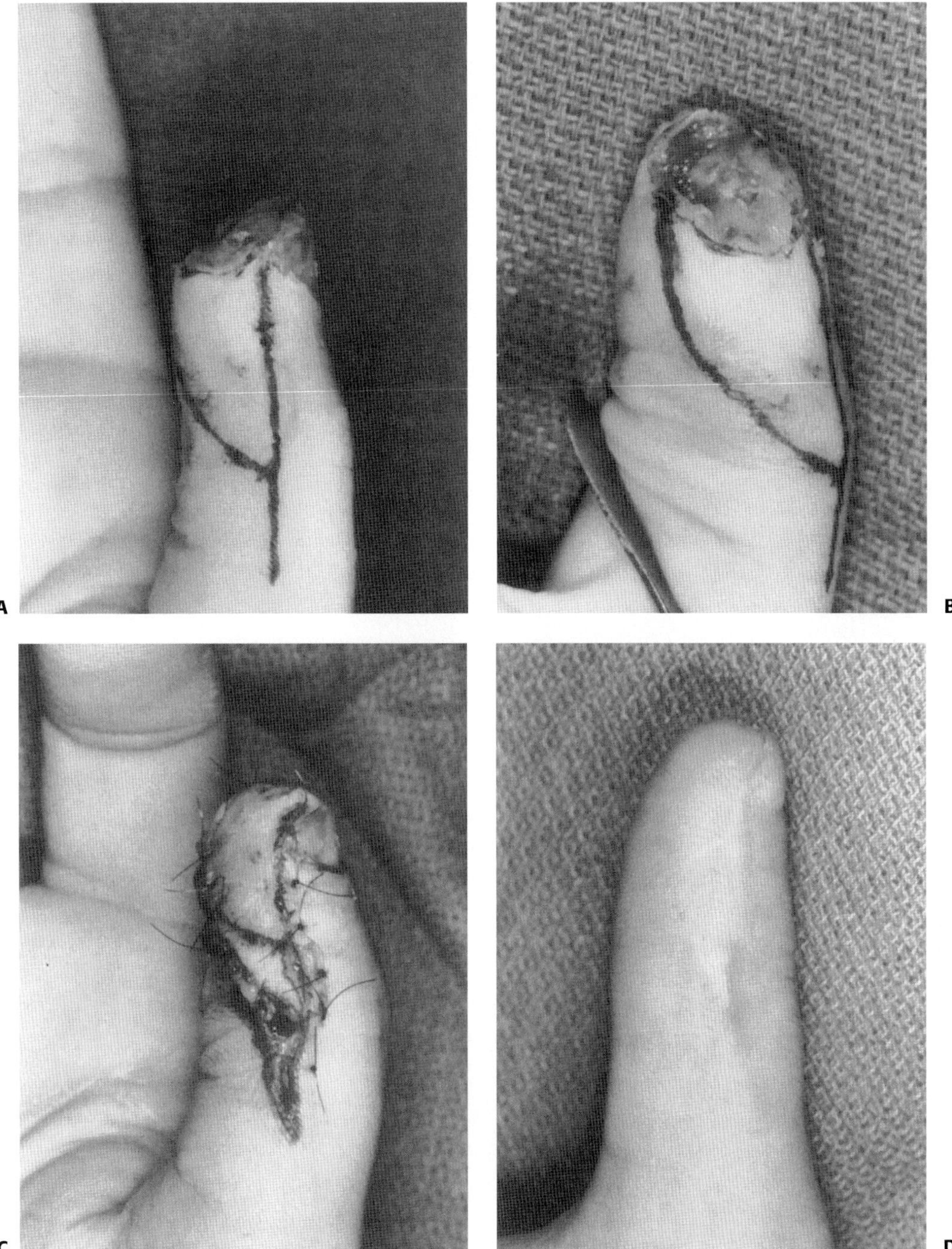

FIGURE 8-24 Pedicle neurovascular island flap for distal thumb coverage. **A.** 16-year-old male with sharp distal tip amputation of the thumb. **B.** A neurovascular island flap based on the radial neurovascular bundle designed in a V-Y fashion. **C.** The flap was mobilized to cover the distal tip. **D.** Restoration of distal thumb contour with intact sensibility. (Courtesy of Richard S. Idler, MD.)

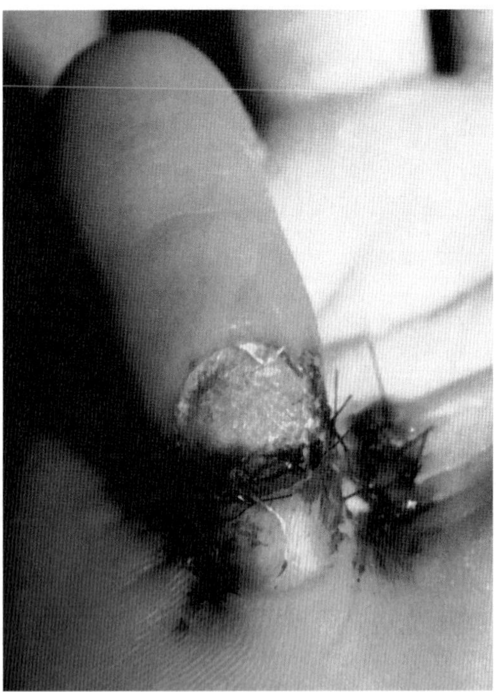

FIGURE 8-25 A thenar H-flap was chosen for this patient.

dorsal fragment can be accomplished with a 0.028-inch smooth Kirschner wire placed parallel to the epiphysis. An irreducible fracture requires open reduction (Fig. 8-25). Fixation techniques vary depending on the age of the child and the fracture configuration. Kirschner wires, however, are the principle means of fixation.

Seymour fractures, physeal fractures with dorsal entrapment of the germinal matrix, require nail plate removal, extrication of the nail bed, and repair. Axial alignment after nail bed repair is maintained with a splint or longitudinal fixation for 4 weeks (Fig. 8-26).

Adolescent mallet fingers with soft-tissue terminal tendon disruption are treated similar to adults with 4 to 6 weeks of dorsal DIP joint splint immobilization. Operative repair of soft tissue or bony mallet fingers rarely is indicated, even for chronic injuries. Most chronic mallet injuries will heal with splint immolization. The loss of digital flexion that can occur with operative intervention can be more disabling than the minor extension lag of an untreated injury (Fig. 8-27).

Jersey Finger

Flexor digitorum profundus avulsion injuries require open repair (Fig. 8-18). Too often this injury is missed in the acute setting. Specific examination for profundus function is necessary for diagnosis. Bone-to-bone fixation is preferred using wires or suture. Fragments that are too small for fixation require bone removal and repair of the tendon directly to the fracture bed. This usually requires transosseous sutures from volar to dorsal, avoiding injury to the nail bed. Repair of long-standing profundus avulsions is controversial.

Amputations

Mild to moderate loss of skin, subcutaneous tissue, and bone is best treated by wound cleansing, dressing changes, and healing by secondary intention. Acceptable functional and cosmetic results are uniform. Skin or composite grafts rarely are necessary for coverage in children and are associated with donor site morbidity, hyperpigmentation and lack of sensibility. Extensive soft-tissue loss with exposed bone requires more innovative coverage. A volar oblique injury usually can be treated with a variety of local flaps, including a V-Y advancement flap, cross finger flap, or thenar flap (Figs. 8-22 and 8-23).

A

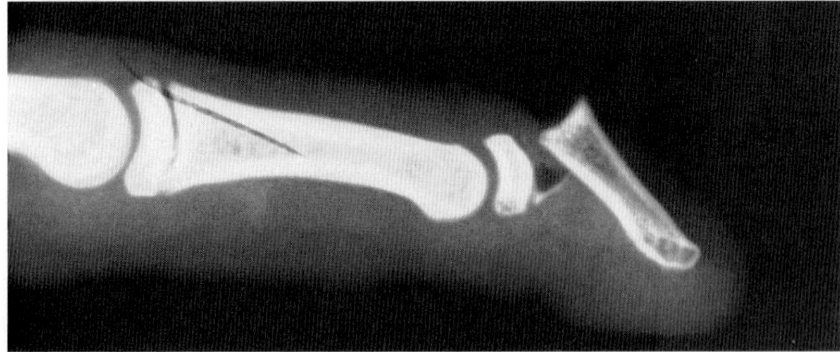

B

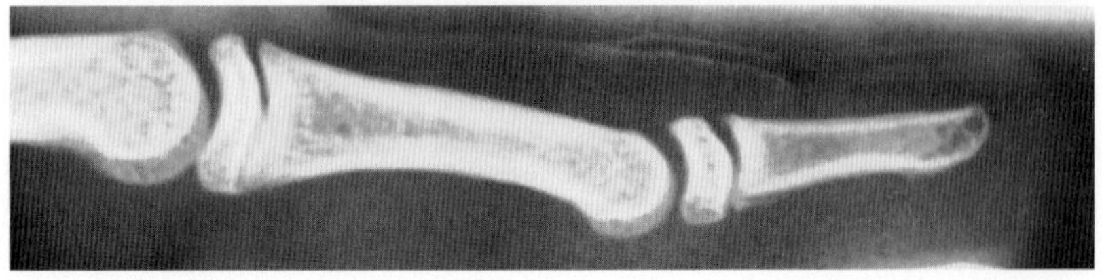

FIGURE 8-26 **A.** A 13-year-old boy sustained an open Salter-Harris type II fracture. **B.** The wound was cleansed, and closed reduction obtained acceptable alignment.

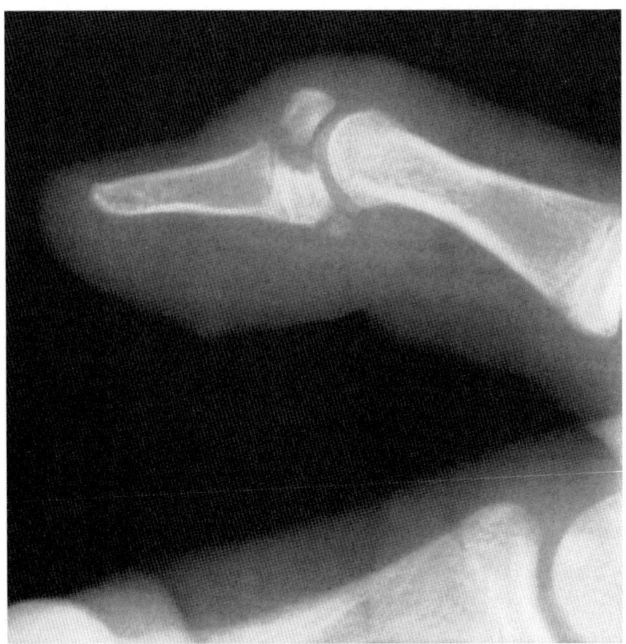

A

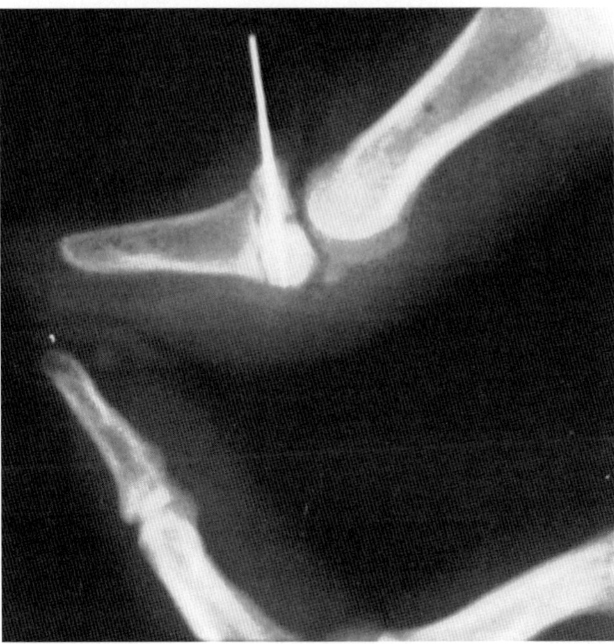

B

FIGURE 8-27 **A.** A 14-year-old boy sustained a displaced Salter-Harris type III fracture of the distal thumb phalanx. **B.** Open reduction was required when manipulation failed to reduce the fracture. Kirschner wire fixation was used to maintain fracture alignment.

Dorsal tissue loss is the more difficult to reconstruct. The nail bed injury adds additional complexity. Mild loss can be treated by local wound care. Moderate to severe loss may require a reverse a cross-finger flap or a more distant flap. Unfortunately, nail bed replacement techniques often result in considerable nail deformity.

Complications

Osseous

Bony complications from distal phalangeal fractures are uncommon. Potential problems include nonunion, malunion, and osteomyelitis. Nonunion and malunion are exceedingly rare, except in open injuries that result in avascular fracture fragments or untreated widely displaced fractures. Osteomyelitis can result from open fractures and requires application of the basic tenets for the treatment of infected bone. Debridement, removal of any sequestrum, and intravenous antibiotics are required to resolve the infection. Additional tissue coverage is necessary in digits with a marginal soft-tissue envelope. These infections are rare due to the robust vascularity of a child's hand.

Soft Tissue

Soft-tissue complications are more prevalent than bony problems. Difficulties may involve the skin, subcutaneous tissue, nail, and tendons. An inadequate soft-tissue envelope can be reconstructed with replacement using a variety of local flaps.

Nail problems depend on the location and degree of nail bed injury. Damage to the germinal matrix produces deficient nail growth and nail ridging. Injury to the sterile matrix causes poor adherence or nail ridging. Treatment options are limited and usually involve resection of the damaged segment and replacement with a full-thickness or split-thickness skin graft (42). Adjacent digits or toes are potential sources of nail bed transfers. The results in children have been superior to those in adults (39,69,77,78). The hook-nail or "parrot's beak" nail is a nail plate complication related to the underlying bony deficit. The nail plate curves over the abbreviated end of the distal phalanx (Fig. 8-28).

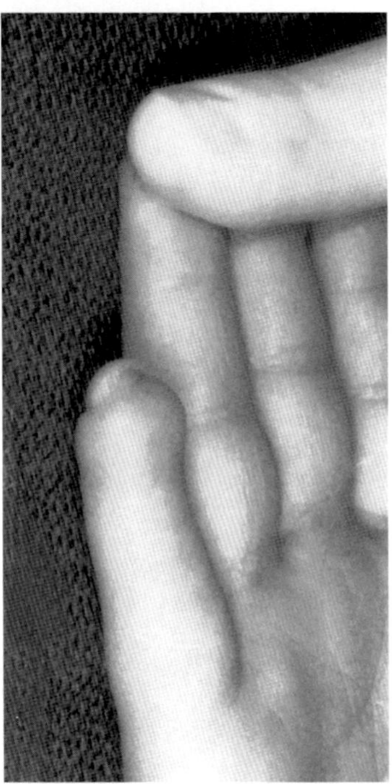

FIGURE 8-28 A hook-nail deformity of the small finger after a distal fingertip amputation.

Treatment requires restoring length to the shortened distal phalanx and creation of an adequate soft-tissue envelope to support the nail plate (Fig. 8-29) (71). Usually a thenar flap or composite graft is used to provide improved support for the nail bed in these situations.

A mild DIP joint or extensor tendon lag can occur after pediatric mallet fracture treatment. No further treatment is warranted. Severe DIP joint deformities are uncommon, but may result in swan-neck positioning of the finger. Reconstruction options are similar to methods used in adults, such as a spiral oblique retinacular ligament reconstruction or central slip tenotomy (25). In a young child untreated lacerations proximal to the terminal tendon insertion may result in an extensor lag that can be repaired successfully with a dermodesis repair (79).

Fractures of the Proximal and Middle Phalanges

Relevant Anatomy

The physes are located in the proximal aspect of the phalanges. The physis of the thumb metacarpal is also located in the proximal portion, whereas the physes of the finger metacarpals are located in the distal segment (Fig. 8-2). The collateral ligaments at the PIP and DIP joints originate from the collateral recesses of the proximal bone and insert onto both the epiphysis and metaphysis of the distal bone (Fig. 8-4). The thumb MCP collateral ligaments resemble those of the interphalangeal joints, having epiphyseal and metaphyseal insertions (Fig. 8-5). The collateral ligaments at the MCP joints of the fingers originate and insert almost exclusively onto the epiphyses of the opposing bones.

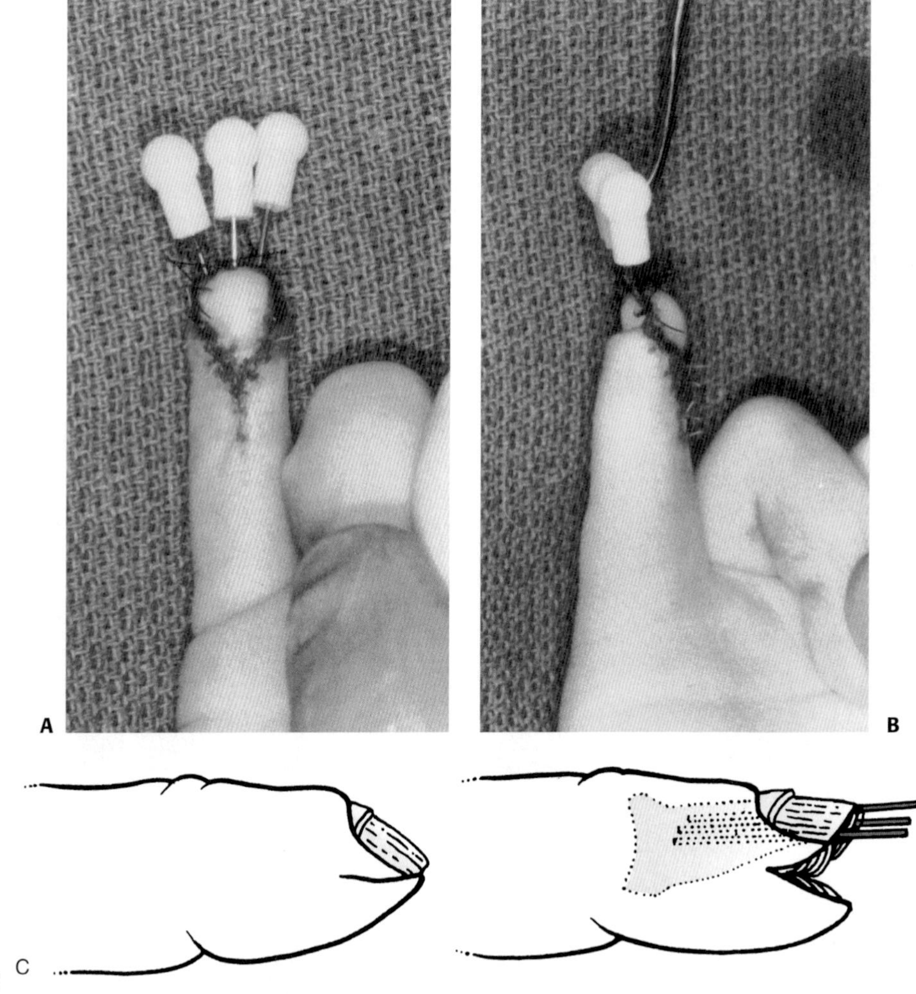

FIGURE 8-29 A,B. Postoperative photographs of the patient shown in Figure 8-25 after the antenna procedure. The procedure involved a volar V-Y advancement flap to cover the distal tip, elevation of the sterile matrix, and the nail supported using three Kirschner wires. **C.** Line drawings demonstrating technique of elevation and support of the sterile matrix with wires. (**A,B** courtesy of William B. Kleinman, MD. **C** reprinted from Atasoy E, Godfrey A, Kalisman M. The "antenna" procedure for the "hook-nail" deformity. *J Hand Surg [Am]* 1983;8:55; with permission.)

TABLE 8-3 Classification of Proximal and Middle Phalanx Fractures

Physeal
Shaft
Phalangeal neck
Intra-articular (condylar)

The extensor tendons insert onto the dorsal aspect of the epiphysis of the middle and distal phalanges. The flexor digitorum superficialis inserts over about two thirds of the central portion of the middle phalanx. The flexor digitorum profundus has a metaphyseal insertion onto the distal phalanx.

Mechanism of Injury

Most fractures of the proximal and middle phalanges result from some form of axial load combined with a torsional or angular force, such as catching a ball or collision in sports. An isolated lateral force across the PIP or MCP joint can lead to a lateral fracture-dislocation. Crush injuries are less common in the proximal and middle phalanges than in the distal phalanx.

Fracture Patterns

The fracture pattern varies with the direction and amount of force incurred. There are four locations: the physis, the shaft, the neck, and the condylar area (Table 8-3).

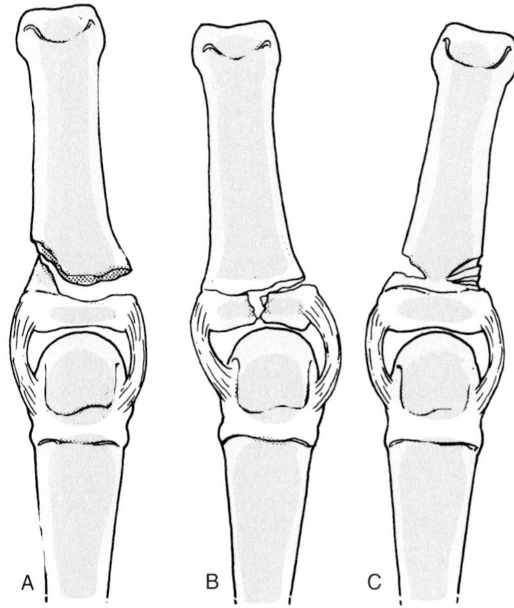

FIGURE 8-30 Salter-Harris fractures of the proximal phalanx. **A.** Salter-Harris type II fracture with the Thurston-Holland fragment. **B.** Intra-articular Salter-Harris type III fracture pattern. **C.** Intra-articular Salter-Harris type IV fracture.

Physeal Fractures. Physeal fractures of the proximal phalanx may be the most common pediatric hand fracture (2,8, 10,30,31). Extraarticular S-H II fractures are most prevalent and intra-articular S-H III and IV fractures less common (Fig. 8-30). In contrast, physeal fractures about the middle phalanx are infrequent. A lateral force across the PIP joint may cause a S-H III or IV fracture or a flexion force may result in a central slip avulsion fracture producing a dorsal S-H III fracture (pediatric boutonniere injury). Small avulsion fragments from the middle phalangeal epiphysis associated with a volar plate injury at the PIP joint are common. However, these bony injuries are not significant in terms of joint stability or growth potential.

The thumb proximal phalanx is susceptible to injury. An ulnar collateral ligament avulsion injury at the base of the thumb proximal phalanx is similar to the adult gamekeeper's or skier's thumb. The fracture pattern usually is an S-H III injury. The ligament usually remains attached to the epiphyseal fracture fragment and may be displaced outside the adductor aponeurosis (80). This "Stener lesion" prohibits healing and requires open reduction to restore articular alignment and joint stability.

Children rarely sustain a comminuted intra-articular fracture of the PIP joint, considered "pilon" fractures or fracture-dislocations (81). These injuries can occur in adolescent athletes and result from an axial load sustained while catching a ball or contacting an opponent. Fracture lines often propagate into the physis. The fracture fragment from the volar side may have the volar plate attached, while the dorsal fragment is likely to have the central slip attached. The central aspect of the joint may be depressed and comminuted (Fig. 8-31). The joint can be unstable and incongruent, requiring careful treatment.

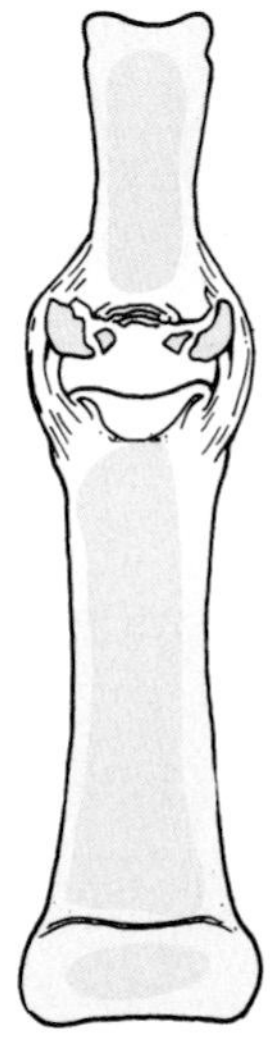

FIGURE 8-31 Pilon fracture of the middle phalanx with comminution and central joint depression of the epiphysis.

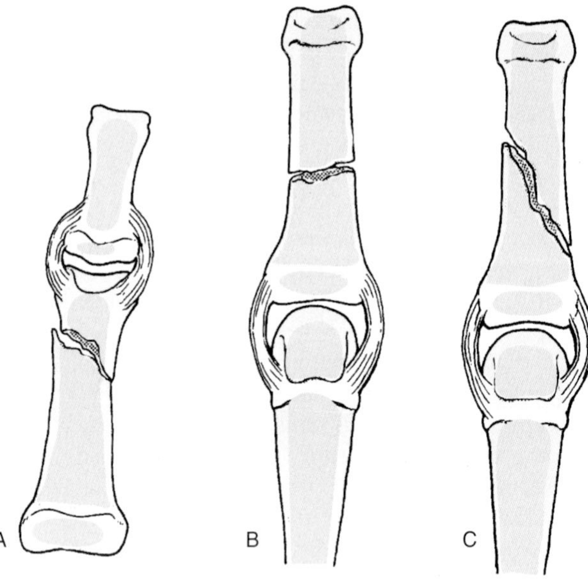

FIGURE 8-32 Shaft fractures. Oblique **(A)**, transverse **(B)**, or spiral **(C)** fractures.

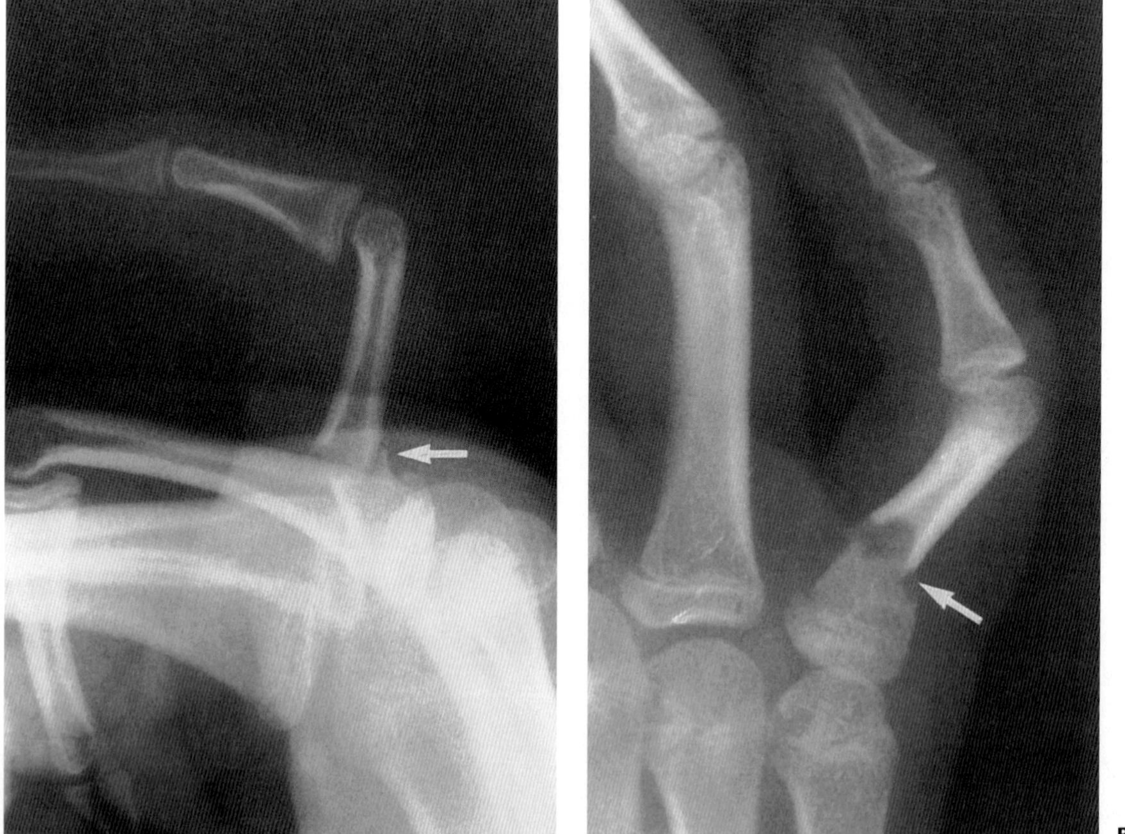

FIGURE 8-33 A,B. Lateral and oblique x-rays of a transverse proximal phalangeal fracture that demonstrates the characteristic apex volar deformity.

Shaft Fractures. Shaft fractures in children are less common. The fracture configuration may be transverse, spiral, or spiral-oblique. The fracture may be comminuted (Fig. 8-32). Proximal phalangeal fractures usually are angulated in an apex volar pattern because the distal fragment is extended by the central slip and lateral band and the proximal fragment is flexed by the intrinsic musculature (Fig. 8-33). Oblique fractures often rotate and shorten. Careful clinical evaluation of rotational alignment is critical. Comminution is secondary to a high-energy injury or direct trauma to the phalanx (Fig. 8-34).

Neck Fractures. Neck fractures of the phalanx are problematic with regards to treatment and functional outcome. Displaced neck fractures also are referred to as subcondylar fractures and often occur in young children as a result of finger entrapment in a closing door. The head fragment remains attached to the collateral ligaments and tends to rotate into extension (82). This displacement disrupts the architecture of the subcondylar fossa, which normally accommodates the volar plate and base of the phalanx during interphalangeal joint flexion. Malunited neck fractures, therefore, result in a mechanical block to interphalangeal joint flexion. Too often these fractures are thought to be nonproblematic and referred late for care.

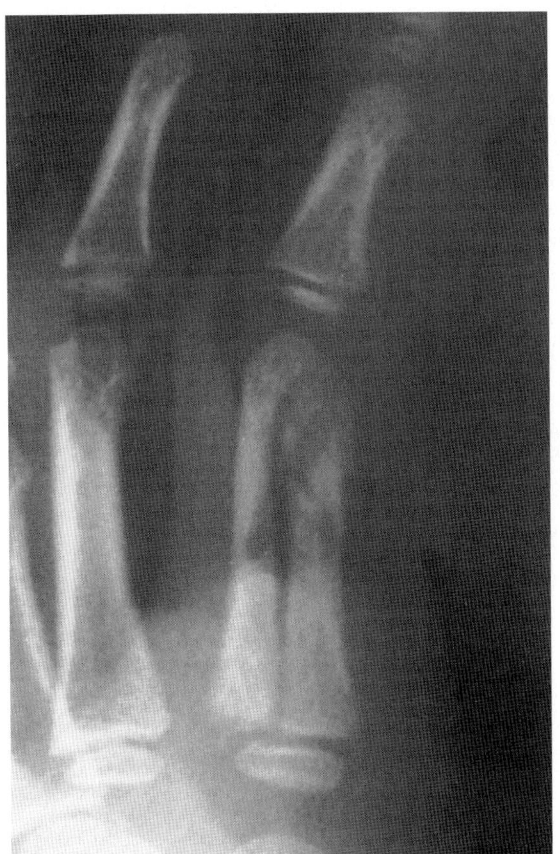

FIGURE 8-34 Comminuted fractures secondary to a crush injury with longitudinal splitting into the physis.

Intra-articular (Condylar) Fractures. Condylar fractures involve the joint and represent a constellation of fracture patterns, including small lateral avulsion fractures, unicondylar or intracondylar fractures, bicondylar or transcondylar fractures, and a rare shearing injury of the entire articular surface and its underlying subchondral bone from the distal aspect of the phalanx. Condylar fractures can be associated with subluxations or dislocations of the joint. Many of these fractures are initially misdiagnosed as sprains (2,8). Restoration of articular alignment and joint stability is critical to a successful outcome.

Diagnosis

Signs and Symptoms

The diagnosis of proximal and middle phalangeal fractures begins with a high index of suspicion based on the history and physical examination. Swelling and eccymosis are the clinical clues to an underlying fracture. The child usually refuses to move the digit and passive motion is resisted. Mild fractures may not be clincially apparent and x-rays should be routinely obtained. Every fracture must be carefully examined for clinical malrotation and rotational deformity regardless of radiographic appearance. Active or passive movement can be used to detect malrotation of the fracture (Fig. 8-35). Active finger flexion will produce deviation of the plane of the nails or frank digital scissoring. Passive wrist extension will induce an abnormal digital cascade through long finger flexor tenodesis.

Radiographic Findings

Anteroposterior and true lateral views are mandatory. Oblique x-rays are often helpful to determine fracture configuration and alignment. Failure to recognize the extent of injury is an ongoing problem, especially with unicondylar and bicondylar fractures. These fractures may appear fairly normal on the anteroposterior view, but a slight overlap of the subchondral surfaces usually is present on the true lateral projection. This "double density" shadow is made by the offset of the displaced condyle and should not be regarded as a normal finding (Fig. 8-36). Questionable x-ray findings can be further evaluated by additional views, tomograms, or fluroscopy (24,44). Phalangeal neck fractures are too often interpreted as benign injuries.

Treatment Options

The treatment of proximal and middle phalangeal fractures varies greatly with the location of injury. Nonoperative treatment is predictable management for most physeal and shaft fractures. Operative treatment is common for neck and condylar fractures, especially fractures that are displaced or unstable.

Physeal Fractures

Most physeal fractures of the proximal and middle phalanges can be managed by simple immobilization. Displaced fractures

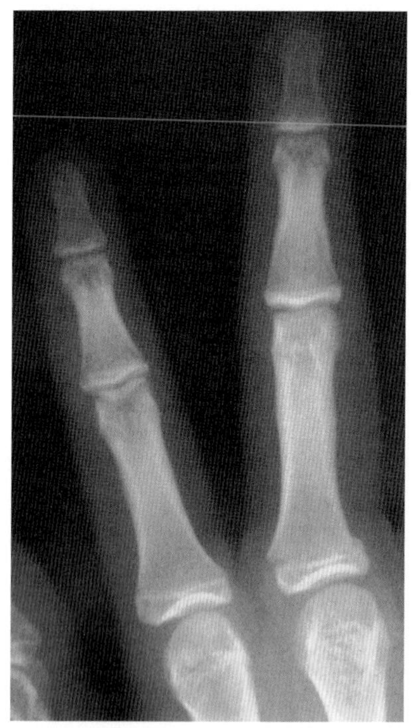

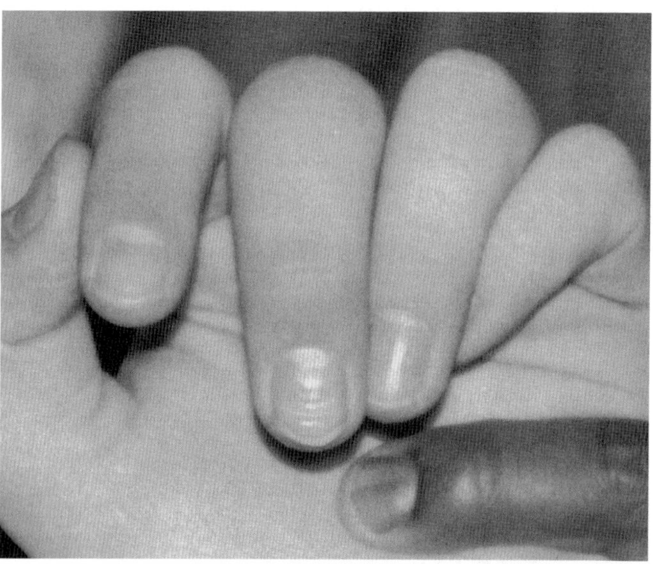

FIGURE 8-35 **A.** Anteroposterior x-ray of a Salter-Harris II fracture at the long finger proximal phalanx. The x-ray reveals slight angulation and can appear benign. Clinical examination must be done to assess the digital cascade for malrotation. **B.** Tenodesis of the wrist with passive extension reveals unacceptable malrotation as evident by the degree of overlap of the middle finger on the ring finger.

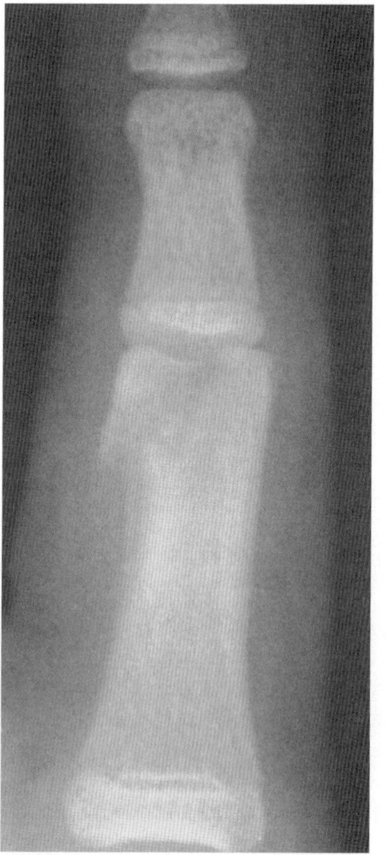

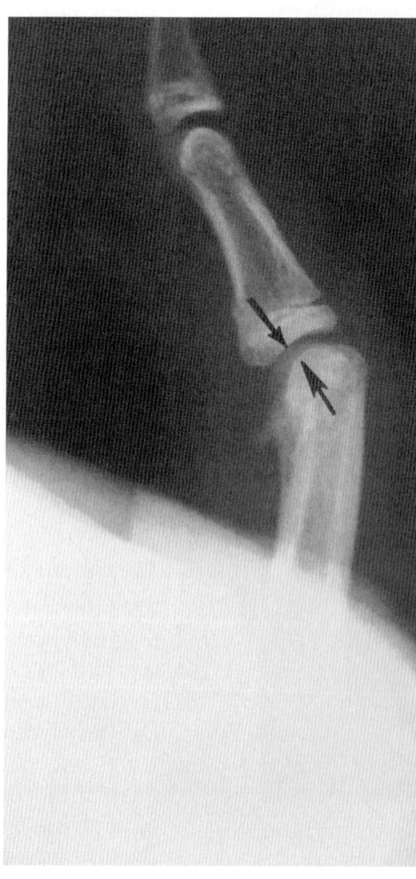

FIGURE 8-36 **A.** Anteroposterior x-ray reveals intra-articular fracture of the small finger. **B.** Lateral view demonstrates double density sign indicative of displacement (*arrows*).

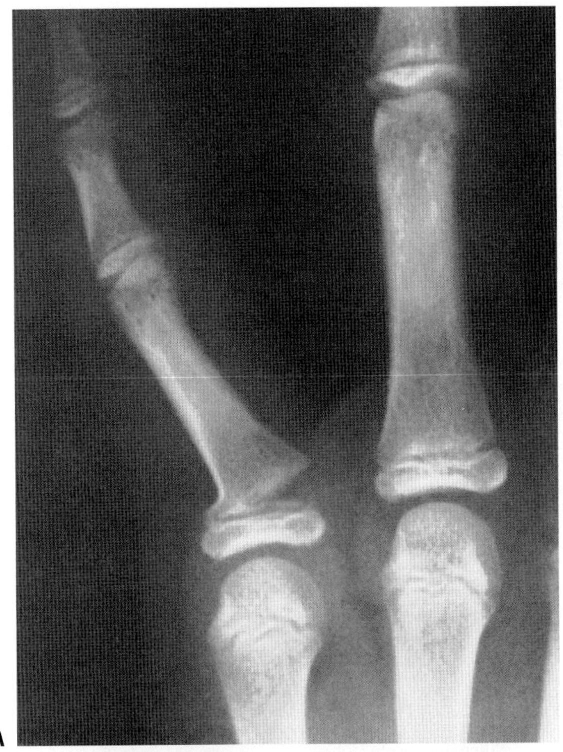

often require closed reduction. A common fracture pattern is a S-H II fracture along the ulnar aspect of the proximal phalanx of the small digit. The small digit is angulated in an ulnar direction. This fracture has been termed the *extra-octave fracture* to denote its potential benefit to the span of a pianist (Fig. 8-37) (41). Minimal displacement is treated with splinting in the safe position for 3 weeks. Moderate displacement requires closed reduction with local anesthesia or conscious sedation. Placing the MCP joint into flexion to tighten the collateral ligaments and angulating the digit into radial deviation reduces the fracture. Placing a pencil or digit in the web space and using it as a fulcrum to assist reduction has been recommended (6). Minimal force is necessary to restore alignment (83,84). Buddy taping and cast immobilization will maintain alignment until healing.

Irreducible fractures of the physis have been reported (8,10,85,86). A variety of tissues, including periosteum and tendons, may prevent reduction. Open treatmnent with removal of the impeding tissue and fracture reduction is required for these rare injuries (Fig. 8-38). In addition, some S-H II fractures may be reducible but unstable after reduction. These frac-

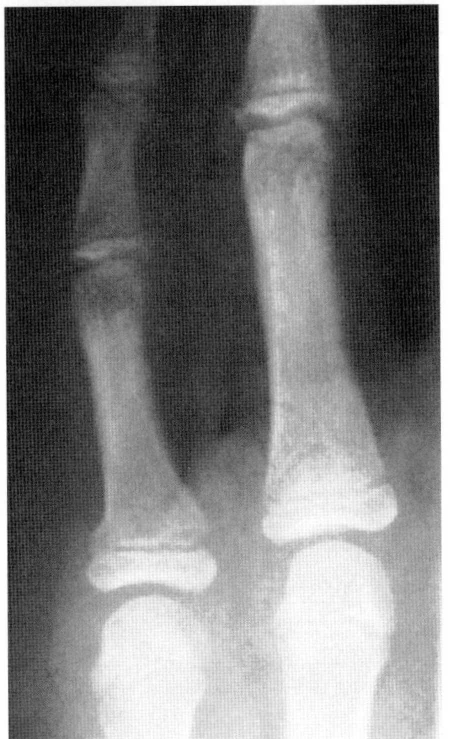

FIGURE 8-37 **A.** An extra-octave fracture in a 12-year-old girl. **B.** The fracture was reduced with the metacarpophalangeal joint in full flexion.

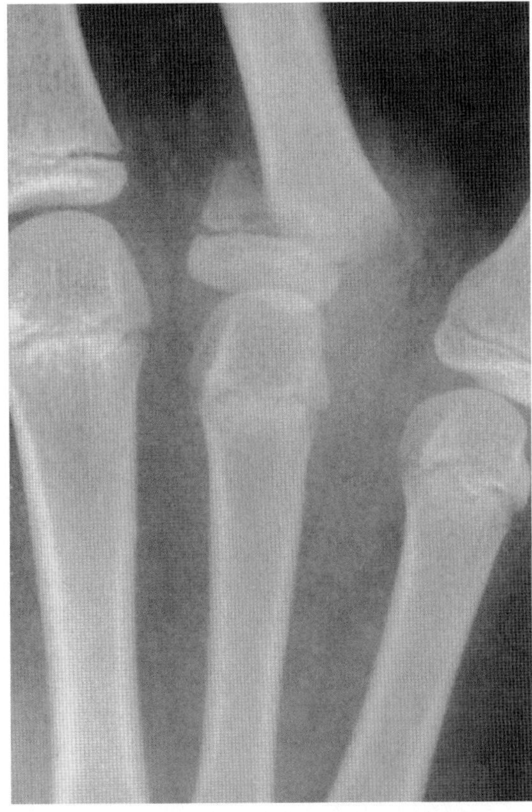

FIGURE 8-38 Displaced Salter-Harris II fracture of the proximal phalanx that was irreducible. The distal fragment was herniated through a rent in the periosteum and extensor mechanism that prohibited reduction.

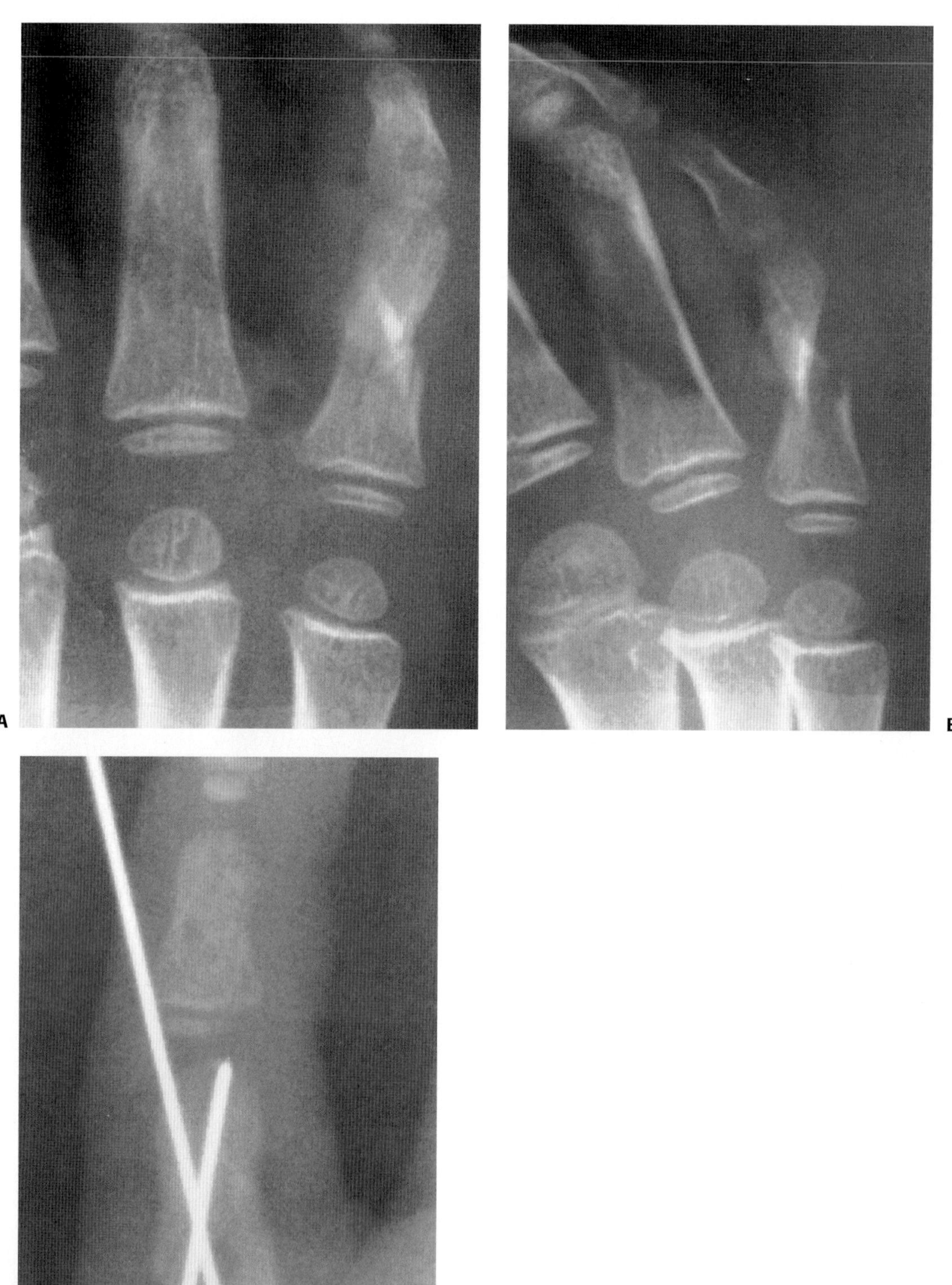

FIGURE 8-39 **A,B.** A minimally comminuted transverse fracture of the proximal phalanx with a short oblique component that was reducible, but reduction was difficult to maintain. **C.** Crossed Kirschner wires were used to stabilize the fracture.

tures tend to be higher energy injuries with more disruption of the supporting soft tissues. Insertion of a smooth Kirschner wire after reduction is required to maintain fracture alignment (85,87). Another indication for operative management is a displaced S-H III fracture of the proximal phalangeal base with a sizable (more than 25%) epiphyseal fragment. Closed or open reduction may be required to restore articular congruity (2,87). Small Kirschner wires can be inserted parallel to the joint surface avoiding the physis (88,89). Tension-bond wiring (90) techniques can be used for S-H III and IV fractures.

Shaft Fractures

Shaft fractures that are nondisplaced and stable can be treated with simple immobilization. Safe position splinting for 3 to 4 weeks should be adequate for clinical union (43). Displaced or angulated fractures require closed reduction. The amount of acceptable angulation in the plane of motion is controversial (26,43). In children less than 10 years of age, 20 to 30 degrees may be acceptable. In children older than 10 years, 10 to 20 degrees is acceptable. Less angulation is acceptable in the coronal plane. Malrotation is not acceptable.

Fractures that are unstable after reduction or irreducible by closed methods require operative intervention. A shaft fracture that is unstable after reduction is managed by Kirschner wire fixation (Fig. 8-39) (91). Open reduction is indicated for fractures that cannot be reduced. A dorsal approach usually is used for exposure. The extensor tendon is split for proximal phalangeal fractures and elevated for middle phalangeal fractures. The choice of implant depends on the age of the patient and the fracture configuration. Smooth wires or screws are preferable to plates to avoid extensor mechanism adherence (92). Bone grafting alone has been described to provide rigid fixation to proximal phalangeal base fractures (93).

Phalangeal Neck Fractures

Closed treatment of fractures of the phalangeal neck is difficult because these fractures often are unstable and displaced (Fig. 8-40). Closed manipulation is done with digital distraction, a volar-directed pressure on the distal fragment, and hyperflexion of the PIP joint. Percutaneous pinning usually is necessary to maintain the reduced position (82). Under fluoroscopy, Kirschner wires are inserted through the collateral recesses and across the fracture. These wires should engage the contralateral cortex proximal to the fracture site. An alternative with a small distal fragment is to insert the pins through the articular surface of the proximal phalanx in a longitudinal fashion, crossing the fracture to engage the proximal fragment.

Intra-articular Fractures

Nondisplaced fractures can be treated by immobilization. Weekly x-rays are necessary to ensure maintenance of reduction. Displaced intra-articular fractures require closed or open reduction (2,87,94). Closed reduction can be accomplished with traction and use of a percutaneous towel clip or reduction clamp to augment fracture reduction. Percutaneous fixation is used to secure the reduction. Fractures not appropriate for closed manipulation require open reduction and internal fixation (Fig. 8-41). A dorsal or lateral incision is used for direct inspection of the fracture and articular surface. Care is taken to preserve the blood supply of the fracture fragments entering through the collateral ligaments. Fracture stabilization is by either Kirschner wires or mini-screws.

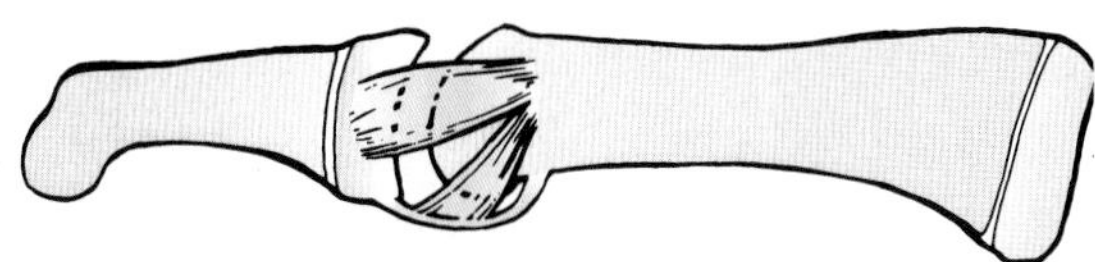

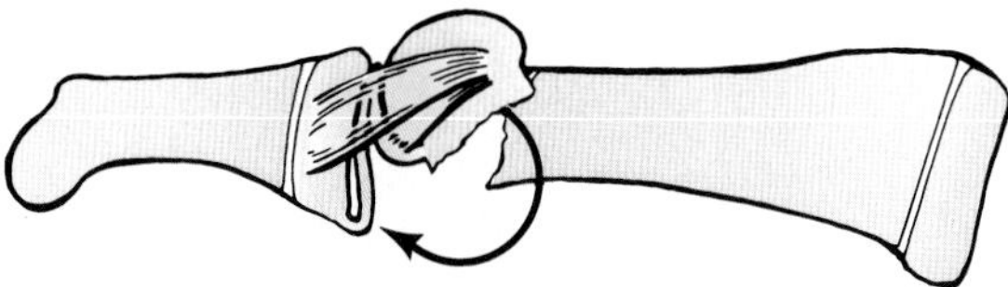

FIGURE 8-40 Phalangeal neck fractures often are unstable and rotated. These fractures are difficult to reduce and control by closed means because of the forces imparted by the volar plate and ligaments. (Reprinted from Wood BE. Fractures of the hand in children. *Orthop Clin North Am* 1976;7:527–534; with permission.)

Certain unusual intra-articular fractures are especially difficult to treat (Fig. 8-42). Shear fractures and osteochondral slice fractures are difficult to recognize. Treatment is open reduction and Kirschner wire fixation. Osteonecrosis, especially of small fragments, is a concern. Some of these fractures require a volar surgical approach.

Comminuted pilon fracture-dislocations of the PIP joint are uncommon in children. Operative intervention usually is required to restore articular congruity. Anatomic reduction is preferred whenever possible (95). Bone grafting may be necessary for stable reduction. Extreme joint comminution may preclude anatomic reduction and alternative treatment options, such as dynamic traction may be necessary (96,97).

Complex Injuries

Combined injuries that affect several tissue systems are common in the digits. Skin, tendon, neurovascular structures, and bone may all be injured in the same digit (Fig. 8-43). Open fracture care is mandatory, followed by establishment of a stable bony foundation. Markedly comminuted fractures or injuries with bone loss may require external fixation followed by delayed bony reconstruction. Neurovascular and tendon reconstruction in children follows the same principles as adults. Rehabilitation of complex injuries in children is complicated by a lack of cooperation. Vascular injuries can affect subsequent growth.

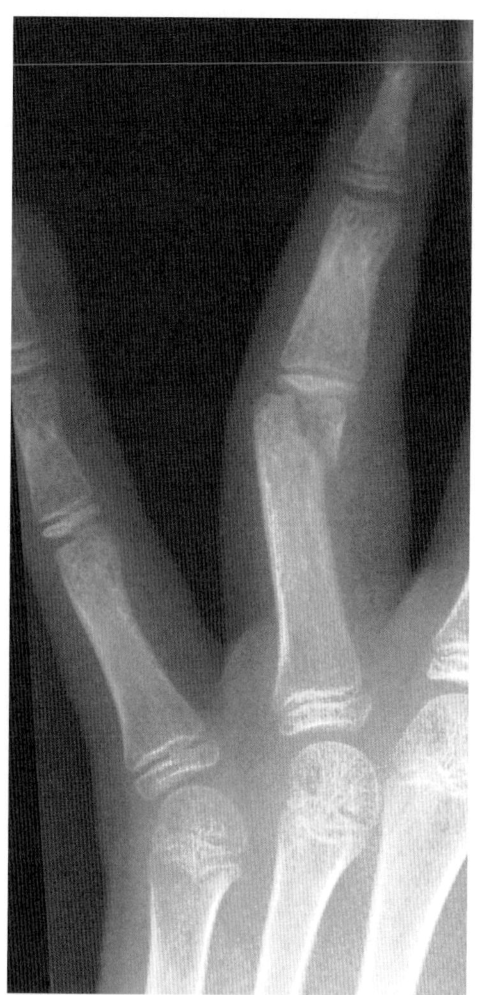

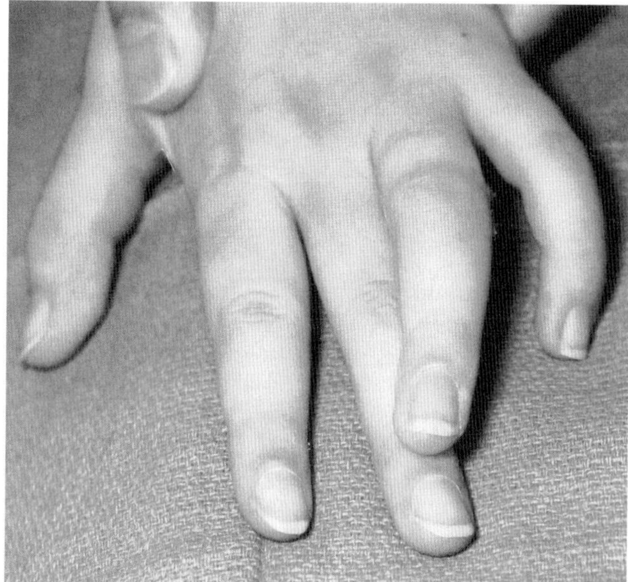

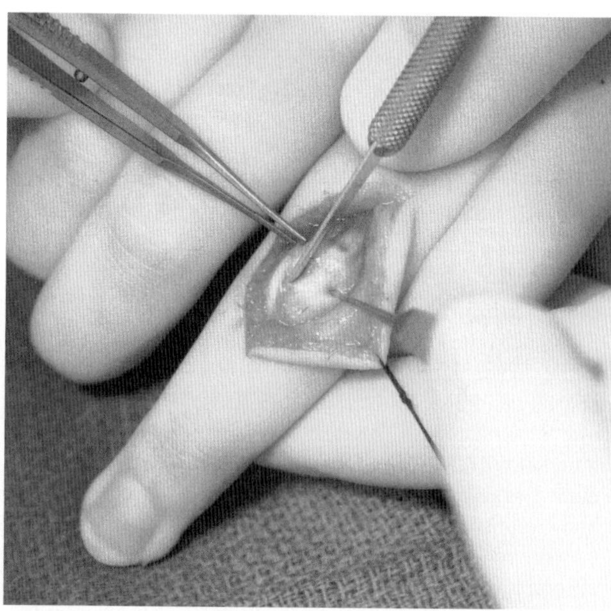

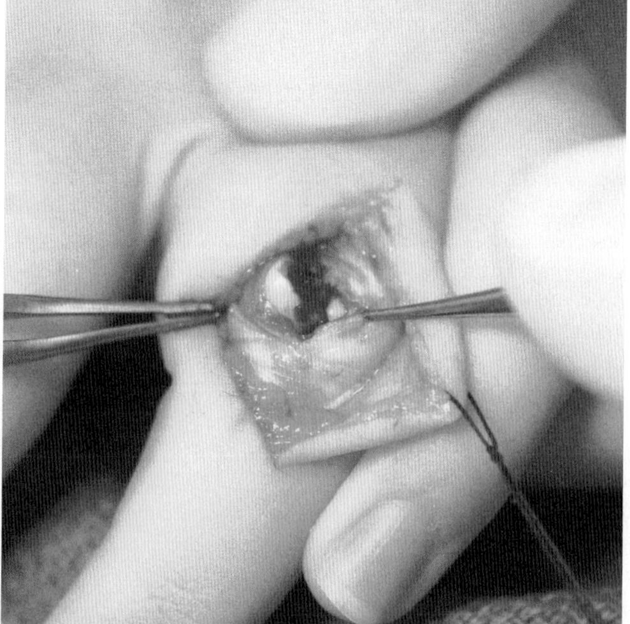

FIGURE 8-41 **A.** A 10 year-old girl with a displaced unicondylar fracture of the ring finger proximal phalanx. **B.** Clinical examination reveals malrotation of the digit. **C.** Dorsal exposure with incision between lateral band and central slip. **D.** Exposure of displaced fracture fragment. *(continues)*

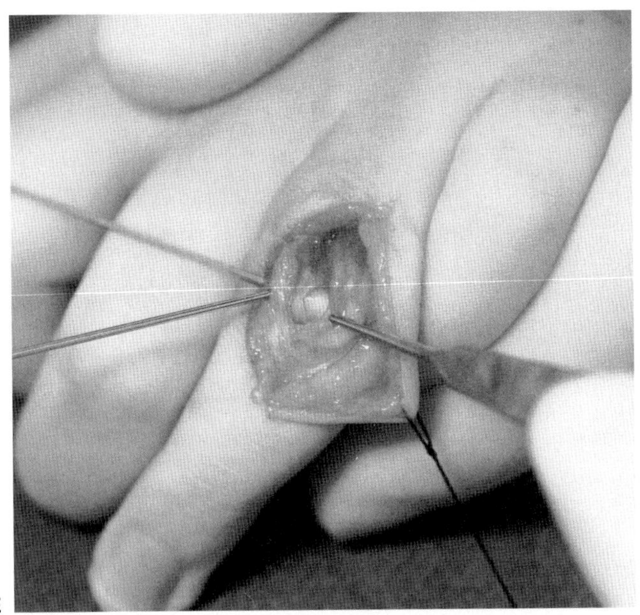

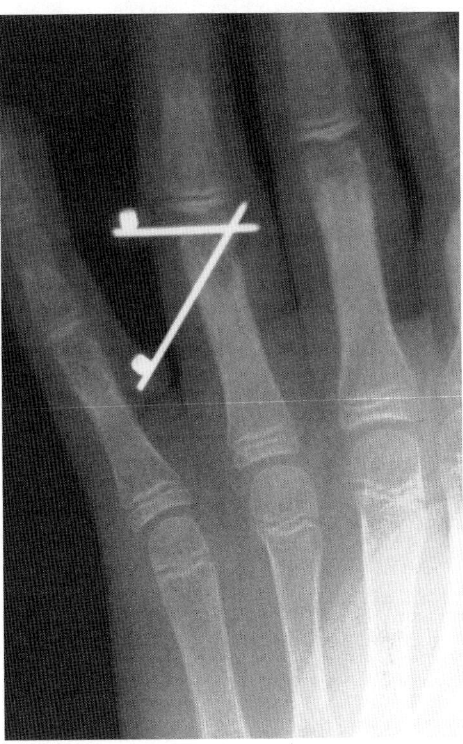

FIGURE 8-41 *(continued)* **E.** Fracture reduced and Kirschner wire fixation. **F.** Postoperative x-ray shows restoration of articular surface. (Courtesy of Shriners Hospital for Children, Philadelphia.)

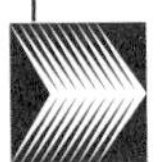

AUTHORS' PREFERRED TREATMENT

Physeal Fractures

Nondisplaced fractures are treated with simple immobilization for 3 weeks. Most displaced S-H I and II fractures can be treated with closed reduction (Fig. 8-44). Alignment is verified clinically by x-rays and rotation is assessed. The hand is immobilized in a safe-position splint, and an x-ray is obtained 5 to 7 days later to ensure maintenance of reduction. When there is doubt about anatomic alignment, the cast is removed for more thorough clinical and x-ray examinations. Immobilization is continued for 3 to 4 weeks. Physeal fractures that are unstable after closed reduction require percutaneous pin fixation. Small smooth wires are used to secure the reduction. Irreducible fractures require open reduction, removal of any interposed tissue, and fixation.

Displaced S-H III fractures of either the middle or proximal phalanges are difficult to reduce and maintain by closed methods. Dorsal S-H III or IV fractures of the middle phalangeal base often require open reduction and fixation to avoid the development of a boutonniere deformity (Fig. 8-45). A dorsal approach, with an incision between the central tendon and the lateral band, is preferred. The PIP joint may require supplemental pin fixation for 3 weeks to permit healing. Lateral S-H III fractures that are displaced more than 1.5 mm or involve more than 25% of the articular surface also may require open reduction and internal fixation. This fracture pattern is especially common in the proximal phalanx of the thumb.

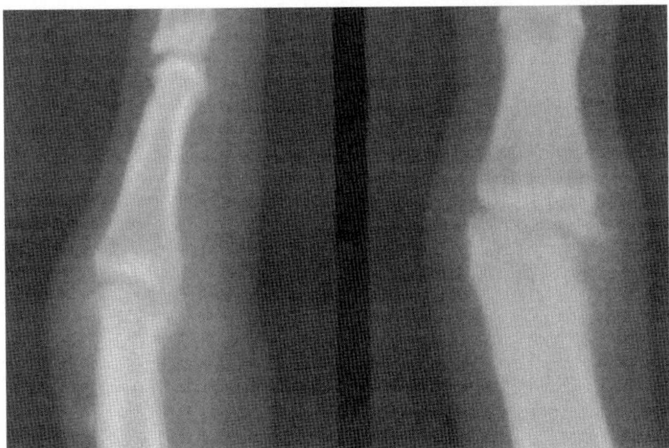

FIGURE 8-42 Intra-articular shearing fracture of the proximal phalanx. There is little bony support for the articular cartilage, which makes fixation difficult.

Shaft Fractures

Nondisplaced fractures are treated with immobilization for 3 to 4 weeks. Displaced fractures are treated with closed

(text continues on page 290)

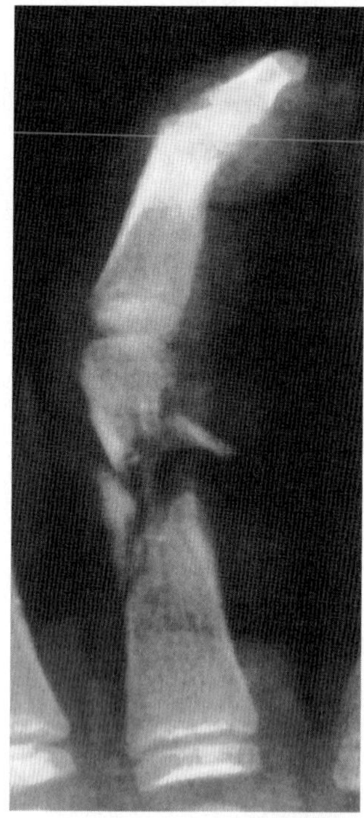
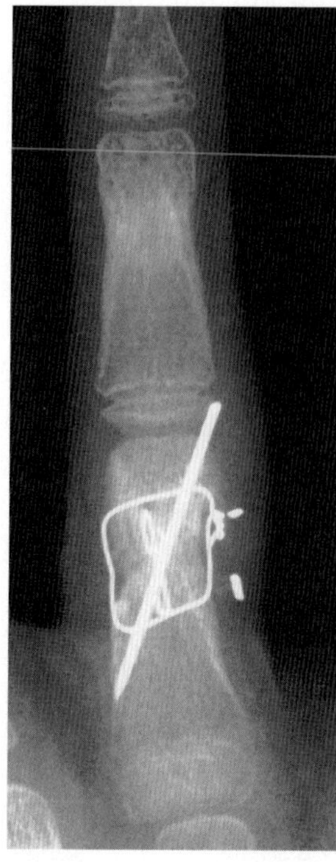

FIGURE 8-43 **A.** A 14-year-old boy sustained a near-amputation of his ring digit with severe soft-tissue injury. **B.** 90-90 intraosseous wiring supplemented with Kirschner wire fixation to provide a stable base for soft tissue repair.

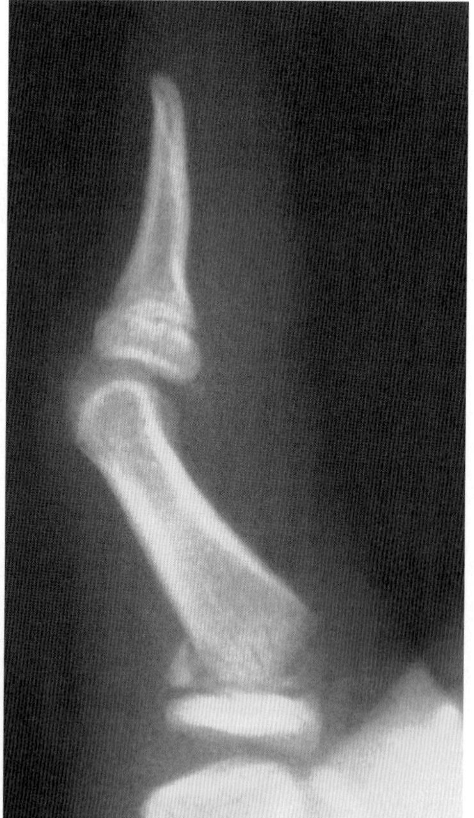
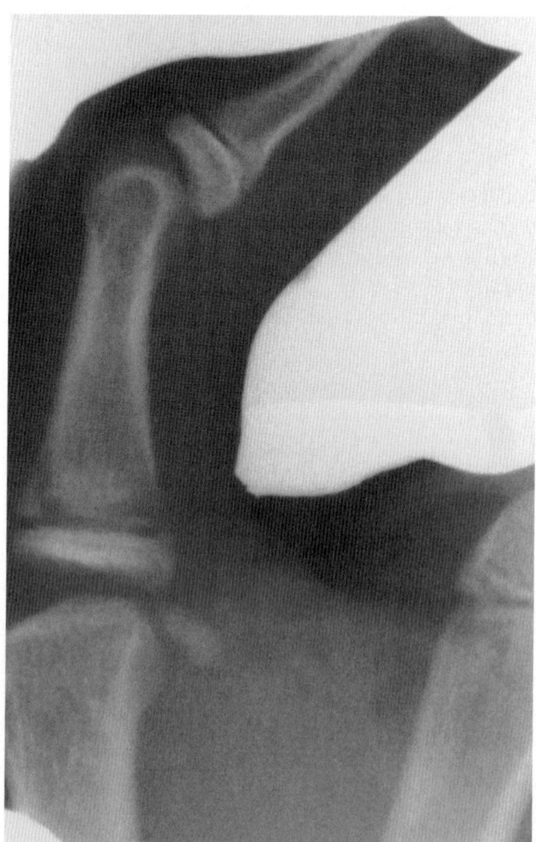

FIGURE 8-44 **A.** Salter-Harris II fracture of the proximal phalanx of the thumb. **B.** Gentle closed reduction, performed under fluoroscopic control, yielded an anatomic reduction.

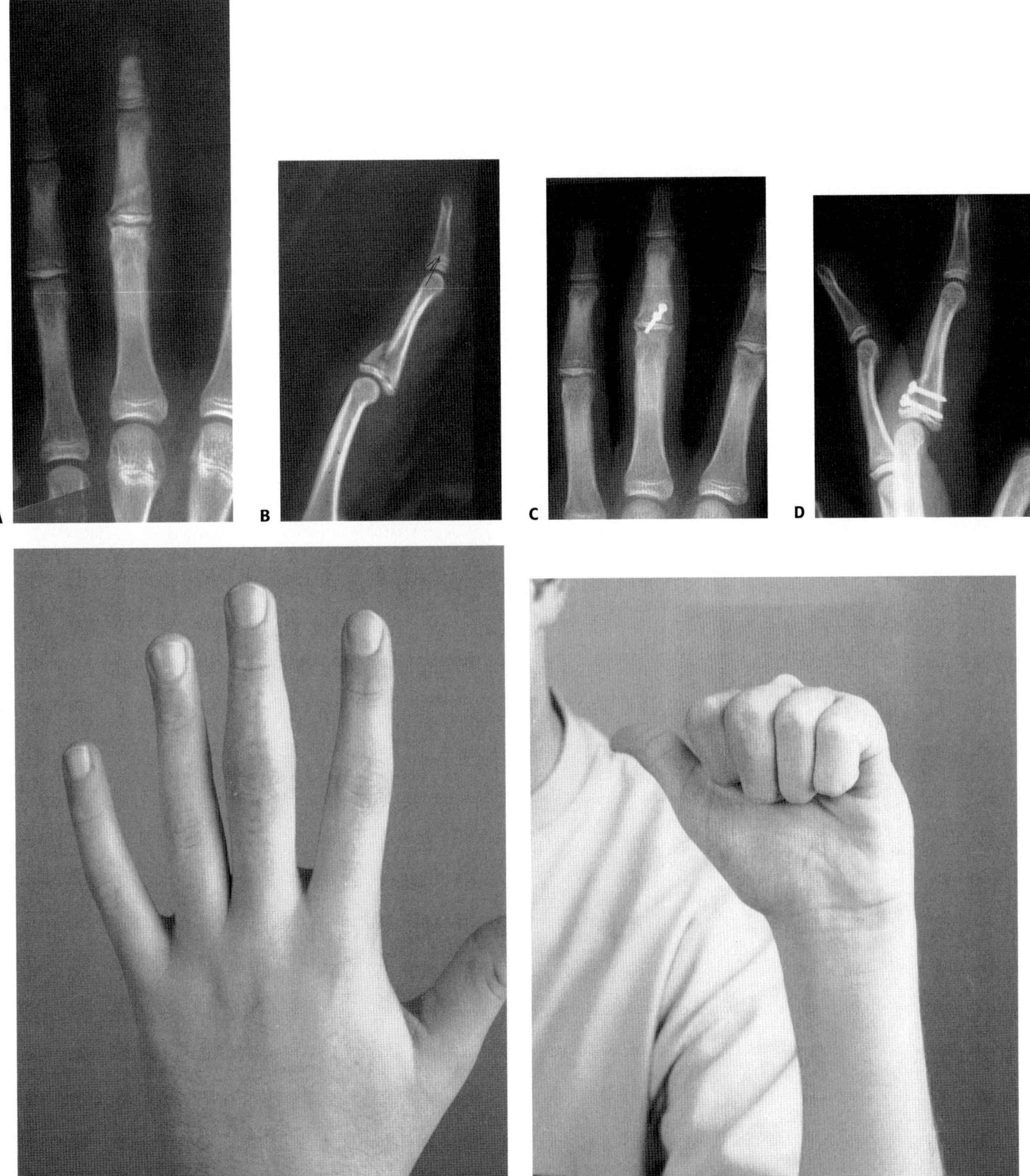

FIGURE 8-45 **A,B.** A 16-year-old male sustained a dorsal Salter-Harris IV fracture of the middle phalanx. **C,D.** Open reduction and internal screen fixation were accomplished through a dorsal approach. X-rays show reduction of joint subluxation and fixation of fracture fragment. **E,F.** Postoperative extension and flexion with near normal motion. (Courtesy of Shriners Hospital for Children, Philadelphia.)

reduction and percutaneous pin fixation (98). Reduction is accomplished with longitudinal traction and rotation of the distal fragment to approximate the proximal fragment. For a proximal phalangeal fracture, the MCP joint is flexed to relax the intrinsic muscle pull and to stabilize the proximal fragment. The fracture orientation dictates the angle of pin insertion. Optimal pin placement is perpendicular to the fracture line. Placement of the pins in the mid-axial line prevents iatrogenic injury of the neurovascular structures or entrapment of the extensor mechanism by the pin. Open reduction is reserved for irreducible fractures.

Neck Fractures

Neck fractures usually require operative intervention. If closed reduction is obtainable, then percutaneous pin fixation is performed. The pins are placed through the collateral recesses to engage the proximal fragment in a crossed fashion. If closed reduction is unsuccessful, open reduction and similar percutaneous pinning are indicated.

Late presentation of a neck fracture requires consideration of the time from injury and fracture displacement. Considerable displacement requires treatment to regain joint flexion (Fig. 8-46). If the fracture line is still visible, a percutaneous pin osteoclasis may be possible. Under fluoroscopy, one or two smooth pins are inserted into the fracture and used to "joystick" the distal fragment into a reduced position (99). The fracture is then stabilized with percutaneous pins. This approach may decrease the risk of osteonecrosis associated with late open reduction. A nascent or established malunion that cannot be reduced by osteoclasis can be treated by late open reduction (Fig. 8-47). The callus is gently removed and the fracture aligned. The risks of osteonecrosis must be weighed against acceptance of the malunion. Mild loss of the condylar recess can be treated with recession of the prominent volar bone rather than risk osteonecrosis associated with extensive fracture mobilization (99,100). In addition, slow remodeling is feasible in very young children without rotational malalignment and with a family that is willing to wait up to 2 years for remodeling (101,102).

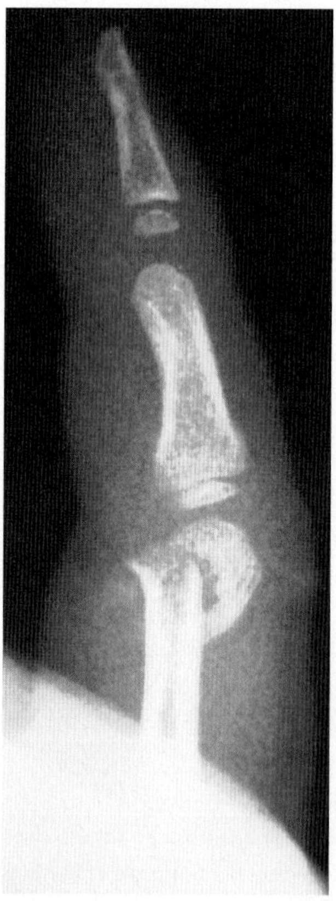

FIGURE 8-46 Displaced phalangeal neck fracture of the proximal phalanx revealing loss of subchondral fossa at the proximal interphalangeal joint joint. If this is not corrected to anatomic alignment, there will be a mechanical block to flexion.

Intra-articular Fractures

Intra-articular fractures of the phalanges usually require percutaneous or open reduction. Unicondylar fractures that are mildly displaced can be treated with closed reduction and percutaneous pinning. Widely displaced unicondylar and bicondylar fractures require open reduction (Fig. 8-41). A dorsal approach is preferred. Fixation usually is obtained with smooth wires. The placement and direction are dictated by the fracture configuration. Rotational control of the fragment may require multiple wires. The fixation device must avoid tethering of the collateral ligament, which will limit motion. Usually a pin is placed parallel to the joint to maintain articular alignment, followed by oblique pins to stabilize the articular fragment(s) to the shaft. In adolescents, miniscrew fixation can be used.

Pilon fractures or intra-articular fracture-dislocations at the proximal phalangeal base present a management dilemma (95). Open reduction is worthwhile when the fragments are large and the epiphysis can be reconstructed. Bone grafting may be necessary for stable reduction. Severe articular damage and communition are treated with dynamic traction.

Postoperative Care and Rehabilitation

The duration of immobilization after surgical intervention for phalangeal fractures is usually 3 to 4 weeks. Percutaneous pins are removed at that time and motion instituted. Formal hand therapy usually is not required, although the child must be encouraged to reestablish a normal usage pattern to improve motion and flexibility. Periarticular fractures are monitored closely for persistent loss of motion that would benefit from formal hand therapy. Patients with complex fractures or replantations are more prone to develop stiffness. In these instances, therapy is prescribed routinely to regain motion. Therapy is directed at both flexion and extension of the injured digit. Static or dynamic splinting may be required after fracture healing.

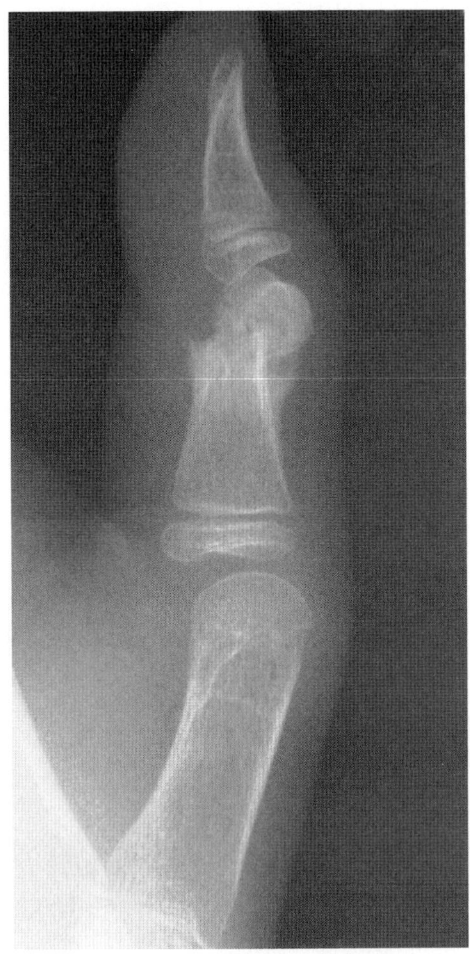

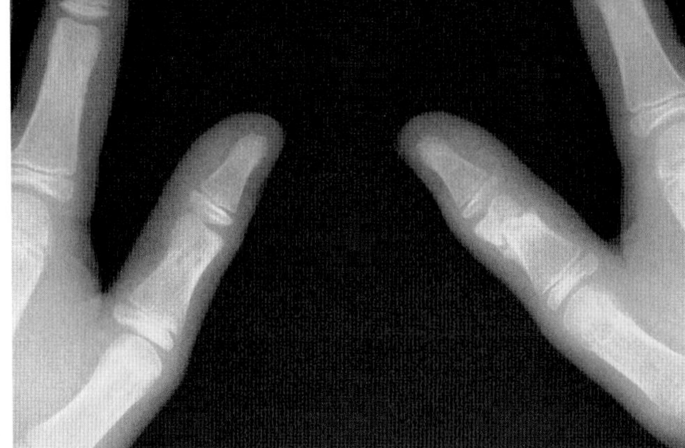

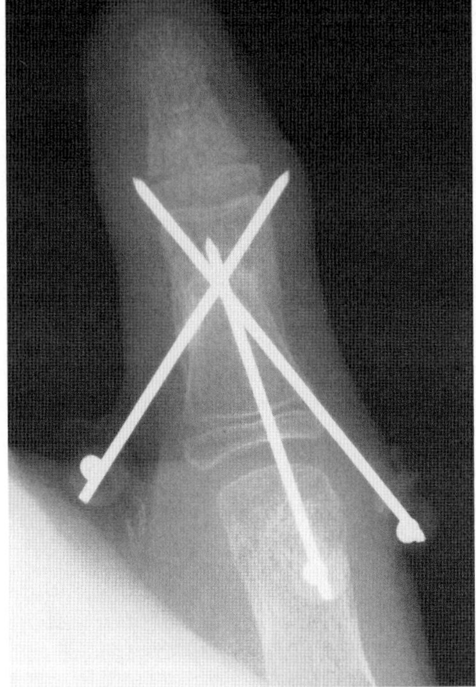

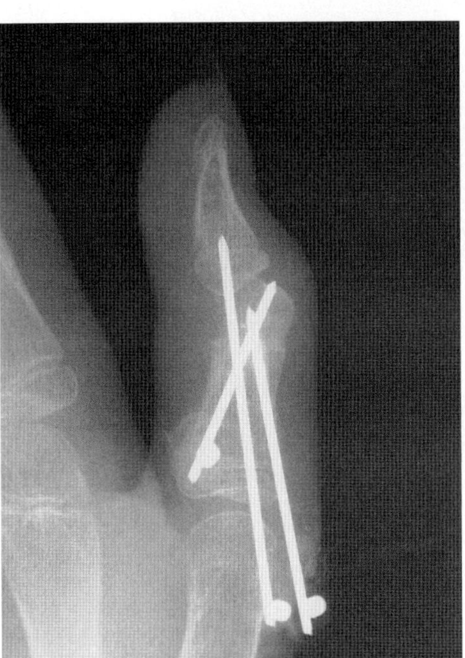

FIGURE 8-47 **A.** A 14-year-old girl with incipient malunion of the right thumb proximal phalanx neck fractures that impedes flexion. **B.** Lateral x-ray reveals loss of the subchondral fossa. **C.** Anteroposterior view after open reduction and Kirschner wire fixation. **D.** Oblique view reveals restoration of subchondral fossa. *(continues)*

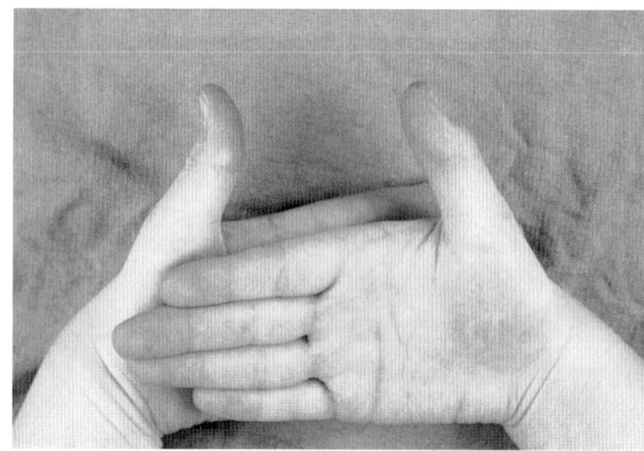

E

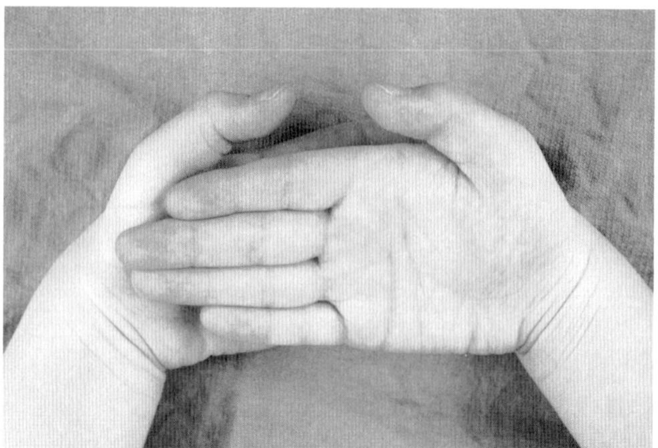

F

FIGURE 8-47 *(continued)* **E,F.** Postoperative flexion and extension compared to the other side. (Courtesy of Shriners Hospital for Children, Philadelphia.)

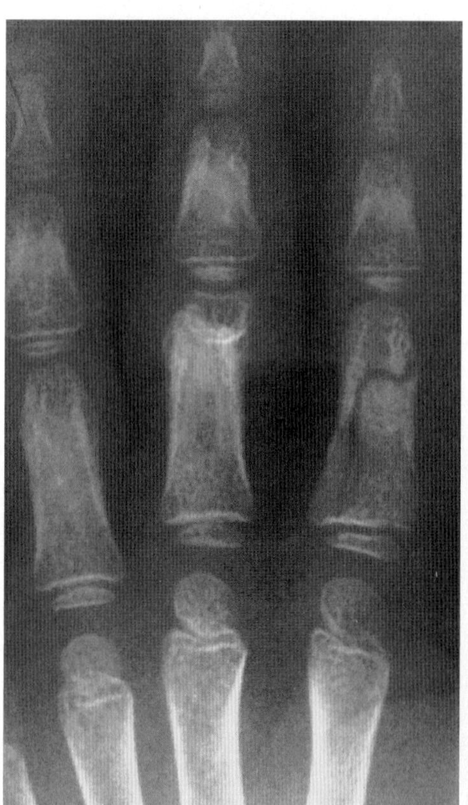

A

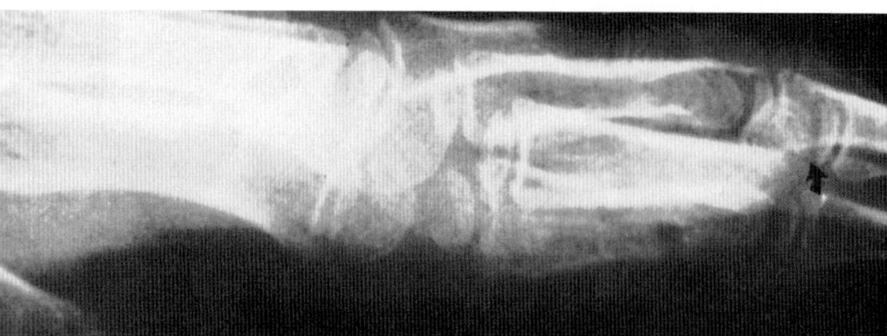

B

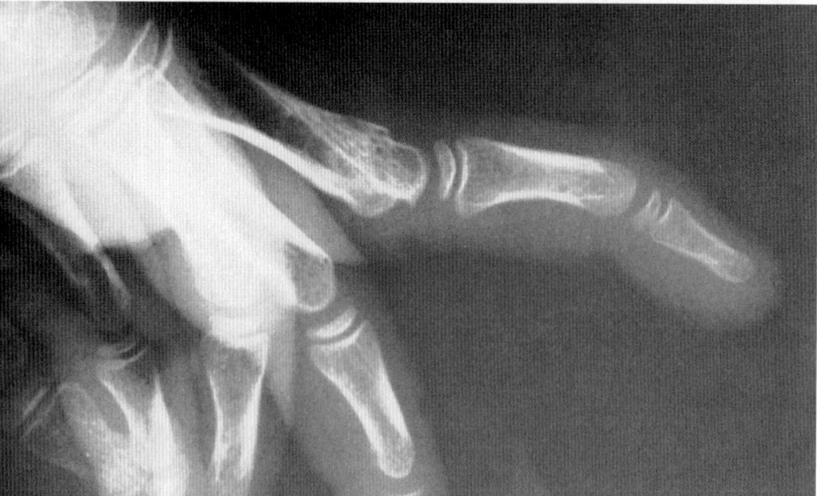

C

FIGURE 8-48 **A.** A 3-year-old girl sustained a fracture of the neck of the proximal phalanx of the index and middle fingers. The displaced fracture in the middle finger appears similar to an epiphysis at the distal end of the phalanx. **B.** No true lateral x-ray of the injured finger was obtained. Close scrutiny of this lateral view shows a dorsally displaced neck fracture, rotated almost 90 degrees (*arrow*). **C.** Eighteen months later, lateral x-ray reveals malunion with hyperextension of the proximal interphalangeal joint and loss of flexion.

Prognosis

The overall results following proximal and middle phalangeal fractures are positive. Considering the frequency of these fractures, the frequency of complications and functional impairment is low. Despite appropriate treatment, however, some children have permanent loss of motion, malunion, or growth disturbance. The major concern is to avoid rotational, articular, or periarticular malunion due to inappropriate diagnosis or treatment.

Complications

Early

Complications associated with proximal and middle phalangeal fractures begin with failure to recognize the injury (Fig. 8-48). Anteroposterior and lateral x-rays must be made correctly and scrutinized for subtle abnormalities. Questionable findings warrant additional views or advanced imaging studies. A misdiagnosis is common in displaced phalangeal neck fractures because the fracture is confused with a minor avulsion fracture.

Another early complication is false interpretation of a "nondisplaced" fracture that is malrotated. All children with phalangeal fractures require careful examination for rotational alignment. The clinical examination is the mainstay for determining fracture rotation. Digital scissoring is indicative of fracture malrotation and requires reduction. Regardless of x-ray appearance, rotational alignment should be evaluated by wrist tenodesis and active motion.

Most phalangeal fractures can be maintained in satisfactory alignment after closed reduction. Certain fractures, however, have a propensity for re-displacement (Fig. 8-49). Oblique shaft fractures, unicondylar articular fractures, and neck fractures are prime examples. Early follow-up to ensure maintenance of reduction is paramount if closed treatment is chosen. Displacement requires repeat manipulation and pin fixation. When in doubt, the digit should be examined carefully for malalignment

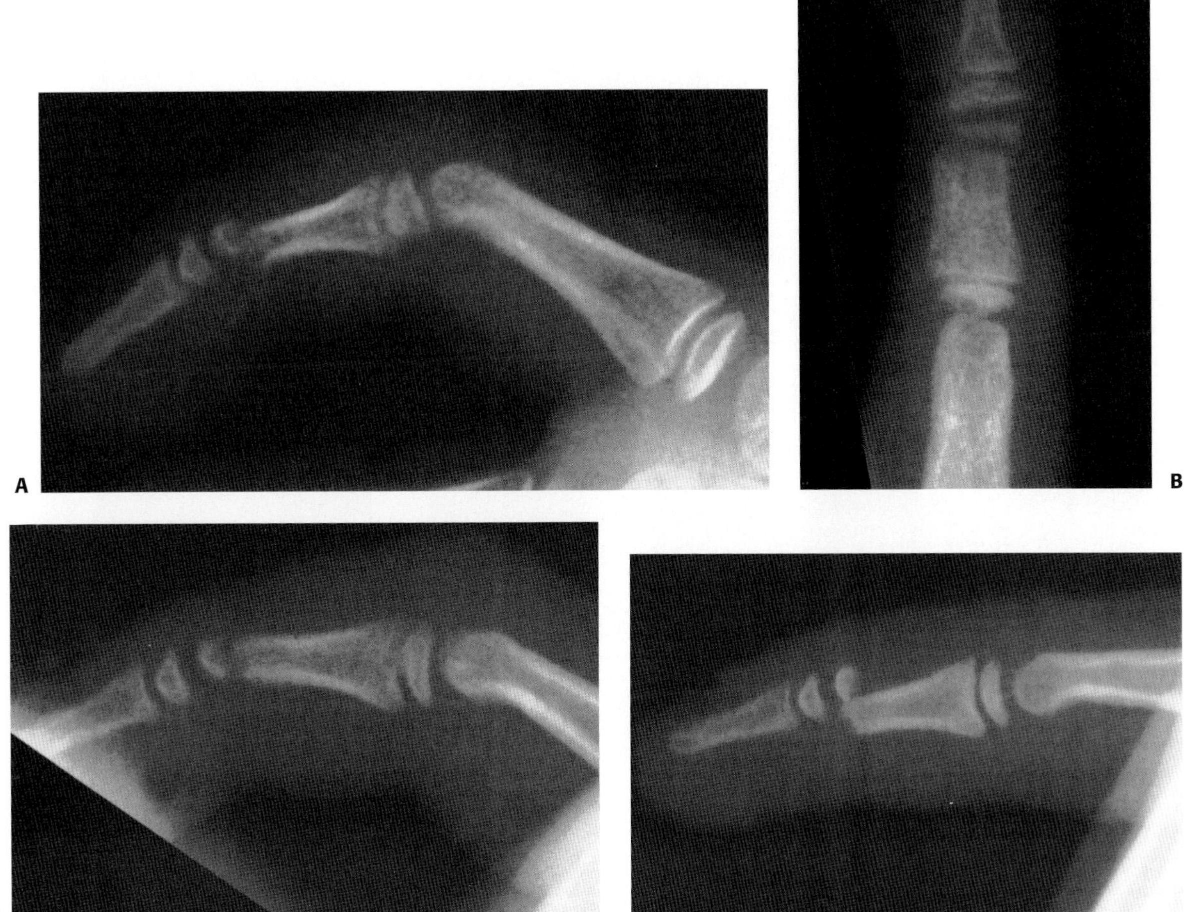

FIGURE 8-49 **A,B.** An 8-year-old girl with a mildly displaced fracture of the neck of the middle phalanx. **C.** Closed reduction was successful on the day of injury and a plaster splint was applied. **D.** Two weeks later, the fracture had markedly re-displaced.

and blocks to motion due to fracture displacement. Most of these fractures do best with pin fixation after stable reduction.

Late

Late complications include nonunion, malunion, osteonecrosis, growth disturbance, and arthritis. Nonunion is rare except in combined injuries with devascularization of the fracture fragments. Bone grafting usually is successful treatment. Malunion can result in angulation or limited motion. Extraarticular malunion can cause angulation or rotational abnormalities. The treatment depends on the child's age and ability to remodel according to fracture location, plane of malunion, and degree of deformity (Fig. 8-50). Considerable deformity may require osteotomy to realign the bone (103). A subcondylar or intra-articular malunion is particularly difficult to treat. Early diagnosis within the first month offers the possibility of fracture realignment through the site of deformity. Treatment of a late diagnosis must consider the risks and benefits associated with extensive surgery. Alternative methods to enhance motion also must be considered. For example, limited flexion from loss of the subcondylar fossa can be remedied by removing the necessary bone to allow joint flexion.

Osteonecrosis usually is related to extensive surgical dissection of a unicondylar or bicondylar fracture fragment. Prevention is the best treatment because reconstruction is limited to some form of joint transfer. Growth disturbance can result from any injury that involves the physis. A shortened or angulated digit may result. It is fortunate that this complication is rare because reconstruction options are limited.

Posttraumatic degenerative joint disease is rare in children, but intra-articular injury and sepsis may result in arthrosis (104). Treatment is directed toward the child's symptoms and not the x-ray findings. Minimal pain and excellent function often accompany considerable arthritic changes on x-rays and warrant no treatment. Pain and functional limitations require treatment; options include a vascularized joint transfer, interposition or distraction arthroplasty, prosthetic joint replacement, and arthrodesis (105).

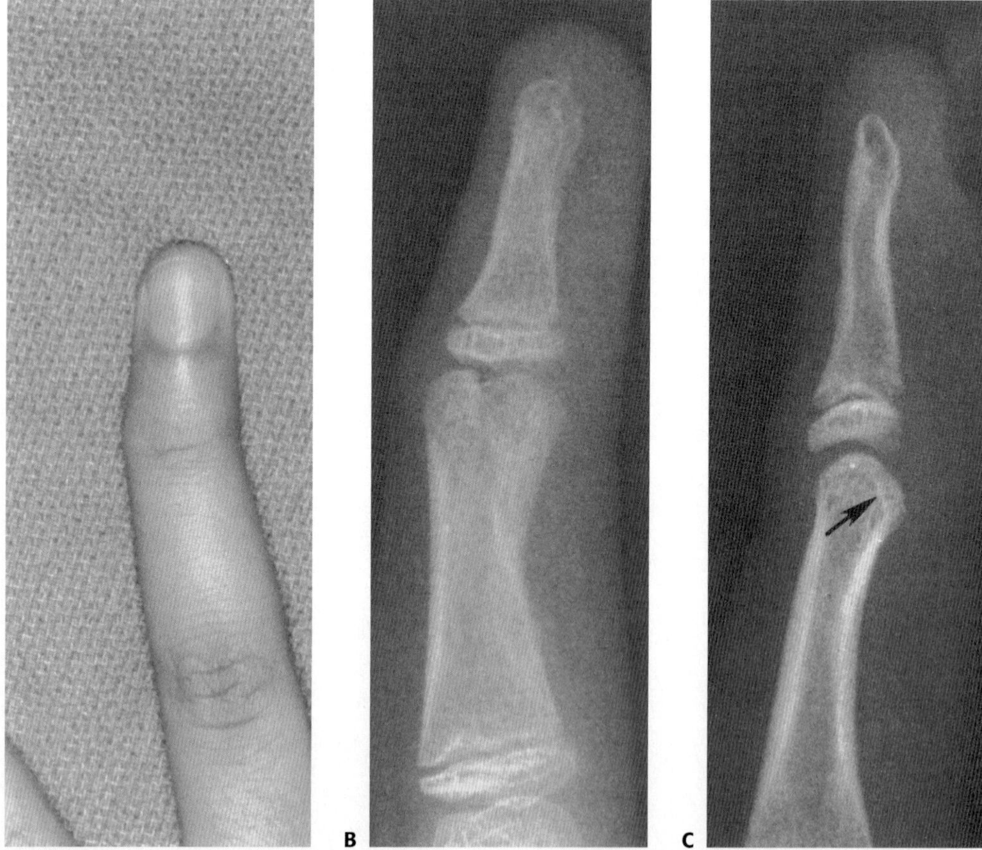

FIGURE 8-50 A. A 13-year-old boy with malunion of the ring finger middle phalanx articular surface. **B,C.** X-rays reveal slight malunion of the radial condyle with mild intra-articular incongruity. The lateral view suggests a double density shadow (*arrow*). The flexion and extension motion of the digit was normal and reconstruction was not recommended.

Fractures of the Metacarpals

Relevant Anatomy

The metacarpals are surrounded by soft tissue and relatively protected within the hand. Considerable variation exists in the relative mobility of the metacarpals through the carpometacarpal (CMC) joints. The index and long rays have minimal CMC joint motion (10–20 degrees). In contrast, the ring and small rays possess more motion (30–40 degrees), and the thumb CMC joint has universal motion.

The neck is the most common site of metacarpal fracture. The metacarpal geometry and composition predispose the metacarpal neck to injury. The distal metacarpal angles as it approaches the MCP joint, and the cortical bone within the subcondylar fossa is relatively thin, which creates a vulnerable area susceptible to injury.

Mechanism of Injury

Direct trauma, rotational forces, and axial loading may all cause fractures of the metacarpal. Contact sports or striking an object are the most common mechanisms.

Fracture Patterns

Fractures of the metacarpals can occur at the epiphysis, physis, neck, shaft, or base (Table 8-4).

Epiphyseal and Physeal Fractures. Epiphyseal and physeal fractures of the metacarpal head are rare but occur most often in the small ray (2,44,106,107). A S-H II fracture of the small metacarpal is most common among patients 12 to 16 years of age (51,76,106,108). Intra-articular, head-splitting fractures at the metacarpal epiphysis and physis consistent with S-H III and IV patterns seldom occur at the metacarpal level (Fig. 8-51).

Metacarpal Neck Fractures. The metacarpal neck is the most frequent site of metacarpal fractures in children. Neck fractures in children are analogous to boxer's fractures in adults (Fig. 8-52). Neck fractures are more common in the small and ring fingers. Fortunately these injuries are juxta-physeal and have significant remodeling potential.

Metacarpal Shaft Fractures. Metacarpal shaft fractures are relatively common. Torsional forces cause oblique and spiral fractures while direct trauma produces transverse fractures. An isolated shaft fracture of a central ray is suspended by the intermetacarpal ligaments, which limit displacement and shortening. In contrast, the border digits (index and small) displace more readily.

TABLE 8-4 Classification of Finger Metacarpal Fractures

Epiphyseal and physeal fractures
Neck fractures
Shaft fractures
Metacarpal base fractures

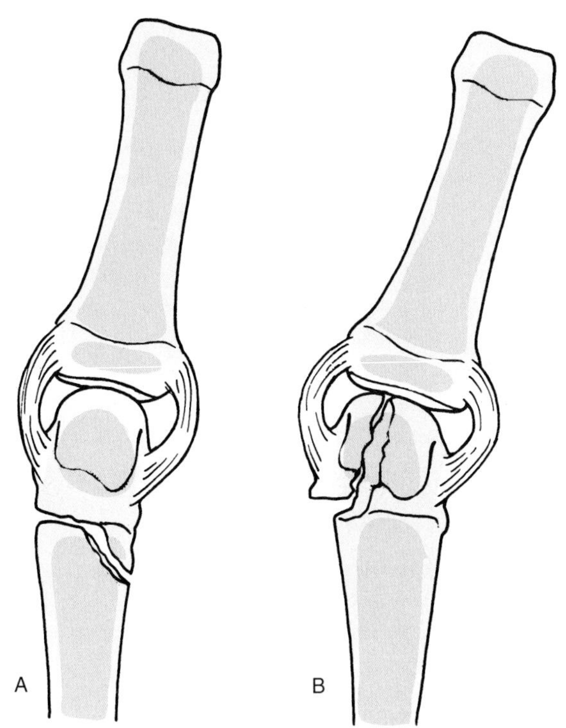

FIGURE 8-51 **A.** A Salter-Harris type II fracture of the metacarpal head. **B.** Head-splitting fracture of the metacarpal epiphysis.

Metacarpal Base Fractures. Metacarpal base fractures are uncommon in children. The base is protected from injury by its proximal location in the hand and the stability afforded by the bony congruence and soft-tissue restraints. Substantial injury to a central metacarpal base usually is from high-energy trauma. The small finger CMC joint is the most prone to injury. Fracture-dislocations often are unstable because of the proximal pull of the extensor carpi ulnaris (reverse Bennett fracture).

Diagnosis

Signs and Symptoms

The diagnosis of metacarpal fracture is based on the history and physical examination. Deformity and swelling may be hidden in the dorsal hand. The child usually avoids active movement and passive motion is resisted. Every metacarpal fracture must be examined for malrotation. Malrotation will result in digital scissoring during active flexion or an abnormal digital cascade with passive tenodesis. Clinical suspicion warrants x-ray examination.

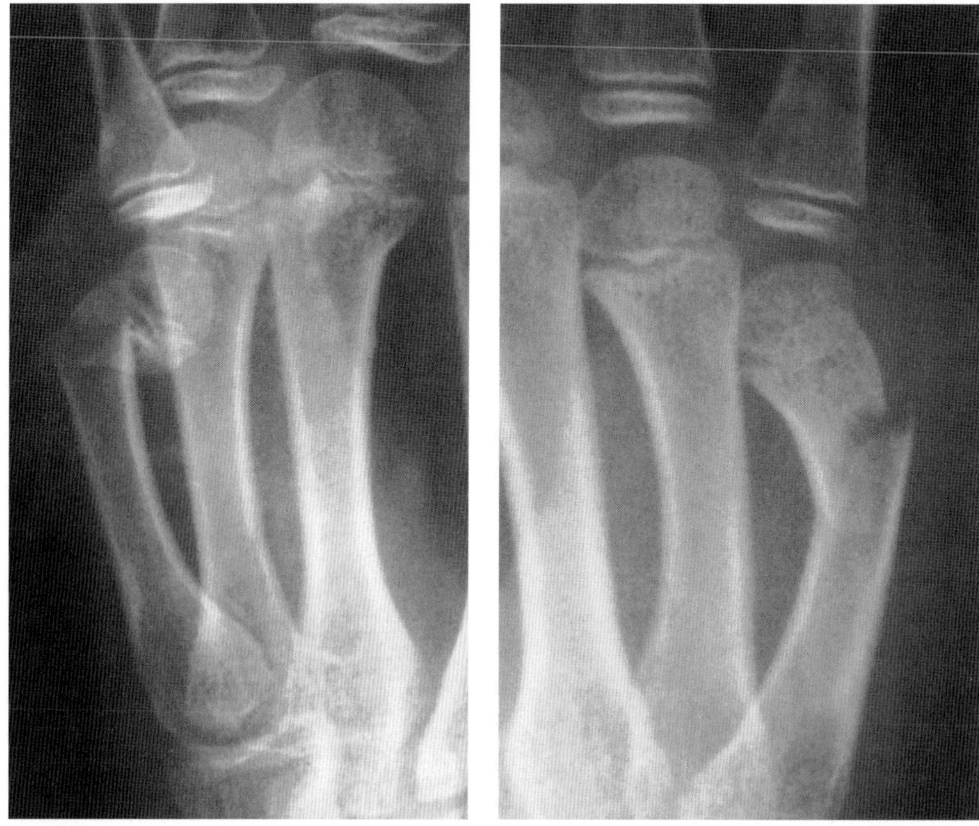

FIGURE 8-52 **A.** A true boxer's fracture of the metacarpal neck of the fifth ray. **B.** This fracture is more in the diaphysis and should not be considered a boxer's fracture.

Radiographic Findings

Metacarpal fractures usually are readily visible on x-rays. Anteroposterior and lateral views may be supplemented by an oblique view to assess fracture configuration. A metacarpal head-splitting fracture may be difficult to detect and requires special views. The Brewerton view is helpful and is made with the dorsum of the hand against the cassette and the MCP joints flexed about 65 degrees. The central beam is angled 15 degrees to the ulnar side of the hand (109). This projection focuses on the metacarpal heads and may highlight subtle bony abnormalities.

Treatment Options

The treatment of metacarpal fractures varies with the location, extent, and configuration of the fracture. Nonoperative or closed treatment is the primary mode of management for most fractures. Operative intervention is used for multiple metacarpal fractures, extensive soft-tissue injury, intra-articular head-splitting fractures, malrotated fractures, and irreducible fractures.

Epiphyseal and Physeal Fractures

Management is based on the amount of displacement and fracture stability. Many of these fractures can be treated by closed methods. Gentle reduction under metacarpal or wrist block anesthesia is followed by application of a splint in the safe position. If the fracture is reducible but unstable, percutaneous pin fixation is recommended. If the Thurston-Holland fragment is large enough, the wire can secure the metaphyseal piece and avoid the physis. Otherwise, the wire must cross the physis to obtain stability. A small-diameter smooth wire is advocated and multiple passes should be avoided.

Displaced intra-articular head-splitting fractures require open reduction and internal fixation to restore articular congruity. Many of these fractures have unrecognized comminution that complicates internal fixation. Wire or screw fixation is used, depending on the age of the patient and size of the fragments. Transosseous suture repair may be necessary. Bone grafting may be necessary for stable reduction. The primary goal of surgical treatment is anatomic reduction. A secondary goal is stable fixation to allow early motion.

Neck Fracture

Metacarpal neck fractures usually are treated by closed methods. The amount of acceptable apex dorsal angulation is controversial. Greater angulation is allowable in the mobile ring and small rays compared to the index and long. Another consideration is the effect of remodeling over time, which is dependent on the age of the child. In general, 10 to 30 degrees of angulation greater than the corresponding CMC joint motion is acceptable.

Considerable angulation can be treated with closed reduction with general anesthesia and splint or cast application. The Jahss maneuver is commonly recommended and involves initial flexion of the MCP joint to 90 degrees to relax the deforming force of the intrinsic muscles and tighten the collateral ligaments (110). Subsequently, upward pressure is applied along the proximal phalanx to push the metacarpal head in a dorsal direction while counter-pressure is applied along the dorsal aspect of the proximal metacarpal fracture. Jahss (110) suggested immobilization with the MCP and PIP joints flexed, but this type of immobilization is no longer advocated for fear of stiffness and skin breakdown. Immobilization in the intrinsic plus or safe position is the appropriate position. A well-molded splint or cast is necessary. The PIP joints may or may not be included in the immobilization depending on the status of the reduction and reliability of the patient.

Uncommonly, a neck fracture may be extremely unstable and require percutaneous pinning (Fig. 8-53). Pins can be inserted in a variety of configurations. Extramedullary techniques include crossed pinning or pinning to the adjacent stable metacarpal. Intramedullary techniques also can be used, similar to those used for metacarpal shaft and neck fractures in adults (111,112). Intramedullary techniques are reserved for patients near physeal closure. Pre-bent Kirschner wires or commercially available implants are inserted through the metacarpal base in an antegrade fashion. The wires can be used to assist in fracture

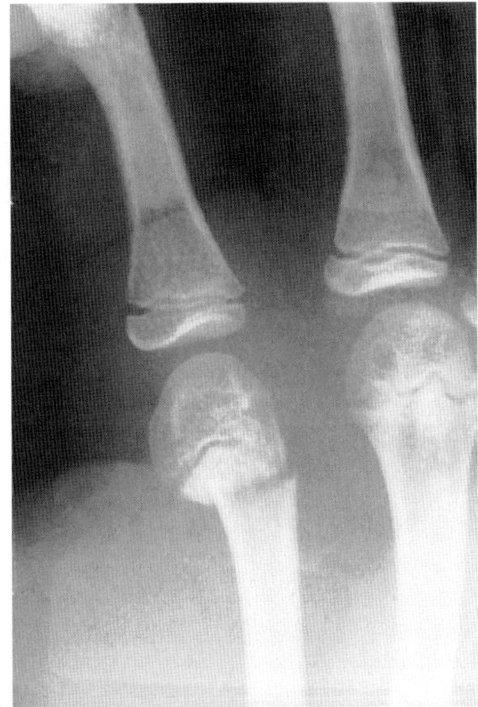

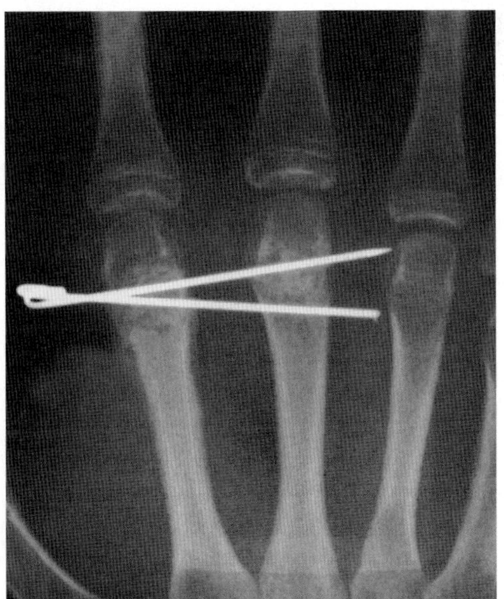

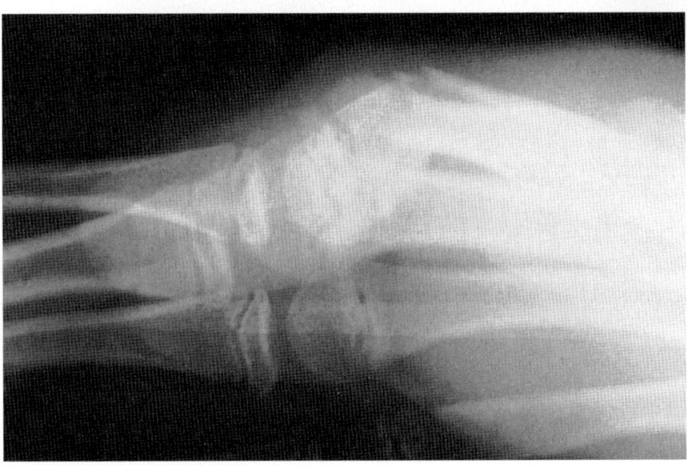

FIGURE 8-53 **A,B.** A 14-year-old boy with a dorsally angulated fracture of the second metacarpal. **C.** Closed reduction was unstable and percutaneous Kirschner wire fixation was performed. (Reprinted from O'Brien ET. Fractures of the hand. In: Green DP, ed. *Operative hand surgery,* 2nd ed. New York: Churchill Livingstone, 1988: 715–716, with permission.)

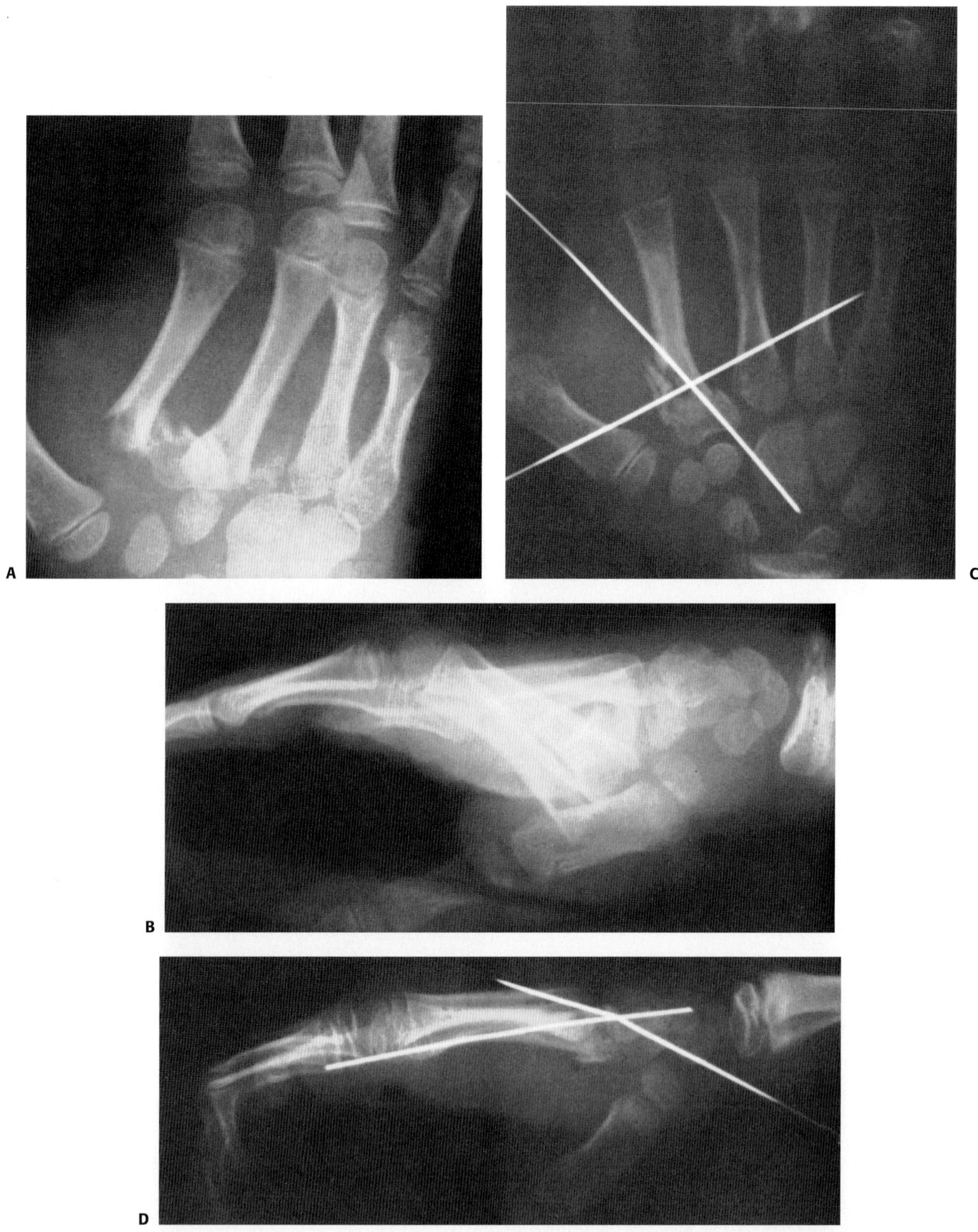

FIGURE 8-54 A,B. An 11-year-old boy sustained a fracture of the proximal shaft of the second metacarpal and a fracture-dislocation of the third carpometacarpal joint. **C,D.** Closed manipulation was unsuccessful and open reduction and Kirschner wire fixation were required.

reduction. Stability is obtained by stacking several wires within the canal and across the fracture site.

Open reduction of metacarpal neck fractures is seldom required in children and is reserved for irreducible fractures, unstable fractures in skeletally mature children, multiple metacarpal fractures, and combination injuries that require a stable bony platform.

Shaft Fractures

An isolated long or ring metacarpal fracture often is minimally displaced because the metacarpals are suspended by the intermetacarpal ligaments. Immobilization for 4 weeks is usually all that is necessary. In contrast, the index and small digits may require additional treatment, such as closed reduction and immobilization. Percutaneous pinning is reserved for unstable shaft fractures. Pins can be inserted with extramedullary or intramedullary techniques.

Open reduction and internal fixation of a metacarpal shaft fracture rarely are indicated in children, unless there are multiple fractures, extensive soft-tissue damage, or the child is skeletally mature. A long spiral-oblique fracture, however, that has substantial malrotation and displacement may require miniscrew fixation to reestablish alignment.

Metacarpal Base Fractures

Fractures of the metacarpal base or fracture-dislocations at the CMC joint are usually high-energy injuries with substantial tissue disruption. Assessment of the muscle compartments for signs of evolving compartment syndrome and careful neurovascular assessment are indicated. Isolated fracture-dislocations of the small ray CMC joint are the most common metacarpal base fractures. Preoperative computed tomographic (CT) scans are appropriate to assess articular congruity and comminution. Closed reduction and percutaneous pinning usually are sufficient to resist the deforming force of the extensor carpi ulnaris (113). The pins can be placed transversely between the metacarpals or across the CMC joint or both.

Open reduction may be necessary to achieve reduction and ensure stable fixation in high-energy injuries (Fig. 8-54) (114,115). A transverse or longitudinal incision can be used for exposure. Longitudinal incisions are recommended in patients with concomitant compartment syndrome to allow for simultaneous decompression. Fixation options are numerous, depending on the fracture configuration. Supplemental bone graft may be necessary to maintain joint congruity.

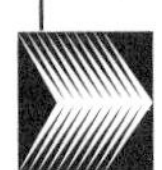

AUTHORS' PREFERRED TREATMENT

Epiphyseal and Physeal Fractures

Most nondisplaced physeal fractures are treated with immobilization. Salter-Harris II metacarpal neck fractures seldom require reduction. These fractures typically occur in adolescents who possess enough remodeling to accept 30 to 35 degrees of sagittal angulation as long as rotation is acceptable and there is sufficient growth remaining. A widely displaced fracture that is reducible requires percutaneous pinning to maintain the reduction (Fig. 8-55). Displaced epiphyseal fractures with considerable intra-articular displacement require open reduction and internal fixation through a dorsal approach and splitting of the extensor apparatus over the MCP joint. Anatomic reduction is the objective and fixation devices vary according to the patient and fracture configuration.

Metacarpal Neck Fractures

Nonoperative and closed methods are the mainstays of treatment. Considerable sagittal angulation is acceptable, especially in the ring and small digits. Small finger angulation up to 30 degrees usually does not necessitate closed reduction as long as there is no malrotation and there is sufficient growth remaining. Greater angulations are treated with closed reduction and cast application. Index and ring finger angulations of more than 20 degrees are treated by closed reduction. Pin fixation is used for unstable fractures that have a tendency to re-displace. Open reduction rarely is necessary.

Metacarpal Shaft Fractures

The number, configuration, and location of the metacarpal shaft fracture(s) dictate treatment. Isolated fractures that are minimally displaced require only immobilization. Isolated fractures that are displaced or malrotated require closed reduction and percutaneous fixation. Rotation is carefully assessed to ensure adequate reduction. An irreducible fracture or multiple fractures usually require open reduction. The fixation technique varies according to the age of the child and fracture pattern. If open fixation is necessary, stable fixation is the goal. Mini-plate and screw fixation is preferred to restore alignment and to allow early mobilization of tendons and soft tissue. The physis should be avoided to prevent growth disturbance. The operative approach and internal fixation principles are similar in children and adults. Long oblique fractures are managed with interfragmentary screw fixation. Short oblique and transverse fractures require a neutralization plate with purchase of four cortices proximal and distal to the fracture.

Metacarpal Base Fractures

Metacarpal base fractures often are displaced or unstable. Extra-articular fractures can be treated by closed reduction with or without percutaneous pinning. Intra-articular fracture-dislocations are more challenging (113–115). Percutaneous pinning often is required to stabilize the fracture and to reduce CMC joint subluxation. The wires are placed between the bases of the adjacent metacarpals or across the CMC joint in isolated injuries. Irreducible or multiple fracture-dislocations require open reduction (Fig. 8-54) (115).

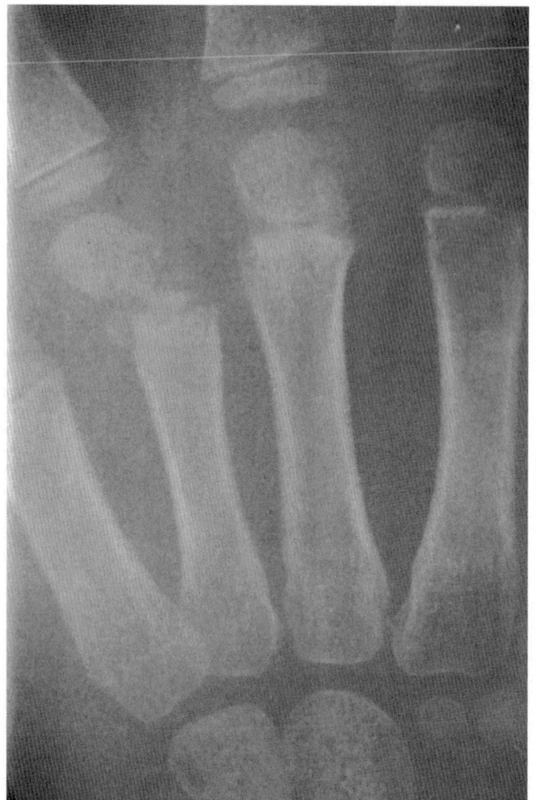

A

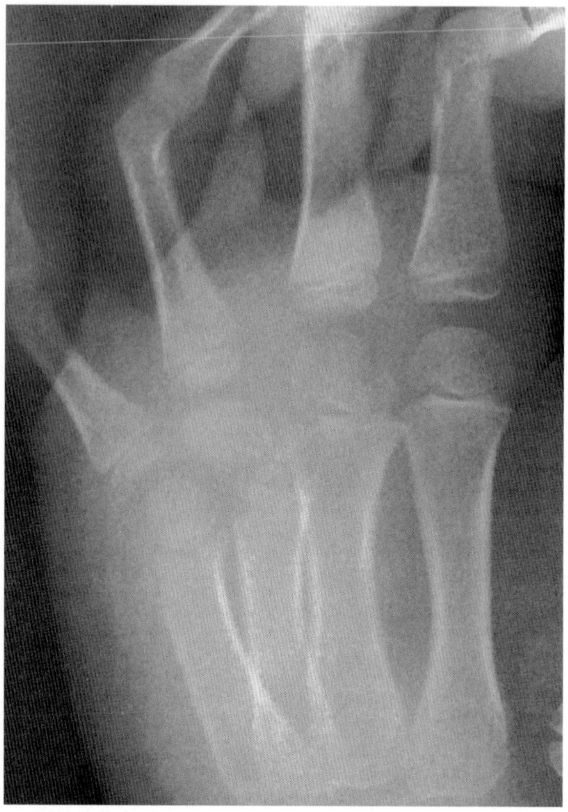

B

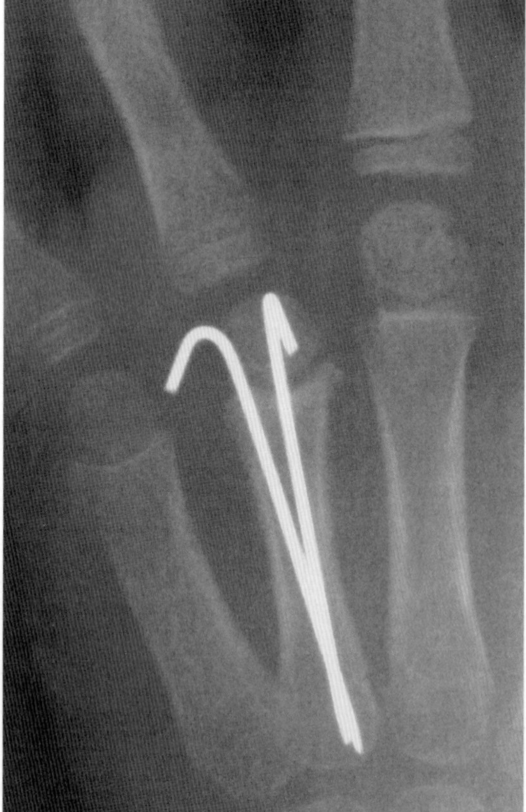

C

FIGURE 8-55 A,B. A 7-year-old boy with a comminuted and displaced physeal fracture of the ring metacarpal. **C.** Closed reduction was successful and percutaneous pinning was used to maintain alignment. The Salter-Harris type II fracture of the small finger metacarpal required no additional treatment.

Postoperative Care and Rehabilitation

Most metacarpal fractures managed by closed treatment are immobilized for 4 weeks. Subsequently, a home program of range of motion exercises is started and formal therapy is not needed. In active children and young athletes, a light splint can be worn for protection from direct trauma and as a warning signal to the patient and his or her peers for an additional few weeks. If percutaneous pin fixation is used, the wires are removed in the office 4 weeks after surgery.

Open fracture reduction depends on the stability of the fixation and the reliability of the patient. Older patients and multiple metacarpal fractures may be best treated with internal fixation. These fractures can be mobilized earlier, usually 5 to 7 days after surgery with a removable splint for protection between exercise sessions for 4 to 6 weeks, provided the patient is reliable.

Prognosis

Most metacarpal fractures heal without substantial sequelae. Mild deformity in the plane of motion is tolerated and may correct with remodeling. Considerable angulation or rotation creates a functional impairment that requires treatment.

Complications

Bony complications include malunion and osteonecrosis (Table 8-5). Nonunion is rare (51,116). Even a small amount (less than 10 degrees) of rotational malalignment may create overlap of the digits during flexion and a functional disturbance (Fig. 8-56). Corrective osteotomy to realign the digit often is necessary with rotational malunions. The ostetotomy can be made at the site of fracture or anywhere along the metacarpal. The proximal shaft or base has certain advantages. This area provides ample bone for healing and offers the opportunity for internal fixation using wires or a plate.

TABLE 8-5 Adverse Factors for Finger Metacarpal Fractures

Epiphyseal and physeal fractures	Avascular necrosis, malreduction/malunion
Neck fractures	Excessive apex dorsal angulation, malrotation
Shaft fractures	Malrotation, soft-tissue interposition, nonunion
Metacarpal base fractures	Loss of reduction, malreduction of articular fragments, late instability

Osteonecrosis of the metacarpal head may occur after an intra-articular frature. Factors include the degree of injury and the intracapsular pressure caused by the hemarthrosis (108,117,118). Theoretically, early joint aspiration may diminish the intra-articular pressure. Fortunately, partial osteonecrosis in a growing child incites remarkable remodeling of the adjacent articular surface and often results in a functional joint. Part-time splint protection during the remodeling phase is recommended. Considerable joint incongruity is rare and reconstructive options are limited (105).

Fractures of the Thumb Metacarpal

Relevant Anatomy

The base of the proximal phalanx and its intimate structures (the volar plate and sesamoid bones) play a role in fracture mechanics. The adductor pollicis, abductor pollicis brevis, and flexor pollicis brevis can displace metcarpal fractures. Their directions of pull dictate the direction of fracture displacement and deformity. The adductor pollicis inserts onto the proximal phalanx and into the extensor apparatus through the adductor aponeurosis. Epiphyseal fragments with the attached ulnar collateral ligament (UCL) may be displaced outside the adductor aponeurosis (206). This pediatric "Stener lesion" prohibits healing and requires open reduction. The abductor pollicis longus inserts onto the metacarpal base and is the primary deforming force in most fracture-dislocations about the thumb CMC joint (119).

Mechanism of Injury

Direct trauma, rotational forces, and axial loading may all cause thumb metacarpal fractures. Sporting endeavors are the prime events causing fractures. A valgus force to the MCP joint usually produces an epiphyseal fracture. Skiing and extreme biking are specific activities that place the thumb MCP joint in a vulnerable position.

Fracture Patterns

Fractures of the thumb metacarpal can occur at the epiphysis, physis, neck, shaft, or base. Fractures of the neck and shaft and their treatment principles are similar to those of the fingers (Table 8-6). Thumb metacarpal base fractures that involve the physis or epiphysis require particular mention (Fig. 8-57).

Thumb Metacarpal Base Fractures. Fractures of the base of the thumb metacarpal are subdivided according to their location. Type A fractures occur between the physis and the junction of the proximal and middle thirds of the bone. They often are transverse or slightly oblique. There often is an element of medial impaction and the fracture is angulated in an apex lateral direction (Fig. 8-58).

Type B and C fractures are S-H II fractures at the thumb metacarpal base. Most patterns have the metaphyseal fragment on the medial side (type B) (Fig. 8-57). The shaft fragment is adducted by the pull of the adductor pollicis and shifted in a

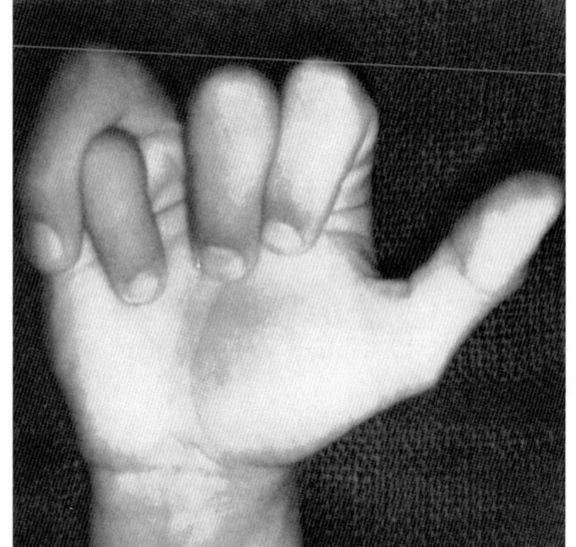

A

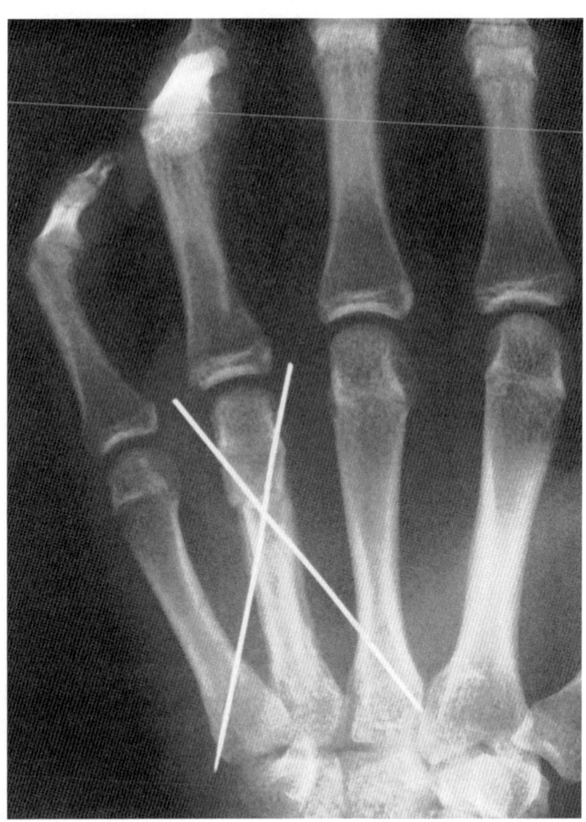

C

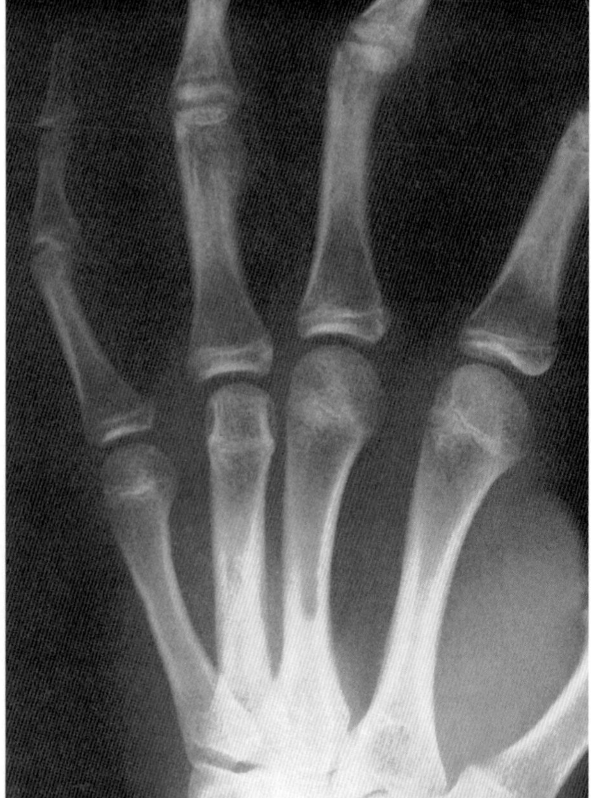

B

FIGURE 8-56 A,B. A 15-year-old boy with severe overlapping of the ring finger on the little finger secondary to rotatory malunion of a spiral fracture of the ring metacarpal. **C.** Distal osteotomy through the deformity stabilized with pin fixation to correct the malrotation. (Reprinted from O'Brien ET. Fractures of the hand. In: Green DP, ed. *Operative hand surgery,* 2nd ed. New York: Churchill Livingstone, 1988:731; with permission.)

TABLE 8-6 Classification of Thumb Metacarpal Fractures

Fractures of the head

Fractures of the shaft

Fractures of the thumb metacarpal base
- Fractures distal to the physis
- Salter-Harris II fractures—metaphyseal medial
- Salter-Harris II fractures—metaphyseal lateral

Intra-articular Salter-Harris III or IV fractures

proximal direction by the pull of the abductor pollicis longus. Although this pattern resembles a Bennett fracture with respect to the deforming forces, there is no intra-articular extension (119). Type C fractures are the least common and have the reverse pattern, with the metaphyseal fragment on the lateral side and the proximal shaft displacement in a medial direction. This pattern often results from more substantial trauma and is not suitable for closed treatment.

A type D fracture is a S-H III or IV fracture that most closely resembles the adult Bennett fracture (7,40,87,120). The deforming forces are similar to a type B injury with resultant adduction and proximal migration of the base-shaft fragment.

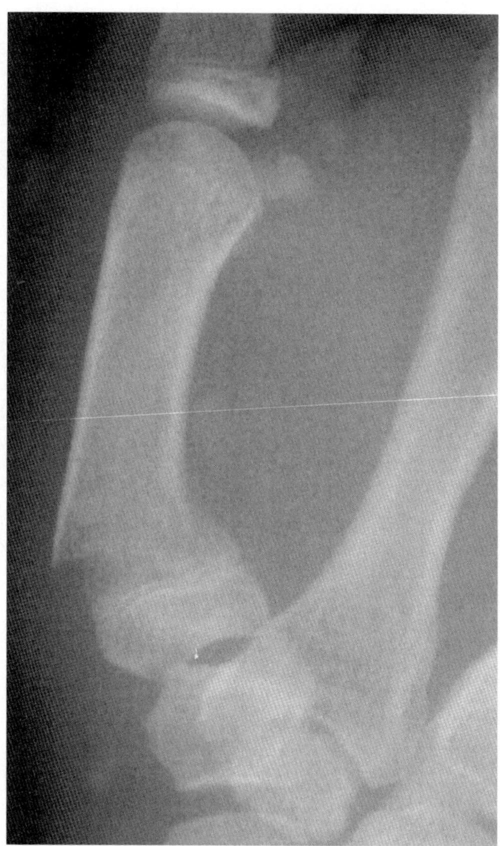

FIGURE 8-58 Metaphyseal thumb metacarpal fracture that does not involve the physis. Treatment was closed reduction and cast immobilization.

Diagnosis

Signs and Symptoms

The diagnosis of thumb metacarpal fracture usually is straightforward. Swelling and ecchymosis are obvious signs of injury. Most of the swelling appears about the thenar eminence. Active thumb motion is limited and passive thumb movement is painful. The thumb may appear angulated or rotated. However, thumb motion is oriented differently than finger movement, which makes angulation and malrotation more difficult to judge.

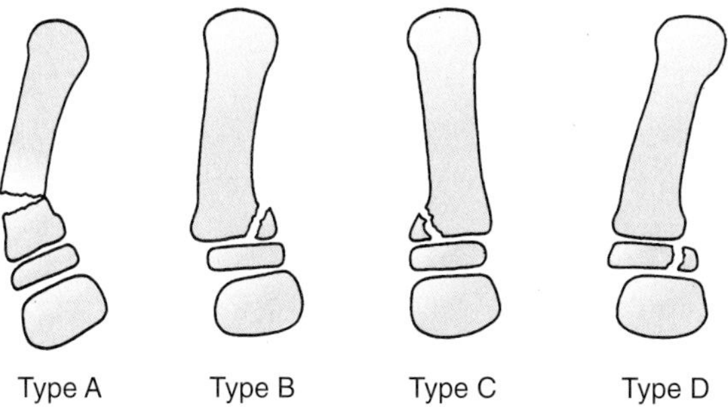

FIGURE 8-57 Classification of thumb metacarpal fractures. Type A: Metaphyseal fracture. Types B and C: Salter-Harris type II physeal fractures with lateral or medial angulation. Type D: Salter-Harris type III fracture (pediatric Bennett's fracture).

Radiographic Findings

Biplanar images of the thumb are mandatory. Anteroposterior and lateral views of the thumb and not the fingers are required. Biplanar x-rays ensure adequate evaluation of fracture position. A hyperpronated view of the thumb accentuates the view of the CMC joint.

Treatment Options

Thumb Metacarpal Base Fractures

Type A. Type A fractures usually can be treated by closed methods (Fig. 8-59). Although swelling about the thenar eminence limits manipulation of the fracture and diminishes the effectiveness of immobilization, most fractures can still be treated successfully by closed reduction and immobilization. The CMC joint has near universal motion, and the physis is proximal in the metacarpal, so remodeling is extensive in young patients. If reduction is attempted, pressure is applied to the apex of the fracture to affect reduction. Since the fracture is close to the

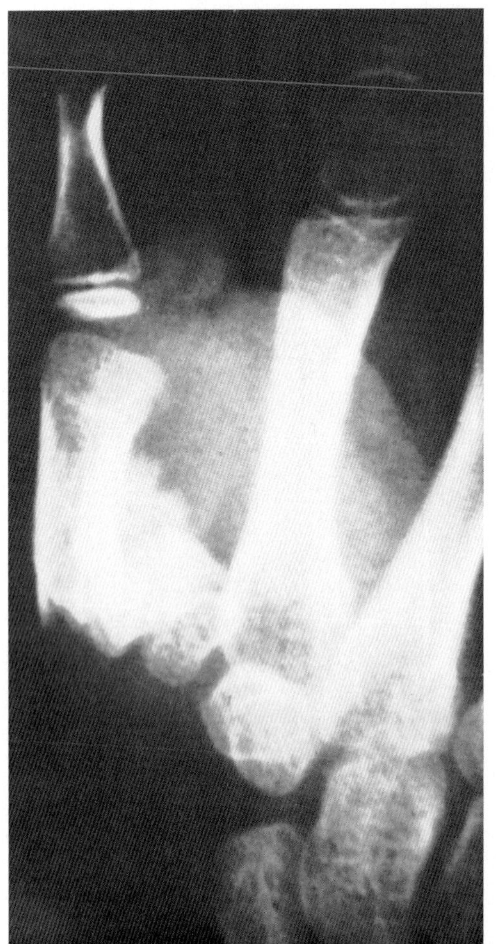

A

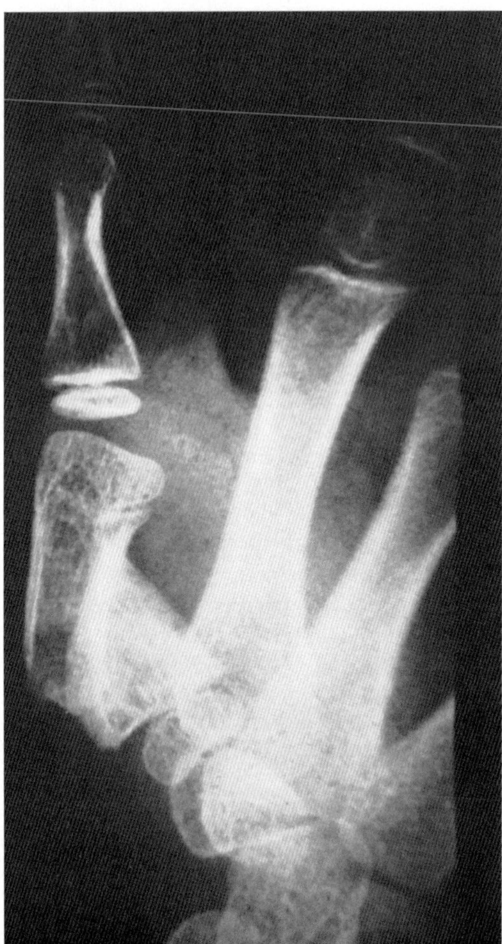

B

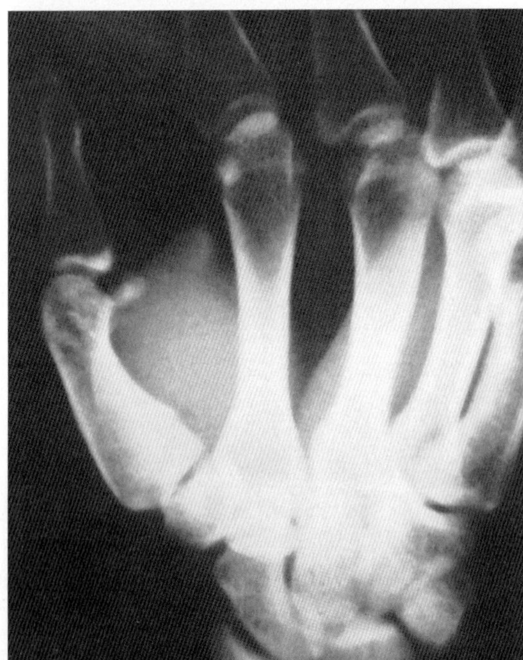

C

FIGURE 8-59 **A.** A 10-year-old boy with a severe head injury sustained a markedly displaced type A fracture of the thumb metacarpal. **B.** One month later, x-ray reveals union of the unreduced fracture with early remodeling. **C.** Seven years later, the x-ray shows substantial remodeling with excellent function. (Remodeling around this multiaxial joint can be compared with that seen in fractures around the proximal humerus.) (Courtesy of Sigurd C. Sandzen, Jr., MD.)

development. This arrangement is thought to provide a unique shelter from injury (7,107). This observation is supported by epidemiologic studies of scaphoid fractures that highlight the infrequent incidence in children younger than 7 years of age and the marked increase in teenagers (137,139).

Force Transmission During Carpal Injury

The mechanisms of injury that create a carpal or distal radial injury are similar. (133,140–143). Concomitant injuries are rare in children, but deserve consideration during the evaluation of the injured child. These combination injuries requires recognition and appropriate treatment to maximize function.

SPECIFIC CARPAL FRACTURES

Scaphoid Fractures

Epidemiology

The scaphoid is the most frequently injured carpal bone in children (107,139,144). Scaphoid fractures are extremely rare during the first decade of life (15,26,137,139,143,145–147). The peak period for scaphoid fractures in skeletally immature children is about 15 years of age, which parallels the evolving ossification of the scaphoid (26). The peak incidence of scaphoid fractures in children and adults is between the late teens and mid-twenties (7,148).

Mechanism of Injury: Differences in Children

The mechanisms and anatomy of scaphoid fractures vary between adults and children (Fig. 8-64). Waist fractures are more common in adults than in children (149,150). However, scaphoid waist fractures are increasing in frequency as participation in contact athletics is occurring at a younger age. These adult-like injuries carry the same risks of nonunion and osteonecrosis as their counterparts in skeletally mature patients (151). In children, fractures of the distal third of the scaphoid have traditionally been the most common injury pattern and often result from direct trauma (137,143,145). Proximal pole fractures are rare in children and often represent an avulsion fracture of the scapholunate ligament. These injuries are at higher risk for non-union and osteonecrosis. The scaphoid also can be fractured as a component of a greater arc perilunar injury (140).

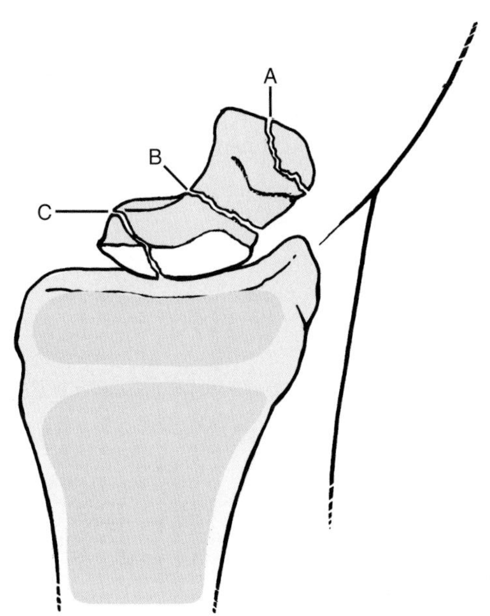

FIGURE 8-64 Three types of scaphoid fractures. *A*, Distal third. *B*, Middle third. *C*, Proximal pole.

Mechanism of Injury: Differences in Location

Distal Scaphoid. Distal pole fractures often are secondary to direct trauma or avulsion with a dorsoradial or dorsovolar fragment. The strong scaphotrapezial ligaments and capsular attachments produce mechanical failure through the bone. Other ligaments can produce additional forces across the distal pole, including the extrinsic volar ligaments and extrinsic dorsal ligaments (Fig. 8-65) (143,152). The fracture line and size of the avulsion fragment vary from an isolated chondral injury that is barely visible on x-ray to a large osteochondral fragment (43).

Middle Third. Middle third fractures do occur in skeletally immature patients. The mechanism of injury usually is wrist dorsiflexion, although alternative mechanisms may lead to fracture (150,153–155). Bony comminution may be present (Fig. 8-66). A careful scrutiny for other injuries about the carpus is mandatory (91,144,146,156).

Proximal Pole. Proximal pole fractures are rare in children but have been reported in competitive adolescent athletes. The mechanism often is unclear, although a dorsiflexion injury may be a precipitating cause. A proximal pole fracture may propagate through the interface between newly ossified tissue and the cartilaginous anlage or the injury may be strictly through the cartilage. Proximal fractures may cause destabilization of the scapholunate joint, as the scapholunate interosseous ligament remains attached to the avulsed fragment (Fig. 8-67).

Fracture Patterns

Fracture patterns are listed in Table 8-7.

Type A: Fractures of the Distal Pole

Type A1: Extra-articular Distal Pole Fractures. The most important prognostic factor is the presence or absence of joint involvement (Fig. 8-68). Extra-articular fractures may be either volar or dorsal avulsions. A volar pattern is more common and is attributed to the stout scaphotrapezial ligaments. A dorsal fracture configuration is less common and is attributed to the

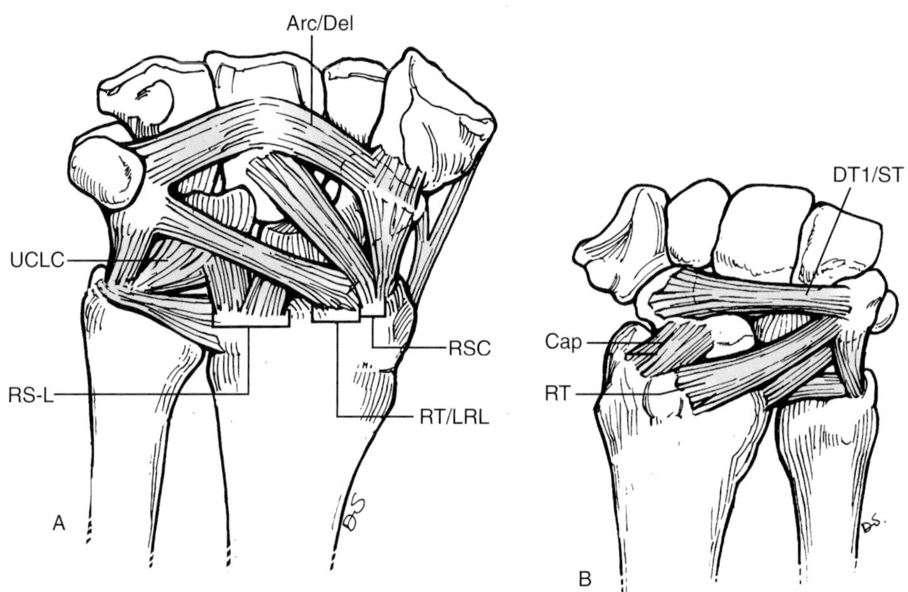

FIGURE 8-65 The volar and dorsal extrinsic and intrinsic carpal ligaments. **A.** Selected volar ligaments about the wrist. *RS-L,* radioscaphoid-lunate; *RT/LRL,* radiotriquetral/long radiolunate; *RSC,* radioscaphocapitate ligament; *Arc/Del,* arcuate or deltoid ligament; *UCLC,* ulnocarpal ligament complex, including ulnocarpal volar ligament, dis-triquetral and disc-lunate ligaments. **B.** Dorsal ligaments about the wrist. *Cap,* capsular attachments; *RT,* radiotriquetral ligament; *DTI/ST,* dorsal transverse intercarpal ligament or scaphotrapezial ligament.

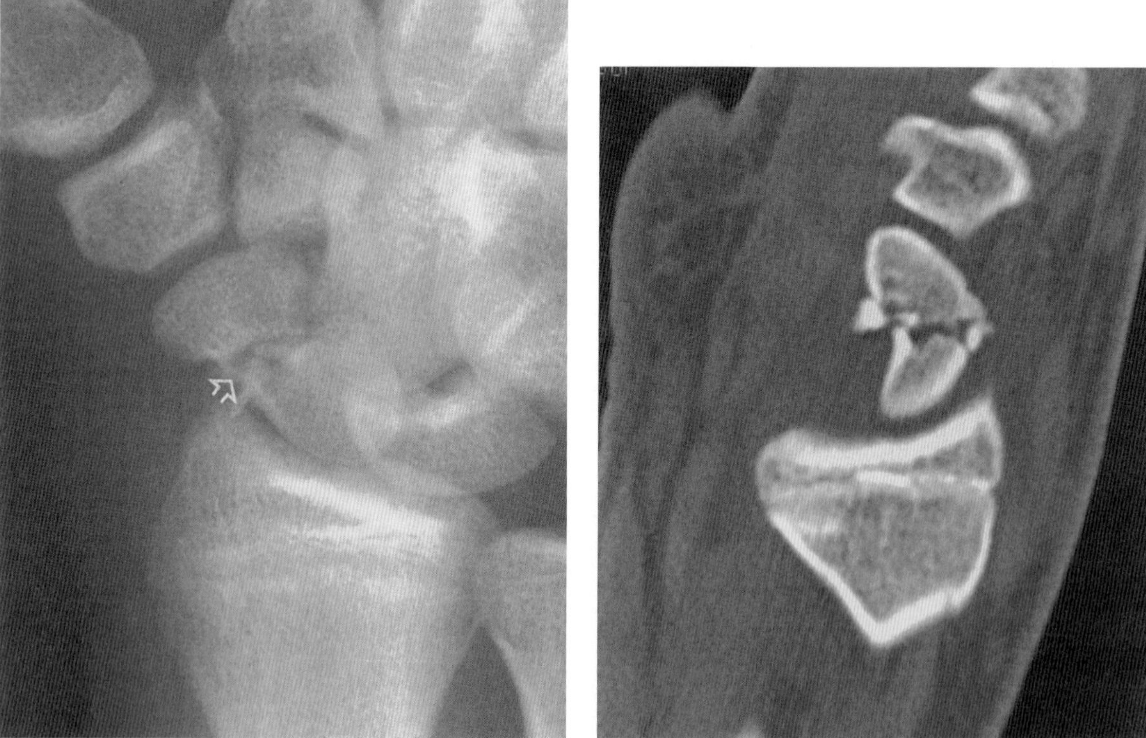

FIGURE 8-66 **A.** A displaced mid-waist scaphoid fracture with comminution, including a butterfly fragment from the volar radial aspect (*arrow*). **B.** Computed tomographic scan demonstrates the comminution. *(continues)*

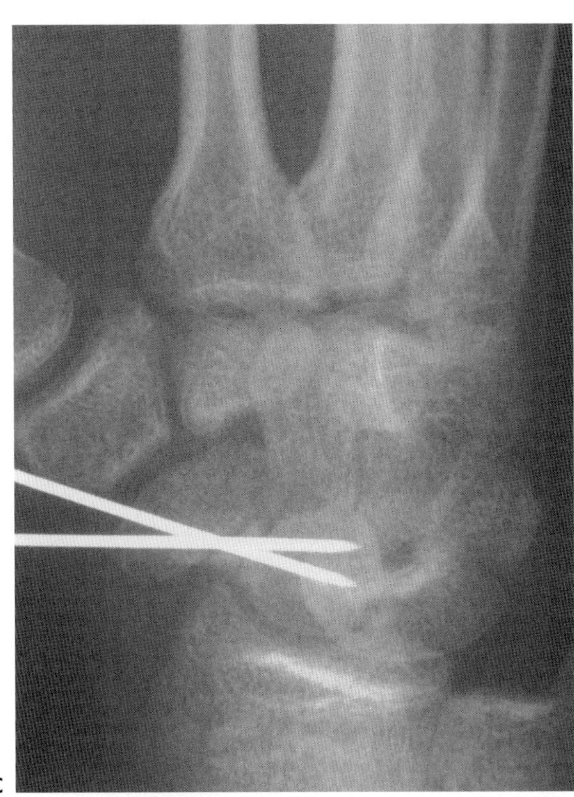

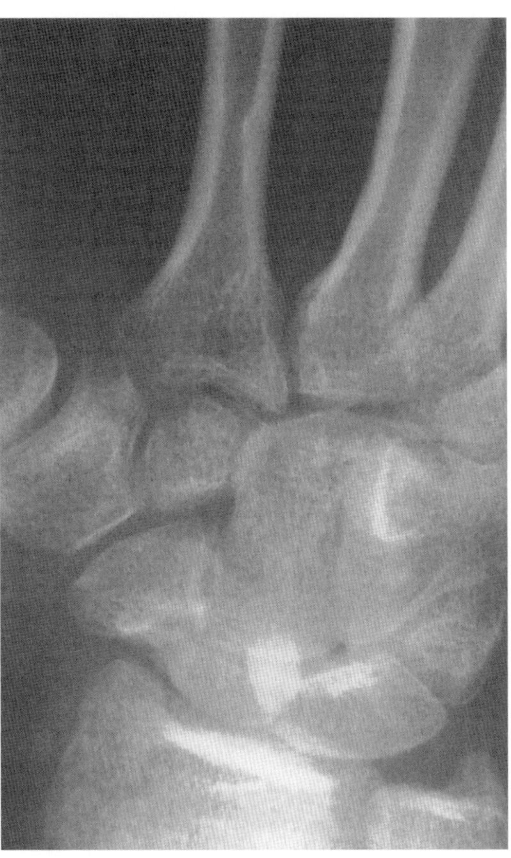

FIGURE 8-66 *(continued)* **C.** Open reduction with internal fixation was performed with two smooth wires and bone graft from the distal radius. **D.** Healing of fracture after pin removal.

dorsal intercarpal ligament. The fragments vary in size and the x-ray appearance is age dependent.

Type A2: Intra-articular Distal Pole Fractures. This type of fracture may be a variation of a type IA fractures with intra-articular extension (Fig. 8-69). Similar types (i.e., volar and dorsal) and mechanisms of injury are possible.

Type B: Middle Third (Waist Fractures). Dividing the bone into thirds or delineating the area bounded by the radioscaphocapitate ligament defines the waist of the scaphoid. Waist fractures occur in many forms (Fig. 8-70). Most children's fractures are incomplete or minimally displaced. Comminuted fractures are rare and associated with higher energy (Fig. 8-66).

Type C: Proximal Fractures. Proximal third fractures present diagnostic and therapeutic dilemmas. The proximal pole is the last to ossify, which further complicates diagnosis. The tenuous blood supply of this region presents the same problems in children as adults in terms of nonunion and osteonecrosis risks.

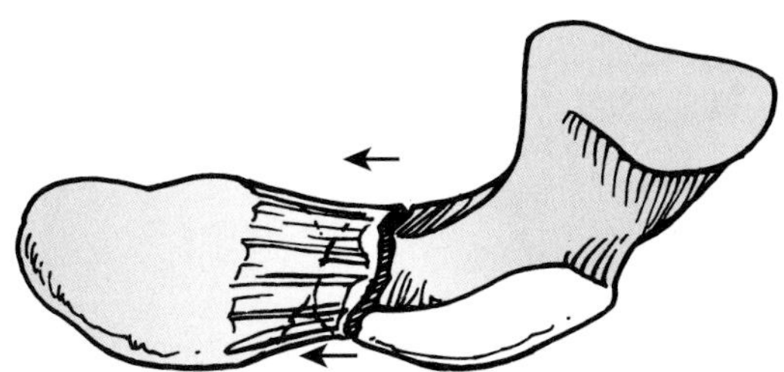

FIGURE 8-67 A proximal pole scaphoid fracture can destabilize the scapholunate articulation. The scapholunate interosseous ligament can avulse a fragment of bone from the proximal pole (*arrows*).

TABLE 8-7 Classification of Scaphoid Fractures

Fractures of the distal pole
Extra-articular distal pole fractures
Intra-articular distal pole fractures
Fractures of the mid-waist
Fractures of the proximal pole

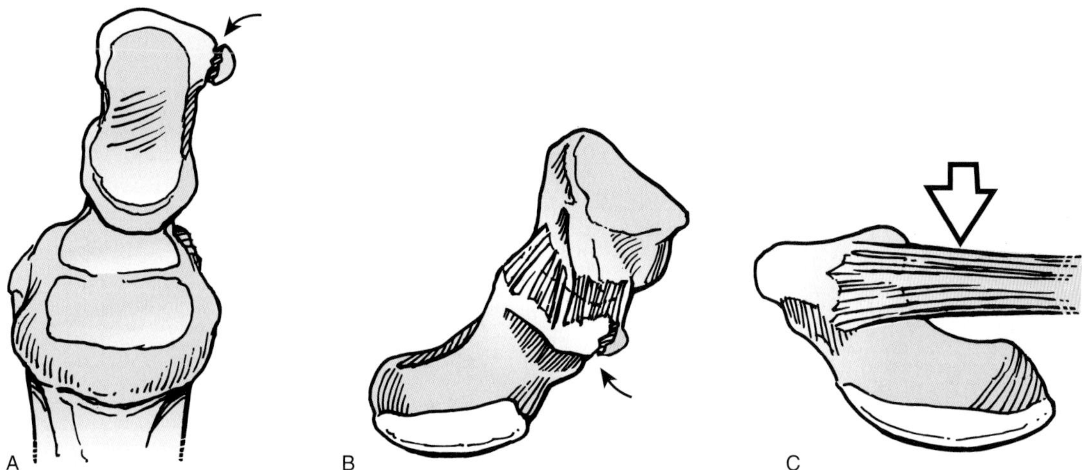

FIGURE 8-68 **A,B.** Small extra-articular distal fractures of the scaphoid (*arrows*) are likely the result of traction forces by the capsule and ligaments. **C.** Extraarticular dorsal fractures can also be the result of capsular attachment (*open arrow*).

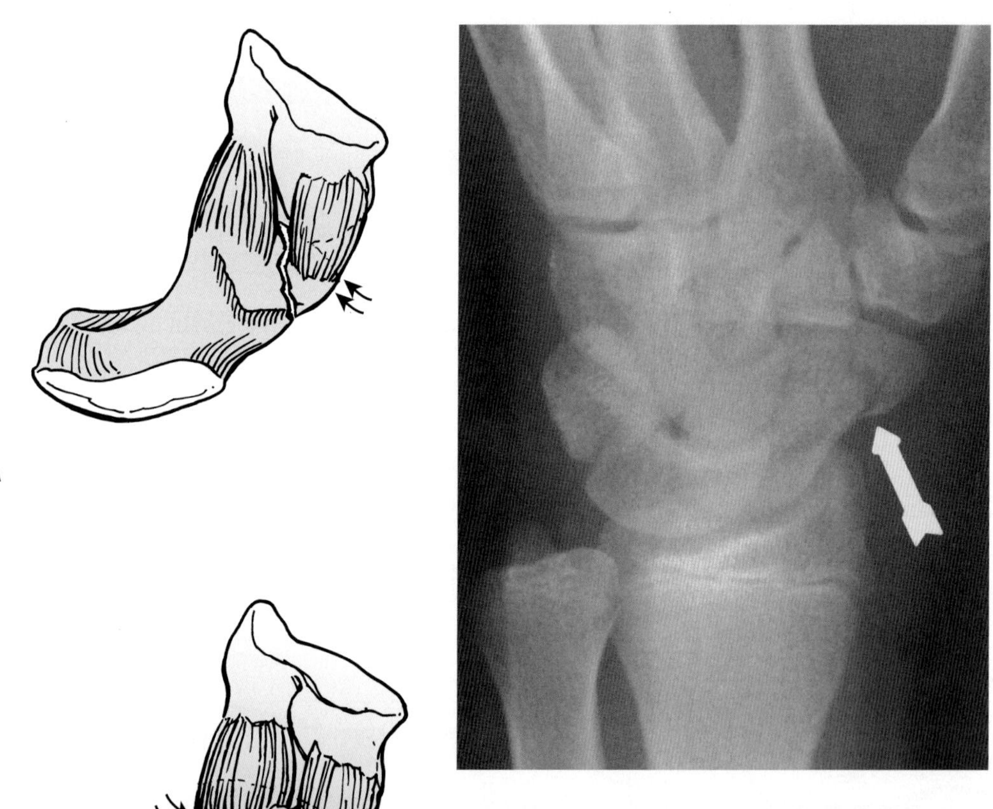

FIGURE 8-69 Two variations of an A2 intra-articular fracture of the scaphoid distal pole. **A.** The more prevalent type is on the radial aspect of the volar distal scaphoid. This fragment is attached to the radial portion of the scaphotrapezial ligament (*arrows*). **B.** The less common type is on the ulnar aspect of the volar distal scaphoid. This fragment is attached to the ulnar portion of the scaphotrapezial ligament (*arrows*). **C.** X-ray of an intra-articular distal pole scaphoid fracture.

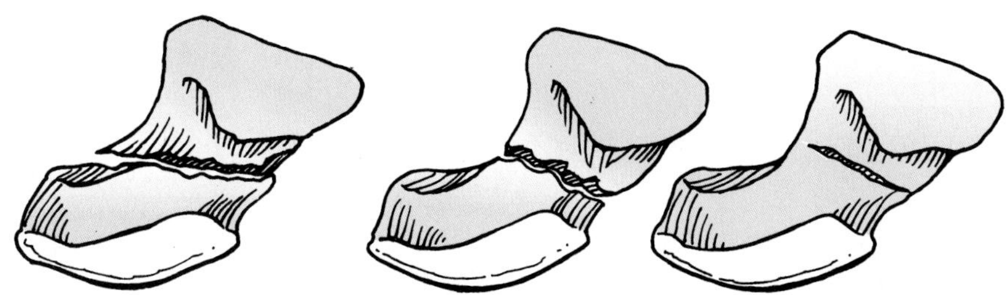

FIGURE 8-70 Mid-waist scaphoid fractures can differ in their location, orientation, and amount of comminution.

Bipartate Scaphoid Controversy: Traumatic Versus Developmental

A bipartite scaphoid probably exists, but is uncommon (Fig. 8-71) (135,138,157,158). Bunnell (159) enumerated five criteria that must be met to diagnose a congenital bipartite scaphoid: (a) similar bilateral appearance, (b) absence of historical or clinical evidence of antecedent trauma, (c) equal size and uniform density of each component, (d) absence of degenerative change between the scaphoid components or elsewhere in the carpus, and (e) smooth, rounded architecture of each scaphoid component. A unilateral "bipartate scaphoid" should be viewed as a post-traumatic scaphoid nonunion.

Diagnosis

Signs and Symptoms

The history, physical examination, and clinical suspicion are the essential elements to diagnosis of a scaphoid fracture (160). While the findings are similar in adults and children, they are more difficult to elicit in children. A consistent history, snuffbox pain, and swelling are indicative of a scaphoid fracture. The distal pole requires careful palpation because of its susceptibility for fracture.

Radiographic Findings

Anteroposterior, lateral, and scaphoid views are routine. The dorsal lip of the radius may obscure a proximal third fracture. Middle third fractures may or may not be evident on initial x-rays. Distal pole fractures are best seen on the lateral view. A pronated oblique view further highlights the CMC joint and distal pole fracture pattern. Advanced imaging studies, such as CT scanning, provide additional detail regarding fracture angulation and displacement (161). The CT images must be made along the longitudinal axis of the scaphoid, which is different than CT imaging of the wrist. Magnetic resonance imaging (MRI) scans recently have been shown to be useful for proper diagnosis of acute scaphoid fractures (162–164).

Variations in the immature carpus may mimic fracture, such as multiple centers of ossification (147). In addition, abnormal scaphoid configurations have been described with certain congenital anomalies (165).

Treatment

Presumed Fracture

Normal x-rays do not exclude the presence of a scaphoid fracture. Clinical suspicion in the presence of normal x-rays warrants immobilization and reevaluation in 2 weeks (144). The cast is removed, the wrist is examined, and x-rays are made. Pain resolution and negative x-rays warrant discontinuation of immobilization and return to normal activities. Persistent pain with normal x-rays requires continued immobilization and advanced imaging studies, such as a bone scan, CT scan, or MRI scan. MRI scans have been shown to be diagnostically useful in this clinical setting to avoid both misdiagnosis and overtreatment (162–164,166). Pain and positive x-ray studies require treatment of the scaphoid fracture.

Confirmed Fracture

X-rays consistent with fracture indicate that immediate treatment is necessary. Nondisplaced fractures are immobilized. The fracture location dictates the type of immobilization. A nondisplaced distal pole fracture is treated with a long- or short-arm thumb spica cast. A nondisplaced waist or proximal pole fracture is treated with long-arm thumb spica cast. The position of casting is controversial. Radial deviation and flexion have been recommended (150,167–171). Conversely, ulnar deviation is contraindicated because this position applies distraction across the fracture site. The elimination of forearm rotation neutralizes the forces across the scaphoid fracture (172,173). The ultimate cast position and the joints immobilized are a matter of individual preference. Most authors favor a long-arm thumb spica cast that permits thumb interphalangeal joint motion (173).

Displaced Fracture

Closed Reduction and Casting. Closed reduction of a displaced scaphoid fracture has been described (170,171,174–176), and a variety of maneuvers and casting techniques have been recommended. Closed reduction is difficult to achieve and maintaining the reduction even more uncertain. Currently, open reduction and internal fixation is a more reliable method for displaced fractures.

Percutaneous Screw Fixation. In adults, percutaneous screw fixation for both nondisplaced and displaced fractures has been

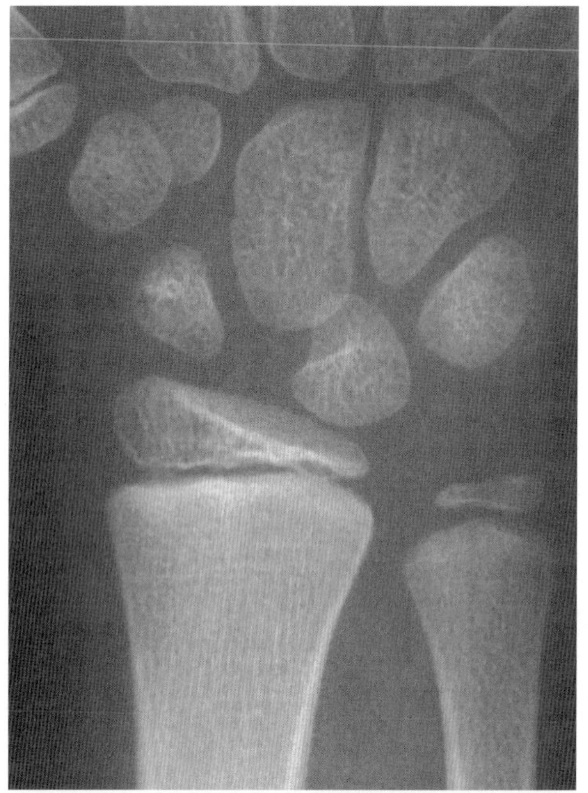

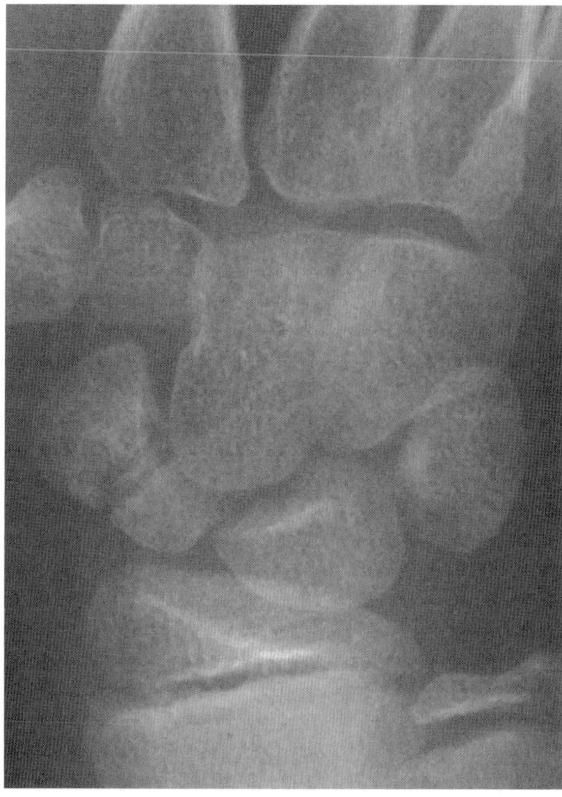

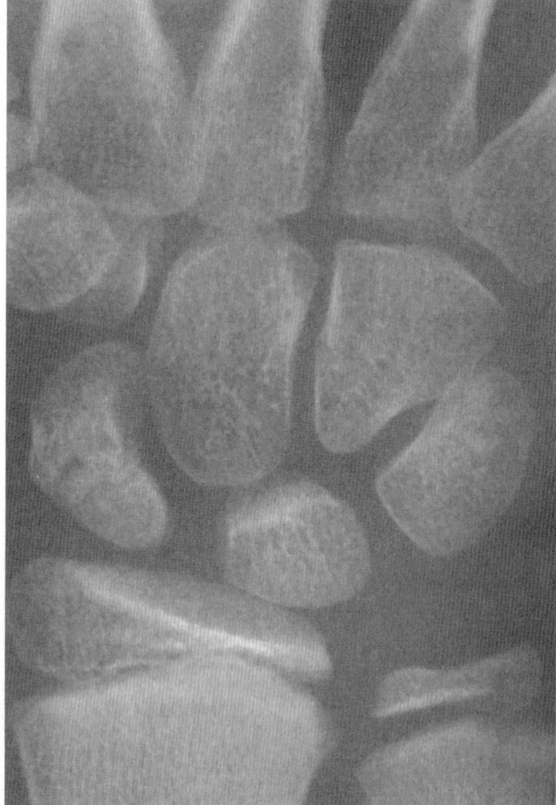

FIGURE 8-71 **A.** A 9-year-old boy who fell on an outstretched writ and had radial-sided pain and tenderness, but original x-rays failed to reveal any bony abnormalities. **B.** About 1.5 years later, the patient had persistent radial-sided wrist pain and x-rays revealed a mid-waist scaphoid nonunion. This would not be considered a bipartite scaphoid, but instead an injury that was sustained when the cartilaginous anlage was present. **C.** After 2 months of casting, early fracture union is present.

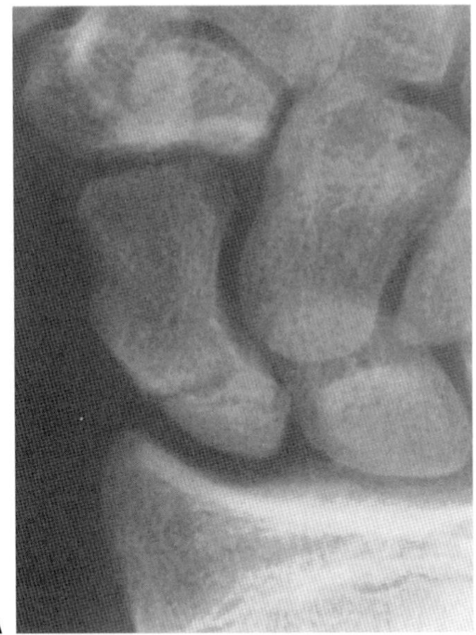
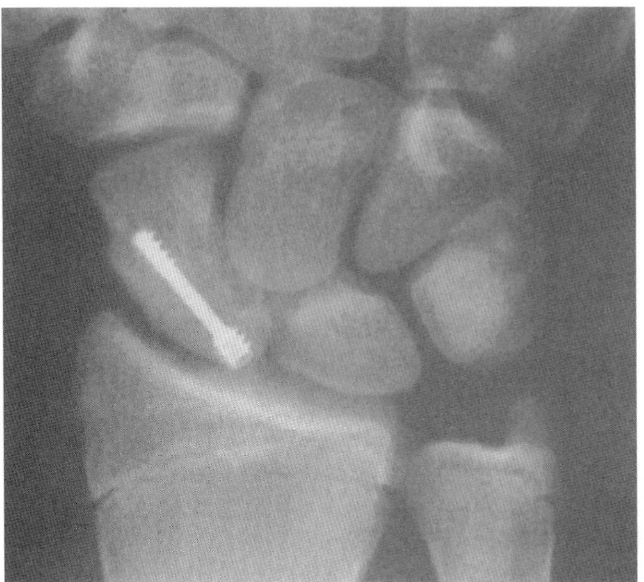

FIGURE 8-72 **A.** Nondisplaced proximal pole scaphoid fracture in a skeletally mature adolescent athlete. **B.** Treatment by percutaneous screw fixation led to healing.

advocated (177,178), and this technique can be used in reliable adolescent patients. Screws can be placed under fluoroscopic control either volarly (distal to proximal) or dorsally (proximal to distal) depending on fracture patterns and surgeon preference (Fig. 8-72).

Open Reduction and Internal Fixation. Displacement of more than 1 mm or intrascaphoid angulation of more than 10 degrees on any image warrants open reduction and internal fixation. Currently, there is no role for open reduction without internal fixation (174). The implant choice is individualized according to the fracture and patient. Kirschner wires and scaphoid screws are the primary fixation techniques (179).

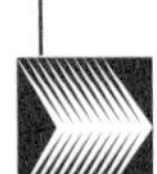

AUTHORS' PREFERRED TREATMENT

Almost all nondisplaced scaphoid fractures are treated with cast immobilization. Indications for open reduction are fractures with more than 1 mm of displacement or an angular deformity of more than 10 degrees. In addition, a transscaphoid perilunate injury is an indication for operative management.

Role of Closed Treatment

The preferred immobilization is a long-arm thumb spica cast for the initial 4 to 6 weeks, followed by a short-arm cast until clinical and radiographic union. X-rays are obtained in the first 7 to 10 days to ensure aligment and then monthly until union. If in doubt regarding anatomic alignment, a CT scan is obtained. A short- or long-arm cast is used for a presumed scaphoid fracture until the diagnosis is delineated. If x-rays do not provide the definitive answer, an MRI scan is obtained.

Open Reduction and Internal Fixation

Displaced fractures are treated with open reduction. Fractures of the middle and distal thirds are exposed through a volar approach. Comminution is treated with bone grafting obtained from the metaphysis of the distal radius or iliac crest. The implant depends on the fracture configuration and age of the child. Smooth wires may be necessary in young children while scaphoid screw fixation is used in adolescents (151,180–182). Wires are buried beneath the skin and removed after union. The postoperative regimen depends on the internal fixation device and stability of the construct. Wires require prolonged immobilization, whereas screws allow early mobilization in reliable patients. Whenever possible, scaphoid screws are advocated.

Fractures of the proximal pole are exposed through a dorsal approach. The proximal pole of the scaphoid is isolated beneath the third dorsal compartment, adjacent to the scapholunate ligament. The fixation device varies according to the fracture configuration and age of the child. Smooth wires and small scaphoid screws are fixation options (183) (Fig. 8-70). In the rare nondisplaced proximal pole fracture, percutaneous screw fixation dorsally is used to provide fracture stability and compression (183). This injury is at high risk for osteonecrosis, nonunion, and collapse without intervention.

Postoperative Care and Rehabilitation

Nondisplaced fractures are treated with immobilization until union. After the cast is removed, a home therapy program is started. Formal therapy usually is not necessary. Displaced fractures that are treated with open reduction and internal fixation require variable periods of immobilization. Fixation with Kirschner wires usually requires prolonged immobilization and often requires formal therapy to recover motion. Stable screw fixation may allow early motion 10 to 14 days after surgery but many adolescents are not reliable in restricting activities. A short-arm thumb spica splint is worn for protection during vigorous activity until union. If patient compliance is doubtful, cast immobilization is continued until the fracture is healed.

Prognosis

Prompt treatment of a nondisplaced scaphoid fracture allows healing in most patients (144). Nondisplaced pediatric scaphoid fractures have a greater than 95% healing rate. A delay in treatment impedes healing and increases the possibility of displacement (87,139,143). Displaced fractures require recognition and open reduction because adequate reduction and fixation result in predictable union.

Complications

The most prevalent complications are missed diagnosis and late presentation. Clinical suspicion must outweigh normal x-rays. Suspected fractures require immobilization and repeat evaluation. Deviation from this paradigm often results in scaphoid displacement or nonunion or both, which necessitate surgical management. Parents, primary care providers, and trainers must be well-informed regarding the subtle symptoms and difficult complications of a fracture nonunion.

Scaphoid nonunion does occur in children (Fig. 8-73), most commonly in adolescents (135–137,144,147,184–187). Open reduction, bone grafting, and internal fixation are the standard procedures for treatment of scaphoid nonunions (Fig. 8-74) (136,147,185,186). The approach varies according to the location of fracture and vascularity of the fracture fragments. The principles of operative scaphoid nonunion treatment in children are similar to those in adults. Scaphoid nonunion results in altered kinematics within the wrist and produces degenerative changes over time (188,189). A child's wrist may be slightly protected from these changes, although this protection should not alter established treatment principles (137,138). It is imperative to achieve union to prevent long-term arthosis.

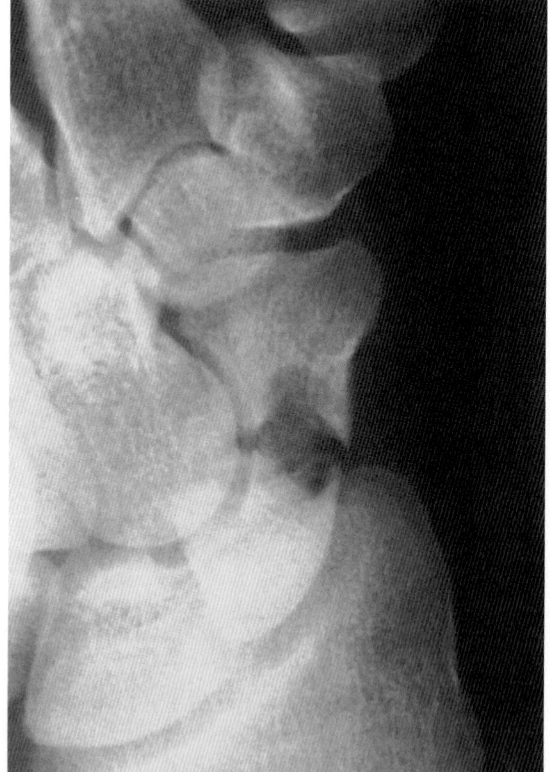

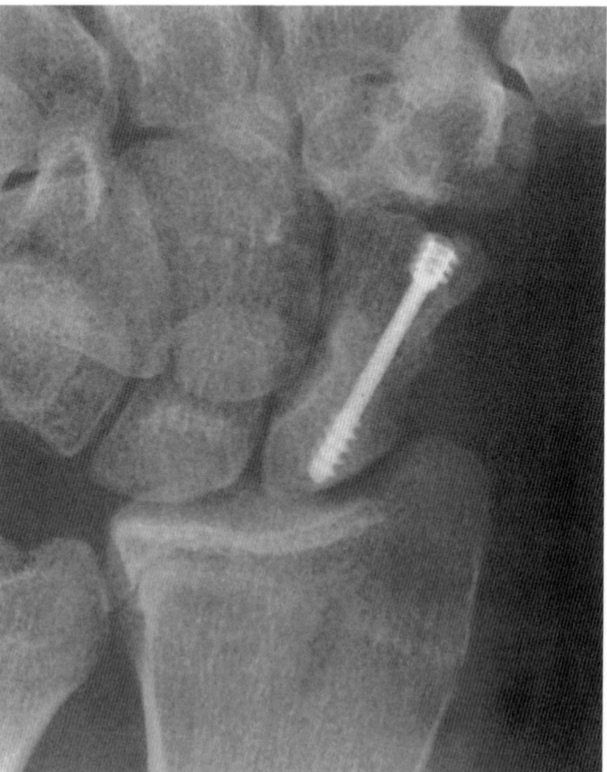

FIGURE 8-73 **A.** A 15-year-old boy developed a nonunion of the scaphoid. A thumb spica cast worn for several months failed to bring about union. The cyst at the mid-waist grew. **B.** Formal takedown of the nonunion through a volar approach plus intercalary bone grafting with Herbert screw fixation resulted in union and excellent function.

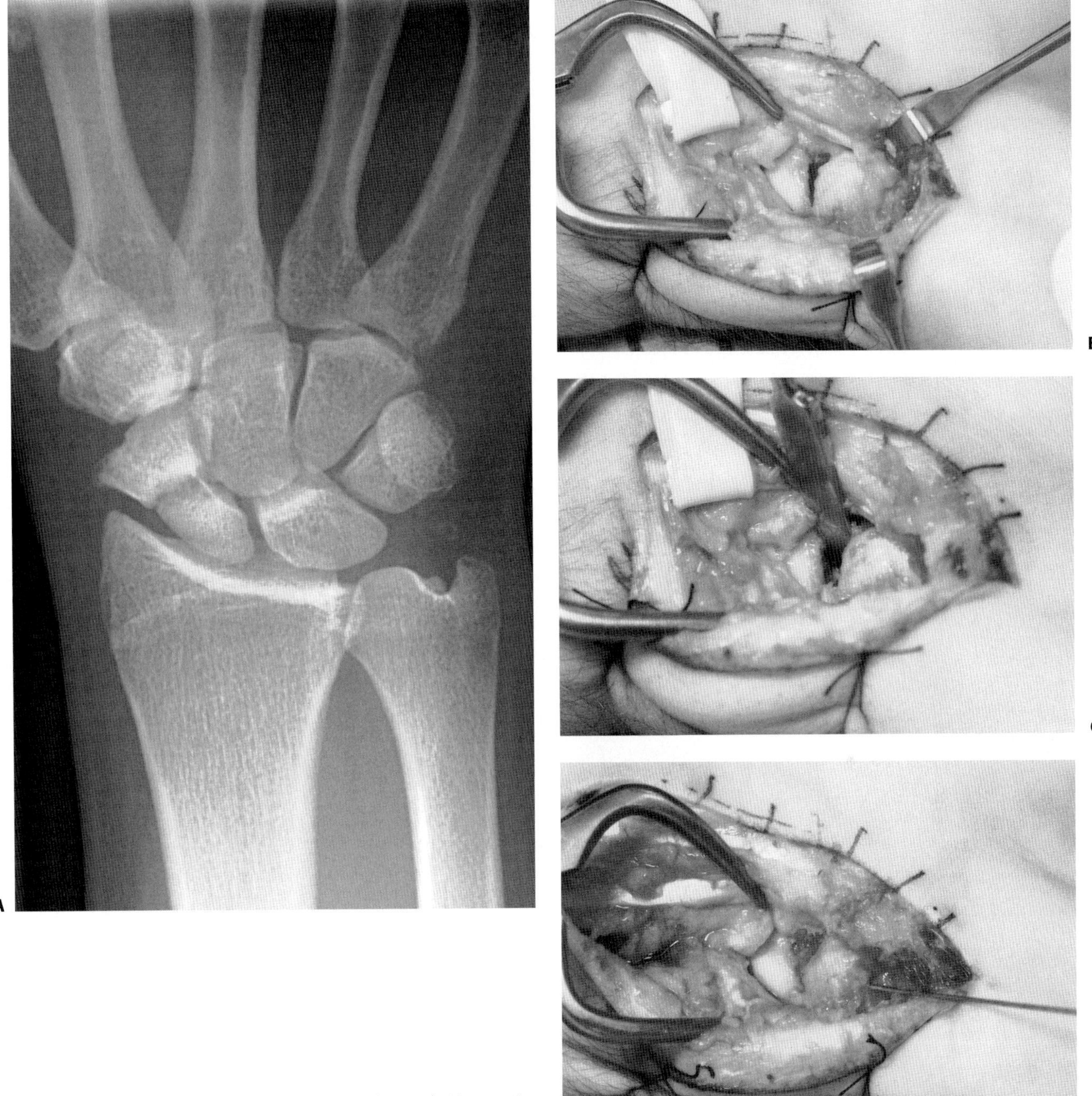

FIGURE 8-74 **A.** A 16-year-old male with a right scaphoid nonunion with resorption at the fracture site. **B.** Volar approach and exposure of the fracture site. **C.** The fracture site was debrided of fibrous material and the hump back deformity was corrected. **D.** The fracture site was packed with bone graft and a guide wire was placed for screw fixation. *(continues)*

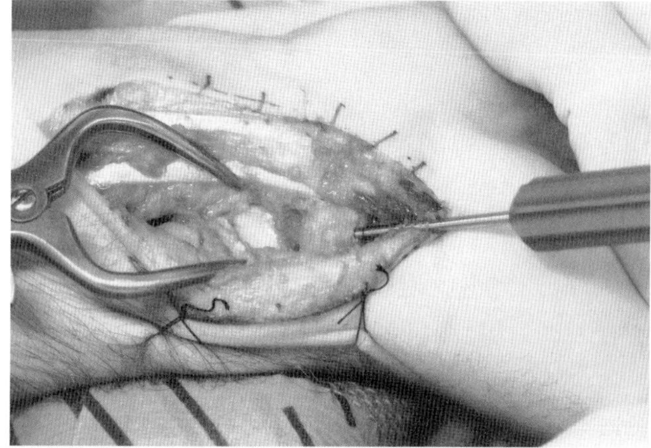

E

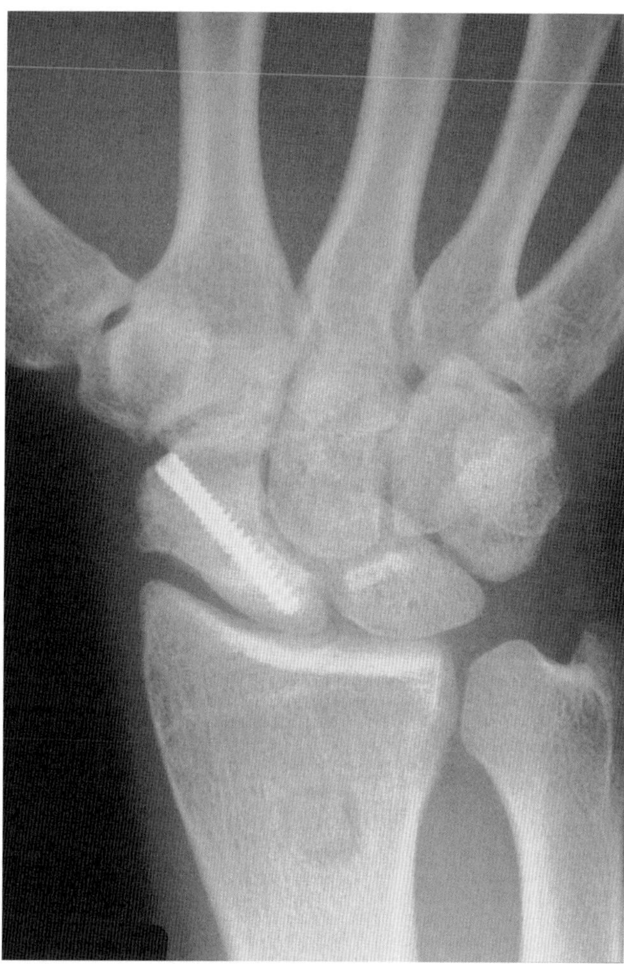

F

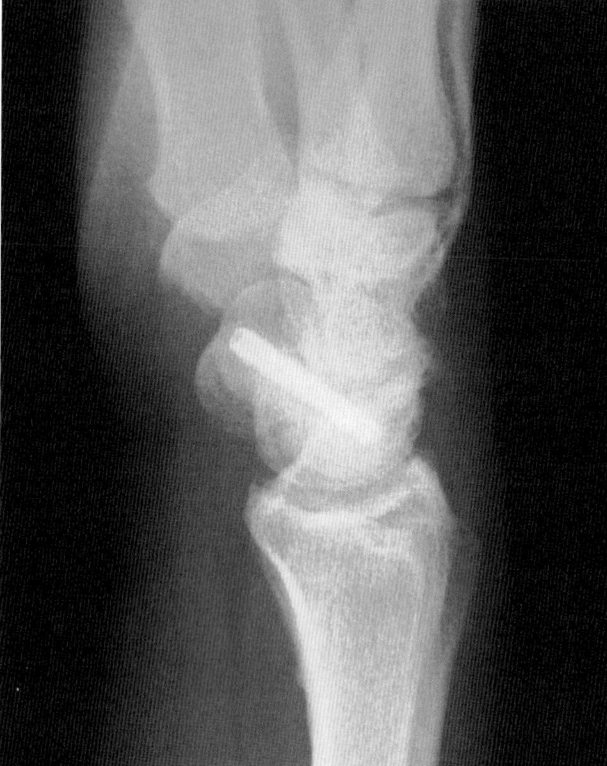

G

FIGURE 8-74 *(continued)* **E.** The screw was inserted over the guide wire. **F,G.** Anteroposterior and lateral x-rays after fracture reduction, bone grafting, and screw placement. (Courtesy of Shriners Hospital for Children, Philadelphia.)

Osteonecrosis may result from a scaphoid fracture. The proximal fragment is more prone to avascular changes. Avascular changes within the proximal fragment do not preclude union after internal fixation. The size of the fragment and the extent of avascularity dictate management. The treatment principles are similar in adults and children. Options to obtain union include conventional or vascularized bone grafting (190). With nonunion and osteonecrosis of the proximal pole, distal radial vascularized grafting has been noted to be successful (190,191).

Capitate Fractures

Epidemiology

Isolated fractures of the capitate are rare and usually result from high-energy trauma (135,192–194). Capitate fractures may represent a form of greater arc perilunar injury (Fig. 8-75). The force can propagate completely around the lunate and cause a perilunate or lunate dislocation (141,144,195). The injury also can halt within the capitate and produce a scaphocapitate syndrome (193,196,197).

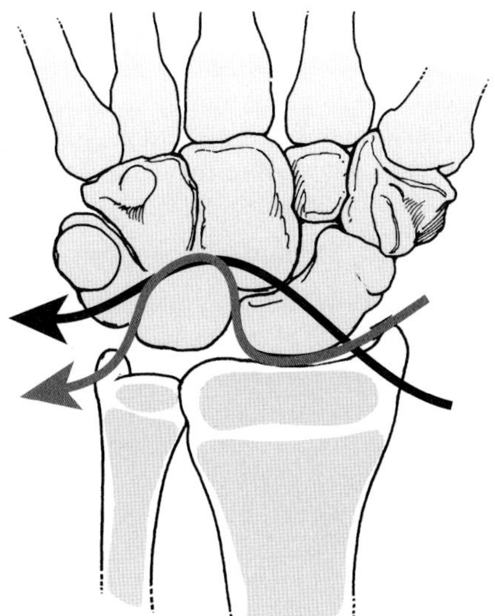

FIGURE 8-75 Progressive perilunar instability. The greater arc (*black arrow*) is associated with fractures of the carpal bones, which may include the scaphoid, lunate, capitate, hamate, and triquetrum. The *blue arrow* depicts the lesser arc, in which forces are transmitted only through soft-tissue structures. (Reprinted from Mayfield JK, Johnson RP, Kilcoyn RK. Carpal dislocations: Pathomechanics and progressive perilunar instability. *J Bone Joint Surg Am* 1980;5:226–241, with permission.)

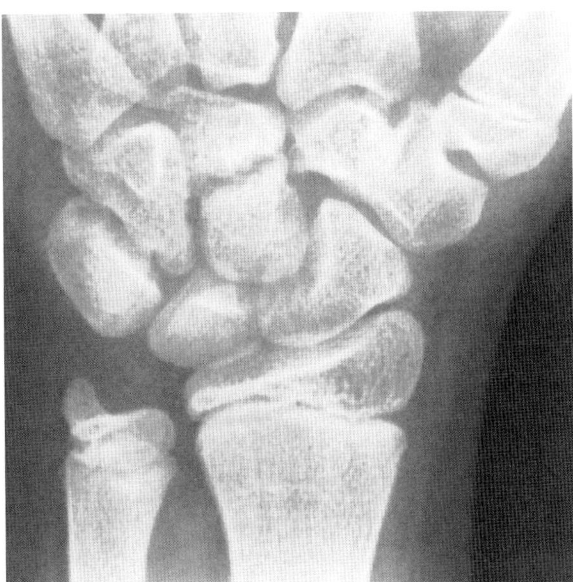

FIGURE 8-76 A 12-year-old boy sustained multiple carpal fractures attributed to a crushing injury. Sixteen months later, an established nonunion of the capitate is present that required bone grafting to obtain union. (Courtesy of James H. Dobyns, MD.)

Mechanism of Injury

Excessive dorsiflexion of the wrist is the most common mechanism. The waist of the capitate abuts against the lunate or dorsal aspect of the radius. The fracture occurs through the waist with variable displacement.

Diagnosis

Signs and Symptoms

The wrist usually is markedly swollen and painful to palpation. The clinical presentation varies with the associated carpal injuries. Median nerve paresthesias may be present secondary to swelling within the carpal tunnel.

Radiographic Findings

Standard anteroposterior and lateral views usually are adequate (Fig. 8-76). Careful scrutiny of the x-rays is necessary. The capitate fracture can be subtle or the proximal capitate fragment can rotate 180 degrees. Either scenario can create a confusing image that often results in misinterpretation. Incomplete ossification further complicates x-ray diagnosis and degree of displacement. Small osteochondral fragments in the mid-carpal region may indicate a greater arc injury or isolated capitate fracture. In these cases, advanced imaging studies, such as MRI or CT may be useful.

Treatment

Treatment depends on the fracture pattern, degree of displacement, and associated injuries. Distraction x-rays, MRI, or CT scans may be necessary to determine the exact pattern of injury.

Nonoperative Treatment

Nondisplaced fractures of the scaphoid and capitate can be treated with a long-arm cast for 6 to 8 weeks (196), as can, isolated nondisplaced capitate fractures. Closed reduction of displaced fractures is not feasible (141).

Operative Treatment

Displaced fractures require open reduction, especially the rotated proximal capitate pole. Associated perilunar injuries also require internal fixation and ligamentous repair. The anatomic relationships within the carpus must be restored. Wire or osseous screw fixation is appropriate stabilization after open reduction.

Prognosis and Complications

The rarity of this injury prevents broad generalizations. Early recognition and appropriate treatment lead to an acceptable outcome. Nonunion is rare and requires bone grafting (198,199) (Fig. 8-76). Despite the considerable rotation of the proximal pole, osteonecrosis of the capitate is rare.

Triquetrum Fractures

Epidemiology

Avulsion fractures of the triquetrum are more common in adults than in children. The injury may occur in adolescents as carpal ossification nears completion. A fracture through the body of the triquetrum is rare and may occur with a perilunar injury as the path of the greater arc injury passes through the triquetrum (137,141,200).

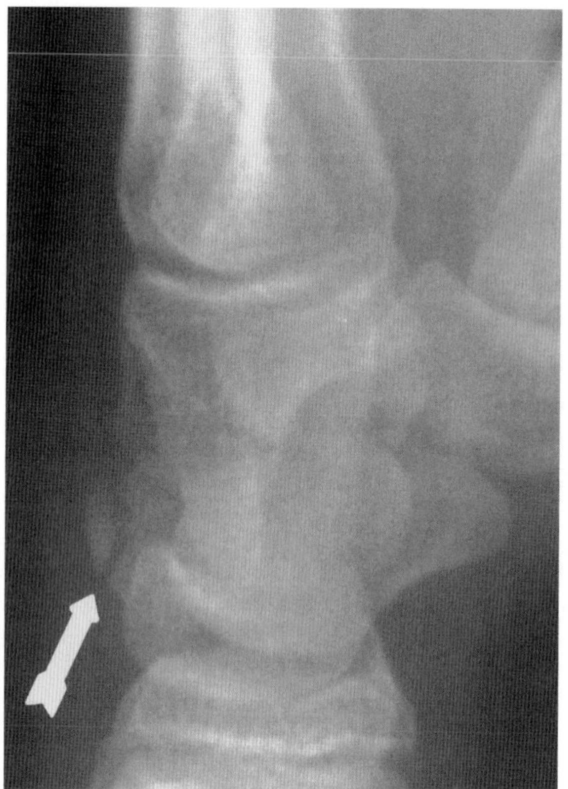

FIGURE 8-77 A minimally displaced dorsal triquetral avulsion fracture (*arrow*) that was treated with short-term immobilization.

Mechanism of Injury

A fall on an outstretched wrist is the common event. The probable mechanism for an avulsion fracture is a pulling force through the dorsal ligaments (Fig. 8-77).

Diagnosis

Signs and Symptoms

The wrist is mildly swollen and painful to palpation over the dorsal triquetrum. The clinical presentation is more severe with associated carpal injuries.

Radiographic Findings

Anteroposterior and lateral views may not show the avulsion fracture. A pronated oblique view highlights the dorsum of the triquetrum and may reveal the avulsed fragment. At times, CT scans are necessary for accurate diagnosis.

Treatment

An avulsion fracture is treated with a short period of immobilization (3 to 6 weeks) followed by motion and return to activities. A fracture through the body of the triquetrum with a perilunar injury requires open reduction and internal fixation.

Prognosis and Complications

Avulsion fractures are relatively minor injuries. Treatment results in prompt and complete recovery. Body fractures associated with perilunar injures have a guarded prognosis, depending on the extent of injury and treatment provided.

Hamate, Pisiform, Lunate, Trapezium Fractures

Pediatric fractures of the hamate, pisiform, lunate, and trapezium are rare (5,23). Hook of the hamate fractures usually occur in adults but may occur in adolescents with traumatic falls. A CT scan may be necessary for diagnosis if the fracture is not visible on the carpal tunnel view. Pisiform fractures are the result of direct trauma. Lunate fractures are associated with Kienböck disease (Fig. 8-78) (201,202), which is uncommon in children. Trapezium fractures can occur with CMC joint injuries about the thumb.

Soft Tissue Injuries About the Carpus

Ligamentous Injuries

Epidemiology. Ligamentous injuries about the pediatric wrist are less common than osseous injuries (156,195,203,204). The immature carpus and viscoelastic ligaments are relatively resistant to injury.

Mechanism of Injury. Fracture-dislocations and isolated ligamentous injuries usually are caused by high-energy trauma (205) (Fig. 8-79). Motor vehicle accidents and sports-related injuries are potential causes of the rare fracture-dislocation.

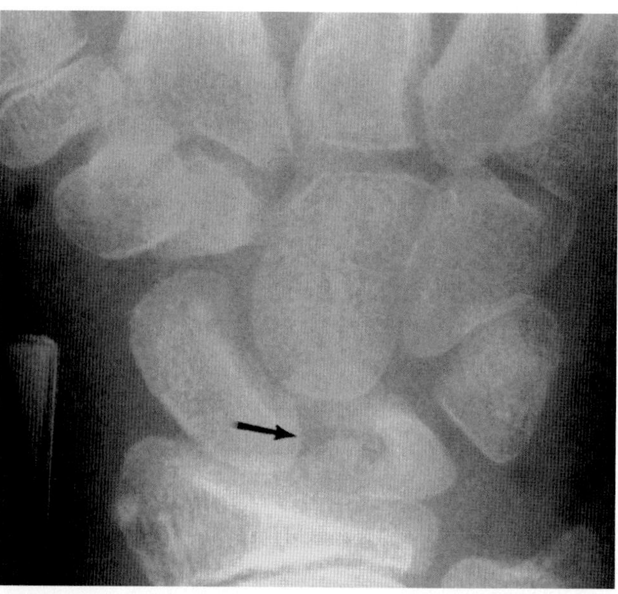

FIGURE 8-78 A 12-year-old boy sustained a wrist injury and developed a small area of segmental rarefaction in the lunate, consistent with osteonecrosis (*arrow*). This may represent a pediatric form of adult Kienböck's lunatomalacia. (Courtesy of Greg Goldsmith, MD.)

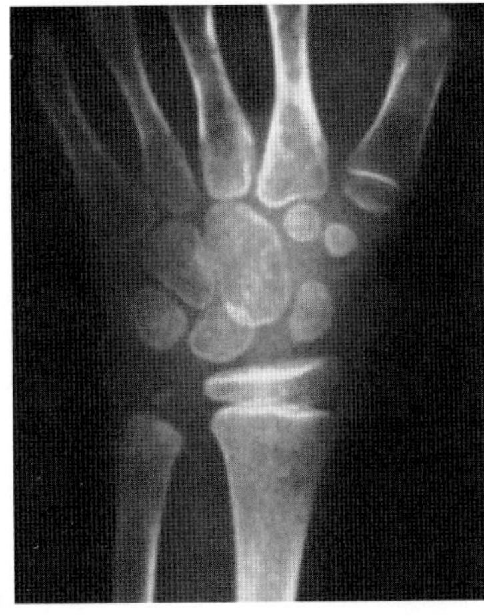

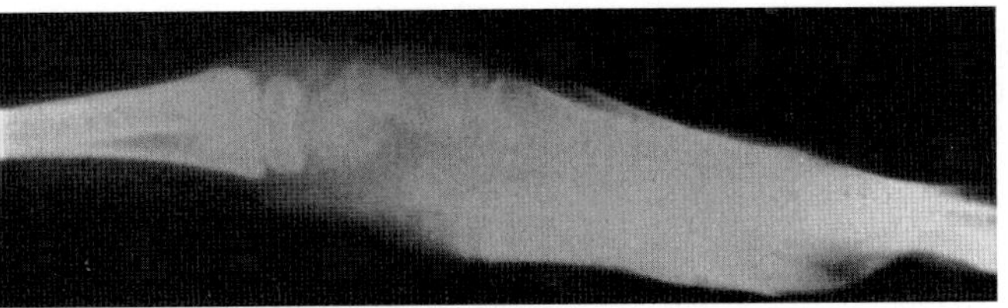

FIGURE 8-79 Anteroposterior **(A)** and lateral **(B)** x-rays of a dorsal perilunar dislocation in a 6-year-old boy. (Courtesy of William F. Benson, MD.)

However, recurrent or chronic wrist pain is not uncommon in adolescents. Most recurrent ligamentous pain results from hypermobility and overuse during the adolescent growth spurt and may result in joint subluxation, chondral impingement, or ligamentous tears similar to patellofemoral injuries in adolescents.

Diagnosis

Signs and Symptoms

A child with an acute traumatic injury avoids use of the wrist and hand. The wrist is swollen and painful to palpation, making isolation of the injured segment difficult except in extremely cooperative children. Provocative maneuvers for carpal instability usually are not possible because of pain in the injured wrist.

Gross instability without pain on stress testing may indicate a hyperelasticity syndrome that is not related to trauma (206). However, recurrent pain does occur in children with hypermobility, overuse, and relative muscular weakness. These children complain of diffuse pain, generalized tenderness, and limited strength on examination. Diagnosis is difficult particularly because of concerns regarding emotional overlay.

Radiographic Findings

Anteroposterior and lateral views are routine. The incomplete ossification complicates x-ray interpretation, especially the assessment of carpal widening. Detection of slight widening or malalignment within the carpus often is difficult. Contralateral views are useful to compare ossification and carpal spacing (207). Suspicion of a fracture warrants advanced imaging studies, such as arthrography, stress x-ray, fluoroscopy, and MRI.

Treatment

General treatment recommendations for rare traumatic dislocation injuries are difficult. Decisive factors include the age of child, degree of clinical suspicion, and extent of injury. Minor injuries are treated with immobilization for 3 to 6 weeks and reexamination. Resolution of symptoms and signs allows return to normal activities. Persistent pain warrants further clinical and x-ray evaluation. Overt ligamentous injuries with static instability and malalignment require accurate diagnosis and appropriate treatment. A complete ligament tear (e.g., an adolescent with a scapholunate injury) is treated with principles similar to those for adults. Open reduction, anatomic reduction, and ligament repair are the basic tenets of treatment.

A child or adolescent with ligamentous laxity and persistent activity-related pain is especially difficult to treat. Discerning focal from nonfocal wrist pathology is imperative. X-rays and MRI scans often are normal. Most of these childrens respond to therapeutic strengthening. Protective sport-specific (e.g., gymnastics) wrist protectors may be appropriate (Fig. 8-80). A small subset of these patients have unresolved pain caused by chondral injuries or ligamentous tears that require arthroscopic treatment (208).

TRIANGULAR FIBROCARTILAGE COMPLEX TEARS

Epidemiology

Tears of the triangular fibrocartilage complex (TFCC) rarely occur in children (209). These tears most often are associated with distal radial fractures, radial growth arrest, ulnar overgrowth, and ulnar carpal impaction, but they may occur in isolation. Most often these patients present late after acute trauma with activity-related pain.

Anatomic Considerations

The TFCC consists of the biconcave triangular fibrocartilage and the volar ulnocarpal ligaments. It spans the sigmoid notch of the radius to the ulnar styloid, providing stability to the distal radioulnar and ulnocarpal joints.

Mechanism of Injury

Rotational forces with axial loading can cause tears of the TFCC. If there is a positive ulnar variance, the resultant ulnar-carpal

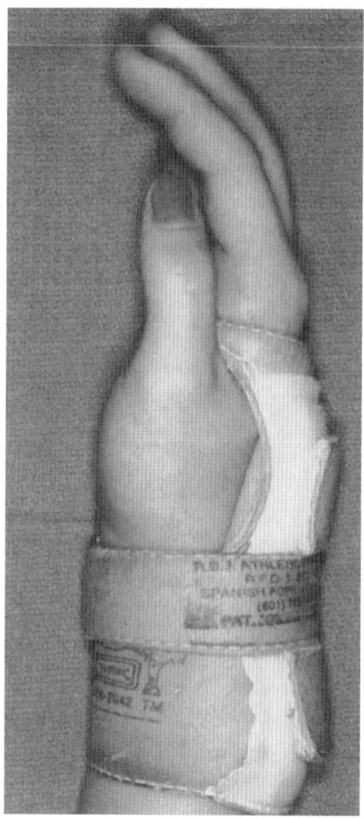
A

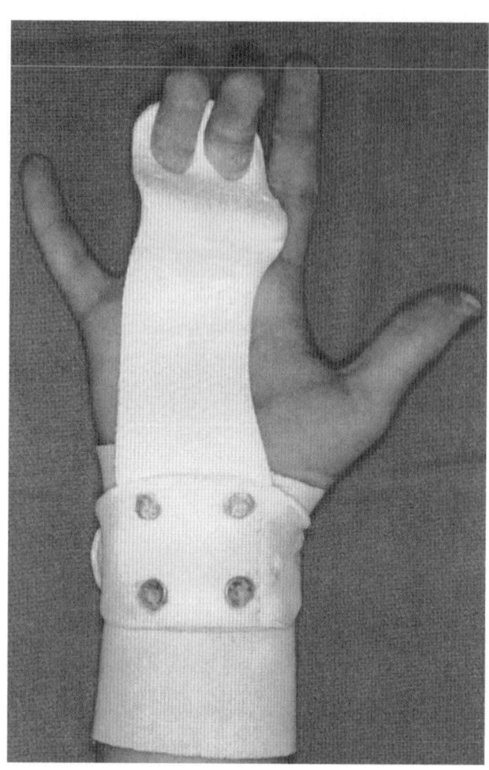
B

FIGURE 8-80 Wrist guards for gymnastics. **A.** The "lion's paw" protector used mainly for vault. **B.** Hand and wrist protectors used primarily for the uneven parallel bars.

impaction predisposes that patient to lunate, triquetral, or TFCC impingement and injuries.

Classification

TFCC tears are classified according to the location of the tear (209). Peripheral tears (type B) are most common in adolescents. Tears from the radial insertion (type D) are next in frequency, while central (type A) and volar (type C) tears are rare (210,211).

Diagnosis

Signs and Symptoms

Pain is localized to the distal ulna and ulnar carpal region. Forearm rotation may be limited and usually reproduces the pain, particularly at the extremes. Compression and ulnar deviation of the carpus against the ulna reproduces the pain and may elicit crepitus. The distal radioulnar joint may be more unstable to stress testing than the contralateral side (209,212).

Radiographic Findings

Plain x-rays may reveal an ulnar styloid avulsion fracture. An acute displaced fracture at the base of the styloid suggests the likelihood of a TFCC tear. Positive ulnar variance is associated with TFCC tears. Hypertrophic healing of ulnar styloid fractures also may result in impingement. Arthrograms and MRI scans may be diagnostic (213,214).

Treatment

The initial approach to adolescents with chronic wrist pain should be a strengthening program. If pain persists after regaining symmetric pinch and grip strength, then further x-ray evaluation is appropriate. If clinical examination or x-ray evaluation is consistent with a TFCC tear or ulnar-carpal impaction, arthroscopy is appropriate. Partial TFCC tears and chondromalacia sites in the carpus are debrided. Full thickness tears are repaired, percutaneously for type B tears and transradially for type D tears.

DISLOCATIONS OF THE HAND AND CARPUS

Dislocations of the Interphalangeal Joints

In children, the soft-tissue stabilizers about the interphalangeal joints are stronger than the physis, which explains the propensity for fracture rather than dislocation. Occasionally, dislocations and fracture-dislocations occur about the interphalangeal and metacarpophalangeal joints (Fig. 8-81).

Distal Interphalangeal Joint

A hyperextension or lateral force may result in dorsal or lateral DIP joint dislocation. The collateral ligaments and volar plate typically detach from the middle phlanx. Most dislocations can be reduced by longitudinal traction, recreation of the dislocation force, and reduction of the distal phalanx. The DIP joint reduction and congruity are confirmed by clinical motion and x-rays.

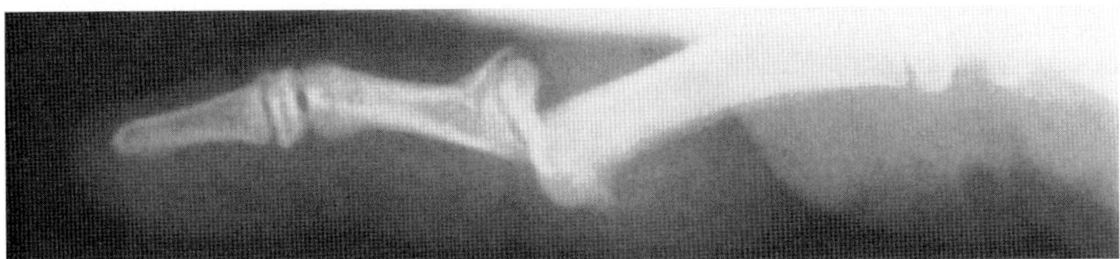

FIGURE 8-81 A dorsal dislocation of the proximal interphalangeal joint with a Salter-Harris type II fracture of the middle phalanx in a 15-year-old boy.

Two to 3 weeks of DIP joint splinting is sufficient, followed by a home program that focuses on DIP joint motion.

Irreducible or complex dislocations of the DIP occur primarily in adults, but can occur in pediatric patients (215–219). Open reduction through a dorsal approach is required for removal of the interposed tissue. The volar plate often is the offending agent, although the collateral ligaments and the flexor digitorum profundus can block reduction (27). A stable DIP joint is treated with DIP joint splinting for 3 to 4 weeks. An unstable DIP joint requires pin fixation for 3 to 4 weeks.

Proximal Interphalangeal Joint

Dislocation of the PIP joint may occur in a variety of directions. Dorsal dislocations are the most common, although lateral and volar dislocations also occur. The differential diagnosis includes adjacent bony and tendon injuries (220). X-rays are required to assess the physis and to confirm joint alignment. The post-reduction lateral x-ray must confirm concentric joint reduction. Subtle joint subluxation is detected by a slight offset between the proximal and middle phalanges along with a dorsal V space instead of smooth articular congruity.

Dorsal PIP Joint Dislocations. The middle phalanx is displaced dorsal to the proximal phalanx (Fig. 8-82). The collateral ligaments and volar plate are disrupted. Many dorsal dislocations probably are joint subluxations that retain some of the collateral ligament or volar plate integrity. Some subluxations are reduced by the patient or trainer and never recieve medical evaluation.

Unreduced dorsal dislocations cause pain and obvious deformity. If necessary, anesthesia usually can be accomplished with a digital block. Sensory exam of the involved digit is important before local anesthesia administration. The dislocation is reduced with longitudinal traction, hyperextension, and palmar translation of the middle phalanx onto the proximal phalanx.

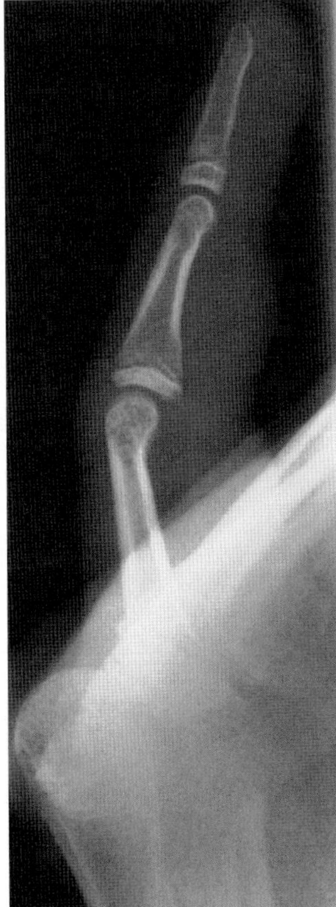

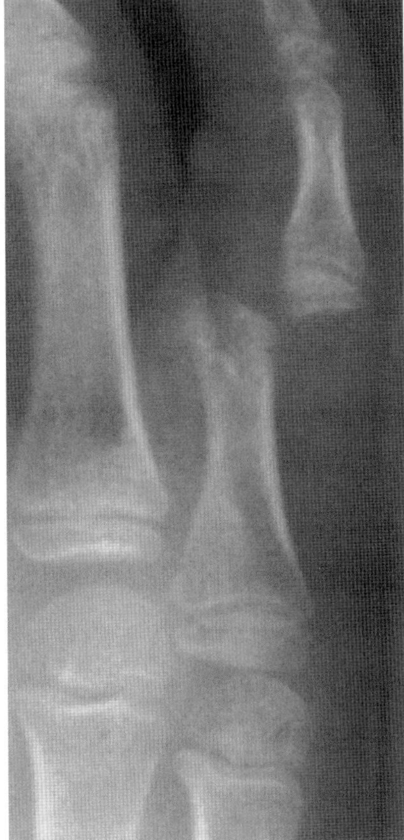

FIGURE 8-82 **A.** Lateral x-ray of a volar plate avulsion injury. There is a small fracture fragment volarly from the ephiphysis of the middle phalanx. Note the associated soft-tissue swelling. These fractures should not be treated with prolonged immobilization. Early buddy taping and motion lessen the risk of a flexion contracture. **B.** Dorsal dislocation of the proximal interphalangeal joint in a 10-year-old girl.

The quality of the reduction and the stability of the joint must be assessed. Asking the patient to flex and extend the digit evaluates active motion (65). Most dislocations are stable throughout the normal range of motion and x-rays confirm a concentric reduction. A stable joint requires a brief period (3–5 days) of splinting for comfort, followed by range of motion and buddy taping. Immediate motion may be started, although pain often prohibits movement. Prolonged immobilization is a concern for the development of PIP joint stiffness.

An unstable reduction tends to subluxate or dislocate during PIP joint extension. The x-rays must be scrutinized for subtle dorsal subluxation and concomitant fracture of the middle phalangeal base. Unstable PIP joint dislocations, with or without small fractures of the middle phalangeal base, have a stable arc of motion that must be defined. This stable arc is typically from full flexion to about 30 degrees of flexion and is used to determine the limits of extension-block splinting (108). A short-arm cast is applied with an aluminum outrigger that positions the MCP joint in flexion and the PIP joint in 10 degrees less than the maximal extension that leads to joint subluxation. This position usually is between 40 and 60 degrees of PIP joint flexion. Reduction is verified by lateral x-rays. The aluminum splint is modified every 7 to 10 days to increase PIP joint extension 10 degrees. A lateral view is taken to confirm concentric reduction. This process in continued over 4 to 5 weeks. The cast and splint are then discontinued and a home therapy program is instituted.

Extremely unstable injuries that dislocate in more than 30 degrees of flexion almost always involve considerable fracture of the middle phalanx. These injuries are regarded as pilon fractures or intra-articular fracture-dislocations. Treatment presents a management dilemma as discussed earlier (95). Options range from open reduction to dynamic traction. Long-term subluxation, stiffness, and arthrosis are concerns.

There is considerable controversy concerning primary repair of torn collateral ligaments associated with PIP joint dislocations in adults (76,149,221–224). There is less debate in children because ligament repair is reserved for specific circumstances, such as an irreducible dislocation or chronic injury (6,40, 224,225).

Volar PIP Joint Dislocations. Volar PIP joint dislocations are uncommon in children (226–228), and the diagnosis often is delayed (226,227). Interposition of soft tissues or bony fragments can render the dislocation irreducible (228). The proximal phalangeal head may herniate between the lateral band and the central tendon. In contrast to dorsal dislocations, long-term results often are suboptimal. This outcome may be related to a delay in treatment or the degree of soft-tissue involvement, especially the central slip.

Volar dislocations require closed or open reduction. Reducible dislocations are treated with 4 weeks of full-time PIP joint extension splinting to promote healing of the central slip (229). X-rays are necessary to confirm concentric reduction. An unstable reduction may require temporary pin fixation across the PIP joint. Irreducible dislocations require open reduction through a dorsal approach to extricate any interposed tissue. The central slip can be repaired to the middle phalanx. Postoperative immobilization consists of 4 weeks of full-time PIP joint extension splinting.

Lateral PIP Joint Dislocations. Pure lateral dislocations are uncommon, although dorsal dislocations may have a lateral component (230). An isolated lateral dislocation represents severe disruption of the collateral ligament complex. The injury is a spectrum of injury, beginning with damage to the proper and accessory collateral ligaments and culminating in volar plate disruption (231). Bony avulsion fragments may accompany the ligamentous failure (86). Closed reduction is uniformly successful. A brief period (5 to 7 days) of immobilization followed by buddy taping to protect the healing collateral ligament complex is the customary treatment.

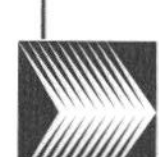

AUTHORS' PREFERRED TREATMENT

Variables that affect treatment of PIP joint dislocations include the extent and anatomic location of soft-tissue disruption, presence or absence of fracture, reducibility, and stability after reduction. The initial treatment of almost all PIP dislocations is an attempt at closed reduction followed by a stability assessment. Early mobilization is important to prevent PIP joint stiffness.

Dorsal Dislocation

A stable reduction is treated with brief immobilization followed by early motion. Coban-wrap buddy taping is used until full stable motion is achieved. Sports are restricted until the patient gains joint stability and full motion and strength. An unstable reduction that can be held reduced in more than 30 to 40 degrees of flexion is treated with extension block splinting. Extremely unstable fracture-dislocations require open treatment, external fixation, or dynamic traction depending on the size of the fracture fragments.

Volar Dislocation

A stable reduction is treated with immobilization for 4 weeks with the PIP joint in extension. Unstable reductions are treated with percutaneous pin fixation to maintain a concentric reduction. Irreducible dislocations require open reduction with repair of the central slip.

Lateral Dislocations

Pure lateral dislocations are rare. Closed reduction usually is obtainable, followed by a brief period of immobilization. Irreducible dislocations require open reduction with or without collateral ligament repair.

Metacarpophalangeal Joint Dislocations

The MCP joint is an uncommon site for dislocation in the child's hand (23,24,232). The dislocation may involve a finger or thumb. The gamekeeper's or skier's thumb can be considered a momentary subluxation or dislocation.

Dorsal Dislocations of the Fingers

The most frequent dislocation of the MCP joint is dorsal dislocation of the index digit (Fig. 8-83), which results from a hyperextension force that ruptures the volar plate (233) and displaces the proximal phalanx dorsal to the metacarpal. The diagnosis is readily apparent because the digit is shortened, supinated, and deviated in an ulnar direction. The interphalangeal joints are slightly flexed. The volar skin is tense over the prominent metacarpal head.

MCP joint dislocations are classified as simple or complex.

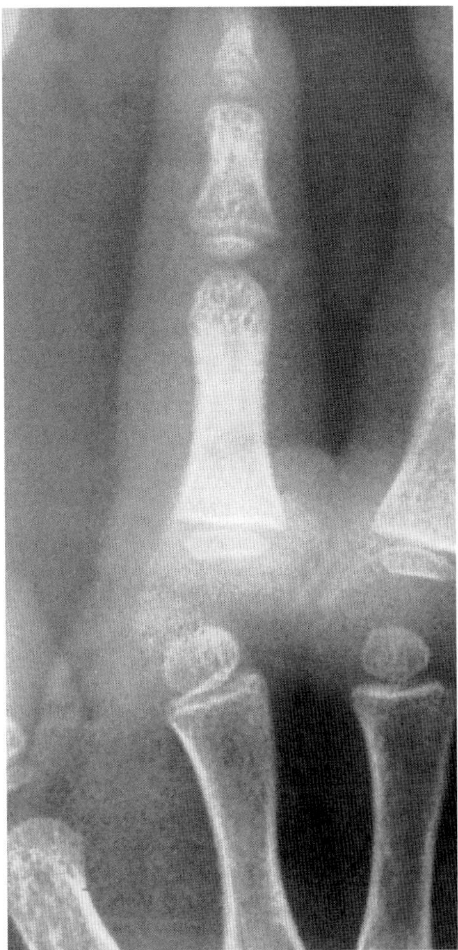

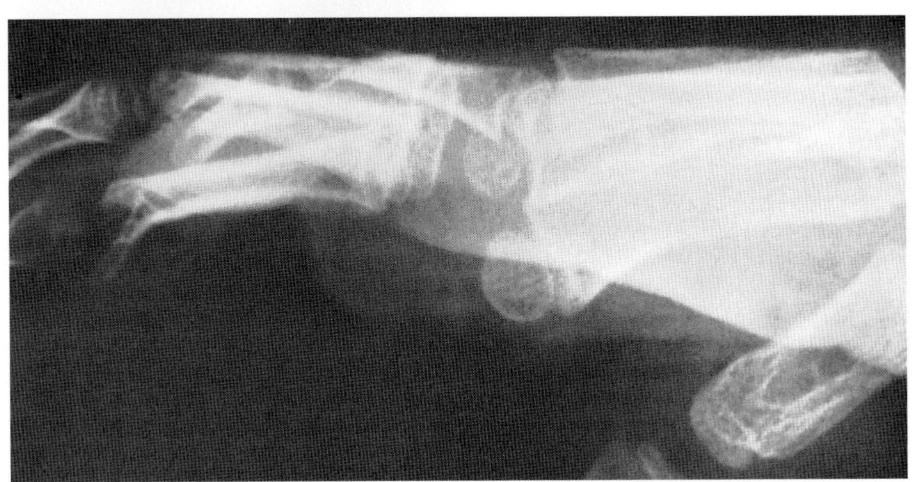

FIGURE 8-83 **A.** A 3-year-old boy with a complete complex dislocation of the index finger metacarpal joint. **B.** Note the parallelism in this lateral view. Open reduction was done through a volar approach.

Complex dislocations are irreducible because of volar plate interposition in the joint. Simple dislocations usually are in a position of hyperextension on x-rays. Irreducible dislocations generally have bayonet apposition of the proximal phalanx dorsal to the metacarpal head. The sesamoid bone(s) of the index or thumb may be seen within the joint. The position of the sesamoid bones is indicative of the site of the volar plate (27,44,234). The most common irreducible dislocation is at the index MCP joint. Multiple structures may impede reduction (235). Most commonly, the metacarpal head becomes "picture-framed" by the flexor tendon on the ulnar side and the lumbrical on the radial side. The superficial transverse metacarpal ligament and the natatory ligaments also can entrap the metacarpal neck. The collar of retraining tissue is tightened by longitudinal traction and this reduction maneuver may convert a dislocation from reducible to irreducible. The volar plate also can be interposed between the metacarpal head and proximal phalanx, which further impedes reduction.

The reduction maneuver involves further hyperextension of the joint and palmar translation of the proximal phalanx. The goal is to extricate the volar plate with the proximal phalanx during palmar translation. Intra-articular infiltration of anesthetic fluid may assist reduction through joint distention and "floating" of the volar plate from its displaced position. The success rate for conversion of an irreducible dislocation to a reducible dislocation is low. Open reduction is necessary in most patients.

Open Reduction

Open reduction can be accomplished through a volar or dorsal approach. The volar approach provides excellent exposure of the metacarpal head and the incarcerated structures (23,24,40,66,235–238). A concern is the proximity of the digital nerves draped over the articular surface of the metacarpal head. A deep skin incision jeopardizes the superficial digital nerves. The skin and soft tissue are gently dissected and the dislocation is exposed. The first annular pulley is incised (2,24). The metacarpal head is extricated from between the flexor tendon and the lumbrical. The joint is evaluated for interposed structures, such as the volar plate and then reduced under direct observation.

The dorsal approach offers a less extensive exposure, but avoids the risk of digital nerve injury (237). Through a dorsal incision the extensor tendon is longitudinally split over the MCP joint. A transverse or longitudinal capsulotomy is made if the injury has not torn the capsule. A Freer elevator is placed within the joint and used to clear the joint of any interposed tissue. Often the interposed volar plate needs to be split longitudinally to reduce the joint. If the flexor tendon is wrapped around the metacarpal, the Freer is used to extricate the metacarpal head.

Regardless of the approach used, early motion is necessary to optimize outcome (235,238). The postoperative regimen is a 3 to 5 day immobilization period, followed by active motion. Rarely, a dorsal blocking splint is needed to prevent hyperextension that may foster repeat dislocation.

Dorsal dislocations of the other fingers are uncommon (Fig. 8-84) (239,240). Lateral fracture-dislocations may often are S-H III fractures involving the base of the proximal phalanx (Fig. 8-85) and require open reduction and internal fixation of the displaced physeal fracture.

Neglected MCP Joint Dislocations

Early treatment is preferred for MCP joint dislocations (241), but delay of a few months may still result in an acceptable outcome. A delay of more than 6 months is associated with joint degeneration and a less predictable result. Late reduction may require a combined dorsal and volar approach for adequate exposure (236,242,243). Collateral ligament resection and temporary MCP joint pin fixation may be necessary.

Dorsal Dislocation of the Thumb Ray

Thumb MCP joint dislocations are similar to those of the fingers and hyperextension is the common mechanism. Thumb dislocations are classified according to the integrity and position of the volar plate, the status of the collateral ligaments, and the

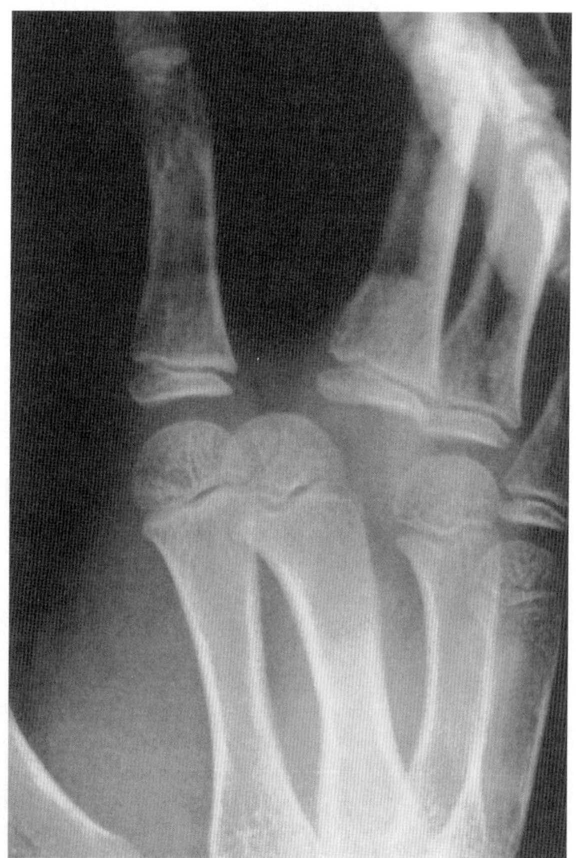

FIGURE 8-84 A rare dorsal dislocation of the long finger that was irreducible by closed means. A dorsal approach permitted inspection of the joint and extrication of the volar plate.

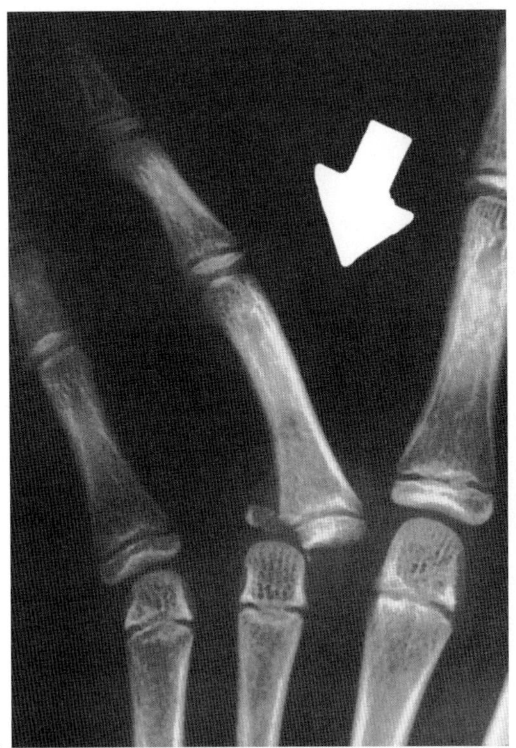
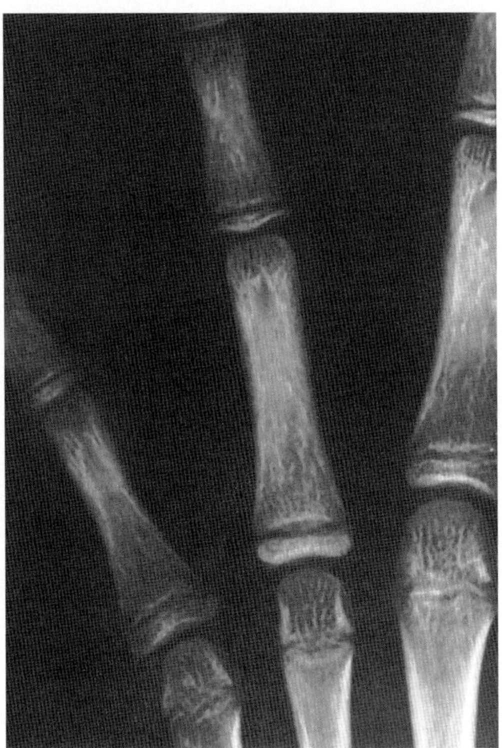

FIGURE 8-85 **A.** A 9-year-old girl sustained this radial fracture-dislocation of the middle fingers. **B.** Closed reduction restorated of joint and fracture alignment.

relative position of the metacarpal and proximal phalanx. The components of the classification are incomplete dislocation, simple complete dislocation, and complex complete dislocation (Fig. 8-86) (244).

Incomplete Thumb MCP Joint Dislocations

An incomplete dislocation implies rupture of the volar plate with partial preservation of the collateral ligament integrity. The proximal phalanx perches on the dorsum of the metacarpal. Closed reduction is easily accomplished and a 3-week course of immobilization is adequate treatment. Return to sports requires an additional 3-week period of protection.

Simple Complete Thumb MCP Dislocation

A simple complete dislocation implies volar plate and collateral ligament disruption. The proximal phalanx is displaced in a dorsal direction and is angulated 90 degrees to the long axis of the thumb metacarpal. Many of these dislocations can be reduced by closed means, although unnecessary longitudinal traction may convert a reducible condition into an irreducible situation (Fig. 8-87) (66,238,245). A successful reduction requires thumb spica immobilization for 3 to 4 weeks to allow healing of the volar plate and collateral ligaments.

Complex Complete Thumb MCP Joint Dislocation

A complete or irreducible dislocation is the most severe type of injury. The long axes of both the proximal phalanx and meta-

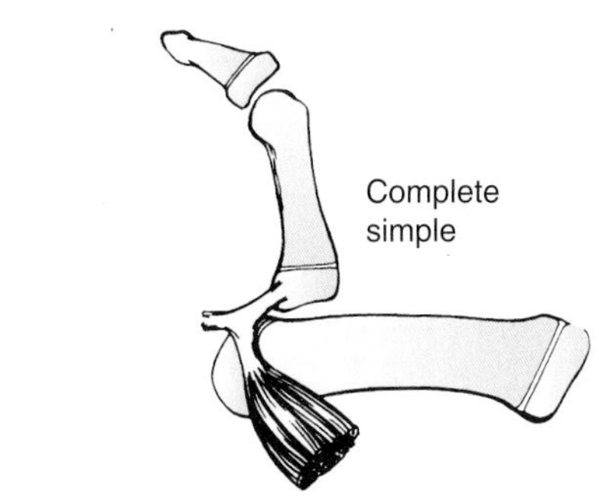

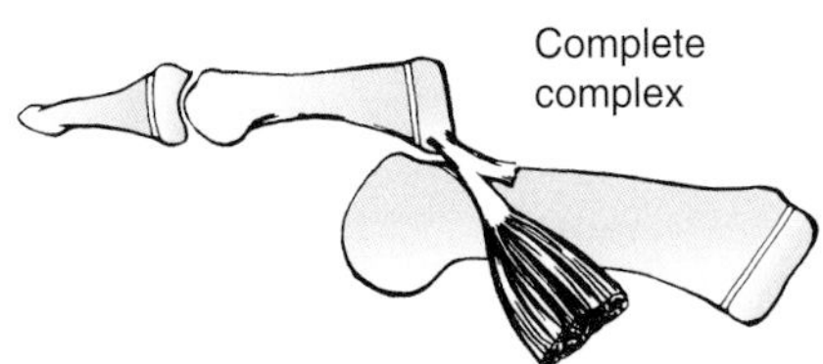

FIGURE 8-86 Simple and complex dorsal dislocations of the thumb metacarpophalangeal joint. Simple **(A)** dislocations are in extension and reducible. Complex dislocations **(B)** are in bayonet apposition and are irreducible because of the interposed volar plate.

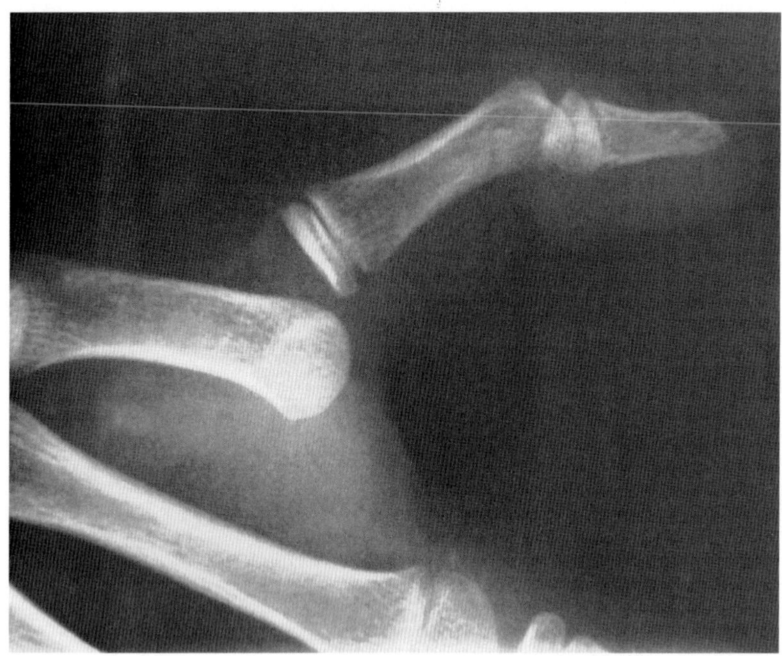

FIGURE 8-87 A 9-year-old boy with a complete simple dorsal dislocation of the thumb metacarpophalangeal joint.

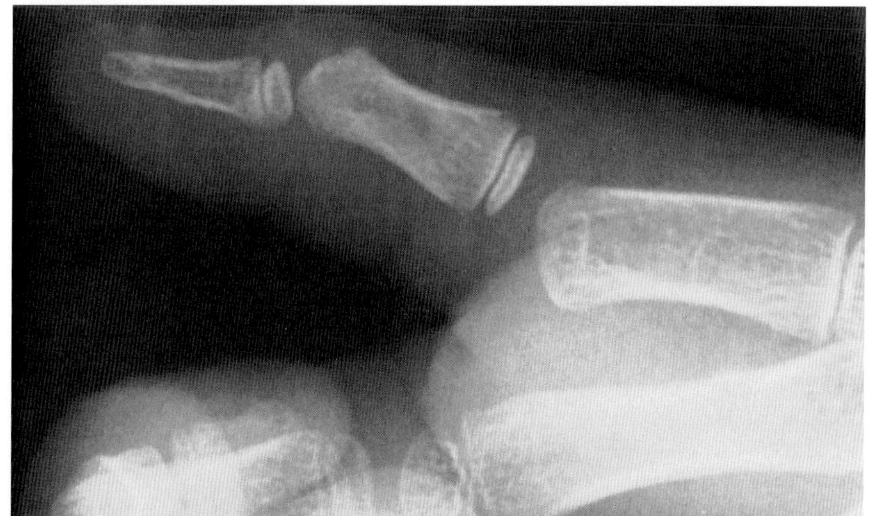

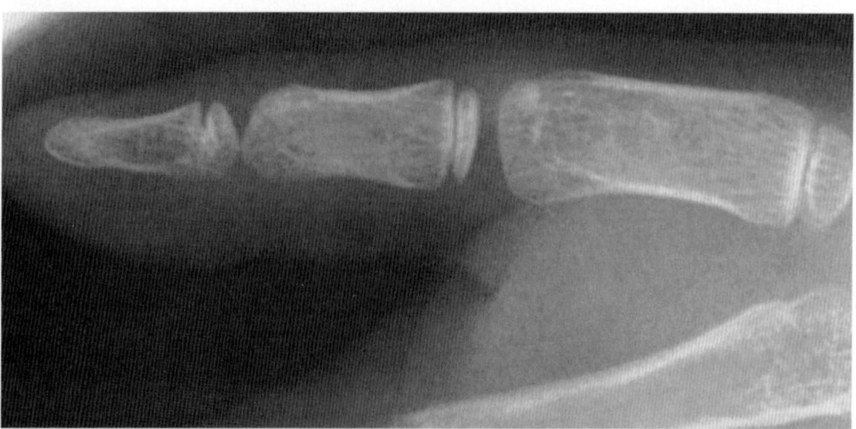

FIGURE 8-88 **A.** Irreducible dorsal metacarpophalangeal dislocation in a 7-year-old boy. **B.** After open reduction through a volar incision.

carpal often are parallel. Open reduction is usually required to extricate the volar plate from within the joint (Fig. 8-88) (232,244,246,247). A dorsal or volar approach is suitable, with concerns similar to those for irreducible index MCP joint dislocations (66,81).

Thumb MCP UCL Injury (Gamekeeper's Thumb)

Ulnar collateral ligament injuries are less prevalent in children than adults. Forced abduction stress at a child's thumb MCP joint results in four types of injury: (a) a simple sprain of the UCL, (b) a rupture or avulsion of the insertion or origin of the ligament, (c) a simple S-H I or II fracture of the proximal physis, or (d) a S-H III avulsion fracture that involves one fourth to one third of the epiphysis of the proximal phalanx (Figs. 8-89, 8-90) (248,249).

The injury is most common in preadolescents and adolescents. A history of trauma is customary, especially sporting endeavors (250). The thumb is swollen about the MCP joint with ecchymosis, and tenderness to palpation is well localized over the UCL. Pain is exacerbated by abduction stress. A complete rupture or displaced fracture lacks a discrete endpoint. Anteroposterior and lateral x-rays are used to diagnosis and delineate fracture configuration. Stress views may be needed if the diagnosis is questionable (Fig. 8-91) (232). MRI can be used to evaluate ligament disruption in complicated injuries.

Cast immobilization for 4 to 6 weeks is adequate for simple sprains, incomplete injuries, and nondisplaced fractures. Complete ruptures or displaced fractures usually require operative intervention. A major concern is displacement of the ligament or fracture fragment behind the adductor aponeurosis, which prohibits healing (80,81). A S-H III fracture of the ulnar corner of the epiphysis of the proximal phalanx is the most common childhood gamekeeper's injury. A displaced fracture (fragment rotated or displaced more than 1.5 mm) requires open reduction and internal fixation to restore the integrity of the UCL and to obtain a congruous joint surface (Fig. 8-92).

Chronic UCL injuries are more difficult to manage (243). Treatment depends on the length of time since original injury, age of the patient, and current level of function. Options range from reconstruction to chondrodesis (105).

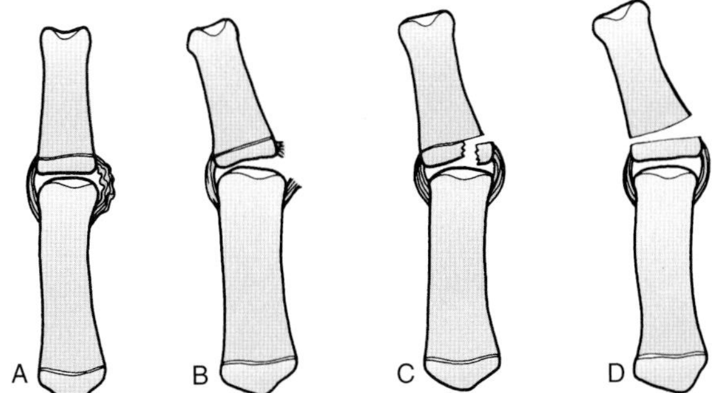

FIGURE 8-89 Ulnar instability of the thumb metacarpal joint. **A.** Simple sprain. **B.** Rupture of the ligament. **C.** Avulsion fracture (Salter-Harris type III). **D.** Pseudo-gamekeeper's injury resulting from a Salter-Harris type I or II fracture of the proximal phalanx.

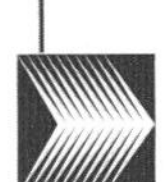

AUTHORS' PREFERRED TREATMENT

The treatment of dorsal MCP joint dislocations of the fingers and thumb should be stepwise and logical. The initial treatment usually is closed reduction for most dislocations. This attempt requires anesthesia to ensure comfort and eliminate resistance. Irreducible dislocations require open reduction. It is important to avoid multiple attempts at closed reduction of an irreducible dislocation. A dorsal or volar approach is used with removal of any interposed structure(s). The volar approach must respect the taut digital nerves overlying the prominent metacarpal head. Postoperative immobilization is used for 3 to 10 days, followed by active motion with splint-protection; athletic activities are restricted until healing is complete.

Ulnar collateral ligament injuries of the thumb are treated according to stability and displacement. Stable ligamentous injuries or minimally displaced fractures are treated with cast immobilization. Unstable ligamentous injuries or displaced fractures are treated with open reduction.

Dislocations of the Carpometacarpal Joints

Closed reduction often is successful, but percutaneous pin fixation is required for unstable reductions. Irreducible dislocations require open reduction. Large avulsion fractures that encompass a considerable part of the joint surface require open reduction to restore articular congruity (Fig. 8-54).

Some children with hypermobility or Ehlers-Danlos syndrome may have recurrent subluxation or dislocation of their CMC joints. Closed treatment is appropriate. Ligamentous reconstruction may be necessary, but the failure rate is high.

Dislocations of the Carpus

Intercarpal dislocations are uncommon in children. The rarity of the injury, small size of the carpal bones, and incomplete ossification promote erroneous diagnosis (51,135,144, 195,203,206,251). The principles of treatment do not differ from those for adults. Delayed diagnosis may require reconstructive surgery to restore stability to the wrist (Fig. 8-93) (251).

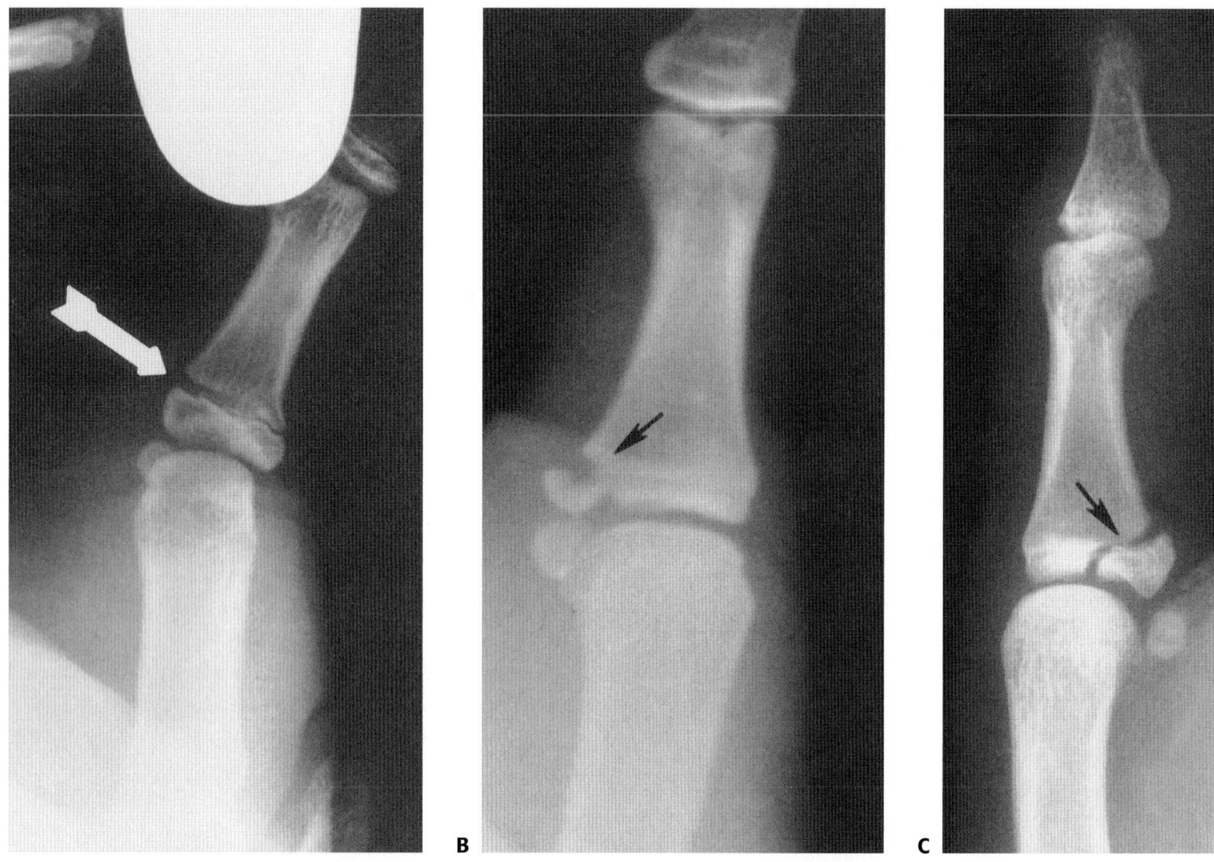

FIGURE 8-90 Spectrum of ulnar collateral ligament injuries of the thumb. **A,B.** On stress examination, a widening of the physis is seen. Varying sizes of fragments **(B,C)** may be associated with ulnar collateral ligament avulsion fractures (*arrows*). The size of the fragment is important with respect to the congruity of the metacarpophalangeal joint.

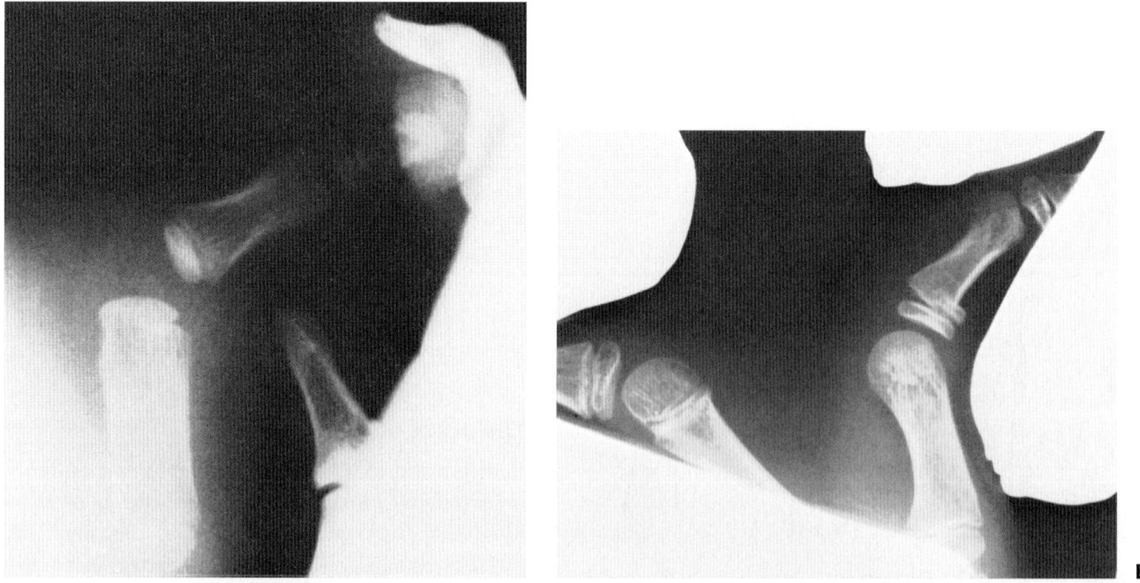

FIGURE 8-91 **A.** Stress x-ray reveals a complete ulnar collateral ligament incompetence. **B.** In this 10-year-old boy, a pseudo-gamekeeper's thumb resulted from a Salter-Harris type II fracture of the proximal phalanx. (**B** courtesy of James H. Dobyns, MD.)

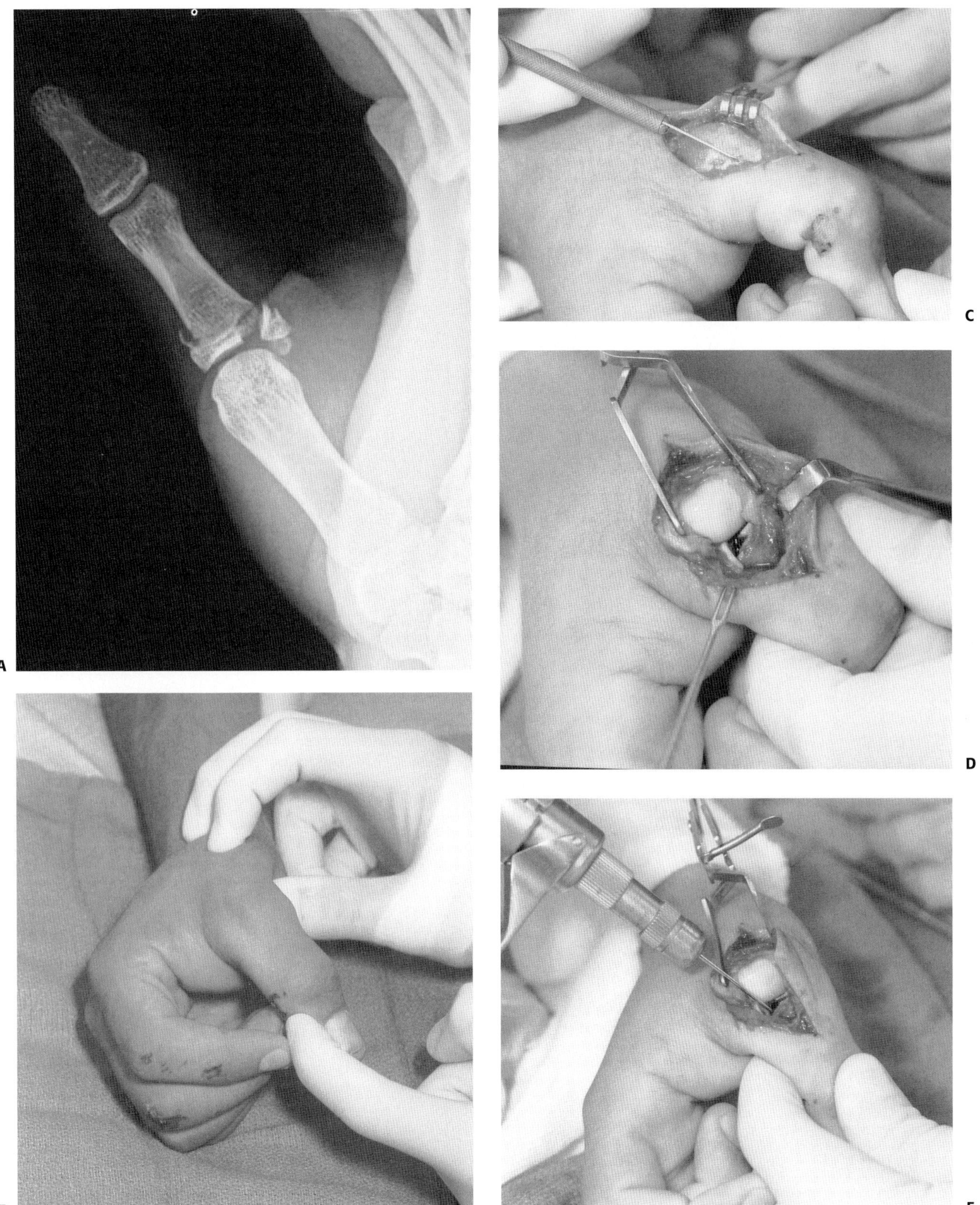

FIGURE 8-92 **A.** A 13-year-old boy with a displaced Salter-Harris III fracture of the right thumb proximal phalanx. **B.** Valgus instability on stress testing. **C.** Exposure through an incision of adductor aponeurosis. **D.** Fracture fragment exposed revealing rotation and displacement. **E.** Antegrade Kirschner wire through fracture site. *(continues)*

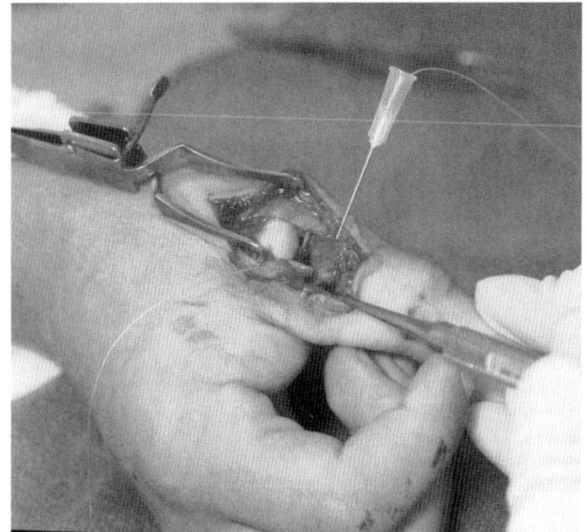

F

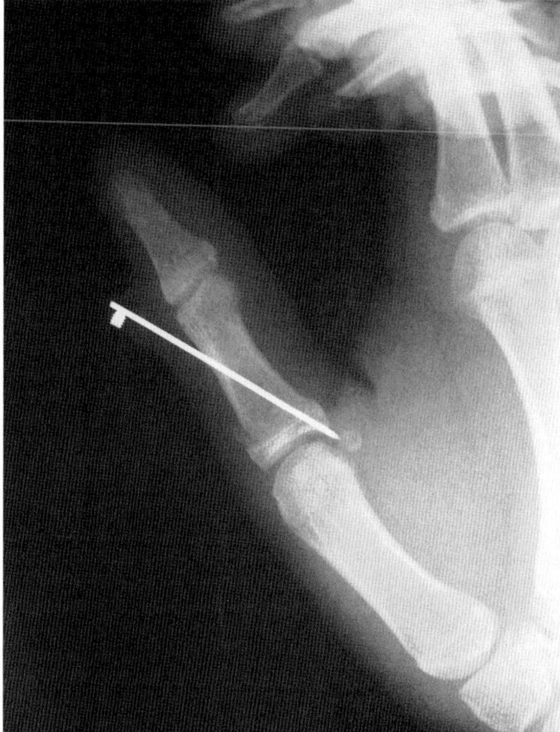

H

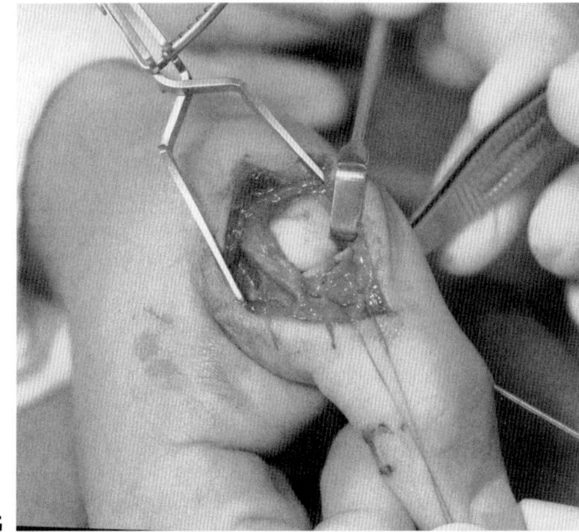

G

FIGURE 8-92 *(continued)* **F.** Thumb is placed into pronation and suture is passed for tension band fixation. **G.** Fracture reduced, Kirschner wire advanced, and suture tied in a figure-of-eight fashion. **H.** After tendon band fixation with resoration of joint and fracture alignment. (Courtesy of Shriners Hospital for Children, Philadelphia.)

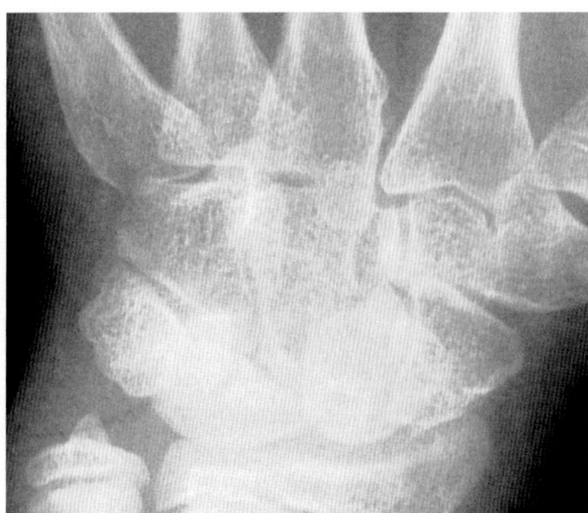

A

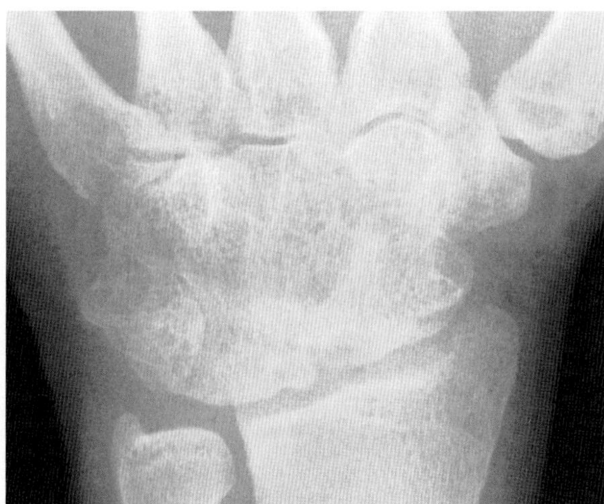

B

FIGURE 8-93 A,B. An 11-year-old girl sustained this injury 7 months previously. Several x-rays had been made, but the correct diagnosis of volar trans-scaphoid perilunate dislocation was not made.

REFERENCES

An asterisk denotes a Level I evidence-based reference.

1. Bhende MS, Dandrea LA, Davis HW. Hand injuries in children presenting to a pediatric emergency department. *Ann Emerg Med* 1993;22:1519–1523.
2. Hastings H 2nd, Simmons BP. Hand fractures in children. A statistical analysis. *Clin Orthop* 1984:120–130.
3. Worlock PH, Stower MJ. The incidence and pattern of hand fractures in children. *J Hand Surg [Br]* 1986;11:198–200.
4. Worlock P, Stower M. Fracture patterns in Nottingham children. *J Pediatr Orthop* 1986; 6:656–660.
5. Benson LS, Waters PM, Kamil NI, et al. Camptodactyly: classification and results of nonoperative treatment. *J Pediatr Orthop* 1994;14:814–819.
6. Wood VE. Fractures of the hand in children. *Orthop Clin North Am* 1976;7:527–542.
7. Grad JB. Children's skeletal injuries. *Orthop Clin North Am* 1986;17:437–449.
8. Leonard MH, Dubravcik P. Management of fractured fingers in the child. *Clin Orthop* 1970;73:160–168.
9. Fischer MD, McElfresh EC. Physeal and periphyseal injuries of the hand. Patterns of injury and results of treatment. *Hand Clin* 1994;10:287–301.
10. Barton NJ. Fractures of the phalanges of the hand in children. *Hand* 1979;11:134–143.
11. Chambers RB. Orthopaedic injuries in athletes (ages 6 to 17). Comparison of injuries occurring in six sports. *Am J Sports Med* 1979;7:195–197.
12. Garrick JG, Requa RK. Injuries in high school sports. *Pediatrics* 1978;61:465–469.
13. Goldberg B, Rosenthal PP, Robertson LS, et al. Injuries in youth football. *Pediatrics* 1988;81:255–261.
14. Markiewitz AD, Andrish JT. Hand and wrist injuries in the preadolescent and adolescent athlete. *Clin Sports Med* 1992;11:203–225.
15. Roser LA, Clawson DK. Football injuries in the very young athlete. *Clin Orthop* 1970; 69:219–223.
16. Weiker GG. Hand and wrist problems in the gymnast. *Clin Sports Med* 1992;11: 189–202.
17. Zaricznyj B, Shattuck LJ, Mast TA, et al. Sports-related injuries in school-aged children. *Am J Sports Med* 1980;8:318–324.
18. Carr D, Johnson RJ, Pope MH. Upper extremity injuries in skiing. *Am J Sports Med* 1981;9:378–383.
19. Blitzer CM, Johnson RJ, Ettlinger CF, et al. Downhill skiing injuries in children. *Am J Sports Med* 1984;12:142–147.
20. Rajesh A, Basu AK, Vaidhyanath R, et al. Hand fractures: a study of their site and type in childhood. *Clin Radiol* 2001;56:667–669.
21. Mahabir RC, Kazemi AR, Cannon WG, et al. Pediatric hand fractures: a review. *Pediatr Emerg Care* 2001;17:153–156.
22. Crick JC, Franco RS, Conners JJ. Fractures about the interphalangeal joints in children. *J Orthop Trauma* 1987;1:318–325.
23. Gilbert A. Dislocation of the MCP joints in children. In: Tubiana R (ed). *The hand*. Philadelphia: WB Saunders, 1985.
24. Light TR, Ogden JA. Complex dislocation of the index metacarpophalangeal joint in children. *J Pediatr Orthop* 1988;8:300–305.
25. Thompson JS, Littler JW, Upton J. The spiral oblique retinacular ligament (SORL). *J Hand Surg [Am]* 1978;3:482–487.
26. Simmons BP, Lovallo JL. Hand and wrist injuries in children. *Clin Sports Med* 1988; 7:495–512.
27. Stuart HC, Pyle SI, Cornoni J, et al. Onsets, completions and spans of ossification in the 29 bonegrowth centers of the hand and wrist. *Pediatrics* 1962;29:237–249.
28. Greulich WW, Pyle SI. *Radiographic atlas of skeletal development of the hand and wrist*, 2nd ed. Stanford, CA: Stanford University Press, 1959.
29. Brighton CT. Clinical problems in epiphyseal plate growth and development. *Instr Course Lect* 1974;3:105–122.
30. Torre BA. Epiphyseal injuries in the small joints of the hand. *Hand Clin* 1988;4: 113–121.
31. Green DP. Hand injuries in children. *Pediatr Clin North Am* 1977;24:903–918.
32. Haines RW. The pseudoepiphysis of the first metacarpal of man. *J Anat* 1974;117: 145–158.
33. Wood VE, Hannah JD, Stilson W. What happens to the double epiphysis in the hand? *J Hand Surg [Am]* 1994;19:353–360.
34. Wakeley CPG. Bilateral epiphysis at the basal end of the second metacarpal. *J Anat* 1974;58:340–345.
35. de Iturriza JR, Tanner JM. Cone-shaped epiphyses and other minor anomalies in the hands of normal British children. *J Pediatr* 1969;75:265–272.
36. Morscher E. Strength and morphology of growth cartilage under hormonal influence of puberty. Animal experiments and clinical study on the etiology of local growth disorders during puberty. *Reconstr Surg Traumatol* 1968;10:3–104.
37. Hankin FM, Janda DH. Tendon and ligament attachments in relationship to growth plates in a child's hand. *J Hand Surg [Br]* 1989;14:315–318.
38. Bogumill GP. A morphologic study of the relationship of collateral ligaments to growth plates in the digits. *J Hand Surg [Am]* 1983;8:74–79.
39. Shepard GH. Nail grafts for reconstruction. *Hand Clin* 1990;6:79–102; discussion 103.
40. Blount WP. Fractures in children. *Schweiz Med Wochenschr* 1954;84:986–988.
41. Rang M. *Children's fractures*, 2nd ed. Philadelphia: JB Lippincott, 1983.
42. Mintzer CM, Waters PM, Brown DJ. Remodelling of a displaced phalangeal neck fracture. *J Hand Surg [Br]* 1994;19:594–596.
43. Coonrad RW, Pohlman MH. Impacted fractures in the proximal portion of the proximal phalanx of the finger. *J Bone Joint Surg Am* 1969;51:1291–1296.
44. Campbell RM Jr. Operative treatment of fractures and dislocations of the hand and wrist region in children. *Orthop Clin North Am* 1990;21:217–243.
45. Kirner J. Doppelseitige Verdrummung des Kleinfingr-grundgleides als Selbstandiges Krankheitsbild. *Fortschr Rontgenstr* 1927;36:804.
46. Dykes RG. Kirner's deformity of the little finger. *J Bone Joint Surg Br* 1978;60:58–60.
47. Hakstian RW. Cold-induced digital epiphyseal necrosis in childhood (symmetric focal ischemic necrosis). *Can J Surg* 1972;15:168–178.
48. Nakazato T, Ogino T. Epiphyseal destruction of children's hands after frostbite: a report of two cases. *J Hand Surg [Am]* 1986;11:289–292.
49. Cullen JC. Thiemann's disease. Osteochondrosis juvenilis of the basal epiphyses of the phalanges of the hand. Report of two cases. *J Bone Joint Surg Br* 1970;52:532–534.
50. Schantz K, Rasmussen F. Thiemann's finger or toe disease. Follow-up of seven cases. *Acta Orthop Scand* 1986;57:91–93.
51. Ogden JA. *Skeletal injury in the child*. Philadelphia: WB Saunders, 1990.
52. Leddy JP, Packer JW. Avulsion of the profundus tendon insertion in athletes. *J Hand Surg [Am]* 1977;2:66–69.
53. Wenger DR. Avulsion of the profundus tendon insertion in football players. *Arch Surg* 1973;106:145–149.
54. Seymour N. Juxta-epiphysial fracture of the terminal phalanx of the finger. *J Bone Joint Surg Br* 1966;48:347–349.
55. Michelinakis E, Vourexaki H. Displaced epiphyseal plate of the terminal phalanx in a child. *Hand* 1980;12:51–53.
56. Savage R. Complete detachment of the epiphysis of the distal phalanx. *J Hand Surg [Br]* 1990;15:126–128.
57. Zook EG, Guy RJ, Russell RC. A study of nail bed injuries: causes, treatment, and prognosis. *J Hand Surg [Am]* 1984;9:247–252.
58. DaCruz DJ, Slade RJ, Malone W. Fractures of the distal phalanges. *J Hand Surg [Br]* 1988;13:350–352.
59. Ersek RA, Gadaria U, Denton DR. Nail bed avulsions treated with porcine xenografts. *J Hand Surg [Am]* 1985;10:152–153.
60. Ruggles DL, Peterson HA, Scott SG. Radial growth plate injury in a female gymnast. *Med Sci Sports Exerc* 1991;23:393–396.
61. Sandzen SC, Oakey RS. Crushing injury of the fingertip. *Hand* 1972;4:253–256.
62. Melone CP Jr, Grad JB. Primary care of fingernail injuries. *Emerg Med Clin North Am* 1985;3:255–261.
63. Al-Qattan MM. Extra-articular transverse fractures of the base of the distal phalanx (Seymour's fracture) in children and adults. *J Hand Surg [Br]* 2001;26:201–206.
64. Crawford RJ, Gupta A, Risitano G, et al. Mucous cyst of the distal interphalangeal joint: Treatment by simple excision or excision and rotation flap. *J Hand Surg [Br]* 1990;15: 113–114.
65. Eaton RG, Dobranski AI, Littler JW. Marginal osteophyte excision in treatment of mucous cysts. *J Bone Joint Surg Am* 1973;55:570–574.
66. Green DP, Terry GC. Complex dislocation of the metacarpophalangeal joint. Correlative pathological anatomy. *J Bone Joint Surg Am* 1973;55:1480–1486.
67. Hamas RS, Horrell ED, Pierret GP. Treatment of mallet finger due to intra-articular fracture of the distal phalanx. *J Hand Surg [Am]* 1978;3:361–363.
68. Kleinman WB, Bowers WH. Fractures, ligamentous injuries to the hand. In: Bora FW Jr, ed. *The pediatric upper extremity: Diagnosis and management*. Philadelphia: WB Saunders, 1988.
69. Zook EG, Russell RC. Reconstruction of a functional and esthetic nail. *Hand Clin* 1990; 6:59–68.
70. Clayburgh RH, Wood MB, Cooney WP 3rd. Nail bed repair and reconstruction by reverse dermal grafts. *J Hand Surg [Am]* 1983;8:594–598.
71. Atasoy E, Ioakimidis E, Kasdan ML, et al. Reconstruction of the amputated finger tip with a triangular volar flap. A new surgical procedure. *J Bone Joint Surg Am* 1970;52: 921–926.
72. Gatewood J. A plastic repair of finger defects without hospitalization. *JAMA* 1926;87: 1479.
73. Kappel DA, Burech JG. The cross-finger flap. An established reconstructive procedure. *Hand Clin* 1985;1:677–683.
74. Moberg E. Aspects of sensation in reconstructive surgery of the upper extremity. *J Bone Joint Surg Am* 1964;46:817–825.
75. Rayan GM, Mullins PT. Skin necrosis complicating mallet finger splinting and vascularity of the distal interphalangeal joint overlying skin. *J Hand Surg [Am]* 1987;12: 548–552.
76. Sandzen SC. *Atlas of wrist and hand fractures*. Littleton, MA: PSG, 1979.
77. Koshima I, Soeda S, Takase T, et al. Free vascularized nail grafts. *J Hand Surg [Am]* 1988;13:29–32.
78. Shibata M, Seki T, Yoshizu T, et al. Microsurgical toenail transfer to the hand. *Plast Reconstr Surg* 1991;88:102–109; discussion 110.
79. De Boeck H, Jaeken R. Treatment of chronic mallet finger deformity in children by tenodermodesis. *J Pediatr Orthop* 1992;12:351–354.
80. Stener B. Displacement of the ruptured ulnar collateral ligament of the MCP joint of the thumb. A clinical and anatomical study. *J Bone Joint Surg Br* 1962;44:869–879.
81. Stener B. Hyperextension injuries to the metacarpophalangeal joint of the thumb: rupture of ligaments, fracture of sesamoid bones, rupture of flexor pollicis brevis. An anatomical and clinical study. *Acta Chir Scand* 1963;125:275–293.
82. Dixon GL Jr, Moon NF. Rotational supracondylar fractures of the proximal phalanx in children. *Clin Orthop* 1972;83:151–156.
83. Al-Qattan MM. Juxta-epiphyseal fractures of the base of the proximal phalanx of the fingers in children and adolescents. *J Hand Surg [Br]* 2002;27:24–30.
84. Ebinger T, Roesch M, Wachter N, et al. Functional treatment of physeal and periphyseal

injuries of the metacarpal and proximal phalangeal bones. *J Pediatr Surg* 2001;36:611–615.
85. Harryman DT 2nd, Jordan TF 3rd. Physeal phalangeal fracture with flexor tendon entrapment. A case report and review of the literature. *Clin Orthop* 1990:194–196.
86. Cowen NJ, Kranik AD. An irreducible juxta-epiphyseal fracture of the proximal phalanx. Report of a case. *Clin Orthop* 1975:42–44.
87. Segmuller G, Schonenberger F. Treatment of fractures in children and adolescents. In: Weber BG, Brunner C, Freuler F (eds). *Fracture of the hand*. New York: Springer-Verlag, 1980:218–225.
88. Freeland AE, Barrett GR, Wheeless GS. Correction of abduction. Deformity of the small finger caused by avulsion of the insertion of the third volar interosseous muscle. *Am J Sports Med* 1985;13:273–276.
89. Butt WD. Rigid wire fixation of fractures of the hand. *Henry Ford Hosp Med Bull* 1956; 4:134–143.
90. Stahl S, Jupiter JB. Salter-Harris type III and IV epiphyseal fractures in the hand treated with tension-band wiring. *J Pediatr Orthop* 1999;19:233–235.
91. Stein F. Skeletal injuries of the hand in children. *Clin Plast Surg* 1981;8:65–81.
*92. Horton TC, Hatton M, Davis TR. A prospective randomized controlled study of fixation of long oblique and spiral shaft fractures of the proximal phalanx: closed reduction and percutaneous Kirschner wiring versus open reduction and lag screw fixation. *J Hand Surg [Br]* 2003;28:5–9.
93. Strickler M, Nagy L, Buchler U. Rigid internal fixation of basilar fractures of the proximal phalanges by cancellous bone grafting only. *J Hand Surg [Br]* 2001;26:455–458.
94. Blair WF, Marcus NA. Extrusion of the proximal interphalangeal joint—case report. *J Hand Surg [Am]* 1981;6:146–147.
95. Stern PJ, Roman RJ, Kiefhaber TR, et al. Pilon fractures of the proximal interphalangeal joint. *J Hand Surg [Am]* 1991;16:844–850.
96. Schenck RR. Dynamic traction and early passive movement for fractures of the proximal interphalangeal joint. *J Hand Surg [Am]* 1986;11:850–858.
97. Agee JM. Unstable fracture dislocations of the proximal interphalangeal joint of the fingers: A preliminary report of a new treatment technique. *J Hand Surg [Am]* 1978; 3:386–389.
98. Green DP, Anderson JR. Closed reduction and percutaneous pin fixation of fractured phalanges. *J Bone Joint Surg Am* 1973;55:1651–1654.
99. Waters PM, Taylor BA, Kuo AY. Percutaneous reduction of incipient malunion of phalangeal neck fractures in children. *J Hand Surg [Am]* 2004;29:707–711.
100. Teoh LC, Yong FC, Chong KC. Condylar advancement osteotomy for correcting condylar malunion of the finger. *J Hand Surg [Br]* 2002;27:31–35.
101. Cornwall R, Waters PM. Remodeling of phalangeal neck fracture malunions in children: Case report. *J Hand Surg [Am]* 2004;29:458–461.
102. Hennrikus WL, Cohen MR. Complete remodelling of displaced fractures of the neck of the phalanx. *J Bone Joint Surg Br* 2003;85:273–274.
103. Gollamudi S, Jones WA. Corrective osteotomy of malunited fractures of phalanges and metacarpals. *J Hand Surg [Br]* 2000;25:439–441.
104. Rank BK, Wakefield AR. *Surgery of repair as applied to hand injuries*. Edinburgh, UK: Livingstone, 1960.
105. Simmons BP, Stirrat CR. Treatment of traumatic arthritis in children. *Hand Clin* 1987; 3:611–627.
106. Light TR, Ogden JA. Metacarpal epiphyseal fractures. *J Hand Surg [Am]* 1987;12: 460–464.
107. Beatty E, Light TR, Belsole RJ, et al. Wrist and hand skeletal injuries in children. *Hand Clin* 1990;6:723–738.
108. McElfresh EC, Dobyns JH. Intra-articular metacarpal head fractures. *J Hand Surg [Am]* 1983;8:383–393.
109. Lane CS. Detecting occult fractures of the metacarpal head: the Brewerton view. *J Hand Surg [Am]* 1977;2:131–133.
110. Jahss SA. Fractures of the metacarpals: a new method of reduction and immobilization. *J Bone Joint Surg* 1938;20:178–186.
111. Foucher G. "Bouquet" osteosynthesis in metacarpal neck fractures: a series of 66 patients. *J Hand Surg [Am]* 1995;20:S86–90.
112. Gonzales MH, Igram CM, Hall RF. Flexible intramedullary nailing for metacarpal fractures. *J Hand Surg [Am]* 1995;20:382–387.
113. Sandzen SC. Fracture of the fifth metacarpal resembling Bennett's fracture. *Hand* 1973; 5:49–51.
114. Kleinman WB, Grantham SA. Multiple volar carpometacarpal joint dislocation. Case report of traumatic volar dislocation of the medial four carpometacarpal joint in a child and review of the literature. *J Hand Surg [Am]* 1978;3:377–382.
115. Whitson RO. Carpometacarpal dislocation: a case report. *Clin Orthop* 1955;(6): 189–195.
116. Ireland ML, Taleisnik J. Nonunion of metacarpal extraarticular fractures in children: Report of two cases and review of the literature. *J Pediatr Orthop* 1986;6:352–355.
117. Prosser AJ, Irvine GB. Epiphyseal fracture of the metacarpal head. *Injury* 1988;19: 34–35.
118. Crock HV, Chari PR, Crock MC. The blood supply of the wrist and hand bones in man. In: Tubiana R, ed. *The hand*, Vol. 1. Philadelphia: WB Saunders, 1981:335–339.
119. Bennett EH. Fractures of the metacarpal bones. *Dublin J Med Sci* 1982;73:72–75.
120. Gedda KO. Studies in Bennett's fracture: Anatomy, roentgenology, and therapy. *Acta Chir Scand* 1954;5:193.
121. Langenskiold A. Surgical treatment of partial closure of the growth plate. *J Pediatr Orthop* 1981;1:3–11.
122. Smith RJ, Peimer CA. Injuries to the metacarpal bones and joints. *Adv Surg* 1977;11: 341–374.
123. Griffiths JC. Bennett's fracture in childhood. *Br J Clin Pract* 1966;20:582–583.
124. Stern PJ. Fractures of the metacarpals and phalanges. In Green DP, ed. *Operative hand surgery*. New York: Churchill Livingstone, 1993:748.
125. Spanberg O, Thoren L. Bennett's fracture: A new method of treatment with oblique traction. *J Bone Joint Surg Br* 1963;45:732–736.
126. Buchler U, McCollam SM, Oppikofer C. Comminuted fractures of the basilar joint of the thumb: combined treatment by external fixation, limited internal fixation, and bone grafting. *J Hand Surg [Am]* 1991;16:556–560.
127. Bergfeld JA, Weiker GG, Andrish JT, et al. Soft playing splint for protection of significant hand and wrist injuries in sports. *Am J Sports Med* 1982;10:293–296.
128. Van Herpe LB. Fractures of the forearm and wrist. *Orthop Clin North Am* 1976;7: 543–556.
129. Mizuta T, Benson WM, Foster BK, et al. Statistical analysis of the incidence of physeal injuries. *J Pediatr Orthop* 1987;7:518–523.
130. Lee BS, Esterhai JL Jr, Das M. Fracture of the distal radial epiphysis. Characteristics and surgical treatment of premature, post-traumatic epiphyseal closure. *Clin Orthop* 1984:90–96.
131. Dicke TE, Nunley JA. Distal forearm fractures in children. Complications and surgical indications. *Orthop Clin North Am* 1993;24:333–340.
132. Crawford AH. Pitfalls and complications of fractures of the distal radius and ulna in childhood. *Hand Clin* 1988;4:403–413.
133. Nafie SA. Fractures of the carpal bones in children. *Injury* 1987;18:117–119.
134. Roy S, Caine D, Singer KM. Stress changes of the distal radial epiphysis in young gymnasts. A report of twenty-one cases and a review of the literature. *Am J Sports Med* 1985;13:301–308.
135. Light TR. Injury to the immature carpus. *Hand Clin* 1988;4:415–424.
136. Pick RY, Segal D. Carpal scaphoid fracture and non-union in an eight-year-old child. Report of a case. *J Bone Joint Surg Am* 1983;65:1188–1189.
137. Larson B, Light TR, Ogden JA. Fracture and ischemic necrosis of the immature scaphoid. *J Hand Surg [Am]* 1987;12:122–127.
138. Louis DS, Calhoun TP, Garn SM, et al. Congenital bipartite scaphoid—fact or fiction? *J Bone Joint Surg Am* 1976;58:1108–1112.
139. Green MH, Hadied AM, LaMont RL. Scaphoid fractures in children. *J Hand Surg [Am]* 1984;9:536–541.
140. Albert MC, Barre PS. A scaphoid fracture associated with a displaced distal radial fracture in a child. *Clin Orthop* 1989:232–235.
141. Compson JP. Trans-carpal injuries associated with distal radial fractures in children: A series of three cases. *J Hand Surg [Br]* 1992;17:311–314.
142. Green WB, Anderson WJ. Simultaneous fracture of the scaphoid and radius in a child. *J Pediatr Orthop* 1982;2:191–194.
143. Vahvanen V, Westerlund M. Fracture of the carpal scaphoid in children. A clinical and roentgenological study of 108 cases. *Acta Orthop Scand* 1980;51:909–913.
144. Christodoulou AG, Colton CL. Scaphoid fractures in children. *J Pediatr Orthop* 1986; 6:37–39.
145. Bloem JJ. Fracture of the carpal scaphoid in a child aged 4. *Arch Chir Neerl* 1971;23: 91–94.
146. Gamble JG, Simmons SC 3rd. Bilateral scaphoid fractures in a child. *Clin Orthop* 1982: 125–128.
147. Southcott R, Rosman MA. Non-union of carpal scaphoid fractures in children. *J Bone Joint Surg Br* 1977;59:20–23.
148. Dunn AW. Fractures and dislocations of the carpus. *Surg Clin North Am* 1972;52: 1513–1538.
149. London PS. Sprains and fractures involving the interphalangeal joints. *Hand* 1971;3: 155–158.
150. Weber ER, Chao EY. An experimental approach to the mechanism of scaphoid waist fractures. *J Hand Surg [Am]* 1978;3:142–148.
151. Mintzer CM, Waters PM. Surgical treatment of pediatric scaphoid fracture nonunions. *J Pediatr Orthop* 1999;19:236–239.
152. Cockshott WP. Distal avulsion fractures of the scaphoid. *Br J Radiol* 1980;53: 1037–1040.
153. Cobey MC, White RK. An operation for nonunions of the carpal navicular. *J Bone Joint Surg* 1946;28:757–764.
154. Fisk GR. Carpal instability and the fractured scaphoid. *Ann R Coll Surg Engl* 1970;46: 63–76.
155. Frykman G. Fracture of the distal radius including sequelae—shoulder-hand-finger syndrome, disturbance in the distal radio-ulnar joint and impairment of nerve function. A clinical and experimental study. *Acta Orthop Scand* 1967:Suppl 108:3+.
156. Aggarwal AK, Sangwan SS, Siwach RC. Trans-scaphoid perilunate dislocation in a child. *Contemp Orthop* 1993;26:172–174.
157. Doman AN, Marcus NW. Congenital bipartite scaphoid. *J Hand Surg [Am]* 1990;15: 869–873.
158. Pfitzner W. Beitrage zure Kenntniss des Menschlichn Extremitatenskelets. VII Die Morphologischen Elemente des Menschlichen Hand-Skelets. *Z Morphol* 1900;2:77–157.
159. Boyes JH. *Bunnell's surgery of the hand*. Philadelphia: JB Lippincott, 1970.
160. Perron AD, Brady WJ, Keats TE, et al. Orthopedic pitfalls in the ED: Scaphoid fracture. *Am J Emerg Med* 2001;19:310–316.
161. Sanders WE. Evaluation of the humpback scaphoid by computed tomography in the longitudinal axial plane of the scaphoid. *J Hand Surg [Am]* 1988;13:182–187.
162. Brydie A, Raby N. Early MRI in the management of clinical scaphoid fracture. *Br J Radiol* 2003;76:296–300.
163. Mack MG, Keim S, Balzer JO, et al. Clinical impact of MRI in acute wrist fractures. *Eur Radiol* 2003;13:612–617.
164. Dorsay TA, Major NM, Helms CA. Cost-effectiveness of immediate MR imaging versus traditional follow-up for revealing radiographically occult scaphoid fractures. *AJR Am J Roentgenol* 2001;177:1257–1263.

165. Poznanski AK, Holt JF. The carpals in congenital malformation syndromes. *Am J Roentgenol Radium Ther Nucl Med* 1971;112:443–459.
166. Johnson KJ, Haigh SF, Symonds KE. MRI in the management of scaphoid fractures in skeletally immature patients. *Pediatr Radiol* 2000;30:685–688.
167. Amadio PC, Berquist TH, Smith DK, et al. Scaphoid malunion. *J Hand Surg [Am]* 1989; 14:679–687.
168. Bora FW Jr, Culp RW, Osterman AL, et al. A flexible wrist splint. *J Hand Surg [Am]* 1989;14:574–575.
169. Yanni D, Lieppins P, Laurence M. Fractures of the carpal scaphoid. A critical study of the standard splint. *J Bone Joint Surg Br* 1991;73:600–602.
170. Hambidge JE, Desai VV, Schranz PJ, et al. Acute fractures of the scaphoid. Treatment by cast immobilisation with the wrist in flexion or extension? *J Bone Joint Surg Br* 1999; 81:91–92.
171. Burge P. Closed cast treatment of scaphoid fractures. *Hand Clin* 2001;17:541–552.
172. Thomaidis VT. Elbow-wrist-thumb immobilisation in the treatment of fractures of the carpal scaphoid. *Acta Orthop Scand* 1973;44:679–689.
173. Gellman H, Caputo RJ, Carter V, et al. Comparison of short and long thumb-spica casts for non-displaced fractures of the carpal scaphoid. *J Bone Joint Surg Am* 1989;71: 354–357.
174. McLaughlin H. Fracture of the carpal navicular (scaphoid) bone; some observations based on treatment by open reduction and internal fixation. *J Bone Joint Surg Am* 1954; 36-A:765–774.
175. Linscheid RL, Dobyns JH, Beabout JW, et al. Traumatic instability of the wrist. Diagnosis, classification, and pathomechanics. *J Bone Joint Surg Am* 1972;54:1612–1632.
176. King RJ, Mackenney RP, Elnur S. Suggested method for closed treatment of fractures of the carpal scaphoid: hypothesis supported by dissection and clinical practice. *J R Soc Med* 1982;75:860–867.
*177. Adolfsson L, Lindau T, Arner M. Acutrak screw fixation versus cast immobilisation for undisplaced scaphoid waist fractures. *J Hand Surg [Br]* 2001;26:192–195.
178. Yip HS, Wu WC, Chang RY, et al. Percutaneous cannulated screw fixation of acute scaphoid waist fracture. *J Hand Surg [Br]* 2002;27:42–46.
179. Mintzer C, Waters PM. Acute open reduction of a displaced scaphoid fracture in a child. *J Hand Surg [Am]* 1994;19:760–761.
180. Herbert TJ, Fisher WE. Management of the fractured scaphoid using a new bone screw. *J Bone Joint Surg Br* 1984;66:114–123.
181. Herbert TJ. Use of the Herbert bone screw in surgery of the wrist. *Clin Orthop* 1986: 79–92.
182. Muramatsu K, Doi K, Kuwata N, et al. Scaphoid fracture in the young athlete—therapeutic outcome of internal fixation using the Herbert screw. *Arch Orthop Trauma Surg* 2002;122:510–513.
183. Rettig ME, Raskin KB. Retrograde compression screw fixation of acute proximal pole scaphoid fractures. *J Hand Surg [Am]* 1999;24:1206–1210.
184. De Boeck H, Van Wellen P, Haentjens P. Nonunion of a carpal scaphoid fracture in a child. *J Orthop Trauma* 1991;5:370–372.
185. Littlefield WG, Friedman RL, Urbaniak JR. Bilateral non-union of the carpal scaphoid in a child. A case report. *J Bone Joint Surg Am* 1995;77:124–126.
186. Maxted MJ, Owen R. Two cases of non-union of carpal scaphoid fractures in children. *Injury* 1982;13:441–443.
187. Onuba O, Ireland J. Two cases of non-union of fractures of the scaphoid in children. *Injury* 1983;15:109–112.
188. Watson HK, Ballet FL. The SLAC wrist: scapholunate advanced collapse pattern of degenerative arthritis. *J Hand Surg [Am]* 1984;9:358–365.
189. Mack GR, Bosse MJ, Gelberman RH, et al. The natural history of scaphoid non-union. *J Bone Joint Surg Am* 1984;66:504–509.
190. Waters PM, Stewart SL. Surgical treatment of nonunion and avascular necrosis of the proximal part of the scaphoid in adolescents. *J Bone Joint Surg Am* 2002;84-A:915–920.
191. Steinmann SP, Bishop AT, Berger RA. Use of the 1,2 intercompartmental supraretinacular artery as a vascularized pedicle bone graft for difficult scaphoid nonunion. *J Hand Surg [Am]* 2002;27:391–401.
192. Gibbon WW, Jackson A. An isolated capitate fracture in a 9-year-old boy. *Br J Radiol* 1989;62:487–488.
193. Vance RM, Gelberman RH, Evans EF. Scaphocapitate fractures. Patterns of dislocation, mechanisms of injury, and preliminary results of treatment. *J Bone Joint Surg Am* 1980; 62:271–276.
194. Young TB. Isolated fracture of the capitate in a 10-year-old boy. *Injury* 1986;17: 133–134.
195. Peiro A, Martos F, Mut T, et al. Trans-scaphoid perilunate dislocation in a child. A case report. *Acta Orthop Scand* 1981;52:31–34.
196. Anderson WJ. Simultaneous fracture of the scaphoid and capitate in a child. *J Hand Surg [Am]* 1987;12:271–273.
197. Gouldesbrough C. A case of fractured scaphoid and os mangum in a bone 10 years old. *Lancet* 1916;2:792.
198. Minami M, Yamazaki J, Chisaka N, et al. Nonunion of the capitate. *J Hand Surg [Am]* 1987;12:1089–1091.
199. Yoshihara M, Sakai A, Toba N, et al. Nonunion of the isolated capitate waist fracture. *J Orthop Sci* 2002;7:578–580.
200. Mayfield JK, Johnson RP, Kilcoyne RK. Carpal dislocations: Pathomechanics and progressive perilunar instability. *J Hand Surg [Am]* 1980;5:226–241.
201. Benz HJ, Blencke BA. [Restitution of lunate bone necrosis in a child (author's trans)]. *Z Orthop Ihre Grenzgeb* 1976;114:819–821.
202. Rasmussen F, Schantz K. Lunatomalacia in a child. *Acta Orthop Scand* 1987;58:82–84.
203. Gerard FM. Post-traumatic carpal instability in a young child. A case report. *J Bone Joint Surg Am* 1980;62:131–133.
204. Giddins GE, Shaw DG. Lunate subluxation associated with a Salter-Harris type 2 fracture of the distal radius. *J Hand Surg [Br]* 1994;19:193–194.
205. Hildebrand KA, Ross DC, Patterson SD, et al. Dorsal perilunate dislocations and fracture-dislocations: questionnaire, clinical, and radiographic evaluation. *J Hand Surg [Am]* 2000;25:1069–1079.
206. Pennes DR, Braunstein EM, Shirazi KK. Carpal ligamentous laxity with bilateral perilunate dislocation in Marfan syndrome. *Skeletal Radiol* 1985;13:62–64.
207. Kaawach W, Ecklund K, Di Canzio J, et al. Normal ranges of scapholunate distance in children 6 to 14 years old. *J Pediatr Orthop* 2001;21:464–467.
208. Earp BE, Waters PM, Wyzykowski RJ. Arthroscopic treatment of post-traumatic wrist instability in pediatric and adolescent patients. *J Bone Joint Surg* (submitted).
209. Terry CL, Waters PM. Triangular fibrocartilage injuries in pediatric and adolescent patients. *J Hand Surg [Am]* 1998;23:626–634.
210. Palmer AK, Werner FW. The triangular fibrocartilage complex of the wrist—anatomy and function. *J Hand Surg [Am]* 1981;6:153–162.
211. Palmer AK. Triangular fibrocartilage complex lesions: a classification. *J Hand Surg [Am]* 1989;14:594–606.
212. Nakamura R. Diagnosis of ulnar wrist pain. *Nagoya J Med Sci* 2001;64:81–91.
213. Cerezal L, del Pinal F, Abascal F, et al. Imaging findings in ulnar-sided wrist impaction syndromes. *Radiographics* 2002;22:105–121.
214. Haims AH, Schweitzer ME, Morrison WB, et al. Limitations of MR imaging in the diagnosis of peripheral tears of the triangular fibrocartilage of the wrist. *AJR Am J Roentgenol* 2002;178:419–422.
215. Palmer AK, Linscheid RL. Irreducible dorsal dislocation of the distal interphalangeal joint of the finger. *J Hand Surg [Am]* 1977;2:406–408.
216. Pohl AL. Irreducible dislocation of a distal interphalangeal joint. *Br J Plast Surg* 1976; 29:227–229.
217. Salamon PB, Gelberman RH. Irreducible dislocation of the interphalangeal joint of the thumb. *J Bone Joint Surg Am* 1978;60:400–401.
218. Selig S, Schein A. Irreducible buttonhole dislocations of the fingers. *J Bone Joint Surg Br* 1940;22.
219. Stripling WD. Displaced intra-articular osteochondral fracture—cause for irreducible dislocation of the distal interphalangeal joint. *J Hand Surg [Am]* 1982;7:77–78.
220. Elson RA. Rupture of the central slip of the extensor hood of the finger. A test for early diagnosis. *J Bone Joint Surg Br* 1986;68:229–231.
221. Borde J, Lefort J. Injuries of the wrist and hand in children. In Tubiana R, ed. *The hand*, Vol. 2. Philadelphia: WB Saunders, 1985:123–145.
222. Bowers WH. The PIP joint volar plate. II: A clinical study of hyperextension injury. *J Hand Surg* 1981;6:77–81.
223. McCue FC, Honner R, Johnson MC, et al. Athletic injuries of the proximal interphalangeal joint requiring surgical treatment. *J Bone Joint Surg Am* 1970;52:937–956.
224. Redler I, Williams JT. Rupture of a collateral ligament of the proximal interphalangeal joint of the fingers. Analysis of eighteen cases. *J Bone Joint Surg Am* 1967;49:322–326.
225. Whipple TL, Evans JP, Urbaniak JR. Irreducible dislocation of a finger joint in a child. A case report. *J Bone Joint Surg Am* 1980;62:832–833.
226. Peimer CA, Sullivan DJ, Wild DR. Palmar dislocation of the proximal interphalangeal joint. *J Hand Surg [Am]* 1984;9A:39–48.
227. Neviaser RJ, Wilson JN. Interposition of the extensor tendon resulting in persistent subluxation of the proximal interphalangeal joint of the finger. *Clin Orthop* 1972;83: 118–120.
228. Jones NF, Jupiter JB. Irreducible palmar dislocation of the proximal interphalangeal joint associated with an epiphyseal fracture of the middle phalanx. *J Hand Surg [Am]* 1985;10:261–264.
229. Thompson JS, Eaton RG. Volar dislocation of the PIP joint. *J Hand Surg* 1977;2:232.
230. Garroway RY, Hurtst LC, Leppard J, et al. Complex dislocations of the PIP joint. A pathoanatomic classification of the injury. *Orthop Rev* 1984;13:21–28.
231. Kiefhaber TR, Stern PJ. Fracture dislocations of the proximal interphalangeal joint. *J Hand Surg [Am]* 1998;23:368–380.
232. Smith RJ. Post-traumatic instability of the metacarpophalangeal joint of the thumb. *J Bone Joint Surg Am* 1977;59:14–21.
233. Burman M. Irreducible hyperextension dislocation of the metacarpophalangeal joint of a finger. *Bull Hosp Joint Dis* 1953;14:290–291.
234. Robins RH. Injuries of the metacarpophalangeal joints. *Hand* 1971;3:159–163.
235. Kaplan EB. Dorsal dislocation of the metacarpophalangeal joint of the index finger. *J Bone Joint Surg Am* 1957;39-A:1081–1086.
236. Barenfeld PA, Weseley MS. Dorsal dislocation of the metacarpophalangeal joint of the index finger treated by late open reduction. A case report. *J Bone Joint Surg Am* 1972; 54:1311–1313.
237. Becton JL, Christian JD Jr, Goodwin HN, et al. A simplified technique for treating the complex dislocation of the index metacarpophalangeal joint. *J Bone Joint Surg Am* 1975; 57:698–700.
238. McLaughlin HL. Complex "locked" dislocation of the metacarpophalangeal joints. *J Trauma* 1965;5:683–688.
239. Nussbaum R, Sadler AH. An isolated, closed, complex dislocation of the metacarpophalangeal joint of the long finger: A unique case. *J Hand Surg [Am]* 1986;11:558–561.
240. Baldwin LW, Miller DL, Lockhart LD, et al. Metacarpophalangeal-joint dislocations of the fingers. *J Bone Joint Surg Am* 1967;49:1587–1590.
241. Hunt JC, Watts HB, Glasgow JD. Dorsal dislocation of the metacarpophalangeal joint of the index finger with particular reference to open dislocation. *J Bone Joint Surg Am* 1967;49:1572–1578.

242. Murphy AF, Stark HH. Cloased dislocation of the metacarpophalangeal joint of the index finger. *J Bone Joint Surg Am* 1967;49:1579–1586.
243. Lipscomb PR, Janes JM. Twenty-year follow-up of an unreduced dislocation of the first metacarpophalangeal joint in a child. Report of a case. *J Bone Joint Surg Am* 1969;51: 1216–1218.
244. Farabeuf LH, Faqb BHL. Dorsal dislocation of the first phalanx of the little finger. Reduction by Farabeuf's dorsal incision. *Lancet* 1901;1:88–90.
245. Burton RI, Eaton RG. Common hand injuries in the athlete. *Orthop Clin North Am* 1973;4:809–838.
246. Weeks PM. *Acute bone and joint injuries of the hand and wrist. A clinical guide to management.* St. Louis, MO: CV Mosby, 1981.
247. Bohart PG, Gelberman RH, Vandell RF, et al. Complex dislocations of the metacarpophalangeal joint. *Clin Orthop* 1982:208–210.
248. White GM. Ligamentous avulsion of the ulnar collateral ligament of the thumb of a child. *J Hand Surg [Am]* 1986;11:669–672.
249. Mintzer CM, Waters PM. Late presentation of a ligamentous ulnar collateral ligament injury in a child. *J Hand Surg [Am]* 1994;19:1048–1049.
250. Winslet MC, Clarke NM, Mulligan PJ. Breakdancer's thumb—partial rupture of the ulnar collateral ligament with a fracture of the proximal phalanx of the thumb. *Injury* 1986;17:201–202.
251. Graham TJ, Jacobson PA. A traumatic palmar midcarpal dislocation in a skeletally immature adolescent with hemiatrophy. *J Hand Surg [Am]* 1999;24:1281–1285.

9

FRACTURES OF THE DISTAL RADIUS AND ULNA

Peter M. Waters and Alexander D. Mih

Forearm fractures in children are the most common long bone fractures, comprising about 40% of all pediatric fractures (1–3). The distal aspect of the radius and ulna is the most common site of fracture in the forearm (2,4–7). These fractures have been reported to be three times more common in boys; however, the increased participation in athletics by girls at a young age may be changing this ratio. Although these fractures occur at any age, they are most frequent during the adolescent growth spurt (8). The fractures are described by location, metaphyseal or physeal, as well as by severity of displacement. The pediatric Galeazzi injury usually involves a distal radial metaphyseal fracture and a distal ulnar physeal fracture that result in a displaced distal radioulnar joint. These injuries are rare, but need to be identified acutely for proper management. The specifics of fracture patterns for individual fracture types are discussed in separate sections of this chapter. Most of these injuries have traditionally been treated with closed reduction and cast immobilization. Indications for percutaneous pinning and open reduction in pediatric patients are evolving and are discussed in each section.

PRINCIPLES OF MANAGEMENT

Mechanism of Injury

A direct fall is the usual mechanism of injury. With the wrist and hand extended, a fracture occurs if the mechanical force is sufficient. Usually this is secondary to a sporting event. Snowboarding, skateboarding, soccer goalkeeping, and horse back riding have been shown to be high-risk-sports (9–15), but a severe enough fall in any recreational activity can lead to a fracture. There is seasonal variation, with an increase in both incidence and severity of fractures in summer (16). Children who are overweight have poor postural balance, ligamentous laxity, or less bone mineralization, and are at increased risk for distal radial fractures (17–19). The fractures generally occur with an extension deformity because of the mechanism of a fall on an outstretched hand. Occasionally a direct blow or a fall onto a flexed wrist and hand causes volar displacement or angulation of the distal fragment. In either case, there may be a rotational component to the fracture pattern.

Repetitive loading of the wrist can lead to physeal stress injuries of the distal radius and, less commonly, the ulna. These injuries are rare, and occur most frequently in gymnasts (20–26). Any patient with chronic physeal region wrist pain who participates in an activity with repetitive axial loading of the wrist, such as gymnastics or break dancing (27), should be examined for a stress injury.

Signs and Symptoms

Regardless of the type, these fractures cause pain in the distal forearm, tenderness directly over the fracture site, and limited motion of the forearm, wrist, and hand. Deformity depends on the degree of fracture displacement. Fractures with marked extension displacement can lead to a silver fork deformity similar to an adult Colles' fracture. Standard anteroposterior (AP) and lateral x-rays are diagnostic of fracture type and displacement. Metaphyseal fractures are most common, followed by physeal fractures (3,28,29); the distal fragment in either usually is extended. Neurovascular examination should be performed before treatment to assess for median or ulnar neuropathy or the rare compartment syndrome. Hand and elbow regions need to be examined clinically and, if appropriate, radiographically for associated injuries.

Associated Injuries

Associated fractures of the hand and elbow regions are rare but need to be assessed because their presence implies more severe trauma. The risk of a compartment syndrome is higher with a "floating elbow" combination of radial, ulnar, and elbow fractures (30). With marked radial or ulnar fracture displacement, neurovascular compromise can occur. Median neuropathy results from contusion at the time of fracture displacement, persistent direct pressure from an unreduced fracture, or an acute compartment syndrome (31). Ulnar neuropathy has been described with similar mechanisms as well as entrapment. Wrist ligamentous and articular cartilage injuries have been described in association with distal radial and ulnar fractures in adults and less commonly in children (32,33). Concomitant scaphoid fractures have occurred (34). Associated wrist injuries need to be treated both in the acute setting and in the patient with persistent pain after fracture healing. Some patients with distal radial and ulnar fractures are multi-trauma victims. Their systemic care modifies their distal forearm fracture care.

Diagnosis and Classification

Distal radial and ulnar fractures are defined by their anatomic relationship to the physis. Transphyseal injuries are classified by the widely accepted Salter-Harris system (35). Metaphyseal injuries may be torus or buckle fractures, greenstick or incomplete fractures, or complete injuries. Pediatric equivalents of adult Galeazzi fracture–dislocations involve a distal radial fracture and either a soft-tissue disruption of the distal radioulnar joint (DRUJ) or a transphyseal fracture of the ulna (Table 9-1). In contrast to adults, skeletally immature patients rarely sustain intra-articular fractures of the distal radius. On occasion, a Salter-Harris type III fracture, a triplane fracture (36), or an adolescent intra-articular Colles' fracture occurs.

Distal radial fracture stability has been more clearly defined in adults (37) than in children. At present, an unstable fracture in a child is often defined as one in which closed reduction cannot be maintained. Pediatric classification systems have yet to more precisely define fracture stability, but this issue is critical in determining proper treatment management. Distal radial metaphyseal fractures have been shown to have a high degree of recurrent displacement and, therefore, inherent instability (38–42).

Fractures also are defined by the degree of displacement and angulation. Static AP and lateral x-rays can be diagnostic of the

TABLE 9-1 Distal Forearm Fractures: General Classification

Physeal fractures
- Distal radius
- Distal ulna

Distal metaphyseal (radius or ulna)
- Torus
- Greenstick
- Complete fractures

Galeazzi fracture–dislocations
- Dorsal displaced
- Volar displaced

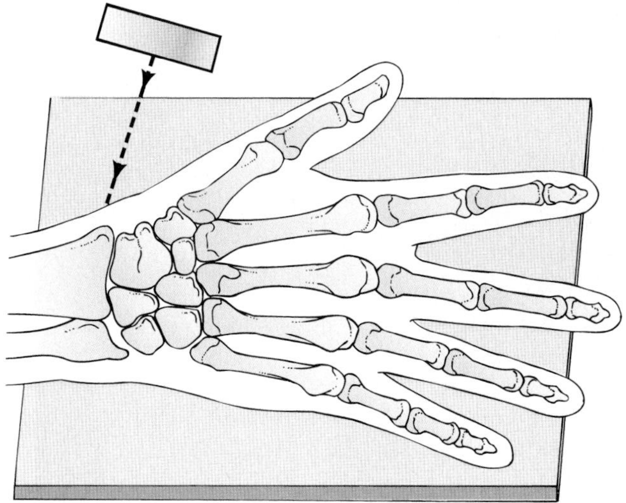

FIGURE 9-1 Angulation of the x-ray beam tangential to the articular surface, provides the optimal lateral view of the distal radius. The wrist is positioned as for the standard lateral x-ray, but the x-ray beam is directed 15° cephalad. (Redrawn from Johnson PG, Szabo RM. Angle measurements of the distal radius: a cadaver study. *Skel Radiol* 1993;22:243; with permission.)

fracture type and degree of deformity (Fig. 9-1). In adults, the distal radial articular alignment averages 22° on the AP view and 11° on the lateral view (43–47). Radial inclination is a goniometric measurement of the angle between the distal radial articular surface and a line perpendicular to the radial shaft on the AP x-ray. Palmar tilt is measured by a line across the distal articular surface and a line perpendicular to the radial shaft on the lateral view. Pediatric values for radial inclination tend to be less, depending on the degree of skeletal maturity of the patient. Palmar tilt tends to be more consistent regardless of the age of the patient.

Rarely, tomographic views are necessary to assess intra-articular involvement or displacement. This can be by AP and lateral tomograms, computerized tomographic (CT) scans, or magnetic resonance imaging (MRI). Dynamic motion studies with fluoroscopy can provide important information on fracture stability and the success of various treatment options. Dynamic fluoroscopy requires adequate pain relief and has been used more often in adult patients with distal radial fractures. Ultrasound has been used to diagnose fractures in some centers (48,49).

SURGICAL AND APPLIED ANATOMY

The distal radial epiphysis normally appears between 0.5 and 2.3 years in boys and 0.4 and 1.7 years in girls (50) . Initially transverse in appearance, it rapidly becomes more adult-like with its triangular shape. The contour of the radial styloid progressively elongates with advancing skeletal maturity. The secondary center of ossification for the distal ulna appears at about age 7. Similar to the radius, the ulnar styloid appears with the adolescent growth spurt. It also becomes more elongated and adult-like until physeal closure. On average, the ulnar physis closes at age 16 in girls and age 17 in boys, whereas the radial physis closes on average 6 months later than the ulnar physis (44,51). The distal radial and ulnar physes contribute approximately 75% to 80% of the growth of the forearm and 40% of the growth of the upper extremity (Fig. 9-2) (52).

The distal radius articulates with the distal ulna at the DRUJ. Both the radius and ulna articulate with the carpus, serving as the support for the hand. The radial joint surface has three concavities for its articulations: the scaphoid and lunate fossa for the carpus and the sigmoid notch for the ulnar head (Fig. 9-3). These joints are stabilized by a complex series of volar and dorsal radiocarpal, ulnocarpal, and radioulnar ligaments. The volar ligaments are the major stabilizers. Starting radially at the radial styloid, the radial collateral, radioscaphocapitate, radiolunotriquetral (long radioulnate), and radioscapholunate (short radioulnate) ligaments volarly stabilize the radiocarpal joint. The dorsal radioscaphoid and radial triquetral ligaments are less important stabilizers.

The triangular fibrocartilage complex (TFCC) is the primary stabilizer of the ulnocarpal and radioulnar articulations. It extends from the sigmoid notch of the radius across the DRUJ and inserts into the base of the ulnar styloid. It also extends distally as the ulnolunate, ulnotriquetral, and ulnar collateral ligaments and inserts into the ulnar carpus and base of the fifth metacarpal (53). The interosseous ligament of the forearm (Fig. 9-4) helps stabilize the radius and ulna more proximally in the diaphysis of the forearm. The ulna remains relatively immobile as the radius rotates around it. The complex structure of ligaments stabilize the radius, ulna, and carpus through the normal wrist motion of 120 degrees of flexion and extension, 50 degrees of radial and ulnar deviation, and 150 degrees of forearm rotation (53).

The length relationship between the distal radius and ulna is defined as ulnar variance. In adults, this is measured by the relationship of the radial corner of the distal ulnar articular surface to the ulnar corner of the radial articular surface (54). However, measurement of ulnar variance in children requires modifications of this technique. Hafner (55) described measuring from the ulnar metaphysis to the radial metaphysis to lessen the measurement inaccuracies related to epiphyseal size and shape (Fig. 9-5). If the ulna and radius are of equal lengths, there is a neutral variance. If the ulna is longer, there is a positive variance, and if the ulna is shorter, there is a negative variance.

Variance is not dependent on the length of the ulnar styloid (56), but the measurement is dependent on forearm positioning and radiographic technique (57–59). X-rays of the wrist to determine ulnar variance should be standardized with the hand and wrist pronated on the cassette, the elbow flexed 90 degrees, and the shoulder abducted 90 degrees (Fig. 9-6). The importance of ulnar variance relates to the force transmission across the wrist with axial loading. Normally the radiocarpal joint bears approximately 80% of the axial load and the ulnocarpal joint bears 20%. Changes in the length relationship of the radius and

(text continues on page 342)

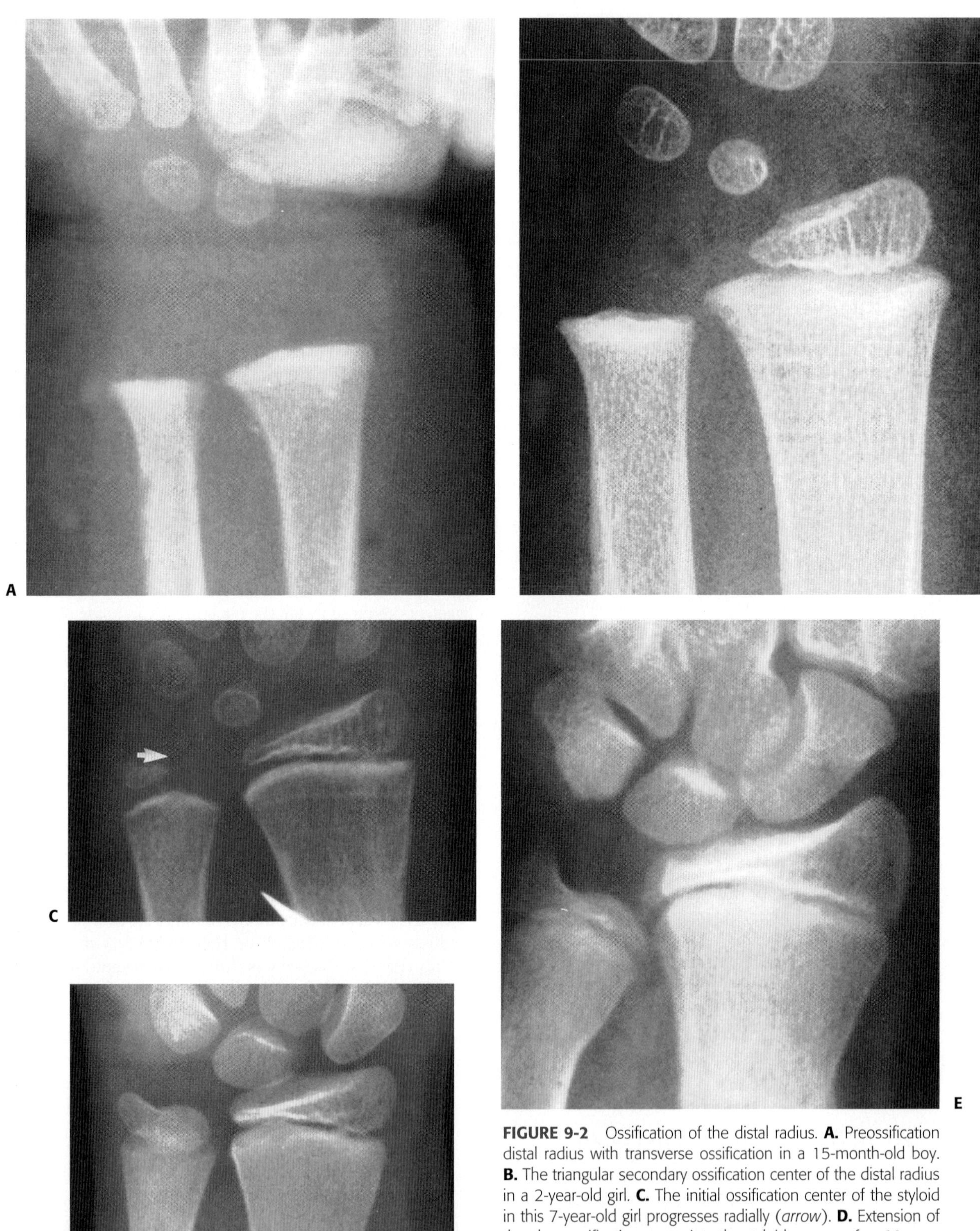

FIGURE 9-2 Ossification of the distal radius. **A.** Preossification distal radius with transverse ossification in a 15-month-old boy. **B.** The triangular secondary ossification center of the distal radius in a 2-year-old girl. **C.** The initial ossification center of the styloid in this 7-year-old girl progresses radially (*arrow*). **D.** Extension of the ulnar ossification center into the styloid process of an 11-year-old. **E.** The styloid is fully ossified and the epiphyses have capped their relative metaphyses in this 13-year-old boy.

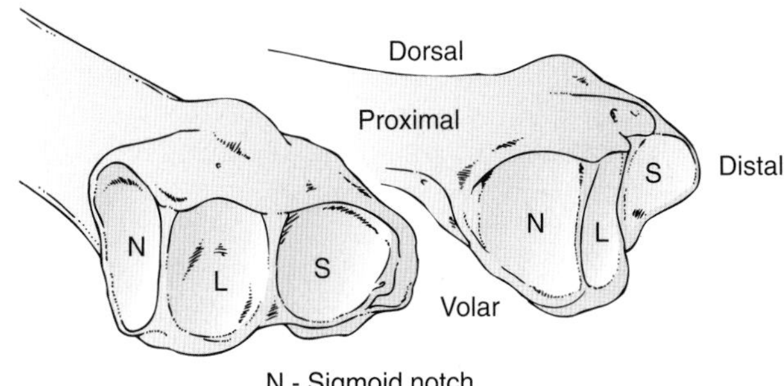

FIGURE 9-3 Articulations of the distal radioulnar joint. (Redrawn from Bowers WH. *Green's operative hand surgery*. New York: Churchill–Livingstone, 1993:988.)

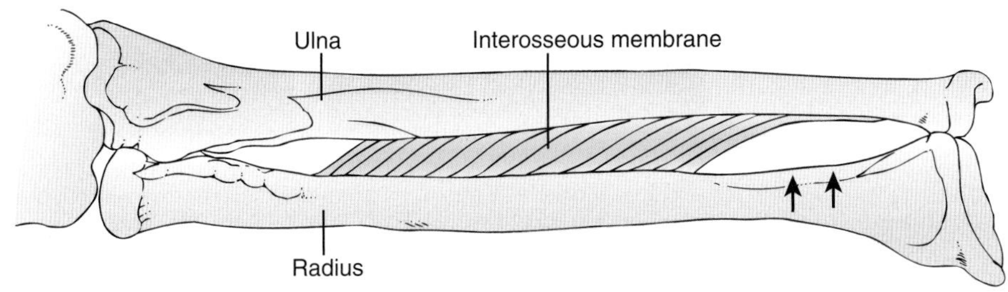

FIGURE 9-4 The attachment and the fibers of the interosseous membrane are such that there is no attachment to the distal radius. (Redrawn from Kraus B, Horne G. Galeazzi fractures. *J Trauma* 1985;25:1094; with permission.)

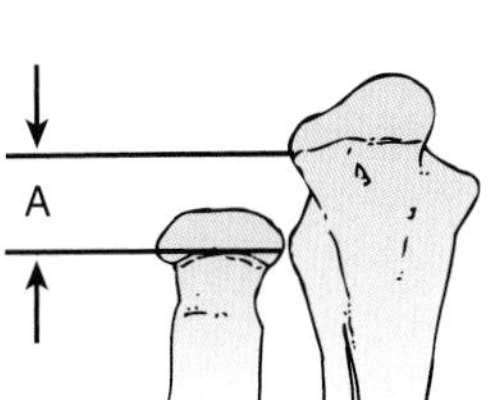

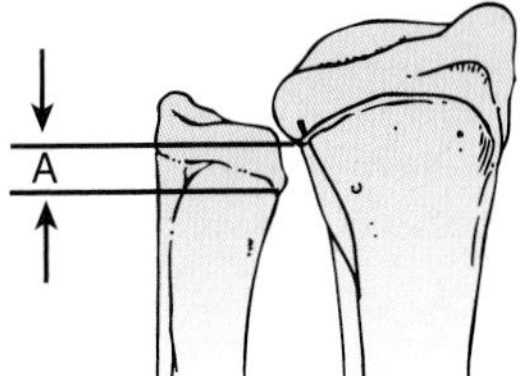

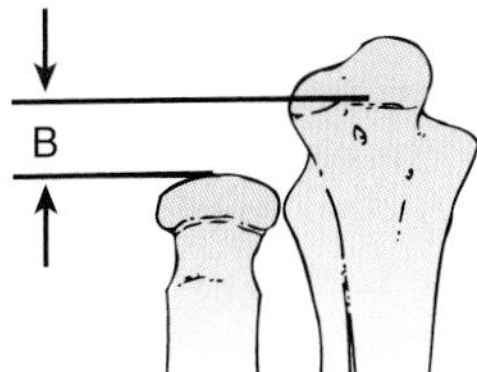

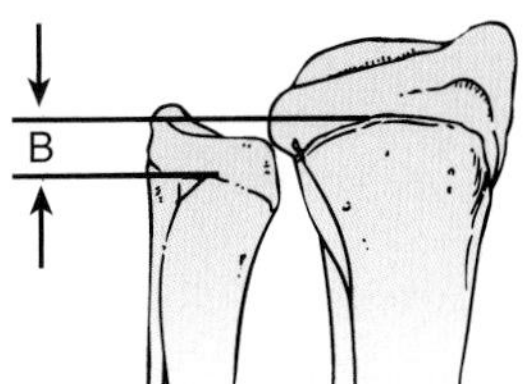

FIGURE 9-5 Hafner's technique to measure ulnar variance. **A.** The distance from the most proximal point of the ulnar metaphysis to the most proximal point of the radial metaphysis. **B.** The distance from the most distal point of the ulnar metaphysis to the most distal point of the radial metaphysis. (From Hafner R, Poznanski AK, Donovan JM. Ulnar variance in children. Standard measurements for evaluation of ulnar shortening in childhood. *Skel Radiol* 1989;18:514; with permission.)

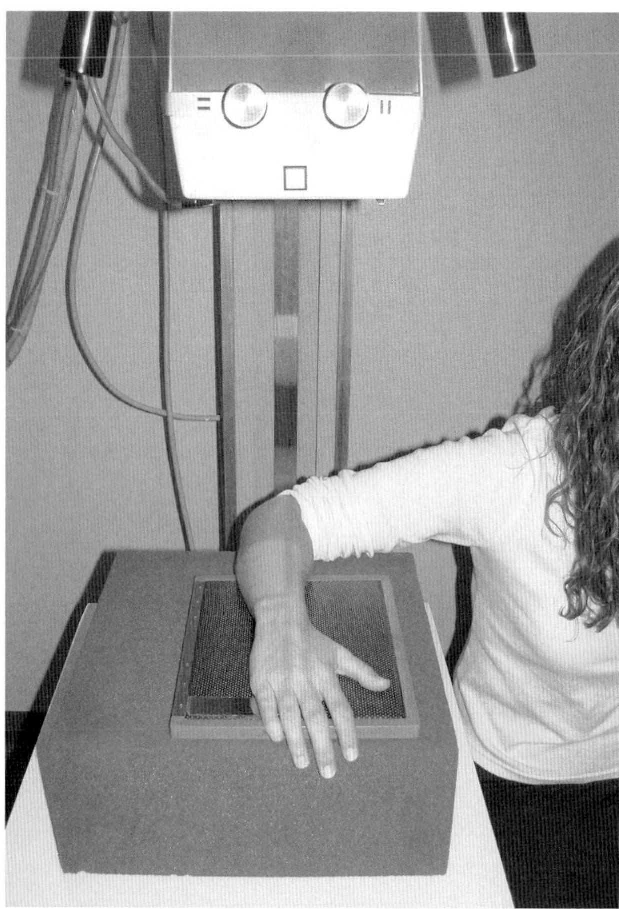

FIGURE 9-6 Technique for neutral rotation x-ray with wrist neutral, forearm pronated, elbow flexed 90 degrees and shoulder abducted 90 degrees.

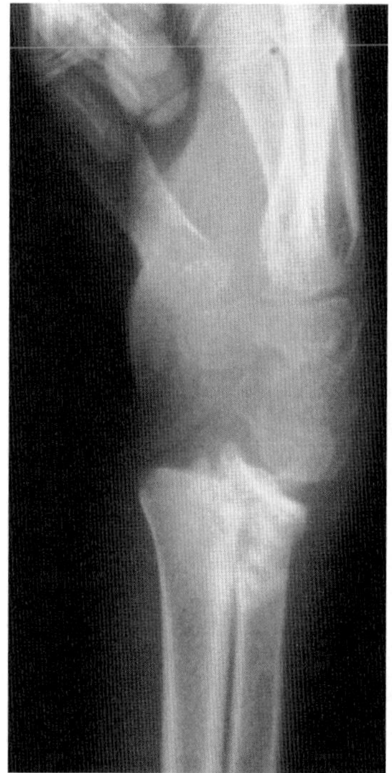

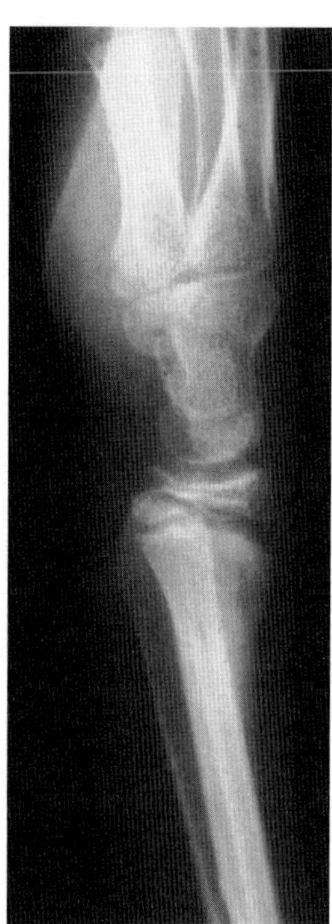

FIGURE 9-7 **A.** A 13-year-old boy presented 1 month after injury with a displaced and healed Salter-Harris type II distal radial fracture with obvious clinical deformity. **B.** Over the next 6 months the patient grew 4 inches and the deformity remodeled without intervention.

ulna alter respective load bearing. Biomechanical and clinical studies have shown that this load distribution is important in fractures, TFCC tears, and Kienbock's disease (26,60,61).

PHYSEAL INJURIES

Distal radial physeal injuries were described more than 100 years ago (62,63), and these early descriptions raised concerns regarding permanent deformity from this injury. In the 1930s, however, Aitken (64,65) concluded from his observations at the Boston City Hospital outpatient clinic that permanent deformity was rare. Instead, he emphasized the remodeling potential of distal radial physeal fractures, even when not reduced. The observations of Aitken have been confirmed throughout the 20th century (Fig. 9-7). Most researchers agree that as long as there is sufficient growth remaining, a distal radial extension deformity from a fracture malunited in extension has the potential to remodel. Permanent deformity, however, can occur in malunited fractures near the end of growth, with rotational deformity, or fractures that cause distal radial growth arrest.

Diagnosis

Distal radial physeal fractures are far more common than distal ulnar physeal fractures (2,29,66–68). The nondominant arm in boys is most commonly injured. The peak incidence is in the preadolescent growth spurt (2,6,69). More than 50% of distal radial physeal fractures have an associated ulnar fracture. This usually is an ulnar styloid fracture but can be a distal ulnar plastic deformation, greenstick, or complete fracture (70–72). The mechanism of injury generally is a fall on an outstretched hand and wrist. Many of the injuries are nondisplaced and present only with pain at the physis (73,74). With displaced fractures, the distal fragment usually moves dorsally, creating an extension deformity that is usually clinically apparent. Patients have pain and tenderness at the fracture site, and the range of motion at the wrist and hand usually is limited by pain. Neurovascular compromise is uncommon but can occur (31). When present, it usually consists of median nerve irritability or dysfunction caused by direct trauma to the nerve at the time of injury or ongoing ischemic compression from the displaced fracture. Thenar muscle function and discriminatory sensibility (two-point discrimination) should be tested before reduction in the emergency setting. Acute carpal tunnel syndrome or forearm compartment syndrome can occur, but more often is caused by marked volar forearm and wrist swelling that occurs after reduction and application of a well-molded, tight cast

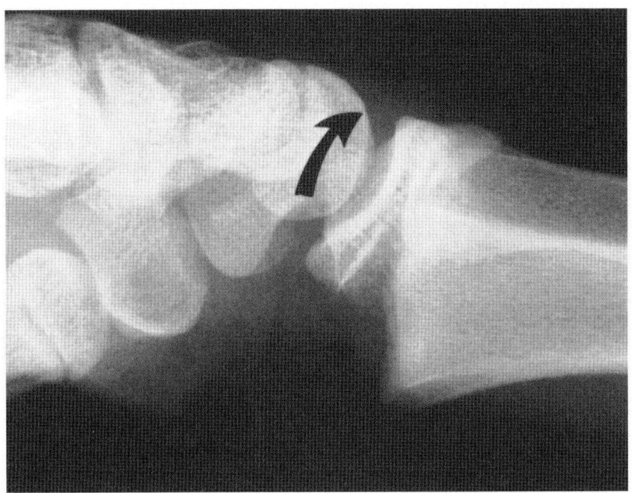

FIGURE 9-8 Dorsally displaced physeal fracture (type A). The distal epiphysis with a small metaphyseal fragment is displaced dorsally (*curved arrow*) in relation to the proximal metaphyseal fragment.

(31,75,76). Open physeal fractures are rare, but the local skin should be examined closely for penetration.

Plain AP and lateral x-rays are diagnostic of the fracture type and deformity. The Salter-Harris system is the basis for classification of physeal fractures (35). Most are Salter-Harris type II fractures. The dorsal displacement of the distal fragment of the epiphysis and dorsal Thurstond-Holland metaphyseal fragment is evident on the lateral view (Fig. 9-8). Salter-Harris type I fractures also usually displace dorsally. Volar displacement of either a Salter-Harris type I or II fracture is less common (Fig. 9-9). Nondisplaced Salter-Harris type I fractures may be indicated only by a displaced pronator fat pad sign (Fig. 9-10) (77,78) or tenderness over the involved physis (70,79). A scaphoid fat pad sign may indicate a scaphoid fracture (Fig. 9-11). If the acute fracture is unrecognized, a late-appearing periosteal reaction may indicate the fracture.

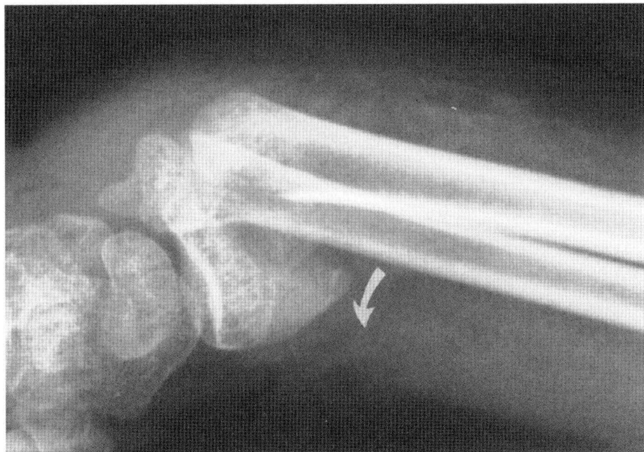

FIGURE 9-9 Volarly displaced physeal fracture (type B). Distal epiphysis with a large volar metaphyseal fragment is displaced in a volar direction (*curved arrow*). (Reprinted from Wilkins KE, ed. *Operative management of upper extremity fractures in children.* Rosemont, IL: American Academy of Orthopaedic Surgeons, 1994:21; with permission.)

Salter-Harris type III fractures are rare and may be caused by a compression injury or an avulsion of the radial origin of the volar radiocarpal ligaments (Fig. 9-12) (71,80). Triplane equivalent fractures (81–83), a combination of Salter-Harris type II and III fractures in different planes, are rare. CT scans may be necessary to define the fracture pattern and degree of intra-articular displacement. Stress injuries to the physis occur most commonly in competitive gymnasts (Fig. 9-13).

Current Treatment Options

Treatment options include no reduction, closed reduction and cast immobilization, closed reduction and pin fixation, and open reduction. Nondisplaced fractures are immobilized until appropriate healing and pain resolution have been achieved (70,79). If there is a question of fracture stability, these fractures should be treated with a well-molded cast and monitored closely during the first 3 weeks of healing to be certain that there is no loss of alignment. Most acute displaced Salter-Harris type I and II fractures can be treated successfully with gentle closed reduction and cast immobilization. There are advocates for both long-arm and short-arm treatment methods (84–90). Closed reduction and percutaneous pin fixation are performed in patients with neurovascular compromise and displaced physeal fractures (31) to lessen the risk of development of a compartment syndrome in the carpal tunnel or forearm. Open reduction is indicated for irreducible fractures, open fractures, displaced Salter-Harris type III and IV fractures, and triplane equivalent fractures. Irreducible fractures usually are due to an entrapped periosteum or pronator quadratus (91). Internal fixation usually is with smooth, small diameter pins to lessen the risk of growth arrest. Plates and screws rarely are used unless the patient is near skeletal maturity because of concerns about further physeal injury. In the rare displaced intra-articular Salter-Harris type III or IV fracture, internal fixation can be intra-epiphyseal without violating the physis. If it is necessary to cross the physis, then smooth, small diameter pins should be used to lessen the risk of iatrogenic physeal injury. Extra-articular external fixation also can be used to stabilize and align the fracture.

Closed Reduction

Most displaced Salter-Harris I and II fractures are treated with closed reduction and cast stabilization. Closed manipulation of the displaced fracture is performed with appropriate conscious sedation, analgesia, or rarely, anesthesia to achieve pain relief and an atraumatic reduction (70,79,92). Most of these fractures involve dorsal and proximal displacement of the epiphysis with an apex–volar extension deformity. Manipulative reduction is by gentle distraction and flexion of the distal epiphysis, carpus,

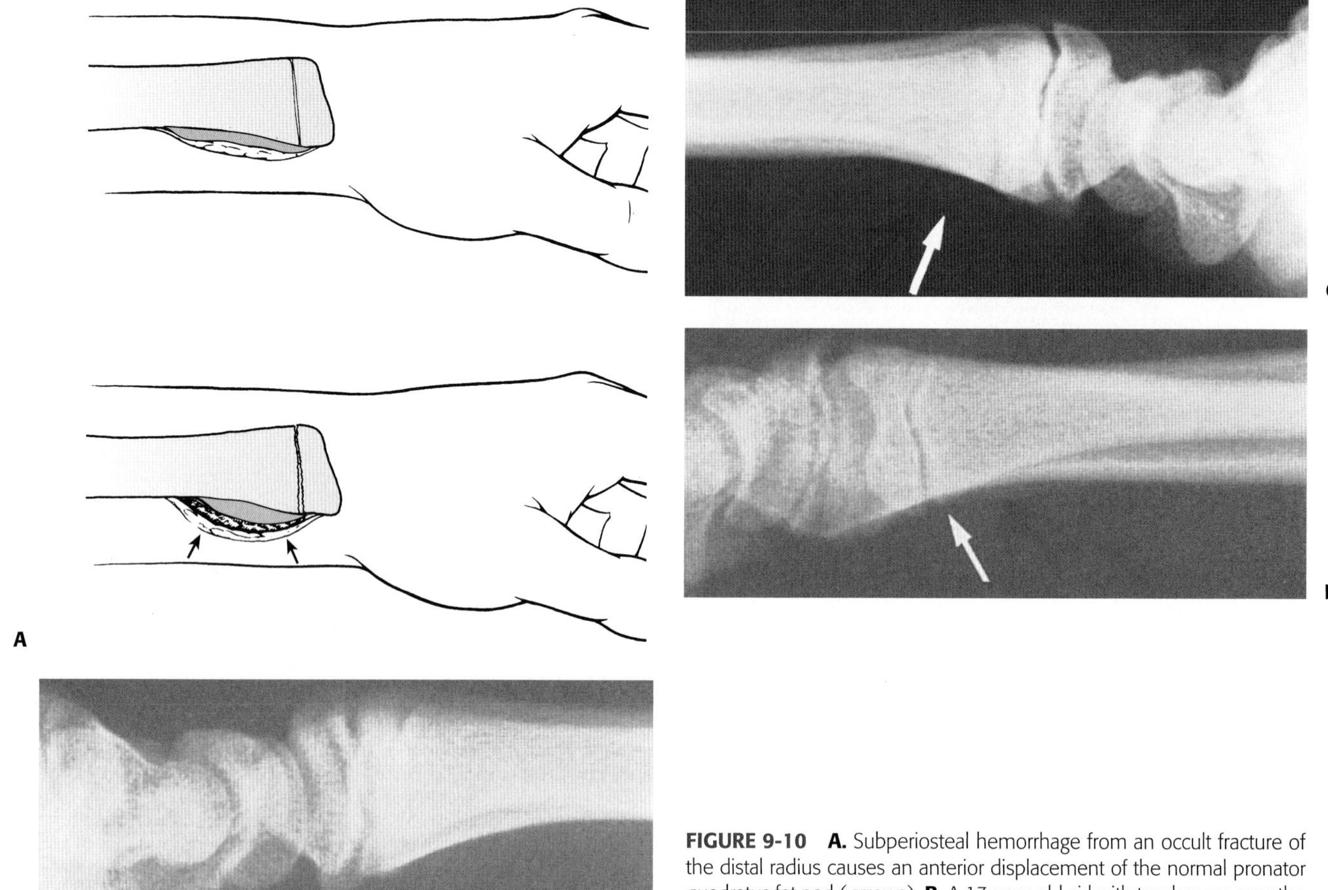

FIGURE 9-10 **A.** Subperiosteal hemorrhage from an occult fracture of the distal radius causes an anterior displacement of the normal pronator quadratus fat pad (*arrows*). **B.** A 13-year-old girl with tenderness over the distal radius after a fall. The only x-ray finding is an anterior displacement of the normal pronator quadratus fat pad (*arrow*). **C.** The opposite normal side (*arrow indicates normal fat pad*). **D.** Two weeks later, there is a small area of periosteal new bone formation (*arrow*) anteriorly, substantiating that bony injury has occurred.

and hand over the proximal metaphysis (Figs. 9-14 and 9-15). The intact dorsal periosteum is used as a tension band to aid in reduction and stabilization of the fracture. Unlike similar fractures in adults, finger trap distraction with pulley weights is often counterproductive. However, finger traps can help stabilize the hand, wrist, and arm for manipulative reduction and casting by applying a few pounds of weight for balance. Otherwise an assistant is helpful to support the extremity in the proper position for casting.

If portable fluoroscopy is available, immediate radiographic assessment of the reduction is obtained. Otherwise, a well-molded cast is applied and AP and lateral x-rays are obtained to assess the reduction. The cast should provide three-point molding over the distal radius to lessen the risk of fracture displacement and should follow the contour of the normal forearm. The distal dorsal mold should not impair venous outflow from the hand, which can occur if the mold is placed too distal and too deep so as to obstruct the dorsal veins. Advocates of short-arm casting (89,90) indicate at least equivalent results with proper casting techniques. Instructions for elevation and close monitoring of swelling and the neurovascular status of the extremity are critical.

The fracture also should be monitored closely with serial x-rays for the first 3 weeks to be certain that there is no loss of anatomic alignment (Fig. 9-16). Generally these fractures are stable after closed reduction and cast immobilization. If there is loss of reduction after 7 days, the surgeon should be wary of repeat reduction because of the risk of physeal arrest (35,70). Fortunately, remodeling of an extension deformity with growth is common if the patient has more than 2 years of growth remaining and the deformity is less than 20 degrees.

Closed Reduction and Percutaneous Pinning

The indications for percutaneous pinning of distal radial physeal fractures are still controversial. The best indication is a displaced

(text continues on page 349)

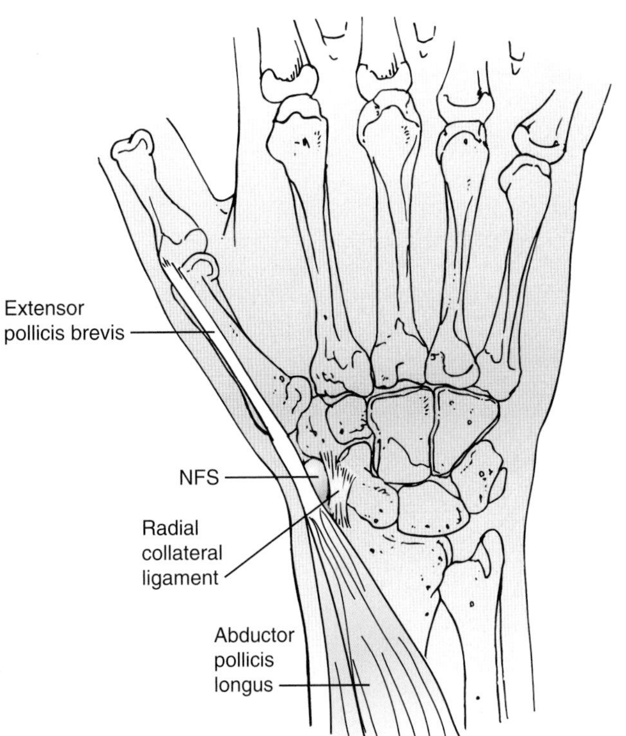

FIGURE 9-11 Anatomic relationships of the navicular fat stripe (*NFS*). The NFS, shaded black, is located between the combined tendons of the abductor pollicis longus and extensor pollicis brevis, and the lateral surface of the carpal navicular. (Reprinted from Terry DW, Ramen JE. The navicular fat stripe. *Ham J Roent Rad Ther Nucl Med* 1975;124:25; with permission.)

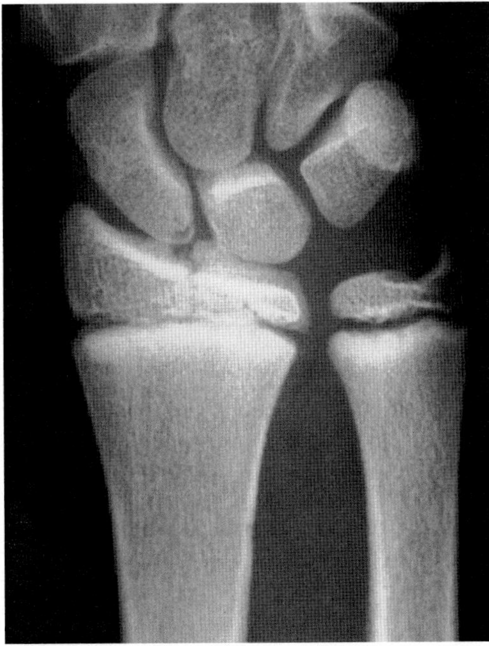

FIGURE 9-12 Anteroposterior x-ray of Salter-Harris type III fracture of the distal radius.

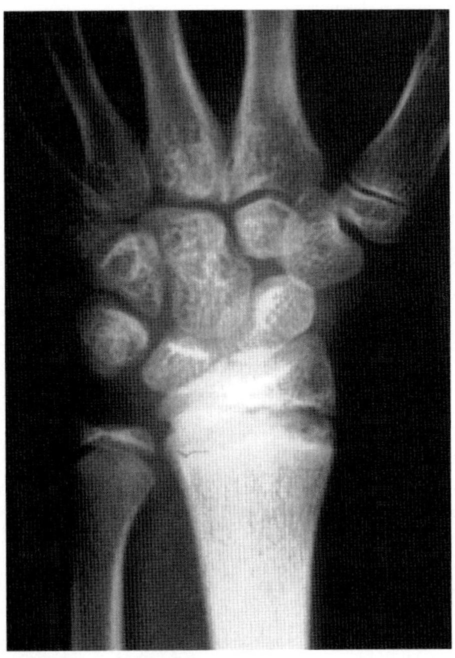

FIGURE 9-13 Stress changes in a female gymnast with widening of the distal radial physis from long-standing high-level performance.

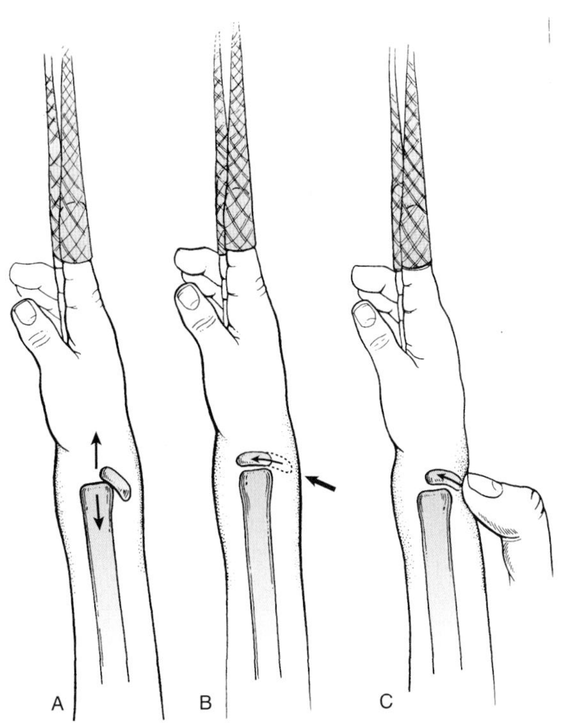

FIGURE 9-14 Acceptable method of closed reduction of distal physeal fractures of the radius. **A.** Position of the fracture fragments as finger trap traction with countertraction is applied (*arrows*). **B.** Often with traction alone the fracture will reduce without external pressure (*arrows*). **C.** If the reduction is incomplete, simply applying direct pressure over the fracture site in a distal and volar direction with the thumb often completes the reduction while maintaining traction. This technique theoretically decreases the shear forces across the physis during the reduction process.

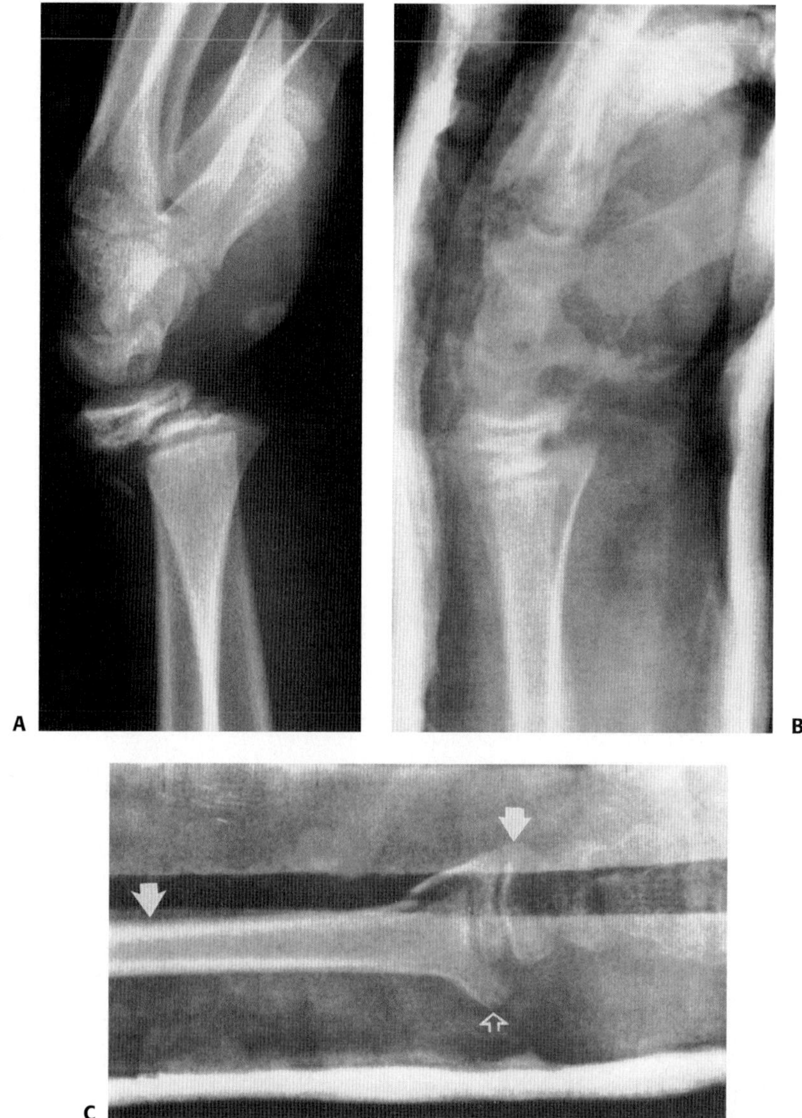

FIGURE 9-15 **A.** Lateral x-ray of dorsally displaced Salter-Harris type II fracture. **B.** Lateral x-ray after closed reduction and cast application. **C.** Reduction of the volar displaced fracture shown in Figure 9-9. The forearm was in supination with three-point molding anterior over the distal epiphysis and proximal shaft (*white arrows*). The third point is placed dorsally over the distal metaphysis (*open arrow*). (The dorsal surface of the cast is oriented toward the bottom of this figure.) (Reprinted from Wilkins KE, ed. *Operative management of upper extremity fractures in children.* Rosemont, IL: American Academy of Orthopaedic Surgeons, 1994:17; with permission.)

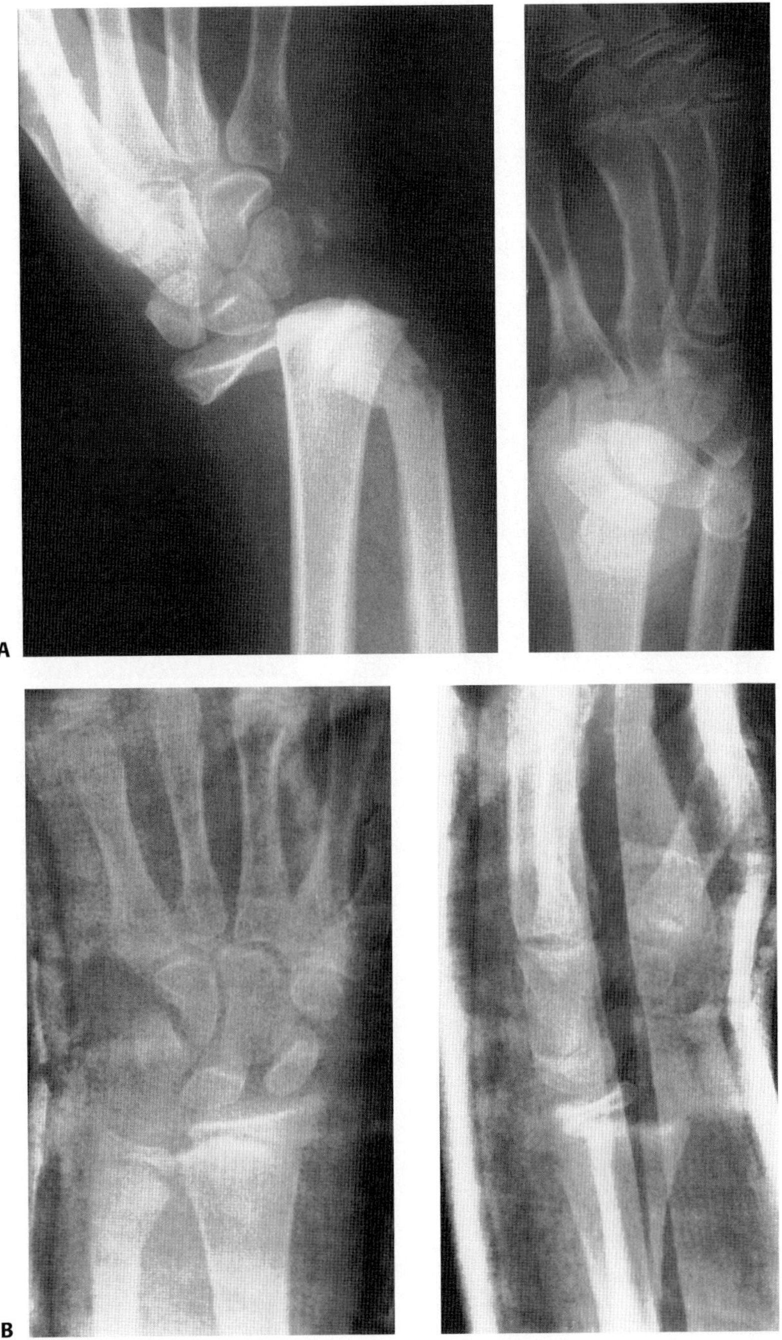

FIGURE 9-16 **A.** Anteroposterior and lateral x-rays of severely displaced Salter-Harris type II fracture of the distal radius. **B.** Closed reduction shows marked improvement but not anatomic reduction. The cast had to be bivalved due to excessive swelling. (*continues*)

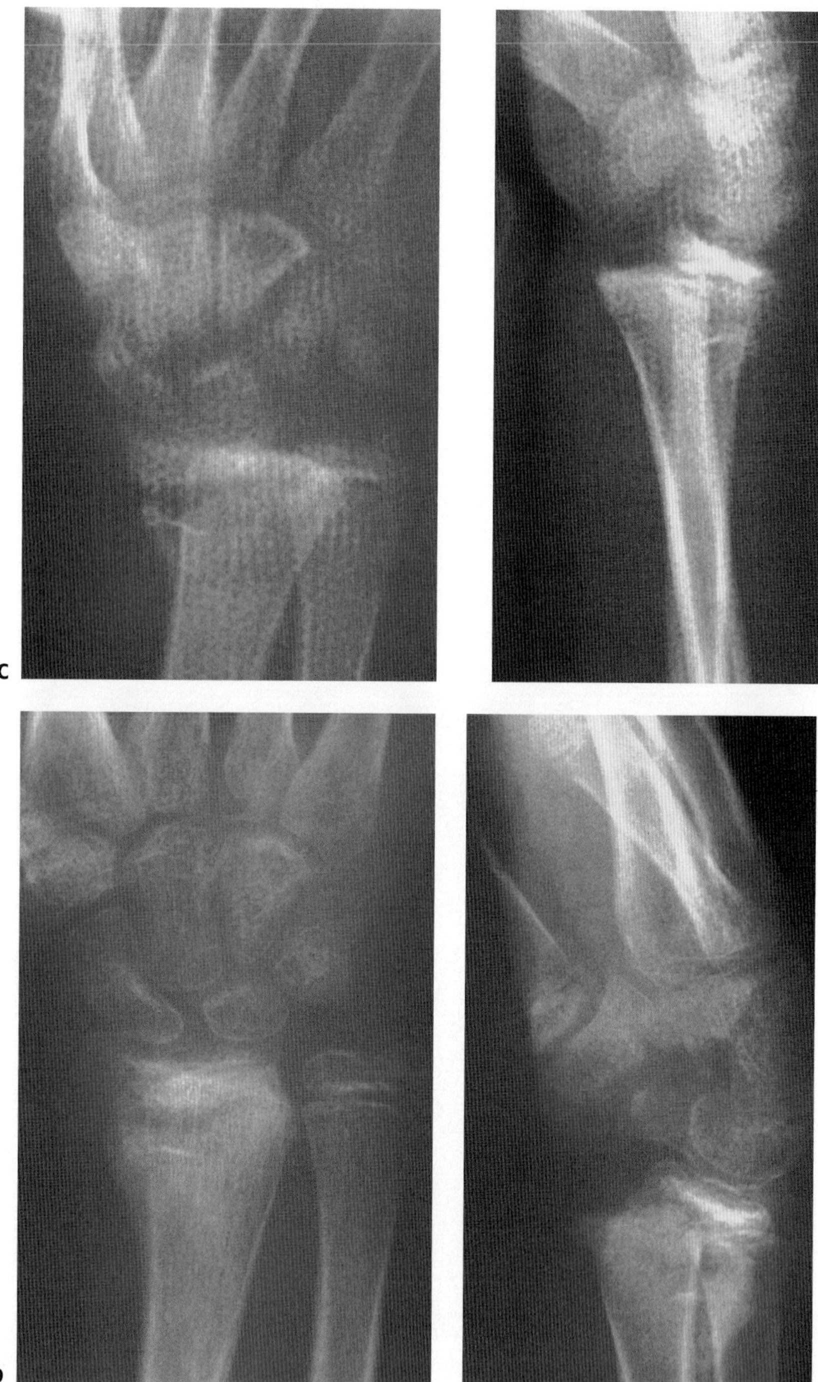

FIGURE 9-16 (*continued*) **C.** Unfortunately, the patient lost reduction after a new fiberglass cast was applied. **D.** Out of cast x-rays show a healed malunion in a similar position to the prereduction x-rays.

radial physeal fracture with median neuropathy and significant volar soft-tissue swelling (31) (Fig. 9-17). These patients are at risk for development of an acute carpal tunnel syndrome or forearm compartment syndrome with closed reduction and well-molded cast immobilization (31,75,76,93). The torn periosteum volarly allows the fracture bleeding to dissect into the volar forearm compartments and carpal tunnel. If a tight cast is applied with a volar mold over that area, compartment pressures can increase dangerously. Percutaneous pin fixation allows the application of a loose dressing, splint, or cast without the risk of loss of fracture reduction.

Pin fixation can be either single or double (Fig. 9-18). Fluoroscopy is used to guide proper fracture reduction and pin placement. Anesthesia is used for adequate pain relief and to lessen the risk of further physeal injury. The fracture is manipulated into anatomic alignment and the initial, and often only, pin is placed from the distal epiphysis of the radial styloid obliquely across the physis into the more proximal ulnar aspect of the radial metaphysis (Fig. 9-19). A sufficient skin incision should be made with pin placement to be certain there is no iatrogenic injury to the radial sensory nerve or extensor tendons. Stability of the fracture should be evaluated with flexion and extension and rotatory stress under fluoroscopy. Often in children and adolescents, a single pin and the reduced periosteum provide sufficient stability to prevent redisplacement of the fracture. If fracture stability is questionable with a single pin, a second pin should be placed. The second pin can either parallel the first pin or, to create cross-pin stability, can be placed distally from the ulnar corner of the radial epiphysis between the fourth and fifth dorsal compartments and passed obliquely to the proximal radial portion of the metaphysis (53,84,94). Again, the skin incisions for pin placement should be sufficient to avoid iatrogenic injury to the extensor tendons.

The pins are bent, left out of the skin, and covered with a sterile dressing. Splint or cast immobilization is used but does not need to be tight because fracture stability is provided by the pins. The pins are left in until there is adequate fracture healing, usually 4 weeks. The pins can be removed in the office without sedation or anesthesia.

One of the arguments against pin fixation is the risk of additional injury to the physis by a pin (36). The risk of physeal arrest is more from the displaced fracture than from a short-term, smooth pin. As a precaution, smooth, small-diameter pins should be used, insertion should be as atraumatic as possible, and removal should be done as soon as there is sufficient fracture healing for fracture stability in a cast or splint alone.

(text continues on page 352)

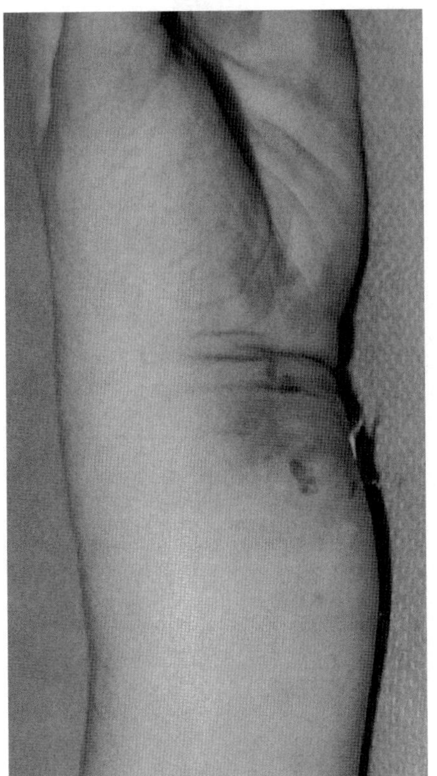
A

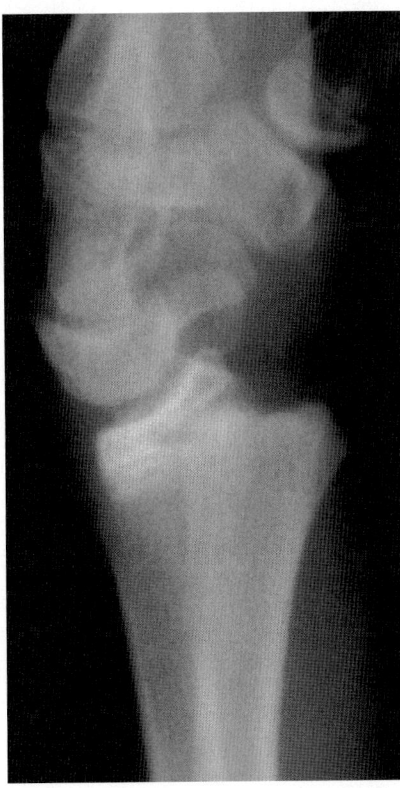
B

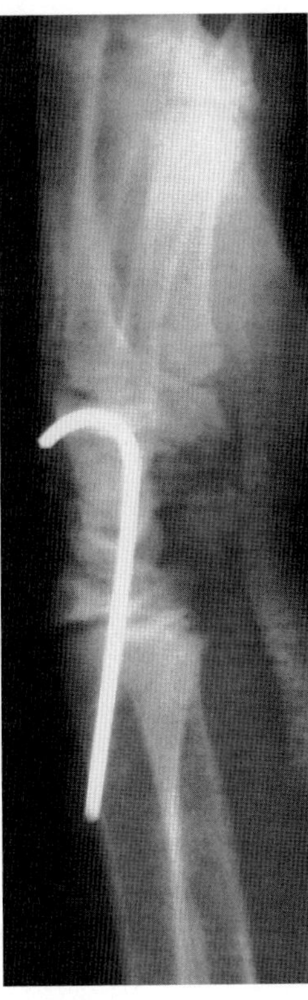
C

FIGURE 9-17 **A.** Clinical photograph of patient with a displaced Salter-Harris type II fracture of the distal radius. The patient has marked swelling volarly with hematoma and fracture displacement. The patient had a median neuropathy upon presentation. **B.** Lateral x-ray of the displaced fracture. **C.** Lateral x-ray in postoperative splint after percutaneous pinning to lessen the risk of neurovascular compromise in a cast.

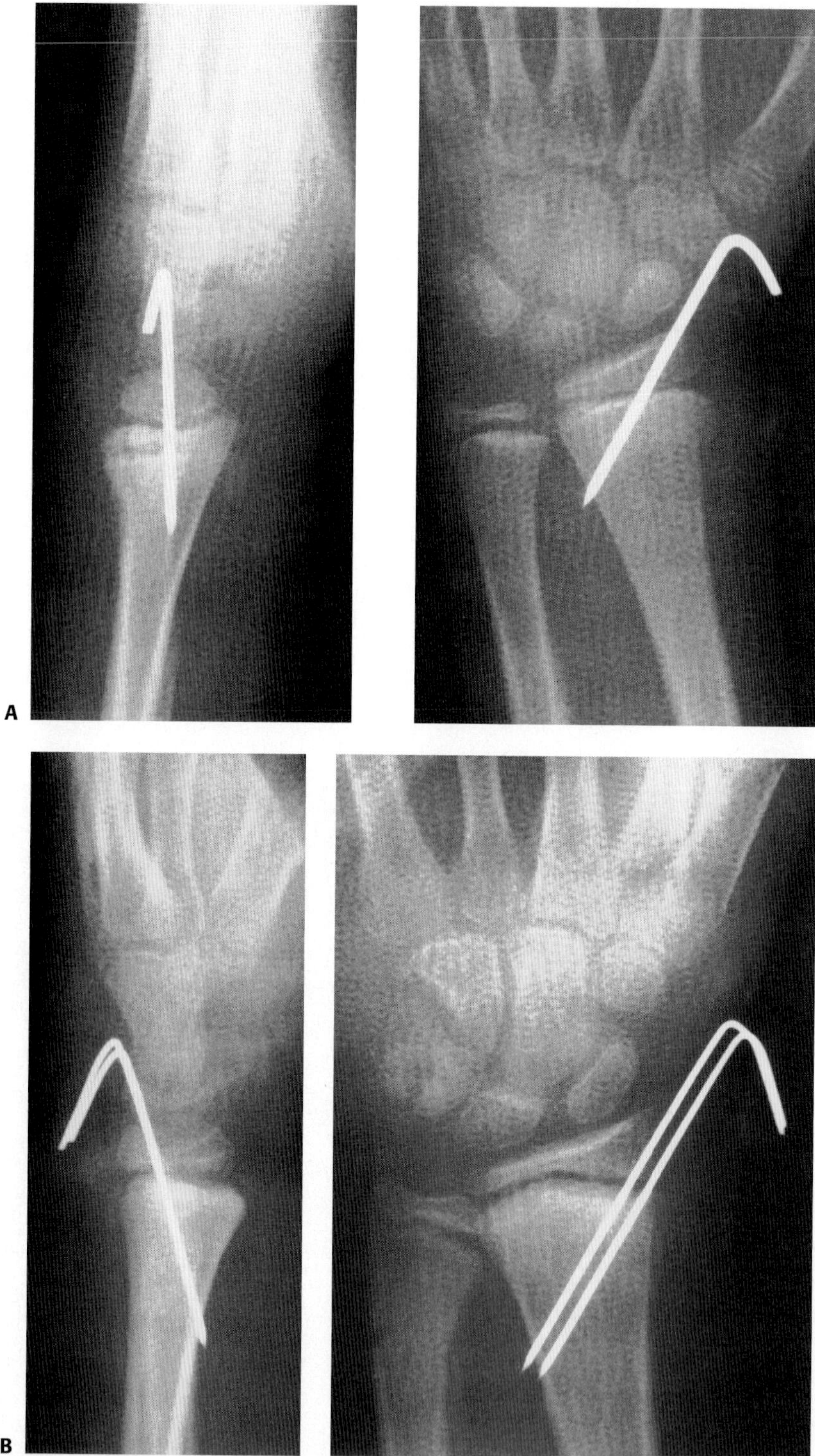

FIGURE 9-18 **A.** Anteroposterior and lateral x-rays of displaced Salter-Harris type II fracture pinned with a single pin. **B.** After reduction and pinning with parallel pins.

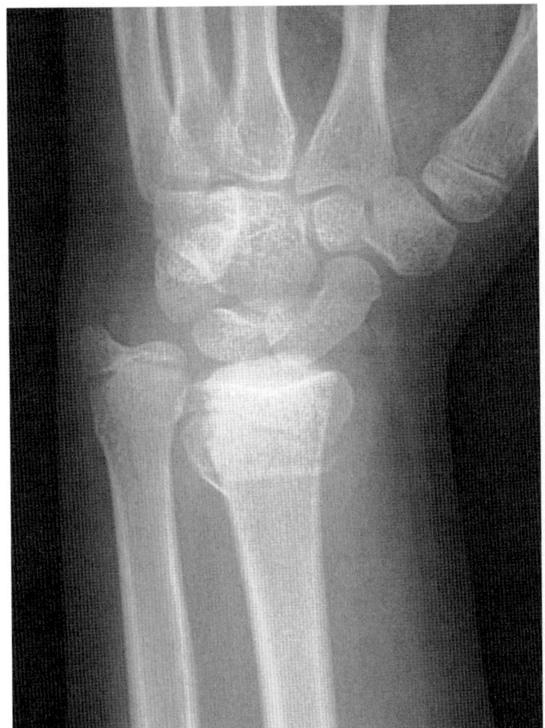

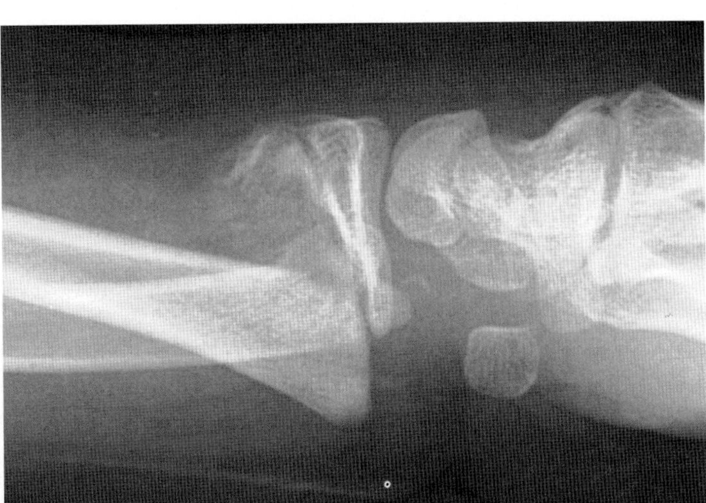

A

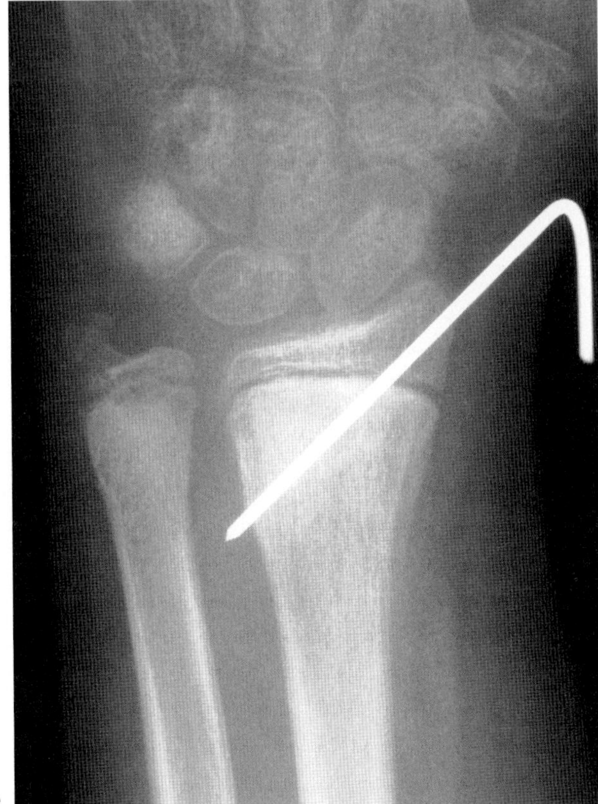

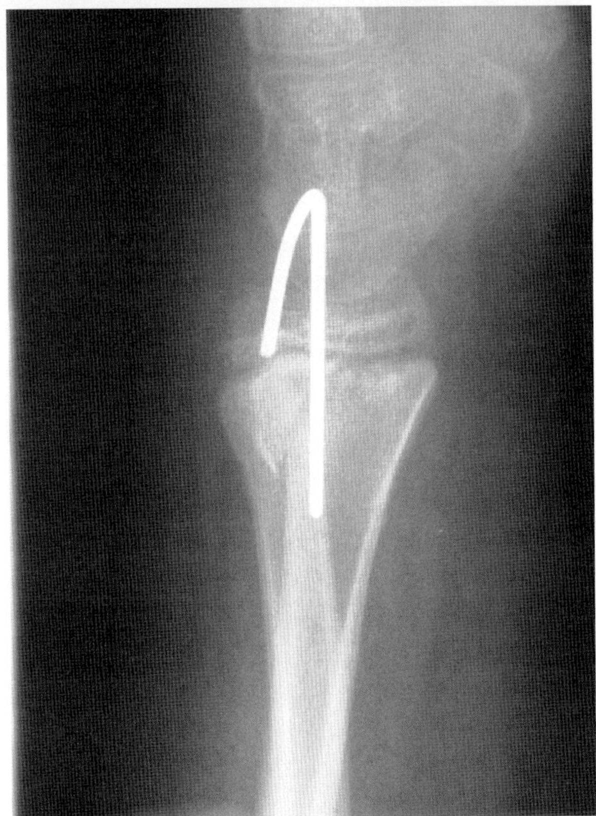

B

FIGURE 9-19 **A.** AP and lateral displaced SH II distal radius. **B.** AP and lateral views 1 month post simple pin fixation of SH II radial physeal fracture.

Open Reduction

The main indication for open reduction of a displaced distal radial Salter-Harris type II physeal fracture is irreducibility. Most often this is caused by interposed periosteum or, less likely, pronator quadratus (91,95,96). Open reduction is done through a volar approach to the distal radial physis. The interval between the radial artery and the flexor carpi radialis is used. This dissection also can proceed directly through the flexor carpi radialis sheath to protect the artery. The pronator quadratus is isolated and elevated from radial to ulnar. Although this muscle can be interposed in the fracture site, the volar periosteum is more commonly interposed. This is only evident after elevation of the pronator quadratus. The periosteum is extracted from the physis with care to minimize further injury to the physis. The fracture can then be easily reduced. Usually a percutaneous smooth pin is used for stabilization of the reduction. The method of pin insertion is the same as after closed reduction.

Open physeal fractures are rare but require irrigation and debridement. Care should be taken with mechanical debridement of the physeal cartilage to avoid further risk of growth arrest. Cultures should be taken at the time of operative debride-

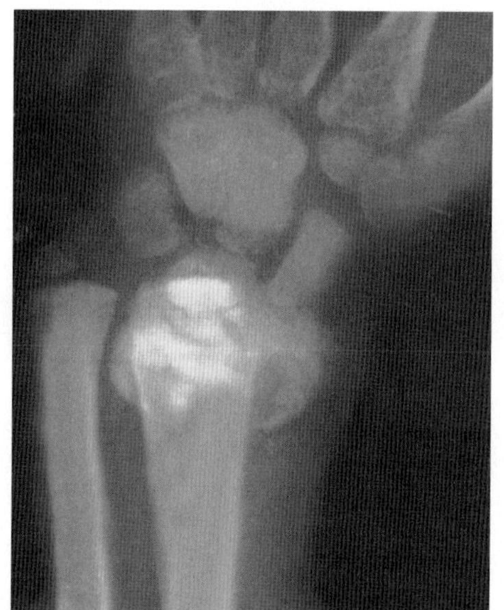

A

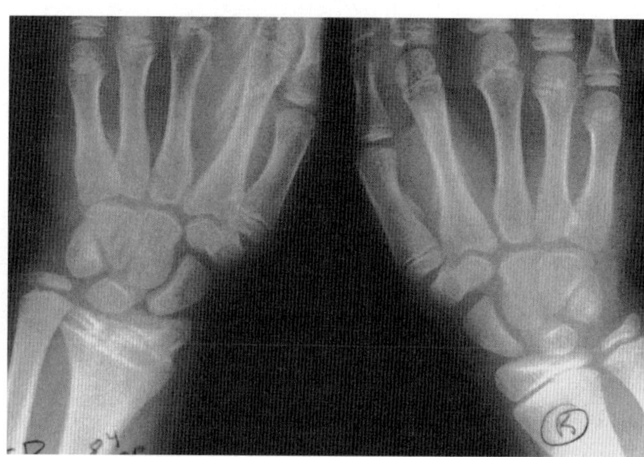

C

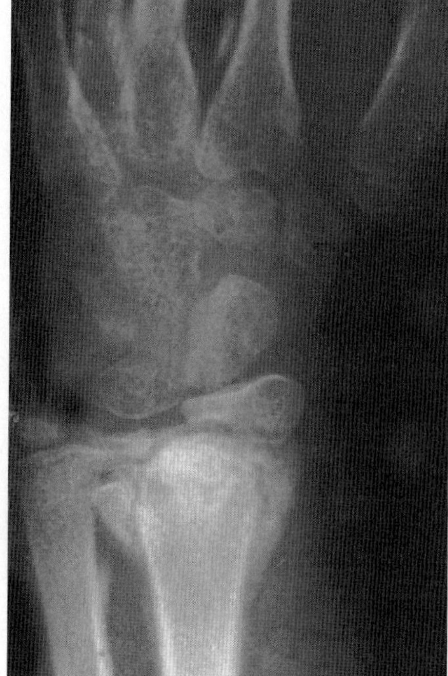

B

FIGURE 9-20 A. A markedly displaced Salter-Harris type IV fracture of the distal radius in an 11-year-old boy who fell from a horse. **B.** X-ray taken 3 weeks after closed reduction demonstrates displacement of the comminuted fragments. **C.** Eighteen months after injury, there was 15 mm of radial shortening, and the patient had a pronounced radial deviation deformity of the wrist.

ment, and appropriate antibiotics are used to lessen the risk of deep space infection.

The rare Salter-Harris type III or IV fracture or triplane fracture (83) may require open reduction if the joint or physis cannot be anatomically reduced closed. The articular and physeal alignment can be evaluated by radiographic tomograms (trispiral or CT), MRI scans, or wrist arthroscopy. If anatomic alignment of the physis and articular surface is not present, the risk of growth arrest, long-term deformity, or limited function is great (Fig. 9-20). Even minimal displacement (more than 1 mm) should not be accepted in this situation. Arthroscopically assisted reduction is helpful to align and stabilize these rare physeal fractures (97,98). Although it is an equipment intensive operation with arthroscopy, external fixation, transphyseal and trans-epiphyseal pin or screw fixation, and fluoroscopy, anatomic reduction and stabilization of the physis and articular surface can be achieved (Fig. 9-21).

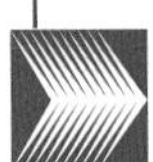

AUTHORS' PREFERRED METHOD OF TREATMENT

Physeal Injuries

Most Salter-Harris type I and II fractures are reduced closed under conscious sedation with the assistance of portable fluoroscopy. A long-arm cast with appropriate three-point molding is applied. This is changed to a short-arm cast when there is sufficient healing for fracture stability, usually after 3 to 4 weeks. Cast immobilization is discontinued when there is clinical and radiographic evidence of fracture healing, generally 4 to 6 weeks after fracture. Range-of-motion and strengthening exercises are begun with a home program. When the child achieves full motion and strength, he or she can return to full activity, including competitive sports. Follow-up x-rays are obtained at 6 to 12 months after fracture to be certain there is no growth arrest.

A patient with a displaced Salter-Harris type I or II physeal fracture associated with significant soft-tissue swelling volarly, median neuropathy, or ipsilateral elbow and radial fractures is treated with closed reduction and percutaneous pinning (Fig. 9-22). This avoids the increased risk of compartment syndrome in the carpal canal or volar forearm that is present if a well-molded, tight cast is applied. In addition, acute percutaneous pinning of the fracture prevents increased swelling, cast splitting, loss of reduction, and concerns about malunion or growth arrest with repeat reduction. Acute pinning of the fracture with one or two smooth pins through the radial epiphysis provides fracture stability without a compressive cast. The risk of growth arrest from a narrow-diameter, smooth pin left in place for 3 to 4 weeks is exceedingly small.

Open reduction is reserved for irreducible Salter-Harris type I and II fractures, open fractures, fractures with associ-

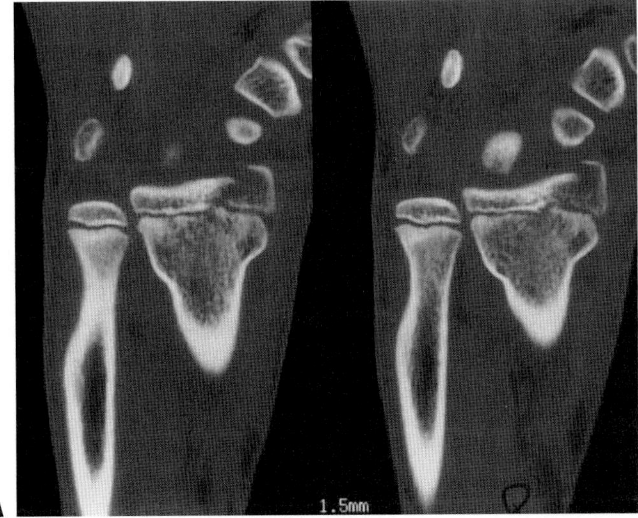

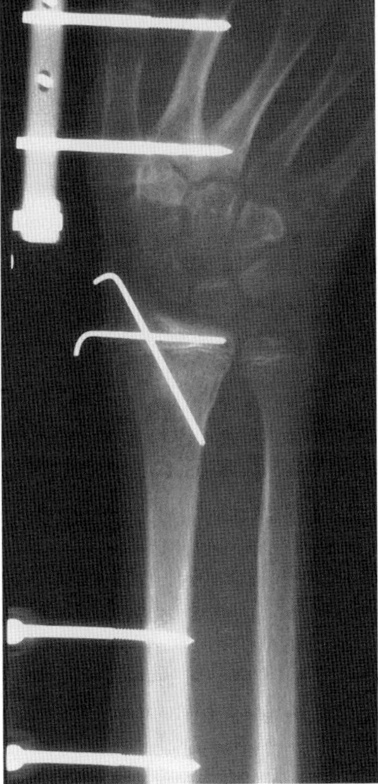

FIGURE 9-21 **A.** Computed tomography scan of displaced Salter-Harris type IV fracture. **B.** Surgical correction included external fixation distraction, arthroscopically assisted reduction, and smooth pin fixation.

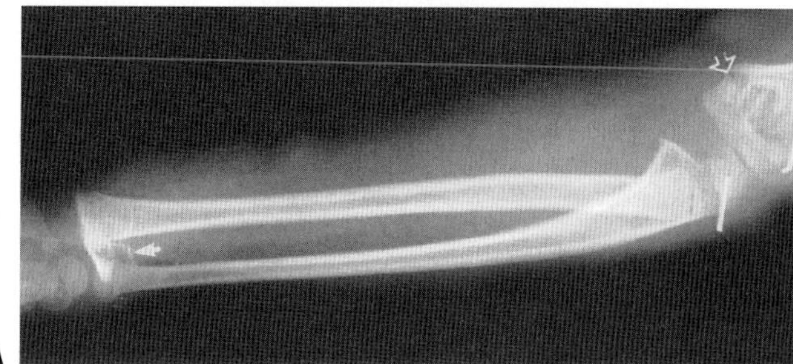

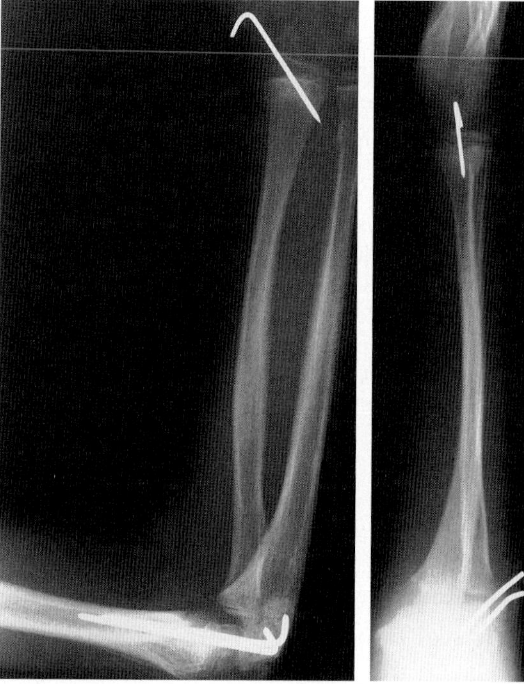

FIGURE 9-22 **A.** Ipsilateral distal radial physeal and supracondylar fractures. This 6-year-old sustained both a dorsally displaced distal radial physeal fracture (*closed arrow*) and a type II displaced supracondylar fracture of the humerus (*open arrows*). **B.** Similar case treated with percutaneous pinning of radial physeal fracture and supracondylar humeral fracture.

ated acute carpal tunnel or forearm compartment syndrome, displaced (more than 1 mm) Salter-Harris type III or IV fractures, or triplane equivalent fractures. For an irreducible Salter-Harris type I or II fracture, exposure is from the side of the torn periosteum. Because these fractures usually are displaced dorsally, a volar exposure is used. Smooth pins are used for stabilization and are left in for 3 to 4 weeks. Open fractures are exposed through the open wound with proximal and distal extension for adequate debridement. All open debridements are performed in the operating room under general anesthesia. Acute compartment syndromes are treated with immediate release of the transverse carpal ligament or forearm fascia. The transverse carpal ligament is released in a Z-plasty fashion to lengthen the ligament and prevent volar bowstringing and scarring of the median nerve against the palmar skin. Displaced intra-articular fractures are best treated with arthroscopically assisted reduction and fixation. Distraction across the joint can be achieved with application of an external fixator or finger traps. Standard dorsal portals (3/4 and 4/5) are used for viewing the intra-articular aspect of the fracture and alignment of the reduction (97,99). In addition, direct observation through the arthroscope can aid in safe placement of the intraepiphyseal pins (98,100). Fluoroscopy is used to evaluate the extra-articular aspects of the fracture (triplane equivalent and type IV fractures), the reduction, and placement of fixation pins.

Complications

Malunion. Complications from physeal fractures are relatively rare. The most frequent problem is malunion. Fortunately, these fractures often occur in children with significant growth remaining. The deformity from a Salter-Harris type I or II fracture is within the plane of motion of the wrist joint and, therefore, will remodel with ensuing growth (Fig. 9-23) (70,79,92). Repeat reduction should not be done more than 7 days after fracture because of the risk of growth arrest. The malunited fracture should be monitored over the next 6 to 12 months for remodeling. If the fracture does not remodel, persistent extension deformity of the distal radial articular surface puts the patient at risk for developing mid-carpal instability (101) or degenerative arthritis of the wrist. Corrective osteotomy with bone grafting and internal fixation is required (102). An opening-wedge dorsal osteotomy is made, iliac crest bone of appropriate trapezoidal shape to correct the deformity is inserted, and either a plate or external fixator is used to maintain correction until healing.

Intra-articular malunion is more worrisome because of the risk of development of degenerative arthritis if the articular stepoff is more than 2 mm (103). MRI or CT scans can be useful in preoperative evaluations. Arthroscopy allows direct examination of the deformity and areas of impingement or potential degeneration. Intra-articular osteotomy with bone grafting in the metaphysis to support the reconstructed articular surface is controversial and risky. However, it has the potential of restoring anatomic alignment to the joint and preventing serious long-term complications. This problem fortunately is uncommon in children because of the rarity of the injury and this type of malunion.

(text continues on page 357)

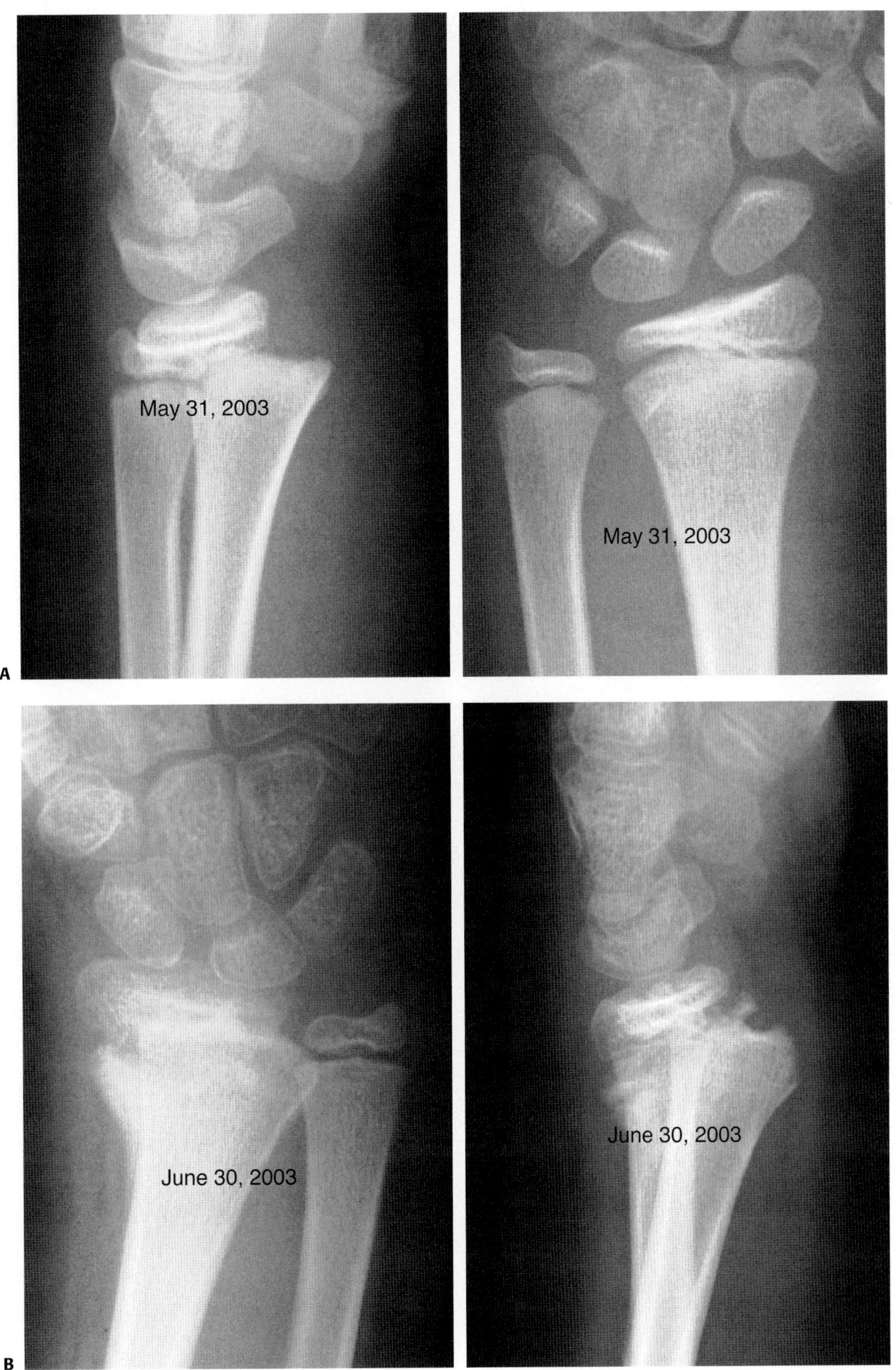

FIGURE 9-23 **A.** Anteroposterior and lateral views of displaced radial physeal fracture. **B.** Healed malunion 1 month after radial physeal fracture. (*continues*)

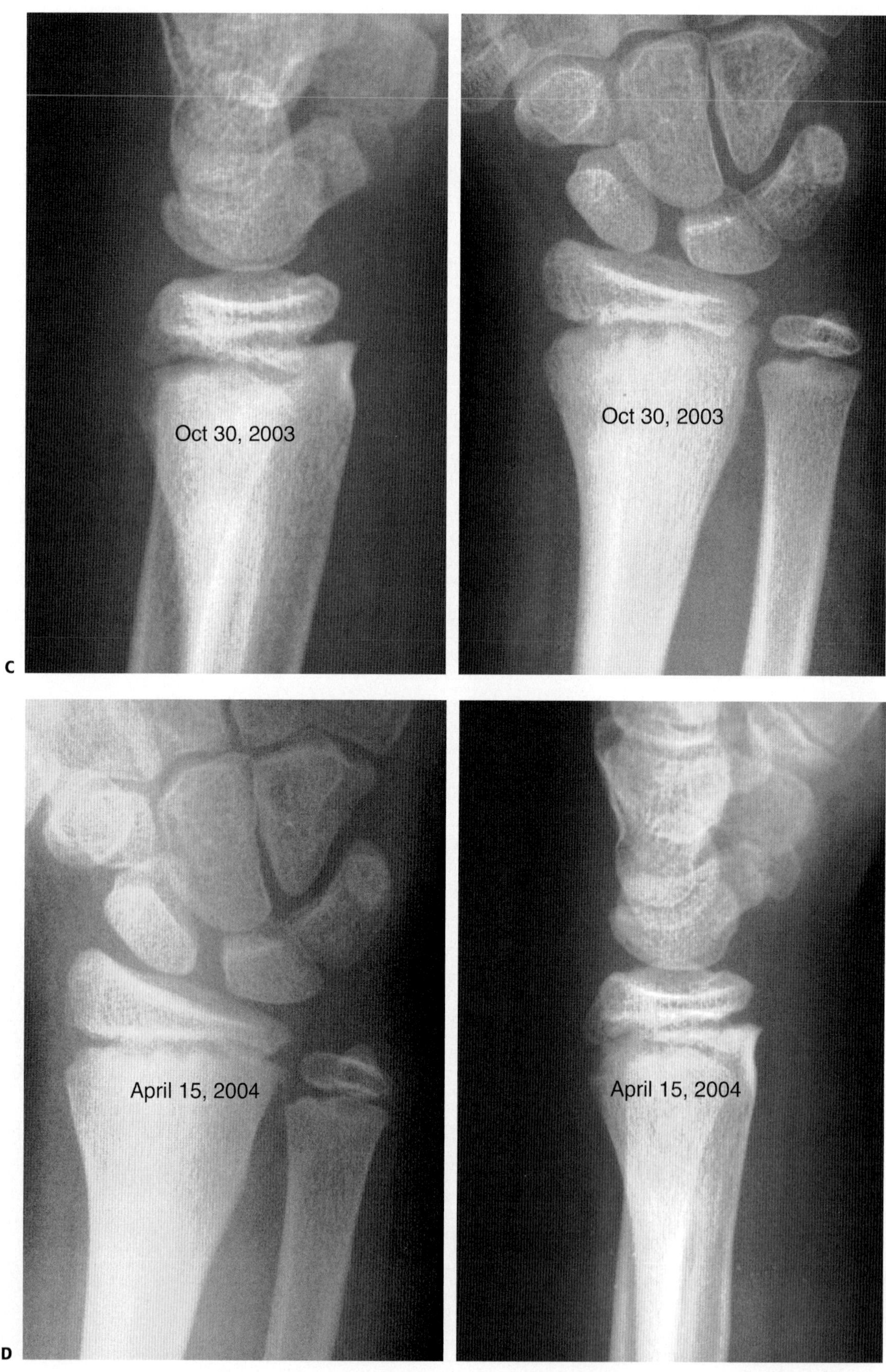

FIGURE 9-23 *(continued)* **C.** Significant remodeling at 5 months after fracture. **D.** Anatomic remodeling with no physeal arrest.

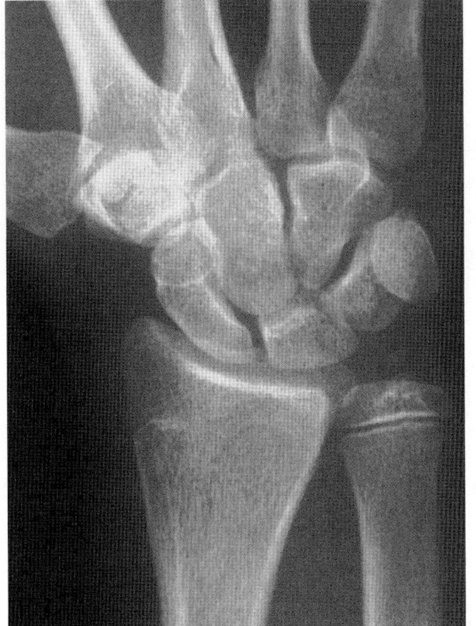

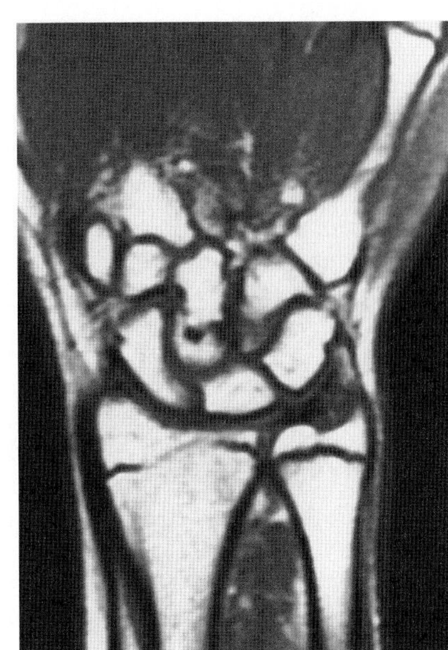

FIGURE 9-24 **A.** Anteroposterior x-ray of growth arrest with open ulnar physis. **B.** Magnetic resonance imaging scan of large area of growth arrest that was not deemed resectable by mapping.

Physeal Arrest. Distal radial physeal arrest can occur from either the trauma of the original injury (Fig. 9-24) (71,85,104) or late (more than 7 days) reduction of a displaced fracture. The incidence of radial growth arrest has been shown to be 4% to 5% of all displaced radial physeal fractures (71,105). The trauma to the physeal cartilage from displacement and compression is a significant risk factor for growth arrest. However, a correlation between the risk of growth arrest and the degree of displacement, type of fracture, or type of reduction has yet to be defined. Similarly, the risk of further compromising the physis with late reduction at various time intervals is still unclear. The current recommendation is for an atraumatic reduction of a displaced physeal fracture less than 7 days after injury.

When a growth arrest develops, the consequences depend on the severity of the arrest and the amount of growth remaining. A complete arrest of the distal radial physis in a skeletally immature patient can be a serious problem. The continued growth of the ulna with cessation of radial growth can lead to incongruity of the DRUJ, ulnocarpal impaction, and development of a TFCC tear (Fig. 9-25). The radial deviation deformity at the wrist can be severe enough to cause limitation of wrist and forearm motion. Pain and clicking can develop at the ulnocarpal or radioulnar joints, indicative of ulnocarpal impaction or a TFCC tear. The deformity will progress until the end of growth. Pain and limited motion and function will be present until forearm length is rebalanced; until the radiocarpal, ulnocarpal, and

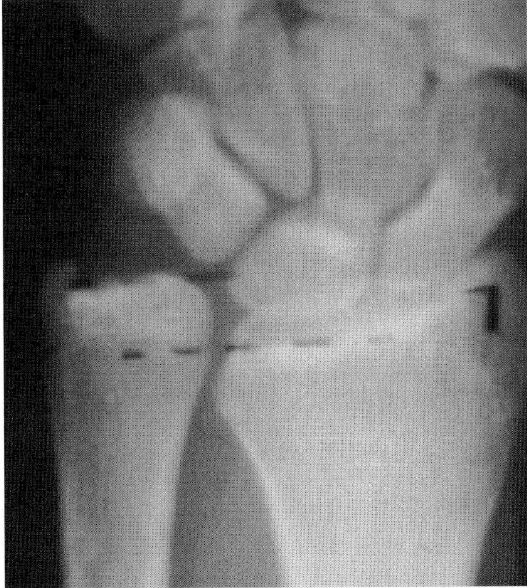

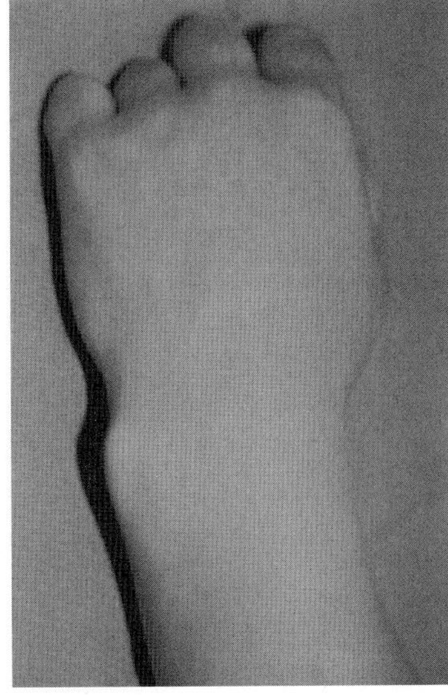

FIGURE 9-25 **A.** Anteroposterior x-ray of radial growth arrest and ulnar overgrowth after physeal fracture. Patient complained of ulnar-sided wrist pain and clicking. **B.** Clinical photograph of ulnar overgrowth and radial deviation deformity.

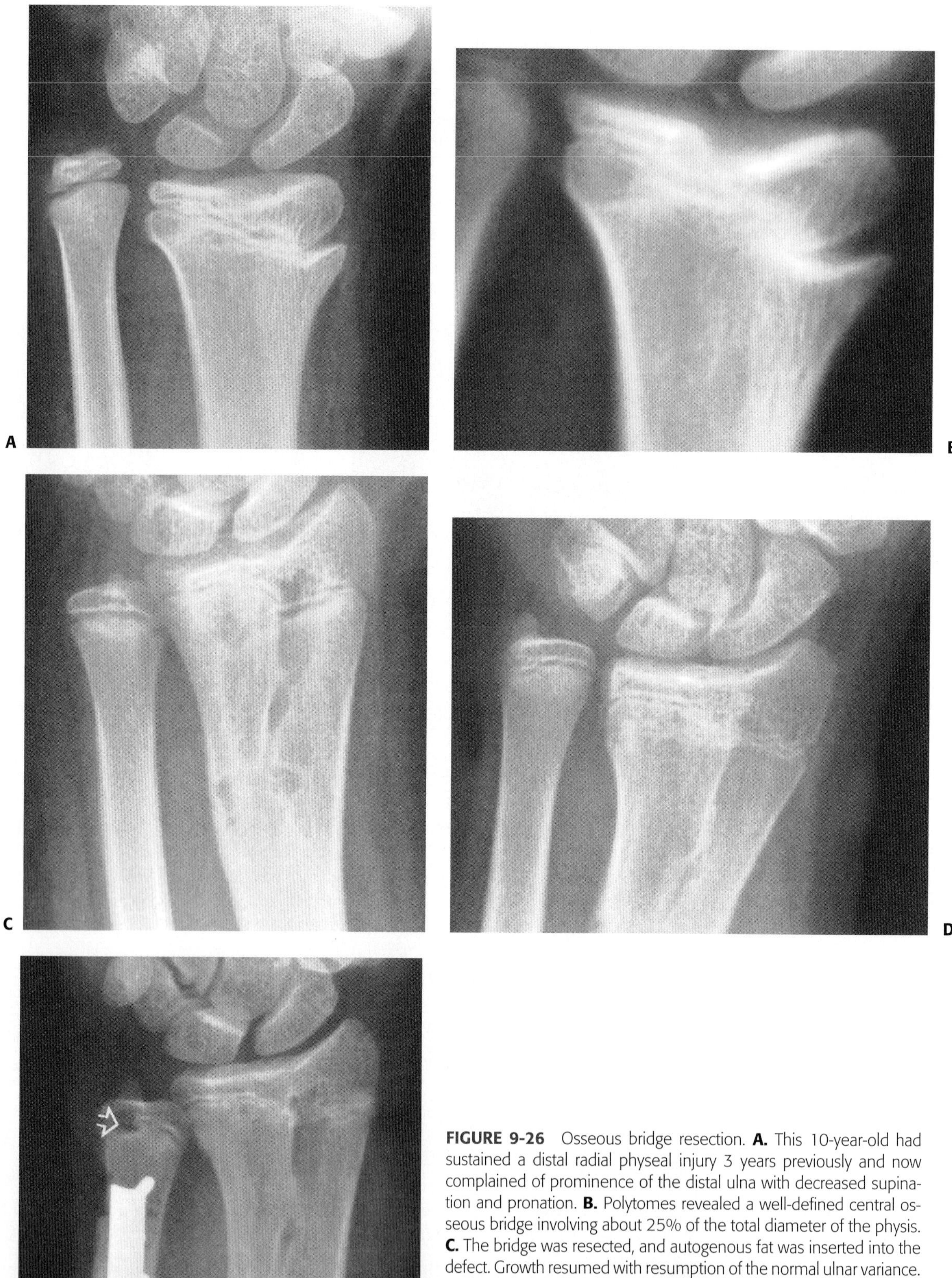

FIGURE 9-26 Osseous bridge resection. **A.** This 10-year-old had sustained a distal radial physeal injury 3 years previously and now complained of prominence of the distal ulna with decreased supination and pronation. **B.** Polytomes revealed a well-defined central osseous bridge involving about 25% of the total diameter of the physis. **C.** The bridge was resected, and autogenous fat was inserted into the defect. Growth resumed with resumption of the normal ulnar variance. Epiphysiodesis of the distal ulna was postponed for 6 months. **D.** Unfortunately, the radius slowed its growth, and a symptomatic positive ulnar variance developed. **E.** This was treated with an epiphysiodesis (*open arrow*) and surgical shortening of the ulna. The clinical appearance and range of motion of the forearm returned to essentially normal.

radioulnar joints are restored; and until the TFCC tear and areas of chondromalacia are repaired or debrided (32,106,107).

Ideally, physeal arrest of the distal radius will be discovered early before the consequences of unbalanced growth develop. Radiographic screening 6 to 12 months after injury can identify the early arrest. A small area of growth arrest in a patient near skeletal maturity may be clinically inconsequential. However, a large area of arrest in a patient with marked growth remaining can lead to ulnocarpal impaction and forearm deformity if intervention is not performed early. An MRI scan can map the area of arrest (108). If it is less than 45% of the physis, a bar resection can be attempted (86,109). This may restore radial growth and prevent future problems (Fig. 9-26). If the bar is larger than 45% of the physis, bar resection is unlikely to be successful. An early ulnar epiphysiodesis will prevent growth imbalance of the forearm (106). The growth discrepancy between forearms in most patients is minor and does not require treatment. However, this is not the case for a patient with an arrest at a very young age, for whom complicated decisions regarding forearm lengthening need to occur.

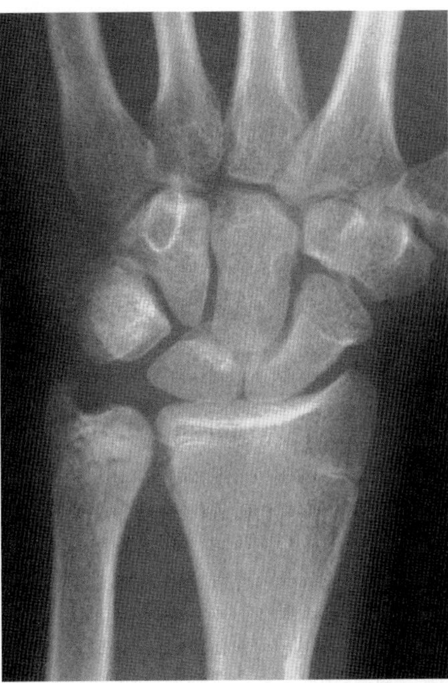

FIGURE 9-27 Anteroposterior x-ray revealing hypertrophic ulnar styloid healing as the source of the ulnar carpal impaction pain in this patient.

Ulnocarpal Impaction Syndrome. The growth discrepancy between the radius and ulna can lead to relative radial shortening and ulnar overgrowth. The distal ulna can impinge on the lunate and triquetrum and cause pain with ulnar deviation, extension, and compression activities (110). This is particularly true in repetitive wrist loading sports such as field hockey, lacrosse, and gymnastics (111). Physical examination loading the ulnocarpal joint in ulnar deviation and compression will recreate the pain. X-rays show the radial arrest, ulnar overgrowth, and distal ulnocarpal impingement. The ulnocarpal impaction also may be caused by a hypertrophic ulnar styloid fracture union (Fig. 9-27) or an ulnar styloid nonunion (112,113). An MRI scan may reveal chondromalacia of the lunate or triquetrum, a tear of the TFCC, and the extent of the distal radial physeal arrest.

Treatment should correct all components of the problem. The ulnar overgrowth is corrected by either an ulnar shortening osteotomy or radial lengthening. Most often a marked degree of positive ulnar variance requires ulnar shortening to neutral or negative variance (Fig. 9-28). If the ulnar physis is still open, a simultaneous arrest should be performed to prevent recurrent deformity. If the degree of radial deformity is marked, this should be corrected by a realignment or lengthening osteotomy. Criteria for radial correction is debatable, but we have used radial inclination of less than 11 degrees on the AP x-ray (Fig. 9-29) (106). In the rare case of complete arrest in a very young patient, radial lengthening is preferable to ulnar shortening to rebalance the forearm.

Triangular Fibrocartilage Complex Tears. Triangular fibrocartilage complex tears should be repaired. The presence of an ulnar styloid nonunion at the base often is indicative of an associated peripheral tear of the TFCC (32,106,107). The symptomatic ulnar styloid nonunion is excised (112–114) and any TFCC tear repaired. If physical examination or preoperative MRI scan indicates a TFCC tear in the absence of an ulnar styloid nonunion, an initial arthroscopic examination can define the lesion and appropriate treatment. Peripheral tears are the most common TFCC tears in children and adolescents and can be repaired arthroscopically by an outside-in suture technique. Tears off the sigmoid notch are the next most common in adolescents and can be repaired with arthroscopic-assisted, transradial sutures. Central tears are rare in children and as opposed to adults with degenerative central tears, arthroscopic debridement usually does not result in pain relief in children. Distal volar tears also are rare and are repaired open, at times with ligament reconstruction (32).

Neuropathy. Median neuropathy can occur from direct trauma from the initial displacement of the fracture, traction ischemia from a persistently displaced fracture, or the development of a compartment syndrome in the carpal canal or volar forearm (Fig. 9-30) (31). All patients with displaced distal radial fractures should undergo a careful motor-sensory examination upon presentation to an acute care facility. The flexor pollicis longus, index flexor digitorum profundus, and abductor pollicis brevis muscles should be tested. Light touch and two-point discrimination sensibility of the thumb and index finger should be tested in any child over 5 years of age with a displaced Salter-Harris type I or II fracture. The presence of median neuropathy and marked volar soft-tissue swelling are indications for percutaneous pin stabilization of the fracture to lessen the risk of compartment syndrome in a cast.

Median neuropathy caused by direct trauma or traction is-

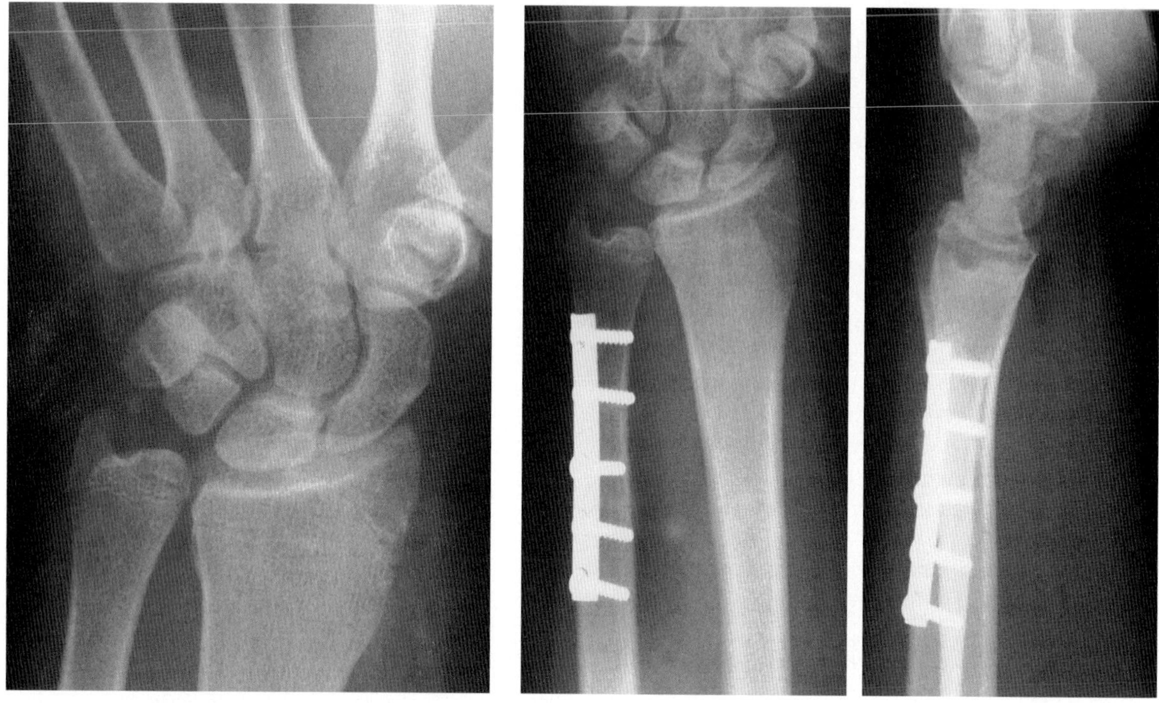

FIGURE 9-28 **A.** Anteroposterior x-ray of distal radial growth arrest, ulnar overgrowth, and an ulnar styloid nonunion. Wrist arthroscopy revealed an intact triangular fibrocartilage complex. **B.** Anteroposterior and lateral x-rays after ulnar shortening osteotomy.

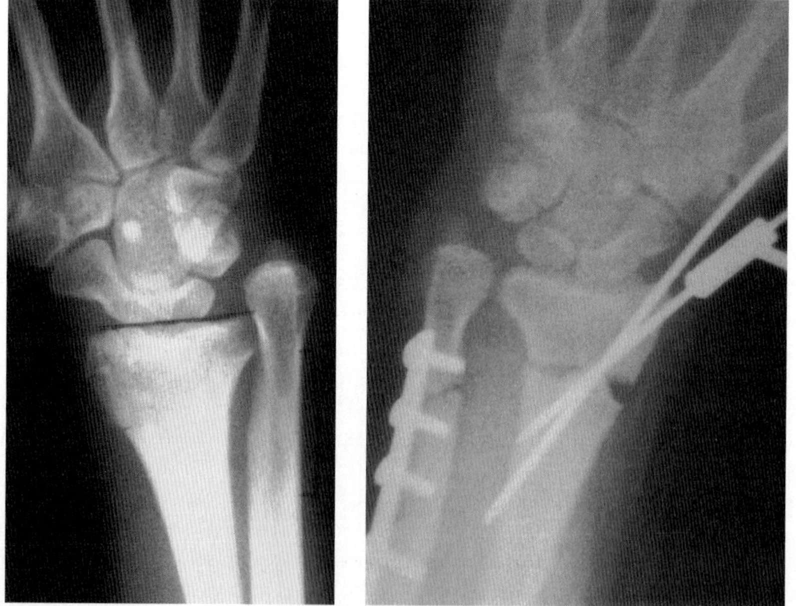

FIGURE 9-29 **A.** More severe ulnar overgrowth with dislocation of the distal radioulnar joint and flattening of the radial articular surface. **B.** Intraoperative fluoroscopic view of ulnar shortening and radial osteotomy to corrective deformities.

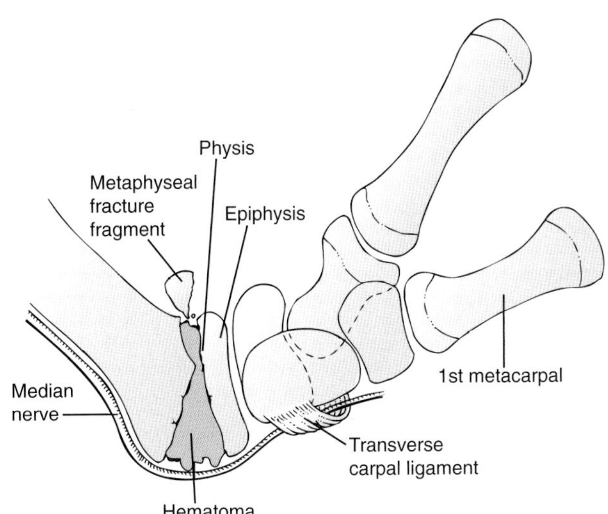

FIGURE 9-30 Volar forearm anatomy outlining the potential compression of the median nerve between the metaphysis of the radius and dorsally displaced physeal fracture. The taut volar transverse carpal ligament and fracture hematoma also are contributing factors. (Redrawn from Waters PM, Kolettis GJ, Schwend R. Acute median neuropathy following physeal fractures of the distal radius. *J Pediatr Orthop* 1994;14:173–177; with permission.)

chemia generally resolves after fracture reduction. The degree of neural injury will determine the length of time to recovery. Recovery can be monitored with an advancing Tinel sign along the median nerve. Motor-sensory testing can define progressive return of neural function.

Carpal Tunnel Syndrome. Median neuropathy caused by a carpal tunnel syndrome will not recover until the carpal tunnel is decompressed. After anatomic fracture reduction and pin stabilization, volar forearm and carpal tunnel pressures are measured. Gelberman (115) recommended waiting 20 minutes or more to allow for pressure-volume equilibration before measuring pressures. If the pressures are elevated beyond 40 mm Hg or the difference between the diastolic pressure and the compartment pressure is less than 30 mm Hg (92), an immediate release of the affected compartments should be performed. The carpal tunnel is released through a palmar incision in line with the fourth ray, with care to avoid injuring the palmar vascular arch and the ulnar nerves exiting the Guyon's canal. The transverse carpal ligament is released with a Z-plasty closure of the ligament to prevent late bow-stringing of the nerve against the palmar skin. The volar forearm fascia is released in the standard fashion.

RADIAL PHYSEAL STRESS FRACTURES

Repetitive axial loading of the wrist in dorsiflexion can lead to physeal stress injuries, almost always involving the radius. Competitive gymnastics is by far the most common cause (21–23,25,116–118). Other activities reported to cause radial physeal stress fractures include break dancing (27). Factors that predispose to this injury include excessive training, poor techniques, and attempts to advance too quickly in competitive level. Proper coaching is important in preventing these injuries.

A child with a radial physeal stress fracture has recurring, activity-related wrist pain, usually aching and diffuse, in the region of the distal radial metaphysis and physis. Extremes of dorsiflexion and palmar flexion reproduce the pain. There is local tenderness over the dorsal, distal radial physis. Resistive contracture strength testing of the wrist dorsiflexors often reproduces the pain. There may be fusiform swelling about the wrist if there is reactive bone formation. The differential diagnosis includes physeal stress injury, ganglion, ligamentous or TFCC injury, tendonitis or muscle-tendon tear, fracture such as a scaphoid fracture, and osteonecrosis of the scaphoid (Preiser's disease) or lunate (Kienbock's disease). X-rays may be diagnostic. Physeal widening and reactive bone formation are indicative of chronic physeal stress fracture. Premature physeal closure indicates long-standing stress (24,119). In this situation, continued ulnar growth leads to an ulnar positive variance and pain from ulnocarpal impaction or a TFCC tear (20,25,111). Normal x-rays may not show an early physeal stress fracture. If the diagnosis is suggested clinically, a bone scan or MRI scan is indicated. Bone scans are sensitive but nonspecific. MRI scans usually are diagnostic.

Treatment first and foremost involves rest. This may be difficult depending on the skill level of the athlete and the desires of the child, coach, and parents to maintain constant training. Education regarding the long-term consequences of a growth arrest is important in this emotionally charged situation. Short-arm cast immobilization for several weeks may be the only way to restrict stress to the radial physis in some patients. Splint protection is appropriate in cooperative patients. Protection should continue until there is resolution of pain with examination and activity. The athlete can maintain cardiovascular fitness, strength, and flexibility while protecting the injured wrist. Once the acute physeal injury has healed, return to weight-bearing activities should be gradual. This requires the cooperation of the coach and parents. Adjustment of techniques and training methods often is necessary to prevent recurrence. The major concern is development of a radial growth arrest in a skeletally immature patient. This is an avoidable complication.

If a radial growth arrest has already occurred upon presentation, treatment depends on the degree of deformity and the patient's symptoms. Physeal bar resection often is not possible because the arrest is too diffuse in stress injuries. If there is no significant ulnar overgrowth, a distal ulnar epiphysiodesis will prevent the development of an ulnocarpal impaction syndrome. For ulnar overgrowth and ulnocarpal pain, an ulnar shortening osteotomy is indicated. Techniques include transverse, oblique, and Z-shortening osteotomies. Transverse osteotomy has a higher risk of nonunion than either oblique or Z-shortening and should be avoided. The status of the TFCC also should be evaluated by MRI scan or wrist arthroscopy. If there is an associated TFCC tear, it should be repaired as appropriate.

ULNAR PHYSEAL FRACTURES

Isolated ulnar physeal fractures are rare injuries. Most ulnar physeal fractures occur in association with radial metaphyseal or physeal fractures. Physeal separations are classified by the standard Salter-Harris criteria. The rare pediatric Galeazzi injury usually involves an ulnar physeal fracture rather than a soft-tissue disruption of the distal radioulnar joint. Another ulnar physeal fracture is an avulsion fracture off the distal aspect of the ulnar styloid (68). Although an ulnar styloid injury is an epiphyseal avulsion, it can be associated with soft-tissue injuries of the TFCC and ulnocarpal joint but does not cause growth-related complications.

Physeal growth arrest is frequent with distal ulnar physeal fractures (Fig. 9-31). Occurring in 21% (120) to 55% (105,121) of patients. It is unclear why the distal ulna has a higher incidence of growth arrest after fracture than does the radius. Ulnae growth arrest in a young child leads to relative radial overgrowth and bowing.

Current Treatment Options

Treatment options are similar to those for radial physeal fractures: immobilization alone, closed reduction and cast immobilization, closed reduction and percutaneous pinning, and open reduction. Often these fractures are minimally displaced or nondisplaced. Immobilization until fracture healing at 3 to 6 weeks is standard treatment. Closed reduction is indicated for displaced fractures with more than 50% translation or 20° angula-

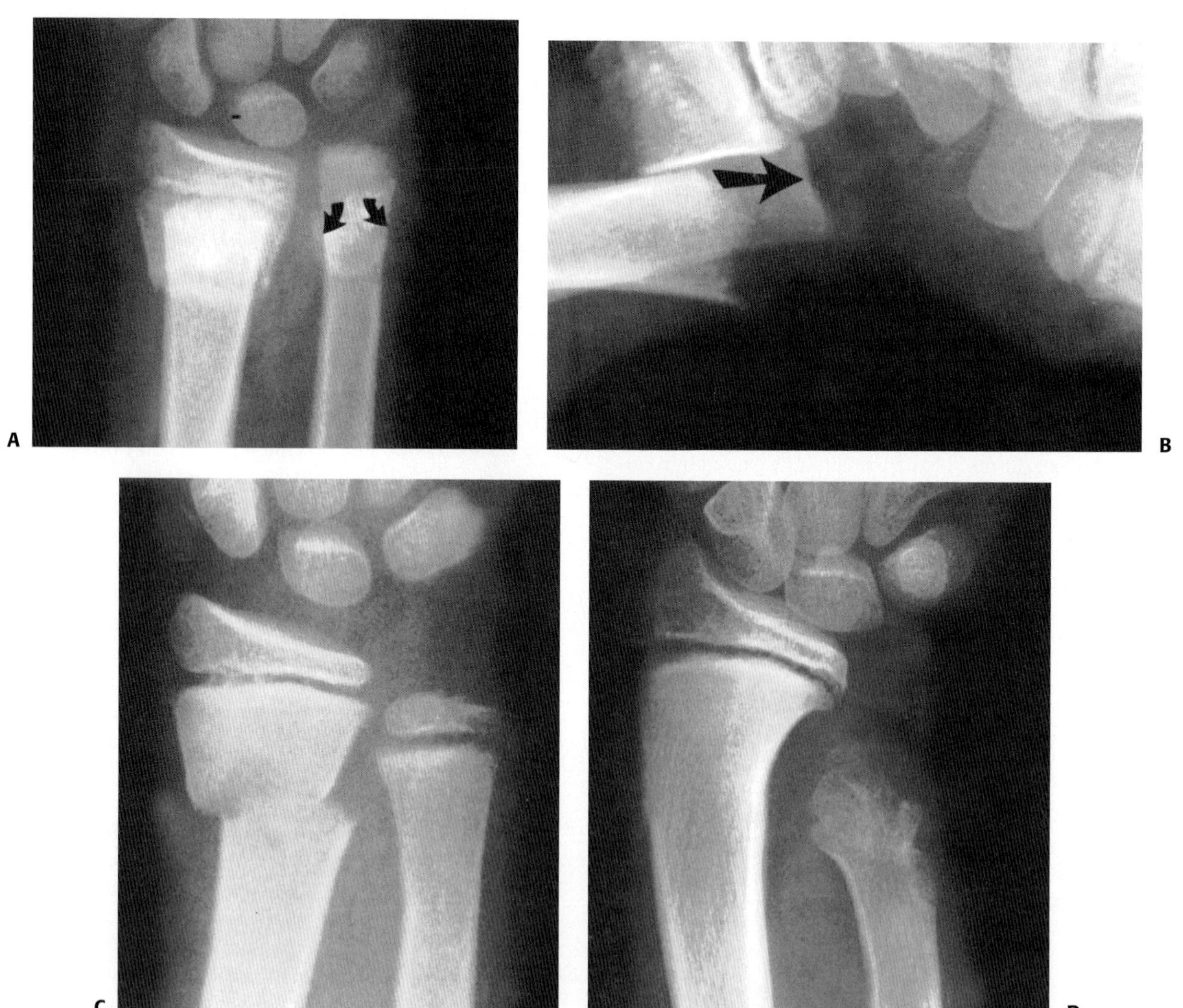

FIGURE 9-31 **A,B.** A 10-year-old boy sustained a closed Salter-Harris type I separation of the distal ulnar physis (*arrows*), combined with a fracture of the distal radial metaphysis. **C.** An excellent closed reduction was achieved atraumatically. **D.** Long-term growth arrest of the distal ulna occurred.

tion. Most ulnar physeal fractures reduce to a near anatomic alignment with reduction of the radial fracture. Failure to obtain a reduction of the ulnar fracture may indicate that there is soft-tissue interposed in the fracture site. This is an indication for open reduction. Exposure should be from the side of the torn periosteum. The interposed soft-tissue (periosteum, extensor tendons, abductor digiti quinti, or flexor tendons) must be extracted from the fracture site (122–124). If reduction is not stable, a small-diameter smooth pin can be used to maintain alignment until healing at 3 to 4 weeks. Further injury to the physis should be avoided during operative exposure and reduction because of the high risk of growth arrest.

ULNAR STYLOID FRACTURES

Ulnar styloid avulsion fractures are common in association with radial fractures (68) and represent a soft-tissue avulsion of the attachment of the TFCC or ulnocarpal ligaments. Treatment consists of immobilization and monitoring of long-term outcome, and most heal without sequelae (125). However, an acute displaced fracture of the base of the styloid represents a disruption of the TFCC. Most of these injuries are caused by high-velocity trauma in adolescents at or near skeletal maturity. Treatment should be open reduction with tension band fixation of the styloid to the metaphysis and repair of the TFCC. The tension band wire is removed at 3 to 6 weeks.

Some ulnar styloid fractures result in nonunion or hypertrophic union (32,112–114). Nonunion may be associated with TFCC tears or ulnocarpal impaction. The hypertrophic healing represents a pseudo-ulnar positive variance and ulnocarpal impaction. Both cause ulnar-sided wrist pain. Compression of the lunate or triquetrum on the distal ulna reproduces the pain. Clicking with ulnocarpal compression or forearm rotation represents either a TFCC tear or chondromalacia of the lunate or triquetrum. Surgical excision of the nonunion or hypertrophic union with repair of the TFCC to the base of the styloid is the treatment of choice. Postoperative immobilization for 4 weeks in a long-arm cast followed by 2 weeks in a short-arm cast protects the TFCC repair.

Complications

Growth Arrest

The most common complication of distal ulnar physeal fractures is growth arrest. Golz (121) described 18 such fractures, with growth arrest in 10%. If the patient is young enough, continued growth of the radius will lead to deformity and dysfunction. The distal ulnar aspect of the radial physis and epiphysis appears to be tethered by the foreshortened ulna (Fig. 9-32). The radial articular surface develops increased inclination toward the foreshortened ulna. This is similar to the deformity Peinado (126) created experimentally with arrest of the distal ulna in rabbits' forelimbs. The distal ulna loses its normal articulation in the sigmoid notch of the distal radius. The metaphyseal-diaphyseal region of the radius often becomes notched from its articulation with the distal ulna during forearm rotation. Frequently, these patients have pain and limitation of motion with pronation and supination (110).

Ideally, this problem is identified before the development of marked ulnar foreshortening and subsequent radial deformity. Because it is well known that distal ulnar physeal fractures have a high incidence of growth arrest, these patients should have serial x-rays for early identification. Unfortunately, in the distal ulnar physis, physeal bar resection generally is unsuccessful. Surgical arrest of the radial physis can prevent radial deformity. Usually this occurs toward the end of growth so that the forearm length discrepancy is not a problem.

Rarely patients present late with established deformity. Treatment involves rebalancing the length of the radius and ulna. The options include hemiphyseal arrest of the radius, corrective radial closing wedge osteotomy, and ulnar lengthening (Figs. 9-32 and 9-33) (110,120,121), or a combination of these procedures (Figs. 9-34 and 9-35). The painful impingement of the radius and ulna with forearm rotation can be corrected with reconstitution of the distal radioulnar joint. If the radial physis has significant growth remaining, a radial physeal arrest should be done at the same time as the surgical rebalancing of the radius and ulna (127). Treatment is individualized depending on the age of the patient, degree of deformity, and level of pain and dysfunction.

METAPHYSEAL FRACTURES

The metaphysis of the distal radius is the most common site of forearm fracture in children and adolescents (2,3,128,129). They occur most commonly in boys in the nondominant arm (130). These fractures have a peak incidence during the adolescent growth spurt, which in girls is age 11 to 12 years and in boys is 12 to 13 years (8). During this time of extensive bone remodeling, there is relative osteoporosis of the distal radial metaphysis, which makes this area more susceptible to fracture with a fall.

Mechanism of Injury

The mechanism of injury generally is a fall on an outstretched hand. The usual dorsiflexion position of the wrist leads to tension failure on the volar side. Fracture type and degree of displacement depend on the height and velocity of the fall (128). These fractures can be nondisplaced torus or buckle injuries (common in younger children with a minimal fall) or dorsally displaced fractures with apex volar angulation (more common in older children with higher velocity injuries) (Fig. 9-33). Displacement may be severe enough to cause foreshortening and bayonet apposition (Fig. 9-34). Rarely, a mechanism such as a fall from a height can cause a distal radial fracture associated with a more proximal fracture of the forearm or elbow (Fig. 9-35) (131–133). These "floating elbow" situations are indicative of higher velocity of trauma and risk of compartment syndrome (30). In addition, a fall with a palmar flexed wrist can produce

(text continues on page 366)

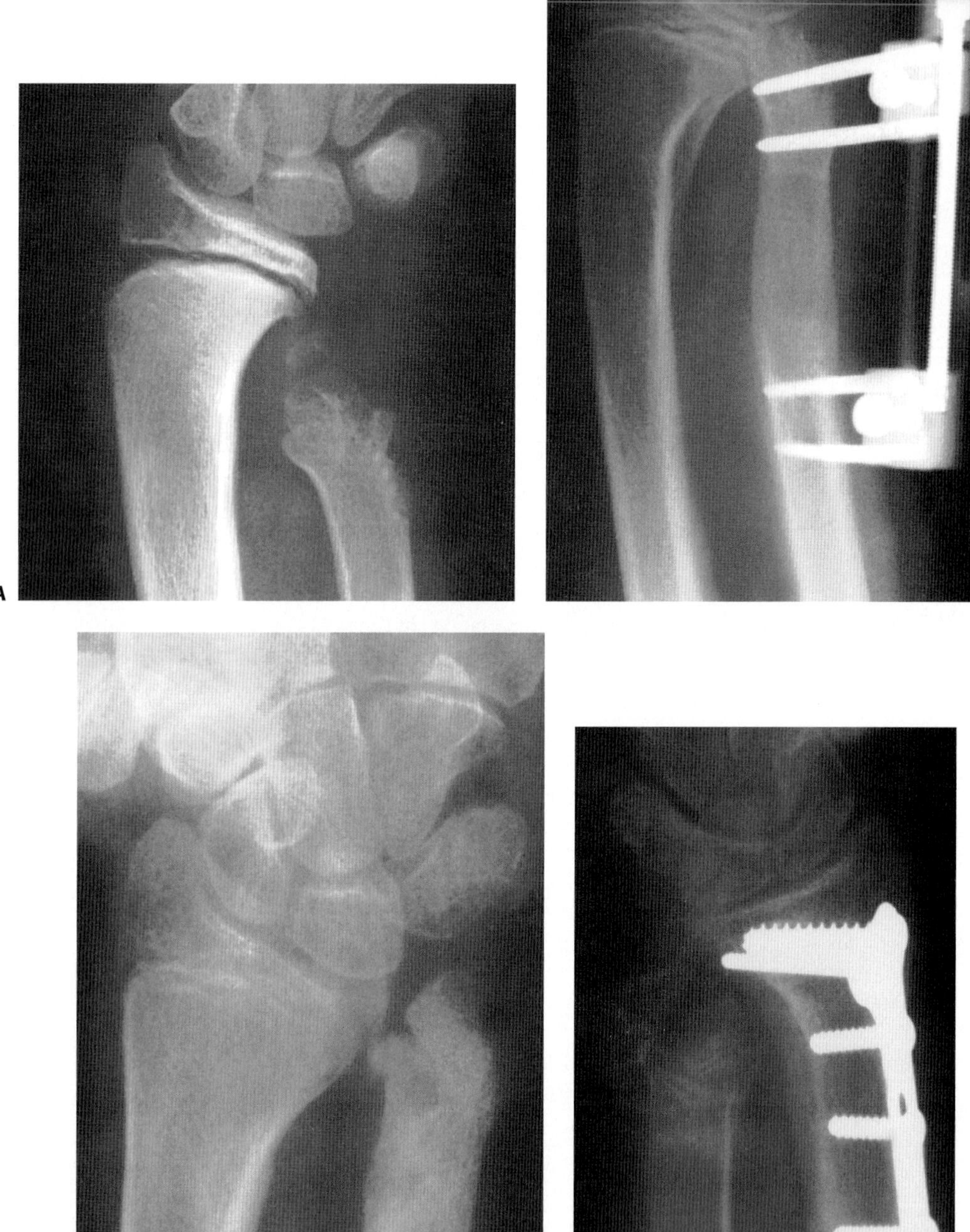

FIGURE 9-32 **A.** The appearance of the distal ulna in the patient seen in Figure 9-21, 3 years after injury, demonstrating premature fusion of the distal ulnar physis with 3.2 cm of shortening. The distal radius is secondarily deformed, with tilting and translocation toward the ulna. **B.** In the patient in Figure 9-21 with distal ulnar physeal arrest, a lengthening of the distal ulna was performed using a small unipolar distracting device. The ulna was slightly overlengthened to compensate for some subsequent growth of the distal radius. **C.** Six months after the lengthening osteotomy, there is some deformity of the distal ulna, but good restoration of length has been achieved. The distal radial epiphyseal tilt has corrected somewhat, and the patient has asymptomatic supination and pronation to 75 degrees. **D.** Similar case to Figure 9-32A–C, but with more progressive distal radial deformity treated with corrective osteotomy and epiphysiodesis of the distal radius.

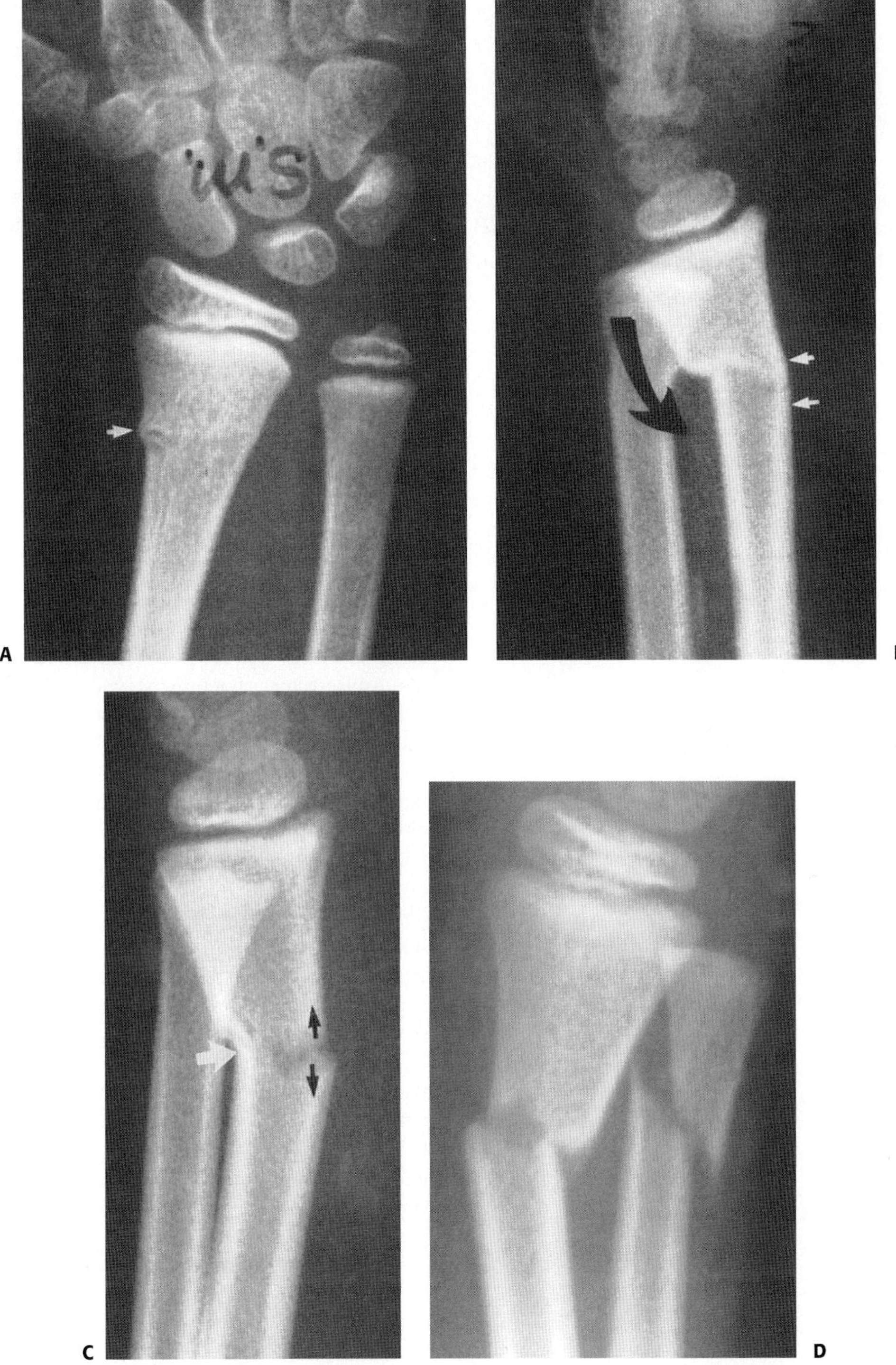

FIGURE 9-33 Metaphyseal biomechanical patterns. **A.** Torus fracture. Simple bulging of the thin cortex (*arrow*). **B.** Compression greenstick fracture. Angulation of the dorsal cortex (*large curved arrow*). The volar cortex is intact but slightly plastically deformed (*small white arrows*). **C.** Tension failure greenstick fracture. The dorsal cortex is plastically deformed (*white arrow*) and the volar cortex is complete and separated (*black arrows*). **D.** Complete length maintained. Both cortices are completely fractured, but the length of the radius has been maintained. (Reprinted from Wilkins KE, ed. *Operative management of upper extremity fractures in children.* Rosemont, IL: American Academy of Orthopaedic Surgeons, 1994:24; with permission.)

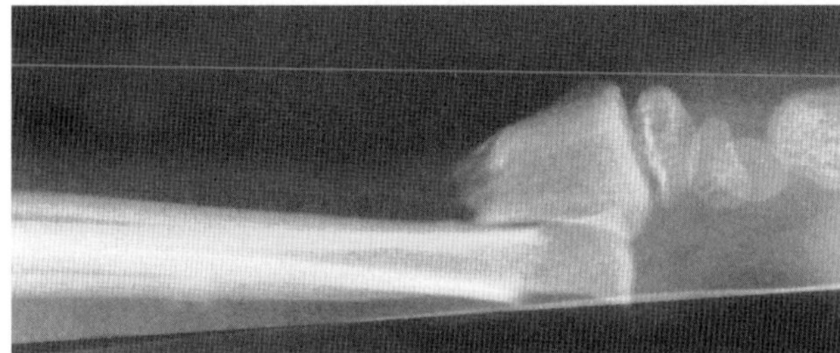

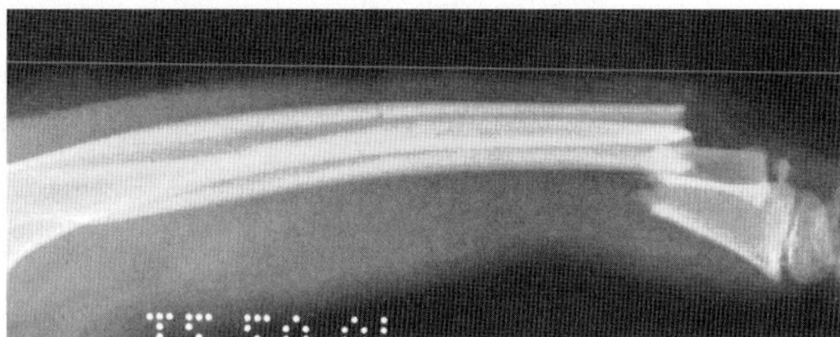

FIGURE 9-34 Complete fractures; bayonet apposition. **A.** Dorsal bayonet. **B.** Volar bayonet.

a volarly displaced fracture with apex dorsal angulation (Fig. 9-36).

Seasonal variation has been noted in these fractures in children younger than 15 years of age. (16). The incidence of wrist and forearm fractures was roughly half (5.7/1000 per year) in the three winter months in Wales compared with the rest of the year (10.7/1000 per year). In addition. the nonwinter month fractures were more severe in terms of requiring reduction and hospitalization in this longitudinal study. Certain sports, such as snowboarding, soccer goalkeeping, and horseback riding, have been shown to have an increased risk of distal radial fracture (11–14,69,134). Protective wrist guards have been shown to decrease the injury rate in snowboarders, especially beginners and persons with rental equipment (13).

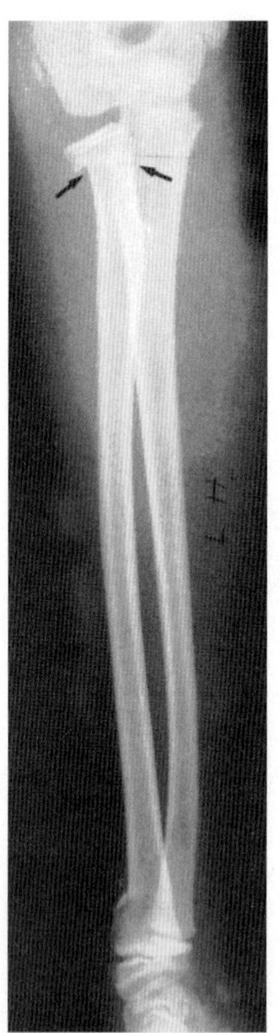

FIGURE 9-35 A 10-year-old girl with an innocuous-appearing distal radial fracture associated with an ipsilateral angulated radial neck fracture (*arrows*).

Signs and Symptoms

Children with distal radial fractures present with pain, swelling, and deformity of the distal forearm (Fig. 9-37). The clinical signs depend on the degree of fracture displacement. With a nondisplaced torus fracture in a young child, medical attention may not be sought until several days after injury, because the intact periosteum is protective in this situation, lessening pain and the child's restriction of activities. Most children with distal radial fractures, however, present acutely after the fall with an obvious deformity. Physical examination is limited by the patient's pain and anxiety, but it is imperative to obtain an accurate examination of the motor and sensory components of the radial, median, and ulnar nerves before treatment. Median nerve motor function is evaluated by testing the abductor pollicis brevis (intrinsic) and flexor pollicis longus (extrinsic) muscles. Ulnar nerve motor evaluation includes testing the first dorsal interosseous (intrinsic), abductor digit quinti (intrinsic), and flexor digitorum profundus to the small finger (extrinsic) muscles. Radial nerve evaluation involves testing the common digital extensors for metacarpophalangeal joint extension. Sensibility to light touch and two-point discrimination should be tested. Normal two-point discrimination is less than 5 mm but is not present until age 5 to 7 years. Pin-prick sensibility testing will only hurt and scare the already anxious child and should be avoided. A prospective study indicated an 8% incidence of nerve injury in children with distal radial fractures (130).

Associated Injuries

The ipsilateral extremity should be carefully examined for fractures of the carpus (34), forearm, or elbow (87,133,135–141) because 3% to 13% of distal radial fractures have associated ipsilateral extremity fractures (133,142), increasing the risk of neurovascular compromise and compartment syndrome (52,132,133). In the multitrauma patient, fracture care is appropriately modified to coincide with appropriate systemic care.

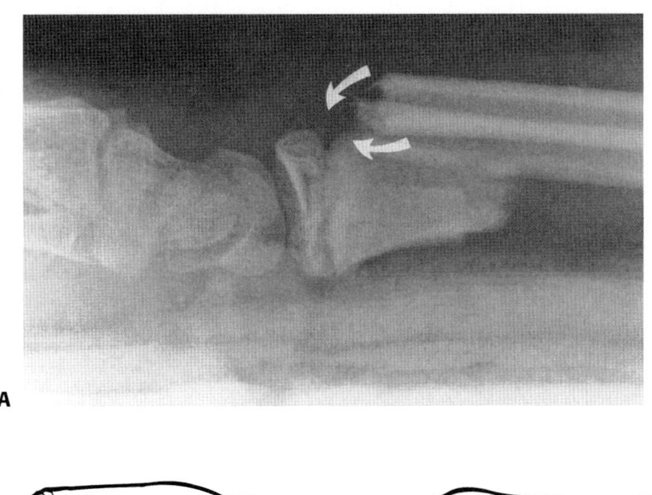

A

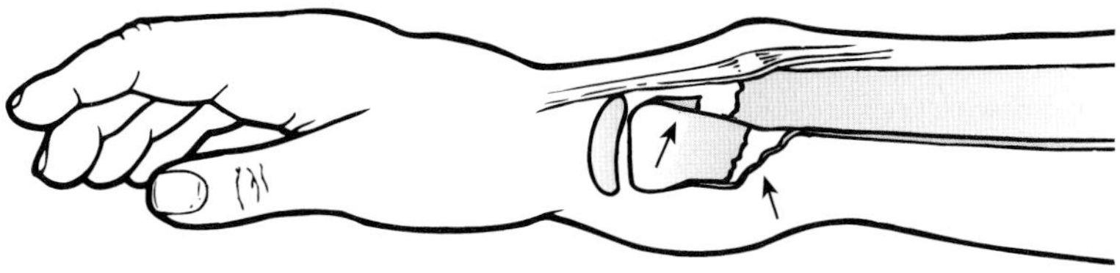

B

FIGURE 9-36 Reverse bayonet. **A.** Typical volar bayonet fracture. Often the distal end of the proximal fragment is buttonholed through the extensor tendons (*arrows*). (Reprinted from Wilkins KE, ed. *Operative management of upper extremity fractures in children.* Rosemont, IL: American Academy of Orthopaedic Surgeons, 1994:27; with permission.) **B.** Intact volar periosteum and disrupted dorsal periosteum (*arrows*). The extensor tendons are displaced to either side of the proximal fragment.

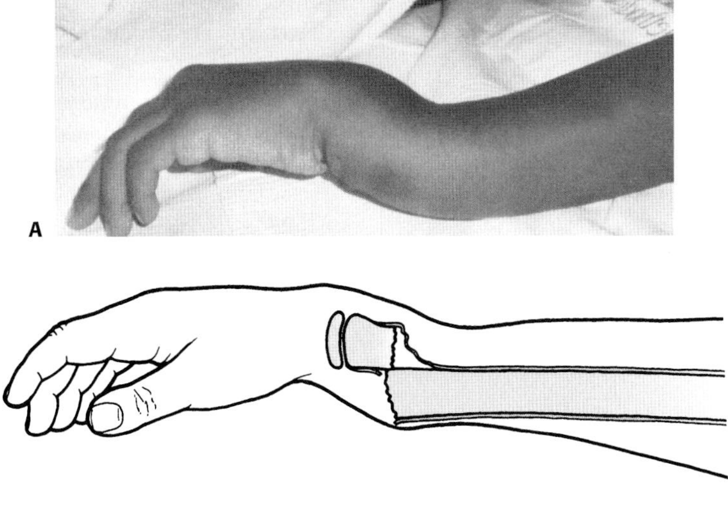

A

B

FIGURE 9-37 Dorsal bayonet deformity. **A.** Typical distal metaphyseal fracture with dorsal bayonet showing a dorsal angulation of the distal forearm. **B.** Usually the periosteum is intact on the dorsal side and disrupted on the volar side.

Diagnosis and Classification

X-rays are diagnostic of the fracture type and degree of displacement. Standard AP and lateral x-rays usually are sufficient. Complete wrist, forearm, and elbow views are necessary for high-velocity injuries or when there is clinical tenderness. More extensive radiographic studies (CT scan, tomograms) usually are not necessary unless there is intra-articular extension of the metaphyseal fracture in a skeletally mature adolescent.

These fractures are classified by fracture pattern, type of associated ulnar fracture, and direction of displacement. Fracture displacement is broadly classified as dorsal or volar. Most distal radial metaphyseal fractures are displaced dorsally with apex volar angulation (3). Volar displacement with apex dorsal angulation can occur with palmar flexion injuries.

Metaphyseal fracture patterns are torus, incomplete or greenstick, and complete fractures. Torus fractures are axial compression injuries. The site of cortical failure is the transition from metaphysis to diaphysis (143). These injuries are stable because of the intact periosteum. Rarely, they may extend into the physis, putting them at risk for growth impairment (81,108). Incomplete or greenstick fractures occur with a combination of compressive and rotatory forces, generally a dorsiflexion force and supination deforming force. This leads to a volar tension-side failure and a dorsal compression injury. The degree of force determines the amount of plastic deformation, dorsal comminution, and fracture angulation and rotation. If the force is sufficient, a complete fracture occurs with disruption of both the volar and dorsal cortices. Length may be maintained with apposition of the proximal and distal fragments. Frequently, the distal fragment lies proximal and dorsal to the proximal fragment in bayonet apposition (Table 9-2).

TABLE 9-2 Classification: Distal Metaphyseal Fractures

Directional displacement
- Dorsal
- Volar

Fracture combinations
- Isolated radius
- Radius with ulna
- Ulnar styloid
- Ulnar physis
- Ulnar metaphysis, incomplete
- Ulnar metaphysis, complete

Biomechanical patterns
- Torus
- Greenstick
- One cortex
- Two cortices
- Complete fracture
- Length maintained
- Bayonet apposition

The ulnar fracture often associated with radial metaphyseal fracture can be metaphyseal or physeal, or an ulnar styloid avulsion. Similar to radial metaphyseal fractures, the ulnar fracture can be complete or incomplete.

Distal radial fractures also can occur in conjunction with more proximal forearm fractures (144), Monteggia fracture–dislocations (145), supracondylar distal humeral fractures (52,132,135), or carpal fractures (34,136–138,140,141,145). The combination of a displaced supracondylar distal humeral fracture and a displaced distal radial metaphyseal fracture has been called the pediatric floating elbow. This injury combination is unstable and has an increased risk for malunion and neurovascular compromise.

Pediatric distal radial metaphyseal fractures are not classified by degree of instability. Unstable fractures have been predominately defined by the failure to maintain a successful closed reduction (Fig. 9-38). This occurs in approximately 30% of complete distal radial metaphyseal fractures (38–40). This high percentage of loss of alignment has been tolerated because of the remodeling potential of the distal radius. Anatomic remodeling is possible because the extension deformity is in the plane of motion of the wrist joint, the metaphyseal fracture is juxtaphyseal, and most of these fractures occur while there is still significant growth remaining. However, concern has increased about the high failure rate of closed reduction to maintain anatomic alignment of these fractures. Factors that have been identified as increasing the risk of loss of reduction with closed manipulation and casting include poor casting, bayonet apposition, translation of more than 50% the diameter of the radius, apex volar angulation of more than 30 degrees, isolated radial fractures, and radial and ulnar metaphyseal fractures at the same level (38–40).

Current Treatment Options

Treatment options are similar to those for radial physeal fractures: immobilization alone, closed reduction and cast immobilization, closed reduction and percutaneous pinning, and open reduction. The fracture type, degree of fracture instability, associated soft-tissue or skeletal trauma, and the age of the patient all influence choice of treatment.

Torus Fractures

Torus fractures are compression injuries with minimal cortical disruption. If only one cortex is violated, the injury is stable. Treatment should consist of protected immobilization to prevent further injury and relieve pain (134,146,147). Once the patient is comfortable, range-of-motion exercises and nontraumatic activities can begin. Fracture healing usually occurs in 2 to 4 weeks (1,70,113,124). Simple torus fractures usually heal without long-term sequelae.

Bicortical disruption on both the AP and lateral views indicates a more severe injury than a stable torus fracture. Splint or limited immobilization in this situation puts the child at risk for displacement. More prolonged, long-arm cast protection in

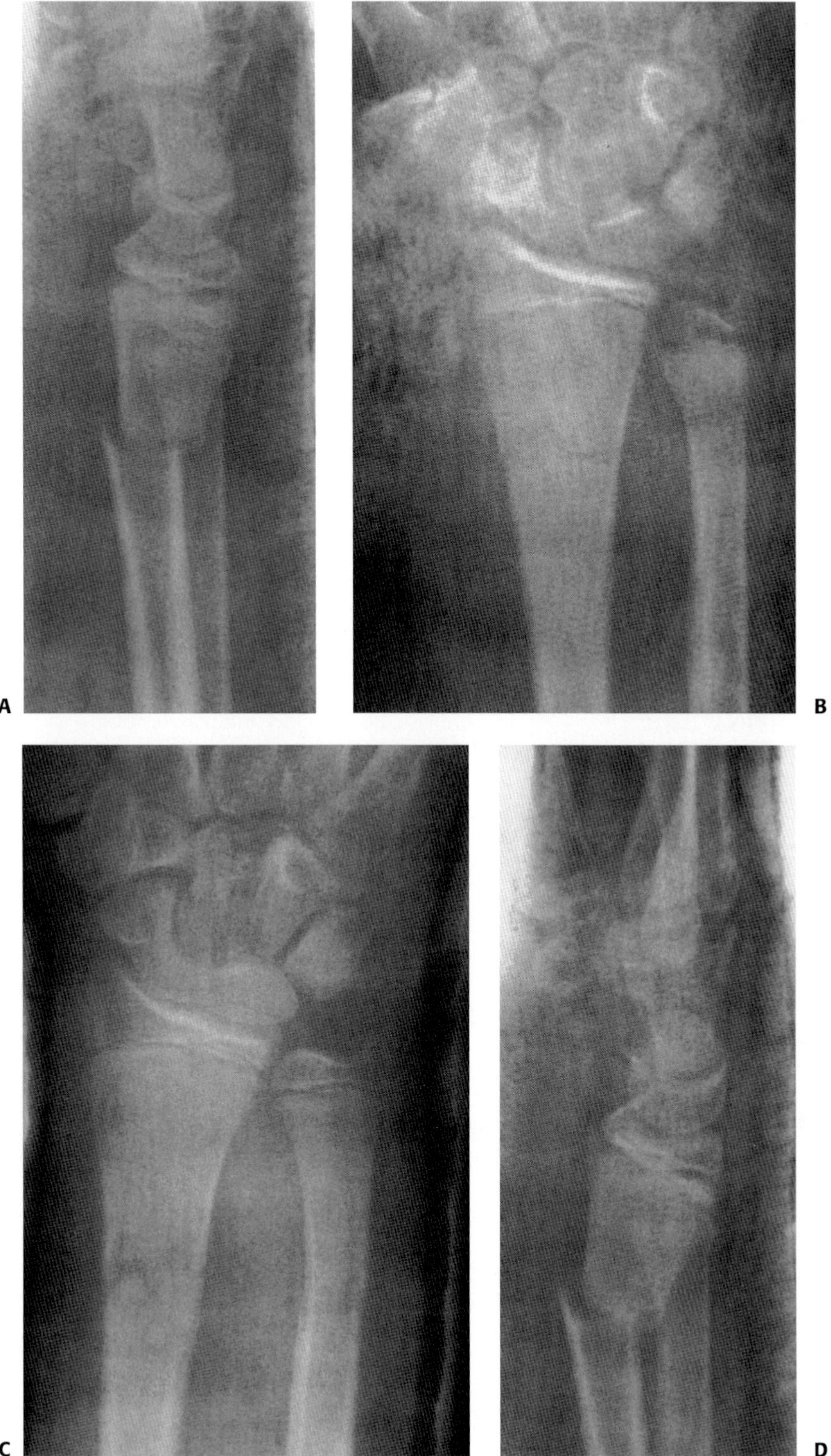

FIGURE 9-38 Serial x-rays at 3 days **(A)** and 10 days **(B)** revealing slow loss of reduction that is common after closed reduction of distal radial metaphyseal fractures.

TABLE 9-3 Acceptable Angular Corrections in Degrees

	Saggital Plane		
Age (yr)	Boys	Girls	Frontal Plane
4–9	20	15	15
9–11	15	10	5
11–13	10	10	0
>13	5	0	0

Acceptable residual angulation is that which will result in total radiographic and functional correction. (Courtesy B. deCourtivron, MD. Centre Hospitalie Universitaire de Tours. Tours, France.)

a young patient who can wiggle out of a short-arm cast and closer follow-up generally are recommended to lessen the risk of malunion. These fractures generally heal in 3 to 6 weeks.

Incomplete/Greenstick Fractures

Immobilization Alone. Treatment of incomplete distal radial and ulnar fractures depends on the age of the patient, the degree and direction of fracture displacement and angulation, the surgeon's biases regarding remodeling, and the surgeon's and community's biases regarding deformity. In younger patients, the remodeling potential of an acute distal radial malunion is extremely high. Acceptable sagittal plane angulation of an acute distal radial metaphyseal fracture has been reported to be from 10 to 35 degrees in patients under 5 years of age (124,130, 148–152). Similarly, in patients under 10 years of age, the degree of acceptable angulation has ranged from 10 to 25 degrees (124,130,148–152). In patients over 10 years of age, acceptable alignment has ranged from 5 to 20 degrees depending on the skeletal maturity of the patient (Table 9-3) (40,124,130, 148–153).

The high potential for remodeling of a distal radial metaphyseal malunion has led some clinicians to recommend immobilization alone. As mentioned, the range of accepted sagittal malalignment has been broad and is age and clinician dependent (Figs. 9-39 and 9-40).

Acceptable frontal plane deformity has been more uniform. The fracture tends to displace radially with an apex ulnar angulation. This does have the potential to remodel (154), but less so than sagittal plane deformity. Most researchers agree that only 10 degrees or less of acute malalignment in the frontal plane should be accepted. More malalignment than this may not remodel and may result in loss of forearm rotation because of the loss of interosseous space between the radius and ulna (Table 9-3) (155).

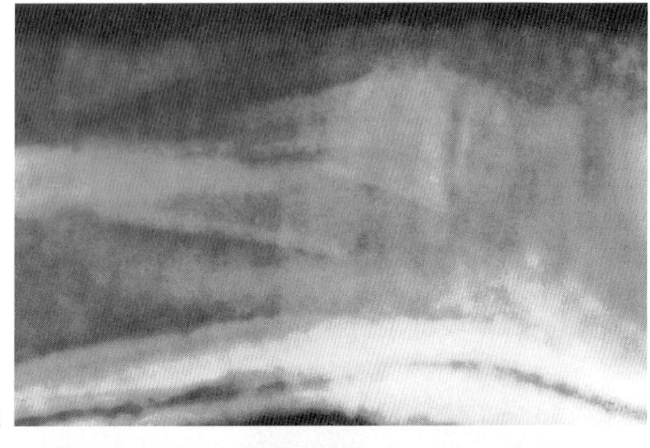
A

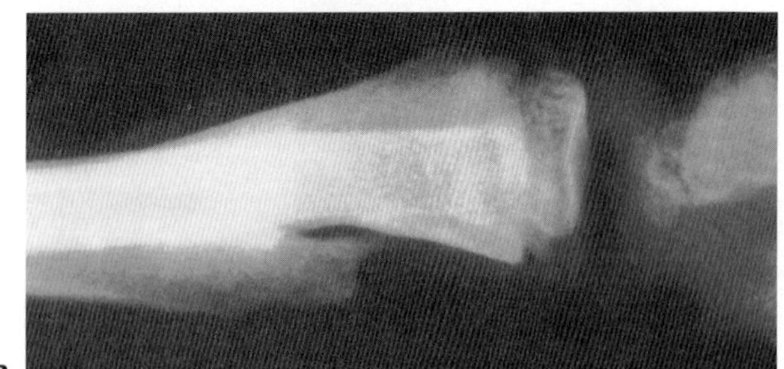
B

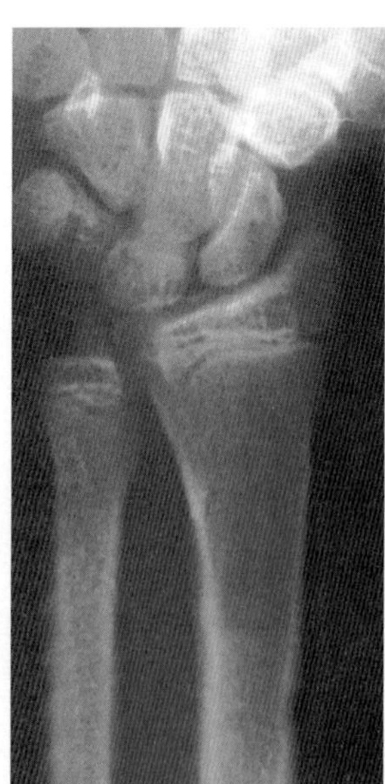
C

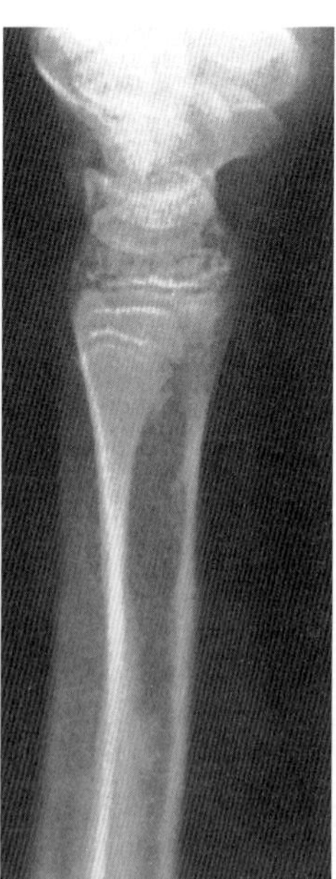
D

FIGURE 9-39 Bayonet remodeling. **A.** After numerous attempts at closed reduction, the best alignment that could be obtained was dorsal bayonet apposition in this 8-year-old. **B.** Three months after fracture, there is good healing and early remodeling. **C,D.** Five years after the injury (age 13), remodeling was complete and the patient had normal appearance and forearm motion.

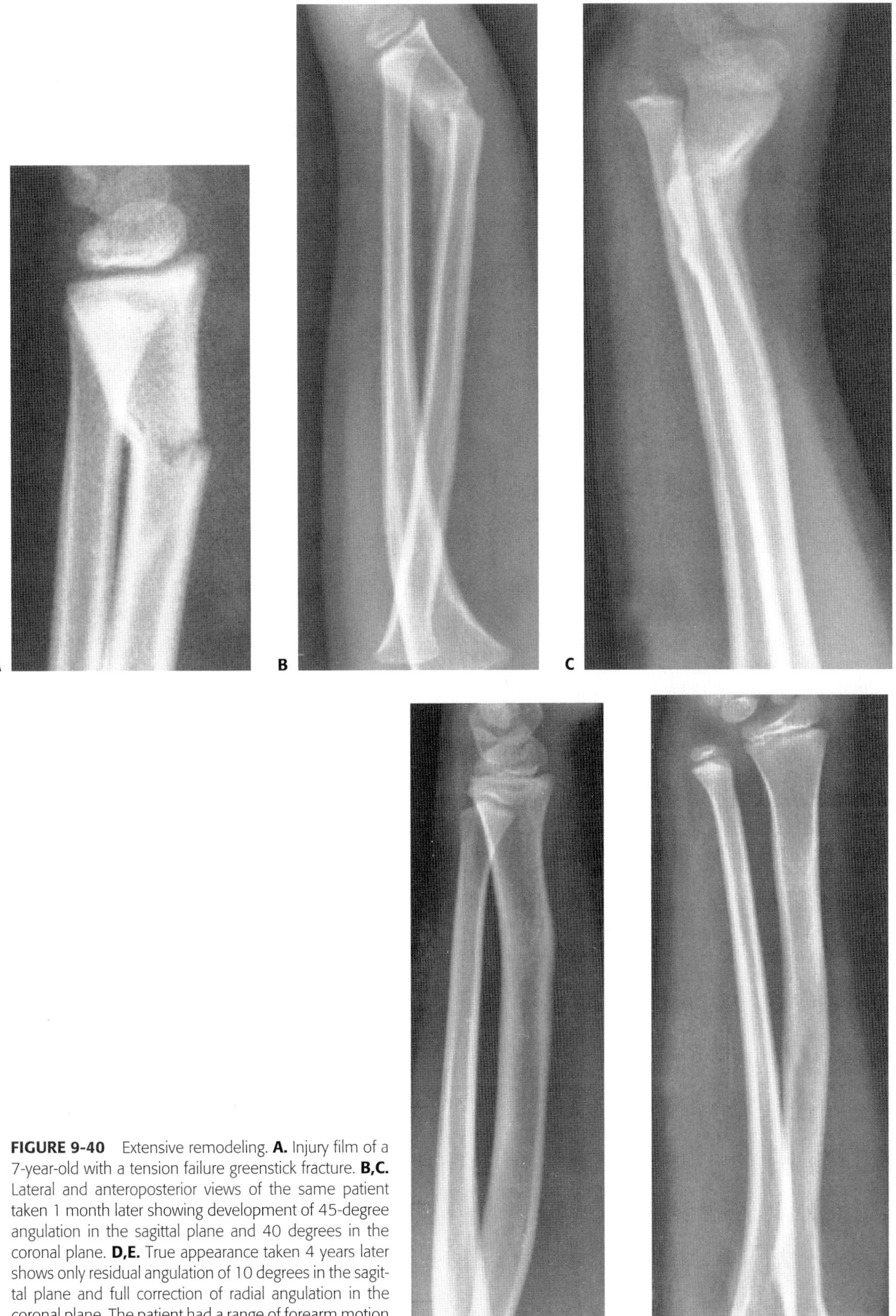

FIGURE 9-40 Extensive remodeling. **A.** Injury film of a 7-year-old with a tension failure greenstick fracture. **B,C.** Lateral and anteroposterior views of the same patient taken 1 month later showing development of 45-degree angulation in the sagittal plane and 40 degrees in the coronal plane. **D,E.** True appearance taken 4 years later shows only residual angulation of 10 degrees in the sagittal plane and full correction of radial angulation in the coronal plane. The patient had a range of forearm motion equal to that of the opposite extremity and was asymptomatic.

Closed Reduction. Most displaced and malaligned incomplete fractures should be reduced closed. The areas of controversy are the degree of acceptable deformity, whether the intact cortex should be fractured, and the position and type of immobilization.

Controversies about acceptable angulation of the fracture after closed reduction involve the same differences discussed in the immobilization section. As mentioned, more malalignment can be accepted in younger patients, in those with sagittal plane deformity, and in those without marked cosmetic deformity. Malaligned apex volar incomplete fractures are less obvious than the less common apex dorsal fractures.

As Evans (156) and Rang (79) emphasized, incomplete forearm fractures have a rotatory component to their malalignment. The more common apex volar fractures represent a supination deformity, whereas the less common apex dorsal fractures are malrotated in pronation. Correction of the malrotation is necessary to achieve anatomic alignment. Controversy exists regarding completion of greenstick fractures (5,79,157–159). Although many researchers advocate completion of the fracture to reduce the risk of subsequent loss of reduction from the intact periosteum and concave deformity acting as a tension band (130,160) to redisplace the fracture, completing the fracture increases the risk of instability and malunion.

The position and type of immobilization also have been controversial. Recommendations for the position of postreduction immobilization include supination, neutral, and pronation. The rationale for immobilization in pronation is that reduction of the more common apex volar fractures requires correction of the supination deformity (156). Following this rationale, apex dorsal fractures should be reduced and immobilized in supination. Pollen (152) believed that the brachioradialis was a deforming force in pronation and was relaxed in supination (Fig. 9-41) and advocated immobilization in supination for all displaced distal radial fractures. Kasser (92) recommended immobilization in slight supination to allow better molding of the volar distal radius. Some researchers advocate immobilization in a neutral position, believing this is best at maintaining the interosseous space and has the least risk of disabling loss of forearm rotation in the long term (150,161,162). Davis and Green (159) and Ogden (124) advocate that each fracture seek its own preferred position of stability. Gupta and Danielsson (88) randomized immobilization of distal radial metaphyseal greenstick fractures in neutral, supination, or pronation to try to determine the best position of immobilization. Their study showed a statistical improvement in final healing with immobilization in supination.

Another area of controversy is whether long-arm or short-arm cast immobilization is better. Most publications on pediatric distal radial fracture treatment advocate long-arm cast treatment for the first 3 to 4 weeks of healing (1,70,92,124,148,162). The rationale is that elbow flexion reduces the muscle forces acting to displace the fracture. In addition, a long-arm cast may further restrict the child's activity and therefore decrease the risk of displacement. However, Chess et al (89,90) reported

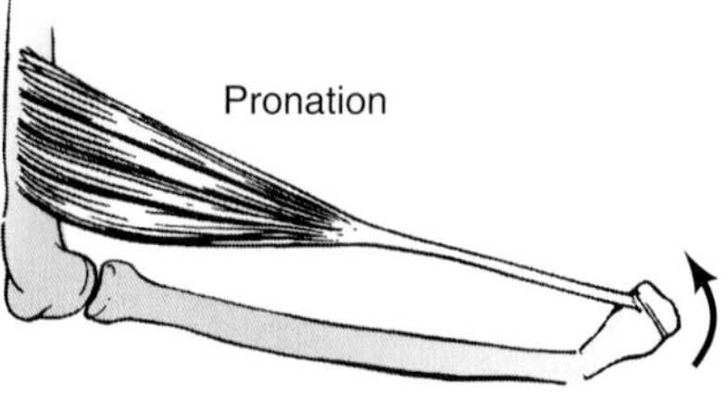

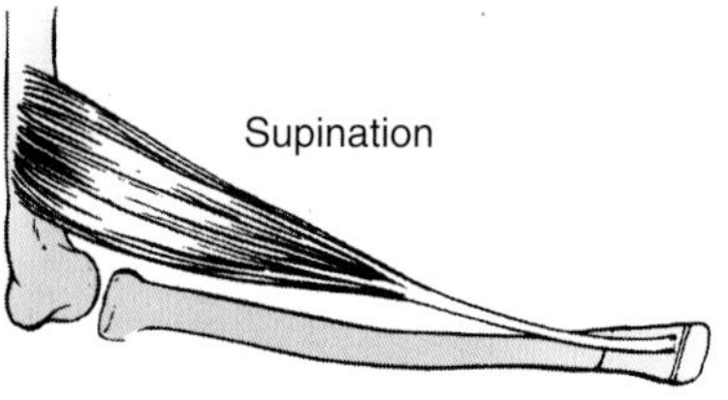

FIGURE 9-41 The brachioradialis is relaxed in supination but may become a deforming force in pronation. (Reprinted from Pollen AG. *Fractures and dislocations in children.* Baltimore: Williams & Wilkins, 1973; with permission.)

redisplacement and reduction rates with well-molded short-arm casts similar to those with long-arm casts. They used a cast index (sagittal diameter divided by coronal diameter at the fracture site) of 0.7 or less to indicate a well-molded cast. Wilkins achieved similar results with short-arm cast treatment (130). The short-arm cast offers the advantage of elbow mobility and better patient acceptance of casting. Despite these data and recommendations, in most centers the standard is long-arm cast immobilization (1,70,148,162,163).

COMPLETE FRACTURES

Complete fractures of the distal radius, with or without an associated displaced ulnar fracture, are unstable fractures. Generally these fractures are displaced dorsally, tearing the volar periosteum and soft-tissues. The distal fragment of epiphysis and metaphysis often is in bayonet apposition with the proximal fragment. Concomitant radial and ulnar fractures at the same level may be more unstable than isolated fractures (40). However, Gibbons reported loss of reduction in 91% of isolated radial fractures after closed reduction. Although a rare fracture with bayonet apposition in a very young patient may remodel (130), the standard treatment for completely displaced fractures is reduction and stabilization. The current controversy is whether cast immobilization alone is adequate stabilization or whether percutaneous pin fixation is more appropriate for displaced, complete, distal radial metaphyseal fractures (164–166).

Reduction Techniques

Techniques of reduction have included initial distraction with finger traps (159,160) followed by direct manipulation of the

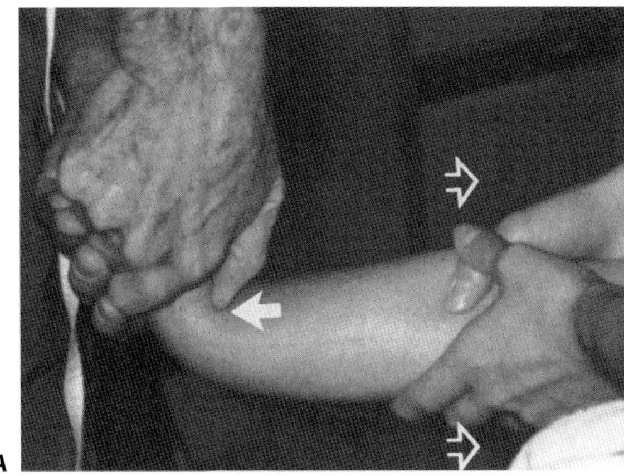

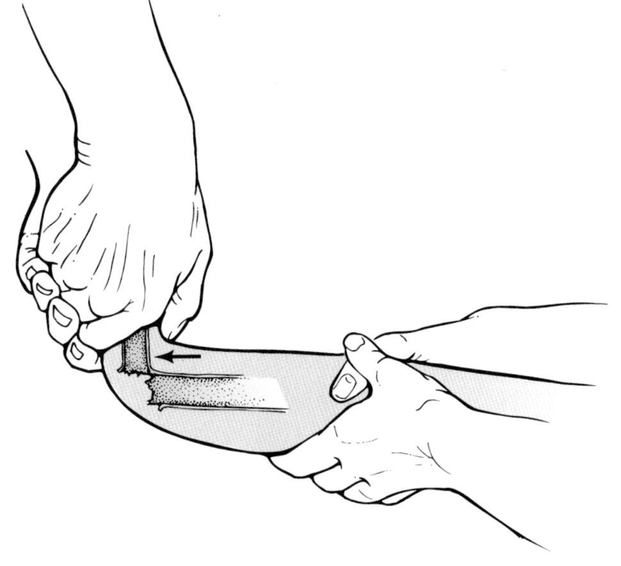

FIGURE 9-42 A,B. Use of the thumb to push the distal fragment hyperdorsiflexed 90 degrees (*solid arrow*) until length is reestablished. Countertraction is applied in the opposite direction (*open arrows*).

fracture by accentuating the deformity. Both Rang (79) and Fernandez (158) expressed concern about the success of finger trap distraction because the intact dorsal periosteum will not stretch adequately to allow reduction. They advocated sequential reduction maneuvers: initial manipulation of the distal fragment dorsally to accentuate the deformity (Fig. 9-42), thumb pressure on the relaxed dorsal edge of the distal fragment to correct the overriding, and reduction of the fracture by forcible application of distal and volar pressure (Fig. 9-43). Anatomic reduction may require repetitive "toggling" of the distal fragment volarly. Reduction is then assessed with fluoroscopic imaging (Fig. 9-44).

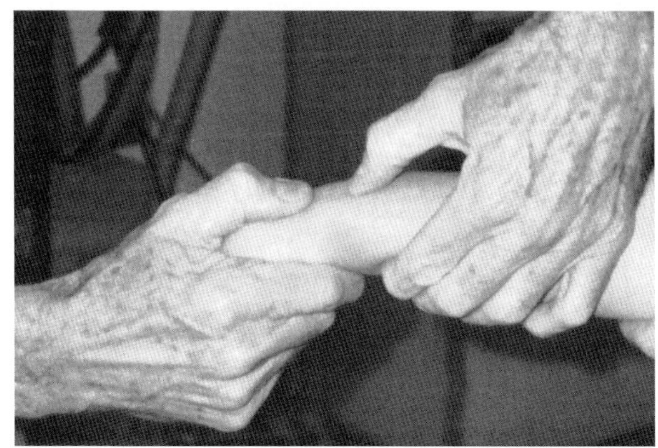

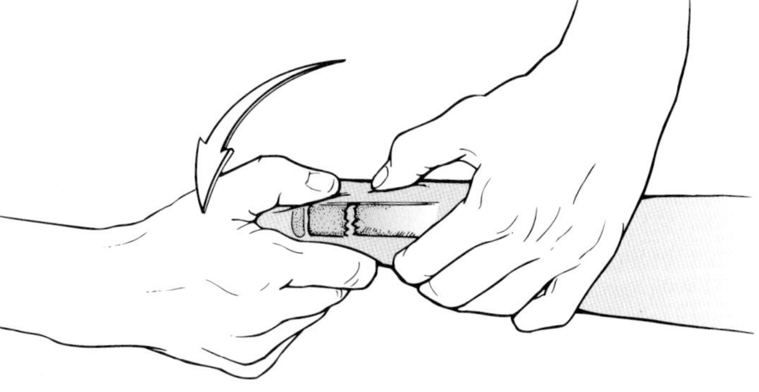

FIGURE 9-43 A,B. Once length has been reestablished, the distal fragment is flexed into the correct position. Alignment is checked by determining the position of the fragments with the thumb and forefingers of each hand.

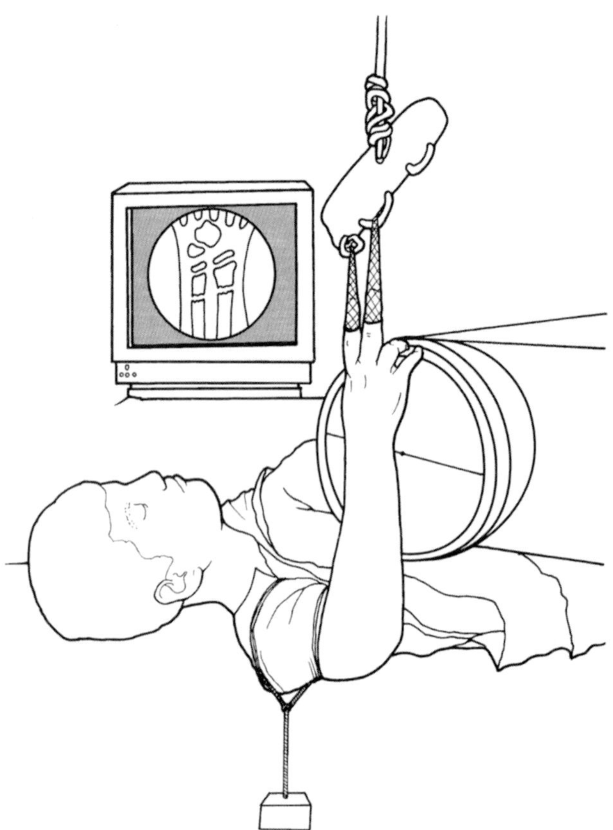

FIGURE 9-44 Once reduced, the fracture is maintained with finger trap traction and countertraction on the arm. The quality of reduction is assessed quickly with the image intensifier.

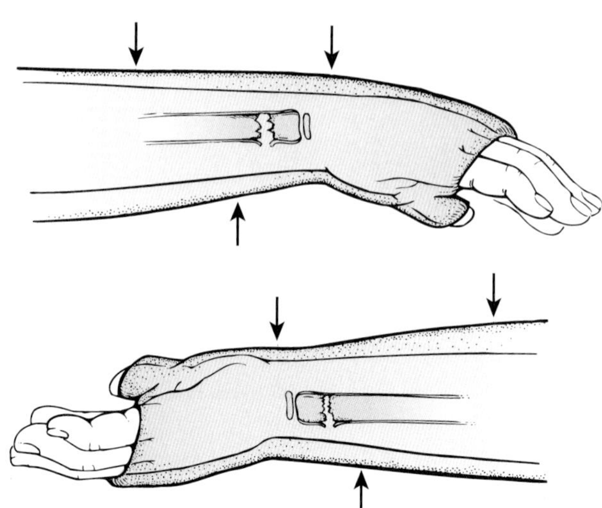

FIGURE 9-45 Three-point molding. **Top.** Three-point molding for dorsally angulated (apex volar) fractures, with the proximal and distal points on the dorsal aspect of the cast and the middle point on the volar aspect just proximal to the fracture site. **Bottom.** For volar angulated fractures, where the periosteum is intact volarly and disrupted on the dorsal surface, three-point molding is performed with the proximal and distal points on the volar surface of the cast and the middle point just proximal to the fracture site on the dorsal aspect of the cast.

There is considerable controversy about what constitutes an acceptable reduction (167–174). This is clearly age dependent, because the younger the patient, the greater the potential for remodeling. Volar-dorsal malalignment has the greatest potential for remodeling because this is in the plane of predominant motion of the joint. Marked radioulnar malalignment is less likely to remodel. Malrotation will not remodel. The ranges for acceptable reduction according to age are given in the immobilization section on incomplete fractures and apply to complete fractures as well.

Cast Immobilization

As discussed earlier, there is some disagreement regarding short-arm or long-arm cast immobilization (89,90,130). However, regardless of the length of the cast, it is imperative to have a well-molded cast over the fracture site (Fig. 9-45). After reduction of a dorsally displaced fracture, three-point fixation is used with dorsal pressure proximal and distal to the fracture site and volar pressure over the reduced fracture (Fig. 9-46). The cast should be molded to the normal contour of the forearm. An extension long-arm cast can be used in younger children to better maintain reduction of the ulnar bow. A thumb spica

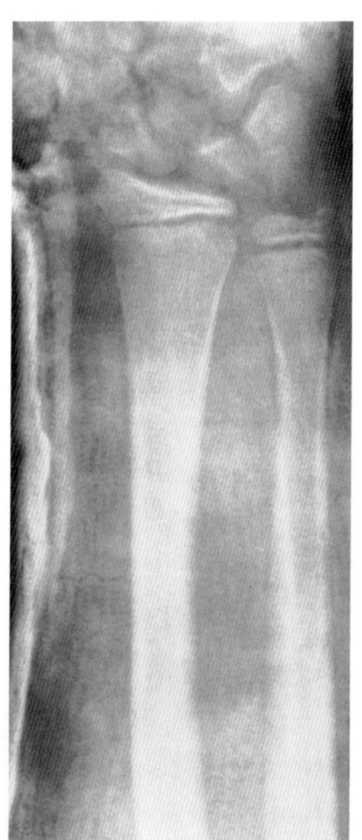

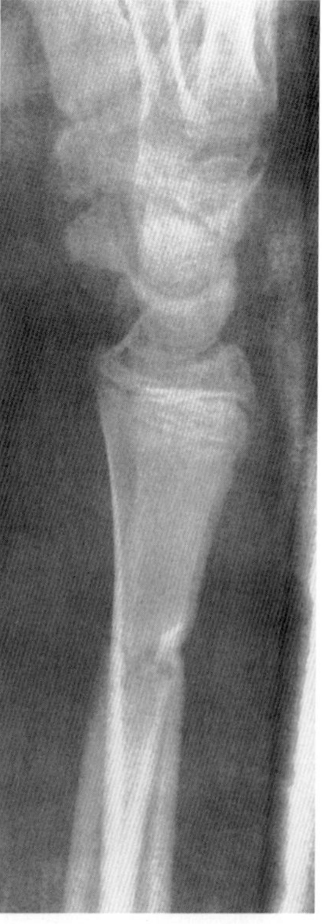

FIGURE 9-46 Anteroposterior and lateral x-rays of anatomic alignment with closed reduction of a distal radial metaphyseal fracture.

component with felt over the dorsum of the thumb and wrist prevents distal migration of cast and skin irritation. Excessive swelling should be monitored due to dependency of the hand. If there is any concern regarding impending compartment syndrome, the cast and Webril should be immediately bivalved and the patient's clinical status monitored closely. In general, closed reduction and well-molded casting will result in successful healing of the fracture in desired alignment (Fig. 9-47).

The primary problem with closed reduction and cast immobilization is loss of reduction (Fig. 9-48). There are many studies that indicate an incidence of loss of reduction in the 20% to 30% range (Fig. 9-48) (38,39,166). Mani et al (38) and Proctor et al (39) described remanipulation rates of 21% and 23%, respectively. Mani et al (38) concluded that initial displacement of the radial shaft of over 50% was the single most reliable predictor of failure of reduction. Proctor et al (39) found that complete initial displacement resulted in a 52% incidence of redisplacement of distal radial fractures in children. Gibbons et al (41) noted that completely displaced distal radial fractures with intact ulnas had a remanipulation rate of 91% after closed reduction and cast immobilization alone compared to a 0% rate of remanipulation when the same fractures were treated with closed reduction, Kirschner wire fixation, and cast immobilization. All three researchers strongly advocated percutaneous pinning of distal radial fractures at risk of redisplacement. Widmann and Waters (40) prospectively studied all distal radial fractures in children requiring reduction over the course of 1 year. Of the 86 distal radial metaphyseal fractures, 31% lost reduction and required further intervention with repeat reduction, casting, or pinning. In patients over 10 years of age with angulation of more than 30 degrees, the remanipulation rate was 75%. These findings led to a prospective, randomized study by Miller et al (175) of distal radial metaphyseal fractures treated by either closed reduction and cast immobilization or closed reduction and percutaneous pinning. Selection criteria were a closed metaphyseal fracture angulated more than 30° in a skeletally immature patient over 10 years of age. To maximize the outcome of the cast immobilization group, these patients were treated by a member of the Pediatric Orthopedic Society of North America with expertise in trauma care. General anesthesia, fluoroscopic control, and a long-arm cast were used. Despite these optimal conditions, 30% of the patients in the cast immobilization group lost reduction and required remanipulation. These findings were similar to McLaughlin's prospective study of pinning and cast treatment of distal radius metaphyseal fractures (166). Again, closed reduction and cast immobilization had a loss of reduction rate of 21% whereas pinning maintained reduction. The authors of these prospective, randomized studies concluded that pinning is a safe effective means of treating distal radial metaphyseal fractures.

The results of all of these studies indicate that distal radial metaphyseal fractures with initial displacement of more than

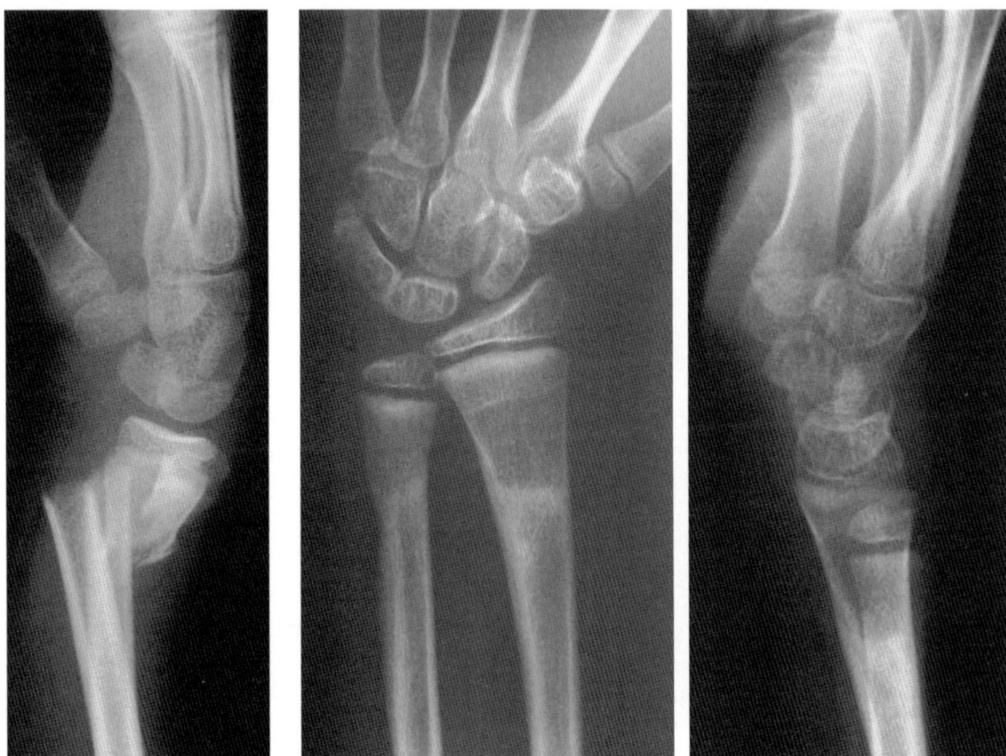

FIGURE 9-47 **A.** Lateral x-ray of displaced metaphyseal radial and ulnae fractures. **B.** Anteroposterior and lateral x-rays show anatomic alignment after closed reduction.

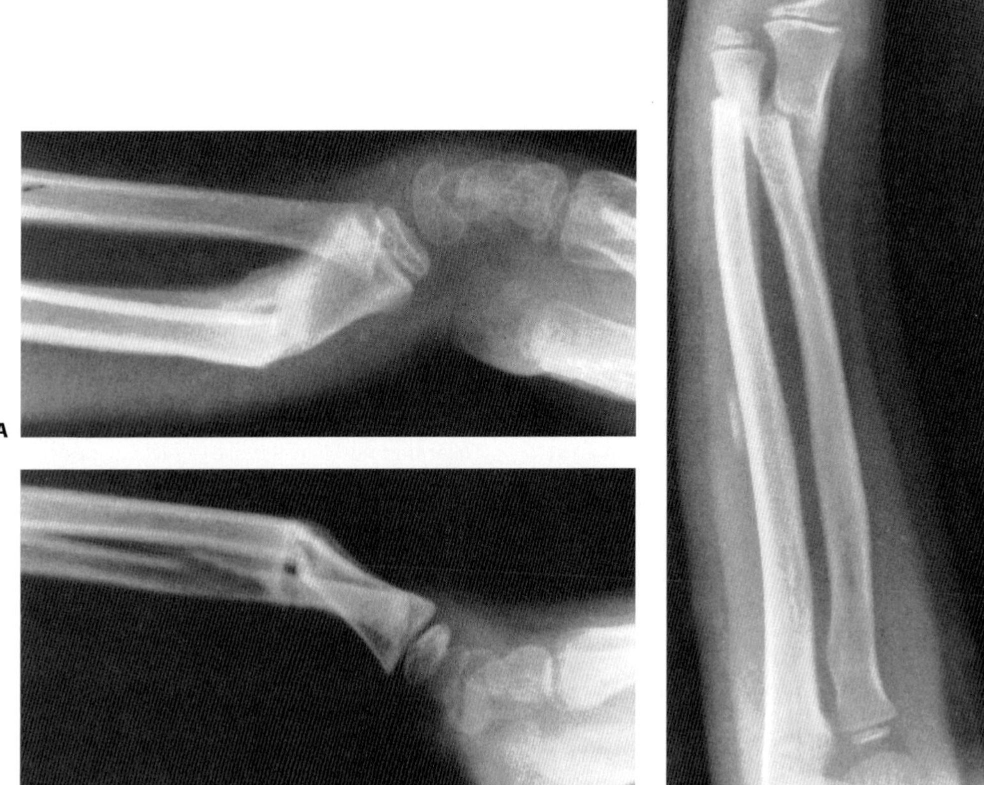

FIGURE 9-48 Results of angulation. **A.** Significant apex volar angulation of the distal fragment. **B.** The appearance was not as apparent cosmetically as in another patient with less angulation that was directed apex dorsally. (Reprinted from Wilkins KE, ed. *Operative management of upper extremity fractures in children.* Rosemont, IL: American Academy of Orthopaedic Surgeons, 1994:27; with permission.) **C.** Radial deviation constricts the interosseous space, which may decrease forearm rotation. (Reprinted from Wilkins KE, ed. *Operative management of upper extremity fractures in children.* Rosemont, IL: American Academy of Orthopaedic Surgeons, 1994:28; with permission.)

30 degrees are inherently unstable. Loss of reduction is common, with the risk in the 20%-to-60% range. Incomplete reduction (38,39) and poor casting techniques (89,90,130) increase the risk of loss of reduction. In addition, the risk of loss of reduction increases with the age of the patient and the degree of initial displacement. Bayonet apposition in a child older than 10 years is the highest risk.

Loss of reduction requires repeat manipulation to avoid a malunion. Although the rate of malunion is frequent after these fractures (70,72,75,76,89,90,92,93,159,176,177), because of the potential for remodeling in skeletally immature patients it has not been considered a serious problem (Fig. 9-49) (43,64,65,148,168,169,178). Distal radial fractures are juxtaphyseal, the malunion often is in the plane of motion of the wrist joint (dorsal displacement with apex volar angulation), and the distal radius accounts for 60% to 80% of the growth of the radius. All these factors favor remodeling of a malunion. However, De Courtivron et al (153) reported that of 602 distal radial fractures, 14% had an initial malunion of more than 5 degrees. Of these, 78% corrected the frontal plane deformity and only 53% remodeled completely in the sagittal plane. In addition, 37% had loss of forearm rotation.

Closed Reduction and Percutaneous Pinning

In the past decade or two, closed reduction and percutaneous pinning have become more common as the primary treatment of distal radial metaphyseal fractures in children and adolescents (38–40,42,179). The indications cited include fracture instability and high risk of loss of reduction (38,39,179), excessive local swelling that increases the risk of neurovascular compromise (31,42,130), ipsilateral fractures of the distal radius and elbow region (floating elbow) that increase the risk of compartment syndrome (133,155), and the likelihood that remanipulation

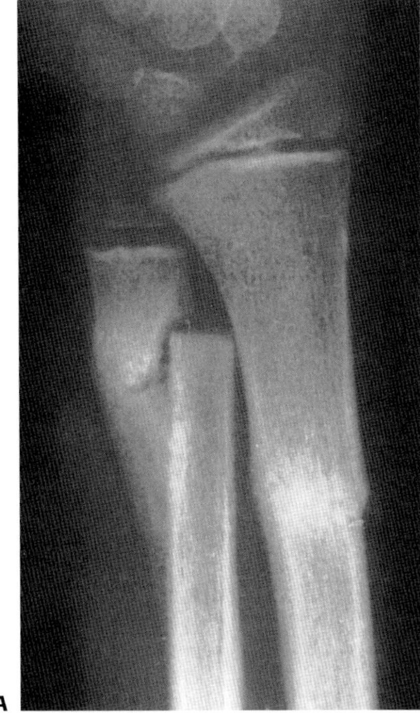

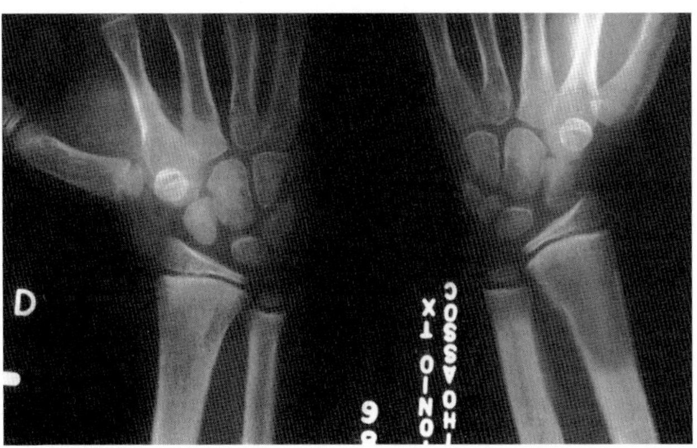

FIGURE 9-49 **A.** Appearance 6 weeks after closed reduction of a distal forearm fracture in an 8½-year-old boy. The radius was reduced, and the ulnar fracture remained overriding. **B.** Eighteen months after injury the ulnar fracture had remodeled completely with symmetric distal radioulnar joints.

will be required (40,130). In addition, surgeon's preference for pinning in a busy office practice has been considered acceptable due to similar complication rates and long-term outcomes with pinning and casting (166,175) obviating the need for remanipulation as alignment is secure.

Pinning usually is done from distal to proximal under fluoroscopic guidance. When possible, the physis is avoided. Adequate exposure should be obtained to avoid radial sensory nerve or extensor tendon injury. Smooth Kirschner or C-wires are used. In younger patients, a single pin with supplemental cast immobilization may be adequate fixation (Fig 9-50). Crossed pins are more stable (Fig. 9-51). The first pin, or single pin, enters from the radial side distal to the fracture and passes obliquely to the ulnar aspect of the radius proximal to the frac-

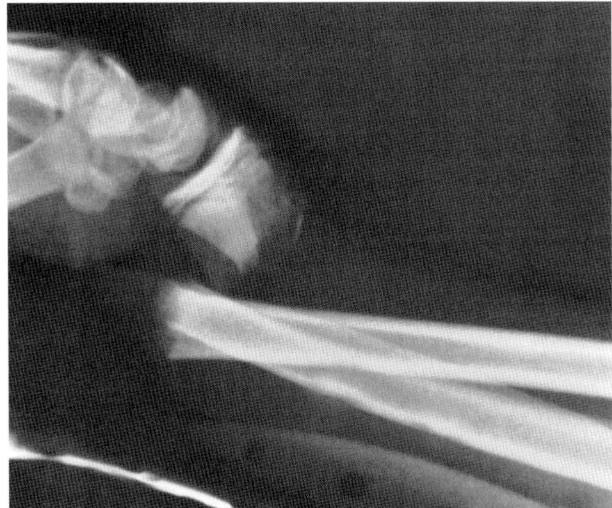

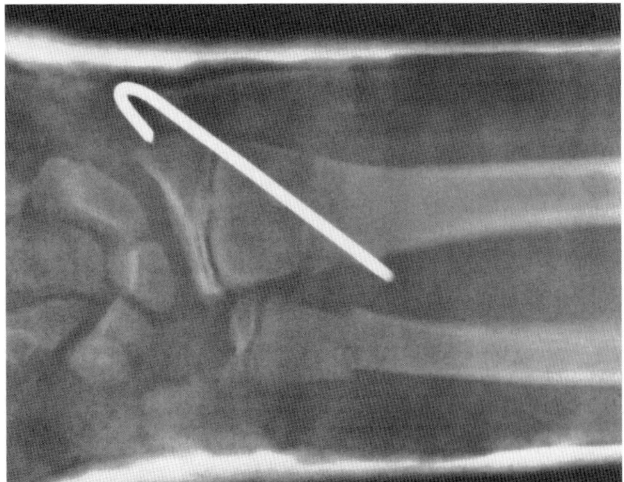

FIGURE 9-50 Severe swelling. **A.** An 11-year-old with marked displacement and severe swelling from a high-energy injury. **B.** Once reduced, the fragment was secured with an oblique percutaneous pin across the fracture site. (Reprinted from Wilkins KE, ed. *Operative management of upper extremity fractures in children.* Rosemont, IL: American Academy of Orthopaedic Surgeons, 1994:29, with permission.)

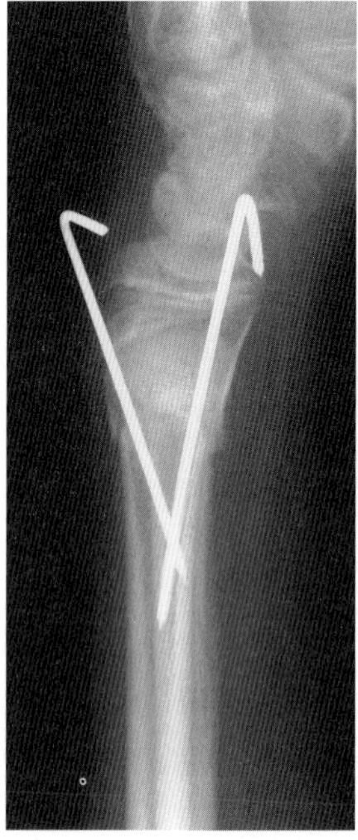
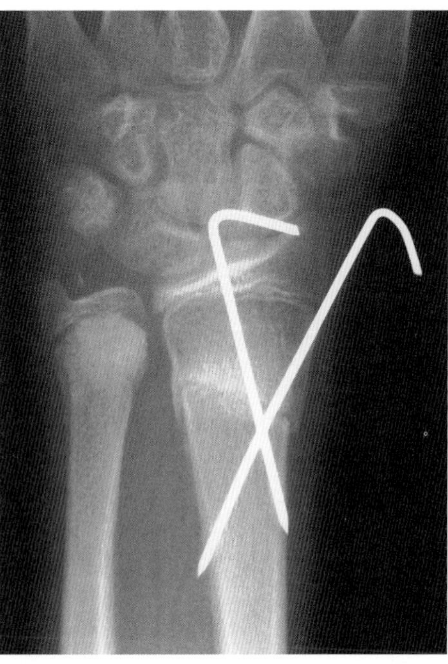

FIGURE 9-51 Crossed pin technique for stabilization of distal radial metaphyseal fracture in skeletally immature patient.

ture. The second pin enters the radius distal to the fracture between the fourth and fifth compartments and passes obliquely across the fracture into the proximal radial side of the radius. The pins are left out through the skin to allow easy removal. Another technique of pinning is intrafocal placement of multiple pins into the fracture site to lever the distal fragment into anatomic reduction (Kapandji technique, Fig. 9-52). The pins are then passed through the opposing cortex for stability (180,181). A supplemental, loose-fitting cast is applied. The advantage of pin fixation is that a tight, well-molded cast is not necessary to maintain reduction. This lessens the risk of neurovascular compromise with associated excessive swelling or ipsilateral fractures. Obviously, pin fixation avoids the risk of loss of reduction in an unstable fracture. Pinning does have the risk of infection and concerns regarding growth injury.

External Fixation

Unlike distal radial fractures in adults, external fixation rarely is indicated for similar fractures in skeletally immature patients. Although it can be used successfully (176,182), the success rates of both closed reduction and percutaneous pinning techniques make it unnecessary for uncomplicated distal radial fractures in children. The best indication is severe associated soft-tissue injuries. A severe crush injury, open fracture, or replantation after amputation that requires extensive soft-tissue care and surgery are all indications for the use of external fixation. Supplemental external fixation also may be necessary for severely comminuted fractures to maintain length and provide additional stability to pin fixation. Standard application of the specific fixator chosen is done with care to avoid injury to the adjacent sensory nerves and extensor tendons.

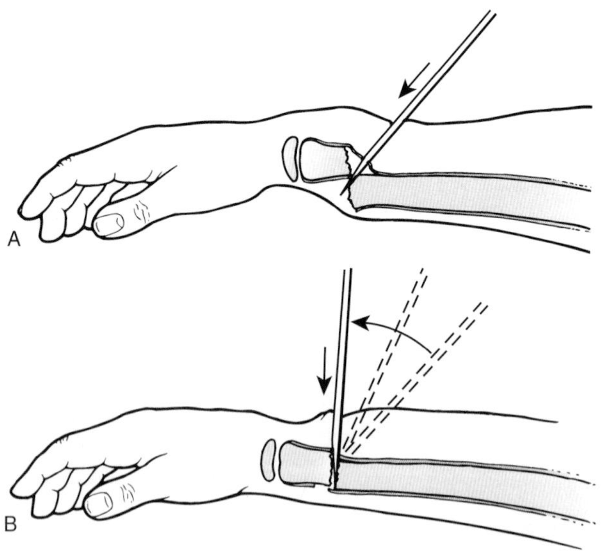

FIGURE 9-52 Pin leverage. **A.** If a bayonet is irreducible, after sterile preparation, a chisel-point Steinmann pin can be inserted between the fracture fragments from a dorsal approach. Care must be taken not to penetrate too deeply past the dorsal cortex of the proximal fragment. **B.** Once the chisel is across the fracture site, it is levered into position and supplementary pressure is placed on the dorsum of the distal fragment (*arrow*) to slide it down the skid into place. This procedure is usually performed with an image intensifier.

Open Reduction

Open reduction is indicated for open or irreducible fractures. Open fractures constitute approximately 1% of all distal radial metaphyseal fractures. All open fractures, regardless of grade of soft-tissue injury, should be irrigated and debrided in the operating room (Fig. 9-53). The open wound should be enlarged adequately to debride the contaminated and nonviable tissues and protect the adjacent neurovascular structures. After thorough irrigation and debridement, the fracture should be anatomically reduced and stabilized, usually with two smooth pins. If the soft-tissue injury is severe, supplemental external fixation allows observation and treatment of the wound without jeopardizing the fracture reduction. The original open wound should not be closed primarily. Appropriate prophylactic antibiotics should be used depending on the severity of the open fracture.

Irreducible fractures are rare (Fig. 9-54) and generally are secondary to interposed soft-tissues. With dorsally displaced fractures, the interposed structure usually is the volar periosteum or pronator quadratus (183) and rarely the flexor tendons or neurovascular structures. In volarly displaced fractures, the periosteum or extensor tendons may be interposed. The fracture should be approached in a standard fashion opposite the side of displacement (i.e., volar approach for an irreducible dorsal fracture). The adjacent neurovascular and tendinous structures are protected and the offending soft-tissue is extracted from the fracture site. Pin stabilization is recommended to prevent problems with postoperative swelling or loss of reduction in cast.

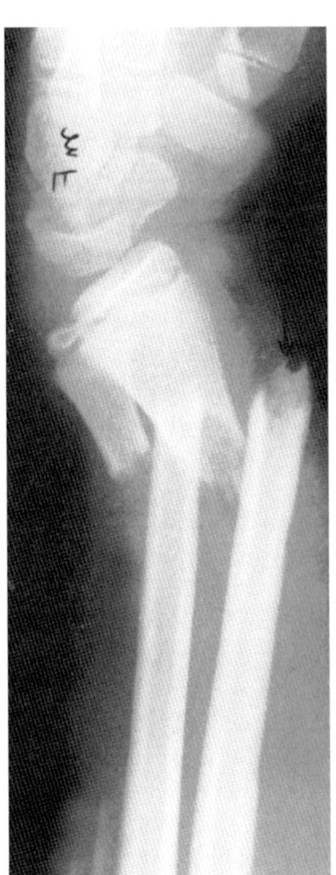

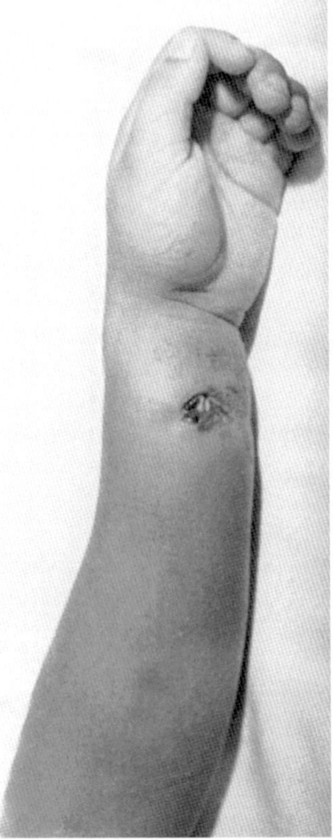

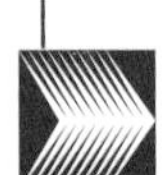

A B

FIGURE 9-53 Open fractures. X-ray **(A)** and clinical photo **(B)** of an open fracture of the distal radius. This patient needs formal irrigation and debridement in the operating room.

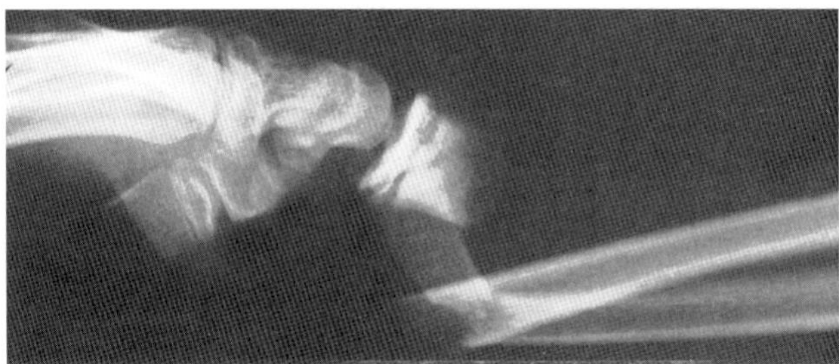

FIGURE 9-54 A 10-year-old girl with a markedly displaced closed fracture of the distal radius with an angulated ulnar fracture. Note the wide separation between the radial fragments. Dimpling of the skin was noted when longitudinal traction was applied and reduction was impossible. At open reduction, the proximal fragment was buttonholed through the forearm fascia and located between the median nerve and finger flexor tendons. The pronator quadratus muscle was also interposed between the two fragments.

Closed reduction rarely fails if there is no interposed soft-tissue. However, occasionally multiple attempts at reduction of a bayonet apposition fracture can lead to significant swelling that makes closed reduction impossible. If the patient is too old to remodel bayonet apposition, open reduction is appropriate. Pin fixation without violating the physis is recommended. Plate fixation can be used in more skeletally mature adolescents. Low profile, fragment specific fixation methods and locking plates also are now commonly used in adult distal radius fractures for internal fixation.

AUTHORS' PREFERRED METHOD OF TREATMENT

Nondisplaced Fractures

Nondisplaced metaphyseal compression fractures, including torus and unicortical compression greenstick fractures, are inherently stable. These include torus and unicortical compression greenstick fractures. Immobilization is used until resolution of pain and x-ray evidence of healing, generally about 3 weeks. Depending on the activity level of the patient, a volar wrist splint or a short-arm cast can be used. Immobilization provides comfort from pain during healing and protects against displacement with secondary injury. It is important that an unstable bicortical fracture not be unrecognized on x-ray. Bicortical fractures need more protection, longer restriction of activity, and closer follow-up to avoid displacement and malunion. A well-molded short- or long-arm cast is applied and x-rays obtained every 7 to 10 days until evidence of early healing is seen. A short-arm cast is then worn until clinical and x-ray healing is complete. Any loss of reduction is treated with repeat reduction. Return to contact sports is restricted until the patient regains full motion and strength.

Minimally Displaced Fractures

Displaced greenstick fractures that are reduced are at risk for redisplacement. If left unreduced or poorly immobilized, a mild deformity can become severe during the course of healing. Therefore, closed anatomic reduction is performed in all bicortical fractures with more than 10 degrees of malalignment. Generally these fractures have apex volar angulation and dorsal displacement. Conscious sedation is used with portable fluoroscopy in the emergency care setting. The distal fragment and hand are distracted and then reduced volarly. With isolated distal radial fractures, it is imperative to reduce the distal radioulnar joint (DRUJ) with appropriate forearm rotation. For apex volar fractures, this usually is with pronation. If the fracture is apex dorsal with volar displacement, the reduction forces are the opposite. A long-arm cast with three-point molding is used for 3 to 4 weeks. X-rays are obtained every 7 to 10 days until there is sufficient callus formation. A short-arm cast or volar wrist splint is used until full healing, generally at 4 to 6 weeks after fracture reduction. The patient is then restricted from contact sports until full motion and strength are regained, which may take up to 3 weeks after cast removal. Formal therapy rarely is required. The patient and parents should be warned at the start of treatment of the risk of redisplacement of the fracture.

Bayonet Apposition

Marked displacement of distal radial metaphyseal fractures usually results in foreshortening and dorsal overlap of the distal fragment on the proximal fragment. This often is associated with a same-level ulnar metaphyseal fracture, similarly in bayonet apposition. Rarely, the distal fragment is in volar bayonet apposition. Both of these situations require more skill of reduction and complete analgesia at the fracture site. At our institution, we reduce this fracture in the emergency room with conscious sedation and supplemental local hematoma block or in the operating room with general anesthesia. In either situation, portable fluoroscopy is used. The fracture usually is reduced in the emergency room in young patients with minimal swelling and no neurovascular compromise and in whom cast treatment will be sufficient. Reduction with general anesthesia is preferred for older patients and for those with marked displacement, swelling, or associated neurovascular compromise in whom percutaneous pin treatment is chosen.

The reduction maneuver is the same regardless of anesthesia type or stabilization method. As opposed to a Colles' fracture in an adult, traction alone will not reduce the fracture because the dorsal periosteum acts as a tension band that does not respond to increasing linear traction with weights. Finger traps with minimal weight (less than 10 lb) can be used to balance the hand and help with rotational alignment (the "steel resident") (see Fig. 9-59). However, applying progressive weight will only distract the carpus and will not alter the fracture alignment.

After applying preliminary traction with either light-weight finger traps or hand traction, a hyperdorsiflexion maneuver is performed. The initial deformity is accentuated and the distal fragment is brought into marked dorsiflexion. The dorsum of the hand should be brought more than 90 degrees and at times parallel to the dorsum of the forearm to lessen the tension on the dorsal forearm. Thumb pressure is used on the distal fragment while still in this deformed position to restore length by bringing the distal fragment beyond the proximal fragment. Reduction is then obtained by flexing the distal fragment while maintaining length. Often this initial reduction maneuver restores length and alignment, but translational reduction is incomplete. The fracture should be completely reduced by toggling the distal fragment all the way volarly by repetitive slight dorsiflexion positioning of the distal fragment followed by volar pressure with the thumbs. It is important to anatomically reduce the fracture. Loss of reduction with cast immobilization is more likely if the fracture remains translated or malaligned.

If the patient presents late with marked swelling and the reduction is difficult, it is useful to try to lever the proximal fragment distally with a percutaneous smooth wire(s). This may prevent an unnecessary open reduction. Percutaneous pin fixation is used after reduction, either by standard pinning or intrafocal techniques.

Cast Treatment

If the patient is under 10 years of age, has no prereduction signs or symptoms of neurovascular impairment, or has minimal swelling, then cast immobilization is used. We use a long-arm cast. The cast is applied with the aid either of an assistant or finger traps and balancing counter weights on the upper arm. The advantage of the finger-trap steel resident is that there is no risk of muscle fatigue, mental distraction, or failure to maintain elbow flexion at 90 degrees that can occur with a human assistant. The cast is applied with the elbow flexed 90 degrees, the wrist in slight palmar flexion, and the forearm in the desired rotation for stability and alignment. This varies with each fracture and each surgeon. Our preference is slight supination (20 to 30 degrees) unless the fracture dictates differently. This allows excellent molding against the volar aspect of the distal radius at the fracture site.

One of the most important elements in a successful long-arm cast for a forearm fracture is the application of the Webril. The Webril should be applied in a continuous roll with overlap of one-third to one-half its width. Extra padding is applied over the olecranon, along the volar and dorsal forearm where the cast may have to be split, and at the ends of the cast to prevent irritation from fraying. Plaster of Paris is used for the cast to obtain the best mold possible. Initially a single layer is applied, followed by splints five layers thick along the volar and dorsal forearm and the extension region of the elbow. This lessens the bulk of the cast and still allows deep molds. The cast is completed with plaster of Paris rolls over the splints. A three-point mold is applied at the fracture site as the cast hardens. In addition, molds are applied to maintain a straight ulnar border, the interosseous space, and straight posterior humeral line. This creates the classic "box" long-arm cast rather than the all too frequent "banana" cast that allows displacement. Final x-rays are obtained, and if the reduction is anatomic, the cast is overwrapped with fiberglass to lessen the weight, increase patient satisfaction, and prevent cast breakdown that could lead to loss of reduction.

Patients are either discharged or admitted to the hospital depending on the degree of concern regarding risk of excessive swelling, neurovascular compromise, and patient and parental reliability. If there is any doubt, the patient is admitted for observation. The cast is split anytime there are signs of neurovascular compromise. The patient is instructed to maintain elevation for at least 48 to 72 hours after discharge and return immediately if excessive swelling or neurovascular compromise occurs. The patient and family are warned of the risk of loss of reduction and the need for close follow-up. We inform our patients and parents that the risk of return to the day surgery unit for repeat reduction or pinning is approximately 20% to 30% during the first 3 weeks.

Follow-up examinations and x-rays are obtained every 7 to 10 days for 3 weeks. If there is loss of reduction, we individualize treatment depending on the patient's age, degree of deformity, time since fracture, and remodeling potential. If restoration of alignment with growth occurs, we reassure the family that the child should achieve anatomic alignment over time with growth. If the child is older, there is risk of further displacement, or the deformity is marked, repeat reduction is done in the day surgery unit with fluoroscopy. Most often, a percutaneous pin is used for the second reduction (Fig. 9-55).

Cast immobilization usually is for 4 to 6 weeks. The long-arm cast is changed to a short-arm cast at 3 to 4 weeks. With clinical and x-ray healing, a protective volar splint is used and activities are restricted until the patient regains full motion and strength, usually in 1 to 3 weeks after cast removal. As with other distal radial fractures, formal physical therapy rarely is required.

Percutaneous Pin Fixation

Percutaneous pinning of distal radial metaphyseal fractures is most often used in patients with excessive swelling or signs of neurologic injury. In these situations, the patient is at risk for

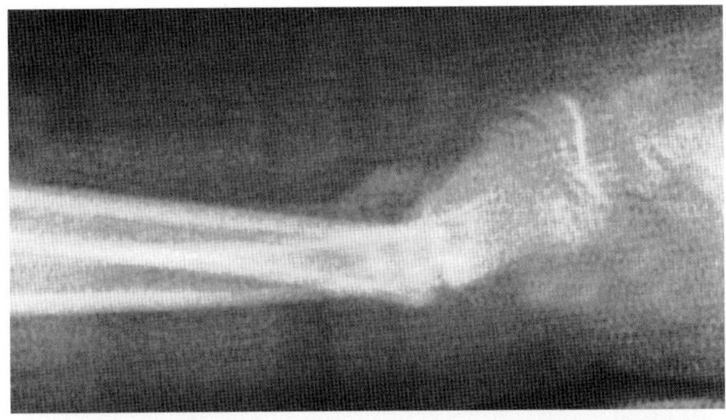

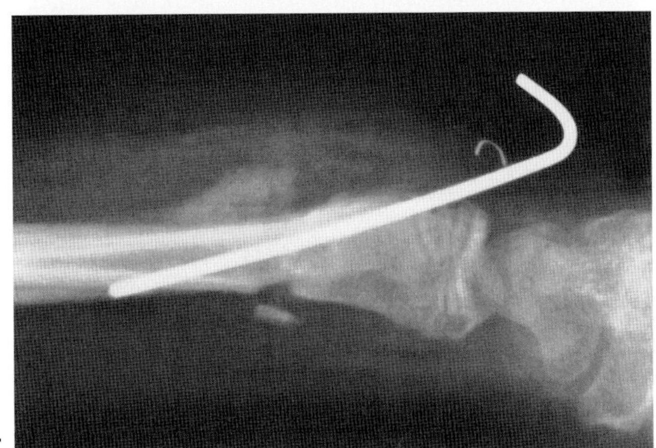

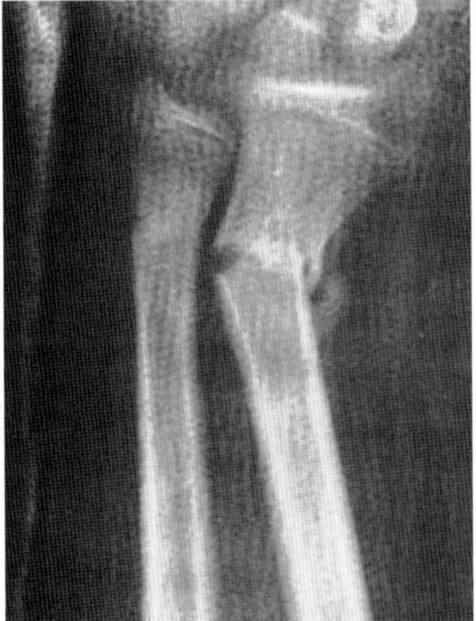

FIGURE 9-55 Remanipulation. **A,B.** Two weeks after what initially appeared to be an undisplaced greenstick fracture, a 14-year-old boy was found to have developed late angulation of 30 degrees in both the coronal and sagittal planes. **C.** Because this was beyond the limits of remodeling, a remanipulation was performed. To prevent reangulation, the fracture was secured with a pin placed percutaneously obliquely through the dorsal cortex.

development of a forearm or carpal tunnel compartment syndrome with a well-molded, tight-fitting cast. Similarly, concurrent displaced supracondylar and distal radial fractures are treated with percutaneous fixation of both fractures to lessen the risk of neurovascular compromise (Fig. 9-56). Older patients near the end of growth with bayonet apposition fractures also are treated with percutaneous pin fixation because they have less ability to remodel and their fractures are very unstable with a high risk of displacement. Finally, open fractures usually are treated with pin fixation.

The pinning technique for the radius is either a single radial-sided pin or crossed radial- and ulnar-sided pins. Fixation of the ulna rarely is necessary. Stability with a single pin is checked with fluoroscopy, and if further fixation is needed, a second pin is added. The physis is avoided if possible. Intrafocal pins are used if reduction is not possible without levering the distal fragment into a reduced position. A small incision is made for the insertion of each pin to protect the radial sensory nerve and adjacent extensor tendons. Smooth pins are used and are removed in the office as soon as there is sufficient healing to make the fracture stable in a cast or splint, usually at 4 weeks. Rehabilitation is similar to that for cast-treated fractures.

Open Reduction

The two most common indications for open reduction are an open fracture and an irreducible fracture. All open fractures are irrigated and debrided in the operating room. The initial open wound is extended adequately to inspect and cleanse the open fracture site. After thorough irrigation and debridement, the fracture is reduced and stabilized. A cast rarely is applied in this situation because of concern about fracture stability, soft-tissue care, and excessive swelling. Crossed-pin fixation often is used with Gustilo grade 1 or 2 open fractures. More severe soft-tissue injuries usually require external fixation with a unilateral frame, with care taken to avoid soft-tissue impingement during pin placement. If flap coverage is necessary for the soft-tissue wounds, the fixator pins should be placed in consultation with the microvascular surgeon planning the soft-tissue coverage.

Irreducible fractures usually are secondary to soft-tissue entrapment. With dorsal displacement, this is most often either the volar periosteum or pronator quadratus, and open reduction through a volar approach is necessary to extract the interposed soft-tissues and reduce the fracture (Fig. 9-57). Percutaneous pin fixation usually is used to stabilize the fracture in patients with open physes. If plate fixation is used, it should avoid violation of the physis (Fig. 9-58). Displaced intra-articular injuries in skeletally immature patients are adult-like and require standard treatment, such as open reduction and internal fixation (Fig. 9-59) or combination treatment with internal and external fixation. Lower profile plating has been used more recently to lessen the incidence of tendon irritation or disruption, especially of the plates that are placed dorsally (Fig. 9-60).

Complications

Distal radial metaphyseal fractures have complications similar to physeal fractures but with different frequencies. Loss of reduction and malunion are the most common problems, and growth-related complications are infrequent. Neurovascular compromise does occur and should be considered in the acute management of this fracture.

Malunion

Loss of reduction is a common complication of distal radial metaphyseal fractures treated with cast immobilization. Because this complication occurs in at least 30% of bayonet apposition fractures (38–42), many surgeons treat this fracture primarily with pin fixation to avoid the problems that can occur with malunion. Otherwise it is clear that patients treated with cast immobilization need to be monitored closely (184).

Fortunately, many angular malunions of the distal radius will remodel (28,114,124,148,154,159,160,168,169,171,173, 185,186) probably because of asymmetric physeal growth (171,187). True growth arrest associated with a distal radial metaphyseal fracture is very rare (188). The younger the patient, the less the deformity, and the closer the fracture is to the physis, the greater the potential for remodeling. It is unclear whether there is any capacity for rotational malunion remodeling

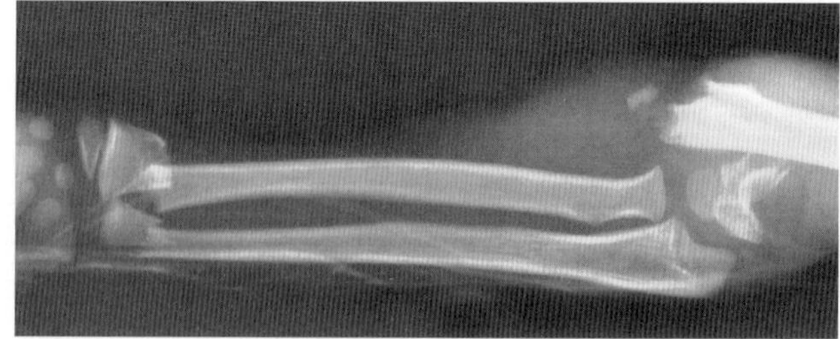
A

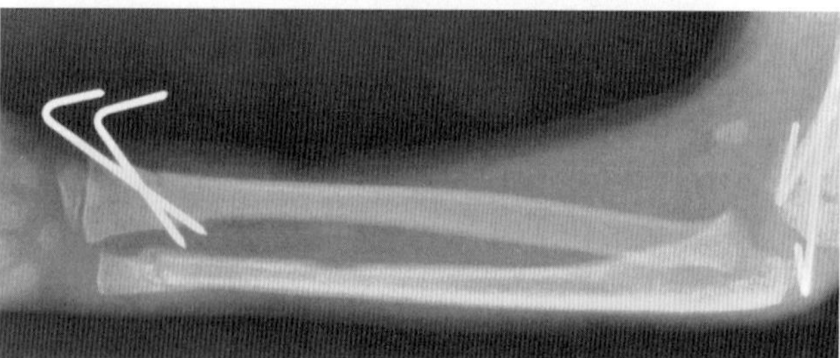
B

FIGURE 9-56 Ipsilateral fractures. **A.** Markedly displaced ipsilateral distal radial and supracondylar fractures. **B.** Both fractures were reduced and stabilized with pins placed percutaneously. (Wilkins KE, ed. *Operative management of upper extremity fractures in children.* Rosemont, IL: American Academy of Orthopaedic Surgeons, 1994:29; with permission.)

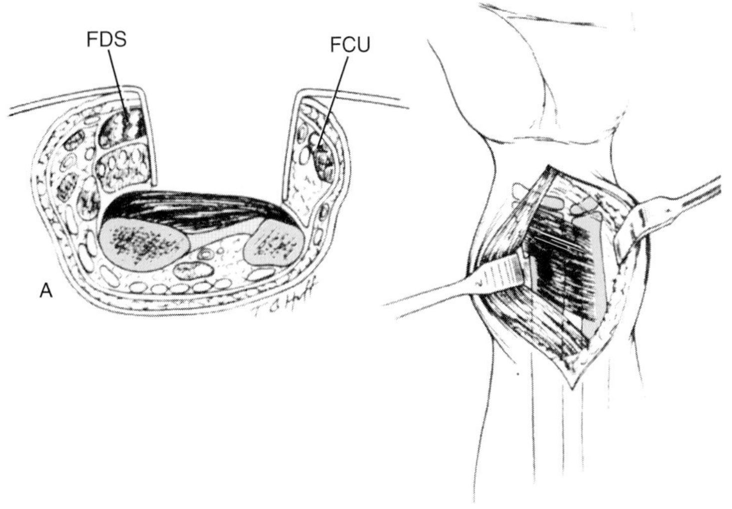

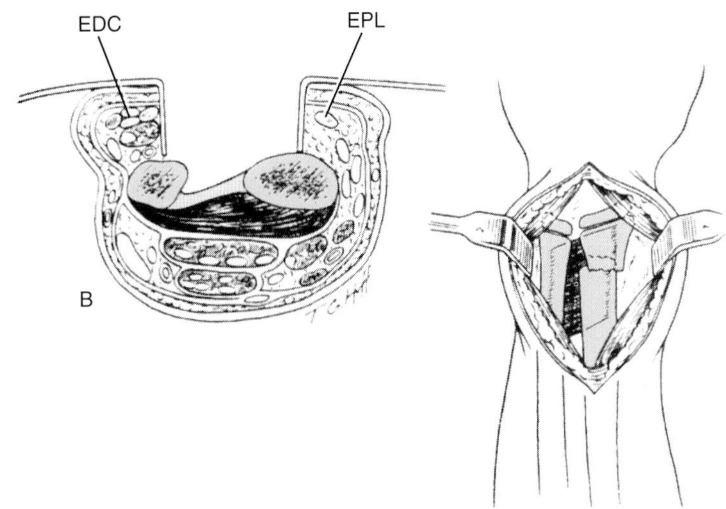

FIGURE 9-57 **A.** Volar approach through the interval between the digital flexors and ulnar neurovascular bundle. *FDS,* flexor digitorum superficialis; *FCU,* flexor carpi ulnaris. **B.** Dorsal approach between the third and fourth dorsal compartments. *EDC,* extensor digitorum communis; *EPL,* extensor pollicis longus. (Reprinted from Holmes JR, Luis DS. Entrapment of pronator quadratus in pediatric distal-radius fractures: recognition and treatment. *J Pediatr Orthop* 1994;14: 498–500; with permission.)

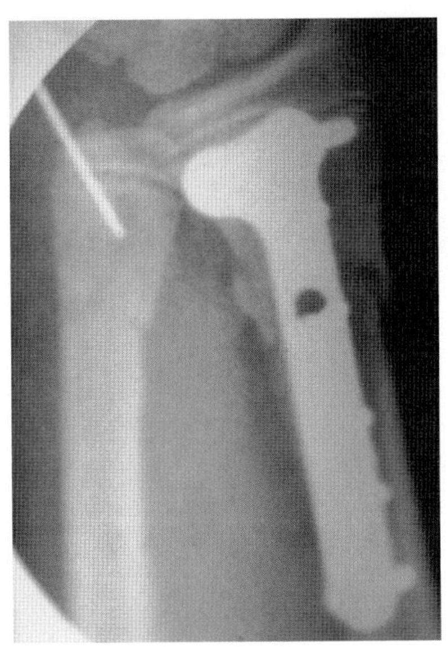

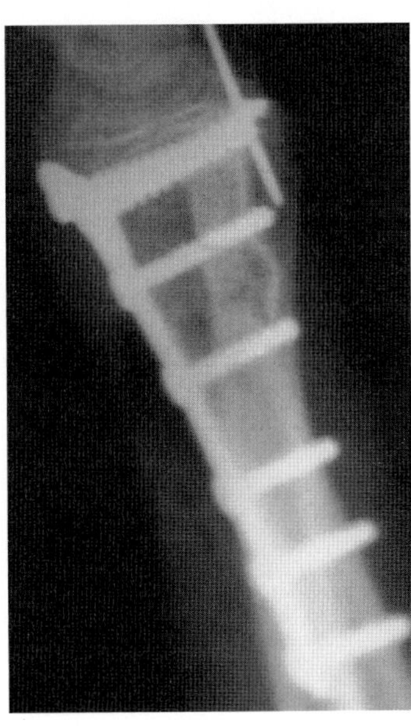

FIGURE 9-58 Open reduction of open radial metaphyseal fracture and ulnar styloid base fracture. After thorough irrigation and debridement of the radius, internal fixation of the radius was performed with care taken to not violate the physis with hardware. The ulna styloid base fracture and TFCC were repaired with an open tension band technique with a suture and smooth wire.

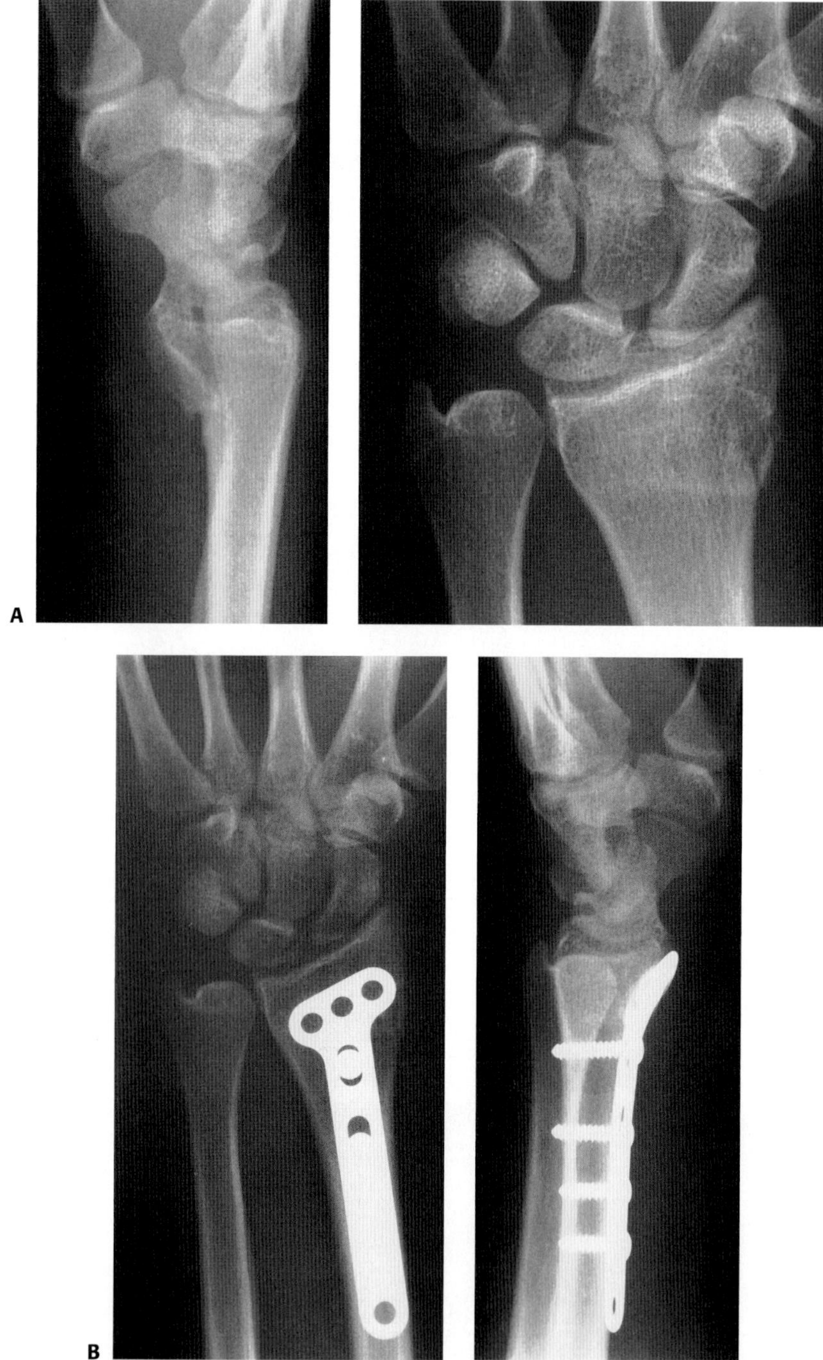

FIGURE 9-59 **A.** Anteroposterior and lateral x-rays of a 15-year-old skeletally mature boy with a displaced intra-articular fracture. **B.** This fracture needs to be treated like an adult's, with open reduction and internal fixation with a volar buttress plate.

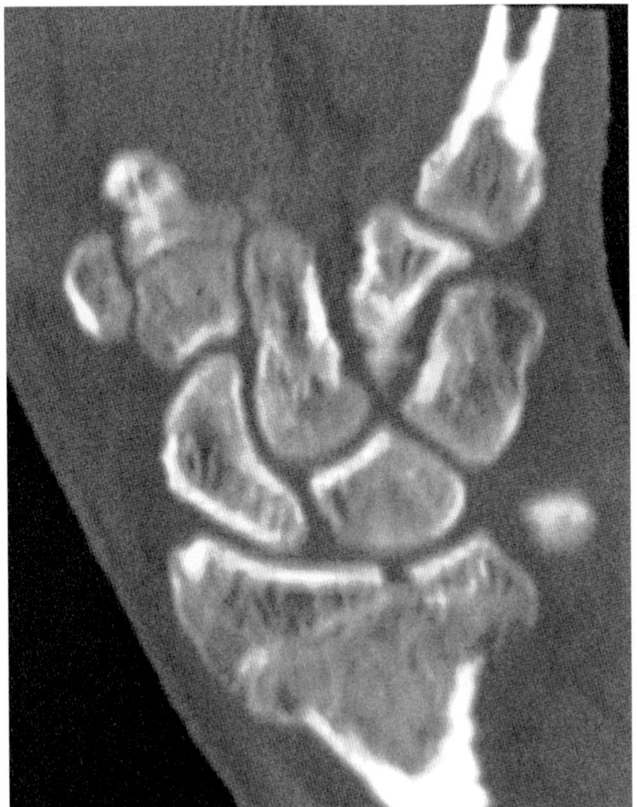

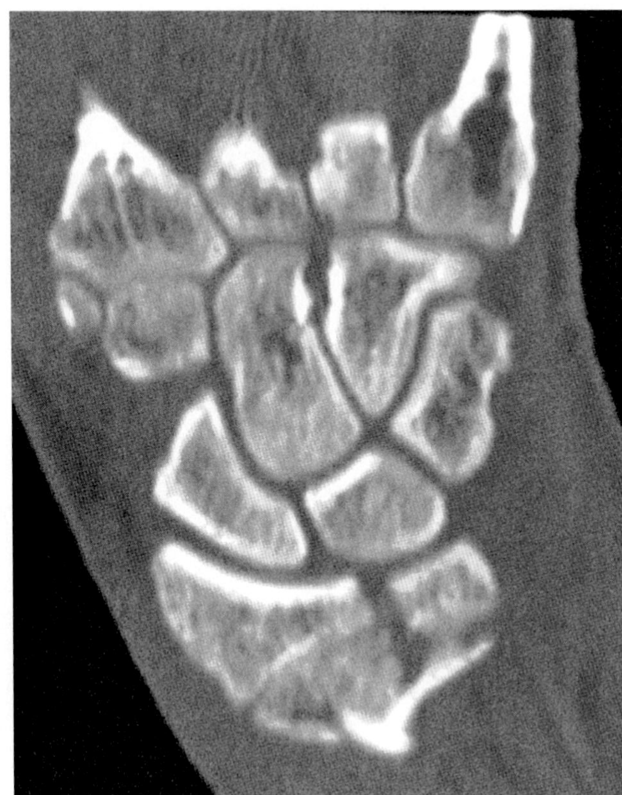

FIGURE 9-60 A. CT scan of a displaced intra-articular fracture of a nearly skeletally mature adolescent. *(continues)*

(178,189). Angular and rotational malunion that does not remodel can lead to loss of motion. The degree and plane of loss of motion, as well as the individual affected, determine if this is functionally significant (184). In cadaveric studies malangulation of more than 20 degrees of the radius or ulna caused loss of forearm rotation (162,190,191), whereas less than 10 degrees of malangulation did not alter forearm rotation significantly. Distal third malunion affected rotation less than middle or proximal third malunion. Radioulnar malunion affected forearm rotation more than volar-dorsal malunion. Excessive angulation may lead to a loss of rotation at a 1:2 degree ratio, whereas malrotation may lead to rotational loss at only a 1:1 degree loss (79). The functional loss associated with rotational motion loss is difficult to predict. This has led some clinicians to recommend no treatment (159,167), arguing that most of these fractures will remodel, and those that do not remodel will not cause a functional problem (192). However, a significant functional problem is present if shoulder motion cannot compensate for loss of supination.

We prefer to reduce forearm fractures to as near to perfect alignment as possible. No element of malrotation is accepted in the reduction. As indicated in the treatment sections, fractures at high risk of loss of reduction and malunion are treated with anatomic reduction and pin or rarely plate fixation. Fractures treated in a cast are followed closely and re-reduced for any loss of alignment of more than 10 degrees. Although loss of forearm rotation can occur with anatomic healing (3,130,193), it is less likely than with malunions.

Unfortunately, not all fractures heal anatomically or remodel to anatomic alignment. Long-term malunion is a concern for mid-carpal instability (101) and long-term arthrosis. A distal radial malunion in a skeletally mature adolescent should be treated with a dorsal open wedge osteotomy, bone graft, and internal fixation (Fig. 9-61) (102,194,195).

Nonunion

Nonunion of a closed radial or ulnar fracture is rare. In children, nonunion has been universally related to a pathologic condition of the bone or vascularity (130). Congenital pseudarthrosis or neurofibromatosis (Fig. 9-62) (196) should be suspected in a patient with a nonunion after a benign fracture. This occurs most often after an isolated ulnar fracture. The distal bone is often narrowed, sclerotic, and plastically deformed. These fractures rarely heal with immobilization. Vascularized fibular bone grafting usually is necessary for healing of a nonunion associated with neurofibromatosis or congenital pseudarthrosis. If the patient is very young, this may include a vascularized epiphyseal transfer to restore distal growth.

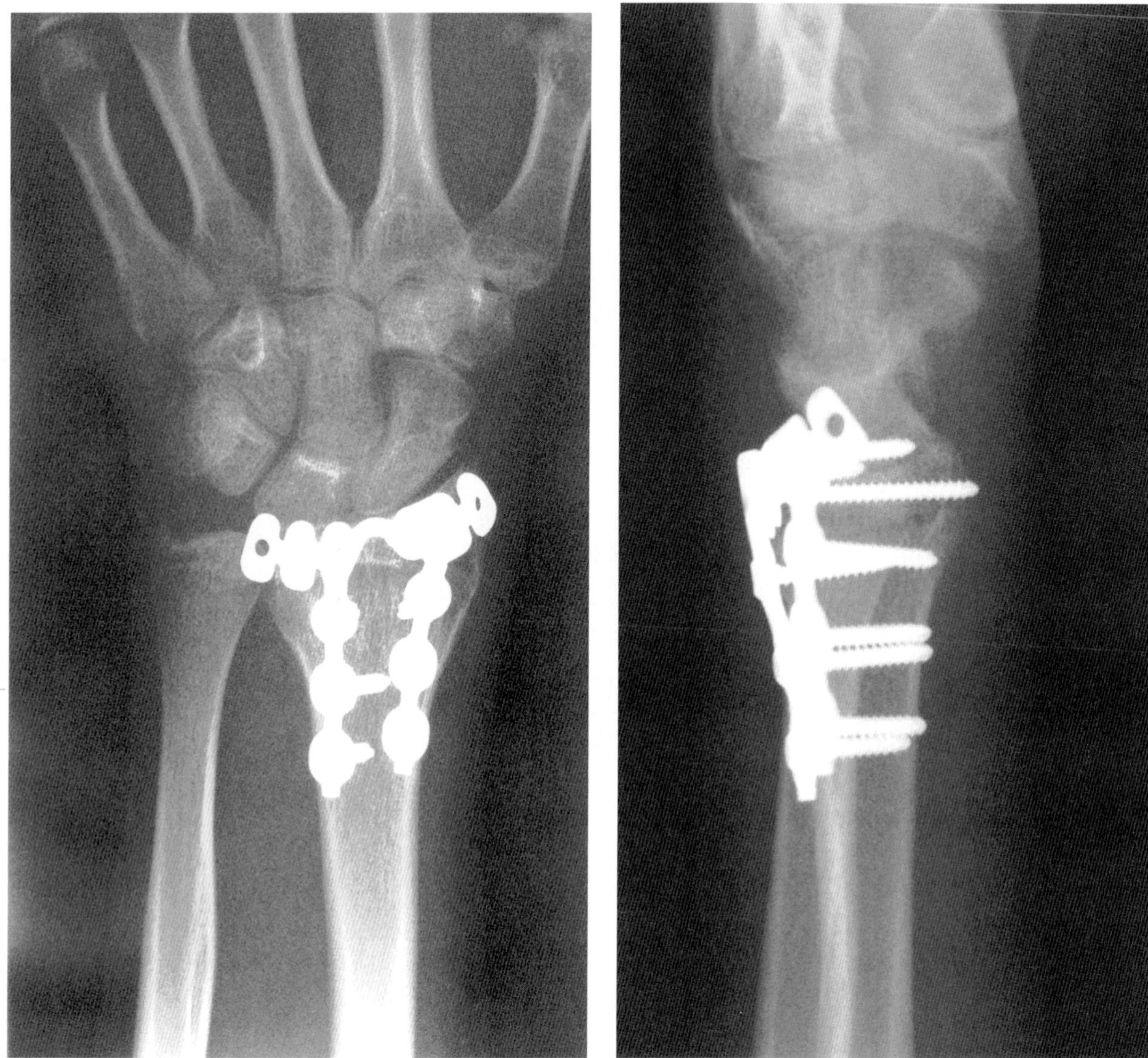

FIGURE 9-60 *(continued)* **B.** Dorsal plating with a low profile system to achieve anatomic reduction and stable fixation.

Vascular impairment also can lead to nonunion. Distal radial nonunion has been reported in a child with an ipsilateral supracondylar fracture with brachial artery occlusion. Revascularization of the limb led to eventual union of the fracture. Nonunion also can occur with osteomyelitis and bone loss (112). Débridement of the necrotic bone and either traditional bone grafting, osteoclasis lengthening, vascularized bone grafting, or creation of a single-bone forearm are surgical options. The choice depends on the individual patient.

Cross-Union

Cross-union is a rare complication of pediatric distal radial and ulnar fractures. It has been described after high-energy trauma and internal fixation (197). A single pin crossing both bones increases the risk of cross-union (197). Synostosis take-down can be performed, but the results usually are less than full restoration of motion. It is important to determine if there is an element of rotational malunion with the cross-union because this will affect the surgical outcome.

Soft-tissue contraction across both bones also has been described (198). Contracture release resulted in restoration of forearm motion.

Refracture

Fortunately, refractures after metaphyseal radial fractures are rare and much less common than after diaphyseal level radial

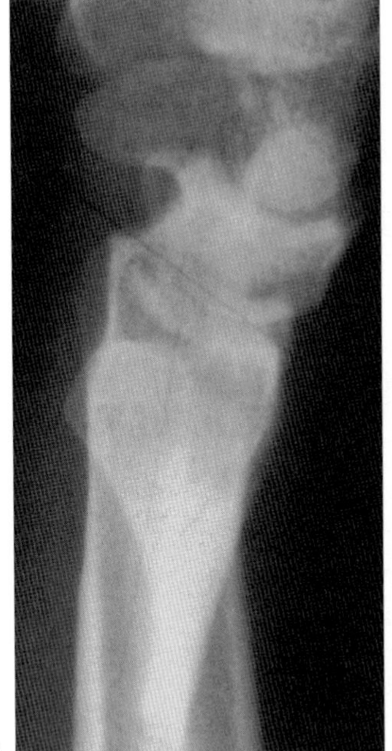
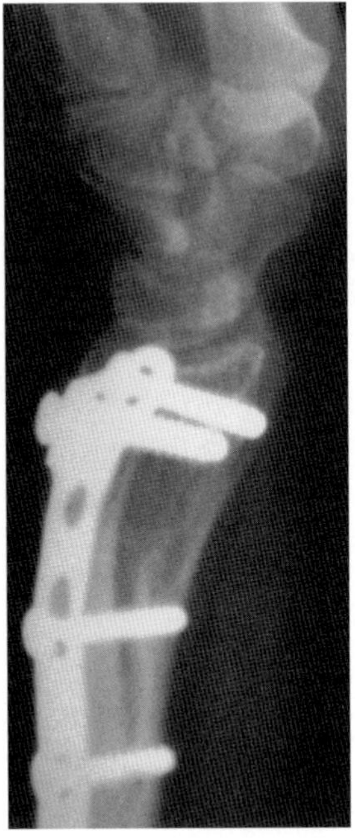

FIGURE 9-61 **A.** Radial metaphyseal fracture that did not remodel in a now 16-year-old skeletally mature boy. **B.** Corrective osteotomy with iliac crest bone graft and internal fixation was performed.

and ulnar fractures. Most commonly, refracture occurs with premature discontinuation of immobilization or early return to potentially traumatic activities. It is advisable to protectively immobilize the wrist until full x-ray and clinical healing (usually 6 weeks) and to restrict activities until full motion and strength are regained (usually an additional 1 to 6 weeks). Individuals involved in high-risk activities, such as downhill ski racing, snowboarding, or skateboarding, should be protected with a splint during those activities for much longer.

Growth Disturbance

Growth arrest of the distal radius after metaphyseal fracture is rare. Abram and Connolly each reported one patient with physeal arrest after nondisplaced torus fractures. Two additional patients were reported in a series of 150 distal radial metaphyseal fractures (199). Wilkins and O'Brien (130) proposed that these arrests may be in fractures that extend from the metaphysis to the physis. This coincides with a Peterson type I fracture (Fig. 9-63) (81,82) and in essence is a physeal fracture. These fractures should be monitored for growth arrest.

Both undergrowth and overgrowth of the distal radius after fracture were described by DePablos (200). The average difference in growth was 3 mm, a range of −5 to +10 mm of growth disturbance compared with the contralateral radius. Maximal overgrowth occurred in the 9- to 12-year-old age group. As long as the patient is asymptomatic, under- or overgrowth is not a problem. If ulnocarpal impaction or DRUJ disruption occurs, then surgical rebalancing of the radius and ulna may be necessary.

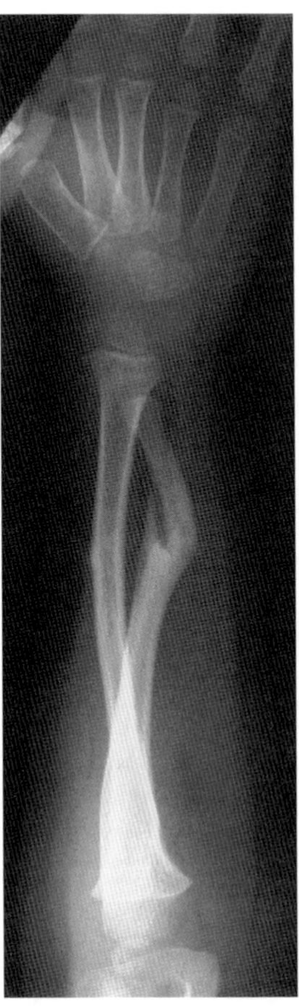

FIGURE 9-62 This 3-year-old presented to the emergency room with pain after an acute fall on his arm. The ulna is clearly pathologic with thinning and deformity before this injury. This represents neurofibromatosis.

Neurovascular Injuries

Both the median and ulnar (174,201) nerves are less commonly injured in metaphyseal fractures than in physeal fractures. The mechanisms of neural injury in a metaphyseal fracture include direct contusion from the displaced fragment, traction ischemia from tenting of the nerve over the proximal fragment (144,154), entrapment of the nerve in the fracture site (70,202), rare laceration of the nerve (Fig. 9-64), and the development of an acute compartment syndrome. If signs or symptoms of neuropathy are present, a prompt closed reduction should be performed. Extreme positions of immobilization should be avoided because this can lead to persistent traction or compression ischemia and increase the risk of compartment syndrome. If there is marked swelling, it is better to percutaneously pin the fracture than to apply a constrictive cast. If there is concern about compartment syndrome, the forearm and carpal canal pressures should be measured immediately. If pressures are markedly elevated, appropriate fasciotomies and compartment releases should be performed immediately. Finally, if the nerve was intact before reduction and is out after reduction, neural entrapment should

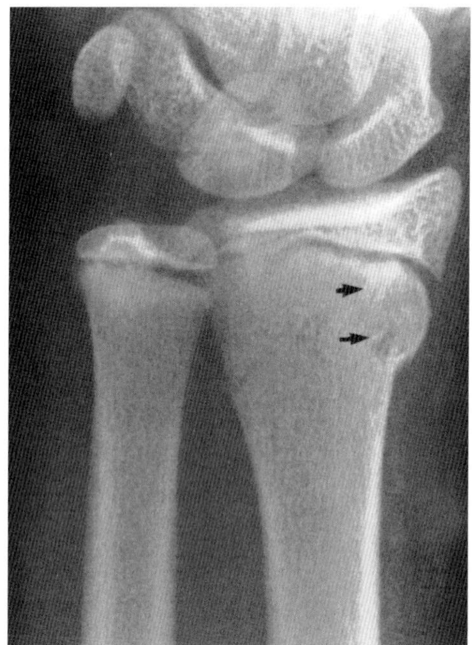

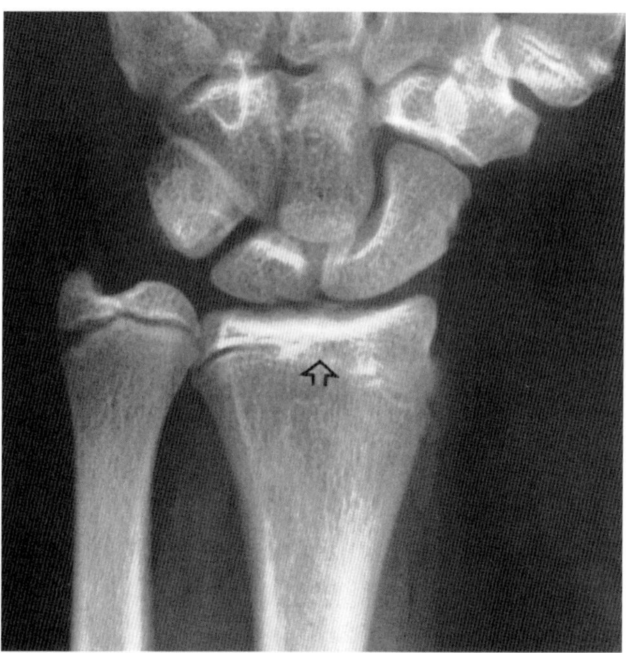

FIGURE 9-63 Physeal arrest in a Peterson type I fracture. **A.** Injury film showing what appears to be a benign metaphyseal fracture. Fracture line extends into the physis (*arrows*). **B.** Two years postinjury, a central arrest (*open arrow*) has developed, with resultant shortening of the radius. (Reprinted from Wilkins KE, ed. *Operative management of upper extremity fractures in children.* Rosemont, IL: American Academy of Orthopaedic Surgeons, 1994:21; with permission.)

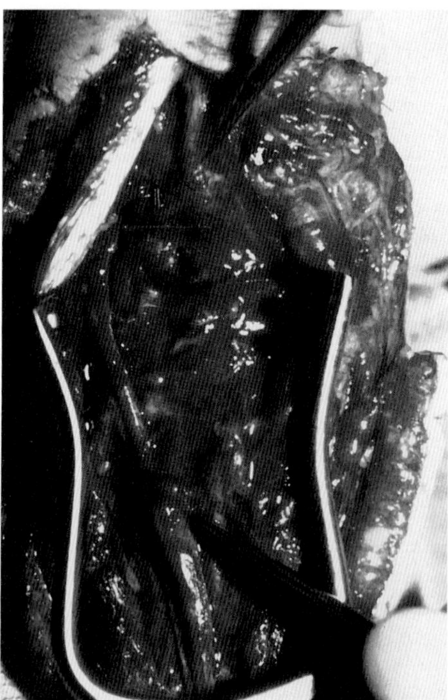

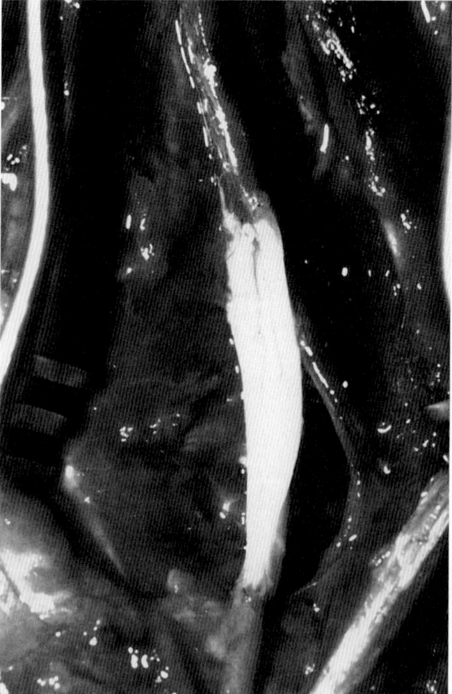

FIGURE 9-64 A grade III open fracture of the radius resulted in complete disruption of the ulnar nerve. Intraoperative photographs of the nerve deficit between the operative jeweler's forceps **(A)** and sural nerve grafting **(B)** after the wound was clean enough to allow for nerve reconstruction.

be considered, and surgical exploration and decompression may be required. Fortunately, most median and ulnar nerve injuries recover after anatomic reduction of the fracture.

Infection

Infection after distal radial fractures is rare and is associated with open fractures or surgical intervention. Fee et al (203) described the development of gas gangrene in four children after minor puncture wounds or lacerations associated with distal radial fractures. Treatment involved only local cleansing of the wound in all four and wound closure in one. All four developed life-threatening clostridial infections. Three of the four required upper limb amputations, and the fourth underwent multiple soft-tissue and bony procedures for coverage and treatment of osteomyelitis.

Infections related to surgical intervention also are rare. Superficial pin site infections can occur and should be treated with pin removal and antibiotics. Deep-space infection from percutaneous pinning of the radius has not been described.

PEDIATRIC GALEAZZI FRACTURES

Fractures of the distal radius associated with DRUJ disruption have been called Galeazzi fracture–dislocations. Although Sir Ashley Cooper is credited with the first description of this injury in 1824, Riccardo Galeazzi (204,205) gave this fracture–dislocation its name with his 1934 report of 18 such injuries. In children, this injury may involve either disruption of the DRUJ ligaments or, more commonly, a distal ulnar physeal fracture (Fig. 9-65) (123,204,206–208). Galeazzi fracture–dislocations are relatively rare injuries in children. Walsh and McLaren (209) cited an occurrence of 3% of pediatric distal radial fractures in their study. Most series of Galeazzi fracture contain a relatively small number of pediatric patients (81,207,209,210).

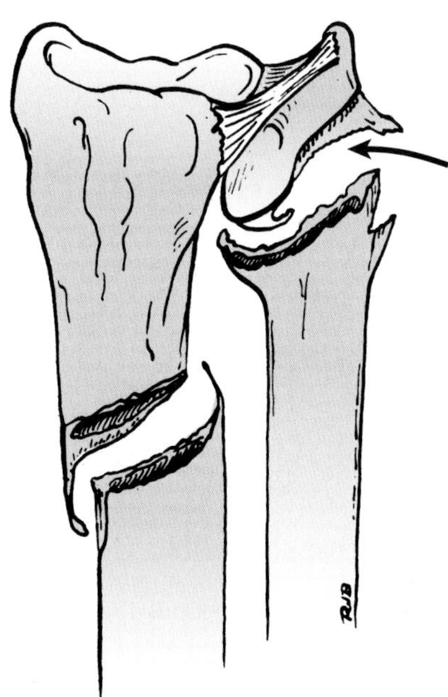

FIGURE 9-65 Galeazzi fracture–dislocation variant. Interposed periosteum can block reduction of the distal ulnar physis (*arrow*). This destabilizes the distal radial metaphyseal fracture. (Reprinted from Lanfried MJ, Stenclik M, Susi JG. Variant of Galeazzi fracture–dislocation in children. *J Pediatr Orthop* 1991;11:333; with permission.)

Mechanism of Injury

The mechanism of injury is axial loading in combination with extremes of forearm rotation (Fig. 9-66) (208,211–213). In adults, the mechanism of injury usually is an axially loading fall with hyperpronation. This results in a distal radial fracture with a dorsal ulnar dislocation. However, in children, both supination (apex volar) and pronation (apex dorsal) deforming forces have been described (207,209,214). The mechanism of injury is most obvious when the radial fracture is an incomplete fracture. With an apex volar (supination) radial fracture, the distal ulna is displaced volarly, whereas with an apex dorsal (pronation) radial fracture, the distal ulna is displaced dorsally (Fig. 9-67). This is evident both on clinical and radiographic examinations. In addition, the radius is foreshortened in a complete fracture, causing more radial deviation of the hand and wrist (Fig. 9-68).

Signs and Symptoms

A child with a Galeazzi injury has pain and limitation of forearm rotation and wrist flexion and extension. Neurovascular impairment is rare. The radial deformity usually is clinically evident. The DRUJ disruption may be obvious by the prominence of the ulnar head. A subtle ligament disruption may be evident only by local tenderness and instability to testing on the DRUJ.

The radial fracture is evident on x-rays and concurrent injuries to the ulna or DRUJ should be identified. A true lateral view is necessary to identify the direction of displacement, which is imperative to determine the method of reduction. Rarely are special x-rays, such as a CT scan, necessary.

Classification

Galeazzi fracture–dislocations are most commonly described by direction of displacement of either the distal ulnar dislocation or the radial fracture. Letts (207,214) preferred to describe the direction of the ulna: volar or dorsal. Walsh and McLaren (209) classified pediatric Galeazzi injuries by the direction of displacement of the distal radial fracture. Dorsal displacement (apex volar) fractures were more common than volar displacement (apex dorsal) fractures in their series. Wilkins and O'Brien (130) modified the Walsh and McLaren method by classifying radial fractures as incomplete and complete fractures and ulnar injuries as true dislocations and physeal fractures (Table 9-4). DRUJ dislocations are called true Galeazzi lesions and distal ulnar physeal fractures are called Galeazzi equivalent lesions (123,207,214,215).

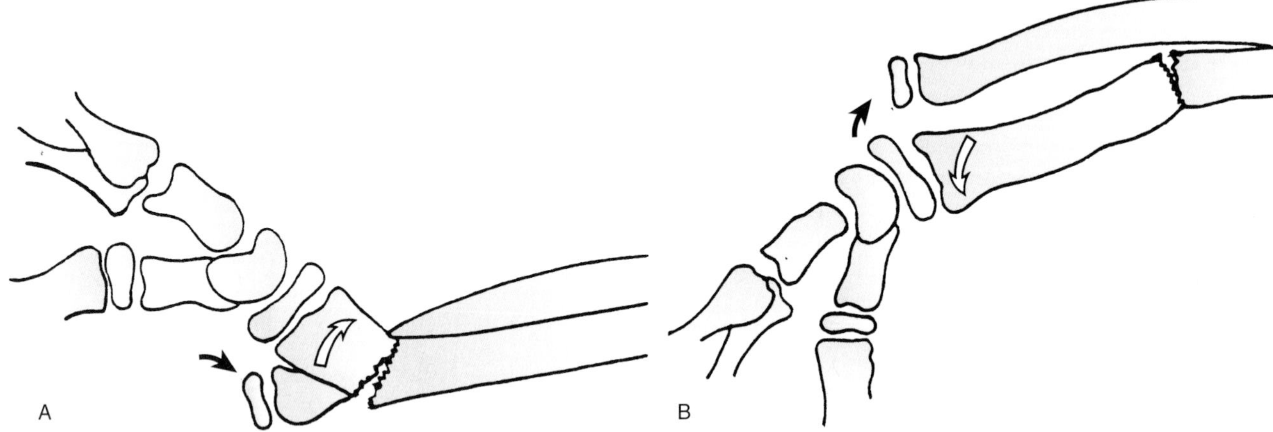

FIGURE 9-66 Walsh's classification. **A.** The most common pattern, in which there is dorsal displacement with supination of the distal radius (*open arrow*). The distal ulna (*black arrow*) lies volar to the dorsally displaced distal radius. **B.** The least common pronation pattern. There is volar or anterior displacement of the distal radius (*open arrow*), and the distal ulna lies dorsal (*black arrow*). (Reprinted from Walsh HPJ, McLaren CANP. Galeazzi fractures in children. *J Bone Joint Surg Br* 1987;69:730–733; with permission.)

Anatomy

The radius normally rotates around the relatively stationary ulna. The two bones of the forearm articulate at the proximal and distal radioulnar joints. In addition, proximally the radius and ulna articulate with the distal humerus and distally with the carpus. These articulations are necessary for forearm pronation and supination. At the DRUJ, the concave sigmoid notch of the radius incompletely matches the convex, asymmetric, semicylindrical shape of the distal ulnar head (56). This allows some translation at the DRUJ with rotatory movements. The ligamentous structures are critical in stabilizing the radius as it rotates about the ulna (Fig. 9-69).

The DRUJ includes multiple soft-tissue attachments, the most important of which is the triangular fibrocartilage complex (TFCC). The TFCC includes the volar and dorsal ligamentous attachments of the distal ulna to the radial sigmoid notch, as well as the distal extension to the ulnar styloid, carpus, and base of the fifth metacarpal. The volar ulnocarpal ligaments (V ligament) from the ulna to the lunate and triquetrum are important ulnocarpal stabilizers (56,216,217). The central portion of the TFCC is the articular disk (Fig. 9-70). The interaction between the bony articulation and the soft-tissue attachments accounts for stability of the DRUJ during pronation and supination. At the extremes of rotation, the joint is most stable. The compression loads between the radius and ulna are aided by the tensile loads of the TFCC to maintain stability throughout rotation.

Throughout the mid-forearm, the interosseous ligament connects the radius to the ulna. It passes obliquely from the proximal radius to the distal ulna. However, the interosseous ligament is not present in the distal radius. Moore et al (218) found that injuries to the TFCC and interosseous ligament were responsible for progressive shortening of the radius with fracture in a cadaveric study. The soft-tissue component to the injury is a major factor in the deformity and instability in a Galeazzi fracture–dislocation.

Current Treatment Options

Pediatric Galeazzi fractures have a higher success rate with nonoperative treatment than similar injuries in adults (208,210). In adults, it is imperative to anatomically reduce and internally fix the distal radial fracture (208,210,218–220). Generally the DRUJ is reduced with reduction and fixation of the radius. In pediatric patients, the distal radial fracture often is a greenstick type that is stable after reduction and cast immobilization is sufficient (209,210). Adolescents with complete fractures should be treated with internal fixation similar to adults.

Closed Reduction

The method of reduction for greenstick radial fractures depends on the type of displacement. With apex volar dorsally displaced fractures of the radius, the rotatory deformity is supination. Pronating the radius and applying a dorsal-to-volar reduction force should align the fracture and reduce the DRUJ. Similarly, if the incomplete radial fracture is an apex dorsal volar displaced fracture, the rotatory deformity is pronation. Supinating the forearm and applying a volar-to-dorsal force should reduce the incomplete fracture of the radius and the DRUJ dislocation (130,207,214,221). In both these situations, portable fluoroscopy can be used to evaluate the fracture–dislocation reduction and to test the stability of the distal ulna. If anatomically reduced and stable, a long-arm cast is applied with appropriate rotation and three-point molds. The cast is left in place for 6 weeks to allow the soft-tissue injuries to heal.

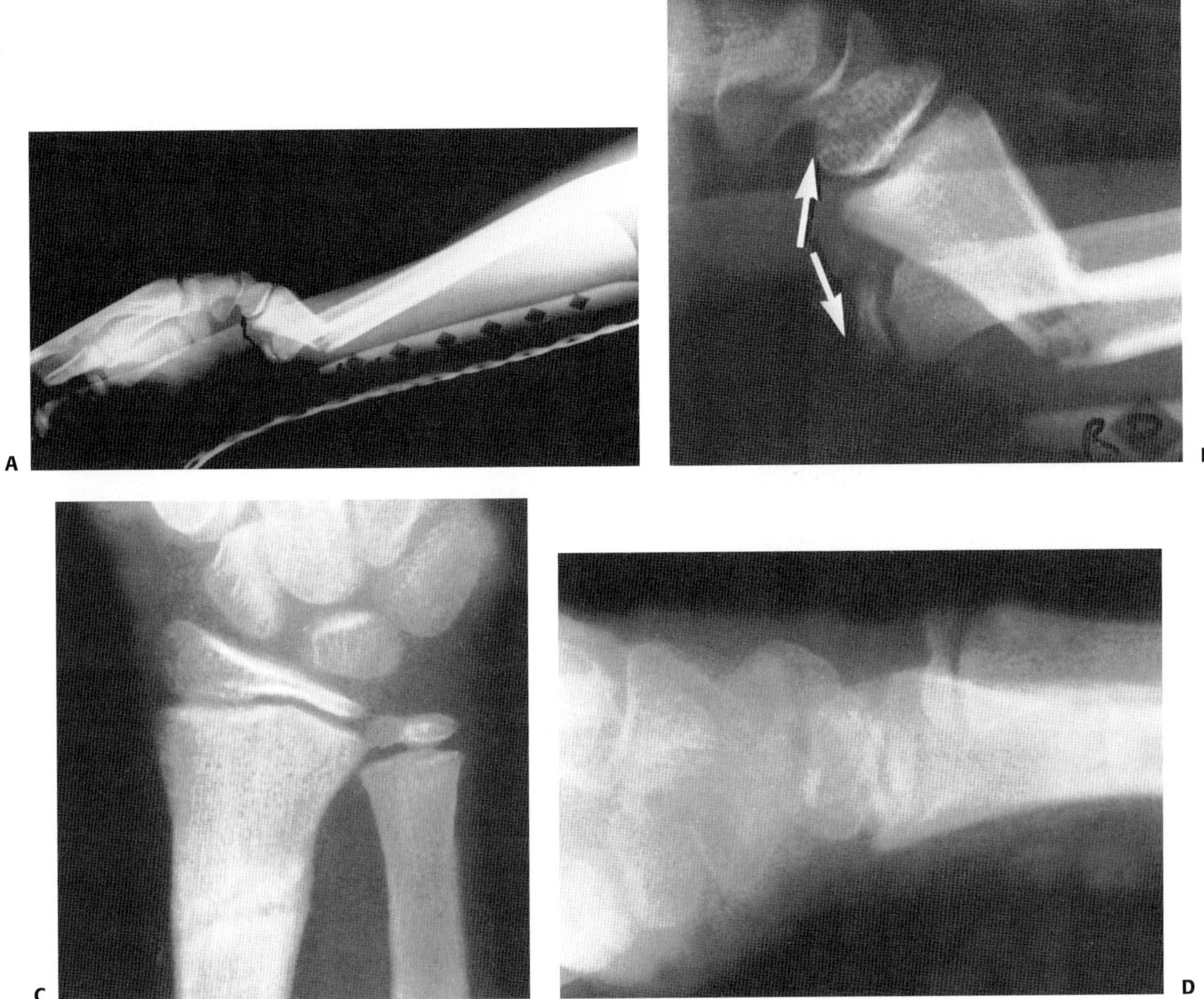

FIGURE 9-67 Supination-type Galeazzi fracture. **A.** View of the entire forearm of an 11-year-old boy with a Galeazzi fracture–dislocation. **B.** Close-up of the distal forearm shows that there has been disruption of the distal radioulnar joint (*arrows*). The distal radial fragment is dorsally displaced (apex volar), making this a supination type of mechanism. Note that the distal ulna is volar to the distal radius. **C,D.** The fracture was reduced by pronating the distal fragment. Because the distal radius was partially intact by its greenstick nature, the length was easily maintained, reestablishing the congruity of the distal radioulnar joint. The patient was immobilized in supination for 6 weeks, after which full forearm rotation and function returned.

In a Galeazzi equivalent injury with a radial fracture and an ulnar physeal fracture, both bones should be reduced. Usually this can be accomplished with the same methods of reduction if the radial fracture is incomplete. The distal ulnar physis can remodel a nonanatomic reduction if there is sufficient growth remaining and the ulnar physis continues to grow normally. Unfortunately, the risk of ulnar growth arrest after a Galeazzi equivalent has been reported to be as high as 55% (121).

Complete fractures of the distal radius have a higher rate of loss of reduction after closed treatment than do incomplete fractures (Fig. 9-71) (130). If not monitored closely and re-reduced if necessary, loss of reduction can lead to malunion with loss of motion and function. These injuries may be best treated with open reduction as in adults.

Open Reduction

The indication for open reduction of the radial fracture is failure to obtain or maintain fracture reduction. This most often occurs with unstable complete fractures. Open reduction and internal fixation of the radius are done through an anterior approach. Standard compression plating is preferred to intramedullary or

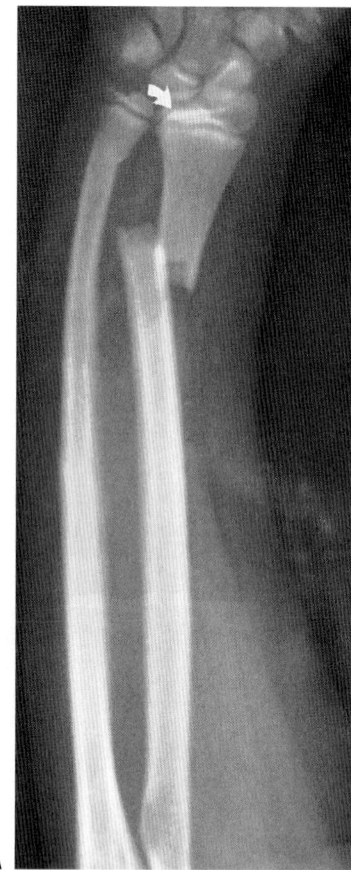

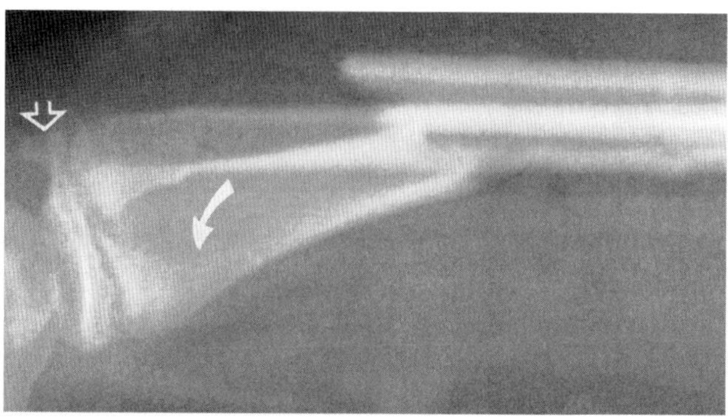

FIGURE 9-68 Pronation Galeazzi. This 8-year-old sustained a pronation Galeazzi fracture. **A.** The anteroposterior view shows some shortening of the distal radius (*arrow*) in relation to the distal ulna, which has a small greenstick component. **B.** The pronation component (*arrow*) is better appreciated on this lateral view. The distal ulna lies dorsal to the distal radius (*open arrow*).

TABLE 9-4 Classification: Galeazzi Fractures in Children

Type I: Dorsal (apex volar) displacement of distal radius
- Radius fracture pattern
  - Greenstick
  - Complete
- Distal ulna physis
  - Intact
  - Disrupted (equivalent)

Type II: Volar (apex dorsal) displacement of distal radius
- Radius fracture pattern
  - Greenstick
  - Complete
- Distal ulna physis
  - Intact
  - Disrupted

Reprinted from Walsh HPJ, McLaren CAN, Owen R. Galeazzi fractures in children. *J Bone Joint Surg Br* 1987;69B:730–733.

cross-pinning techniques (Fig. 9-72). Stable, anatomic reduction of the radius almost always leads to stable reduction of the DRUJ dislocation. A long-arm cast is used for 6 weeks to allow fracture and soft-tissue healing.

Occasionally, the DRUJ dislocation cannot be reduced (Fig. 9-73) because of interposed soft-tissues, most commonly the periosteum, extensor tendons (extensor carpi ulnaris, extensor digit quinti), TFCC, or other ligamentous structures (207, 222–224). The easiest approach for open reduction of the DRUJ is an extended ulnar approach. Care should be taken to avoid injury to the ulnar sensory nerve. This approach allows exposure both volarly and dorsally to extract the interposed soft-tissues and repair the torn structures. Smooth pin fixation of the DRUJ can be used to maintain reduction and allow application of a loose-fitting cast. The pin is removed in the office at 4 weeks with continuation of the cast for 6 weeks.

Similarly, the ulnar physeal fracture can be irreducible in a Galeazzi equivalent injury. This also has been reported to be secondary to interposed periosteum (123,208), extensor tendons (95,122,148,225), or joint capsule (226). Open reduction must be executed with care to avoid further violating the physis.

Incomplete Fractures

Incomplete fractures of the distal radius with either a true dislocation of the DRUJ or an ulnar physeal fracture are treated with

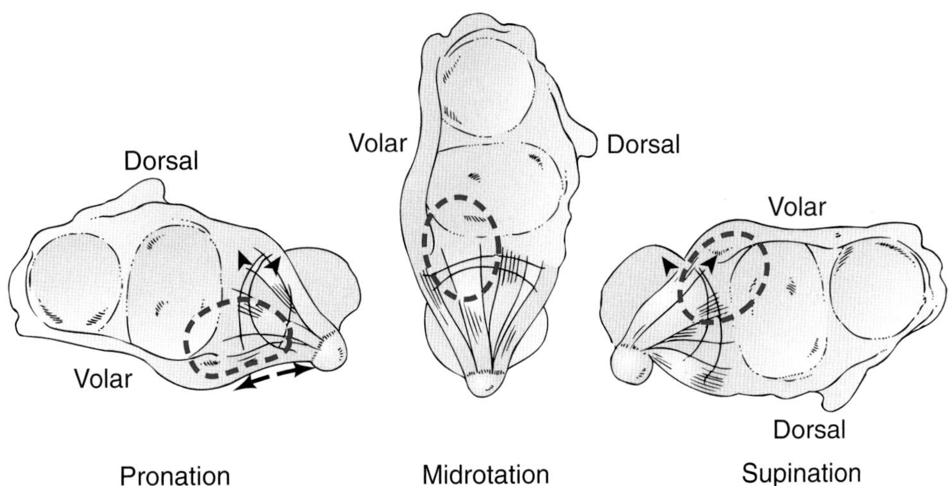

FIGURE 9-69 Distal radioulnar joint stability in pronation (*left*) is dependent on (a) tension developed in the volar margin of the triangular fibrocartilage (TFCC, *small arrows*) and (b) compression between the contact areas of the radius and ulna (volar surface of ulnar articular head and dorsal margin of the sigmoid notch, *large arrows*). Disruption of the volar TFCC would therefore allow dorsal displacement of the ulna in pronation. The reverse is true in supination, where disruption of the dorsal margin of the TFCC would allow volar displacement of the ulna relative to the radius as this rotational extreme is reached. The dark area of the TFCC emphasizes the portion of the TFCC that is not supported by the ulnar dome. The dotted circle is the arc of load transmission (lunate to TFCC) in that position. (Redrawn from Bowers WH. *Green's operative hand surgery*. New York: Churchill–Livingstone, 1993.)

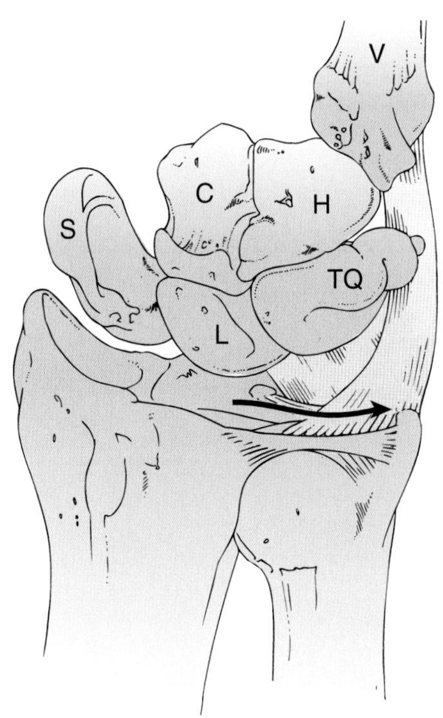

FIGURE 9-70 Diagrammatic drawing of the TFCC and the prestyloid recess. The meniscal reflection runs from the dorsoulnar radius to the ulnovolar carpus. The arrow denotes access under the reflection to the tip of the styloid—the so-called prestyloid recess. (Redrawn from Bowers WH. *Green's operative hand surgery*. New York: Churchill–Livingstone, 1993.)

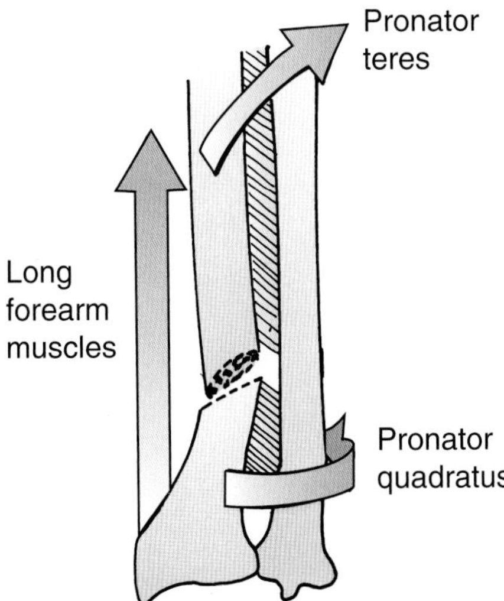

FIGURE 9-71 Fractures of the distal radius are angulated toward the ulna due to the pull of the long forearm muscles and the pronator quadratus. (Redrawn from Cruess RL. The management of forearm injuries. *Orthop Clin North Am* 1973;4:969–982; with permission.)

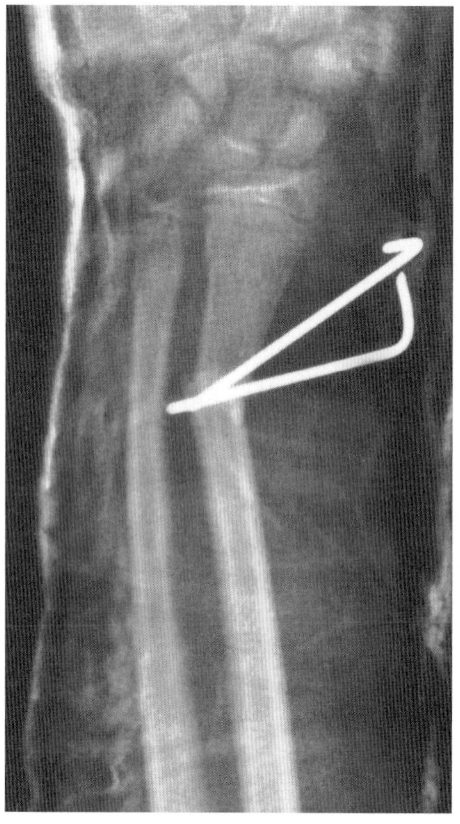

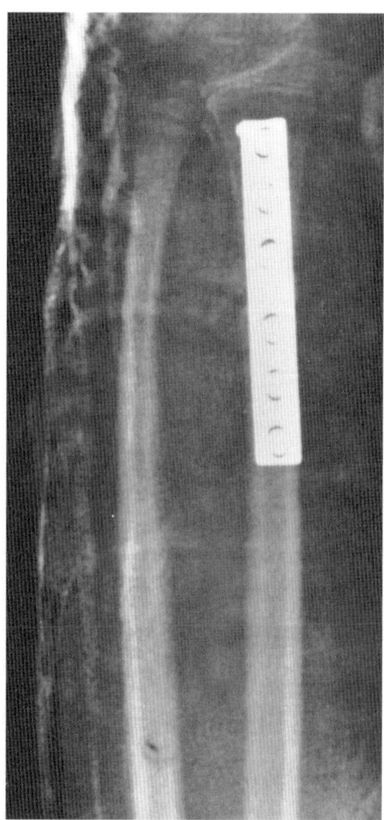

FIGURE 9-72 **A.** The patient with the pronation injury shown in Figure 9-68 had a closed reduction and attempted fixation with pins placed percutaneously across the fracture site. However, this was inadequate in maintaining the alignment and length of the fracture of the distal radius. **B.** The length of the radius and the distal radioulnar relationship were best reestablished after internal fixation of the distal radius with a plate placed on the volar surface. The true amount of shortening present on the original injury film (see Fig. 9-68A) is not really appreciated until the fracture of the distal radius is fully reduced. (Reprinted from Wilkins KE, ed. *Operative management of upper extremity fractures in children.* Rosemont, IL: American Academy of Orthopaedic Surgeons, 1994: 34; with permission.)

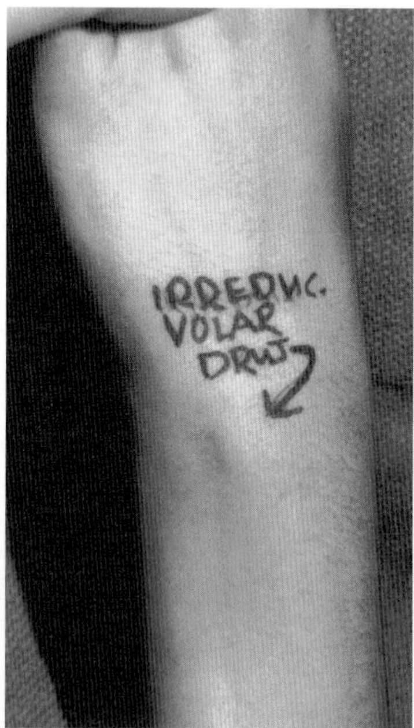

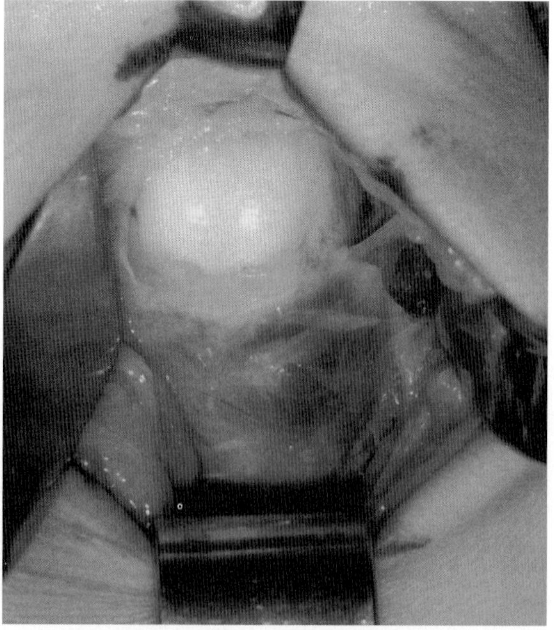

FIGURE 9-73 An adolescent girl presented 4 weeks after injury with a painful, stiff wrist. **A.** By examination, she was noted to have a volar distal radioulnar dislocation that was irreducible even under general anesthesia. **B.** At the time of surgery the distal ulna was found to have buttonholed out of the capsule, and there was entrapped triangular fibrocartilage and periosteum in the joint.

closed reduction and long-arm cast immobilization. This can be done in the emergency room with conscious sedation or in the operating room with general anesthesia. Portable fluoroscopy is used. If the fracture is apex volar with dorsal displacement of the radius and volar dislocation of the DRUJ, then pronation and volar-to-dorsal force on the radial fracture is used for reduction. If the fracture is apex dorsal with volar displacement of the radius and dorsal dislocation of the DRUJ, then supination and dorsal-to-volar force is applied to the distal radius for reduction. The reduction and stability of the fracture and DRUJ dislocation are checked on dynamic fluoroscopy before long-arm cast immobilization. If both are anatomically reduced and stable, the cast is used for 6 weeks to allow soft-tissue and fracture healing. In a Galeazzi equivalent injury, there is potential for remodeling of the physeal fracture if sufficient growth remains. As long as the DRUJ is reduced, malalignment of less than 10 degrees can remodel in a young child. The risk of physeal growth arrest is high with this physeal injury, and operative exposure may increase the risk of growth impairment. If the fracture is severely malaligned, the DRUJ cannot be reduced, or the patient is older and remodeling is unlikely, open reduction and smooth pin fixation are indicated (130).

Complete Fractures

Open reduction and internal fixation with an anterior plate and screws are used for complete Galeazzi fractures of the radius. The DRUJ usually reduces anatomically and is stable with reduction and fixation of the radius. The patient is immobilized in a long-arm cast for 4 weeks and a short-arm cast for 2 more weeks. Return to unrestricted activities and sports depends on restoration of full motion and strength.

Irreducible Dislocations

Irreducible dislocations are treated with open reduction. Extensile exposure is necessary to define the pathologic anatomy and carefully reduce the DRUJ. The interposed soft-tissues are extracted and repaired. Depending on the stability of the reduction and repair, a supplemental smooth pin may be used across the DRUJ for 4 weeks to maintain the joint reduction. This is particularly true if the patient presents late.

Complications

Malunion and DRUJ Subluxation

Malunion of the radius can lead to subluxation of the DRUJ, limited forearm rotation, and pain, usually secondary to persistent shortening and malrotation of the radial fracture. Most often this occurs when complete fractures are treated with closed reduction and there is failure to either obtain or maintain reduction of the radial fracture. The ulna remains subluxed and heals with an incongruent joint. Treatment of this requires proper recognition and corrective osteotomy. If physical examination is not definitive for diagnosis, then a CT scan in pronation, neutral rotation, or supination may be helpful. An MRI scan or wrist arthroscopy will aid in the diagnosis and management of associated ligamentous, chondral, or TFCC injuries that will benefit from debridement or repair. It is important to understand that if the DRUJ subluxation is caused by a radial malunion, a soft-tissue reconstruction of the DRUJ alone will fail (56). In the true soft-tissue disruption, often repair of the TFCC will stabilize the DRUJ. If there is no TFCC tear, soft-tissue reconstruction of the DRUJ ligaments with extensor retinaculum or local tendon is appropriate.

Ulnar Physeal Arrest

Golz et al (121) cited ulnar physeal arrest with in 55% of Galeazzi equivalent fractures. If the patient is young enough, this ulnar growth arrest in the presence of ongoing radial growth will lead to deformity. Initially there will be ulnar shortening. Over time, the foreshortened ulna can act as a tether, causing asymmetric growth of the radius. There will be increased radial articular inclination on the AP x-ray and subluxation of the DRUJ. Operative choices include ulnar lengthening, radial closing wedge osteotomy, radial epiphysiodesis, and a combination of the above procedures that is appropriate for the individual patient's age, deformity, and disability.

Nerve Injury

Injuries to the ulnar nerve (210) and anterior interosseous nerve (227,228) have been described with Galeazzi fracture–dislocations. These injuries have had spontaneous recovery. Moore et al (229) described an 8% rate of injury to the radial nerve with operative exposure of the radius for internal fixation in their series. Careful surgical exposure, dissection, and retraction can decrease this risk.

REFERENCES

1. Lawton L. Fractures of the distal radius and ulna in management of pediatric fractures. In Letts M, ed. *Management of pediatric fractures*. New York: Churchill-Livingstone, 1994:345–368.
2. Landin LA. Fracture patterns in children: analysis of 8682 fractures with special reference to incidence, etiology, and secular changes in a Swedish urban population, 1950–1979. *Acta Chir Scand Suppl* 1983;202:1–109.
3. Thomas EM, Tuson KW, Browne PS. Fractures of the radius and ulna in children. *Injury* 1975;7:120–124.
4. Cheng JC, Shen WY. Limb fracture pattern in different pediatric age groups: a study of 3,350 children. *J Orthop Trauma* 1993;7:15–22.
5. Johnson PG, Szabo RM. Angle measurements of the distal radius: a cadaver study. *Skeletal Radiol* 1993;22:243–246.
6. Worlock P, Stower M. Fracture patterns in Nottingham children. *J Pediatr Orthop* 1986; 6:656–660.
7. Reed MH. Fractures and dislocations of the extremities in children. *J Trauma* 1977; 17:35.
8. Bailey DA, Wedge JH, McCulloch RG, et al. Epidemiology of fractures of the distal end of the radius in children as associated with growth. *J Bone Joint Surg Am* 1989;71: 1225–1231.
9. Kocher MS, Waters PM, Micheli LJ. Upper extremity injuries in the paediatric athlete. *Sports Med* 2000;30:117–135.
10. Sasaki K, Takagi M, Ida H, et al. Severity of upper limb injuries in snowboarding. *Arch Orthop Trauma Surg* 1999;119:292–295.
11. Sasaki K, Takagi M, Kiyoshige Y, et al. Snowboarder's wrist: its severity compared with Alpine skiing. *J Trauma* 1999;46:1059–1061.
12. Matsumoto K, Sumi H, Sumi Y, et al. Wrist fractures from snowboarding: a prospective study for 3 seasons from 1998 to 2001. *Clin J Sport Med* 2004;14:64–71.
13. Ronning R, Ronning I, Gerner T, et al. The efficacy of wrist protectors in preventing snowboarding injuries. *Am J Sports Med* 2001;29:581–585.
14. Kyle SB, Nance ML, Rutherford GW Jr, et al. Skateboard-associated injuries: participation-based estimates and injury characteristics. *J Trauma* 2002;53:686–690.
15. Boyd KT, Brownson P, Hunter JB. Distal radial fractures in young goalkeepers: a case for an appropriately sized soccer ball. *Br J Sports Med* 2001;35:409–411.

16. Wareham K, Johansen A, Stone MD, et al. Seasonal variation in the incidence of wrist and forearm fractures, and its consequences. *Injury* 2003;34:219–222.
17. Ma D, Jones G. The association between bone mineral density, metacarpal morphometry, and upper limb fractures in children: a population-based case-control study. *J Clin Endocrinol Metab* 2003;88:1486–1491.
18. Goulding A, Jones IE, Taylor RW, et al. Dynamic and static tests of balance and postural sway in boys: effects of previous wrist bone fractures and high adiposity. *Gait Posture* 2003;17:136–141.
19. Nork SE, Hennrikus WL, Loncarich DP, et al. Relationship between ligamentous laxity and the site of upper extremity fractures in children: extension supracondylar fracture versus distal forearm fracture. *J Pediatr Orthop B* 1999;8:90–92.
20. Albanese SA, Palmer AK, Kerr DR, et al. Wrist pain and distal growth plate closure of the radius in gymnasts. *J Pediatr Orthop* 1989;9:23–28.
21. Caine D, Roy S, Singer KM, et al. Stress changes of the distal radial growth plate. A radiographic survey and review of the literature. *Am J Sports Med* 1992;20:290–298.
22. De Smet L, Claessens A, Lefevre J, et al. Gymnast wrist: an epidemiologic survey of ulnar variance and stress changes of the radial physis in elite female gymnasts. *Am J Sports Med* 1994;22:846–850.
23. Meeusen R, Borms J. Gymnastic injuries. *Sports Med* 1992;13:337–356.
24. Roy S, Caine D, Singer KM. Stress changes of the distal radial epiphysis in young gymnasts. A report of twenty-one cases and a review of the literature. *Am J Sports Med* 1985;13:301–308.
25. Tolat AR, Sanderson PL, De Smet L, et al. The gymnast's wrist: acquired positive ulnar variance following chronic epiphyseal injury. *J Hand Surg [Br]* 1992;17:678–681.
26. Ekenstrom F. The anatomy of the distal radioulnar joint. *Clin Orthop Rel Res* 1992; 275:14–18.
27. Gerber SD, Griffin PP, Simmons BP. Break dancer's wrist. *J Pediatr Orthop* 1986;6: 98–99.
28. Gandhi RK, Wilson P, Mason Brown JJ, et al. Spontaneous correction of deformity following fractures of the forearm in children. *Br J Surg* 1962;50:5–10.
29. Mizuta T, Benson WM, Foster BK, et al. Statistical analysis of the incidence of physeal injuries. *J Pediatr Orthop* 1987;7:518–523.
30. Ring D, Waters PM, Hotchkiss RN, et al. Pediatric floating elbow. *J Pediatr Orthop* 2001;21:456–459.
31. Waters PM, Kolettis GJ, Schwend R. Acute median neuropathy following physeal fractures of the distal radius. *J Pediatr Orthop* 1994;14:173–177.
32. Terry CL, Waters PM. Triangular fibrocartilage injuries in pediatric and adolescent patients. *J Hand Surg [Am]* 1998;23:626–634.
33. Earp BE, Waters PW, Wyzokowski RJ. Arthroscopic treatment of partial scapholunate tears in pediatric and adolescent patients with chronic wrist pain. *J Bone Joint Surg Am* (submission).
34. Smida M, Nigrou K, Soohun T, et al. Combined fracture of the distal radius and scaphoid in children. Report of 2 cases. *Acta Orthop Belg* 2003;69:79–81.
35. Salter RB, Harris WR. Injuries involving the epiphyseal plate. *J Bone Joint Surg Am* 1963;45:587–622.
36. Boyden EM, Peterson HA. Partial premature closure of the distal radial physis associated with Kirschner wire fixation. *Orthopedics* 1991;14:585–588.
37. Waters PM, Mintzer CM, Hipp JA, et al. Noninvasive measurement of distal radius instability. *J Hand Surg [Am]* 1997;22:572–579.
38. Mani GV, Hui PW, Cheng JC. Translation of the radius as a predictor of outcome in distal radial fractures of children. *J Bone Joint Surg Br* 1993;75:808–811.
39. Proctor MT, Moore DJ, Paterson JM. Redisplacement after manipulation of distal radial fractures in children. *J Bone Joint Surg Br* 1993;75:453–454.
40. Widmann R, Waters PM, Reeves S. Complications of closed treatment of distal radius fractures in children. POSNA Annual Meeting. Miami, 1995.
41. Gibbons CL, Woods DA, Pailthorpe C, et al. The management of isolated distal radius fractures in children. *J Pediatr Orthop* 1994;14:207–210.
42. Waters PM, Miller B, Taylor B, et al. Prospective study of displaced radius fractures in adolescents treated with casting vs. percutaneous pinning. AAOS Annual Meeting, 2000.
43. Hughston JC. Fractures of the forearm. *J Bone Joint Surg Am* 1962;44:1664–1667.
44. Mino DE, Palmer AK, Levinsohn EM. Radiography and computerized tomography in the diagnosis of incongruity of the distal radio-ulnar joint. A prospective study. *J Bone Joint Surg Am* 1985;67:247–252.
45. Morton R. A radiographic survey of 170 clinically diagnosed as "Colles" fracture. *Lancet* 1907;1:731–732.
46. Short WH, Palmer AK, Werner FW, et al. A biomechanical study of the distal radius. *J Hand Surg Am* 1897;12:529–534.
47. van der Linden W, Ericson R. Colles' fracture. How should its displacement be measured and how should it be immobilized? *J Bone Joint Surg Am* 1981;63:1285–1288.
48. Eksioglu F, Altinok D, Uslu MM, et al. Ultrasonographic findings in pediatric fractures. *Turk J Pediatr* 2003;45:136–140.
49. Hubner U, Schlicht W, Outzen S, et al. Ultrasound in the diagnosis of fractures in children. *J Bone Joint Surg Br* 2000;82:1170–1173.
50. Garn SM, Rohmann CG, Silverman FN. Radiographic standards for postnatal ossification and tooth calcification. *Med Radiogr Photogr* 1967;43:45–66.
51. Greulich W, Pyle SI. *Radiographic atlas of skeletal development of the hand and wrist*. Stanford: Stanford University Press, 1959.
52. Ogden JA, Beall JK, Conlogue GJ, et al. Radiology of postnatal skeletal development. IV. Distal radius and ulna. *Skeletal Radiol* 1981;6:255–266.
53. Fernandez DL, Palmer AK. Fractures of the distal radius. In: Green D, Hotchkiss R, Pederson W, eds. *Green's operative hand surgery*. New York: Churchill-Livingstone, 1999:929–985.
54. Hulten O. Uber anatomische variationen der hand-gelenkknochen. *Acta Radiol* 1928; 9:155–168.
55. Hafner R, Poznanski AK, Donovan JM. Ulnar variance in children—standard measurements for evaluation of ulnar shortening in juvenile rheumatoid arthritis, hereditary multiple exostosis and other bone or joint disorders in childhood. *Skel Radiol* 1989; 18:513–516.
56. Bowers W. The distal radioulnar joint. In: Green D, Hotchkiss R, Pederson W, eds. *Green's operative hand surgery*. New York: Churchill-Livingstone, 1999:986–1032.
57. Epner RA, Bowers WH, Guilford WB. Ulnar variance—the effect of wrist positioning and roentgen filming technique. *J Hand Surg Am* 1982;7:298–305.
58. Friedman SL, Palmer AK, Short WH, et al. The change in ulnar variance with grip. *J Hand Surg Am* 1993;18:713–716.
59. Steyers CM, Blair WF. Measuring ulnar variance: a comparison of techniques. *J Hand Surg Am* 1989;14:607–612.
60. Gelberman RH, Salamon PB, Jurist JM, et al. Ulnar variance in Kienbock's disease. *J Bone Joint Surg Am* 1975;57:674–676.
61. Palmer AK, Werner FW. The triangular fibrocartilage complex of the wrist—anatomy and function. *J Hand Surg Am* 1981;6:153–162.
62. Bruns. *Dislocations in joint fractures*. Philadelphia: WB Saunders, 1924:370.
63. Poland J. *Traumatic separation of the epiphysis*. London: Smith, Elder & Co., 1898.
64. Aitken AP. Further observations on the fractured distal radial epiphysis. *J Bone Joint Surg Am* 1935;17:922–927.
65. Aitken AP. The end results of the fractured distal radial epiphysis. *J Bone Joint Surg Am* 1935;17:302–308.
66. Peterson CA, Peterson HA. Analysis of the incidence of injuries to the epiphyseal growth plate. *J Trauma* 1972;12:275–281.
67. Peterson HA, Madhok R, Benson JT, et al. Physeal fractures: Part 1. Epidemiology in Olmsted County, Minnesota, 1979–1988. *J Pediatr Orthop* 1994;14:423–430.
68. Stansberry SD, Swischuk LE, Swischuk JL, et al. Significance of ulnar styloid fractures in childhood. *Pediatr Emerg Care* 1990;6:99–103.
69. Jones IE, Williams SM, Dow N, et al. How many children remain fracture-free during growth? A longitudinal study of children and adolescents participating in the Dunedin Multidisciplinary Health and Development Study. *Osteoporos Int* 2002;13:990–995.
70. Armstrong P, Joughlin J, Clarke H. Pediatric fractures of the forearm, wrist, and hand in skeletal trauma in children. In: Green N, Swiontkowski M, eds. *Skeletal trauma in children*. Philadelphia: WB Saunders, 1994:161–257.
71. Lee BS, Esterhai JL Jr, Das M. Fracture of the distal radial epiphysis. Characteristics and surgical treatment of premature, post-traumatic epiphyseal closure. *Clin Orthop* 1984:90–96.
72. Lesko PD, Georgis T, Slabaugh P. Irreducible Salter-Harris type II fracture of the distal radial epiphysis. *J Pediatr Orthop* 1987;7:719–721.
73. Pershad J, Monroe K, King W, et al. Can clinical parameters predict fractures in acute pediatric wrist injuries? *Acad Emerg Med* 2000;7:1152–1155.
74. Musharafieh RS, Macari G. Salter-Harris I fractures of the distal radius misdiagnosed as wrist sprain. *J Emerg Med* 2000;19:265–270.
75. Santoro V, Mara J. Compartmental syndrome complicating Salter-Harris type II distal radius fracture. *Clin Orthop* 1988:226–229.
76. Crawford AH. Pitfalls and complications of fractures of the distal radius and ulna in childhood. *Hand Clin* 1988;4:403–413.
77. Sasaki Y, Sugioka Y. The pronator quadratus sign: its classification and diagnostic usefulness for injury and inflammation of the wrist. *J Hand Surg Br* 1989;14:80–83.
78. Zammit-Maempel I, Bisset RA, Morris J, et al. The value of soft-tissue signs in wrist trauma. *Clin Radiol* 1988;39:664–668.
79. Rang M. *Children's fractures*. Philadelphia: JB Lippincott, 1983.
80. Arima J, Uchida Y, Miura H, et al. Osteochondral fracture in the distal end of the radius. *J Hand Surg Am* 1993;18:489–491.
81. Peterson HA. Physeal fractures: Part 3. Classification. *J Pediatr Orthop* 1994;14: 439–448.
82. Peterson HA. Physeal fractures: Part 2. Two previously unclassified types. *J Pediatr Orthop* 1994;14:431–438.
83. Peterson HA. Triplane fracture of the distal radius: case report. *J Pediatr Orthop* 1996; 16:192–194.
84. Stein AH Jr, Katz SF. Stabilization of comminuted fractures of the distal inch of the radius: percutaneous pinning. *Clin Orthop* 1975:174–181.
85. Horii E, Tamura Y, Nakamura R, et al. Premature closure of the distal radial physis. *J Hand Surg Br* 1993;18:11–16.
86. Langenskiold A, Osterman K. Surgical treatment of partial closure of the epiphysial plate. *Reconstr Surg Traumatol* 1979;17:48–64.
87. Compson JP. Trans-carpal injuries associated with distal radial fractures in children: a series of three cases. *J Hand Surg Br* 1992;17:311–314.
88. Gupta RP, Danielsson LG. Dorsally angulated solitary metaphyseal greenstick fractures in the distal radius: results after immobilization in pronated, neutral, and supinated position. *J Pediatr Orthop* 1990;10:90–92.
89. Chess DG, Hyndman JC, Leahey JL. Short-arm plaster for paediatric distal forearm fractures. *J Bone Joint Surg Br* 1987;69:506.
90. Chess DG, Hyndman JC, Leahey JL, et al. Short-arm plaster cast for distal pediatric forearm fractures. *J Pediatr Orthop* 1994;14:211–213.
91. Manoli A 2nd. Irreducible fracture-separation of the distal radial epiphysis. Report of a case. *J Bone Joint Surg Am* 1982;64:1095–1096.
92. Kasser JR. Forearm fractures. In MacEwen GD, Kasser JR, Heinrich SD, eds. *Pediatric fractures: a practical approach to assessment and treatment*. Baltimore: Williams & Wilkins, 1993:165–190.
93. Hernandez J Jr, Peterson HA. Fracture of the distal radial physis complicated by compartment syndrome and premature physeal closure. *J Pediatr Orthop* 1986;6:627–630.

94. Lenoble E, Dumontier C, Goutallier D, et al. Fracture of the distal radius. A prospective comparison between trans-styloid and Kapandji fixations. *J Bone Joint Surg Br* 1995; 77:562–567.
95. Karlsson J, Appelqvist R. Irreducible fracture of the wrist in a child. Entrapment of the extensor tendons. *Acta Orthop Scand* 1987;58:280–281.
96. Young TB. Irreducible displacement of the distal radial epiphysis complicating a fracture of the lower radius and ulna. *Injury* 1984;16:166–168.
97. Geissler W, Freeland A, Weiss A-P, et al. Techniques of wrist arthroscopy. Instructional course lecture. *J Bone Joint Surg Am* 1999;81:1184–1197.
98. Doi K, Hattori Y, Otsuka K, et al. Intra-articular fractures of the distal aspect of the radius: arthroscopically assisted reduction compared with open reduction and internal fixation. *J Bone Joint Surg Am* 1999;81:1093–1110.
99. Freeland AE, Geissler WB. The arthroscopic management of intra-articular distal radius fractures. *Hand Surg* 2000;5:93–102.
100. Lindau T. Wrist arthroscopy in distal radial fractures using a modified horizontal technique. *Arthroscopy* 2001;17:E5.
101. Watson K, Talesnik J. Midcarpal instability caused by malunited fracture of the distal radius. *J Hand Surg Am* 1984:350.
102. Fernandez DL. Correction of post-traumatic wrist deformity in adults by osteotomy, bone-grafting, and internal fixation. *J Bone Joint Surg Am* 1982;64:1164–1178.
103. Knirk JL, Jupiter JB. Intra-articular fractures of the distal end of the radius in young adults. *J Bone Joint Surg Am* 1986;68:647–659.
104. Valverde JA, Albinana J, Certucha JA. Early posttraumatic physeal arrest in distal radius after a compression injury. *J Pediatr Orthop B* 1996;5:57–60.
105. Cannata G, De Maio F, Mancini F, et al. Physeal fractures of the distal radius and ulna: long-term prognosis. *J Orthop Trauma* 2003;17:172–179; discussion 179–180.
106. Waters PM, Bae DS, Montgomery KD. Surgical management of posttraumatic distal radial growth arrest in adolescents. *J Pediatr Orthop* 2002;22:717–724.
107. Palmer AK, Glisson RR, Werner FW. Relationship between ulnar variance and triangular fibrocartilage complex thickness. *J Hand Surg Am* 1984;9:681–682.
108. Peterson HA. Partial growth plate arrest and its treatment. *J Pediatr Orthop* 1984;4: 246–258.
109. Langenskiold A. Surgical treatment of partial closure of the growth plate. *J Pediatr Orthop* 1981;1:3–11.
110. Bell MJ, Hill RJ, McMurtry RY. Ulnar impingement syndrome. *J Bone Joint Surg Br* 1985;67:126–129.
111. DiFiori JP, Puffer JC, Aish B, et al. Wrist pain, distal radial physeal injury, and ulnar variance in young gymnasts: does a relationship exist? *Am J Sports Med* 2002;30: 879–885.
112. Burgess RC, Watson HK. Hypertrophic ulnar styloid nonunions. *Clin Orthop* 1988: 215–217.
113. Maffulli N, Fixsen JA. Painful hypertrophic non-union of the ulnar styloid. *J Hand Surg Br* 1990;15:355–357.
114. Onne L, Sandblom PH. Late results in fractures of the forearm in children. *Acta Chir Scand Suppl* 1949;98:549–567.
115. Gelberman RH. Acute carpal tunnel syndrome. In Gelbern AN, ed. *Operative nerve repair and reconstruction*. Philadelphia: JB Lippincott, 1991:937–948.
116. Dobyns JH, Gabel GT. Gymnast's wrist. *Hand Clin* 1990;6:493–505.
117. Mandelbaum BR, Bartolozzi AR, Davis CA, et al. Wrist pain syndrome in the gymnast. Pathogenetic, diagnostic, and therapeutic considerations. *Am J Sports Med* 1989;17: 305–317.
118. Ruggles DL, Peterson HA, Scott SG. Radial growth plate injury in a female gymnast. *Med Sci Sports Exerc* 1991;23:393–396.
119. Yong-Hing K, Wedge JH, Bowen CV. Chronic injury to the distal ulnar and radial growth plates in an adolescent gymnast. A case report. *J Bone Joint Surg Am* 1988;70: 1087–1089.
120. Nelson DA, Buchanan JR, Harrison CS. Distal ulnar growth arrest. *J Hand Surg Am* 1984;9:164–171.
121. Golz RJ, Grogan DP, Greene TL, et al. Distal ulnar physeal injury. *J Pediatr Orthop* 1991;11:318–326.
122. Evans DL, Stauber M, Frykman GK. Irreducible epiphyseal plate fracture of the distal ulna due to interposition of the extensor carpi ulnaris tendon. A case report. *Clin Orthop* 1990;251:162–165.
123. Landfried MJ, Stenclik M, Susi JG. Variant of Galeazzi fracture-dislocation in children. *J Pediatr Orthop* 1991;11:332–335.
124. Ogden JA. *Skeletal injury in the child*. Philadelphia: WB Saunders, 1990.
125. Langenberg R. [Fracture of the ulnar styloid process. Effect on wrist function in the presence of distal radius fracture]. *Zentralbl Chir* 1989;114:1006–1011.
126. Peinado A. Distal radial epiphyseal displacement after impaired distal ulnar growth. *J Bone Joint Surg Am* 1979;61:88–92.
127. Noonan KJ. Pediatric upper extremity fractures. In: Price CT, ed. *Complication in orthopaedics*. Rosemont, IL: American Academy of Orthopaedic Surgeons, 2004.
128. Skillern PGJ. Complete fracture of the lower third of the radius in childhood with greenstick fracture of the ulna. *Ann Surg* 1915;61:209–225.
129. Kiely PD, Kiely PJ, Stephens MM, et al. Atypical distal radial fractures in children. *J Pediatr Orthop B* 2004;13:202–205.
130. Wilkins KE, O'Brien E. Distal radius and ulnar fractures. In: Bucholz RW, Heckman JD, eds. *Rockwood and Green's Fractures in Adults*. Philadelphia: Lippincott Williams & Wilkins, 2002.
131. Weiker GG. Hand and wrist problems in the gymnast. *Clin Sports Med* 1992;11: 189–202.
132. Papavasiliou V, Nenopoulos S. Ipsilateral injuries of the elbow and forearm in children. *J Pediatr Orthop* 1986;6:58–60.
133. Stanitski CL, Micheli LJ. Simultaneous ipsilateral fractures of the arm and forearm in children. *Clin Orthop* 1980:218–222.
134. Symons S, Rowsell M, Bhowal B, et al. Hospital versus home management of children with buckle fractures of the distal radius. A prospective, randomised trial. *J Bone Joint Surg Br* 2001;83:556–560.
135. Roposch A, Reis M, Molina M, et al. The floating forearm: supracondylar fractures of the humerus associated with ipsilateral forearm fractures in children. *J Pediatr Orthop* 2001;21(3):307–312.
136. Hove LM. Simultaneous scaphoid and distal radial fractures. *J Hand Surg Br* 1994;19: 384–388.
137. Grundy M. Fractures of the carpal scaphoid in children. A series of eight cases. *Br J Surg* 1969;56:523–524.
138. Greene WB, Anderson WJ. Simultaneous fracture of the scaphoid and radius in a child. *J Pediatr Orthop* 1982;2:191–194.
139. Templeton PA, Graham HK. The 'floating elbow' in children. Simultaneous supracondylar fractures of the humerus and of the forearm in the same upper limb. *J Bone Joint Surg Br* 1995;77:791–796.
140. Trumble TE, Benirschke SK, Vedder NB. Ipsilateral fractures of the scaphoid and radius. *J Hand Surg Am* 1993;18:8–14.
141. Vahvanen V, Westerlund M. Fracture of the carpal scaphoid in children. A clinical and roentgenological study of 108 cases. *Acta Orthop Scand* 1980;51:909–913.
142. Fowles JV, Kassab MT. Displaced supracondylar fractures of the elbow in children. A report on the fixation of extension and flexion fractures by two lateral percutaneous pins. *J Bone Joint Surg Br* 1974;56B:490–500.
143. Light TR, Ogden DA, Ogden JA. The anatomy of metaphyseal torus fractures. *Clin Orthop* 1984;188:103–111.
144. Banas MP, Dalldorf PG, Marquardt JD. Skateboard and in-line skate fractures: a report of one summer's experience. *J Orthop Trauma* 1992;6:301–305.
145. Biyani A. Ipsilateral Monteggia equivalent injury and distal radial and ulnar fracture in a child. *J Orthop Trauma* 1994;8:431–433.
146. Solan MC, Rees R, Daly K. Current management of torus fractures of the distal radius. *Injury* 2002;33:503–505.
147. Davidson JS, Brown DJ, Barnes SN, et al. Simple treatment for torus fractures of the distal radius. *J Bone Joint Surg Br* 2001;83:1173–1175.
148. Blount WP. *Fractures in children*. Baltimore: Williams & Wilkins, 1955.
149. Cooper RR. Management of common forearm fractures in children. *J Iowa Med Soc* 1964;54:689–698.
150. MacLaughlin HL. *Trauma*. Philadelphia: WB Saunders, 1959.
151. Sharrard WJW. *Paediatric orthopaedics and fractures*. Oxford: Blackwell Scientific Publications, 1971.
152. Pollen AG. *Fractures and dislocations in children*. Baltimore: Williams & Wilkins, 1973.
153. De Courtivron B. Spontaneous correction of the distal forearm fractures in children. European Pediatric Orthopaedic Society Annual Meeting. Brussels, Belgium, 1995.
154. Perona PG, Light TR. Remodeling of the skeletally immature distal radius. *J Orthop Trauma* 1990;4:356–361.
155. Wilkins KE. Operative management of upper extremity fractures in children. American Academy of Orthopaedic Surgeons. Rosemont, Illinois, 1994.
156. Evans EM. Fractures of the radius and ulna. *J Bone Joint Surg Br* 1951;33-B:548–561.
157. Schranz PJ, Fagg PS. Undisplaced fractures of the distal third of the radius in children: an innocent fracture? *Injury* 1992;23:165–167.
158. Fernandez DL. Conservative treatment of forearm fractures in children. In: Chapchal G, ed. *Fractures in children*. New York: Thieme-Stratton, 1981.
159. Davis DR, Green DP. Forearm fractures in children: pitfalls and complications. *Clin Orthop* 1976;120:172–183.
160. Stuhmer KG. Fractures of the distal forearm. In: Weber BG, Burner C, Freuler F, eds. *Treatment of fractures in children and adolescents*. New York: Springer-Verlag, 1980: 203–217.
161. Deffer PA, Schonholtz G, Litchman HM. Displaced distal forearm fractures in children. *Bull Hosp Joint Dis* 1963;24:42–47.
162. Tachdjian MO. *Pediatric orthopedics*, 2nd ed. Philadelphia: WB Saunders, 1990.
163. Kasser JR. Fractures. In MacEwen GD, Kasser JR, Heinrich SD, eds. *A practical approach to assessment and treatment*. Baltimore: Williams & Wilkins, 1993:165–190.
164. Carpenter C, Williams P. Management of completely displaced metaphyseal fractures of the distal radius in children. *J Bone Joint Surg Br* 2003;85:933; author reply 933–934.
165. Gambhir AK, Fischer J, Waseem M. Management of completely displaced metaphyseal fractures of the distal radius in children. *J Bone Joint Surg Br* 2003;85:463; author reply 463.
166. McLauchlan GJ, Cowan B, Annan IH, et al. Management of completely displaced metaphyseal fractures of the distal radius in children. A prospective, randomised controlled trial. *J Bone Joint Surg Br* 2002;84:413–417.
167. Daruwalla JS. A study of radioulnar movements following fractures of the forearm in children. *Clin Orthop* 1979;139:114–120.
168. Friberg KS. Remodelling after distal forearm fractures in children. I. The effect of residual angulation on the spatial orientation of the epiphyseal plates. *Acta Orthop Scand* 1979;50:537–546.
169. Friberg KS. Remodelling after distal forearm fractures in children. II. The final orientation of the distal and proximal epiphyseal plates of the radius. *Acta Orthop Scand* 1979; 50:731–739.
170. Hogstrom H, Nilsson BE, Willner S. Correction with growth following diaphyseal forearm fracture. *Acta Chir Scand* 1976;47:229–303.
171. Larsen E, Vittas D, Torp-Pedersen S. Remodeling of angulated distal forearm fractures in children. *Clin Orthop Rel Res* 1988;237:190–195.
172. Roberts JA. Angulation of the radius in children's fractures. *J Bone Joint Surg Br* 1986; 68:751–754.
173. Roy DR. Completely displaced distal radius fractures with intact ulnas in children. *Orthopedics* 1989;12:1089–1092.

174. Vance RM, Gelberman RH. Acute ulnar neuropathy with fractures at the wrist. *J Bone Joint Surg Am* 1978;60:962–965.
175. Miller BS, Taylor B, Widmann R, et al. Cast immobilization versus percutaneous pin fixation of displaced distal radius fractures in children: a prospective, randomized study. *J Pediatr Orthop,* in press.
176. Voto SJ, Weiner DS, Leighley B. Redisplacement after closed reduction of forearm fractures in children. *J Pediatr Orthop* 1990;10:79–84.
177. Creasman C, Zaleske DJ, Ehrlich MG. Analyzing forearm fractures in children. The more subtle signs of impending problems. *Clin Orthop* 1984;188:40–53.
178. Fuller DJ, McCullough CJ. Malunited fractures of the forearm in children. *J Bone Joint Surg Br* 1982;64:364–367.
179. Guero S. Fractures and epiphyseal fracture separation of the distal bones of the forearm in children. In: Saffar P, Cooney WP, eds. *Fractures of the distal radius*, vol. 280. Philadelphia: JB Lippincott, 1995.
180. Trumble TE, Wagner W, Hanel DP, et al. Intrafocal (Kapandji) pinning of distal radius fractures with and without external fixation. *J Hand Surg Am* 1998;23:381–394.
181. Low CK, Liau KH, Chew WY. Results of distal radial fractures treated by intra-focal pin fixation. *Ann Acad Med Singapore* 2001;30:573–576.
182. Schuind F, Cooney WP 3rd, Burny F, et al. Small external fixation devices for the hand and wrist. *Clin Orthop* 1993;293:77–82.
183. Holmes JR, Louis DS. Entrapment of pronator quadratus in pediatric distal-radius fractures: recognition and treatment. *J Pediatr Orthop* 1994;14:498–500.
184. Younger AS, Tredwell SJ, Mackenzie WG, et al. Accurate prediction of outcome after pediatric forearm fracture. *J Pediatr Orthop* 1994;14:200–206.
185. Friberg KS. Remodelling after distal forearm fractures in children. III. Correction of residual angulation in fractures of the radius. *Acta Orthop Scand* 1979;50:741–749.
186. Qairul IH, Kareem BA, Tan AB, et al. Early remodeling in children's forearm fractures. *Med J Malaysia* 2001;56[Suppl D]:34–37.
187. Karaharju EO, Ryoppy SA, Makinen RJ. Remodelling by asymmetrical epiphysial growth. An experimental study in dogs. *J Bone Joint Surg Br* 1976;58:122–126.
188. Tang CW, Kay RM, Skaggs DL. Growth arrest of the distal radius following a metaphyseal fracture: case report and review of the literature. *J Pediatr Orthop B* 2002;11:89–92.
189. Ryoppy S, Karaharju EO. Alteration of epiphyseal growth by an experimentally produced angular deformity. *Acta Orthop Scand* 1974;45:490–498.
190. Tarr RR, Garfinkel AI, Sarmiento A. The effects of angular and rotational deformities of both bones of the forearm. An in vitro study. *J Bone Joint Surg Am* 1984;66:65–70.
191. Matthews LS, Kaufer H, Garver DF, et al. The effect on supination-pronation of angular malalignment of fractures of both bones of the forearm. *J Bone Joint Surg Am* 1982;64:14–17.
192. Johari AN, Sinha M. Remodeling of forearm fractures in children. *J Pediatr Orthop B* 1999;8:84–87.
193. Nilsson BE, Obrant K. The range of motion following fracture of the shaft of the forearm in children. *Acta Orthop Scand* 1977;48:600–602.
194. Meier R, Prommersberger KJ, van Griensven M, et al. Surgical correction of deformities of the distal radius due to fractures in pediatric patients. *Arch Orthop Trauma Surg* 2004;124:1–9.
195. Prommersberger KJ, Van Schoonhoven J, Lanz UB. Outcome after corrective osteotomy for malunited fractures of the distal end of the radius. *J Hand Surg Br* 2002;27:55–60.
196. Kameyama O, Ogawa R. Pseudarthrosis of the radius associated with neurofibromatosis: report of a case and review of the literature. *J Pediatr Orthop* 1990;10:128–131.
197. Vince KG, Miller JE. Cross-union complicating fracture of the forearm. Part II: Children. *J Bone Joint Surg Am* 1987;69:654–661.
198. Fatti JF, Mosher JF. An unusual complication of fracture of both bones of the forearm in a child. A case report. *J Bone Joint Surg Am* 1986;68:451–453.
199. Fodden DI. A study of wrist injuries in children: the incidence of various injuries and of premature closure of the distal radial growth plate. *Arch Emerg Med* 1992;9:9–13.
200. de Pablos J, Franzreb M, Barrios C. Longitudinal growth pattern of the radius after forearm fractures conservatively treated in children. *J Pediatr Orthop* 1994;14:492–495.
201. Clarke AC, Spencer RF. Ulnar nerve palsy following fractures of the distal radius: clinical and anatomical studies. *J Hand Surg Br* 1991;16:438–440.
202. Wolfe JS, Eyring EJ. Median-nerve entrapment within a greenstick fracture; a case report. *J Bone Joint Surg Am* 1974;56:1270–1272.
203. Fee NF, Dobranski A, Bisla RS. Gas gangrene complicating open forearm fractures. Report of five cases. *J Bone Joint Surg Am* 1977;59:135–138.
204. Reckling FW, Peltier LF. Riccardo Galeazzi and Galeazzi's fracture. *Surgery* 1965;58:453–459.
205. Galeazzi R. Di una particulare sindrome, traumatica delle scheletro dell avambraccio. *Attie Mem Soc Lombardi Chir* 1934;2:12.
206. Bley L, Seitz WH, Jr. Injuries about the distal ulna in children. *Hand Clin* 1998;14:231–237.
207. Letts RM. Monteggia and Galeazzi fractures. In: Letts RM, ed. *Management of pediatric fractures*. New York: Churchill-Livingstone, 1994:313–321.
208. Reckling FW, Cordell LD. Unstable fracture-dislocations of the forearm. The Monteggia and Galeazzi lesions. *Arch Surg* 1968;96:999–1007.
209. Walsh HP, McLaren CA, Owen R. Galeazzi fractures in children. *J Bone Joint Surg Br* 1987;69:730–733.
210. Mikic ZD. Galeazzi fracture-dislocations. *J Bone Joint Surg Am* 1975;57:1071–1080.
211. Dameron TB Jr. Traumatic dislocation of the distal radio-ulnar joint. *Clin Orthop* 1972;83:55–63.
212. Rose-Innes AP. Anterior dislocation of the ulna at the inferior radio-ulnar joint. Case report, with a discussion of the anatomy of rotation of the forearm. *J Bone Joint Surg Br* 1960;42-B:515–521.
213. Snook GA, Chrisman OD, Wilson TC, et al. Subluxation of the distal radio-ulnar joint by hyperpronation. *J Bone Joint Surg Am* 1969;51:1315–1323.
214. Letts M, Rowhani N. Galeazzi-equivalent injuries of the wrist in children. *J Pediatr Orthop* 1993;13:561–566.
215. Homans J, Smith JA. Fracture of the lower end of the radius associated with fracture or dislocation of the lower end of the ulna. *Boston Med Surg J* 1922;187:401–407.
216. Schuind F, An KN, Berglund L, et al. The distal radioulnar ligaments: a biomechanical study. *J Hand Surg Am* 1991;16:1106–1114.
217. Werner FW, Palmer AK, Fortino MD, et al. Force transmission through the distal ulna: effect of ulnar variance, lunate fossa angulation, and radial and palmar tilt of the distal radius. *J Hand Surg Am* 1992;17:423–428.
218. Moore TM, Klein JP, Patzakis MJ, et al. Results of compression-plating of closed Galeazzi fractures. *J Bone Joint Surg Am* 1985;67:1015–1021.
219. Mohan K, Gupta AK, Sharma J, et al. Internal fixation in 50 cases of Galeazzi fracture. *Acta Orthop Scand* 1988;59:318–320.
220. Kraus B, Horne G. Galeazzi fractures. *J Trauma* 1985;25:1093–1095.
221. Vesely DG. The distal radio-ulnar joint. *Clin Orthop* 1967;51:75–91.
222. Cetti NE. An unusual cause of blocked reduction of the Galeazzi injury. *Injury* 1977;9:59–61.
223. Biyani A, Bhan S. Dual extensor tendon entrapment in Galeazzi fracture-dislocation: a case report. *J Trauma* 1989;29:1295–1297.
224. Itoh Y, Horiuchi Y, Takahashi M, et al. Extensor tendon involvement in Smith's and Galeazzi's fractures. *J Hand Surg Am* 1987;12:535–540.
225. Ooi LH, Toh CL. Galeazzi-equivalent fracture in children associated with tendon entrapment—report of two cases. *Ann Acad Med Singapore* 2001;30:51–54.
226. Engber WD, Keene JS. Irreducible fracture-separation of the distal ulnar epiphysis. Report of a case. *J Bone Joint Surg Am* 1985;67:1130–1132.
227. Warren JD. Anterior interosseous nerve palsy as a complication of forearm fractures. *J Bone Joint Surg Br* 1963;45:511–512.
228. Stahl S, Freiman S, Volpin G. Anterior interosseous nerve palsy associated with Galeazzi fracture. *J Pediatr Orthop B* 2000;9:45–46.
229. Moore TM, Lester DK, Sarmiento A. The stabilizing effect of soft-tissue constraints in artificial Galeazzi fractures. *Clin Orthop* 1985;194:189–194.

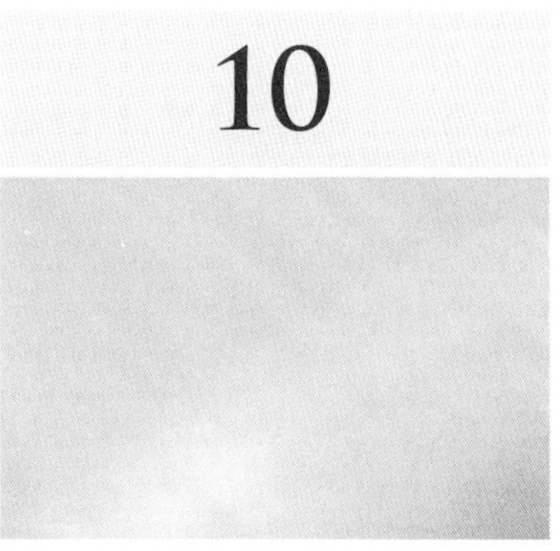

10

INJURIES TO THE SHAFTS OF THE RADIUS AND ULNA

Charles T. Mehlman and Eric J. Wall

Injuries to the shafts of the radius and ulna are one of the most common reasons for children to receive orthopaedic care (1–3) and are among the most challenging to the orthopaedist because of their treatment complexity and frequent complications (4–6). Because of numerous differences in both treatment and prognosis, shaft fractures are considered to be clinically distinct from fractures of the distal (metaphyseal fractures and physeal fractures) and proximal (radial neck fractures and physeal fractures) ends of the same bones (7–13). Most shaft injuries present no unusual challenges and require nothing more than skillful closed fracture care (14–16). The remainder constitute a mixture of crooked bones, anxious parents, and hyperkinetic children that may truly test the orthopaedist's entire skill set (including psychosocial skills). Issues regarding reduction, remanipulation, recasting, remodeling, and refracture must be mastered. Shaft fractures of the forearm also are the most common reason for orthopaedic surgery of the forearm in children (1,17). Thus, it is very important for orthopaedic surgeons who treat children to master both the cognitive and technical aspects of operative treatment for injuries to the shafts of the radius and ulna.

HISTORY

Forearm fractures in children are common both in contemporary and ancient terms. In one of the oldest examples, the remains of a 15-year-old from the Paleolithic period (the Stone Age) demonstrate post-traumatic forearm deformity (18). Among the skeletons of children from medieval England (circa 950 A.D.) acute trauma and new bone formation were most common in 6- to 10-year-olds (19). Other archeological reports from the medieval period (circa 1100–1550 A.D.) indicate that forearm fractures were not only common but also presumably well treated, based on absence of substantial deformity (20). This latter finding may simply be an early testament to pediatric remodeling potential.

The contemporary history of pediatric forearm fracture care bears the marks of many orthopaedic icons. The Austrian surgeon Lorenz Böhler (1885–1973) had a world-wide impact on fracture care (21,22). In the late 1920s he published his important book *The Treatment of Fractures*, and it flourished for nearly three decades. It was translated into eight different languages and published in 13 German and 5 English editions (22). Böhler recognized that reduction tactics that used exaggeration of the deformity and re-engagement of the bone ends often were effective in distal-third forearm fractures, but longitudinal traction was his main tool for reducing fractures in the middle and proximal thirds (23) (Fig. 10-1). His protocol for forearm fracture reduction included belted countertraction of the humerus above the flexed elbow while exerting "steady (not jerky) strong traction by pulling on the thumb with one hand and on the second to fourth fingers with the other hand. Traction on the thumb must be stronger than that on the other fingers" (Fig. 10-2) (23). Böhler believed that forearm fracture reduction would occur within 5 to 10 minutes when using this technique, and he favored skin-tight plasters (i.e., form-fitting casts with little to no padding) for immobilization (22,24). He stated that "it is unimportant whether lateral displacement of half or even of the entire width of the diaphysis is corrected, because such

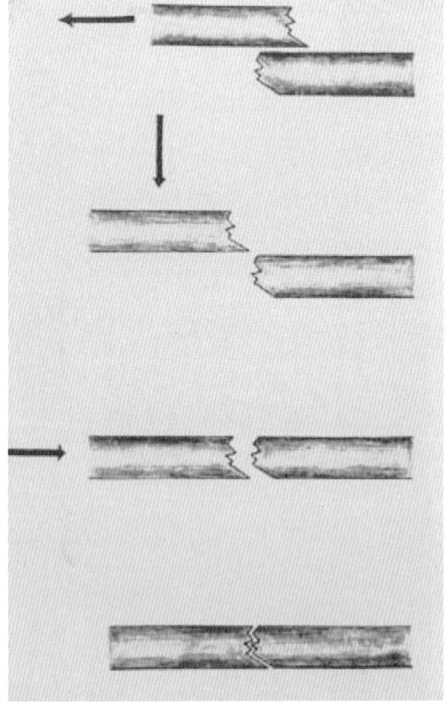

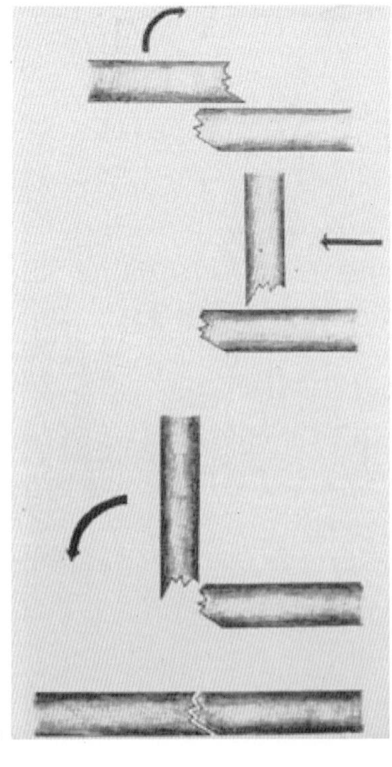

FIGURE 10-1 Fracture reduction techniques for complete fractures from Böhler's original textbook. **A.** Longitudinal traction method. **B.** Exageration of deformity method. (Reproduced from Böhler L. *The treatment of fractures*, 5th English edition. New York: Grune & Stratton, 1956.)

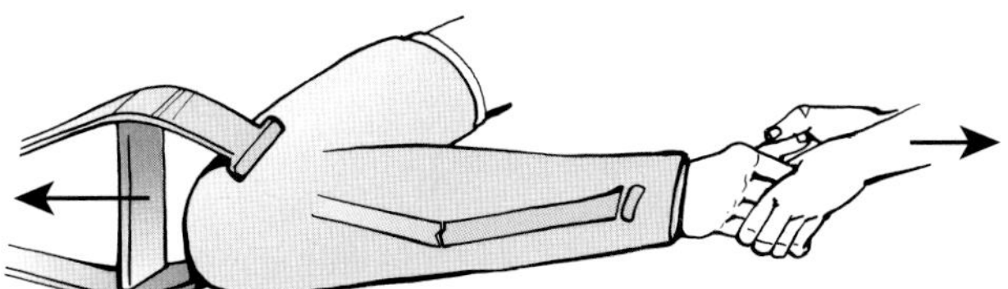

FIGURE 10-2 Böhler's horizontal traction/countertraction method.

displacement usually disappears within a year. The same is true of angulation up to 10 or 15 degrees. More marked angulation and rotation must be corrected. Shortening is of no importance. There is never any necessity in adolescents to reduce closed forearm fractures operatively, or to unite the fragments with nails, wires or plates and screws" (23). Böhler's outspoken criticism of pediatric forearm surgery continued, "Operative treatment, as bourne out by x-ray pictures in the literature, is very often practiced in children, and consists of osteosynthesis of different types as well as open reduction. It is superfluous, because conservative treatment is always successful. Moreover, operative treatment is dangerous in that infection with all its consequences may ensue. Pseudarthroses have also been reported following operative treatment, which are unknown in children" (23).

Despite high-profile critics such as Böhler, enthusiasm for internal fixation in children grew, reflecting the resurgent interest in osteosynthesis in adults that occurred in the late 1930s (25). With the publication of his highly regarded textbook *Operative Orthopaedics* in 1939, the American Willis Campbell (1880–1941) tacitly approved operations on children's forearm fractures by illustrating open reduction and internal fixation of a distal-third forearm shaft fracture in a patient who was perhaps as young as 11 or 12 years of age (Fig. 10-3). He stated, "When satisfactory alignment or fixation in fractures of both bones of the forearm is not possible by conservative measures, skeletal traction or open reduction is required. This is particularly true of oblique or spiral fractures. Internal fixation, preferably by a vitallium plate, should be applied to prevent bowing" (26). Later advocates of osteosynthesis such as the Belgian Jean Verbrugge (1896–1964) also reported on internal fixation for fractures in children, listing forearm fractures as one of the most common indications (27). The rather indiscriminate application of surgical techniques (by some surgeons of the day) to children helps explain the criticism from Böhler and other authors who followed (23,28–31).

In the 1950s two important authors influenced pediatric forearm fracture care. The Englishman Sir John Charnley (1911–1982) in his textbook *The Closed Treatment of Common Fractures* challenged the utility of Böhler's horizontal traction approach to forearm reduction and advocated his preferred method of vertical traction (Fig. 10-4) (32). Charnley did not accept Böhler's concept of skin-tight plasters and favored padded plasters with three-point molding instead (Fig. 10-5). This concept was embodied by Charnley's maxim: "A curved plaster is necessary in order to make a straight limb" (32).

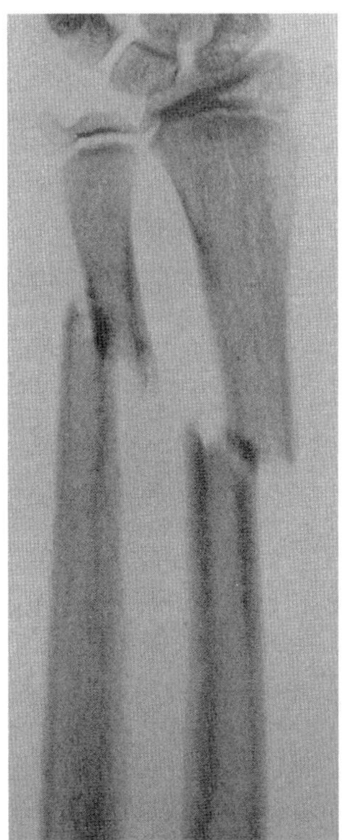

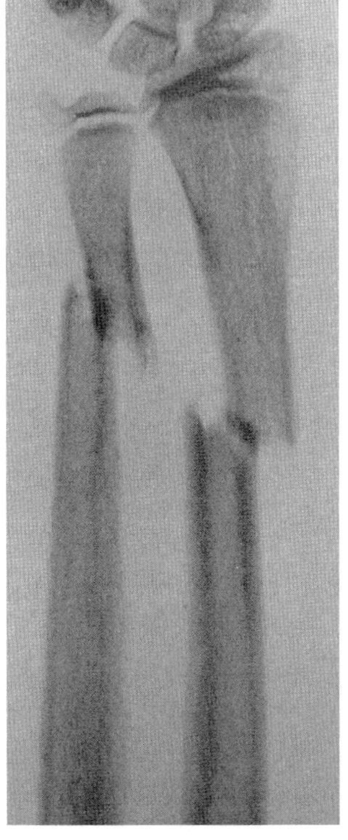

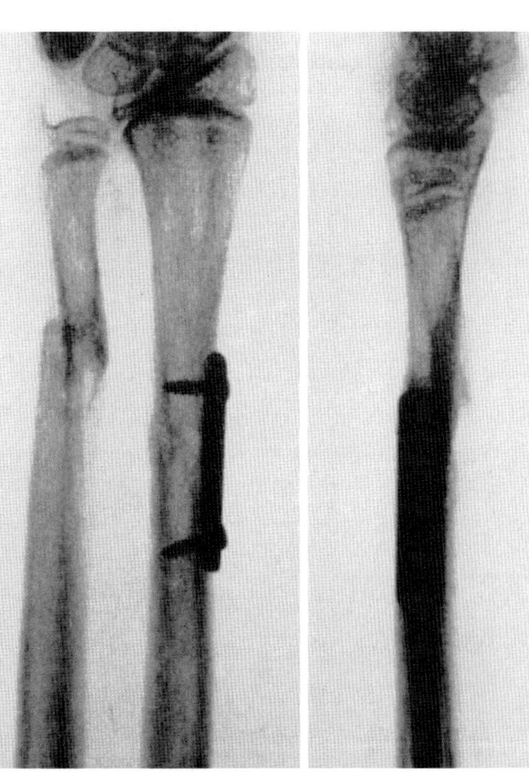

FIGURE 10-3 Original illustration from Campbell's 1939 textbook. **A.** Approximately 12-year-old patient with distal-third radius and ulna shaft fracture. **B.** Postoperative x-rays after plate fixation of radius.

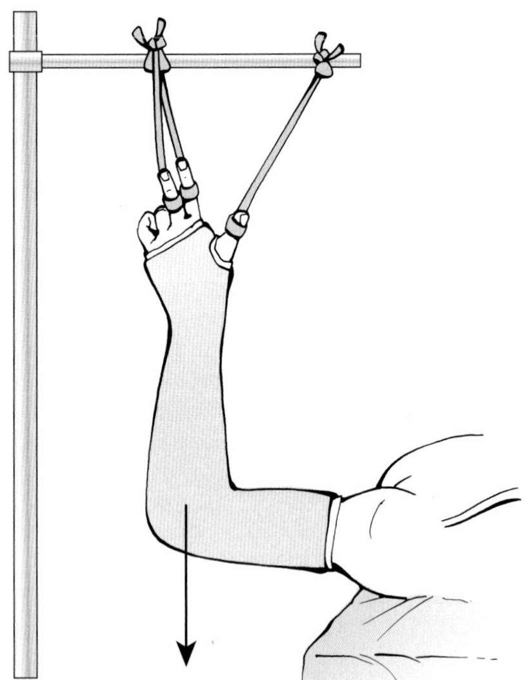

FIGURE 10-4 Charnley's vertical traction.

The American Walter Blount (1900–1992), in his book on children's fractures (33), offered strong recommendations for nonoperative treatment of nearly all children's fractures (especially fractures of the middle third of the forearm). He was an outspoken critic of most surgical treatment of children's fractures and offered impressive illustrations of successful nonoperative care of forearm shaft fractures in children (Fig. 10-6) (33). Blount's frustration regarding the state of affairs of children's fractures is captured in this 1967 quote: "The ever-changing crop of fledgling surgeons of trauma must learn anew that fractures in children are different from those in adults. This is particularly true of fractures of the forearm" (29). The reduction technique he advocated was one of manually exaggerating the fracture deformity while simultaneously applying traction and using the surgeon's thumbs as a fulcrum. Regarding forearm fractures in children Blount also stated, "Bayonet apposition in good alignment is not to be confused with angular deformity. . . . Too many men treat roentgenograms instead of children" (33).

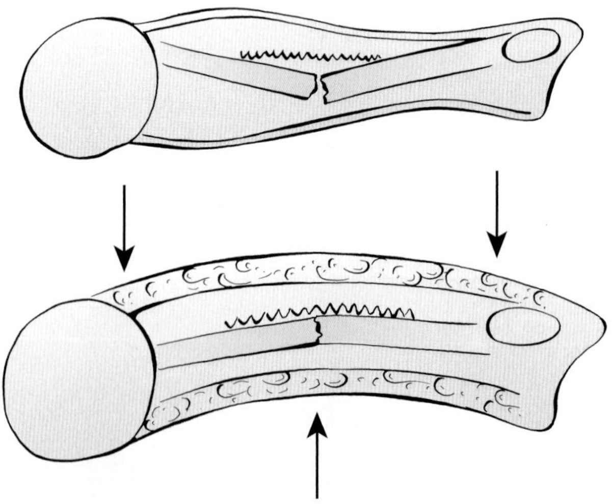

FIGURE 10-5 Charnley's three-point mold illustration.

By the mid-1960s another important personality entered the world of pediatric fractures: the Englishman Mercer Rang (1933–2003). Rang first published a book entitled *The Growth Plate and Its Disorders*, which was aimed at orthopaedists who cared for children, and later (1974) his classic text *Children's Fractures*, in which he highlighted many of the practical aspects of caring for children's fractures, including forearm fractures. Contrary to the forearm shaft fracture rotational dogma of others, Rang said, "Immobilize the fracture in the position—any position—in which the alignment is correct and the reduction feels stable" (34). He also discussed the value of single-bone internal fixation with a Kirschner wire in selected patients when open reduction was preferable to malunion (34). The bulk of his discussion of reduction techniques and casting techniques was not new (it reflected the work of those who had come before him), but it was effectively illustrated (with his own artwork) and communicated to generations of orthopaedic surgeons around the world (35).

EPIDEMIOLOGY

Risk is a central concept in clinical epidemiology (36). Landin has shown that the overall risk of fracture in children slowly increases for both boys and girls until they are 11 or 12 years old and then drops for girls and increases further for boys (37) (Fig. 10-7). This risk difference is starkly illustrated by the fact that boys who are 13 or older have approximately double the fracture rate of their female peers (37). Forearm fractures have been reported to be the most common pediatric fracture associated with backyard trampoline (38) use and the second most common one (supracondylar humeral fractures were first) associated with monkeybars (39). Using a national database, Chung and Spilson looked at the frequency of upper extremity fractures in the United States and found that the single largest demographic group was fractures of the radius and ulna in children aged 14 years or less, with a rate approaching 1 in 100 (3).

Large studies that distinguish distal radial fractures from forearm shaft fractures indicate that overall, radial shaft injuries rank as the third most common fracture of childhood (behind distal radial and supracondylar humeral fractures) (1). Open fractures in children are most often fractures of the shaft of the radius and ulna or tibial shaft fractures (1). Forearm shaft injuries are the most common site of refracture (37). Forearm shaft fractures have been shown to occur most commonly in the 12- to 16-year-old age group, a challenging age group to treat (1).

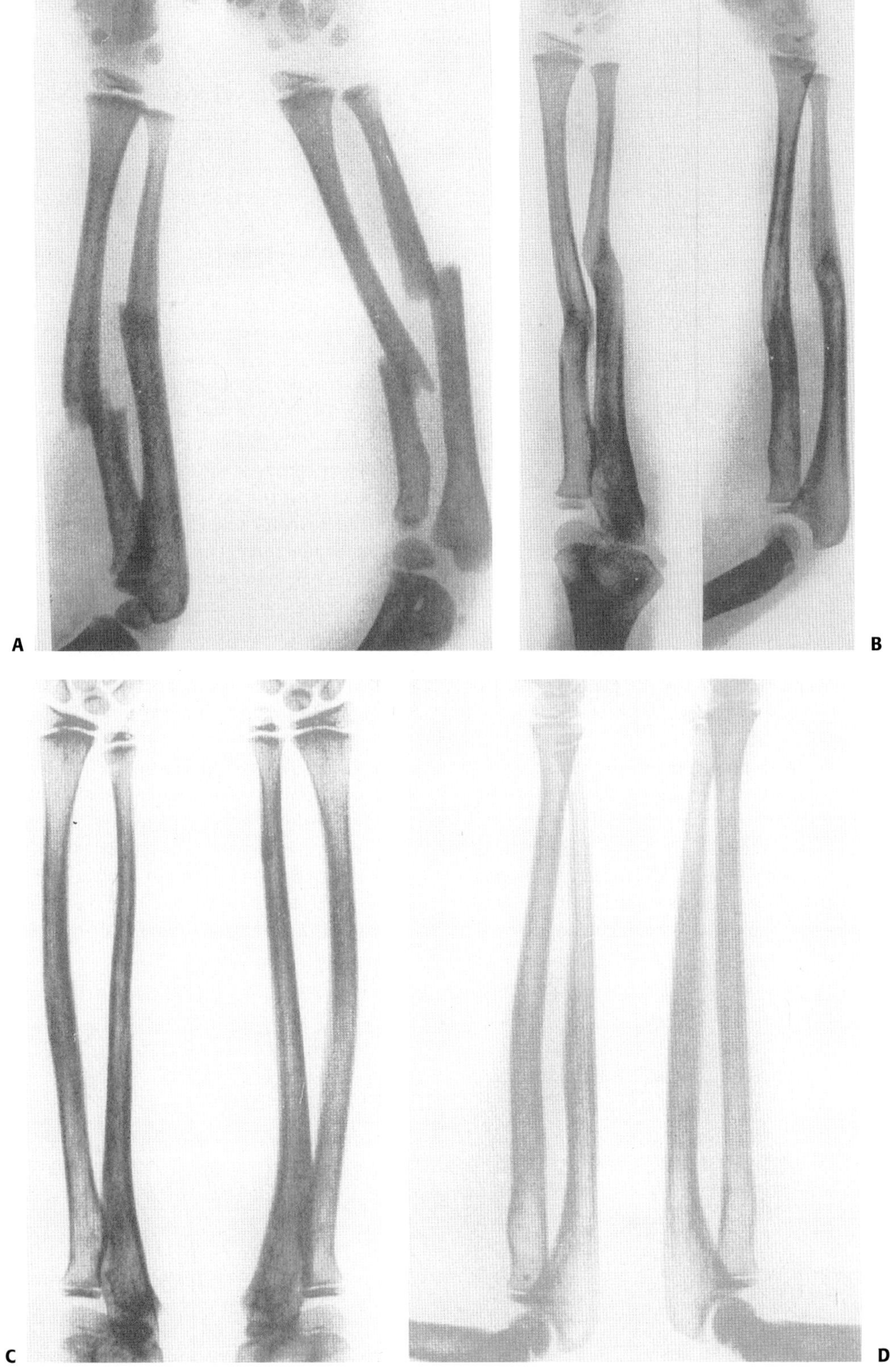

FIGURE 10-6 Case illustration from Blount's original work showing dramatic remodeling. **A.** Six-year-old boy with both-bone forearm fracture. **B.** Six months after injury. Comparison of AP x-rays **(C)** and lateral x-rays **(D)** of both forearms at 5-years follow-up.

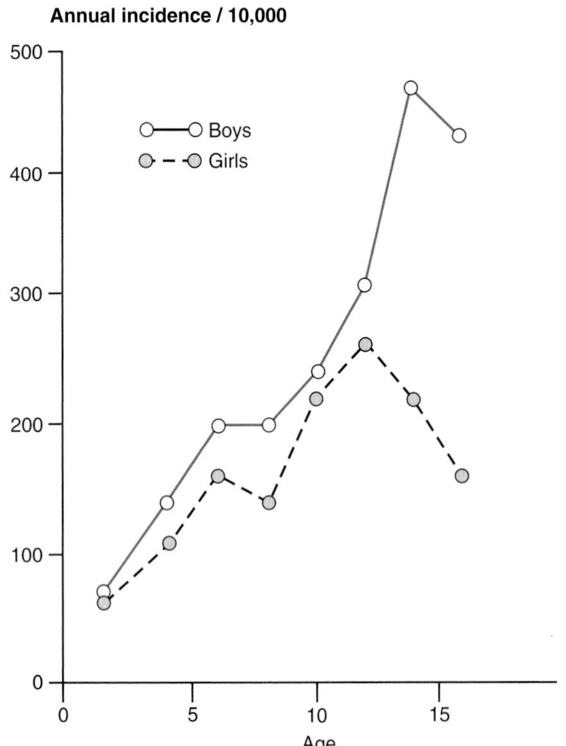

FIGURE 10-7 Annual incidence of all fractures in children. (From Landin LA. Epidemiology of children's fractures. *J Pediatr Orthop B* 1997;6: 79–83.)

The impact of increasing age on fracture incidence is further illustrated by Worlock and Stower, who showed that the rate of forearm shaft fractures in school-age children (more than 5 years old) is more than double that in toddlers (1.5 to 5 years old) (40). Age also may have an effect on injury severity. Many experienced clinicians have pointed out the increasing level of treatment difficulty as the level of forearm fracture moves proximally (9–12,41), and more proximal fractures tend to occur in older patients (12).

PRINCIPLES OF MANAGEMENT

Mechanism of Injury

The primary mechanism of injury associated with radial and ulnar shaft fractures is a fall on an outstretched hand that transmits indirect force to the bones of the forearm (42–44). Biomechanical studies have suggested that the junction of the middle and distal thirds of the radius and a substantial portion of the shaft of the ulna have an increased vulnerability to fracture (45). Often a significant rotational component is associated with the fall, causing the radius and ulna to fracture at different levels (Fig. 10-8) (46,47). If the radial and ulnar fractures are near the same level, a minimal torsional component can be inferred (Fig. 10-9). If comminution is present, higher-energy trauma should be suspected (48). Significant hyperpronation forces are associated with isolated shaft fractures of either the radius or the ulna and concomitant dislocation of either the distal or the proximal radioulnar joint. Thus, in any single-bone forearm shaft fracture, these important joints need to be closely scrutinized. Galeazzi and Monteggia fracture–dislocations are discussed in Chapter 12. A direct force to the arm (such as being hit by a baseball bat) can fracture a single bone (usually the ulna) without injury to the adjacent distal or proximal radioulnar joints (30). Isolated ulnar shaft fractures have been referred to as "nightstick fractures." Alignment of the radial head should be confirmed in any child with such a fracture to avoid a "missed Monteggia" injury (49). Isolated radial shaft fractures are rare but notoriously difficult to reduce with closed methods (50,51). Rang referred to appex volar greenstick fractures of the distal radial shaft near the metaphysis as "the slipper" because of its annoying tendency to lose position after otherwise satisfactory reduction (52).

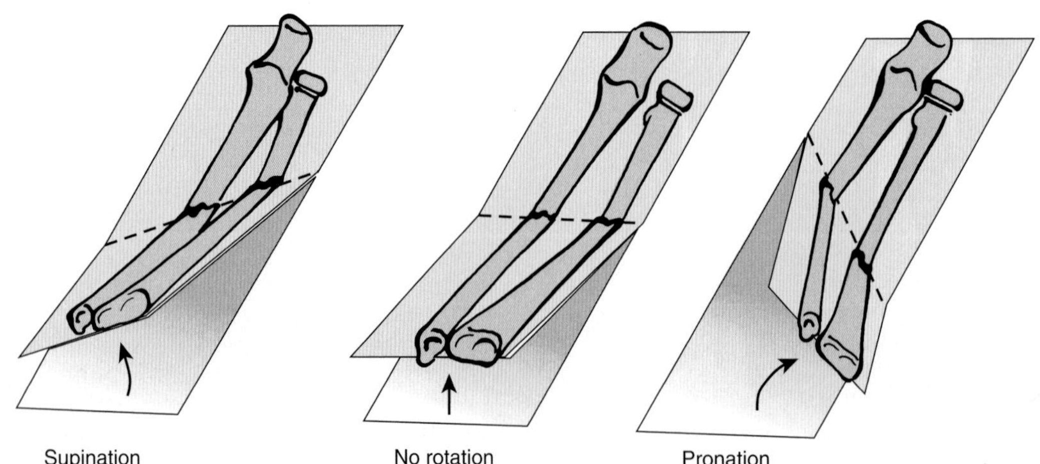

FIGURE 10-8 Radius and ulna shaft fractures occurring at different levels, implying rotational mechanism.

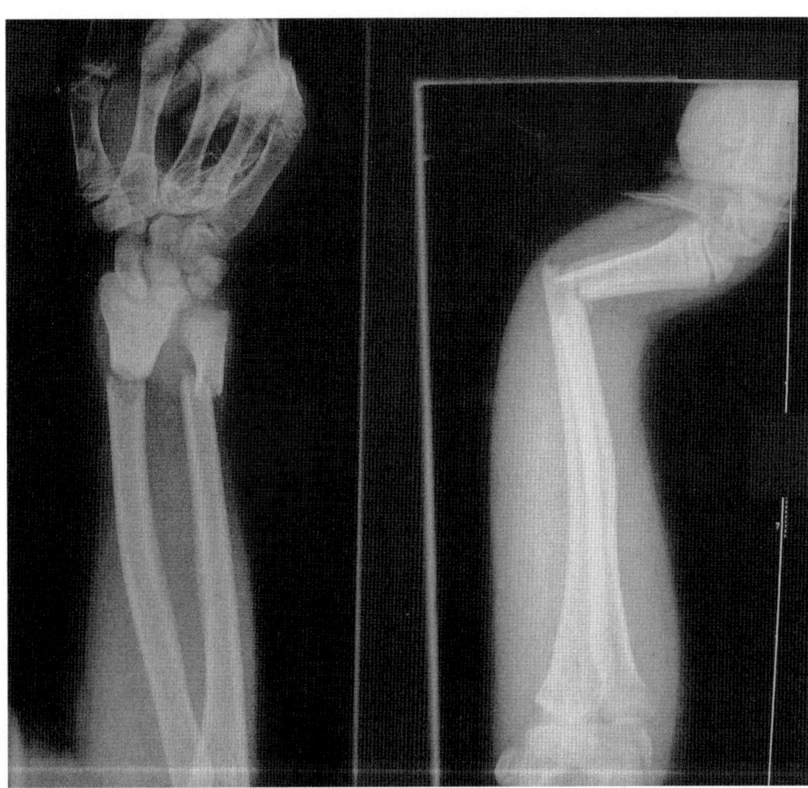

FIGURE 10-9 Radius and ulna shaft fractures occurring at same level, implying no significant rotation.

The mechanisms of injury of two particular forearm fracture patterns, traumatic bowing (53) (also known as bow fractures or plastic deformation) and greenstick fracture, also bear mentioning. Bone behaves differently based on the direction of the forces applied to it. This is the so-called anisotropic property of bone, and it can be simply explained as follows: bone is more resistant to axial forces than to bending and rotational forces (54). Pediatric bone also is much more porous than its adult counterpart and behaves somewhat differently from a biomechanical standpoint (55,56). Because of its porosity, pediatric bone absorbs significantly more energy prior to failure than does adult bone (57). When relatively slowly applied longitudinal forces bend immature bone beyond its elastic limits and into its plastic zone, traumatic bowing results (58,59). Thus, when a bending force is applied relatively slowly, many microfractures occur along the length of the bone, leading to macroscopic deformity without discernible radiographic fracture.

Greenstick fractures represent an intermediate step between plastic deformation and complete fractures (60). On anteroposterior (AP) and lateral x-rays, greenstick fractures show cortical violation of one, two, or three of their radiographic cortices, and thus some bony continuity is preserved. Rotational deformity is considered to be intimately related to the clinical deformity seen with greenstick fractures of the forearm, and the analogy of a cardboard tube that tends to bend as it is twisted has been offered by Holdsworth (10). Specifically, hyperpronation injuries usually are associated with apex-dorsal greenstick fractures of the forearm, and hypersupination injuries usually are associated with exactly the opposite (35,51). The treatment of these greenstick fractures often requires a derotation maneuver in addition to correction of any angulation (51,61).

Signs and Symptoms

The signs and symptoms indicating fracture of the shafts of the radius and ulna usually are not subtle. Deformity and pain are the classic findings. Patients typically experience exquisite pain emanating from the involved area. Decreased pronation and supination motion are also usually noted (62). Neither practitioners nor parents are always reliable assessors of children's pain, and ideally patients should rate their own pain (63,64). Significant anxiety and muscle spasm almost always amplify a child's painful experience (65,66). It has been suggested that muscle spasm is a protective effort by the body to splint or otherwise protect the injured body part (66). When such muscle spasm occurs in association with certain fracture patterns (e.g., a radial shaft fracture proximal to the pronator teres insertion), it produces predictable fracture displacement (e.g., a pronated distal radial fragment and a supinated proximal fragment).

More subtle fractures present special diagnostic challenges. Certain pathologic fractures of the forearm may occur in the absence of overt trauma (67,68). Many minimally displaced fractures of the shafts of the radius and ulna can be mistaken for a "sprain" or "just a bruise" for several days to several weeks.

This usually occurs in young children who continue to use the fractured arm during low-level play activities. As a general rule, a fracture should be suspected if the child has not resumed all normal arm function within 1 or 2 days of injury.

Associated Injuries

Most fractures of the shafts of the radius and ulna occur as isolated injuries, but wrist and elbow fractures may occur in conjunction with forearm fractures, and the elbow and wrist region needs to be included on standard forearm x-rays (44,69–72). If clinical suspicion is high, then dedicated wrist and elbow films are necessary. The so-called floating elbow injury (fracture of the bones of the forearm along with ipsilateral supracondylar humeral fracture) is a well-described entity that must not be missed (70–73). Surgical stabilization of both the supracondylar fracture and the forearm fractures has been recommended by multiple authors in recent years (73–77). Galeazzi and Monteggia fracture–dislocations also must be ruled out (see Chap. 12). Compartment syndrome also can occur in conjunction with a floating elbow injury (78) or with isolated forearm shaft fractures (79,80). This rare but potentially devastating complication can lead to Volkmann contracture, which has been shown to occur after forearm shaft fractures almost as often as it does after supracondylar humeral fractures in children (81). Patients with severe pain unrelieved by immobilization and mild narcotic medication should be reassessed for excessive swelling and tight forearm compartments. If loosening of the splint, cast, and underlying cast materials fails to relieve pain, then measurement of compartment pressures and subsequent fasciotomy may be necessary.

Abrasions or seemingly small unimportant lacerations that occur in conjunction with forearm fractures must be carefully evaluated, because they may be an indication of an open fracture. Clues to the presence of an open fracture include persistent slow bloody ooze from a small laceration near the fracture site, and subcutaneous emphysema on injury films. Careful evaluation and in some situations sterile probing of suspicious wounds will be necessary. Open forearm fractures are discussed later in this chapter.

Vascular or neurological injuries rarely are associated with forearm shaft fractures, but the consequences of such injuries are far-reaching. Serial neurovascular examinations should be performed and documented. Radial and ulnar pulses along with distal digital capillary refill should be routinely evaluated. Davis and Green reported nerve injuries in 1% (5/547) of their pediatric forearm fracture patients, with the most commonly injured nerve being the median nerve (6). Combined data from three large series of pediatric open forearm fractures reveal an overall nerve injury rate at presentation of 10% (17/173), with the median nerve once again being the one most commonly injured (17,82,83). To screen for these rare but significant injuries, every child with a forearm fracture should routinely have evaluation of the radial, ulnar, and median nerves (RUM testing) (50). Nerve injuries occurring at the time of injury must be differentiated from treatment-related or iatrogenic neurologic deficits.

Davidson suggested using the game of "rock-paper-scissors" for testing the median, radial, and ulnar nerves (Fig. 10-10) (84). The pronated fist is the rock and tests median nerve function. The extended fingers and wrist depict paper and test radial nerve function. Fully flexed small and ring fingers, an adducted thumb, and spreading the index and ring fingers mimics scissors and tests ulnar nerve function. Further focused testing should also be done on two important nerve branches: the anterior interosseous nerve (branch of median nerve), and the posterior interosseous nerve (branch of radial nerve). The anterior interosseous nerve provides motor function to the index flexor digitorum profundus, the flexor pollicis longus, and pronator quadratus and is best tested by having the patient make an "OK" sign. The posterior interosseous nerve typically innervates the extensor carpi ulnaris, extensor digitorum communis, extensor digiti minimi, extensor indicis, and the three out-cropping muscles (85). Its function is best documented by full extension of the phalangeal and metacarpophalangeal joints. This is especially difficult to test in a patient in a cast or splint that partially covers the fingers. Most injuries that occur in association with forearm fractures are true neurapraxias and typically resolve over the course of days to weeks (6,80).

Diagnosis and Classification

Fractures of the shafts of the radius and ulna often are described in rather imprecise terms such as "both-bone forearm fracture" and "greenstick fracture." X-rays confirm the diagnosis of forearm shaft fracture and are the basis for most classification systems. The most comprehensive classification of forearm fractures is the one adopted by the Orthopaedic Trauma Association (86). Although this system is sound in concept, its 36 discrete subtypes (86) make it impractical for everyday clinical use, and it has not been widely used by clinical researchers (87). Despite its complexity, the OTA classification does not account for one of the most important prognostic factors in pediatric forearm shaft fracture: location of the fracture in the distal, middle, or proximal third of the shaft.

Clinicians and clinical researchers have favored simpler descriptions of forearm shaft fractures. An orderly and practical approach to forearm shaft fracture classification should provide information about the bone (single bone, both bones), the level (distal, middle, or proximal third), and the pattern (plastic deformation, greenstick, complete, comminuted). Bone involvement is important because it not only indicates the severity of injury but also influences suspicion regarding additional soft tissue injury (e.g., single-bone injury increases the likelihood of a Monteggia or Galeazzi injury) (88) and affects reduction tactics (unique single-bone fracture reduction strategies can be used) (Fig. 10-11). Single-bone shaft fractures occur, but both-bone fractures are more common. Level is important for anatomic reasons relative to muscle and interosseous ligament attachments, as well as differences in prognosis for distal-, middle-,

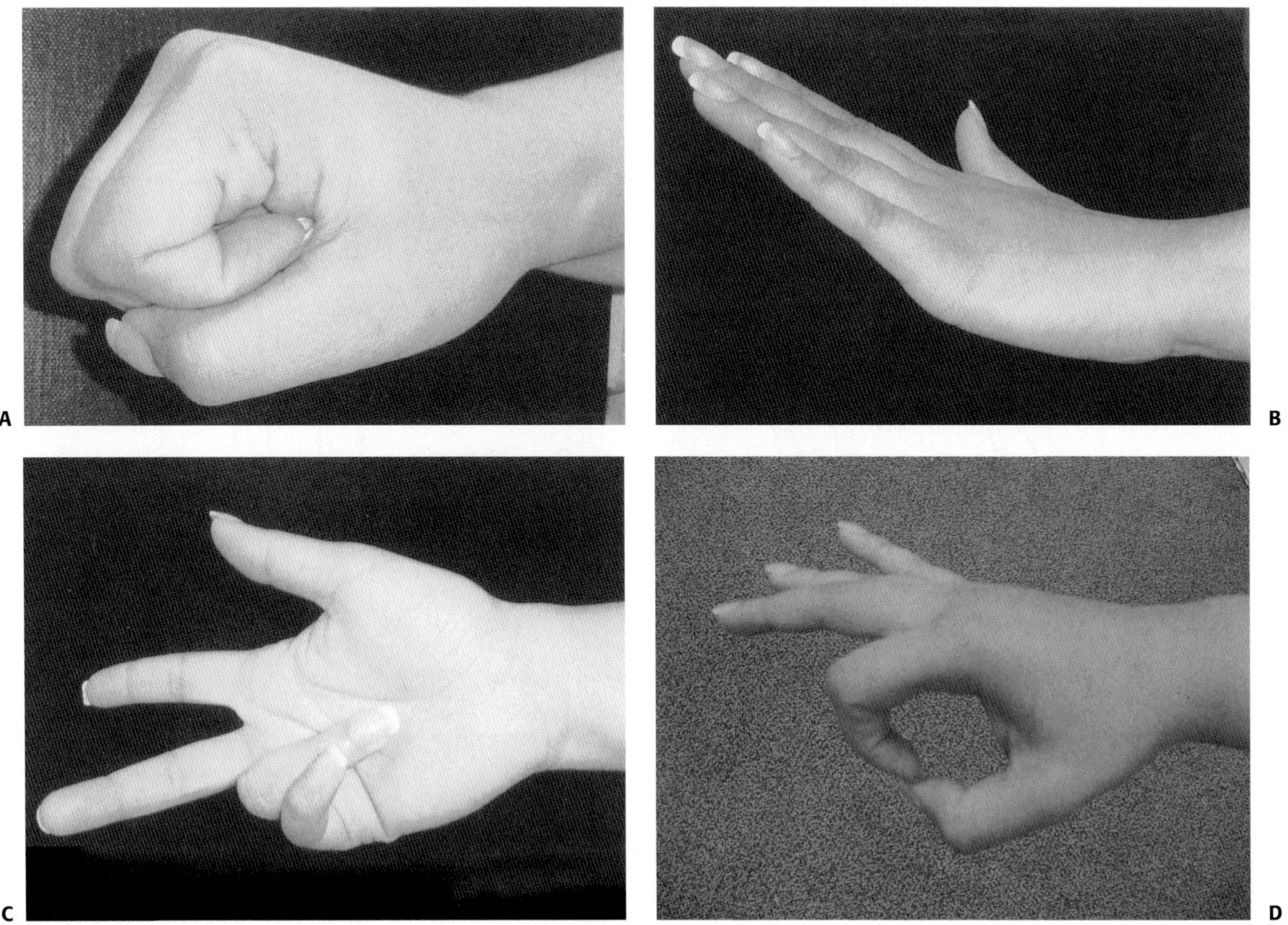

FIGURE 10-10 Upper extremity motor nerve physical examination. **A.** Rock position demonstrates median nerve motor function. **B.** Paper position demonstrates radial nerve motor function. **C.** Scissor position demonstrates ulnar nerve motor function. **D.** "OK" sign demonstrates function of anterior interosseus nerve.

and proximal-third shaft fractures. Pattern is important because it significantly alters the treatment approach. For example, the primary reduction strategy is very different for greenstick fractures (rotation) from for complete fractures (vertical traction). Certain comminuted fractures (e.g., comminution of both bones) may preclude reduction and casting and require plate fixation (89,90). Fortunately, comminuted fracture patterns are rare in children. For all practical purposes, the buckle fracture pattern that is common in the distal radial metaphysis never occurs in isolation in the shaft region. The typical buckle fracture "speed bump" may accompany either plastic deformation or greenstick fractures. Thus, there are two bones, three levels, and four common fracture patterns (Fig. 10-12). We believe this is a practical and clinically relevant way to describe forearm shaft fractures.

Once the forearm fracture has been described in the terms of this practical classification, fracture displacement must be evaluated. Fracture displacement can occur as angulation, rotation, shortening, or translation. Angulation is important in treatment decision-making and can be measured with reasonable reliability (91,92). Rotation is a simple concept, but it is difficult to assess clinically (5,93). The best that usually can be done is to roughly estimate rotation within a 45-degree margin of error (5,12). Based on available clinical studies it appears that less than 1 cm of shortening should be accepted in either single-bone or both-bone fracture patterns (94–98). It also has been suggested that the shortening that accompanies displaced fractures may help preserve future motion through interosseous membrane relaxation (5). Translation also is a simple concept and can be easily measured. Completely (100%) translated fractures of the middle third (5,12) and distal third (96–98) of the forearm have been shown to reliably remodel. Certain situations may raise concern regarding complete translation, such as isolated middle-third radial fractures with medial (ulnar) displacement that significantly narrows the interosseous space and translation in children who have less than 2 full years of growth remaining, because remodeling of the translated fracture site is less predictable than in younger children (4,56).

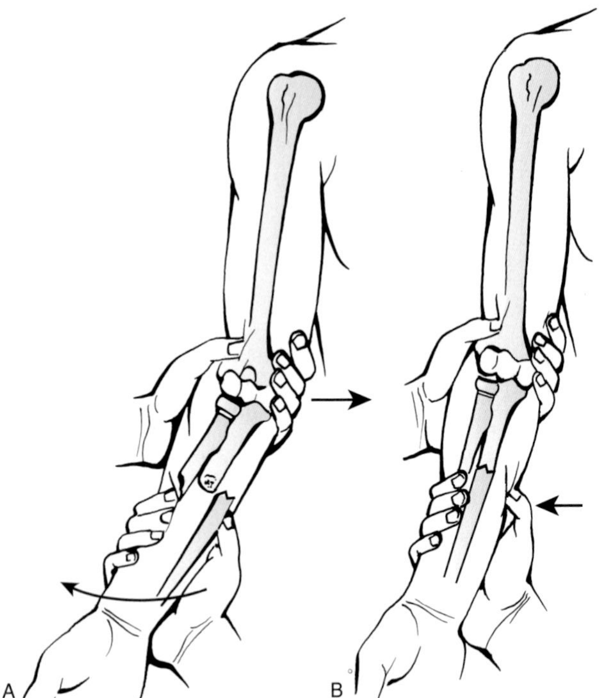

FIGURE 10-11 Isolated ulnar shaft reduction technique (Blount). Valgus force applied to fracture site and direct thumb pressure over distal ligament.

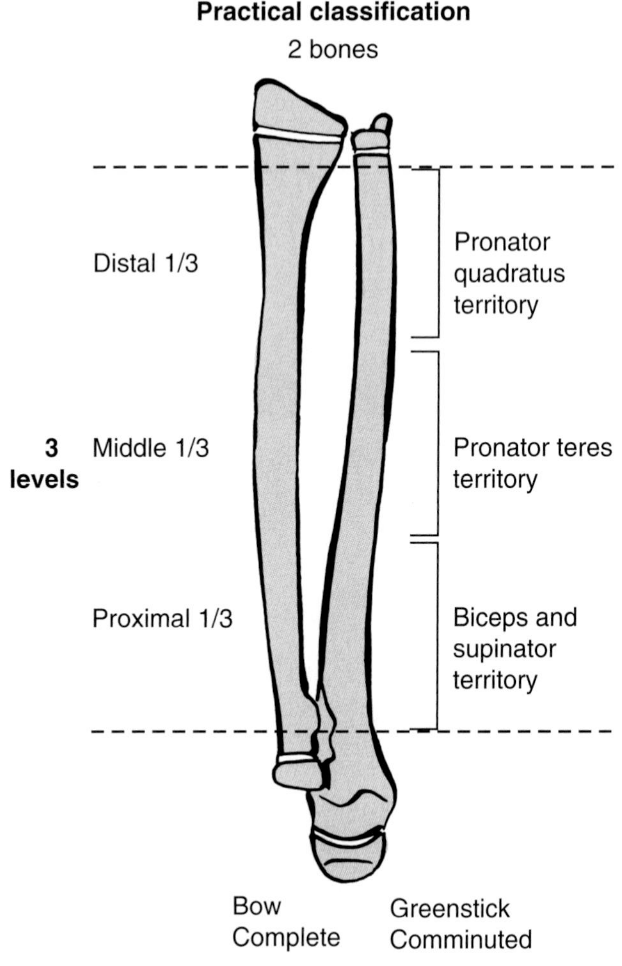

FIGURE 10-12 Practical classification of forearm shaft fractures. (Distal dotted line defined by proximal extent of Lister's tubercle and proximal dotted line defined by proximal extent of bicipetal tuberosity.)

Rationale

The fundamental reason for treating fractures of the shafts of the radius and ulna relates to the likelihood of bad results in the absence of adequate care. Data from certain developing countries may be as close as we come to natural history studies of untreated fractures. Archibong and Onuba reported on 102 pediatric fracture patients treated in southeastern Nigeria. Their patients most commonly had upper extremity fractures and they frequently experienced significant delays in seeking medical treatment, which led to high rates of malunion requiring surgical treatment (99). Other Nigerian authors have found that young age was not protective against fracture malunion (more than 50%) and nonunion (25%) following traditional bonesetter treatment (100). It is unclear whether children treated in this fashion are better or worse off than if they had received no treatment at all. The rationale for treating pediatric forearm shaft fractures is thus based on the premise that the results of modern orthopaedic treatment will far exceed "pseudo-natural histories" such as these.

The consequences of excessively crooked (and malrotated) forearm bones are both cosmetic and functional (Fig. 10-13) (10,11,101–105). Despite their great concern to parents, cosmetic issues have not been formally studied, and as a result the practitioner must interpret forearm cosmetic issues on a case-by-case basis. Clinical experience has shown that the ulna appears to be less forgiving from a cosmetic standpoint because of its long subcutaneous border. Early and repeated involvement of the parents (or other legal guardians) in an informed and shared decision-making process is essential.

Bony malunion and soft tissue fibrosis have both been implicated as causes of limited forearm motion after forearm shaft fractures (102,106). Limited forearm pronation and supination can have significant effects on upper extremity function (5,70,107). Inability to properly pronate often can be compensated for with shoulder abduction, but no easy compensatory mechanism exists for supination deficits (5,10,50,107). Daruwalla identified a nearly 53% rate of limited forearm rotation (subtle in some, dramatic in others) in his series of 53 children with forearm fractures and attributed it to angular deformity and rotational malalignment (69). Several patients in Price's series of pediatric forearm malunions had severe forearm range-of-motion losses that significantly limited vocational and avocational activities (5). Trousdale and Linscheid reported range-of-motion losses severe enough to prompt corrective osteoto-

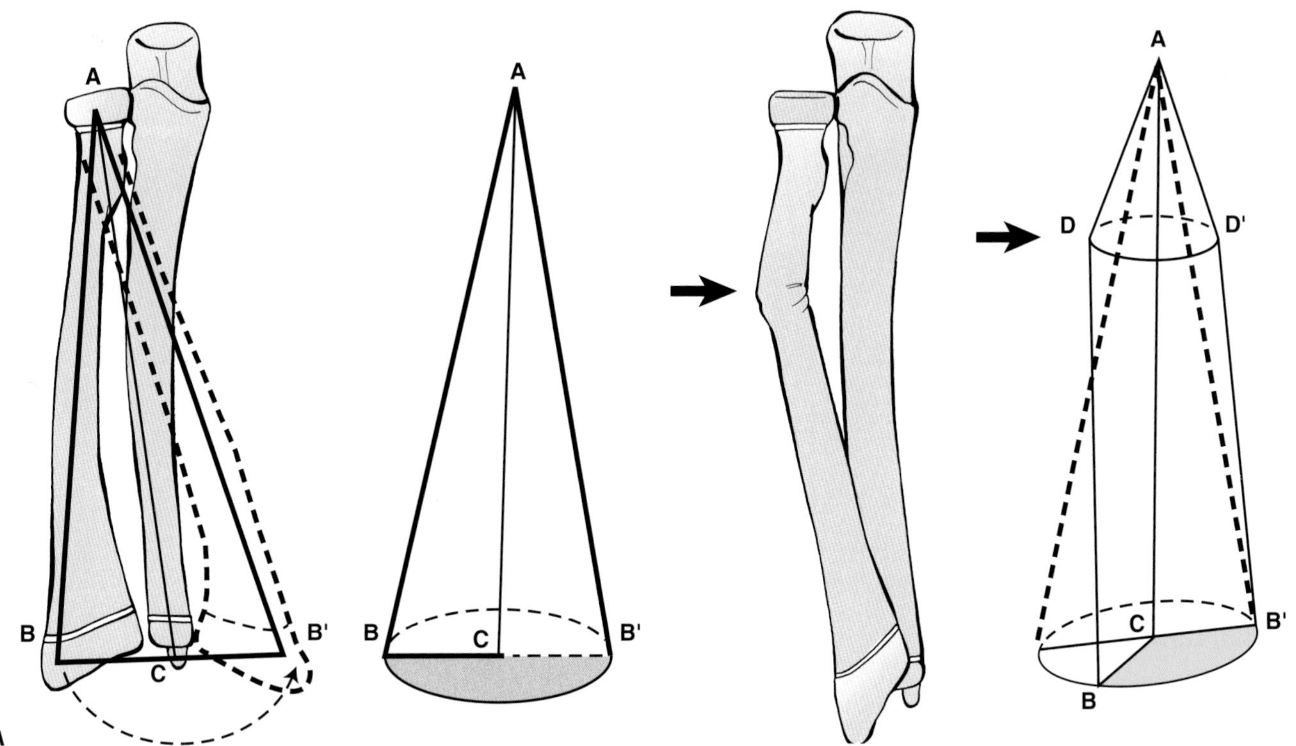

FIGURE 10-13 Effect of forearm malunion on forearm motion. **A.** Normal arc of forearm motion. **B.** Angulated radius leads to diminished arc of forearm motion. (Ogden JA. *Skeletal injury in the child*. Philadelphia: Lea & Febiger, 1982.)

mies in many of their predominantly pediatric (less than 14 years old at time of injury) patients with forearm malunions (11). Meier also reported significant range-of-motion deficits in association with pediatric forearm malunion (108).

Range-of-motion losses due to deformity have been studied by numerous authors using adult cadaveric forearm specimens. Matthews et al studied 10-degree and 20-degree midshaft angular deformities of the radius and ulna in 10 forearm specimens (101). They found that 10-degree deformities of either bone individually resulted in little or no measurable motion loss (in the range of 3 degrees or less). When both bones were angulated 10 degrees dorsal, volar, or toward the interosseous membrane, larger motion losses were documented (approximately 10 degrees pronation and 20 degrees supination). Significantly greater losses of motion occurred when one or both bones were angulated 20 degrees (approximately 40 degrees for both pronation and supination). Some of the 10-degree angulated specimens demonstrated "cosmetically unacceptable deformity" (101). These findings indicate that relatively small angular deformities can be clinically significant.

Additional important information about the influence of fracture level on forearm motion was provided by a series of experiments conducted by Sarmiento et al (109,110). They found that fracture angulation of 15 to 30 degrees led to greater supination losses when the deformity was in the middle third of the forearm (40 to 90 degrees) and greater pronation losses when in the distal third (30 to 80 degrees) (109). Fracture angulation of 10 degrees or less in the proximal or middle forearm rarely resulted in more than 15 degrees of motion loss (109,110), but the same angulation in the distal third of the forearm was at times (usually with isolated radius fracture) associated with pronation losses of 20 degrees (109,110). These findings challenge commonly held beliefs that the distal third of the forearm is the most forgiving. These same authors asserted that rotational malalignment led to rotational motion losses that usually were equal in magnitude and opposite in direction to the deformity (e.g., a 10-degree pronation deformity led to a 10-degree loss of supination) (109).

Rotational malalignment of the forearm has been studied in greater detail in recent years (111–113). In isolated midshaft radial fractures, more than 30 degrees of malrotation was a threshold for significant losses in motion (approximately 15 degrees) (111). Isolated midshaft ulnar fracture malrotation did not alter the total arc of forearm motion but did change the set point (e.g., a 30-degree pronation deformity took away 30 degrees of pronation and added 30 degrees of supination) (113). Larger ulnar axial malalignment of 45 degrees decreased overall forearm rotation by no more than 20 degrees (113). Large residual ulnar shaft translation has similarly been found to have little impact on forearm rotation (114). Simulated combined radial and ulnar midshaft rotational malunions resulted in the worst motion (more than 50% losses of pronation and supination)

TABLE 10-1 Condensed Range-of-Motion Information

	Ulna 40 degrees Pronated	Ulna 0 degrees Neutral	Ulna 40 degrees Supinated
Radius 40 degrees pronated	102/52	105/57	62/65
Radius neutral	97/58	90/90	69/107
Radius 40 degrees supinated	53/55	52/95	46/110

Numerator is pronation while denominator is supination.
From Dumont CE, Thalmann R, Macy JC. The effect of rotational malunion of the radius and ulna on supination and pronation. *J Bone Joint Surg [Br]* 2002;84:1070–1074.

when 60-degree rotational malunions were in opposite directions (112). Rotational malunions that approximated recommended limits in the literature (45 degrees) (5) produced less extreme but real limitations of motion (Table 10-1) (112). From these studies and our clinical experience, it appears that the radius is more sensitive to rotational problems and less sensitive regarding cosmetic issues, while the ulna is exactly the opposite.

The goal of treatment is to achieve satisfactory healing of the forearm injury within established anatomical and functional guidelines while also taking into account the reasonable degree of remodeling that can be expected in growing children. Most of the time these goals can be achieved with closed fracture care, and little or no radiographic or clinical abnormality can be detected following healing. A paradox exists in pediatric forearm fractures whereby anatomical radiographic alignment is not always associated with normal motion, and normal motion often is associated with nonanatomical radiographic healing (5,102,106,109). Herein lays the inherent controversy between operative and nonoperative treatment approaches (Table 10-2). In patients with anatomical x-rays, range-of-motion problems usually have been attributed to scarring of the interosseous membrane (5,107,115). With nonanatomical x-rays (incomplete remodeling), range-of-motion deficits usually are attributed to the radiographic abnormalities. Thus, treatment of forearm shaft fracture must balance the risk of allowing stiffness to occur secondary to malunion against the risk of creating stiffness secondary to surgical procedures.

The rationalization for remodeling of pediatric forearm fractures has strong historical support (21,23,30,116), but knowledge of the limits of remodeling must be taken into consideration. Established reduction criteria state that complete (100%) translation is acceptable (5,97), as well as up to 15 degrees of angulation and up to 45 degrees of malrotation (5). Because important forearm fracture treatment decisions frequently are based on radiographic measurement of angular deformities, it must be remembered that these angles are projected shadows that are affected by rotation (117). If angulation is present on both AP and lateral views (commonly called two orthogonal views), the true deformity is out of the plane of the x-rays and its true magnitude is greater than that measured on each individual view. Certain forearm shaft fracture deformities are clearly "two-plane deformities" whose maximal angular magnitude is in some plane other than the standard AP or lateral plane (Fig. 10-14) (118). Bär and Breitfuss produced a table (based on the Pythago-

TABLE 10-2 Pros and Cons of Cast Versus Surgical Treatment

	Pro	Con
Cast treatment	Long track record Negligible infection risk Fine-tuning possible	Anatomic reduction rare Stiffness may still occur Frequent follow-up visits
Surgical treatment	Anatomic reduction Minimize immobilization Fewer follow-up visits	Risk of infection Need for implant removal Stiffness from surgery

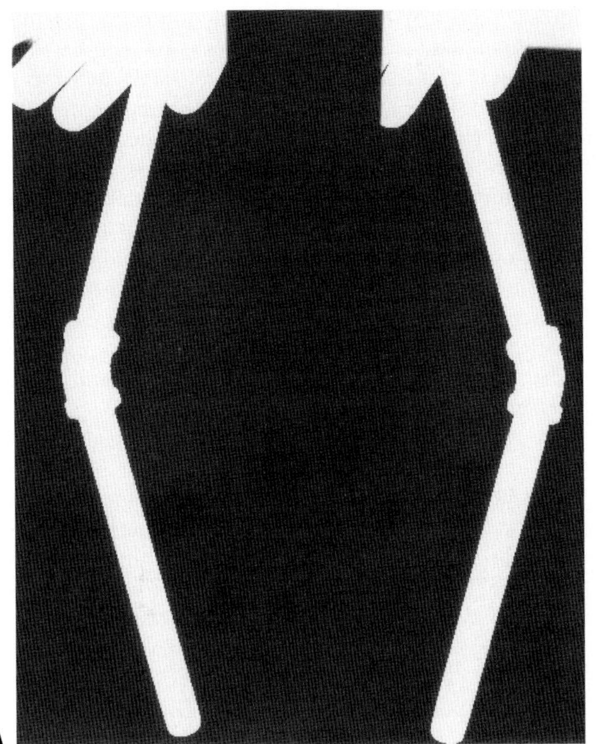
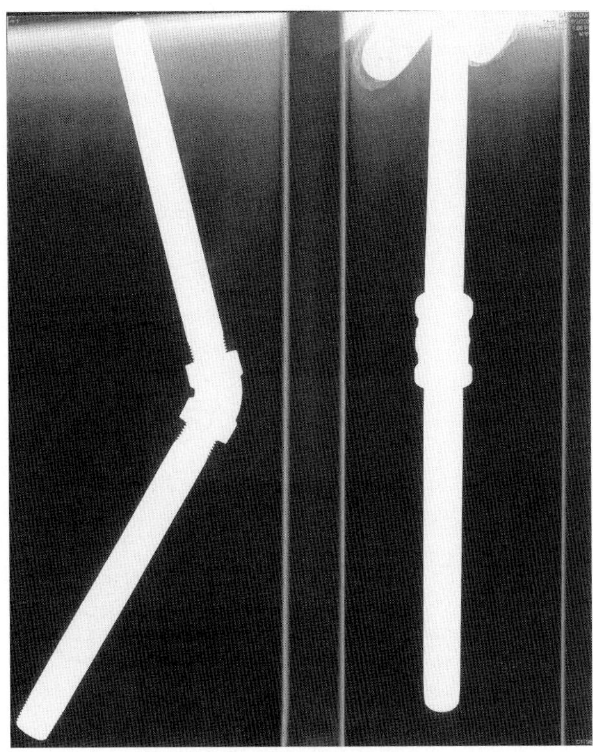

FIGURE 10-14 Underestimation of true angulation. **A.** "Out of the AP and lateral plane" underestimates angulation at 30 degrees. **B.** True AP and lateral demonstrates that true maximal angulation is 40 degrees.

rean theorem) that predicts the true maximal angulation (118). Accurate deformity measurement can be made when angulation is seen on only one view and there is no angulation on the other orthogonal view. A cast change with molding, remanipulation under analgesia or anesthesia, or surgical fixation may become necessary, but even with anatomical reduction patients may not regain full pronation and supination (102,107). Most series of pediatric forearm fractures document excellent subjective results, and only with special goniometric testing is a decreased range of motion detected objectively (12).

Published clinical studies have shown that pediatric forearm shaft fractures have great remodeling potential that occurs through several mechanisms (119). The distal radial epiphysis will redirect itself toward normal at about 10 degrees per year. As long as the physis is open, this rate is independent of age. Although the epiphysis will return to normal direction, it will have little effect on correcting an angular deformity at the midshaft compared to fractures at the subphyseal level. Remodeling also occurs with lengthening of the bone through growth, which produces an apparent decrease in angulation, especially if measured as the difference between the proximal and distal ends of the bone. Bone also remodels by intramembranous apposition on the concave side and resorption on the convex side (57,119). This occurs throughout life, but more rapidly when driven by the thick periosteum found in children. Larsen (120) found that although the epiphyseal angle realigns quickly, children older than 11 years correct bone angulation less than the younger children. Thomas stated the following regarding pediatric forearm remodeling potential: "We should not fail to recall that the remodeling capabilities of the bones of children have not changed in the last million years and that open reduction and internal fixation must be undertaken only after due deliberation" (8).

SURGICAL AND APPLIED ANATOMY

Bony Anatomy and Static Restraints

The forearm is a large nonsynovial joint with nearly a 180-degree arc of motion. Its bones, the radius and ulna, are not simple straight bony tubes. The shaft of the radius is a three-sided structure with two prominent curvatures. One major gradual convexity (approximately 10 degrees with its apex lateral-radial) is present along its midportion; a second, more acute curve of approximately 15 degrees with its apex medial occurs proximally near the bicipital tuberosity (121–123). The deviation along the midportion is commonly referred to as the radial bow, and maintenance of this normal contour is a goal of forearm shaft fracture care (124–126). The most important bony landmarks of the radius are the radial styloid (lateral prominence) and the bicipital tuberosity (anteromedial prominence), which are oriented somewhat less than 180 degrees away from

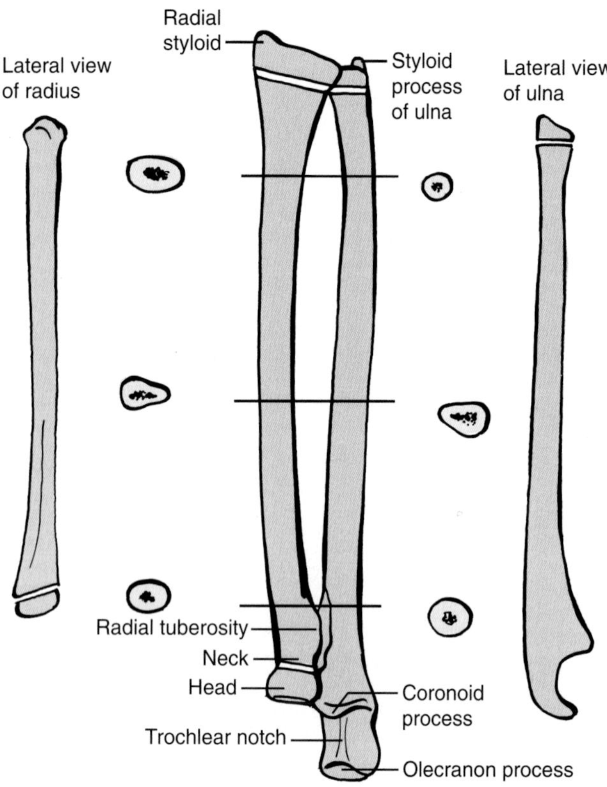

FIGURE 10-15 Radius and ulna anatomy.

each other (Fig. 10-15) (127). Anthropologists consider a full 180-degree relationship to be characteristic of Neanderthal osteology (128). Maintenance of the styloid-tuberosity rotational relationship is another forearm shaft fracture principle. The nutrient artery of the radius enters the bone in its proximal half and courses anterior to ulnar (medial) (129). Such nutrient vessels typically are seen on only one orthogonal view and should not be confused with fracture lines.

In cross-section most of the shaft of the ulna also is shaped like a classic three-sided prism, while its more distal and proximal portions are much more circular. The most important bony landmarks of the ulna are its styloid process (distally) and its coronoid process (proximally). These two landmarks are oriented nearly 180 degrees from one another, with the styloid aimed in a posterior (dorsal) direction and the coronoid in an anterior (volar) direction (127). Tracking styloid-coronoid rotational alignment of the ulna is another part of forearm shaft fracture care. The ulnar shaft has mild curvatures in both its proximal (apex lateral/radial) and distal (apex medial/ulnar) portions but is otherwise relatively straight (121,122). The nutrient artery to the ulna enters it in its proximal half and courses anterior to radial (lateral) (129).

The classic works of Evans helped focus attention on rotational deformity associated with fractures of both bones of the forearm (46,51,130). Evans stated, "The orthodox position in which to immobilize these fractures is that of full supination for the upper third, and the midposition for fractures of the middle and lower thirds, these positions being based on the anatomical arrangement of the pronators and supinators of the forearm. However, it is unreasonable to suppose that all fractures at a given level will present the same degree of rotational deformity" (130). He pointed out the importance of tracking the rotational alignment of the free-moving radial fragment by ascertaining the relative location of the bicipital tuberosity. This was a major step forward in refining the orthopaedic care of these forearm injuries. On a fully supinated AP x-ray of an unfractured forearm, the bicipital tuberosity points predominantly in a medial direction (nearly 180 degrees opposite of the radial tuberosity) (130). The radius and ulna also are nearly parallel to each other on such a view. On a fully pronated AP x-ray of an unfractured forearm, the bicipital tuberosity points in a lateral direction and the radial tuberosity is situated medially (130). The radius also crosses over the ulna in a pronated AP view. Mercer Rang noted that in an unfractured limb, the bicipital tuberosity tended to align with a point near the thenar eminence (Fig. 10-16) (34), more nearly a 165-degree relationship than a true 180-degree one. These relationships are best assessed on standard x-rays that include the entire forearm on one film (5,11,69) rather than the specialized bicipital tuberosity view originally suggested by Evans (130).

Some generalities regarding the appearance and closure of secondary ossification centers of the radius and ulna should be kept in mind, because these growth areas must be respected during both surgical and nonsurgical fracture care (131–134). The secondary center (epiphysis) of the distal radius is the first to appear, at around 1 year of age (135,136). Next are the epiphyses of the proximal radius and distal ulna, which appear by about 4 to 6 years of age (137). The proximal ulna is last and appears at around 9 years of age (138). Physeal closure occurs in two stages, with the proximal radius and proximal ulna closing by about 15 years of age and the distal radius and ulna by about 18 years of age (139). It must be remembered that girls' physes close 1–2 years before their male counterparts.

The radius and ulna are joined by three major passive restraints: the proximal radioulnar joint (PRUJ), the distal radioulnar joint (DRUJ), and the interosseous membrane complex, all of which have important stabilizing and load-transferring functions. These structures allow rotation of the radius about the ulna along an axis that runs approximately from the center of the radial head to the center of the distal ulna (107,140). The PRUJ and DRUJ are discussed elsewhere in this book. The structure and biomechanical function of the interosseous membrane have been studied extensively in recent years. Hotchkiss et al showed that the central band of the interosseous membrane (the interosseous ligament) courses from a point near the junction of the proximal and middle thirds of the radius to a point near the junction of the middle and distal thirds of the ulna. It is an important longitudinal stabilizer of the forearm in that 71% of forearm longitudinal stiffness is provided by the interosseous ligament after radial head excision (141). Transverse vectors also have been identified (142) and reflect the stabilizing effect of the interosseous ligament during pronation and supination

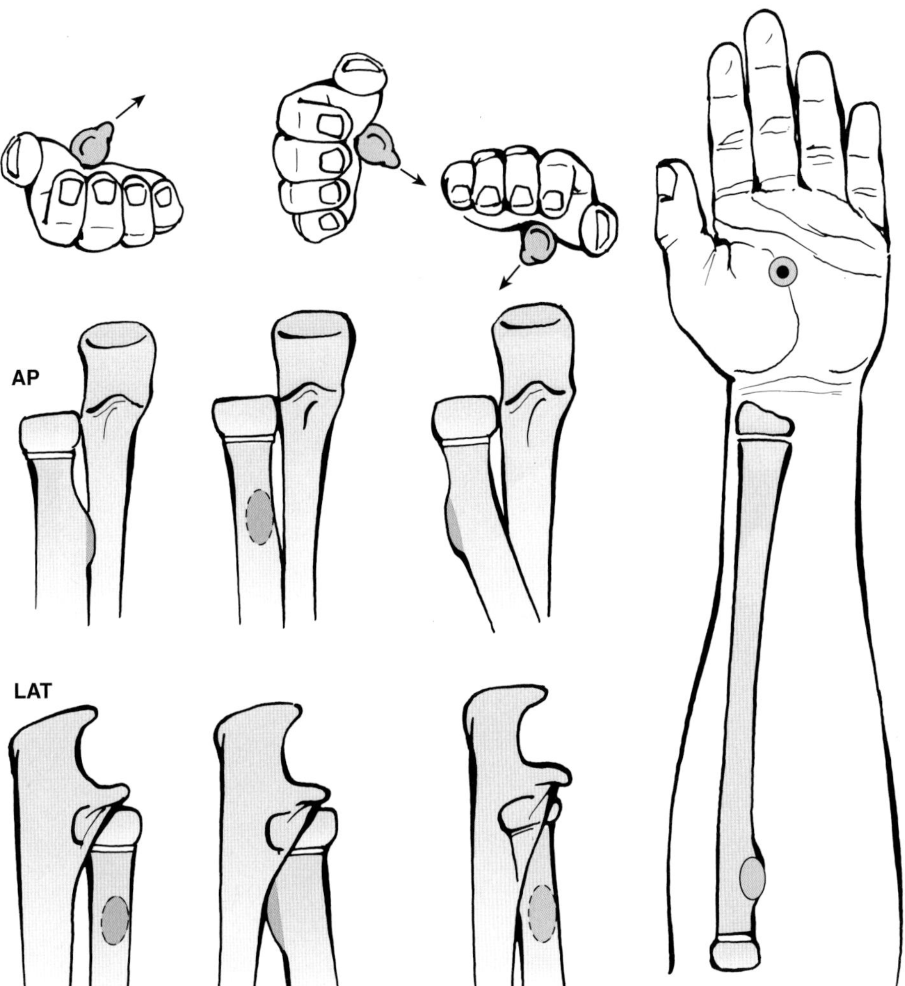

FIGURE 10-16 Rang's illustration depicting the position of the bicipital tuberosity on AP and lateral views with the forearm in pronation, supination and neutral position. (From Rang M. *Children's fractures*. Philadelphia: JB Lippincott, 1974.)

movements. The interosseous ligament demonstrates tensile properties comparable to the patellar tendon and the anterior cruciate ligament (143), indicative of the magnitude of the arm forces to which this structure is subjected.

Although some difference of opinion still exists (144–146), multiple studies have shown that the most strain in the central band of the interosseous membrane is generated when the forearm is in the neutral position (145,147,148). These findings of maximal strain in neutral in cadaver studies also are consistent with radiographic measurement studies (12) and dynamic magnetic resonance imaging studies of the forearm showing that the interosseous space is maximal near a neutral position (149). This may help explain certain pathologic situations such as the fixed supination deformity of neonatal brachial plexus palsy (150) as well as limitations of pronation and supination that occur after fractures, induced by encroachment on the interosseous space from all angulated fractures (Fig. 10-17) (151). The interosseous membrane also serves as an important anchoring point for at least six forearm muscles: the flexor digitorum profundus, flexor pollicis longus, extensor indicis, and the three outcropping muscles.

Pertinent Anatomy of the Muscles and Nerves

The paired and seemingly balanced radial and ulnar bones have an unbalanced number of muscular connections. The ulna typically has 14 attached muscles and the radius only 9 (Tables 10-3 and 10-4) (121,152). Powerful supinators attach to the proximal third of the forearm, while important pronators attach to its middle and distal thirds (Fig. 10-18). The accompanying vasculature of the forearm is complex: these muscles are supplied by more than 248 vascular pedicles arising from the brachial artery, its branches, or other collateral vessels (153). The radial, ulnar, and median nerves (or their branches) along with the musculocutaneous nerve provide all of the key innervations to the motors that attach to the forearm bones. As mentioned earlier, the median nerve is the most commonly injured (6,17,83,84).

The radial nerve proceeds from a posterior to anterior direction and enters the forearm after passing the lateral epicondyle. Near this same level, it divides into superficial and deep terminal branches. The deep motor branch of the radial nerve also is known as the posterior interosseous nerve. Most commonly

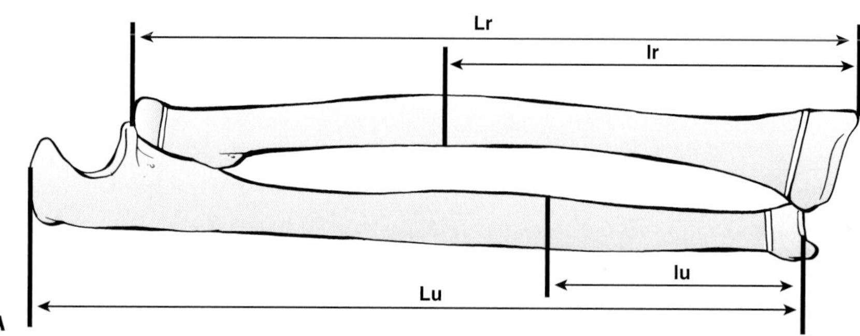

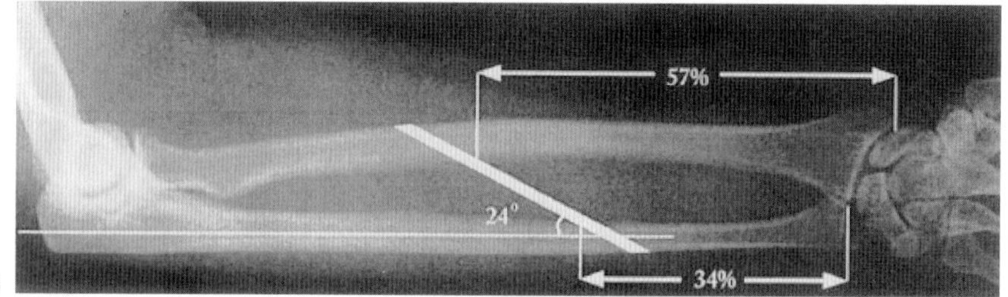

FIGURE 10-17 Anatomy of interosseous ligament. **A.** Central oblique orientation of interosseous ligament. **B.** Interosseous ligament attachment in terms of percentage forearm length. (From Skahen JR 3rd, Palmer AK, Werner FW, Fortino MD. Reconstruction of the interosseous membrane of the forearm in cadavers. *J Hand Surg [Am]* 1997; 22:986–994.)

(55% of the time) a motor branch arises from the radial nerve proper or its superficial terminal branch to innervate the extensor carpi radialis brevis, while the rest of the time (45%) this motor branch comes from the posterior interosseous nerve (154). The superficial branch travels along with and beneath the brachioradialis. The posterior interosseous nerve enters the supinator muscle, passing the fibrous thickening called the arcade of Frohse shortly after branching from the radial nerve proper. It courses within the supinator past the proximal radius, later exiting this muscle dorsally (posteriorly) near the junction of the proximal and middle thirds of the radius. Following its emergence from the supinator, the posterior interosseous nerve branches repetitively to the superficial extensors and the deeper outcropping muscles. The ulnar nerve enters the forearm between the two heads of the flexor carpi ulnaris (155). It traverses the forearm between the flexor carpi ulnaris and the flexor digitorum profundus. In the distal forearm it lies just beneath the flexor carpi ulnaris. The median nerve enters the forearm as it passes between the two heads of the pronator teres (156). It next passes beneath the archway created by the two heads of the flexor digitorum superficialis. The median nerve then continues down the course of the forearm nestled between the flexor digitorum superficialis and the flexor digitorum profundus. It becomes much more superficial as it nears the level of the carpal tunnel. The anterior interosseous branch arises from the median nerve at a level roughly corresponding to the junction of the proximal and middle thirds of the radius. Abundant muscle shields the radial, ulnar, and median nerves from the shafts of the radius and ulna through most of the forearm.

TABLE 10-3 Nine Muscles That Attach to the Radius (and their innervation)

1. Abductor pollicis longus (PIN)
2. Biceps (musculocutaneous nerve)
3. Brachioradialis (radial nerve)
4. Extensor pollicis longus (PIN)
5. Flexor digitorum superficialis (median nerve)
6. Flexor pollicis longus (AIN)
7. Pronator quadratus (AIN)
8. Pronator teres (median nerve)
9. Supinator (PIN)

Common Surgical Approaches

The large exposure required for plate fixation of pediatric forearm fractures can be achieved with three surgical approaches: the Henry (anterior) and Thompson (posterior) approaches to the radial shaft and the direct (medial) approach to the ulnar shaft (157,158). Compartment syndrome release usually requires the serpentine incision of McConnell's combined approach (159). These approaches and their variations are well described and illustrated in detail elsewhere (160–164). For open reduction of both the radius and the ulna, most authors favor separate incisions to minimize the possibility of communicating hematoma and synostosis (124,165,166). The Thompson approach to the radius generally is used for fractures of its proximal third (167) but requires special care to protect the posterior interosseous nerve (168–170). Other authors have emphasized

TABLE 10-4 14 Muscles That Attach to the Ulna (and their innervation)

1. Abductor pollicis longus (PIN)
2. Anconeus (radial nerve)
3. Biceps (musculocutaneous nerve)
4. Brachialis (musculocutaneous + small branches median and radial nerves)
5. Extensor carpi ulnaris (PIN)
6. Extensor indicis proprius (PIN)
7. Extensor pollicis longus (PIN)
8. Flexor carpi ulnaris (ulnar nerve)
9. Flexor digitorum profundus (AIN, index & long; ulnar nerve, ring & small)
10. Flexor digitorum superficialis (median nerve)
11. Pronator teres (median nerve)
12. Pronator quadratus (AIN)
13. Supinator (PIN)
14. Triceps (radial nerve)

Occasionally the accessory head flexor pollicis longus (aka Gantzer's muscle; from coronoid region in 15% of specimens) is innervated by AIN.

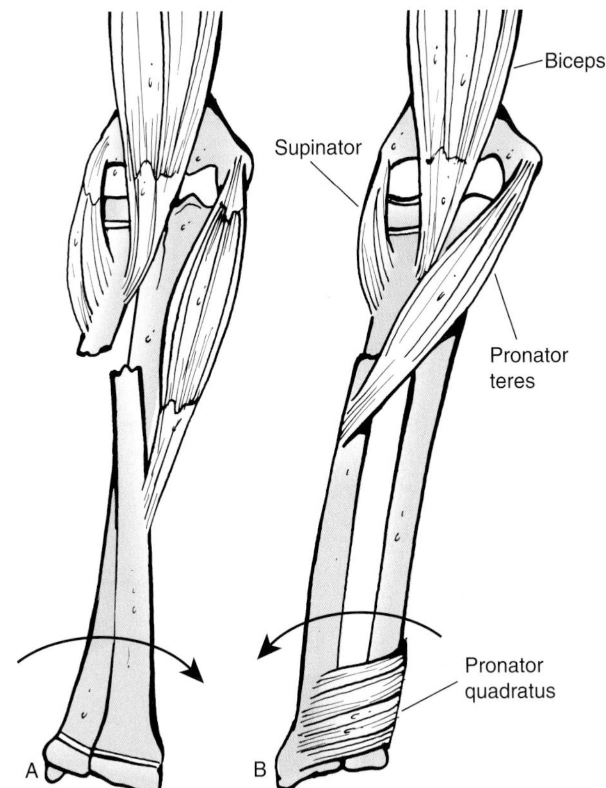

FIGURE 10-18 Muscle forces acting in proximal, middle, and distal thirds.

the utility of the Henry approach for plating of the proximal radius (170). When open reduction is done in conjunction with other internal fixation techniques (e.g., intramedullary fixation), limited versions of the same surgical approaches are used.

Indirect reduction and internal fixation of forearm fractures requires knowledge of appropriate physeal-sparing entry portals about the distal and proximal forearm. Because of the relative inaccessibility of its proximal end, the radius usually is approached only distally through either a dorsal or radial entry point. The dorsal entry point is near the proximal base of Lister's tubercle or just lateral to it in a small bare area between the second and third dorsal compartments. This location is a short distance proximal to the physis of the distal radius. Another dorsal alternative is pin entry just medial to Lister's tubercle, between the third and fourth dorsal compartments (171), but this may entail greater tendon risk. The most commonly used radial entry point is located in line with the styloid process just proximal to the physis (16). Entry in this area passes through the floor of the first dorsal compartment, and thus the tendons of abductor pollicis longus and extensor pollicis brevis (as well as branches of the superficial radial nerve) must be protected (Fig. 10-19). Because of its extensive branching pattern, portions of the superficial branch of the radial nerve may be at risk when dorsal or radial intramedullary entry points are used (172,173).

Both distal and proximal intramedullary entry sites for the ulna have been described (15,174–177). In the distal portion of the ulna an entry site can be made proximal to the physis and in the interval between the extensor carpi ulnaris and flexor carpi ulnaris tendons. Care must be taken to avoid branches of the dorsal cutaneous sensory nerve. Ulnar entry is most easily accomplished in the proximal portion of the bone along its lateral metaphyseal border (just distal to the olecranon apophysis), piercing peripheral fibers of the anconeus (Fig. 10-20) (178–180). This anconeus entry site described by the Nancy group avoids the physis and avoids the painful bursa that tends to form over "tip of the olecranon" pins.

Transphyseal approaches to both the distal radius (133, 134,176) and the proximal ulna (170,175,181) have been suggested by some authors. Significant growth potential exists at the distal radius (approximately 10 mm per year), while there is proportionately less from the olecranon apophysis (approximately 2 mm per year). Although clinical studies have seemed

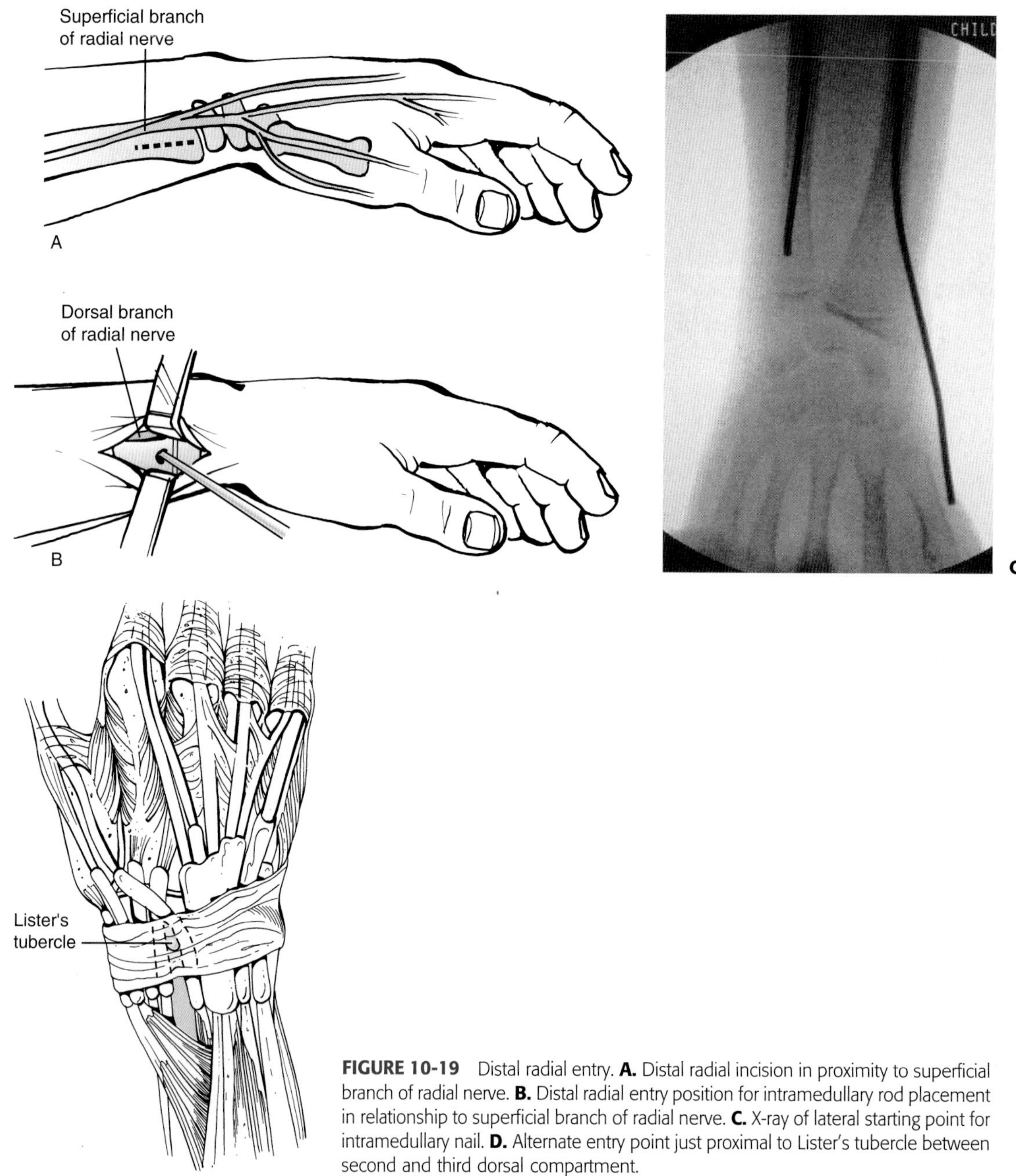

FIGURE 10-19 Distal radial entry. **A.** Distal radial incision in proximity to superficial branch of radial nerve. **B.** Distal radial entry position for intramedullary rod placement in relationship to superficial branch of radial nerve. **C.** X-ray of lateral starting point for intramedullary nail. **D.** Alternate entry point just proximal to Lister's tubercle between second and third dorsal compartment.

to indicate that both of these physes can be transgressed, such practices still entail unnecessary risk to the physis because there are few if any technical advantages to transphyseal entry of either bone (especially the radius).

CURRENT CLOSED TREATMENT OPTIONS

Overview of Closed Fracture Treatment

Most pediatric radial and ulnar shaft fractures can be treated by nonoperative methods. Low-energy, undisplaced, and minimally displaced forearm fractures (most bow, greenstick, complete, and comminuted fractures) can be immediately immobilized in a properly molded (three-point mold concept of Charnley) above-elbow cast (181). If posttraumatic tissue swelling is a concern, noncircumferential splint immobilization (e.g., sugar tong splint) can be used initially (50,182,183). For fractures in the distal third of the forearm, below-elbow casting has been shown to be as effective as above-elbow casting in maintenance of satisfactory fracture alignment (184,185). Appropriate follow-up is important for these undisplaced fractures (an initial screening x-ray usually is taken 7 to 14 days after injury) because displacement

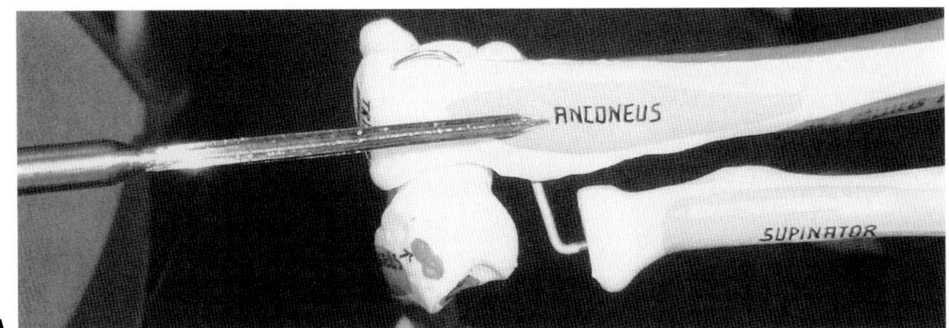

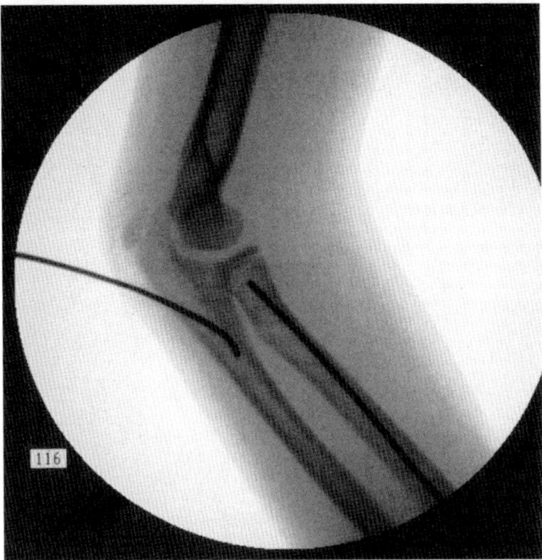

FIGURE 10-20 Proximal ulna entry. **A.** Anconeus entry point (first ulna proximal to growth plate). **B.** X-ray of proximal ulna entry point.

may still occur for a variety of reasons: new trauma to the extremity, male gender, missed follow-up appointments, and poor casting technique (50,182,186,187).

Good casting technique is infrequently discussed in contemporary orthopaedic textbooks and sometimes is underemphasized during orthopaedic residency training. The principles of good forearm casting technique include: (a) interosseous molding, (b) supracondylar molding, (c) appropriate padding, (d) evenly distributed cast material, (e) straight ulnar border, and (f) three-point molding (Fig. 10-21). The risk of excessive cast tightness can be minimized through the use of the stretch-relax fiberglass casting technique described by Davids et al (188). Chess et al described a cast index for distal radial fractures defined as the sagittal cast width divided by the coronal cast width at the level of the fracture site; a normal ratio is considered to be 0.70 (184). The cast index has not been validated for forearm shaft fractures, but it embodies the sound concept of good interosseous molding. Advanced techniques such as pins and plaster and cast wedging also have a role to play (189,190). Cast wedging is almost always done with an opening wedge technique because this entails less risk of soft tissue impingement (191).

Displaced fractures usually require reduction following appropriate analgesia (98,192). Options include hematoma block (193–195), regional intravenous anesthesia (196–198), and inhalational methods (195,199,200). After informed consent for the sedation and reduction is obtained, monitored sedation can be used in the emergency department with a combination of narcotics and anxiolytics (201). This typically requires a dedicated nurse to administer oxygen and perform appropriate monitoring functions (vital signs, continuous EKG, and pulse oximetry) (202–204). Ketamine protocols also are being used with increased frequency (201,205). Young children with less than 5 or 10 degrees of angulation in the plane of wrist and elbow motion probably do not require the additional trauma, time, expense, and sedation risk involved in a formal reduction because of the predictable remodeling in this age group (99). It has been shown that the more displaced the fracture, the more likely that formal monitored sedation techniques will be used for pediatric forearm fracture reduction as opposed to other techniques (192).

More specific closed treatment options are discussed for pediatric forearm injuries in terms of their common fracture patterns: bow (plastic deformation), greenstick, complete, and comminuted.

Traumatic Bowing/Plastic Deformation

Although traumatic bowing was described by Rauber in 1876 (206), it was not widely recognized until Spencer Borden's clas-

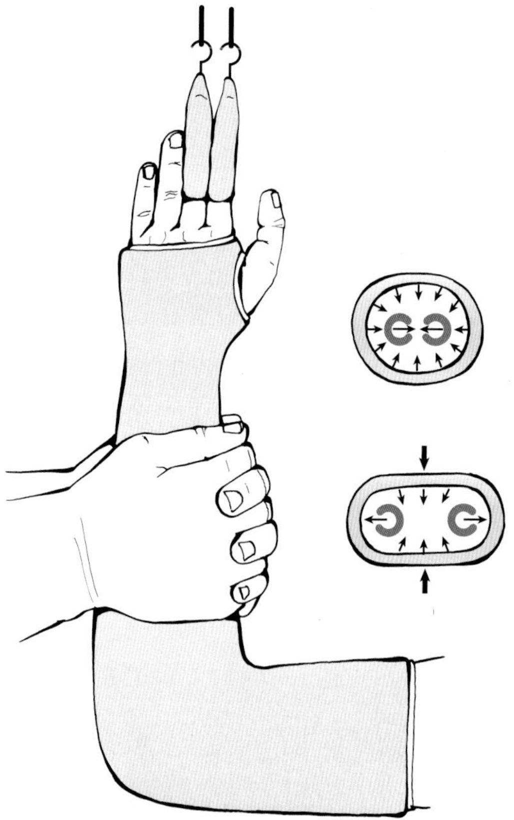

FIGURE 10-21 Interosseous mold technique.

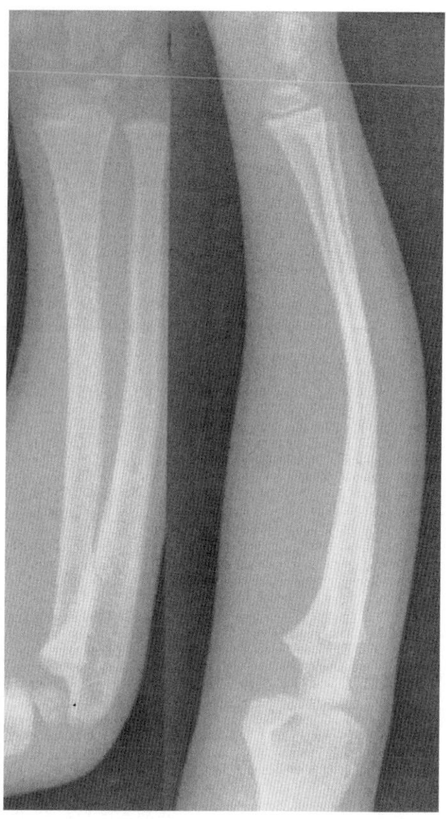

FIGURE 10-22 Bow fracture: approximately 15 degrees of apex dorsal bowing of radius and ulna shaft.

sic paper was published in 1974 (58). This injury occurs almost exclusively with children's forearm fractures (207). Bow fractures (Fig. 10-22) show no obvious macroscopic fracture line or cortical discontinuity, but they do demonstrate multiple microfractures (slip lines) along the length of the bow (208). At times a nearly classic buckle fracture (torus fracture) coexists with a bow fracture. The most common clinical scenario is a plastically deformed ulna along with a more typical fracture of the radius (59).

Borden and subsequent authors stressed the importance of natural remodeling potential in these injuries but voiced concern about this approach in older children (especially those over 10 years of age) (58,59,208). Vorlat and DeBoeck reported incomplete remodeling in 3 of 11 children at long-term follow-up (average 6.7 years) after traumatic bowing of the forearm (209). Because these three children were between the ages of 7 and 10 at the time of injury, the authors recommended more aggressive efforts at reduction in all patients with clinically significant deformity (more than 10 degrees) older than 6 years of age (209). Traumatic bowing that causes cosmetically or functionally unacceptable angular deformity (210) must be manipulated under general anesthesia or deep sedation because strong (20 to 30 kg) gradual force applied over 2 to 3 minutes is required to obtain acceptable alignment (Fig. 10-23) (208). Application of this reductive pressure over a rolled towel fulcrum followed by a three-point molded cast can substantially (although at times still incompletely) correct the deformity. Care must be taken to avoid direct pressure over adjacent epiphyses for fear of creating a physeal fracture.

Greenstick Fractures

Greenstick fractures present special issues in terms of diagnosis and treatment. Angulated greenstick fractures of the shafts of the radius and ulna at different levels indicate a significant rotational component to the injury (see Fig. 10-8). Evans, Rang, and others have stated that the apex-volar angulation pattern usually is associated with a supination-type injury mechanism, while most apex-dorsal greenstick fractures involve a pronation-type injury mechanism (Fig. 10-24) (4,34,51,130), although exceptions certainly occur (51,211). Often the apparent angular deformity can be corrected by simply reversing the forearm rotational forces (e.g., reducing an apex-dorsal pronation-type injury with supination). Noonan and Price observed that it is difficult to remember whether to use pronation or supination reductive forces and suggested that most fractures can be reduced by rotating the palm toward the deformity (4). They also noted that most greenstick fractures are supination injuries with apex-

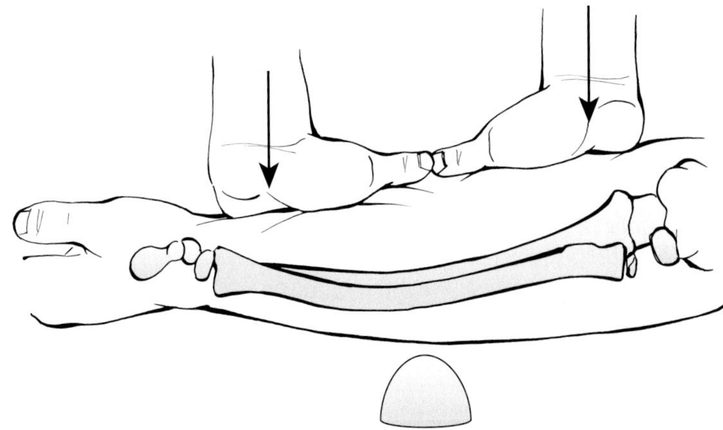

FIGURE 10-23 Reduction technique of bow fracture over fulcrum. (From Sanders WE, Heckman JD. Traumatic plastic deformation of the radius and ulna: a closed method of correction of deformity. *Clin Orthop* 1984;188:58–67.)

volar angulation and thus can be reduced by a pronation movement (4).

Greenstick fractures that occur near the same level probably have little to no rotational component and are best corrected by manipulative reduction and three-point molding techniques (see Fig. 10-9). Charnley believed that greenstick fractures of the forearm in children perfectly illustrated his dictum that "a curved plaster is necessary in order to make a straight limb" (32). He also stated that "the unsuspected recurrence of angular deformity in greenstick fractures of the forearm, while concealed in plaster, is an annoying event if it takes the surgeon by surprise and is not discovered until the plaster is removed. Parents, quite understandably, may be more annoyed about this happening to their children than if it had happened to themselves, and do not easily forgive the surgeon" (32). Despite these concerns, it is clear from large published reports that greenstick fractures can almost always be successfully treated with nonoperative methods (134).

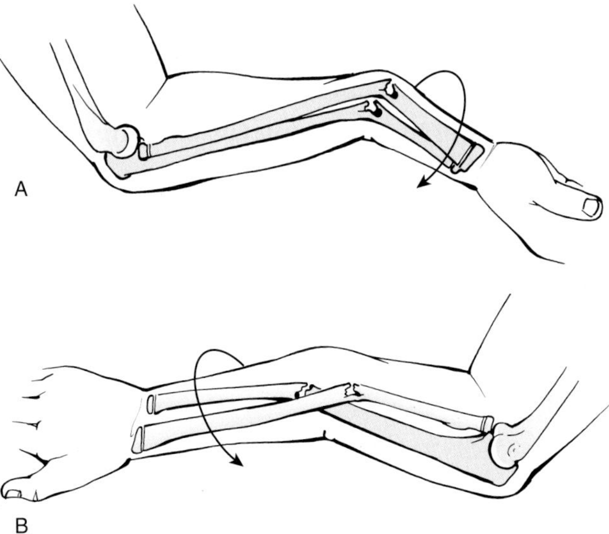

FIGURE 10-24 Shaft fractures at different levels implies rotational mechanism. **A.** Apex-volar angulation with supination deformity of the forearm. **B.** Apex-dorsal angulation with pronation deformity of forearm.

Two philosophies are reflected in the literature regarding greenstick fracture reduction: one in which the greenstick fracture is purposely completed and another in which it is not. Those who favor completing the fracture (dating back at least to the 1859 work of Malgaigne) cite concerns about lostreduction and recurrent deformity that can be prevented only by converting the greenstick into a complete fracture (28,30,31,89). Others prefer to maintain and perhaps exploit some of the inherent stability of the greenstick fracture (6,8,51,184,212). In addition to the traditional view that loss of reduction is less likely if a greenstick fracture is completed, there also is the theoretical advantage of a lower refracture rate because of more exuberant callus formation (4,184). To the best of our knowledge these theories have not been validated in any controlled clinical studies. Davis and Green advocated a derotational approach to greenstick fracture reduction and reported a 10% (16/151) reangulation rate in their series of patients with greenstick fracture (6). They compared this to the 25% (12/47) reangulation rate in patients with complete fractures and questioned the wisdom of routinely completing greenstick fractures (6). In a prospective study, Boyer et al showed statistically that greenstick fractures maintain their reduction better than complete forearm fractures (213).

Complete Fractures

Complete fractures in different regions of the shaft of the forearm behave differently from a clinical perspective and have classically been divided into distal-, middle-, and proximal-third fractures. Single-bone complete fractures usually are caused by direct trauma (nightstick fracture) and are difficult to reduce. Blount described a reduction technique that may be effective for reduction of a displaced single-bone shaft fracture. The intact bone is used as a lever to re-establish length of the fractured bone, and then transverse forces are applied to realign the bone ends (Fig. 10-11). Both-bone complete fractures (often with bayonet shortening) are common and are best treated with finger-trap or arm traction applied over 5 to 10 minutes. This stretches out the soft tissue envelope and aids in both reduction and cast or splint application. Traction allows complete fractures to "seek their own level of rotation" and allows correction of rotational malalignment by the orthopaedist (6).

The position of immobilization for forearm fractures has been an area of debate since the days of Hippocrates (30). Theoretically the position of forearm rotation in an above-elbow cast or splint affects rotational alignment of complete fractures at all levels; however, a study of distal-third forearm fractures found no significant effect of forearm rotation position on ultimate alignment (213). We are aware of no similar studies analyzing the effects of forearm position on middle- or proximal-third shaft fractures, and treatment is influenced by certain anatomical considerations. Because of the strong supination pull of the biceps, aided by the supinator, complete proximal radial fractures may be best immobilized in supination so that the distal forearm rotation matches that of the proximal forearm (see Fig. 10-18). The position of immobilization of fractures in the middle third of the forearm commonly is dictated by whether the radial fracture occurs distal or proximal to the insertion of the pronator teres. Fractures proximal to its insertion are best treated by fully supinating the distal fragment, while those distal to its insertion are probably best treated in a neutral position.

Manipulated fractures should be evaluated weekly for the first 2 to 3 weeks, because most position loss can be recognized and corrected during this time (214,215). Any significant shift in position between visits necessitates cast wedging or a cast change, with remolding and possible fracture remanipulation if unacceptable displacement is present. Voto et al found that in general 7% of forearm fractures redisplace; this can occur up to 24 days after the initial manipulation (215). Davis reported a 25% reangulation rate in complete fractures (6). Remanipulation can be done in the office following administration of oral analgesics. Judicious use of benzodiazepines may also be valuable because of their anxiolytic effects.

Although in adults the above-elbow cast generally is changed to a below-elbow cast after 3 to 4 weeks, this is unnecessary in most children because they heal more quickly and permanent elbow stiffness is rare (216). A cast change at week 3 or 4 also can be traumatic to a young child and carries the additional small risk of cast saw injury. Once the fracture shows good callus formation, the cast can be removed. Because shaft fractures of the radius and ulna in children have a significant rate of refracture (9,37,217), they should be splinted for an additional period of time (218). Parents should be warned of the risk of refracture.

Above-elbow casting with the elbow in extension has been suggested for some complete fractures of the middle and proximal thirds (219–221). The supination moment exerted by the biceps has been shown to be diminished when the elbow is extended (222). Walker and Rang reported successful treatment of 13 middle- or proximal-third forearm shaft fractures with this method (some following failed flexed-elbow casting) (220). They suggested that the "short fat forearms" of some young children prevented successful flexed-elbow casting (220). Turco et al also reported 20 children treated with this method and emphasized full supination of the forearm (221). Three of their patients required cast wedging, but at final follow-up 19 of the 20 patients had excellent results (221). One patient who was lost to follow-up for 6 months (presumably removing his own cast) did suffer "mild residual deformity" (221). Rang recommended that benzoin be applied to the skin, in addition to creation of an adequate supracondylar mold, to further secure the cast (220). Casting the thumb in abduction with extra pudding may prevent the cast from sliding. Turco suggested that reduction should be obtained with horizontal traction applied to the extended upper extremity, followed by additional steps outlined in Table 10-5. Based on published clinical results, concerns related to cast slippage and elbow stiffness appear to have been overstated (220,221). The main drawback of this technique is its awkwardness as compared to flexed-elbow casting (220).

Comminuted Fractures

Although comminuted forearm fractures are less common in children than in adults (8), they do occur (28,89,90,166,167,223). Comminuted fractures tend to occur in conjunction with high-energy injuries, such as open fractures (28,224). Comminuted forearm fractures deserve special attention because they often require specially tailored treatment approaches. If satisfactory reduction cannot be achieved or maintained by closed methods, then other treatment alternatives should be considered.

One option is to accept some shortening; according to Price, this may help maintain motion through interosseous membrane slackening (5). Shortening of more than 1 cm is unacceptable in either single-bone or both-bone comminuted patterns. Standard closed fracture treatment generally is unsuccessful when both bones are comminuted, and surgical stabilization may be necessary (89). Bellemans and Lamoureux reported intramedullary

TABLE 10-5 Turco Technique for Extended Elbow Cast Treatment

1. Closed reduction under sedation
   a. Supine patient, fully supinated forearm
   b. Abducted shoulder
   c. Elbow extended (approx. 170 degrees)
2. Above-elbow cast applied
   a. Interosseous mold
   b. Supracondylar mold
3. Weekly x-rays first 3 weeks
4. Cast changes based on "Rule of 3's"
   a. 3 weeks at 170 degrees
   b. 3 weeks at 135 degrees
   c. 3 weeks at 90 degrees

nailing of all comminuted forearm fractures in their pediatric series (223). Other reported fixation methods for comminuted forearm fractures in children include plate-and-screw devices (89,90), flexible intramedullary nailing for single-bone comminution (87), and pins-and-plaster techniques (225). Bone grafting is rarely if ever indicated in acute comminuted forearm features in children.

CURRENT SURGICAL TREATMENT OPTIONS

Overview of Surgical Treatment

Duncan and Weiner cited an "aggressive surgical mentality" as the reason for frequent operative treatment of pediatric forearm fractures (190), and Wilkins expressed concern about "impetuous" surgeons who are too eager to operate (226). Cheng et al documented a more than 10-fold increase in the rate of operative treatment of forearm shaft fractures in children (1), but it is unclear as to whether this increase in operative treatment has led to a commensurate improvement in clinical outcomes.

Operative treatment of radial and ulnar shaft fractures usually is reserved for open fractures, those associated with compartment syndrome, floating elbow injuries, and fractures that develop unacceptable displacement during nonoperative management. Residual angulation after closed treatment is much better tolerated by younger children than older adolescents and adults because of the increased remodeling potential in the younger age group (115). As a consequence, adolescents are more likely to benefit from surgical treatment of their forearm fractures than are younger children. Although internal fixation is the standard of care for displaced forearm fractures in adults, the success of nonoperative methods and the complications associated with internal fixation have tempered enthusiasm for its application to pediatric forearm fractures. Compared to closed treatment methods, healing is slower after open reduction and internal fixation (223), no matter what type of implant is used (89). Crossed Kirschner wire fixation techniques that often are used successfully in the distal radius are technically difficult in the shaft region of the radius and ulna. In rare situations, external fixation has been used for pediatric forearm fixation (227).

Preoperative planning is essential regardless of which surgical technique is chosen. Assessment of the fracture, including rotation and the presence or absence of comminution, is important. Bone–plate mismatch (due to narrow bones and wide plates) and extensive soft tissue dissection are risks when adult-sized plates are applied to pediatric bones (16). Before intramedullary nailing of fractures, the forearm intramedullary canal diameter should be measured, especially at the narrowest canal dimension; typically this is the central portion of the radius (228) and the distal portion of the ulna. Precise canal measurement can be difficult (122,229), and the consequences of a nail or pin that is too large are probably worse than those of a nail or pin that is too small (230). Modern digital radiography systems have made these measurements easier (231).

Plate Fixation

Open reduction and internal fixation of pediatric forearm shaft fractures with plates and screws is a well-documented procedure in both pediatric series (165,232–234) and adult series that include patients as young as 13 (235) and even 7 (236) years of age. In one of the early series of pediatric forearm fractures fixed with plates (237), dynamic compression plates (DCP) and one-third tubular plates applied with standard AO technique (six cortices above and below the fracture site) obtained good results (237). Four-cortex fixation on either side of the fracture site has been shown to be equally effective in pediatric forearm fractures (167).

Plate fixation uses the standard adult approach and technique except that smaller plates (2.7 mm compression and one-third tubular), fewer screws, and single-bone fixation often are acceptable (167). Plate fixation may allow more anatomic and stable correction of rotational and angular abnormalities and restoration of the radial bow than with noncontoured intramedullary rods; however, the larger incisions and extensive surgical exposures required for plate fixation have raised concerns regarding unsightly scars (16,165,171) and muscle fibrosis with consequent motion loss (167). While the cosmetic concerns seem valid, ultimate forearm motion is similar with the two techniques, with only minor losses reported in the literature after both plating and intramedullary nailing (80,115,176,238).

Open reduction and internal fixation with plates and screws may be appropriate in the management of fractures with delayed presentation or fractures that angulate late in the course of cast care (83,167), when significant fracture callus makes closed reduction and percutaneous passage of intramedullary nails difficult or impossible (239). Other indications for plate fixation include shaft fractures with significant comminution (89) and impending or established malunion (11) or nonunion (230,240,241). Several authors have reported good results with plate fixation of the radius only (26,34,234,242) or the ulna only (Fig. 10-25) (243). Bhaskar and Roberts compared 20 children with both-bone plate fixation to 12 with ulna-only fixation and found significantly more complications in the dual plating group, although motion was equal at 1-year follow-up (243). Single-bone fixation requires satisfactory reduction of both bones. Flynn and Waters stated that they would preferentially plate the radius only when the fracture could not be reduced by closed means (242). Two patients in Bhaskar and Roberts' study required open reduction and internal fixation of the radius when it was not adequately reduced after plate fixation of the ulna (243).

Kirschner Wire, Rush Rod, and Steinmann Pin Intramedullary Fixation

Currently, intramedullary fixation is the preferred method for internal fixation of forearm fractures in children (124,134,166, 174,175,177,178,181,244). Intramedullary fixation of children's forearm fractures dates back at least to Fleischer's 1975 report in the German literature in which he called it "marrow wiring" (245). Closed intramedullary nailing (also

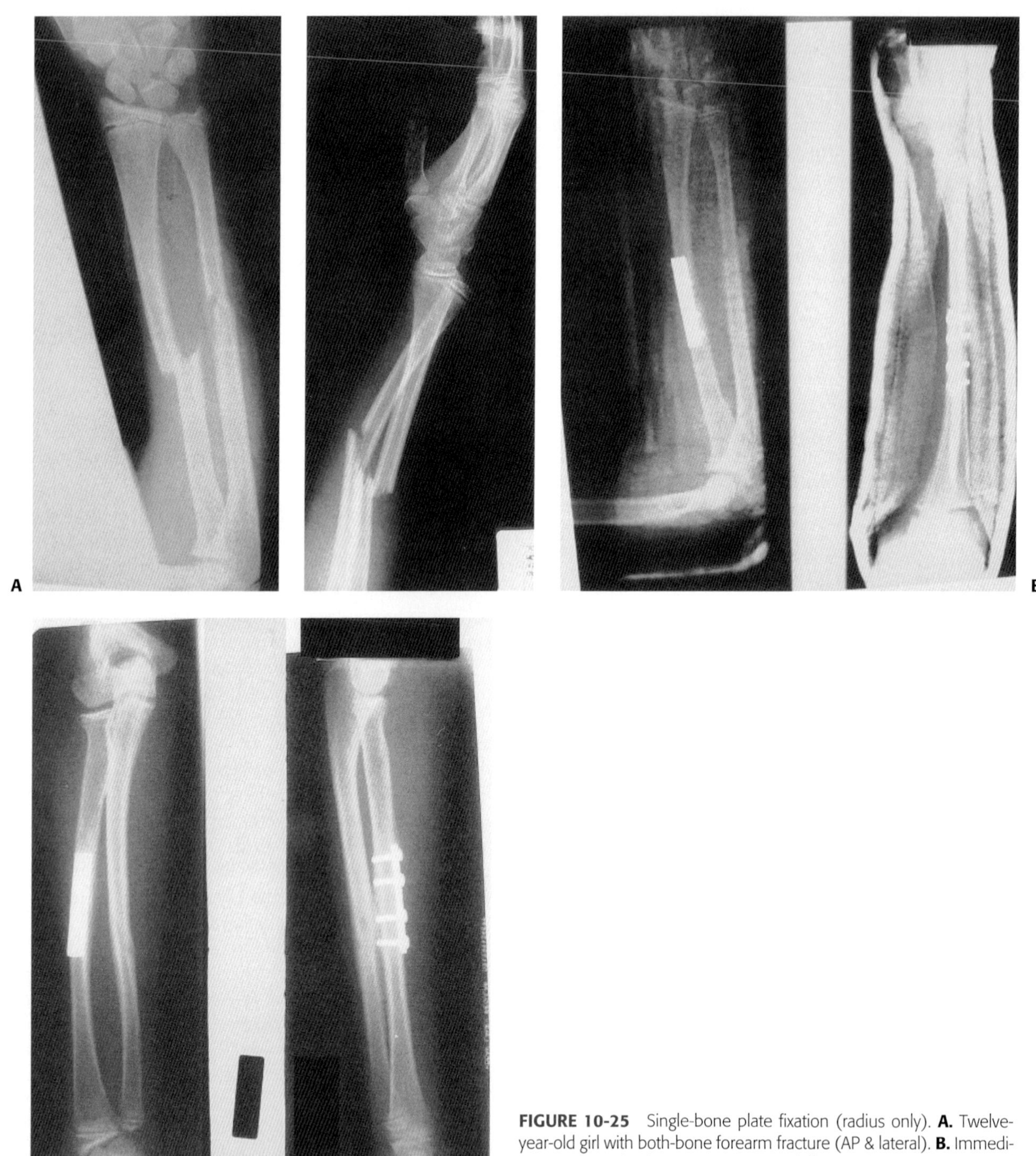

FIGURE 10-25 Single-bone plate fixation (radius only). **A.** Twelve-year-old girl with both-bone forearm fracture (AP & lateral). **B.** Immediate postoperative images. **C.** Two-year follow-up images. (Courtesy of Tom Welle, DO.)

known as indirect reduction and internal fixation) of diaphyseal forearm fractures in adolescents was later reported in the English language literature by Ligier et al (179), Amit et al (181), and others (16,180,246). A variety of implants have been used for forearm intramedullary nailing, including Kirschner wires, Rush rods, and Steinmann pins.

Intramedullary fixation has several advantages over plate fixation, including improved cosmesis because of smaller incisions and less deep tissue dissection (leading to a lower risk of stiffness) (16,80,166,176). Contoured pins are used in the radius to preserve its natural anatomical bow (80,124,181,247); contoured pins are not necessary for the ulna (181). Although the rotational stability of pediatric forearm fractures treated with intramedullary fixation has been questioned, Blasier and Salaman suggested that the strong periosteum in children resists torsional stresses (246). In a cadaver study of the rotational stability of fractures of the ulna and radius treated with Rush rods, Ono et al found that intramedullary fixation of both bones reduced fracture rotation to one eighth of that in unfixed fractures (248).

Elastic Stable Intramedullary Nailing

In the early 1980s Metaizeau et al described elastic stable intramedullary nailing (ESIN) of pediatric forearm fractures (249) with small-diameter (1.5 to 2.5 mm) contoured implants (179). No effort was made to fill the medullary canal as with other intramedullary nailing techniques (87), and the "summit of the curve must be calculated preoperatively to lie at the level of the fracture" (180). The prebent flexible rods (known as Nancy nails) were reported to maintain satisfactory fracture alignment while encouraging development of normal physiologic fracture callus (179,249,250). Good results with this technique have been reported by numerous authors (87,251–257).

Because the ESIN technique emphasizes the interdependence of the radius and ulna, if both bones are fractured, both bones are internally fixed (180). It also is dependent on anchorage of the nails in the upper and lower metaphyseal portions of the bone to produce an internal three-point fixation construct (180). Technique principles include fixing first the bone that is easiest to reduce, using physeal-sparing entry points, and using small nails varying in diameter from 1.5 to 2.5 mm (180). A nail that is too large may lead to nail incarceration and distraction at the fracture site, especially in the ulna (230). Contouring of both nails is recommended, with particular attention to restoration of the appropriate radial bow (Fig. 10-26). Initially, nails were removed by about the fourth postoperative month, but several refractures led the originators of the technique to delay nail removal until 1 full year after surgery (180). Pin ends should be cut short and buried to maintain prolonged fixation.

Immediate motion has been recommended by some authors after ESIN of pediatric forearm fractures (177,180,223,251), while others have recommended immobilization for variable periods of time (178). Early refracture with nails in place has been reported. Bellemans and Lamoureux considered displaced oblique or comminuted midshaft forearm fractures in children older than 7 years of age to be an indication for ESIN (223). They considered bayonet apposition (overriding) to be unacceptable at any age because of concerns about rotational malalignment and frequent narrowing of the interosseous space (223). Their fixation technique involved passage of the intramedullary nails followed by rotation of each nail until the greatest distance between the two bones was achieved in full supination (223).

Management of Open Fractures

In one large epidemiologic study, open fractures of the shafts of the radius and ulna and open tibial shaft fractures occurred with equal frequency, making them the most common open fractures

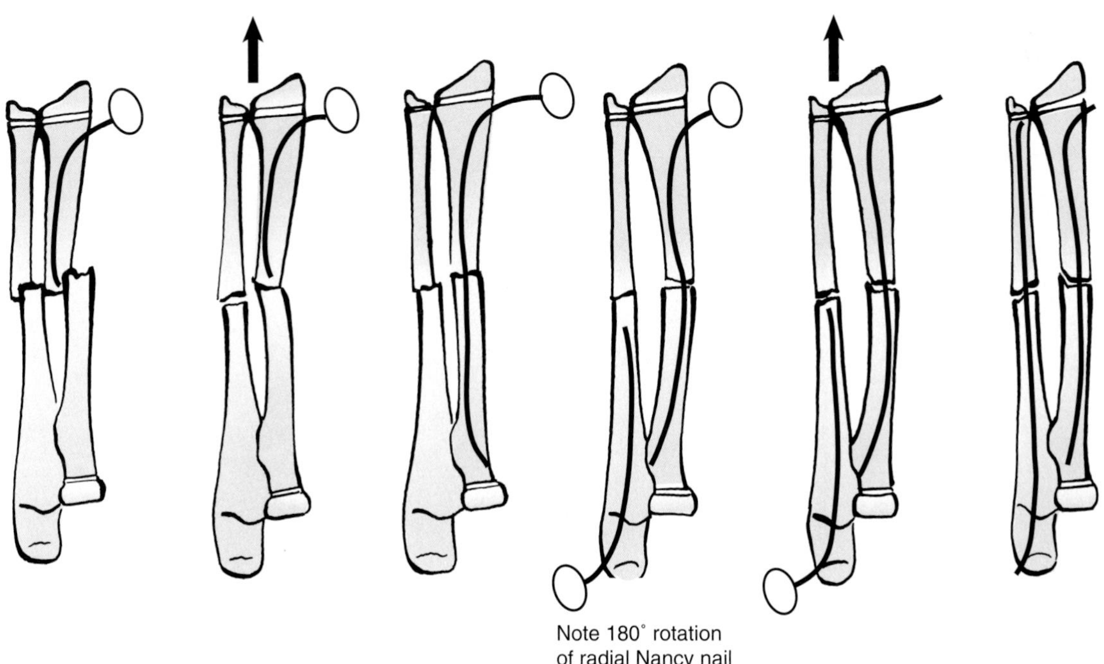

FIGURE 10-26 Metaizeau elastic stable intramedullary nailing technique. The radial rod is twisted 180 degrees in step 4 to re-establish the radial bow.

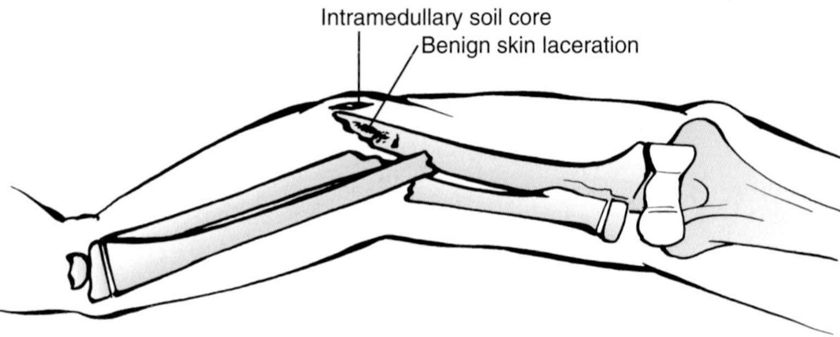

FIGURE 10-27 Intramedullary organic contamination of an open forearm fractures.

in children (1). Although the infection rate is extremely low for open fractures, even grade I open forearm fractures in children have been associated with serious complications such as gas gangrene (258). Early irrigation and debridement (259,260) are indicated for open forearm fractures, and care should be taken to inspect and properly clean the bone ends (44). Roy and Crawford recommended routinely inspecting both of the bone ends (171) for the presence of intramedullary foreign material (Fig. 10-27). Once debrided, open forearm fractures can be stabilized by any of the available internal fixation methods without undue risk of infection (Fig. 10-28) (17,82,83). Open fractures tend to be more unstable than closed fractures (because of soft tissue stripping and comminution) and require internal fixation more commonly. Internal fixation also may facilitate soft tissue management and healing (167). The amount of periosteal stripping and possible foreign body reaction associated with open forearm fractures may produce an unusual radiographic appearance, the "ruffled border sign" (Fig. 10-29). Usually this seems to represent a normal healing response in growing children, but occasionally it is an early sign of osteomyelitis. The infection rate ranges from 0% to 33% for open fractures in children (5,6,17,80,82,83, 167,214,234). Even grade I open forearm fractures in children can be complicated by gas gangrene or osteomyelitis, and therapeutic amputation has been reported (6,28,258). Open fracture

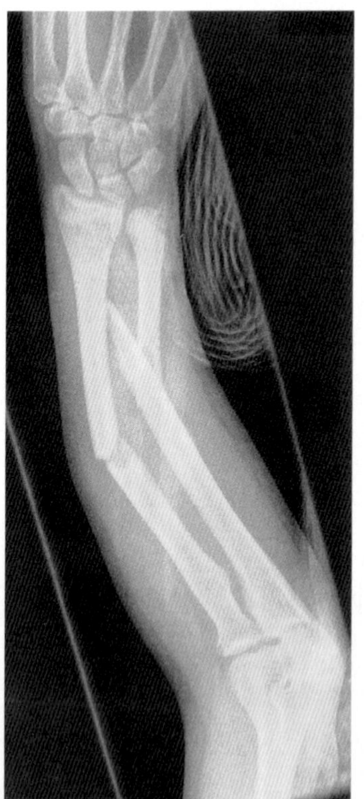
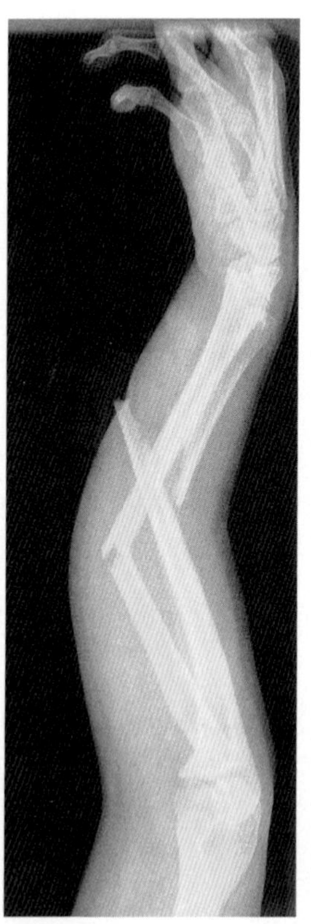
A
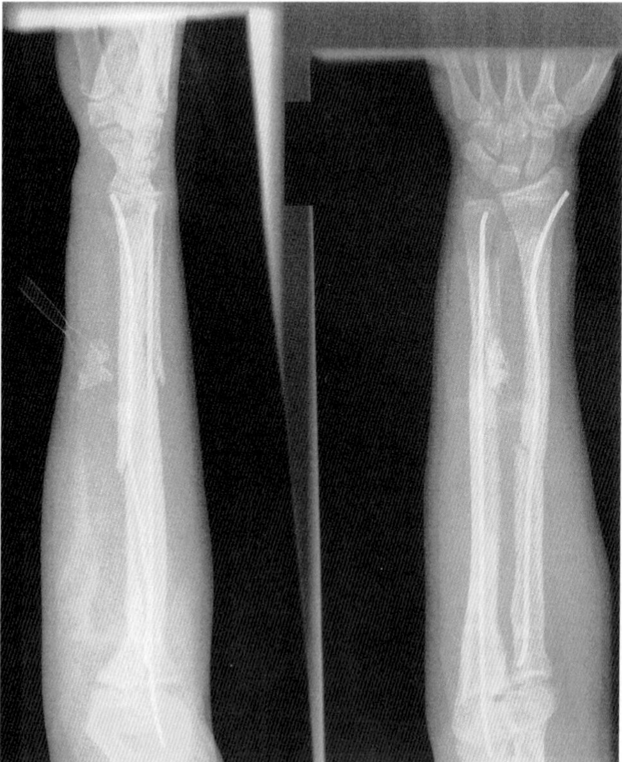
B

FIGURE 10-28 Thirteen-year-old girl with open forearm fracture. **A.** AP and lateral x-rays; note extrusion of ulna on lateral view. **B.** After irrigation and debridement and flexible nail internal fixation. Note the Penrose drain in the ulnar wound.

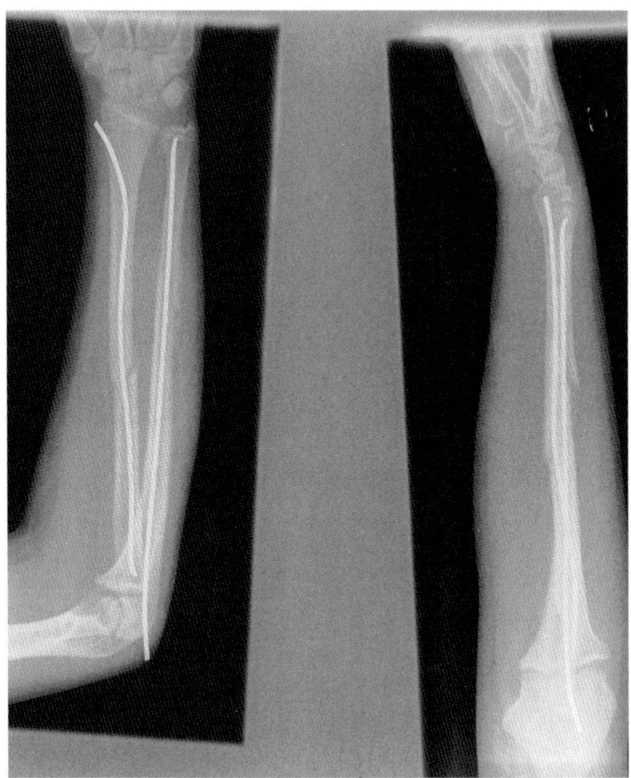

FIGURE 10-29 Ruffled border sign at the site of previous open fracture of ulna; same patient from Figure 10-28 at 1-month follow-up.

grade does not appear to correlate with the infection rate in childhood forearm fractures, with most of the serious forearm infections reported in the literature occurring after grade I fractures.

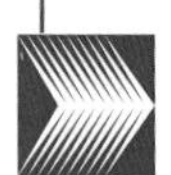

AUTHORS' PREFERRED METHOD OF TREATMENT

Closed Fracture Care

We agree with Jones and Weiner that "closed reduction still remains the gold standard for closed isolated pediatric forearm fractures" (14). Most nondisplaced and minimally displaced radial and ulnar shaft fractures can be splinted in the emergency department and referred for orthopaedic follow-up within 1 week. X-rays are repeated at the first orthopaedic visit and a cast is applied. During warmer weather, when fracture incidence peaks, we tend to use waterproof cast liners. We avoid flexing the elbow past 80 to 90 degrees in waterproof casts because the soft tissue crease that forms in the antecubital fossa tends to trap moisture. Because waterproof cast lining alone does not shield the skin from cast saw cuts and burns as well as traditional padding does, specialized material may be added along the anticipated course of the cast saw to protect the skin during cast removal. Two such materials are blue cast strips (De-Flex Strip Cast Removal Aid, WL Gore & Associates, Flagstaff, AZ) and a plastic zipstrip (inserted between the skin and cast liner). We prefer an above-elbow cast for all forearm fractures in children under the age of 4 years, because young children tend to lose or remove a below-elbow cast due to soft tissue differences (baby fat) common to the age group (98). Most older children with forearm shaft fractures also are treated with above-elbow casting, except for those with stable distal-third fractures. Good forearm casting technique should focus on the principles outlined earlier in this chapter. Patients with nondisplaced fractures usually are re-evaluated radiographically in 1 to 2 weeks after initial immobilization to check for fracture displacement. Forearm shaft fractures heal more slowly than metaphyseal and physeal fractures of the distal radius and ulna (6,217). The cast is removed in 6 to 8 weeks if adequate healing is present. Because of the significant refracture rate after forearm shaft fractures, we splint these fractures for another several weeks until all transverse lucency of the original fracture disappears and all four cortices are healed. Fractures that heal in bayonet apposition (complete translation and some shortening) can take longer to heal than those with end-to-end apposition and may require prolonged splinting to prevent refracture (96,98).

Fracture Reduction/Conscious Sedation Protocol

Significantly displaced forearm shaft fractures are usually manipulated in the emergency department using a conscious sedation protocol. After obtaining informed consent for conscious sedation and fracture manipulation, an intravenous line is started, and the child's blood pressure, pulse, respirations, EKG, and peripheral oxygen level are monitored during the procedure and for about 30 minutes after the procedure. We use fentanyl and midazolam (Versed) administered intravenously in divided doses. Although many children moan or cry briefly during the manipulation, very few recall pain. Reductions are done under mini-C-arm (fluoroscopy) control. The initial position of forearm rotation is based on the level of the fracture, and the final position is based on the best reduction under fluoroscopy. Small portable fluoroscopy units save time and money (estimated to be 10% of the cost of conventional x-rays). Finger-trap traction with 10 to 15 pounds of counterweight frequently is used for completely displaced both-bone forearm fractures (especially those with shortening). We do not complete greenstick fractures because the partial bone continuity adds stability.

Because of concerns about soft tissue swelling, manipulated fractures are placed into a plaster sugar-tong splint (incorporating the elbow). Before manipulation, the sugar-tong splint is prepared by laying out 7 to 10 layers of appropriate-length 3-inch plaster casting material on top of a work surface. A four-layer matched length of cotton cast padding also is laid out and will form the inner padding (skin side) of the splint. A final single layer of cast padding is laid out and will form the outer layer of the splint to prevent elastic wrap adherence to the plaster. Once manipulation is completed the plaster is dipped, wrung out, smoothed, and then sandwiched between the dry four-ply and one-ply cotton padding. This splint is then placed with the four-ply cotton side against the skin and secured with an elastic bandage. We prefer to avoid the circumferential application of cotton padding because it may limit splint expansion during follow-up swelling. If necessary, parents also can unwrap and loosen the elastic bandage at home to relieve pressure if swelling makes the splint too tight. Patients are given discharge instructions and a prescription for mild narcotic analgesics.

Patients usually return to the office within a week for repeat x-rays and clinical assessment. Provided that satisfactory alignment has been maintained, we remove the elastic wrap but leave the plaster sugar-tong splint in place. The splint is "boxed in" by applying cotton cast padding over the splint and the exposed upper arm, and by wrapping with fiberglass to convert the splint into an above-elbow cast. Follow-up x-rays are taken of manipulated fractures at about 1-week intervals for the next 2 weeks. Fractures that are losing position but are still in acceptable alignment usually require removal and remolding of a new cast to prevent further position deterioration. Minor remanipulations can be done in the office after appropriate administration of oral analgesics and anxiolytics. Major remanipulations are best done with general anesthesia. The decision regarding remanipulation may be aided by viewing of the cosmetic deformity by the parents and physician after all splint and cast materials are removed.

By the end of the fourth week after injury, many above-elbow casts can be converted to below-elbow casts (often a waterproof cast in warm weather). This step may be omitted in younger children because of their faster healing and their minimal inconvenience from temporary elbow immobilization (216). Patients can return to sports after conversion to a below-elbow cast as long as the cast is padded during play and league rules allow casts. Patients usually are required to have a physician's note allowing sports participation with a cast. Adequate fracture healing (bridging callus of four cortices) usually has occurred after several more weeks of cast treatment but should be confirmed by radiographic and physical examination before unlimited athletic participation. Older children are given home elastic band strengthening exercises and allowed to participate in normal activities while they continue to be protected in either a removable Velcro fracture brace or a customized thermoplastic forearm gauntlet brace. Formal physical therapy rarely is required. This fracture protocol is aimed at minimizing refracture risk.

Acceptable Limits of Angulation

Based on available evidence in the literature, we accept approximately 20 degrees of angulation in distal-third shaft fractures of the radius and ulna, 15 degrees at the midshaft level, and 10 degrees in the proximal third (provided the child has at least 2 years of growth remaining) (261). We accept 100% translation if shortening is less than 1 cm. Although other authors recommend accepting up to 45 degrees of rotation, we find this is extremely difficult to measure accurately using the bicipital tuberosity and radial styloid as landmarks because of the lack of anatomical distinction in younger children. Bow fractures seem to have less remodeling potential than other fractures, and radiographically or cosmetically unacceptable angulation may require gradual, forceful manipulation under sedation or general anesthesia. Children approaching skeletal maturity (less than 2 years of remaining growth) should be treated using adult criteria because of their reduced remodeling potential. Parents should be cautioned that even mild angulation of the ulna, especially posterior sag, will produce an obvious deformity after cast removal because of the bone's subcutaneous location (Fig. 10-30). This cosmetic deformity is exacerbated by abundant callus formation, but it will ultimately remodel if it falls within acceptable angulation criteria. Ulnar sag may be countered by placing the child in a extended elbow cast. Mild to moderate angulation of the radius usually produces much less cosmetic deformity (Fig. 10-31).

Surgical Treatment

Most forearm shaft fractures continue to be successfully treated with closed methods at our institution. Our top two indications for surgical treatment of these injuries are open shaft fractures and shaft fractures that exceed our stated reduction limits. If surgical treatment is deemed necessary,

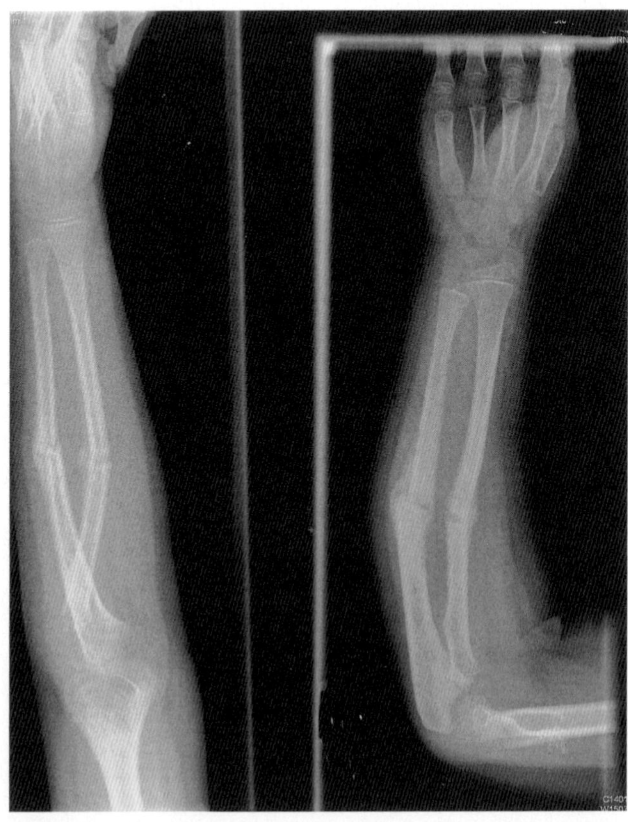

FIGURE 10-30 Ulnar sag on serial x-rays. Note the prominent ulnar fracture callus.

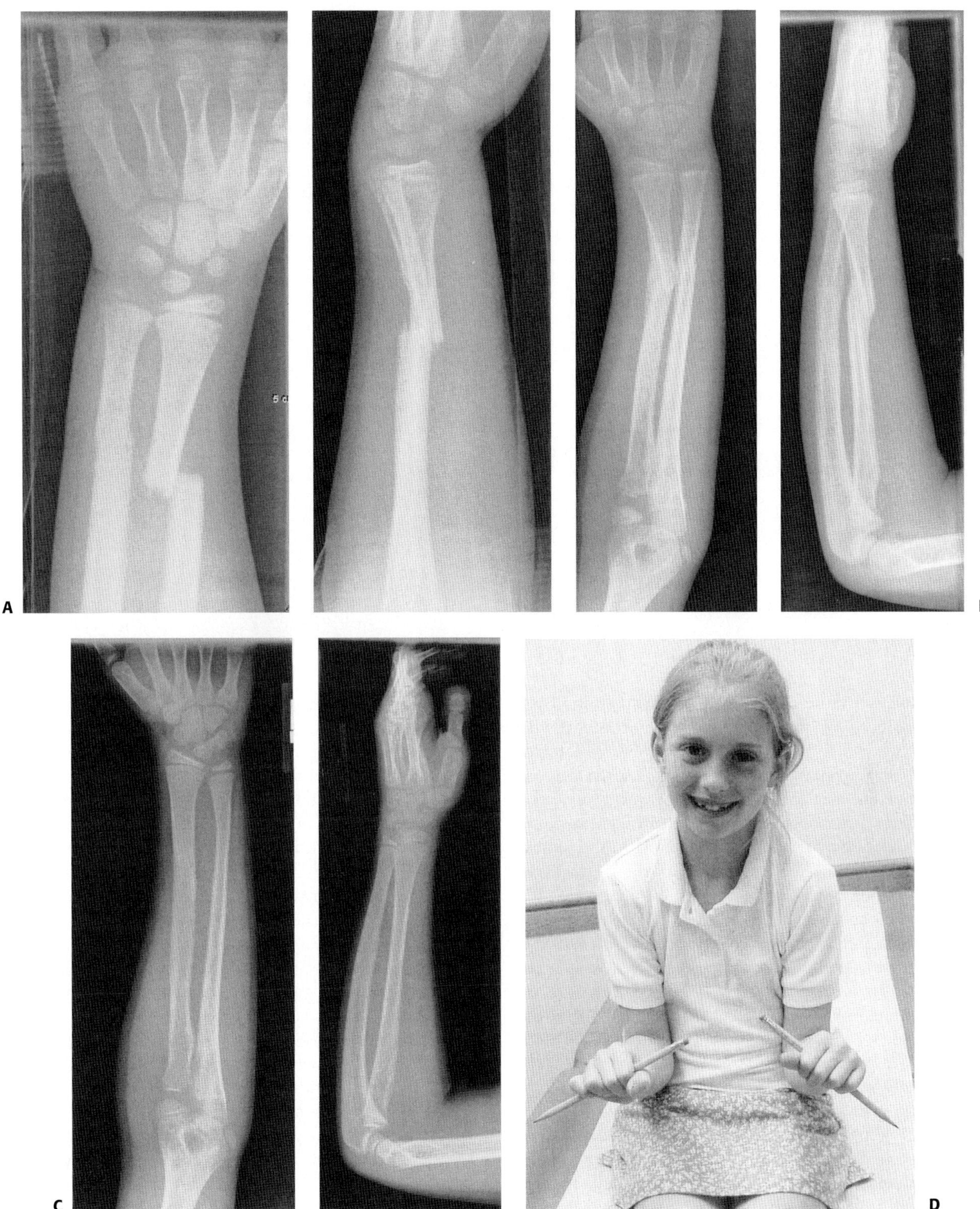

FIGURE 10-31 Seven-year-old girl with both-bone complete forearm fracture. **A.** AP and lateral injury x-rays. **B.** Two-month follow-up x-rays. **C**. Two-year follow-up x-ray shows mild residual deformity. **D.** Pronation. (*continues*)

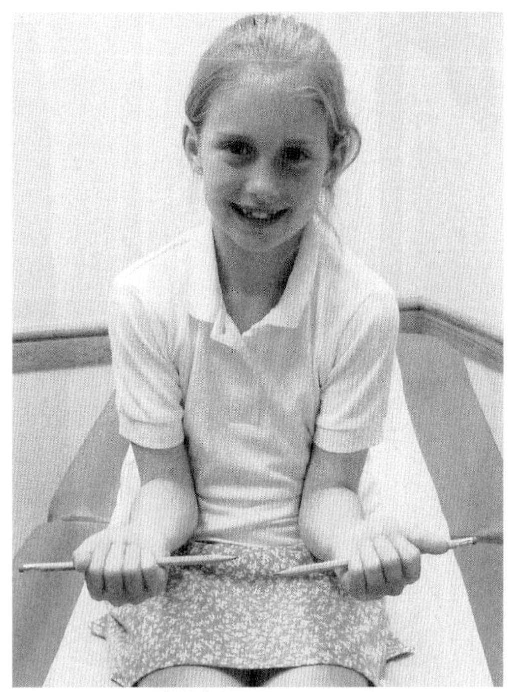

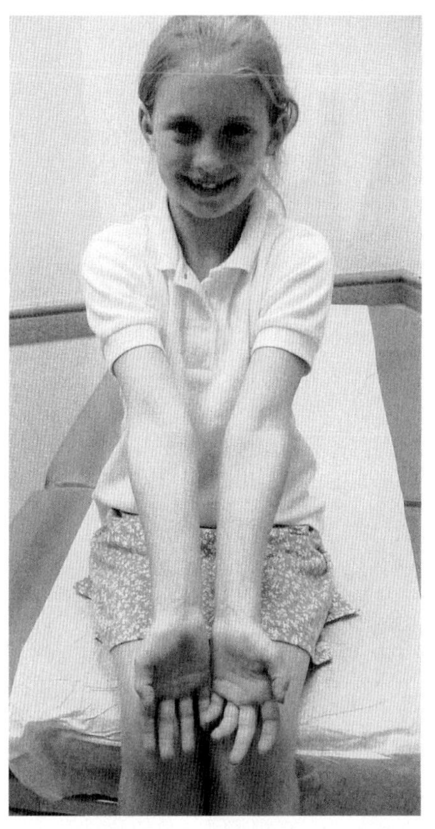

FIGURE 10-31 (continued) **E.** Supination. **F.** Axial alignment at 2-year follow-up.

intramedullary fixation is preferred over plate fixation because of reduced soft tissue disruption. We occasionally fix one bone when both bones are fractured if overall forearm alignment is acceptable and stable after single-bone fixation.

If single-bone fixation is done, the ulna usually is treated first because of its more benign entry site, subcutaneous location, and relatively straight canal compared to the radius. Our preferred intramedullary ulnar entry site is just distal to the olecranon apophysis (anconeus starting point), just anterior to the subcutaneous border of the proximal ulna on its lateral side. Care is taken not to enter the ulna more than 5 mm anterior to its subcutaneous crest to avoid encroachment into the region of the proximal radioulnar joint. Pins placed directly through the tip of the olecranon apophysis have a strong tendency to cause bursitis and significant pain until removal. We prefer to open the cortex with an awl because it tends to wander less than motorized drills and it allows ulnar entry with little or no formal incision. The awl technique also simplifies operating room setup in that no pneumatic hose hookups or battery packs are necessary.

If dual bone fixation is elected, then the radius is fixed first as it is usually more difficult. The distal radial entry site can be either through a physeal-sparing direct lateral approach through the floor of the first dorsal compartment or dorsally near the proximal extent of Lister's tubercle between the second and third dorsal compartments. Both of these entry points are approximately 1 cm proximal to the physis of the distal radius. We insert the radial nail through a 1- to 2-cm incision, protecting the superficial radial nerve and the dorsal tendons with small blunt retractors. An awl is used to gain intramedullary access to the radius. We typically use small intramedullary nails (2.0 to 2.5 mm in diameter) to maintain some flexibility at the fracture site and stimulate appropriate callus formation. Larger nails may become incarcerated in either the narrow central canal of the radius or that of the distal third of the ulna. Failure to pass the intramedullary nail across the fracture site after several attempts may necessitate a limited open reduction through a 1- to 2-cm incision to directly pass the rod across the fracture site (Fig. 10-32). Persistence in attempting to achieve closed reduction and rodding has been associated with compartment syndrome (79).

We prefer to leave the nails buried beneath the skin because complete fracture healing takes at least 2 months, often more. Because refracture can even occur with nails in place, we protect children for at least the first month with a removable fracture brace. If a single bone of a both-bone fracture is fixed, above-elbow cast immobilization usually is necessary instead of a below-elbow cast or brace, as is used after dual-bone fixation. After the appearance of satisfactory callus, splint and activity restrictions are progressively relaxed. We recommend nail removal after complete four-cortex healing of each bone (6 to 12 months in some patients).

Plating is preferred to intramedullary nailing when early

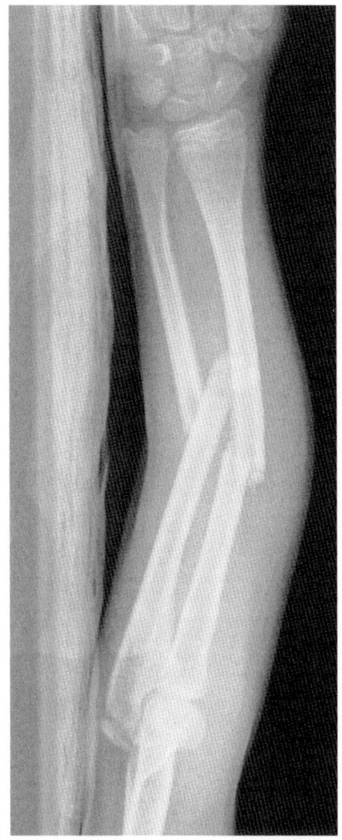

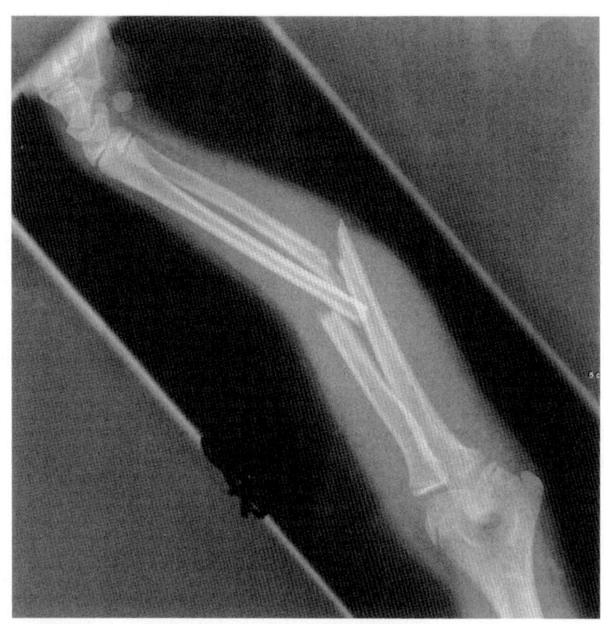

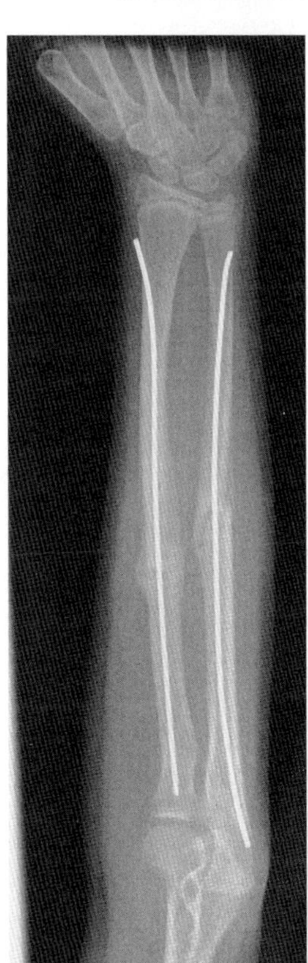

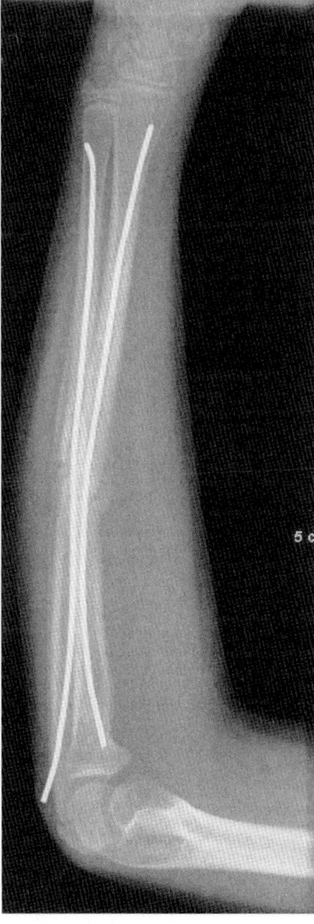

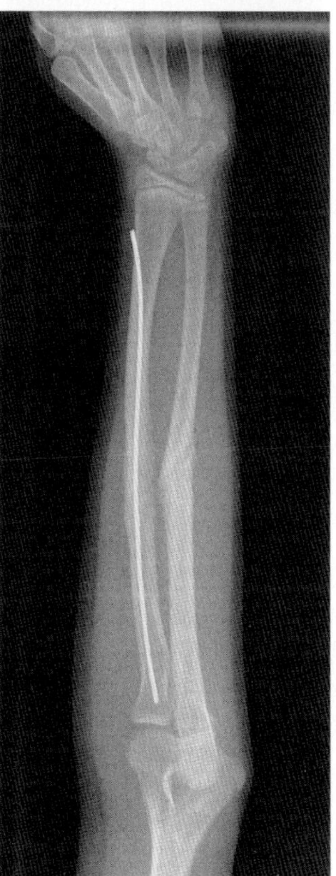

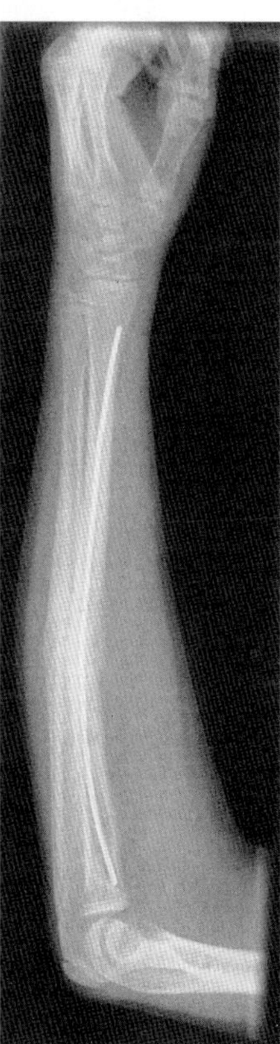

FIGURE 10-32 Twelve-year-old girl with midshaft both-bone complete forearm fracture. **A.** AP and lateral injury x-rays. **B.** Two-month follow-up x-rays. **C.** Six-month follow-up x-rays (ulnar nail removed). (*continues*)

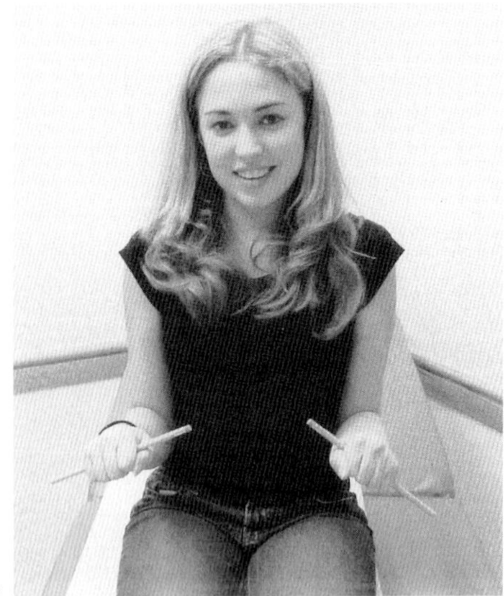
D

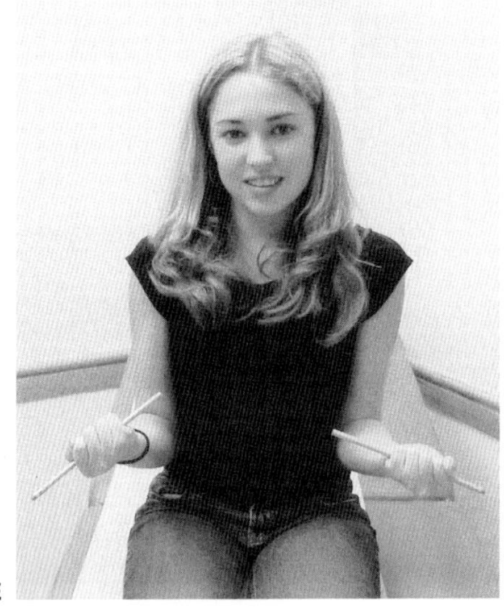
E

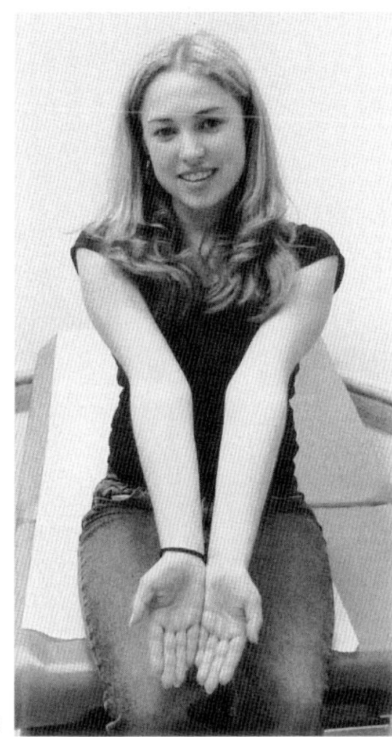
F

FIGURE 10-32 *(continued)* **D.** Pronation. **E.** Supination. **F.** Axial alignment.

malunion is present and callus formation is noted radiographically. Plating allows open osteoclasis and reduction. The plating technique is similar to that used in adults, except that smaller plates can be used and fewer cortices (often only four cortices above and below the fracture) are required for adequate fixation. In children with both-bone forearm fractures, plating of a single bone may be adequate and reduce the morbidity associated with dual-bone plating (243). Significant comminution of both bones also may be an indication for plate fixation.

COMPLICATIONS

Redisplacement/Malalignment

The most common short-term complication of forearm shaft fracture treatment is loss of satisfactory reduction in a previously well-reduced and well-aligned fracture, a complication that occurs in 10% (6,14,184,225,262) to 25% of patients (6,262). Initial follow-up x-rays are a screening test aimed at identifying redisplacement. Kramhoft and Solgaard recommended that children with displaced diaphyseal forearm fractures have screening radiography at 1 and 2 weeks after reduction (214). Voto also pointed out that most fractures that redisplace do so within the first 2 weeks after injury (216). Inability to properly control fracture alignment with closed methods is the most commonly reported indication for operative intervention (124, 134,171,174,176).

The most common explanations for loss of fracture reduction are cast-related (poor casting technique, no evidence of three-point molding) (184,225). The more experienced the surgeon, the greater the likelihood of successful reduction (262). Other factors that have been found to be associated with forearm fracture redisplacement are quality of initial reduction (182), missed follow-up appointments (50), proximal-third fractures (12), and failure of the doctor to respond to early warning signs such as slight loss of reduction at 1-week follow-up (187). Strategies for dealing with redisplacement include (a) allowing the deformity to remodel (106), (b) cast wedging (28,189,191), (c) rereduction and recasting (6,225), (d) pins and plaster (29,190,225), (e) indirect reduction and internal fixation (181), and (f) open reduction and internal fixation (167). Reports in the literature suggest that most forearm shaft fractures that redisplace can be successfully managed with repeat closed reduction and casting (6,225).

Forearm Stiffness

The forearm is a predominantly nonsynovial joint with high-amplitude motion as its main function. The most common long-term complication of forearm shaft fracture treatment is significant forearm stiffness (106), with pronation loss occurring almost twice as frequently as supination loss (10). Loss of pronation or supination motion sometimes occurs despite perfectly normal-appearing x-rays (5,102,115). Abnormal bony alignment of the forearm bones leads to predictable motion deficits (263). Stiffness that exceeds that expected from bony malalignment alone (263) and stiffness that occurs with normal x-rays are indications of fibrosis of the interosseous membrane or contracture of the interosseous ligament (5,115).

With focused testing of forearm motion, between 18% (93) and 72% (10) of patients show at least some minor deficits after nonsurgical treatment. Most minor deficits are not even noticed by patients and rarely are associated with functional limitations (69,93,102). More severe losses of forearm rotation have far greater impact (264). In their series (5) of malunited forearm fractures (thus strongly weighted to demonstrate forearm stiffness), Price et al reported a 15% (6/39) rate of mild stiffness (up to 25-degree loss) and an 8% (3/39) rate of severe forearm stiffness (loss of 45 degrees or more of either pronation or supination). Holdsworth's series (10) of malunited pediatric forearm fractures had a similar rate (6%) of severe forearm stiffness. Holdsworth told the classic story of a girl whose inability to properly pronate caused her to elbow her neighbors when eating at the table (10). Patrick pointed out that it is possible to compensate for pronation losses with shoulder abduction, but no similar compensation mechanism exists for supination losses (107). Such severe motion loss is a very undesirable outcome. For surgical treatment of these injuries to be a rational choice, the rates of stiffness after surgery must be lower than those after cast treatment.

Bhaskar and Roberts published one of the only studies of plated pediatric forearm fractures to report goniometric pronation and supination data. Both their single-bone (ulna) and both-bone plated patients showed mild forearm motion losses (maximal 18% loss of pronation) (265). Variable rates of mild forearm range-of-motion losses have been reported after intramedullary fixation. Amit et al reported a 40% rate of mild stiffness (5 to 10 degrees) in 20 pediatric patients after Rush rod fixation of forearm fractures (181). Combined data from five series of the flexible intramedullary nailing (Kirschner wires, Steinmann pins, Nancy nails) reveal a 1.6% rate (2/128) of mild forearm stiffness (up to a 20-degree loss) and a 0% (0/128) rate of severe motion loss (40 degrees or more loss of either pronation or supination) (134,166,176,181,223,266). No published series of nonoperatively treated forearm shaft fracture patients has exceeded these results relative to preservation of forearm motion.

Refracture

Refracture occurs more often after forearm shaft fractures in children than after any other fracture (37). Tredwell found that forearm refractures occurred at an average of 6 months after original injury and were more common in boys (3:1) and in older children (approximately 12 years old) (9). Refracture rates of 4% (266) to 8% (267) have been reported in pediatric diaphyseal forearm fractures. Bould and Bannister reported that diaphyseal forearm fractures were eight times more likely to refracture than metaphyseal fractures (268). Schwarz et al found that 84% (21/28) of the forearm refractures in their series had initially presented as greenstick fractures (269). Based on the stage of bony healing, refractures may occur through the original fracture site, through both the original site and partially through intact bone, or completely through intact bone (270), but most seem to occur through the original fracture site.

Several authors have suggested that internal fixation is necessary after refracture (87,217,271), but Schwarz et al reported good results with repeat closed reduction and casting in 14 of 17 patients with refractures (269). Closed reduction also has been shown to be effective for forearm refractures that occur with flexible nails in place (272). The best treatment of refracture is prevention, and patients should be splint-protected (removable forearm splint or thermoplastic gauntlet) for a period of two months depending on activity after initial bone healing (4,6). Refracture is rare during splint wear. Parents must be cautioned about the risk of refracture despite apparently adequate bone healing on x-rays.

Refracture after plate removal has been discussed frequently in the literature (15,89,236–238) and appears to be associated with decreased bone density beneath the plate (273). This has led many authors to question the routine use of plate fixation for pediatric forearm fractures (15,50,165,246). Refractures also have been reported after removal of intramedullary forearm fixation in children (80,83,115,133,176,180,253). The main strategies aimed at decreasing the risk of refractures after implant removal are documentation of adequate bony healing before implant removal, and an additional period of splint protection after implant removal until the holes have filled in.

Malunion

Evaluation of pediatric forearm fracture malunion must take into account established malreduction limits and expected pediatric remodeling potential. Thus, a malunion of 30 degrees may become less than 10 degrees during the course of follow-up. The level of the malunited fracture also must be considered, because the consequences of malreduction vary according to level (110,261). More deformity in the predominant plane of motion is acceptable in fractures near the very end of long bones than in diaphyseal fractures. Often normal motion is preserved despite persistent radiographic abnormality (Fig. 10-33).

Malunion of radial and ulnar shaft fractures can lead to cosmetic deformity and loss of motion; however, significant loss of function occurs in only a small percentage of patients (69,93,102). Some authors have recommended more aggressive efforts at correction of forearm fracture malunions (108). Early malunions (up to 4 or 5 weeks after injury) can be treated with closed osteoclasis under anesthesia. If closed osteoclasis fails to adequately mobilize the fracture, a minimally invasive drill osteoclasis can be done (104). A small-diameter drill (or Kirschner wire) is used to make multiple holes in the region of the malunion before forcefully manipulating the bone back into alignment (104). Internal fixation is rarely if ever needed.

Once significant callus is present, indirect reduction and internal fixation with flexible intramedullary nails can be difficult or impossible because the fracture site is now blocked with callus. Thus, established or impending malunions that cannot be adequately controlled with a cast may require formal open reduction and plate fixation. Most fractures that heal with angulation or rotation of more than the established criteria regain full motion and have an excellent cosmetic outcome. Fractures may require corrective osteotomy if they fail to remodel after an adequate period of observation or if adequate motion fails to return (11,108). Such corrective osteotomies have been done

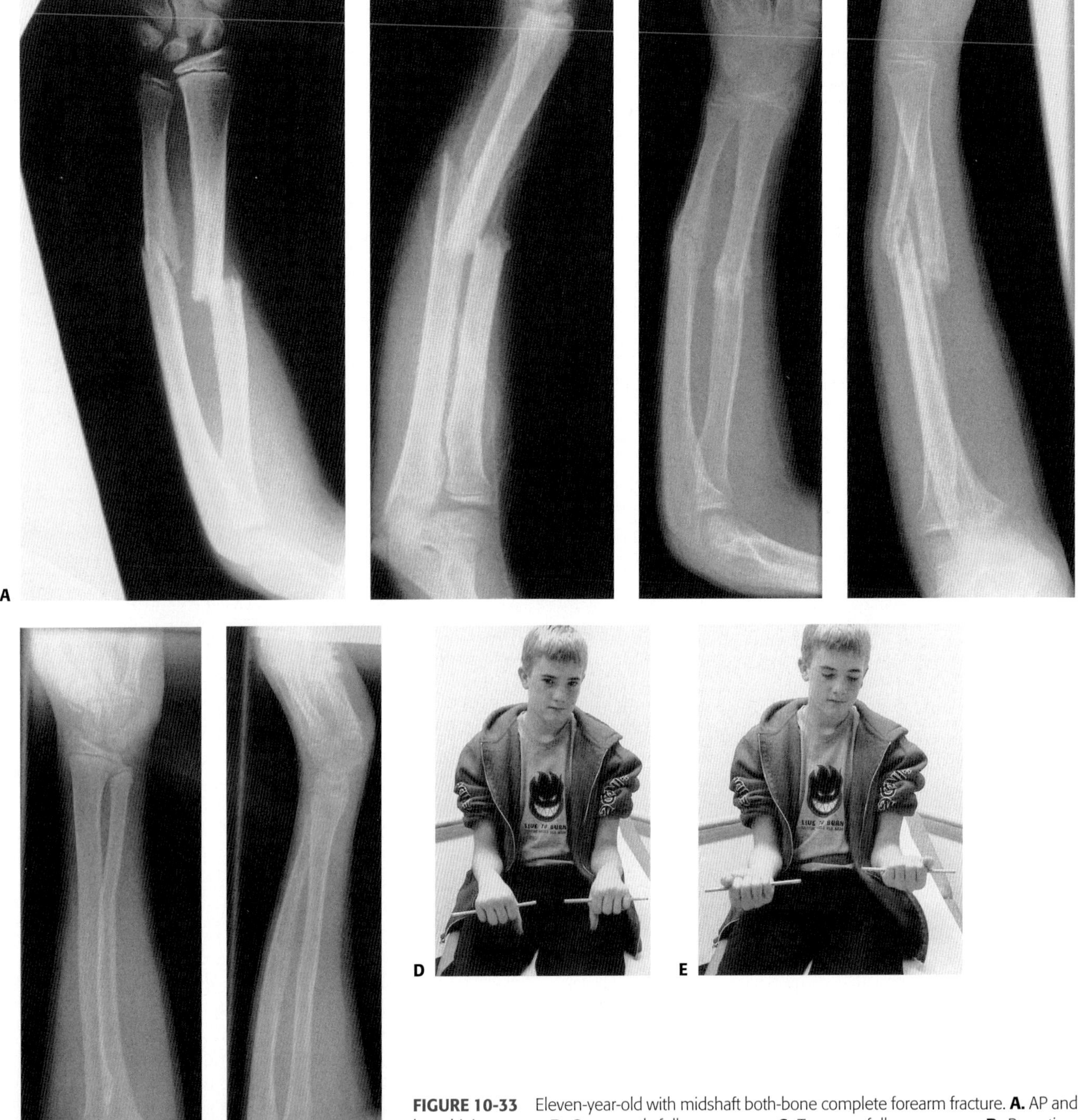

FIGURE 10-33 Eleven-year-old with midshaft both-bone complete forearm fracture. **A.** AP and lateral injury x-rays. **B.** One-month follow-up x-rays. **C.** Two-year follow-up x-rays. **D.** Pronation. **E.** Supination. *(continues)*

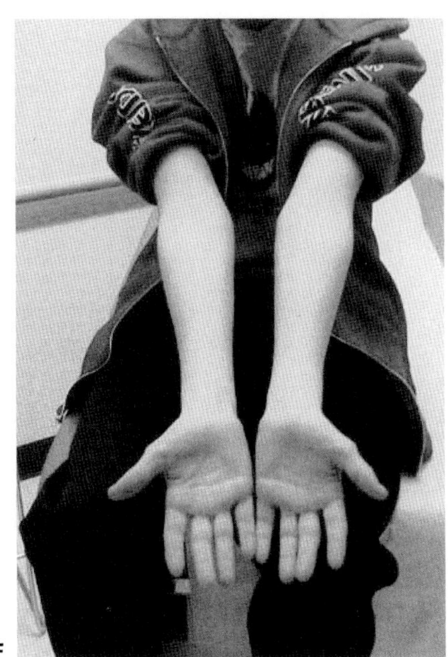

F

FIGURE 10-33 (*continued*) **F.** Axial alignment.

long after injury (up to 27 years) and additional motion has still been regained (11), but most malunions do not require osteotomy, especially in younger children with tremendous remodeling potential.

Delayed Union/Nonunion

The diagnosis of delayed union is based on documentation of slower-than-normal progression toward union (241). Daruwalla stated that normal healing of closed pediatric forearm shaft fractures occurs at an average of 5.5 weeks (range 2 to 8 weeks) (69). Delayed union can be practically defined as a failure to demonstrate complete healing (four cortices) on sequential x-rays by 12 weeks after injury, which exceeds the upper limit of normal healing by about 1 month. Nonunion can be defined as absence of complete bony union by 6 months after injury, which exceeds the upper limit of normal healing by about 4 months.

Delayed unions and nonunions are rare after closed forearm shaft fractures in children (241,274,275). In six large series of pediatric diaphyseal forearm fractures treated by closed methods, a less than 0.5% rate (1/263) of delayed union and no nonunions were reported (5,10,69,93,115,214). Delayed unions and nonunions are more common after open reduction and internal fixation and open fractures. Particular concern has been raised about the potential of antegrade ulnar nailing (olecranon starting point) to distract the fracture site (230). Combined data from four series of plated pediatric forearm fractures indicated a 3% (3/89) nonunion rate (165,167,237,265); 24% (21/89) of these were open fractures and at least one (167) of the three nonunions occurred after a grade III open fracture (165,237). Large series of open pediatric forearm fractures (treated by a variety of internal fixation methods) reported comparable numbers: 5% (8/173) delayed union rate and 1% (2/173) nonunion rate (17,83,84). In a series of 30 nonunions in children, only 6 were in the forearm, and half of these were after open fractures (241).

Because of the overall rarity of nonunions in children, the possibility of unusual diagnoses such as neurofibromatosis must be considered (276–279). After open injury or surgical intervention for other reasons, the possibility of septic nonunion must be ruled out. In the absence of such extraneous factors, nonunion of pediatric forearm fractures seems to be related to surgical treatment (275–279). Weber and Cech divided nonunions into atrophic and hypertrophic types (280). Atrophic nonunions probably are best treated with bone grafting and compression plating. Compression plating or other stable internal fixation without grafting usually is sufficient for hypertrophic nonunions (281).

Cross-Union/Synostosis

Posttraumatic radioulnar synostosis results in complete loss of forearm rotation. Most cross-unions that form after pediatric forearm shaft fractures are type 2 lesions (diaphyseal cross-unions), as described by Vince and Miller (282) (Fig. 10-34). Although some series of adult forearm fractures reported synostosis rates of 6% to 9% (283,284), posttraumatic radioulnar synostosis is a rare complication of pediatric forearm shaft fractures (282). In children, it usually is associated with high-energy injuries (282), radial neck fractures (285), and surgically treated forearm fractures (80,286). Some have suggested a familial predisposition to this complication (287). Postoperative synostosis after forearm fractures in children is almost exclusively associated with plate fixation (103,167). The risk of cross-union is increased when open reduction and internal fixation of both-bone fractures are done through one incision (50,283).

Both osseous and nonosseous cross-unions may form in the forearm (288–290), but the more common type is osseous. After a synostosis matures (6 to 12 months), it can be excised, along with any soft tissue interposition (139,282). The results of synostosis resection may be better in adults than children (282), perhaps because of the more biologically active periosteum in children (48,282). Interposition of inert material (such as Gore-tex or bone wax) has been used to decrease the chances of recurrent synostosis (282,286,288,291). Nonsteroidal anti-inflammatory drugs and radiation treatment have been reported after synostosis excision in adults, but their use in children remains undefined.

Infection

Infection occurs only in surgically treated forearm shaft fractures and open fractures. Appropriately timed preoperative antibiotic prophylaxis is believed to diminish the risk of infection. Children with open forearm fractures are considered to be at high risk for infection, and early (usually less than 24 hours) (259) irrigation and debridement are indicated (171). Whether the backyard or the barnyard, the football field or the hay field,

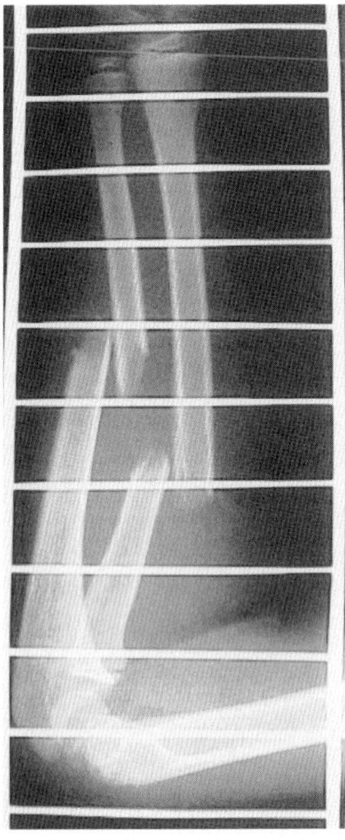
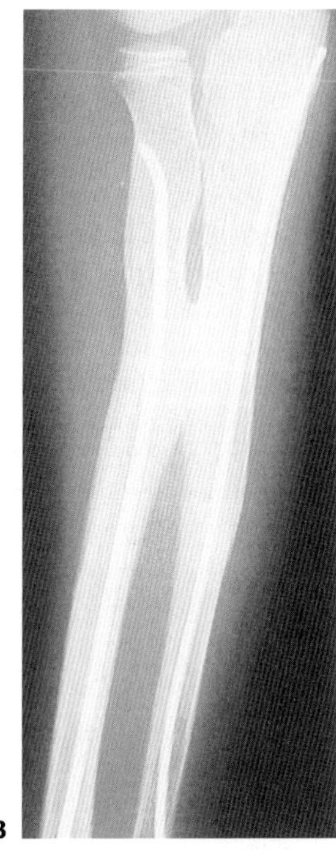
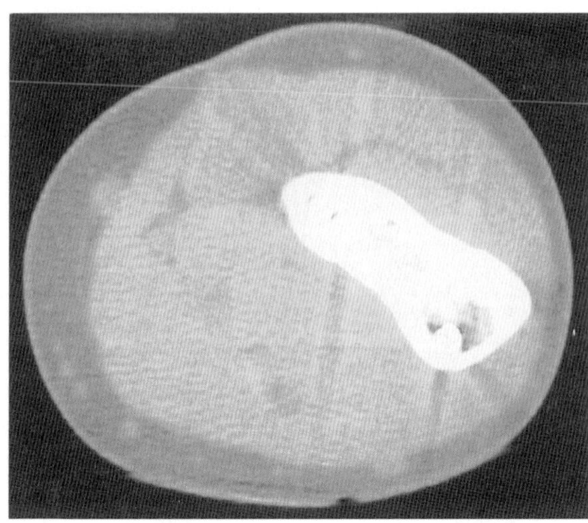

FIGURE 10-34 Radioulnar synostosis following closed injury. **A.** Injury x-rays. **B.** Plain x-rays showing synostosis. **C.** CT scan showing synostosis. (Courtesy of Alan Aner, MD.)

open forearm fractures that occur in organic settings are best treated with early irrigation and debridement with inspection of the intramedullary canal of both bone ends, where soil contamination tends to occur during injury (see Fig. 10-27). Soil contamination has been reported to lead to gas gangrene and subsequent upper extremity amputation in children with grade I open forearm fractures (258).

In four published series of plated pediatric forearm fractures (25% open fractures), deep infection (osteomyelitis) occurred in 5% (4/83) (165,167,237,264). Such deep infections usually require extensive additional surgical treatment to eradicate them. Combined data from 12 series of similar pediatric forearm fractures (15% open fractures) treated with intramedullary Kirschner wires, Steinmann pins, or Rush rods revealed a deep infection rate of 0.46% (2/437) (80,124,134,166,175,176,178, 181,244,247,292) and a superficial infection rate of 2.5% (11/ 437). Six studies of ESIN fixation reported a 0.2% (1/370) deep infection rate and a 3% (12/370) superficial infection rate (87,177,178,251,293,294). Superficial infections may require oral antibiotics, pin removal, or both.

Open forearm fractures clearly are at increased risk for infection. Most (96%) open forearm fractures in children are Gustilo and Anderson (295) grade I or II (17,82,83). Two studies specifically investigated the relationship between the time from injury until irrigation and debridement and the risk of later infection. Luhmann et al reported on 65 fractures (52 type I, 12 type II, 1 type III) that were irrigated and debrided an average of 5.6 hours (range 1.5 to 24 hours) after injury (82), and Greenbaum et al reported 62 fractures (58 type I, 4 type II) that were irrigated and debrided an average of 14.6 hours (range 1.7 to 37.8 hours) after injury (17). No statistically significant association was found in either of these studies; however, most (87%) of these fractures were grade I injuries. Pooled data revealed an overall 1.2% rate (2/173) of deep infection and a 0.6% rate (1/ 173) of superficial infection after current open fracture treatment protocols (17,82,83).

Neurapraxia

The median nerve is the most commonly injured nerve with forearm shaft fractures (whether closed or open injuries) (6,17,82,83), but any peripheral nerve and at times multiple nerves may be involved (80). Most of these injuries are simple neurapraxias that occur at the time of injury and resolve spontaneously over weeks to months (6,295,296). Actual nerve entrapment within or perforation by the bony fragments has been reported (297–304), most often with greenstick fractures (300–303). Constricting fracture callus and fibrous tissue also have been known to cause nerve palsies (297,300). In patients who fail to recover normal nerve function within a satisfactory time period (299), nerve exploration, decompression, and possible nerve repair should be considered. If signs of progressive nerve recovery (e.g., advancing Tinel's sign, return of function) are not present by the end of the third month after injury, further diagnostic work-up (EMG with nerve conduction studies) is indicated.

Nerve injury after internal fixation is always a concern. Operative treatment of pediatric forearm fractures by either indirect reduction and internal fixation techniques or classic open reduction and internal fixation techniques requires fracture manipulation and soft tissue retraction, which have the potential to worsen existing subclinical nerve injury or to create a new injury. Such injuries are rare and almost certainly underreported. Nerve injury after pediatric forearm plate fixation has been alluded to but not discussed extensively (166). Luhmann et al reported an 8% (2/25) iatrogenic nerve injury rate after fixation with intramedullary Kirschner wires or Rush rods (175); both were ulnar nerve injuries that resolved in 2 to 3 weeks. Cullen et al reported one ulnar nerve injury that took 3 months to resolve in a group of 20 patients treated with Kirschner wires or Rush rods (80).

Certain sensory nerves also are at risk for iatrogenic damage during surgical forearm fracture treatment, especially the superficial branch of the radial nerve (175,178,292). Pooled data from six series that included 370 ESIN procedures revealed a 2% (7/370) rate of injury to the superficial branch of the radial nerve (87,177,178,251,293,294). The branching pattern of this sensory nerve is complex, and efforts must be taken to protect it during insertion of intramedullary nails through distal radial entry points (172,173).

Muscle or Tendon Entrapment/Tendon Rupture

Severely displaced forearm fractures may trap portions of muscle between the fracture fragments (124,305). Often interposed tissue can be effectively removed during standard fracture reduction, but the muscle may become an obstacle to successful closed reduction. Much of the volar aspects of the shafts of the radius and ulna is covered by the flexor pollicis longus and flexor digitorum profundus, respectively. Many displaced forearm shaft fractures also have apex volar angulation (4). As a result, portions of these muscles (or their tendons) are particularly prone to fracture site incarceration (Fig. 10-35). The pronator quadratus also is vulnerable to fracture site entrapment in the distal third of the radius and ulna, and it can block reduction of distal-third forearm fractures (305).

Flexor digitorum profundus entrapment within ulnar (306–309) and radial (310) shaft fractures has been reported. Entrapment of the flexor digitorum profundus typically causes an inability to fully extend the involved finger (usually index, long, or ring fingers alone or in combination) (308,309). Even if identified early, this complication rarely responds to occupational or physical therapy. Surgical intervention is the preferred treatment and requires only a small incision (usually over the ulna) through which the adherent tissue is elevated with a blunt instrument from the bone at the site of the fracture. Excellent restoration of finger motion can be achieved, even when the release is done up to 2 years after the fracture (306).

Extensor tendon injury has been reported after intramedullary nailing of pediatric forearm shaft fractures (124,251, 294,311). Primary tendon disruption may be caused by direct trauma during either nail insertion or extraction. Delayed tendon disruption may be caused by slow erosion of the tendon as it glides past a sharp nail edge. The possibility of this complication can be minimized by using surgical incisions large enough to allow insertion of small blunt retractors to protect adjacent tendons during nail insertion and extraction. Avoidance of tendon erosion requires pin lengths that extend beyond the tendon level into either the subcutaneous tissues (80,176) or through the skin (external pins) (124). Conceivably the pins could be buried completely within the bone, but this would require either accepting them as permanent implants (something not commonly practiced at this time) or significantly increasing the level of difficulty of nail removal.

Compartment Syndrome

Compartment syndrome is rare after closed forearm fractures in children, but its consequences can be devastating. Yuan et al found no compartment syndromes in 205 closed forearm injuries (79), and Jones and Weiner reported no compartment syndromes in their series of 730 closed forearm injuries (14). A single compartment syndrome that developed during cast treatment of a 12-year-old girl with a closed both-bone forearm fracture was reported by Cullen et al (80). Because the diagnosis of compartment syndrome can be difficult in children (312), the index of suspicion must be high.

Compartment syndrome should be suspected in any child who is not reasonably comfortable 3 to 4 hours after adequate reduction and immobilization of a forearm fracture (313). The risk of compartment syndrome is higher with open fractures (79,83) and fractures that are difficult to reduce and require extended operative efforts (79). Yuan et al voiced concern that the 10% (3/30) rate of compartment syndrome in their patients with closed fractures might be due to multiple passes or "misses" with intramedullary devices during efforts at indirect reduction and internal fixation (79). Compartment syndrome was reported by Haasbeek and Cole in 5 (11%) of 46 open forearm fractures in their series (83). The so-called floating elbow injury has been associated with a rate of compartment syndrome as high as 33% (78). Forearm compartment syndrome is best treated with fasciotomy, releasing both the superficial and deep volar compartments and the mobile wad. Both the lacertus fibrosis and the carpal tunnel should be released as part of the procedure.

Complex Regional Pain Syndromes

Complex regional pain syndromes such as reflex sympathetic dystrophy are uncommon complications after pediatric forearm shaft fractures (165). Paradoxically, relatively minor injuries seem to place patients at greatest risk (314,315). The most reliable sign in children is true allodynia: significant reproducible pain with light touch on the skin. Swelling and other vasomotor changes often are accompanying signs (316). The diagnosis in children is made based almost exclusively on the history and physical examination, with little reliance on studies such as bone scans (314). These pain syndromes are best treated initially with physical therapy aimed at range of motion and desensitiza-

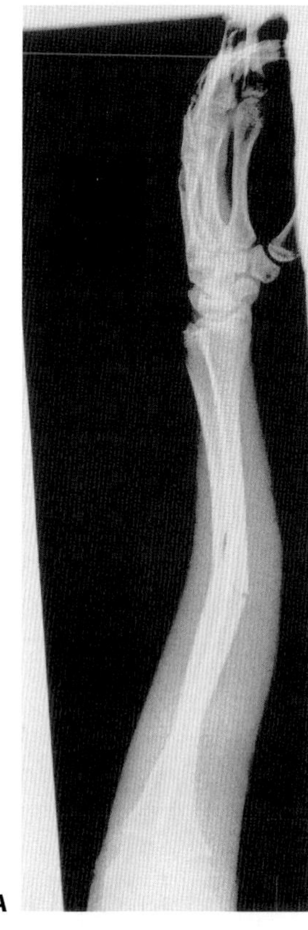

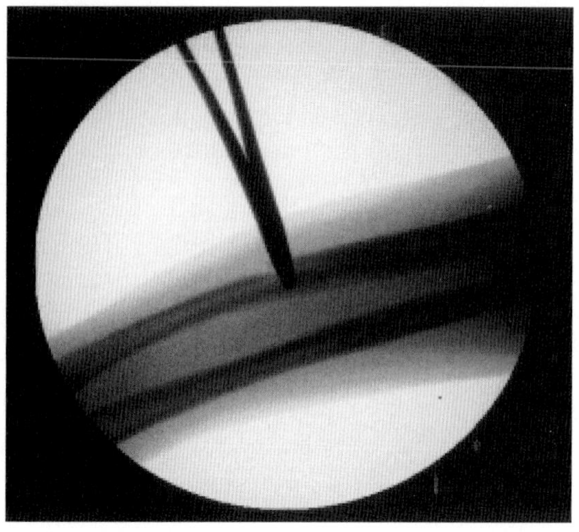

FIGURE 10-35 Muscle/tendon incarceration. **A.** Injury x-ray showing mild apex-volar fracture angulation. **B.** Flexor digitorum profundus entrapment in the ulnar fracture site required surgical extirpation.

tion (314,315). Failure to respond to physical therapy may warrant a referral to a qualified pediatric pain specialist (316,317).

CONTROVERSIES/FUTURE DIRECTIONS

Fracture Risk/Fracture Prevention

Over the past three decades, the rate of forearm fractures has increased dramatically in the United States: 33% higher for boys and 56% higher for girls (318). Certain risk-taking behaviors demonstrated by children, as well as increased use of motorized vehicles like all-terrain vehicles, may be at least partly to blame (319,320). Increased general physical activity patterns and decreased calcium intake also have been suggested as explanations (318), but gaps persist in our epidemiologic understanding. Preventing these injuries remains an admirable but elusive goal. Two main avenues of research have been explored: optimizing safety during activities known to be associated with forearm fractures, and investigating biologic mechanisms related to fracture risk.

The relationship between in-line skating (rollerblading) and pediatric forearm fractures has been shown (321,322), with one in eight children sustaining a fracture on his or her first skating attempt (322). Prevention efforts have focused largely on protective gear. Wrist guards have been shown to decrease distal forearm bone strain (323) and injury rates (324). Similar protective effects of wrist guards in snowboarders have been shown (325). Trampolines are another target of injury prevention efforts aimed at a specific play activity (326). Dramatic increases in trampoline-related injuries were reported during the 1990s, with rates doubling (327) or even tripling (328). Safety recommendations have ranged from constant adult supervision and one-child-at-a-time use (329) to outright bans on public trampoline use (327,328).

A variety of biologic risk factors have been studied relative to forearm fractures. Children who avoid drinking milk have been shown to have increased fracture risk (330), as well as those who prefer to drink fruit juice and soda (331). Several studies have shown an increased risk of fractures in girls aged 3 to 15 years with low bone density (332,333). Diet, nutrition, and exercise are being explored as causative factors, but the precise reason for the low bone density has not been confirmed. Too little physical activity (as measured by television, computer, and video viewing) has been associated with increased fracture risk, presumably because of decreased bone mineral density (334). Caution also must be exercised when obtaining dual-energy x-ray absorptiometry (DEXA) data in children, as up to 88% of scans may be misinterpreted (335). Childhood obesity is a growing problem in our society (336,337). Increased body weight and decreased cross-sectional dimensions of the forearm bones also have been found in girls who fracture their forearms (338). Other researchers have found an increased risk of forearm fracture in obese children (339,340).

Parental Presence During Fracture Reduction

Parental presence is becoming increasingly popular for pediatric emergency department procedures. Several studies on chest tubes, intravenous cannulation, lumbar puncture, and urethral catheterization have shown increased parental satisfaction when parents are allowed to stay for these procedures (341–343). Parental presence during induction of anesthesia also has been shown to have favorable effects on children older than 4 years of age (344). To the best of our knowledge there are no published studies on parental presence during orthopaedic procedures performed in the emergency department setting. There also are no parental presence studies on any emergency department procedures performed on children who are under sedation, when the child is probably not aware of the parent's presence.

Certain relationships between perceived procedural invasiveness and parental presence have been borne out in the literature. Four hundred parents from the Indiana area were surveyed, and with increasing invasiveness, the parents' desire to be present decreased (345). A survey of academic emergency medicine attendings, residents, and nurses from across the country also showed that there is an inverse relationship between increasing invasiveness and support for parental presence (346). Boudreaux et al published their critical review of the parental presence literature and concluded that "randomized controlled trials are mixed regarding whether family presence actually helps the patient" (347).

Extrapolation of information from the previously mentioned studies to pediatric orthopaedic settings should be done with caution. We typically allow parents to be present for the induction of sedation, and once the patient is sedated the parents are asked to wait in a designated area. If parents are allowed to be present, we strongly recommend a dedicated employee to attend to the parent or parents (a "spotter"). Several parents (typically fathers) have fainted during such orthopaedic procedures and injured themselves. Parents who stay for a reduction also should be counseled that the patient may moan or cry during reduction but will not remember it. Parents who are not present during reduction should be asked to wait far enough away from the procedure room so they cannot hear the child.

ACKNOWLEDGMENTS

The authors wish to acknowledge the priceless teaching and constructive feedback afforded us by our senior partner, Alvin H. Crawford, MD, FACS, as well as the skilled assistance of Ms. Kelli Israel and Ms. Tiffany Whatley in the preparation of this chapter.

REFERENCES

An asterisk denotes a Level I evidence-based reference.

1. Cheng JCY, Ng BKW, Ying SY, Lam PKW. A 10-year study of the changes in the pattern and treatment of 6,493 fractures. *J Pediatr Orthop* 1999;19:344–350.
2. Mann DC, Rajmaira S. Distribution of physeal and nonphyseal fractures in 2,650 long-bone fractures in children aged 0–16 years. *J Pediatr Orthop* 1990;10:713–716.
3. Chung KC, Spilson SV. The frequency and epidemiology of hand and forearm fractures in the United States. *J Hand Surg [Am]* 2001;26:908–915.
4. Noonan KJ, Price CT. Forearm and distal radius fractures in children. *J Am Acad Orthop Surg* 1998;6:146–156.
5. Price CT, Scott DS, Kurzner ME, Flynn JC. Malunited forearm fractures in children. *J Pediatr Orthop* 1990;10:705–712.
6. Davis DR, Green DP. Forearm fractures in children: pitfalls and complications. *Clin Orthop* 1976;120:172–183.
7. Sauer HD, Mommsen U, Bethke K, Langendorff HU. Fractures of the proximal and middle third of the lower arm in children. *Z Kinderchir Grenzgeb* 1980;29:357–363.
8. Thomas EM, Tuson KWR, Browne PSH. Fractures of the radius and ulna in children. *Injury* 1975;7:120–124.
9. Tredwell SJ, Van Peteghem K, Clough M. Pattern of forearm fractures in children. *J Pediatr Orthop* 1984;4:604–608.
10. Holdsworth BJ, Sloan JP. Proximal forearm fractures in children: residual disability. *Injury* 1982;14:174–179.
11. Trousdale RT, Linscheid RL. Operative treatment of malunited fractures of the forearm. *J Bone Joint Surg [Am]* 1995;77:894–902.
12. Creasman C, Zaleske DJ, Ehrlich MG. Analyzing forearm fractures in children: the more subtle signs of impending problems. *Clin Orthop* 1984;188:40–53.
13. Vittas D, Larsen E, Torp-Pederson S. Angular remodeling of midshaft forearm fractures in children. *Clin Orthop Relat Res* 1991;265:261–264.
14. Jones K, Weiner DS. The management of forearm fractures in children: a plea for conservatism. *J Pediatr Orthop* 1999;19:811–815.
15. Price CT, Mencio GA. Injuries to the shafts of the radius and ulna. In: Beaty JH, Kasser JR, eds. *Rockwood & Wilkins fractures in children,* 5th ed. Philadelphia: Lippincott Williams & Wilkins, 2001:452–460.
16. Wright J, Rang M. Internal fixation for forearm fractures in children. *Techniques Orthop* 1989;4:44–47.
17. Greenbaum B, Zionts LE, Ebramzadeh D. Open fractures of the forearm in children. *J Orthop Trauma* 2001;15:111–118.
18. Formicola V, Pontrandolfi A, Svoboda J. The Upper Paleolithic Triple Burial of Dolni Vestonice: pathology and funerary behavior. *Am J Phys Anthropol* 2001;115:372–379.
19. Lewis ME. Impact of industrialization: comparative study of child health in four sites from medieval and postmedieval England (A.D. 850–1859). *Am J Phys Anthropol* 2002; 119:211–223.
20. Grauer AL, Roberts CA. Paleoepidemiology, healing, and possible treatment of trauma in the medieval cemetery population of St Helen-on-the-Walls, York, England. *Am J Phys Anthropol* 1996;100:531–544.
21. Önne L, Sandblom PH. Late results in fractures of the forearm in children. *Acta Chir Scand* 1949;98:549–567.
22. Sop AL, Mehlman CT, Meiss L. Hyphenated-history: The Böhler-Braun frame. *J Orthop Trauma* 2003;17:217–221.
23. Böhler L. *The treatment of fractures,* 5th English ed. New York: Grune & Stratton, 1956: 21–23.
24. Rang M. *The story of orthopaedics.* Philadelphia: WB Saunders, 2000:472.
25. Schlich T. *Surgery, science and industry: a revolution in fracture care, 1950s–1990s.* New York: Palgrave-Macmillan, 2002:21.
26. Campbell WC. *Campbell's Operative Orthopaedics,* 1st ed. St Louis: The CV Mosby Company, 1939.
27. Verbrugge J. Clinical survey of 163 cases of internal fixation with metal in fractures in children. *J Bone Joint Surg [Am]* 1956;38:1384–1385.
28. Hughston JC. Fractures of the forearm in children. *J Bone Joint Surg [Am]* 1962;44: 1678–1693.
29. Blount WP. Frearm fractures in children. *Clin Orthop* 1967;51:93–107.
30. Blount WP, Schaefer AA, Johnson JH. Fractures of the forearm in children. *JAMA* 1942; 120:111–116.
31. Beekman F, Sullivan JE. Some observations on fractures of long bones in children. *Am J Surg* 1941;51:722–738.
32. Charnley J. *The closed treatment of common fractures.* Edinburgh: Livinstone, 1957.
33. Blount WP. *Fractures in children.* Baltimore: Williams & Wilkins, 1955:78.
34. Rang M. *Children's fractures.* Philadelphia: JB Lippincott, 1974:126.
35. Moseley CF. Obituary: Mercer Rang, FRCSC (1933–2003). *J Pediatr Orthop* 2004;24: 446–447.
36. Mehlman CT. Clinical epidemiology. In: Koval KJ, ed. *Orthopaedic Knowledge Update,* 7. Rosemont, IL: AAOS, 2002:82.
37. Landin LA. Epidemiology of children's fractures. *J Pediatr Orthop B* 1997;6:79–83.
38. Black GB, Amadeo R. Orthopedic injuries associated with backyard trampoline use in children. *J Pediatr Surg* 2004;39:653.
39. Waltzman ML, Shannon M, Bowen AP, Bailey MC. Monkeybar injuries: complications of play. *Pediatrics* 1999;103:e58.
40. Worlock P, Stower M. Fracture patterns in Nottingham children. *J Pediatr Orthop* 1986; 6:656–660.
41. Ostermann PAW, Richter D, Meccklenburg K, et al. Pediatric forearm fractures: indications, technique, and limits of conservative management. *J Orthop Trauma* 2000;14: 73.
42. Aktas S, Saridogan K, Moralar U, Ture M. Patterns of single segment non-physeal extremity fractures in children. *Int Orthop* 1999;23:345–347.
43. Crawford AH, Cionni AS. Management of pediatric orthopedic injuries by the emergency medicine specialist. In: *Pediatric critical illness and injury: assessment and care.* Rockville: Aspen System Publications, 1984:213–225.
44. Kasser JR. Forearm fractures. *AAOS Instructional Course Lect* 1992;41:391–396.
45. Hsu ES, Patwardhan AG, Meade KP, et al. J. Cross-sectional geometrical properties and bone mineral content of the human radius and ulna. *Biomechanics* 1993;26:1307–1318.

46. McGinley JC, Hopgood BC, Gaughan JP, et al SH. Forearm and elbow injury: the influence of rotational position. *J Bone Joint Surg [Am]* 2003;85:2403–2409.
47. Evans EM. Pronation injuries of the forearm with special reference to the anterior Monteggia fracture. *J Bone Joint Surg [Br]* 1949;31:578–588.
48. Do T. Forearm. In: Cramer KE, Scherl SA, eds. *Orthopaedic surgery essentials.* Philadelphia: Lippincott Williams & Wilkins, 2004:125–130.
49. Hoppenfeld S, Zeide MS. *Orthopaedic dictionary.* Philadelphia: JB Lippincott, 1994:275.
50. Crawford AH. Pitfalls and complications of fractures of the distal radius and ulna in childhood. *Hand Clin* 1988;4:403–413.
51. Evans EM. Fractures of the radius and ulna. *J Bone Joint Surg [Br]* 1951;33:548–561.
52. Rang M. *Children's fractures,* 2nd ed. Philadelphia: JB Lippincott, 1982:203.
53. Border S. Roentgen recognition of acute plastic bowing of the forearm in children. *Am J Roentgenol Radium Ther Nucl Med* 1975;125:524–530.
54. Carter DR, Spengler DM. Mechanical properties and composition of cortical bone. *Clin Orthop* 1978;135:192–217.
55. Chamay A. Mechanical and morphological aspects of experimental overload and fatigue in bone. *J Biomechanics* 1970;3:263–270.
56. Ogden JA. Uniqueness of growing bones. In: Rockwood CA, Wilkins KE, King RE, eds. *Fractures in children.* Philadelphia: JB Lippincott, 1991:10–14.
57. Curry JD, Butler G. The mechanical properties of bone tissue in children. *J Bone Joint Surg [Am]* 1975;57:810–814.
58. Borden S. Traumatic bowing of the forearm in children. *J Bone Joint Surg [Am]* 1974; 56:611–616.
59. Mabrey JD, Fitch RD. Plastic deformation in pediatric fractures: mechanism and treatment. *J Pediatr Orthop* 1989;9:310–314.
60. Casey PJ, Moed BR. Greenstick fractures of the radius in adults: a report of two cases. *J Orthop Trauma* 1996;10:209–212.
*61. Gupta RP, Danielsson LG. Dorsally angulated solitary metaphyseal greenstick fractures in the distal radius: results after immobilization in pronated, neutral, and supinated position. *J Pediatr Orthop* 1990;10:90–92.
*62. Soong C, Rocke LG. Clinical predictors of forearm fracture in children. *Arch Emerg Med* 1990;7:196–199.
*63. Kelly AM, Powell CV, Williams A. Parent visual analogue scale ratings of children's pain do not reliably reflect pain reported by child. *Pediatr Emerg Care* 2002;18:159–162.
*64. Singer AJ, Gulla J, Thode HC Jr. Parents and practitioners are poor judges of young children's pain severity. *Acad Emerg Med* 2002;9:609–612.
65. Cameron ML, Sponseller PD, Rossberg MI. Pediatric analgesia and sedation for the management of orthopedic conditions. *Am J Orthop* 2000;29:665–672.
66. Gartland JJ. *Fundamentals of orthopaedics,* 4th ed. Philadelphia: WB Saunders, 1987: 34.
67. Koo WW, Sherman R, Succop P, et al. Fractures and rickets in very low birth weight infants: conservative mangement and outcome. *J Pediatr Orthop* 1989;9:326–330.
68. Jacobsen ST, Hull CK, Crawford AH. Nutritional rickets. *J Pediatr Orthop* 1986;6: 713–716.
69. Daruwalla JS. A study of radioulnar movements following fractures of the forearm in children. *Clin Orthop* 1979;139:114–120.
70. Biyani A, Gupta SP, Sharma JC. Ipsilateral supracondylar fractures of the humerus and forearm bone in children. *Injury* 1989;20:203–207.
71. Williamson DM, Cole WG. Treatment of ipsilateral supracondylar and forearm fractures in children. *Injury* 1992;23:159–161.
72. Stanitski CL, Micheli LJ. Simultaneous ipsilateral fractures of the arm and forearm in children. *Clin Orthop* 1980;153:218–222.
73. Roposch A, Reis M, Molina M, et al. Supracondylar fractures of the humerus associated with ipsilateral fractures in children: a report of forty-seven cases. *J Pediatr Orthop* 2001;21:307–312.
74. Tabak AY, Celebi L, Murath HH, et al. Closed reduction and percutaneous fixation of supracondylar fracture of the humerus and ipsilateral fracture of the forearm in children. *J Bone Joint Surg [Br]* 2003;85:1169–1172.
75. Templeton PA, Graham HK. The floating elbow in children: simultaneous supracondylar fractures of the humerus and of the forearm in the same upper limb. *J Bone Joint Surg [Br]* 1995;77:791–796.
76. Ring D, Waters PM, Hotchkiss RN, Kasser JR. Pediatric floating elbow. *J Pediatr Orthop* 2001;21:456–459.
77. Harrington P, Sharif I, Fogarty EE, et al. Management of the floating elbow injury in children. *Arch Orthop Trauma Surg* 2000;120:205–208.
78. Blakemore LC, Cooperman DR, Thompson GH, et al. Compartment syndrome in ipsilateral humerus and forearm fractures in children. *Clin Orthop* 2000;376:32–38.
79. Yuan PS, Pring ME, Gaynor TP, et al. Compartment syndrome following intramedullary fixation of pediatric forearm fractures. *J Pediatr Orthop* 2004;24:370–375.
80. Cullen MC, Roy DR, Giza E, Crawford AH. Complications of intramedullary fixation of pediatric forearm fractures. *J Pediatr Orthop* 1998;18:14–21.
81. Mubarak SJ, Carroll NC. Volkmann's contracture in children: aetiology and prevention. *J Bone Joint Surg [Br]* 1979;61:285–293.
82. Luhmann SJ, Schootman M, Schoenecker PL, et al. Complications and outcomes of open pediatric forearm fractures. *J Pediatr Orthop* 2004;24:1–6.
83. Haasbeek JF, Cole WG. Open fractures of the arm in children. *J Bone Joint Surg [Br]* 1995;77:576–581.
84. Davidson AW. Rock, paper, scissors. *Injury* 2003;34:61–63.
85. Branovacki G, Hanson M, Cash R, Gonzalez M. The innervation of the radial nerve at the elbow and in the forearm. *J Hand Surg [Br]* 1998;23:167–169.
86. Anonymous. Fracture and Dislocation Compendium: Orthopaedic Trauma Association Committee for Coding and Classification. *J Ortho Trauma* 1996;10:1–153.
87. Richter D, Ostermann PAW, Ekkernkamp A, et al. Elastic intramedullary nailing: a minimally invasive concept in the treatment of unstable forearm fractures in children. *J Pediatr Orthop* 1998;18:457–461.
88. Van Herpe LB. Fractures of the forearm and wrist. *Orthop Clin North Am* 1976;7: 543–556.
89. Flynn JM. Pediatric forearm fractures: decision making, surgical techniques, and complications. *AAOS Instructional Course Lect* 2002;51:355–360.
90. Flynn JM, Sarwark JF, Waters PM, et al. The surgical management of pediatric fractures of the upper extremity. *AAOS Instructional Course Lect* 2003;52:635–645.
91. Lautman S, Bergerault F, Saidani N, Bonnard C. Roentgenographic measurement of angle between shaft and distal epiphyseal growth plate of radius. *J Pediatr Orthop* 2002; 22:751–753.
92. Tachakra S, Doherty S. The accuracy of length and angle measurement in videoconferencing teleradiology. *J Telemed Telecare* 2002;8 (suppl 2):85–87.
93. Carey PJ, Alburger PD, Betz RR, et al. Both-bone forearm fractures in children. *Orthopedics* 1992;15:1015–1019.
94. Carsi B, Abril JC, Epeldegui T. Longitudinal growth after nonphyseal forearm fractures. *J Pediatr Orthop* 2003;23:203–207.
95. Depablos J, Franzreb M, Barrios C. Longitudinal growth pattern of the radius after forearm fractures conservatively treated in children. *J Pediatr Orthop* 1994;14:492–495.
96. Roy DR. Completely displaced distal radius fractures with intact ulnas in children. *Orthopedics* 1989;12:1089–1092.
97. Mehlman CT, O'Brien MS, Crawford AH, et al. Irreducible fractures of the distal radius in children. Presented at Pediatric Orthopaedic Society of North America 2001 Annual Meeting, Cancun, May 1–5, 2001.
98. Do TT, Strub WM, Foad SL, et al. Reduction versus remodeling in pediatric distal forearm fractures: a preliminary cost analysis. *J Pediatr Orthop B* 2003;12:109–115.
99. Archibong AE, Onuba O. Fractures in children in South Eastern Nigeria. *Cent Afr J Med* 1996;42:340–343.
100. OlaOlorun DA, Oladiran IO, Adeniran A. Complications of fracture treatment by traditional bonesetters in Southwest Nigeria. *Fam Pract* 2001;18:635–637.
101. Matthews LS, Kaufer H, Garver DF, Sonstegard DA. The effect on supination-pronation of angular malalignment of fractures of both bones of the forearm: an experimental study. *J Bone Joint Surg [Am]* 1982;64:14–17.
102. Nilsson BE, Obrant K. The range of motion following fracture of the shaft of the forearm in children. *Acta Orthop Scand* 1977;48:600–602.
103. Wilson JC Jr, Krueger JC. Fractures of the proximal and middle thirds of the radius and ulna in children: study of the end results with analysis of treatment and complications. *Am J Surg* 1966;112:326–332.
104. Blackburn N, Ziv I, Rang M. Correction of the malunited forearm fracture. *Clin Orthop* 1984;188:54–57.
105. Blount WP. Osteoclasis for supination deformities in children. *J Bone Joint Surg* 1940; 22:300–314.
106. Högström H, Nilsson BE, Willner S. Correction with growth following diaphyseal forearm fracture. *Acta Orthop Scand* 1976;47:299–303.
107. Patrick J. A study of supination and pronation with especial reference to the treatment of forearm fractures. *J Bone Joint Surg* 1946;28:737–748.
108. Meier R, Prommersberger KJ, Lanz U. Surgical correction of malunited fractures of the forearm in children. *Z Orthop Ihre Grenzgeb* 2003;141:328–335.
109. Tarr RR, Garfinkel AI, Sarmiento A. The effects of angular and rotational deformities of both bones of the forearm: an in vitro study. *J Bone Joint Surg [Am]* 1984;66:65–70.
110. Sarmiento A, Ebramzadeh E, Brys D, Tarr R. Angular deformities and forearm function. *J Orthop Res* 1992;10:121–133.
111. Kasten P, Krefft M, Hesselbach J, Weinberg AM. How does torsional deformity of the radial shaft influence the rotation of the forearm? A biomechanical study. *J Orthop Trauma* 2003;17:57–60.
112. Dumont CE, Thalmann R, Macy JC. The effect of rotational malunion of the radius and ulna on supination and pronation. *J Bone Joint Surg [Br]* 2002;84:1070–1074.
113. Tynan MC, Fornalski S, McMahon PJ, et al. The effects of ulnar axial malalignment on supination and pronation. *J Bone Joint Surg [Am]* 2000;82:1726–1731.
114. McHenry TP, Pierce WA, Lais RL, Schacherer TG. Effect of displacement of ulna-shaft fractures on forearm rotation: a cadaveric model. *Am J Orthop* 2002;31:420–424.
115. Kay S, Smith C, Oppenheim WL. Both-bone midshaft forearm fractures in children. *J Pediatr Orthop* 1986;6:306–310.
116. Campbell WC. *Orthopedics of childhood.* New York: Appleton and Company, 1930: 154–156.
117. Floyd AS. Is the measurement of angles on radiographs accurate? Brief report. *J Bone Joint Surg [Br]* 1988;70:486–487.
118. Bär HF, Breitfus H. Analysis of angular deformities on radiographs. *J Bone Joint Surg [Br]* 1989;71:710–711.
119. Schock CC. "The crooked straight": distal radial remodeling. *J Ark Med Soc* 1987;84: 97–100.
120. Larsen E, Vittas D, Torp-Pederson S. Remodeling of angulated distal forearm fractures in children. *Clin Orthop Res* 1988;237:190–195.
121. Gray H. *Gray's anatomy: the classic collector's edition.* New York: Bounty, 1977:152–157.
122. Sage FP. Medullary fixation of fractures of the forearm: a study of the medullary canal of the radius and a report of fifty fractures of the radius treated with a prebent triangular nail. *J Bone Joint Surg [Am]* 1959;41:1489–1516.
123. Firl M, Wünsch L. Measurement of bowing of the radius. *J Bone Joint Surg [Br]* 2004; 86:1047–1049.
124. Pugh DMW, Galpin RD, Carey TP. Intramedullary Steinmann pin fixation of forearm fractures in children: long-term results. *Clin Orthop* 2000;376:39–48.
125. Schemitsch EH, Richards RR. The effect of malunion on functional outcome after plate fixation of fractures of both bones of the forearm in adults. *J Bone Joint Surg Am* 1992; 74:1068–1078.
126. Schemitsch EH, Jones D, Henley MB, et al. A comparison of malreducation after plate and intramedullary nail fixation of forearm fractures. *J Orthop Trauma* 1995;9:8–16.

127. Milch H. Roentenographic diagnosis of torsional deformities in tubular bones. *Surgery* 1944;15:440–450.
128. Trinkaus E, Churchill SE. Neanderthal radial tuberosity orientation. *Am J Phys Anthropol* 1988;75:15–21.
129. Giebel GD, Meyer C, Koebke J, Giebel G. Arterial supply of forearm bones and its importance for the operative treatment of fractures. *Surg Radiol Anat* 1997;19:149–153.
130. Evans EM. Rotational deformity in the treatment of fractures of both bones of the forearm. *J Bone Joint Surg* 1945;27:373–379.
131. Paul AS, Kay PR, Haines JF. Distal ulnar growth plate arrest following a diaphyseal fracture. *J R Coll Surg Edinb* 1992;37:347–348.
132. Pritchett JW. Does pinning cause distal radial growth plate arrest? *Orthopaedics* 1994; 17:550–551.
133. Yung SH, Lam CY, Choi KY, et al. Percutaneous intramedullary Kirschner wiring for displaced diaphyseal forearm fractures in children. *J Bone Joint Surg* 1998;80:91–94.
134. Yung PSH, Lam CY, Ng BKW, et al. Percutaneous transphyseal intramedullary Kirschner wire pinning: a safe and effective procedure for treatment of displaced forearm fracture in children. *J Pediatr Orthop* 2004;24:7–12.
135. Ogden JA, Beall JK, Conlogue GL, Light TR. Radiology of postnatal skeletal development, IV: distal radius and ulna. *Skel Radiol* 1981;6:255–266.
136. Bley L, Seitz WH. Injuries about the distal ulna in children. *Hand Clin* 1998;14: 231–237.
137. Silberstein MJ, Brodeur AE, Graviss ER. Some vagaries of the radial head and neck. *J Bone Joint Surg [Am]* 1982;64:1153–1157.
138. Silberstein MJ, Brodeur AE, Graviss ER, Luisiri A. Some vagaries of the olecranon. *J Bone Joint Surg [Am]* 1981;63:722–725.
139. Ogden JA. *Skeletal injury in the child*. Philadelphia: Lea & Febiger, 1982:56–57.
140. Hollister AM, Gellman H, Waters RL. The relationship of the interosseous membrane to the axis of rotation of the forearm. *Clin Orthop* 1994;298:272–276.
141. Hotchkiss RN, An KN, Sowa DT, et al. An anatomic and mechanical study of the interosseous membrane of the forearm: pathomechanics of proximal migration of the radius. *J Hand Surg [Am]* 1989;14:256–261.
142. Pfaeffle HJ, Kischer KJ, Manson TT, et al. Role of the forearm interosseous ligament: is it more than just longitudinal load transfer? *J Hand Surg [Am]* 2000;25:680–688.
143. Pfaeffle HJ, Tomaino MM, Grewal R, et al. Tensile properties of the interosseous membrane of the human forearm. *J Orthop Res* 1996;14:842–845.
144. Gabriel MT, Pfaeffle HJ, Stabile KJ, et al. Passive strain distribution in the interosseous ligament of the forearm: implications for injury reconstruction. *J Hand Surg [Am]* 2004; 29:293–298.
145. Skahen JR 3rd, Palmer AK, Werner FW, Fortino MD. Reconstruction of the interosseous membrane of the forearm in cadavers. *J Hand Surg [Am]* 1997;22:986–994.
146. DeFrate LE, Li G, Zayontz SJ, Herndon JH. A minimally invasive method for the determination of force in the interosseous ligament. *Clin Biomech* 2001;16:895–900.
147. Manson TT, Pfaeffle HJ, Herdon JH, et al. Forearm rotation alters interosseous ligament strain distribution. *J Hand Surg [Am]* 2000;25:1058–1063.
148. Markolf KL, Lamey D, Yang S, et al. Radioulnar load-sharing in the forearm: a study in cadavers. *J Bone Joint Surg [Am]* 1998;80:879–888.
149. Nakamura T, Yabe Y, Horiuchi Y. In vivo MR studies of dynamic changes in the interosseous membrane of the forearm during rotation. *J Hand Surg [Br]* 1999;24:245–248.
150. McGinley JC, Kozin SH. Interosseous membrane anatomy and functional mechanics. *Clin Orthop* 2001;383:108–122.
151. Yasutomi T, Nakatsuchi Y, Koike H, Uchiyama S. Mechanism of limitation of pronation/ supination of the forearm in geometric models of deformities of the forearm bones. *Clin Biomech* 2002;17:456–463.
152. Doyle JR, Botte MJ. *Surgical anatomy of the hand & upper extremity*. Philadelphia: Lippincott Williams & Wilkins, 2003:34–40.
153. Revol MP, Lantieri L, Loy S, Guerin-Surville H. Vascular anatomy of the forearm muscles: a study of 50 dissections. *Plast Reconstr Surg* 1991;88:1026–1033.
154. Abrams RA, Ziets RJ, Lieber RL, Botte MJ. Anatomy of the radial nerve motor branches in the forearm. *J Hand Surg [Am]* 1997;22:232–237.
155. Gonzalez MH, Lotfi P, Bendre A, et al. The ulnar nerve at the elbow and its local branching: an anatomic study. *J Hand Surg [Br]* 2001;26:142–144.
156. Chantelot C, Feugas C, Guillem P, et al. Innervation of the medial epicondylar muscles: an anatomic study in 50 cases. *Surg Radiol Anat* 1999;21:165–168.
157. Crenshaw AH Jr. Surgical approaches. In: Canale ST, ed. *Campbell's operative orthopaedics*,10th ed. St. Louis: CV Mosby, 2003:107–109.
158. Müller ME, Allgower M, Schneider R, Willenegger H. *Manual of internal fixation: techniques recommended by the AO-ASIF Group,* 3rd ed. Berlin: Springer-Verlag, 1991: 454–467.
159. Henry AK. *Extensile exposure*, 2nd ed. Edinburgh: Churchill Livingstone, 1966: 107–108.
160. Bass RL, Stern PJ. Elbow and forearm anatomy and surgical approaches. *Hand Clin* 1994;10:343–356.
161. Hoppenfeld S. *Surgical exposures in orthopaedics,* 3rd ed. Philadelphia: Lippincott Williams & Wilkins, 2003.
162. Allen PE, Vickery CW, Atkins RM. A modified approach to the flexor surface of the distal radius. *J Hand Surg [Br]* 1996;21:303–304.
163. Elgafy H, Ebraheim NA, Yeasting RA. Extensile posterior approach to the radius. *Clin Orthop* 2000;373:252–258.
164. Shenoy RM. Biplanar exposure of the radius and ulna through a single incision. *J Bone Joint Surg [Br]* 1995;77:568–570.
165. VanderReis WL, Otsuka NY, Moroz P, Mah J. Intramedullary nailing versus plate fixation for unstable forearm fractures in children. *J Pediatr Orthop* 1998;18:9–13.
166. Kucukkaya M, Kabukcuoglu Y, Tezer M, et al. The application of open intramedullary fixation in the treatment of pediatric radial and ulnar shaft fractures. *J Orthop Trauma* 2002;16:340–344.
167. Wyrsch B, Mencio GA, Green NE. Open reduction and internal fixation of pediatric forearm fractures. *J Pediatr Orthop* 1996;16:644–650.
168. Strauch RJ, Rosenwasser MP, Glazer PA. Surgical exposure of the dorsal proximal third of the radius: how vulnerable is the posterior interosseous nerve? *J Shoulder Elbow Surg* 1996;5:342–346.
169. Dilberti T, Botte MJ, Abrams RA. Anatomical considerations regarding the posterior interosseous nerve during posterolateral approaches to the proximal part of the radius. *J Bone Joint Surg [Am]* 2000;82:809–813.
170. Mekhail AO, Ebraheim NA, Jackson WT, Yeasting RA. Vulnerability of the posterior interosseous nerve during proximal radius exposures. *Clin Orthop* 1995;315:199–208.
171. Roy DR, Crawford AH. Operative management of fractures of the shaft of the radius and ulna. *Orthop Clin North Am* 1990;21:245–250.
172. Abrams RA, Brown RA, Botte MJ. The superficial branch of the radial nerve: an anatomic study with surgical implications. *J Hand Surg [Am]* 1992;17:1037–1041.
173. Auerbach DM, Collins ED, Kunkle KL, Monsanto EH. The radial sensory nerve: an anatomic study. *Clin Orthop* 1994;308:241–249.
174. Lee S, Nicol RO, Stott NS. Intramedullary fixation for pediatric unstable forearm fractures. *Clin Orthop* 2002;402:245–250.
175. Luhmann SJ, Gordon JE, Schoenecker PL. Intramedullary fixation of unstable both-bone forearm fractures in children. *J Pediatr Orthop* 1998;18:451–456.
176. Shoemaker SD, Comstock CP, Mubarak SJ, et al. Intramedullary Kirschner wire fixation of open or unstable forearm fractures in children. *J Pediatr Orthop* 1999;19:329–337.
177. Verstreken L, Delronge G, Lamoureux J. Shaft forearm fractures in children: intramedullary nailing with immediate motion: a preliminary report. *J Pediatr Orthop* 1988;8: 450–453.
178. Calder PR, Achan P, Barry M. Diaphyseal forearm fractures in children treated with intramedullary fixation: outcome of K-wires versus elastic stable intramedullary nail. *Injury* 2003;34:278–282.
179. Ligier JN, Metaizeau JP, Prevot J, Lascombes P. Elastic stable intramedullary pinning of long bone shaft fractures in children. *Z Kinderchir* 1985;40:209–212.
180. Lascombes P, Prevot J, Ligier JN, et al. Elastic stable intramedullary nailing in forearm shaft fractures in children. *J Pediatr Orthop* 1990;10:167–171.
181. Amit Y, Salai M, Chechik A, et al. Closing intramedullary nailing for the treatment of diaphyseal forearm fractures in adolescence: a preliminary report. *J Pediatr Orthop* 1985;5:143–146.
182. Younger ASE, Tredwell SJ, Mackenzie WG. Factors affecting fracture position at cast removal after pediatric forearm fracture. *J Pediatr Orthop* 1997;17:332–336.
183. Thorndike AaDC. Fractures of the forearm and elbow in children. *N Engl J Med* 1941; 225:475–480.
184. Chess DG, Hyndman JC, Leahey JL, et al. Short arm plaster cast for distal pediatric forearm fractures. *J Pediatr Orthop* 1994;14:211–213.
*185. Galpin RD, Webb GR, Armstrong DG, Schlatterer D. A comparison of short and long-arm plaster casts for displaced distal-third pediatric forearm fractures: a prospective randomized trial. Presented at Pediatric Orthopaedic Society of North America 2004 Annual Meeting, St Louis, MO, April 27–May 1, 2004.
186. Schranz PJ, Fagg PS. Undisplaced fractures of the distal third of the radius in children: an innocent fracture? *Injury* 1992;23:165–167.
187. Gandhi RK, Wilson P, Mason-Brown JJ, Macleod W. Spontaneous correction of deformity following fractures of the forearm in children. *Br J Surg* 1962;50:5–10.
188. Davids JR, Frick SL, Skewes E, Blackhurst DW. Skin surface pressure beneath an above-the-knee cast: plaster casts compared with fiberglass casts. *J Bone Joint Surg [Am]* 1997; 79:565–569.
189. Bartl V, Gal P, Skotakova J, Kmostak P. Treatment of redislocated fragments of long bones using plaster cast wedging. *Rozhl Chir* 2002;81:415–420.
190. Duncan J, Weiner D. Unstable pediatric forearm fractures: use of "pins and plaster." *Orthopedics* 2004;27:267–269.
191. Keenan WNW, Clegg J. Intraoperative wedging of casts: correction of residual angulation after manipulation. *J Pediatr Orthop* 1995;15:826–829.
192. Vanderbeek BL, Mehlman CT, Foad SL, et al. The use of conscious sedation for forearm fracture reduction in children: does race matter? Presented at American Academy of Pediatrics 2003 Annual Meeting, New Orleans, Oct. 31–Nov. 5, 2003.
*193. Johnson PQ, Noffsinger MA. Hematoma block of distal forearm fractures: is it safe? *Orthop Rev* 1991;20:977–979.
194. Furia JP, Alioto RJ, Marquardt JD. The efficacy and safety of the hematoma block for fracture reduction in closed isolated fractures. *Orthopaedics* 1997;20:423–426.
*195. Hennrikus WL, Shin AY, Klingelberger CE. Self-administered nitrous oxide and a hematoma block for analgesia in the outpatient reduction of fractures in children. *J Bone Joint Surg [Am]* 1995;77:335–339.
196. Juliano PJ, Mazur JM, Cummings RJ, McCluskey WP. Low-dose lidocaine intravenous regional anesthesia for forearm fractures in children. *J Pediatr Orthop* 1992;12:633–635.
*197. Bratt HD, Eyres RL, Cole WG. Randomized double-blind trial of low and moderate dose lidocaine regional anesthesia for forearm fractures in dhildhood. *J Pediatr Orthop* 1996;16:660–663.
*198. Davidson AJ, Eyres RL, Cole WG. A comparison of prilocaine and lidocaine for intravenous regional anaesthesia for forearm fracture reduction in children. *Paediatr Anaesth* 2002;12:146–150.
*199. Evans JK, Buckley SL, Alexander AH, Gilpin AT. Analgesia for the reduction of fractures in children: a comparison of nitrous oxide with intramuscular sedation. *J Pediatr Orthop* 1995;15:73–77.
*200. Gregory PR, Sullivan JA. Nitrous oxide compared with intravenous regional anesthesia in pediatric forearm fracture manipulation. *J Pediatr Orthop* 1996;16:187–191.
*201. Kennedy RM, Porter FL, Miller JP, Jaffe DM. Comparison of fentanyl/midazolam with

ketamine/midazolam for pediatric orthopedic emergencies. *Pediatrics* 1998;102: 956–963.

*202. Hoffman GM, Nowakowski R, Troshynski TJ, et al. Risk reduction in pediatric procedural sedation by application of an American Academy of Pediatrics/American Society of Anesthesiologists process model. *Pediatrics* 2002;109:236–243.

203. American Academy of Pediatrics Committee on Drugs. Guidelines for monitoring of pediatric patients during and after sedation for diagnostic and therapeutic procedures: addendum. *Pediatrics* 2002;110:836–838.

204. American Academy of Pediatrics Committee on Drugs. Guidelines for monitoring and management of pediatric patients during and after sedation for diagnostic and therapeutic procedures. *Pediatrics* 1992;89:1110–1115.

*205. Godambe SA, Elliot V, Matheny D, Pershad J. Comparison of propofol/fentanyl versus ketamine/midazolam for brief procedural sedation in a pediatric emergency department. *Pediatrics* 2003;112:116–123.

206. Simonian PT, Hanel DP. Traumatic plastic deformity of an adult forearm: case report and literature review. *J Orthop Trauma* 1996;10:213–215.

207. Kienitz R, Mandell R. Traumatic bowing of the forearm in children: report of a case. *J Am Osteopath Assoc* 1985;85:565–568.

208. Sanders WE, Heckman JD. Traumatic plastic deformation of the radius and ulna: a closed method of correction of deformity. *Clin Orthop* 1984;188:58–67.

209. Vorlat P, DeBoeck H. Bowing fractures of the forearm in children: a long-term followup. *Clin Orthop* 2003;413:233–237.

210. Rydholm U, Nilsson JE. Traumatic bowing of the forearm: a case report. *Clin Orthop* 1979;139:121–124.

211. Griffin PP, Green DP. Forearm fractures in children [letter]. *Clin Orthop* 1977;129: 320–321.

212. Alpar EK, Thompson K, Owen R, Taylor JF. Midshaft fractures of forearm bones in children. *Injury* 1981;13:153–158.

213. Boyer BA, Overton B, Schraeder W, et al. Position of immobilization for pediatric forearm fractures. *J Pediatr Orthop* 2002;22:185–187.

214. Kramhoft M, Solgaard S. Displaced diaphyseal forearm fractures in children: classification and evaluation of the early radiographic prognosis. *J Pediatr Orthop* 1989;9: 586–589.

215. Voto SJ, Weiner DS, Leighley B. Redisplacement after closed reduction of forearm fractures in children. *J Pediatr Orthop* 1990;10:79–84.

216. Kelly JP, Zionts LE. Economic considerations in the treatment of distal forearm fractures in children. Presented at American Academy of Orthopaedic Surgeons 68th Annual Meeting, San Francisco, Feb. 28–March 4, 2001.

217. Arunachalam VSP, Griffiths JC. Fracture recurrence in children. *Injury* 1975;7:37–40.

218. Crawford AH. Orthopedics. In: Rudolph CD, Rudolph AM, Hostetter MK, et al, eds. *Rudolph's pediatrics*, 21st ed. New York: McGraw Hill, 2002:2451.

219. Watson-Jones R. *Fractures and other bone and joint injuries*, 1st ed. Edinburgh: Livingstone, 1940:379–380.

220. Walker JL, Rang M. Forearm fractures in children: cast treatment with the elbow extended. *J Bone Joint Surg [Br]* 1991;73:299–301.

221. Shaer JA, Smith B, Turco VJ. Mid-third forearm fractures in children: an unorthodox treatment. *Am J Orthop* 1999;28:60–63.

222. Murray WM, Delp SL, Buchanan TS. Variation of muscle moment arms with elbow and forearm position. *J Biomechanics* 1995;28:513–525.

223. Bellemans M, Lamoureux J. Indications for immediate percutaneous intramedullary nailing of complete diaphyseal forearm shaft fractures in children. *Acta Orthop Belg* 1995;61(suppl I):169–172.

224. Martin J, Marsh JL, Nepola JV, et al. Radiographic fracture assessments: which ones can we reliably make? *J Orthop Trauma* 2000;14:379–385.

225. Voto SJ, Weiner DS, Leighley B. Use of pins pnd Plaster in the treatment of unstable pediatric forearm fractures. *J Pediatr Orthop* 1990;10:85–89.

226. Wilkins KE. Operative management of children's fractures: is it a sign of impetuousness or do the children really benefit? *J Pediatr Orthop* 1998;18:1–3.

227. Schranz PJ, Gultekin C, Colton CL. External fixation of fractures in children. *Injury* 1982;23:80–82.

228. Smith H, Sage FP. Medullary fixation of forearm fractures. *J Bone Joint Surg [Am]* 1957; 39:91–98.

229. Soeur R. Intramedullary pinning of diaphyseal fractures. *J Bone Joint Surg* 1946;28: 309–331.

230. Ogonda L, Wong-Chung J, Wray R, Canavan B. Delayed union and nonunion of the ulna following intramedullary nailing in children. *J Pediatr Orthop B* 2004;13:330–333.

231. Parikh SN, Brody AS, Crawford AH. Use of a Picture Archiving and Communication System (PACS) and computed plain radiography in preoperative planning. *Am J Orthop* 2004;33:62–64.

232. Spiegel PG, Mast JM. Internal and external fixation of fractures in children. *Orthop Clin North Am* 1980;11:405–421.

233. Thompson GH, Wilbur JH, Marcus RE. Internal fixation of fractures in children and adolescents: a comparative analysis. *Clin Orthop* 1984;188:10–20.

234. Ortega R, Loder RT, Louis DS. Open reduction and internal fixation of forearm fractures in children. *J Pediatr Orthop* 1996;16:651–654.

235. Chapman MW, Gordon E, Zissimos AG. Compression-plate fixation of acute fractures of the diaphysis of the radius and ulna. *J Bone Joint Surg [Am]* 1989;71:159–169.

236. Deluca PA, Lindsey RW, Ruwe PA. Refracture of bones of the forearm after the removal of compression plates. *J Bone Joint Surg [Am]* 1988;70:1372–1376.

237. Nielson AB, Simonsen O. Displaced forearm fractures in children treated with AO plates. *Injury* 1984;15:393–396.

238. Vainionpaa S, Bostman O, Patiala H, Rokkanen P. Internal fixation of forearm fractures in children. *Acta Orthop Scand* 1987;58:121–123.

239. Schöne G. The classic: the treatment of forearm fractures with pins. *Clin Orthop* 1988; 234:2–4.

240. Hahn MP, Richter D, Muhr G, Ostermann PA. Pediatric forearm fractures: diagnosis, therapy and possible complications. *Unfallchirurg* 1997;100:760–769.

241. Lewallen RP, Peterson HA. Nonunion of long bone fractures in children: a review of 30 cases. *J Pediatr Orthop* 1985;5:135–142.

242. Flynn JM, Waters PM. Single-bone fixation of both-bone forearm fractures. *J Pediatr Orthop* 1996;16:655–659.

243. Bhaskar AR, Roberts JA. Treatment of unstable fractures of the forearm in children: is plating of a single bone adequate? *J Bone Joint Surg [Br]* 2001;83:253–258.

244. Qidwai SA. Treatment of diaphyseal forearm fractures in children by intramedullary Kirschner wires. *J Trauma* 2001;50:303–307.

245. Fleischer H. Marrow wiring in lower-arm fractures of children. *Dtsch Med Wochenschr* 1975;100:1278–1279.

246. Blaiser RD, Salamon PB. Closed intramedullary rodding of pediatric adolescent forearm fractures. *Oper Tech Orthop* 1993;3:128–133.

247. Waseem M, Paton RW. Percutaneous intramedullary elastic wiring of displaced diaphyseal forearm fractures in children. A modified technique. *Injury* 1999;30:21–24.

248. Ono M, Bechtold JE, Merkow RL, et al. Rotational stability of diaphyseal fractures of the radius and ulna fixed with Rush pins and/or fracture bracing. *Clin Orthop* 1989; 240:236–243.

249. Metaizeau JP, Ligier JN. Surgical treatment of fractures of the long bones in children: interference between osteosynthesis and the physiological processes of consolidations: therapeutic indications. *J Chir (Paris)* 1984;121:527–537.

250. Prevot J, Guichet JM. Elastic stable intramedullary nailing for forearm fractures in children and adolescents. *J Bone Joint Surg* 1996;20:305.

251. Griffet J, El Hayek T, Baby M. Intramedullary nailing of forearm fractures in children. *J Pediatr Orthop B* 1999;8:88–89.

252. Wurfel AM, Voigt A, Linke F, Hofmann von Kap-Herr S. New aspects in the treatment of complete and isolated diaphyseal fractures of the forearm in children. *Unfallchirurgie* 1995;21:70–76.

253. Toussaint D, Vanderlinden C, Bremen J. Stable elastic nailing applied to diaphyseal fractures of the forearm in children. *Acta Orthop Belg* 1991;57:147–153.

254. Shah MH, Heffernan G, McGuinness AJ. Early experiences with titanium elastic nails in a trauma unit. *Ir Med J* 2003;96:213–214.

255. Till H, Huttl B, Knorr P, Dietz HG. Elastic stable intramedullary nailing (ESIN) provides good long-term results in pediatric long-bone fractures. *Eur J Pediatr Surg* 2000;10: 319–322.

256. Myers GJC, Gibbons PJ, Glithero PR. Nancy nailing of diaphyseal forearm fractures: single bone fixation for fractures of both bones. *J Bone Joint Surg [Br]* 2004;86:581–584.

257. Schlickewei W, Salm R. Indications for intramedullary stabilization of shaft fractures in childhood: what is reliable and what is an assumption? *Kongressbd Dtsch Ges Kongr* 2001;118:431–434.

258. Fee NF, Dobranski A, Bisla RS. Gas gangrene complicating open forearm fractures: report of five cases. *J Bone Joint Surg [Am]* 1977;59:135–138.

259. Skaggs DL, Kautz KM, Kay RM, Tolo VT. Effect of delay of surgical treatment on rate of infection in open fractures in children. *J Pediatr Orthop* 2000;20:19–22.

260. Mehlman CT, Crawford AH, Roy DR, et al. Undisplaced fractures of the distal radius and ulna in children: risk factors for displacement. Presented at American Academy of Orthopaedic Surgeons 2002 Annual Meeting, Dallas, Feb. 13–17, 2001.

261. Younger ASE, Tredwell SJ, Mackenzie WG, et al. Accurate prediction of outcome after pediatric forearm fracture. *J Pediatr Orthop* 1994;14:200–206.

262. Chan CF, Meads BM, Nicol RO. Remanipulation of forearm fractures in children. *N Z Med J* 1997;110:249–250.

263. Kasten P, Krefft M, Hesselbach J, Weinberg AM. Computer simulation of forearm rotation in angular deformities: a new therapeutic approach. *Injury* 2002;33:807–813.

264. Morrey BF, Askew LJ, Chao EY. A biomechanical study of normal functional elbow motion. *J Bone Joint Surg [Am]* 1981;63:872–877.

265. Bhaskar AR, Roberts JA. Treatment of unstable fractures of the forearm in children. Is plating of a single bone adequate? *J Bone Joint Surg Br* 2001;83:253–258.

266. Fiala M, Carey TP. Paediatric forearm fractures: an analysis of refracture rate. *Orthop Trans* 1994–1995;18:1265–1266.

267. Litton LO, Adler F. Refracture of the forearm in children: a frequent complication. *J Trauma* 1963;3:41–51.

268. Bould M, Bannister GC. Refractures of the radius and ulna in children. *Injury* 1999; 30:583–586.

269. Schwarz N, Pienaar S, Schwarz AF, et al. Refracture of the forearm in children. *J Bone Joint Surg [Br]* 1996;78:740–744.

270. White AA, Panjabi MM, Southwick WO. The four biomechanical stages of fracture repair. *J Bone Joint Surg [Am]* 1977;59:188–192.

271. Prevot J, Lascombes P, Guichet JM. Elastic stable intramedullary nailing for forearm fractures in children and adolescents. *Orthop Trans* 1996;20:305.

272. Muensterer OJ, Regauer MP. Closed reduction of forearm refractures with flexible intramedullary nails in situ. *J Bone Joint Surg [Am]* 2003;85:2152–2155.

273. Kettunen J, Kroger H, Bowditch M, et al O. Bone mineral density after removal of rigid plates from forearm fractures: preliminary report. *J Orthop Sci* 2003;8:772–776.

274. Fike EA, Bartal E. Delayed union of the distal ulna in a child after both-bone forearm fracture. *J South Orthop Assoc* 1998;7:113–116.

275. Song KS, Kim HKW. Nonunion as a complication of an open reduction of a distal radial fracture in a healthy child: a case report. *J Orthop Trauma* 2003;17:231–233.

276. Crawford AH, Schorry EK. Neurofibromatosis in children: the role of the orthopaedist. *J Am Acad Orthop Surg* 1999;7:217–230.

277. Crawford AH, Bagamery N. Osseous manifestations of neurofibromatosis in childhood. *J Pediatr Orthop* 1986;6:672–688.

278. Jacobsen FS, Crawford AH. Complications in neurofibromatosis. In: Epps CH, Bowen JR, eds. *Complications in pediatric orthopaedic surgery*. Philadelphia: JB Lippincott, 1995: 678–680.
279. Manske PR. Forearm pseudarthrosis-neurofibromatosis: a case report. *Clin Orthop* 1979;139:125–127.
280. Weber BG, Cech O. *Pseudarthrosis*. Bern, Switzerland: Hans Huber, 1976.
281. Lavelle DG. Delayed union and nonunion of fractures. In: Canale ST, ed. *Campbell's operative orthopaedics,* 10th ed. St Louis: Mosby, 2003:3125–3127.
282. Vince KG, Miller JE. Cross-union complication fracture of the forearm: part II, children. *J Bone Joint Surg [Am]* 1987;69:654–660.
283. Bauer G, Arand M, Mutschler W. Posttraumatic synostosis after forearm fracture osteosynthesis. *Arch Orthop Trauma Surg* 1991;110:142–145.
284. Stern PJ, Drury WJ. Complications of plate fixation of forearm fractures. *Clin Orthop* 1983;175:25–29.
285. Roy DR. Radioulnar synostosis following proximal radial fracture in child. *Orthop Rev* 1986;15:89–94.
286. Ogun TC, Sarlak A, Arazi M, Kapicioglu MIS. Posttraumatic distal radioulnar synostosis and distal radial epiphyseal arrest. *Ulusal Travma Dergisi* 2002;8:59–61.
287. Maempel FZ. Post-traumatic radioulnar synostosis. A report of two cases. *Clin Orthop Relat Res* 1984;186:182–185.
288. Aner A, Singer M, Feldbrin Z, et al. Surgical treatment of posttraumatic radioulnar synostosis in children. *J Pediatr Orthop* 2002;22:598–600.
289. Cleary JE, Omer GE. Congenital proximal radioulnar synostosis: natural history and functional assessment. *J Bone Joint Surg [Am]* 1985;76:539–545.
290. Vu L, Mehlman CT. Tarsal coalition. eMedicine Orthopaedics. Available at: http://www.emedicine.com/orthoped/topic326.htm. Accessed September 1, 2005.
291. Batz W, Hoffman V, Kap-Herr S, Pistor G. Posttraumatic radioulnar synostoses in childhood. *Aktuelle Tramatol* 1986;16:13–16.
292. Stanley EA. Treatment of midshaft fractures of the radius and ulna utilizing percutaneous intramedullar pinning. *Ortho Trans* 1996;20:305.
293. Mann D, Schnabel M, Baacke M, Gotzen L. Results of elastic stable intramedullary nailing (ESIN) in forearm fractures in childhood. *Unfallchirurg* 2003;106:102–109.
294. Lascombes P, Prevot J, Ligier JN, et al. Elastic stable intramedullary nailing in forearm shaft fractures in children: 85 case. *J Pediatr Ortho* 1990;10:167–171.
295. Gustilo RB, Anderson JT. Prevention of infection in the treatment of one thousand and twenty-five open fractures of long bones: retrospective and prospective analyses. *J Bone Joint Surg [Am]* 1976;58:453–458.
296. Nieman R, Maiocco B, Deeney VF. Ulnar nerve injury after closed forearm fractures in children. *J Pediatr Orthop* 1998;18:683–685.
297. Stahl S, Rozen N, Michaelson M. Ulnar nerve injury following midshaft forearm fractures in children. *J Hand Surg [Br]* 1997;22:788–789.
298. Gainor BJ, Olson S. Combined entrapment of the median and anterior interosseous nerves in a pediatric both-bone forearm fracture. *J Orthop Trauma* 1990;4:197–199.
299. Al-Qattan MM, Clarke HM, Zimmer P. Radiological signs of entrapment of the median nerve in forearm shaft fractures. *J Hand Surg [Br]* 1994;19:713–719.
300. Proubasta IR, De Sena L, Caceres EP. Entrapment of the median nerve in a greenstick forearm fracture: a case report and review of the literature. *Bull Hosp Jt Dis* 1999;58: 220–223.
301. Prosser AJ, Hooper G. Entrapment of the ulnar nerve in a greenstick fracture of the ulna. *J Hand Surg [Br]* 1986;11:211–212.
302. Huang K, Pun WK, Coleman S. Entrapment and transection of the median nerve associated with greenstick fractures of the forearm: a case report and review of the literature. *J Trauma* 1998;44:1101–1102.
303. Genelin F, Karlbauer AF, Gasperschitz F. Greenstick fracture of the forearm with median nerve entrapment. *J Emerg Med* 1988;6:381–385.
304. Geissler WB, Fernandez DL, Graca R. Anterior interosseous nerve palsy complicating a forearm fracture in a child. *J Hand Surg [Am]* 1990;15:44–47.
305. Holmes JR, Louis DS. Entrapment of pronator quadratus in pediatric distal radius fractures: recognition and treatment. *J Pediatr Orthop* 1994;14:498–500.
306. Rayan GM, Hayes M. Entrapment of the flexor digitorum profundus in the ulna with fracture of both bones of the forearm: report of a case. *J Bone Joint Surg [Am]* 1986; 68:1102–1103.
307. Kolkman KA, Von Niekerk JL, Rieu PN, Festen C. A complicated forearm greenstick fracture: case report. *J Trauma* 1992;32:116–117.
308. Shaw BA, Murphy KM. Flexor tendon entrapment in ulnar shaft fractures. *Clin Orthop* 1996;330:181–184.
309. Hendel D, Aner A. Entrapment of the flexor digitorum profundus of the ring finger at the site of an ulnar fracture: a case report. *Ital J Orthop Traumatol* 1992;18:417–419.
310. Watson PA, Blair W. Entrapment of the index flexor digitorum profundus tendon after fracture of both forearm bones in a child. *Iowa Orthop J* 1999;19:127–128.
311. Ponet M, Jawish R. [Stable flexible nailing of fractures of both bones of the forearm in children]. *Chir Pediatr* 1989;30:117–120.
312. Rang M, Armstrong P, Crawford AH, et al. Symposium: management of fractures in children and adolescents, parts I & II. *Contemp Orthop* 1991;23:517–548, 621–644.
313. Crawford AH. Orthopedic injury in children. In: Callaham ML, ed. *Current practice of emergency medicine,* 2nd ed. Philadelphia: BC Decker, 1991:1232–1233.
314. Stanton RP, Malcolm JR, Wesdock KA, Singsen BH. Reflex sympathetic dystrophy in children: an orthopaedic perspective. *Orthopaedics* 1993;16:773–780.
315. Wilder RT, Berde CB, Wolohan M, et al. Reflex sympathetic dystrophy in children. *J Bone Joint Surg [Am]* 1992;74:910–919.
316. Lee BH, Scharff L, Sethna NF, et al. Physical therapy and cognitive-behavioral treatment for complex regional pain syndromes. *J Pediatr* 2002;141:135–140.
317. Kemper KJ, Sarah R, Silver-Highfield E, et al. On pins and needles? Pediatric pain patients' experience with acupuncture. *Pediatrics* 2000;105:941–947.
318. Khosla S, Melton LJ, Dekutoski MB, et al. Incidence of childhood distal forearm fractures over 30 years: a population-based study. *JAMA* 2003;290:1479–1485.
319. Brown RL, Koepplinger ME, Mehlman CT, et al. All-terrain vehicle and bicycle crashes in children: epidemiology and comparison of injury severity. *J Pediatr Surg* 2002;37: 375–380.
320. Ma D, Morley R, Jones G. Risk-taking coordination and upper limb fractures in children: population-based case-control study. *Osteoporos Int* 2004;15:633–638.
321. Powell EC, Tanz RR. In-line skate and rollerskate injuries in childhood. *Pediatr Emerg Care* 1996;12:259–262.
322. Mitts KG, Hennrikus WL. In-line skating fractures in children. *J Pediatr Orthop* 1996; 16:640–643.
323. Staebler MP, Moore DC, Akelman E, et al. The effect of wrist guards on bone strain in the distal forearm. *Am J Sports Med* 1999;27:500–506.
324. Scheiber RA, Branche-Dorsey CM, Ryan GW, et al. Risk factors for injuries from in-line skating and the effectiveness of safety gear. *N Engl J Med* 1996;335:1630–1635.
325. O'Neil DF. Wrist injuries in guarded versus unguarded first-time snowboarders. *Clin Orthop* 2003;409:91–95.
326. Esposito PW. Trampoline injuries. *Clin Orthop* 2003;409:43–52.
327. Smith GA. Injuries to children in the United States related to trampolines 1990–1995: a national epidemic. *Pediatrics* 1998;101:406–412.
328. Furnival RA, Street KA, Schunk JE. Too many pediatric trampoline injuries. *Pediatrics* 1999;103:e57.
329. Larson BJ, Davis JW. Trampoline-related injuries. *J Bone Joint Surg [Am]* 1995;77: 1174–1178.
330. Goulding A, Rockell JE, Black RE, et al. Children who avoid drinking cow's milk are at increased risk for prepubertal bone fractures. *J Am Diet Assoc* 2004;104:250–253.
331. Petridou E, Karpathios T, Dessypris N, et al. The role of dairy products and non-alcoholic beverages in bone fractures among schoolage children. *Scand J Soc Med* 1997; 25:119–125.
332. Goulding A, Cannan R, Williams SM, et al. Bone mineral density in girls with forearm fractures. *J Bone Miner Res* 1998;13:143–148.
333. Goulding A, Jones IE, Taylor RW, et al. More broken bones: a four-year double cohort study of young girls with and without distal forearm fractures. *J Bone Miner Res* 2000; 15:2011–2018.
334. Ma D, Jones G. Television, computer and video viewing/physical activity and upper limb fracture risk in children: a population-based case control study. *J Bone Miner Res* 2003;18:1970–1977.
335. Gafni RI, Baron J. Overdiagnosis of osteoporosis in children due to misinterpretation of DEXA. *J Pediatr* 2004;144:253–257.
336. Inge TH, Krebs NF, Garcia VF, et al. Bariatric surgery for severely overweight adolescents: concerns and recommendations. *Pediatrics* 2004;114:217–223.
337. Garcia VF, Langford L, Inge TI. Application of laparoscopy for bariatric surgery. *Curr Opin Pediatr* 2003;15:248–255.
338. Skaggs DL, Loro ML, Pitukcheewanont P, et al. Increased body weight and decreased radial cross-sectional dimensions in girls with forearm fractures. *J Bone Miner Res* 2001; 16:1337–1342.
339. Jones IE, Williams SM, Goulding A. Associations of birth weight and length, childhood size, and smoking with bone fractures during growth: evidence from a birth cohort study. *Am J Epidemiol* 2004;159:343–350.
340. Goulding A, Jones IE, Taylor RW, et al. Bone mineral density and body composition in boys with distal forearm fractures: a dual-energy x-ray absorptiometry study. *J Pediatr* 2001;139:509–515.
341. Powers KS, Rubenstein JS. Family presence during invasive procedures in the pediatric intensive care unit: a prospective study. *Arch Pediatr Adolesc Med* 1999;153:955–958.
342. Bauchner H, Vinci R, Bak S, et al. Parents and procedures: a randomized controlled trial. *Pediatrics* 1996;98:861–867.
343. Haim-Cohen Y, Amir J, Harel L, et al. Parental presence during lumbar puncture: anxiety and attitude toward the procedure. *Clin Pediatr (Phila)* 1996;35:2–4.
344. Kain ZN, Mayes LC, Caramico LA, et al. Parental presence during induction of anesthesia: a randomized controlled trial. *Anesthesiology* 1996;84:1060–1067.
345. Boie ET, Moore GP, Brummett C, Nelson DR. Do parents want to be present during invasive procedures performed on their children in the emergency department? A survey of 400 parents. *Ann Emerg Med* 1999;34:70–74.
346. Beckman AW, Sloan BK, Moore GP, et al. Should parents be present during emergency department procedures on children and who should make the decision? A survey of emergency physician and nurse attitudes. *Acad Emerg Med* 2002;9:154–158.
347. Boudreaux ED, Francis JL, Loyacano T. Family presence during invasive procedures and resuscitations in the emergency department: a critical review and suggestions for future research. *Ann Emerg Med* 2002;40:193–205.

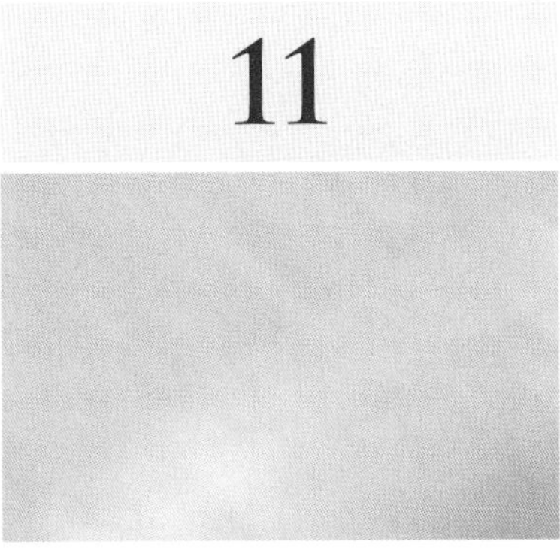

FRACTURES OF THE PROXIMAL RADIUS AND ULNA

Robert E. Eilert and Mark A. Erickson

Fractures of the proximal radius in skeletally immature patients usually involve the metaphysis or physis. True isolated radial head fractures are rare. In the proximal ulna, the olecranon, which biomechanically is a metaphysis, often fails with a greenstick pattern. Fractures in this area also may involve the physis. Fractures of the olecranon associated with proximal radioulnar joint disruption are considered part of the Monteggia fracture–dislocation complex and are discussed in Chapter 12.

FRACTURES OF THE PROXIMAL RADIUS

Incidence

Fractures of the radial neck account for slightly more than 1% of all children's fractures (1). In skeletally immature children, the radial head or epiphysis rarely is fractured, probably because of the large amount of cartilage in the radial head. If the fracture involves the epiphysis, it usually is part of a Salter-Harris type IV fracture pattern. In 90% of proximal radial fractures, the fracture line involves either the physis or the neck (2). In six large series of elbow fractures, the incidence of fracture of the radial neck was remarkably consistent, varying only from 5% to 8.5% (2–7). Fractures of the radial neck and head in skeletally immature patients account for only 14% to 20% of the total injuries of the proximal radius (5,8).

In most series, the age of occurrence varies from 4 to 14 years of age, with the median age ranging from 9 to 10 years (2,9–15). There is little difference in the occurrence rates between boys and girls (2,9,11); however, this injury seems to occur in girls approximately 2 years earlier than in boys (13).

Anatomy

Ossification Process

In the embryo, the proximal radius is well defined by 9 weeks of gestation. By 4 years of age, the radial head and neck have the same contours as in an adult (7). Ossification of the proximal radius epiphysis begins at approximately 5 years of age as a

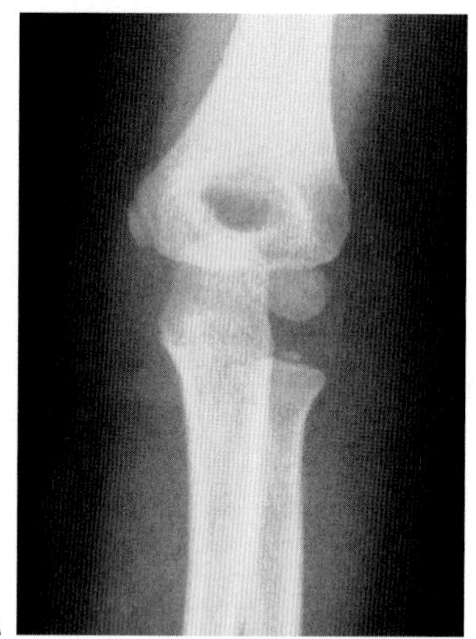
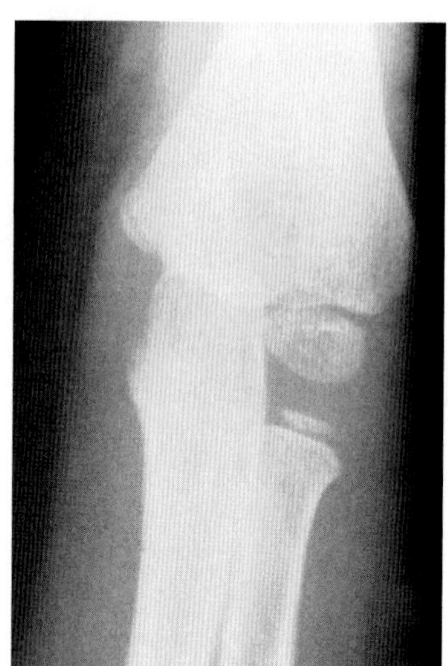
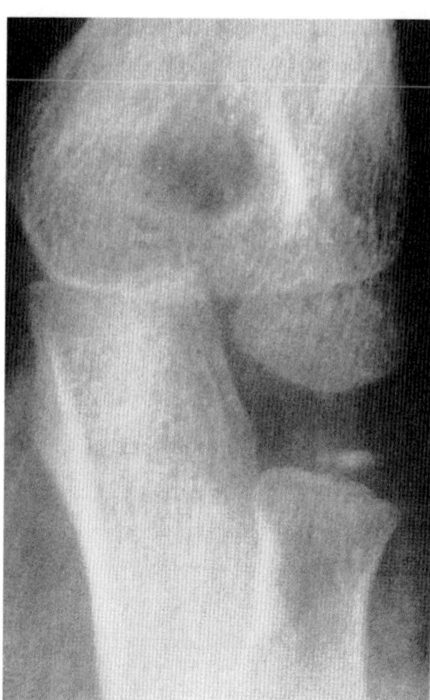

FIGURE 11-1 Ossification pattern. **A.** At 5 years, ossification begins as a small oval nucleus. **B.** As the head matures, the center widens but remains flat. **C.** Double ossification centers in developing proximal radial epiphysis. (**C** reprinted with permission from The Journal of Bone and Joint Surgery, Inc.)

small, flat nucleus (Fig. 11-1). This ossific nucleus can originate as a small sphere or it can be bipartite, which is a normal variation and should not be misinterpreted as a fracture (16–18).

Angulation Normal. In the preossification stage, on the anteroposterior (AP) projection x-ray, the edge of the metaphysis of the proximal radius slopes distally on its lateral border. This angulation is normal and not a fracture.

In the AP view, the lateral angulation varies from 0 to 15 degrees, with the average being 12.5 degrees (15). In the lateral view, the angulation can vary from 10 degrees anterior to 5 degrees posterior, with the average being 3.5 degrees anterior (15).

Soft Tissue Attachments. No ligaments attach directly to the radial neck or head. The radial collateral ligaments attach to the orbicular ligament, which originates from the radial side of the ulna. The articular capsule attaches to the proximal third of the neck. Distally, the capsule protrudes from under the orbicular ligament to form a pouch (recessus sacciformis). Thus, only a small portion of the neck lies within the articular capsule (19). Because much of the neck is extracapsular, fractures involving only the neck may not produce an intraarticular effusion, and the fat pad sign may be negative with fracture of the radial neck (16,18,20).

The "Cam" Effect. The proximal radioulnar joint has a precise congruence. The axis of rotation of the proximal radius is a line through the center of the radial head and neck. When a displaced fracture disrupts the alignment of the radial head on the center of the radial neck, the arc of rotation changes. Instead of rotating smoothly in a pure circle, the radial head rotates with a "cam" effect. This disruption of the congruity of the proximal radioulnar joint results in a loss of the range of motion in supination and pronation (Fig. 11-2) (21).

Diagnosis

Clinical Findings

Following a fracture, palpation over the radial head or neck is painful. The pain usually is increased more with passive forearm

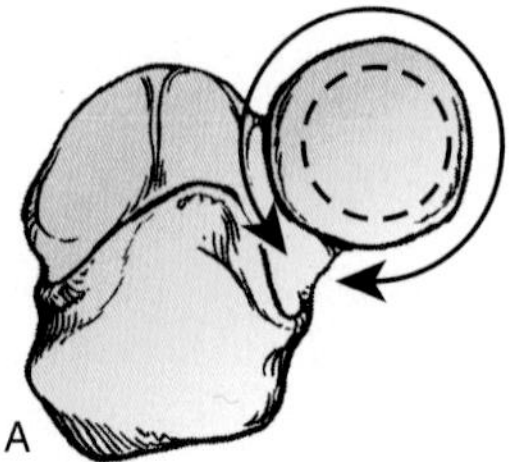

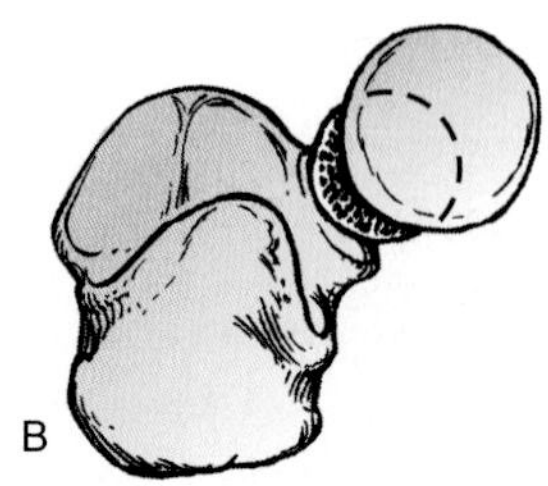

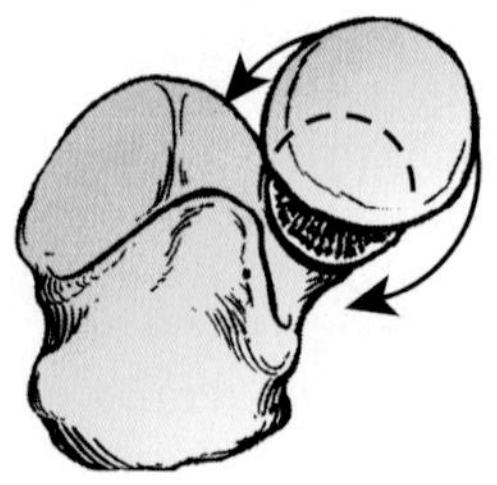

FIGURE 11-2 **A.** Normal rotation of the forearm causes the radial head to circumscribe an exact circle within the proximal radioulnar joint. **B.** Any translocation of the radial head limits rotation because of the "cam" effect described by Wedge and Robertson (21).

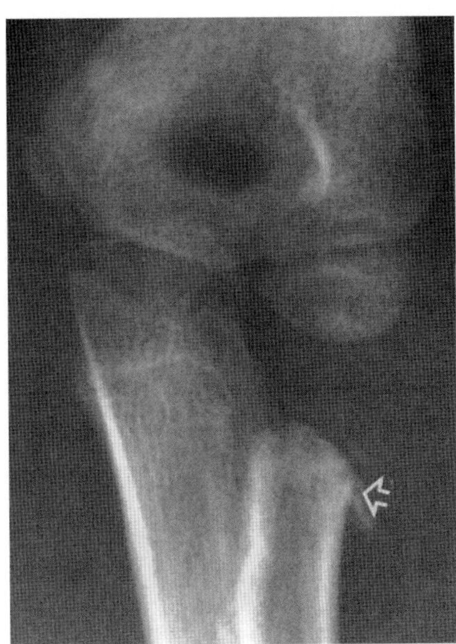

FIGURE 11-3 Preosseous fracture. The only clue to the presence of a fracture of the radial neck with displacement of the radial head was loss of smoothness of the metaphyseal margin (*arrow*).

supination and pronation than with elbow flexion and extension. In a young child, the primary complaint may be wrist pain (22), and pressure over the proximal radius may accentuate this referred wrist pain. The wrist pain may be secondary to radial shortening and subsequent distal radioulnar joint dysfunction. The misdirection of such a presentation reinforces the principle of x-raying both ends of a fractured long bone.

Radiographic Evaluation

Supination–Pronation Views. The fracture usually is easy to see on both AP and lateral x-ray views. Occasionally, oblique views with the forearm both supinated and pronated will reveal the fracture line clearly.

Some variants in the ossification process can resemble a fracture. Most of these involve the radial head, although a step-off also can develop as a normal variant of the metaphysis. There may be a persistence of the secondary ossification centers of the epiphysis. Comparison views are useful for evaluation of unusual ossification centers after an acute elbow injury.

The diagnosis of a partially or completely displaced fracture of the radial neck may be difficult in the preosseous age group. The only clue may be a little irregularity in the smoothness of the proximal metaphyseal margin (Fig. 11-3). Rokito et al (23) reported complete displacement of the radial head in a 5-year-old boy, in whom the only clue on radiography was a small speck of ossification in the elbow joint (Fig. 11-4A). The full extent of the injury was appreciated when the radial head was outlined with MRI (see Fig. 11-4B).

Perpendicular Views. If the elbow cannot be extended because of pain, special views are necessary to see the elbow in full AP profile. One view is taken with the beam perpendicular to the distal humerus, and the other with the beam perpendicular to the proximal radius. A regular AP view with the elbow flexed may not show the fracture because of obliquity of the beam. The perpendicular views show the physeal line of the radius in clear profile.

With a minimally displaced fracture, the fracture line may be difficult to see because it is superimposed on the proximal ulna, and oblique views of the proximal radius may be helpful (16,19). One oblique view that is especially helpful is the radiocapitellar view suggested by Greenspan et al and Hall-Craggs et al (24–26). This view projects the radial head anterior to the coronoid process (Fig. 11-5) and is especially helpful if full supination and pronation views are difficult to obtain because of acute injury (Fig. 11-6).

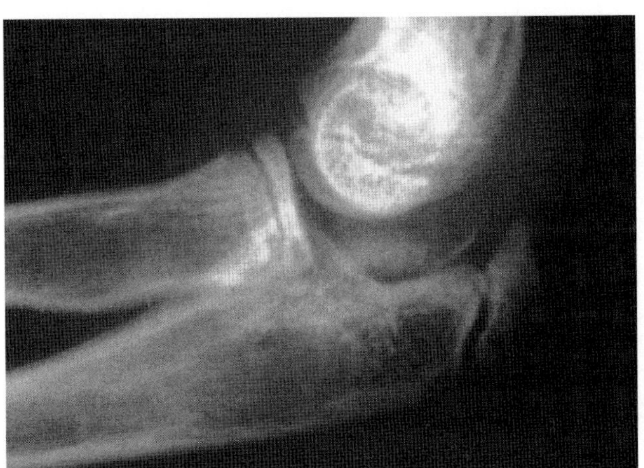

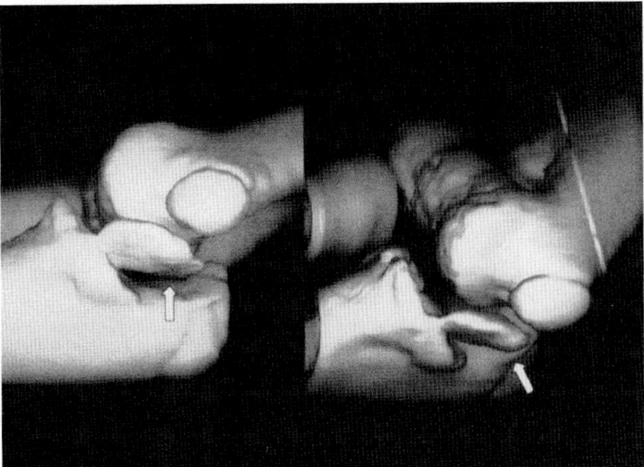

FIGURE 11-4 Unappreciated diagnosis. Osteochondral flap fracture of proximal ulna. **A.** X-ray. **B.** 3D CT. (**B** Reprinted with permission from the Journal of Orthopaedic Trauma.)

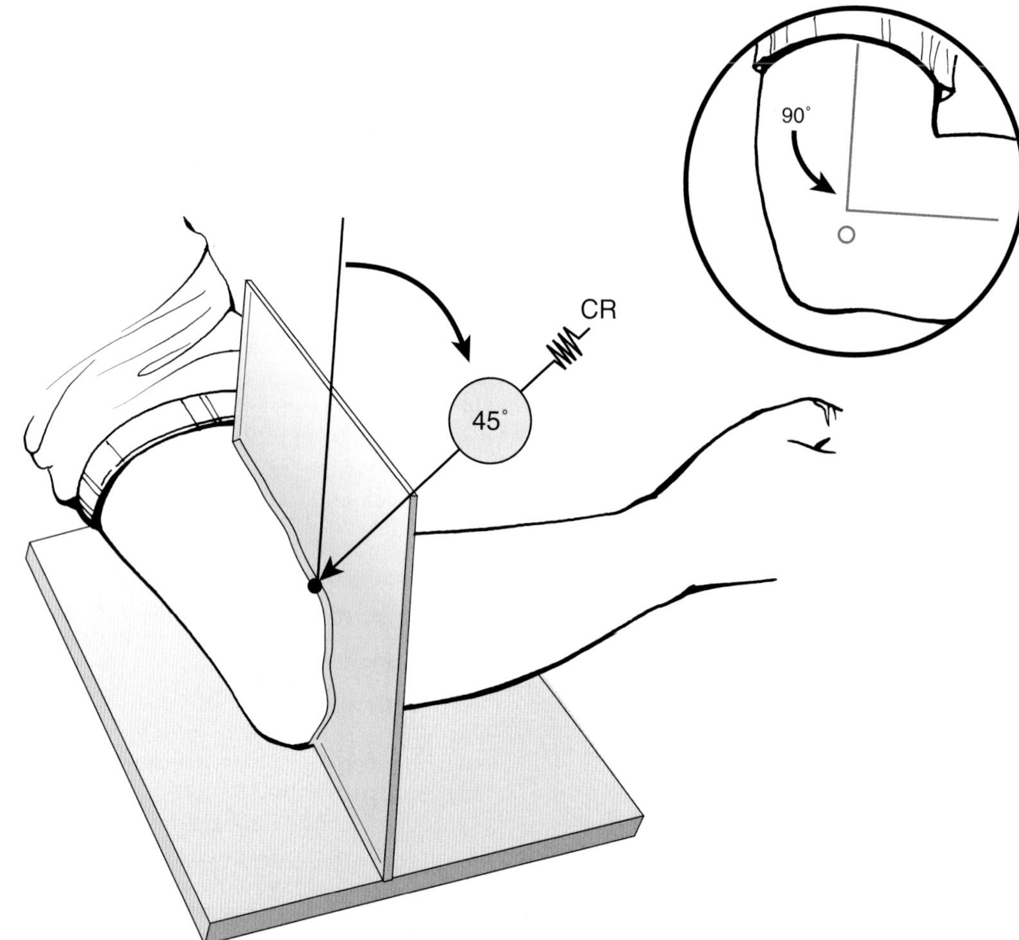

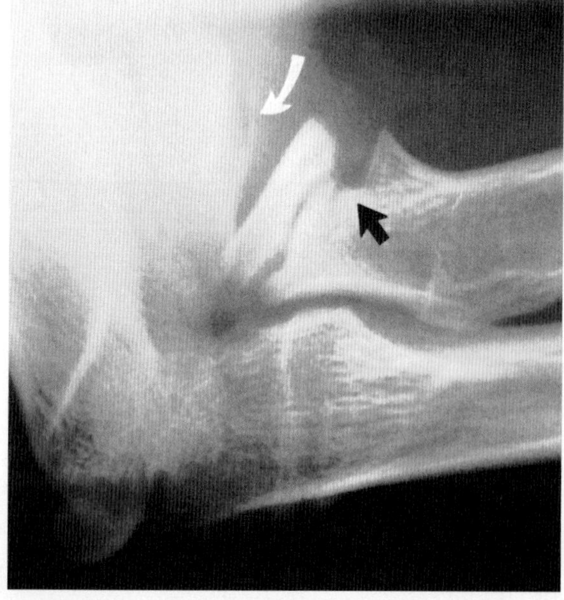

FIGURE 11-5 **A.** Radiocapitellar view. Center of x-ray beam is directed at 45 degrees to separate proximal radius and ulna on the x-ray. (Reprinted from Long BW. *Orthopaedic Radiography*. Philadelphia: W.B. Saunders; 1995:152; with permission.) **B.** Angular stress deformity: anterior angulation of the radial head and neck in a 12-year-old baseball pitcher. There is evidence of some disruption of the normal growth of the anterior portion of the physis (*black arrow*). The capitellum also shows radiographic signs of osteochondritis dissecans (*white arrow*). (Courtesy of Kenneth P. Butters, MD.)

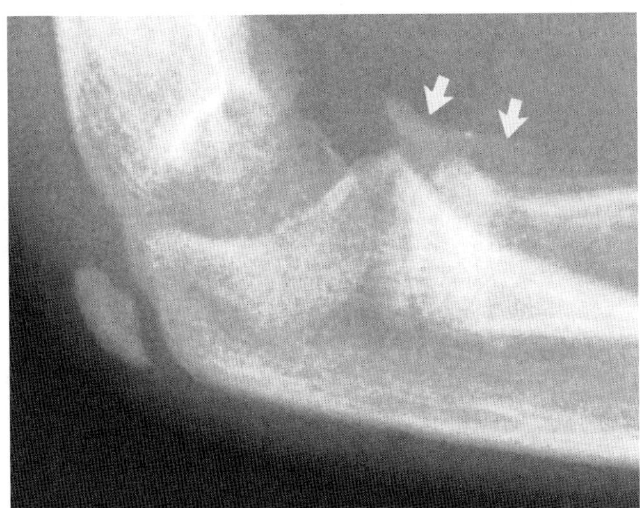

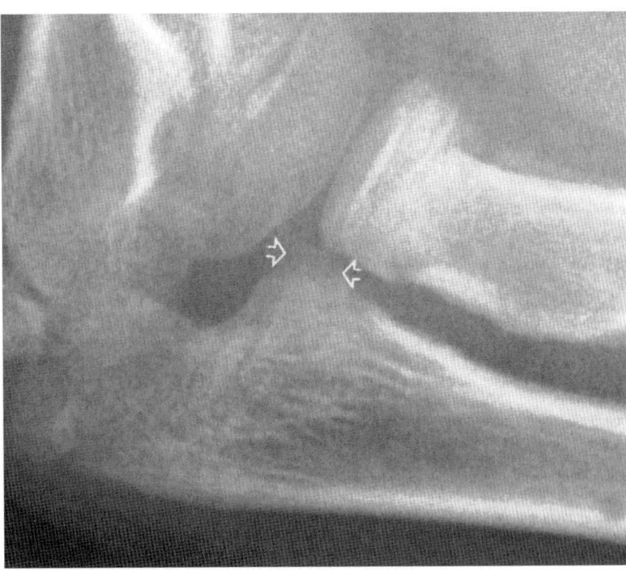

FIGURE 11-6 The radiocapitellar view. **A.** X-rays of a 13-year-old girl who had sustained a radial neck fracture associated with an elbow dislocation. There is ectopic bone formation (*arrows*). In this view, it is difficult to tell the exact location of the ectopic bone. **B.** The radiocapitellar view separates the radial head from the coronoid process and shows that the ectopic bone is from the coronoid process (*arrows*) and not the radial neck.

If the epiphysis is ossified, displacement of the radial head usually is obvious on an x-ray, but a minimally displaced fracture is difficult to diagnose before ossification has begun (27). The loss of the smoothness of the metaphyseal margin may be the only finding. Ultrasonography can be used to evaluate for hemarthrosis and displacement of the fracture and allows a dynamic range-of-motion evaluation (28).

The supinator fat pad is a small layer of fat that overlies the supinator muscle in the proximal forearm. Displacement of the supinator fat pad may indicate fracture of the proximal radius (29). The supinator fat pad and distal humeral anterior and posterior fat pads are not always displaced with occult fractures of the radial neck or physis (18,20,30).

If there is localized tenderness of the radial head and neck, special studies may be necessary. Arthrography, MRI, and ultrasound (28) are options for determining any displacement of the unossified radial head.

Classification

Chambers classified proximal radial fractures into three major groups based on the mechanism of injury and displacement of the radial head (Table 11-1):

- Group I: The radial head is primarily displaced (most proximal radial injuries are in this group).
- Group II: The radial neck is primarily displaced.
- Group III: Stress injuries.

Head-Displaced Fractures (Group I)

To describe head-displaced fractures, Chambers combined the classifications of Jeffrey (5) and Newman (11) to produce a new

TABLE 11-1 Classification of Fractures Involving the Proximal Radius

Group I: Primary displacement of the radial head

A. Valgus fractures
1. Type A—Salter-Harris type I and II injuries of the proximal radial physis
2. Type B—Salter-Harris type IV injuries of the proximal radial physis
3. Type C—Fractures involving only the proximal radial metaphysis

B. Fractures associated with elbow dislocation
1. Type D—Reduction injuries
2. Type E—Dislocation injuries

Group II: Primary displacement of the radial neck

A. Angular injuries (Monteggia type III variant)

B. Torsional injuries

Group III: Stress injuries

A. Osteochondritis dissecans of the radial head

B. Physeal injuries with neck angulation

classification based primarily on the mechanism of injury. The two subclasses of fractures in group I are valgus injuries and those associated with elbow dislocations. Valgus injuries are subdivided into three types based on the location of the fracture line (Fig. 11-7). Fractures associated with an elbow dislocation are subdivided into two types. The first is based on the original concept proposed by Jeffrey (5) that the fracture occurs during spontaneous reduction (Fig. 11-8A). In this case, the radial head lies proximal to the posterior aspect of the joint. The second is based on Newman's concept (11) that the fracture and displacement occur during the process of dislocation of the elbow. In this type, the radial head lies distal to the anterior portion of the joint (see Fig. 11-8B). Most radial head fractures in children described in the literature have been Salter-Harris type IV injuries containing portions of both the epiphysis and metaphysis, and there is no need to further subclassify them.

Neck-Displaced Fractures (Group II)

For the neck-displaced fractures, there are two subgroups, angular and torsional. An angular fracture of the radial neck may be associated with a proximal ulnar fracture. This association is recognized as a Monteggia variant.

Stress Injuries (Group III)

The final group, stress injuries, includes osteochondritis of the radial head and physeal injuries of the neck that produce angular deformities.

Mechanisms of Injury

Table 11-2 lists the proposed mechanisms for fractures of the radial head and neck in children.

Primary Displacement of the Radial Head (Group I)

In general, these fractures are caused by a force that is applied to the radial head and is secondarily transmitted to the radial neck, which fractures because it is metaphyseal bone with a thinner cortex. Angulation, rotation, translocation, or complete separation of the radial head from the neck can displace the radial head. This displacement of the radial head produces an incongruity of the proximal radioulnar joint, which is the major cause of dysfunction. For displaced radial head fractures, the treatment goal is to reduce the proximal radioulnar joint to its normal congruous position and restore range of motion.

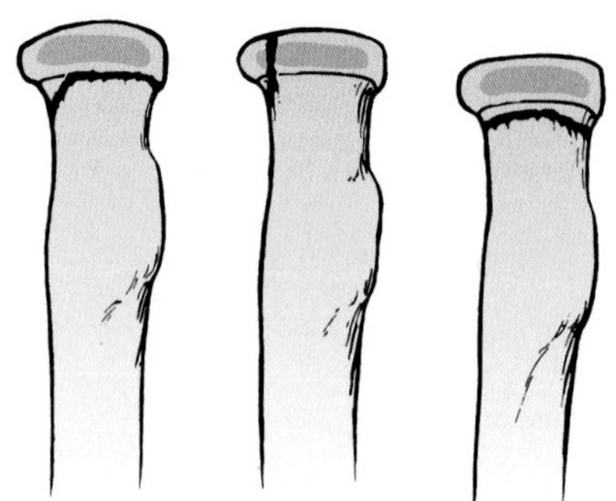

FIGURE 11-7 Types of valgus injuries. *Left*: Type A: Salter-Harris type I or II physeal injury. *Center*: Type B: Salter-Harris type IV injury. *Right*: Type C: Total metaphyseal fracture pattern.

Valgus Injuries

Angular Force on the Neck. Most of these injuries occur in a fall on the outstretched arm with the elbow in extension (2,5,7,11,19,31). An associated valgus thrust to the forearm (Fig. 11-9) compresses the radiocapitellar joint. The cartilaginous head absorbs the force and transmits it to the weaker physis or metaphysis of the neck (19). These fractures characteristically produce an angular deformity of the head with the neck (see Fig. 11-9A). The direction of angulation depends on whether the forearm is in a supinated, neutral, or pronated position at the time of the fall. Vostal (19) showed that in neutral, the pressure is concentrated on the lateral portion of the head and neck. In supination, the pressure is concentrated anteriorly, and in pronation it is concentrated posteriorly.

Associated Injuries. This valgus stress pattern causes associated injuries about the elbow (5,7,13,31,32) (see Fig. 11-9B,C) such as greenstick fracture of the olecranon (Fig. 11-10), which Bado (33) considered an equivalent of a type I Monteggia lesion. An avulsion fracture of the medial epicondylar apophysis also may occur (34). In Fowles and Kassab's series of patients with radial neck fractures (4), more than 61% had one of these associated injuries.

Children with an increased carrying angle may be predisposed to injury of the proximal radius. Henrikson (2) found that the degree of cubitus valgus in patients who sustained this injury was greater than in patients with other types of elbow fractures.

Fracture Patterns in Valgus Injuries. With valgus elbow injuries, the fracture pattern can be one of three types (A, B, C) (Fig. 11-11). In the first two types, the fracture line involves the physis. Type A represents either a Salter-Harris type I or II physeal injury. In a Salter-Harris type II injury, the metaphyseal fragment is triangular and lies on the compression side. In type B fractures, the fracture line courses vertically through the metaphysis, physis, and epiphysis to produce a Salter-Harris type IV fracture pattern (see Fig. 11-11). This is the only fracture type that involves the articular surface of the radial head. In type C fractures, the fracture line lies completely within the metaphysis (Fig. 11-12), and the fracture can be transverse or oblique. Type B fractures are rare. The incidences of types A and C fractures are approximately equal (13).

Displacement Patterns. Regardless of the type of fracture pattern, displacement can vary from minimal angulation to complete separation of the radial head from the neck (Fig. 11-13). With minimal angulation, the congruity of the proximal radioulnar

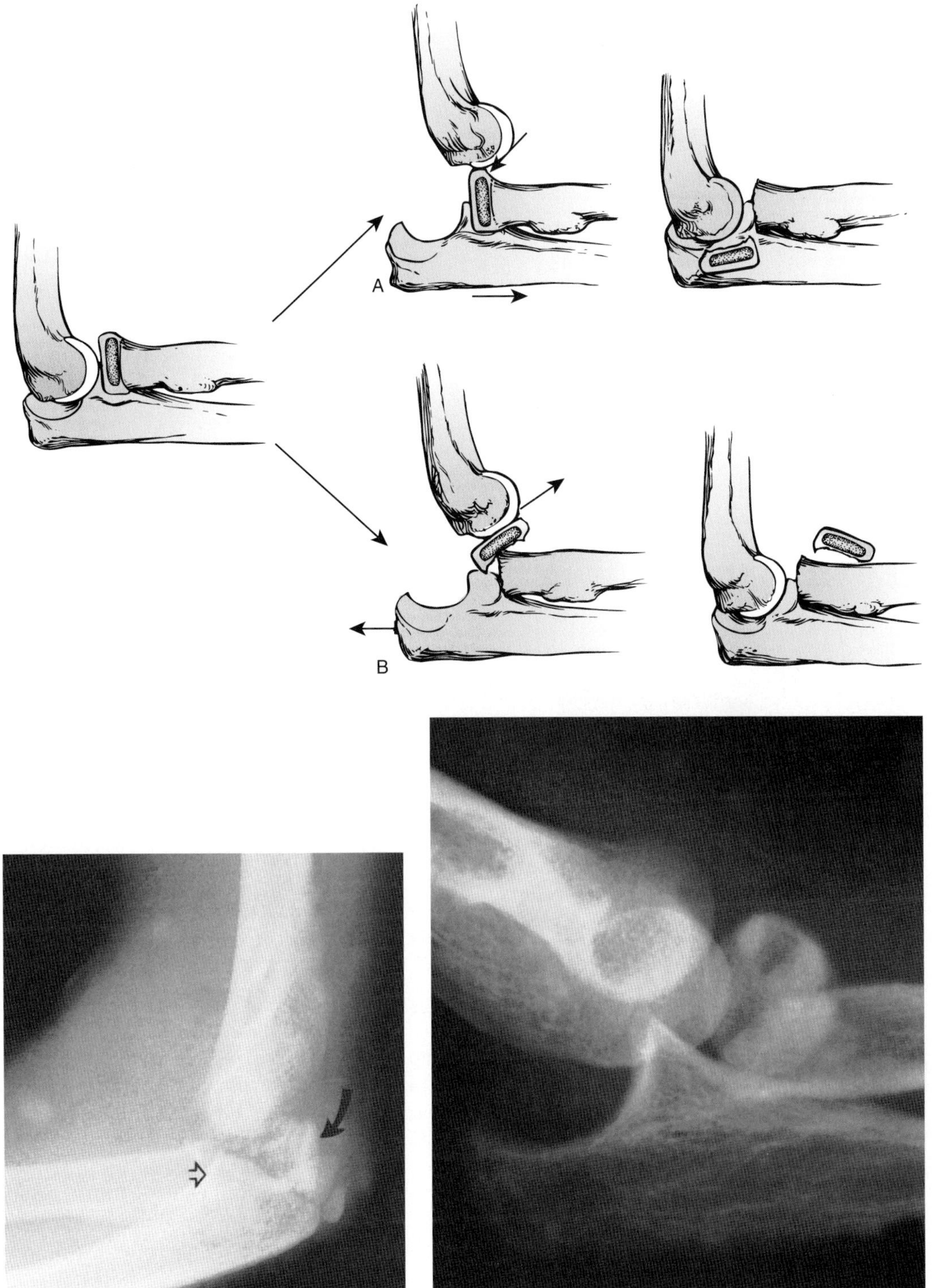

FIGURE 11-8 Dislocation fracture patterns. **A.** Type D: The radial neck is fractured during the process of reduction by the capitellum pressing against the distal lip of the radial head (41). **B.** Type E: The radial neck is fractured during the process of dislocation by the capitellum pressing against the proximal lip of the radial head (67). **C.** X-rays of a radial head that was fractured during the reduction of the dislocation (type D). The radial head (*solid arrow*) lies posterior to the distal humerus, and the distal portion of the neck (*open arrow*) is anterior. (Courtesy of Richard E. King, MD.) **D.** X-ray of the dislocated elbow in which the fracture of the radial neck occurred during the process of dislocation (type E).

TABLE 11-2 Fractures of the Radial Head and Neck: Proposed Mechanisms in Children

I. Primary displacement of the head (incongruous)
   A. Valgus injuries
   B. Associated with dislocation of the elbow
      1. During reduction
      2. During dislocation

II. Primary displacement of the neck
   A. Angular forces
   B. Rotational forces

III. Chronic stress forces

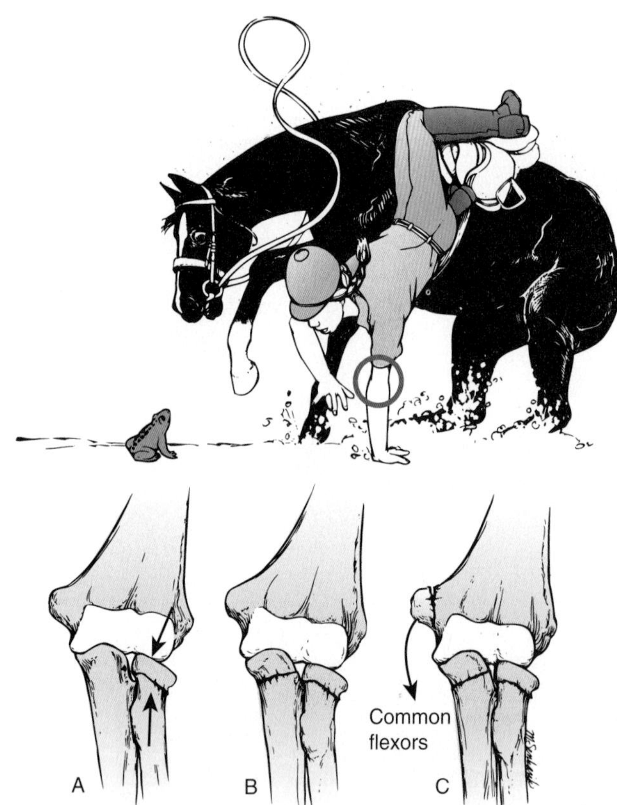

FIGURE 11-9 The most common mechanism of radial neck fractures involves a fall on the outstretched arm. This produces an angular deformity of the neck **(A)**. Further valgus forces can produce a greenstick fracture of the olecranon **(B)** or an avulsion of the medial epicondylar apophysis **(C)**. (Redrawn with permission from Jeffery CC. Fracture of the head of the radius in children. *J Bone Joint Surg [Br]* 1950;32:314–324.)

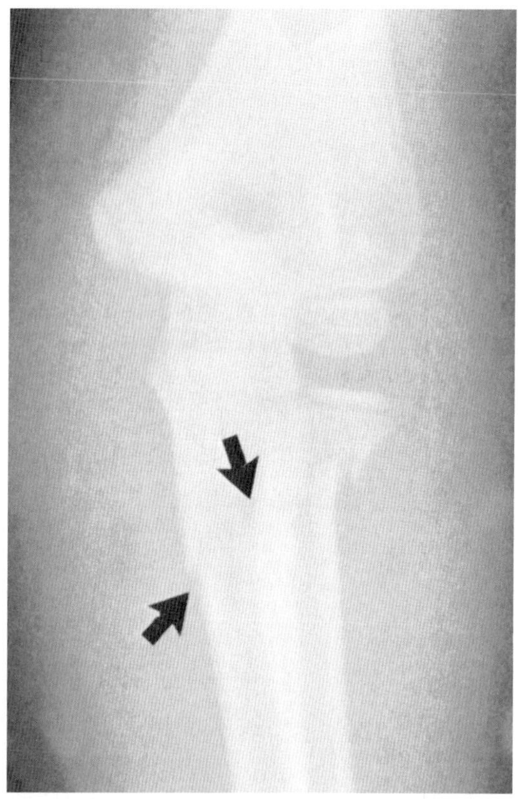

FIGURE 11-10 Associated fractures of valgus stress. Anteroposterior view of a fracture of the radial neck associated with a greenstick fracture of the olecranon (*arrows*).

joint usually is retained. If the radial head is displaced in relation to the radial neck, the congruity of the proximal radioulnar joint is lost, producing the cam effect. Completely displaced fractures often are associated with more severe injuries.

Neck Migration. Patterson (35) believed that once the stabilizing effect of the radial head is lost, the radial metaphyses migrate proximally. This proximal migration of the distal fragment tends to be ulnarward because of muscle pull by the supinator and biceps muscles (Fig. 11-14). Patterson attempted to counteract these forces in his manipulative technique (see section on Patterson's Manipulative Technique). When there is a strong valgus component, the proximal portion of the distal fragment of the radius can get locked medial to the coronoid process, making a closed reduction almost impossible (36,37).

Associated with Elbow Dislocation. In two rare types of fractures of the radial neck associated with elbow dislocation, the head fragment is totally displaced from the neck (5,11, 34,38–40). The proposed mechanism is a fall on the hand with the elbow flexed, which causes a momentary partial dislocation of the elbow and forces the radial head posterior to the capitellum.

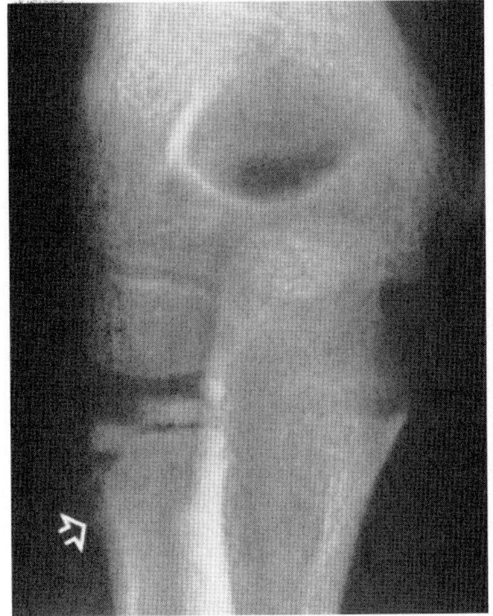

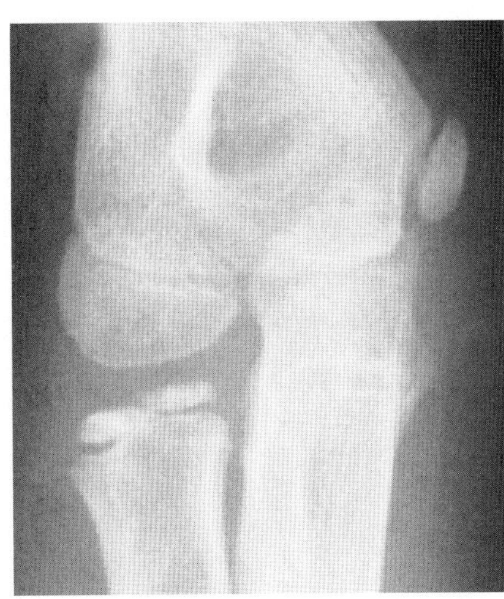

FIGURE 11-11 Valgus (type B) injury. **A.** Three weeks after the initial injury, there was evidence of distal migration of this Salter-Harris type IV fracture fragment. Periosteal new bone formation has already developed along the distal metaphyseal fragment (*arrow*). **B.** Six months after the initial injury, there is evidence of an osseous bridge formation between the metaphysis and the epiphysis. Subsequently, the patient had secondary degenerative arthritis with loss of elbow motion and forearm rotation.

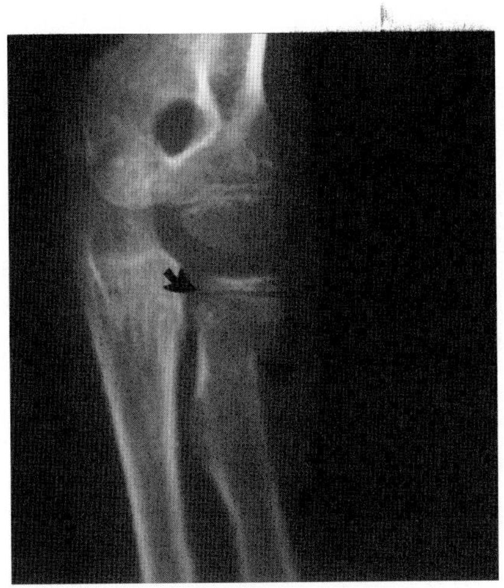

FIGURE 11-12 Valgus type C injury. The fracture line is totally metaphyseal and oblique (*arrows*).

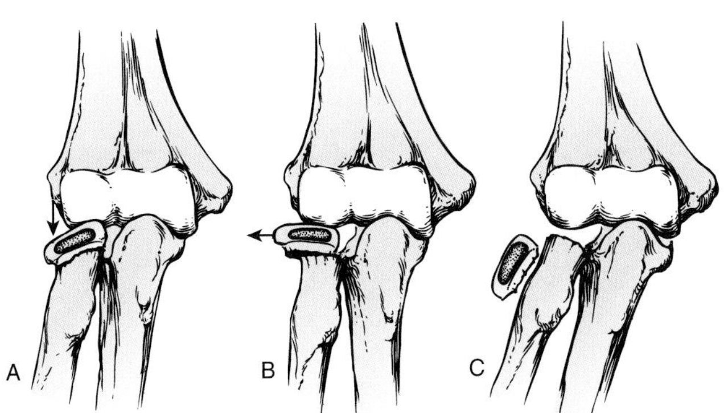

FIGURE 11-13 Displacement patterns. The radial head can be angulated **(A)**, translated **(B)**, or completely displaced **(C)**.

During Reduction (Type D). In the original description of this injury, Jeffrey (5) suggested that displacement and fracture occurred during spontaneous reduction of the transiently dislocated elbow. During this reduction process, the capitellum applies a proximal force to the distal lip of the radial head, causing it to separate as the forearm and distal radius are reduced distally (see Fig. 11-8A). The radial neck and olecranon return to their anatomic locations while the radial head remains in the posterior aspect of the joint (40).

During Dislocation (Type E). Newman (11) described a type of radial head fracture in which the fracture occurs during the process of dislocation. In this case, the capitellum applies a distally directed force to the proximal lip of the radial head as the elbow is dislocated (see Fig. 11-8B). The elbow may remain dislocated with the radial head lying anterior and often parallel to the long axis of the neck fragment. If the dislocation is reduced, either by manipulation or spontaneously, the radial head lies free in the anterior portion of the elbow joint (11,15,40).

Primary Displacement of the Radial Neck (Group II)

Rarely, angular or torsional forces cause a primary disruption or deformity of the neck while the head remains congruous within the proximal radioulnar joint. Treatment of these fractures is manipulation of the distal neck fragment to align it with the head.

Angular Forces. Angular forces always produce type III Monteggia equivalents. A Monteggia type III fracture pattern is created when a varus force is applied across the extended elbow, resulting in a greenstick fracture of the olecranon or proximal ulna and a lateral dislocation of the radial head (41). Occasionally, however, the failure occurs at the radial neck (Monteggia III equivalent) and the radial neck displaces

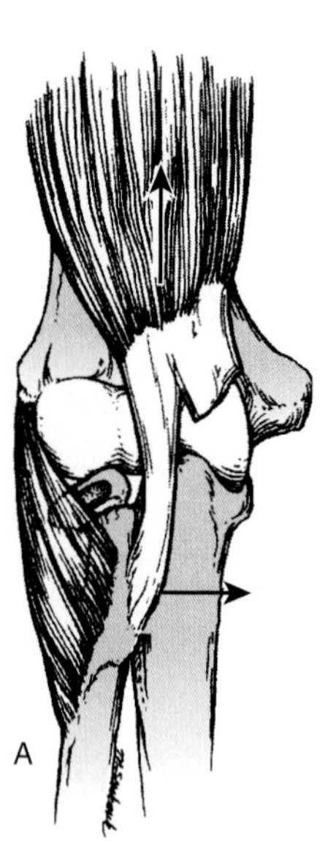

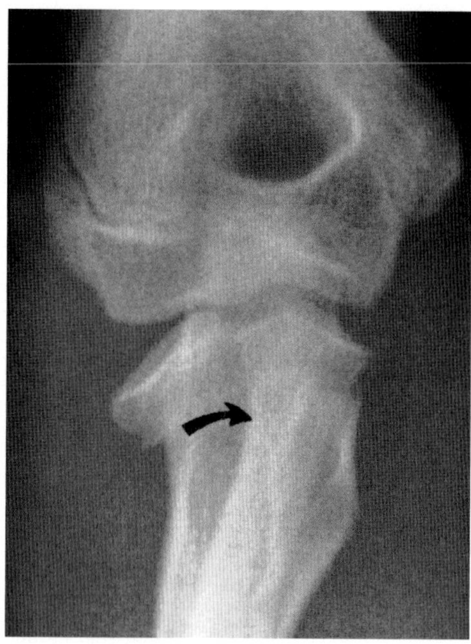

FIGURE 11-14 **A.** Forces producing displacement. Once the stabilizing effect of the radial head is lost, the distal fragment (radial neck and proximal shaft) is displaced ulnarward and proximally by the unopposed biceps and supinator muscles (*arrows*). (Redrawn with permission from Patterson RF. Treatment of displaced transverse fractures of the neck of the radius in children. *J Bone Joint Surg* 1934;16:695.) **B.** X-ray showing proximal and medial (ulnar) displacement of distal neck fragment (*arrow*). (From Wilkins KE, ed. *Operative management of upper extremity fractures in children*. Rosemont, IL: American Academy of Orthopaedic Surgeons, 1994:55.)

laterally, leaving the radial head and proximal neck fragment in anatomic position under the orbicular ligament (Fig. 11-15) (42).

Rotational Forces. Rotational forces may fracture the radial neck in young children before ossification of the proximal radial epiphysis. Both reports of this injury are in the European literature (2,31), and in both the initial rotational force was in supination. Reduction was achieved by pronation of the forearm. Diagnosis of these injuries is difficult and may require arthrography or an examination under general anesthesia. This injury should be differentiated from the more common subluxation of the radial head (pulled elbow syndrome), in which the forearm usually is held in pronation with resistance to supination. In addition, on radiography there usually are no signs of hemarthrosis, as is seen in the torsional fractures.

Stress Injuries (Group III)

A final mechanism of injury is chronic repetitive stress, both longitudinal and rotational, on either the head or the proximal radial physis. These injuries usually are the result of athletic activity in which the upper extremity is required to perform repetitive motions. Repetitive stresses disrupt growth of either the neck or the head, with eventual deformity. A true stress fracture is not present.

In the United States, the popularity of organized sports has produced a number of unique injuries in children related to repetitive stress applied to growth centers. This is especially true in the immature elbow. Most injuries are related to throwing sports, primarily Little League baseball. Most of this "Little League pathology" involves tension injuries on the medial epicondyle. In some athletes, however, the lateral side is involved as well because of the repetitive compressive forces applied to the capitellum and radial head and neck. In the radial head, lytic lesions similar to osteochondritis dissecans may occur (43–45) (Figs. 11-16 and 11-17). If the stress forces are transmitted to the radial neck, the anterior portion of the physis may be injured, producing an angular deformity of the radial neck (see Fig. 11-5) (46).

Treatment

The options for treatment for radial head fractures include:

1. Immobilization with no manipulation
2. Manipulative closed reduction
3. Percutaneous pin reduction
4. Intramedullary pin reduction
5. Open reduction with or without internal fixation
6. Excision of either the entire head or a small head fragment

Several factors must be considered in choosing a method of treatment, including the degree of angulation and displacement, the association of other injuries, the age of the patient, and the time elapsed since the injury.

Prognostic Factors

Some factors may be more important than the type of treatment in determining the final result. A poor result is more likely if the fracture is associated with other injuries, such as an elbow dislocation, a fracture of the olecranon, or avulsion of the medial epicondylar apophysis (4,30). The magnitude of force to the elbow is a major factor in determining the quality of the result (6,13).

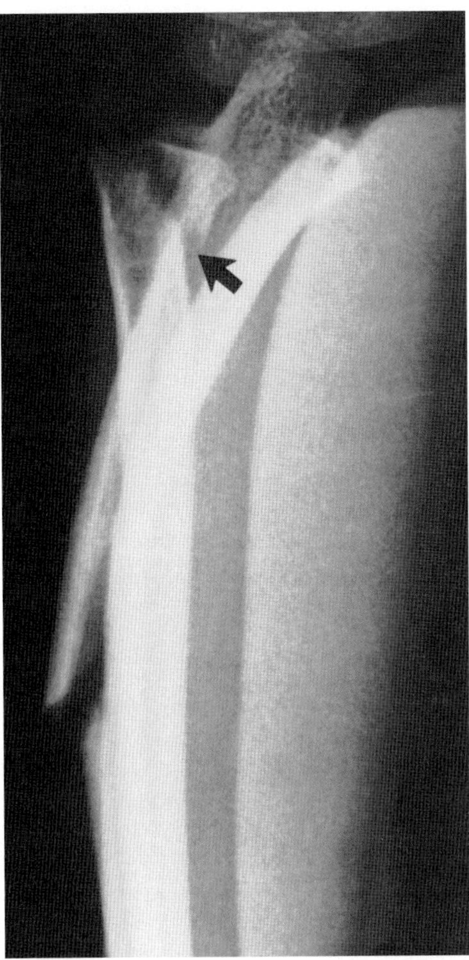

FIGURE 11-15 Angular forces. This 8-year-old sustained a type III Monteggia equivalent in which the radial neck fractured (*arrow*), leaving the radial head reduced proximally. (Courtesy of Ruben D. Pechero, MD.)

Initial Angulation and Displacement. Tibone and Stoltz (14) reported that the number of good results decreased if the initial angulation exceeded 30 degrees or the amount of displacement exceeded 3 mm. Newman (11,13) found that more than 4 mm of initial displacement increased the frequency of poor results and the risk of synostosis with the proximal ulna.

Angulation and Displacement After Reduction. Residual tilt of the radial head is better tolerated than displacement. Pollen (47) believed that in older children, only 15 degrees of angulation should be accepted without attempting manipulation. The spontaneous correction that can be expected to occur with growth in younger children is approximately 10 degrees. Some clinicians accept up to 30 degrees of residual angulation (6,11,15,17,48), whereas others believe that up to 45 degrees of residual angulation can yield a satisfactory result (7,9,49,50).

Age Effect. It is still controversial whether age has a favorable or unfavorable effect on the outcome (13). The cam effect will limit supination and pronation if there is significant displacement of the proximal fragment. However, adequate remodeling with a functional range of motion can occur with as much as 40% displacement (Fig. 11-18) in a young child.

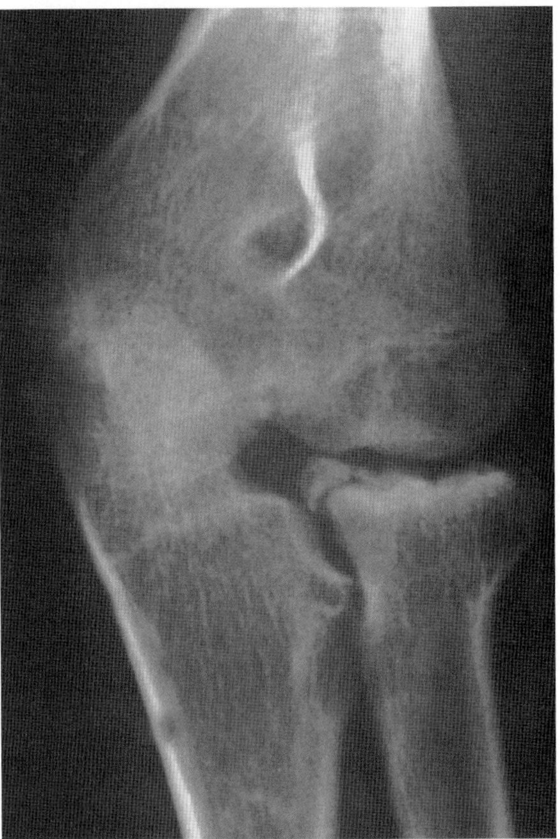

FIGURE 11-16 Osteochondritis dissecans. X-ray of this 11-year-old Little League pitcher's elbow shows fragmentation of the subchondral surfaces of the radial head. These changes and the accelerated bone age are evidence of overuse.

Timing. Surgery should be done as soon as possible after the injury; the later the surgical intervention, the poorer the result. McBride and Monnet (51) described three patients in whom an osteotomy of the neck was done for residual angulation 3 to 5 weeks after injury. All had further loss of range of motion because of the development of a proximal cross-union. Blount (49) set a limit of 5 days, after which surgical intervention is more likely to produce a poorer result than if the fracture is left untreated.

Outcomes

In general, a closed reduction will yield a better result than an open reduction. This may be true because injuries that can be managed by closed methods are the result of less severe trauma than those requiring open reduction. The poor results in those managed with open methods may be due

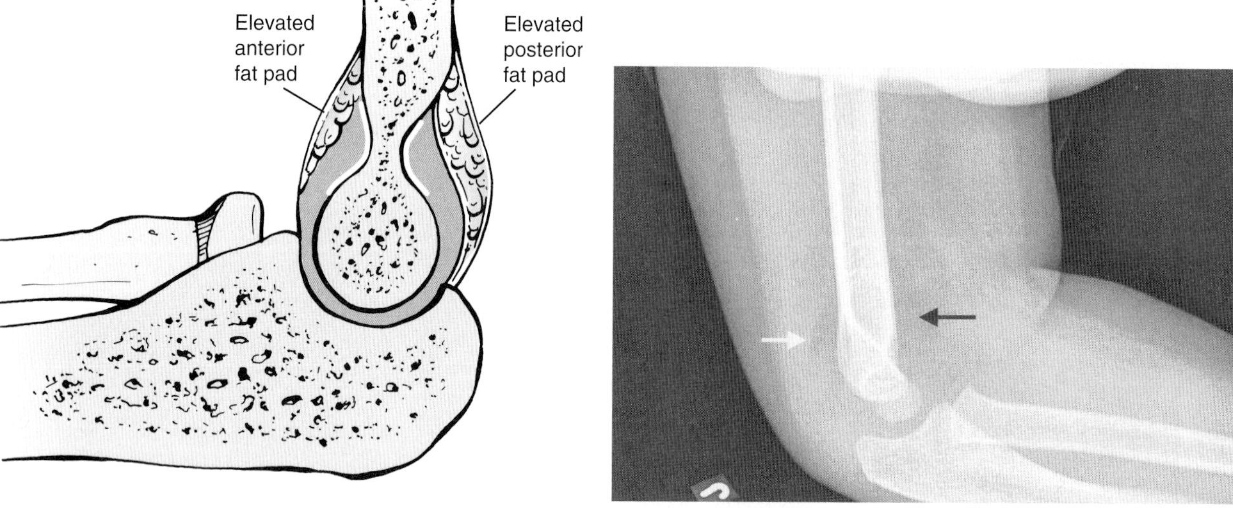

FIGURE 11-17 Elevated anterior and posterior fat pads. **A.** Illustration (adapted with permission from The Journal of Bone and Joint Surgery, Inc.). **B.** *White arrow*: posterior fat pad sign. *Black arrow*: anterior fat pad sign.

just as much to the associated soft tissue injuries as to the surgical insult.

The overall incidence of poor results in large series varies from 15% to 33% (2,4,13,15,32). Considering only severely displaced fractures, the incidence of poor results was as high as 50% (13). Thus, at least one in five or six children can be expected to have a poor result despite adequate treatment. It is wise to counsel the parents before beginning treatment, if poor prognostic factors are present. Very little improvement in motion occurs after 6 months. Steinberg et al (13) found that range of motion in their patients at 6 months was almost equal to that when the patients were examined years later.

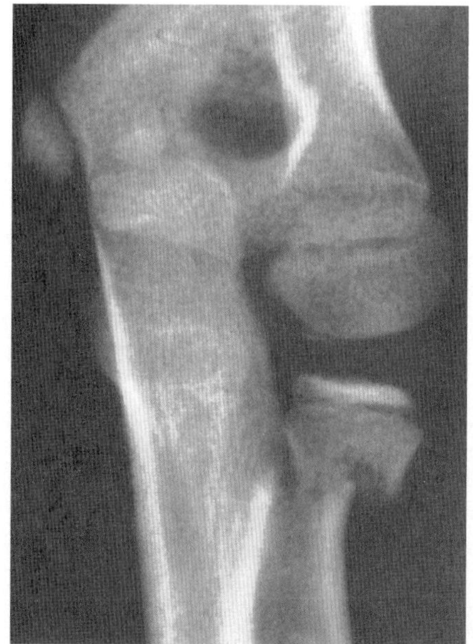

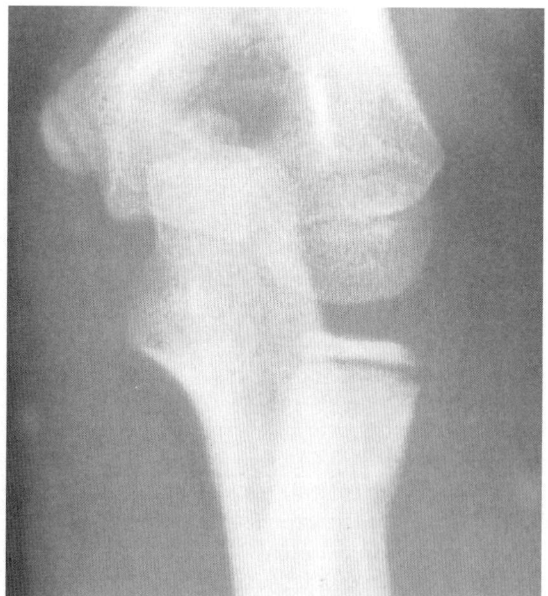

FIGURE 11-18 Translocation remodeling. **A.** Injury film of a 9-year-old who had 60 degrees of supination and pronation by clinical examination with local anesthesia into the elbow joint. Because range of motion was functional, the position was accepted. **B.** Two months after fracture, there was almost complete remodeling of the translocation. The patient's forearm rotation was 75 degrees in both directions. (Courtesy of Earl A. Stanley, Jr., MD.)

Nonoperative Methods

Immobilization (Up to 30 Degrees of Angulation). Immobilization is the treatment of choice for fractures in younger children in which the angulation of the radial head is less than 20 to 30 degrees. A collar and cuff, a posterior splint, or a light long-arm cast is sufficient to provide comfort and protection from further injury. Aspiration of the intraarticular hematoma may decrease pain.

Manipulative Closed Reduction (30 to 60 Degrees of Angulation). Although acceptable results can be obtained with angulation of up to 45 degrees, closed reduction should be attempted for fractures with more than 30 degrees of angulation. A closed reduction usually is satisfactory for fractures with angulation up to 60 degrees. The chance of achieving a satisfactory closed reduction is much less when the initial angulation exceeds 60 degrees.

Patterson's Manipulative Technique. Many authors (17,52) advocate manipulative reduction with the elbow in extension, as described by Patterson (35). General or regional anesthesia can provide adequate relaxation. The orbicular ligament should be intact to stabilize the proximal radial head fragment (17). In Patterson's technique, an assistant grasps the arm proximal to the elbow joint with one hand (Fig. 11-19, left) and places the other hand medially over the distal humerus to provide a medial fulcrum for the varus stress applied across the elbow. The surgeon applies distal traction with the forearm supinated to relax the supinators and biceps. A varus force is then placed on the elbow to overcome the ulnar deviation of the distal fragment so that it can be aligned with the proximal fragment. This varus force also helps open up the lateral side of the joint, which facilitates manipulation of the head fragment.

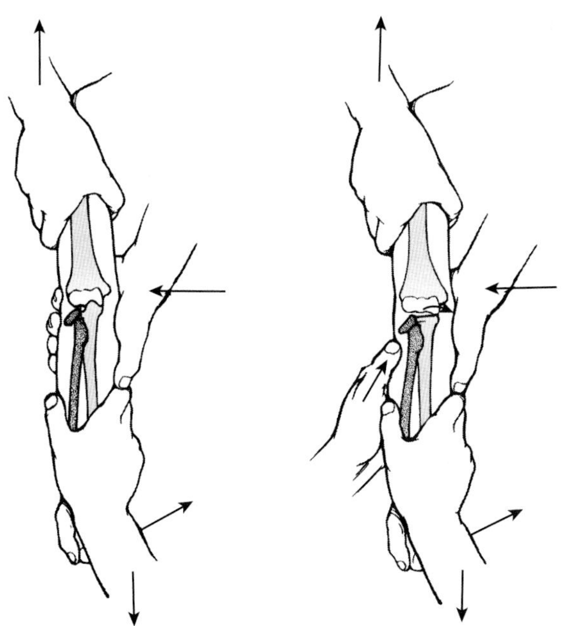

FIGURE 11-19 Patterson's manipulative technique. *Left*: An assistant grabs the arm proximally with one hand placed medially against the distal humerus. The surgeon applies distal traction with the forearm supinated and pulls the forearm into varus. *Right*: Digital pressure applied directly over the tilted radial head completes the reduction. (Redrawn with permission from Patterson RF. Treatment of displaced transverse fractures of the neck of the radius in children. *J Bone Joint Surg* 1934;16:696–698.)

Although forearm supination relaxes the supinator muscle, supination may not be the best position for manipulation of the head fragment. Jeffrey (5) pointed out that the tilt of the radial head can be anterior or posterior depending on the position of the forearm at the time of injury. With this degree of rotation, the prominent tilt of the proximal fragment can be felt laterally. The direction of maximal tilt can be confirmed by x-ray. The best position for reduction is the degree of rotation that places the radial head most prominent laterally. If the x-ray beam is perpendicular to the head in maximal tilt, it casts an oblong or rectangular shadow; if not, the shadow is oval or almost circular (5). With a varus force applied across the extended elbow, the maximal tilt directed laterally, and the elbow in varus, the radial head can be reduced with the pressure of a finger (see Fig. 11-19, *right*).

Kaufman et al (53) proposed another technique in which the elbow is manipulated in the flexed position. The surgeon presses his or her thumb against the anterior surface of the radial head with the forearm in pronation.

Most authors recommend immobilization in pronation after reduction because it is the forearm motion most often restricted after fracture (21). Some have recommended supination because they believe it is easier for the patient to regain active pronation than active supination during rehabilitation. Whether pronation or supination is chosen, they recommend 90 degrees of flexion for the elbow. Fluoroscopy can determine whether pronation or supination results in the optimal reduction of the fracture.

In uncommon circumstances, the head fragment may lie proximal to the neck and parallel to its long axis. In four reports since 1960, the authors accepted the result of closed reduction (39,54,55). On closer inspection the head was rotated 180 degrees so that the articular surface of the head was facing the fracture surface of the radial neck.

Operative Techniques

Although most fractures are stable after reduction, redisplacement can occur, especially if the initial tilt was more than 60 degrees (32,56). Fractures with more than 90 degrees of angulation, especially those in which the head fragment is lying free in the joint, are almost impossible to reduce by closed methods.

Percutaneous Pin Reduction. The use of percutaneous pin reduction with an image intensifier is a popular method of satisfactorily reducing moderately to severely displaced fractures (52,57–60). Various authors have used an awl, a Steinmann pin (61), a periosteal elevator (62), or a double-pointed "bident"

(57) that in theory controls rotation better. Pesudo et al, in their series of 22 displaced radial neck fractures, found that the results after percutaneous pin reduction were superior to those after open reduction (59).

Biyani et al (63) described driving the pin used to reduce the radial head across the fracture site to stabilize it. The pin is removed and motion is allowed after 3 weeks.

Intramedullary Pin Reduction. In 1980, Metaizeau et al (64) proposed reducing severely tilted radial neck fractures with an intramedullary wire passed from the distal metaphysis. A report 13 years later (65) demonstrated the effectiveness of this technique. A wire is inserted into the medullary canal through an entrance hole in the distal metaphysis (Fig. 11-20). Once the wire reaches the fracture site, the angulation at the tip enables it to engage the proximal fracture site at the neck. Once engaged, the wire is twisted to reduce the head and neck fragment. This technique has produced results superior to open reduction with fewer complications (66,67).

Wallace Method for Reduction of Radial Neck Fracture. Fluoroscopy in an AP projection is used to determine the forearm rotation that exposes the maximal amount of deformity of the fracture, and the level of the bicipital tuberosity of the proximal radius is marked. A 1-cm dorsal skin incision is made at that level just lateral to the subcutaneous border of the ulna. A Joker Elevator is gently inserted between the ulna and the radius, with care not to disrupt the periosteum of the radius or the ulna. The radial shaft usually is much more ulnarly displaced than expected, and the radial nerve is lateral to the radius at this level. While counterpressure is applied against the radial head, the distal fragment of the radius is levered away from the ulna. An assistant can aid in this maneuver by gently applying traction and rotating the forearm back and forth to disimpact the fracture fragments. If necessary to correct angulation, a percutaneous Kirschner wire can be inserted into the fracture site, parallel to the radial head, to lever the physis perpendicular to the axis of the radius.

Once an adequate reduction has been obtained, an oblique Kirschner wire is inserted to provide fracture fixation. The wire is removed 3 weeks after surgery (Figs. 11-21 and 11-22).

Open Reduction. With valgus injuries, a residual tilt of 45 degrees probably produces as good a result as trying to achieve a perfect reduction surgically. An acceptable closed reduction can produce a better result than an anatomically perfect open surgical reduction (Table 11-3).

Early reviews reported poor results with significant loss of range of motion in patients treated operatively (9,11,14,21) but more recently Steinberg et al (13) combined their results of open reduction of severely displaced fractures with those of five other series (5,14,32,59) and reported 49% good results after operative treatment compared to 25% after nonoperative treatment. None of these authors used percutaneous pin reduction. The results of moderately displaced fractures treated operatively were equal to the results of those treated nonoperatively.

If the head of the radius is completely displaced, results usually are better with surgical intervention. Some authors have

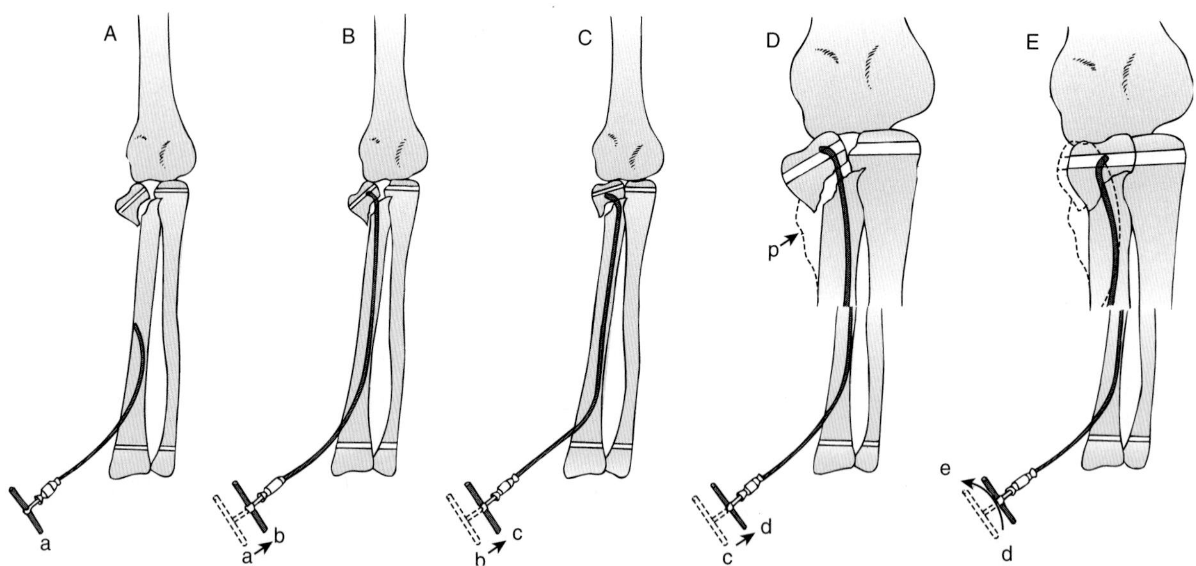

FIGURE 11-20 Intramedullary pin reduction. **A.** The insertion point for the curved flexible pin is in the metaphysis. **B.** The curved end of the rod passes in the shaft and engages the proximal fragment. **C.** Manipulation of the rod disimpacts the fracture. **D,E.** Once disimpacted, the head fragment is rotated into position with the intramedullary rod. (From Metaizeau JP, Lascombes P, Lemelle JL, et al. Reduction and fixation of displaced radial neck fractures by closed intramedullary pinning. *J Pediatr Orthop* 1993;13:355–356; with permission.)

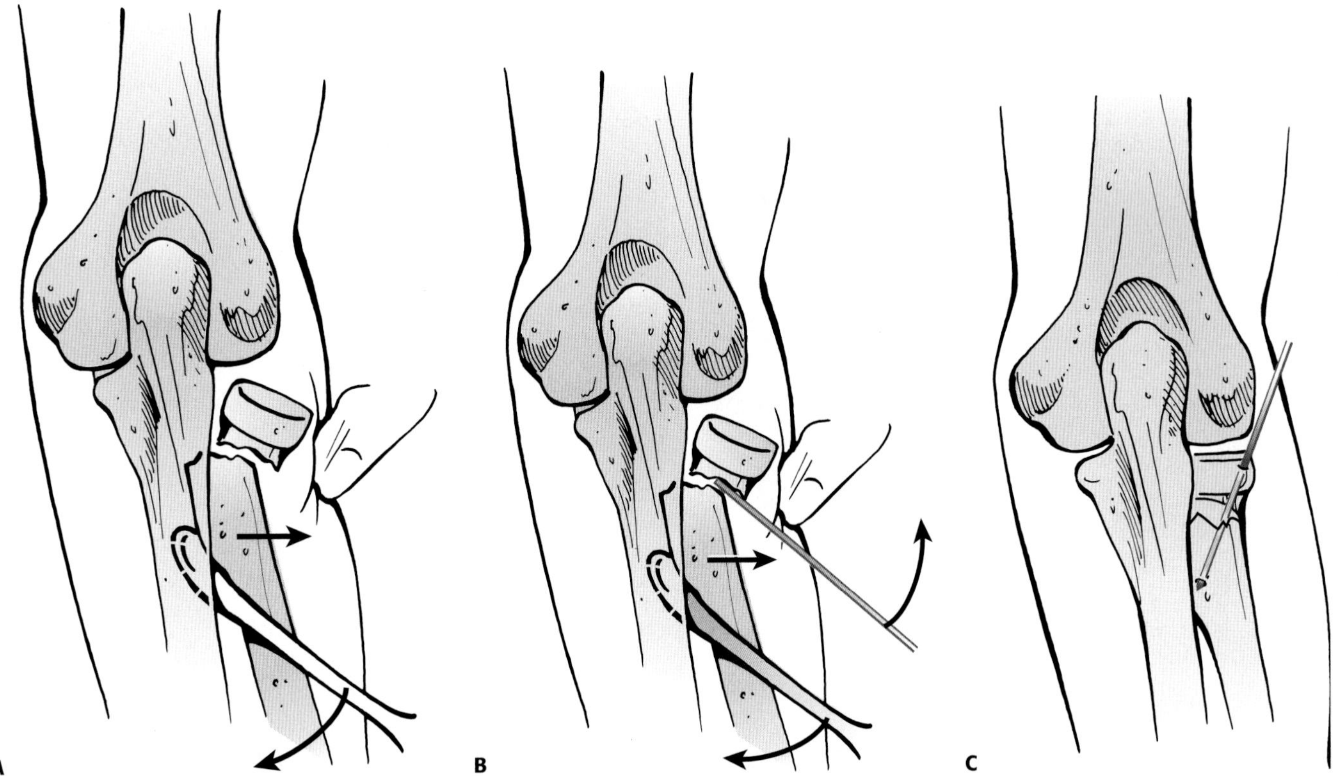

FIGURE 11-21 Wallace radial head reduction technique. **A.** A Joker Elevator is used to lever the distal fragment laterally while the thumb pushes the proximal fragment medially. **B.** Kirschner wires are used to assist the reduction if necessary. **C.** The position of the reduction can be fixed with an oblique Kirschner wire.

shown that a completely separated radial head remains viable if surgically replaced as late as 48 hours after injury (8,68).

Some fractures may be irreducible by closed means because interposition of the capsule or annular ligament between the head and neck blocks reduction (19). Strong et al (69) described an unusual fracture pattern in which the radial head was trapped by the orbicular ligament. They found that these fractures were irreducible by closed methods and required open reduction.

Fixation Methods. Some authors have recommended inserting a small wire through the capitellum across the radial head and into the neck to fix radial head fractures (17,27,61), but this technique has a high incidence of complications (4,11,21,30). Even in a long-arm cast, the elbow joint has slight motion, which can cause the pin to fatigue and break (Fig. 11-23). The retrieval of the remaining portion of the pin from the proximal radius is almost impossible without imposing considerable trauma. Even if the pin does not break, the motion of the pin may erode the joint surface and fragment the radial head (11,21).

Other suggested methods of fixing the displaced radial neck after open reduction include intramedullary bone pegs, direct pin insertion through the head by way of an olecranon osteotomy (70), or with a forked plate (71).

The most common technique in current use involves placement of a pin obliquely across the fracture site into the radial head (4,32,52). The pin can be placed either proximal to distal (Fig. 11-24) or, preferably, distal to proximal. The protruding pin is easy to remove after the fracture heals.

Some believe that internal fixation is unnecessary after open reduction (11,21,49). Wedge and Robertson (21) found that patients without internal fixation had more good results than those with internal fixation. Use of internal fixation does not guarantee that the fragment will not slip. Newman (11) described two patients in whom the head slipped postoperatively despite Kirschner wire fixation.

One complication of open reduction is injury to the posterior interosseous nerve. To avoid this complication, Jones and Esah (32) recommended identifying the nerve as it courses through the supinator muscle. Kaplan (72) and Strachan and Ellis (73) demonstrated that with the forearm in pronation, the posterior interosseous nerve displaces ulnarward, out of the way of the surgical dissection. They also recommended that the patient be prone during exploration of the proximal radius to help keep the forearm pronated.

The orbicular ligament should be left intact if possible. If dividing it is necessary for reduction, it should be repaired (4).

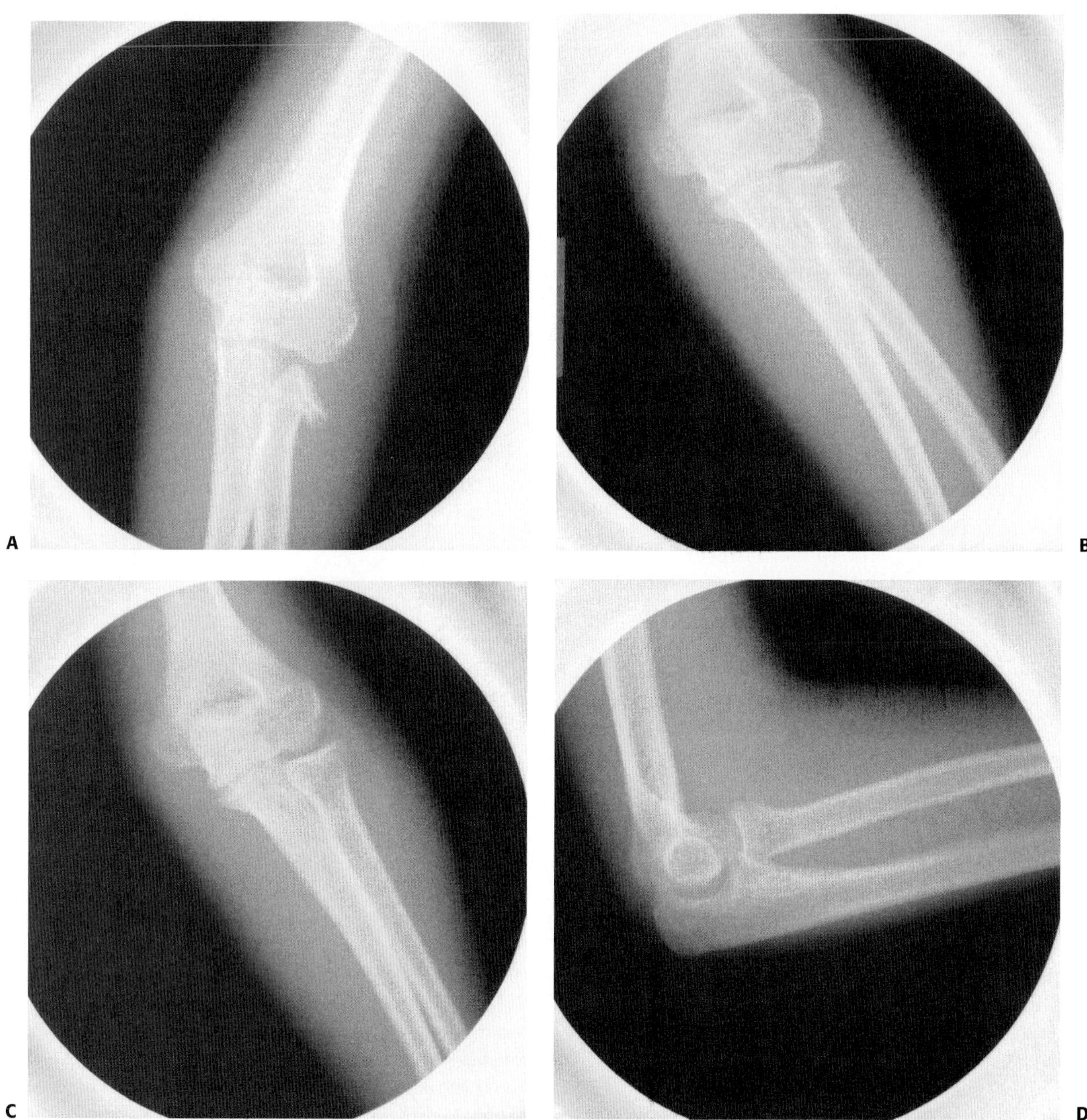

FIGURE 11-22 **A.** Radial neck fracture angulated 45 degrees in a 14-year-old girl. **B.** X-ray after closed reduction using thumb pressure on the radial head. **C.** Final reduction after manipulation of the distal fragment with an elevator using the Wallace technique. **D.** Lateral view of the elbow after reduction.

TABLE 11-3 Acceptable Reduction

Less than 45 degrees of angulation
No translation
50 to 60 degrees of pronation and supination on clinical examination

Type B Injuries. For type B (Salter-Harris type IV) fractures, a small marginal fragment can be safely removed and the remaining large portion of the head reduced without internal fixation (21).

Radial Head Fractures. Pelto et al (74) reported good to excellent results with the use of absorbable polyglycolide pins in patients older than 13 years of age. "Transient local abacterial tissue reaction" occurred but did not lead to any long-term negative effects. There was no comment on the effect on the physis.

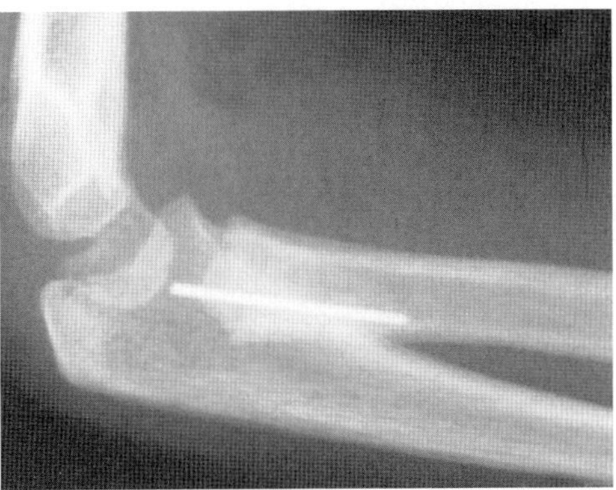

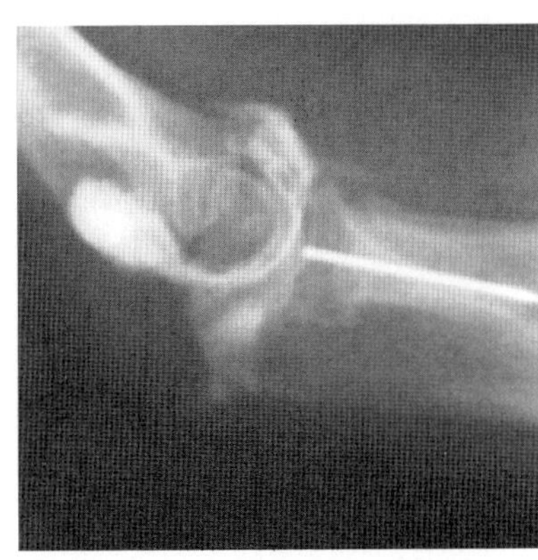

FIGURE 11-23 Transcapitellar pin in a 4-year-old with a completely displaced fracture of the radial neck. **A.** Three weeks after injury, when the pin was removed, it had fractured and a portion remained in the proximal radius. **B.** An arthrogram revealed that the fractured end was at the joint surface of the radial head. The piece was left in place, with subsequent resumption of normal elbow motion.

To fix a large displaced head fragment in a Salter-Harris type III or IV fracture, a transepiphyseal screw is useful (Fig. 11-25).

Radial Head Excision. Resection of the radial head fragment was popular in the 1920s and 1930s, but reported results have been uniformly poor (2,32,56). Cubitus valgus and radial deviation at the wrist are common sequelae. The procedure is contraindicated in a growing child.

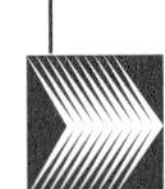

AUTHORS' PREFERRED TREATMENT

We tend to be as conservative as possible in treating these fractures (Table 11-4). Although they may appear reasonably minor both radiographically and clinically, we initially emphasize to the parents that some loss of motion may occur even with an anatomic reduction. The problem is usually a loss of range of motion in supination and pronation. Little pain or loss of upper extremity function occurs despite the residual loss of forearm rotation.

Nonoperative Methods

Moderate Tilt (30 to 60 Degrees). If the radial head is tilted more than 30 degrees, we attempt a manipulative closed reduction. If there is a great amount of pain or resistance to pronation and supination, we aspirate the elbow after a sterile preparation and frequently inject 2 to 3 mL of 1% lidocaine (75), but a general anesthetic is preferable for full relaxation. We prefer the Israeli technique for simple, moderately

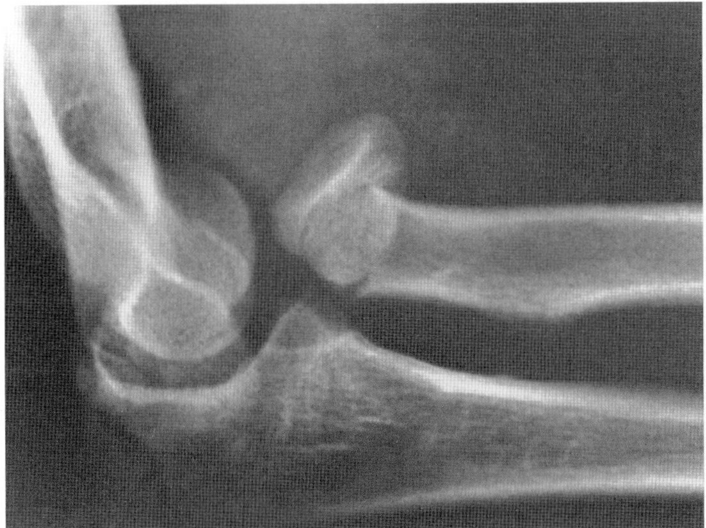

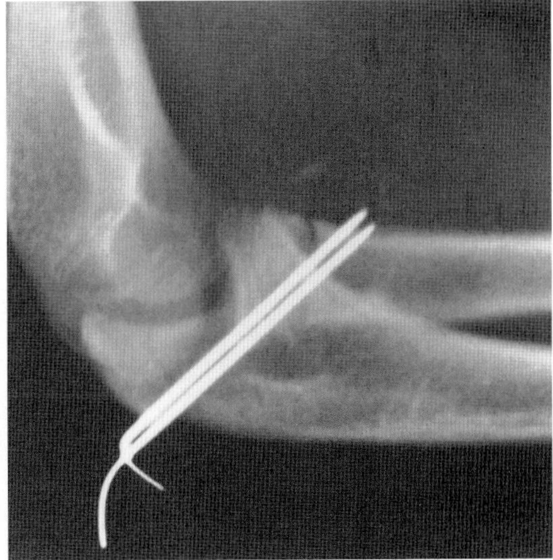

FIGURE 11-24 Oblique pin. **A.** Displaced fracture of the radial neck in a 10-year-old. **B.** A closed reduction was performed, and to stabilize the head fragment two pins were placed percutaneously and obliquely across the fracture site from proximal to distal. If open reduction and pinning are done, the preferred alignment is obliquely across the fracture site from distal to proximal. (From Wilkins KE, ed. *Operative management of upper extremity fractures in children.* Rosemont, IL: American Academy of Orthopaedic Surgeons, 1994:57; with permission.)

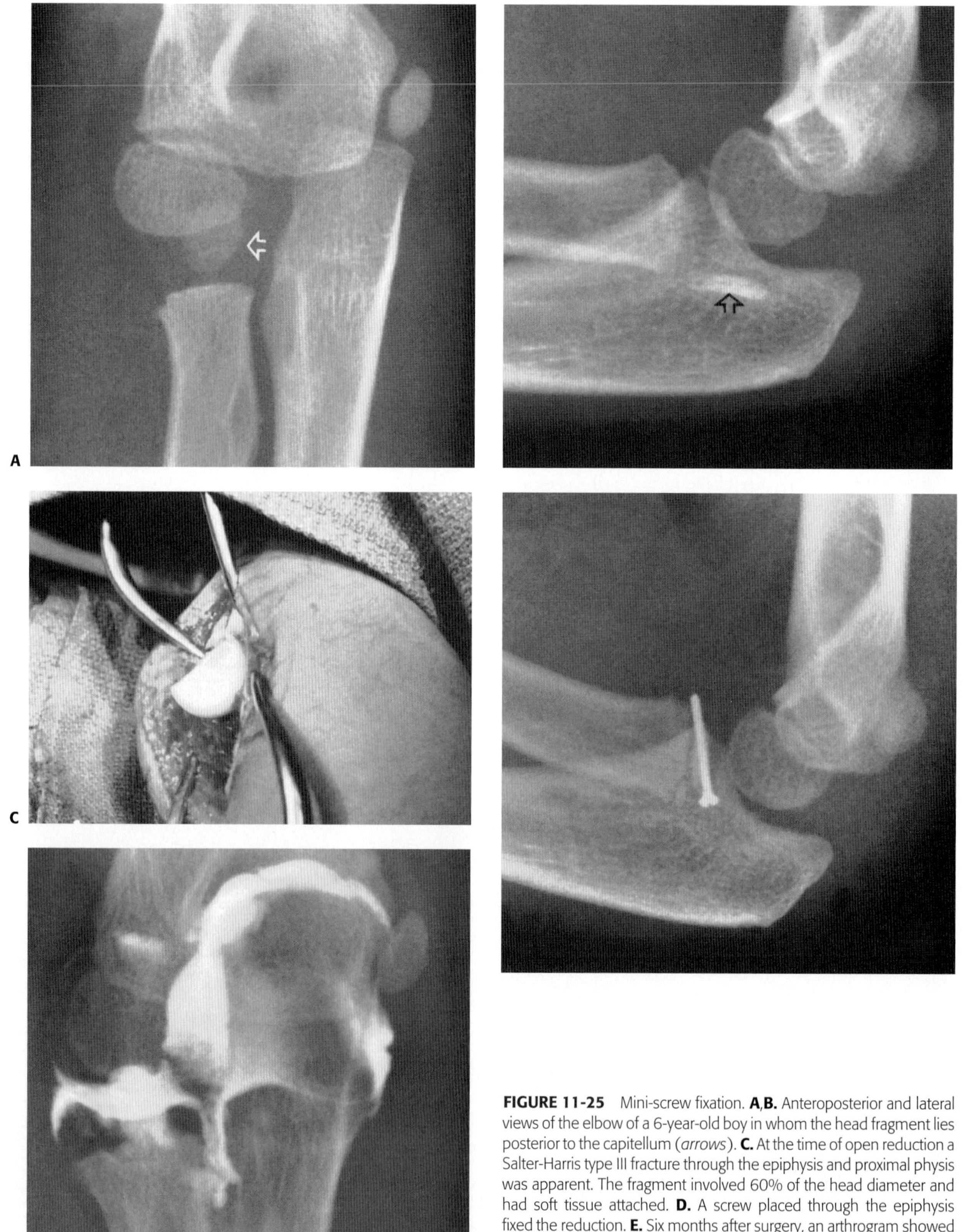

FIGURE 11-25 Mini-screw fixation. **A,B.** Anteroposterior and lateral views of the elbow of a 6-year-old boy in whom the head fragment lies posterior to the capitellum (*arrows*). **C.** At the time of open reduction a Salter-Harris type III fracture through the epiphysis and proximal physis was apparent. The fragment involved 60% of the head diameter and had soft tissue attached. **D.** A screw placed through the epiphysis fixed the reduction. **E.** Six months after surgery, an arthrogram showed maintenance of the architectural structure of the medial head after screw removal. The patient had 60 degrees of supination and pronation. (From Wilkins KE, ed. *Operative management of upper extremity fractures in children.* Rosemont, IL: American Academy of Orthopaedic Surgeons, 1994:58; with permission.)

TABLE 11-4 Treatment of Radial Head Fractures

Fracture Status	Treatment
Minimally displaced (<30 degrees angulation, no translation)	Long-arm cast or posterior splint (7–10 days) Early motion
Angulation >30 degrees	Closed reduction under general anesthesia using flexion–pronation (Israeli) technique Long-arm cast (10–14 days)
Angulation >45 degrees	Elastic bandage wrap reduction Flexion–pronation (Israeli) reduction technique Percutaneous pin reduction Long-arm cast (10–14 days)
Angulation fixed at >40 degrees, translation >3 mm	Percutaneous wire reduction
Displacement, with <60 degrees supination–pronation, radial head completely displaced	Open reduction (± internal fixation)

displaced radial head fractures (Fig. 11-26). The important aspect is to ensure that the elbow is flexed at 90 degrees for the manipulation. Usually there is resistance to pronation (Fig. 11-27). With thumb pressure applied to the radial head, the opposite hand forces the forearm into full pronation (see Fig. 11-27). After reduction, the range of motion should be at least 60 degrees of supination and pronation (see Fig. 11-26B). If the range of supination and pronation is adequate, we accept the reduction regardless of the x-ray appearance. We attempt closed reduction first even with completely displaced radial neck fractures. Occasionally a surprisingly satisfactory reduction can be obtained (Fig. 11-28).

Elastic Bandage Wrap. If we cannot obtain an adequate reduction using the Patterson or Israeli technique, we try some other techniques before surgical intervention. Serendipitously, Chambers found that he could reduce the fracture by wrapping the extremity tightly from distal to proximal with an elastic Esmarch bandage (Fig. 11-29).

Operative Techniques

Percutaneous Pin Reduction. We try every manipulative technique before we resort to open reduction. For most moderately or severely displaced fractures, we attempt a semiclosed reduction using the percutaneous pin reduction technique (Fig. 11-30). A good image intensifier is essential. We have found that a single-point awl or the blunt end of a Steinmann pin is adequate. If the radial head is small or soft, we use a small Craig biopsy needle or the blunt end of the Steinmann pin to prevent penetration of the radial head with a sharp end of a Steinmann pin.

To avoid injury to the posterior interosseous nerve, we insert the pin as closely as possible to the lateral aspect of the olecranon (see Fig. 11-30A). Again, we accept 45 to 60 degrees of angulation as long as the displacement is small and the patient has at least 50 to 60 degrees of supination and pronation after reduction.

Elevator Reduction Technique. We have found the Wallace method for manipulating the distal fragment useful for displaced fractures (see Figs. 11-21 and 11-22).

Open Reduction

If an adequate closed reduction is not possible and loss of motion is significant, we prefer an open reduction with as little dissection as possible. We approach the fracture with the patient prone and the forearm pronated. After making the skin incision, we dissect between the anconeus and extensor carpi ulnaris muscles to reach the orbicular ligament and reposition the head as gently as possible. Usually, the head fragment is stable after reduction. If it is not, we stabilize the reduction with a small pin placed obliquely through a separate stab incision from distal to proximal across the fracture site.

Delayed Reduction

If the fracture is more than 4 days old and there is no significant supination or pronation forearm motion, we reduce the head surgically, if reduction is not possible closed. However, we warn the parents of the possibility for myositis ossificans and proximal radioulnar synostosis.

Immobilization After Reduction

After the reduction, we prefer to immobilize the upper extremity with the elbow in 90 degrees of flexion and the forearm in slight pronation. The patient starts active motion as soon as possible. After a closed reduction, we start gradual active motion at 10 to 14 days, depending on the initial displacement and the degree of stability of reduction. We prefer to use a long-arm cast. The bivalved cast is useful as a splint during rehabilitation.

Associated Injuries and Complications

Complications of fractures of the radial neck and head, especially those associated with other fractures or a dislocation of the elbow, range from the most common problem of loss of motion to rare nerve injuries (Table 11-5). The most complete reviews of these complications are by Steinberg et al (13) and D'Souza et al (9).

(text continues on page 465)

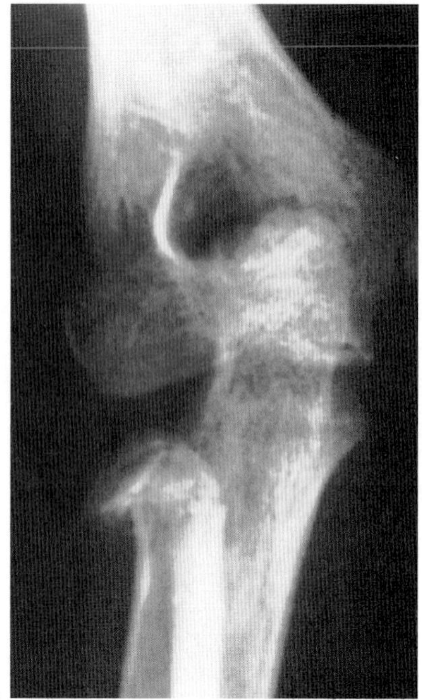

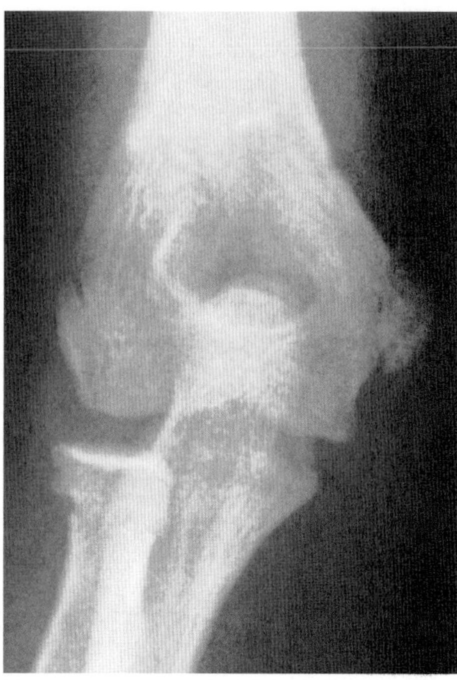

FIGURE 11-26 Flexion–pronation (Israeli) reduction technique. **A.** X-ray of the best reduction obtained by the Patterson method. **B.** Position of the radial head after the flexion–pronation method. (Courtesy of Gerald R. Williams, MD.)

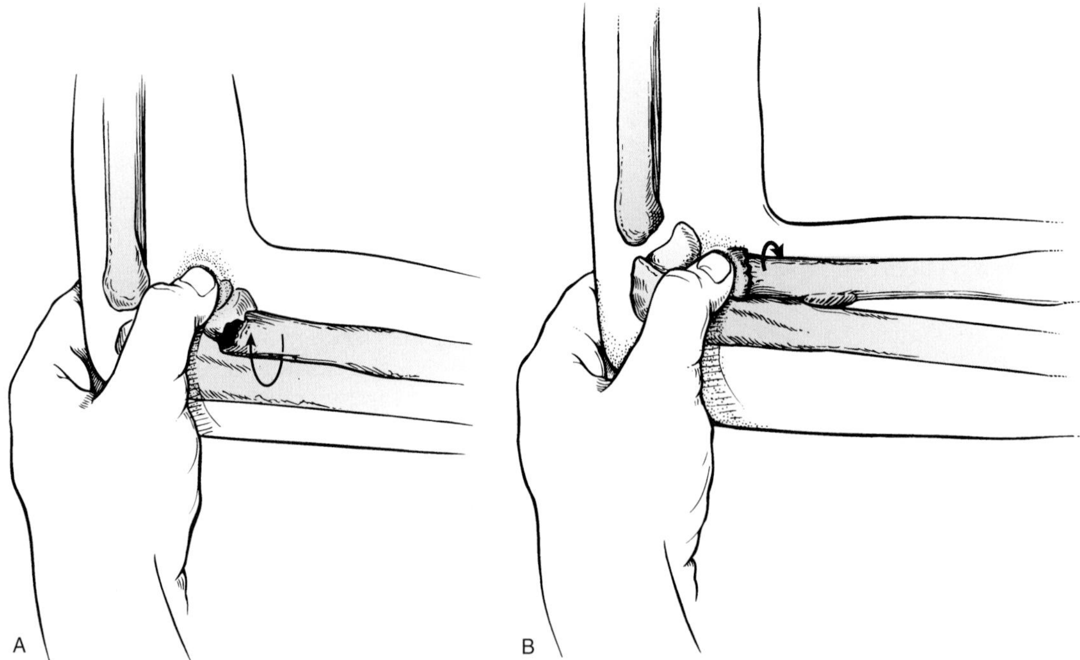

FIGURE 11-27 Flexion–pronation (Israeli) reduction technique. **A.** With the elbow in 90 degrees of flexion, the thumb stabilizes the displaced radial head. Usually the distal radius is in a position of supination. The forearm is pronated to swing the shaft up into alignment with the neck (*arrow*). **B.** Movement is continued to full pronation for reduction (*arrow*). (See also Fig. 11-18.)

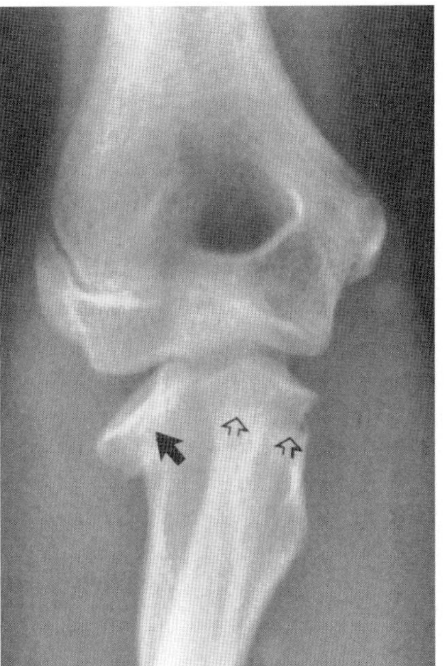

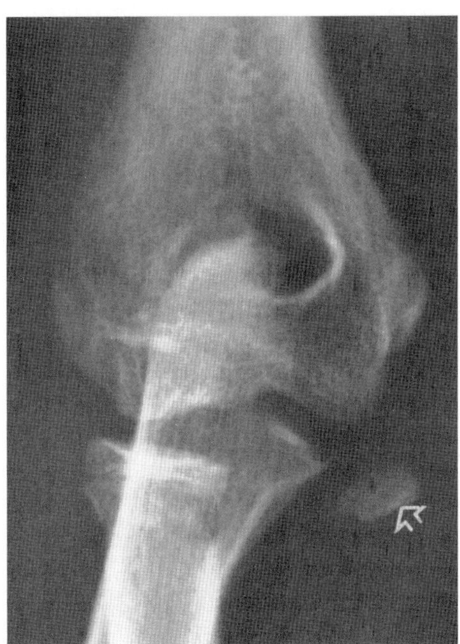

FIGURE 11-28 Widely displaced fracture of the radial head in a 9-year-old girl. **A.** The neck fragment (*open arrows*) was medial and the head fragment (*closed arrow*) remained within the orbicular ligament. **B.** Reduction was satisfactory using the flexion–pronation method. The small fragment medially (*arrow*) is from the metaphysis. The patient resumed full rotation of the forearm after reduction. (From Wilkins KE, ed. *Operative management of upper extremity fractures in children.* Rosemont, IL: American Academy of Orthopaedic Surgeons, 1994:55; with permission.)

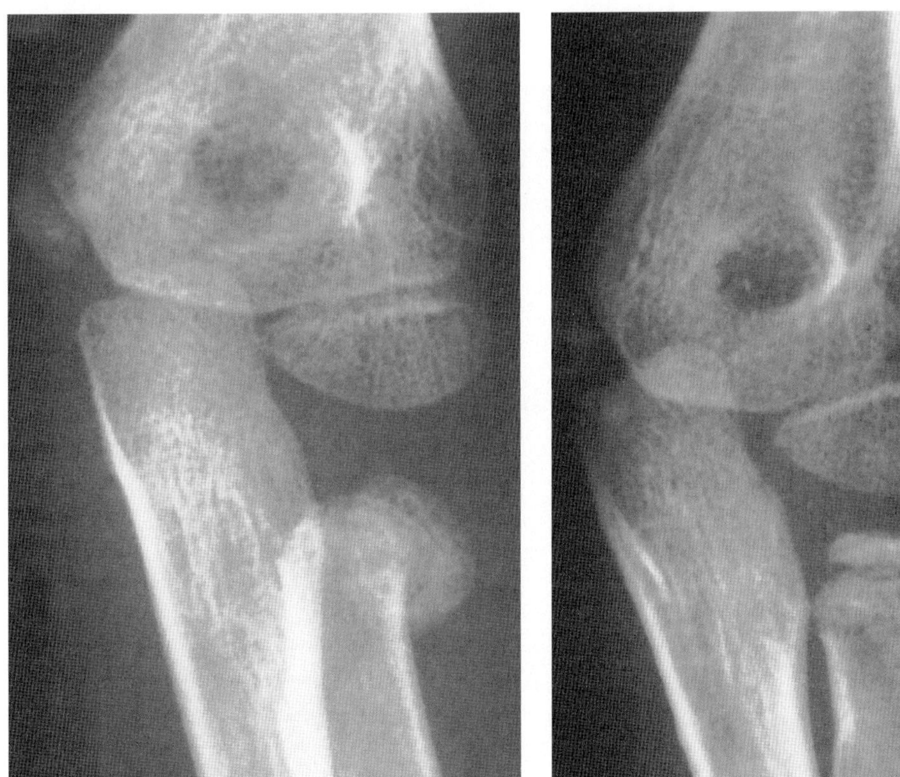

FIGURE 11-29 Elastic bandage wrap reduction. **A.** The final position achieved after manipulation by the Patterson method. **B.** Position of the radial head after applying an elastic bandage to exsanguinate the extremity.

FIGURE 11-30 Percutaneous pin reduction. **A.** Image intensification shows the awl inserted next to the olecranon and directed proximally toward the radial head fragment. This is to avoid injury to the posterior interosseous nerve. **B.** Totally displaced valgus injury. **C.** Position of the Steinmann pin during reduction. **D.** Appearance 2 months after surgery. The patient has 60 degrees of supination and pronation with full elbow extension and flexion.

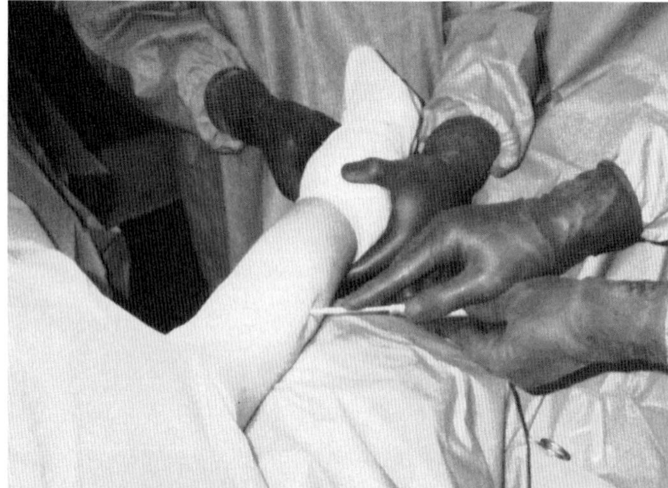
A

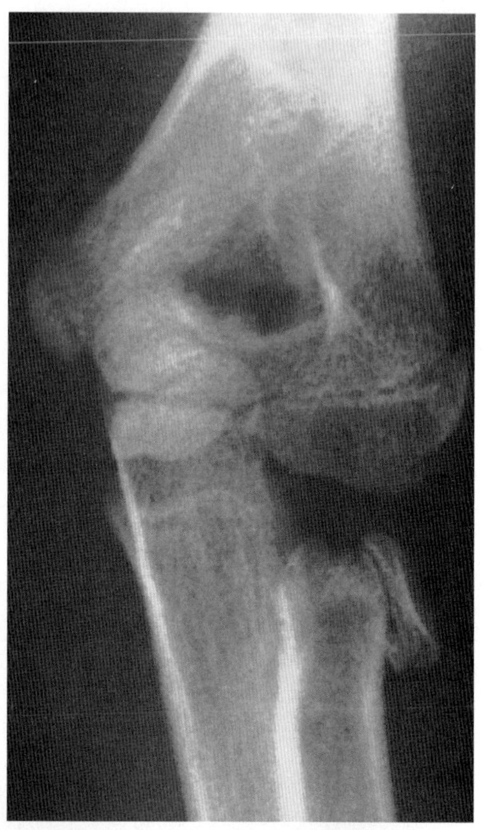
B

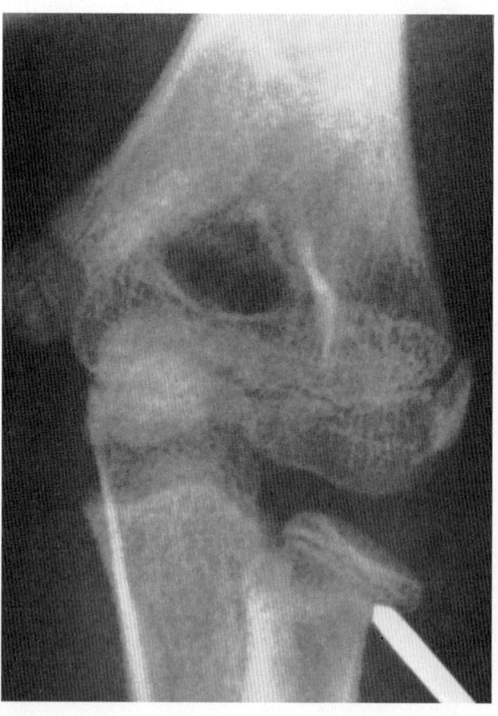
C

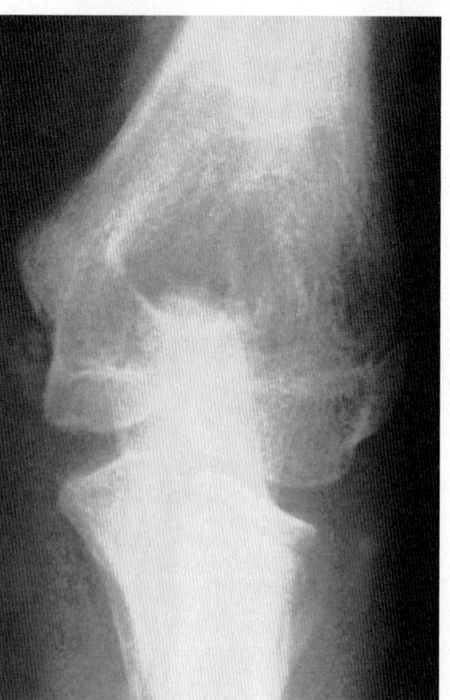
D

TABLE 11-5 Complications of Radial Head and Neck Fractures

Failure to obtain acceptable reduction
Loss of motion (expected)
Radial head overgrowth
Notching of the radial neck
Premature physeal closure
Angular deformities
Nonunion
Osteonecrosis
Radioulnar synostosis
Problems with initial diagnosis

Loss of Motion

Loss of motion is secondary to a combination of loss of joint congruity and fibrous adhesions. Loss of pronation is more common than loss of supination. Flexion and extension rarely are significantly limited. Enlargement of the radial head, a common sequela, can contribute to the subsequent loss of elbow motion (8).

Radial Head Overgrowth

Next to loss of range of motion of the elbow and forearm, radial head overgrowth is probably the most common sequela (20% to 40%) (9,15). The increased vascularity from the injury probably stimulates epiphyseal growth. Radial head overgrowth usually does not compromise functional results (32,52), but it may produce some crepitus or clicking with forearm rotation (9).

Notching of the Radial Neck

O'Brien (7) suggested that notching of the radial head in several patients was secondary to scar tissue forming around the neck from the orbicular ligament. It did not result in any functional deficit. Notching may be a normal variant of radial head anatomy.

Premature Physeal Closure

Many series report premature physeal closure (4,7,8,11,13,21) after fractures of the radial head and neck. This complication did not appear to affect the overall results significantly, except in one patient described by Fowles and Kassab (4), who had a severe cubitus valgus. Newman (11) found that shortening of the radius was never more than 5 mm compared with the opposite uninjured side.

Nonunion of the Radial Neck

Nonunion of the radial neck is rare; union may occur (30) after prolonged treatment (Fig. 11-31).

Osteonecrosis of the Radial Head

The incidence of osteonecrosis is probably higher than recognized. D'Souza et al (9) reported the frequency to be 10% to

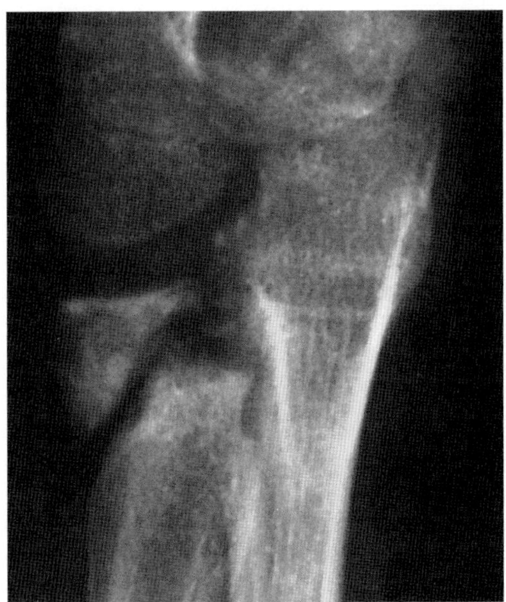

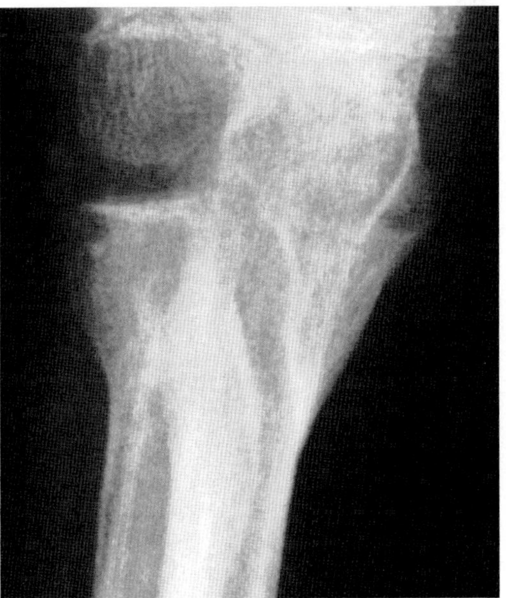

FIGURE 11-31 Nonunion. **A.** Eight months after radial neck fracture in an 8.5-year-old girl. Patient had mild aching pain, but no loss of motion. There was some suggestion of proximal subluxation of the distal radioulnar joint. **B.** Three months later, the fracture is united after long-arm cast immobilization and external electromagnetic stimulation. (Courtesy of Charles T. Price, MD.)

20% in their patients, 70% of whom had open reductions. In patients with open reduction, the overall rate of osteonecrosis was 25%. Jones and Esah (32) and Newman (11) found that patients with osteonecrosis had poor functional results. It has been our experience, however, that revascularization can occur without any significant functional loss. Only in those in whom a residual functional deficit occurs is osteonecrosis considered a problem (Fig. 11-32).

Changes in Carrying Angle (Cubitus Valgus)

In patients who have fractures of the radial neck, the carrying angle often is 10 degrees more (increased cubitus valgus) than on the uninjured side (9,32). The increase in carrying angle appears to produce no functional deficit and no significant deformity.

Vascular Injuries

There are no reports of major vascular injuries with isolated fractures of the proximal radius.

Nerve Injuries

Partial ulnar nerve injury (2) and posterior interosseous nerve injury may occur as a direct result of the fracture, but most injuries to the posterior interosseous nerves are caused by surgical exploration (9) or percutaneous pin reduction (38). These posterior interosseous nerve injuries usually are transient.

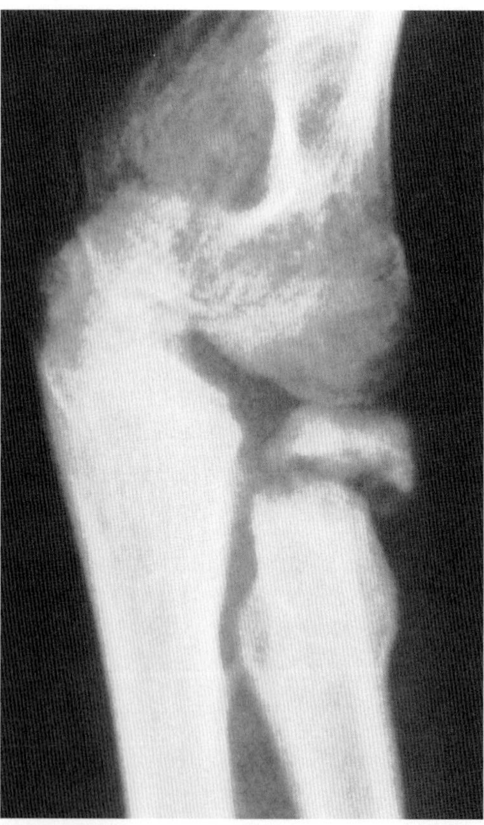

FIGURE 11-32 Osteonecrosis with nonunion in a radial head 1 year after open reduction. Both nonunion and osteonecrosis of the radial neck and head are present. Severe degenerative arthritis developed subsequently. (Courtesy of Richard E. King, MD.)

Compartment Syndrome

Peters and Scott (76) described three patients with volar forearm compartment syndrome after minimally displaced or angulated fractures of the radial head. All required volar fasciotomy.

Radioulnar Synostosis

Proximal synostosis is the most serious complication that can occur after radial head fracture (Fig. 11-33). It occurs most often after open reduction of severely displaced fractures (2,8,11,60), but it can occur after closed reduction. Delayed treatment increases the likelihood of this complication. All three patients described by Gaston et al (8) had treatment initiated more than 5 days after injury.

Myositis Ossificans

Myositis ossificans is relatively common but usually does not impair function. Vahvanen (15) noted that some myositis ossificans occurred in 32% of his patients. In most, it was limited to the supinator muscle. If ossification was more extensive and was associated with a synostosis, the results were poor.

Osteomyelitis

Veranis reported a rare case of hematogenous osteomyelitis after a closed fracture of the radial neck (77). The diagnosis was delayed despite the fact that the child had fever and continuous pain after the fracture.

Malunion

Failure to reduce a displaced and angulated proximal radial fracture in a young child often results in an angulated radial neck with subsequent incongruity of both the proximal radioulnar joint and the radiocapitellar joint (Fig. 11-34). Partial physeal arrest also can create this angulation (see Fig. 11-5).

In our experience, this malunion, because of the incongruity of the radiocapitellar joint, often results in erosion of the articular surface of the capitellum, with subsequent degenerative joint disease. In the English literature, there is little information about using osteotomies of the radial neck to correct this deformity.

Summary

Results after open reduction of radial head fractures are less favorable than those after closed reduction. However, fractures requiring open reduction usually are the result of a more severe injury. Closed reductions with angulations of up to 45 degrees produce clinical results as good as those with a more anatomic reduction after operation. The surgeon should warn the parents of the likelihood of residual loss of motion after open reduction. Whenever possible, internal fixation should be avoided.

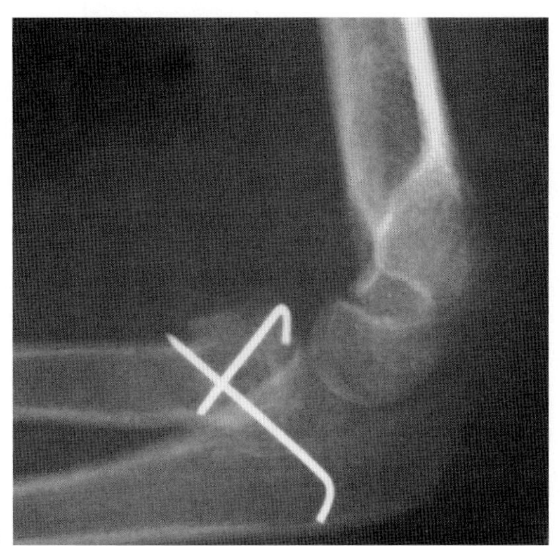
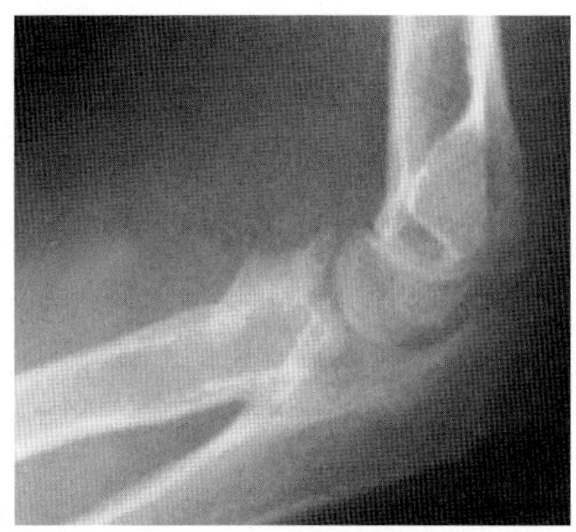
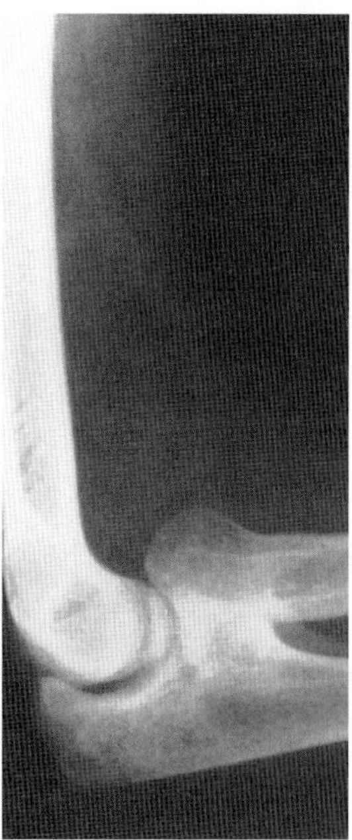

FIGURE 11-33 Radioulnar synostosis. **A.** Surgical intervention with wire fixation was necessary for a satisfactory reduction in this patient who had a totally displaced radial neck fracture. **B.** Six weeks after surgery, there was evidence of a proximal radioulnar synostosis. **C.** X-ray taken 6 months after reduction shows a solid synostosis with anterior displacement of the proximal radius. (Courtesy of R. E. King, MD.)

FRACTURES OF THE PROXIMAL ULNA (OLECRANON)

Fractures Involving the Proximal Apophysis

Incidence

"Separation of the olecranon epiphysis is the rarest form of epiphyseal detachment" (78). This quote from Poland's 1898 textbook on epiphyseal fractures is still true. Only 16 acute fractures of the ulnar apophysis are mentioned in the recent English literature (78–81). In addition to these acute injuries in children, seven have been described in young adults with open physes (82–85). In the French literature, Bracq (86) described 10 patients in whom the fracture extended distal and parallel to the apophyseal line and then crossed it at the articular surface.

Anatomy

The Ossification Process. At birth, the ossification of the metaphysis of the proximal ulna extends only to the midportion of the semilunar notch. At this age, the leading edge of the metaphysis usually is perpendicular to the long axis of the olecranon (Fig. 11-35A,B). As ossification progresses, the proximal border of the metaphysis becomes more oblique. The anterior margin extends proximally and to three fourths of the width of the semilunar notch by 6 years of age. At this age, the physis extends distally to include the coronoid process (see Fig. 11-35C). A secondary center of ossification never in the coronoid process. Just before the development of the secondary center of ossification in the olecranon, the leading edge of the metaphysis develops a well-defined sclerotic margin (80). Ossification of the olecranon occurs in the area of the triceps insertion at approximately 9 years of age (see Fig. 11-35D) (80). Ossification of the coronoid process is completed about the time that the olecranon ossification center appears (78). The term "apophysis" usually is applied to an epiphysis that is subjected to traction by a muscle insertion. "Apophysis" and "epiphysis" are used interchangeably in this chapter to describe the olecranon secondary growth center because it contributes to length and articular surface as well.

Bipartite Centers. The secondary ossification center of the olecranon may be bipartite (87) (see Fig. 11-35E). The major center within the tip of the olecranon is enveloped by the triceps insertion. This was referred to by Porteous (87) as a *traction center*. The second and smaller center, an articular center, lies under the proximal fourth of the articular surface of the semilunar notch.

Closure Process. Fusion of the olecranon epiphysis with the metaphysis, which progresses from anterior to posterior, occurs at approximately 14 years of age. The sclerotic margin that defines the edge of the metaphysis may be mistaken for a fracture (see Fig. 11-35F) (80). Rarely, the physeal line persists into adulthood (82,83,85), usually in athletes who have used the extremity in repetitive throwing activities (84,88–91). The chronic tension forces applied across the apophysis theoretically prevent its normal closure.

(text continues on page 470)

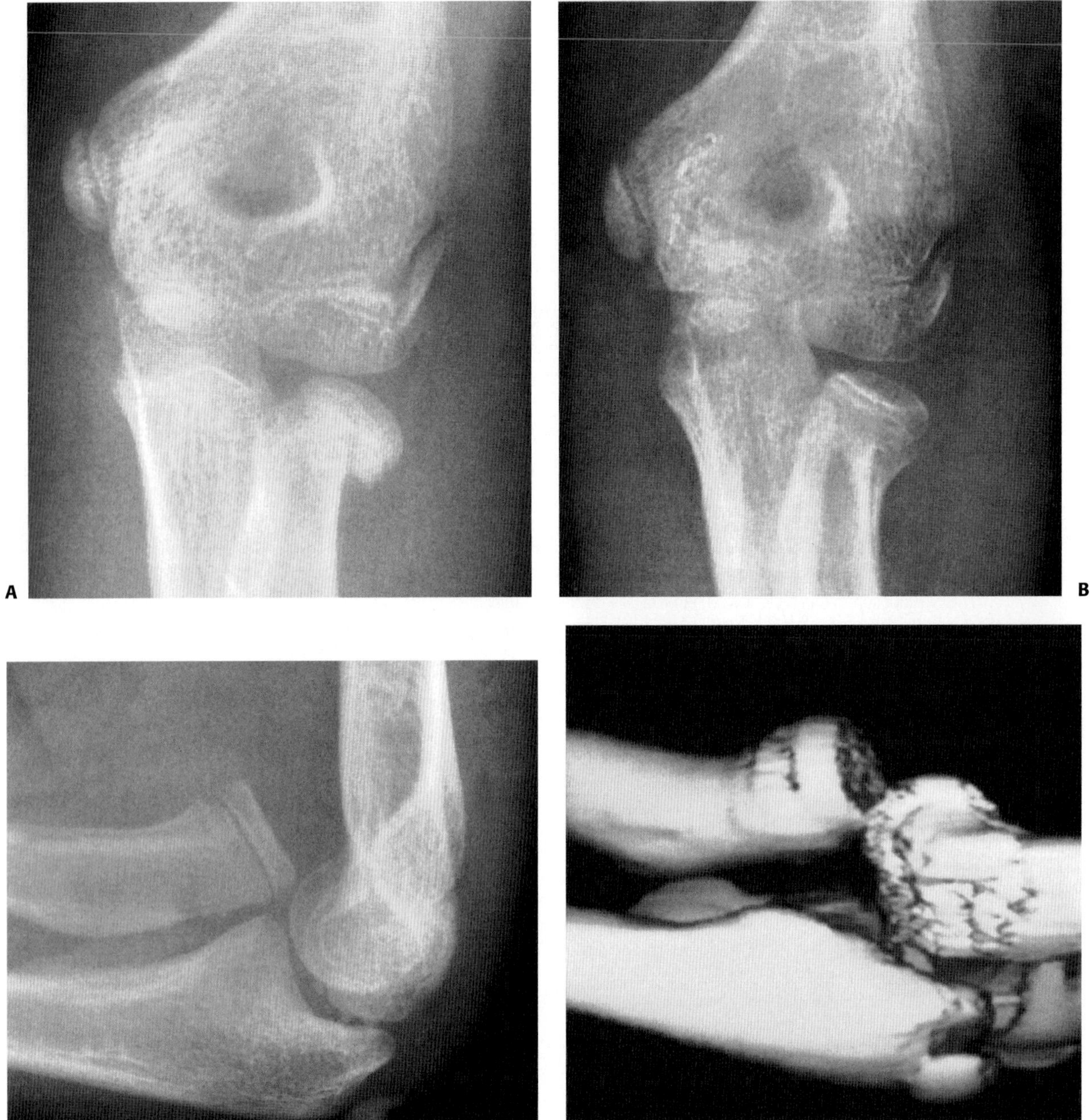

FIGURE 11-34 Angulation. **A.** Injury film showing 30 degrees of angulation and 30% lateral translocation of a radial neck fracture in a 10-year-old. **B.** X-ray appearance of the proximal radius taken about 5 months later, showing lateral angulation of the neck. **C.** Lateral view showing the anterior relationship of the radial neck with proximal migration. At this point the patient had full supination and pronation but a clicking sensation with forearm rotation in the area of the radial head. **D.** 3D reconstruction showing the incongruity of the proximal radiocapitellar joint. (Courtesy of Vince Mosca, MD.)

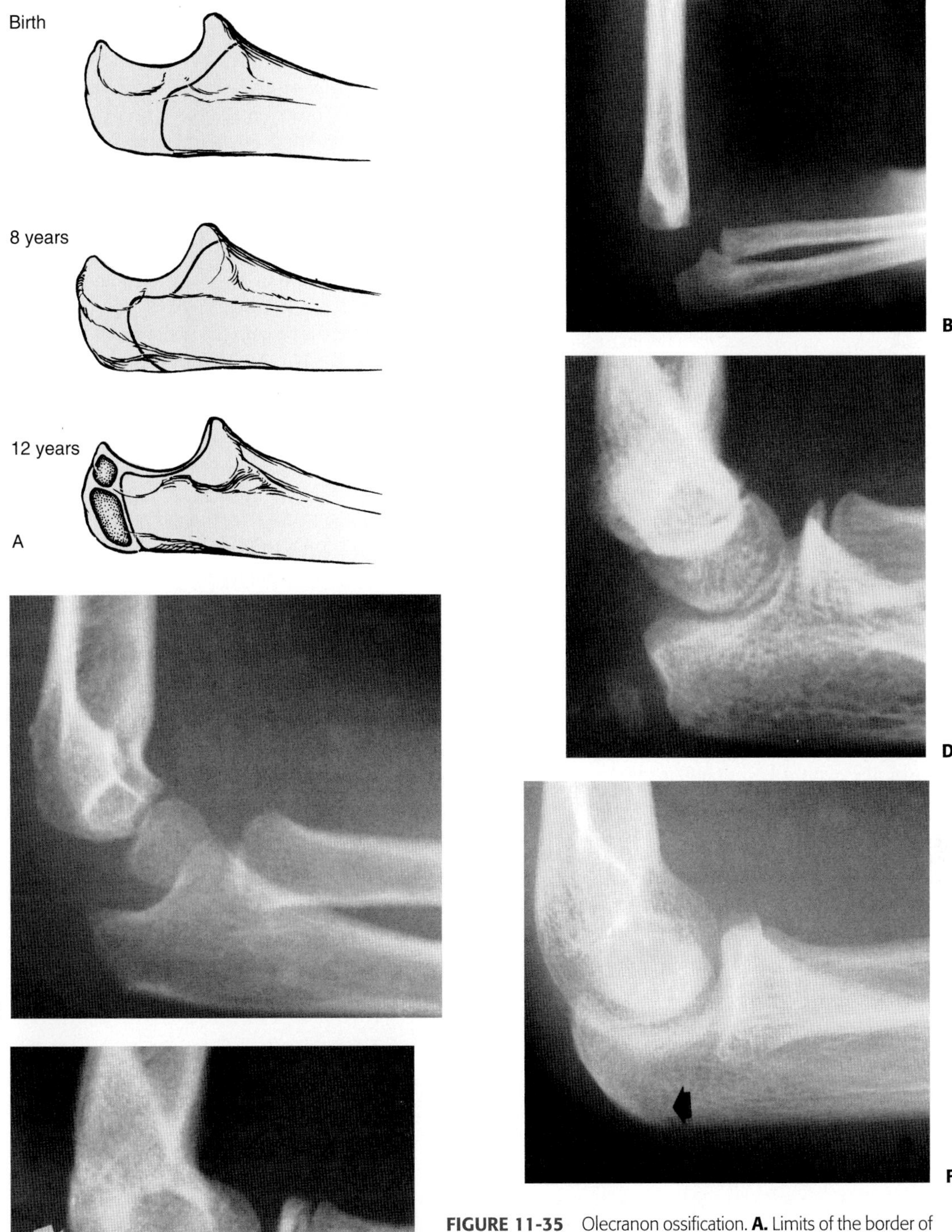

FIGURE 11-35 Olecranon ossification. **A.** Limits of the border of ossification at birth, 8 years, and 12 years. **B.** Lateral view of olecranon at 6 months of age. The proximal margin is perpendicular to the long axis of the ulna. **C.** Lateral view of the olecranon at 6 years of age. The proximal margin is oblique. **D.** Secondary ossification center developing in the olecranon in a 10-year-old. A sclerotic border has developed on the proximal metaphyseal margin. **E.** Bipartite secondary ossification center. The larger center is the traction center (*open arrow*). The smaller, more proximal center is the articular center (*white arrow*). **F.** Before complete fusion, a partial line remains (*arrow*), bordered by a sclerotic margin.

Patella Cubiti. Occasionally, a separate ossification center called a *patella cubiti* develops in the triceps tendon at its insertion on the tip of the olecranon (92). This ossicle is completely separate and can articulate with the trochlea. It usually is unilateral, unlike other persistent secondary ossification centers, which are more likely to be bilateral and familial. Zeitlin (93) believed that the patella cubiti was a traumatic ossicle rather than a developmental variation.

Signs and Symptoms

Clinical: Swelling Plus Defect. The primary clinical findings of an olecranon fracture are tenderness and swelling. If the fragment is completely displaced, the child cannot extend the elbow. A palpable defect may be present between the apophysis and the proximal metaphysis. Poland (78) described the crepitus between the fragments as being muffled because cartilage covers the fracture surfaces.

Radiography: Proximal Metaphyseal Displacement. The radiographic diagnosis may be difficult before ossification of the olecranon apophysis. The only clue may be a displacement of the small ossified metaphyseal fragment (Fig. 11-36), and the diagnosis may be based only on the clinical sign of tenderness over the epiphyseal fragment. If there is any doubt about the degree of displacement, injection of radiopaque material into the joint may delineate the true nature of the fracture.

Mechanism of Injury

The location of the triceps expansion insertion on the metaphysis distal to the physis probably accounts for the rarity of fracture along the physeal line. Only a few reports mention the mechanism of these physeal injuries. In most of the fractures reported by Poland (78), three of which were confirmed by amputation specimens, the force of the injury was applied directly to the elbow. The force may be applied indirectly, producing an avulsion type of fracture. In our experience, this fracture usually is caused by avulsion forces across the apophysis with the elbow flexed, similar to the more common flexion metaphyseal injuries. Children with osteogenesis imperfecta (usually the tarda form) seem especially predisposed to this injury (94,95).

Stress fractures of the olecranon apophysis can occur in athletes (especially baseball players) who place considerable recurrent tension forces on the olecranon (96). Stress injuries also have been reported in elite gymnasts (97) and tennis players (89). If the recurring activity persists, a symptomatic malunion can develop (83,85,89–91).

Classification

Injuries to the apophysis of the olecranon can be classified as one of three types (Table 11-6). Type I is a simple apophysitis in which there is irregularity in the secondary ossification center (88,97) (Fig. 11-37A). The apophyseal line may widen. Type II is an incomplete stress fracture that involves primarily the apophyseal line, with widening and irregularity (see Fig. 11-37B). A small adjacent cyst may form, but usually the architecture of the secondary ossification center is normal. These injuries occur primarily in sports requiring repetitive extension of the elbow, such as baseball pitching (96), tennis (89), or gymnastics (97). Type III injuries involve complete avulsion of the apophysis. True apophyseal avulsions (type IIIA) occur in younger children as a fracture through the apophyseal plate (see Fig. 11-37A,B). In some of his amputation specimens, Poland (78) found that the proximal apophyseal fragment included the distal tongue, which extended up to the coronoid process. Apophyseal–metaphyseal combination fractures (type IIIB), in which metaphyseal fragments are attached to the apophysis (see Fig. 11-37C,D), usually occur in older children. Grantham and Kiernan (79) likened it to a Salter-Harris type II physeal injury. Proximal displacement of the fragment is the only clue seen on an x-ray.

Treatment

There is no standard method of treatment, because few such fractures have been described. For fractures with significant

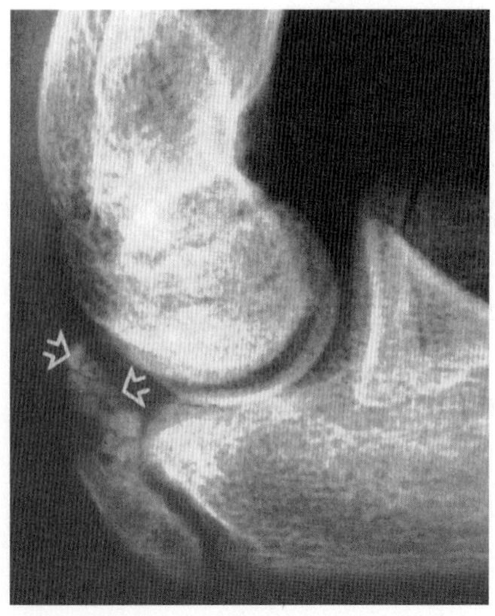

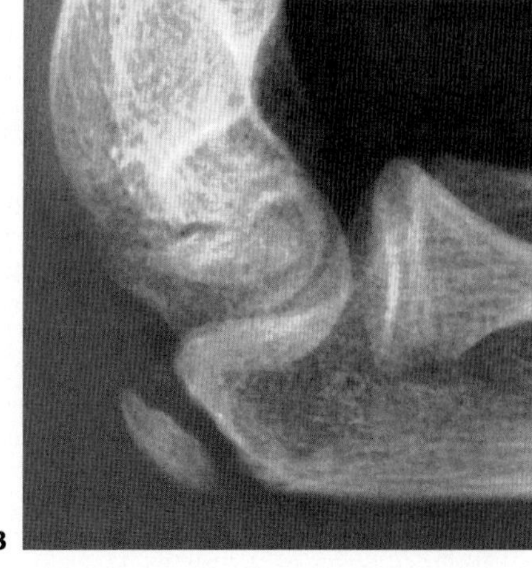

FIGURE 11-36 Apophysitis. **A.** Chronic stimulation with irregular ossification of the articular apophyseal center (*arrows*) in a basketball player who practiced dribbling 3 hours per day. **B.** Normal side for comparison.

TABLE 11-6 Classification of Apophyseal Injuries of the Olecranon

Type I: Apophysitis

Type II: Incomplete stress fracture

Type III: Complete fractures
A. Pure apophyseal avulsions
B. Apophyseal–metaphyseal combinations

displacement, treatment usually is open reduction with internal fixation using a combination of axial pins and tension-band wiring (Fig. 11-38) (78,79,81). There has been concern that applying compressive forces across the apophysis might cause growth arrest. In our experience, fusion of the apophysis to the metaphysis is accelerated. Apophyseal fractures usually occur when the physis is near natural closure. The growth proximally is appositional rather than lengthwise across the apophyseal plate itself. As a result, we have not found any functional shortening of the olecranon because of the early fusion of the apophysis to the metaphysis (see Fig. 11-38D). In practice, the use of a compression screw across an ossified olecranon fracture causes no loss of ulna length. Children who sustain injuries before the development of the secondary ossification center may develop a deformity that is visible on x-rays (Fig. 11-39). Although there may be shortening of the olecranon, it does not appear to produce functional problems. There are no reports of the effects of this injury in very young children or infants. Most stress injuries respond to simple rest from the offending activity. However, a chronic stress fracture can result in a symptomatic nonunion. Use of a compressive screw alone across the nonunion often is sufficient (97), but supplemental bone grafting may be necessary to achieve union (82,83).

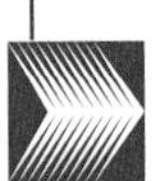

AUTHORS' PREFERRED TREATMENT

Undisplaced Fractures

For apophysitis and undisplaced stress fractures, we ask the patient to cease the offending activity. During this period of rest, the patient should maintain upper extremity strength with a selective muscle exercise program as well as maintain cardiovascular conditioning. When a persistent nonunion of

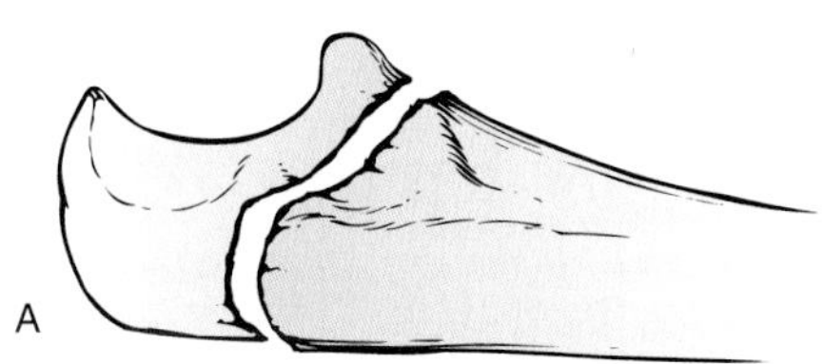

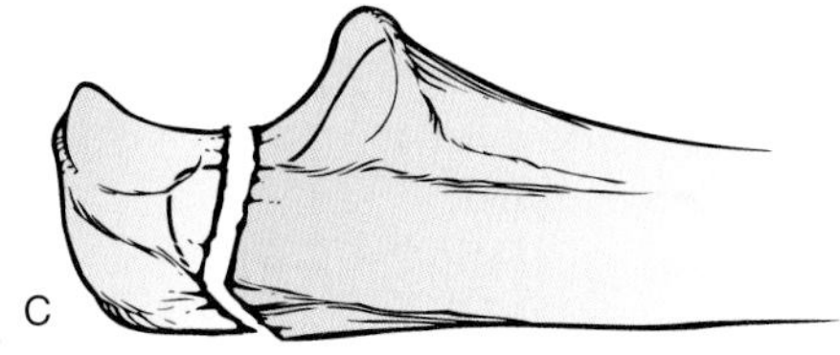

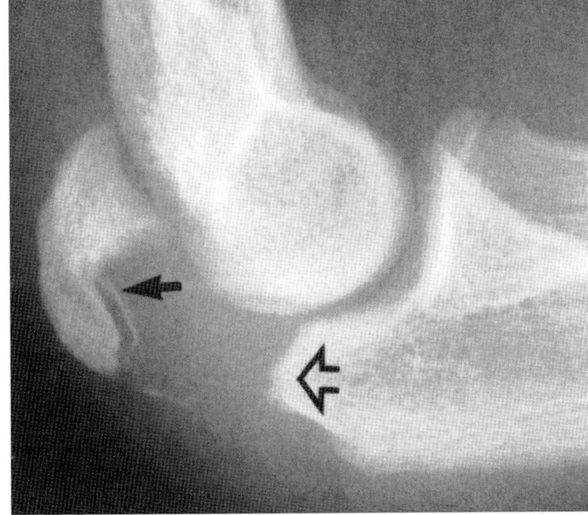

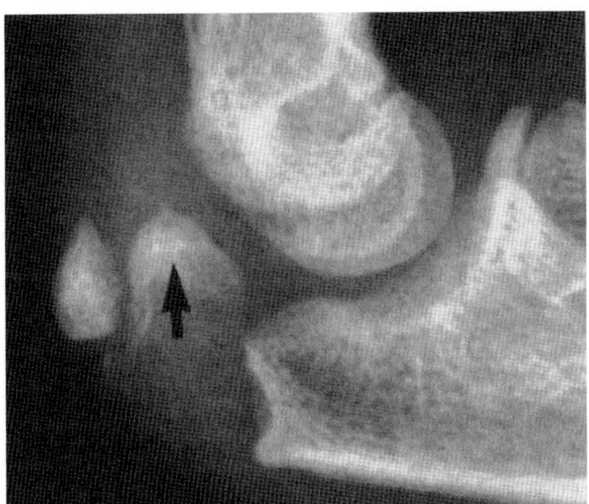

FIGURE 11-37 Apophyseal avulsions. *Pure apophyseal avulsions.* **A.** The fracture follows the contour of the apophyseal line. **B.** The distal fracture line is in the shape of the apophyseal line (*open arrow*) with a small metaphyseal flake attached to the apophysis (*solid arrow*). *Apophyseal–metaphyseal combination.* **C.** The fracture line follows the line of tension stress. **D.** A large portion of the metaphysis (*arrow*) is often with the proximal metaphyseal fragment.

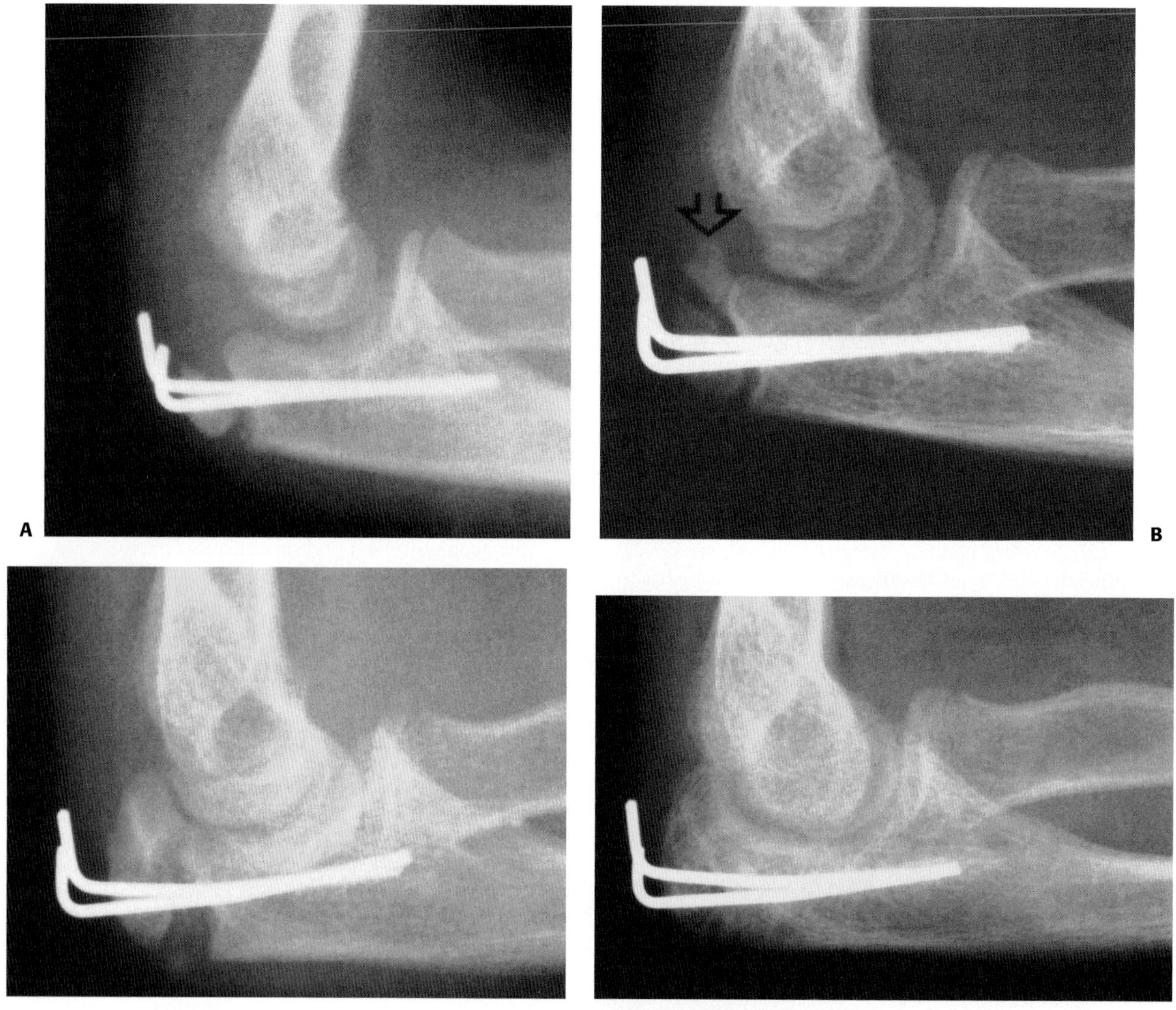

FIGURE 11-38 Operative treatment of an apophyseal fracture. **A.** Postoperative x-ray of the fracture shown in Figure 11-40D, which was stabilized with small Steinmann pins alone. **B.** Five months later, growth has continued in the traction center and the articular center is ossified (*arrow*). **C.** One year after injury, the apophysis was partially avulsed a second time. The two secondary ossification centers are now fused. **D.** Three months after the second fracture, the fracture gap has filled in, producing a normal olecranon.

the olecranon in an adolescent does not demonstrate healing after a reasonable period of simple rest, we place a cannulated compression screw across the apophysis to stimulate healing.

Displaced Fractures

With minimal displacement of the fracture, satisfactory closed reduction can be obtained with the elbow extended. We usually immobilize the elbow in a long-arm cast in extension. Percutaneous pinning will stabilize the reduction if there is any concern about loss of reduction. Completely displaced fractures are treated operatively using a tension-band technique. In young children, we use small Steinmann or Kirschner pins. The tension band is a strong absorbable suture of one of the polyglycolic acid substances. Alternatively, standard 16- to 18-gauge wire can be used in older adolescents. Patients with large ossification centers are treated with a compression screw similar to those with metaphyseal fractures.

Associated Injuries and Complications

Spur Formation

Smith (81) noted that overgrowth of the epiphysis proximally may produce a bony spur. In some patients these proximal spurs became symptomatic and were removed.

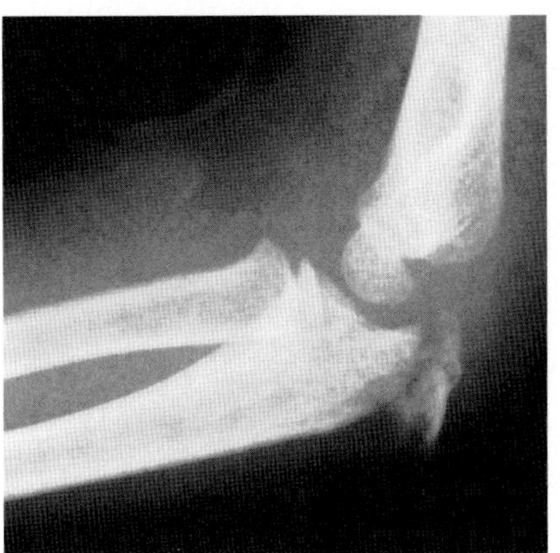
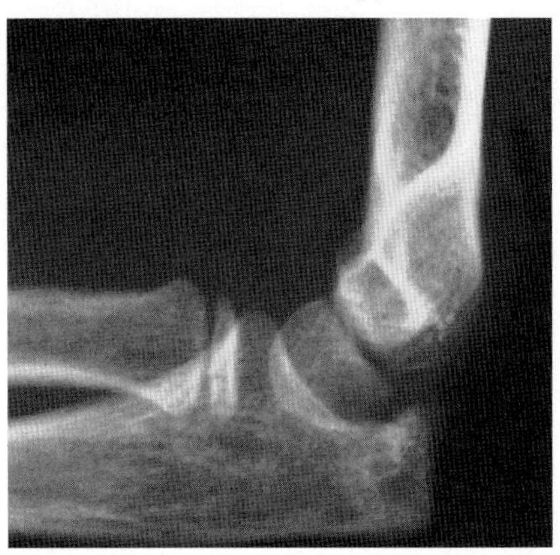
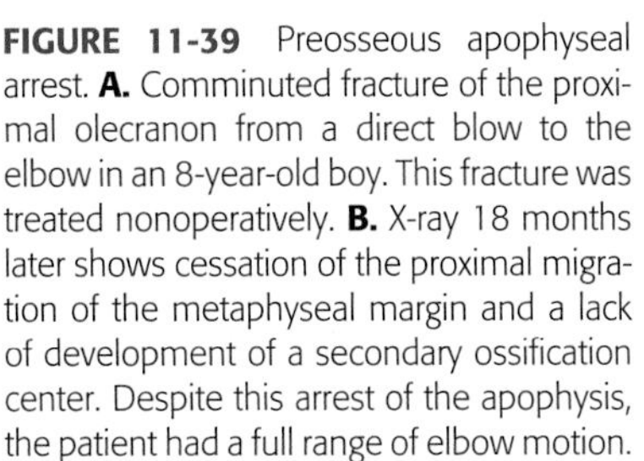

FIGURE 11-39 Preosseous apophyseal arrest. **A.** Comminuted fracture of the proximal olecranon from a direct blow to the elbow in an 8-year-old boy. This fracture was treated nonoperatively. **B.** X-ray 18 months later shows cessation of the proximal migration of the metaphyseal margin and a lack of development of a secondary ossification center. Despite this arrest of the apophysis, the patient had a full range of elbow motion.

Nonunion

The cause and treatment of nonunion are discussed in the previous section.

Apophyseal Arrest

Apophyseal arrest appears to have no significant effect on elbow function (see Fig. 11-39).

Metaphyseal Fractures of the Olecranon

Incidence

Isolated metaphyseal fractures of the olecranon are relatively rare (Table 11-7). They often are associated with other fractures about the elbow. In the combined series of 4,684 elbow fractures reviewed, 230 were olecranon fractures, for an incidence of 4.9%. This agrees with the incidence of 4% to 6% in the major series reported (98–100). Only 10% to 20% of the total fractures reported in these series required an operation. Six reports totaling 302 patients with fractures of the olecranon in children are in the English literature (79,99,101,102). Considering all age groups, 25% of olecranon fractures in these reports occurred in the first decade and another 25% in the second decade (10). During the first decade, the peak age for olecranon fracture was between age 5 and 10 years (102,103). Approximately 20% of patients had an associated fracture or dislocation of the elbow, most involving the proximal radius. Only 10% to 20% required an operation.

TABLE 11-7 Incidence of Metaphyseal Fractures of the Olecranon

Age distribution: 1st decade, 25%; 2nd decade, 25%; 3rd decade, 50%

Peak age: 5–10 yr

Extremity predominance: left (55%)

Sex predominance: male (65%)

Associated elbow injuries: 20%

Requiring surgical intervention: 19%

Anatomic Considerations

Because the olecranon is a metaphyseal area, the cortex is relatively thin, allowing for the development of greenstick-type fracture deformities. The periosteum is immature and thick, which may prevent the degree of separation seen in adults. Likewise, the larger amount of epiphyseal cartilage in children may serve as a cushion to lessen the effects of a direct blow to the olecranon. In the production of supracondylar fractures, ligamentous laxity in this age group tends to force the elbow into hyperextension when the child falls on the outstretched upper extremity. This puts a compressive force across the olecranon and locks it into the fossa in the distal humerus, where it is protected. An older person, whose elbow does not go into hyperextension, is more likely to fall with the elbow semiflexed. This unique biomechanical characteristic of the child's olecranon predisposes it to different fracture patterns than those in adults.

Signs and Symptoms

Flexion injuries cause soft tissue swelling over the olecranon fracture. The abrasion or contusion associated with a direct blow to the posterior aspect of the elbow provides a clue as to the mechanism the injury. If there is wide separation, a defect can be palpated between the fragments. In addition, there may be weakness or even lack of active extension of the elbow, which is difficult to evaluate in an anxious young child with a swollen elbow.

On x-ray, the fracture lines associated with flexion injuries usually are perpendicular to the long axis of the olecranon. This differentiates them from the residual physeal line, which is oblique and directed proximal and anterior (80). In extension injuries, the longitudinally directed greenstick fracture lines may be difficult to appreciate, and x-rays should be scrutinized

TABLE 11-8 Classification of Metaphyseal Fractures of the Olecranon

Group A: Flexion injuries

Group B: Extension injuries
1. Valgus pattern
2. Varus pattern

Group C: Shear injuries

to detect associated fractures of the proximal radius or distal humerus.

Classification

Papavasiliou et al (100) defined two major groups of olecranon fractures in which the fracture line is either intraarticular or extraarticular. The degree of displacement defines subclassifications in each group. We prefer to classify these fractures based on the mechanism of injury (Table 11-8): those associated with flexion injuries, those associated with extension injuries, and shear injuries. Extension injuries are further divided into varus and valgus patterns.

Mechanism of Injury

Three main mechanisms produce metaphyseal olecranon fractures, depending on whether the elbow is flexed or extended at the time of injury. First, in injuries occurring with the elbow flexed, posterior tension forces play an important role. Second, in injuries in which the fracture occurs with the elbow extended, the varus or valgus bending stress across the olecranon is responsible for the typical fracture pattern. Third, a less common mechanism involves a direct blow to the elbow that produces an anterior bending or shear force across the olecranon. In this type, the tension forces are concentrated on the anterior portion of the olecranon.

Flexion Injuries. A fall with the elbow semiflexed places considerable tension forces across the posterior aspect of the olecranon process. Proximally, the triceps applies a force to the tip of the olecranon process. Distally, there is some proximal pull by the insertion of the brachialis muscle. Thus, the posterior cortex is placed in tension. This tension force alone, if applied rapidly enough and with sufficient force, may cause the olecranon to fail at its midportion (Fig. 11-40). A direct blow applied to the posterior aspect of the stressed olecranon makes it more vulnerable to failure. With this type of mechanism, the fracture line usually is transverse and perpendicular to the long axis of the olecranon (Fig. 11-41). Because the fracture extends into the articular surface of the semilunar notch, it is classified as intraarticular.

The degree of separation of the fracture fragments depends on the magnitude of the forces applied versus the integrity of the soft tissues. The low incidence of displaced olecranon fractures indicates that the soft tissues are quite resistant to these avulsion forces. In flexion injuries, there are relatively few associated soft tissue injuries or other fractures (102).

Extension Injuries. Because the ligaments are more flexible in children, the elbow tends to hyperextend when a child breaks

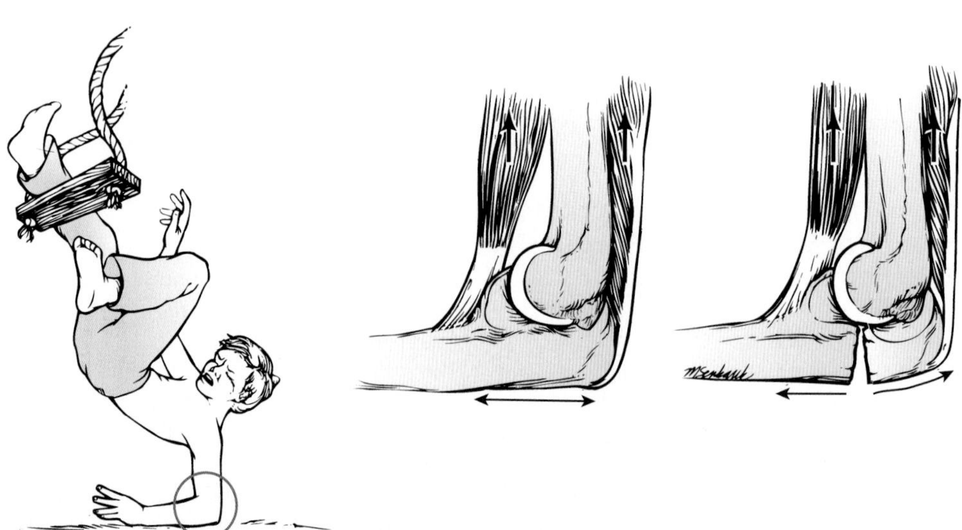

FIGURE 11-40 Mechanism of flexion injuries. *Center.* In the flexed elbow, a tension force develops on the posterior aspect of the olecranon (*small double arrow*) because of the pull of the brachialis and triceps muscles (*large arrows*). *Right.* Failure occurs on the tension side, which is posterior as a result of the muscle pull or a direct blow to the prestressed posterior olecranon.

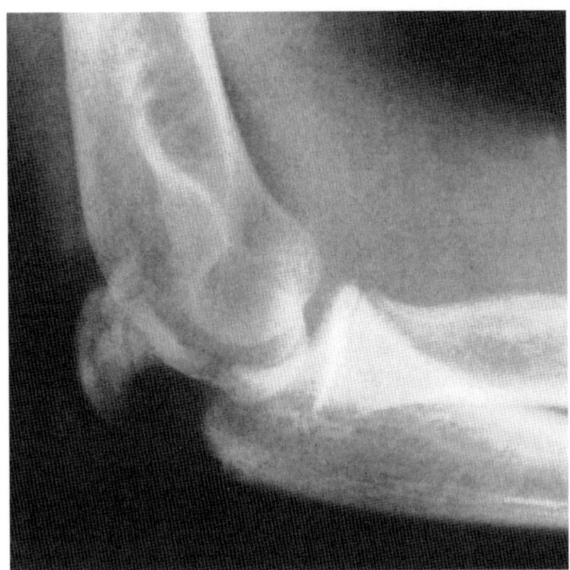

FIGURE 11-41 X-ray of flexion injury showing greater displacement on the posterior surface.

a fall with the outstretched upper extremity. In this situation, the olecranon may be locked into the olecranon fossa. If the elbow goes into extreme hyperextension, usually the supracondylar area fails. If, however, the major direction of the force across the elbow is abduction or adduction, a bending moment stresses the olecranon. Most of this force concentrates in the distal portion of the olecranon. Because the olecranon is metaphyseal bone, the force produces greenstick-type longitudinal fracture lines (Fig. 11-42). Most of these fracture lines are linear and remain extraarticular. In addition, because the fulcrum of the bending force is more distal, many of the fracture lines may extend distal to the coronoid process and into the proximal ulnar shaft regions. The major deformity of the olecranon with this type of fracture usually is an angulated greenstick type of pattern.

Many of these fractures are associated with other injuries in the elbow region, which depend on whether the bending force is directed toward varus or valgus. If a child falls with the forearm in supination, the carrying angle tends to place a valgus stress across the elbow. The result may be a greenstick fracture of the ulna with an associated fracture of the radial neck or avulsion of the medial epicondylar apophysis (Fig. 11-43). If the fracture involves the radial neck, Bado (33) classified it as an equivalent of the type I Monteggia lesion.

If the body falls against the inner aspect of the elbow or if the forearm is pronated, a varus force is placed across the elbow (Fig. 11-44). The major injury associated with this varus force is a partial or total lateral dislocation of the radial head. Bado (33) classified this as a type III Monteggia lesion. In this type of fracture, the posterior interosseous nerve may be injured.

Shear Injuries. Anterior tension failure is a rare injury that can occur when a direct blow to the proximal ulna causes it to fail with an anterior tension force; the proximal radioulnar joint maintains its integrity. The most common type of shear injury is caused by a shear force applied directly to the posterior aspect of the olecranon, with the distal fragment displacing anteriorly (Figs. 11-45 and 11-46). The intact proximal radioulnar joint displaces with the distal fragment. In this type of injury, the elbow may be either flexed or extended when the direct shear force impacts the posterior aspect of the olecranon. These fractures are due to a failure in tension, with the force concentrated along the anterior cortex. This is opposite to the tension failure occurring on the posterior aspect of the cortex in the more common flexion injuries. In the shear-type injury, the fracture line may be transverse or oblique. The differentiating feature from the more common flexion injury is that the thick posterior periosteum usually remains intact. The distal fragment is displaced anteriorly by the pull of the brachialis and biceps

(text continues on page 478)

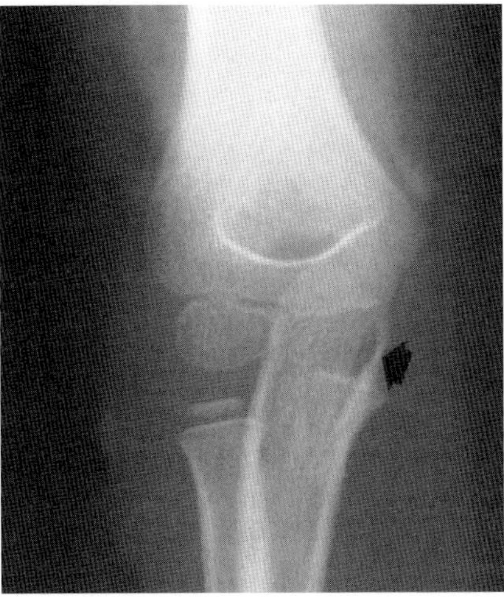

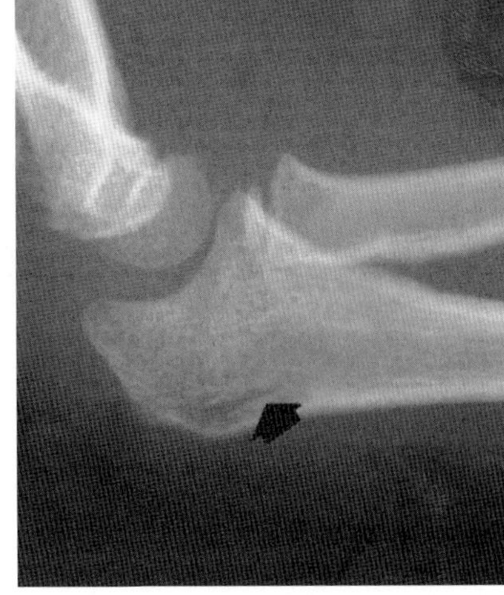

FIGURE 11-42 **A.** Anteroposterior view of a linear greenstick fracture line (*arrow*) in the medial aspect of the olecranon. **B.** Lateral view showing the posterior location of the fracture line (*arrow*).

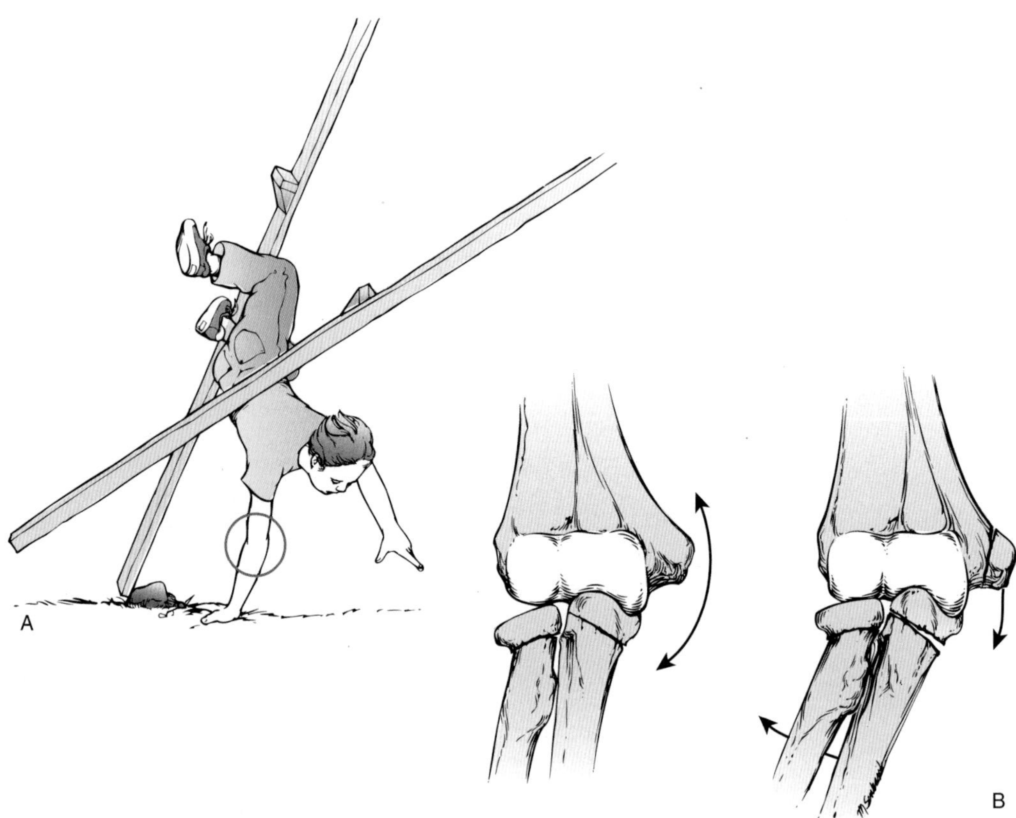

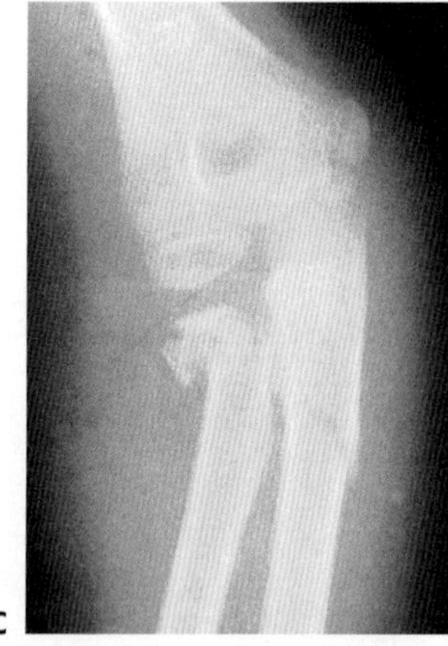

FIGURE 11-43 Valgus pattern of an extension fracture. **A.** A fall with the elbow extended places a valgus stress on the forearm. **B.** With increased valgus, a greenstick fracture of the olecranon can occur with or without a fracture of the radial neck or avulsion of the medial epicondylar apophysis. **C.** X-ray of a valgus extension fracture of the olecranon with an associated fracture of the radial neck.

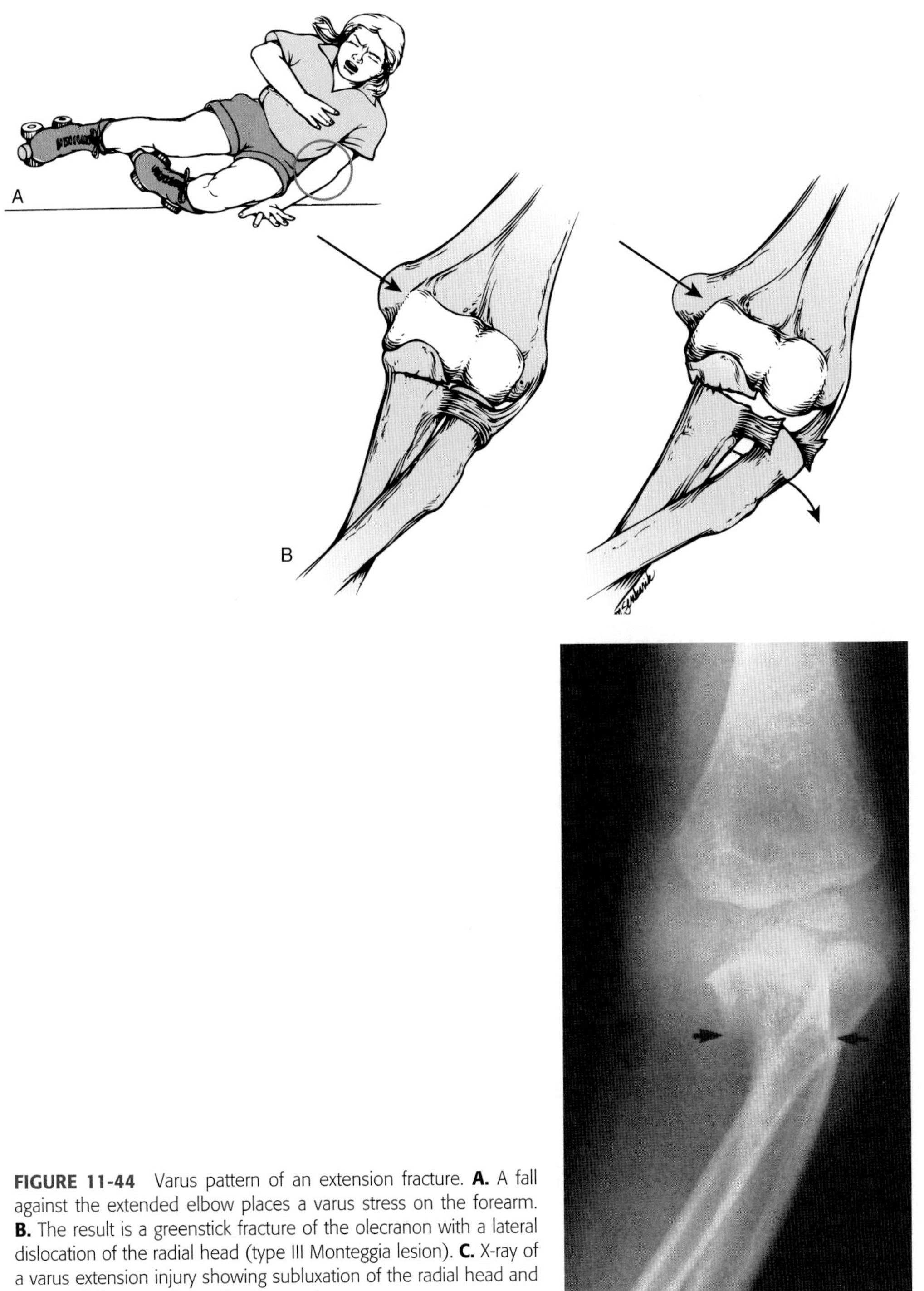

FIGURE 11-44 Varus pattern of an extension fracture. **A.** A fall against the extended elbow places a varus stress on the forearm. **B.** The result is a greenstick fracture of the olecranon with a lateral dislocation of the radial head (type III Monteggia lesion). **C.** X-ray of a varus extension injury showing subluxation of the radial head and greenstick fracture of the ulna (*arrows*).

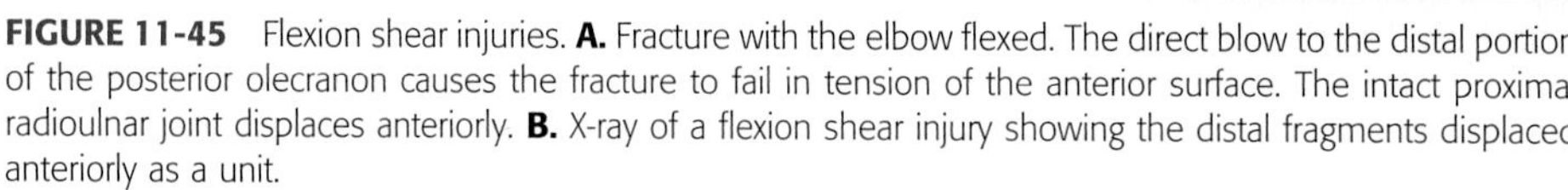

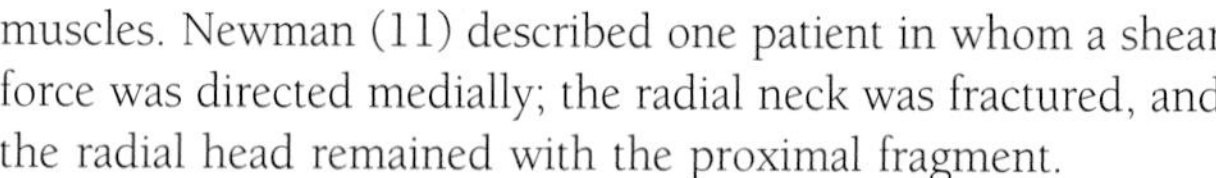

FIGURE 11-45 Flexion shear injuries. **A.** Fracture with the elbow flexed. The direct blow to the distal portion of the posterior olecranon causes the fracture to fail in tension of the anterior surface. The intact proximal radioulnar joint displaces anteriorly. **B.** X-ray of a flexion shear injury showing the distal fragments displaced anteriorly as a unit.

muscles. Newman (11) described one patient in whom a shear force was directed medially; the radial neck was fractured, and the radial head remained with the proximal fragment.

Associated Injuries

Associated injuries occur in 48% to 77% of patients with olecranon fractures (100,103–105), especially varus and valgus greenstick extension fractures, in which the radial head and neck most commonly fracture (see Fig. 11-43). Other associated injuries include fractures of the ipsilateral radial shaft (106), Monteggia type I lesions with fractures of both the ulnar shaft and olecranon (42), and fractures of the lateral condyle (Fig. 11-47) (86).

Treatment

The mechanism of injury can serve as a useful guide in choosing the proper treatment method.

Flexion Injuries. Flexion injuries are the most common type of olecranon fractures. Most displace minimally and require immobilization with the elbow in no more than 75 to 80 degrees of flexion (Fig. 11-48). Even if the fracture displaces severely, immobilization in full or partial extension usually allows the olecranon to heal satisfactorily (81,98,107).

If the fracture is significantly displaced or comminuted, open reduction with internal fixation usually is required. Recommended fixation devices vary from catgut or absorbable suture (108) to an axial screw (70), tension-band wiring with axial pins (79,81,107–111) or a plate (112). Internal fixation allows early motion. No one has reported significant growth disturbances from internal fixation of metaphyseal olecranon fractures.

Murphy et al (113) compared the failure of various fixation devices under rapid loading: (a) figure-of-eight wire alone, (b) cancellous screw alone, (c) AO tension band, and (d) cancellous screw with a figure-of-eight wire combination. The cancellous screw alone and figure-of-eight wire alone were by far the weakest. The greatest resistance to failure was found in the combination of a screw plus figure-of-eight wire, followed closely by the AO tension-band fixation. In their clinical evaluation of patients, comparing the AO tension band and combination screw and figure-of-eight wire, they found more clinical problems associated with the AO technique (114). The main problem with the AO technique is the subcutaneous prominence of the axial wires (115). To prevent proximal migration of these wires, Montgomery (116) devised a method of making eyelets in the proximal end of the wires through which he passed the figure-of-eight fixation wire.

Extension Injuries. Treatment of extension injuries requires both adequate realignment of the angulation of the olecranon and treatment of the secondary injuries. Often in varus injuries,

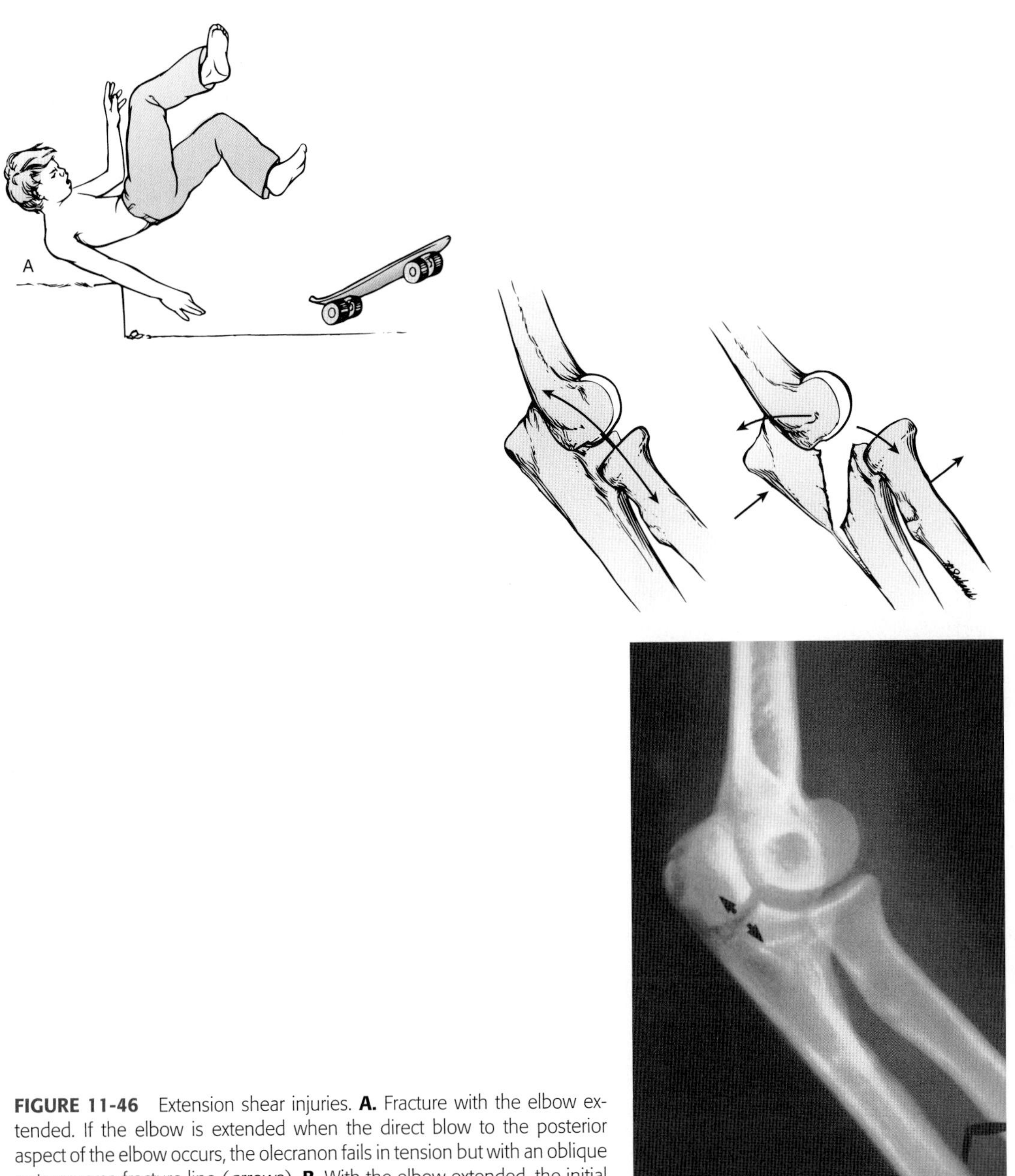

FIGURE 11-46 Extension shear injuries. **A.** Fracture with the elbow extended. If the elbow is extended when the direct blow to the posterior aspect of the elbow occurs, the olecranon fails in tension but with an oblique or transverse fracture line (*arrows*). **B.** With the elbow extended, the initial failure is in the anterior articular surface (*arrows*).

correction of the alignment of the olecranon also reduces the radial head. The olecranon angulation corrects with the elbow in extension. This locks the proximal olecranon into the olecranon fossa of the humerus so that the distal angulation can be corrected at the fracture site with a valgus force applied to the forearm. Occasionally, in extension fractures, complete separation of the fragments requires open reduction and internal fixation (Fig. 11-49).

Zimmerman (107) reported that the original angulation tends to redevelop in some fractures. If a varus force produced the fracture, the proximal ulna or olecranon may drift back into varus, which can cause a painful subluxation of the radial head. A secondary osteotomy of the proximal ulna or olecranon may be necessary if the angulation is significant.

Shear Injuries. For anterior shear fractures, the key to management is recognition that the distal fragment is displaced anteriorly and the posterior periosteum remains intact. The intact posterior periosteum can serve as an internal tension band to facilitate reduction.

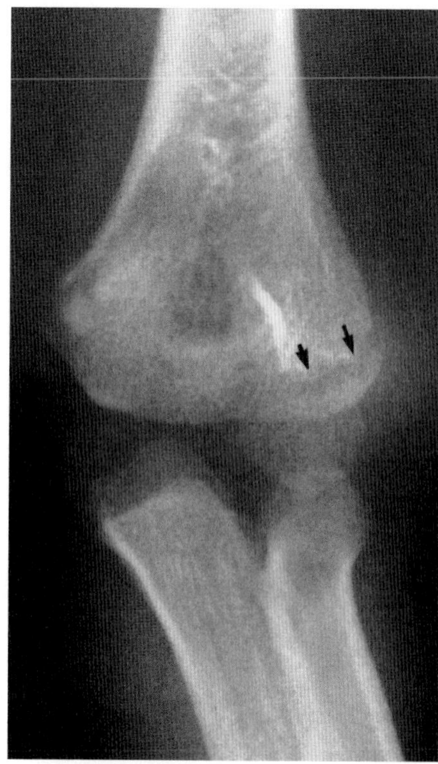

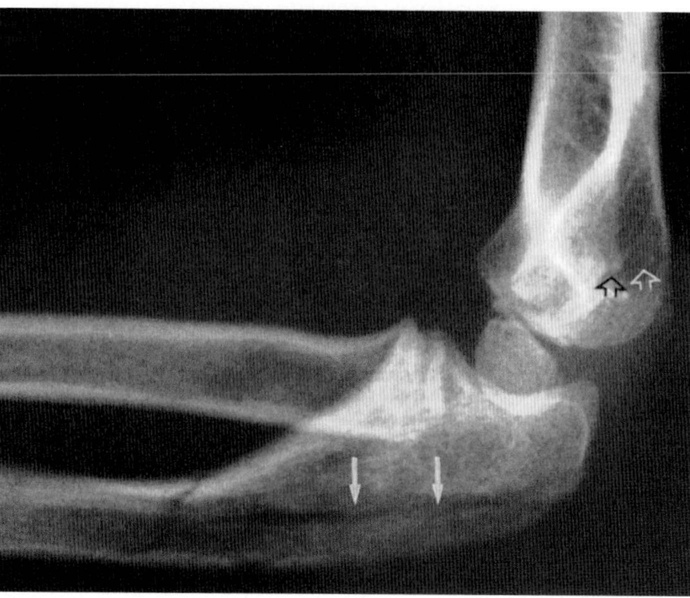

FIGURE 11-47 **A.** Undisplaced fracture of the lateral condyle (*arrows*) associated with a varus greenstick fracture of the olecranon. **B.** Lateral view showing greenstick fractures in the olecranon (*solid arrows*) and a nondisplaced fracture of the lateral condyle (*open arrows*).

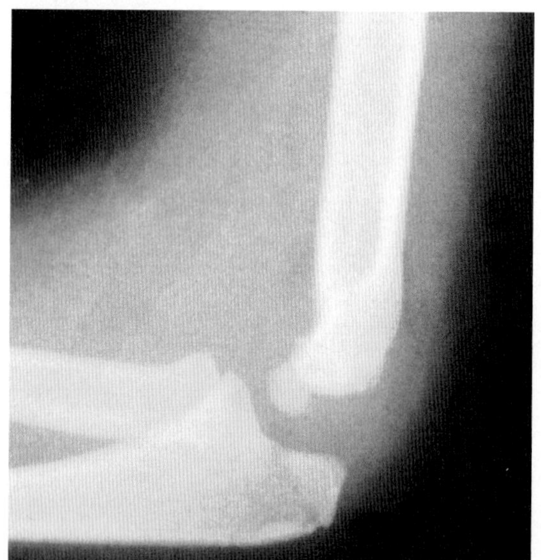

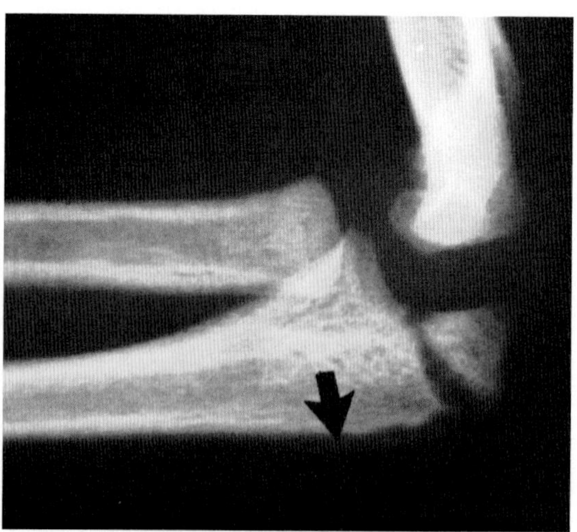

FIGURE 11-48 Simple immobilization of a flexion injury. **A.** Injury film, lateral view, showing minimal displacement. **B.** Three weeks later, the fracture has displaced further. Periosteal new bone is along the posterior border of the olecranon (*arrow*). Healing was complete with a normal range of motion. (Courtesy of Jesse C. DeLee, MD.)

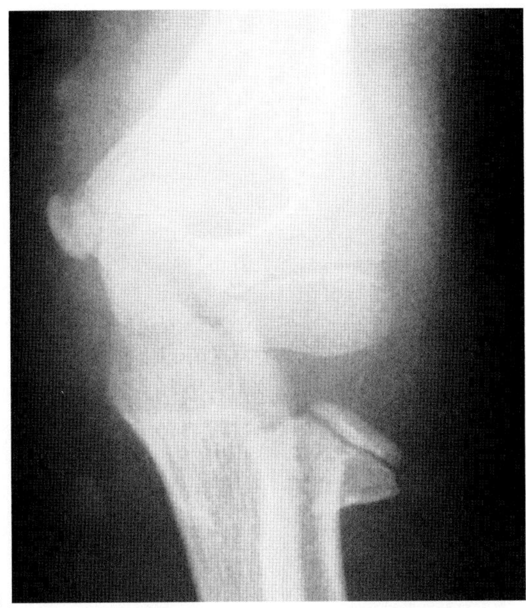

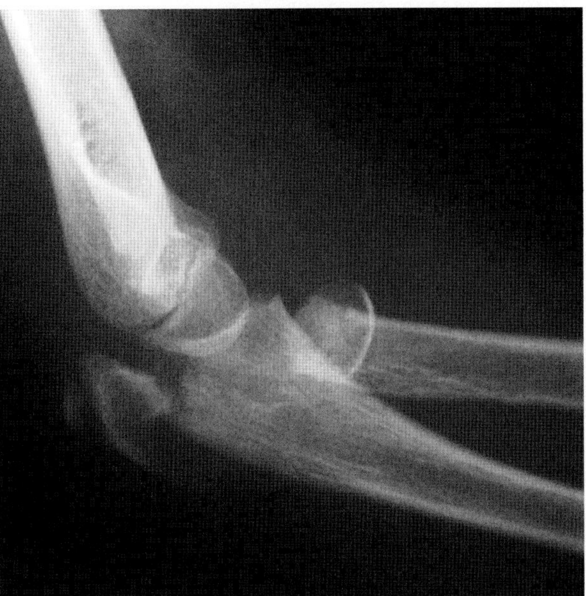

FIGURE 11-49 Open reduction of a valgus extension injury. **A.** Anteroposterior injury film shows complete displacement of the radial head. **B.** Lateral view also shows the degree of displacement of the olecranon fracture. This patient required surgical intervention with internal fixation to achieve a satisfactory reduction.

Some of these fractures are reduced better in flexion, and the posterior periosteum serves as a compressive force to maintain the reduction. Smith (81) reported treatment of this fracture using an overhead sling placed to apply a posteriorly directed force against the proximal portion of the distal fragment. The weight of the arm and forearm helps supplement the tension-band effect of the posterior periosteum.

If the periosteum is torn or early motion is desirable, Zimmerman (107) advocated internal fixation of the two fragments with an oblique screw perpendicular to the fracture line (Fig. 11-50).

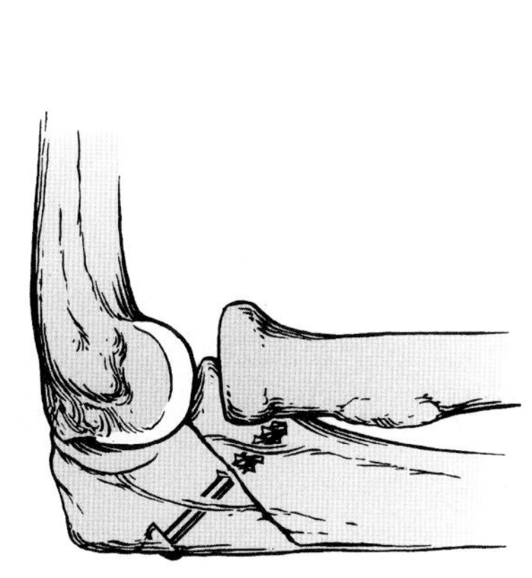

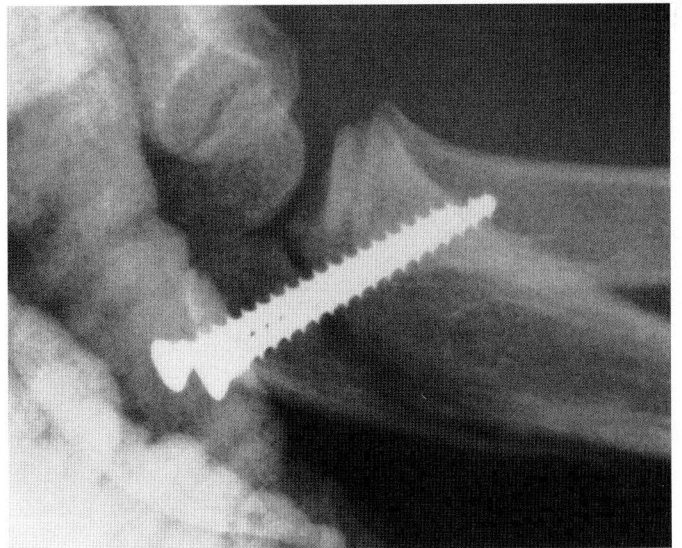

FIGURE 11-50 Operative treatment of extension shear fractures. **A.** If the periosteum is insufficient to hold the fragments apposed, an interfragmentary screw can be used, as advocated by Zimmerman (122). **B.** An extension shear type of fracture secured with two oblique interfragmentary screws.

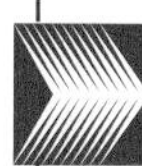

AUTHORS' PREFERRED TREATMENT

We use a classification based on the mechanism of injury in choosing the method of treatment (see Table 11-8).

Flexion Injuries

Nonoperative. We immobilize most nondisplaced flexion injuries with the elbow in 5 to 10 degrees of flexion for approximately 3 weeks. It is important to obtain x-rays of these fractures after approximately 5 to 7 days in the cast to ensure that there has not been any significant displacement of the fragment.

Operative: Tension Band. To determine which injuries need internal fixation, we palpate the fracture for a defect and flex the elbow to determine the integrity of the posterior periosteum. If the fragments separate with either of these maneuvers, they are unstable and are fixed internally so that active motion can be started as soon as possible.

We prefer a modification of the tension-band technique. Originally we used the standard AO technique with axial

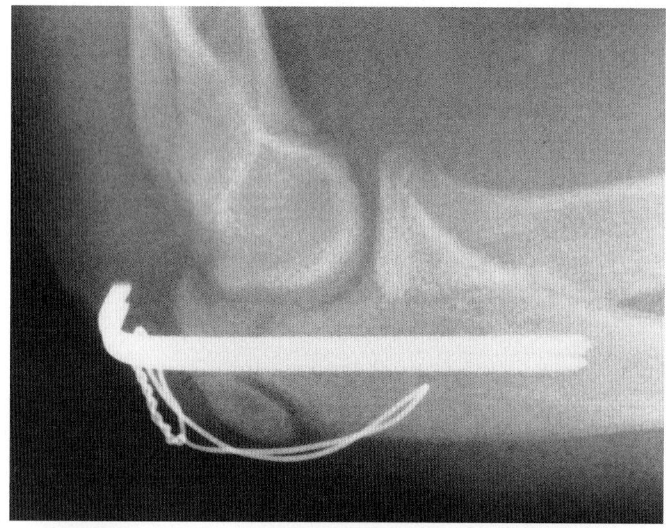

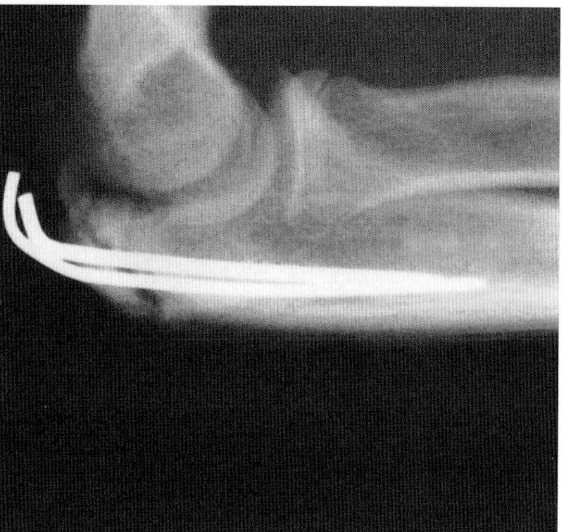

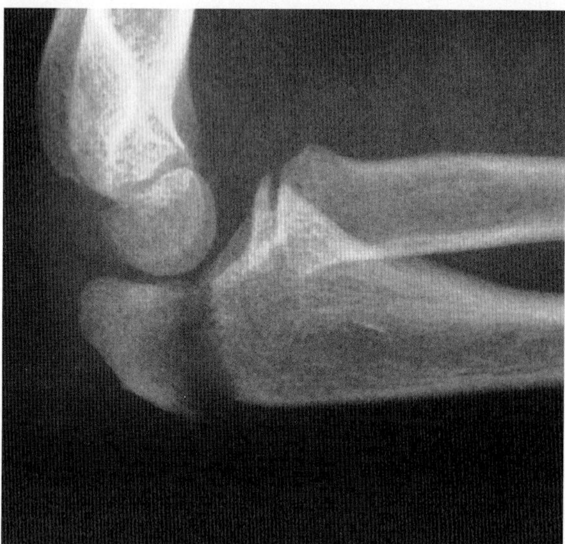

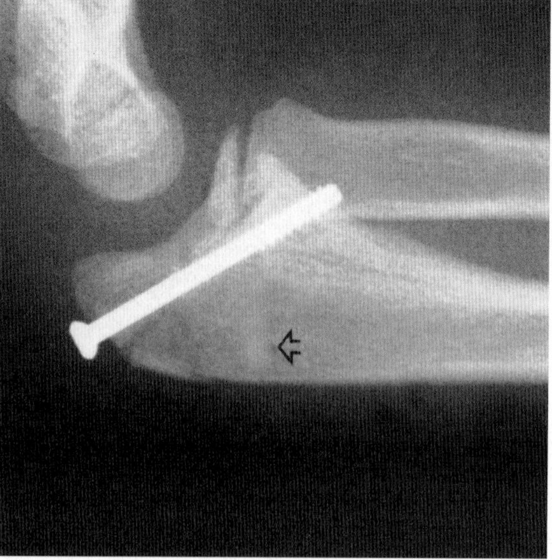

FIGURE 11-51 Internal tension-band techniques. **A.** Standard AO technique with stainless steel wire. The wire can be prominent in the subcutaneous tissues. **B.** Axial wires plus polydioxanone sutures (PDS) 6 weeks after surgery. **C.** A displaced flexion-type injury in an 11-year-old boy. There is complete separation of the fracture fragments. **D.** A cancellous lag screw plus PDS. The screw engages the anterior cortex of the coronoid process. The PDS passes through a separate drill hole in the olecranon (*open arrow*) and crosses in a figure-of-eight manner over the fracture site and around the neck of the screw.

Kirschner wires or Steinmann pins and figure-of-eight stainless steel as the tension band (Fig. 11-51A). Because removal of the wire often required reopening the entire incision, we now use an absorbable suture for the figure-of-eight tension band. Number 1 polydioxanone (PDS) suture, which is slowly absorbed over a few months, is ideal (see Fig. 11-51B). When rigid internal fixation is applied, rapid healing at the fracture site produces internal stability before the PDS absorbs. We prefer Kirschner wires in patients who are very young and have very little ossification of the olecranon apophysis (see Fig. 11-38). If the axial wires become a problem, we remove them through a small incision. Most recently, we have used a combination of an oblique cortical screw with PDS as the tension band (see Fig. 11-51C,D) and are pleased with the results. In the past we had to remove almost all the axial wires; very few of the screws cause enough symptoms to require removal. Occasionally, we use the tension-band wire technique with 16- or 18-gauge wire in a heavier patient.

Extension Injures

For extension injuries, we anesthetize the patient to allow a forceful manipulation of the olecranon while it is locked inits fossa in extension. Because this is a greenstick fracture, we slightly overcorrect to prevent the development of reangulation. These fractures may require manipulation/remanipulation in 1 to 2 weeks if the original angulation recurs. Associated fractures are treated as if they were isolated injuries.

Shear Injuries

Most shear fractures can be treated nonoperatively. We usually immobilize them in enough hyperflexion to hold the fragments together, if the posterior periosteum is intact (Fig. 11-52). If the periosteum is torn, an oblique screw is an excellent way to secure the fracture (see Fig. 11-50). If considerable swelling prevents the elbow from being hyperflexed enough to use the posterior periosteum as a tension band, an oblique screw is a good choice.

Postoperative Care

The elbow is placed at a 70- to 80-degree angle and held in a long-arm cast. The cast should be bivalved if there is excessive swelling. The cast or posterior splint is worn for 3 weeks, at which time the patient begins active range of motion.

Associated Injuries and Complications

Relatively few complications arise from the olecranon fracture itself.

Irreducibility. An and Loder (117) reported inability to reduce the fracture in one of their patients because the proximal fragment was entrapped in the joint.

Nonunion. Nonunion is unusual and should not be confused with congenital pseudarthrosis of the ulna, which is rare (Fig. 11-53). In the latter condition, there is no antecedent trauma.

Delayed Union. Delayed radiographic union usually is asymptomatic (108). In Mathews' series (108), one fracture treated with catgut ultimately progressed to a nonunion. Despite this, the patient had only a 10-degree extension lag and grade 4 triceps strength. An accessory ossicle, such as a patella cubiti, is not a nonunion.

Compartment Syndrome. Mathews (108) described one patient with Volkmann ischemic contracture after an undisplaced linear fracture in the olecranon.

Nerve Injuries. Zimmerman (107) reported ulnar nerve neuropraxia from the development of a pseudarthrosis of the olecranon where inadequate fixation was used.

Elongation. Elongation of the tip of the olecranon may complicate healing of a fracture. Figure 11-54 illustrates a delayed union in which the apophysis became elongated to the point that it limited extension. This proximal overgrowth of the tip of the apophysis has occurred in olecranon fractures after routine open reduction and internal fixation (100).

Loss of Reduction. Apparently stable fractures treated with external immobilization may lose reduction, which results in a significant loss of elbow function (Fig. 11-55).

Fractures of the Coronoid Process

Anatomy

Up to age 6 years, the coronoid process consists of epiphyseal and physeal cartilage at the distal end of a tongue extending from the apophysis of the olecranon. The coronoid process does not develop a secondary center of ossification, but instead ossifies along with the advancing edge of the metaphysis (see Fig. 11-35).

Incidence

The incidence of fracture of the coronoid varies from less than 1% to 2% (99) of elbow fractures. Because most fractures of the coronoid process occur with dislocations of the elbow, it seems logical that they would happen in older children. However, in a review of 23 coronoid fractures in children, Bracq (11) found that the injuries occurred in two peak age groups: one was between 8 and 9 years of age and the other between 12 and 14 years.

Although most coronoid fractures are associated with elbow dislocations, fractures of the olecranon, medial epicondyle, and lateral condyle also can occur (11). The fracture of the coronoid may be part of a greenstick olecranon fracture (i.e., the extension-type metaphyseal fracture; Fig. 11-56). Isolated coronoid fractures theoretically are caused by avulsion by the brachialis or secondary to an elbow dislocation that reduced spontaneously,

(text continues on page 488)

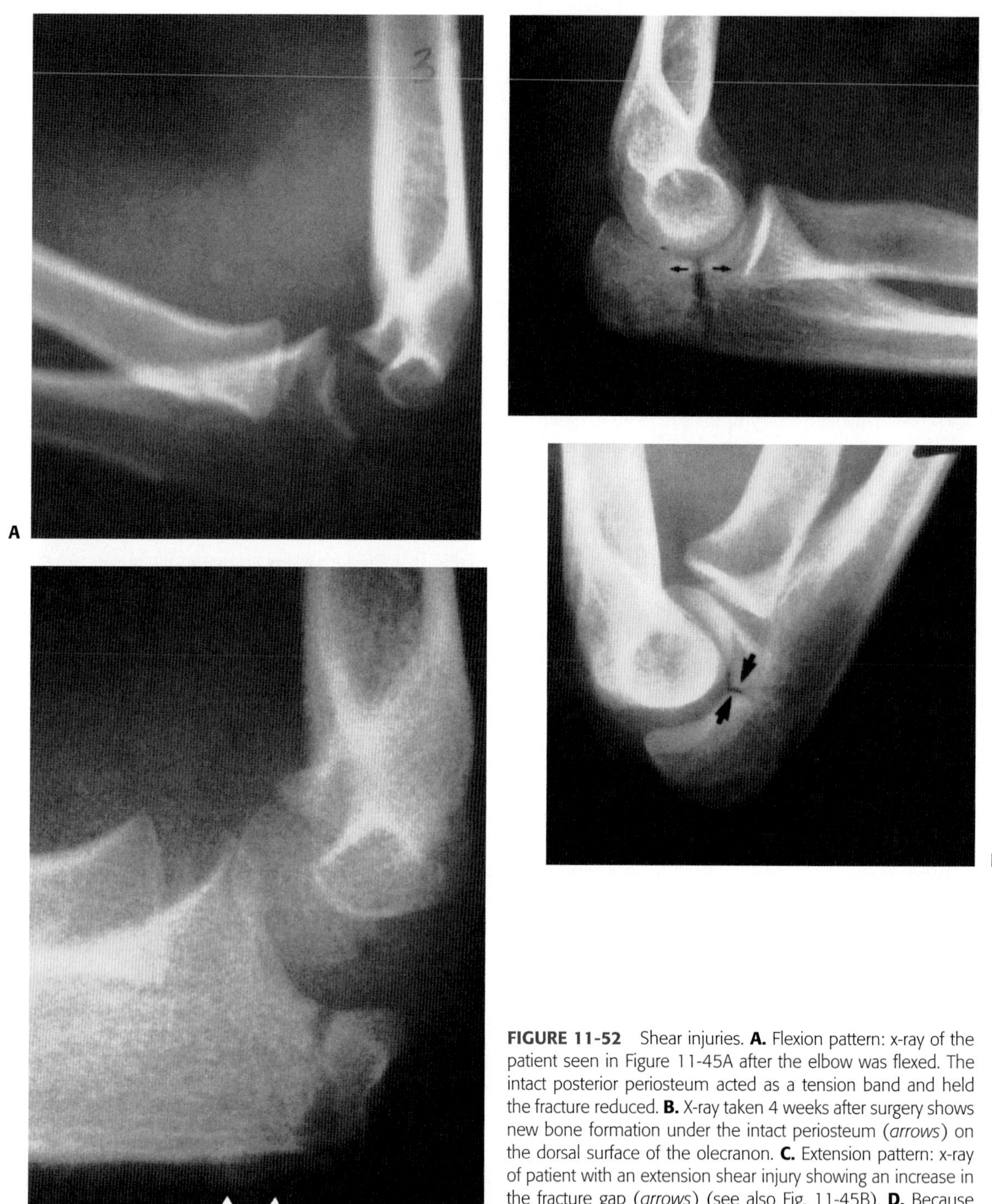

FIGURE 11-52 Shear injuries. **A.** Flexion pattern: x-ray of the patient seen in Figure 11-45A after the elbow was flexed. The intact posterior periosteum acted as a tension band and held the fracture reduced. **B.** X-ray taken 4 weeks after surgery shows new bone formation under the intact periosteum (*arrows*) on the dorsal surface of the olecranon. **C.** Extension pattern: x-ray of patient with an extension shear injury showing an increase in the fracture gap (*arrows*) (see also Fig. 11-45B). **D.** Because the dorsal periosteum and cortex were intact, the fracture gap (*arrows*) closed with flexion of the elbow.

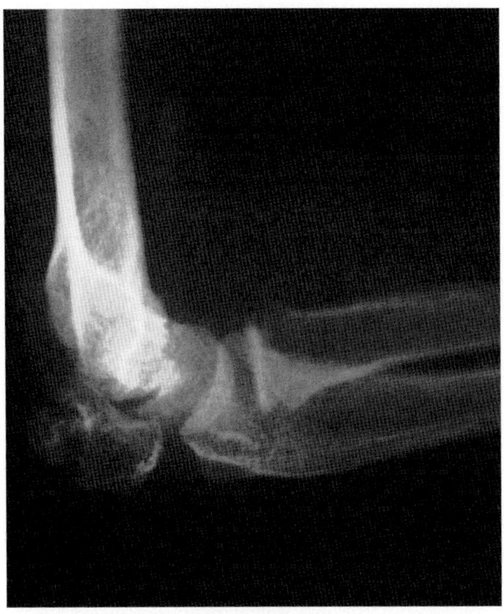

FIGURE 11-53 Congenital pseudarthrosis of the olecranon in a 9-year-old girl who had limited elbow extension and no antecedent trauma. The edges of the bone were separated by thick fibrous tissue. (Courtesy of Michael J. Rogal, MD.)

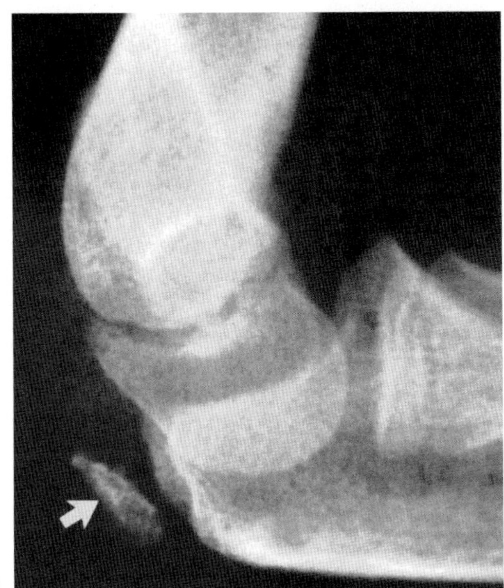

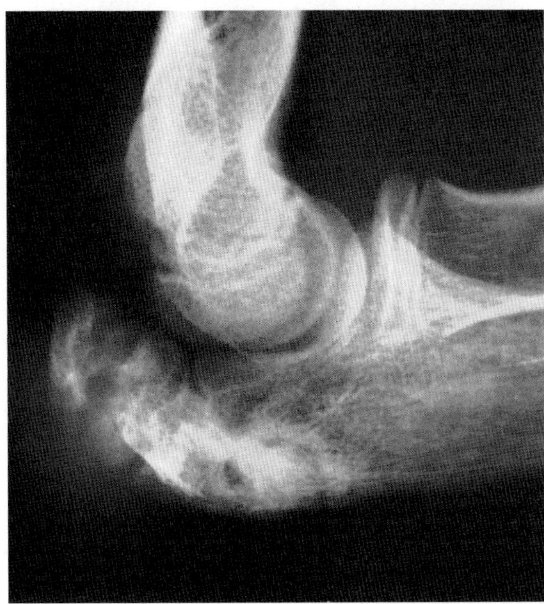

FIGURE 11-54 **A.** Injury film showing partial avulsion of the tip of the olecranon apophysis (*arrow*). **B.** X-ray taken 4 years later shows a marked elongation and irregular ossification of the apophysis. (Courtesy of Joel Goldman, MD.)

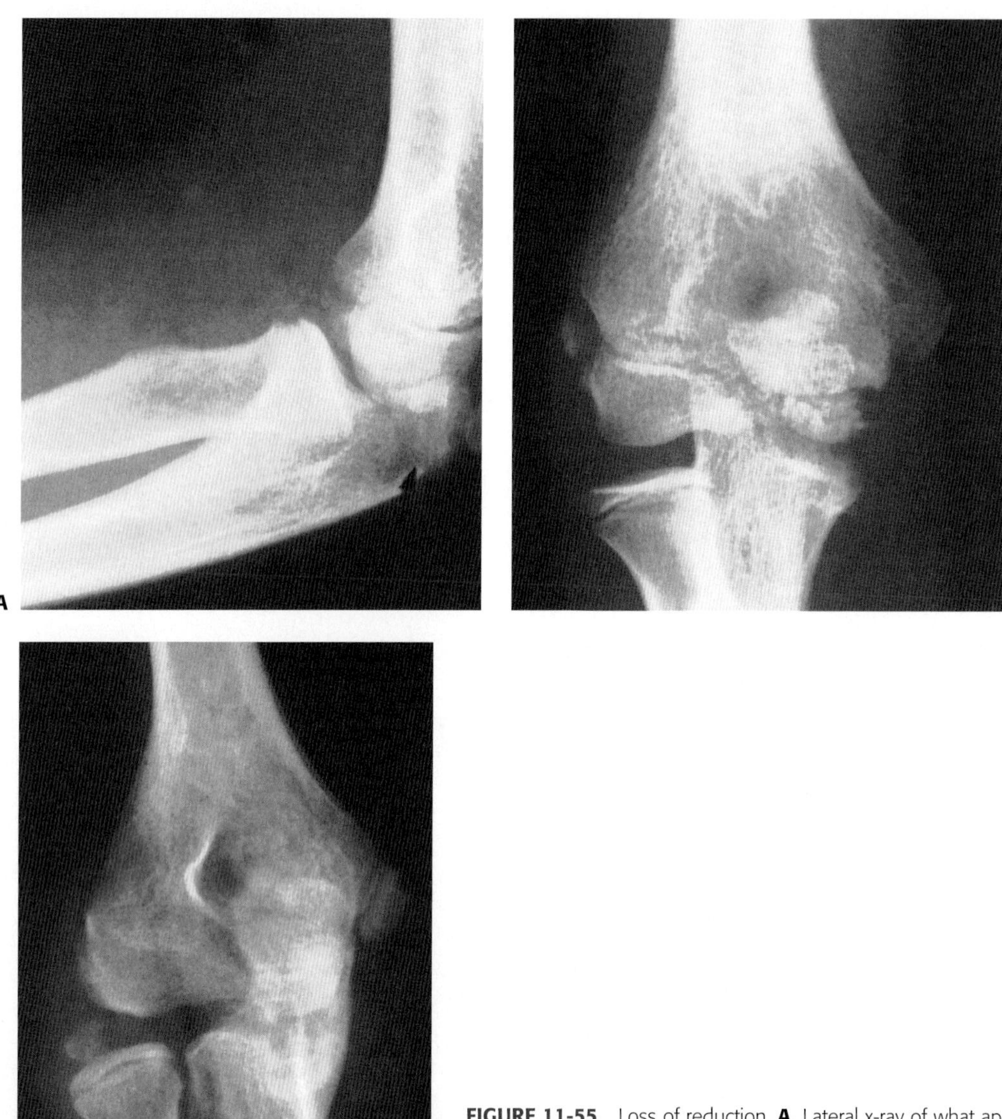

FIGURE 11-55 Loss of reduction. **A.** Lateral x-ray of what appeared to be a simple undisplaced fracture (*arrow*) of the olecranon in a 13-year-old girl. **B.** On the anteroposterior film, the fracture also appears undisplaced. The mild lateral subluxation of the radial head was not recognized. **C.** X-rays taken 5 months later showed further lateral subluxation with resultant incongruity of the elbow joint. (Courtesy of Richard W. Williamson, MD.)

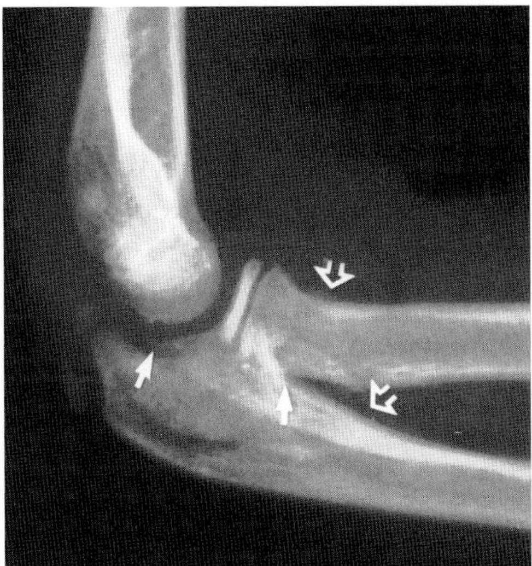

FIGURE 11-56 Fracture of the coronoid (*arrow*) as part of an extension valgus olecranon fracture pattern. There was an associated fracture of the radial neck. Both the neck fracture and the distal portion of the coronoid process show periosteal new bone formation (*open arrows*).

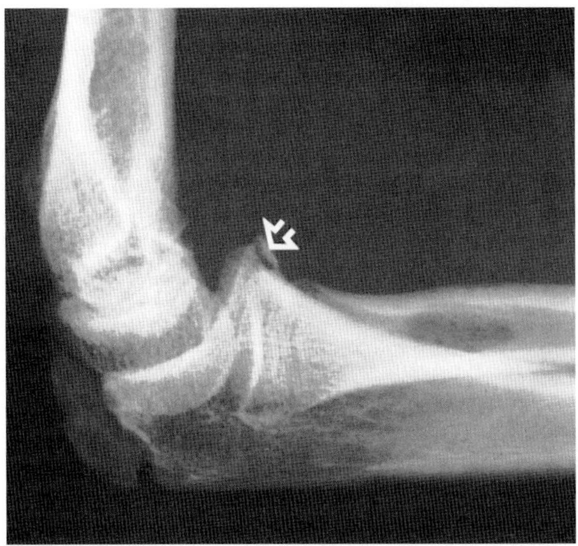

FIGURE 11-57 Lateral x-ray of an 11-year-old boy who injured his left elbow. Displaced anterior and posterior fat pads, plus a small fracture of the coronoid (*arrow*), indicate a probable partially dislocated elbow as the primary injury.

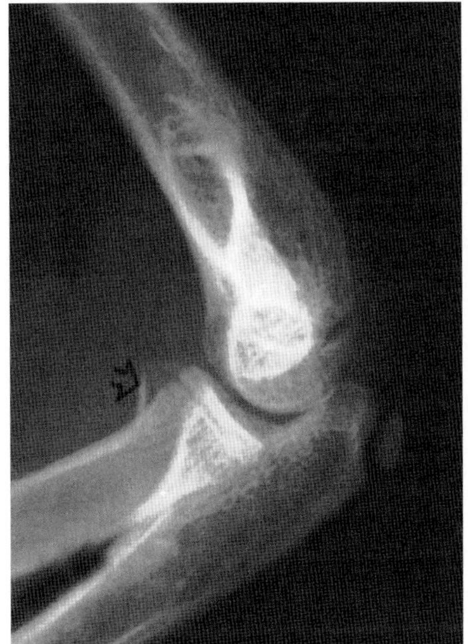

A

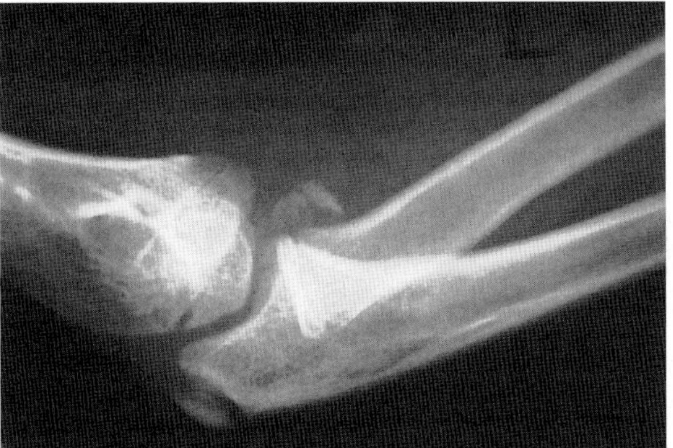

B

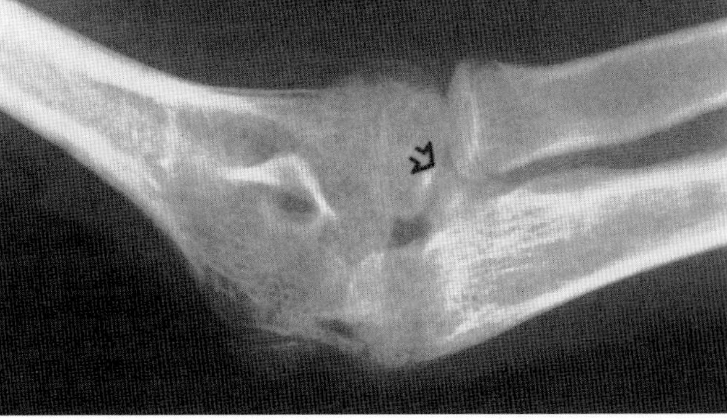

C

FIGURE 11-58 **A.** Based on this original lateral x-ray, a 12-year-old boy with a swollen elbow was thought to have a fracture of the radial neck (*arrow*). **B.** With an oblique view, it is now obvious that the fragment is from the coronoid process. **C.** Five months later, the protuberant healed coronoid process (*arrow*) is seen on this radiocapitellar view.

which usually is associated with hemarthrosis and a small avulsion of the tip of the olecranon process (Fig. 11-57).

Diagnosis

The x-ray diagnosis of this fracture often is difficult because on the lateral view the radial head is superimposed over the coronoid process. Evaluation of a minimally displaced fracture may require oblique views (13) (Fig. 11-58). The radiocapitellar view (see Fig. 11-6) shows the profile of the coronoid process.

In young children, in whom the coronoid process contains mostly cartilage, an unusual flap injury may occur (8). In this rare injury, the elbow dislocates and the articular surface flips back into the joint. The only clue to this fracture may be the presence of a small flake of bone in the anterior part of the joint on the lateral x-ray.

Classification

Regan and Morrey (82) classified coronoid fractures into three types based on the amount of the coronoid process involved (Table 11-9). This classification is useful in predicting the outcome and in determining the treatment. Type I fractures involve only the tip of the process (see Fig. 11-57), type II fractures involve more than just the tip but less than 50% of the process (see Fig. 11-58), and type III fractures involve more than 50% of the process.

Treatment

The degree of displacement or the presence of elbow instability guides the treatment. The associated injuries also are a factor in treatment. Regan and Morrey (81,82) treated types I and II fractures with early motion if there were no contradicting associated injuries. For initial immobilization, if the fracture is associated with an elbow dislocation, the elbow is placed in approximately 100 degrees of flexion, with the forearm in full supination (11). Occasionally, in partial avulsion fractures, the fracture reduces more easily with the elbow in extension. In these rare cases, the brachialis muscle may be an aid in reducing the fragment in extension (102). Regan and Morrey (81) found that the elbow often was unstable in type III fractures, and they secured these fractures with internal fixation. They had satisfactory results with type I and II fractures, but in only 20% of type III fractures were the results satisfactory.

TABLE 11-9 Classification of Fractures of the Coronoid Process

Type I: Avulsion of the tip of the coronoid process only

Type II: A single or comminuted fragment involving ≤50% of the coronoid process

Type III: A single or comminuted fragment involving >50% of the coronoid process

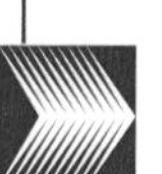

AUTHORS' PREFERRED TREATMENT

We usually treat coronoid fractures with early motion, much as we do elbow dislocations. The presence of a coronoid fracture alerts us to be especially thorough in looking for other injuries. In children, surgery rarely is necessary. If there is a large fragment and marked displacement, open reduction is done through a Henry anterior approach to the elbow. The fragment is fixed with a mini-fragment screw or sewn in place through two drill holes in the posterior aspect of the ulna.

Associated Injuries and Complications

Complications are rare. In fractures with a large fragment (type III), the elbow may be unstable and prone to recurrent dislocations. Nonunion with the production of a free fragment in the joint occurs rarely in children (96).

REFERENCES

1. Landin LA. Fracture patterns in children. *Acta Paediatr Scand Suppl* 1983;54:192.
2. Henrikson B. Isolated fracture of the proximal end of the radius in children. *Acta Orthop Scand* 1969;40:246–260.
3. Boyd HB, Altenberg AR. Fractures about the elbow in children. *Arch Surg* 1944;49: 213–224.
4. Fowles JV, Kassab MT. Observations concerning radial neck fractures in children. *J Pediatr Orthop* 1986;6:51–57.
5. Jeffrey CC. Fracture of the head of the radius in children. *J Bone Joint Surg [Br]* 1950; 32:314–324.
6. Lindham S, Hugasson C. Significance of associated lesions including dislocation of fracture of the neck of the radius in children. *Acta Orthop Scand* 1979;50:79–83.
7. O'Brien PI. Injuries involving the radial epiphysis. *Clin Orthop* 1965;41:51–58.
8. Gaston SR, Smith FM, Boab OD. Epiphyseal injuries of the radial head and neck. *Am J Surg* 1953;85:266–276.
9. D'Souza S, Vaishya R, Klenerman L. Management of radial neck fractures in children. A retrospective analysis of 100 patients. *J Pediatr Orthop* 1993;13:232–238.
10. Landin LA, Danielsson LG. Elbow fractures in children: an epidemiological analysis of 589 cases. *Acta Orthop Scand* 1986;57:309.
11. Newman JH. Displaced radial neck fractures in children. *Injury* 1977;9:114–121.
12. Robert M, Moulies D, Longis B, et al. Les fractures de l'extremite superieure du radius chez l'enfant. *Chir Pediatr* 1986;27:318–321.
13. Steinberg EL, Golomb D, Salama R, et al. Radial head and neck fractures in children. *J Pediatr Orthop* 1988;8:35–40.
14. Tibone JE, Stoltz M. Fracture of the radial head and neck in children. *J Bone Joint Surg [Am]* 1981;63:100–106.
15. Vahvanen V. Fracture of the radial neck in children. *Acta Orthop Scand* 1978;49:32–38.
16. Brodeur AE, Silberstein JJ, Graviss ER. *Radiology of the pediatric elbow*. Boston: GK Hall, 1981.
17. McCarthy SM, Ogden JA. Radiology of postnatal skeletal development. *Skeletal Radiol* 1982;9:17–26.
18. Silberstein MJ, Brodeur AE, Graviss ER. Some vagaries of the radial head and neck. *J Bone Joint Surg [Am]* 1982;64:1153–1157.
19. Vostal O. Fracture of the neck of the radius in children. *Acta Chir Orthop Traumatol Cech* 1970;37:294–301.
20. Irshad F, Shaw NJ, Gregory RJ. Reliability of fat-pad sign in radial head/neck fractures of the elbow. *Injury* 1997;28:433–435.
21. Wedge JH, Robertson DE. Displaced fractures of the neck of the radius. *J Bone Joint Surg [Br]* 1982;64:256.
22. Anderson TE, Breed AL. A proximal radial metaphyseal fracture presenting as wrist pain. *Orthopedics* 1982;5:425–428.
23. Rokito SE, Anticevic D, Strongwater AM, et al. Case report and review of the literature: chronic fracture-separation of the radial head in a child. *J Orthop Trauma* 1995;9: 259–262.

24. Greenspan A, Norman A. The radial head-capitellum view: useful technique in elbow trauma. *AJR Am J Roentgenol* 1982;138:1186–1188.
25. Greenspan A, Norman A, Rosen H. Radial head-capitellum view in elbow trauma: clinical application and radiographic-anatomic correlation. *AJR Am J Roentgenol* 1984; 143:355–359.
26. Hall-Craggs MA, Shorvon PJ, Chapman M. Assessment of the radial head-capitellum view and the dorsal fat-pad sing in acute elbow trauma. *AJR Am J Roentgenol* 1985; 145:607–609.
27. Rodriguez-Merchan EC. Percutaneous reduction of displaced radial neck fractures in children. *J Trauma* 1994;37:812–814.
28. Lazar RD, Waters PM, Jaramillo D. The use of ultrasonography in the diagnosis of occult fracture of the radial neck: a case report. *J Bone Joint Surg [Am]* 1998;80:1361–1364.
29. Rogers SL, Mac Ewan DW. Changes due to trauma in the fat plane overlying the supinator muscle: a radiologic sign. *Radiology* 1969;92:954–958.
30. Scullion JE, Miller JH. Fracture of the neck of the radius in children: prognostic factors and recommendations for management. *J Bone Joint Surg [Br]* 1985;67:491.
31. Gille P, Mourot M, Aubert F, et al. Fracture par torsion du col du radius chez l'enfant. *Rev Chir Orthop* 1978;64:247–248.
32. Jones ERW, Esah M. Displaced fracture of the neck of the radius in children. *J Bone Joint Surg [Br]* 1971;53:429–439.
33. Bado JL. The Monteggia lesion. *Clin Orthop* 1967;50:71–86.
34. Carl AL, Ain MC. Complex fracture of the radial neck in a child: an unusual case. *J Orthop Trauma* 1994;8:255–257.
35. Patterson RF. Treatment of displaced transverse fractures of the neck of the radius in children. *J Bone Joint Surg* 1934;16:695–698.
36. Fogarty EE, Blake NS, Regan BF. Fracture of the radial neck with medial displacement of the shaft of the radius. *Br J Radiol* 1983;56:486–487.
37. Manoli A II. Medial displacement of the shaft of the radius with a fracture of the radial neck. *J Bone Joint Surg [Am]* 1979;61:788–789.
38. Baehr FH. Reduction of separated upper epiphysis of the radius. *N Engl J Med* 1932; 24:1263–1266.
39. Fraser KE. Displaced fracture of the proximal end of the radius in a child. A case report of the deceptive appearance of a fragment that had rotated 180°. *J Bone Joint Surg [Am]* 1995;77:782–783.
40. Ward WT, Williams JJ. Radial neck fracture complicating closed reduction of a posterior elbow dislocation in a child: case report. *J Trauma* 1991;31:1686–1688.
41. Wright PR. Greenstick fracture of the upper end of the ulna with dislocation of the radio-humeral joint or displacement of the superior radial epiphysis. *J Bone Joint Surg [Br]* 1963;45:727–731.
42. Olney BW, Menelaus MB. Monteggia and equivalent lesions in childhood. *J Pediatr Orthop* 1989;9:219–223.
43. Ellman H. Osteochondrosis of the radial head. *J Bone Joint Surg [Am]* 1972;54:1560.
44. Tullos HS, King JW. Lesions of the pitching arm in adolescents. *JAMA* 1972;220: 264–271.
45. Woods GW, Tullos HS, King JW. The throwing arm: elbow joint injuries. *J Sports Med* 1973;1:43–47.
46. Ellman H. Anterior angulation deformity of the radial head. *J Bone Joint Surg [Am]* 1975;57:776–778.
47. Pollen AG. *Fractures and dislocations in children.* Baltimore: Williams & Wilkins, 1973.
48. Radomisli TE, Rosen AL. Controversies regarding radial neck fractures in children. *Clin Orthop* 1998;353:30–39.
49. Blount WP. Fractures in children. *AAOS Instr Course Lect* 1950;7:194–202.
50. Vocke AK, Von Laer L. Displaced fractures of the radial neck in children: long-term results and prognosis of conservative treatment. *J Pediatr Orthop B* 1998;7:217–222.
51. McBride ED, Monnet JC. Epiphyseal fracture of the head of the radius in children. *Clin Orthop* 1960;16:264–271.
52. Dormans JP, Rang M. Fractures of the olecranon and radial neck in children. *Orthop Clin North Am* 1990;21:257–268.
53. Kaufman B, Rinott MG, Tanzman M. Closed reduction of fractures of the proximal radius in children. *J Bone Joint Surg [Br]* 1989;71:66–67.
54. Wood SK. Reversal of the radial head during reduction of fractures of the neck of the radius in children. *J Bone Joint Surg [Br]* 1969;51:707–710.
55. Wray CC, Harper WM. The upside-down radial head: brief report. *Injury* 1989;20: 241–242.
56. Dougall AJ. Severe fracture of the neck of the radius in children. *J R Coll Surg Edinb* 1969;14:220.
57. Angelov AA. New method for treatment of the dislocated radial neck fracture in children. In: Chapchal G, ed. *Fractures in children.* New York: Georg Thieme, 1981: 192–194.
58. Bernstein SM, McKeever P, Bernstein L. Percutaneous pinning for radial neck fractures. *J Pediatr Orthop* 1993;13:84–88.
59. Pesudo JV, Aracil J, Barcelo M. Leverage method in displaced fractures of the radial neck in children. *Clin Orthop* 1982;169:215–218.
60. Steele JA, Graham HK. Angulated radial neck fractures in children: a prospective study of percutaneous reduction. *J Bone Joint Surg [Br]* 1992;74:760–764.
61. Rodriguez-Merchan EC. Displaced fractures of the head and neck of the radius in children: open reduction and temporary transarticular internal fixation. *Orthopedics* 1991;14:697–700.
62. Futami T, Tsukamoto Y, Itoman M. Percutaneous reduction of displaced radial neck fractures. *J Shoulder Elbow Surg* 1995;4:162–167.
63. Biyani A, Mehara A, Bhan S. Percutaneous pinning of radial neck fractures. *Injury* 1994; 25:169–171.
64. Metaizeau JP, Prevot J, Schmitt M. Reduction et fixation des fractures et decollements epiphysaires de la tete radiale par broche centromedullaire. *Rev Chir Orthop* 1980;66: 47–49.
65. Metaizeau JP, Lascombes P, Lemelle JL, et al. Reduction and fixation of displaced radial neck fractures by closed intramedullary pinning. *J Pediatr Orthop* 1993;13: 355–360.
66. Gonzalez-Herranz P, Alvarez-Romera A, Burgos J, et al. Displaced radial neck fractures in children treated by closed intramedullary pinning (Metaizeau technique). *J Pediatr Orthop* 1997;17:325–331.
67. Sessa S, Lascombes P, Prevot J, et al. Fractures of the radial head and associated elbow injuries in children. *J Pediatr Orthop B* 1996;5:200–209.
68. Key AJ. Survival of the head of the radius in a child after removal and replacement. *J Bone Joint Surg* 1946;28:148–149.
69. Strong ML, Kropp M, Gillespie R. Fracture of the radial neck and proximal ulna with medial displacement of the radial shaft. Report of two cases. *Orthopedics* 1989;12: 1577–1579.
70. Mac Lennan A. Common fractures about the elbow joint in children. *Surg Gynecol Obstet* 1937;64:447–453.
71. Leung KS, Tse PYT. A new method of fixing radial neck fractures: brief report. *J Bone Joint Surg [Br]* 1989;71:326–327.
72. Kaplan EB. Surgical approach to the proximal end of the radius and its use in fractures of the head and neck of the radius. *J Bone Joint Surg* 1941;23:86–92.
73. Strachan JCH, Ellis BW. Vulnerability of the posterior interosseous nerve during radial head resection. *J Bone Joint Surg [Br]* 1971;53:320–323.
74. Pelto K, Hirvensalo E, Bostman O, et al. Treatment of radial head fractures with absorbable polyglycolide pins: a study on the security of the fixation in 38 cases. *J Orthop Trauma* 1994;8:94–98.
75. Dooley JF, Angus PD. The importance of elbow aspiration when treating radial head fractures. *Arch Emerg Med* 1991;8:117–121.
76. Peters CL, Scott SM. Compartment syndrome in the forearm following fractures of the radial head or neck in children. *J Bone Joint Surg [Am]* 1995;77:1070–1074.
77. Veranis N, Laliotis N, Vlachos E. Acute osteomyelitis complicating a closed radial fracture in a child: a case report. *Acta Orthop Scand* 1992;63:341–342.
78. Poland J. *A practical treatise on traumatic separation of the epiphyses.* London: Smith, Elder & Co, 1898.
79. Granthan SA, Kiernan HA. Displaced olecranon fractures in children. *J Trauma* 1975; 15:197–204.
80. Saberstein MJ, Brodeur AE, Graviss ER, et al. Some vagaries of the olecranon. *J Bone Joint Surg [Am]* 1981;63:722–725.
81. Smith FM. *Surgery of the elbow.* Philadelphia: WB Saunders, 1972.
82. Kovach JI, Baker BE, Mosher JF. Fracture-separation of the olecranon ossification center in adults. *Am J Sports Med* 1985;13:105–111.
83. Pavlov H, Torg JS, Jacobs B, et al. Nonunion of olecranon epiphysis: two cases in adolescent baseball pitchers. *AJR Am J Roentgenol* 1981;136:819–820.
84. Skak SV. Fracture of the olecranon through a persistent physis in an adult: a case report. *J Bone Joint Surg [Am]* 1993;75:272–275.
85. Torg JS, Moyer R. Nonunion of a stress fracture through the olecranon epiphyseal plate observed in an adolescent baseball pitcher. *J Bone Joint Surg [Am]* 1977;59: 264–265.
86. Bracq H. Fractures de l'olecrane. *Rev Chir Orthop* 1987;73:469–471.
87. Porteous CJ. The olecranon epiphyses. *Proc J Anat* 1960;94:286.
88. Danielson LG, Hedlund ST, Henricson AS. Apophysitis of the olecranon: a report of four cases. *Acta Orthop Scand* 1983;54:777–778.
89. Retrum RK, Wepfer JF, Olen DW, et al. Case report 355: delayed closure of the right olecranon epiphysis in a right-handed tournament-class tennis player. *Skeletal Radiol* 1986;15:185–187.
90. Turtel AH, Andrews JR, Schob CJ, et al. Fractures of unfused olecranon physis: a re-evaluation of this injury in three athletes. *Orthopedics* 1995;18:390–394.
91. Wilkerson RD, Johns JC. Non-union of an olecranon stress fracture in an adolescent gymnast: a case report. *Am J Sports Med* 1990;18:432–434.
92. Thijn CJP, van Ouwerkerk WPL, Scheele PM, et al. Unilateral patella cubiti: a probable post-traumatic disorder. *Eur J Radiol* 1992;14:60–62.
93. Zeitlin A. The traumatic origin of accessory bones at the elbow. *J Bone Joint Surg* 1935; 17:933–938.
94. Di Cesare PE, Sew-Hoy A, Krom W. Bilateral isolated olecranon fractures in an infant as presentation of osteogenesis imperfecta. *Orthopedics* 1992;15:741–743.
95. Mudgal CS. Olecranon fractures in osteogenesis imperfecta: a case report. *Acta Orthop Belg* 1992;58:453–456.
96. Pappas AM. Elbow problems associated with baseball during childhood. *Clin Orthop* 1982;164:30–41.
97. Maffulli N, Chan D, Aldridge MJ. Overuse injuries of the olecranon in young gymnasts. *J Bone Joint Surg [Br]* 1992;74:305–308.
98. Fahey JJ. Fractures of the elbow in children. *AAOS Instr Course Lect* 1980;17:13–46.
99. Maylahn DJ, Fahey JJ. Fractures of the elbow in children. *JAMA* 1958;166:220–228.
100. Papavasiliou VA, Beslikas TA, Nenopoulos S. Isolated fractures of the olecranon in children. *Injury* 1987;18:100–102.
101. Gaddy BC, Strecker WB, Schoenecker PL. Surgical treatment of displaced olecranon fractures in children. *J Pediatr Orthop* 1997;17:321–324.
102. Newell RLM. Olecranon fractures in children. *Injury* 1975;7:33–36.
103. Graves SC, Canale ST. Fractures of the olecranon in children: long-term follow-up. *J Pediatr Orthop* 1993;13:239–241.

104. Burge P, Benson M. Bilateral congenital pseudoarthrosis of the olecranon. *J Bone Joint Surg [Br]* 1987;69:460–462.
105. Theodorou SD, Ierodiaconou MN, Roussis N. Fracture of the upper end of the ulna associated with dislocation of the head of the radius in children. *Clin Orthop* 1988; 228:240–249.
106. Suprock MD, Lubahn JD. Olecranon fracture with unilateral closed radial shaft fracture in a child with open epiphysis. *Orthopedics* 1990;13:463–465.
107. Zimmerman H. Fractures of the elbow. In: Weber BG, Brunner C, Freuler F, eds. *Treatment of fractures in children and adolescents.* New York: Springer-Verlag, 1980.
108. Mathews JG. Fractures of the olecranon in children. *Injury* 1981;12:207–212.
109. Fan G-F, Wu C-C, Shin C-H. Olecranon fractures treated with tension band wiring techniques: Comparisons among three different configurations. *Chang Keng I Hsueh* 1993;16:231–238.
110. Roe SC. Tension band wiring of olecranon fractures: a modification of the AO technique. *Clin Orthop* 1994;308:284–286.
111. Rowland SA, Burkhart SS. Tension band wiring of olecranon fractures. A modification of the AO technique. *Clin Orthop* 1992;277:238–242.
112. Teasdall R, Savoie FH, Hughes JL. Comminuted fractures of the proximal radius and ulna. *Clin Orthop* 1993;292:37–47.
113. Murphy DF, Greene WB, Dameron TB. Displaced olecranon fractures in adults. *Clin Orthop* 1987;224:215–223.
114. Murphy DF, Greene WB, Gilbert JA, et al. Displaced olecranon fractures in adults. biomedical analysis of fixation methods. *Clin Orthop* 1987;224:210–214.
115. Macko D, Azabo RM. Complications of tension band wiring of olecranon fractures. *J Bone Joint Surg [Am]* 1985;67:1396–1401.
116. Montgomery RJ. A secure method of olecranon fixation: a modification of tension band wiring technique. *J R Coll Surg Edinb* 1986;31:179–182.
117. An HS, Loder RT. Intra-articular entrapment of a displaced olecranon fracture. *Orthopedics* 1989;12:289–291.
118. Bracq H. Fracture de l'apophyse coronoide. *Rev Chir Orthop* 1987;73:472–473.
119. Blasier RD. Intra-articular flap fracture of the olecranon in a child. *J Bone Joint Surg [Am]* 1989;71:945–947.
120. Regan W, Morrey BF. Classification and treatment of coronoid process fractures. *Orthopedics* 1992;15:845–848.
121. Regan W, Morrey B. Fractures of the coronoid process of the ulna. *J Bone Joint Surg [Am]* 1989;71:1348–1354.
122. Tanzman M, Kaufman B. Fracture of the coronoid process of the ulna requiring reduction in extension. *J Hand Surg [Am]* 1988;13:741–742.

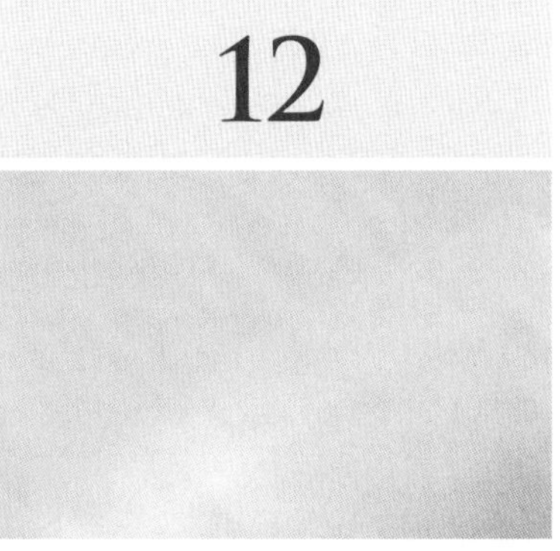

MONTEGGIA FRACTURE–DISLOCATION IN CHILDREN

José F. de la Garza

Monteggia fracture–dislocations involve an ulna fracture in association with a radial head dislocation. The main problem with this injury has been a failure to correctly diagnose the injury. The original description of an anterior dislocation of the proximal radius and fracture of the proximal ulna has been expanded to include dislocations of the radial head in multiple directions and combinations of injuries to the ulna and distal humerus. Fortunately, if the injury is recognized, a successful outcome generally occurs if the principles outlined in this chapter are followed. Treatment results are better in children than in adults.

HISTORICAL BACKGROUND

"I unhappily remember the case of a girl who, after a fall, seemed to me to have sustained a fracture of the ulna in its upper third. It might have been that some commotion of the dislocated bone misled me at the beginning of treatment, or else it might have been that there really was a fracture of the ulna with a dislocation of the radius, as I undoubtedly found in another case. The fact is that at the end of the month, when the bandage was removed and all the swelling had disappeared, I found that on extending the forearm the head of the radius jumped outwards, forming a hard ugly prominence on the anterior surface of the elbow, showing in an extremely obvious way that this was a true anterior dislocation of the head of the radius. When compressed it went back into place, but left to itself it came out again, especially on extension of the forearm. I applied compresses and a new bandage to hold it in but it would not stay in place." This was the original description by Giovanni Monteggia in 1814 (1).

Giovanni Batista Monteggia, a surgical pathologist and public health official in Milan, first described Monteggia fractures. He observed the original two injuries in cadavers and provided the description: "A traumatic lesion distinguished by a fracture of the proximal third of the ulna and an anterior dislocation of the proximal epiphysis of the radius."

Authors such as Smith (2), Speed and Boyd (3), Tompkins (4), Evans (5), Penrose (6), and Wright (7) in the beginning of the last century made important contributions in understanding the mechanism of this injury.

The classic monograph of Jose Luis Bado (8), written in Spanish in 1958 and in English (9) in 1962, coined the term "Monteggia lesion" and made an important contribution to understanding the complexity of this injury.

Jose Luis Bado, while Chief Director of the Instituto de Orthopedia y Traumatologia in Montevideo, Uruguay, studied proximal radial dislocations in association with fractures of the ulna. In his monograph, Bado defined the Monteggia lesion as an association of a radial head fracture or dislocation with a fracture of the middle or proximal ulna.

CLASSIFICATION

Numerous classification schemes have been developed, but Bado's classification has stood the test of time. Bado's classification divides Monteggia fractures into four types of true Monteggia lesions and equivalent lesions (Fig. 12-1).

True Monteggia Lesions (The Originals)

Type I

A type I lesion is an anterior dislocation of the radial head with a fracture of the ulnar diaphysis. The ulnar fracture can be at any level, but usually it is midshaft. This is the most common Monteggia injury in children, representing around 70% in most series.

Type II

Type II in most cases is an adult injury. The main characteristic of this injury is the posterior dislocation of the radial head with an associated ulnar diaphyseal or metaphyseal fracture with posterior angulation. This lesion is uncommon in children. Peiró et al (10) reported 1 type II lesion in their series of 25 acute Monteggia lesions in children. In 1965, Pavel et al (11), in their review of a series of posterior Monteggia fracture dislocations, reported only one type II lesion in a child. In both series, the children were older, approximately 13 years of age. Although reported as high as 6% by some authors, the overall prevalence of type II fractures in children is 3% when all studies are considered. In their series of 36 consecutive Monteggia fracture–dislocations in children, Ring and Waters found only 1 (3%) type II injury (12).

Type III

A type III lesion consists of a lateral or anterolateral dislocation of the radial head associated with a fracture of the ulnar metaphysis. The ulnar metaphyseal fracture usually is a greenstick type in children. This is the second most common type of Monteggia

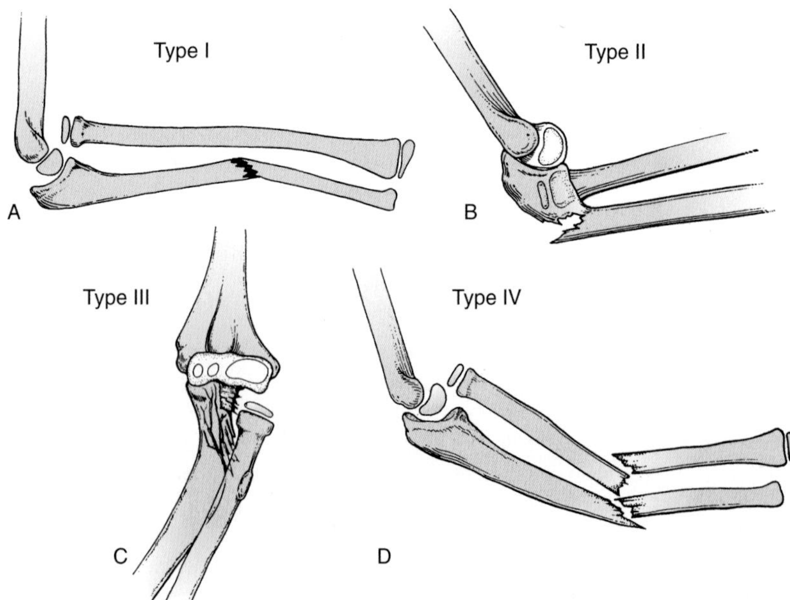

FIGURE 12-1 Bado's classification. **A.** Type I (anterior dislocation): the radial head is dislocated anteriorly and the ulna has a short oblique or greenstick fracture in the diaphyseal or proximal metaphyseal area. **B.** Type II (posterior dislocation): the radial head is posteriorly and posterolaterally dislocated; the ulna is usually fractured in the metaphysis in children. **C.** Type III (lateral dislocation): there is lateral dislocation of the radial head with a greenstick metaphyseal fracture of the ulna. **D.** Type IV (anterior dislocation with radius shaft fracture): the pattern of injury is the same as with a type I injury, with the inclusion of a radius shaft fracture below the level of the ulnar fracture.

fracture–dislocation in children (23%). This fracture pattern often is associated with radial nerve injuries and a coexisting intra-articular obstruction to radial head reduction, which requires surgical reduction of the radial head.

Extension of the ulnar fracture into the olecranon leads some investigators to classify this type of fracture–dislocation as a different lesion (12–16). If there is no concurrent radioulnar disassociation with the proximal ulnar fracture and radiocapitellar dislocation, the injury should be considered a fracture–dislocation of the elbow, not strictly a Monteggia fracture. This lesion is included by others in series of Monteggia fractures, classifying them by the direction of the radial head dislocation, usually lateral and anterolateral (17–20).

Type IV

Type IV Monteggia lesions are the least common (1%) in both children and adults. They are characterized by anterior dislocation of the radial head with fractures of the ulna and radius at the same level or with the radial fracture distal to the ulnar fracture (see Fig. 12-1). Wiley and Galey (20), Olney and Menelaus (18), and Dormans and Rang (21) all reported an average frequency of approximately 1% for type IV lesions. Ring and Waters, however, reported 4 type IV fractures (11%) in 36 consecutive Monteggia fracture–dislocations in children; they recorded any otherwise unclassified fracture of both bones of the forearm with proximal radioulnar dislocation as type IV lesions (12).

Monteggia Equivalent Injuries

Bado classified certain injuries as equivalents to the classic or true Monteggia lesions because of their similar mechanism of injuries, radiographic pattern, or methods of treatment.

Type I Equivalents

Type I equivalents (Fig. 12-2) include isolated anterior dislocation of the radial head; however, because minimal plastic deformation of the ulna accompanies the radial head dislocation, "isolated" dislocation probably is a misnomer. The best way to identify plastic deformation of the ulna is with the Mubarack line (the ulnar bow line) (see Fig. 12-41). Also included in this subclassification is the "pulled elbow" syndrome. The typical mechanism of longitudinal traction with pronation, possibly combined with hyperextension of the elbow joint, makes the pulled elbow syndrome similar to type I Monteggia fractures, even though there is no radiographic evidence of ulnar fracture or radial dislocation. Another type I equivalent lesion is fracture of the ulnar diaphysis with fracture of the radial neck. Fracture of the radial and ulnar shafts may be considered a type I equivalent if the radial fracture is above the junction of the middle and proximal thirds. Two additional type I equivalents are fracture of the ulnar diaphysis with either anterior dislocation of the radial head or olecranon fracture and posterior dislocation of the ulnohumeral joint with or without fracture of the proximal radius. Another type I equivalent not described before is elbow subluxation in addition to the anterior dislocation of the radius and the fracture of the ulna (Fig. 12-3).

Type II Equivalents

In his original classification, Bado stated that there were no equivalents to type II Monteggia lesions other than epiphyseal fracture of the radial head or fracture of the radial neck. Considering the mechanism of this injury as defined by Penrose (6), a posterior elbow dislocation could be considered a type II equivalent in children.

Types III and IV Equivalents

Bado also stated that there were no equivalents for types III and IV lesions. More recent reviews, however, have described fracture patterns that, because of the mechanism of injury, might be classified as type III or IV equivalents. Ravessoud reported an oblique fracture of the ulna with varus malalignment and a displaced lateral condylar fracture in a 13-year-old patient

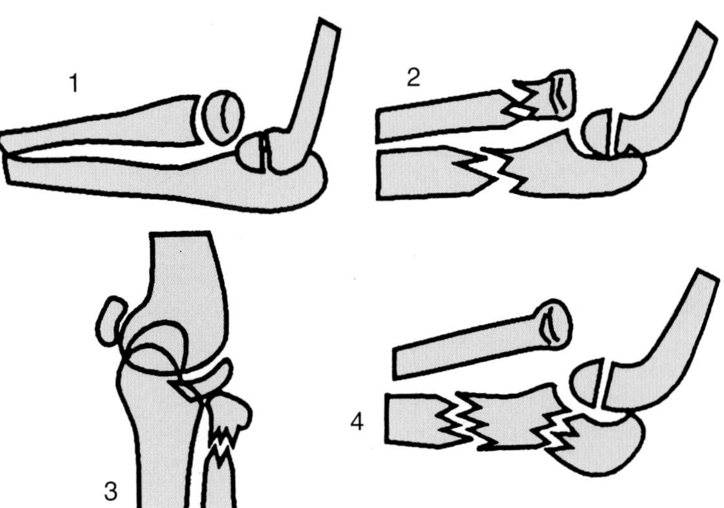

FIGURE 12-2 Type I Monteggia equivalents. 1: Isolated anterior radial head dislocation. 2: Ulnar fracture with fracture of the radial neck. 3: Isolated radial neck fractures. 4: Elbow (ulnohumeral) dislocation with or without fracture of the proximal radius.

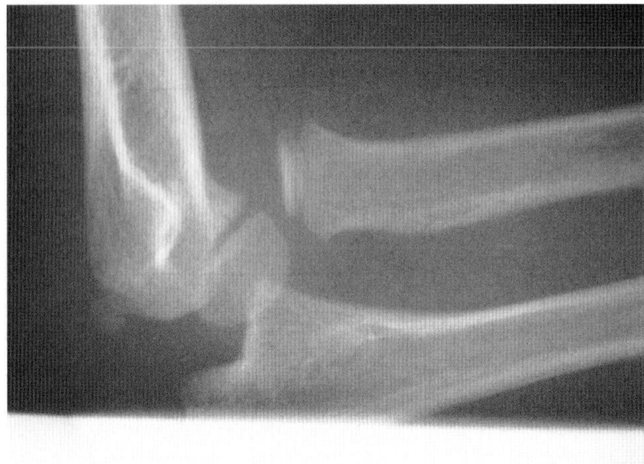
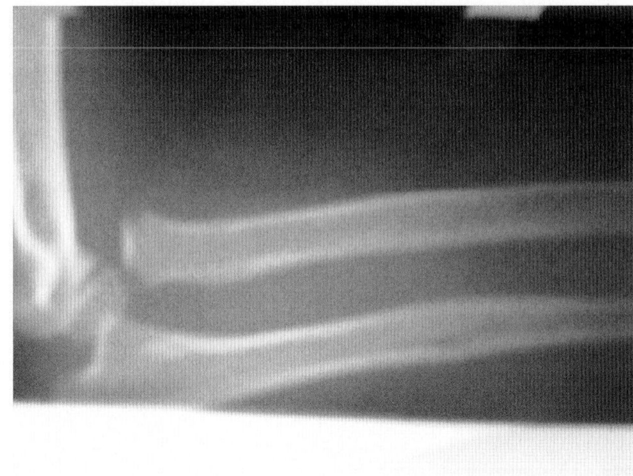

FIGURE 12-3 Type I Monteggia equivalent that includes elbow subluxation in addition to the radioulnar dislocation.

(Fig. 12-4) (22). This fracture pattern, which suggests hyperextension of the elbow combined with varus force, is produced by the same mechanism of injury as a type III lesion, as described by Wright (7).

We have classified fractures of the distal humerus, ulnar diaphysis, and radial neck (see Fig. 12-4) as equivalent to a type IV Monteggia fracture–dislocation because of the mechanism of injury. Bhandari and Jindal described a type IV variant that included a fracture of the mid-third radial shaft, an anterolaterally angulated fracture of the proximal ulna, and a posterior lateral dislocation of the radial head. A similar lesion was reported by Givon et al (23).

Hybrid Lesion

A hybrid lesion similar to a type III Monteggia lesion has been described in which anterior dislocation of the radial head was associated with a fracture of the metaphyseal region of the ulna that extended into the olecranon. Other studies have reported dislocation of the radial head in multiple directions. The treatment and outcome of each fracture are determined by the direction of the radial head dislocation combined with the pattern of the ulnar fracture.

Other Classifications

Dormans and Rang (21) extended Bado's classification by adding a type V, intermittent and habitual dislocation of the radiocapitellar joint and proximal radioulnar joint. Others (20,24) have considered the Bado type IV lesion to be a variant of type I and have excluded it from their classifications.

Letts et al (25) devised a classification of Monteggia fractures in children based on both the direction of the radial head dislocation and the type of ulnar fracture (Fig. 12-5). The Bado type I class was subdivided into three subtypes. Letts type A is anterior bowing of the ulna due to plastic deformation with anterior

FIGURE 12-4 Type III equivalent described by Ravessou: an oblique fracture of the ulna with varus alignment and a displaced lateral condylar fracture. Type IV equivalent described by Arazi: fractures of the distal humerus, ulnar diaphysis, and radial neck.

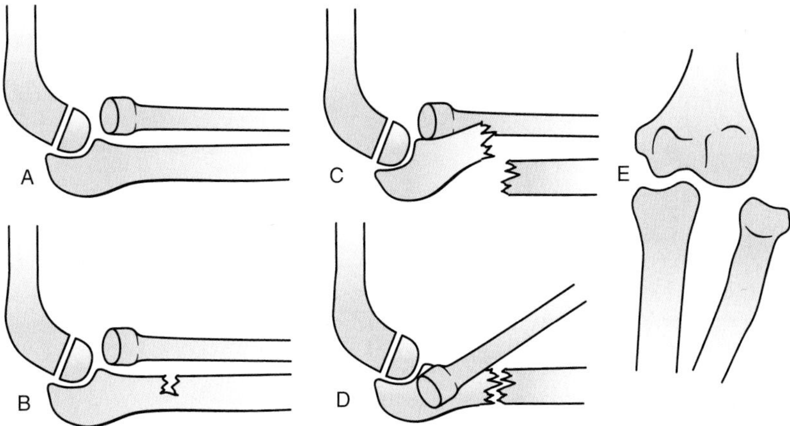

FIGURE 12-5 Pediatric Monteggia fracture classification by Letts et al. **A.** Anterior dislocation of the radial head with plastic deformation of the ulna. **B.** Anterior dislocation of the radial head with greenstick fracture of the ulna. **C.** Complete fracture of the ulna with anterior dislocation of the radial head. **D.** Posterior dislocation of the radial head with fracture of the ulnar metaphysis. **E.** Lateral dislocation of the radial head and metaphyseal greenstick fracture of the ulna.

dislocation of the radial head. Type B includes a greenstick fracture of the ulna, and type C has a complete ulnar fracture. Letts types D and E correspond, respectively, to Bado types II and III.

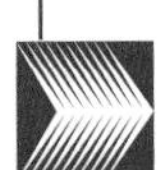

AUTHOR'S PREFERRED CLASSIFICATION

We prefer to use Bado's classification in evaluating and treating Monteggia lesions (Table 12-1). Although recognizing the contributions of other researchers, we believe that treatment principles are better determined by the direction of the radial head dislocation than the pattern of the ulnar fracture. Further, it is important not to exclude a type IV lesion from any classification scheme because the recognition and proper management of the radial fracture are important to the success of its treatment.

We also recognize a hybrid lesion consisting of a radial head dislocation and metaphyseal ulnar fracture extending into the olecranon. In this fracture–dislocation pattern, there may or may not be disassociation of the proximal radioulnar complex.

TABLE 12-1 Authors' Classification of Monteggia Fracture–Dislocations

Type	Dislocation	Fracture
True lesions		
I	Anterior	Metaphysis–diaphysis
II	Posterior	Metaphysis–diaphysis
III	Lateral	Metaphysis
IV	Anterior	Radial diaphysis, ulnar diaphysis
Hybrid lesion	Anterior, posterior, or lateral	Metaphysis or olecranon

Type	Description
Equivalent lesions	
I	Isolated dislocation of radial head Radial neck fracture (isolated) Radial neck fracture in combination with a fracture of the ulnar diaphysis Radial and ulnar fractures with the radial fracture above the junction of the middle and proximal thirds Fracture of ulnar diaphysis with anterior dislocation of radial head and an olecranon fracture
II	Posterior dislocation of the elbow
III	Ulnar fracture with displaced fracture of the lateral condyle
IV	None described

ANATOMY AND BIOMECHANICS

In addition to osseous injury of the Monteggia lesion, one must recognize the effect on ligaments, muscles, and nerves. Certain anatomic relations between the proximal radius and ulna and their surrounding structures must be taken into account in the management of Monteggia fractures. These can be divided into ligaments, bones, muscles, and nerves.

Ligaments

Annular Ligament

Stability of the proximal radioulnar joint is provided by the surrounding ligaments, primarily the annular ligament. The annular ligament maintains the position of the radial head within the radial notch of the ulna through the entire range of rotation, becoming tighter in supination because of the shape of the radial head. The substance of the annular ligament is reinforced by the radial collateral ligament at the elbow joint (see Fig. 12-3).

Quadrate Ligament

The quadrate ligament (26), or ligament of Denucé (27), is located between the radius and ulna distal to the annular ligament (Fig. 12-6). It consists of a dense anterior border and a thinner posterior border with an even thinner central portion. The two borders limit rotation and stabilize the radial head at limits of supination and pronation. The anterior border becomes tight in supination, adding stability to the proximal radioulnar joint. Excessive pronation causes the posterior border to fail, producing instability of the radial head.

Oblique Ligament

The oblique ligament, or ligament of Weitbrecht (28), extends from the ulna proximally to the radius distally (Fig. 12-7). It begins below the radial notch of the ulna and ends just below the biceps tuberosity on the radius. The bow of the radius tightens the oblique ligament when the radius is in supination and provides additional stability to the proximal radioulnar joint.

Interosseous Membrane

The interosseous membrane is distal to and separate from the oblique ligament, with its fibers running in the opposite direction (see Fig. 12-7). It acts in concert with the oblique ligament to approximate the radioulnar joint. The fibers of both the oblique and interosseous membranes tighten with supination of the radius.

Osseous Relations

There is little inherent osseous stability in the proximal radioulnar joint. The shape of the radial head contributes to tightness of the ligaments as the radius rotates.

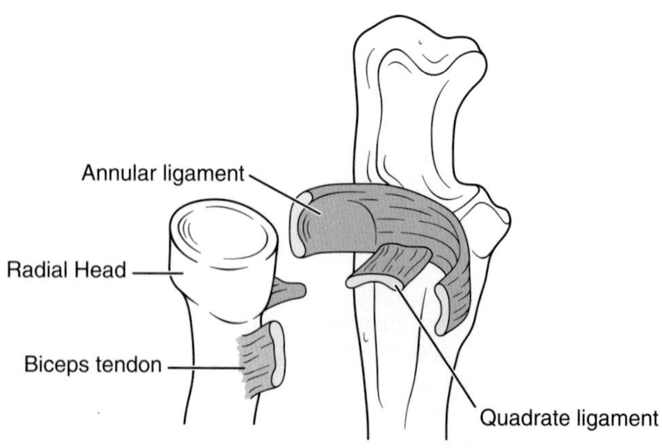

FIGURE 12-6 Ligamentous anatomy of the proximal radioulnar joint.

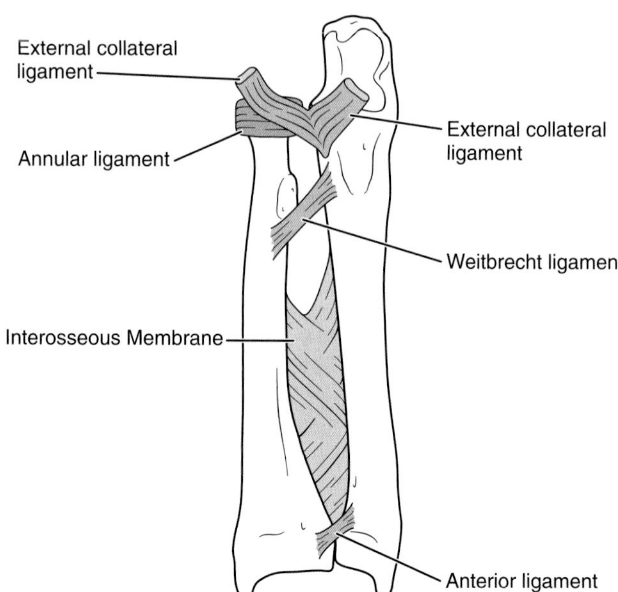

FIGURE 12-7 Ligaments of the forearm. In supination, the annular ligament, quadrate ligament, oblique ligament, and interosseous membrane are taut, stabilizing the radial head.

Shape of the Radial Head

The head of the radius is elliptical in its cross-section (Fig. 12-8). In supination, the long axis of the ellipse is perpendicular to the ulna, causing the annular ligament and the anterior border of the quadrate ligament to stabilize the proximal radioulnar joint further by tightening.

The contact area between the radius and the radial notch is greater in supination because of the broadened surface area of the circumference of the radial head in that position. The portion of the radial head circumference adjacent to the radial notch, when supinated, is less curved and is longer, proximal to distal, than other portions of the circumference. This provides a minimal increase in stability as the ligaments tighten.

Bow of the Radius

In the anatomic position, the apex of the radial bow is lateral (see Fig. 12-7). This curvature allows increased range of pronation as the radius rotates along the axis between the proximal and distal radioulnar joints. When the radius is in supination, the bow tightens the oblique and interosseous ligaments and increases proximal radioulnar stability.

Muscles

Whereas the ligaments stabilize the humeral–radioulnar complex, the muscles play an active role in the mechanism of injury that produces Monteggia fracture–dislocations.

Biceps Brachii

The biceps, inserting into the biceps tuberosity on the proximal radius, is a major deforming force. It is active in the pathome-

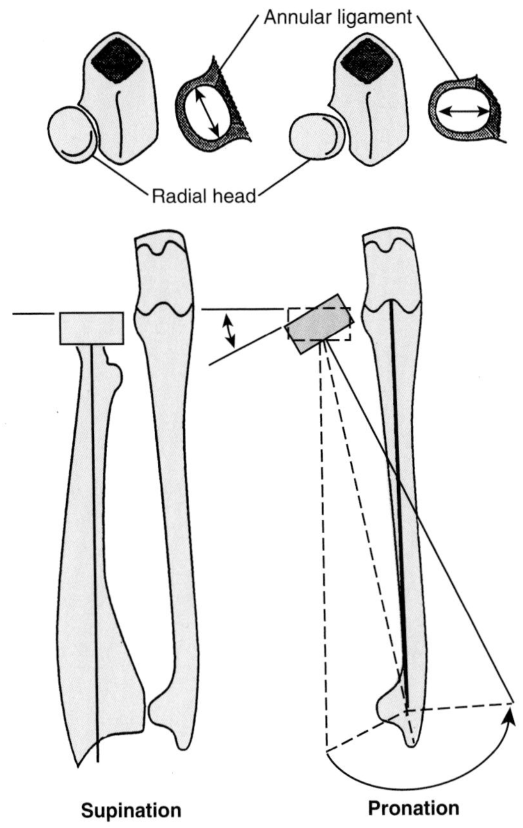

FIGURE 12-8 The radial head is an elliptical structure secured by the annular ligament, which allows movement and gives stability. Because of the shape of the radial head, the stability provided by the annular ligament is maximized in supination.

chanics of Monteggia fracture–dislocation, violently pulling the proximal radius away from the capitellum as the elbow goes into extension. During treatment, the effect of the biceps must be regulated by elbow flexion to prevent recurrence of the radial head dislocation.

Anconeus and Forearm Flexors

The anconeus and forearm flexors act together to create a radially angulated bow in the ulna in a Monteggia fracture–dislocation. The normal function of the anconeus is unclear. Electromyographic studies show that it helps stabilize the elbow as it goes into extension, creating a valgus moment at the joint, and during forearm pronation counteracts the varus moment produced by the pronator teres against an intact ulna (4,29).

The forearm flexors create a bowstring effect, producing a tendency for the fractured ulna to shorten and angulate radially after reduction (4).

Nerves

Posterior Interosseous Nerve

There is a close relation between the posterior interosseous nerve and the proximal radius, with the nerve coursing anterior and anterolateral to the radial head and neck on its path through the supinator muscle. With anterolateral dislocations of the radial head, direct trauma may cause paresis of the nerve. In adults, there is a more discrete organization of the proximal border of the superficial head of the supinator, forming the arcade of Frohse (Fig. 12-9) (30). This band is not as well defined in children, which may partially account for the lower incidence of permanent injury to the posterior interosseous nerve in children, as well as the high incidence of resolution once reduction of the radius is obtained (31).

Ulnar Nerve

The ulnar nerve, relatively tethered by the cubital tunnel, can be at risk in Monteggia fractures involving the proximal end of the ulna, particularly type II injuries (32).

CHARACTERISTICS AND MANAGEMENT OF MONTEGGIA INJURIES

Type I Lesions

Clinical Findings

Bado, in his original description, provided an accurate clinical picture of Monteggia fracture–dislocations. In general, there is fusiform swelling about the elbow. The child has significant pain and cannot move the elbow in either flexion and extension or pronation and supination. Usually an angular change in the forearm itself is evident, with the apex shifted anteriorly. There may be tenting of the skin or an area of ecchymosis on the volar aspect of the forearm. Later, as the swelling subsides, anterior fullness may remain in the cubital fossa. If the injury is seen late, as in a Monteggia fracture with only plastic deformation of the ulna but complete dislocation of the radial head, there is a persistent anterior prominence at the elbow and loss of full flexion at the elbow. The child may not be able to extend the digits at the metacarpophalangeal joint or at the interphalangeal joint of the thumb because of a paresis of the posterior interosseous nerve.

Radiographic Evaluation

The standard evaluation of a type I Monteggia fracture includes anteroposterior (AP) and lateral x-rays of the forearm. Any disruption of the ulna, especially an apparently innocuous bowing, should alert the physician to look for a disruption of the joints at either end of the forearm, particularly the position of the radial head (33–35).

Radiocapitellar Relation. The radiocapitellar relation is particularly important and is best defined by a true lateral view of the elbow. This relation in a type I Monteggia fracture may appear normal on an AP x-ray despite obvious disruption on the lateral view (Fig. 12-10). If there is doubt regarding the radiocapitellar relation, a true lateral view of the opposite elbow should be

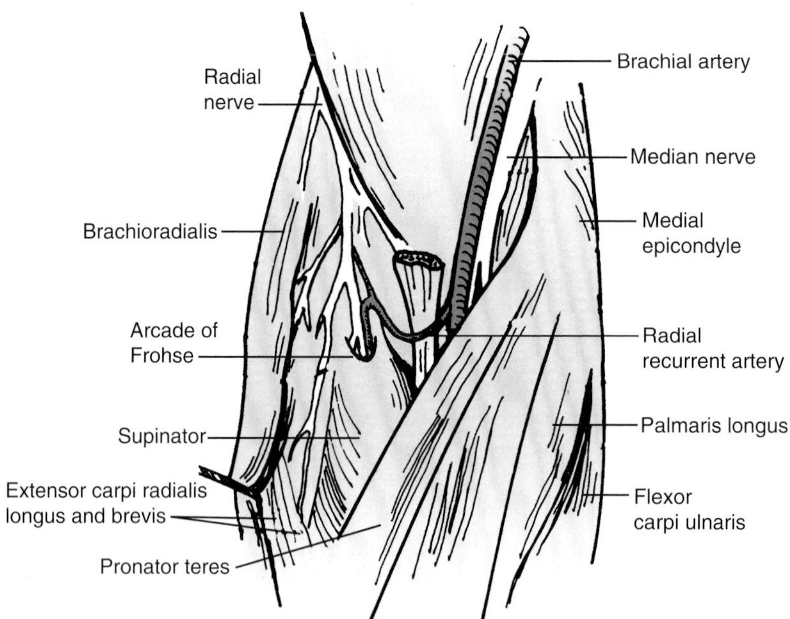

FIGURE 12-9 Dissection of the forearm at the level of the elbow.

obtained for comparison. Smith (2) and later Storen (36) noted that a line drawn through the center of the radial neck and head should extend directly through the center of the capitellum. This alignment should remain intact regardless of the degree of flexion or extension of the elbow (Fig. 12-11). In some instances, there is disruption of the radiocapitellar line in a normal elbow. Miles and Finlay (37) pointed out that the radiocapitellar line passes through the center of the capitellum only on a true lateral projection. They reported five patients in whom the elbow was clinically normal but the radiocapitellar line appeared disrupted. In analyzing the x-rays, they found that the radiographic projection of the elbow usually was an oblique view or that the forearm was pronated in the x-ray. If this disruption appears on x-rays in a child with an acute injury, however, it is the treating surgeon's responsibility to ensure that it is an insignificant finding.

A

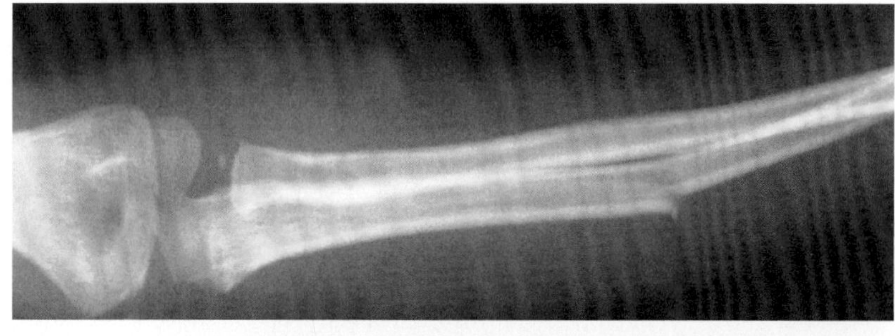

B

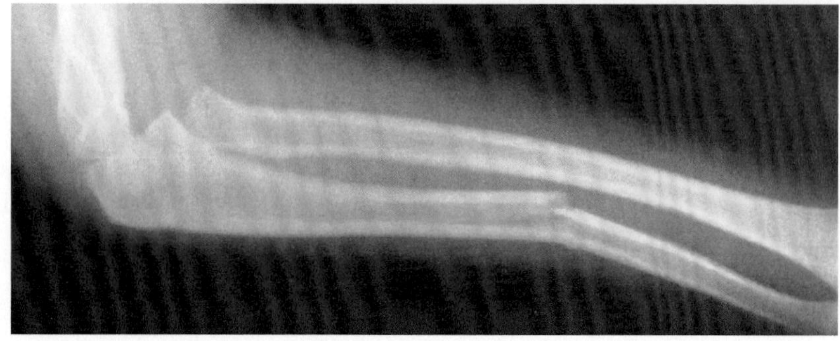

FIGURE 12-10 The AP view **(A)** demonstrates an apparently located radial head, but the lateral view **(B)** shows an anterior dislocation of the radial head. Note the disruption of the radiocapitellar line.

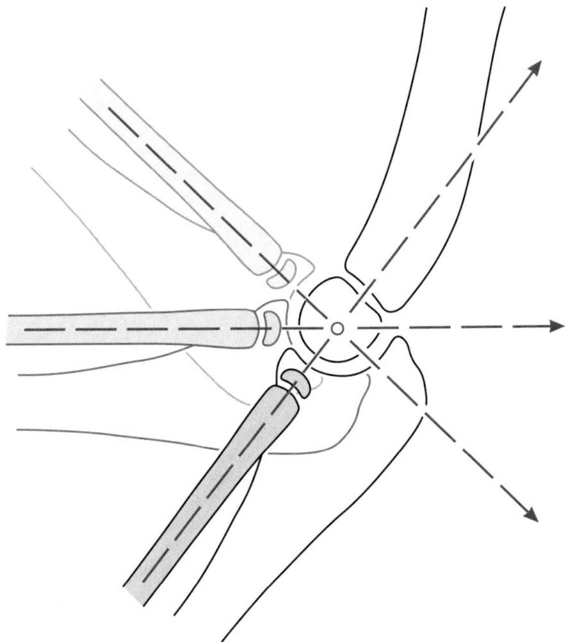

FIGURE 12-11 Composite drawing with the elbow in various degrees of flexion. A line drawn down the long axis of the radius bisects the capitellum of the humerus regardless of the degree of flexion or extension of the elbow.

Traumatic Versus Congenital Dislocation. When the radiocapitellar relation is disrupted, radiographic evaluation of the shape of the radial head and neck helps determine the cause of the disruption, especially if there is no history of trauma or the significance of the trauma is questioned. Bucknill (38) suggested that McFarland's (39) classic description of congenital radial head dislocation with an atypical deformed radial head, dysplastic capitellum, concavity of the posterior border of the proximal ulna, and para-articular ossifications probably represented old traumatic dislocations. Lloyd-Roberts and Bucknill (40) noted that many unilateral anterior dislocations probably were old traumatic dislocations rather than congenital dislocations. Caravias (41) recognized that the existence of a congenital anterior dislocation as a separate entity was doubtful and that true congenital dislocation of the head was rare. True congenital dislocation usually is bilateral and posterior and often is associated with various syndromes such as Ehlers-Danlos, nail-patella, and Silver syndrome (Fig. 12-12) (40,42). Therefore, all isolated anterior and anterolateral dislocations of the radial head, regardless of symptoms, should be considered as having a traumatic origin. Severe abnormalities in the form and size of the radial head can make it difficult to differentiate between congenital malformation and an undetected traumatic dislocation (Fig. 12-13). Regardless of the etiology, congenital or traumatic, treatment is the same as that for an undetected posterior dislocation of the radial head.

Mechanism of Injury

Three separate mechanisms of type I lesions have been described: direct trauma (3–5,9,43–47), hyperpronation, and hyperextension (43,47).

Direct Blow Theory. The first theory proposed in the English literature was the direct blow mechanism described by Speed and Boyd (3) (Fig. 12-14) and confirmed by Smith (2). This theory actually was proposed by Monteggia (48), who noted that the fracture occurs when a direct blow on the posterior aspect of the forearm first produces a fracture through the ulna. Then, either by continued deformation or direct pressure, the radial head is forced anteriorly with respect to the capitellum, causing the radial head to dislocate. Monteggia explained that these injuries sometimes resulted from a blow by a staff or cudgel on the forearm raised to protect the head (49). Another eponym for the Monteggia fracture–dislocation, the *parry fracture,* has been mentioned in the literature. During the American Civil War, Monteggia fractures were frequent because of direct blows on the forearm received while attempting to parry the butt of a rifle during hand-to-hand combat. The major argument against this theory as the sole mechanism is that in the usual clinical situation there rarely is evidence of a direct blow to the posterior aspect of the forearm, such as a contusion or laceration (4,5).

Hyperpronation Theory. In 1949, Evans (5) published his observations regarding anterior Monteggia fractures. Previous investigators had based their direct blow theory purely on clinical observation, but Evans used cadaveric experiments to support his hypothesis. He demonstrated that hyperpronation of the forearm produced a fracture of the ulna with a subsequent dislocation of the radial head. He postulated that during a fall, the outstretched hand, initially in pronation, is forced into further pronation as the body twists above the planted hand and forearm (Fig. 12-15). This hyperpronation causes the radius to be crossed over the mid-ulna, resulting in anterior dislocation of the radial head or fracture of the proximal third of the radius and fracture of the ulna. In the patients reported in Evans' article, the ulnar fractures demonstrated a pattern consistent with anterior tension and shear or longitudinal compression. His cadaveric studies, however, showed the ulna fracture pattern to be consistent with a spiral or torsional force. This theory also was supported by Bado (50).

Two arguments have been used to dispute the hyperpronation mechanism (4). First, the ulnar fracture rarely presents clinically in a spiral pattern; it usually is oblique, indicating an initial force in tension with propagation in shear rather than rotation. Second, Evans' experiments, which were done on totally dissected forearms, did not take into consideration the dynamic muscle forces at play during a fall on an outstretched hand in vivo.

Hyperextension Theory. In 1971, Tompkins (4) analyzed both theories and presented good clinical evidence that type I

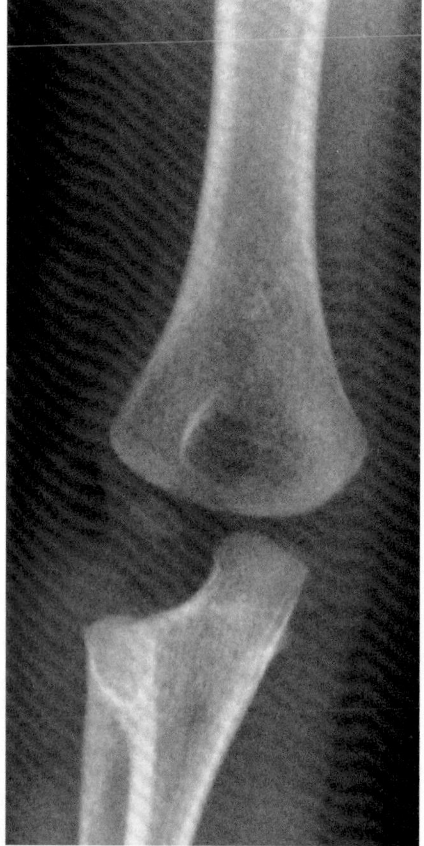

FIGURE 12-12 Congenital versus traumatic dislocation. **A.** AP view of the elbow of a 7-year-old who presented with limited forearm rotation. **B.** Lateral x-ray of the same child. Note dysplastic radial head. Anterior bowing of the ulna and a hypoplastic capitellum also are evident. Is this congenital or old trauma? **C.** AP x-ray of congenital synostosis. **D.** Lateral x-ray of congenital synostosis and posterior dislocation. Note posterior bow of the ulna and hypoplasia of the capitellum. This is congenital. (Interestingly, these are opposite elbows of the same child.)

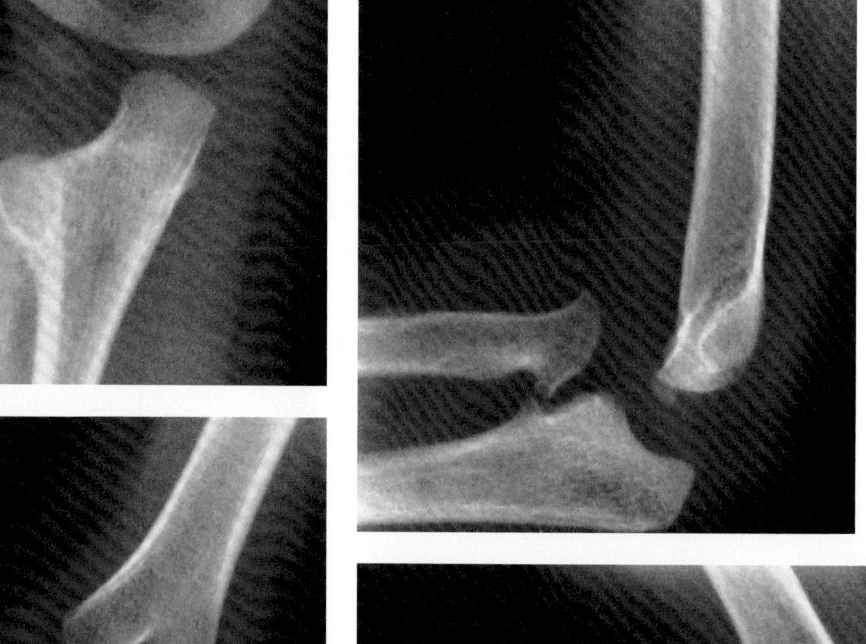

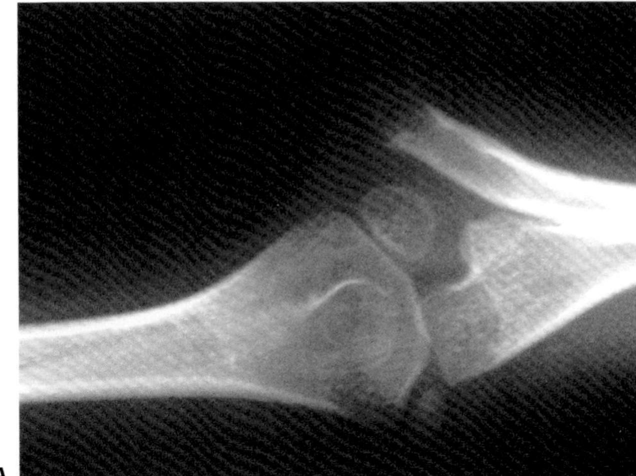

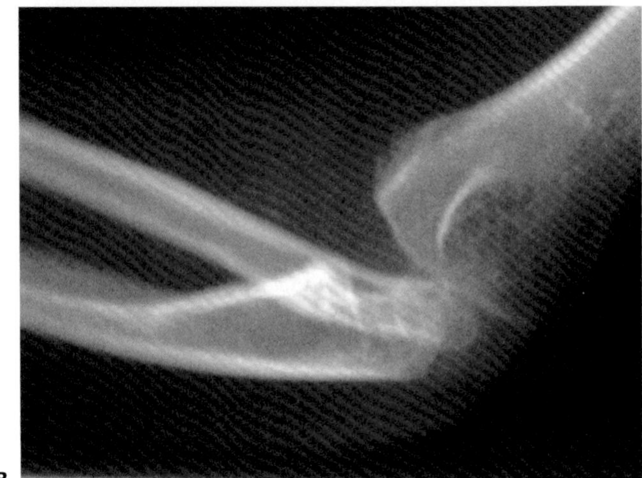

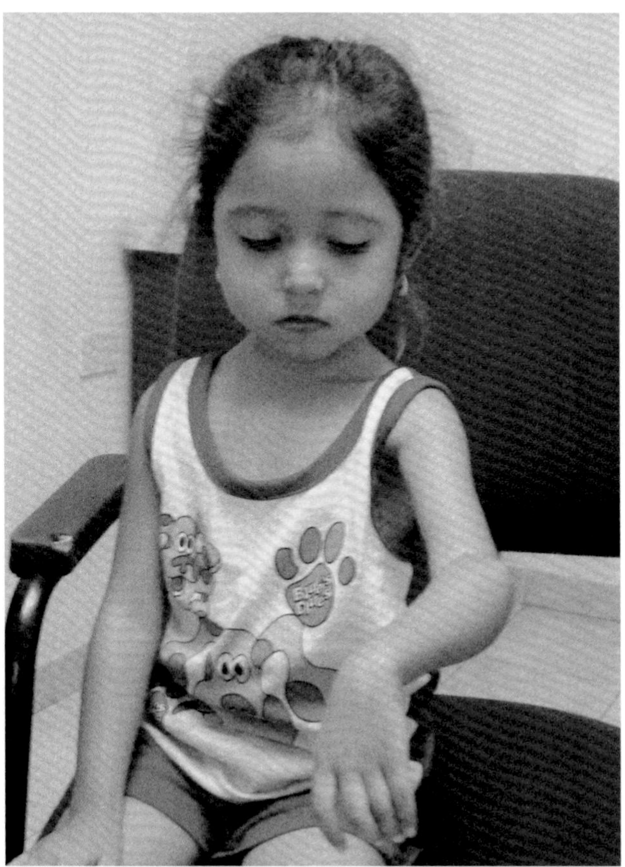

FIGURE 12-13 Congenital versus traumatic dislocation. **A.** AP view of the elbow joint shows complete dislocation and angulation and loss of the shape of the radial head. **B.** Lateral view shows posterior dislocation and hypoplastic radial head. **C.** Clinical photograph shows protrusion of the radial head dislocation.

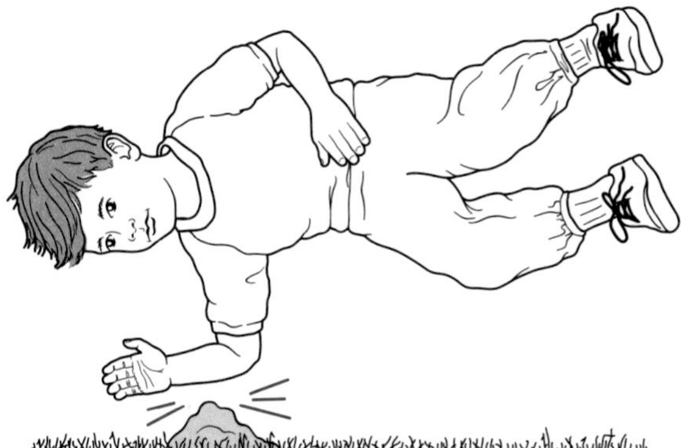

FIGURE 12-14 The fracture–dislocation is sustained by direct contact on the posterior aspect of the forearm, either by falling onto an object or by the object striking the forearm. The continued motion of the object forward dislocates the radial head after fracturing the ulna.

Monteggia fractures were caused by a combination of dynamic and static forces. His study postulated three steps in the fracture mechanism (Fig. 12-16): hyperextension, radial head dislocation, and ulnar fracture. The patient falls on an outstretched arm with forward momentum, forcing the elbow joint into hyperextension. The radius is first dislocated anteriorly by the violent reflexive contracture of the biceps, forcing the radius away from the capitellum. Once the radius is dislocated, the weight of the body is transferred to the ulna. Because the radius usually is the main weight-transmitting bone in the forearm, the ulna cannot handle the longitudinal force and subsequently fails in tension. This tension force produces an oblique fracture line, often with a butterfly fragment, or a greenstick fracture in the ulnar diaphysis or diaphyseal–metaphyseal junction. In addition to the momentum of the injury, the anterior angulation of the ulna results from the pull of the intact interosseous membrane on the distal fragment, causing it to follow the radius. The brachialis muscle causes the proximal ulnar fragment to flex at the elbow.

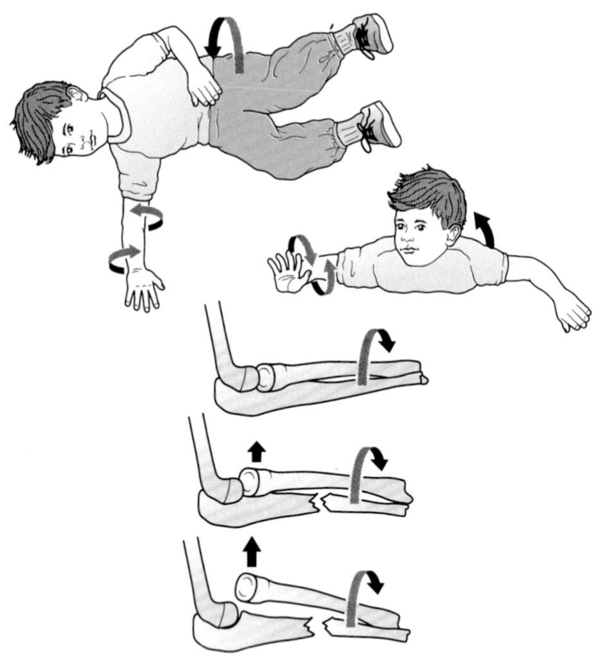

FIGURE 12-15 Hyperpronation theory (Evans). Rotation of the body externally forces the forearm into pronation. The ulnar shaft fractures with further rotation, forcibly dislocating the radial head.

Summary of Mechanisms of Injury

The Monteggia lesion probably can be caused by any of the three proposed mechanisms, but the most common mechanism is a fall on an outstretched hand that forces the elbow into complete extension, locking the olecranon into the humerus.

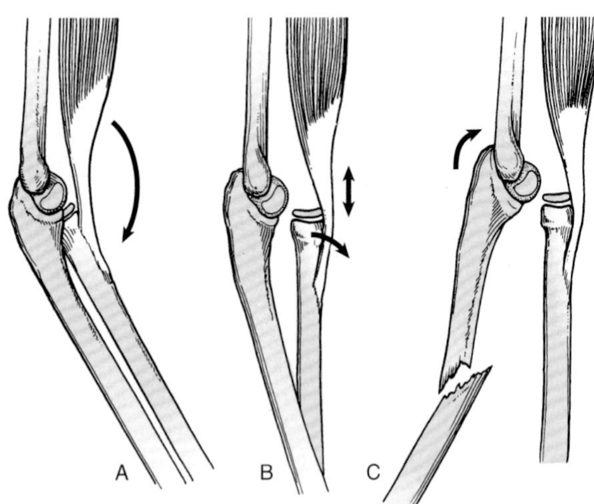

FIGURE 12-16 Hyperextension theory. **A.** Hyperextension: forward momentum caused by a fall on an outstretched hand forces the elbow into extension. **B.** Radial head dislocation: the biceps contracts, forcibly dislocating the radial head. **C.** Ulnar fracture: forward momentum causes the ulna to fracture because of tension on the anterior surface.

The forearm is in a rotational position of neutral to mid-pronation. As the ulna locks into the humerus, the bending force stresses the radioulnar joint. Because of the relatively pronated position of the joint, the ligamentous restraints are lax, providing only tenuous stability for the radial head. The anterior bending force, combined with a reflexive contraction of the biceps, violently dislocates the radial head anteriorly.

The radioulnar joint and its ligamentous complex are at risk because of the ligamentous laxity and decreased contact area between the proximal radius and ulna created by the rotation of the forearm. At mid-rotation, the short axis of the elliptical radial head is perpendicular to the ulna, causing the annular ligament and the dense anterior portion of the quadrate ligament to be relaxed. The contact area of the proximal radioulnar joint, because of the shape of the radial head, also is decreased, further reducing the stability of the joint. The ulna, now the main weight-bearing structure of the forearm, is loaded by a continued bending moment, causing tension on the anterior cortex and producing failure. The force at the site of failure is propagated in shear at approximately 45 degrees to the long axis of the ulna. This mechanism may produce plastic deformation with an anterior bow, a greenstick fracture, or an oblique fracture pattern, all of which are seen clinically. As the anterior bending movement continues, the vector of the biceps changes and acts as a tether and resists any further advance of the proximal radius. The distal fragment of the ulna continues to advance, acting as a fulcrum against the radial shaft. The anteriorly directed force of the distal ulnar fragment, combined with the retrograde resistance of the biceps, may create a fracture of the radius, or a type IV Monteggia lesion.

Treatment

Although most treatment recommendations are based on the Bado classification, Ring and Waters based their treatment choices on the type of ulnar fracture rather than on the Bado type. *Plastic deformation* of the ulna is treated with reduction (with general anesthesia) of the ulnar bow to obtain stable reduction of the radioulnar joint. *Incomplete (greenstick or buckle) fractures* are treated with closed reduction and casting. They suggested that almost all Monteggia fractures in children (types I and III) are most stable when immobilized in 100 to 110 degrees of flexion and full supination. For a *nearly complete* greenstick fracture or one associated with a radial fracture (type IV), intramedullary Kirschner wire fixation is considered for more stability. For *complete transverse* or *short oblique fractures,* which often are in bayonet apposition with malalignment or shortening, Kirschner wires are used to manipulate the proximal fragment into a reduced position and to hold the reduction. Long oblique or comminuted fractures, which may develop shortening and malalignment even with intramedullary fixation, are stabilized with a short plate and screws. Using this treatment protocol, Ring and Waters reported excellent results in all 28 patients treated within 24 hours of injury (Table 12-2). Two poor results occurred in patients who were referred late with persistent radial head dislocations.

TABLE 12-2 Treatment of Monteggia Fracture–Dislocations in Children According to Ulnar Injury

Type of Ulnar Injury	Treatment
Plastic deformation	Closed reduction of the ulnar bow and cast immobilization
Incomplete (greenstick or buckle) fracture	Closed reduction and cast immobilization
Complete transverse or short oblique fracture	Closed reduction and intramedullary Kirschner wire fixation
Long oblique or comminuted fracture	Open reduction and internal fixation with plate and screws

From Ring D, Jupiter JB, Waters PM, Monteggia fractures in children and adults. *J Am Acad Orthop Surg* 1998;6:215–224; with permission.

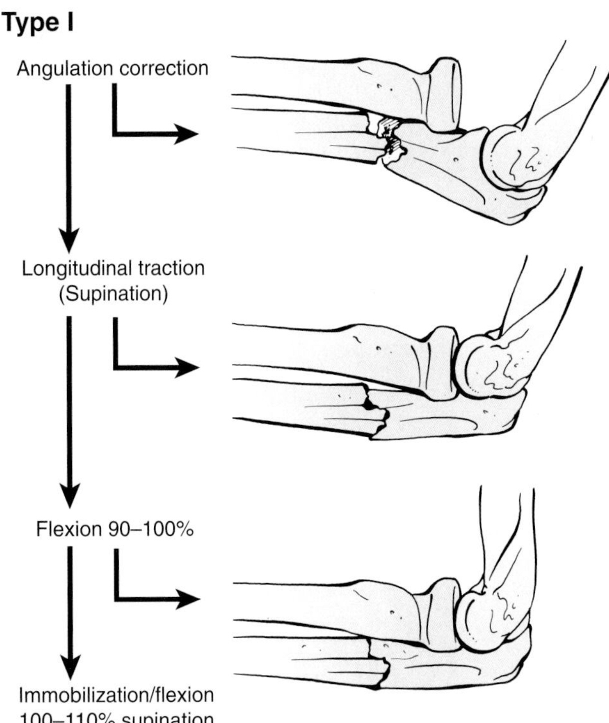

FIGURE 12-17 Reduction of a type I Monteggia fracture–dislocation.

Nonoperative Treatment. In all series (2,10,17,18,20,21,25, 43,47,51–53), anterior Monteggia lesions in children have uniformly good results when treated by manipulative closed reduction if the radial head is properly aligned and the ulna fracture is reduced with length preserved.

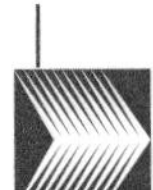

AUTHOR'S PREFERRED TREATMENT

Nonoperative treatment should generally involve three steps: correcting the ulnar deformity, providing a stable reduction of the radial head, and relieving the deforming muscle forces to prevent recurrent radial head dislocation and ulnar angulation (Fig. 12-17). Following is a step-by-step description of the different maneuvers for reduction of type I of Monteggia fractures.

Reduction of the Ulnar Fracture. The first step is to reestablish the length of the ulna by longitudinal traction and manual correction of any angular deformities present. The forearm is held in relaxed supination as longitudinal traction is applied, with manual pressure directed over the apex until the angular deformity is corrected clinically and radiographically (Fig. 12-18). With greenstick fractures, the plastic deformity must be corrected or the fracture completed to prevent recurrence of the angular deformity and, possibly, dislocation of the radial head (Fig. 12-19). Up to 10 degrees of angulation is acceptable in a complete fracture, providing a concentric radial head reduction is maintained (54). Angulation up to 25 degrees was noted in one series (17) to be compatible with full elbow and forearm motion. This degree of deformity usually remodels with time (46) (Fig. 12-20). In general, ulnar alignment should be nearly anatomic.

Reduction of the Radial Head. Once ulnar length and alignment have been reestablished, the radial head can be relocated. This often is accomplished simply by flexing the elbow to 90 degrees or more, thus producing spontaneous reduction (Fig. 12-21). Occasionally, posteriorly directed pressure over the anterior aspect of the radial head is necessary for reduction of the radial head. Flexion of the elbow to 110 to 120 degrees stabilizes the reduction. Once the radial head position is thought to be established, it should be scrutinized radiographically in numerous views to ensure a concentric reduction. With a type I fracture, the optimal radiographic view is a true lateral of the elbow with the forearm held in supination. The longitudinal axis of the radius should pass directly through the center of the capitellum (Fig. 12-22).

Alleviation of Deforming Forces. Once the concentric reduction of the radial head is confirmed, the elbow should be placed at approximately 110 to 120 degrees of flexion to alleviate the force of the biceps, which could redislocate the radial head (see Fig. 12-21). The forearm is placed in a position of mid-supination to neutral rotation to alleviate the forces of the supinator muscle and the anconeus, as well as the forearm flexors, which tend to produce radial angulation of the ulna.

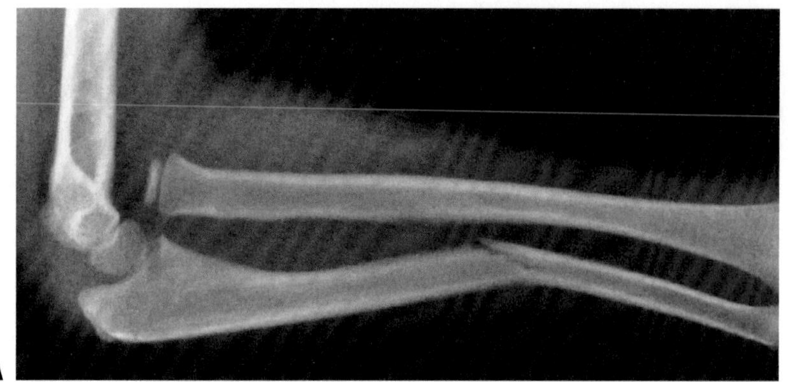

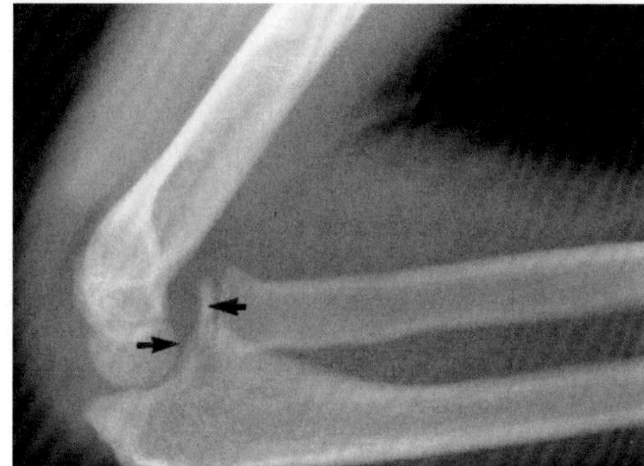

FIGURE 12-18 Closed reduction, type I lesion. **A.** Typical type I lesion in a 7-year-old. **B.** The deformity of the ulna is corrected first, and then the elbow is hyperflexed. However, the radial head is still anteriorly subluxed (*arrows*), and the ulna still has some anterior plastic deformation.

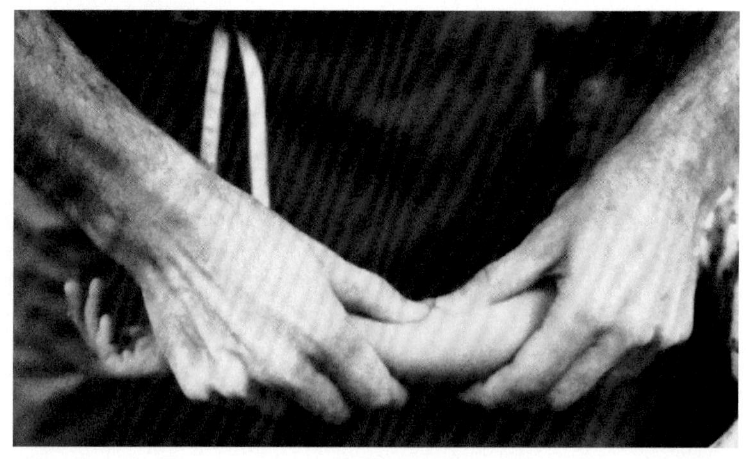

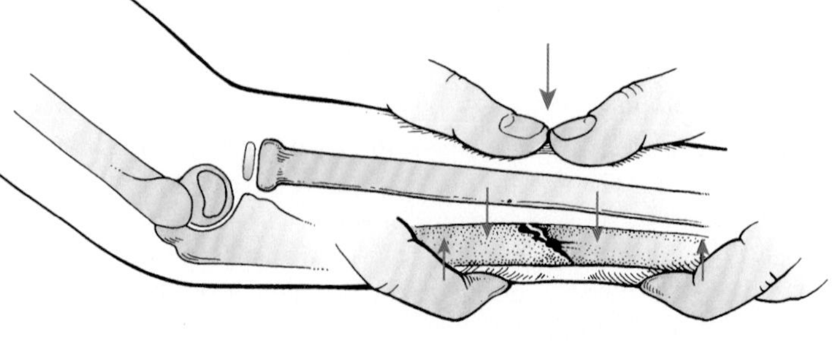

FIGURE 12-19 **A,B.** Correction of plastic deformation. Plastic deformation of the ulna must be corrected to prevent recurrence of the angular deformity. This allows reduction of the radial head and prevents its late subluxation. (From Wilkins KE, ed. *Operative management of upper extremity fractures in children*. Rosemont, IL: American Academy of Orthopaedic Surgeons, 1994, with permission.)

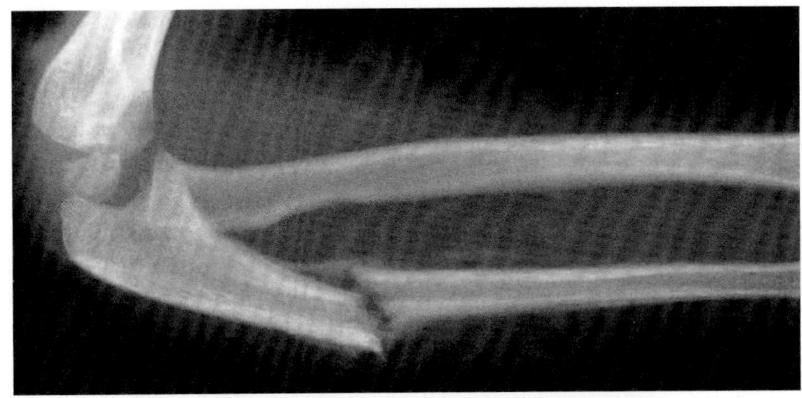

A

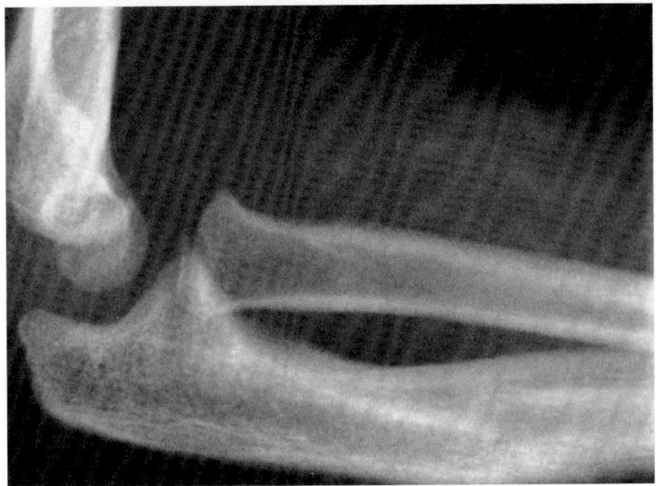

B

FIGURE 12-20 **A.** Type I Monteggia fracture–dislocation with posterior angulation of the ulna at 3 weeks after injury. **B.** Lateral x-ray at 3 months after injury shows remodeling.

Immobilization. Once the fracture is reduced and the neutralization position is established, a molded long-arm splint or cast is applied (Fig. 12-23) to hold the elbow joint in the appropriate amount of flexion, usually 110 to 120 degrees. Once the cast is completed, careful radiographic assessment should establish the concentric reduction of the radial head with respect to the capitellum, as well as satisfactory alignment of the ulna.

After Care. The patient is followed at 7- to 10-day intervals to confirm continued satisfactory reduction by radiography. At 4 to 6 weeks after the initial reduction, if there is radiographic evidence of consolidation of the ulnar fracture and stability of the radial head, the long-arm cast can be removed, with progressive guarded return to full activity.

Operative Treatment

Indications. Although uncommon, there are two indications for operative treatment of type I fracture–dislocations: failure of ulnar reduction and failure of radial head reduction.

Failure of Ulnar Reduction. If the ulnar fracture cannot be reduced or held in satisfactory alignment by closed treatment, operative intervention is indicated. The quality of the ulnar reduction affects the ability to reduce the radial head, which is of primary importance. Watson and Singer (55) reported median nerve entrapment that prevented ulnar reduction in a greenstick fracture in a 6-year-old with a type I Monteggia lesion. If the ulnar fracture can be reduced but not maintained because of the obliquity of the fracture, internal fixation combined with open or closed reduction may be necessary (17,18). Intramedullary fixation, rather than fixation with a plate, is standard in most series of Monteggia fracture–dislocations in children (9,10,17,18,20,21,36,56,57). This method of fixation can be accomplished percutaneously, using image intensification and flexible nails or Kirschner wires; this avoids the potential complications of open reduction and plate fixation (58–62).

Failure of Radial Head Reduction. The second indication is failure to reduce the radial head satisfactorily by closed means. This is more common in type III Monteggia lesions, but it also can occur in type I lesions. It results from the interposition of material, including torn fragments of the ruptured orbicular ligament and capsule or an entrapped orbicular ligament pulled over the radial head (4,63). Interposed cartilaginous or osteochondral fractures (Fig. 12-24) in the radiocapitellar joint or radial notch in the ulna may prevent complete reduction of the radial head

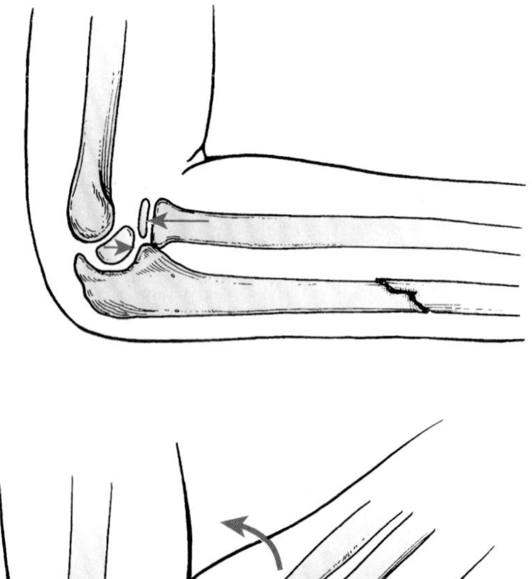

FIGURE 12-21 Reduction of the radial head. Flexing the elbow spontaneously reduces the radial head. Occasionally, manual pressure is required in combination with flexion.

(4,24). Morris (64) described a patient in whom reduction of the radial head was obstructed by radial nerve entrapment between the radial head and ulna (Fig. 12-25).

Surgical Approach. The most direct approach to the radiocapitellar joint is from the posterolateral aspect of the elbow. The interval between the anconeus and the extensor carpi ulnaris, using the distal portion of a Kocher J incision, provides sufficient exposure of the radial head and the interposed structures (65,66). This approach protects the posterior interosseous nerve when the forearm is pronated. A more extensile approach was described by Boyd (67). This exposure is begun by making an incision following the lateral border of the triceps posteriorly to the lateral condyle and extending it along the radial side of the ulna (Fig. 12-26). The incision is carried under the anconeus and extensor carpi ulnaris in an extraperiosteal manner, elevating the fibers of the supinator from the ulna. This carries the approach down to the interosseous membrane, allowing exposure of the radiocapitellar joint, excellent visualization of the orbicular ligament, access to the proximal fourth of the entire radius, and approach to the ulnar fracture, all through the same incision (3,52,67).

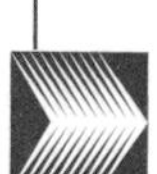

AUTHOR'S PREFERRED TREATMENT

The importance of radial head reduction should be emphasized because failure of reduction affects the long-term outcome. Ulnar reduction directly affects the surgeon's ability to reduce the radial head. In children, the preferred treatment is closed manipulative reduction. If, however, reduction of the

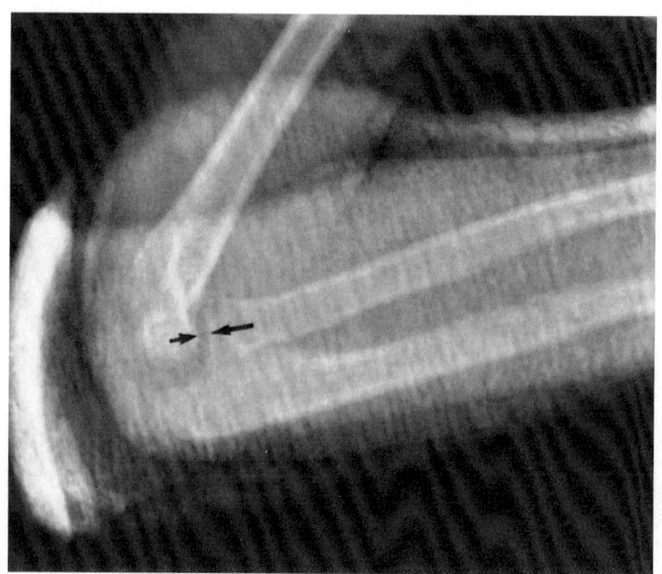

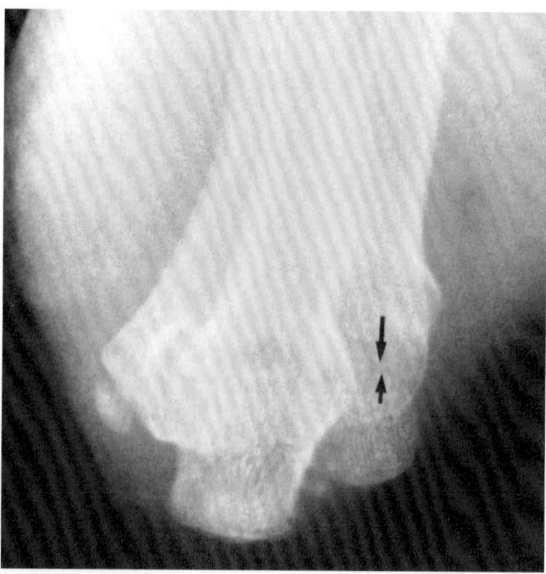

FIGURE 12-22 Once the reduction is complete, x-rays should be analyzed for reestablishment of the radiocapitellar line (*arrows*) and ulnar alignment on both the lateral **(A)** and Jones **(B)** views.

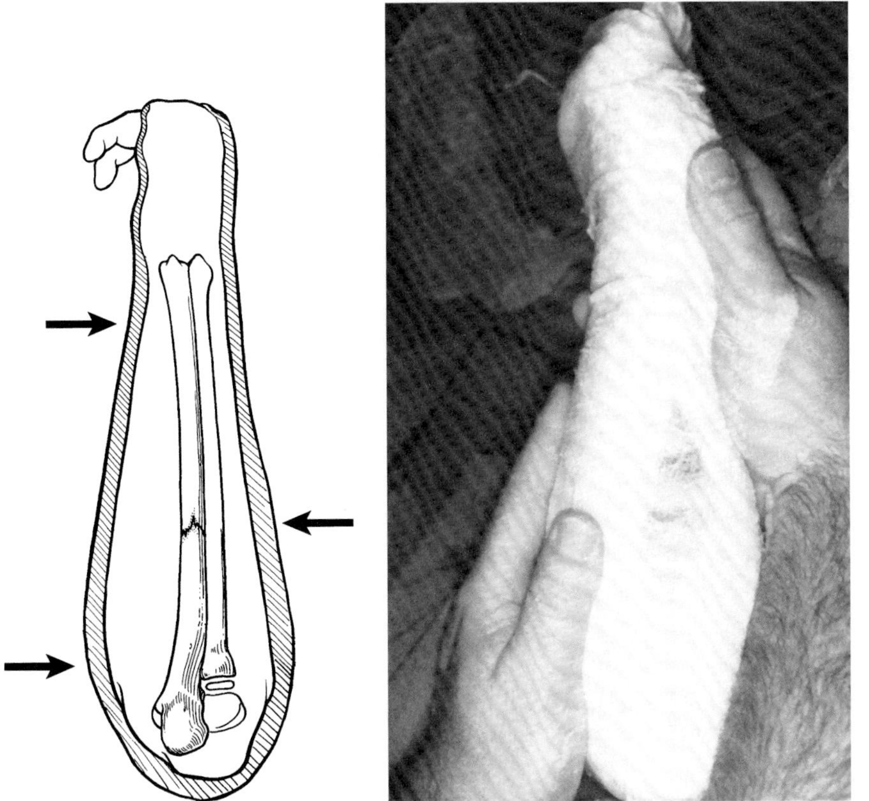

FIGURE 12-23 Immobilization after reduction. **A.** After reduction, the forearm is immobilized with three-point molding (*arrows*) to maintain ulnar alignment. **B.** The forearm component is incorporated into a long-arm cast with the elbow flexed to 110 to 120 degrees of flexion.

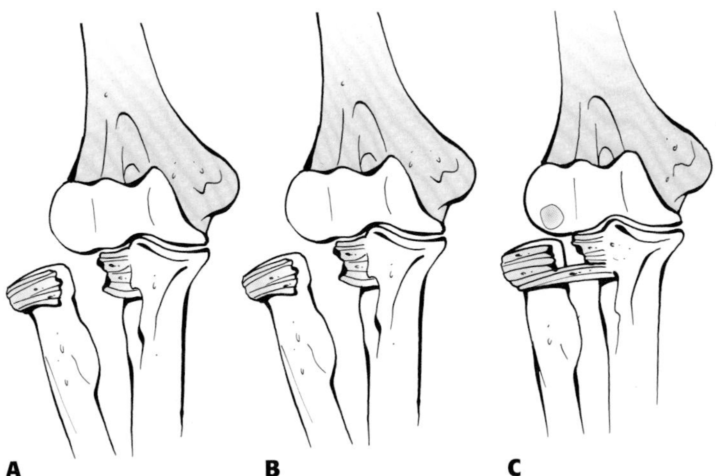

FIGURE 12-24 Radial head/annular ligament. **A.** Radial head dislocation and complete annular ligament tear. **B.** Radial head dislocation and partial ligament tear. **C.** Radial head dislocation and partial or complete annular ligament tear and osteochondral fragment.

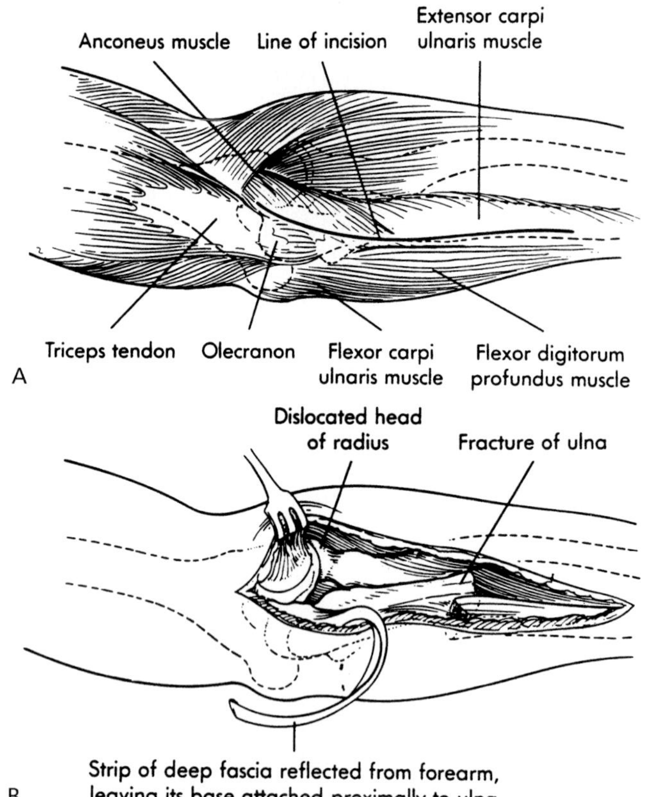

FIGURE 12-25 Surgical approach. **A.** The incision is carried under the anconeus and extensor carpi ulnaris to expose the radial head and orbicular ligament. **B.** The incision can be extended distally to allow exposure of the ulnar fracture and proximally to facilitate harvesting of the tendinous strip for orbicular ligament reconstruction, if necessary.

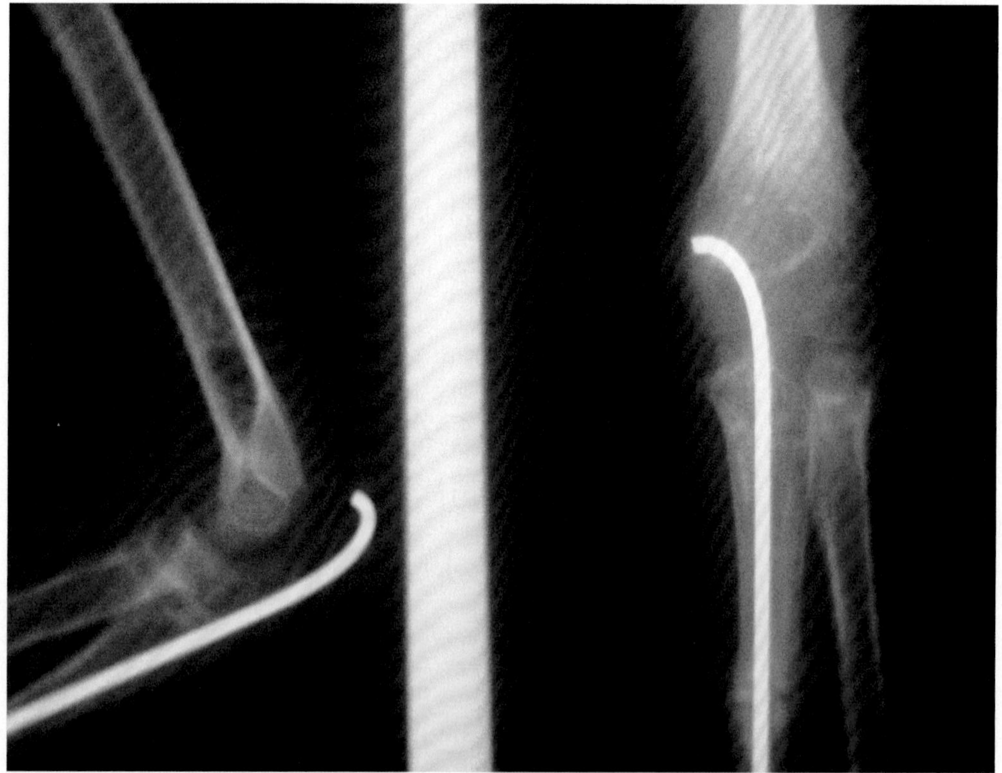

FIGURE 12-26 Stabilization of the ulna. Unstable fractures or those in children 12 years of age or older can be immobilized using a percutaneous pinning technique.

radial head or ulnar fracture cannot be obtained or if instability of the ulnar fracture threatens the radial reduction, operative treatment is always indicated.

Surgical Approach. We prefer to use the Boyd approach because of its extensile nature (see Fig. 12-26).

Treatment of the Annular Ligament. Once the reduction is obtained through this approach, we repair the annular ligament, providing it can be done simply. If the ligament has been pulled over the radial head, it should be incised, replaced in its normal location, and repaired. Immediate reconstruction of the annular ligament usually is unnecessary because the radial head usually maintains its stability once the ulnar fracture is reduced to a satisfactory position.

If the reduction is unstable, we repair or reconstruct the annular ligament, combining it with the use of a transcapitellar Steinmann pin or transmetaphyseal pin from the radial neck to the ulnar proximal metaphysis (see Fig. 12-43); this is a safe way to maintain the reduction and to avoid the elbow joint with the transcapitellar Steinmann pin. The details of annular ligament reconstruction are discussed later in the section on old, undetected Monteggia lesions.

Treatment of the Ulnar Fracture. The ulnar fracture usually is treated closed, provided satisfactory alignment can be obtained. If the fracture seems to be unstable on the initial films or at the initial reduction, or if the child is younger than 12 years of age, internal fixation using an intramedullary pinning technique is done (58–60,62). This can be accomplished by using a single pin of sufficient size or multiple small pins, nesting them within the medullary canal to provide stability (see Fig. 12-26). This technique is minimally invasive and provides adequate stability in most fractures. It also allows easy retrieval of the instrumentation and has an overall low complication rate (61).

After Care (Same as Closed Reduction). Once reduction is obtained, a long-arm cast is applied with the elbow flexed 90 to 100 degrees and the forearm in neutral position.

Type II Monteggia Fracture–Dislocations

Incidence

Posterior Monteggia fracture–dislocations are uncommon, accounting for 6% in most series of Monteggia lesions in children (68), usually in older patients (approximately 13 years) (11) who have sustained significant trauma (47,69,70). However, type II Monteggia lesions are probably more common than reported because they often go unrecognized, being classified as type III lesions with posterolateral radial head dislocations.

Clinical Findings

As with type I Monteggia lesions, the elbow region is swollen but exhibits posterior angulation of the proximal forearm and a marked prominence in the area posterolateral to the normal location of the radial head. The entire upper extremity should be examined because of the frequency of associated fractures (11,71).

Radiographic Evaluation

Standard radiographic views of the forearm demonstrate the pertinent features for classifying this fracture. The typical finding is a proximal metaphyseal fracture of the ulna with possible extension into the olecranon (Fig. 12-27) (18,69,72). Midshaft fractures also occur, with an oblique fracture pattern (8,18,69). The radial head is dislocated posteriorly or posterolaterally (9) and should be carefully examined for other injuries. Accompanying fractures of the anterior margin of the radial head have been noted in adults (11,69) but not in children.

Mechanism of Injury

The cause of the type II Monteggia lesion is subject to debate. Bado thought the lesion was caused by direct force and sudden rotation and supination (9). Penrose analyzed seven fractures in adults (6) and noted that a proximal ulnar fracture was the typical pattern. He postulated that the injury occurred by longitudinal loading rather than direct trauma (3). Olney and Menelaus (18) reported four type II lesions in their series of children's Monteggia fractures. Three of these patients had proximal ulnar fractures and one an oblique midshaft fracture, suggesting two different mechanisms of injury.

The mechanism proposed and experimentally demonstrated by Penrose (6) was that type II lesions occur when the forearm is suddenly loaded in a longitudinal direction with the elbow flexed 60 degrees. He showed that a type II lesion occurred consistently if the anterior cortex of the ulna was weakened; otherwise, a posterior elbow dislocation was produced (Fig. 12-28). A possible difference in bony anatomy of the ulna suggested a reason for the high incidence of type II Monteggia fractures in older adults and their rarity in children. Penrose further noted that the rotational position of the forearm did not seem to affect the type of fracture produced.

Haddad et al (73) described type II Monteggia injuries caused by low-velocity injuries in six adults, five of whom were on long-term corticosteroid therapy. They suggested that this supports the theory that the type II (posterior) Monteggia injury is a variant of posterior elbow dislocation, in that it occurs when the ulna is weaker than the ligaments surrounding the elbow joint, resulting in an ulnar fracture before the ligament disruption associated with dislocation occurs.

Treatment

Nonoperative. As with type I injuries, type II lesions usually have a satisfactory result after closed reduction (10,18,20, 25,46). The ulnar fracture is reduced by longitudinal traction in line with the long axis of the forearm while the elbow is held at 60 degrees of flexion (Fig. 12-29). The radial head may reduce spontaneously or may require gentle, anteriorly directed pressure applied to its posterior aspect. The elbow is extended once

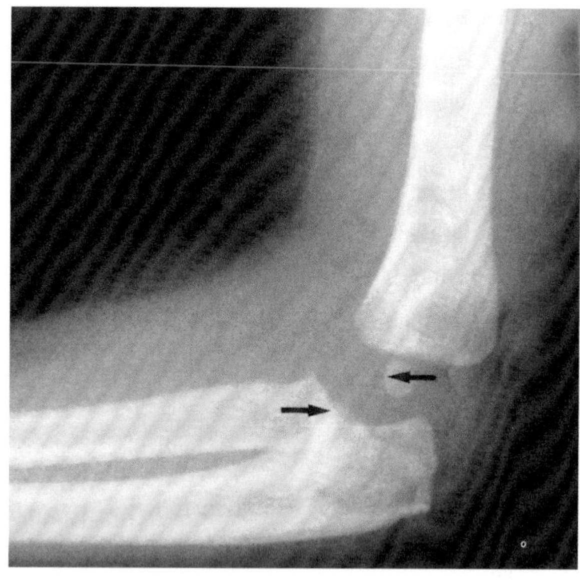

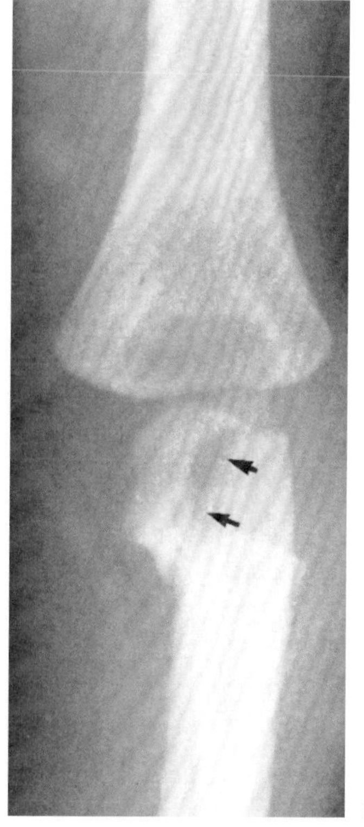

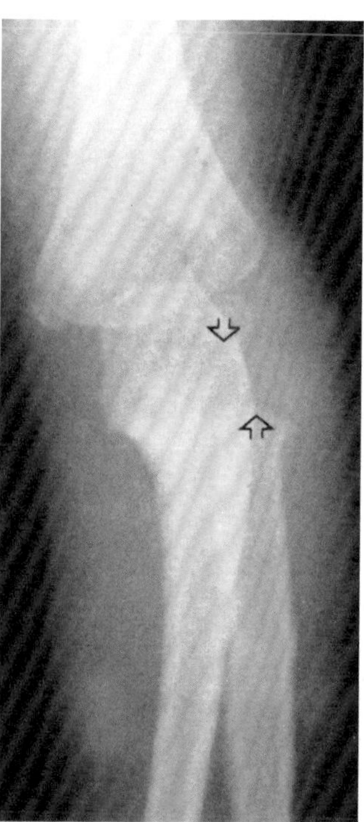

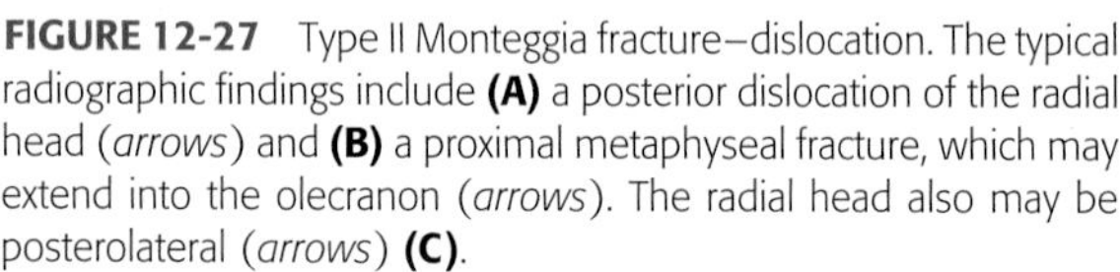

FIGURE 12-27 Type II Monteggia fracture–dislocation. The typical radiographic findings include **(A)** a posterior dislocation of the radial head (*arrows*) and **(B)** a proximal metaphyseal fracture, which may extend into the olecranon (*arrows*). The radial head also may be posterolateral (*arrows*) **(C)**.

the radial head is reduced and is immobilized in that position to stabilize the radial head and allow molding posteriorly to maintain the ulnar reduction (Fig. 12-30) (10,21,74,75). If the ulna alignment cannot be maintained, an intramedullary Kirschner wire should be used.

Operative. Because of the rarity of the lesion, there are no established indications for operative treatment. Treatment goals are stable concentric reduction of the radial head and alignment of the ulnar fracture. The radial head should be reduced by open technique if there is interposed tissue or if it is accompanied by a fractured capitellum or radial head. The ulnar fracture is exposed along its subcutaneous border if necessary and fixed internally. Fixation can be accomplished by plating or intramedullary fixation. Because of children's ability to heal rapidly, intramedullary fixation is adequate and sometimes can be done percutaneously after a closed reduction of the ulna (59,60).

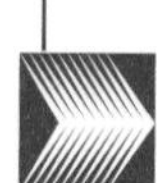

AUTHOR'S PREFERRED TREATMENT

First, ulnar length is reestablished by applying longitudinal traction and straightening the angular deformity. The radial head may reduce spontaneously or with gentle, anteriorly directed force directly over the radial head. Once reduced, the position of the head can be stabilized by holding the elbow in extension. The alignment of the ulnar fracture can be maintained by applying a cast with the elbow in extension or by using percutaneous intramedullary fixation. If intramedullary pinning is used, the elbow may be flexed to 80 degrees and a cast applied. X-rays should be taken after cast application and approximately every 7 to 10 days to confirm continued reduction of the radial head.

The Boyd approach can be used to obtain reduction of the radial head if it cannot be obtained through closed manipulation. Management of the annular ligament is the same as described for type I Monteggia lesions.

The cast, either in full extension or flexed 80 degrees at the elbow, is maintained for 3 to 4 weeks, and then changed to a removable splint. This allows early intermittent range of motion in a protected manner for 3 to 4 more weeks. At 6 to 8 weeks after injury, the patient can be released to full activities. This protocol may avoid the necessity for formal physical therapy (10).

Type III Monteggia Fracture–Dislocations

Clinical Findings

Lateral swelling, varus deformity of the elbow, and significant limitation of motion, especially supination, are the hallmarks of lateral (type III) Monteggia fracture–dislocations.

Incidence

Type III lesions are common in children, second in frequency to anterior type I Monteggia fracture–dislocations (9,10,18,

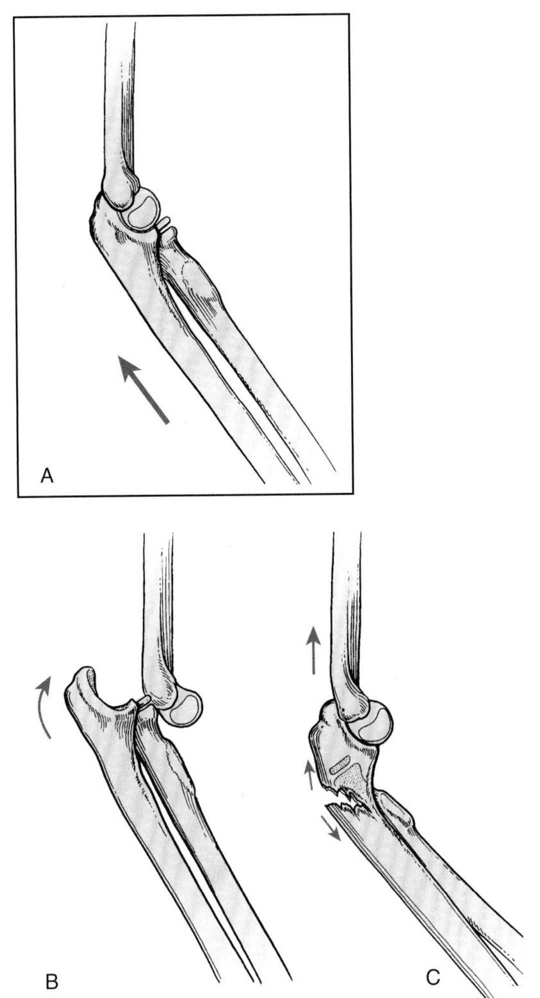

FIGURE 12-28 Mechanism of injury for type II Monteggia fracture–dislocation. **A.** The elbow is flexed approximately 60 degrees; a force is applied longitudinally, parallel to the long axis of the forearm. **B.** A posterior elbow dislocation may occur. **C.** If the integrity of the anterior cortex of the ulna is compromised, a type II fracture–dislocation occurs.

20,76). Injuries to the radial nerve, particularly the posterior interosseous branch, occur frequently with this lesion (12,13,77). Open reduction of the radial head often is necessary because of interposition of soft tissue between it and the ulna or capitellum (7,12,13,15,63,78).

Radiographic Evaluation

The radial head may be displaced laterally or anterolaterally (10,59). The ulnar fracture often is in the metaphyseal region (7,9,10,12,13,15,63), but it can occur more distally (18,20,63). Radial angulation at the fracture site is common to all lesions, regardless of the level. X-rays of the entire forearm should be obtained because of the association of distal radial and ulnar fractures with this elbow injury complex (72).

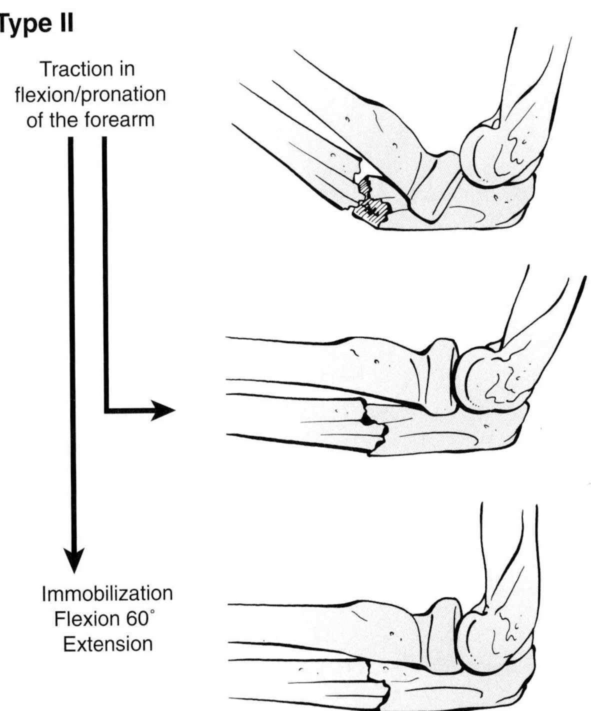

FIGURE 12-29 Longitudinal traction and pronation of the forearm and immobilization in 60 degrees flexion or complete extension.

Mechanism of Injury

Wright (7) studied fractures of the proximal ulna with lateral and anterolateral dislocations of the radial head and concluded that the mechanism of injury was varus stress at the level of the elbow, in combination with an outstretched hand planted firmly against a fixed surface (Fig. 12-31). This usually produces a greenstick ulnar fracture with tension failure radially and compression medially. The radial head dislocates laterally, rupturing the annular ligament. Hume (15) suggested that the injury may be the result of hyperextension of the elbow combined with pronation of the forearm. Other authors confirmed the mechanism of varus force at the elbow as the cause of these injuries (9,10,16,21,76). The direction of the radial head dislocation is probably determined by the rotation and angulation force applied simultaneously with the varus moment at the elbow (76).

Treatment

Nonoperative. Nonoperative treatment is effective in nearly all patients (7,9,10,15,16,18,20,21,25,76,79), although the rate of operative treatment has been reported to be as high as 12% (18).

Focus on Ulnar Reduction. Reduction is carried out by reversing the mechanism of injury (10,21,72,76). The elbow is held in extension with longitudinal traction. Valgus stress is placed on the ulna at the site of the fracture, producing clinical realign-

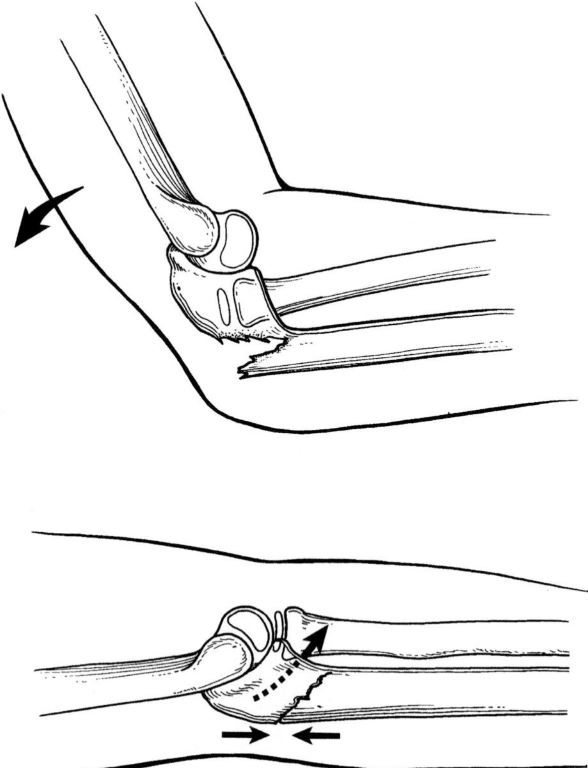

FIGURE 12-30 Reduction of type II lesion. The elbow is held at 60 degrees of flexion; traction is applied in line with the forearm and the elbow is extended. It may be necessary to apply pressure over the radial head to complete the reduction.

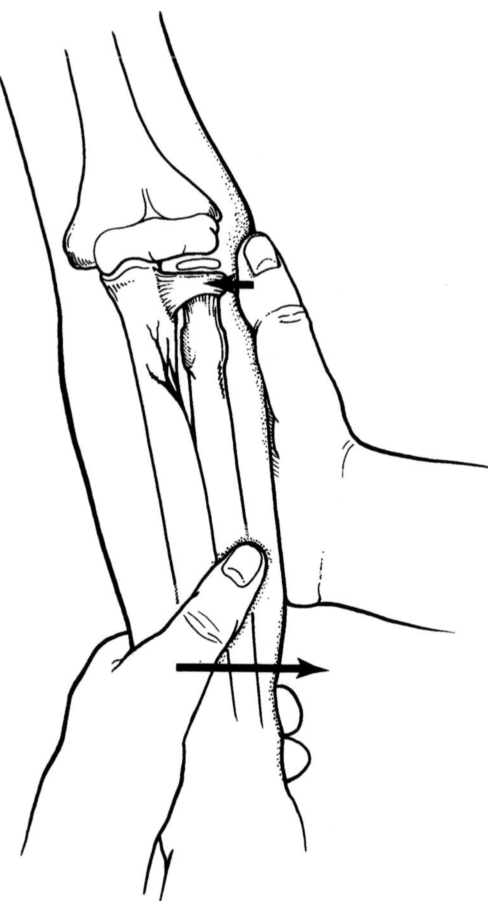

FIGURE 12-32 Reduction of type III lesion. Valgus stress is placed on the ulna at the fracture site (*arrows*), producing clinical realignment. The radial head may spontaneously reduce.

ment. The radial head may spontaneously reduce or need assistance with gentle pressure applied laterally (Fig. 12-32). Reduction sometimes produces a palpable click (72). Ulnar length and alignment must be maintained to ensure a stable radial head.

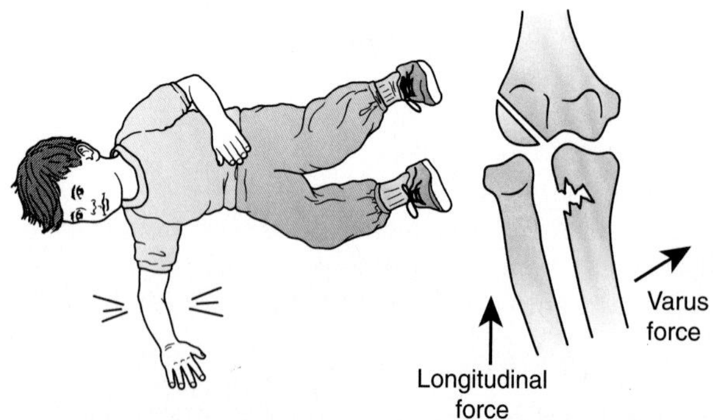

FIGURE 12-31 Mechanism of injury for type III lesions. A forced varus stress causes a greenstick fracture of the proximal ulna and a true lateral or anterolateral radial head dislocation.

Confirm Radial Head Reduction. X-rays are obtained in the standard views (37). The position of the radial head is important. Any malalignment in either view implies the possibility of interposed tissue or persistent malalignment of the ulna. The angular alignment of the ulna must be as straight as possible to allow and maintain reduction of the radial head (17).

Maintenance of Reduction. Reduction is maintained by a long-arm cast with the elbow in flexion. The degree of flexion varies depending on the direction of the radial head dislocation. When the radius is in a straight lateral or anterolateral position, flexion to 110 to 120 degrees improves stability (20,21,46,76). If there is a posterolateral component to the dislocation, a position of only 70 to 80 degrees of flexion has been recommended (72).

Forearm Rotation. Forearm rotation usually is in supination, which tightens the interosseous membrane and further stabilizes the reduction (9,20,21,76). Over the years, one researcher has changed the suggested position of immobilization from pronation (16) to semisupination (72). Ramsey and Pedersen (46) recommended neutral as the best position of rotation to avoid loss of motion; their patients showed no loss of reduction using that position.

Operative. Surgical intervention has two goals: reduction and stabilization of the radial head and the ulnar fracture.

Radial Head Reduction. The radial head is reduced through a Boyd approach (63,67). This allows removal of the interposed tissues (4,24,63) and repair or reconstruction of the annular ligament if necessary (Fig. 12-33) (3,17,38,78–80). The surgical technique is essentially the same as previously described for a type I Monteggia fracture–dislocation.

Ulnar Stabilization. Stabilization of the ulna is necessary to prevent recurrent lateral dislocation of the radial head. Varus alignment or radial bow, particularly with oblique fractures, may lead to subluxation of the radius (Fig. 12-34) (17,18).

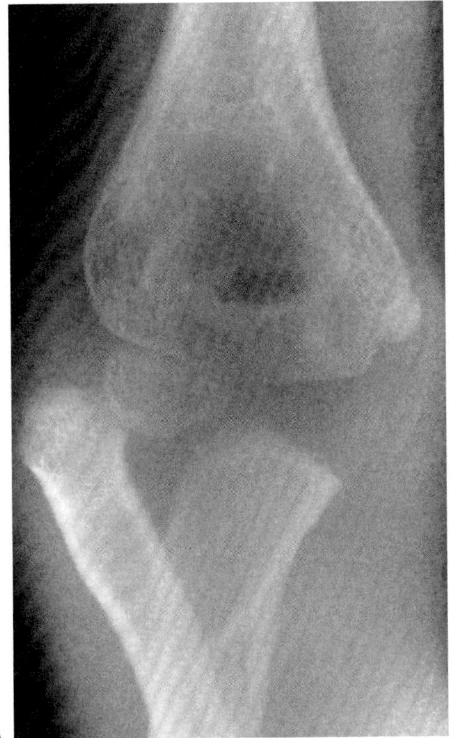
A

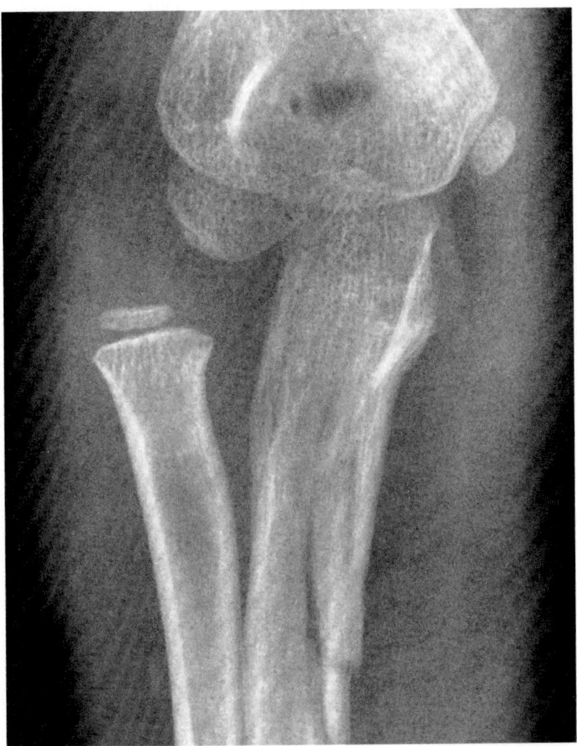
B

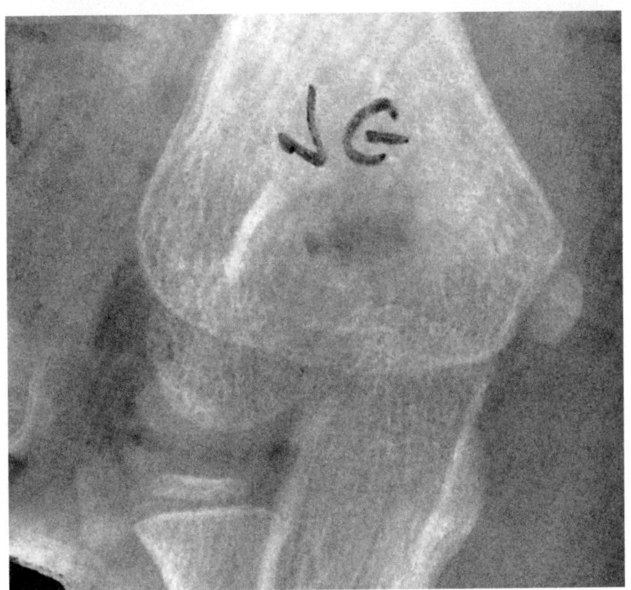

C

FIGURE 12-33 Irreducible type III lesion. **A.** Injury films showing typical greenstick olecranon fracture and lateral dislocation of a type III Monteggia lesion. **B.** After manipulation and correction of the ulnar deformity, the radial head still was not reduced. **C.** Open reduction was performed to extract the interposed torn orbicular ligament.

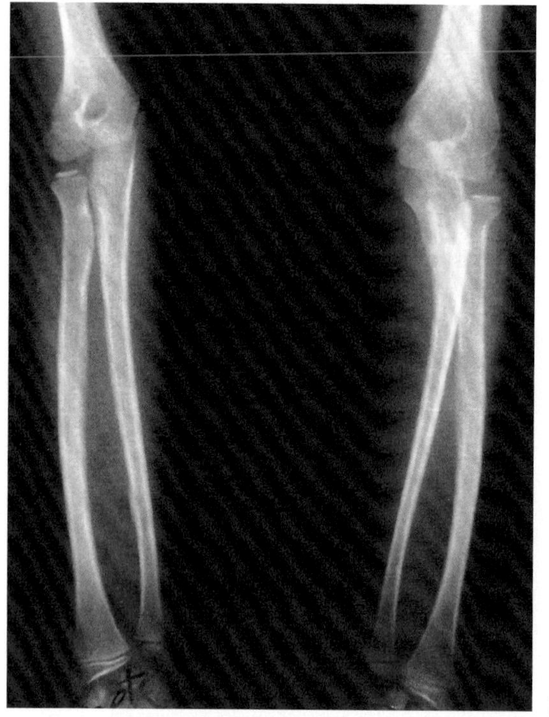

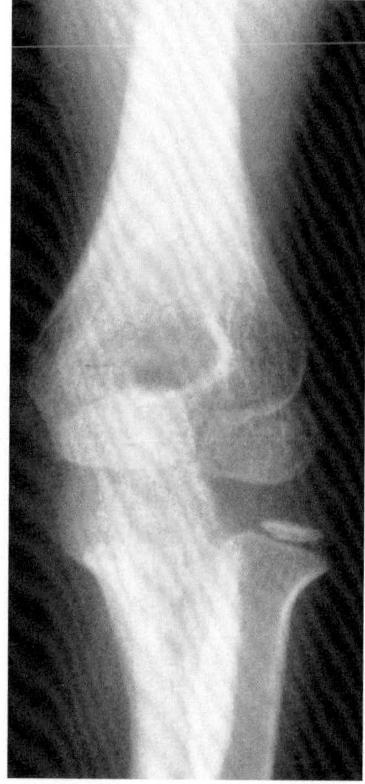

FIGURE 12-34 Radial bow of the ulna. **A.** AP views of both elbows showing residual radial bow of the proximal ulna after an incompletely reduced Monteggia type III lesion. **B.** This bow has produced a symptomatic lateral subluxation of the radial head.

Fixation with plates (17) and Kirschner wires (8) obtained satisfactory results. Up to 25 degrees of varus angulation is consistent with normal alignment and function (18), and any residual deformity decreases with time (46).

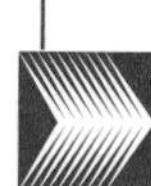

AUTHOR'S PREFERRED TREATMENT

We concur with Cunningham, who believed that reduction of the dislocated radial head is an important part of the management of the Monteggia fracture–dislocation. Our method of treatment is aimed primarily at obtaining and maintaining reduction of the radial head, either by open or closed technique. The type of treatment of the ulnar fracture is determined by its effect on the primary goal, radial head reduction.

Nonoperative. The reduction maneuvers for nonoperative type III lesions are shown in Figure 12-35.

Reduction Technique. The elbow is held in extension to control the proximal fragment by locking the olecranon into the humerus. Longitudinal traction is applied in line with the forearm with valgus stress applied at the ulnar fracture site (see Fig. 12-32). This usually allows the radial head to become reapposed to the capitellum, but pressure laterally over the prominence of the radial head may be necessary.

Radiographic Evaluation. X-rays are taken in the AP and lateral planes to confirm the reduction of the radial head and assess the ulnar alignment. Up to 10 degrees of ulnar angulation is acceptable in younger children, provided the radial head reduction is concentric and stable.

Immobilization. A long-arm cast is applied in two portions. First, a Muenster type of short-arm cast is applied with the

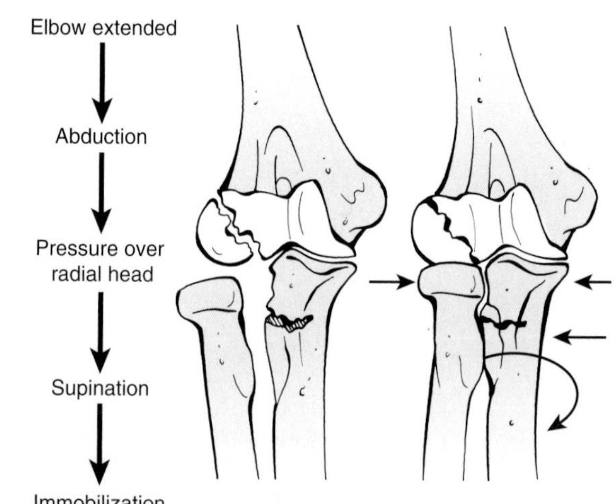

FIGURE 12-35 Schematic reduction maneuvers for nonoperative type III Monteggia fracture.

forearm in neutral rotation. This allows careful molding of the cast to maintain the alignment of the ulnar fracture. The elbow is then flexed to approximately 110 degrees in lateral or anterolateral dislocations and the cast is completed to the axilla. In younger children, where the cast may be hard to mold, a loop sling is incorporated into the cast to prevent it from migrating distally. Although we have no experience with the method, treatment of a posterolateral dislocation with an extended elbow cast with valgus molding seems logical.

After Care. X-rays should be taken in the completed cast to confirm continued reduction of the radial head and satisfactory ulnar alignment. The cast is left in place for 3 to 4 weeks, depending on the age of the child. A removable splint is worn for an additional 3 to 4 weeks while early ranging of the elbow is begun. Restoration of rotation is particularly important at this time. Before application of the splint 3 to 4 weeks after injury and when the splint is discontinued at 6 to 8 weeks, x-rays are taken to assess the reduction. At 6 to 8 weeks after injury, sufficient healing usually has occurred to allow gradual return to full activities.

Operative Treatment. The indication for operative treatment is failure to obtain or maintain reduction of the radial head and alignment of the ulnar fracture.

Reducing the Radial Head. Failed closed reduction of the radial head implies interposition of soft tissue, which is removed through a Boyd approach (see Fig. 12-25). If possible, the annular ligament is repaired, but formal reconstruction usually is unnecessary if the radiocapitellar relation is restored and stable. If stability is in question, the annular ligament is reconstructed as described for a type I Monteggia lesion.

Ulnar Realignment. Before a formal annular ligament reconstruction, ulnar alignment must be evaluated critically. Ulnar malalignment may prevent relocation of the radial head. The ulnar fracture can usually be reduced closed, but open reduction may be necessary because of interposed tissue. Once reduced, the ulna can be maintained by the insertion of intramedullary pins. The ends of the pins can be buried subcutaneously and removed later with minimal surgery.

After Care. Postoperative care is the same as for a fracture treated nonoperatively, with emphasis on early motion.

Type IV Lesions

Clinical Findings

The appearance of the limb with a type IV lesion is similar to that of a type I lesion. More swelling and pain are present because of the magnitude of force required to create this complex injury. Particular attention should be given to the neurovascular status of the limb, anticipating the possible increased risk for a compartment syndrome. Although this injury is uncommon in general and rare in children, the radiocapitellar joint should be examined in all midshaft forearm fractures to avoid missing this injury complex (Fig. 12-36). Failure to recognize the radial head dislocation is the major complication of this fracture (81).

Radiographic Evaluation

The anterior radial head dislocation is similar to that in a type I Monteggia lesion (Fig. 12-37). The radial and ulnar fractures usually are in the middle third (82), with the radial fracture usually distal to the ulnar injury. They may be complete or greenstick.

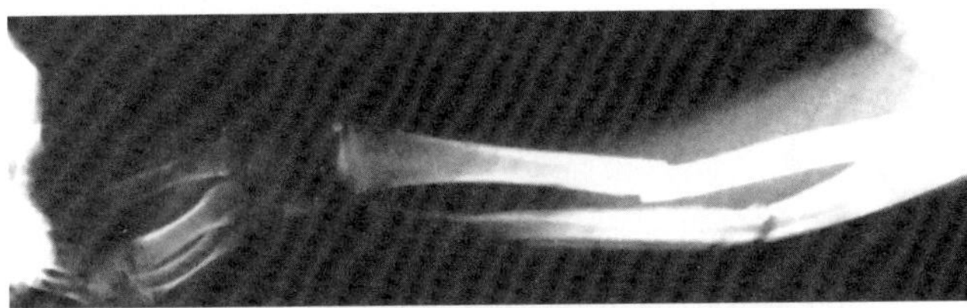

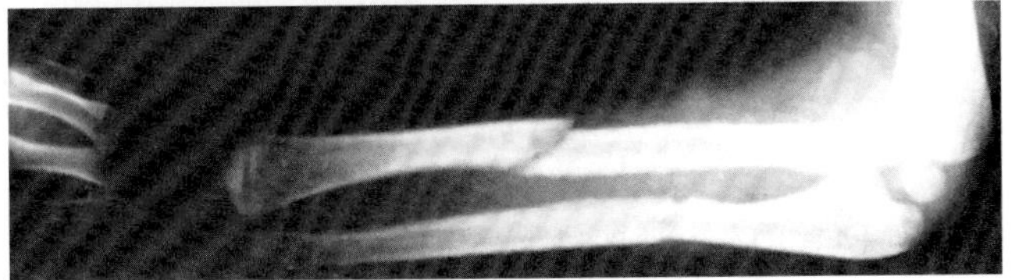

A

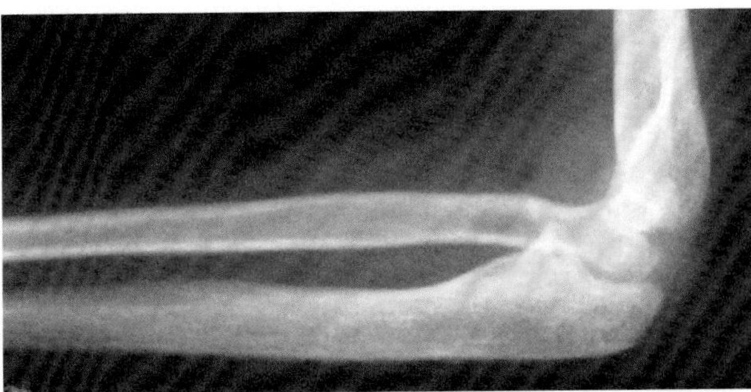

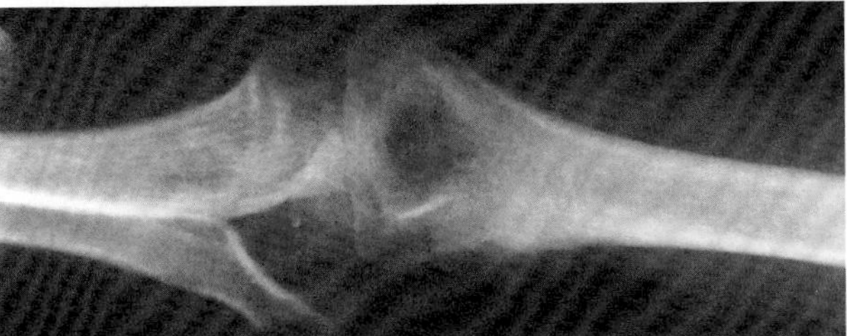

B

FIGURE 12-36 Type IV Monteggia lesion. **A.** Anterior dislocation of the head of the radius with fracture of the upper third of the radial shaft with the ulna angulated anteriorly. The dislocation of the radial head was not recognized. **B.** Five years later, the radial head was still dislocated, misshapen, and prominent. A full range of motion was present, with the exception of a loss of 10 degrees of full supination. The patient had no pain, but generalized weakness was noted in this extremity, especially in throwing motions.

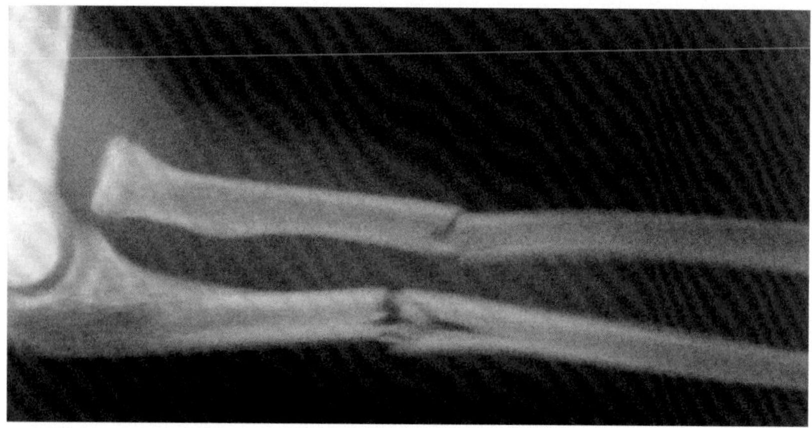

FIGURE 12-37 Type IV lesion. There is an anterior dislocation of the radial head. The radial and ulnar fractures usually are in the middle third of the shaft, with the radial fracture distal to the ulnar fracture.

Mechanism of Injury

Bado proposed that a type IV lesion is caused by hyperpronation (8). Of two case reports discussing the mechanism of injury, one implies that the injury is due to hyperpronation (17), and the other to a direct blow (83). Olney and Menelaus (18) reported a single type IV lesion in their series but did not discuss the mechanism. We believe type IV lesions are caused by the mechanism described for type I lesions.

Treatment

This complex lesion has been treated by both closed (18) and open (9) techniques. Percutaneous intramedullary fixation of the radial and ulnar fractures with flexible pins and closed reduction of the radial head also have been described (83,84).

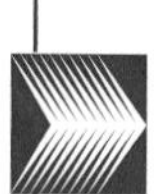

AUTHOR'S PREFERRED TREATMENT

The goals of treatment for a type IV Monteggia lesion are similar to those of other types. The presence of the free-floating proximal radial fragment hampers the ability to reduce the radial head. Stabilization of the radial fracture converts a type IV lesion to a type I lesion, making treatment easier.

Nonoperative. Closed reduction should be attempted initially, with the aim of transforming the type IV lesion to a type I lesion (Fig. 12-38), especially if the radial and ulnar fractures have greenstick patterns. Use of the image intensifier allows immediate confirmation of reduction, especially of the radial head. Closed treatment of unstable ulnar lesions should not be attempted. If the initial reduction cannot be obtained, we prefer intramedullary fixation to maintain the reduction (Fig. 12-39).

Operative. Type IV fractures usually are unstable, and the reduction of the radial head is easy to obtain and maintain after intramedullary pinning of the radius; in children older than 12 years, plating of the radius through a Henry extensile approach (85) provides more rigid stabilization (Fig. 12-40). Once stability is achieved, a closed reduction of the radial head is attempted. This usually is successful, but any intra-articular obstruction can be removed through a Boyd approach.

After Care. The elbow is immobilized in a long-arm cast for 4 weeks in 110 to 120 degrees of flexion with the forearm in neutral rotation. A short-arm cast is used for an additional 4 weeks while early range of motion at the elbow and forearm is begun. Forearm rotation, within the limits of cast restric-

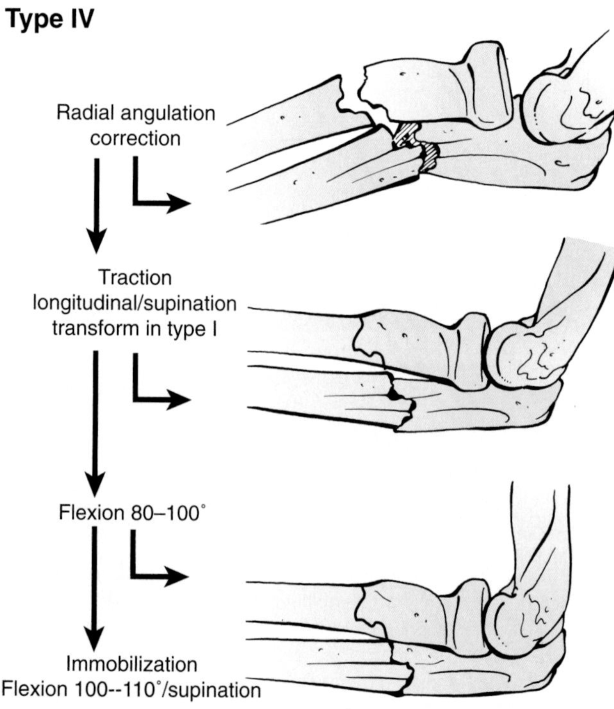

FIGURE 12-38 Reduction schematic for type IV Monteggia fracture.

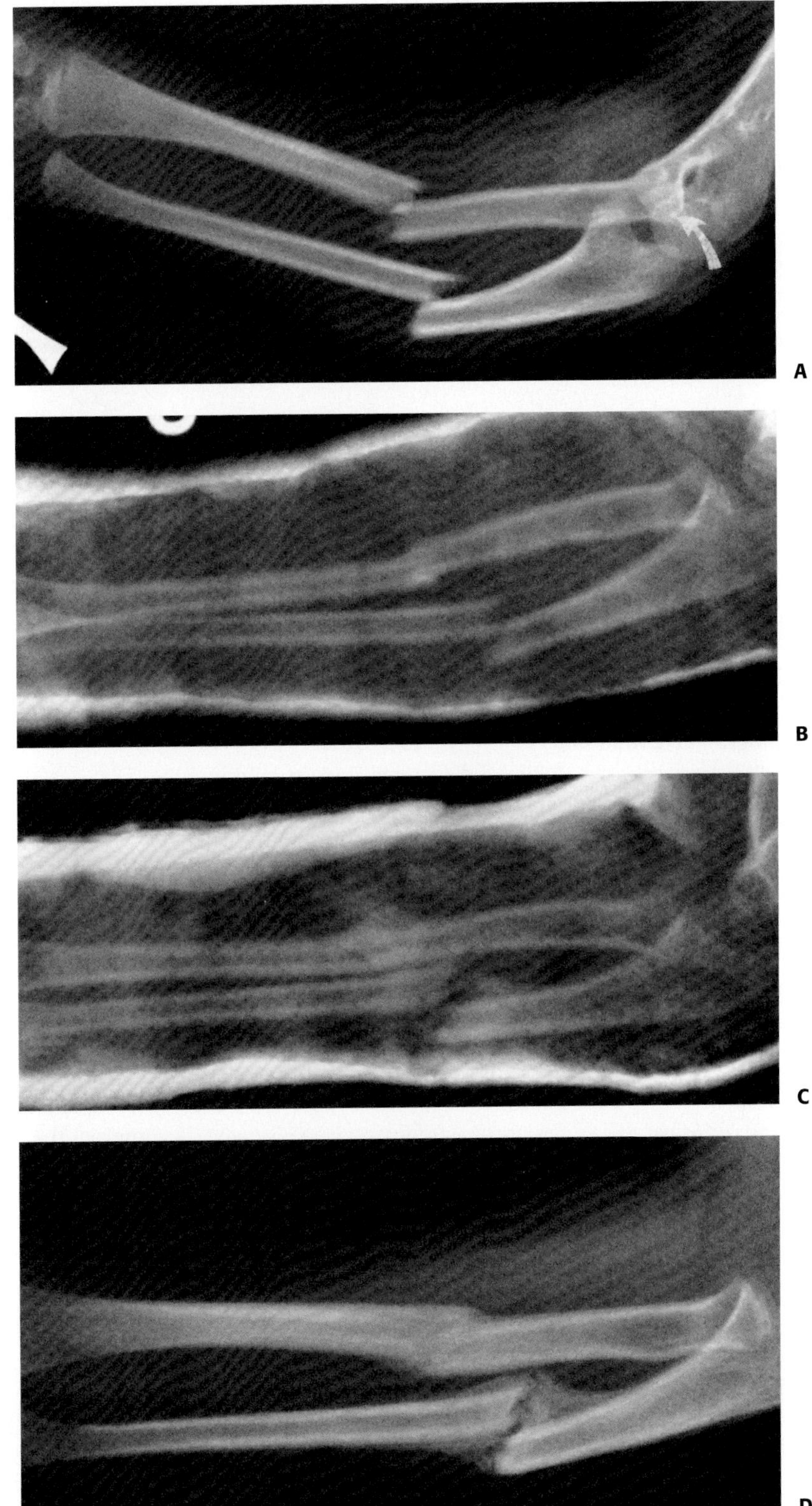

FIGURE 12-39 Type IV closed reduction. **A.** Injury film of a 7-year-old with fractures of the shafts of the radius and ulna and associated dislocation of the radial head. **B.** Initial closed reduction with some residual posterior angulation. **C.** At 3 weeks after injury, the forearm was remanipulated to correct the posterior angulation. **D.** Appearance 8 weeks after reduction, still with slight posterior angulation. *(continues)*

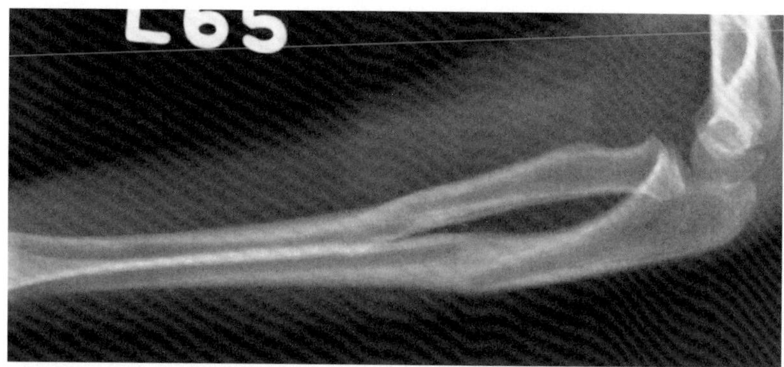

FIGURE 12-39 (*continued*) **E.** Six months later, there has been considerable remodeling.

tions, is specifically encouraged to avoid permanent loss of rotation. At 8 weeks after injury, gradual return to full activities is allowed.

Monteggia Equivalent Lesions

Clinical Findings

Clinical findings are similar to those for the corresponding Bado lesion, with the common triad of pain, swelling, and deformity.

Radiographic Evaluation

As with the Bado types, careful radiographic study should be made with at least two orthogonal views. Special views such as obliques should be obtained to clearly delineate the associated injuries (e.g., radial head or neck fractures, lateral humeral condyle fractures) and allow adequate pretreatment planning.

Mechanism of Injury

The mechanism of injury by which the fracture occurs helps define its equivalent type and is discussed in the sections on the relevant Bado type.

Treatment

As with the other Bado types, treatment focuses on two general components of the lesion: ulnar fracture and associated injury.

Ulnar Fracture. This fracture is treated as are other Bado types. The method is dictated by the fracture pattern and location and its stability after reduction.

Associated Injury. These associated fractures and dislocations are evaluated and treated using principles based on the particular injury. They are discussed thoroughly in other sections of this chapter.

COMPLICATIONS

Old Undetected Fracture–Dislocations

An undetected dislocation of the radial head is uncommon (2,21,84,86). Isolated radial head dislocations with no apparent lesion of the ulna associated with remote trauma have been mistaken for congenital radial head dislocations (39,87), although the existence of a unilateral congenital dislocation of the radial head (40). The shape of the ulna in patients with a seemingly isolated dislocation of the radial head indicates persistent plastic deformation of the ulna and a traumatic etiology to this radial lesion (Figs. 12-41 and 12-42) (35). The diagnosis of radial head dislocation can be confirmed by evaluation of the radiocapitellar line (see Fig. 12-11) (2,36,37).

Natural History

Recognition of a dislocated radial head at the time of injury can prevent the difficult problem of persistent radial head dislocation. When a previously undetected dislocation is encountered, the natural history of the untreated lesion should be considered in determining the method of treatment. The belief that many children with persistent dislocation of the radial head do well has been supported by several investigators (44,88–90). Fahey

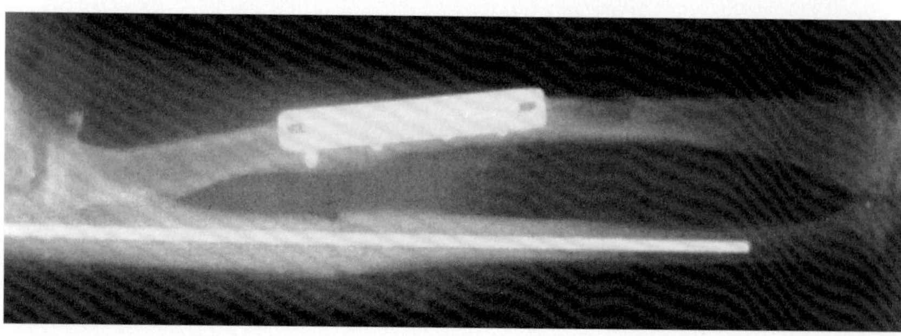

FIGURE 12-40 Operative treatment, type IV lesion. The initial goal is to stabilize the radius. In older children, a plate may be indicated. Intramedullary pinning usually is adequate. (See Fig. 12-31 for injury film.)

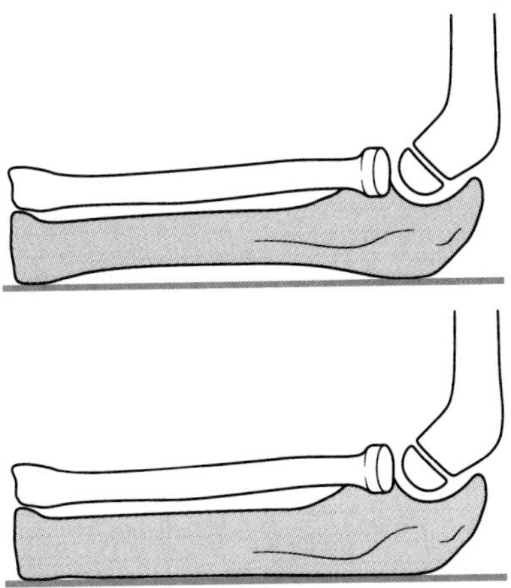

FIGURE 12-41 The ulnar bow line. This line, drawn between the distal ulna and the olecranon, defines the ulna bow. The ulnar bow sign is deviation of the ulnar border from the reference line of more than 1 mm.

(91) suggested that although in the short term persistent dislocations do well, they cause problems later. Other reports support the view that the natural history of persistent dislocation is not benign and is associated with restricted motion, deformity, functional impairment (weakness, instability), pain, degenerative arthritis, and late neuropathy (15,23,26,35,41,80,92–97). Kalamchi (96) reported pain, instability, and restricted motion, especially loss of pronation and supination. He also noted that children have a valgus deformity and a prominence on the anterior aspect of the elbow. Tardy nerve palsies have been reported subsequent to long-standing unrecognized Monteggia lesions (40,92,97,98).

Indications for Treatment

Blount (99), in his classic monograph, and Fowles et al (17) suggested that reconstruction provides the best results in patients who have had a dislocation for 3 to 6 months or less. If radial head reduction is necessary, an ulnar osteotomy is done, the radial head is reduced, and reduction is maintained with fixation between the ulnar metaphysis and the radial neck with-

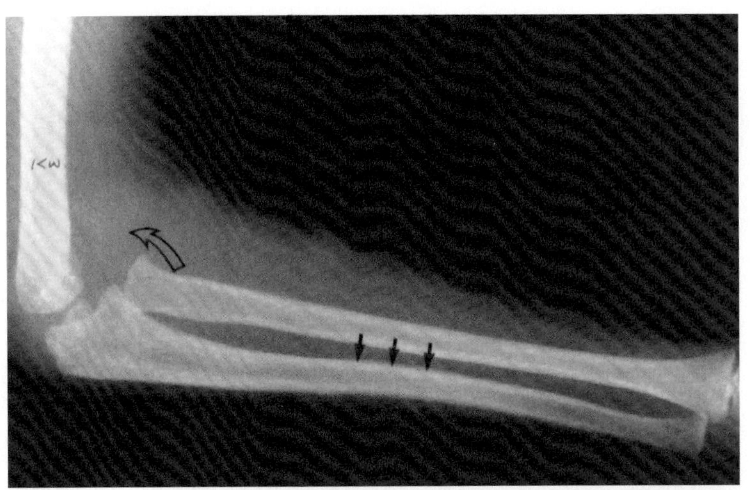

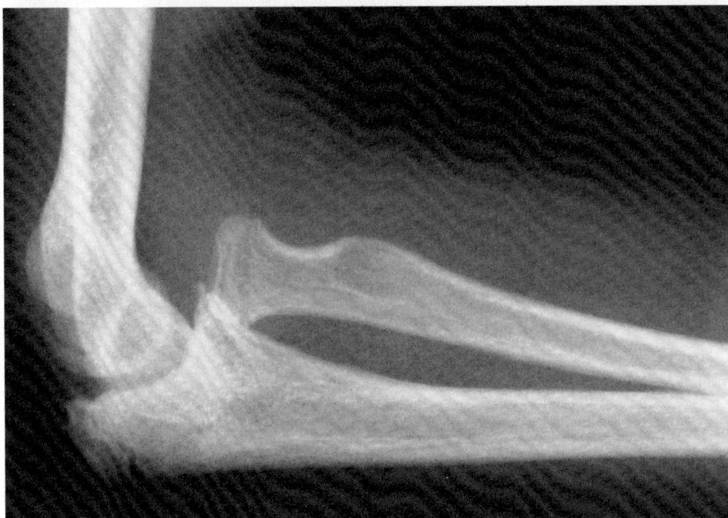

FIGURE 12-42 Ulnar bow line. **A.** The injury film of an 8-year-old girl who fell, spraining her arm. Note anterior bow of the ulna (*black arrows*) and loss of the radiocapitellar relation (*open arrow*). **B.** Film at time of diagnosis. Note persistent ulnar bow and overgrowth of radius.

out ligament reconstruction (Fig. 12-43). Fowles et al reported successful relocations up to 3 years after injury, Freedman et al (80) up to 6 years after injury. Throughout the literature, the appropriate age for radial head reduction seems to be younger than 10 years (100). Hirayama et al (101) suggested that the procedure not be performed if there is significant deformity of the radial head, flattening of the capitellum, or valgus deformity of the neck of the radius.

In a more recent report, however, Seel and Peterson (102) suggested that the age of the patient and the duration of the dislocation are unimportant. Their criteria for surgical repair were (a) normal concave radial head articular surface and (b) normal shape and contour of the ulna and radius (deformity of either was corrected by osteotomy). They treated seven patients (all girls) ranging in age from 5 to 13 years for chronic dislocations that had been present from 3 months to 7 years. All seven were fully active with no elbow pain or instability at an average of 4 years after surgery.

Although they recommended surgical treatment of chronic Monteggia lesions in children because of the long-term sequelae, Rodgers et al (83) cautioned that the results of reconstructive procedures are unpredictable and associated with a number of serious complications. Fourteen complications occurred in their seven patients (11 months to 12 years of age) treated from 5 weeks to 39 months after injury, including malunion of the ulnar shaft, residual radiocapitellar subluxation, radiocapitellar dislocation, transient ulnar nerve palsy, partial laceration of the radial nerve, loss of fixation, nonunion of the ulnar osteotomy, compartment syndrome, conversion reaction, and possible fibrous synostosis.

Historical Development of Surgical Repair

The technique for delayed reduction of the radial head in a Monteggia fracture–dislocation is attributed to Bell-Tawse (79), who used the surgical approach described by Boyd (67). Other surgical approaches have been developed but are not as adaptable to annular ligament reconstruction (65,66).

Annular Ligament Reconstruction

Once the capsule has been debrided from the joint, consideration is given as to whether the annular ligament needs to

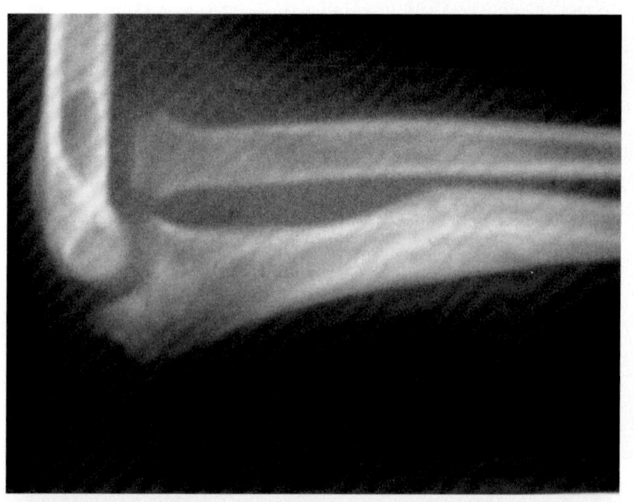
A

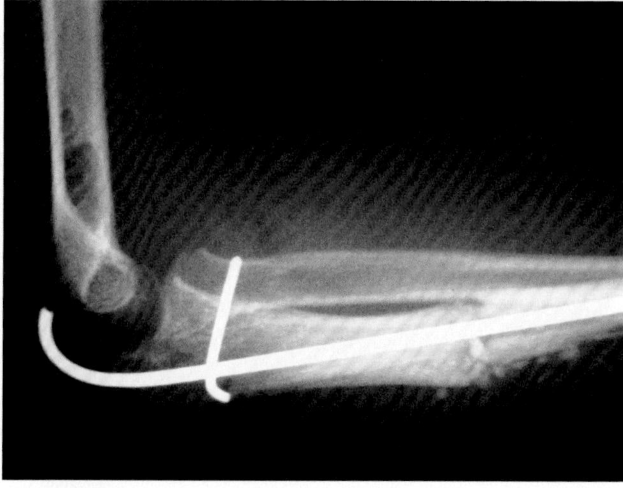
B

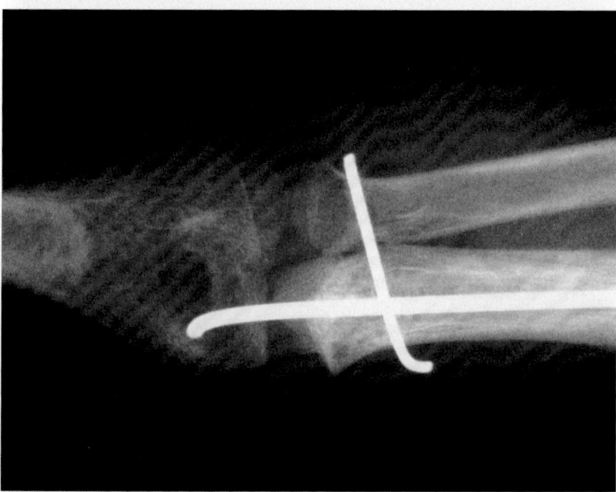
C

FIGURE 12-43 Old Monteggia fracture–dislocation treated with an ulnar osteotomy and reduction of the radial head using a transmetaphyseal pin from the radial neck to the ulnar proximal metaphysis.

be reconstructed. Kalamchi (96) restored stability after open reduction and osteotomy by reefing the remnants of the annular ligament, but most authors have considered reconstruction necessary, probably because of insufficiency of the natural structure. Although Bell-Tawse (79) used a strip of triceps tendon, other authors have tried other materials, including the lacertus fibrosus (103), a strip of the forearm fascia (104), a strip of palmaris longus tendon (55), and chromic ligature (105). Bell-Tawse (79) used the central portion of the triceps tendon passed through a drill hole and around the radial neck to stabilize the reduction and immobilized the elbow in a long-arm cast in extension. Bucknill (38) and Lloyd-Roberts (40) modified the Bell-Tawse procedure by using the lateral portion of the triceps tendon, with a transcapitellar pin for stability. The elbow was immobilized in flexion. Hurst and Dubrow (95) used the central portion of the triceps tendon, but carried the dissection of the periosteum distally along the ulna to the level of the radial neck, which provided more stable fixation than stopping dissection at the olecranon as described by Bell-Tawse. They also used a periosteal tunnel rather than a drill hole for fixation of the tendinous strip to the ulna. Thompson and Lipscomb (106) used a fascia lata graft passed through a hole drilled in the ulna.

Osteotomy

For a Monteggia lesion with a mildly displaced ulnar fracture but persistent dislocation of the radial head, an osteotomy of the ulna usually is not indicated (40). However, various types of osteotomies have been used to facilitate reduction of the radial head and prevent recurrent subluxation after annular ligament reconstruction (Fig. 12-44). Kalamchi (96) reported using a "drill hole" ulnar osteotomy to obtain reduction of the radial head in two patients. Minimal periosteal stripping with this technique allowed the osteotomy to heal rapidly. Hirayama et al (101) used a 1-cm distraction ulnar osteotomy approximately 5 cm distal to the tip of the olecranon, with plate-and-screw fixation, but complications with loosening and plate breakage occurred. Mehta (107,108) used an osteotomy of the proximal ulna stabilized with bone graft. In neither series was annular ligament repair done. Oner and Diepstraten (109) suggested that ulnar osteotomy is not necessary in type I lesions (anterior dislocation), but in type III lesions (anterolateral dislocation) recurrent subluxation is likely without osteotomy (see Fig. 12-27). Freedman et al (80) reported a delayed open reduction of a type I Monteggia lesion without annular ligament reconstruction but with ulnar osteotomy, radial shortening, and deepening of the radial notch of the ulna.

Inoue and Shionoya (110) compared the results of simple corrective ulnar osteotomy in six patients with those of posterior angular (overcorrected) osteotomy in six others and found that better clinical outcomes were obtained with the angular osteotomy. Tajima and Yoshizu (111), in a series of 23 neglected Monteggia fractures, found that the best results were obtained by opening wedge osteotomy of the proximal ulna without ligament reconstruction.

Exner (112) reported that in patients with chronic dislocation of the radial head after missed type I Monteggia lesions, reduction was successfully obtained with ulnar corticotomy and gradual lengthening and angulation of the ulna using an external fixator. Another option for type IV old Monteggia fracture is a shortening osteotomy of the radius, usually indicated for angulation of the radius without angulation of the ulna (Fig. 12-45).

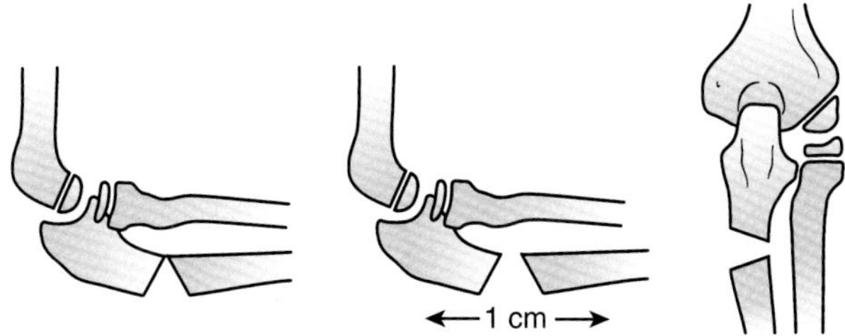

FIGURE 12-44 Ulnar osteotomies. *Left.* Floating open osteotomy without fixation or bone graft. *Center.* Hirayama distraction osteotomy, grafted and fixed with a plate and screws. Mehta osteotomy is similar but is held with a bone graft only. *Right.* Valgus osteotomy for a type III lesion: floating osteotomy with bone graft. This osteotomy can be stabilized with an intramedullary pin.

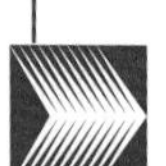

AUTHOR'S PREFERRED TREATMENT

Indications. In patients younger than 12 years of age with delayed diagnosis of a Monteggia lesion, the radial head should be replaced in its appropriate relation with the capitellum. Even though the child may do well in the short term without reduction of the radial head, problems usually develop in adolescence or adulthood, when progressive instability, pain, weakness of the forearm, and restriction of motion are likely to occur. There also is a risk of tardy radial or ulnar nerve palsies.

Surgical Approach. The skin incision begins approximately halfway between the central portion of the triceps and the lateral border, beginning proximal enough to obtain 6 to 7 cm of tendinous strip. The incision continues distally along the lateral border of the ulna just past the level of the radial neck. Dissection is carried deep, lifting the anconeus off the ulna extraperiosteally. The capsule is entered and any interposed capsule, old ligament, or osteochondral fragment is removed from the joint. The radial notch of the ulna also is cleaned to allow the radial head to fall into place once reduced. Capsular adhesions are removed from the radial head to allow it to fall away from the anterior capsule.

Radial Head Reduction. Radial head reduction is then attempted. If it is accomplished, it is scrutinized for congruity

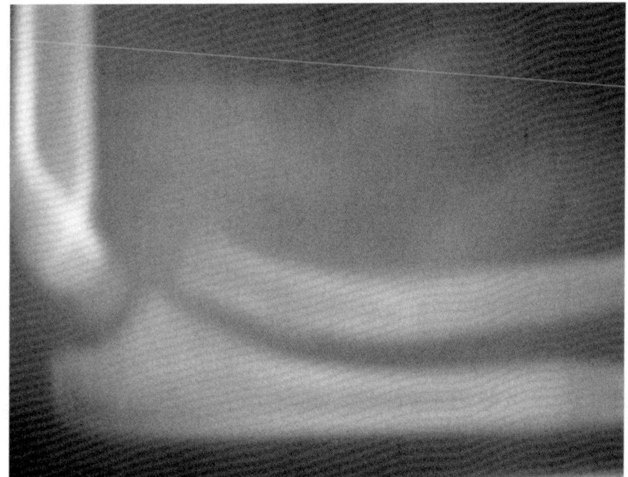

A

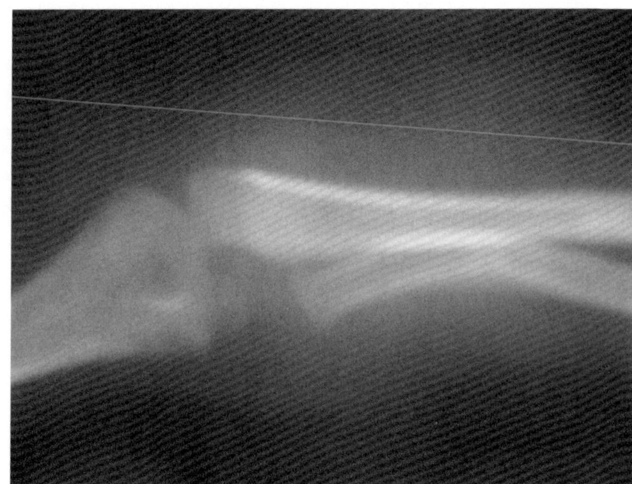

B

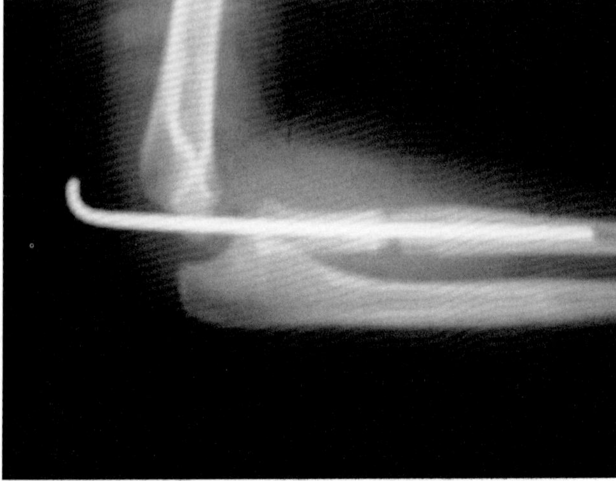

C

FIGURE 12-45 Type IV old Monteggia fracture treated by a shortening osteotomy of the radius.

between the radial head and the capitellum. If this is satisfactory, a ligamentous reconstruction can be done. If the radius cannot be reduced, an ulnar osteotomy is made at the site of maximal deformity through a small incision, leaving the periosteum as undisturbed as possible. If reduction of the radial head still cannot be achieved, radial shortening can be considered (see Fig. 12-45).

After ligament reconstruction, the ulnar osteotomy can be stabilized or left to "float." Stabilization can be obtained by plating, bone grafting, or intramedullary fixation. Percutaneous intramedullary fixation with flexible Kirschner wires allows self-adjustment and adds stability to the entire reconstruction; it is our preferred fixation method.

Annular Ligament Reconstruction. At the time of exposure, the triceps aponeurosis and tendon are examined to locate their thickest portion. A 1 × 6-cm strip is developed and carried distally, carefully elevating the periosteum from the proximal ulna down to the level of the radial neck. In the Bell-Hawse technique, a hole slightly larger than the strip of tendon is drilled in the ulna. The strip of tendon is then passed around the radial neck and through the hole in the ulna. The ligament is then brought back and sutured to itself (Fig. 12-46).

More recently, Seel and Peterson (102) described the use of two holes drilled in the proximal ulna. The holes are placed at the original attachments of the annular ligament and allow repair of the annular ligament (frequently avulsed from one attachment and trapped within the joint) or reconstruction of the annular ligament with whatever material is desired (they suggested triceps tendon). This technique secures the radial head in its normal position from any dislocated position and allows osteotomy for correction of any accompanying deformity of the ulna or radius. Seel and Peterson noted that the Bell-Tawse procedure tends to pull the radius posterolaterally (Fig. 12-47, left) and possibly constricts the neck of the radius, thereby potentially limiting the growth of the radial neck ("notching") and reducing forearm

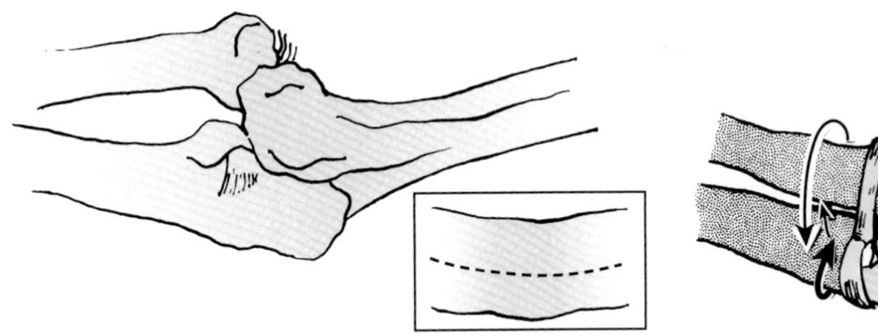

FIGURE 12-46 The central slip of the triceps is used to reconstruct an annular ligament.

rotation. Seel and Peterson placed a single drill hole obliquely across the ulna to exit medially at the site of the medial attachment of the annular ligament on the coronoid process of the ulna (see Fig. 12-47, center). The tendon was routed through the tunnel, brought around the neck, and sutured to the lateral side of the ulna. With this construct, the direction of stability was posteromedial. The use of two drill holes to secure the annular ligament or other reconstructive tendon at both normal attachments of the annular ligament on the ulna achieved a more normal posteromedial holding force on the neck of the radius (see Fig. 12-47, right).

Alternatives to holes drilled in the bone are small bone staples and bone-anchoring devices (Fig. 12-48). De Boeck (113) reported a 9-year-old boy who had ON and bone resorption of the radial neck after a late annular ligament reconstruction using a sling of triceps tendon for an unrecognized radial head dislocation.

Stabilizing the Radial Head. Once concentric reduction is achieved, the radiocapitellar relation is secured by passing a transcapitellar Steinmann pin through the posterior aspect of the capitellum into the radial head and neck with the elbow at 90 degrees and the forearm in supination (see Fig. 12-48). A pin of sufficient size is mandatory to avoid pin failure (114); a small pin will fatigue (Fig. 12-49). Alternative techniques to secure the reduction of the radius include transversely pinning the radius to the ulna (25) and immobilizing the elbow in extension (79).

After Care. After wound closure, a long-arm cast is applied with the forearm in 60 to 90 degrees of supination. The position of the elbow is predetermined by the transcapitellar Steinmann pin. This position relaxes the biceps and maintains the ulna in neutral position. The cast is maintained for 6 weeks, after which the cast and pin are removed and active motion is begun, especially pronation and supination. Elbow flexion and extension return rapidly but rotary motion of the forearm may take 6 to 9 months to improve, with pronation possibly limited permanently (83).

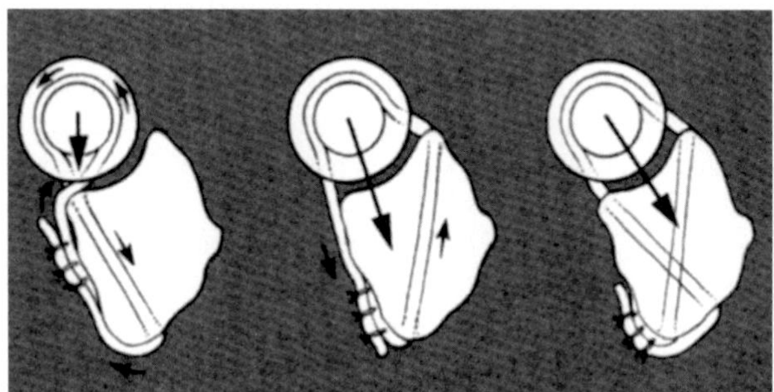

FIGURE 12-47 Drawings of transverse cuts of the proximal right radius and ulna (viewed distally) at the level of the radial head. *Left.* Route of the triceps tendon in Bell-Tawse reconstruction. The direction of stability is posterior (*large arrow*). *Center.* Drill hole placed obliquely to exit the ulna at the site of the medial annular ligament attachment. The direction of stability is posteromedial (*large arrow*). *Right.* Two drill holes exit the ulna at sites of medial and lateral annular ligament attachments. The direction of stability is anatomic (*arrow*).

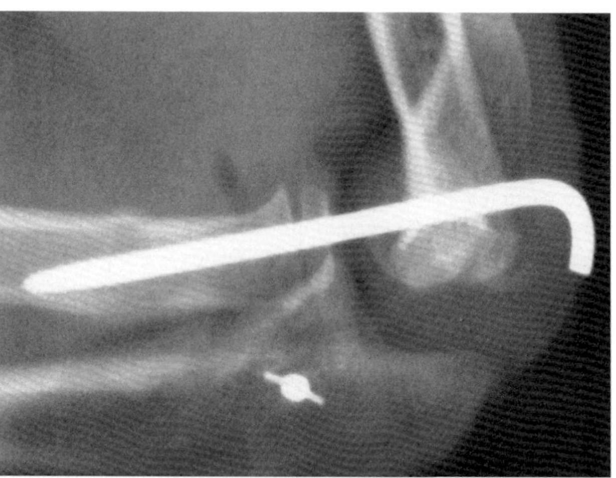

FIGURE 12-48 Fixation of radial head. After the ligament is reconstructed, the radial head is stabilized with a transcapitellar pin. Note the use of a bone anchor as an alternative to the drill hole.

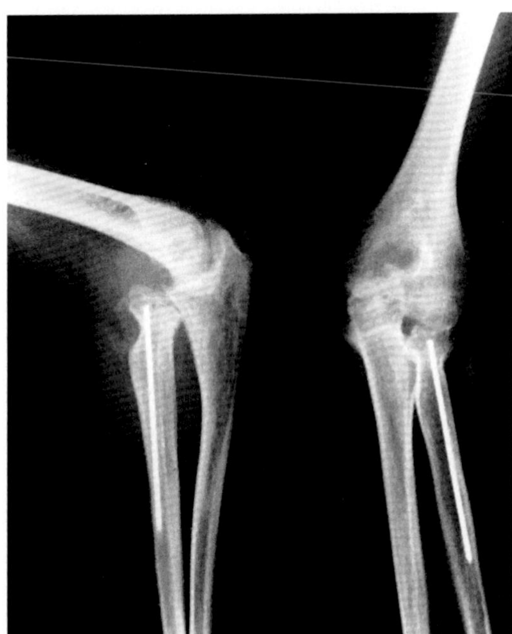

FIGURE 12-49 X-ray showing a broken transcapitellar wire with subsequent dislocation of the radial head. A pin of sufficient size is mandatory to avoid pin failure. It is better to avoid the transcapitellar fixation and use the radioulnar fixation.

Nerve Injuries

Radial Nerve

The literature reflects a 10% to 20% incidence of radial nerve injury, making it the most common complication associated with Monteggia fractures (15). It is most commonly associated with types I and III injuries (2,44,79). The posterior interosseous nerve is most commonly injured because of its proximity to the radial head and its intimate relation to the arcade of Frohse (see Fig. 12-9). The arcade may be thinner and therefore more pliable in children (30). This may account in part for the rapid resolution of the nerve injury in children.

Such a lesion in a child is treated expectantly. Nerve function usually returns by approximately 9 weeks after reduction, if not sooner (31,32). It has been recommended that the nerve be explored if there is no clinical or electromyographic return of neurologic function by 12 weeks (31,32). These recommendations are drawn from series of adult patients and may be premature and unnecessary in children. A review of a series of children's Monteggia lesions (18) recommends waiting 6 months before intervention in a posterior interosseous nerve injury. Most series report 100% resolution in both fractures treated promptly and those treated late (92,97,115).

Spinner (30) reported three posterior interosseous nerve injuries in children. All function returned spontaneously, but he recommended that if no clinical or electromyographic return occurs in approximately 6 weeks, exploration and neurolysis of the nerve should be done. Two reports (64,104) of irreducible Monteggia fractures caused by interposition of the radial nerve posterior to the radial head documented return of function approximately 4 months after the nerve was replaced to its normal anatomic position and the radial head was reduced. Morris (64), in cadaveric studies, showed that significant anterior dislocation of the radial head and varus angulation of the elbow allowed the radial nerve to slide posterior to the radial head and, with subsequent reduction of the radial head, become entrapped.

Ulnar Nerve

Bryan (43) reported one adult with an ulnar nerve lesion associated with a type II Monteggia lesion, with spontaneous resolution. Stein et al (32) reported three combined radial and ulnar nerve injuries, two of which required exploration for functional return of the nerve.

Median Nerve

Median nerve injuries are uncommon with Monteggia fractures, but injury to the anterior interosseous nerve has been reported (20,55). Stein et al (32), in their report specifically examining nerve injuries in Monteggia lesions, reported no median nerve deficits. Watson and Singer (55) reported entrapment of the main trunk of the median nerve in a greenstick ulnar fracture in a 6-year-old girl. Completion of the fracture was necessary for release of the nerve. At 6 months after surgery, there was full motor recovery but sensation was slightly reduced in the tips of the index finger and thumb.

Tardy Nerve Palsy

Tardy radial nerve palsy associated with radial head dislocation has been infrequently reported (92,97,98,115,116). Although reported treatment has varied, excision of the radial head with exploration and neurolysis of the nerve generally produced good results (92,97), while exploration of the nerve alone produced variable results (98,115). Yamamoto et al (116) combined radial head resection and nerve exploration with tendon transfers, producing good results in two patients.

Associated Fractures and Unusual Lesions

Monteggia lesions have been associated with fractures of the wrist and the distal forearm (9), most often distal radial and ulnar joint dislocation and sprain or fracture of the distal radius through the physis or distal metaphysis (Fig. 12-50) (9,83,95,96,117). Galeazzi fractures also may occur with Monteggia lesions (9,45). Radial head and neck fractures commonly are associated with type II fractures (9,69) but may occur with other types (97,118,119). With a type II lesion, the radial head fracture usually is at its anterior rim (69). Strong et al (120) reported two type I equivalent lesions consisting of a fractured radial neck and midshaft ulnar fracture. This injury was unique because of significant medial displacement of the distal radial fragment. Obtaining and maintaining reduction of the radius was difficult with a closed technique.

Fractures of the lateral condyle also have been associated with Monteggia fractures (10). Ravessoud (22) reported an ipsilateral ulnar shaft lesion and a lateral condylar fracture without

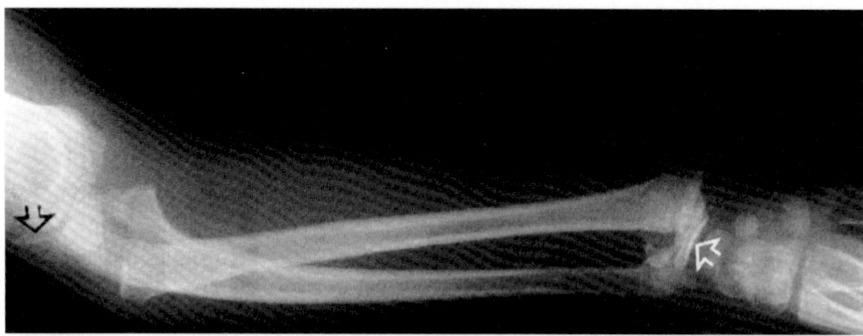

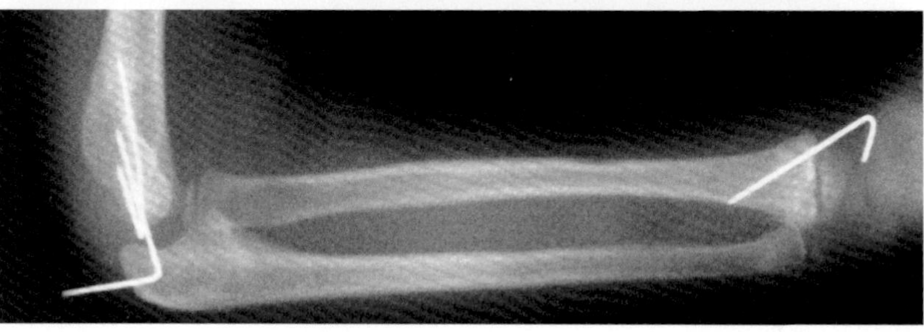

FIGURE 12-50 Associated injuries. An 8-year-old child with a high-velocity injury to the entire forearm. **A.** Type III Monteggia fracture and associated lateral condylar (*black arrow*) and distal radial physeal (*white arrow*) fractures. **B.** After reduction and percutaneous pin fixation.

loss of the radiocapitellar relation, suggesting a Monteggia type II equivalent. Kloen et al (121) reported an unusual bilateral Monteggia fracture and described the operative technique for this treatment. Despite surgical and rehabilitative challenges, excellent results were obtained in both elbows.

Periarticular Ossification

Two patterns of ossification after Monteggia fracture–dislocations have been noted radiographically: around the radial head and myositis ossificans. Ossification around the radial head and neck (15,36,40,79,90,115) appears as a thin ridge of bone in a caplike distribution and may be accompanied by other areas resembling sesamoid bones (Fig. 12-51); they resorb with time. Ossification also may occur in the area of the annular ligament (122). Elbow function generally is not affected by the formation of these lesions (15,36,40,79,90).

The other form of ossification is true myositis ossificans, reported to occur in approximately 3% of elbow injuries and 7%

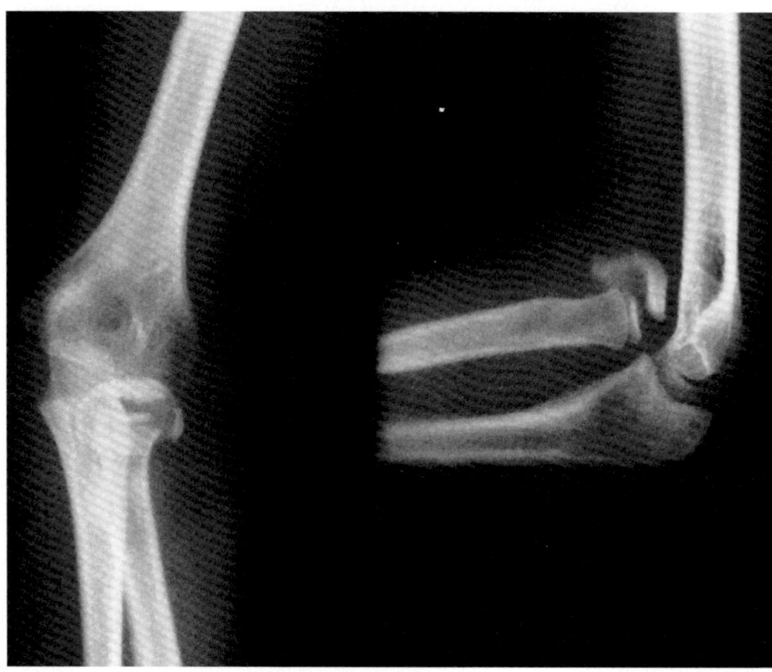

FIGURE 12-51 Periarticular ossification. Persistent dislocations of the radial head are frequently accompanied by a thin cap of bone and other areas resembling sesamoid bones.

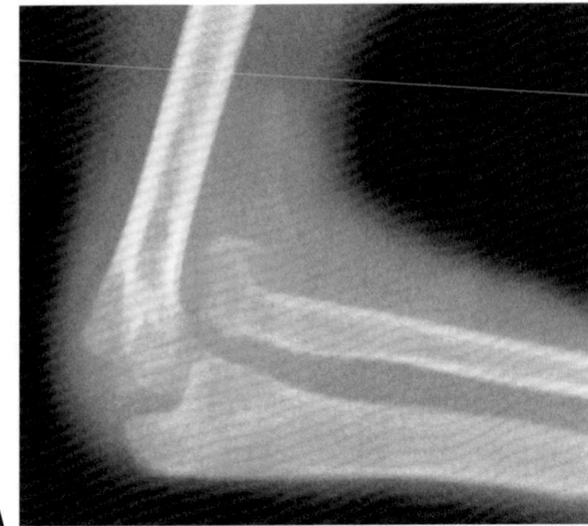

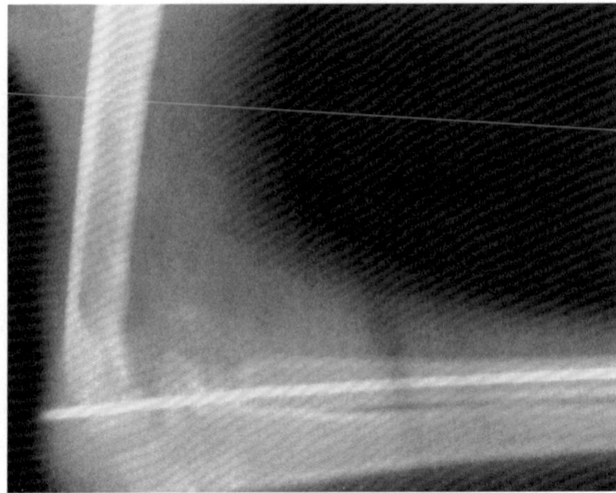

FIGURE 12-52 Periarticular ossification. **A.** Lateral x-ray of an old anterior dislocated radial head. **B.** Two months after treatment, with resolution of ossification.

of Monteggia lesions in adults and children (124). Myositis ossificans has a good prognosis in patients younger than 15 years of age, appearing at 3 to 4 weeks after injury and resolving in 6 to 8 months (Fig. 12-52). Its occurrence is related to the severity of the initial injury, association with a fractured radial head, the number of remanipulations during treatment, and passive motion of the elbow during the postoperative period (123,124).

SUMMARY

Adherence to several fundamental principles helps ensure a good outcome after Monteggia fracture–dislocations in children:

1. Evaluation of the radial head location requires an AP view of the proximal forearm and a true lateral view of the elbow.
2. The radiocapitellar line must be intact in all views.
3. If the radial head is dislocated, always look for ulnar fracture or plastic deformation.
4. Stability of the ulnar reduction is required to maintain reduction of the radial head. Stability may be inherent to the fracture pattern or achieved by internal fixation.
5. Radial head reduction confirmed by an intact radiocapitellar line must be achieved by open or closed means.
6. If the radial head is unstable, reconstruction of the annular ligament and/or removal of interposed soft tissue is required.

REFERENCES

1. Rang M. *The story of orthopaedics*. Philadelphia: Saunders, 2000.
2. Smith FM. Monteggia fractures: an analysis of 25 consecutive fresh injuries. *Surg Gynecol Obstet* 1947;85:630–640.
3. Speed JS, Boyd HB. Treatment of fractures of ulna with dislocation of head of radius: Monteggia fracture. *JAMA* 1940;125:1699.
4. Tompkins DG. The anterior Monteggia fracture. *J Bone Joint Surg [Am]* 1971;53:1109–1114.
5. Evans M. Pronation injuries of the forearm. *J Bone Joint Surg [Br]* 1949;31:578–588.
6. Penrose JH. The Monteggia fracture with posterior dislocation of the radial head. *J Bone Joint Surg [Br]* 1951;33:65–73.
7. Wright PR. Greenstick fracture of the upper end of the ulna with dislocation of the radio-humeral joint or displacement of the superior radial epiphysis. *J Bone Joint Surg [Br]* 1963;45:727.
8. Bado JL. *La lesion de Monteggia*. Inter-Medica Sarandi 328 S.R.L, 1958.
9. Bado JL. The Monteggia lesion. *Clin Orthop* 1967;50:71–86.
10. Peiró A, Andres F, Fernandez-Esteve F. Acute Monteggia lesions in children. *J Bone Joint Surg [Am]* 1977;59:92–97.
11. Pavel A, Pitman J, Lance E, et al. The posterior Monteggia fracture: a clinical study. *J Trauma* 1965;5:185.
12. Ring D, Waters PM. Operative fixation of Monteggia fractures in children. *J Bone Joint Surg [Br]* 1996;78:734–739.
13. Beddow FH, Corkery PH. Lateral dislocation of the radio-humeral joint with greenstick fracture of the upper end of the ulna. *J Bone Joint Surg [Br]* 1960;42:782–784.
14. Bruce HE, Harvey JP, Wilson JC. Monteggia fracture. *J Bone Joint Surg [Am]* 1974;56:1563–1576.
15. Hume AL. Anterior dislocation and fracture of olecranon. *J Bone Joint Surg [Br]* 1957;39:508–512.
16. Theodorou SD. Dislocation of the head of the radius associated with fracture of the upper end of ulna in children. *J Bone Joint Surg [Br]* 1969;51:700–706.
17. Fowles JV, Sliman N, Kassah MT. The Monteggia lesion in children. *J Bone Joint Surg [Am]* 1983;65:1276–1283.
18. Olney B, Menelaus M. Monteggia and equivalent lesions in childhood. *J Pediatr Orthop* 1989;9:219.
19. Papavasilou V, Nenopoulos S. Monteggia-type elbow fracture in childhood. *Clin Orthop* 1988;233:230–233.
20. Wiley JJ, Galey JP. Monteggia injuries in children. *J Bone Joint Surg [Br]* 1985;67:728–731.
21. Dormans JP, Rang M. The problem of Monteggia fracture–dislocations in children. *Orthop Clin North Am* 1990;21:251.
22. Ravessoud F. Lateral condyle fracture and ipsilateral ulnar shaft fracture: Monteggia equivalent lesions. *J Pediatr Orthop* 1985;5:364–366.
23. Givon U, Pritsch M, Levy O, et al. Monteggia and equivalent lesions: a study of 41 cases. *Clin Orthop* 1997;337:208–215.
24. Ogden JA. *Skeletal injury in children*. Baltimore: Lea & Febiger, 1990:478.
25. Letts M, Locht R, Wiens J. Monteggia fracture–dislocations in children. *J Bone Joint Surg [Br]* 1985;67:724–727.
26. Kaplan EB. The quadrate ligament of the radio-ulnar joint in the elbow. *Bull Hosp Joint Dis* 1964;25:126–130.
27. Denucé A. *Mémoire sun les luxations du coude*. Thèse de Paris, 1854.
28. Weitbrecht J. *Syndesmologia sive historia ligamentorum corporis humani*. Petropoli Typographia Academiae Sclantiarum, Brecht, 1742.
29. Basmajian JV, Griffen WR. Function of anconeus muscle. *J Bone Joint Surg [Am]* 1972;54:1712–1714.
30. Spinner M. The arcade of Frohse and its relationship to P.I.N. paralysis. *J Bone Joint Surg [Br]* 1968;50:809.
31. Spinner M, Freundlich B, Teicher J. Posterior interosseous nerve palsy as a complication of Monteggia fracture in children. *Clin Orthop* 1968;58:141.
32. Stein F, Grabias S, Deffer P. Nerve injuries complicating Monteggia lesions. *J Bone Joint Surg [Am]* 1971;53:1432.
33. Curry GJ. Monteggia fracture. *Am J Surg* 1947;123:613–617.
34. Karachalios T, Smith EJ, Pearse MF. Monteggia equivalent injury in a very young patient. *Injury* 1992;23:419–420.

35. Lincoln TL, Mubarak SJ. "Isolated" traumatic radial head dislocation. *J Pediatr Orthop* 1994;14:454–457.
36. Storen G. Traumatic dislocation of radial head as an isolated lesion in children. *Acta Chir Scand* 1958–1959;116:144–147.
37. Miles KA, Finlay DBL. Disruption of the radio-capitellar line in the normal elbow. *Injury* 1989;20:365–367.
38. Bucknill TM. The elbow joint. *Proc R Soc Med* 1977;70:620.
39. McFarland B. Congenital dislocation of the head of the radius. *Br J Surg* 1936;24: 41–49.
40. Lloyd-Roberts GC, Bucknill TM. Anterior dislocation of the radial head in children. *J Bone Joint Surg [Br]* 1977;59:402–406.
41. Caravias DE. Some observations on congenital dislocation of the head of the radius. *J Bone Joint Surg [Br]* 1957;39:86–90.
42. Almquist EE, Gordon LH, Blue AI. Congenital dislocation of the head of the radius. *J Bone Joint Surg [Am]* 1969;51:1118–1127.
43. Bryan RS. Monteggia fracture of the forearm. *J Trauma* 1971;11:992–998.
44. Naylor A. Monteggia fractures. *Br J Surg* 1942;29:323.
45. Odena IC [Milch H, transl]. Bipolar fracture–dislocation of the forearm. *J Bone Joint Surg [Am]* 1952;34:968–976.
46. Ramsey R, Pedersen H. The Monteggia fracture–dislocation in children. *JAMA* 1962; 82:115.
47. Reckling F. Unstable fracture–dislocations of the forearm: Monteggia and Galeazzi lesions. *J Bone Joint Surg [Am]* 1982;64:857–863.
48. Monteggia GB. *Instituzioni chirurgiche.* Milan: Maspero, 1814.
49. Peltier LF. Eponymic fractures: Giovanni Battista Monteggia and Monteggia's fracture. *Surgery* 1957;42:585–591.
50. Bado JL. *The Monteggia lesion.* Springfield, IL: Charles C Thomas, 1962.
51. Anderson HJ. Monteggia fractures. *Adv Orthop Surg* 1989;4:201–204.
52. Boyd HB, Boals JC. The Monteggia lesion: a review of 159 cases. *Clin Orthop* 1969; 66:94.
53. Rodgers WB, Waters PM, Hall JE. Chronic Monteggia lesions in children: complications and results of reconstruction. *J Bone Joint Surg [Am]* 1996;78:1322–1329.
54. Price CT, Scott D, Kurener M, et al. Malunited forearm fracture in children. *J Pediatr Orthop* 1990;10:705–712.
55. Watson JAS, Singer GC. Irreducible Monteggia fracture: beware nerve entrapment. *Injury* 1994;25:325–327.
56. Lambrinudi C. Intramedullary Kirschner wires in the treatment of fractures. *Proc R Soc Med* 1940;33:153.
57. Thompson HA, Hamilton AT. Monteggia fracture: internal fixation of fractured ulna with I.M. Steinmann pin. *Am J Surg* 1950;79:579–584.
58. Lascombes P, Prevot J, Ligen JN, et al. Elastic stable intramedullary nailing in forearm shaft fractures in children: 85 cases. *J Pediatr Orthop* 1990;10:167–171.
59. Parsch K. Die Morote-Drahtung bei proximalen und mittleren Unterarm Schaft Frakturen des Kindes. *Oper Orthop Traumatol* 1990;2:245–255.
60. Perez Sicialia JE, Morote Jurado JL, Corbach Girones JM, et al. Osteosintesis percuntabea eu fracturas diafisaris de ante brazo en ninos y adolescentes. *Rev Esp Cir Ost* 1977; 12:321–334.
61. Thompson GH, Wilber J, Marcus R. Internal fixation of fractures in children and adolescents. *Clin Orthop* 1984;188:10.
62. Verstreken LG. Shaft forearm fractures in children. intramedullary nailing with immediate motion: a preliminary report. *J Pediatr Orthop* 1988;8:450–453.
63. Wise RA. Lateral dislocation of the head of radius with fracture of the ulna. *J Bone Joint Surg* 1941;23:379.
64. Morris A. Irreducible Monteggia lesion with radial nerve entrapment. *J Bone Joint Surg [Am]* 1974;56:1744–1746.
65. Gorden ML. Monteggia fracture: a combined surgical approach employing a single lateral incision. *Clin Orthop* 1967;50:87–93.
66. Strachen JCH, Ellis BW. Vulnerability of the posterior interosseous nerve during radial head reduction. *J Bone Joint Surg [Br]* 1971;53:320–332.
67. Boyd HB. Surgical exposure of the ulna and proximal one-third of the radius through one incision. *Surg Gynecol Obstet* 1940;71:86–88.
68. Landin LA. Fracture patterns in children. *Acta Paediatr Scand Suppl* 1983;54:192.
69. Edwards EG. The posterior Monteggia fracture. *Am Surg* 1952;18:323–337.
70. Reckling FW, Cordell LD. Unstable fracture–dislocations of the forearm. *Arch Surg* 1968;96:999.
71. Kristiansen B, Eriksen AF. Simultaneous type II Monteggia lesion and fracture separation of the lower radial epiphysis. *Injury* 1986;17:51–62.
72. Theodorou SD, Ierodiaconou MD, Rousis N. Fracture of the upper end of the ulna associated with dislocation of the head of the radius in children. *Clin Orthop* 1988; 228:240–249.
73. Haddad ES, Manktelow ARJ, Sarkar JS. The posterior Monteggia: a pathological lesion? *Injury* 1996;27:101–102.
74. King RE. The Monteggia lesion. In: Rockwood CA Jr, Wilkins KE, King RE, eds. *Fractures in children,* 3rd ed. Philadelphia: JB Lippincott, 1991:453–497.
75. Walker J, Rang M. Forearm fractures in children. *J Bone Joint Surg [Br]* 1991;73:299.
76. Mullick S. The lateral Monteggia fracture. *J Bone Joint Surg [Am]* 1977;57:543–545.
77. Spinner M, Kaplan E. The quadrate ligament of the elbow. *Acta Orthop Scand* 1970; 41:632–647.
78. Thakore HKD. Lateral Monteggia fracture in children. *Int J Orthop Trauma* 1983:55.
79. Bell-Tawse AJS. The treatment of malunited anterior Monteggia fractures in children. *J Bone Joint Surg [Br]* 1965;47:718–723.
80. Freedman L, Luk K, Leong JC. Radial head reduction after a missed Monteggia fracture: brief report. *J Bone Joint Surg [Br]* 1988;70:846–847.
81. Beaty JH. Fractures and dislocations about the elbow in children: section on Monteggia fractures. *AAOS Instr Course Lect* 1991;40:373–384.
82. Eady JL. Acute Monteggia lesions in children. *J S C Med Assoc* 1975;71:107–112.
83. Rodgers WB, Smith BG. A type IV Monteggia injury with a distal diaphyseal radius fracture in a child: case report. *J Orthop Traumatol* 1993;7:84–86.
84. Gibson WK, Timperlake RW. Orthopedic treatment of 4 type IV Monteggia fracture-dislocations in a child. *J Bone Joint Surg [Br]* 1992;74:780–781.
85. Henry AK. *Extensile exposure.* Baltimore: Williams & Wilkins, 1970.
86. Tait G, Sulaiman SK. Isolated dislocation of the radial head: a report of two cases. *Injury* 1988;19:125.
87. Duverney JG. *Traité des maladies de os.* Paris: De Bure l'Aire, 1751.
88. Pollen AG. *Fractures and dislocations in children.* Edinburgh: Churchill Livingstone, 1973:67.
89. Salter RB, Zaltz C. Anatomic investigations of the mechanism of injury and pathologic anatomy of "pulled elbow" in young children. *Clin Orthop* 1971;77:134.
90. Stelling F, Cote R. Traumatic dislocation of head of radius in children. *JAMA* 1956; 160:732–736.
91. Fahey JJ. Fractures of the elbow in children: Monteggia's fracture–dislocation. *AAOS Instr Course Lect* 1960;17:39.
92. Austin R. Tardy palsy of the radial nerve from a Monteggia fracture. *Injury* 1926;7: 202–204.
93. Best TN. Management of old unreduced Monteggia fracture dislocations of the elbow in children. *J Pediatr Orthop* 1994;14:193–199.
94. Blasier D, Trussell A. Ipsilateral radial head dislocation and distal fractures of both forearm bones in a child. *Am J Orthop* 1995;24:498–500.
95. Hurst LC, Dubrow EN. Surgical treatment of symptomatic chronic radial head dislocation: a neglected Monteggia fracture. *J Pediatr Orthop* 1983;3:227–230.
96. Kalamchi A. Monteggia fracture–dislocation in children. *J Bone Joint Surg [Am]* 1986; 68:615–619.
97. Adams JR, Rizzoli H. Tardy radial and ulnar nerve palsy: a case report. *J Neurosurg* 1959;16:342.
98. Holst-Nielson F, Jensen V. Tardy posterior interosseus nerve palsy. *J Hand Surg [Am]* 1984;9:572–575.
99. Blount WP. *Fractures in children.* Baltimore: Williams & Wilkins, 1955.
100. Stoll TN, Baxter Nillis R, Paterson DC. Treatment of the missed Monteggia fracture in the child. *J Bone Joint Surg [Br]* 1992;74:436–440.
101. Hirayama T, Takemitsu Y, Yagihara K, et al. Operation for chronic dislocation of the radial head in children. *J Bone Joint Surg [Br]* 1987;69:639–642.
102. Seel MJ, Peterson HA. Management of chronic posttraumatic radial head dislocation in children. *J Pediatr Orthop* 1999;19:306–312.
103. Corbett CH. Anterior dislocation of the radius and its recurrence. *Br J Surg* 1931;19: 155.
104. Spar I. A neurologic complication following Monteggia fracture. *Clin Orthop* 1977;122: 207–209.
105. May Y, Mauck W. Dislocation of the radial head with associated fracture of the ulna. *South Med J* 1961;54:1255–1261.
106. Thompson D, Lipscomb B. Recurrent radial head subluxation treated with annular ligament reconstruction. *Clin Orthop* 1989;246:131–135.
107. Mehta SD. Flexion osteotomy of ulna for untreated Monteggia fracture in children. *Indian J Surg* 1985;47:15–19.
108. Mehta SD. Missed Monteggia fracture. *J Bone Joint Surg [Br]* 1993;75:337.
109. Oner FC, Diepstraten AFM. Treatment of chronic post-traumatic dislocation of the radial head in children. *J Bone Joint Surg [Br]* 1993;75:577–581.
110. Inoue G, Shionoya K. Corrective ulnar osteotomy for malunited anterior Monteggia lesions in children: 12 patients followed for 1–12 years. *Acta Orthop Scand* 1998;69: 73–76.
111. Tajima T, Yoshizu T. Treatment of long-standing dislocation of the radial head in neglected Monteggia fractures. *J Hand Surg [Am]* 1995;20:S91–S94.
112. Exner GU. Missed chronic anterior Monteggia lesion. Closed reduction by gradual lengthening and angulation of the ulna. *J Bone Joint Surg [Br]* 2001;83(4):469–470.
113. De Boeck H. Radial neck osteolysis after anular ligament reconstruction a case report. *Clin Orthop* 1997;342:94–98.
114. King RE. Letter to the editors. *J Pediatr Orthop* 1983;3:623.
115. Lichter R, Jackson T. Tardy palsy of posterior interosseous nerve with Monteggia fracture. *J Bone Joint Surg [Am]* 1975;57:124–125.
116. Yamamoto K, Yoshiaki Y, Tomihara M. Posterior interosseous nerve palsy as a complication of Monteggia fractures. *Arch Jpn Chin* 1977;46:46–56.
117. Kamali M. Monteggia fracture. *J Bone Joint Surg [Am]* 1974;56:841–843.
118. Fahmy NRM. Unusual Monteggia lesions in kids. *Injury* 1980;12:399–404.
119. Frazier JL, Buschmann WR, Insler HP. Monteggia type I equivalent lesion: diaphyseal ulna and proximal radius fracture with a posterior elbow dislocation in a child. *J Orthop Trauma* 1991;5:373–375.
120. Strong M, Kopp M, Gillespie R. Fracture of the radial neck and proximal ulna with medial displacement of the radial shaft. *Orthopedics* 1989;12:1577.
121. Kloen P, Rubel IF, Farley TD, Weiland AJ. Bilateral Monteggia fractures. *Am J Orthop* 2003;32(2):98–100.
122. Earwaker J. Post-traumatic calcification of the annular ligament of the radius. *Skeletal Radiol* 1992;21:149–154.
123. Thompson HC, Garcia R. Myositis ossificans: aftermath of elbow injuries. *Clin Orthop* 1967;50:129–134.
124. Neviaser RJ, LeFevre GW. Irreducible isolated dislocation of the radial head: a case report. *Clin Orthop* 1971;80:72–74.

THE ELBOW REGION: GENERAL CONCEPTS IN THE PEDIATRIC PATIENT

James H. Beaty and James R. Kasser

At the turn of the century, Sir Robert Jones (1) echoed the opinion of that era about elbow injuries: "The difficulties experienced by surgeons in making an accurate diagnosis; the facility with which serious blunders can be made in prognosis and treatment; and the fear shared by so many of the subsequent limitation of function, serve to render injuries in the neighborhood of the elbow less attractive than they might otherwise have proved." These concerns are applicable even today. In other bones, good results can often be obtained with minimal treatment, but in the elbow, more aggressive treatment is often required to avoid complications. An understanding of the basic anatomy and x-ray landmarks of the elbow is essential in choosing appropriate treatment.

EPIDEMIOLOGY

Because children tend to protect themselves with their outstretched arms when they fall, upper-extremity fractures account for 65% to 75% of all fractures in children. The most common area of the upper extremity injured is the distal forearm (2,3); 7% to 9% of upper-extremity fractures involve the elbow.

The distal humerus accounts for approximately 86% of fractures about the elbow region. Supracondylar fractures are the most frequent elbow injuries in children, reported to occur in 55% to 75% of patients with elbow fractures. Lateral condylar fractures are the second most common, followed by medial epicondylar fractures. Fractures of the olecranon, radial head and neck, and medial epicondyle and T-condylar fractures are much less common.

Elbow injuries are much more common in children and adolescents than in adults (4,5). The peak age for fractures of the distal humerus is between 5 and 10 years old (6). Houshian et al reported that the average age of 355 children with elbow fractures was 7.9 years (7.2 years in boys, 8.5 years in girls). Contrary to most reports, these investigators found elbow fractures more frequent in girls (54%) than in boys. In a study of 450 supracondylar humeral fractures, Cheng et al found a median age of 6 years (6.6 years in boys and 5 years in girls) and a predominance of injuries (63%) in boys.

Physeal injuries in most parts of the body occur in older children between the ages of 10 and 13; however, the peak age for injuries to the distal humeral physes is 4 to 5 years in girls and 5 to 8 years in boys. In most physeal injuries, the increased incidence with advanced age is believed to be due to weakening of the perichondrial ring as it matures (see Chap. 5). Thus, some different biomechanical forces and conditions must exist about the elbow to make the physis more vulnerable to injuries at an earlier age. (For more data on the relationship of fractures about the elbow to all types of fractures, see Chap. 1).

TABLE 13-1 Sequence and Timing of Ossification in the Elbow

	Girls (y)	Boys (y)
Capitellum	1.0	1.0
Radial head	5.0	6.0
Medial epicondyle	5.0	7.5
Olecranon	8.7	10.5
Trochlea	9.0	10.7
Lateral epicondyle	10.0	12.0

Data from Cheng JC, Wing-Man K, Shen WY, et al. A new look at the sequential development of elbow-ossification centers in children. *J Pediatr Orthop* 1998;18:161–167.

ANATOMY

The elbow is a complex joint composed of three individual joints contained within a common articular cavity. Several anatomic concepts are unique to the growing elbow.

The Ossification Process

The process of differentiation and maturation begins at the center of the long bones and progresses distally. The ossification process begins in the diaphyses of the humerus, radius, and ulna at the same time. By term, ossification of the humerus has extended distally to the condyles. In the ulna, it extends to more than half the distance between the coronoid process and the tip of the olecranon. The radius is ossified proximally to the level of the neck. The bicipital tuberosity remains largely unossified (Table 13-1) (7). Brodeur et al compiled a complete atlas of ossification of the structures about the elbow (8), and their work is an excellent reference source for finer details of the ossification process about the elbow.

Distal Humerus

Ossification of the distal humerus proceeds at a predictable rate. In general, the rate of ossification in girls exceeds that of boys (9–11). In some areas, such as the olecranon and lateral epicondyle, the difference between boys and girls in ossification age may be as great as 2 years (10). During the first 6 months, the distal humerus' ossification border is symmetric (Fig. 13-1).

Lateral Condyle

On average, the ossification center of the lateral condyle appears just before 1 year of age but may be delayed as late as 18 to 24 months (4). When the lateral condyle's ossific nucleus first appears, the distal humeral metaphyseal border becomes asymmetric. The lateral border slants and becomes straight to conform with the ossification center of the lateral condyle (Fig. 13-2). By the end of the second year, this border becomes well defined, possibly even slightly concave. This ossification center

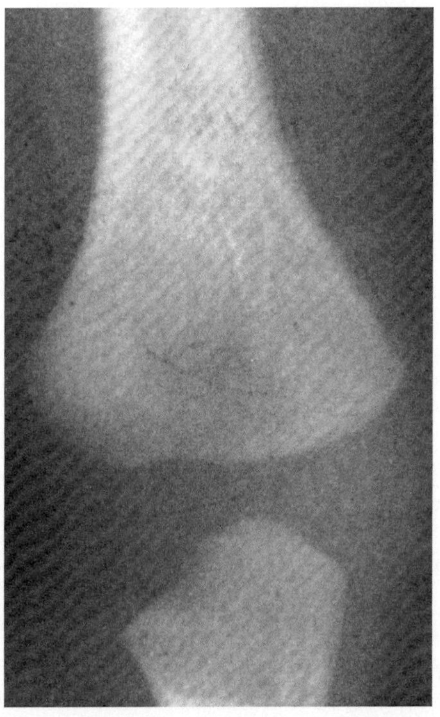

FIGURE 13-1 During the first 6 months, the advancing ossifying border of the distal humerus is symmetric.

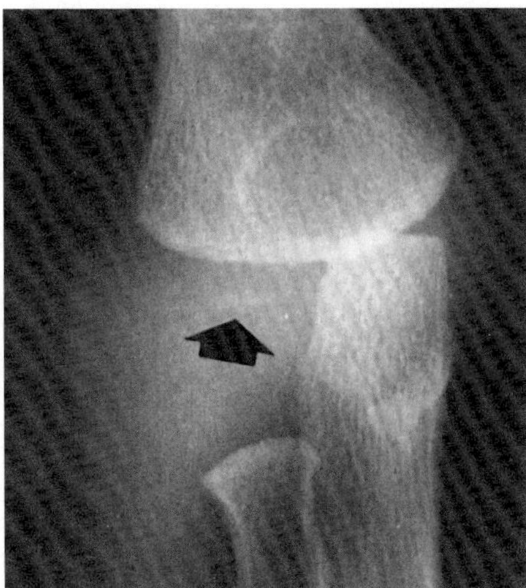

FIGURE 13-2 Ossification at 12 months. As the ossification center of the lateral condyle develops (*arrow*), the lateral border of the metaphysis becomes straighter.

is usually spherical when it first appears. It becomes more hemispherical as the distal humerus matures (12) and the ossific nucleus extends into the lateral ridge of the trochlea (Fig. 13-3). On the lateral view, the physis of the capitellum is wider posteriorly. This is a normal variation and should not be confused with a fracture (12).

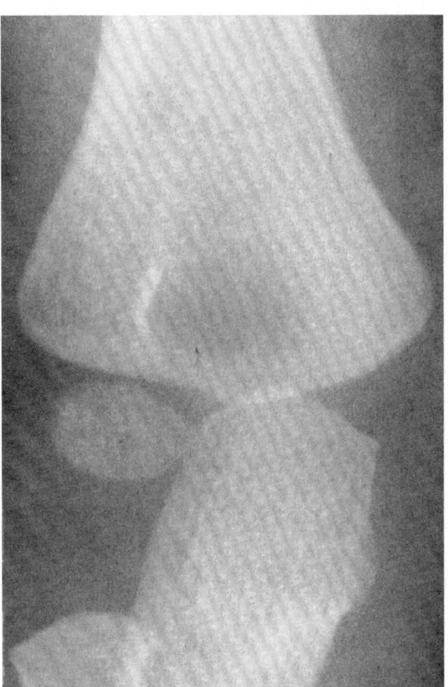

FIGURE 13-3 At 24 months, the oval-shaped secondary ossification center of the lateral condyle extends into the lateral crista of the trochlea. The lateral border of the neck (metaphysis) of the radius is normally angulated both anteriorly and laterally.

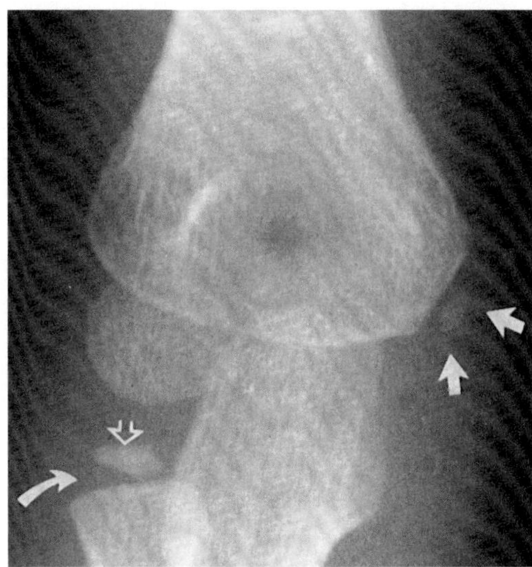

FIGURE 13-4 At about 5 or 6 years of age, a secondary center develops in the medial epicondylar apophysis (*white arrows*). At this same time, the ossification center of the radial head also develops (*open arrow*). Note that the physis of the proximal radius is widened laterally (*curved arrow*).

Medial Epicondyle

At about 5 to 6 years of age, a small concavity develops on the medial aspect of the metaphyseal ossification border. In this area, a medial epicondyle begins to ossify (Fig. 13-4).

Trochlea

At about 9 to 10 years of age, the trochlea begins to ossify. Initially, it may be irregular with multiple centers (Fig. 13-5).

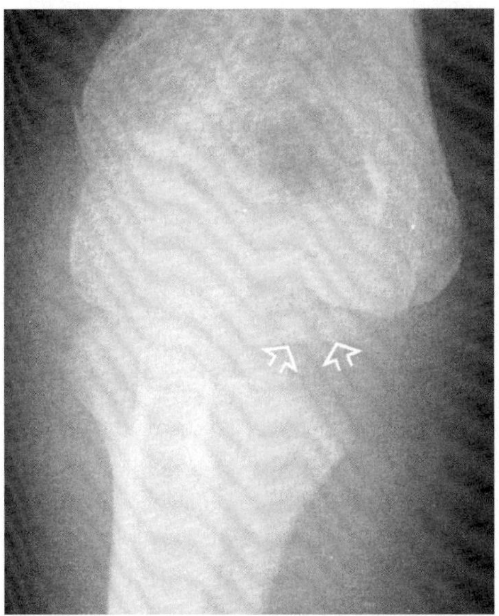

FIGURE 13-5 At about 9 years of age, the ossification of the medial crista of the trochlea may begin as two well-defined centers (*arrows*). These multiple centers can give the trochlea a fragmented appearance.

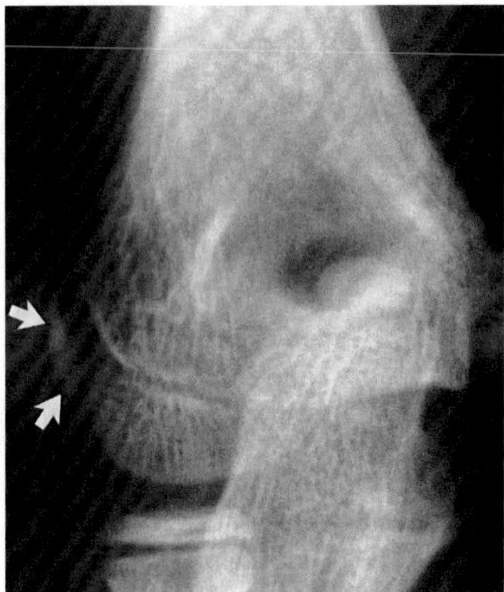

FIGURE 13-6 The apophysis of the lateral epicondyle ossifies as either an oblong or a triangular center (*arrows*). The wide separation of this center from the metaphyseal and epiphyseal borders of the lateral condyle is normal.

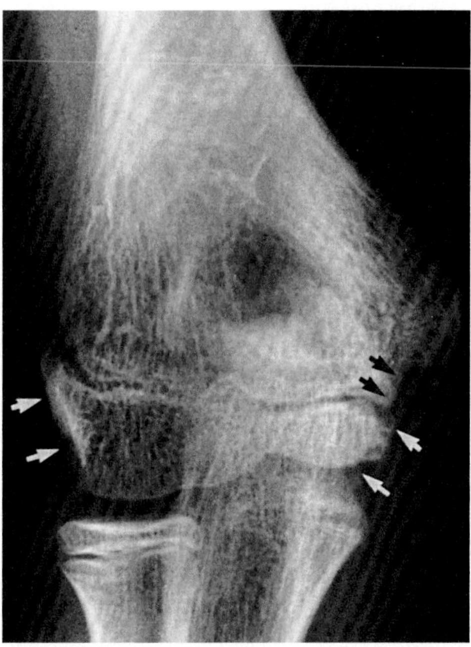

FIGURE 13-7 The secondary ossification centers of the lateral condyle, trochlea, and lateral epicondylar apophysis fuse to form one center (*white arrows*). This common center is separated from the medial epicondylar apophysis by advancing metaphyseal bone (*black arrows*).

Lateral Epicondyle

The lateral epicondyle is last to ossify and is not always visible (Fig. 13-6). At about 10 years of age, it may begin as a small, separate oblong center, rapidly fusing with the lateral condyle (12).

The Fusion Process

Just before completion of growth, the capitellum, lateral epicondyle, and trochlea fuse to form one epiphyseal center. Metaphyseal bone separates the extra-articular medial epicondyle from this common humeral epiphyseal center (Fig. 13-7). The common epiphyseal center ultimately fuses with the distal humeral metaphysis. The medial epicondyle may not fuse with the metaphysis until the late teens.

Proximal Radius

The head of the radius begins to ossify at about the same time as the medial epicondyle (Fig. 13-4). The ossification center is present in at least 50% of girls by 3.8 years of age, but may not be present in the same proportion of boys until around 4.5 years (9). Initially, the ossification center is elliptical, and the physis is widened laterally due to the obliquity of the proximal metaphysis. The ossification center flattens as it matures. At about age 12, it develops a concavity opposite the capitellum (12).

Ossification of the radial head may be bipartite or may produce an irregularity of the second center. These secondary or irregular ossification centers should not be interpreted as fracture fragments.

Olecranon

There is a gradual proximal progression of the proximal ulnar metaphysis. At birth, the ossification margin lies halfway between the coronoid process and the tip of the olecranon. By about 6 or 7 years of age, it appears to envelop about 66% to 75% of the capitellar surface. The final portion of the olecranon ossifies from a secondary ossification center that appears around 6.8 years of age in girls and 8.8 years in boys (Fig. 13-8A). Peterson (13) described two separate centers: one articular and the other a traction type (Fig. 13-8B). This secondary ossification center of the olecranon may persist late into adult life (14).

Fusion of the Ossification Centers

The epiphyseal ossification centers of the distal humerus fuse as one unit and then fuse later to the metaphysis. The medial epicondyle is the last to fuse to the metaphysis. The ranges of onset of the various centers' ossification and their fusion to other centers or the metaphysis are summarized in Figure 13-9. Each center contributes to the overall architecture of the distal humerus (Fig. 13-9C).

Fusion of the proximal radial and olecranon epiphyseal centers with their respective metaphyses occurs at around the same time that the common distal humeral epiphysis fuses with its metaphysis (i.e., between 14 and 16 years of age) (8,15,16).

Noting that the pattern and ossification sequence of the six secondary ossification centers around the elbow were mainly derived from studies conducted more than 30 years ago, Cheng et al evaluated elbow x-rays of 1,577 Chinese children (17).

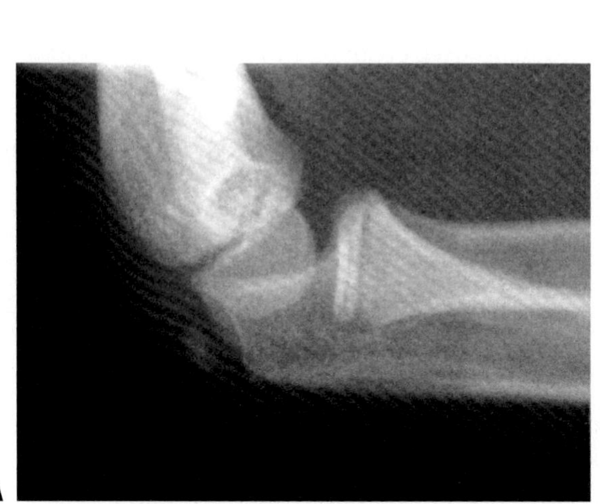

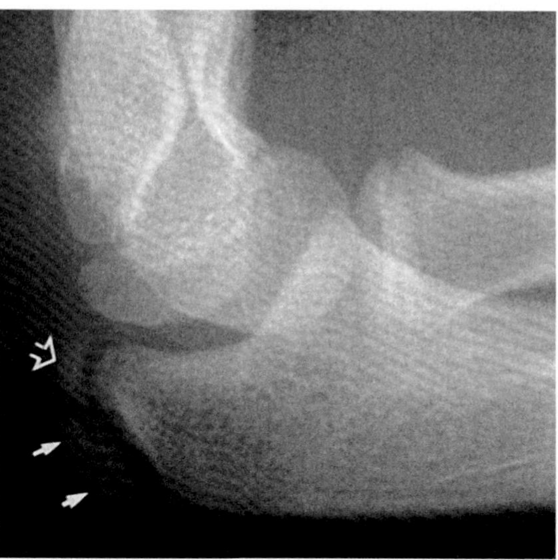

FIGURE 13-8 Ossification of the olecranon. **A.** Secondary ossification begins as an oblique oblong center at about 6 to 8 years of age. **B.** It may progress as two separate ossification centers: articular (*open arrow*) and traction (*closed arrows*).

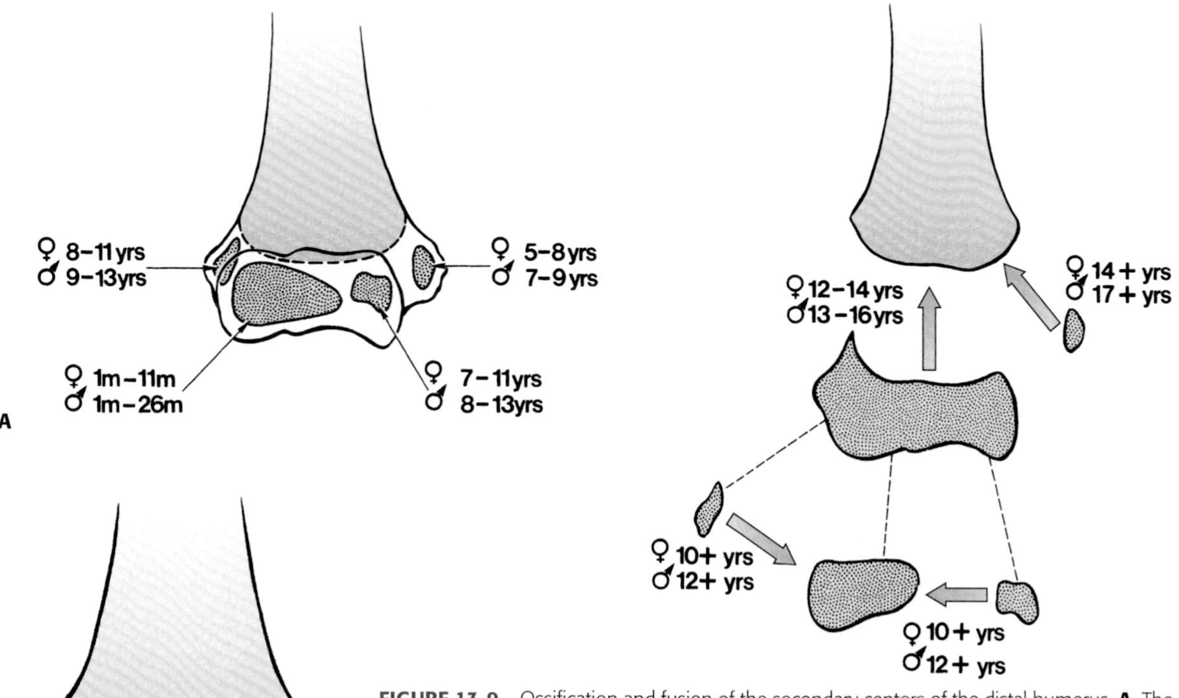

FIGURE 13-9 Ossification and fusion of the secondary centers of the distal humerus. **A.** The average ages for the onset of ossification of the various ossification centers are shown for both boys and girls. **B.** The ages at which these centers fuse with each other are shown for both boys and girls. (Modified and reprinted with permission from Haraldsson S. On osteochondrosis deformans juvenilis capituli humeri including investigation of the intra-osseous vasculature in the distal humerus. *Acta Orthop Scand* 1959;38[suppl].) **C.** The contribution of each secondary center to the overall architecture of the distal humerus is represented by the stippled areas.

They found that the sequence of ossification was the same in boys and girls—capitellum, radial head, medial epicondyle, olecranon, trochlea, and lateral epicondyle—but ossification was delayed by about 2 years in boys in all ossification centers except the capitellum (Table 13-1).

Blood Supply

Extraosseous

There is a rich arterial network around the elbow (Fig. 13-10) (18). The major arterial trunk, the brachial artery, lies anteriorly in the antecubital fossa. Most of the intraosseous blood supply of the distal humerus comes from the anastomotic vessels that course posteriorly.

Three structural components govern the location of the entrance of the vessels into the developing epiphysis. First, there is no communication between the intraosseous metaphyseal vasculature and the ossification centers. Second, vessels do not penetrate the articular surfaces. The lateral condyle is nonarticular only at the origin of the muscles and collateral ligaments. Third, the vessels do not penetrate the articular capsule except at the interface with the surface of the bone. Thus, only a small portion of the lateral condyle posteriorly is both nonarticular and extracapsular (Fig. 13-11) (19).

Intraosseous

The most extensive study of the intraosseous blood supply of the developing distal humerus was conducted by Haraldsson (Fig. 13-12) (11,19), who demonstrated that there are two types of vessels in the developing lateral condyle. These vessels enter the posterior portion of the condyle just lateral to the origin of

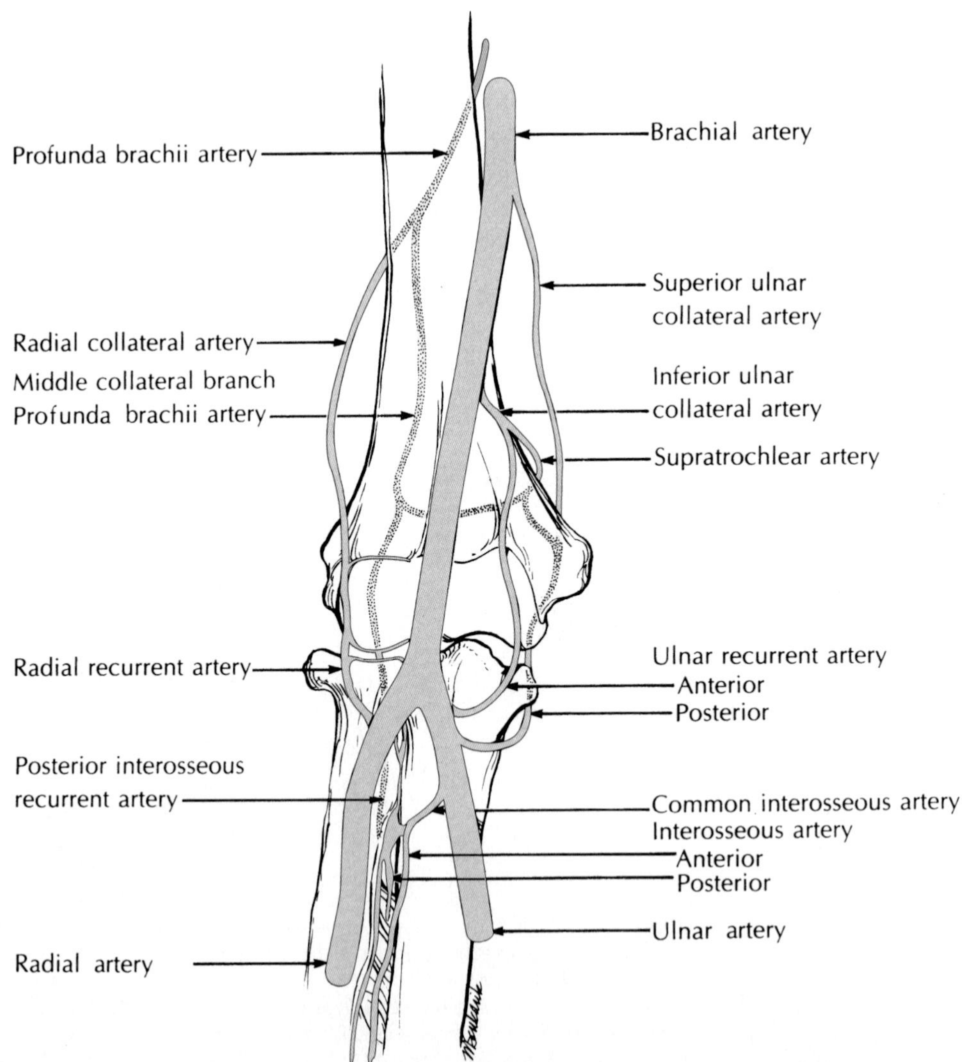

FIGURE 13-10 The major arteries about the anterior elbow.

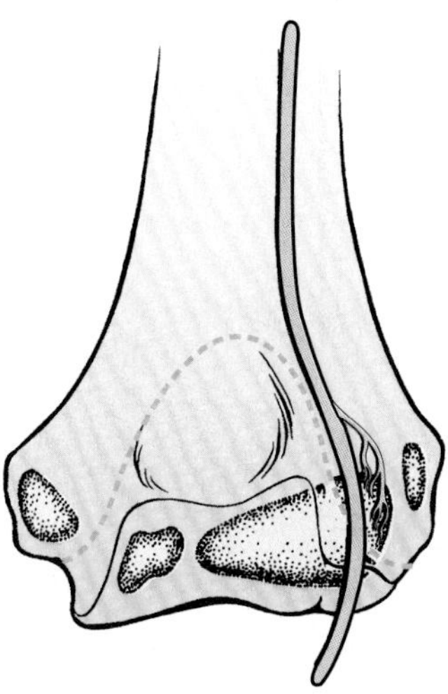

FIGURE 13-11 The vessels supplying the lateral condylar epiphysis enter the posterior aspect of the condyle, which is extra-articular. (Modified and reprinted with permission from Haraldsson S. On osteochondrosis deformans juvenilis capituli humeri including investigation of the intra-osseous vasculature in the distal humerus. *Acta Orthop Scand* 1959; 38[suppl]:1–232.)

the capsule and proximal to the articular cartilage near the origin of the anconeus muscle. They penetrate the nonossified cartilage and traverse it to the developing ossific nucleus. In a young child, this is a relatively long course (Fig. 13-12A). These vessels communicate with one another within the ossific nucleus but do not communicate with vessels in either the metaphysis or nonossified chondroepiphysis. Thus, for practical purposes, they are end vessels.

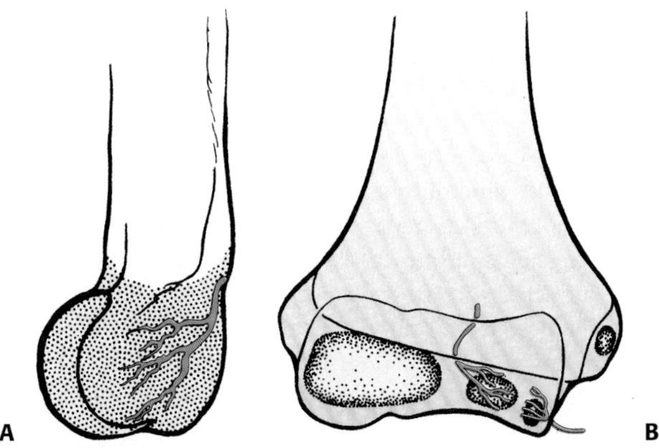

FIGURE 13-12 Intraosseous blood supply of the distal humerus. **A.** The vessels supplying the lateral condylar epiphysis enter on the posterior aspect and course for a considerable distance before reaching the ossific nucleus. **B.** Two definite vessels supply the ossification center of the medial crista of the trochlea. The lateral vessel enters by crossing the physis. The medial one enters by way of the nonarticular edge of the medial crista. (Modified and reprinted with permission from Haraldsson S. On osteochondrosis deformans juvenilis capituli humeri including investigation of the intra-osseous vasculature in the distal humerus. *Acta Orthop Scand* 1959;38[suppl]:1–232.)

The lateral condyle's ossification center extends into the lateral portion of the trochlea. Thus, the lateral crista or ridge of the trochlea derives its blood supply from these condylar vessels. The medial ridge or crista remains unossified for a longer period of time.

The trochlea is covered entirely by articular cartilage and lies totally within the confines of the articular capsule. The vessels that supply the nucleus of the ossific centers of the trochlea must therefore traverse the periphery of the physis to enter the epiphysis.

Haraldsson's (19) studies have shown two sources of blood supply to the ossific nucleus of the medial portion of the trochlea (Fig. 13-12B). The lateral vessel, on the posterior surface of the distal humeral metaphysis, penetrates the periphery of the physis and terminates in the trochlear nucleus. Because this vessel supplying the trochlea is an end vessel, it is especially vulnerable to injury by a fracture that courses through either the physis or the very distal portion of the humeral metaphysis. Injury to this vessel can markedly decrease the nourishment to the developing lateral ossific nucleus of the trochlea. The medial vessel penetrates the nonarticulating portion of the medial crista of the trochlea. This multiple vascular source may account for the development of multiple ossification centers in the maturing trochlea, giving it a fragmented appearance (Fig. 13-5).

When growth is complete, metaphyseal and epiphyseal vessels anastomose freely. The blood supply from the central nutrient vessel of the shaft reaches the epicondylar regions in the skeletally mature distal humerus (20).

Intra-Articular Structures

The articular surface lies within the confines of the capsule, but nonarticulating areas involving the coronoid and radial fossae anteriorly and the olecranon fossa posteriorly are also within the confines of the articular cavity (21). The capsule attaches just distal to the coronoid and olecranon processes. Thus, these processes are intra-articular (22). The entire radial head is intra-articular, with a recess or diverticulum of the elbow's articular cavity extending distally under the margin of the orbicular ligament. The medial and lateral epicondyles are extra-articular.

The anterior capsule is thickened anteriorly. These longitudinally directed fibers are very strong and become taut with the elbow in extension. In hyperextension, the tight anterior bands of the capsule force the ulna firmly into contact with the humerus. Thus, the fulcrum of rotation becomes transmitted proximally into the tip of the olecranon in the supracondylar area. This is an important factor in the etiology of supracondylar fractures.

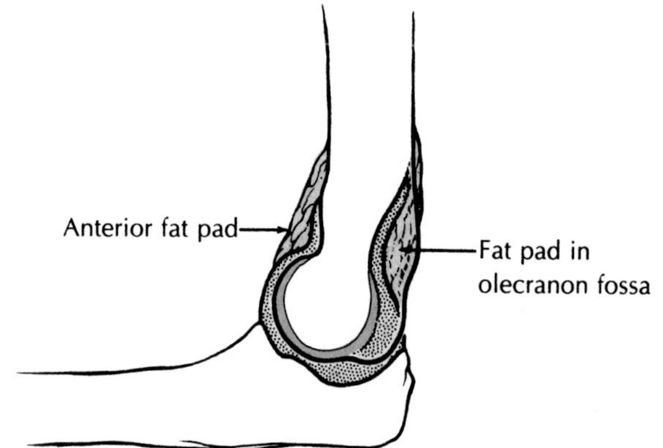

FIGURE 13-13 The elbow fat pads. Some of the coronoid fat pad lies anterior to the shallow coronoid fossa. The olecranon fat pad lies totally within the deeper olecranon fossa.

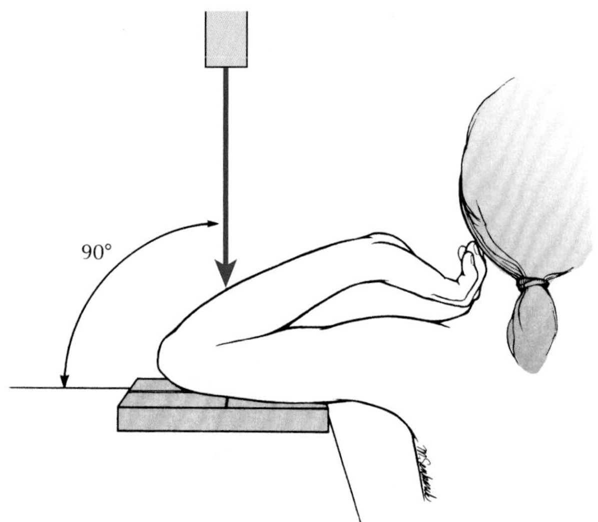

FIGURE 13-14 Jones axial x-ray view of the elbow.

Fat Pads

At the proximal portion of the capsule, between it and the synovial layer, are two large fat pads (Fig. 13-13). The posterior fat pad lies totally within the depths of the olecranon fossa when the elbow is flexed. The anterior fat pad extends anteriorly out of the margins of the coronoid fossa. The significance of these fat pads in the interpretation of x-rays of the elbow is discussed later.

Ligaments

The pertinent ligamentous anatomy involving the orbicular and collateral ligaments is discussed in the sections on the specific injuries involving the radial neck, medial epicondyle, and elbow dislocations.

X-RAY FINDINGS

Because of the ever-changing ossification pattern, identification and delineation of fractures about the elbow in the immature skeleton may be subject to misinterpretation. The variables of ossification of the epiphyses should be well known to the orthopaedic surgeon who treats these injuries.

Standard Views

The standard x-rays of the elbow include an anteroposterior (AP) view with the elbow extended and a lateral view with the elbow flexed to 90 degrees and the forearm neutral.

Jones View

It is often difficult for a child to extend the injured elbow, and an axial view of the elbow, the Jones view, may be helpful (Fig. 13-14). The distal humerus is normally difficult to interpret due to the superimposed proximal radius and ulna. There is often a high index of suspicion for a fracture, but none is visible on routine AP and lateral x-rays. In this case, internal and external oblique views may be helpful. This is especially true in identifying fractures of the radial head and coronoid process.

AP Landmarks

Baumann Angle

In the standard AP view, the major landmark is the angulation of the physeal line between the lateral condyle and the distal humeral metaphysis. The ossification center of the lateral condyle extends into the radial or lateral crista of the trochlea (Fig. 13-9C). This physeal line forms an angle with the long axis of the humerus. The angle formed by this physeal line and the long axis of the humerus is the Baumann angle (Fig. 13-15A) (23). The Baumann angle is not equal to the carrying angle of the elbow in older children (12). This is a consistent angle when both sides are compared and the x-ray beam is directed perpendicular to the long axis of the humerus. Acton and McNally reviewed the descriptions of the Baumann angle in a number of commonly used textbooks and discovered three variations of measurement technique. They recommended that the angle should always be measured between the long axis of the humerus and the inclination of the capitellar physis, as Baumann described, and that it should be called the "shaft-physeal" angle to avoid confusion.

Caudad-cephalad angulation of the x-ray tube or right or left angulation of the tube by as much as 30 degree changes the Baumann angle by less than 5 degrees. If, however, the tube becomes angulated in a cephalad-caudad direction by more than 20 degrees, the angle is changed significantly and the measurement is inaccurate.

In their cadaver studies, Camp et al (24) found that rotation of the distal fragment or the entire reduced humerus can also alter the projection of the Baumann angle. They found that to be accurate, the humerus must be parallel to the x-ray plate, with the beam directed perpendicular to the film as well.

Thus, in the routine AP x-rays of the distal humerus, including the Jones view, the Baumann angle is a good measurement of any deviation of the distal humerus' angulation (25).

Other Angles

Two other angles measured on AP x-rays are commonly used to determine the proper alignment of the distal humerus or carrying angle. The humeral-ulnar angle is determined by lines longitudinally bisecting the shaft of the humerus with the shaft of the ulna (Fig. 13-15B) (14,26,27). The metaphyseal-diaphyseal angle is determined by a line that longitudinally bisects the shaft of the humerus with a line that connects the widest points of the metaphysis of the distal humerus (see Fig. 13-15C) (28). The humeral-ulnar angle is the most accurate in determining the true carrying angle of the elbow. The Baumann angle also has a good correlation with the clinical carrying angle, but it may be difficult to measure in adolescents in whom the ossification center of the lateral condyle is beginning to fuse with other centers. The metaphyseal-diaphyseal angle is the least accurate of the three (29).

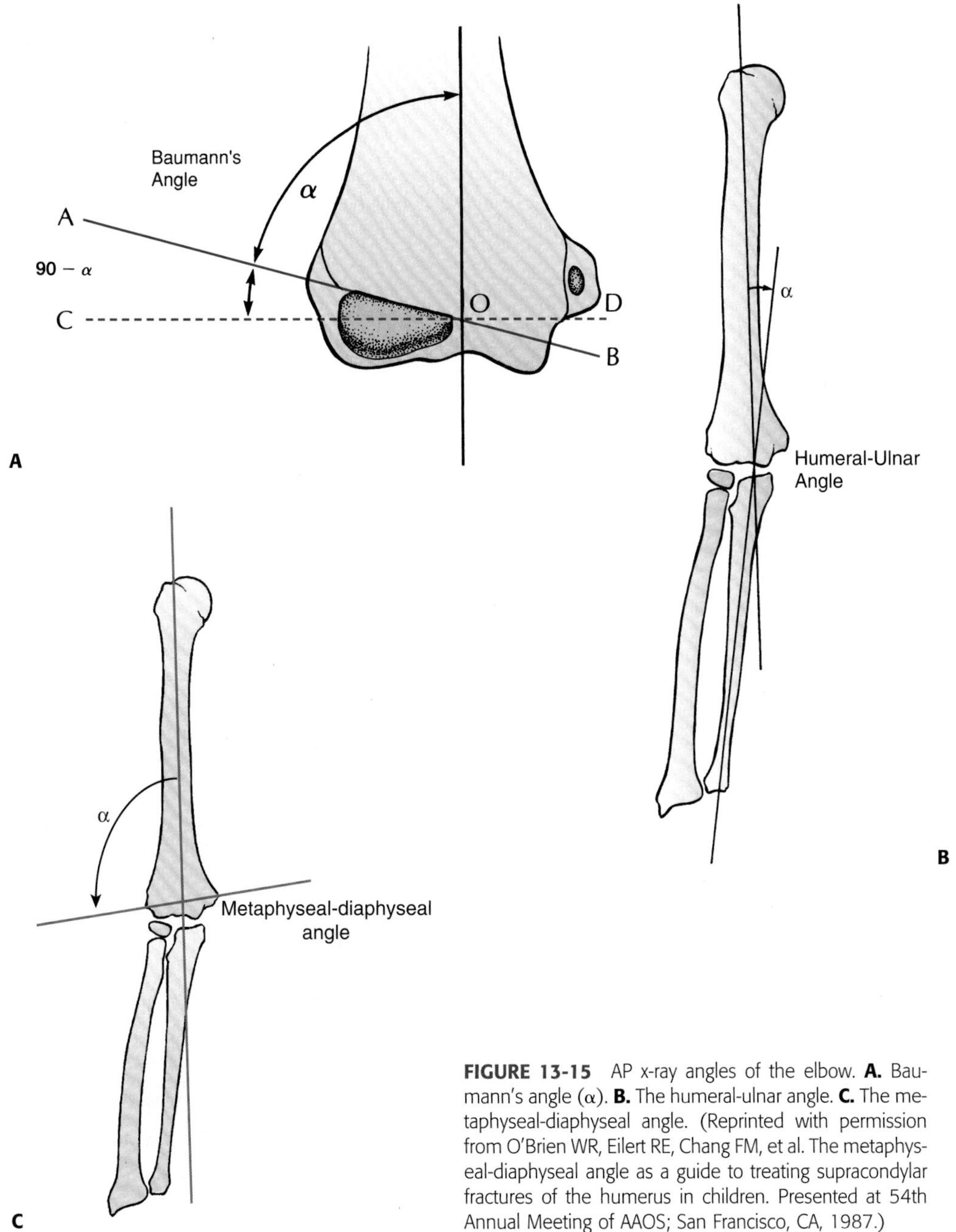

FIGURE 13-15 AP x-ray angles of the elbow. **A.** Baumann's angle (α). **B.** The humeral-ulnar angle. **C.** The metaphyseal-diaphyseal angle. (Reprinted with permission from O'Brien WR, Eilert RE, Chang FM, et al. The metaphyseal-diaphyseal angle as a guide to treating supracondylar fractures of the humerus in children. Presented at 54th Annual Meeting of AAOS; San Francisco, CA, 1987.)

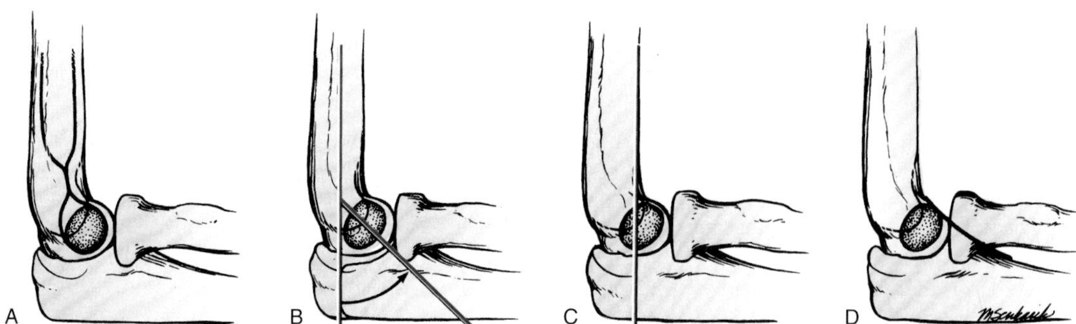

FIGURE 13-16 Lateral x-ray lines of the distal humerus. **A.** The teardrop of the distal humerus. **B.** The angulation of the lateral condyle with the shaft of the humerus. **C.** The anterior humeral line. **D.** The coronoid line.

Lateral Landmarks

Teardrop

The lateral projection of the distal humerus presents a teardrop-like shadow above the capitellum (16). The anterior dense line making up the teardrop represents the posterior margin of the coronoid fossa. The posterior dense line represents the anterior margin of the olecranon fossa. The inferior portion of the teardrop is the ossification center of the capitellum. On a true lateral projection, this teardrop should be well defined (Fig. 13-16A).

Shaft-Condylar Angle

On the lateral x-ray, there is an angulation of 40 degrees between the long axis of the humerus and the long axis of the lateral condyle (Fig. 13-16B). This can also be measured by the flexion angle of the distal humerus, which is calculated by measuring the angle of the lateral condylar physeal line with the long axis of the shaft of the humerus (31).

Anterior Humeral Line

If a line is drawn along the anterior border of the distal humeral shaft, it should pass through the middle third of the ossification center of the capitellum. This is referred to as the *anterior humeral line* (Fig. 13-16C). Passage of the anterior humeral line through the anterior portion of the lateral condylar ossification center or anterior to it indicates the presence of posterior angulation of the distal humerus. In a large study of minimally displaced supracondylar fractures, Rogers et al (32) found that this anterior humeral line was the most reliable factor in detecting the presence or absence of occult fractures.

Coronoid Line

A line directed proximally along the anterior border of the coronoid process should barely touch the anterior portion of the lateral condyle (Fig. 13-16D). Posterior displacement of the lateral condyle projects the ossification center posterior to this coronoid line (16).

Pseudofracture

Some vagaries of the ossification process about the elbow may be interpreted as a fracture (16). For example, the ossification of the trochlea may be irregular, producing a fragmented appearance (Fig. 13-5). This fragmentation can be misinterpreted, especially if the distal humerus is slightly oblique or tilted. These secondary ossification centers may be mistaken for fracture fragments lying between the semilunar notch and lateral condyle (Fig. 13-17).

On the lateral view, the physeal line between the lateral condyle and the distal humeral metaphysis is wider posteriorly. This appearance may give a misinterpretation that the lateral condyle is fractured and tilted (12).

On the AP view before the radial head ossifies, there is normally some lateral angulation to the radial border of the neck of the radius that may give the appearance of subluxation (Fig.

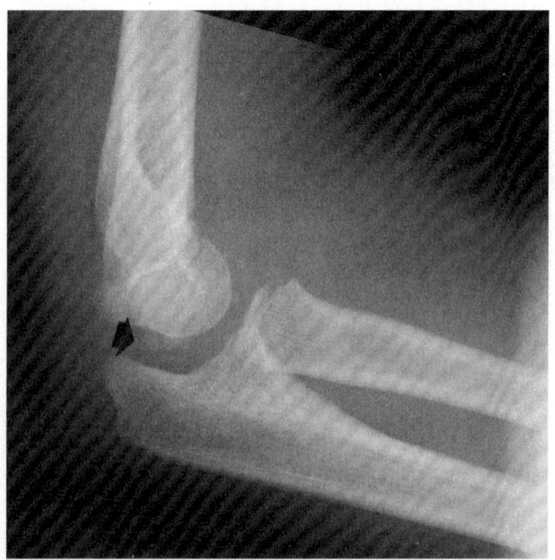

FIGURE 13-17 Pseudofracture of the elbow. The trochlea with its multiple ossification centers may be misinterpreted as fracture fragments lying between the joint surfaces (*arrow*).

13-3). The true position of the radial head can be confirmed by noting the relationship of the proximal radius to the ossification center of the lateral condyle on the lateral projection (32).

Fat Pad Signs of the Elbow

There are three areas in which fat pads overlie the elbow's major structures. Displacement of any of the fat pads can indicate an occult fracture. The first two areas are the fat pads that overlie the capsule in the coronoid fossa anteriorly and the olecranon fossa posteriorly. Displacement of either or both of these fat pads is usually referred to as the *classic elbow fat pad sign*. A third accumulation of fat overlies the supinator muscle as it wraps around the proximal radius.

Olecranon (Posterior) Fat Pad

Because the olecranon fossa is deep, the fat pad here is totally contained within the fossa. It is not visible on a normal lateral x-ray of the elbow flexed to 90 degrees (Fig. 13-18A). Distention of the capsule with an effusion, as occurs with an occult intra-articular fracture, a spontaneously reduced dislocation, or even an infection, can cause the dorsal or olecranon fat pad to be visible (33).

Coronoid (Anterior) Fat Pad

Likewise, the ventral or coronoid fat pad may be displaced anteriorly (Fig. 13-18B) (34). Because the coronoid fossa is shallow, the fat pad in this area projects anterior to the bony margins and can be seen normally as a triangular radiolucency anterior to the distal humerus. Although displacement of the classic elbow fat pads is a reliable indication of an intra-articular effusion, there may be instances in which only one of the fat pads is displaced. Brodeur et al (12) and Kohn (20) have shown that the coronoid fat pad is more sensitive to small effusions than the olecranon fat pad. It can be displaced without a coexistent displacement of the olecranon fat pad (Fig. 13-18C).

Supinator Fat Pad

A layer of fat on the anterior aspect of the supinator muscle wraps around the proximal radius. This layer of fat or fat pad may normally bow anteriorly to some degree. Brodeur et al (12) stated that displacement may indicate the presence of an occult fracture of the radial neck. Displacement of the fat line or pad is often difficult to interpret; in a review of fractures involving the proximal radius, Schunk et al (16) found it to be positive only 50% of the time.

Fat Pad Variations

For the fat pads to be displaced, the capsule must be intact. This can explain why there may be no displacement of the fat

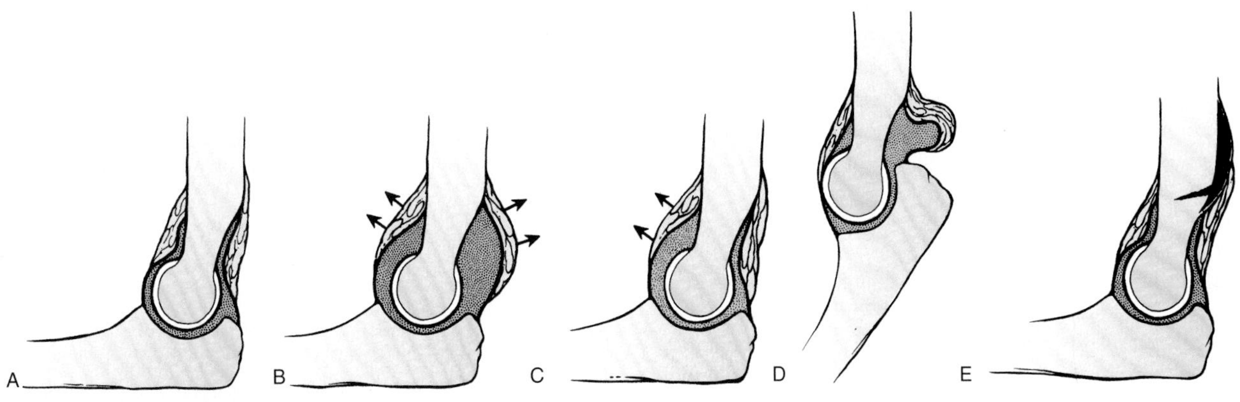

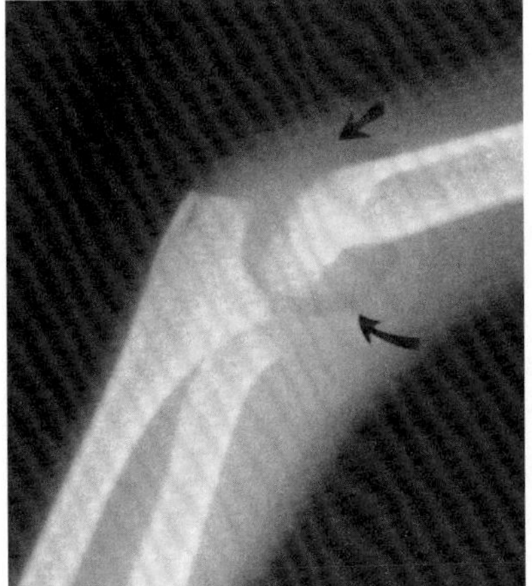

FIGURE 13-18 X-ray variations of the elbow fat pads. **A.** Normal relationships of the two fat pads. **B.** Displacement of both fat pads (*arrows*) with an intra-articular effusion. **C.** In some cases, the effusion may displace only the anterior fat pad (*arrows*). **D.** In extension, the posterior fat pad is normally displaced by the olecranon. **E.** An extra-articular fracture may lift the distal periosteum and displace the proximal portion of the posterior fat pad. **F.** An x-ray showing displacement of both fat pads (*arrows*) from an intra-articular effusion. (Modified and reprinted with permission from Murphy WA, Siegel MJ. Elbow fat pads with new signs and extended differential diagnosis. *Radiology* 1977;124:656–659.)

pads with an elbow dislocation that has spontaneously reduced due to capsule rupture. Murphy and Siegel (28) described other variations of classic fat pad displacement. If the elbow is extended, the fat pad is normally displaced from the olecranon fossa by the olecranon (Fig. 13-18D). Distal humeral fractures may cause subperiosteal bleeding and may lift the proximal portion of the olecranon fat pad without the presence of an effusion (Fig. 13-18E). These false-negative and false-positive findings must be kept in mind when interpreting the presence or absence of a fat pad with an elbow injury.

Corbett's (25) review of elbow injuries indicated that if a displacement of the posterior fat pad existed, a fracture was almost always present. Displacement of the anterior fat pad alone, however, could occur without a fracture. Corbett also determined that the degree of displacement bore no relation to the fracture's size. Skaggs and Mirzayan (35) reported that 34 of 45 children (76%) with a history of elbow trauma and an elevated posterior fat pad had x-ray evidence of elbow fractures at an average of 3 weeks after injury, although AP, lateral, and oblique x-rays at the time of injury showed no other evidence of fracture. They recommended that a child with a history of elbow trauma and an elevated fat pad should be treated as if a nondisplaced elbow fracture were present. Donnelly et al (36), however, found evidence of fracture in only 9 of 54 children (17%) who had a history of trauma and elbow joint effusion but no identifiable fracture on initial x-rays. They concluded that joint effusion without a visible fracture on initial x-rays does not correlate with the presence of occult fracture in most patients (83%). Persistent effusion did correlate with occult fracture: 78% of those with occult fractures had persistent effusions, compared with 16% of those without fractures.

Comparison X-Rays

Although it is often tempting to order comparison x-rays in a child with an injured elbow due to the difficulty evaluating the irregularity of the ossification process, the indications for ordering comparison x-rays are rare. Kissoon et al (37) found that using routine comparison x-rays in children with injured elbows did not significantly increase the accuracy of diagnosis, regardless of the interpreter's training. Petit et al reviewed 3,128 x-rays of 2,470 children admitted to a pediatric emergency department for osteoarticular trauma and found that only 22% of the x-rays revealed abnormal findings; 33.3% of elbow x-rays revealed abnormalities. Fewer than half of clinically suspected fractures were confirmed by x-ray.

Magnetic Resonance Imaging

Major and Crawford used magnetic resonance imaging (MRI) to evaluate seven children who had x-rays that showed effusion but no fractures; four of the children had fractures identified by MRI. These investigators suggested that an occult fracture is usually present when effusion occurs, even if a fracture is not visible on x-ray. Griffith et al reviewed the x-rays and MRI scans of 50 children with elbow trauma. X-rays identified effusions in 34% of the children and fractures in 52%; MRI identified effusions in 96% and fractures in 74%. Although MRI revealed a broad spectrum of bone and soft tissue injury beyond that shown on x-rays (bone bruising, muscle and ligament injuries, physeal injury, fracture), the additional information provided by MRI had little influence on patient treatment and no value in predicting clinical outcome. We have found MRI to be helpful in evaluating articular fractures to identify fracture pattern and extent, fragment position, and any interposed structure.

REFERENCES

1. Johansson O. Capsular and ligament injuries of the elbow joint. *Acta Chir Scand* 1962; 287(suppl).
2. Beekman F, Sullivan JE. Some observations on fractures of long bones in children. *Am J Surg* 1941;51:722–738.
3. Landin LA, Danielsson LG. Elbow fractures in children: an epidemiological analysis of 589 cases. *Acta Orthop Scand* 1986;57:309.
4. Buhr AJ, Cooke AM. Fracture patterns. *Lancet* 1959;1:531–536.
5. Wilkins KE. Fractures and dislocations of the elbow region. In: Rockwood CA Jr, Wilkins KE, Beaty JH, eds. *Fractures in children,* 4th ed. Philadelphia: Lippincott-Raven, 1996: 653–904.
6. Henrikson B. Supracondylar fracture of the humerus in children. *Acta Chir Scand* 1966; 369(suppl).
7. Gray DJ, Gardner E. Prenatal development of the human elbow joint. *Am J Anat* 1951; 88:429–469.
8. Brodeur AE, Silberstein JJ, Graviss ER. *Radiology of the Pediatric Elbow.* Boston: GK Hall, 1981.
9. Elgenmark O. The normal development of the ossific centers during infancy and childhood. *Acta Paediatr Scand* 1946;33(suppl).
10. Francis CC. The appearance of centers of ossification from 6-15 years. *Am J Phys Anthropol* 1940;27:127–138.
11. Haraldsson S. The intraosseous vasculature of the distal end of the humerus with special reference to capitulum. *Acta Orthop Scand* 1957;27:81–93.
12. Brodeur AE, Silberstein JJ, Graviss ER, et al. The basic tenets for appropriate evaluation of the elbow in pediatrics. In: *Current problems in diagnostic radiology.* Chicago: Year Book Medical, 1983.
13. Peterson CA, Peterson HA. Analysis of the incidence of injuries to the epiphyseal growth plate. *J Trauma* 1972;12:275–281.
14. O'Brien WR, Eilert RE, Chang FM, et al. The metaphyseal diaphyseal angle as a guide to treating supracondylar fractures of the humerus in children. Presented at 54th Annual Meeting of AAOS; San Francisco, CA, 1987.
15. Blount WP, Cassidy RH. Fractures of the elbow in children. *JAMA* 1951;146:699–704.
16. Schunk VK, Grossholz M, Schild H. Der Supinatorfettkorper bei Frakturen des Ellbogengelenkes. *ROFO* 1989;150:294–296.
17. Cheng JC, Wing-Man K, Shen WY, et al. A new look at the sequential development of elbow-ossification centers in children. *J Pediatr Orthop* 1998;18:161–167.
18. Wilson PD. Fractures and dislocations in the region of the elbow. *Surg Gynecol Obstet* 1933;56:335–359.
19. Haraldsson S. On osteochondrosis deformans juvenilis capituli humeri including investigation of intra-osseous vasculature in distal humerus. *Acta Orthop Scand* 1959;38(suppl).
20. Kohn AM. Soft tissue alterations in elbow trauma. *AJR* 1959;82:867–874.
21. William PL, Warwick R. *Gray's anatomy.* Philadelphia: WB Saunders, 1980.
22. Jenkins F. The functional anatomy and evolution of the mammalian humeroulnar articulation. *Am J Anat* 1973;137:281–298.
23. Baumann E. Beitrage zur Kenntnis dur Frackturen am Ellbogengelenk. *Bruns Beitr F Klin Chir* 1929;146:1–50.
24. Camp J, Ishizue K, Gomez M, et al. Alteration of Baumann's angle by humeral position: implications for treatment of supracondylar humerus fractures. *J Pediatr Orthop* 1993; 13:521–555.
25. Corbett RH. Displaced fat pads in trauma to the elbow. *Injury* 1978;9:297–298.
26. Beals RK. The normal carrying angle of the elbow. *Clin Orthop* 1976;19:194–196.
27. Ippolito E, Caterini R, Scola E. Supracondylar fractures of the humerus in children. Analysis at maturity of 53 patients treated conservatively. *J Bone Joint Surg (Am)* 1986; 68:333–344.
28. Murphy WA, Siegel MJ. Elbow fat pad with new signs and extended differential diagnosis. *Radiology* 1977;124:659–665.
29. Smith L. Deformity following supracondylar fractures of the humerus. *J Bone Joint Surg (Am)* 1960;42:235–252.

30. D'Arienzo M, Innocenti M, Pennisi M. The treatment of supracondylar fractures of the humerus in childhood (cases and results). *Arch Putti Chir Organi Mov* 1983;33:261–269.
31. Porteous CJ. The olecranon epiphyses. *J Anat* 1960;94:286.
32. Sandegrad E. Fracture of the lower end of the humerus in children: treatment and end results. *Acta Chir Scand* 1944;89:1–16.
33. Yang Z, Wang Y, Gilula LA, et al. Microcirculation of the distal humeral epiphyseal cartilage: implications for post-traumatic growth deformities. *J Hand Surg (Am)* 1998; 23:165–172.
34. Bohrer SP. The fat pad sign following elbow trauma: its usefulness and reliability in suspecting "invisible" fractures. *Clin Radiol* 1970;21:90–94.
35. Skaggs DL, Mirzayan R. The posterior fat pad sign in association with occult fracture of the elbow in children. *J Bone Joint Surg (Am)* 1999;81:1429–1433.
36. Donnelly LF, Klostermeier TT, Klosterman LA. Traumatic elbow effusions in pediatric patients: are occult fractures the rule? *AJR* 1998;171:243–245.
37. Kissoon N, Galpin R, Gayle M, et al. Evaluation of the role of comparison radiographs in the diagnosis of traumatic elbow injuries. *J Pediatr Orthop* 1995;15:449–453.

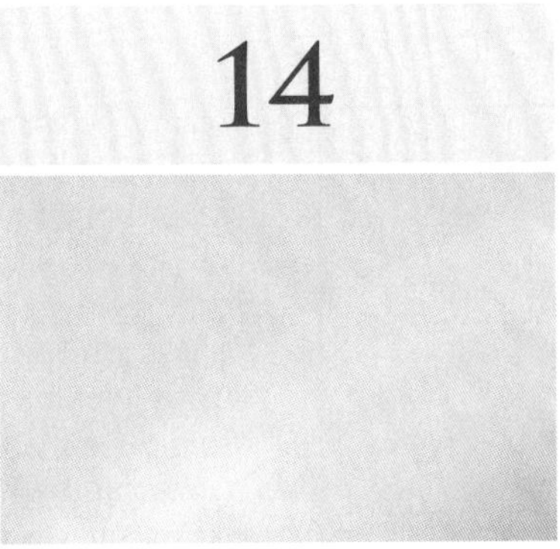

SUPRACONDYLAR FRACTURES OF THE DISTAL HUMERUS

James R. Kasser and James H. Beaty

Between the mid-20th century, when early reports of pinning distal humeral fractures first appeared, and the present, treatment of supracondylar fractures has evolved tremendously. Blount's caution against operative management (1) has given way to modern concepts of treatment involving skeletal stabilization and soft tissue management, which have greatly improved outcomes (2–6). The improvement in stabilization techniques and the efficient application of such therapy represents further advancements in this area.

Both treatment costs and clinical results have been significantly affected over the past 25 years (7). Problems of vascular compromise, Volkmann ischemic contracture, and neurovascular entrapment in the fracture callus have been greatly decreased, but not eliminated.

INCIDENCE AND GENERAL CONSIDERATIONS

The peak age at which supracondylar fractures occur is between 5 and 7 years. The rate of occurrence increases steadily in the first 5 years of life, and traditionally boys have had a higher incidence of this fracture than girls. Combining 64 reports of supracondylar fractures totaling 8,361 displaced fractures of the distal humerus yields a consistent pattern, as shown in Table 14-1. Boys have historically outnumbered girls by about three to two, although the added series since the last publication of this text (8–10) have resulted in an increasing ratio of girls sustaining supracondylar fractures. It makes sense that we will see a continued movement toward equal incidence in girls and boys given trends in activity. The average age at fracture is 6.7

TABLE 14-1 Incidence of Supracondylar Fractures

	Percentage of Total Number of Fractures (%)
Side involved	
Right	39.2
Left	60.8
Gender incidence	
Male	59.5
Female	40.5
Ipsilateral fractures	1.0
Open fractures	1.0
Volkmann contracture	<0.5
Flexion type	2.0
Fractures with nerve injuries[a]	7.7
Radial nerve	41.2[b]
Median nerve	36.0[b]
Ulnar nerve	22.8[b]
Vascular injury	1.0

Data were compiled from 8361 fractures occurring in 64 major series.
[a] Average age was 6.7 years.
[b] Percentage of total nerve injuries.

years. The left or nondominant side predominates in almost all studies. Two thirds of children hospitalized with elbow injuries have supracondylar fractures. Nerve injury occurs in at least 7% and significant vascular injury in 1%. The radial nerve has been the most frequently involved nerve in older studies; however, the median nerve is much more commonly injured, particularly the anterior interosseous nerve (AIN), in more recent studies (11,12). The ulnar nerve is most commonly injured iatrogenically during pinning or in a flexion-type of supracondylar fracture. It is possible that there has been a change in the displacement pattern of these fractures, accounting for the change in frequency of median nerve injuries, but it is more likely that the subtle loss of thumb and finger flexion that indicates an AIN injury is more frequently recognized.

Increased ligamentous laxity (Fig. 14-1) has been correlated with the occurrence of supracondylar fractures (13,14) and with ulnar nerve subluxation (15). Unfortunately, the common association with ligamentous laxity places the nerve at risk for iatrogenic injury from medial pinning in the group most likely to sustain this fracture.

Almost all supracondylar fractures are caused by accidental trauma rather than abuse. A fall from a height accounts for 70% of all supracondylar fractures (9). In children under 3 years of age, the fracture usually occurs in a fall from a bed, from furniture, or down stairs. In children over 3 years of age, the fracture generally results due to a fall from monkey bars, swings, or other playground equipment. In one study of 99 patients with supracondylar fractures seen over a 15-month period, only one was secondary to abuse (16). When a child under 15 months of age has a supracondylar fracture of the distal humerus, a nonaccidental cause should be considered; with a reasonable history, however, such a cause is unlikely.

The most commonly associated fractures are distal radial fractures, but fractures of the scaphoid and proximal humerus do occur. Monteggia fractures (17) have also been reported in association with supracondylar fractures. Pulse is absent at presentation in 12% to 15% of patients, but vascular insufficiency

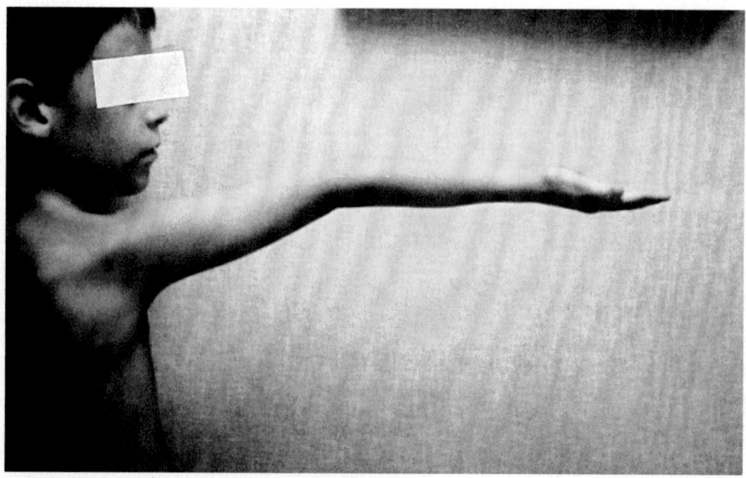

FIGURE 14-1 Hyperflexibility. At the peak age for supracondylar fractures, there is a naturally occurring hyperextension of the elbow, which predisposes the distal humerus to this type of fracture. (From Wilkins KE. The operative management of supracondylar fractures. *Orthop Clin N Am* 1990;21:269–289, with permission.)

requiring operative intervention is relatively rare (1% to 2%) (18–21). Volkmann ischemic contracture is rare, occurring in about 0.5% of patients. Most distal humeral supracondylar fractures are displaced in extension, and flexion-type injuries are seen infrequently.

EXTENSION-TYPE SUPRACONDYLAR FRACTURES

Mechanism of Injury

Supracondylar fractures generally occur as a result of a fall onto the outstretched hand with the elbow in full extension (Fig. 14-2) (22). The flexed elbow may be stabilized by the biceps, brachialis, and triceps muscles, but once extended beyond neutral, the elbow flexor muscles are at a poor mechanical advantage, and there is little resistance to injury. The olecranon in its fossa in the distal humerus acts as a fulcrum, whereas the capsule transmits an extension force to the distal humerus just proximal to the physis as the elbow hyperextends. The capsular insertion, distal to the olecranon fossa and proximal to the physis, is critical in producing a consistent failure pattern of a transcondylar fracture in children. In full extension, the elbow becomes tightly interlocked, concentrating bending forces in the distal humerus (23). Given a similar fall on the outstretched arm from a height, several investigators have tried to differentiate between distal radial injuries and supracondylar fracture occurrence based on ligamentous laxity. Nork (24) concluded that a patient with ligamentous laxity is more likely to have a supracondylar than a distal radial fracture. In a similar analysis by McLauchlan (25), however, it was felt that the degree of ligamentous laxity was not the differentiating factor determining which bone is fractured.

Posterior displacement of the distal fragment occurs with the proximal or metaphyseal fragment impaling the anterior soft tissue structures. The fracture in the sagittal plane was classically described by Kocher (26) as extending obliquely from anterior and distal to posterior and proximal. Clinical studies by Holmberg (27) and Nand (28), however, have demonstrated that the fracture pattern is transverse on lateral x-rays in more than 80% of patients (Fig. 14-3). The fracture line in the anteroposterior (AP) view extends transversely across both the medial and lateral columns of the distal humerus at the middle level of the olecranon fossa.

Role of the Periosteum

As the supracondylar fracture displaces posteriorly, the anterior periosteum fails and tears away from the displaced distal fragment. The anterior loss of periosteal integrity leads to frequent failure of anterior callus formation in early fracture healing, which is of little significance clinically (Fig. 14-4). Further fracture displacement is accompanied by corresponding increased periosteal disruption with decreased fracture stability.

Intact medial or lateral periosteum, the periosteal hinge, has been said to provide stability after fracture reduction (29–31). Forearm pronation (32,33) after reduction of a posteromedially displaced supracondylar fracture is said to stabilize reduction by closing the fracture gap laterally, tensioning the medial periosteal hinge, and tightening the lateral ligaments of the elbow (Fig. 14-5). Conversely, a laterally displaced supracondylar fracture is more stable in supination. Experimental data by Abraham

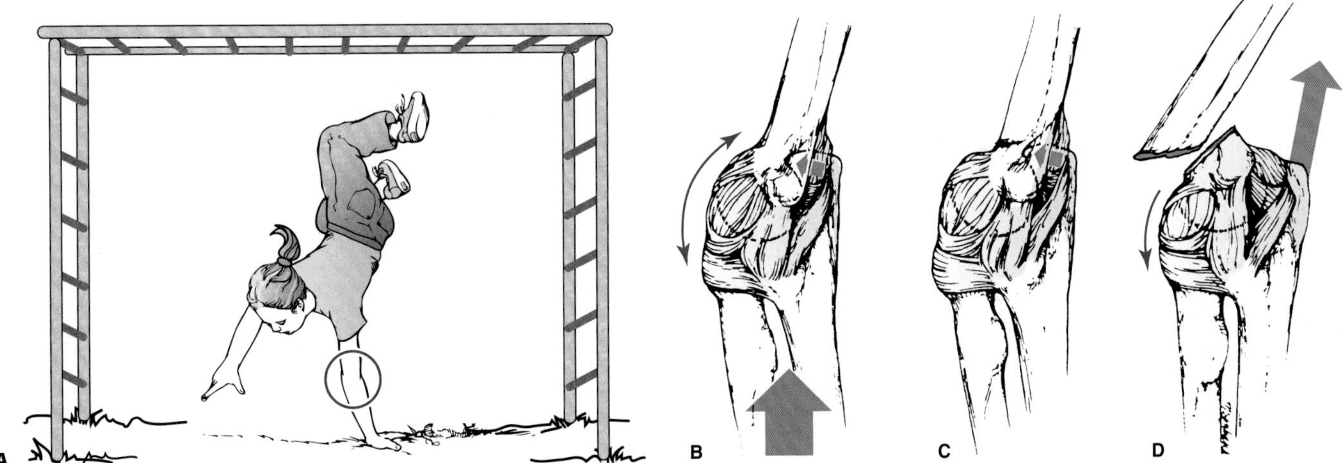

FIGURE 14-2 Hyperextension forces. **A.** Most young children attempt to break their falls with the upper extremity extended. Because of the laxity of the ligaments, the elbow becomes locked into hyperextension. **B.** This converts the linear applied force (*large arrow*) to an anterior tension force. Posteriorly, the olecranon is forced into the depths of the olecranon fossa (*small arrow*). **C.** As the bending force continues, the distal humerus fails anteriorly in the supracondylar area. **D.** When the fracture is complete, the distal fragment becomes posteriorly displaced. The strong action of the triceps (*large arrow*) produces proximal displacement of the distal fragment.

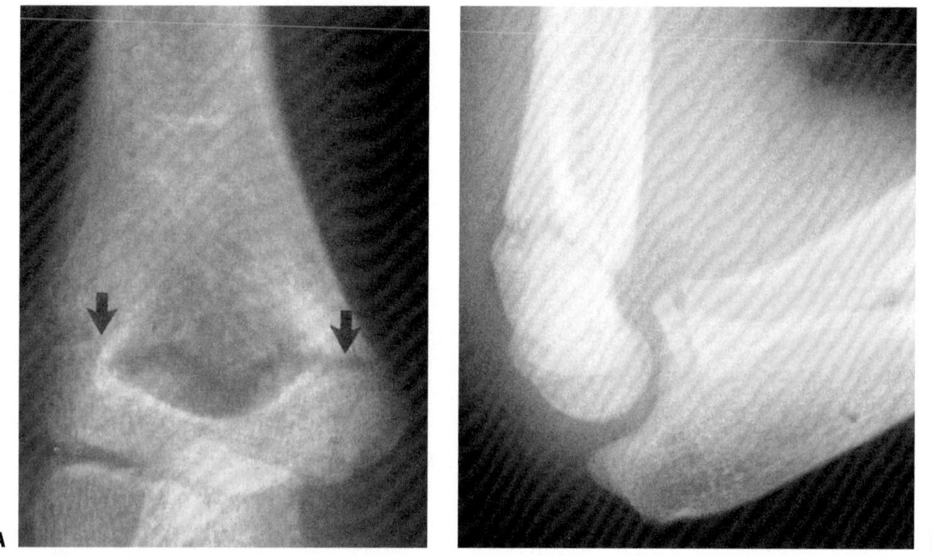

FIGURE 14-3 Orientation of fracture lines. **A.** The typical transverse fracture line originates just above the epicondyles and courses through the supracondylar area (*arrows*). **B.** In the lateral projection, the fracture line is usually also transverse.

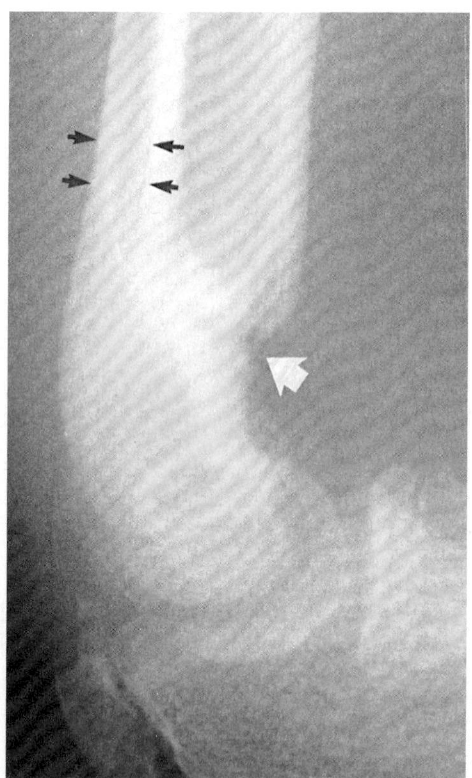

FIGURE 14-4 Periosteal changes. In these x-rays taken 2 months after fracture, the lateral view demonstrates a persistent gap (*white arrow*) in the anterior cortical margin where interposed periosteum prevented anatomic reduction. Note the absence of periosteal new bone anteriorly on the proximal fragment, although there is abundant periosteal new bone (*black arrows*) on the posterior surface.

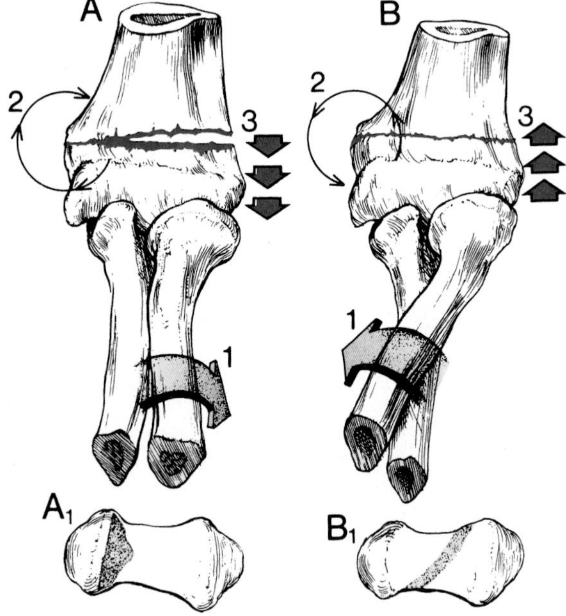

FIGURE 14-5 Intra-articular stabilizing forces. **A.** Supination of the forearm (*1*) creates a downward lateral tilt of the distal fragment (*3*). This produces compressive forces between the articulating surface of the ulna and the trochlea's medial border (*A1, stippled area*), which in turn, generates clockwise forces (*2*) about the medial side of the fracture. **B.** Pronation of the forearm (*1*) creates an upward tilt of the distal fragment (*3*) due to the compressive forces between the articulating surface of the ulna and the lateral border of the trochlea (*B1, stippled area*), which in turn, generates counterclockwise forces (*2*) about the medial side of the fracture. (From Abraham E, Powers T, Witt P, et al. Experimental hyperextension supracondylar fractures in monkeys. *Clin Orthop* 1982;171: 309–318, with permission.)

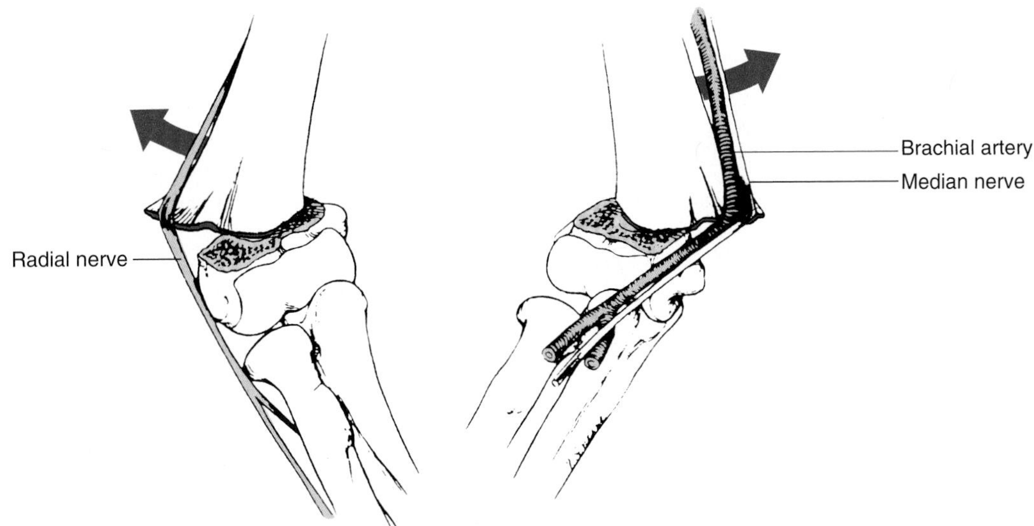

FIGURE 14-6 Neurovascular relations. If the distal spike penetrates the brachialis muscle laterally (posteromedial fractures), the radial nerve may be tethered (*left*). If the spike penetrates medially (posterolateral fractures), both the median nerve and brachial artery can be tethered (*right*).

(34) questioned this generally accepted concept, suggesting that little stability results from an intact periosteal hinge. If the periosteum is intact medially and laterally in a supracondylar fracture with pure posterior displacement, it may yield a very stable reduction. After reduction and fracture pinning, however, the forearm position is not an issue clinically.

Posteromedial Versus Posterolateral Displacement of Extension-Type and Supracondylar-Type Fractures

Generally, medial displacement of the distal fragment is more common than lateral displacement, occurring in approximately 75% of patients in most series (35). The biceps tendon insertion and axis of muscle pull lies medial to the shaft of the humerus, and Holmberg (27) suggested that this anatomic location of muscle pull created a force that tended to displace the distal humeral fragment medially. Hyperextension of the elbow negates the dynamic protective role of the biceps/triceps in stabilizing the elbow at impact compounded by the olecranon acting as a fulcrum in the fossa leading to this fracture. In one series with a high preponderance of median nerve and brachial artery injuries, however, 47% of patients had posterolateral displacement of the distal humeral fragment (19).

The position of the hand and forearm at the time of injury plays a role in the direction of the distal humeral fragment's displacement. In a patient who falls onto an outstretched supinated arm, the forces applied tend to disrupt the posteromedial periosteum first and displace the fragment posterolaterally. Conversely, if a patient falls with the arm pronated, the distal fragment tends to become displaced posteromedially. Whether the displacement is medial or lateral is important because it determines which soft tissue structures are at risk from the penetrating injury of the proximal metaphyseal fragment. Medial displacement of the distal fragment places the radial nerve at risk, and lateral displacement of the distal fragment places the median nerve and brachial artery at risk (Fig. 14-6). The brachial artery and median nerve may become entrapped in the fracture site with lateral displacement, but they are highly unlikely to become entrapped with the distal fragment displaced medially. The brachial artery is placed further at risk by the ulnar-sided tether of the supratrochlear artery (Fig. 14-7).

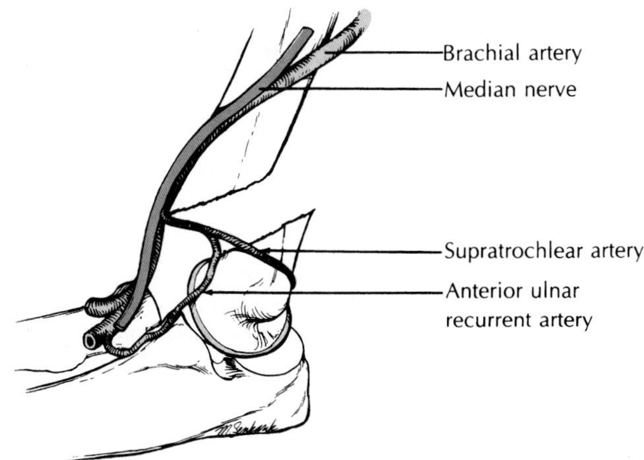

FIGURE 14-7 Arterial pathology. The supratrochlear branch that arises from the anterior ulnar recurrent artery may bind the main trunk of the brachial artery against the sharp end of the proximal fragment. (Modified and reprinted with permission from Rowell PJW. Arterial occlusion in juvenile humeral supracondylar fracture. *Injury* 1974;6:254–256.)

TABLE 14-2 Classification of Supracondylar Fractures

Type I	Undisplaced
Type II	Displaced (with intact posterior cortex)
Type III	Displaced (no cortical contact) Posteromedial Posterolateral

The Gartland classification of supracondylar fractures is currently the most commonly used system based on its prevalence in the literature. It is easy to use and facilitates treatment decisions as well as communication. The Gartland (36) classification (Table 14-2) is based on the x-ray appearance of fracture displacement. A type I or nondisplaced fracture (Fig. 14-8) has an anterior humeral line that intersects the capitellum, an intact olecranon fossa, no medial or lateral displacement, no medial column collapse, and a normal Baumann angle. A type II fracture is extended but not completely translated with some cortical contact. The anterior humeral line does not intersect the capitellum. Some rotational displacement and tilt into varus, as determined by the Baumann angle, may be present. A type III fracture has a circumferential break in the cortex with displacement of the fracture fragments. In the common extension-type supracondylar fracture, the distal fragment is displaced posteriorly with the metaphyseal fragment impaled into the brachialis muscle and anterior soft tissues. The distal fragment's x-ray appearance may be highly variable depending on (a) the degree of ossification of the distal humeral epiphysis, (b) the size of the ossified metaphyseal fragment, and (c) the distal humeral fragment's position of flexion and rotation. Always be aware of the possibility of a "T" type fracture in the type III with an intracondylar split.

Signs and Symptoms

An elbow or forearm fracture should be suspected in a child with elbow pain or failure to use the upper extremity after a fall. Initial x-rays should include the entire extremity, because multiple fractures may be present even with an injury that seems like minor trauma. In children with elbow pain and failure to use the upper extremity, the differential diagnosis should include occult fracture, nursemaid's elbow, and infection. With a clear history of a "pulling type" of injury, manipulation for a nursemaid's elbow may be performed before an x-ray is obtained. In general, if the history is not clear or if there is any question of a fall onto an outstretched hand as the mechanism of injury, an x-ray should always be obtained before elbow manipulation. With a type I supracondylar fracture, there may be distal humeral tenderness, distension or swelling in the anconeus soft spot (elbow effusion), restriction of motion, and evidence of bruising. X-rays may be negative except for a posterior fat pad sign. In a series of patients presenting with elbow pain postinjury with a posterior fat pad sign, Skaggs (37) found that 53% had a supracondylar fracture. In type III fractures, gross displacement (Fig. 14-9) of the elbow is evident. An anterior pucker sign (35) may be present if the proximal fragment has penetrated the brachialis and the anterior fascia of the elbow (Fig. 14-10). When the proximal fragment is disengaged from its pucker in the skin, there is sometimes bleeding as a definitive sign of a grade I open fracture. Careful motor, sensory, and vascular examinations should be performed in all patients; this may be quite difficult in a young child but should be attempted. Sensation should be tested in discrete sensory areas of the radial nerve (dorsal first web space), medial nerve (palmar index finger), and ulnar nerve (palmar little finger). Motor examination should include finger, wrist, and thumb extension (radial nerve), index distal interphalangeal flexion and thumb interphalangeal flexion (AIN), thenar strength (median), and interossei (ulnar nerve) muscle function. The vascular examination should include determining the presence of pulse, as well as warmth, capillary refill, and color of the hand. Tenseness of the volar compartment should be evaluated, and the amount of swelling about the elbow should be noted. Passive finger extension and flexion should be tested and the findings should be accurately recorded. In the initial examination of a child with a severe supracondylar fracture with high parental and patient anxiety, it is easy to overlook vital information. Because further decision making depends on an accurate initial assessment, care should always be taken to obtain all of the previously mentioned information as accurately as possible. When the elbow injury is obvious, examination should follow the proximal humerus and distal radius looking for signs of associated or occult fractures.

Radiologic Evaluation

All patients with a history of a fall onto an outstretched hand as well as pain and inability to use the extremity should undergo a thorough radiologic evaluation. This may include obtaining AP and lateral views of the entire upper extremity (Fig. 14-11). Comparison views are rarely required by an experienced physician, but occasionally may be needed to evaluate an ossifying epiphysis. The AP x-ray should always be taken as an AP of the distal humerus rather than an AP of the elbow in which the elbow is held in flexion. This allows more accurate evaluation of the distal humerus and decreases the error in determining angular malalignment in the distal humerus. It also allows better evaluation of the olecranon fossa as an indication of injury in the distal humerus. The lateral film should be taken as a true lateral with the humerus held in the anatomic position and

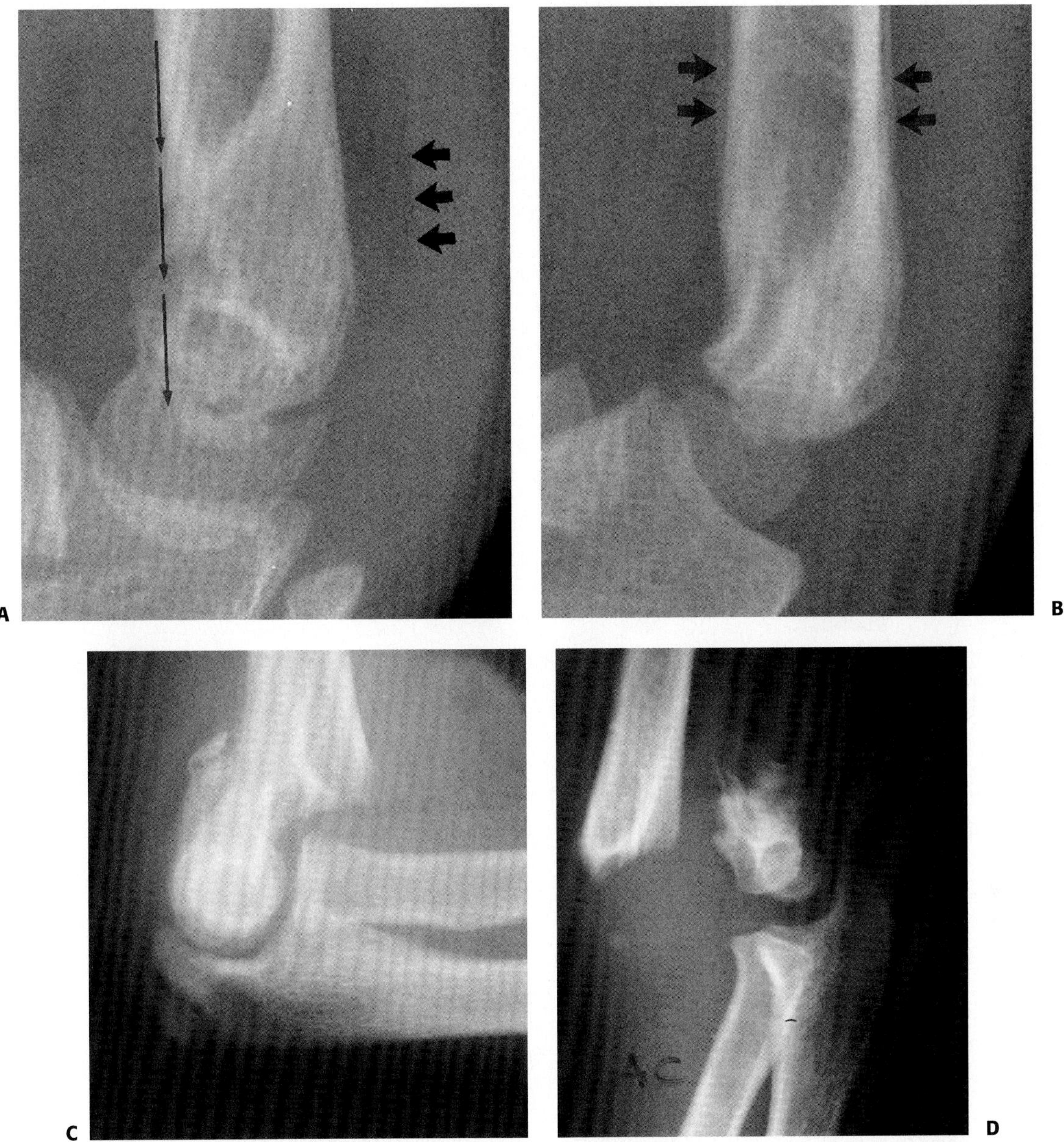

FIGURE 14-8 Types of supracondylar fractures. **A.** Type I fracture, where the anterior humeral line (*long arrows*) crosses through the ossification center of the capitellum. There is also posterior displacement of the olecranon fat pad (*large arrows*). **B.** Three weeks postinjury, there is evidence of new periosteal bone formation from both the anterior and posterior cortices (*arrows*). Because a definite fracture line was not seen in the original x-rays, this new bone formation confirms the original suspicion of a fracture. **C.** Type II. Lateral view of a displaced supracondylar fracture with the posterior cortex intact. There is both rotation and angulation of the distal fragment. **D.** Type III. Totally displaced fracture. There is no contact between the fragments.

not externally rotated (Fig. 14-12). Oblique views of the distal humerus (Fig. 14-13) occasionally may be helpful when a supracondylar fracture or occult condylar fracture is suspected but not seen on standard AP and lateral views, but should not be routinely ordered to evaluate an elbow injury. In the absence of a clear osseous injury, always look for a posterior fat pad sign or an elevated anterior fat pad, as this is an important indicator of an occult intra-articular elbow injury or more frequently a type I supracondylar fracture.

If the AP and lateral views show a displaced type II or III supracondylar fracture but do not show full detail of the distal humeral fragment, we usually obtain further x-ray evaluation in the operating room with the patient anesthetized. Repeat trips for x-ray evaluation in the emergency setting

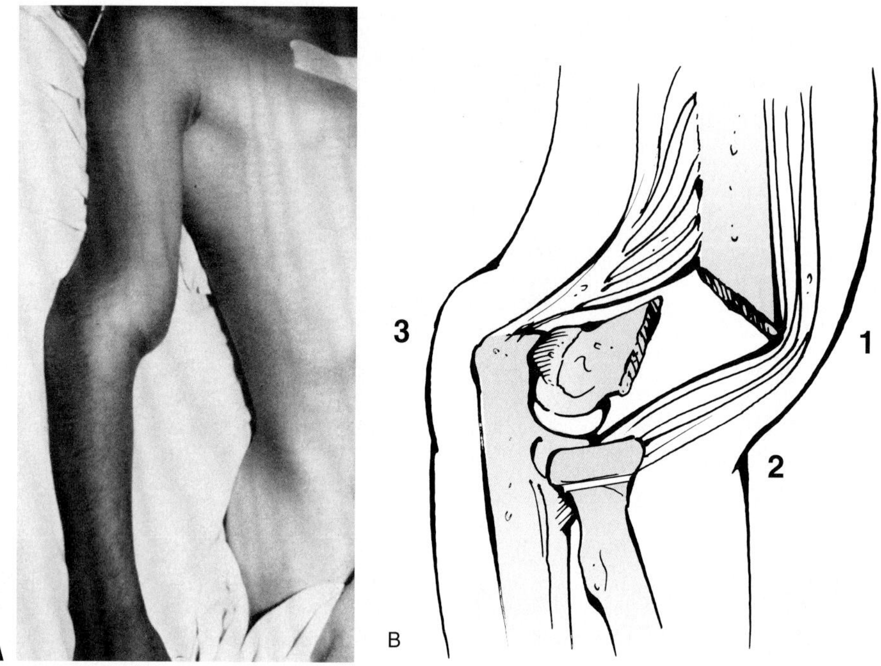

FIGURE 14-9 **A.** Clinical appearance. **B.** The S-shaped configuration is created by the prominence of the proximal fragment's spike (*1*), flexion of the distal fragment (*2*), and the posterior prominence of the olecranon (*3*).

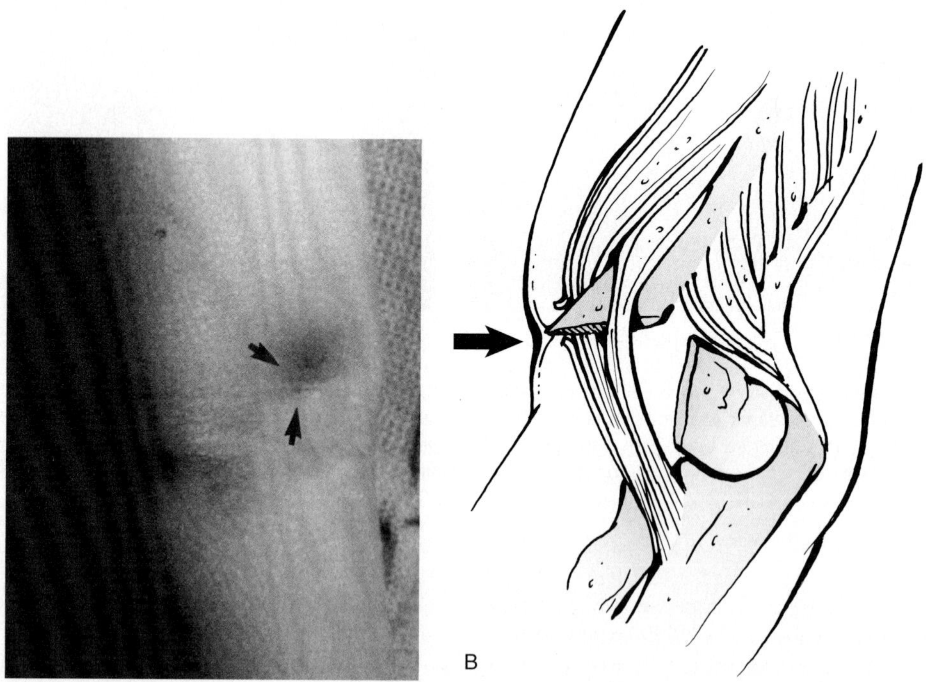

FIGURE 14-10 The pucker sign. This patient had penetration of the proximal fragment's spike into the subcutaneous tissue. In the AP view **(A)**, there is a large puckering or defect in the skin where the distal fragment has pulled the skin inward. Laterally **(B)**, there is puckering of the skin (*arrow*) in the area where the spike has penetrated into the subcutaneous tissue.

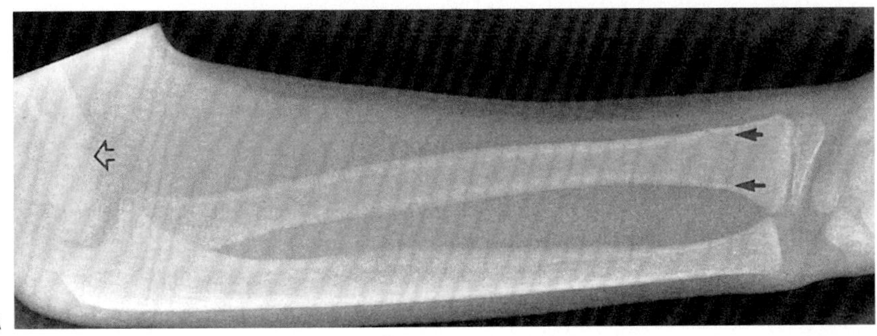

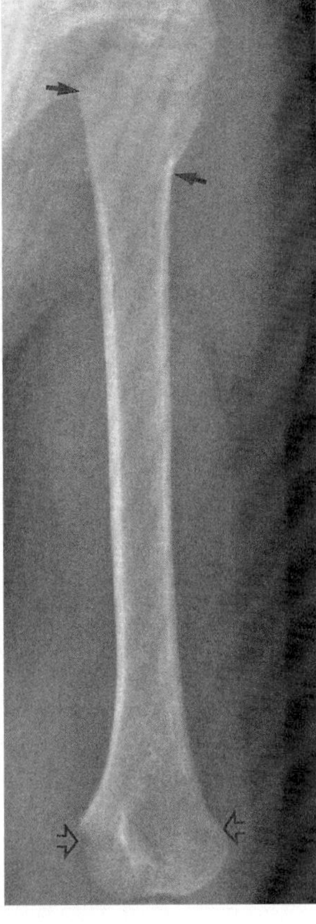

FIGURE 14-11 Occult ipsilateral fractures. **A.** Type II supracondylar fracture (*open arrow*) with an occult distal radial fracture (*solid arrows*). **B.** Type II supracondylar fracture (*open arrows*) with an occult proximal humeral fracture (*solid arrows*).

generally result in increased pain without significant improvement in x-ray quality. Detailed x-rays need to be obtained at some point, however, to define the fracture anatomy with particular emphasis on (a) impaction of the medial column, (b) supracondylar comminution, and (c) vertical split of the epiphyseal fragment. T-condylar fractures (Fig. 14-14) can initially appear to be supracondylar fractures, but these generally occur in children over 10 years of age, in whom supracondylar fractures are less likely.

In a young child, an epiphyseal separation (38) can mimic an elbow dislocation. In an epiphyseal separation, the fracture propagates through the physis without a metaphyseal fragment. This fracture occurs in very young children with primarily chondral epiphyses. On physical examination, the patient appears to have a supracondylar fracture with gross swelling about the elbow and marked discomfort. The key to making the diagnosis and differentiating this injury from an elbow dislocation is seeing that the capitellum remains aligned with the radial head. Sometimes, a supracondylar fracture with a small metaphyseal fragment can mimic a lateral condylar fracture (Fig. 14-15). In such cases, more data are required to initiate treatment. An arthrogram may be helpful to determine the extent of the elbow injury. In selected patients, magnetic resonance imaging or ultrasonography (38) may also aid in evaluating the injury to the unossified epiphysis.

Treatment

General Principles

Initial management of all patients suspected of having an elbow injury is splinting in a comfortable position, generally 20 to 30 degrees of elbow flexion, pending careful physical examination and x-ray evaluation. The initial responder to a child with an elbow injury and polytrauma should assess the neurovascular status and other injuries, including but not limited to head injury and general cardiorespiratory status. Tight bandaging or splinting, excessive flexion or forced extension should be avoided, as they may compromise vascularity.

Type I (Nondisplaced)

The distal humeral injury may not be the primary problem: neurologic compromise has been reported with nondisplaced supracondylar fractures (39). X-rays of the entire extremity should be reviewed to be sure that there is no injury in other parts of the humerus or in the forearm bones. On x-ray, a type I supracondylar fracture generally has a visible fracture line traversing the medial and lateral columns at the level of the olecranon fossa without displacement. The anterior humeral line transects the capitellum. In general, in a type I fracture, the periosteum is intact with significant inherent stability of the fracture. A type I fracture may only become apparent with repeat x-rays at 1- to 2-week follow-up after presentation with elbow

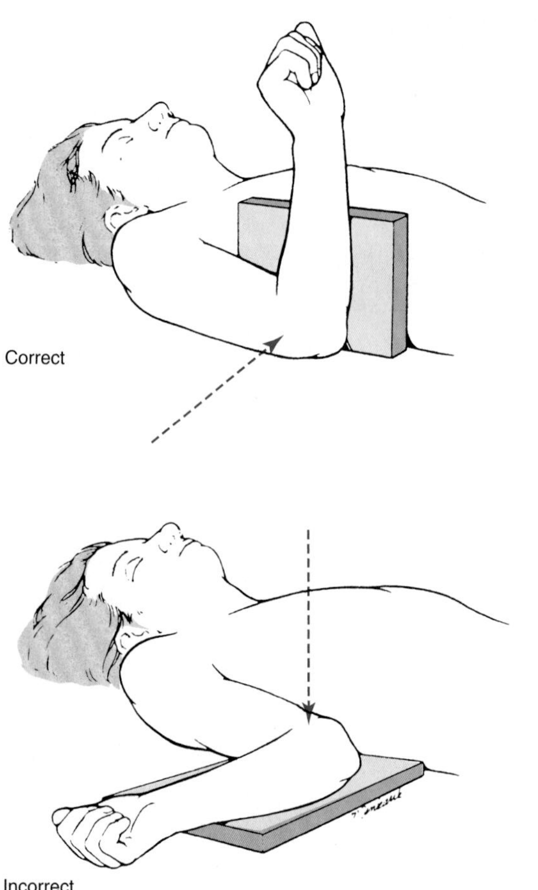

FIGURE 14-12 X-ray positioning. The correct method of taking a lateral view is with the upper extremity directed anteriorly rather than externally rotated.

pain posttrauma and initial x-ray findings limited to a posterior fat pad sign. Periosteal reaction in the distal humerus may be all that is visible on x-ray.

Simple immobilization with a posterior splint applied at 60 to 90 degrees of elbow flexion with side supports or a simple collar and cuff is all that is necessary (22,40). This arrangement allows swelling to occur and does not put the brachial artery at risk of compression. Using Doppler examination of the brachial artery after supracondylar fractures, Mapes and Hennrikus (41) found that flow was decreased in the brachial artery in positions of pronation and increased flexion. A simple splint with the forearm in neutral position and the elbow flexed no more than 90 degrees should be used initially. Before the splint is applied, it should be confirmed that the pulse is intact and that there is good capillary refill. A circumferential cast may be applied if additional fractures require treatment, but careful observation is necessary to avoid any risk of compartment syndrome.

X-rays are obtained 3 to 7 days after fracture to document lack of displacement, and a long arm cast can be applied with a ring over the distal portion of the cast and a sling around the neck to support the weight of the cast (Fig. 14-16). Without support, the cast's weight applies an extension torque about the distal humerus, and can lead to fracture displacement (although this is rare). If there is any evidence of distal fragment extension, as judged by lack of intersection of the anterior humeral line with the capitellum, the fracture should be reduced and placed in a cast or treated with percutaneous pinning to secure the reduction. The most common cause of cubitus varus deformity is inadequate treatment of types I and II fractures, rather than the deformity complicating type III fractures.

An acceptable position is determined by the anterior humeral line transecting the capitellum on the lateral x-ray, a Baumann angle of 70 to 78 degrees or equal to the other side, and an

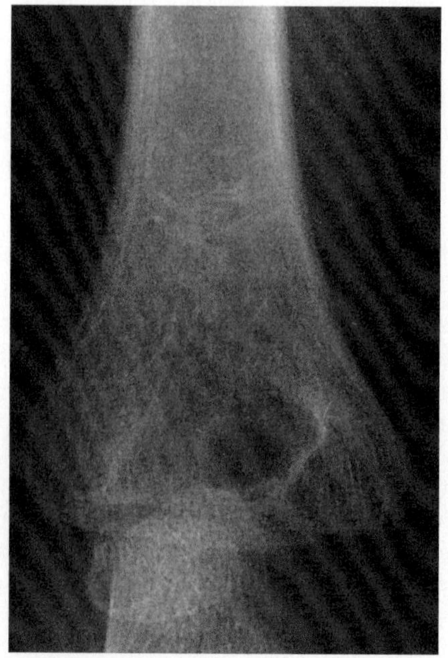

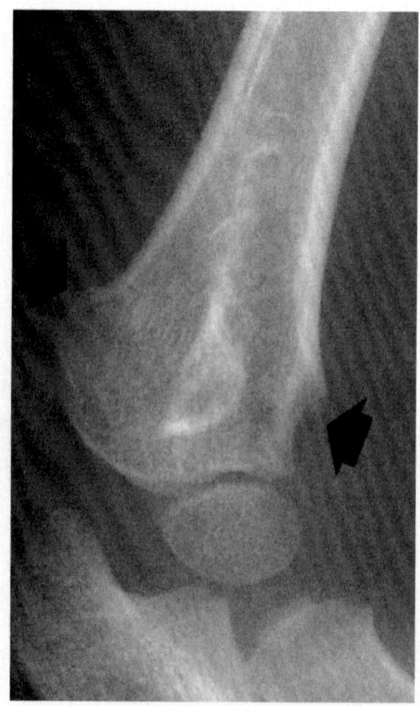

FIGURE 14-13 Oblique views. Often, the fracture line is not visualized on any of the lateral or anteroposterior views **(A)**. An oblique view **(B)** of the distal humerus may demonstrate the extent of the fracture line (*arrows*).

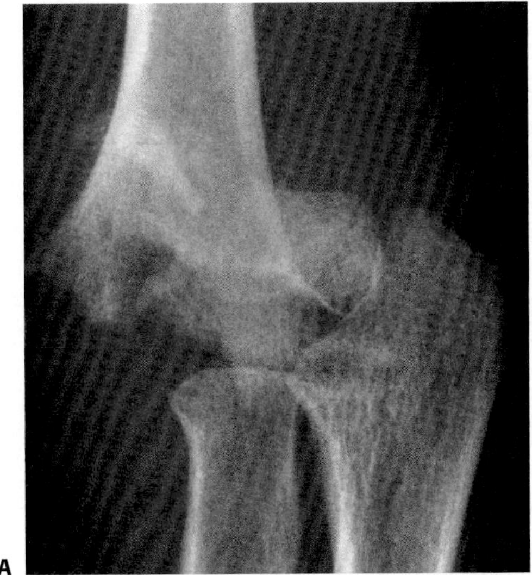

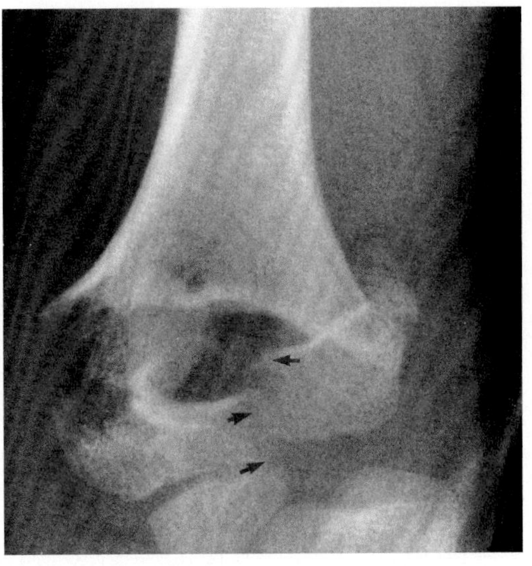

FIGURE 14-14 Occult T-condylar. **A.** Original x-rays appear to show a type III posteromedial supracondylar fracture. **B.** After manipulation, the vertical intercondylar fracture line (*arrows*) was visualized.

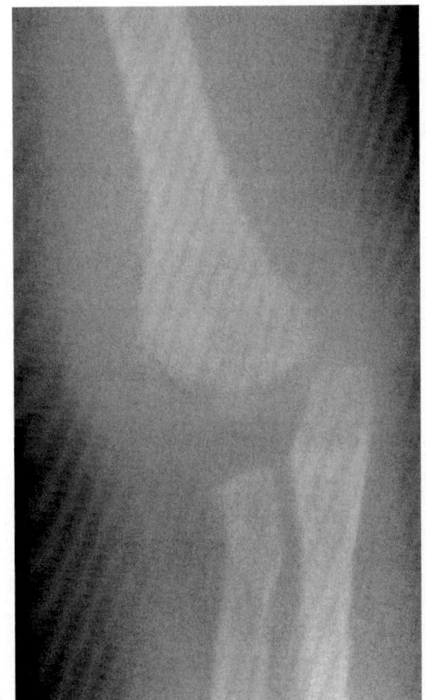

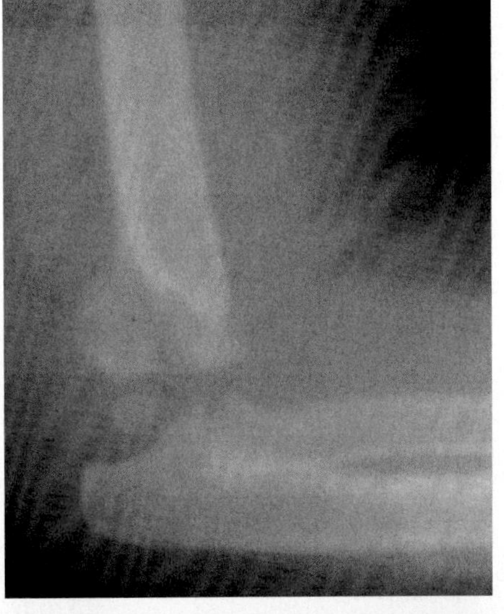

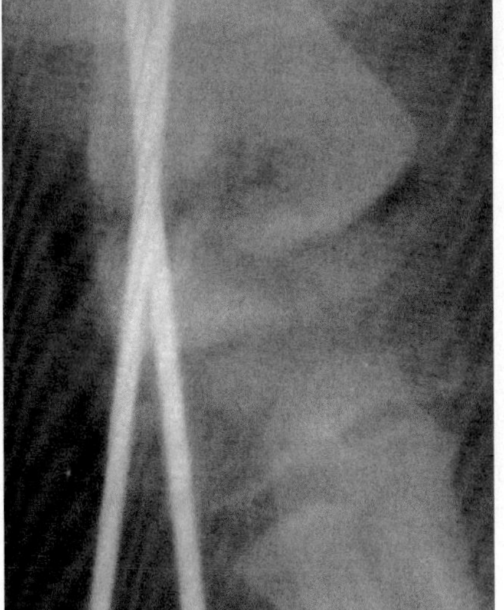

FIGURE 14-15 This 1.2-year-old girl sustained a fracture that on the anteroposterior view **(A)** appears like an elbow dislocation and on the lateral view **(B)** has the appearance of a lateral condyle fracture. **C.** Arthrography showed the outline of the entire cartilaginous epiphysis. This is an epiphyseal separation with a metaphyseal fragment (Salter II).

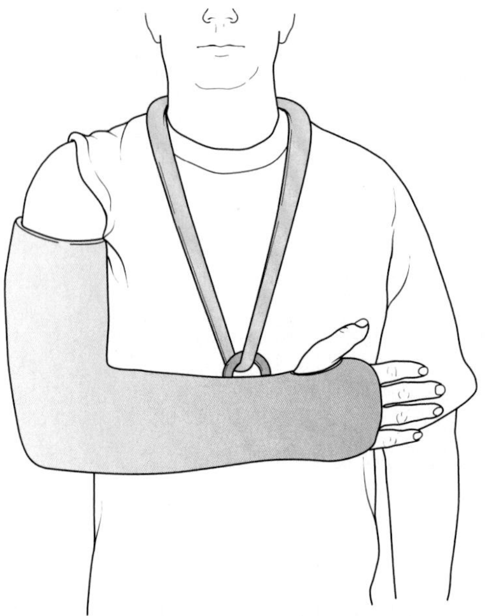

FIGURE 14-16 Because the cast's weight can produce an extension movement about the distal humerus, a ring and padded strap around the neck are necessary to support the weight of the cast.

intact olecranon fossa. Medial column collapse can lead to varus deformity in an otherwise minimally displaced and normally healing distal humeral fracture. The duration of immobilization for supracondylar fractures is 3 to 4 weeks, whether type I, II, or III. In general, no physical therapy is required after this injury. Patients may be seen 4 weeks after immobilization is removed to ensure that range of motion and strength are returning normally. As the outcome in type I fractures is predictably excellent if alignment is maintained at the time of early healing, cast removal follow-up visits are optional depending on family and medical circumstances.

Remember that the initial x-ray is a static representation of the actual injury that may involve soft tissue disruption much greater than one might expect from the minimal bony abnormality. Excessive swelling, nerve or vascular disruption, or excessive pain are indicative of this mismatch. Periosteal disruption may render this fracture inherently unstable. Type I supracondylar fractures require follow-up and careful treatment.

Type II Fracture (Displaced With an Intact Cortical Contact)

This fracture category encompasses a broad array of distal humeral hyperextension injuries, depending on the degree of rotation. Even greater than the variation in fracture stability is the spectrum of soft tissue injuries with type II supracondylar fractures. Careful assessment of the soft tissue injury is critical in treatment decision making. Radiologic definition of this injury demonstrates an incomplete osseous separation with some posterior cortical contact. Therefore, good stability should be obtained with closed reduction. Medial column collapse (Fig. 14-17) must be identified because a varus deformity may result from a simple closed reduction without stabilization when these are present. In such cases, recognizing the medial collapse, a selection for skeletal stabilization with pinning will avoid malunion (42).

Significant swelling, obliteration of pulse with flexion, neu-

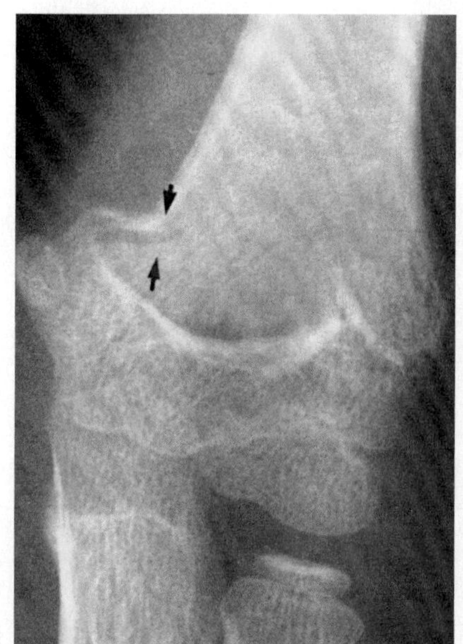

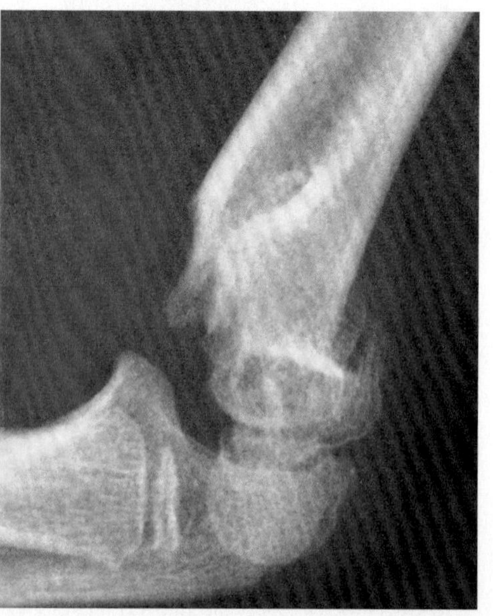

FIGURE 14-17 Greenstick medial collapse. **A.** An anteroposterior view of a type II fracture shows greater collapse of the weaker medial column (*arrows*). **B.** The lateral view shows that the posterior cortex is still partially intact. (From Wilkins KE. The management of severely displaced supracondylar fractures of the humerus. *Techniques Orthop* 1989;4:12–24, with permission.)

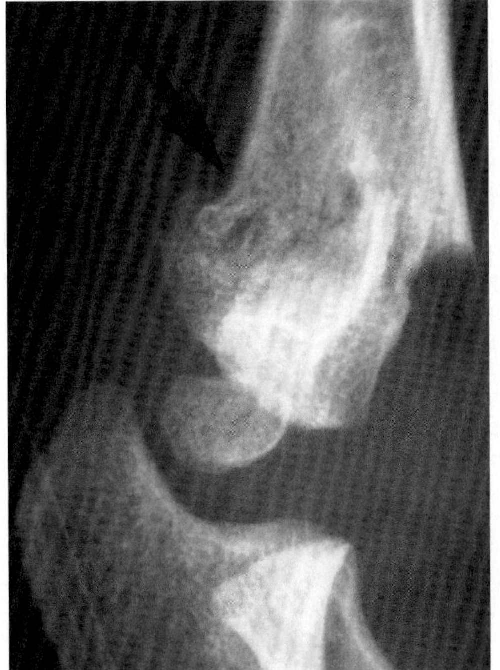

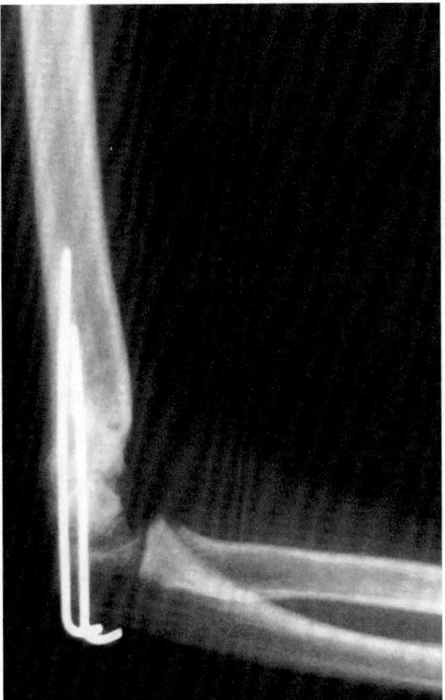

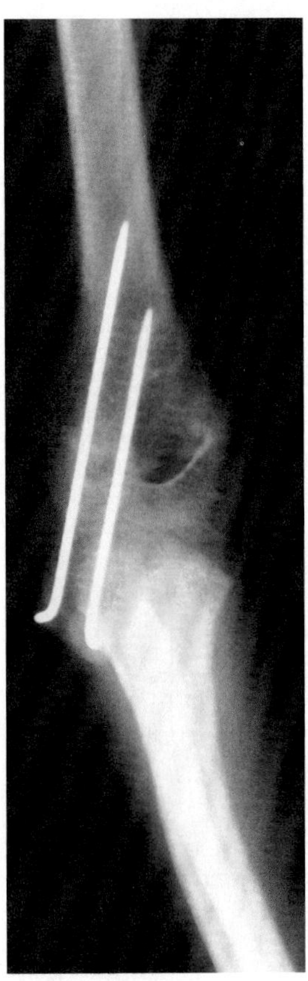

FIGURE 14-18 This type II supracondylar fracture **(A)** is stable after closed reduction and is ideal for pinning with two lateral pins **(B,C)**. The pins should be placed slightly divergent and should engage the opposite cortex for maximum stability.

rovascular injuries, excessive angulation, and other injuries in the same extremity are indications for pin stabilization of most type II fractures. If pinning is chosen, two lateral pins (6,43) through the distal humeral fragment, engaging the opposite cortex of the proximal fragment, are generally sufficient to maintain fracture alignment (Fig. 14-18). The posterior cortex and the intact periosteum provide some degree of inherent stability. Cross pinning of this fracture is generally not needed. The techniques for crossed and lateral pinning are described later on in this chapter. If pin stabilization is used, the pins are left protruding through the skin and are removed at 3 to 4 weeks after fixation, generally without the need for sedation or anesthesia.

Recently, researchers have proposed "selective pinning" for type II fractures. They proposed reduction, splinting in flexion, and a nonmovable collar and cuff with careful early follow-up. Fractures that displace or angulate may require pin stabilization at 5 to 7 days. Any type II fracture with unacceptable initial alignment or for which there is concern about displacement or noncompliant follow-up should be reduced and pinned. All attempts should be made to prevent angular deformity because the remodeling potential of the distal humerus is very limited.

Type III Extension Supracondylar Fracture

In this fracture, the periosteum is torn, there is no cortical contact between the fragments, and soft tissue injury may accompany the fracture. Careful preoperative evaluation is mandatory. If circulatory compromise is indicated by absent pulse and a pale hand, or if compartment syndrome is suspected, emergent reduction and skeletal stabilization are mandatory. Alternative methods of management, including traction and closed reduction with collar and cuff (Fig. 14-19) or casting, can be used in the absence of acute vascular insufficiency in rare circumstances. There are two viable alternatives for achieving fracture alignment: acute manipulative reduction and traction.

Technique of Reduction

For closed reduction, traction is applied first, followed by correction of rotational deformity. The extension deformity is corrected with pressure by the surgeon's thumb over the olecranon and posterior humeral condyles. The distal humeral fragment's alignment is verified in AP and lateral views. With the elbow held in hyperflexion, Jones' views, rotating the arm slightly to expose the medial and lateral column of the distal humerus, are valuable to document reduction.

Whether a fracture is held in place with pins or a cast, realigning the humerus is necessary, and the technique of manipulative reduction is the same (Fig. 14-20). The patient is anesthetized, and the affected arm is extended over the screen of the C-arm fluoroscopic unit. Longitudinal traction is applied first to dislodge the proximal fragment, which may be entrapped in

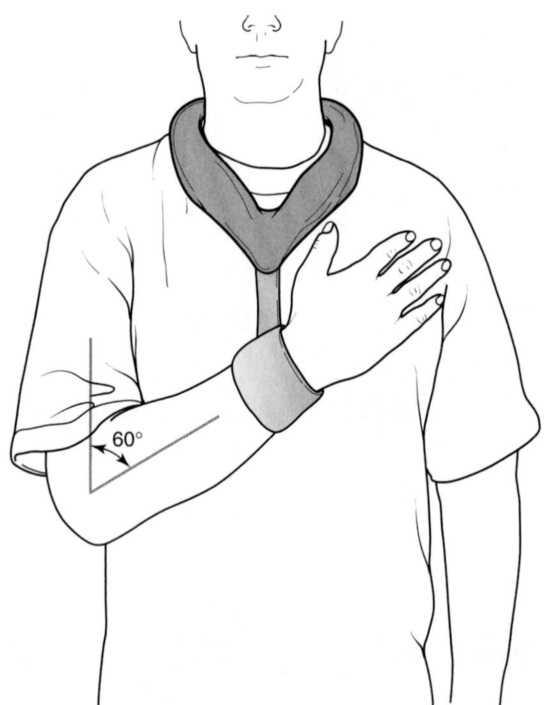

FIGURE 14-19 A collar and cuff is a safe treatment option that can be used to maintain reduction in hyperflexion.

the brachialis muscle, the antecubital fascia, or the superficial fat and skin. If traction does not restore length and alignment, a "milking maneuver" has been described by Archibeck (44) and Peters (45) to disengage the proximal fragment from the soft tissue. This maneuver is carried out by manipulating the soft tissue over the fracture to pull the soft tissue away from the proximal fragment rather than simply applying traction on the bones, which may not allow reduction of a buttonholed proximal fragment. Once length is restored, medial or lateral translation is corrected. The image intensifier is helpful for this because the medial and lateral columns should be realigned on the AP image. Rotation is corrected simultaneously, but in general, malrotation resolves as traction is applied and as the medial and lateral alignment is corrected, due to the effect of the surrounding soft tissue. A flexion reduction maneuver is then performed with pressure of the thumb over the olecranon and to a variable degree, over the distal condyles of the humerus. Generally, the fracture reduction can be felt, and the elbow is then held in hyperflexion and pronation to achieve a stable reduction. The pulse is usually obliterated in this position, and the hand is pale. Circulation will be restored once the fracture is stabilized, and the elbow will be extended in nearly all cases.

AP and lateral views are obtained using the image intensifier. With the elbow flexed, a pure AP view is difficult to interpret, so the actual AP view is taken by rotating the arm slightly medially and laterally to view the columns of the distal humerus and the reduction of the fracture (Fig. 14-21). The arm is then externally rotated to obtain a lateral view of the distal humerus. The surgeon rotates the entire arm by placing one hand on the proximal humerus while the other holds the wrist pronated with the elbow hyperflexed. This is generally a stable position that will allow rotation of a reduced supracondylar fracture. The lateral image is then evaluated for restoration of the distal humerus' cortical contour, fracture gap reduction, and presence of the anterior humeral line intersecting the capitellum.

Rotating the arm with the fracture reduced and held in a stable position is possible in nearly all posteromedially displaced supracondylar fractures (Fig. 14-22). In posterolaterally displaced supracondylar fractures, however, the reduction is frequently unstable in hyperflexion and may be less stable in pronation. If the fracture reduction is unstable, the C-arm should be rotated to obtain AP and lateral views rather than attempting to rotate the arm and losing a tenuous reduction. An anatomic or nearly anatomic reduction is a prerequisite for skeletal stabilization.

If this type of stabilization cannot be achieved by closed reduction or traction, open reduction can be used. Failure to achieve accurate alignment with closed means is an indication for open reduction.

In patients in whom a closed reduction cannot be obtained, there is risk that entrapment of neurovascular structures prevents realignment and open reduction is indicated. In a study by Letts (46) in which closed reduction could not be obtained in 41 patients, 15 were found to have either the median nerve and brachial artery or the radial nerve entrapped in the fracture site. Preoperative neurovascular deficit was not predictive of this.

Cast Immobilization Technique

Because type III fractures are intrinsically unstable, the elbow must be held in extreme flexion to prevent the distal fragment from rotating; these fractures tend to rotate with flexion of less than 120 degrees (47). Usually, however, severe swelling prevents the elbow from being kept in hyperflexion. When the swelling subsides, the distal fragment tends to rotate horizontally, making it susceptible to varus angulation, particularly if the fracture line is angulated (Fig. 14-23). In most series (3,48–50), the results of type III fractures treated with closed reduction and cast immobilization are not as good as those treated with pinning. Hadlow et al (51), however, suggested that selective use of casting is beneficial, reporting that in their series, 61% of type III and 77% of type II fractures were successfully treated without pinning.

A figure-of-eight cast (Fig. 14-24) is used to maintain flexion of at least 120 degrees. If the arm can be flexed to 120 degrees with an intact pulse, casting can be used as primary treatment. Alburger et al (52) reported that using skin traction initially until swelling decreases allowed successful use of casting without pinning. Although a number of historic series used casting as primary treatment, most recent reports favor pinning of this fracture due to concerns about vascular compromise, compartment syndrome, and malunion. When a cast is used as primary treatment, it should be worn for 3 to 4 weeks. After cast removal, motion is encouraged, and the patient is placed in a sling until comfortable, which may vary from hours to days. Physical ther-

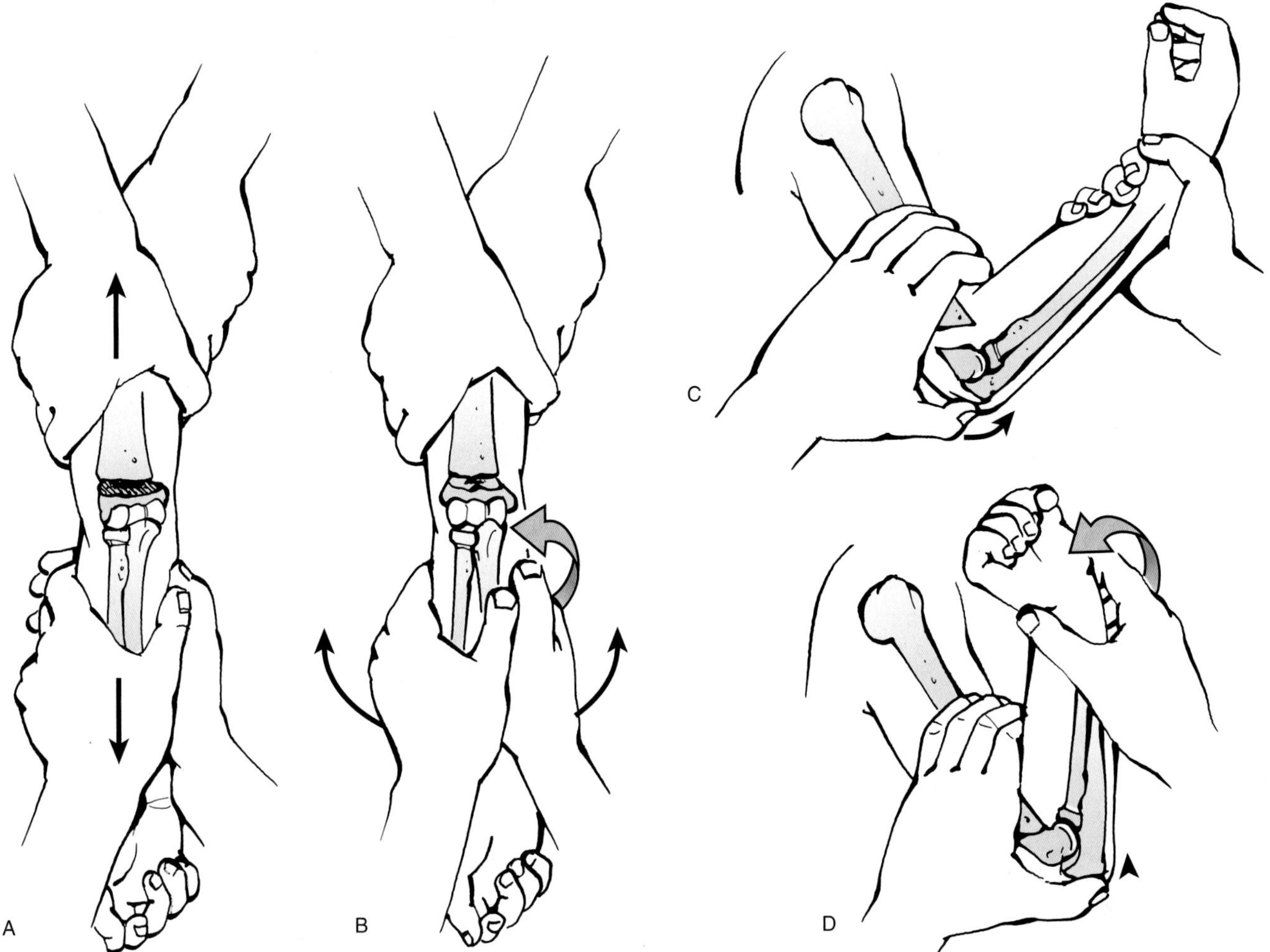

FIGURE 14-20 Manipulative closed reduction. **A.** Traction is applied with the elbow in extension and the forearm in supination. The assistant stabilizes the proximal fragment. After traction has been applied and the length regained, the fracture is hyperextended to obtain apposition of the fragments. **B.** While traction is maintained, the varus or valgus angulation along with the rotation of the distal fragment is corrected. **C.** Once the length and alignment have been corrected, the elbow is flexed. Pressure is applied over the posterior aspect of the olecranon to facilitate reduction of the distal fragment. **D.** The distal fragment is finally secured to the proximal fragment by pronating the forearm.

apy usually is not required, because simple active motion is encouraged and typically is sufficient.

Technique of Pin Fixation

Pin fixation of humeral supracondylar fractures has been performed for more than 50 years (53–55). Before the development of the fluoroscopic unit, blind pinning (27) was performed; Jones noted that even the "average surgeon" could do this without complications. Modern imaging techniques and improved power equipment have made percutaneous pinning the standard treatment for this difficult fracture. Flynn (56,57) and later Wilkins (35,58), among others (2,5,49,59,60) popularized modern pinning techniques and documented their value. Present controversy includes (a) crossed pins (Fig. 14-25) or two or more lateral pins; (b) burying pins or leaving them out through the skin; (c) timing of pinning, that is, emergent, urgent, or elective; and (d) the role of open reduction. Absorbable polyglycolide pins have not been found suitable for fixation of supracondylar fractures (61).

Zionts (62) evaluated the torsional strength of pin configurations in an adult humeral cadaver model. The maximal strength was gained by using two crossed pins with one placed through the medial condyle and one through the lateral condyle, extending up the corresponding columns and engaging the opposite cortex. The torque required to produce 10 degrees of rotation averaged 37% less with two lateral pins parallel and 80% less with two lateral pins crossed than with medial and lateral crossed pins. Thus, lateral pinning required significantly less

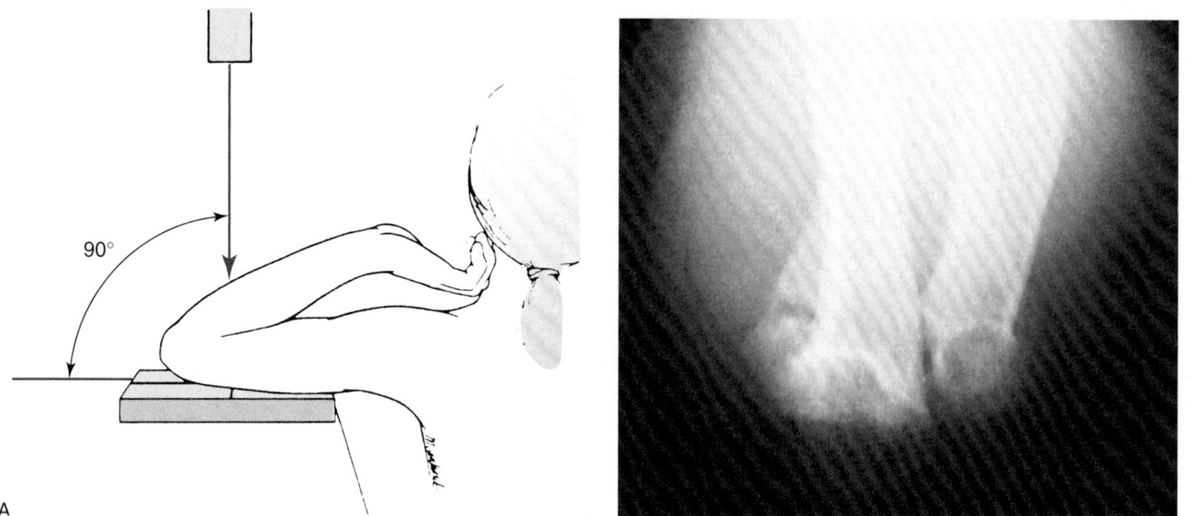

FIGURE 14-21 Jones view. **A.** The proper elbow position and tube direction for the Jones view. **B.** X-ray of an elbow taken with the tube 90 degrees to the film. Rotating the arm slightly medially and laterally will expose the humeral columns more clearly.

force to produce 10 degrees of displacement than did crossed pinning (Fig. 14-26). The question, however, is whether the resistance to torque provided by lateral pinning is sufficient to allow fracture healing without displacement, if supplemented by cast immobilization in the clinical setting. In addition, the experimental models have no intact periosteum, which will provide further fracture stability, nor do they have pediatric cancellous bone, which may be quite different in terms of pin fixation mechanics. In a biomechanical analysis of lateral pinning versus crossed pinning, Newton et al (63) found that divergence of two lateral pins was superior to parallel configuration. They found crossed pins provided significantly more strength in axial rotation. Newton recommended divergent placement of two lateral pins and a determination of rotational stability before medial pin placement.

Onwuanyi (64), in a clinical series, also concluded that there was greater stability or ability to maintain reduction with the crossed pinning technique. Cheng (43) reported 180 type III

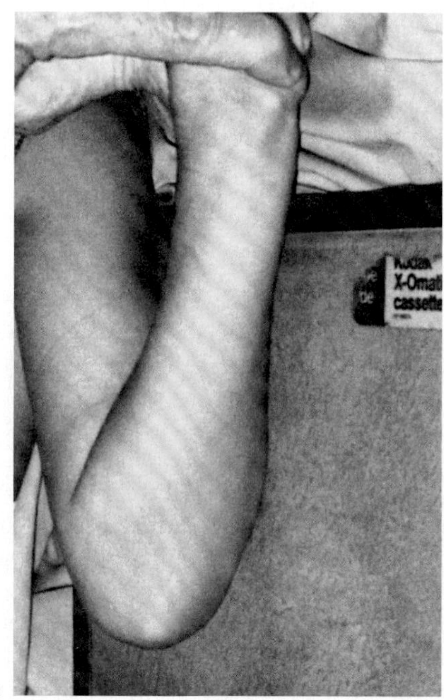

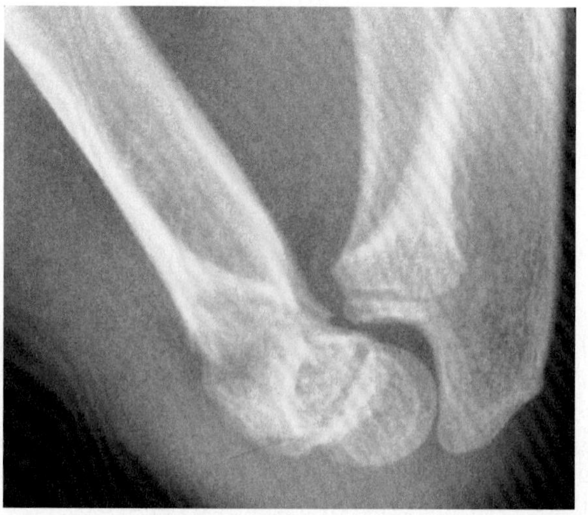

FIGURE 14-22 Stability in external rotation. **A.** Hyperflexion of the elbow will allow external rotation of the arm to a position where a lateral view **(B)** of the distal humerus can be taken without moving the fluoroscopy unit or x-ray.

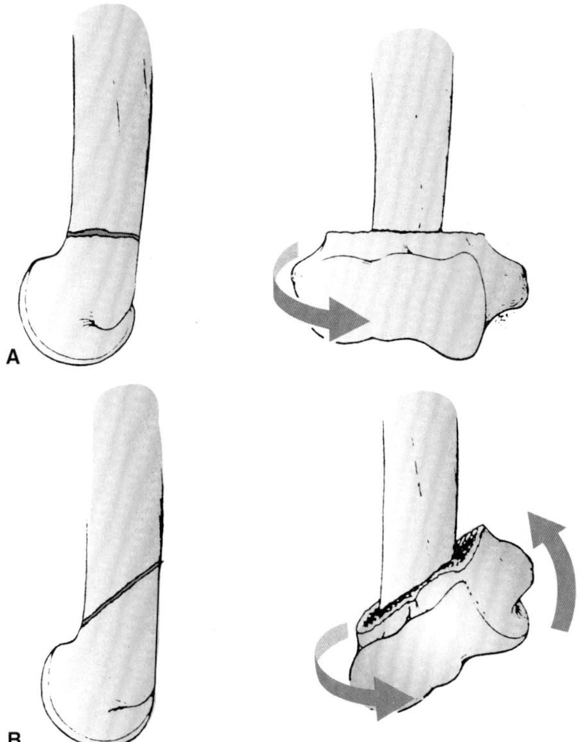

FIGURE 14-23 Effects of obliquity of the fracture line. If the fracture line is transverse **(A)**, pure rotation does not produce angulation. If the fracture line is oblique **(B)**, rotation of the distal fragment produces a secondary distal angulation.

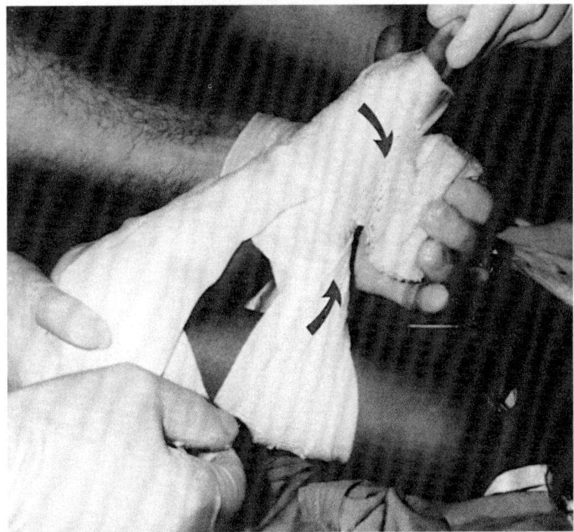

FIGURE 14-24 Figure-of-eight wrap. In the figure-of-eight cast, both the padding and the plaster are wrapped in a figure-of-eight manner (*arrows*). (From Wilkins KE. The management of severely displaced supracondylar fractures of the humerus. *Techniques Orthop* 1989;4:5–24, with permission.)

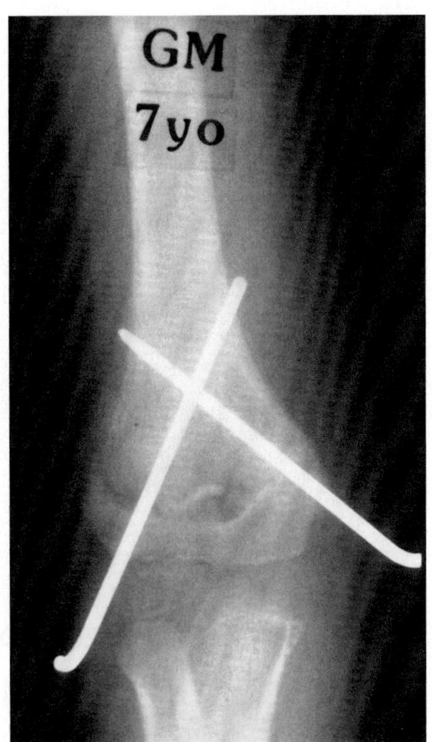

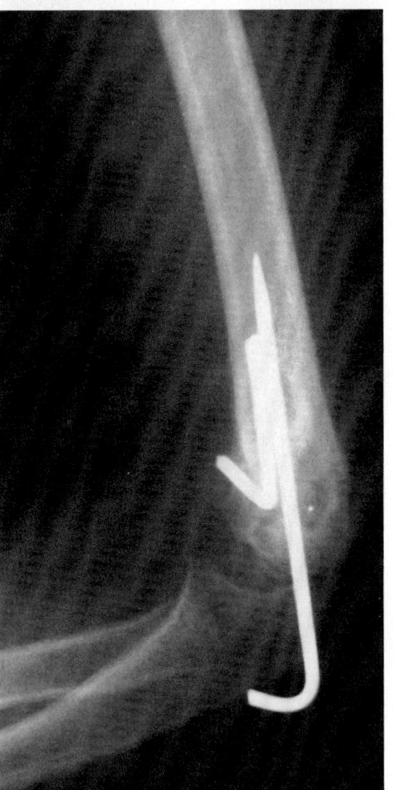

FIGURE 14-25 Crossed pinning is a more stable configuration than two lateral pins. The lateral pin is placed at the border of the ossified lateral condyle. The medial pin enters the medial epicondyle and is generally more transverse than the lateral pin.

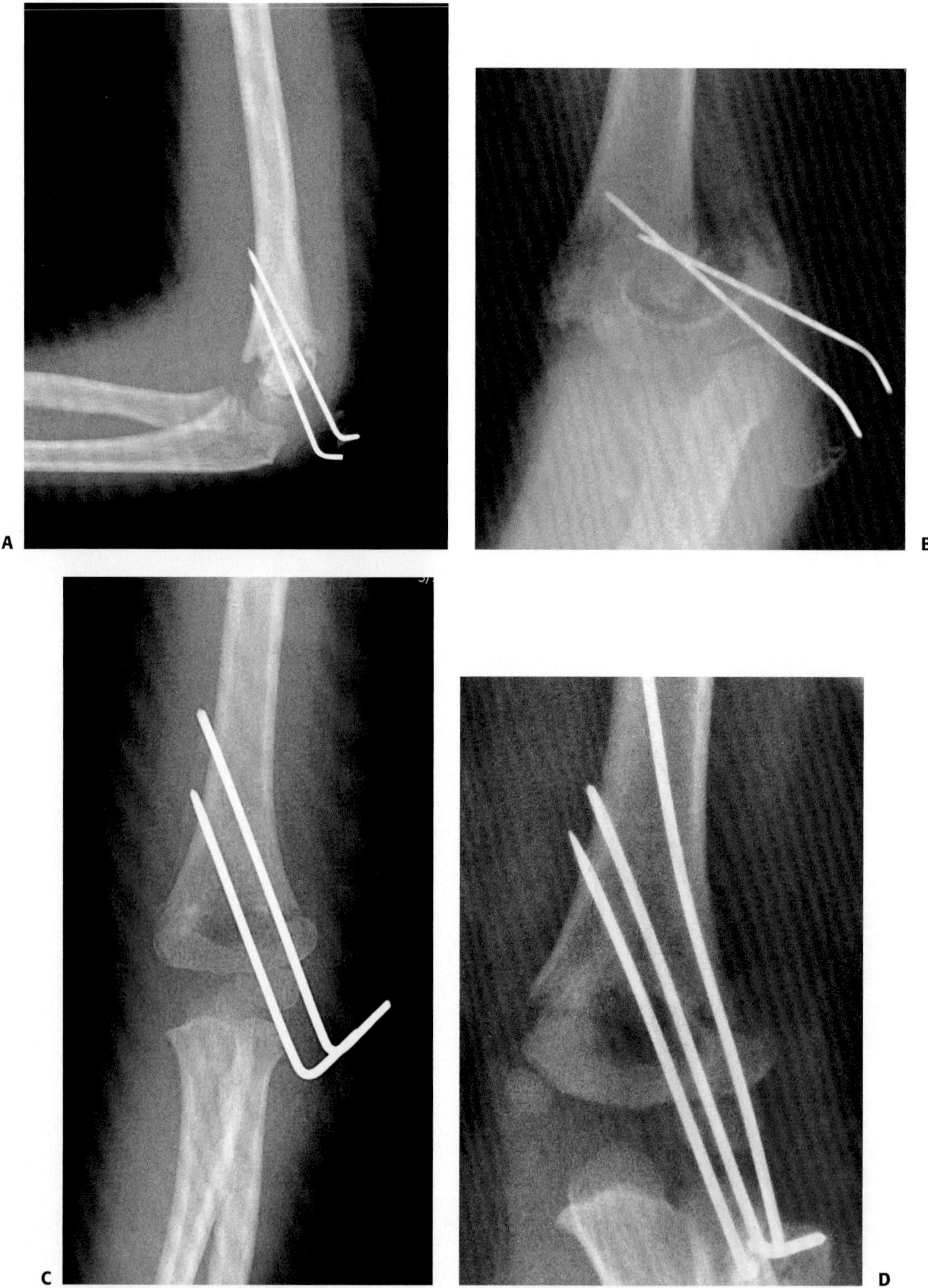

FIGURE 14-26 Lateral pin constructs. **A.** Two lateral pins optimally placed, widely spaced, and divergent will secure both columns. Crossing the olecranon fossa is allowable. **B.** Small convergent wires may be unstable and should not be used. **C.** Rotational instability is commonly seen if fixation is not stable. **D.** A third lateral or medial wire may be added if instability is detected at surgery.

supracondylar fractures treated with lateral pinning as primary treatment in nearly all. He reported very low incidences of cubitus varus deformity and loss of reduction and concluded that in actual practice, there was no difference between two lateral pins and crossed pins. He recommended lateral pins as the treatment of choice because there is less risk of ulnar nerve injury with this technique.

Skaggs (65) reviewed 345 supracondylar fractures treated by pinning of which 204 were type III. Of these, 153 fractures were treated by crossed pins and 51 were treated with two lateral pins. In the 141 type II fractures, 74 were treated with lateral pins, and 67 were managed by crossed pins. The medial pin was associated with a 4% risk of ulnar nerve injury when the medial pin was placed without hyperflexion and 15% if the medial pin was placed with hyperflexion. Solak, however, found no difference in complication rates with two lateral pins versus crossed pins (66).

The primary risk with crossed pinning is injury to the ulnar nerve by a medial pin. The frequency of ulnar nerve injury in reported series ranges from 0% to 15% (35,67–70). Because the ulnar nerve may sublux anteriorly when the elbow is hyperflexed in as many as 30% of patients (15), it is at significant risk in the crossed pinning technique. Locating the ulnar nerve with a nerve stimulator has been suggested (71). Making a small 1.5-cm incision over the medial epicondyle for placement of the medial pin has also been proposed as a way to locate and protect the ulnar nerve. This technique works well and may avert the problem of iatrogenic ulnar nerve injury when crossed pinning is required for very unstable fractures. Also, placing the lateral side pin first with the elbow hyperflexed and then placing the medial pin with the elbow in only 90 degrees of flexion lessens this risk. Some individuals believe that they can palpate the ulnar nerve at the time of pinning and avoid it. Schwend (72) demonstrated that the location of the ulnar nerve cannot be adequately determined by palpation to allow blind medial pinning.

Crossed Pins Technique

Steel pins 0.062 mm or 0.075 mm (5/64 inches) in diameter are used in the crossed pins technique (Fig. 14-27). After reduction of the fracture and with the C-arm screen used as an operating table, the arm is held with the elbow hyperflexed and the forearm pronated to maintain the reduction. Anatomic reduction is confirmed with the image intensifier before pinning. The lateral pin is always inserted first. The insertion site is made so that the pin will traverse the lateral portion of the ossified capitellum, cross the physis, proceed up the lateral column, and always engage the opposite medial cortex proximally. Using a Kirschner wire (K-wire) or a radiodense object, the position for inserting the pin is documented on AP and lateral views. A small incision is made in the skin. The pin is placed using a power drill and a sharp K-wire. Provisional stability is achieved with the first pin. Then, the elbow is gently extended to about 45 degrees of flexion to allow a perfect AP x-ray of the distal humerus to ensure anatomic alignment. The elbow is then flexed to 120 degrees and externally rotated and a lateral image is obtained with fluoroscopy. A second pin is then placed medially. A small 1.5-cm incision is made over the medial epicondyle, and dissection is performed down to the level of the medial epicondyle. If the ulnar nerve has subluxed over the medial epicondyle, sometimes blunt dissection stimulates the nerve and the fingers will move slightly. If the ulnar nerve is found, it should be retracted posteriorly and a pin should be placed through the medial epicondyle under direct vision. The position of the K-wire from the medial side is confirmed with fluoroscopy. The pin should enter the medial epicondyle and not the

A 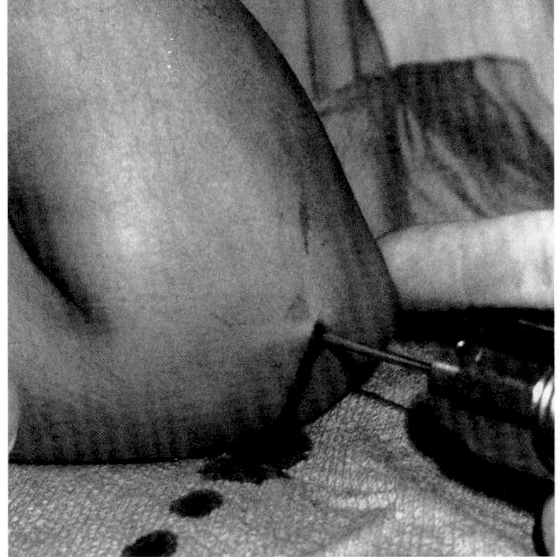

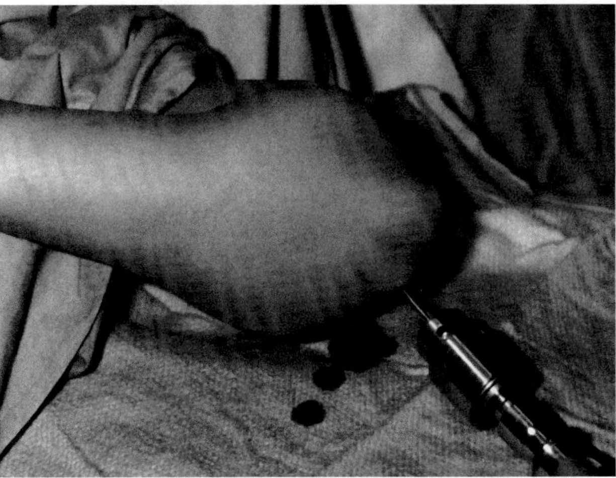 B

FIGURE 14-27 Lateral pin placement. **A.** The lateral pin is placed first using the C-arm screen as an operating room table. The elbow is held in hyperflexion in order to place the lateral pin. **B.** The lateral view is obtained by externally rotating the arm, holding the elbow in hyperflexion for stability.

ulnar groove. The medial pin is generally more horizontal than the lateral pin and should traverse the medial column and engage the opposite lateral cortex.

Variations in the crossed pinning technique include (a) no medial incision (Fig. 14-28), (b) maintenance of reduction by strapping the arm in a position of hyperflexion before pinning, (c) using a bar as a fulcrum to facilitate reduction, as described by Flynn (56), and (d) pinning the medial side first with the elbow in hyperflexion. If no medial incision is used, the ulnar nerve is palpated and pushed posteriorly as the pin is inserted. Pinning medially with the elbow in hyperflexion has the benefit of holding the fracture in a stable position while pinning, but places the ulnar nerve at higher risk, and should therefore be avoided.

Lateral Pin Technique

Two or three lateral pins (0.062 mm or 0.75 mm) (43,64,73,74) provide less stability than crossed pins, but there is no risk to the ulnar nerve, which is a significant benefit of this technique. Skaggs et al (74) evaluated lateral pin fixation in a consecutive

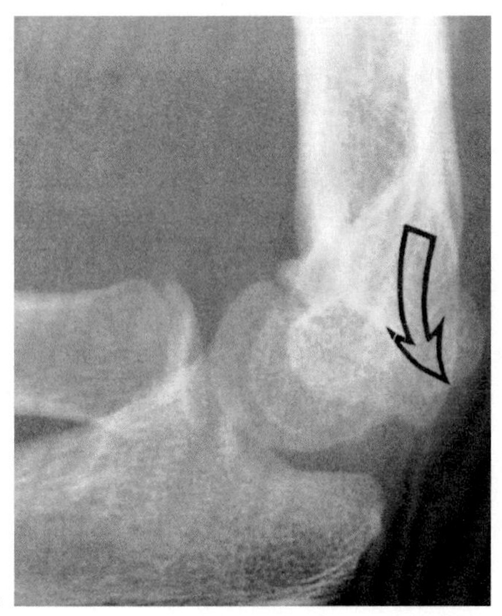

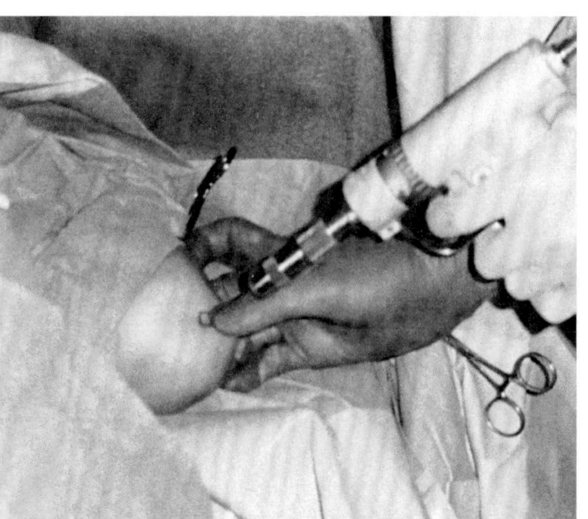

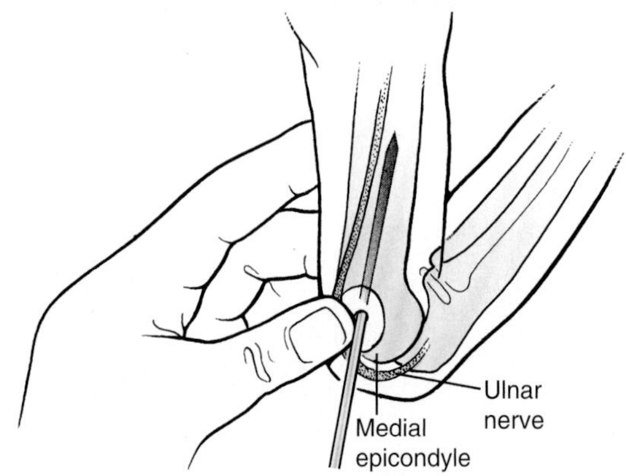

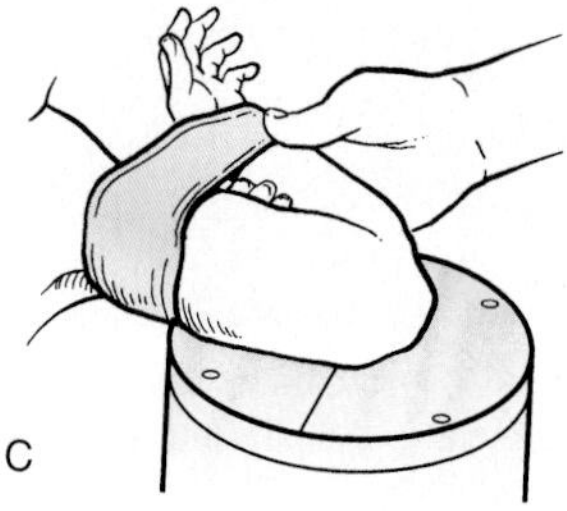

FIGURE 14-28 Medial pin placement. **A.** The medial epicondyle is posteromedial (*arrow*). **B.** The medial pin is placed directly through the medial epicondyle, using the opposite thumb to pull posterior the soft tissues, thus protecting the ulnar nerve. **C.** The relationship of vital structures during medial pin placement. The pin is directed from posteromedial to anterolateral directly through the medial epicondyle's center under control of the image intensifier, with the upper extremity fully externally rotated.

series of 124 fractures with 69 type II and 55 type III injuries. They found no malunions and no iatrogenic nerve injuries in their series. One patient had a pin track infection. They concluded that lateral pinning could be done with safety and security if the following steps were taken: (a) maximize pin separation at the fracture site; (b) engage the medial and lateral columns; (c) be sure that the pins engage sufficient bone in both the proximal and distal fragments; and (d) have a low threshold for placing a third lateral pin to increase stability.

Technique of Lateral Pin Fixation

The operating room set up for two lateral pins is exactly the same as that for crossed pins. After achieving closed reduction and confirming the position on AP and lateral views, the first pin site should be chosen with the second pin in mind. The goal is to have two pins that are divergent on the AP and lateral views. If the pins are placed so that they cross well proximal to the fracture, this positioning may be satisfactory, but is not as secure as parallel pins and is much less stable than a divergent alignment. Two pins crossing at the fracture is unsatisfactory because torque will not be satisfactorily resisted, and a rotational deformity may result.

In choosing a site for the first pin, we generally place it through the center of the ossified capitellum, cross the olecranon fossa, giving it greater stability, and then further penetrate the medial cortex. A second pin is placed through the distal humeral epiphysis lateral to the capitellum but clearly within the epiphysis. The pin proceeds up the lateral column and engages the opposite cortex. If the first pin is placed centrally in the lateral column, the second pin will nearly always cross the first just above the fracture, which will be a less satisfactory lateral pinning. Maximal pin separation increases the stability with this technique.

Gentle stress can be used to test the stability of two lateral pins. If the arm can be grasped by the proximal humerus and stressed mildly without displacing the fracture, the fixation is satisfactory. If displacement occurs, it is generally rotational with loss of reduction of the medial column. We simply reduce the fracture to an anatomic position and place either a medial pin as described in the technique for crossed pinning or a third lateral pin (75).

After pinning by any technique, the patient is placed in a splint or bivalved long arm cast with the forearm in neutral and the elbow flexed 60 to 90 degrees. Although this flexion position is chosen as a general rule, it is imperative that the elbow is placed in a position that is most favorable for neurovascular structures. If the pulse becomes weak or obliterated at 80 degrees of flexion, the arm should be put in a position where the pulse is strongest. The study by Mapes and Hennrikus (41), using Doppler evaluation of the brachial artery, showed that with progressive flexion and pronation, the pulse pressure (and therefore, flow) was incrementally diminished. Fracture stability is gained by skeletal stabilization, and the splint or cast is simply placed to protect the patient. If a circular cast is used, it should be bivalved and spread to prevent constriction. A child should never be in a circular cast with the elbow hyperflexed following this procedure.

Iyengar et al compared early and delayed pinning to determine whether fractures treated more than 8 hours after trauma had higher incidences of open reductions and complications (76). They concluded that there was no difference. Keep in mind that this was a retrospective review, and it is possible that severe fractures were treated emergently, which would bias the conclusion. Subsequently, in a group of 198 fractures of which 52 were treated early and 146 were delayed greater than 8 hours, Mehlman (77) found that elective treatment appeared not to increase risk. They could find no negative effect in delayed treatment in selected cases of type II and III supracondylar fractures. Leet (78) and Gupta (79) both showed no increase in open reduction with selective delay in treating displaced supracondylar fractures.

With smooth pins left out through the skin, there is rarely a need for anesthesia during pin removal. A very low infection rate accompanies pinning (less than 1%) because they are in place only 3 to 4 weeks.

Intramedullary Pin Fixation

Prevot et al (80) reported their experience with intramedullary fixation of supracondylar fractures in children. After closed reduction, the pins were inserted proximally at the junction of the middle and proximal third and were passed distally in the shaft, diverging in each of the supracondylar columns. Their laboratory experiments comparing this type of fixation with medial-lateral and lateral pins showed that proximally placed pins diverging in the distal fragment were more stable than other percutaneous pin fixation methods.

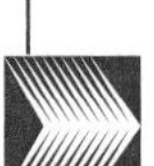

AUTHORS' PREFERRED TREATMENT

For nondisplaced or type I fractures, a splint or cast with a collar and cuff is reasonable. With this course, follow-up in less than 1 week is mandatory with x-ray evaluation. We prefer closed reduction and pinning of most type II and all type III supracondylar fractures. Two lateral pins are chosen as the initial postreduction fixation method in nearly all cases. The decision whether to place a third lateral pin or a medial pin if two lateral pins fail to provide acceptable fixation is not clearly data driven at this time. The determination of instability is based on the inadequacy of two lateral pins to hold the distal fragment securely. If one chooses a medial pin, a small incision over the medial epicondyle to visualize and protect the ulnar nerve is mandatory. In a study of 121 practicing pediatric orthopaedic surgeons regarding pin configuration, Kim (81) resolved that most surgeons (93.4%) in the UK use medial and lateral pinning, known as *crossed pinning*. We are not aware of a similar study in the US, but there is mounting evidence that lateral pinning is safer than crossed pinning and that there is increasing enthusiasm for this safer configuration.

The use of "systematic pinning" (82) reported by Mazda has yielded superior results to those achieved with less invasive interventions. Although some investigators have criticized this approach as overtreatment, it clearly decreases the risks associated with this injury, and has improved outcomes. The timing of treatment needs to be individualized based on the surgeon, institution, and patient. No statement including "all" should be applied to supracondylar fractures. An increasing number of supracondylar fractures are being treated with closed reduction and pinning the day after injury in the absence of neurovascular injury without any harm to the patient. We endorse this concept, provided close monitoring is performed before surgical stabilization.

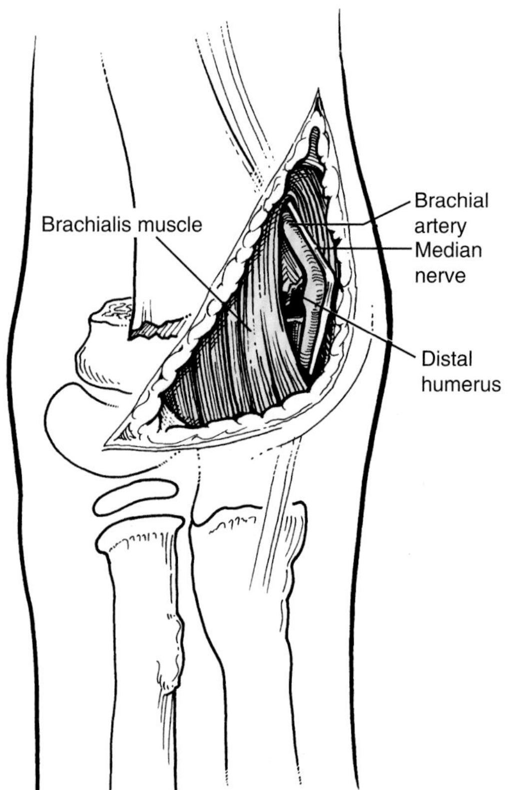

FIGURE 14-29 Tenting of neurovascular bundle. With posterolateral fractures, the neurovascular structures are often tented over the medial spike of the proximal fragment. This fragment can be "buttonholed" through the brachialis muscle.

Open Reduction

Closed reduction may not be possible because of interposed soft tissue, especially in posterolaterally displaced supracondylar fractures. Open reduction is indicated to obtain alignment if closed reduction is unsuccessful. Irreducibility generally results from the proximal fragment being buttonholed through soft tissue or interposition of the biceps or neurovascular structures. An open reduction is also indicated if there is an open fracture that requires irrigation and debridement or simply if a satisfactory closed reduction cannot be performed.

During the early part of this century, there was a reluctance to recommend open reduction of supracondylar fractures. With improvement in operative techniques and more experience with surgical intervention, open reduction of acute supracondylar fractures has become widely accepted. With primary treatment of displaced supracondylar fractures remains closed reduction and percutaneous pinning. The role of open reduction and the frequency of open surgery has been evaluated (46). In a study by Reitman (83), the rate of open reduction was 8% with 65 open cases in 862 fractures. These figures are in keeping with comparable data and clinical results with the closed treatment. Oh (84) and Kaewpornsawan (85) similarly demonstrated that selective open reduction produces results that are as good as closed treatment and pinning, with a very low complication rate.

The high incidence of entrapment of neurovascular structures in individuals skilled in closed reduction supports using open reduction in irreducible fractures. The approach for open reduction has been somewhat controversial. Anterior, medial, lateral, and posterior approaches have all been recommended. Those who advocate medial and lateral approaches (86) operate through the side in which the periosteal hinge is torn; that is, a lateral approach is used for posteromedial displacement or a medial approach is used for posterolateral displacement. The posterior approach (87) to the elbow through the triceps muscle and tendon has been used with excellent results. Our preference is the direct anterior approach (88,89) through a transverse anterior incision in the antecubital fossa, extending proximally, medially as needed. Gennari (89) compared the anterior and posterior approach with the conclusion that the posterior approach is easier but may result in circulatory compromise to the lateral condyle and stiffness. The proximal humeral fragment generally transects the brachialis muscle. The structures remaining intact anteriorly are the biceps tendon and neurovascular bundle (Fig. 14-29). The anteromedial approach provides easy access to an entrapped neurovascular bundle and allows anatomic reduction of the humeral fracture under direct vision by simply placing a retractor on the remaining portion of the brachialis muscle. Koudstaal (90) demonstrated that the anterior approach was preferable when compared to a historic group of open reductions through other approaches.

After open reduction of the fracture, pins are then placed either medially and laterally or two pins are placed laterally as just described, to provide stable fixation. After open reduction, pins may be left in place slightly longer than after closed reduction, but there are no firm data on this approach. Good callus should be observed at the fracture before pin removal, generally 3 to 4 weeks after injury. Prolonged pin fixation is not necessary. Ponce (91) studied the benefit of a 7- to 10-day follow-up to ensure that the fracture did not fall into unacceptable alignment, finding that it was rarely necessary.

We prefer anteromedial open reduction if it is required after attempted closed reduction. Pin fixation can be either crossed or using two lateral pins. With an anteromedial approach to the fracture, the ulnar nerve can be visualized and protected when the medial pin is inserted.

Incidence of Complications Lessened

Open reduction has been increasingly accepted because there are relatively few complications with this method. Surgical experience (3,46,83–85,90,92–96) has dispelled the fears of infection, myositis ossificans, and neurovascular injury (36, 97–99). In a combined series of 470 fractures treated by open reduction, the incidence of infection was 2.5%, all of which resolved (29,30,49,50,86,88,100–109). The incidence of neurovascular complications from the procedure itself was essentially zero. Four patients with myositis ossificans (1.4%) were reported, all in a single series (29).

The most frequent complication of surgical management appears to be a loss of range of motion. One of the reasons given in the past for loss of motion was the use of a posterior approach. It has been stated that approaching the fracture through the relatively uninvolved posterior tissues induces added scar leading to stiffness. In earlier reported series using a posterior approach, loss of range of motion was significant. Preferred use of the anterior approach has resulted in a lower stiffness rate and complications similar to closed treatment. Residual cubitus varus occurred in as many as 33% of patients in some of the earlier series (29,86,110,111), most due to inadequate surgical reduction. When good reduction was obtained, the incidence of cubitus varus deformity was low. Surgical intervention alone does not guarantee an anatomic reduction; the quality of the reduction achieved at the time of surgery is important.

Lal and Bahn (112) reported that delayed open reduction 11 to 17 days after injury, did not increase the frequency of myositis ossificans. If a supracondylar fracture is unreduced or poorly reduced, delayed open reduction and pin fixation appear to be justified. Agus (113) showed that delay in reduction and pinning can be safely accomplished after skeletal traction and malreduction.

Open supracondylar fractures generally have an anterior puncture wound where the metaphyseal spike penetrates the skin. Even if the open wound is only a small puncture in the center of an anterior pucker, open irrigation and debridement are indicated. The anterior approach, using a transverse incision with medial or lateral extension as needed, is recommended. The neurovascular bundle is directly under the skin and tented over the metaphyseal fragment, so care should be taken in approaching this fracture surgically. The skin incision can be extended medially proximally and laterally distally. Often, only the transverse portion of the incision is required, which gives a better cosmetic result. The brachialis muscle is usually transected because it is a muscle belly to its insertion on the coronoid attachment and is highly vulnerable to trauma from the proximal metaphyseal fragment. The fracture surfaces are examined and washed, and a curette is used to remove any dirt or entrapped soft tissue. Once the debridement and washing are complete, the fracture is stabilized with K-wires. All patients with open fractures are also treated with antibiotics: generally, cephalothin for Gustilo types I, II, and IIIA injuries, with the addition of an aminoglycoside for types IIIB and C fractures.

Traction Management of Type III Supracondylar Fractures

Traction can be used to manage type III supracondylar fractures by allowing swelling to decrease and facilitating closed reduction, as described by Alburger et al (52) and others (114,115). In this technique, patients are placed in sidearm or overhead skin traction for 3 to 5 days until elbow hyperflexion can be tolerated for closed reduction. Alburger et al reported 92% good or excellent results in 39 patients treated in this manner.

Definitive treatment of the fracture with 14 days of traction or until healing has occurred historically has led to a very low incidence of cubitus varus deformity, as documented by Smith (24,30,114–116). In a series of supracondylar fractures treated with overhead skeletal traction, D'Ambrosia (111) found no cubitus varus deformities; with sidearm or skin traction for definitive treatment, the rate of varus deformity was 33%. Piggot (117) documented the efficacy of straight lateral skin traction with a report of only 4% cubitus varus deformities and no vascular complications. A comparison by Prietto (118) of pinning and Dunlop's traction demonstrated the relative benefits of pinning in decreased costs and shorter hospital stays in addition to a lower cubitus varus rate. He reported a 5% rate of cubitus varus deformity in the pinning group and 33% in the Dunlop's traction group. Palmer (119), Worlock (115), and Badhe (120) have advocated skeletal traction overhead with use of an olecranon wing nut (Fig. 14-30). Overhead traction was superior to sidearm traction and had a low incidence of cubitus varus (2% to 9%) in these series. The olecranon wing nut is a simple device

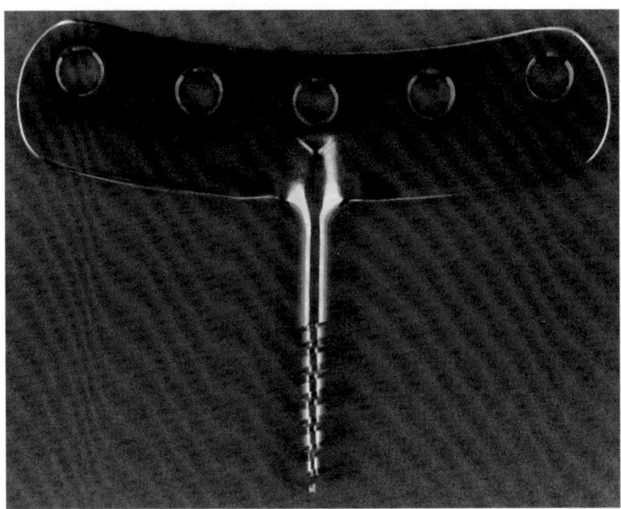

FIGURE 14-30 The olecranon wing nut is a simple skeletal traction device. Varying the insertion point of the rope alters torque about the distal fragment.

that can be placed in the proximal ulna without risk of injury to the ulnar nerve, as might occur in placing a transverse traction pin. The wing nut offers the advantage of applying a torque about the distal humeral fragment by changing the traction rope's position into the holes in the wing nuts.

The indications for traction as the definitive management of a supracondylar fracture are (a) an unstable comminuted fracture reduction or pattern that cannot be pinned and (b) supracondylar comminution or medial column comminution that is not suitable for pinning and would certainly collapse with simple casting after reduction. The duration of traction is usually about 14 days before cast immobilization in this rapidly healing fracture. Prolonged traction may be necessary if poor reduction is obtained in traction, because significant callus must be present for fracture stability before casting.

Technique of Traction Wing Nut Insertion

With the arm prepped in a sterile manner, a hole is drilled in the cortex opposite the coronoid process of the ulna. A 3.2-mm drill bit is used, and a hole is made through both cortices just distal to the coronoid process. A wing nut is then placed through the small incision. The wing nut engages the opposite cortex but does not penetrate it. A sterile dressing is placed around the interface between the wing nut and skin. Next, a traction rope and weights are applied (Fig. 14-31). A sling is used to support the hand and forearm. Initially, traction of about 5 pounds is applied, depending on the patient's size. The shoulder should be lifted just off the bed (119). AP and lateral x-rays should be taken in traction to judge the adequacy of reduction. After there is good callus formation (generally after 10 to 15 days), the patient is removed from traction and placed in a long arm cast, which is worn for about 2 weeks.

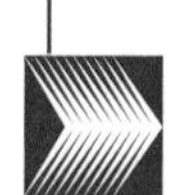

AUTHORS' PREFERRED TREATMENT

For supracondylar comminution (Fig. 14-32) in which stable pinning is impossible to achieve, we have uniformly chosen traction using the olecranon wing nut. Although these fractures are relatively rare, they do occur, and orthopaedic surgeons should be familiar with using traction as a technique to manage this fracture. Anatomic reduction of the fracture is not critical with traction, but maintaining alignment is vital. Callus formation is rapid in the area of the fracture, and the distal fragment should be confirmed as neither hyperextended nor rotated into varus or valgus malalignment, based on x-ray evaluation while in traction. After good callus formation (generally after about 14 days), the patient can be removed from traction and placed in a long arm cast.

For irreducible fractures, we prefer open reduction to simply placing the child in traction to maintain alignment until healing has occurred. Data from Leet et al (78) indicate the high frequency of neurovascular entrapment as well as

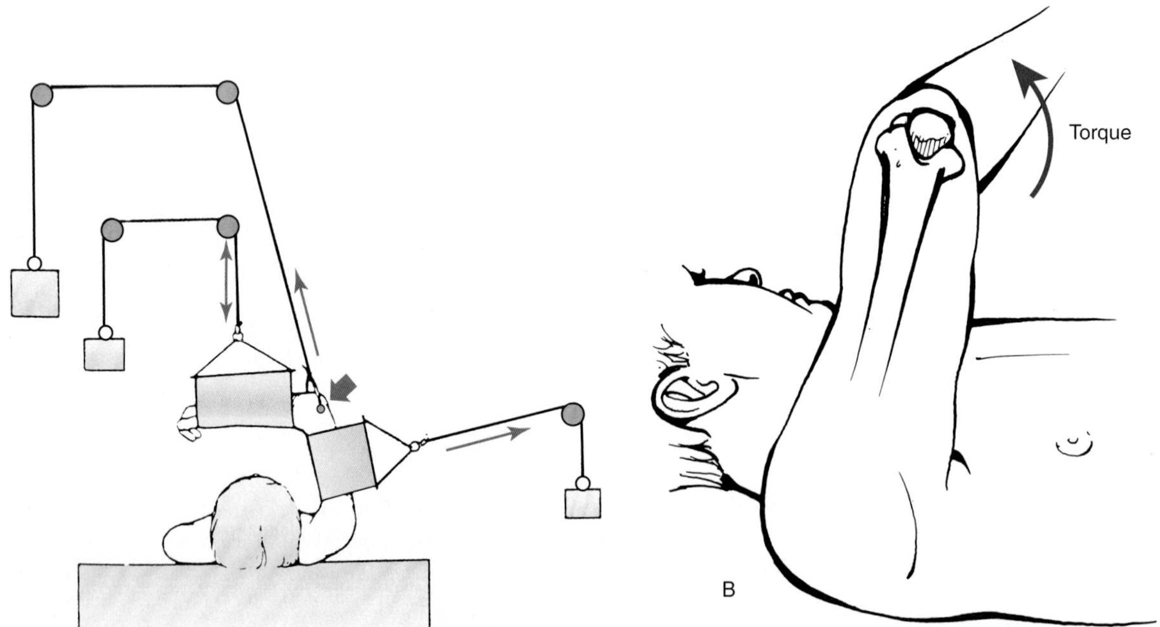

FIGURE 14-31 Overhead olecranon wing nut traction. The arm is suspended by a threaded wing nut through the olecranon (*short arrow*). The forces maintaining the reduction (*long arrows*) are exerted upward **(A)** through the pin and sideways through a counter-sling against the arm. The forearm is supported with a small sling (*double arrow*). By placing the traction rope eccentric to the screw's axis, a torque can be created to correct varus or valgus alignment **(B)**.

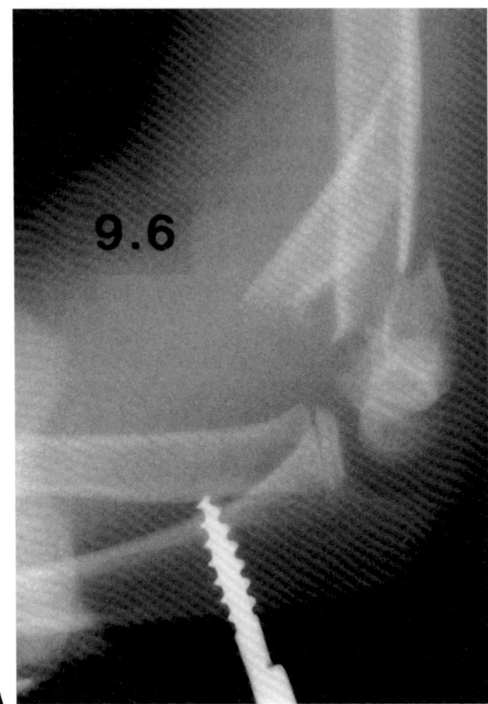

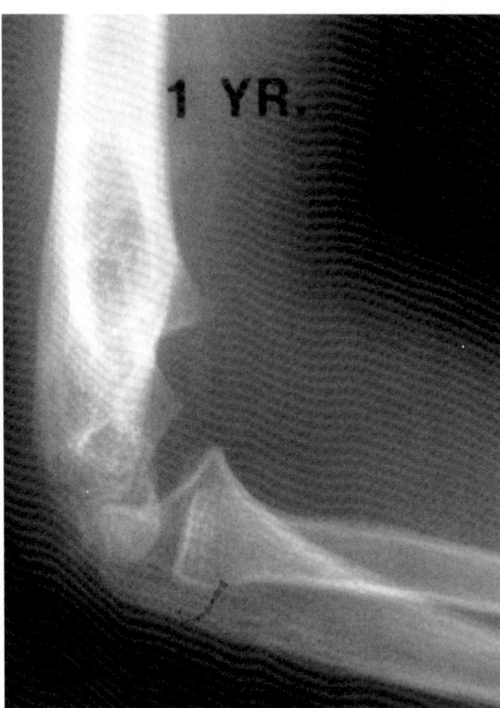

FIGURE 14-32 **A.** Because of supracondylar comminution, stable pinning could not be achieved, and traction was chosen. **B.** Remodeling occurred over 1 year, and the patient regained full motion with normal alignment.

the outstanding results from open reduction in all modern series. Our approach is anterior with medial extension proximally and laterally distally as needed. Pin fixation is accomplished with either two lateral pins or crossed pins as needed to render the fracture stable.

Vascular Injury

Type III supracondylar fractures have significant incidences of brachial artery injury, vascular insufficiency, and compartment syndrome, each of which should be evaluated separately in a patient with a severe elbow injury.

Brachial Artery Injuries and Vascular Insufficiency

About 10% to 20% of patients with type III supracondylar fractures present with an absent pulse (20,121,122). In the emergency management of a patient with a type III supracondylar fracture, the arm should be splinted with the elbow in about 30 degrees of flexion. This configuration will facilitate transporting the patient to the appropriate facility for care and x-ray evaluation. The presence of a pulse and perfusion of the hand should be documented. Perfusion is estimated by color, warmth, and capillary refill. The question sometimes raised in the emergency room evaluation of a patient with supracondylar fracture and poor blood flow to the hand is whether an arteriogram should be performed as part of the preoperative evaluation. The answer is an emphatic "no" (122). The initial approach to managing a patient with vascular compromise secondary to a supracondylar fracture should be immediate closed reduction and stabilization with K-wires. If an anatomic reduction cannot be obtained closed, open reduction through an anterior approach (46,93) with medial extension allows evaluation of the brachial artery and removal of the neurovascular bundle entrapped within the fracture site or repair of the brachial artery.

After closed reduction and stabilization, the pulse and perfusion of the hand should be evaluated. Most extension-type supracondylar fractures are reduced and pinned with the elbow in hyperflexion. With more than 120 degrees of elbow flexion, the radial pulse generally is lost, even in patients with an initially intact pulse. After pinning when the arm is extended, the pulse frequently does not return immediately. This is presumably secondary to arterial spasm, aggravated by swelling about the artery and decreased peripheral perfusion in the anesthetized, somewhat cool intraoperative patient.

Because of this phenomenon, 10 to 15 minutes should be allowed for recovery of perfusion in the operating room before any decision is made regarding the need for exploring the brachial artery and restoring flow to the distal portion of the extremity. Because most patients without a palpable pulse maintain adequate distal perfusion, the absence of a palpable pulse alone is not an indication for exploring a brachial artery. Gillingham and Rang (123) recommended observing patients with absent pulse, because most pulses returned within 10 days. The decision to explore a brachial artery needs to be based on objective criteria.

Traditionally, the decision has been based only on whether the hand was warm and pink. The following case indicates the difficulty with these criteria. A 2-year-old girl was injured in a fall from a couch (Fig. 14-33). A type III supracondylar fracture and a pale, cool hand were documented on presentation to a local emergency department. Two hours later, the patient was brought to the operating room, where a cool, pale hand with poor capillary refill and an absent pulse was noted. Immediate closed reduction and pinning was performed with nearly anatomic reduction. The hand felt warmer, and capillary refill was present. The pulse was not palpable, but because of the improved state of the patient's hand, no exploration of the brachial artery was performed. During the next 4 hours, the patient was observed closely with increasing fussiness, a nonpalpable pulse, and slow capillary refill. An arteriogram was performed, showing brachial artery obstruction. Compartment pressures were measured, and increased pressure was noted in the volar compartment. A decision was made to return to the operating room for exploration, repair of the brachial artery, and forearm fasciotomy. Whereas the outcome in this case was satisfactory with no long-term sequelae other than scarring, the question is whether the low perfusion with subsequent ischemia and compartment syndrome could have been identified at the time of the closed reduction and immediate repair done.

What would happen if no repair had been performed in the preceding case? Had a repair been performed immediately, could the development of a compartment syndrome have been averted? What is the relationship between compartment syndrome and perfusion? Is there a way to determine when flow is insufficient in a more objective way?

Several investigators have attempted to provide criteria for repair in addition to warmth and color in the patient with absence of a palpable pulse. Two groups have studied the use of simple Doppler ultrasonography in the operating room (21,122). In the absence of a palpable pulse, a Doppler device can be used to measure lower flow states with small-pulse amplitude. Shaw (122) found no false-positive explorations when patients with pulses that could not be palpated but were identified on Doppler evaluation were observed, and exploration was performed in those in whom no pulse was found with either palpation or Doppler. The brachial artery was either transected or entrapped in all patients with surgical exploration, and none with "spasm" underwent surgery. Using the same criteria, Schoenecker et al (21) identified six patients for exploration. Three had a damaged or transected brachial artery with no flow, and three had an artery kinked or trapped in the fracture. At follow-up, all patients with vascular repair had a radial pulse. One patient with more than 24 hours of vascular insufficiency had an unsatisfactory outcome. Copley et al (20) reported that of 17 patients with type III supracondylar fractures and no palpable pulse at presentation, 14 recovered pulse after reduction. The three explorations identified significant vascular injury, and the brachial artery was repaired. Most significantly in their series was the finding of increasing vascular insufficiency during postoperative observation in some cases. If one finds the hand to be well perfused despite not having a palpable pulse, close follow-up in the hospital is mandatory. The patient should be observed for increasing narcotic requirements, increasing pain, and decreased passive finger motion. A very low threshold for returning to the operating room for exploration and fasciotomy must be maintained rather than assuming that perfusion from collaterals is sufficient.

Some surgeons recommend pulse oximetry (33,124) for evaluating postreduction circulation. Our experience with the use of a Nelkor system for this technique is that when used in the operating room, false positive or underestimation of perfusion often occurs. We believe this is secondary to its use in an anesthetized person with low blood pressure and peripheral vasoconstriction. As a patient is waking up and pulse pressure and peripheral circulation are increased, pulse oximetry becomes a more valid way to determine perfusion. We have found pulse oximetry useful for evaluating patients after vascular repair or pinning but not for intraoperative decision making. Copley and Dormans (20) reported that some patients who initially had good perfusion and an intact pulse lost both in the postoperative period. Two of 14 patients showed signs of increased vascular insufficiency over a 48-hour period and required subsequent reconstruction. Data such as these support in-hospital observation of patients with supracondylar fractures, especially those with evidence of vascular compromise.

Obliteration of the intact preoperative radial pulse after closed reduction and pinning is a strong indication for brachial artery exploration only when accompanied by evidence of impaired circulation to the hand. After 10 to 15 minutes is allowed for resolution of arterial spasm as a cause for loss of pulse, the brachial artery should be explored if the hand is not warm and pink. Either direct arterial entrapment at the fracture or arterial compression by a fascial band pulling across the artery may cause loss of pulse after fracture reduction. As described earlier, the other indication for brachial artery exploration is persistent vascular insufficiency after reduction and pinning.

Exploration of the Brachial Artery

The orthopaedic surgeon and vascular surgeon need to work together in order to manage this problem emergently. Often, the release of a fascial band or an adventitial tether resolves the problem of obstructed flow. This is a simple procedure performed at the time exploring the antecubital fossa and identifying the brachial artery. In some patients, however, a formal vascular repair and vein graft are required. The brachial artery should be approached through a transverse incision across the antecubital fossa, with a medial extension turning proximally at about the level of the medial epicondyle (Fig. 14-34). After reduction and pinning the fracture, care must be taken because the neurovascular bundle may be difficult to identify when it is surrounded by hematoma, but it may lie in a very superficial position. At the level of the fracture, the artery may seem to disappear into the fracture site, covered with shredded brachialis muscle. This occurs when the artery is tethered by a fascial

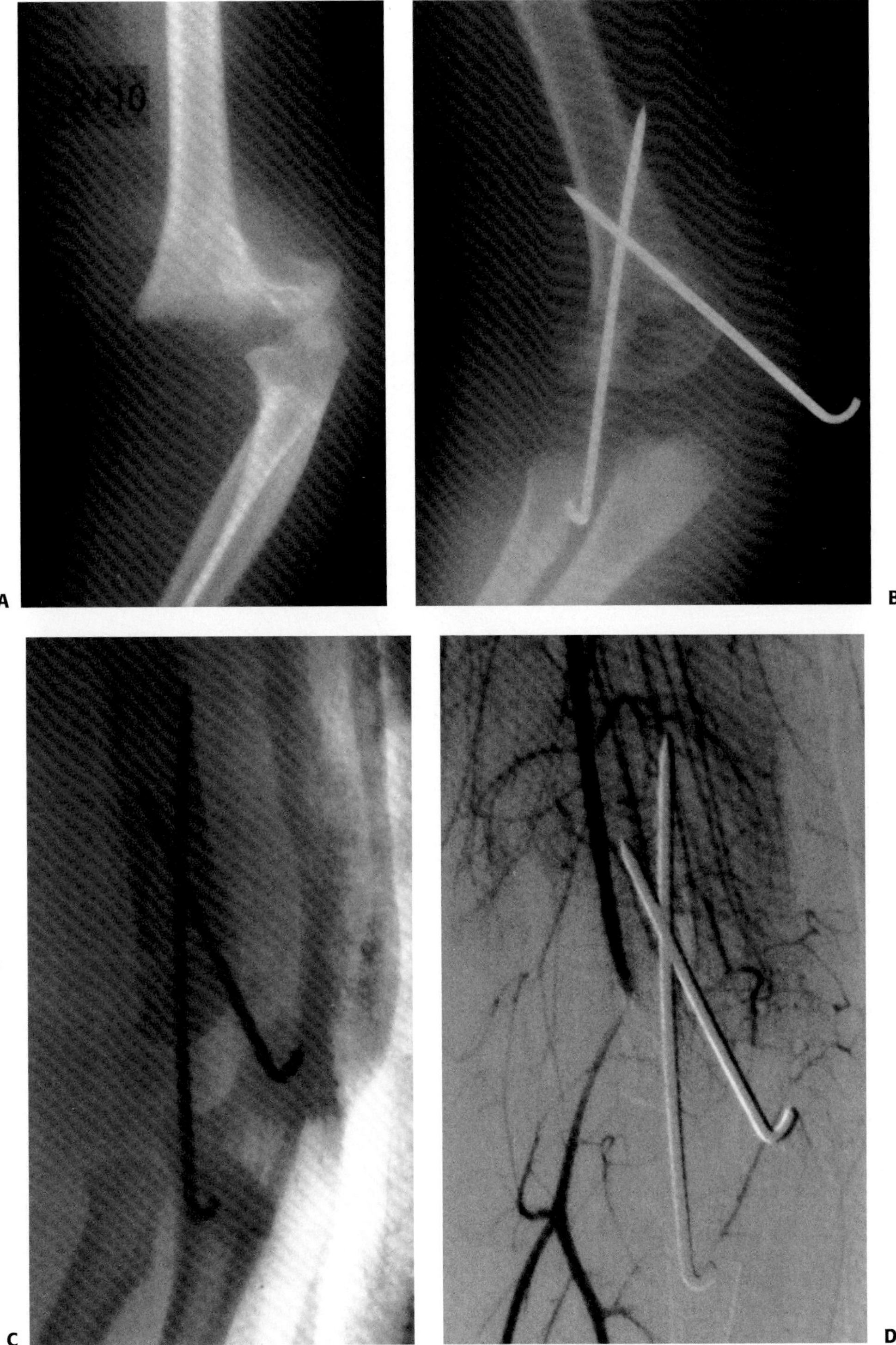

FIGURE 14-33 **A.** This 2-year-old patient sustained a type III supracondylar fracture with vascular compromise. **B.** Pinning was performed in a nearly anatomic position. **C,D.** Six hours postoperatively, increasing pain, a pale hand, and evolving compartment syndrome prompted arteriography, showing brachial artery occlusion.

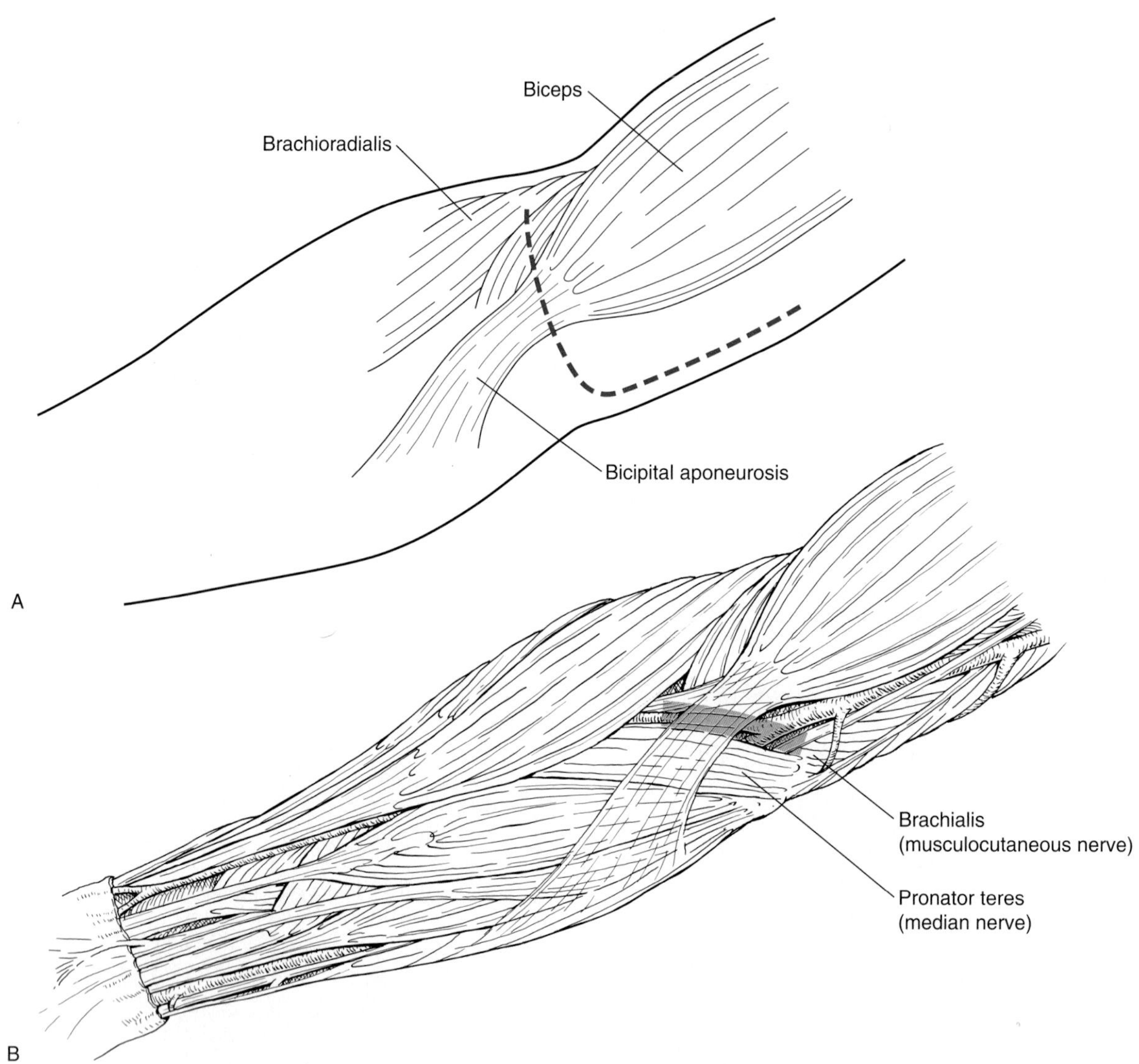

FIGURE 14-34 Brachial artery exploration through anteromedial approach. (*continues*)

band or arterial adventitia attached to the proximal metaphyseal spike pulling the artery in the fracture site. Dissection should occur proximally to distally, along the brachial artery, identifying both the artery and the median nerve. Arterial injury is generally at the level of the supratrochlear artery (Fig. 14-7), which provides a tether, making the artery vulnerable at this location. Arterial transection or direct arterial injury can be identified at this level. Entrapment of the neurovascular bundle in the fracture is best identified by proximal to distal dissection.

The vascular surgeon generally makes the decision to repair a damaged artery or use a vein graft. If spasm is the cause of arterial insufficiency, several techniques have been recommended. If arterial spasm is the cause of inadequate flow, and collateral flow is not sufficient to maintain the hand, attempts to relieve the spasm may be tried. Both stellate ganglion block and application of Papaverine or local anesthetic to the artery have been found to be beneficial in this situation. If these techniques do not relieve the spasm, and if collateral flow is insufficient, the injured portion of the vessel is excised and a vein graft is inserted. When flow is restored, the wound is closed, the patient is placed in a splint with the elbow flexed less than 90 degrees, and the forearm is supinated. Postoperative monitoring should include temperature, pulse oximetry, and frequent examinations for signs of compartment syndrome or ischemia. Although injecting urokinase has been suggested to increase flow (125), we have had no experience with this technique.

Sabharwal et al (126) documented that 3.2% of patients with type III supracondylar fractures have an absent pulse at presentation, for which they recommended noninvasive monitoring. Magnetic resonance angiography and color-flow duplex Doppler were helpful in deciding whether or not to explore the bra-

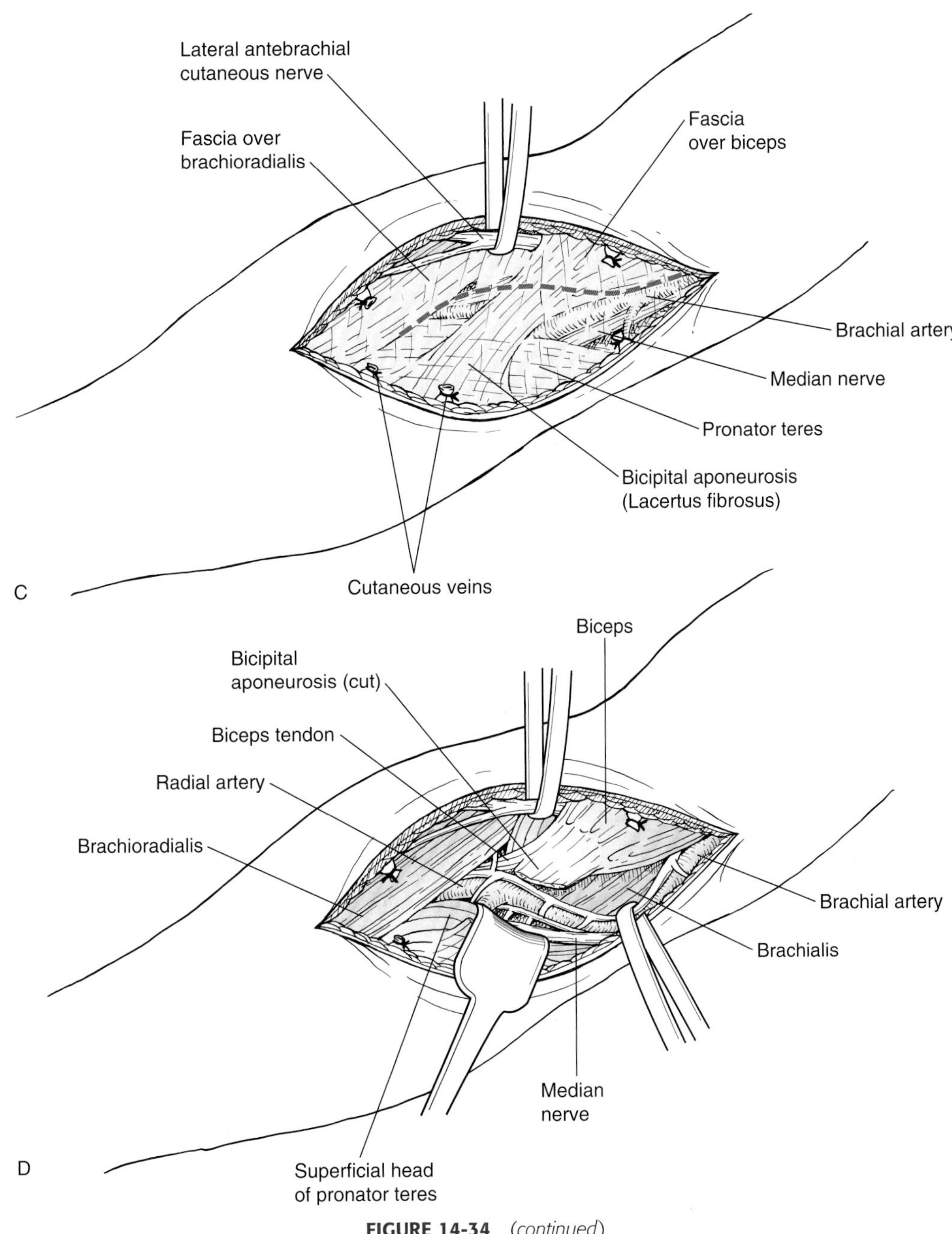

FIGURE 14-34 *(continued)*

chial artery. Although repair is technically feasible, Sabharwal et al cautioned that high rates of reocclusion and residual stenosis argued against early revascularization if not absolutely necessary. Early reocclusion, however, was not reported by Schoenecker et al (21) or Shaw et al (122).

The necessity of early treatment of vascular compromise was emphasized by Ottolenghi (127) who found no Volkmann ischemic contractures (128) in patients in whom vascular compromise was treated within 12 hours. The frequency of this complication increased steadily with repair between 12 and 24 hours; after 24 hours of delay in treatment, outcomes were uniformly poor. This series presents convincing evidence that prompt exploration of arterial insufficiency markedly decreases the incidence of Volkmann ischemic contracture. Note that brachial artery obstruction and compartment syndrome, although related, are not equivalent, and both are fortunately rare problems. Ischemia will lead to a compartment syndrome, but the presence of a radial pulse does not preclude it.

Compartment Syndrome

In acute compartment syndrome (128,129), increased pressure in a closed fascial space causes muscle ischemia. With untreated ischemia, muscle edema increases, further increasing pressure, decreasing flow, and leading to muscle necrosis, fibrosis, and death of involved muscles. Forearm compartment syndrome occurs after 1% or fewer supracondylar fractures. A compartment syndrome of the forearm may occur with or without brachial artery injury and in the presence or absence of a radial pulse. The diagnosis of a compartment syndrome is based on resistance to passive finger movement and dramatically increasing pain after fracture. The classic five "P's" for the diagnosis of compartment syndrome—pain, pallor, pulselessness, paresthesias, and paralysis—are poor indicators of a compartment syndrome.

Mubarak and Carroll (128) recommended forearm fasciotomy if clinical signs of compartment syndrome are present or if intracompartmental pressure is greater than 30 mm Hg. Heppenstal et al (130) suggested that a difference of 30 mm Hg between diastolic blood pressure and compartment pressure should be the threshold for release. If pain is increasing and finger extension is decreasing, fasciotomy is clearly indicated. Measuring compartment pressures in a terrified, crying child is difficult, and if clinical signs of compartment syndrome are present, a trip to the operating room for evaluation and possible fasciotomy is often a better course of action than pressure measurement and observation.

Clinical conditions that contribute to the development of compartment syndrome are direct muscle trauma at the time of injury, swelling with intracompartmental fractures (associated forearm fracture), decreased arterial inflow, restricted venous outflow, and elbow position. The supracondylar fracture's mechanism of injury is critical. An associated forearm fracture or forearm crush injury significantly increases the likelihood of compartment syndrome. Blakemore (131) found a 7% incidence of forearm compartment syndrome (three of 33 patients) with the combined injury of supracondylar fracture and radial fracture. An arterial injury in association with multiple injuries or crush injury further diminishes blood flow to the forearm musculature and increases the probability of a compartment syndrome. Interestingly, Battaglia (132) documented the relationship between increasing elbow flexion above 90 degrees and increasing volar compartment pressure. In a patient with an evolving postoperative compartment syndrome, not only should the dressings be loosened, but the elbow should be extended to a position well below 90 degrees.

Even if distal pulse is found by palpation or Doppler examination, an evolving compartment syndrome may be present. Increased swelling over the compartment, increased pain, and decreased finger mobility are cardinal signs of an evolving compartment syndrome. Evaluation of possible compartment syndrome cannot be based on the presence or absence of a radial pulse alone. If a compartment syndrome does appear to be evolving, initial management includes removing all circumferential dressings. The volar compartment should be palpated, and the elbow should be extended. We believe that the fracture should be immediately stabilized with K-wires to allow proper management of the soft tissues.

Another factor that contributes to the development of compartment syndrome is warm ischemic time after injury. When blood flow is compromised and the hand is pale with no arterial flow, muscle ischemia is possible, depending on the time of oxygen deprivation. After fracture reduction and flow restoration, the warm ischemic time should be noted. If this time is more than 6 hours, compartment syndrome secondary to ischemic muscle injury is likely. Prophylactic volar compartment fasciotomy can be performed at the time of arterial reconstruction. The exact indication for prophylactic fasciotomy in the absence of an operative revascularization is uncertain. Even when the diagnosis is delayed or the if compartment syndrome is chronic, fasciotomy has been shown to be of some value.

Technique for Volar Fasciotomy

The volar compartment of the forearm can be approached through the classic Henry approach or the ulnar approach (Fig. 14-35). If the compartment syndrome is associated with a brachial artery and median nerve injuries, we generally use the Henry approach as an extension of the vascular repair. The advantage of the ulnar approach, as described by Willis and Rorabeck (133) is that it produces a more cosmetically pleasing scar. A volar fasciotomy involves opening the volar compartment from the carpal tunnel distally to the lacertus fibrosa and antecubital fascia proximally. The fascia over the deep flexors is opened, as is the superficial fascia, to decompress the deep volar compartment of the forearm. Failure to release the deep volar fascia may cause contracture of the deep finger flexors. Generally, only the volar compartment is released, with an associated decrease in pressure in the dorsal or extensor compartment. If the volar Henry approach is used, the interval between the brachioradialis, the flexor carpi radialis, and the radial artery are retracted ulnarward. The deep volar compartment is exposed. The flexor digitorum profundus and flexor pollicis longus are exposed along with the pronator teres proximally and the pronator quadratus distally.

If the ulnar approach is used, as described by Willis and Rorabeck (133), the release is performed from the carpal canal to the antecubital fossa, as with the Henry approach. The skin incision begins above the elbow crease, medial to the biceps tendon (Fig. 14-35); it crosses the elbow crease and extends distally along the ulnar border to the volar wrist, where it courses radially across the carpal canal. The fascia over the flexor carpi ulnaris is incised, and the interval between the flexor carpi ulnaris and the flexor digitorum sublimis is identified. The ulnar nerve and artery are retracted, exposing the deep flexor compartment of the forearm. The deep flexor fascia is incised. The ulnar nerve and artery, as well as the carpal tunnel, are decompressed distally.

After fasciotomy, the wound is generally left open. An effective way to manage the wound is with a criss-crossed rubber band technique, securing the rubber bands in place with skin

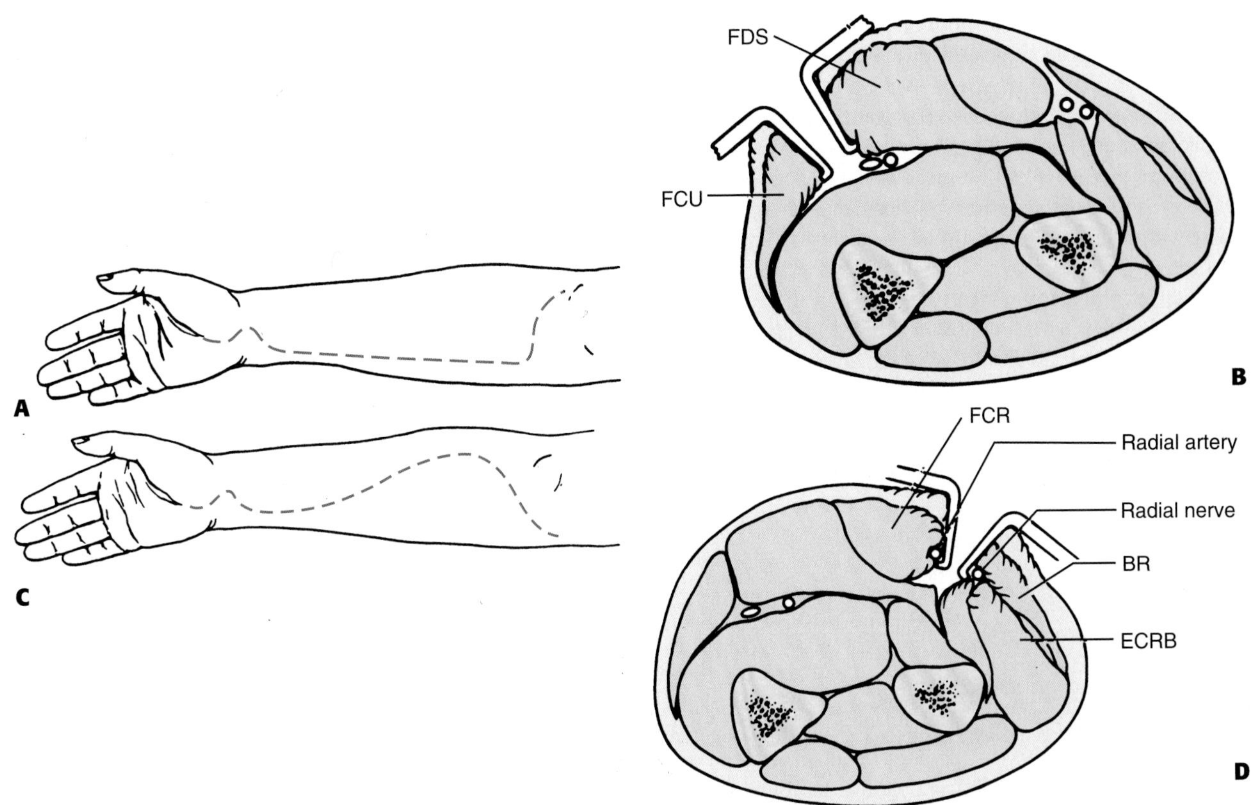

FIGURE 14-35 Surgical approach for forearm fasciotomy. **A.** Ulnar approach, skin incision. **B.** Ulnar approach, intermuscular interval (FDS, flexor digitorum sublimis; FCU, flexor carpi ulnaris). **C.** Henry approach, skin incision. **D.** Henry approach, FCR, flexor carpi radialis interval (BR, brachioradialis; ECRB, extensor carpi radialis brevis). (From Willis RB, Rorabeck CH. Treatment of compartment syndrome in children. *Orthop Clin N Am* 1990; 21:407–408, with permission.)

staples. An alternative is to simply place a sterile dressing over the open wound, but this makes wound closure difficult and probably increases the need for skin grafting. Definitive closure or skin grafting is generally performed within 5 to 7 days. Skeletal stabilization of the supracondylar and forearm fractures is important to properly manage compartment syndrome.

Neurologic Deficit

In most modern series, the incidence of neurologic deficit with supracondylar fractures is 10% to 20% (39,59) with an incidence as high as 49% in one series (19). Reports differ as to whether the radial or median nerve is the most frequently injured. In modern series, the AIN appears to be the most commonly injured (11,121,134), with loss of motor power to the flexor pollicis longus and the deep flexor to the index finger as first described by Spinner in 1969 (135). The direction of the fracture's displacement determines the nerve most likely to be injured. If the distal fragment is displaced posteromedially, the radial nerve is more likely to be injured. Conversely, if the displacement of the distal fragment is posterolateral, the neurovascular bundle is stretched over the proximal fragment, injuring the median nerve or AIN or both. In a flexion type of supracondylar fracture, which is rare, the ulnar nerve is the most likely nerve to be injured.

In general, if the nerve deficit is present when the patient arrives in the emergency department and if the fracture is reducible, open reduction of the fracture and exploration of the injured nerve are not indicated. In most series, nerve recovery, whether radial, median, or ulnar, generally occurs at an average of 2 to 2½ months. Culp et al (136) reported identification of eight injured nerves in five patients in which spontaneous recovery did not occur by 5 months after injury. Neurolysis was successful in restoring nerve function in all but one patient. Nerve grafting may be indicated for nerves not in continuity at the time of exploration. Neurolysis for perineural fibrosis is generally successful in restoring nerve function. There is no indication for early electromyographic analysis or treatment other than observation for nerve deficit until 6 months after fracture.

In their series of radial nerve injuries with humeral fractures, Amillo et al (137) reported that of 12 injuries that did not spontaneously recover within 6 months of injury, only one was associated with a supracondylar fracture. Perineural fibrosis was present in four patients, three nerves were entrapped in callus, and five were either partially or totally transected.

In the supracondylar area, perineural fibrosis appears to be the most common cause of prolonged nerve deficit. Although nerve injury is related to fracture displacement, a neural deficit can exist with even minimally displaced fractures. Sairyo et al (39) reported one patient in whom radial nerve palsy occurred with a slightly angulated fracture that appeared to be a purely extension type fracture on initial x-rays. Even in patients with mild injuries, a complete neurologic examination should be performed before treatment. An irreducible fracture with nerve deficit is an indication for open reduction of the fracture to ensure that there is no nerve entrapment. Chronic nerve entrapment in healed callus can give the appearance of a hole in the bone, Metev's sign. Nerve transection is rare, and almost always involves the radial nerve (134,136,138–140).

Iatrogenic injury to the ulnar nerve has been reported to occur in 1% to 15% of patients with supracondylar fractures (65,67–70). In a large series of type III supracondylar fractures, the rate of iatrogenic injury to the radial nerve was less than 1%. The course of the ulnar nerve through the cubital tunnel, between the medial epicondyle and the olecranon, makes it vulnerable when a medial pin is placed. The ulnar nerve generally is injured by direct trauma from the medial pin, with or without actual penetration of the nerve. If the pin is placed in the ulnar groove rather than in the medial epicondyle, injury is likely. The ulnar nerve may sublux over the medial epicondyle in as many as 30% of patients; this is usually bilateral and associated with ligamentous laxity. Ulnar nerve subluxation occurs most commonly with hyperflexion of the elbow, and injury to the nerve is most likely when a medial pin is placed with the elbow in hyperflexion.

If an ulnar neuropathy is documented postoperatively when one was not present preoperatively and a medial pin has been placed, what is the appropriate treatment? Brown and Zinar (67) reported four ulnar nerve injuries associated with pinning of supracondylar fractures, all of which resolved spontaneously 2 to 4 months after pinning. Lyons et al (141) documented ulnar nerve injuries associated with pinning in 19 of 375 patients who had cross-pinning of supracondylar fractures. The medial pin was removed in only four patients. Two patients had explorations, which found no nerve transection. These researchers recommended leaving the medial pin in place until the fracture heals. Rasool (69) reported six patients with ulnar nerve injuries in whom early exploration was performed. In two patients, the nerve was penetrated, and in three, it was constricted by a retinaculum over the carpal tunnel, aggravated by the pin. In one patient, the nerve was subluxed and was fixed anterior to the cubital tunnel by the pin. Full recovery occurred in three patients, partial recovery in two, and no recovery in two. Royce et al (70) reported spontaneous recovery of ulnar nerve function in three patients. One nerve that was explored had direct penetration, and the pin was replaced in the proper position. Two patients had late-onset ulnar nerve palsies discovered during healing, and the medial pin was removed.

If an immediate postoperative neural injury is documented, we prefer to explore the ulnar nerve and to replace the pin in the proper position or convert to a lateral pin construct. If an ulnar nerve lesion is documented weeks later in the course of fracture healing, we remove the pin but do not explore the nerve.

Preventing ulnar nerve injury is obviously more desirable than treating ulnar neuropathy. Due to the frequency of ulnar nerve injury with crossed pinning, most surgeons prefer to use two lateral pins if possible and no medial pin. Keep in mind that two lateral pins are about 30% less resistant to torque than crossed pins. Successful maintenance of alignment of type III supracondylar fractures with two lateral pins has been reported, however (43). If cross-pinning is to be used, nerve penetration and indirect trauma to the nerve can be prevented by making a 1.5-cm incision over the medial epicondyle and being certain that the ulnar nerve is protected when the medial pin is placed. Michael and Stanislas described another alternative for protecting the ulnar nerve; they attached a nerve stimulator to a needle, which was used for localizing the ulnar nerve (71). Once the ulnar nerve was identified, a standard pinning technique was used, placing the medial pin 0.5 mm to 0.75 mm anterior to the nerve. We have no experience with this technique. The contralateral elbow should always be examined for ulnar nerve subluxation in flexion because it is usually bilateral and associated with ligamentous laxity. Some surgeons palpate the ulnar nerve and push it posteriorly (Fig. 14-28). Schwend, however, showed this method to be unreliable (72).

Radial nerve injuries are rare complications of supracondylar fracture pinning. The most common cause is probably a direct piercing injury to the radial nerve, as the medial pin exits the anterolateral cortex of the humerus. To prevent this type of injury, ensure that pin penetration in the opposite cortex is limited to 1 mm to 2 mm. The medial pin should be backed out slightly if it protrudes significantly beyond the cortex. Spontaneous recovery of radial nerve function generally occurs.

Elbow Stiffness

Loss of motion after extension-type supracondylar fractures is rare in children. Two series analyzed this complication in detail (142,143) and found that fractures treated closed had an average loss of motion of 4 degrees. In those treated with open reduction, the loss of flexion was 6.5 degrees and the flexion contracture was 5 degrees. Loss of motion has been reported with the posterior triceps splitting incision for open reduction (29,104,144).

Although motion loss is usually minimal, significant loss of flexion can occur. This problem is generally caused by either posterior distal fragment angulation, posterior translation of the distal fragment with anterior impingement, or medial rotation

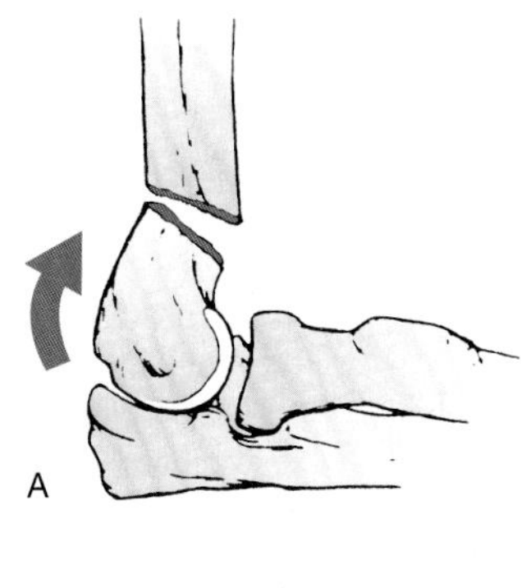

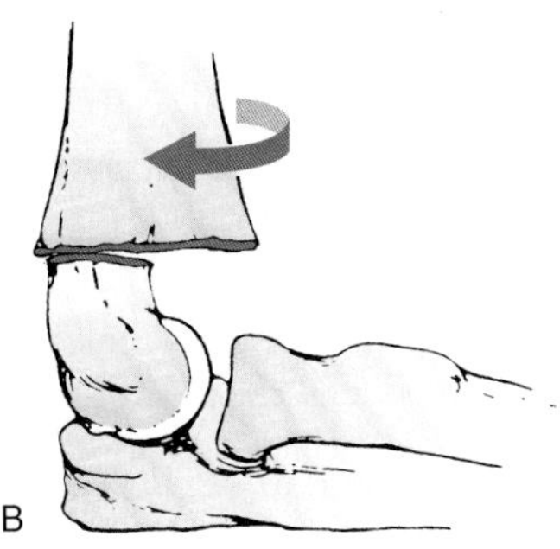

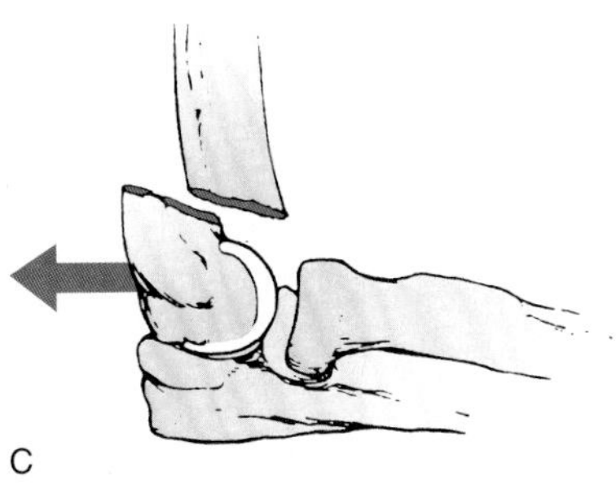

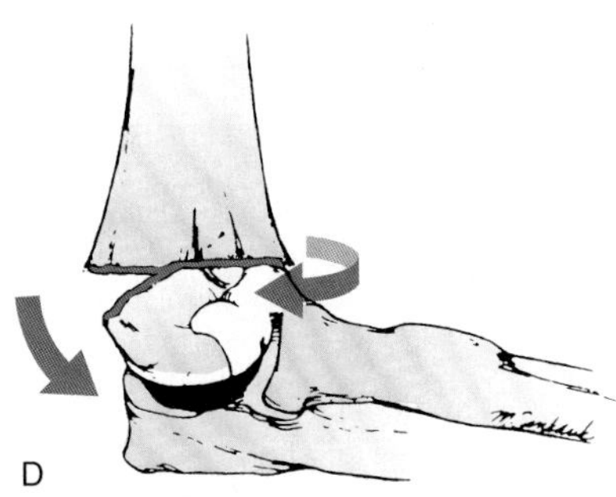

FIGURE 14-36 Distal fragment rotation. **A.** Posterior angulation only of the distal fragment. **B.** Pure horizontal rotation without angulation. **C.** Pure posterior translocation without rotation or angulation. **D.** Horizontal rotation with coronal tilting, producing a cubitus varus deformity. There is a positive crescent sign. (Modified and reprinted with permission from Marion J, LaGrange J, Faysse R, et al. Les fractures de l'extremite inferieure de l'humerus chez l'enfant. *Rev Chir Orthop* 1962;48:337–413.)

of the distal fragment with a protruding medial metaphyseal spike proximally (Fig. 14-36). In young children with significant growth potential, there may be significant remodeling of anterior impingement, and any corrective surgery should be delayed at least 1 year. Although anterior impingement can significantly remodel, there is little remodeling to persistent posterior angulation or hyperextension.

Myositis Ossificans

Myositis ossificans is often mentioned as a possible complication (145) of supracondylar fractures, but it is remarkably rare (Fig. 14-37). This complication has been described after open reduction, but vigorous postoperative manipulation or physical therapy is believed to be the most commonly associated factor (49,146–148).

In a report of two patients with myositis ossificans after closed reduction of supracondylar fractures, Aitken (149) noted that limitation of motion and calcification disappeared after 2 years. Postoperative myositis ossificans can be observed with the expectation of spontaneous resolution of both restricted motion and the myositis ossificans. There is no indication for early excision. Spinner (135) reported a single case of myositis ossificans associated with sudden onset of pain posttrauma in which a 1-year-old lesion of myositis ossificans was fractured. With excision, the pain was relieved, and full range of motion returned.

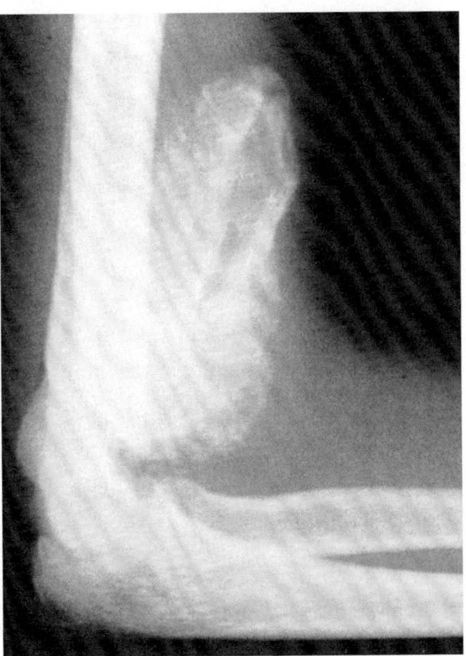

FIGURE 14-37 Myositis ossificans. Ossification of the brachialis muscle developed in this 8-year-old who had undergone multiple attempts at reduction. (Courtesy of John Schaeffer, MD.)

Nonunion

The distal humeral metaphysis is a well-vascularized area with remarkably rapid healing, and nonunion of a supracondylar fracture is rare, with only a single case described by Wilkins and Beaty after open reduction (35). We have not seen nonunion of this fracture. With infection, devascularization, and soft tissue loss, the risk of nonunion increases.

Avascular Necrosis

Avascular necrosis of the trochlea after supracondylar fracture has been reported. The blood supply of the trochlea's ossification center is fragile, with two separate sources. One small artery is lateral and courses directly through the physis of the medial condyle. It provides blood to the medial crista of the trochlea. If the fracture line is very distal, this artery can be injured, producing avascular necrosis of the ossification center and resulting in a classic fishtail deformity (Fig. 14-38). Kim (150) identified 18 children with trochlear abnormalities after elbow injuries, five of which were supracondylar fractures. MRI indicated low-signal intensity on T2 indicative of cartilage necrosis. Cubitus varus deformity developed in all cases.

Symptoms of avascular necrosis of the trochlea do not occur for months or years. Healing is normal and motion is regained, but mild pain and occasional locking develop with characteristic radiologic findings. Routine long-term follow-up radiographs of supracondylar fractures are not necessary because this complication is highly unusual, and the fishtail deformity of the distal humerus does not compromise function.

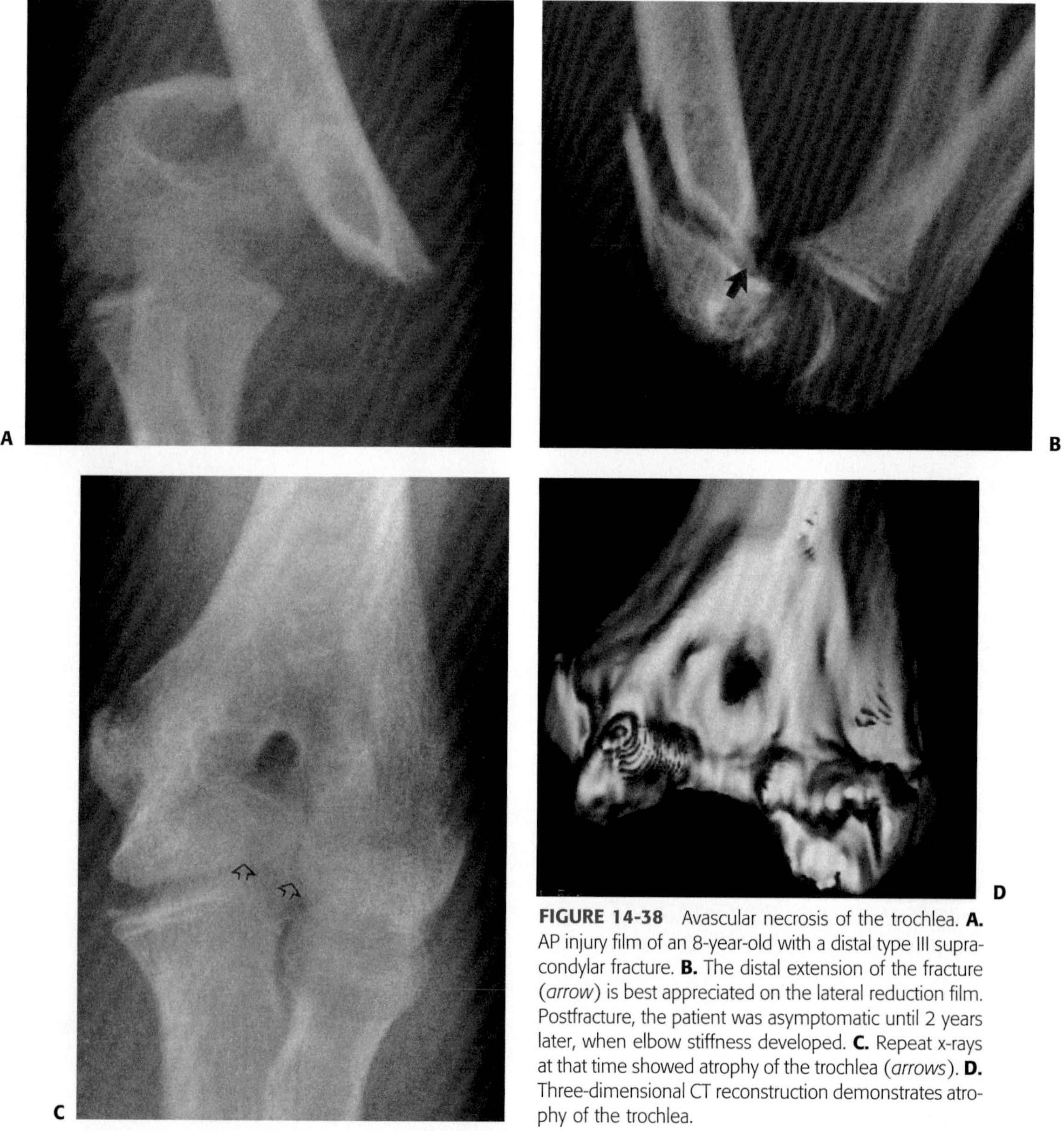

FIGURE 14-38 Avascular necrosis of the trochlea. **A.** AP injury film of an 8-year-old with a distal type III supracondylar fracture. **B.** The distal extension of the fracture (*arrow*) is best appreciated on the lateral reduction film. Postfracture, the patient was asymptomatic until 2 years later, when elbow stiffness developed. **C.** Repeat x-rays at that time showed atrophy of the trochlea (*arrows*). **D.** Three-dimensional CT reconstruction demonstrates atrophy of the trochlea.

Angular Deformity

Angular deformities of the distal humerus after supracondylar fractures are much less common since the development of modern techniques of skeletal stabilization. In the past, the incidence of cubitus varus deformity after supracondylar fractures ranged from 9% to 58% (144,151–153). Pirone et al (49) reported cubitus varus deformities in 14% of patients treated with cast immobilization compared with 3% in patients with percutaneous pin fixation. A decrease in frequency of cubitus varus deformity after the use of percutaneous pin fixation has been reflected in other recent series (2,5,49,56,57,60,61,154). The usual etiology of cubitus varus deformity is malunion of the distal humeral fragment rather than growth disturbance (19). Distal humeral varus is generally believed to be a result of residual coronal angulation aggravated by malrotation and hyperextension. Osteonecrosis with or without growth arrest is a rare but very important cause of varus deformity (150).

Malunion of the distal humerus usually creates a static deformity (Fig. 14-39), which becomes evident as the patient gains full motion. A flexion deformity obscures the true varus deformity, which is generally associated with hyperextension. Although some investigators have proposed that unequal growth in the distal humerus causes varus deformity (27,119,148, 153,155,156), this is unlikely to cause a significant varus deformity in the first few months after fracture. The distal humerus' growth is 20% of that of its overall length. In a 5-year-old, therefore, the amount of distal humeral growth in 1 year is approximately 2 mm, making it unlikely that growth asymmetry is a significant cause of varus deformity that occurs within the first 6 to 12 months after fracture. Avascular necrosis of the trochlea or medial portion of the distal humeral fragment can result in progressive varus deformity, however. In a series of 36 varus deformities reported by Voss et al (157), four patients had medial growth disturbance and distal humeral avascular necrosis as a cause of progressive varus deformity.

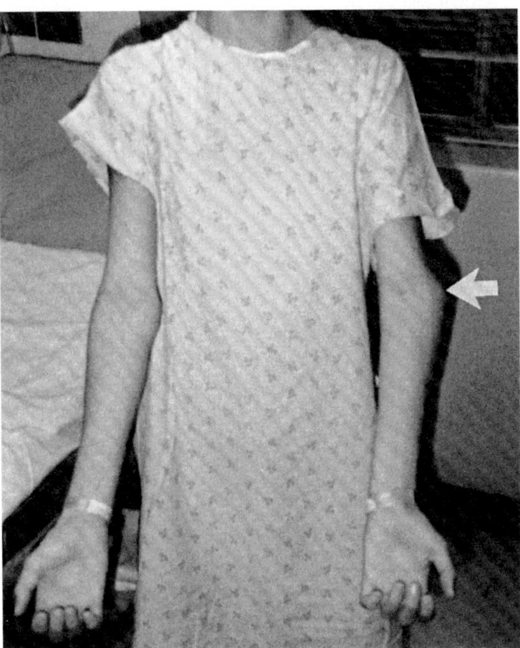

FIGURE 14-39 Cosmetic effects. A combination of varus coronal rotation and medial horizontal rotation of the distal fragment causes the lateral condyle to be unduly prominent (*arrow*). This accentuates the unpleasant appearance of the cubitus varus deformity. (From Wilkins KE. Residuals of elbow trauma in children. *Orthop Clin N Am* 1990;21:291–314, with permission.)

Horizontal rotation (35,56,158) in a medial direction or internal rotation of the distal fragment is believed to predispose to distal fragment varus angulation (Fig. 14-36). Eccentric position of the biceps has been suggested as a cause of varus tilting by the distal fragment. Chess et al (159) evaluated the clinical appearance of cubitus varus in an anatomic study of 256 combinations of varus angulation, internal rotation, and posterior angulation. They found that the major component of cubitus varus deformity was true varus angulation in the coronal plane. Internal rotation appeared to worsen the deformity. In a clinical study (160,161), the true distal humeral rotation was measured on wedges removed from osteotomies of the distal humerus; the horizontal rotation of the distal humerus did not correlate with the severity of cubitus varus (157). Horizontal rotation may accentuate the clinical varus deformity, but it is not the primary cause. Coronal plane deformity and hyperextension are the factors in cubitus varus deformity and are important in planning surgical correction.

Some researchers have suggested that cubitus varus deformity may produce weakness, but most believe that the effects are primarily cosmetic. An increased risk of fracture (162), especially of the lateral condyle, has been linked with cubitus varus deformity (Fig. 14-40). Takahara (163) reported nine patients with distal humeral fractures complicating varus deformity. Supracondylar fractures as well as epiphyseal separations were included in these nine fractures. Further problems complicating varus deformity involved the shoulder. Gurkan showed a relationship between varus deformity and posterior shoulder instability in three patients (164). Tardy ulnar nerve palsy has also been associated with varus and internal rotational malalignment (164,165). Although varus angulation may complicate throwing, the functional effects of cubitus varus deformity are generally less significant than the increased incidence of subsequent fracture and the deformity's cosmetic effect.

The appearance of cubitus varus deformity is distinctive upon x-ray. On the AP view, the angle of the physis of the lateral condyle (Baumann's angle) is more horizontal than normal. Keenan (115) showed that there was insignificant variation in Baumann's angle between boys and girls. On the lateral view, the superimposition of the capitellum on the olecranon produces a crescent sign (Fig. 14-41).

Cubitus varus deformity is also associated with a significant increase in late ulnar nerve palsies, as reported in the Japanese literature (167–169). With a cubitus varus deformity, the olecranon fossa moves to the ulnar side of the distal humerus (170), and the triceps shifts a bit ulnarward. Investigators theorized that this ulnar shift might compress the ulnar nerve against the

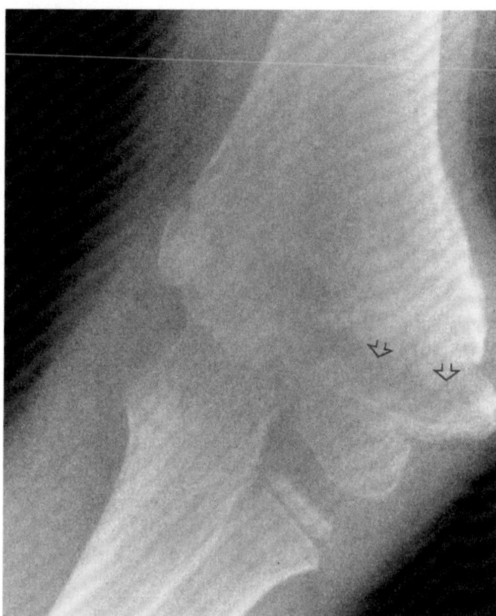

FIGURE 14-40 Predisposition to lateral condyle fracture. This 5-year-old sustained a supracondylar fracture of this extremity 1 year before this acute stage II fracture of the lateral condyle (*arrows*). It was thought that the cubitus varus deformity predisposed the patient to this second fracture. (Courtesy of Kenneth P. Butters, MD.)

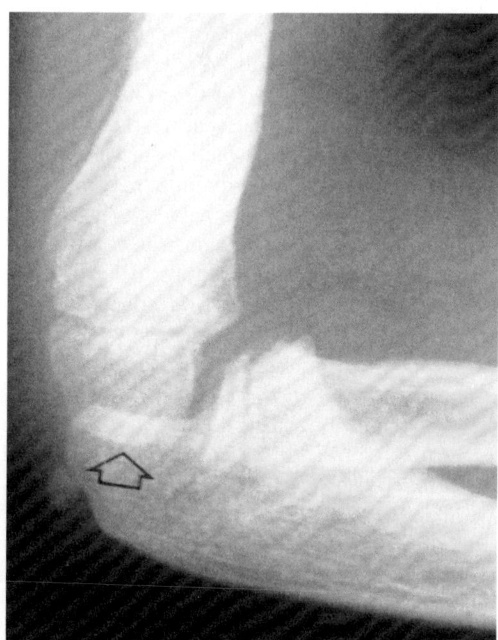

FIGURE 14-41 A patient with cubitus varus shows overlapping of the distal humerus, with the olecranon (*arrow*) producing the typical crescent sign.

medial epicondyle, narrowing the cubital tunnel and resulting in chronic neuropathy. In a recent report (167), a fibrous band running between the heads of the flexor carpi ulnaris was thought to cause ulnar nerve compression.

Treatment of Cubitus Varus Deformity

As for the treatment of any posttraumatic malalignment, options include (a) observation with expected remodeling, (b) hemiepiphysiodesis and growth alteration, and (c) corrective osteotomy. Observation is generally not appropriate because although hyperextension may remodel to some degree in a young child (Fig. 14-42), in an older child, little remodeling occurs even in the joint's plane of motion.

Hemiepiphysiodesis of the distal humerus may rarely be of value, but only to prevent cubitus varus deformity from developing in a patient with clear medial growth arrest or trochlear avascular necrosis. If untreated, medial growth disturbance will lead to lateral overgrowth and progressive deformity. Lateral epiphysiodesis will not correct the deformity, but will prevent it from increasing. Voss et al (157) used hemiepiphysiodesis with osteotomy in two patients with growth arrest and varus deformity. The humerus varies in length by a few centimeters from one individual to another, but in general, it is about 30 cm long at skeletal maturity. Approximately 65% of the length of the humerus is achieved by age 6 years. A 6-year-old child has approximately 10 cm of growth left in the entire humerus, with only approximately 2 cm provided by the distal physis. Growth arrest, in the absence of avascular necrosis or collapse, will be a very slowly evolving phenomenon, and epiphysiodesis in a child older than 6 years will have little effect on longitudinal growth. In general, prevention of increasing deformity from medial growth arrest is the only role for lateral epiphysiodesis. Because of the slow growth rate in the distal humerus, we do not believe there is any role for lateral epiphysiodesis in correcting a varus deformity in a child with otherwise normal physis.

Osteotomy

Osteotomy is the only way to correct a cubitus varus deformity with a high probability of success. A variety of corrective osteotomies have been described, almost all with significant complications (Table 14-3). Stiffness, nerve injury, and recurrent deformities are the most commonly reported complications. An overall complication rate approaching 25% in many series has led to some controversy about the value of a distal humeral corrective osteotomy for cubitus varus deformity.

To choose an appropriate osteotomy, the deformity's exact location must be determined. Because malunion is the cause of most cubitus varus deformities, the angular deformity usually occurs at the level of the fracture. Rotation and hypertension contribute to the deformity, but varus is the most significant factor (159). Hyperextension can produce a severe deformity in some patients. After determining the location and cause of the deformity, the appropriate osteotomy can be chosen. In general, a lateral closing wedge osteotomy with a medial hinge will correct the varus deformity, with some minor correction of hyperextension (157,171–181).

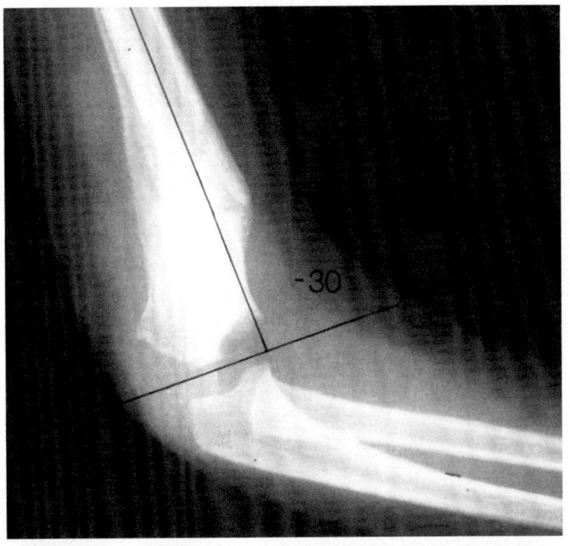

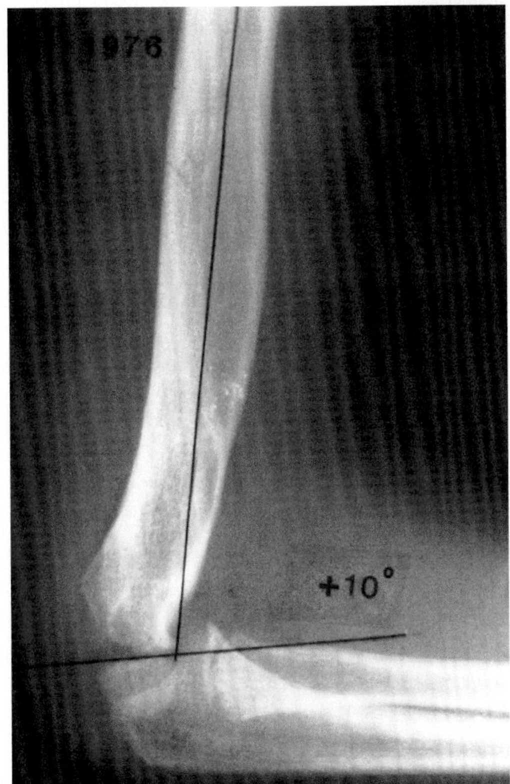

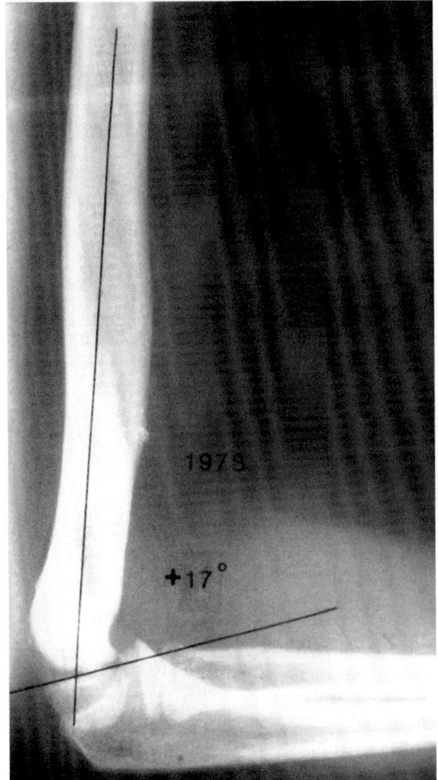

FIGURE 14-42 A hyperextension deformity in the distal humerus may remodel somewhat, whereas varus and valgus deformity do not. Hyperextension deformity in the distal humerus after fracture **(A)**. Four years later **(B)**, a more normal distal humeral anatomy is seen with remodeling of the hyperextension deformity; 2 years later, **(C)**, a normal distal humeral anatomy is reconstituted.

An oblique configuration (Fig. 14-43) places the corrective osteotomy's center of rotation as close to the actual level of the deformity as possible. Oppenheim et al recommended osteotomy at a higher level, emphasizing that the length of the cuts should be equal (Fig. 14-44) (182). The higher the osteotomy is, the more translation is produced in correcting the angular deformity. Proper preoperative planning places the osteotomy's apex close to the level of the deformity and obtains the best anatomic result.

On an AP x-ray of the humerus with the forearm in full supination, the size of the wedge and the angular correction needed are determined. An "incomplete" lateral closing wedge osteotomy is performed, leaving a small medial hinge of bone intact. The osteotomy usually is fixed with two K-wires placed laterally. In the absence of an intact medial hinge, two lateral wires probably are not sufficient to secure this osteotomy (157). Wilkins and Beaty (35) recommended crossed wires in this situation.

TABLE 14-3 Results of Several Studies Using Various Osteotomies

Study (Ref.)	Cases	Type Fixation	Complications
Incomplete Osteotomies			
Ring and Secor	15	MOW, Riedel clamp, tibial graft	Three neutral Three ulnar palsies
Rang (191)	20	LCW, K-wires	One aneurysm One skin slough One nerve palsy Six varus Two stiff
Carlson et al	12	LCW, staple	None
Bellemore et al (172)	27	LCW, K-wire, French technique	Four infections Four loss of fixation Three varus Four poor scars Five prominent condyles
Gao	15	LCW, suture	Three undercorrected
McCoy and Piggot	20	LCW, French technique	Four neutral Two varus Two stiff One poor scar
Graham et al (176)	16	LCW, cast	Two varus
Danielsson et al	11	LCW, staple	None
Mixed Osteotomies			
Oppenheim et al (182)	4 incomplete, 31 complete	LCW, K-wires, French technique	Five nerve palsies Three infections Twelve varus One stiff Two poor scars
Unspecified Osteotomies			
Sweeney (180)	15	LCW, K-wires Complete osteotomies	Five varus
Langenskiöld and Kivilaakso	11	LCW, unicortical plate, rot.	Two varus Two neutral Two reoperations
Labelle et al (179)	15	LCW, K-wires, rot.	Three loss of fixation Three nerve palsies
DeRosa and Graziano (184)	11	SC, screw	One loss of fixation, varus
Kanaujia et al	11	Dome K wires	Two stiff
Laupattarakasem et al	57	SC, screws	Three loss of fixation Two reoperations Two prominent condyles
Uchida et al (169)	12	SC, screws	None
Voss and Kasser (157)	34	K-wires	No nerve palsies, One loss of fixation

MOW, medial opening wedge; LCW, lateral closing wedge; rot., rotational correction; SC, step-cut osteotomy.

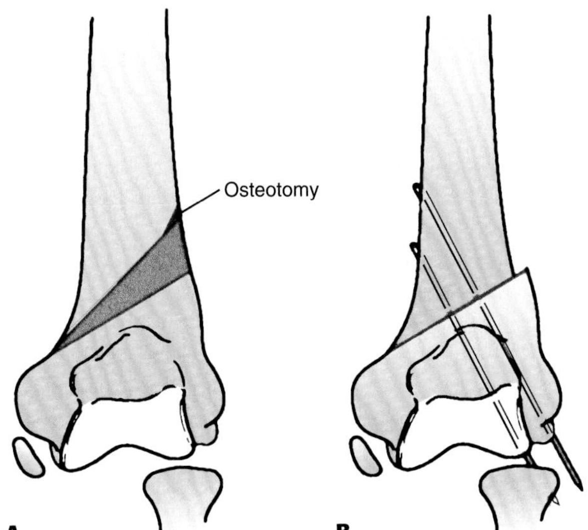

FIGURE 14-43 **A.** By moving the apex of the closing wedge distally, the osteotomy's center of rotation is moved closer to the deformity. **B.** Upon closing a distally based wedge osteotomy, there is less translational effect than in a more proximally based osteotomy.

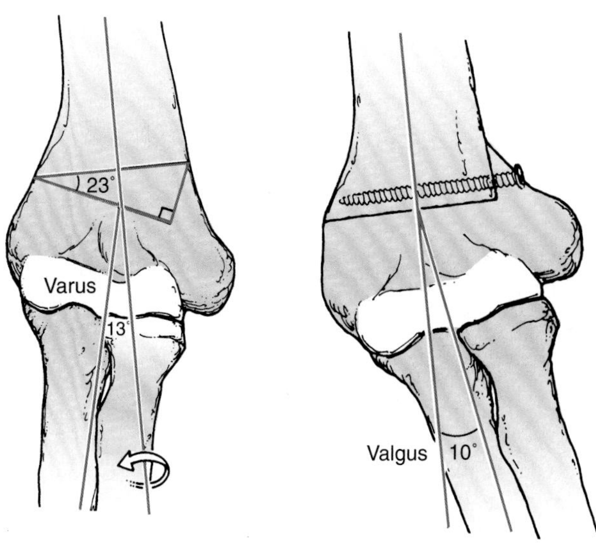

FIGURE 14-45 The step-cut osteotomy. The distal fragment can be rotated in the horizontal plane (*circular arrow*) to correct that part of the deformity. (From De Rosa GP, Graziano CP. A new osteotomy for cubitus varus. *Clin Orthop* 1988;236:160–165, with permission.)

With this incomplete osteotomy, rotation cannot be corrected, but rotational deformity was not found to be a significant problem in studies by Voss (157) and Oppenheim (182).

Japanese surgeons (183) described a dome osteotomy in which a curved osteotomy is made in the supracondylar area.

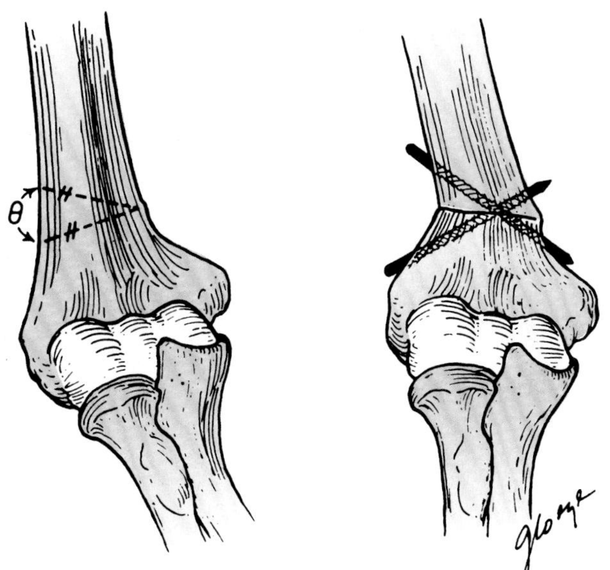

FIGURE 14-44 Technique of the lateral closing wedge osteotomy. The limbs should be of equal length, and the medial cortex should remain intact. (From Oppenheim WL, Clader TJ, Smith C, et al. Supracondylar humeral osteotomy for traumatic childhood cubitus varus deformity. *Clin Orthop* 1984;188:36, with permission.)

Proponents of this osteotomy suggest that multiplane correction is possible without inducing translation in the distal fragment and that rotation can be corrected. This osteotomy is best performed through a posterior approach.

DeRosa and Graziano (184) described a step-cut osteotomy (Fig. 14-45) in which the distal fragment is slotted into the proximal fragment and the osteotomy is secured with a single screw. Multiple osteotomies with varying degrees of complexity have been recommended. In general, increasing complexity means increasing complications. No series of osteotomies has been reported without some significant complications.

Results of Osteotomy

Functional outcomes are generally good, but the preoperative functional deficit is nearly always minor in patients with cubitus varus deformities. Complications of humeral osteotomy include stiffness, nerve injury, and persistent deformity (Table 14-3); however, with a properly performed osteotomy, complications are relatively few. Ippolito et al (185) reported long-term follow-up of patients with supracondylar osteotomies, 50% of whom had poor results. Increasing deficit has been reported after osteotomy in young children, but this did not occur in the series reported by Voss et al (157) in which four patients had growth arrest and avascular necrosis; lateral epiphysiodesis was performed to prevent recurrent deformity in two of these patients.

Hyperextension deformity may remodel over time (Fig. 14-42), but correction is slow and inconsistent. In one series (157), hyperextension deformities remodeled as much as 30 degrees in very young children, but in older children, there was no significant remodeling in the flexion/extension plane. If hyperextension appears to be a major problem, osteotomy should also be directed at this deformity rather than simple correction of the varus deformity; this situation requires a multiplane osteotomy.

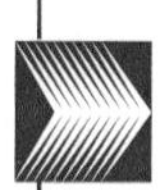

AUTHORS' PREFERRED TREATMENT

We prefer an incomplete lateral closing wedge osteotomy to correct most cubitus varus deformities. It is a simple procedure with a very low complication rate. A lateral approach is used rather than a posterior approach, and it is a muscle-preserving osteotomy that allows rapid rehabilitation after healing. Stiffness and nerve injury are rare complications of this procedure. Performing the procedure with the patient supine allows easy observation of the correction achieved. K-wire fixation can be used in the juvenile age group and screw fixation can be used in adolescents. By taking this route as an oblique osteotomy, the apex, or center of rotation is closer to the deformity resulting in less translation of the distal fragment. The distal cut should be just proximal to the olecranon and coronoid fossa.

There is no reason to mobilize the ulnar nerve, but care is taken not to penetrate the medial cortex with a saw. The radial nerve's position limits proximal lateral dissection. Symeonides et al (186) reported finding a radial nerve entrapped within fracture callus in the lateral aspect of the metaphysis. With severe deformity or neurologic abnormality, anatomy of neurovascular structures is unlikely to be normal and nerve exploration is necessary.

Wilkins recommended combining dome and lateral closing wedge osteotomies through a posterior approach for multiplanar correction. This procedure is performed with the patient prone. For patients with significant hyperextension deformity, we would choose this approach and procedure for multiplanar correction.

FLEXION-TYPE SUPRACONDYLAR FRACTURE

Flexion-type supracondylar humeral fractures account for about 2% of humeral fractures. A flexion pattern of injury may not be recognized until reduction is attempted because initial radiographs are inadequate. A key to recognizing a flexion-type supracondylar fracture is that it is unstable in flexion, whereas extension-type fractures generally are stable in hyperflexion. A laterally displaced supracondylar fracture may actually be a flexion-type injury.

Etiology and Pathology

The mechanism of injury is generally believed to be a fall directly onto the elbow rather than a fall onto the outstretched hand with hyperextension of the elbow (Fig. 14-46). The distal fragment is

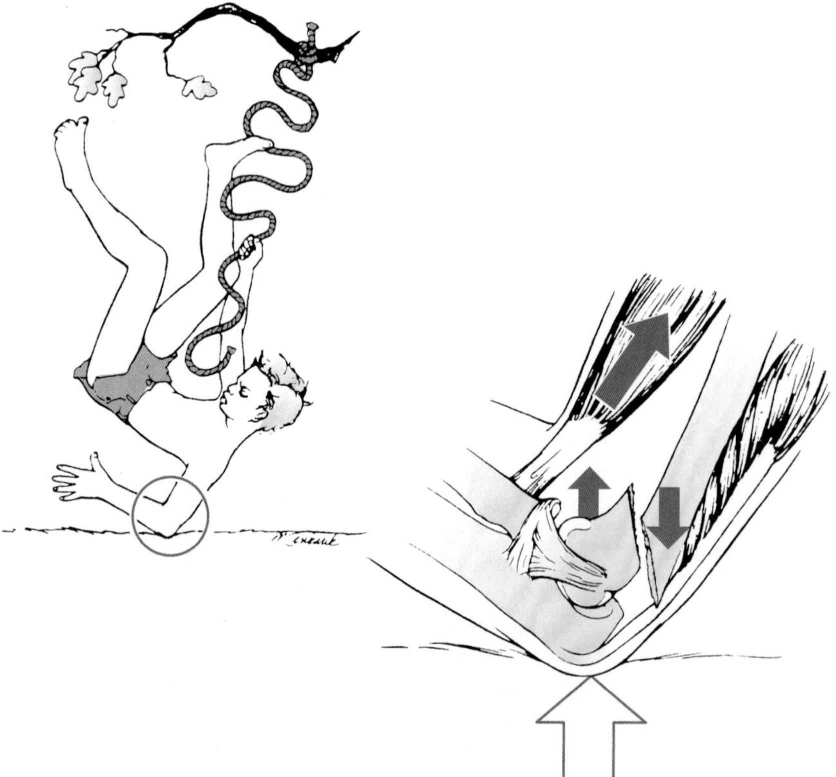

FIGURE 14-46 Flexion mechanism. Flexion-type fractures usually result from a blow to the posterior aspect of the elbow. The obliquity of the fracture line may be opposite that of an extension type. The large black arrows demonstrate the usual direction of fragment displacement.

displaced anteriorly and may migrate proximally in a totally displaced fracture. The ulnar nerve is vulnerable in this fracture pattern (149,152,187,188), and it may be entrapped in the fracture or in the healing callus (189).

X-Ray Findings

The x-ray appearance of the distal fragment varies from mild angular deformity to complete anterior displacement. Anterior displacement is often accompanied by medial or lateral translation (Fig. 14-47). Associated fractures of the proximal humerus and radius mandate full x-ray evaluation of the upper extremity. Fracture classification is the same as for extension-type supracondylar fractures (36): type I, nondisplaced fracture; type II, minimally angulated with cortical contact; and type III, totally unstable displaced distal fracture fragment.

Treatment

In general, type I flexion-type supracondylar fractures are stable nondisplaced fractures that can simply be protected in a long-arm cast (28,190,191). If mild angulation, as in a type II fracture, requires some reduction in extension, the arm can be immobilized with the elbow fully extended. X-ray evaluation with the elbow extended is easily obtained and accurate in determining the adequacy of reduction. Reduction is assessed by evaluat-

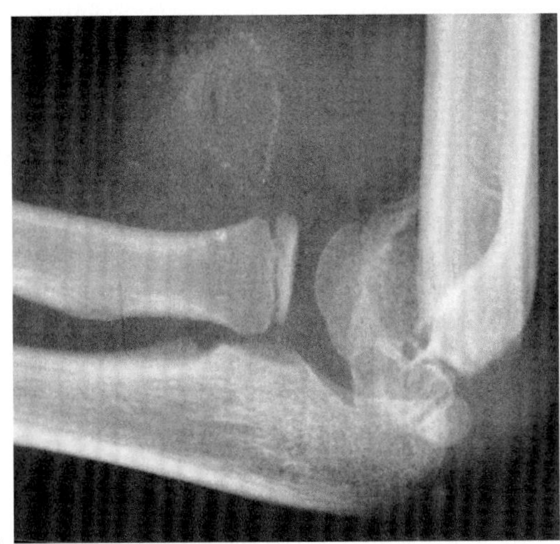

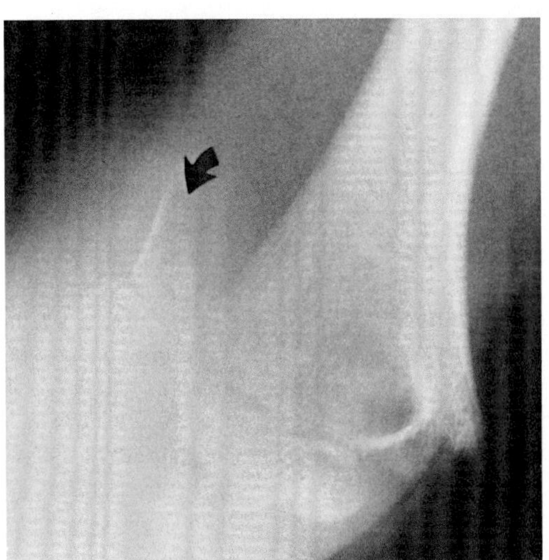

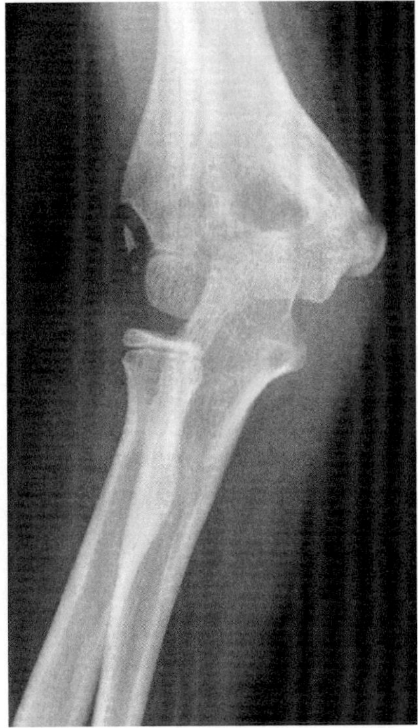

FIGURE 14-47 Flexion valgus deformity. Lateral **(A)** and AP views **(B)** of a flexion-type supracondylar fracture. The distal fragment (*arrow*) is laterally displaced in the coronal plane as well. Despite aggressive treatment, there was mild residual cubitus valgus plus a flexion contracture when the fracture healed **(C)**. (From Wilkins KE. Residuals of elbow trauma in children. *Orthop Clin N Am* 1990;21:291–314, with permission.)

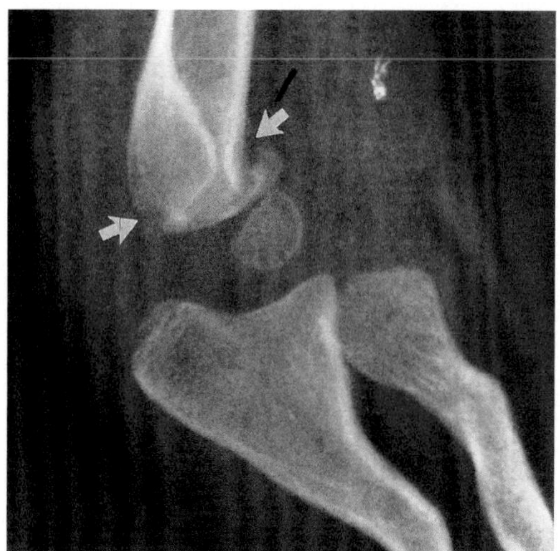

FIGURE 14-48 Type I flexion injury. A type I flexion supracondylar fracture pattern (*arrows*) in a 6-year-old below-the-elbow amputee. There is only about a 10 degree increase in the shaft condylar angle. The patient was treated with a simple posterior splint.

ing the olecranon fossa, Baumann's angle, and the anterior humeral line intersecting the lateral condyle. If reduction cannot be obtained, as is often the case, or if rotation persists, soft tissue interposition, possibly the ulnar nerve, should be suspected. DeBoeck studied 22 flexion-type supracondylar fractures (192). He found cast treatment to be satisfactory in nondisplaced cases, as one would expect. In the other 15 cases, closed reduction and percutaneous pinning was successful in most patients.

A problem with type III flexion supracondylar fractures is that reduction is not easy to achieve and when achieved, the elbow is usually in extension, making it quite difficult to stabilize the distal fragment using pins.

Type I and II fractures (Figs. 14-48 and 14-49) are generally reduced if any angular displacement is seen on fluoroscopic intraoperative evaluation. Type II fractures can be immobilized in an extension cast with the elbow fully extended (Fig. 14-49). A ring is applied so that a sling around the neck can support the cast's weight. The cast is removed at 3 weeks. If closed reduction is performed without skeletal stabilization, follow-up x-rays usually are taken at 1 week and when the cast is removed at 3 weeks.

Pinning is generally required for unstable type II and III flexion supracondylar fractures. The pinning technique described for extension-type supracondylar fractures is not appropriate for this fracture, because its instability in flexion precludes pinning with the elbow hyperflexed. Pinning should be performed after closed reduction with the elbow in mild flexion or full extension.

In a flexion-type supracondylar fracture, if reduction can be obtained in extension, it is rarely, if ever, stable in flexion. Sometimes, the soft tissue injury is so severe that the distal fragment may be manipulated in almost any direction, demonstrating significant instability. In general, a slightly less-than-anatomic reduction can be accepted as long as (a) there is no soft tissue interposition of tissue, (b) Baumann's angle is close to the other side, and (c) neither flexion nor extension is seen on the lateral view. Although rotating the arm is often possible for a lateral view of extension supracondylar fracture, the C-arm must be moved to obtain satisfactory x-ray results when pinning a flexion-type supracondylar fracture, because they are usually rotationally unstable even when reduced.

Pinning is generally performed with the elbow in approximately 30 degrees of flexion, holding the elbow in a reduced position (Fig. 14-50). If closed reduction can be obtained, pinning can be accomplished in this position. Placing a trac-

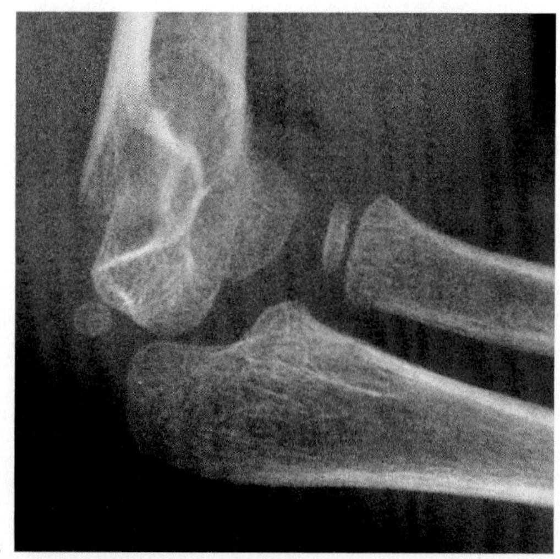

A

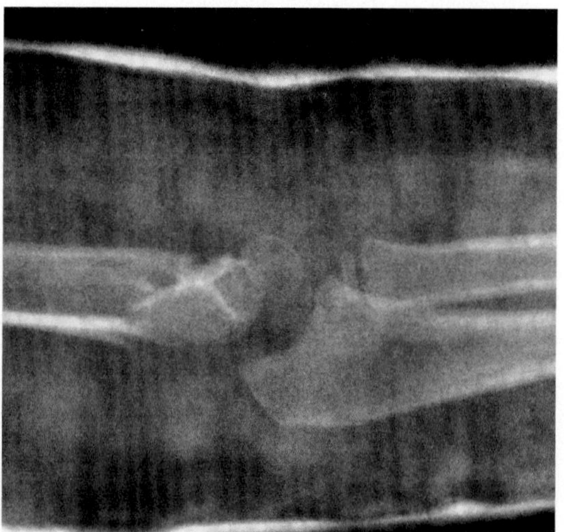

B

FIGURE 14-49 Closed reduction, extension cast. **A.** A 5-year-old girl sustained a type II flexion pattern. **B.** She was manipulated into extension and found to be stable, and thus was maintained in a long-arm cast in extension.

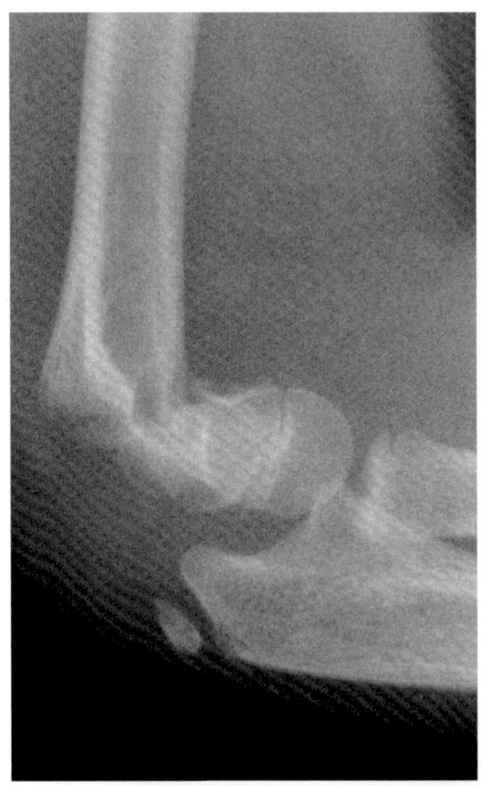

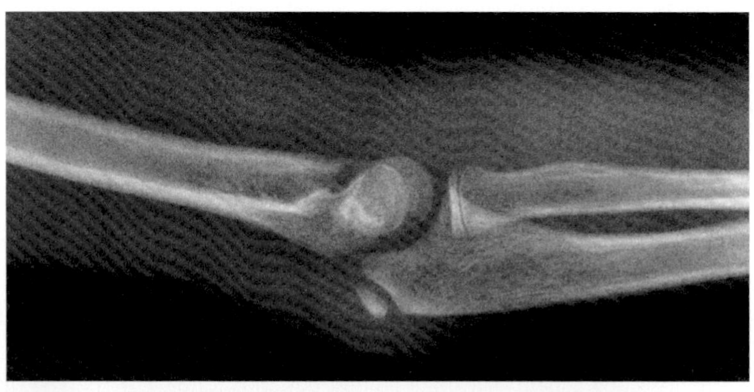

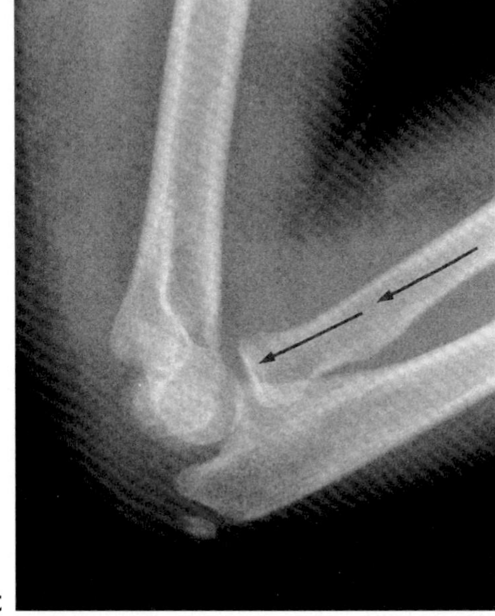

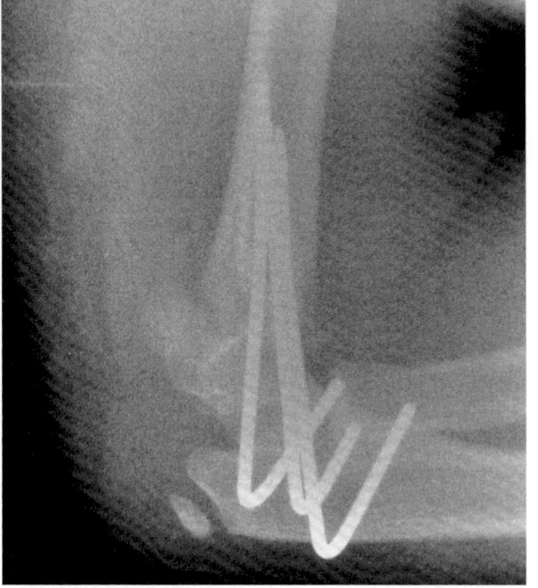

FIGURE 14-50 Closed reduction, pin fixation. **A.** Injury film of a 9-year-old with a type II flexion injury. **B.** A satisfactory reduction was achieved by fully extending the elbow. **C.** The elbow was then gradually flexed to full flexion, maintaining pressure proximally through the forearm (*arrows*) to keep the distal humeral fragment extended. **D.** The distal fragment was then secured with three pins placed laterally.

tion-type of olecranon wing nut through the proximal ulna to give a better grip on the distal fragment may facilitate reduction.

The lateral pin is generally placed first through the lateral condyle, extending through the proximal fragment and engaging the opposite cortex. The medial pin is then placed through the medial epicondyle. We make a small incision over the medial epicondyle to ensure that the ulnar nerve is not entrapped in the fracture.

After pinning a flexion-type supracondylar fracture, the arm should be placed in a bivalved cast. If the fracture is held in anatomic position with pins, a flexed-arm cast can be used to provide better patient comfort, but a cast with the elbow in almost full extension is acceptable.

Open reduction may be required for flexion-type supracondylar fractures. Open reduction is best performed through an anteromedial or posterior approach, rather than an anterior approach, as is used for extension-type supracondylar fractures. With flexion-type fractures, brachialis remains intact and must be retracted in order to expose the fracture, necessitating a medial extension to the anterior approach. To ensure that the ulnar nerve is not entrapped in the fracture site, exploring the ulnar nerve or at least identification is probably advisable with this fracture, which is another reason for a medial approach to open reduction.

Anteromedial Open Reduction of Flexion-Type Supracondylar Fractures

The surgeon makes a transverse incision across the antecubital fossa, curving proximally posterior to the neuromuscular bundle. Dissection is carried down to the level of the superficial fascia of the forearm and antecubital fossa. The neurovascular bundle is identified and retracted medially. The brachialis and biceps tendons are retracted laterally to expose the fracture site and facilitate reduction. If there is medial soft tissue impingement or a question of ulnar nerve entrapment within the fracture, the dissection should be carried around posterior to the medial epicondyle, so the ulnar nerve and fracture can be identified.

Postoperative immobilization is maintained for 3 or 4 weeks until good callus formation is present. Pins are generally left out through the skin and removed in the office without the need for anesthetic. No immediate rehabilitation is given, but the patient is encouraged to begin gentle activities with the arm and to begin regaining motion without a stressful exercise program.

Traction

Traction is used very rarely for this type of fracture, but the elbow is generally unstable in increased flexion, which is a comfortable position for the patient in traction. Although overhead traction works best for extension-type supracondylar fractures, we think that side arm traction might be better for this fracture; however, we are not aware of any data on this issue. X-ray evaluation in traction is mandatory to confirm the adequacy of reduction. After approximately 14 days in traction, with a stable distal humeral fracture and good callus formation, the arm is immobilized in a cast with the elbow in extension, and x-rays are obtained. We prefer wing nut–type traction for this to apply skeletal traction with the elbow flexed 30 to 40 degrees for comfort. This method may require some sling suspension, as well as a skeletal traction pin or wing nut. If an ulnar neuropathy develops in traction, the nerve is probably trapped in the fracture, and open reduction as well as ulnar nerve exploration are indicated.

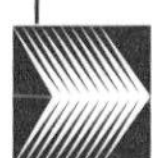

AUTHORS' PREFERRED TREATMENT

In general, we treat type I flexion supracondylar fractures with a splint or cast with the elbow flexed for comfort. Minimally displaced type II fractures that reduce in extension are treated in an extension cast. Unstable types II and III fractures are pinned. We make a small incision over the medial epicondyle if a medial pin is placed. Open reduction through an anteromedial or posterior approach is used if an anatomic closed reduction cannot be obtained.

ACKNOWLEDGMENTS

The authors thank Kaye Wilkins for his past contributions to this chapter, his work in developing effective management methods, and his efforts in communicating this information to the orthopaedic community.

REFERENCES

1. Blount WP. *Fractures in Children.* Baltimore: Williams & Wilkins, 1955:26–42.
2. Boyd DW, Aronson DD. Supracondylar fractures of the humerus: a prospective study of percutaneous pinning. *J Pediatr Orthop* 1992;12(6):789–794.
3. Cramer KE, Devito DP, Green NE. Comparison of closed reduction and percutaneous pinning versus open reduction and percutaneous pinning in displaced supracondylar fractures of the humerus in children. *J Orthop Trauma* 1992;6(4):407–412.
4. France J, Strong M. Deformity and function in supracondylar fractures of the humerus in children variously treated by closed reduction and splinting, traction, and percutaneous pinning. *J Pediatr Orthop* 1992;12(4):494–498.
5. Pirone AM, Krajbich JI, Graham HK. Management of displaced supracondylar fractures of the humerus in children [letter]. *J Bone Joint Surg (Am)* 1989;71:313.
6. Topping RE, Blanco JS, Davis TJ. Clinical evaluation of crossed-pin versus lateral-pin fixation in displaced supracondylar humerus fractures. *J Pediatr Orthop* 1995;15(4): 435–439.
7. Sutton WR, Greene WB, Georgopoulos G, et al. Displaced supracondylar humeral fractures in children. A comparison of results and costs in patients treated by skeletal traction versus percutaneous pinning. *Clin Orthop Relat Res* 1992;(278):81–87.
8. Cheng JC, Lam TP, Maffulli N. Epidemiological features of supracondylar fractures of the humerus in Chinese children. *J Pediatr Orthop B* 2001;10(1):63–67.
9. Farnsworth CL, Silva PD, Mubarak SJ. Etiology of supracondylar humerus fractures. *J Pediatr Orthop* 1998;18(1):38–42.
10. Houshian S, Mehdi B, Larsen MS. The epidemiology of elbow fracture in children: analysis of 355 fractures, with special reference to supracondylar humerus fractures. *J Orthop Sci* 2001;6(4):312–315.
11. Cramer KE, Green NE, Devito DP. Incidence of anterior interosseous nerve palsy in supracondylar humerus fractures in children. *J Pediatr Orthop* 1993;13(4):502–505.
12. Spinner M, Schreiber SN. Anterior interosseous-nerve paralysis as a complication of supracondylar fractures of the humerus in children. *J Bone Joint Surg (Am)* 1969;51(8): 1584–1590.
13. Blount WP. Volkmann's ischemic contracture. *Surg Gynecol Obstet* 1950;90:244–246.
14. Nassar A, Chater E. Open reduction and Kirschner wire fixation for supracondylar fracture of the humerus (Scientific Exhibit). In American Orthopaedic Association Meeting. Toronto, 1992.
15. Zaltz I, Waters PM, Kasser JR. Ulnar nerve instability in children. *J Pediatr Orthop* 1996; 16(5):567–569.
16. Strait RT, Siegel RM, Shapiro RA. Humeral fractures without obvious etiologies in children less than 3 years of age: when is it abuse? *Pediatrics* 1995;96(4 Pt 1):667–671.
17. Powell RS, Bowe JA. Ipsilateral supracondylar humerus fracture and Monteggia lesion: a case report. *J Orthop Trauma* 2002;16(10):737–740.
18. Bristow WR. Myositis ossificans and Volkmann's paralysis: notes on two cases, illustrating the rarer complications of supracondylar fracture of the humerus. *Br J Surg* 1923; 10:475–481.
19. Campbell CC, Waters PM, Emans JB, et al. Neurovascular injury and displacement in type III supracondylar humerus fractures. *J Pediatr Orthop* 1995;15(1):47–52.
20. Copley LA, Dormans JP, Davidson RS. Vascular injuries and their sequelae in pediatric supracondylar humeral fractures: toward a goal of prevention. *J Pediatr Orthop* 1996; 16(1):99–103.

21. Schoenecker PL, Delgado E, Rotman M, et al. Pulseless arm in association with totally displaced supracondylar fracture. *J Orthop Trauma* 1996;10(6):410–415.
22. Charnley J. *Closed Treatment of Common Fractures*. Edinburgh: Churchill Livingstone, 1961:105–115.
23. Minkowitz B, Busch MT. Supracondylar humerus fractures. Current trends and controversies. *Orthop Clin N Am* 1994;25(4):581–594.
24. Nork SE, Hennrikus WL, Loncarich DP, et al. Relationship between ligamentous laxity and the site of upper extremity fractures in children: extension supracondylar fracture versus distal forearm fracture. *J Pediatr Orthop B* 1999;8(2):90–92.
25. McLauchlan GJ, Walker CR, Cowan B, et al. Extension of the elbow and supracondylar fractures in children. *J Bone Joint Surg (Br)* 1999;81(3):402–405.
26. Kocher T. *Beitrage zur Kenntniss Einiger Praktisch Wichtiger Fracturformen*. Edited by Sallmann C, Basil, 1895.
27. Holmberg L. Fractures in the distal end of the humerus in children. *Acta Chir Scand* 1945;92:(Suppl 103):1–69.
28. Nand S. Management of supracondylar fracture of the humerus in children. *Int Surg* 1972;57(11):893–898.
29. Godley DR, Leong JCY, Yau A. Open reduction and internal fixation of supracondylar fractures of the humerus in children in Hong Kong: long-term results. *Abbot Proc* 1978; 9:30–34.
30. Kekomaki M, Luoma R, Rikalainen H, et al. Operative reduction and fixation of a difficult supracondylar extension fracture of the humerus. *J Pediatr Orthop* 1984;4(1): 13–15.
31. Salter RB. *Textbook of Disorders and Injuries of the Musculoskeletal System*. Baltimore: Williams & Wilkins, 1970.
32. Arnold JA, Nasca RJ, Nelson CL. Supracondylar fractures of the humerus: the role of dynamic factors in prevention of deformity. *J Bone Joint Surg (Am)* 1977;59(5):589–595.
33. Khare GN, Gautam VK, Kochhar VL, et al. Prevention of cubitus varus deformity in supracondylar fractures of the humerus. *Injury* 1991;22(3):202–206.
34. Abraham E, Powers T, Witt P, et al. Experimental hyperextension supracondylar fractures in monkeys. *Clin Orthop Relat Res* 1982;(171):309–318.
35. Wilkins KE, Beaty J. *Fractures in Children*. Philadelphia: Lippincott-Raven, 1996.
36. Gartland JJ. Management of supracondylar fractures of the humerus in children. *Surg Gynecol Obstet* 1959;109(2):145–154.
37. Skaggs DL, Mirzayan R. The posterior fat pad sign in association with occult fracture of the elbow in children. *J Bone Joint Surg (Am)* 1999;81(10):1429–1433.
38. Ziv N, Litwin A, Katz K, et al. Definitive diagnosis of fracture-separation of the distal humeral epiphysis in neonates by ultrasonography. *Pediatr Radiol* 1996;26(7): 493–496.
39. Sairyo K, Henmi T, Kanematsu Y, et al. Radial nerve palsy associated with slightly angulated pediatric supracondylar humerus fracture. *J Orthop Trauma* 1997;11(3): 227–229.
40. Williamson DM, Cole WG. Treatment of selected extension supracondylar fractures of the humerus by manipulation and strapping in flexion. *Injury* 1993;24(4):249–252.
41. Mapes RC, Hennrikus WL. The effect of elbow position on the radial pulse measured by Doppler ultrasonography after surgical treatment of supracondylar elbow fractures in children. *J Pediatr Orthop* 1998;18(4):441–444.
42. De Boeck H, De Smet P, Penders W, et al. Supracondylar elbow fractures with impaction of the medial condyle in children. *J Pediatr Orthop* 1995;15(4):444–448.
43. Cheng JC, Lam TP, Shen WY. Closed reduction and percutaneous pinning for type III displaced supracondylar fractures of the humerus in children. *J Orthop Trauma* 1995; 9(6):511–515.
44. Archibeck MJ, Scott SM, Peters CL. Brachialis muscle entrapment in displaced supracondylar humerus fractures: a technique of closed reduction and report of initial results. *J Pediatr Orthop* 1997;17(3):298–302.
45. Peters CL, Scott SM, Stevens PM. Closed reduction and percutaneous pinning of displaced supracondylar humerus fractures in children: description of a new closed reduction technique for fractures with brachialis muscle entrapment. *J Orthop Trauma* 1995; 9(5):430–434.
46. Fleuriau-Chateau P, McIntyre W, Letts M. An analysis of open reduction of irreducible supracondylar fractures of the humerus in children. *Can J Surg* 1998;41(2):112–128.
47. Millis MB, Singer IJ, Hall JE. Supracondylar fracture of the humerus in children. Further experience with a study in orthopaedic decision-making. *Clin Orthop Relat Res* 1984; 188:90–97.
48. Kurer MH, Regan MW. Completely displaced supracondylar fracture of the humerus in children. A review of 1708 comparable cases. *Clin Orthop Relat Res* 1990;(256): 205–214.
49. Pirone AM, Graham HK, Krajbich JI. Management of displaced extension-type supracondylar fractures of the humerus in children. *J Bone Joint Surg (Am)* 1988;70(5): 641–650.
50. Walloe A, Egund N, Eikelund L. Supracondylar fracture of the humerus in children: review of closed and open reduction leading to a proposal for treatment. *Injury* 1985; 16(5):296–299.
51. Hadlow AT, Devane P, Nicol RO. A selective treatment approach to supracondylar fracture of the humerus in children. *J Pediatr Orthop* 1996;16(1):104–106.
52. Alburger PD, Weidner PL, Betz RR. Supracondylar fractures of the humerus in children. *J Pediatr Orthop* 1992;12(1):16–19.
53. Jones KG. Percutaneous pin fixation of fractures of the lower end of the humerus. *Clin Orthop Relat Res* 1967;50:53–69.
54. Miller OL. Blind nailing of the T fracture of the lower end of the humerus which includes the joint. *J Bone Joint Surg* 1939;21:933–938.
55. Swenson AL. The treatment of supracondylar fractures of the humerus by Kirschner wire transfixion. *J Bone Joint Surg (Am)* 1948;30:993–997.
56. Flynn JC, Matthews JG, Benoit RL. Blind pinning of displaced supracondylar fractures of the humerus in children. Sixteen years' experience with long-term follow-up. *J Bone Joint Surg (Am)* 1974;56(2):263–272.
57. Flynn JC, Zink WP. Fractures and dislocations of the elbow. In: MacEwen GD, Kasser JR, Heinrich SD, eds. *Pediatric Fractures: A Practical Approach to Assessment and Treatment*. Baltimore: Williams & Wilkins, 1993:133–164.
58. Wilkins KE. Supracondylar fractures: what's new? *J Pediatr Orthop B* 1997;6(2): 110–116.
59. Mehlman CT, Crawford AH, McMillion TL, et al. Operative treatment of supracondylar fractures of the humerus in children: the Cincinnati experience. *Acta Orthop Belg* 1996; 62(Suppl 1):41–50.
60. Mehserle WL, Meehan PL. Treatment of the displaced supracondylar fracture of the humerus (type III) with closed reduction and percutaneous cross-pin fixation. *J Pediatr Orthop* 1991;11(6):705–711.
61. Bostman O, Makela EA, Sodergard J, et al. Absorbable polyglycolide pins in internal fixation of fractures in children. *J Pediatr Orthop* 1993;13(2):242–245.
62. Zionts LE, McKellop HA, Hathaway R. Torsional strength of pin configurations used to fix supracondylar fractures of the humerus in children. *J Bone Joint Surg (Am)* 1994; 76(2):253–256.
63. Lee SS, Mahar AT, Miesen D, et al. Displaced pediatric supracondylar humerus fractures: biomechanical analysis of percutaneous pinning techniques. *J Pediatr Orthop* 2002;22(4):440–443.
64. Onwuanyi ON, Nwobi DG. Evaluation of the stability of pin configuration in K-wire fixation of displaced supracondylar fractures in children. *Int Surg* 1998;83(3):271–274.
65. Skaggs DL, Hale JM, Bassett J, et al. Operative treatment of supracondylar fractures of the humerus in children. The consequences of pin placement. *J Bone Joint Surg (Am)* 2001;83A(5):735–740.
66. Solak S, Aydin E. Comparison of two percutaneous pinning methods for the treatment of the pediatric type III supracondylar humerus fractures. *J Pediatr Orthop B* 2003; 12(5):346–349.
67. Brown IC, Zinar DM. Traumatic and iatrogenic neurological complications after supracondylar humerus fractures in children. *J Pediatr Orthop* 1995;15(4):440–443.
68. Ikram MA. Ulnar nerve palsy: a complication following percutaneous fixation of supracondylar fractures of the humerus in children. *Injury* 1996;27(5):303–305.
69. Rasool MN. Ulnar nerve injury after K-wire fixation of supracondylar humerus fractures in children. *J Pediatr Orthop* 1998;18(5):686–690.
70. Royce RO, Dutkowsky JP, Kasser JR, et al. Neurologic complications after K-wire fixation of supracondylar humerus fractures in children. *J Pediatr Orthop* 1991;11(2): 191–194.
71. Michael SP, Stanislas MJ. Localization of the ulnar nerve during percutaneous wiring of supracondylar fractures in children. *Injury* 1996;27(5):301–302.
72. Wind WM, Schwend RM, Armstrong DG. Predicting ulnar nerve location in pinning of supracondylar humerus fractures. *J Pediatr Orthop* 2002;22(4):444–447.
73. Arino VL, Lluch EE, Ramirez AM, et al. Percutaneous fixation of supracondylar fractures of the humerus in children. *J Bone Joint Surg (Am)* 1977;59(7):914–916.
74. Skaggs DL, Cluck MW, Mostofi A, et al. Lateral-entry pin fixation in the management of supracondylar fractures in children. *J Bone Joint Surg (Am)* 2004;86A(4):702–707.
75. Gordon JE, Patton CM, Luhmann SJ, et al. Fracture stability after pinning of displaced supracondylar distal humerus fractures in children. *J Pediatr Orthop* 2001;21(3): 313–318.
76. Iyengar SR, Hoffinger, SA, Townsend DR. Early versus delayed reduction and pinning of type III displaced supracondylar fractures of the humerus in children: a comparative study. *J Orthop Trauma* 1999;13(1):51–55.
77. Mehlman CT, Strub WM, Roy DR, et al. The effect of surgical timing on the perioperative complications of treatment of supracondylar humeral fractures in children. *J Bone Joint Surg (Am)* 2001;83A(3):323–327.
78. Leet AI, Frisancho J, Ebramzadeh E. Delayed treatment of type 3 supracondylar humerus fractures in children. *J Pediatr Orthop* 2002;22(2):203–207.
79. Gupta N, Kay RM, Leitch K, et al. Effect of surgical delay on perioperative complications and need for open reduction in supracondylar humerus fractures in children. *J Pediatr Orthop* 2004;24(3):245–248.
80. Prevot J, Lascombes P, Metaizeau JP, et al. Supracondylar fractures of the humerus in children: treatment by downward nailing. *Rev Chir Orthop Reparatrice Appar Mot* 1990; 76(3):191–197.
81. Kim WY, Chandru R, Bonshahi A, et al. Displaced supracondylar humeral fractures in children: results of a national survey of paediatric orthopaedic consultants. *Injury* 2003; 34(4):274–277.
82. Mazda K, Boggione C, Fitoussi F, et al. Systematic pinning of displaced extension-type supracondylar fractures of the humerus in children. A prospective study of 116 consecutive patients. *J Bone Joint Surg (Br)* 2001;83(6):888–893.
83. Reitman RD, Waters P, Millis M. Open reduction and internal fixation for supracondylar humerus fractures in children. *J Pediatr Orthop* 2001;21(2):157–161.
84. Oh CW, Park BC, Kim PT, et al. Completely displaced supracondylar humerus fractures in children: results of open reduction versus closed reduction. *J Orthop Sci* 2003;8(2): 37–41.
85. Kaewpornsawan K. Comparison between closed reduction with percutaneous pinning and open reduction with pinning in children with closed totally displaced supracondylar humeral fractures: a randomized controlled trial. *J Pediatr Orthop B* 2001;10(2): 131–137.
86. Weiland AJ, Meyer S, Tolo VT, et al. Surgical treatment of displaced supracondylar fractures of the humerus in children. Analysis of fifty-two cases followed for five to fifteen years. *J Bone Joint Surg (Am)* 1978;60(5):657–661.
87. Sibly TF, Briggs PJ, Gibson MJ. Supracondylar fractures of the humerus in childhood: range of movement following the posterior approach to open reduction. *Injury* 1991; 22(6):456–458.

88. Danielsson L, Pettersson H. Open reduction and pin fixation of severely displaced supracondylar fractures of the humerus in children. *Acta Orthop Scand* 1980;51(2): 249–255.
89. Gennari JM, Merrot T, Piclet B, et al. Anterior approach versus posterior approach to surgical treatment of children's supracondylar fractures: comparative study of thirty cases in each series. *J Pediatr Orthop B* 1998;7(4):307–313.
90. Koudstaal MJ, De Ridder VA, De Lange S, et al. Pediatric supracondylar humerus fractures: the anterior approach. *J Orthop Trauma* 2002;16(6):409–412.
91. Ponce BA, Hedequist DJ, Zurakowski D, et al. Complications and timing of follow-up after closed reduction and percutaneous pinning of supracondylar humerus fractures: follow-up after percutaneous pinning of supracondylar humerus fractures. *J Pediatr Orthop* 2004;24(6):610–614.
92. Archibald DA, Roberts JA, Smith MG. Transarticular fixation for severely displaced supracondylar fractures in children. *J Bone Joint Surg (Br)* 1991;73(1):147–149.
93. Aronson DC, van Vollenhoven E, Meeuwis JD. K-wire fixation of supracondylar humeral fractures in children: results of open reduction via a ventral approach in comparison with closed treatment. *Injury* 1993;24(3):179–181.
94. Celiker O, Pestilci FI, Tuzuner M. Supracondylar fractures of the humerus in children: analysis of the results in 142 patients. *J Orthop Trauma* 1990;4(3):265–269.
95. Furrer M, Mark G, Ruedi T. Management of displaced supracondylar fractures of the humerus in children. *Injury* 1991;22(4):259–262.
96. Gehling H, Gotzen L, Giannadakis K, et al. Treatment and outcome of supracondylar humeral fractures in childhood. *Unfallchirurg* 1995;98(2):93–97.
97. Sharrad WJW. *Pediatric Orthopaedics and Fractures*. Oxford: Blackwell Scientific, 1971.
98. Smith FM. *Surgery of the Elbow*. Philadelphia: WB Saunders, 1972.
99. Watson-Jones R. *Fractures and Joint Injuries*. Edinburgh: ES Livingstone, 1956.
100. Alcott WH, Bowden BW, Miller PR. Displaced supracondylar fractures of the humerus in children: long-term follow-up of 69 patients. *J Am Osteopath Assoc* 1997;76(12): 910–915.
101. Bender J. Cubitus varus after supracondylar fracture of the humerus in children: can this deformity be prevented? *Reconstr Surg Traumatol* 1979;17:100–106.
102. Carcassonne M, Bergoin M, Hornung H. Results of operative treatment of severe supracondylar fractures of the elbow in children. *J Pediatr Surg* 1972;7(6):676–679.
103. Gates DJ. Supracondylar fracture of humerus: problem in children managed with open reduction. *Orthop Rev* 1982;11:91–98.
104. Gruber MA, Hudson OC. Supracondylar fracture of the humerus in childhood. End-result study of open reduction. *J Bone Joint Surg (Am)* 1964;46:1245–1252.
105. Hart GM, Wilson DW, Arden GP. The operative management of the difficult supracondylar fracture of the humerus in the child. *Injury* 1977;9(1):30–34.
106. Krebs B. Surgical treatment of supracondylar humeral fractures in children. *Ugeskr Laeger* 1980;142(14):871–872.
107. Nassar A, Chater E. Open reduction and Kirschner wire fixation for supracondylar fracture of the humerus. *J Bone Joint Surg (Br)* 1976;58:135–136.
108. Ramsey RH, Griz J. Immediate open reduction and internal fixation of severely displaced supracondylar fractures of the humerus in children. *Clin Orthop Relat Res* 1973; 90:131–132.
109. Shifrin PG, Gehring HW, Iglesias LJ. Open reduction and internal fixation of displaced supracondylar fractures of the humerus in children. *Orthop Clin N Am* 1976;7(3): 573–581.
110. Alonso-Llames M. Bilaterotricipital approach to the elbow. Its application in the osteosynthesis of supracondylar fractures of the humerus in children. *Acta Orthop Scand* 1972;43(6):479–490.
111. D'Ambrosia RD. Supracondylar fractures of humerus—prevention of cubitus varus. *J Bone Joint Surg (Am)* 1972;54(1):60–66.
112. Lal GM, Bhan S. Delayed open reduction for supracondylar fractures of the humerus. *Int Orthop* 15(3):189–191.
113. Agus H, Kalenderer O, Kayali C, Eryanilmaz G. Skeletal traction and delayed percutaneous fixation of complicated supracondylar humerus fractures due to delayed or unsuccessful reductions and extensive swelling in children. *J Pediatr Orthop B* 2002;11(2): 150–154.
114. Smith L. Deformity following supracondylar fractures of the humerus. *Am J Orthop* 1960;42A:235–252.
115. Worlock PH, Colton C. Severely displaced supracondylar fractures of the humerus in children: a simple method of treatment. *J Pediatr Orthop* 1987;7(1):49–53.
116. Smith L. Supracondylar fractures of the humerus treated by direct observation. *Clin Orthop Relat Res* 1967;50:37–42.
117. Piggot J, Graham HK, McCoy GF. Supracondylar fractures of the humerus in children. Treatment by straight lateral traction. *J Bone Joint Surg (Br)* 1986;68(4):577–583.
118. Prietto CA. Supracondylar fractures of the humerus. A comparative study of Dunlop's traction versus percutaneous pinning. *J Bone Joint Surg (Am)* 1979;61(3):425–428.
119. Palmer EE, Niemann KM, Vesely D, Armstrong JH. Supracondylar fracture of the humerus in children. *J Bone Joint Surg (Am)* 1978;60(5):653–656.
120. Badhe NP, Howard PW. Olecranon screw traction for displaced supracondylar fractures of the humerus in children. *Injury* 1998;29(6):457–460.
121. Dormans JP, Squillante R, Sharf H. Acute neurovascular complications with supracondylar humerus fractures in children. *J Hand Surg (Am)* 1995;20(1):1–4.
122. Shaw BA, Kasser JR, Emans JB, et al. Management of vascular injuries in displaced supracondylar humerus fractures without arteriography. *J Orthop Trauma* 1990;4(1): 25–29.
123. Gillingham BL, Rang M. Advances in children's elbow fractures. *J Pediatr Orthop* 1995; 15(4):419–421.
124. Ray SA, Ivory JP, Beavis, JP. Use of pulse oximetry during manipulation of supracondylar fractures of the humerus. *Injury* 1991;22(2):103–104.
125. Cairns RA, MacKenzie WG, Culham JA. Urokinase treatment of forearm ischemia complicating supracondylar fracture of the humerus in three children. *Pediatr Radiol* 1993; 23(5):391–394.
126. Sabharwal S, Tredwell SJ, Beauchamp RD, et al. Management of pulseless pink hand in pediatric supracondylar fractures of humerus. *J Pediatr Orthop* 1997;17(3):303–310.
127. Ottolenghi CE. Acute ischemic syndrome: its treatment prophylaxis of Volkmann's syndrome. *Am J Orthop* 1960;2:312–316.
128. Mubarak SJ, Carroll NC. Volkmann's contracture in children: aetiology and prevention. *J Bone Joint Surg (Br)* 1979;61B(3):285–293.
129. Holden CE. The pathology and prevention of Volkmann's ischaemic contracture. *J Bone Joint Surg (Br)* 1979;61-B(3):296–300.
130. Heppenstall RB, Sapega AA, Scott R, et al. The compartment syndrome. An experimental and clinical study of muscular energy metabolism using phosphorus nuclear magnetic resonance spectroscopy. *Clin Orthop Relat Res* 1988;(226):138–155.
131. Blakemore LC, Cooperman DR, Thompson GH, et al. Compartment syndrome in ipsilateral humerus and forearm fractures in children. *Clin Orthop Relat Res* 2000;(376): 32–38.
132. Battaglia TC, Armstrong DG, Schwend RM. Factors affecting forearm compartment pressures in children with supracondylar fractures of the humerus. *J Pediatr Orthop* 2002;22(4):431–439.
133. Willis RB, Rorabeck CH. Treatment of compartment syndrome in children. *Orthop Clin N Am* 1990;21(2):401–412.
134. McGraw JJ, Akbarnia BA, Hanel DP, et al. Neurological complications resulting from supracondylar fractures of the humerus in children. *J Pediatr Orthop* 1986;6(6): 647–650.
135. Spinner RJ, Jacobson SR, Nunley JA. Fracture of a supracondylar humeral myositis ossificans. *J Orthop Trauma* 1995;9(3):263–265.
136. Culp RW, Osterman AL, Davidson RS, et al. Neural injuries associated with supracondylar fractures of the humerus in children. *J Bone Joint Surg (Am)* 1990;72(8): 1211–1215.
137. Amillo S, Barrios RH, Martinez-Peric R, et al. Surgical treatment of the radial nerve lesions associated with fractures of the humerus. *J Orthop Trauma* 1993;7(3):211–215.
138. Banskota A, Volz RG. Traumatic laceration of the radial nerve following supracondylar fracture of the elbow. A case report. *Clin Orthop Relat Res* 1984;(184):150–152.
139. Boyd HB, Altenberg AR. Fractures about the elbow in children. *Arch Surg* 1944;49: 213–224.
140. Martin DF, Tolo VT, Sellers DS, et al. Radial nerve laceration and retraction associated with a supracondylar fracture of the humerus. *J Hand Surg (Am)* 1989;14(3):542–545.
141. Lyons JP, Ashley E, Hoffer MM. Ulnar nerve palsies after percutaneous cross-pinning of supracondylar fractures in children's elbows. *J Pediatr Orthop* 1998;18(1):43–45.
142. Coventry MB, Henderson CC. Supracondylar fractures of the humerus: 49 cases in children. *Rocky Mt Med J* 1956;53(5):458–465.
143. Henrikson B. Supracondylar fracture of the humerus in children. A late review of end-results with special reference to the cause of deformity, disability and complications. *Acta Chir Scand* 1966;369(Suppl):1–72.
144. Marion J, LaGrange J, Faysse R, et al. Les fractures de l'extremite inferieure de l'humerus chez enfant. *Rev Chir Orthop* 1962;48:337–413.
145. Smith FM. Kirschner wire traction in elbow and upper arm injuries. *Am J Surg* 1947; 74:700–707.
146. Allison N. Fractures about the elbow. *J Am Med Assoc* 1927;89:1568–1572.
147. Kramhoft M, Keller IL, Solgaard S. Displaced supracondylar fractures of the humerus in children. *Clin Orthop Relat Res* 1987;(221):215–220.
148. Siris IE. Supracondylar fracture of the humerus. *Surg Gynecol Obstet* 1939;68:201–220.
149. Aitken AP, Smith L, Blackette CW. Supracondylar fractures in children. *Am J Surg* 1943;59:161–171.
150. Kim HT, Song MB, Conjares JN, et al. Trochlear deformity occurring after distal humeral fractures: magnetic resonance imaging and its natural progression. *J Pediatr Orthop* 2002;22(2):188–193.
151. Edman P, Loehr G. Supracondylar fractures of the humerus treated with olecranon traction. *Acta Chir Scand* 1963;126:505–516.
152. Fowles JV, Kassab MT. Displaced supracondylar fractures of the elbow in children. A report on the fixation of extension and flexion fractures by two lateral percutaneous pins. *J Bone Joint Surg (Br)* 1974;56B(3):490–500.
153. Hoyer A. Treatment of supracondylar fracture of the humerus by skeletal traction in an abduction splint. *J Bone Joint Surg (Am)* 1952;24-A-3:623–637.
154. Kallio PE, Foster BK, Paterson DC. Difficult supracondylar elbow fractures in children: analysis of percutaneous pinning technique. *J Pediatr Orthop* 1992;12(1):11–15.
155. Bailey GG Jr. Nerve injuries in supracondylar fractures of the humerus in children. *N Engl J Med* 1939;221:260–263.
156. Brewster AH. Fractures in the region of the elbow in children: an end-result study. *Surg Gynecol Obstet* 1940;71:643–649.
157. Voss FR, Kasser JR, Trepman E, et al. Uniplanar supracondylar humeral osteotomy with preset Kirschner wires for posttraumatic cubitus varus. *J Pediatr Orthop* 1994; 14(4):471–478.
158. Dowd GS, Hopcroft PW. Varus deformity in supracondylar fractures of the humerus in children. *Injury* 1979;10(4):297–303.
159. Chess DG, Leahey JL, Hyndman JC. Cubitus varus: significant factors. *J Pediatr Orthop* 1994;14(2):190–192.
160. Mahaisavariya B, Laupattarakasem W. Rotational deformity of the distal humerus in cubitus varus. *J Med Assoc Thai* 1994;77(1):19–24.
161. Mahaisavariya B, Laupattarakasem W. Supracondylar fracture of the humerus: malrotation versus cubitus varus deformity. *Injury* 1993;24(6):416–418.
162. Davids JR, Maguire MF, Mubarak SJ, et al. Lateral condylar fracture of the humerus following posttraumatic cubitus varus. *J Pediatr Orthop* 1994;14(4):466–470.

163. Takahara M, Sasaki I, Kimura T, et al. Second fracture of the distal humerus after varus malunion of a supracondylar fracture in children. *J Bone Joint Surg (Br)* 1998;80(5): 791–797.
164. Gurkan I, Bayrakci K, Tasbas B, et al. Posterior instability of the shoulder after supracondylar fractures recovered with cubitus varus deformity. *J Pediatr Orthop* 2002;22(2): 198–202.
165. Mitsunari A, Muneshige H, Ikuta Y, et al. Internal rotation deformity and tardy ulnar nerve palsy after supracondylar humeral fracture. *J Shoulder Elbow Surg* 1995;4(1 Pt 1):23–29.
166. Keenan WN, Clegg J. Variation of Baumann's angle with age, sex, and side: implications for its use in radiological monitoring of supracondylar fracture of the humerus in children. *J Pediatr Orthop* 1996;16(1):97–98.
167. Abe M, Ishizu T, Shirai H, et al. Tardy ulnar nerve palsy caused by cubitus varus deformity. *J Hand Surg (Am)* 1995;20(1):5–9.
168. Bindra RR. Brachial artery aneurysm following supracondylar fracture of the humerus (unpublished data; edited, 1990).
169. Uchida Y, Sugioka Y. Ulnar nerve palsy after supracondylar humerus fracture. *Acta Orthop Scand* 1990;61(2):118–119.
170. Ogino T, Minami A, Fukuda K. Tardy ulnar nerve palsy caused by cubitus varus deformity. *J Hand Surg (Br)* 1986;11(3):352–356.
171. Amspacher JC, Messenbaugh JF Jr. Supracondylar osteotomy of the humerus for correction of rotational and angular deformities of the elbow. *South Med J* 1964;7:846–850.
172. Bellemore MC, Barrett IR, Middleton RW, et al. Supracondylar osteotomy of the humerus for correction of cubitus varus. *J Bone Joint Surg (Br)* 1984;66(4):566–572.
173. Cotton FJ. Elbow fractures in children. *Ann Surg* 1902;35:252–269.
174. French PR. Varus deformity of the elbow following supracondylar fractures of the humerus in children. *Lancet* 1959;2:439–441.
175. Gaddy BC, Manske PR, Pruitt DL, et al. Distal humeral osteotomy for correction of posttraumatic cubitus varus. *J Pediatr Orthop* 1994;14(2):214–219.
176. Graham B, Tredwell SJ, Beauchamp RD, et al. Supracondylar osteotomy of the humerus for correction of cubitus varus. *J Pediatr Orthop* 1990;10(2):228–231.
177. Johnson E, Oppenheim WL. The problem: cubitus varus after elbow fracture. *Orthop Consultation* 1985;8–12.
178. Kagan N, Herold HZ. Correction of axial deviations after supracondylar fractures of the humerus in children. *Int Surg* 1973;58(10):735–737.
179. Labelle H, Bunnell WP, Duhaime M, et al. Cubitus varus deformity following supracondylar fractures of the humerus in children. *J Pediatr Orthop* 2(5):539–546, 1982.
180. Sweeney JG. Osteotomy of the humerus for malunion of supracondylar fractures. *J Bone Joint Surg (Br)* 1975;57:117.
181. Wong HK, Balasubramaniam P. Humeral torsional deformity after supracondylar osteotomy for cubitus varus: its influence on the postosteotomy carrying angle. *J Pediatr Orthop* 1992;12(4):490–493.
182. Oppenheim WL, Clader TJ, Smith C, et al. Supracondylar humeral osteotomy for traumatic childhood cubitus varus deformity. *Clin Orthop Relat Res* 1984;(188):34–39.
183. Higaki T, Ikuta Y. The new operation method of the domed osteotomy for 4 children with varus deformity of the elbow joint. *J Jpn Orthop* 1982;31:300–335.
184. DeRosa GP, Graziano GP. A new osteotomy for cubitus varus. *Clin Orthop Relat Res* 1988;236:160–165.
185. Ippolito E, Moneta MR, D'Arrigo C. Post-traumatic cubitus varus. Long-term follow-up of corrective supracondylar humeral osteotomy in children. *J Bone Joint Surg (Am)* 1990;72(5):757–765.
186. Symeonides PP, Paschaloglou C, Pagalides T. Radial nerve enclosed in the callus of a supracondylar fracture. *J Bone Joint Surg (Br)* 1975;57(4):523–524.
187. Hagen R. Skin-traction-treatment of supracondylar fractures of the humerus in children. A ten-year review. *Acta Orthop Scand* 1964;35:138–148.
188. Royle SG, Burke D. Ulna neuropathy after elbow injury in children. *J Pediatr Orthop* 1990;10(4):495–496.
189. Lalanandham T, Laurence WN. Entrapment of the ulnar nerve in the callus of a supracondylar fracture of the humerus. *Injury* 1984;16(2):129–130.
190. el-Ahwany MD. Supracondylar fractures of the humerus in children with a note on the surgical correction of late cubitus varus. *Injury* 1974;6(1):45–56.
191. Rang M. *Children's Fractures*. Philadelphia: JB Lippincott, 1974.
192. DeBoeck H. Flexion-type supracondylar elbow fractures in children. *J Pediatr Orthop* 2001;21(4):460–463.

SUGGESTED READING

Bakalim G, Wilppula E. Supracondylar humeral fractures in children. Causes of changes in the carrying angle of the elbow. *Acta Orthop Scand* 1972;43(5):366–374.

Berghausen T, Leslie BM, Ruby LK, Zimbler S. The severely displaced pediatric supracondylar fracture of humerus treated by skeletal traction with olecranon pin. *Orthop Rev* 1986; 15(8):510–515.

Bosanquet JS, Middleton RW. The reduction of supracondylar fractures of the humerus in children treated by traction-in-extension. A review of 18 cases. *Injury* 1983;14(4): 373–380.

Carlson CS Jr, Rosman MA. Cubitus varus: a new and simple technique for correction. *J Pediatr Orthop* 1982;2(2):199–201.

Chattoadhyay A. Suggested method of fixation in supracondylar fracture. *J Ind Med Assoc* 1984;82:204–205.

Chen RS, Liu CB, Lin XS, et al. Supracondylar extension fracture of the humerus in children. Manipulative reduction, immobilisation and fixation using a U-shaped plaster slab with the elbow in full extension. *J Bone Joint Surg (Br)* 2001;83(6):883–887.

Corkery PH. The management of supracondylar fractures of the humerus in children. *Br J Clin Pract* 1964;18:583–591.

Danielsson LG, Hussein S, el-Haddad I, Gupta RP. Staple fixation of osteotomy for cubitus varus. A simple technique used in 11 children. *Acta Orthop Scand* 1991;62(1): 55–57.

Eid AM. Reduction of displaced supracondylar fracture of the humerus in children by manipulation in flexion. *Acta Orthop Scand* 1978;49(1):39–45.

El-Sharkawi AH, Fattah HA. Treatment of displaced supracondylar fractures of the humerus in children in full extension and supination. *J Bone Joint Surg (Br)* 1965;47:273–279.

Gao GX. A simple technique for correction of cubitus varus. *Chin Med J (Engl)* 1986; 99(10): 853–854.

Hart VL. Reduction of supracondylar fractures in children. *Surgery* 1942;11:33–37.

Ippolito E, Caterini R, Scola E. Supracondylar fractures of the humerus in children. Analysis at maturity of fifty-three patients treated conservatively. *J Bone Joint Surg (Am)* 1986;68(3): 333–344.

Jefferiss CD. "Straight lateral traction" in selected supracondylar fractures of the humerus in children. Injury 1977;8(3):213–220.

Kanaujia RR, Ikuta Y, Muneshige H, et al. Dome osteotomy for cubitus varus in children. *Acta Orthop Scand* 1988;59(3):314–317.

Kennedy JG, El Abed K, Soffe K, et al. Evaluation of the role of pin fixation versus collar and cuff immobilisation in supracondylar fractures of the humerus in children. *Injury* 2000;31(3):163–167.

Kristensen JL, Vivild O. Supracondylar fractures of the humerus in children. *Acta Orthop Scand* 1976;47:375–380.

Langenskiold A, Kivilaakso R. Varus and valgus deformity of the elbow following supracondylar fractures of the humerus. *Acta Orthop Scand* 1967;38:313–320.

Laupattarakasem W, Mahaisavariya B, Kowsuwon W, Saengnipanthkul S. Pentalateral osteotomy for cubitus varus. Clinical experiences of a new technique. *J Bone Joint Surg (Br)* 1989;71(4):667–670.

Laurence W. Supracondylar fractures of the humerus in children. A review of 100 cases. *Br J Surg* 1957;44:143–147.

Lipscomb PR. Vascular and neural complications in supracondylar fractures of the humerus in children. *J Bone Joint Surg (Am)* 1955;37A(3):487–492.

Matsuzaki K, Nakatani N, Harada M, Tamaki T. Treatment of supracondylar fracture of the humerus in children by skeletal traction in a brace. *J Bone Joint Surg (Br)* 2004;86(2): 232–238.

Maylahn DJ, Fahey JJ. Fractures of the elbow in children: review of three hundred consecutive cases. *J Am Med Assoc* 1958;166(3):220–228.

McCoy GF, Piggot J. Supracondylar osteotomy for cubitus varus. The value of the straight arm position. *J Bone Joint Surg (Br)* 1988;70(2):283–286.

Miller HG, Wilkins KE. The supracondylar fracture of the humerus in children. An analysis of complications. San Antonio, Texas, University of Texas Medical School, 1979 (unpublished data).

Mitchell WJ, Adams JP. Fractures and dislocations of the elbow in children. *Curr Pract Orthop Surg* 1964;23:102–124.

Nacht JL, Ecker ML, Chung SM, et al. Supracondylar fractures of the humerus in children treated by closed reduction and percutaneous pinning. *Clin Orthop Relat Res* 1983;177: 203–209.

Parikh SN, Wall EJ, Foad S, et al. Displaced type II extension supracondylar humerus fractures: do they all need pinning? *J Pediatr Orthop* 2004;24(4):380–384.

Reed FE Jr, Apple DF Jr. Ipsilateral fractures of the elbow and forearm. *South Med J* 1976; 69(2):149–151.

Reinaerts HH, Cheriex EC. Assessment of dislocation in the supracondylar fracture of the humerus, treated by overhead traction. *Reconstr Surg Traumatol* 1979;17:92–99.

Ring D, Secor C. Bow elbow (cubitus varus). *J Bone Joint Surg (Am)* 1951;33A(3):572–576.

Skolnick MD, Hall JE, Micheli LJ. Supracondylar fractures of the humerus in children. *Orthopaedics* 1980;3:395–406.

Sorrel E. Les lesions nerveuses dans les fractures fermies recentes de l'extremite inferieure de l'humerus. *Rev Ortho* 1938;25:609–647.

te Slaa RL, Faber FW, Nollen AJ, van Straaten T. Supracondylar fractures of the humerus in children; a long-term follow-up study. *Neth J Surg* 1988;40(4):100–103.

Vahvanen V, Aalto K. Supracondylar fracture of the humerus in children. A long-term follow-up study of 107 cases. *Acta Orthop Scand* 1978;49(3):225–233.

van Egmond DB, Tavenier D, Meeuwis JD. Anatomical and functional results after treatment of dislocated supracondylar fractures of the humerus in children. *Neth J Surg* 1985;37(2): 45–49.

Webb AJ, Sherman FC. Supracondylar fractures of the humerus in children. *J Pediatr Orthop* 1989;9(3):315–325.

THE ELBOW: PHYSEAL FRACTURES, APOPHYSEAL INJURIES OF THE DISTAL HUMERUS, OSTEONECROSIS OF THE TROCHLEA, AND T-CONDYLAR FRACTURES

James H. Beaty and James R. Kasser

PHYSEAL FRACTURES

All the physes of the distal humerus are vulnerable to injury, each with a distinct fracture pattern. This vulnerability of the various physes to injury is altered by age and injury mechanism. Next to those of the distal radius, injuries to the distal humeral physes are the most common physeal injuries. In general, the physes of the major long bones are most vulnerable to fracture just before puberty, when the perichondral ring is weakest (1). Fractures involving the medial epicondylar apophysis are most common in preadolescents (peak ages, 11 to 15 years), probably because many avulsions of this apophysis are associated with posterolateral dislocations, which are also common in this age group. Fractures involving the lateral condylar physis occur early, with the average age around 6 years (1,2–5). Fractures concerning the medial condylar physis are rare and occur most often in children 8 to 12 years of age (2,4,5). Fractures involving the total distal humeral physis may occur in neonates or within the first 2 to 3 years of life (6,7).

The specific fracture patterns, incidence, and mechanism of injury are discussed in detail in the following sections dealing with these specific fractures.

Fractures Involving the Lateral Condylar Physis

Incidence and Outcome

Fractures involving the lateral condylar region in the immature skeleton either cross the physis or follow it for a short distance into the trochlea. Fractures of the lateral condylar physis constitute 16.9% of distal humeral fractures.

Fractures of the lateral condylar physis are only occasionally associated with injuries outside the elbow region (8–10). Within the elbow region, the associated injuries that can occur with this fracture include dislocation of the elbow (which may be a result of the injury to the lateral condylar physis rather than a separate injury), radial head fractures, and fractures of the olecranon, which are often greenstick fractures. Acute fractures involving only the anatomic capitellum are rare in the immature skeleton.

The diagnosis of lateral condylar physeal injuries may be less obvious both clinically and on x-ray than that of supracondylar fractures, especially if the fracture is minimally displaced. Functional loss of range of motion in the elbow is much more frequent with lateral condylar physis fractures because the fracture line often extends into the articular surface. Malunion of a supracondylar fracture that results in cubitus varus is likely to result in a surgically correctable cosmetic deformity with an essentially normal range of motion in the elbow. A poorly treated lateral condylar physeal injury, however, is likely to result in a significant loss of range of motion that is not as responsive to surgical correction. The complications of supracondylar fractures are usually evident in the immediate postinjury period. The poor outcome of a lateral condylar physeal fracture may not be obvious until months or even years later (11–13). Ippolito et al (11) evaluated 49 individuals with humeral condylar fractures 18 to 45 years after the injury. Twenty fractures with displacement of 2 mm to 10 mm with no tilting of the osteochondral fragment had been treated without reduction, and 16 fractures with marked displacement and fragment tilting had been treated surgically; all 36 had good results. All 13 patients treated operatively or nonoperatively for old, displaced fractures had poor results. Nonunion developed in four patients, and osteonecrosis occurred in six. Arthrosis of the elbow was found in fractures complicated by osteonecrosis and nonunion and in old fractures when the humeral condyle was resected, but it was not observed in uncomplicated fractures.

Fracture Anatomy and Classification

Milch (14) defined fractures that exited through the trochleo-capitellar groove as type I and those that exited through the trochlea as type II. Around the same time, Cotton (15) described more details of the various subluxations of both the fragment and elbow joint that occurred with this type of fracture. He noted that because the fragment was usually still attached to the proximal radius, both the radius and ulna were subluxed. The most common displacement was "outward and backward"; "inward and forward" displacement was rare. Cotton also noted that the main pathology was associated with condylar fragment rotation. He observed that this fracture often resulted in limited extension, had some local lateral outgrowth at the fracture site, and rarely resulted in axial deviation of the elbow unless there was a resultant nonunion. More recent investigators have added little to his description of this lesion's pathology.

Lateral condylar physeal fractures can be classified by either the fracture line's anatomic location or by the stage of displacement, as described by Wilkins.

Anatomic Location. Salter and Harris classified lateral condylar physeal injuries as type IV injuries in their classification of physeal fractures (16). A true Salter-Harris type IV injury through the ossific nucleus of the lateral condyle is rare. Although lateral condylar fractures are similar to Salter-Harris type II and IV fractures, treatment guidelines follow those of a type IV injury: open reduction and internal fixation of displaced intra-articular fractures, with the potential for mild growth disturbance of the distal humeral physis. There is no contact between the trochlea's ossification center and the exposed bone in the metaphyseal fragment.

Because the fracture line starts in the metaphysis and then courses along the physeal cartilage, it has some of the characteristics of both type II and IV injuries according to the Salter-Harris classification. This fracture classification is debatable, because the fracture exits the joint in the not-yet-ossified cartilage of the trochlea.

Mirsky, Karas, and Weiner (17) compared intraoperative findings to preoperative x-ray classification in 25 displaced fractures of the lateral condyle and found that in 13 (52%), the Milch classification did not correlate with intraoperative findings. Eight of 17 fractures (47%) classified preoperatively as Milch type I fractures (Fig. 15-1) were unstable, and five of eight fractures classified preoperatively as Milch type II fractures (Fig. 15-2) were extra-articular, extending across the distal humeral physis medially. Mirsky et al (17) identified three distinct fracture patterns: nine fractures exited the distal humeral epiphysis just medial to the capitellum, 11 exited through the trochlear epiphysis, and five extended across the physis medially. No fracture appeared to traverse the ossified portion of the capitellum (Milch type I).

Stage of Displacement

Displacement has been described as occurring in three stages (Fig. 15-3) (18,19). In the first stage, the fracture is relatively undisplaced, and the articular surface is intact (Fig. 15-3A,B).

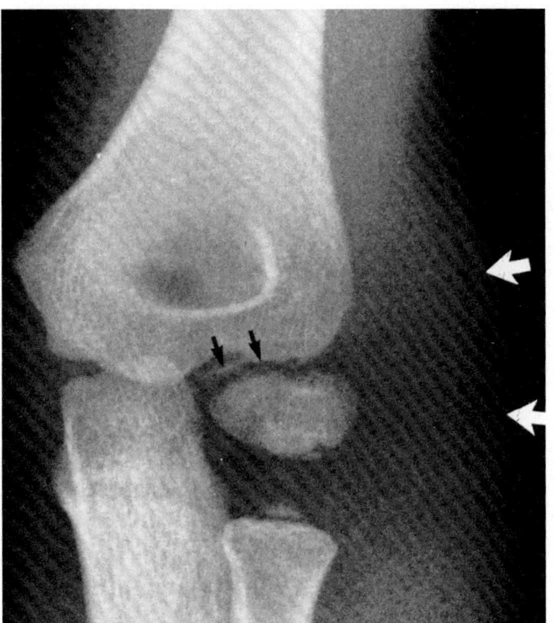

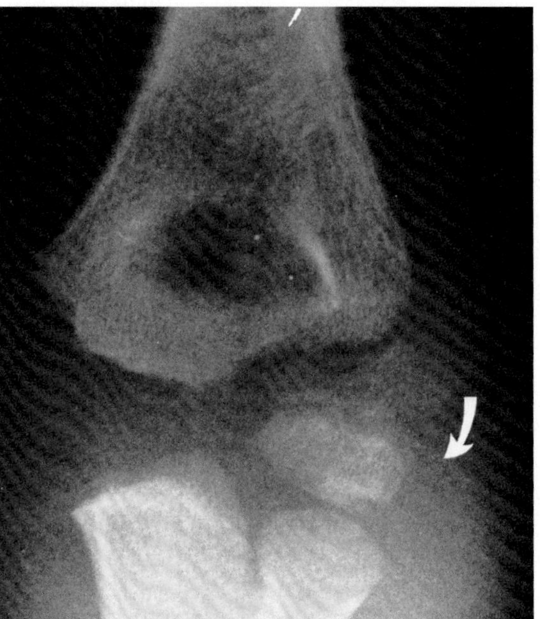

FIGURE 15-1 **A.** Injury film of a 7-year-old with an undisplaced fracture of the lateral condyle (*small arrows*). Attention was drawn to the fracture's location due to extensive soft tissue swelling on the lateral aspect (*white arrows*). **B.** Because of the extensive soft tissue injury, there was little intrinsic stability, allowing the fracture to become displaced at 7 days (*arrow*).

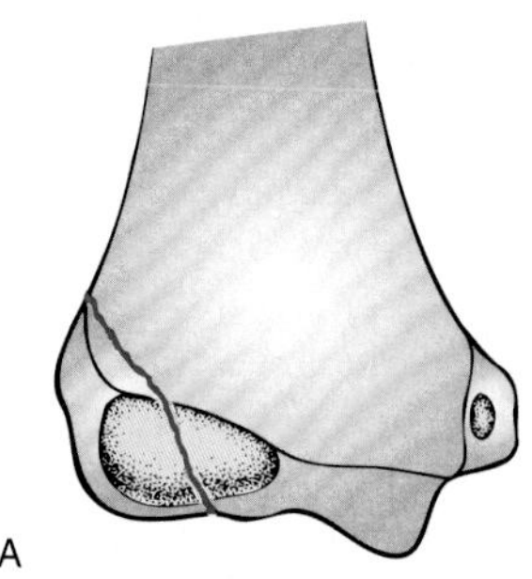

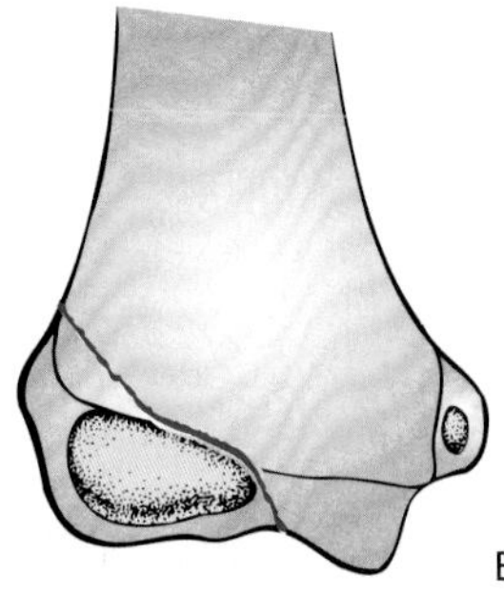

FIGURE 15-2 Physeal fractures of the lateral condyle. **A.** Physeal injury (Milch type II) through the nonossified trochlea. **B.** Physeal injury (Milch type I) through the ossific nucleus of the lateral condyle. (Adapted and reprinted with permission from Milch HE. Fractures and fracture–dislocations of the humeral condyles. *J Trauma* 1964;4:592–607.)

Because the trochlea is intact, there is no lateral shift of the olecranon.

In the second stage, the fracture extends completely through the articular surface (Fig. 15-3C,D). This allows the proximal fragment to become more displaced and can allow lateral displacement of the olecranon. In the third stage, the condylar fragment is rotated and totally displaced laterally and proximally, which allows translocation of both the olecranon and the radial head (Fig. 15-3E,F).

Badelon et al (20) modified the description of stage I displacement to include fractures with less than 2 mm of displacement seen on the anteroposterior (AP) or lateral x-ray only or seen on both views.

Soft Tissue Injuries

The fracture line usually begins in the posterolateral metaphysis, with a soft tissue tear in the area between the origins of the extensor carpi radialis longus and the brachioradialis muscle. The extensor carpi radialis longus and brevis muscles remain attached to the free distal fragment, along with the lateral collateral ligaments of the elbow. If there is much displacement, both the anterior and posterior aspects of the elbow capsule are usually torn. This soft tissue injury, however, is usually localized to the lateral side and may help identify a minimally displaced fracture. More extensive soft tissue swelling at the fracture site may indicate more severe soft tissue injury (21,22), which may indicate that the fracture is prone to late displacement.

Displacement of the Fracture and Elbow Joint

The degree of displacement varies according to the magnitude of the force applied and whether the cartilaginous hinge of the articular surface remains intact. If the articular surface is intact, the resultant displacement of the condylar fragment is simply a lateral tilt hinging on the intact medial articular surface. Horn et al (23) studied 16 lateral humeral condylar fractures with x-ray and magnetic resonance imaging (MRI) and determined that all fractures unstable on x-ray had disruption of the cartilage hinge on MRI, confirming the relation of the cartilage hinge on fracture stability. If the fracture is complete, the fragment can be rotated and displaced varying degrees; in the most severe fractures, rotation is almost the full 180 degrees, so that the lateral condylar articular surface opposes the denuded metaphyseal fracture surface. Wilson (24) showed that in addition to this coronal rotation of the distal fragment, rotation can also occur in the horizontal plane. The lateral margin is carried posteriorly, and the medial portion of the distal fragment rotates anteriorly.

Because the usual fracture line disrupts the lateral crista of the trochlea, the elbow joint is unstable, creating the possibility of posterolateral subluxation of the proximal radius and ulna. Thus, the forearm rotates along the coronal plane into valgus, and there may also be lateral translocation of the lateral condyle with the radius and ulna (Fig. 15-4). This concept of lateral translocation is important in the late reconstruction of untreated fractures.

In physeal fractures, where the fracture line traverses the lateral condylar epiphysis, the elbow remains reasonably stable because the trochlea remains intact. Total coronal rotation of the condylar fragment can occur with this injury. The axial deformity that results is pure valgus without translocation (Fig. 15-4).

This posterolateral elbow instability with the lateral condylar physeal injury has led to the mistaken concept that this injury is associated with a primary dislocation of the elbow (25), which is rarely the case. The posterolateral instability of the elbow is usually a result of the injury, not a cause of it (26).

Mechanism of Injury

As Heyl (27) stated, the local biomechanics of the distal humerus must be different in children because this injury is rare in adults. Two mechanisms have been suggested: "push-off" and "pull-off."

The pull-off or avulsion theory has more advocates than the push-off mechanism (18,28). In early studies (28), this injury was consistently produced in young cadavers by adducting the forearm with the elbow extended and the forearm supinated. The work of Jakob and Fowles (18) confirmed the results of these studies. Some of Stimson's (28) work strengthens the push-off theory. In his cadaver studies, he produced the injury by applying a sharp blow to the palm when the elbow was flexed (15); other investigators have speculated that because the forearm goes into valgus when extended, the radial head can push off the lateral condyle or that the injury can result from a direct blow to the olecranon.

It is likely that both mechanisms can produce this injury. The more common type of fracture, which extends to the apex of the trochlea, is probably a result of avulsion forces on the condyle, with the olecranon's sharp articular surface serving to direct the force along the physeal line into the trochlea. When a child falls forward on his or her palm with the elbow flexed, the radial head is forced against the capitellum and may cause

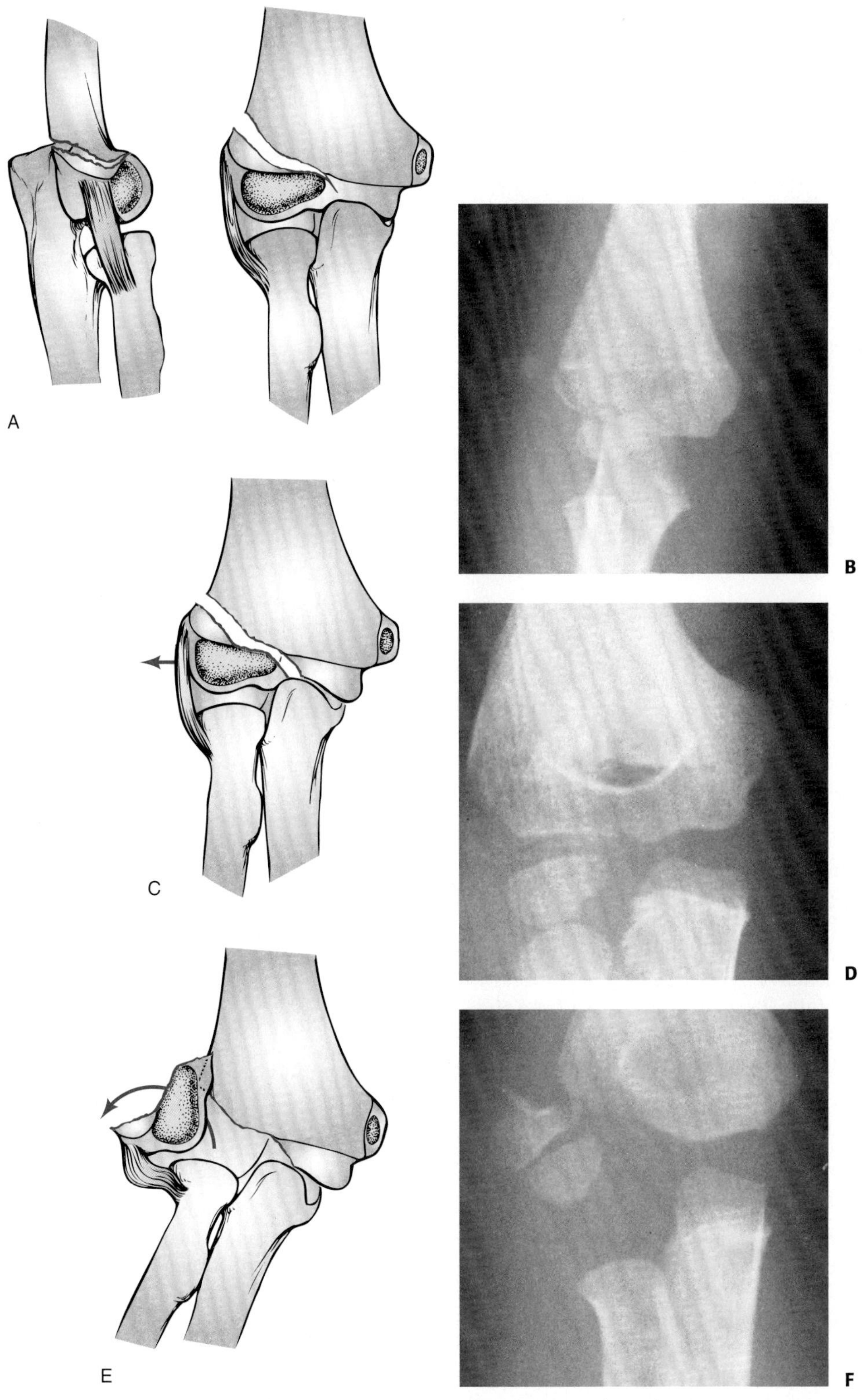

FIGURE 15-3 Stages of displacement. **A,B.** Stage I displacement—articular surface intact. **C,D.** Stage II displacement—articular surface disrupted. **E,F.** Stage III displacement—fragment rotated. (A, C, and E: Reprinted with permission from Jakob R, Fowles JV, Rang M, et al. Observations concerning fractures of the lateral humeral condyle in children. *J Bone Joint Surg (Br)* 1975;57:430–436.)

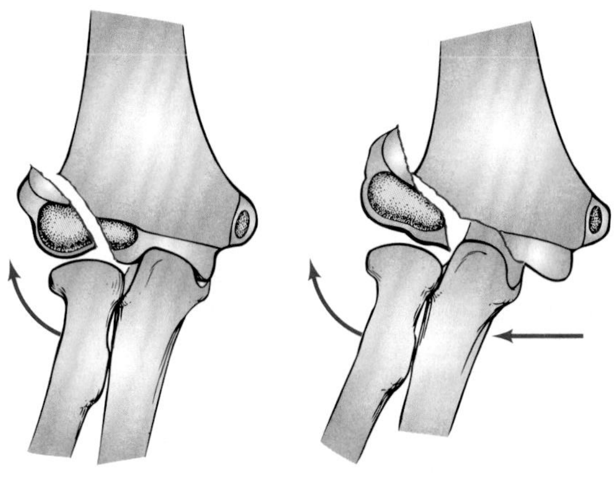

FIGURE 15-4 Angular deformities. **A.** Milch type I fractures tend only to angulate. **B.** Milch type II fractures are unstable with lateral translocation in addition to angulation. (Modified and reprinted with permission from Milch HE. Fractures and fracture–dislocations of the humeral condyles. *J Trauma* 1964;4:592–607.)

the less common Milch type I physeal fracture that courses through the ossific nucleus of the capitellum.

Signs and Symptoms

Compared with the marked distortion of the elbow that occurs with displaced supracondylar fractures, little distortion of the elbow, other than that produced by the fracture hematoma, may be present with lateral condylar fractures. The key to the clinical evaluation of this fracture is the location of soft tissue swelling concentrated over the lateral aspect of the distal humerus (21). Stage I displacement may produce only local tenderness at the condylar fracture site, which may be increased by forcibly flexing the wrist. Stage II or III displacement may result in some local crepitus with motion of the lateral condylar fragment. The benign appearance of the elbow with some stage I and II displacements may account for the delay of parents seeking treatment for a child with a minimally displaced fracture.

X-Ray Findings

The x-ray appearance varies according to the fracture line's anatomic location and the displacement stage. In the AP view, the metaphyseal flake may be small and seemingly minimally displaced. The degree of displacement can often be better appreciated on the true lateral view. In determining whether the articular hinge is intact (i.e., stage I vs stage II), the relationship of the proximal ulna to the distal humerus is evaluated for the presence of lateral translocation. Oblique views are especially helpful in patients in whom a stage I displacement is suspected.

In a prospective study of 112 children with nondisplaced and minimally displaced fractures of the lateral condyle, Finnbogason et al (29) identified three groups of fractures: stable fractures, fractures with an undefinable risk, and fractures with a high risk of later displacement. Stable fractures had no gap or a small gap and did not extend all the way to the epiphyseal cartilage; most of these 65 fractures were in younger children and none had later displacement. Fractures with undefinable risk of displacement were the same type as stable fractures, but the fracture could be clearly observed extending all the way to the epiphyseal cartilage; displacement occurred in 6 (17%) of these 35 fractures. High-risk fractures had a gap that was as wide or almost as wide laterally as medially; displacement occurred in five of 12 (42%) of these fractures.

Kamegaya et al (30) reported that MRI evaluation of 12 minimally displaced (less than 2 mm on x-ray) lateral condylar fractures identified five fractures that crossed the physis into the joint space and were unstable fractures. One of five fractures with 1-mm displacement was unstable, and four fractures of seven with 2-mm displacement were unstable. These investigators suggested that MRI evaluation might prevent late displacement or delayed union by identifying those minimally displaced fractures that required percutaneous pin fixation rather than cast immobilization.

A major diagnostic difficulty lies in differentiating this fracture from a fracture of the entire distal humeral physis. In a young child in whom the condyle is unossified, an arthrogram or MRI may be helpful (Figs. 15-5, 15-6, and 15-7) (8). Potter (31) recommended MRI with thin (1.5 mm to 2 mm) sections and appropriate pulse sequencing to provide differential contrast between subchondral bone, cartilage, and joint fluid.

In fractures of the entire distal humeral physis, the proximal radius and ulna are usually displaced posteromedially (Fig. 15-8A). The relationship of the lateral condylar ossification center to the proximal radius remains intact. In true fractures involving only the lateral condylar physis, the relationship of the condylar ossification center to the proximal radius is lost (Fig. 15-8B). In addition, any displacement of the proximal radius and ulna is more likely to be lateral due to the loss of stability provided by the lateral crista of the distal humerus.

Treatment Methods

Fractures involving the lateral condylar physis can be treated with simple immobilization alone, closed reduction and percutaneous pinning, or open surgical reduction.

Immobilization

Minimally displaced fractures are stable and have considerable intrinsic soft tissue attachments that prevent displacement of the distal fragment. About 40% of lateral condylar physeal fractures are sufficiently undisplaced so that they can be treated by simple immobilization without surgical intervention (18). If the fracture line is barely perceptible on the original x-ray (stage I displacement), the degree of displacement is usually minimal and the chance for subsequent displacement is low. X-rays should be obtained weekly for the first 3 weeks after injury to ensure that late displacement does not occur.

Undisplaced fractures can usually be treated via simple immobilization with good results. Speed and Macey (32) reported

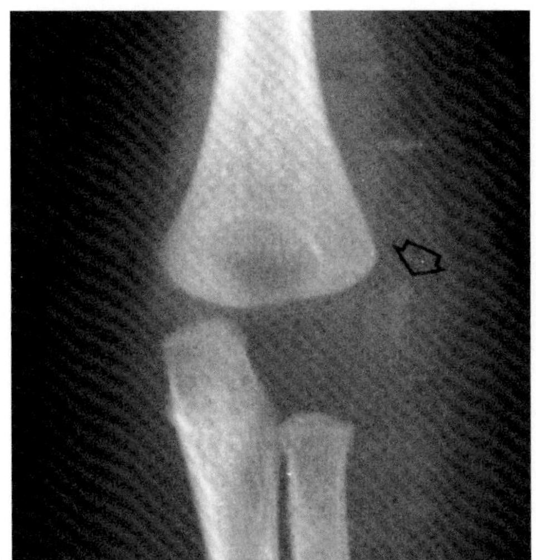
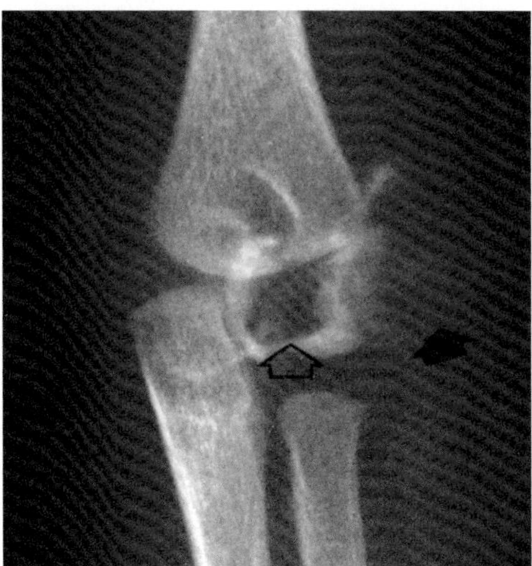

FIGURE 15-5 Unossified lateral condyle. **A.** AP view. A small ossific nucleus can barely be seen (*arrow*) in the swollen lateral soft tissues. **B.** An arthrogram shows the defect left by the displaced lateral condyle (*open arrow*). The displaced condyle is outlined in the soft tissues (*solid arrow*).

uniformly excellent results both anatomically and functionally in patients with undisplaced fractures, none of whom had any abnormalities of growth or premature physeal fusion. Simple immobilization of nondisplaced or minimally displaced (less than 2 mm) fractures in a sling, collar and cuff, or posterior splint appears adequate (20,32–35). Close follow-up and repeat x-rays to detect any late displacement are mandatory if this method is used.

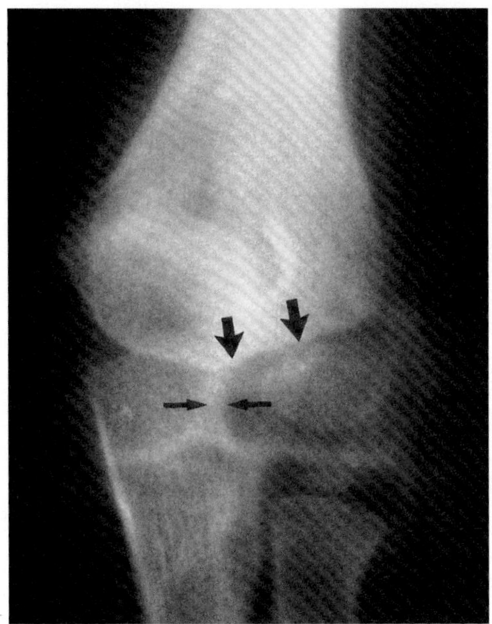

FIGURE 15-6 Arthrogram of stage I fracture of the lateral condyle (*large arrows*). Articular surface is intact with no displacement (*small arrows*).

In their long-term study of fractures treated nonoperatively, Badelon et al (20) determined that only fractures with type I displacement (i.e., the fracture line is seen on only one x-ray view) can be safely treated nonoperatively. In their experience, any fracture with displacement, even of less than 2 mm, can displace later in the cast or splint. In a review of 57 fractures of the lateral condyle, Beaty and Wood (34) found that two of 24 fractures with stage I displacement displaced late. Bast, Hoffer, and Aval (33) reported a union rate of 98% after nonoperative treatment of 95 nondisplaced or minimally displaced fractures of the lateral humeral condyle. Their criteria for nonoperative treatment were acute fracture (less than 24 hours at initial evaluation) and displacement of less than 2 mm in three x-ray planes (AP, lateral, and internal oblique). Two fractures that displaced 6 and 9 days after closed reduction required open reduction and internal fixation before they united without complications.

Late Displacement

Careful clinical examination is important in predicting which fractures will displace later. The potential to displace often depends more on the degree of associated soft tissue injury and whether the articular cartilage of the trochlea is intact, rather than on the amount of initial displacement. Considerable soft tissue swelling on the lateral aspect of the distal humerus, which can be appreciated both clinically and on x-rays, should alert the physician to the fact that the fracture may be unstable and has the potential to displace. If crepitus between the fragments is detected with motion of the forearm or elbow, significant loss of soft tissue attachments and a potentially unstable fracture should be suspected (15).

Closed Reduction and Percutaneous Pinning

Several techniques have been described for initial reduction, with the recommended elbow position ranging from hyperflex-

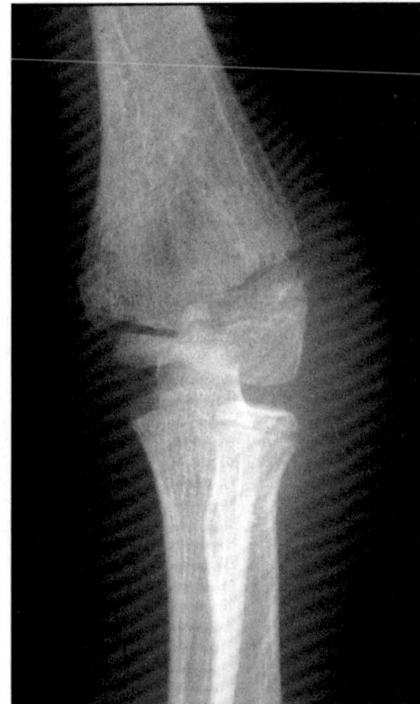

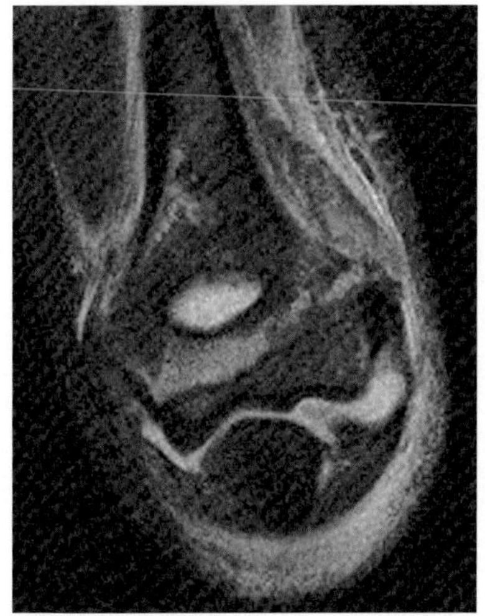

FIGURE 15-7 A. X-ray of a stable type II fracture of the lateral condyle in a 10-year-old child. **B.** Gradient-echo MRI clearly differentiates this fracture from a fracture of the entire distal humeral physis.

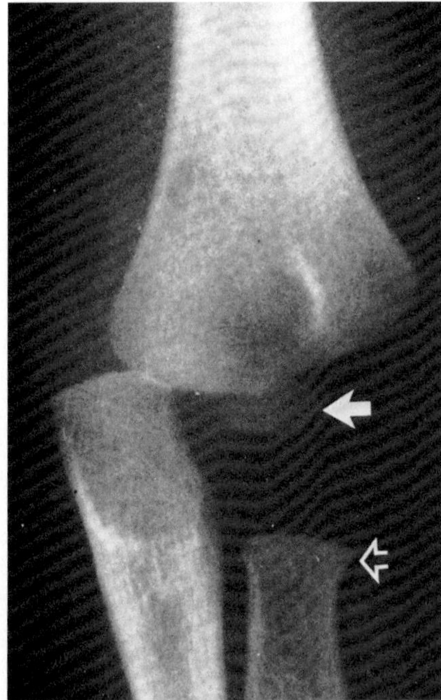

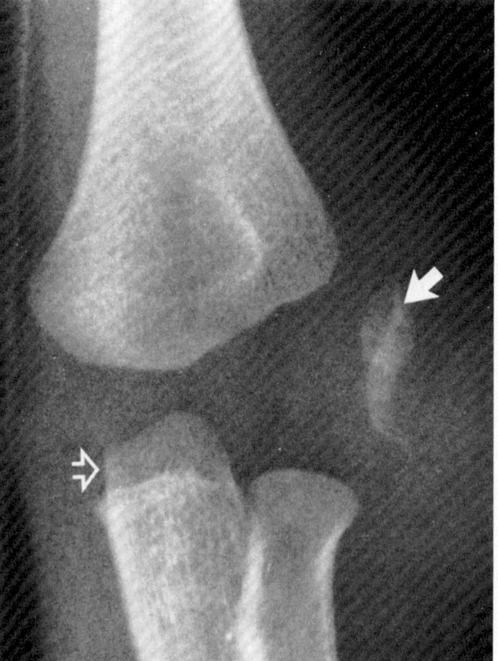

FIGURE 15-8 A. Total distal humeral physeal fracture in a 2-year-old. The lateral condyle (*closed arrow*) has remained in line with the proximal radius. The proximal radius, ulna, and lateral condyle have all shifted medially (*open arrow*). **B.** Displaced fracture of the lateral condyle in a 2-year-old. The relationship of the lateral condyle (*closed arrow*) to the proximal radius is lost. Both the proximal radius and ulna (*open arrow*) have shifted slightly laterally.

ion to full extension; however, it appears from clinical experience and experimental studies that reduction is best achieved with the forearm supinated and the elbow extended. Placing a varus stress on the extended elbow allows further room for manipulation of the fragment. Unfortunately, it is difficult to maintain reduction of a displaced lateral condylar fracture with closed techniques, and closed reduction is not recommended for treating stage III displaced lateral condylar fractures. Minimally displaced fractures can be stabilized with percutaneous pins across the fracture. In lateral condylar physeal fractures with moderate displacement, confirmation of fracture stability by stress testing and arthrography may precede percutaneous pin fixation. Mintzer et al (36) reported good results after percutaneous pin fixation of 12 lateral condylar fractures with displacement of more than 2 mm. They believed this method is appropriate for selected fractures with 2 mm to 4 mm of displacement and an arthrographically demonstrated congruent joint surface. If a satisfactory reduction cannot be obtained, then reduction should be achieved and maintained by open reduction and internal fixation.

Open Reduction and Internal Fixation

Because of the high incidence of poor functional and cosmetic results with closed reduction methods, open reduction has become the most widely advocated method for unstable fractures with stage II displacement and fractures with stage III displacement (18,19,25,35,37–45). In a study of 97 children with minimally displaced lateral condylar fractures, Launay et al (46) found that immobilization alone resulted in additional displacement and more nonunions than did operative treatment. About 60% of all fractures involving the lateral condylar physis require open reduction and internal fixation (18). There is uniform agreement regarding the need for open reduction of displaced fractures of the lateral condylar physis. Most investigators recommend fixation with smooth Kirschner wire (K-wires) in children or screws in adolescents nearing skeletal maturity.

Pin and Screw Fixation

Smooth pins are the most frequently used method of fragment fixation (18,19,32,34,44,45,47). Blount et al (37) believed that at least two pins were necessary to prevent rotation. The passage of a smooth wire through the physis does not result in any growth disturbance (48,49), which is of note because only 20% of the humerus' growth occurs through the distal humeral physis. It also appears that the wires can be placed either parallel or crossed in the distal fragments.

The ideal place for the pins is in the metaphyseal fragment. They should cross at the lateral aspect of the metaphysis and diverge as much as possible to enhance the stability of fixation. If there is only a small metaphyseal fragment, the pins can be placed across the physis without concern.

When adequate reduction and internal fixation are carried out early (i.e., within the first few days after the injury), the results are uniformly good. The key, however, is to be sure that the reduction is adequate. Hardacre et al (39) found that poor results after open reduction occurred when the reduction was incomplete. Surgery alone does not ensure a good result unless the reduction is nearly anatomic and the fixation is secure.

Early surgical intervention is essential, because organization of the clot with early fibrin development makes it difficult to achieve a reduction without extensive soft tissue dissection in fractures that are treated late. The pins can be buried or left protruding through the skin with a low incidence of infection. Leaving pins buried requires a second operative procedure, even though it usually can be accomplished with a local anesthetic. The fracture generally is sufficiently stable to allow pin removal by 3 to 4 weeks and to allow the patient to begin protected active range of elbow motion at 2 to 3 weeks.

Screw fixation has been used less frequently in children, although Jeffrey (40) recommended it in 1958. Sharma et al (50) reported painless, full range of elbow motion in 36 of 37 children who had displaced (more than 2 mm in any direction) lateral condylar fractures fixed with partially threaded 4-mm AO cancellous screws. One patient had delayed union, with loss of 10 degrees of elbow motion.

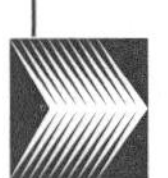

AUTHORS' PREFERRED TREATMENT

Immobilization

If the fracture is minimally displaced on x-ray (i.e., the metaphyseal fragment is less than 2 mm from the proximal fragment on AP and lateral views) and the clinical signs also indicate there is reasonable soft tissue integrity, we simply immobilize the elbow in a long-arm cast with the forearm in neutral rotation and the elbow flexed 60 to 90 degrees. X-rays are taken within the first 3 to 5 days after the fracture with the cast removed and the elbow comfortably extended. If there is no displacement, the x-rays are repeated in another 3 to 5 days. If the x-rays again show no displacement, then another long-arm cast is applied and is worn for about 3 to 5 weeks, or until fracture union is apparent.

In some fractures with more than the allowable 2 mm of displacement (type II injury), the fracture pattern is such that the articular cartilage appears intact. If there is any question about the stability at the time of the fracture, MRI can be obtained or the extremity can be examined with the patient under general anesthesia. Gentle varus stress views with the forearm supinated and the elbow extended should be taken to determine if the fracture displaces significantly. Preoperative MRI or intraoperative arthrography can be used to determine the stability of the nonossified articular cartilage of the trochlea.

Percutaneous Pins

For fractures with stage II displacement (2 mm to 4 mm), varus stress views should be obtained and arthrography should be

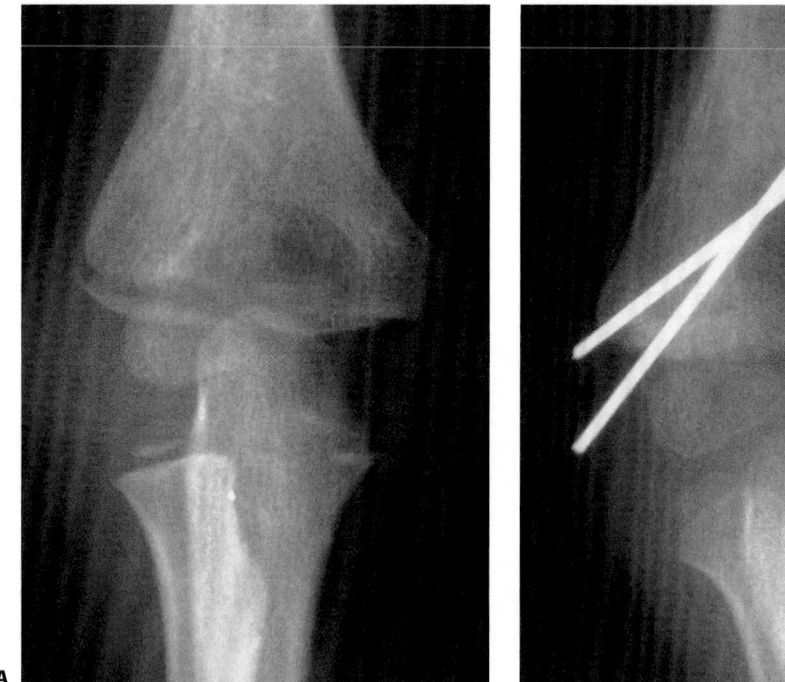

FIGURE 15-9 Stage II fracture of the lateral condyle. **A.** AP x-ray shows 4 mm of displacement of the metaphyseal segment; however, the fracture was stable by stress examination and arthrography. **B.** Four weeks after percutaneous pinning, the fracture is healed.

done with the patient under anesthesia. If the fracture is stable, percutaneous pinning is indicated (Fig. 15-9).

Open Reduction

If the fracture is grossly unstable, open reduction and internal fixation are indicated. We prefer open reduction and internal fixation of all fractures with stage III displacement. It is important that open reduction is performed as soon as possible after the injury. The standard lateral Kocher approach provides sufficient exposure of the fragment. Often, a tear in the aponeurosis of the brachioradialis muscle laterally leads directly to the fracture site. Extreme care must be taken to avoid dissecting near the posterior portion of the fragment, because this is the entrance of the blood supply of the lateral condylar epiphysis.

Mohan, Hunter, and Colton (51) recommended a posterolateral approach because of the excellent exposure it provides with minimal dissection. Another suggested advantage is the improved cosmetic results by more posterior placement of the surgical scar. Mohan et al (51) reported no complications in 20 patients in whom this approach was used.

The quality of the reduction is determined by evaluating the fracture line along the articular surface's anterior aspect. This usually can be determined either by direct vision or by digital palpation. We prefer to use smooth K-wires that cross just medial to the condylar fragment to maintain the reduction (Fig. 15-10). The wires penetrate the skin through a separate stab incision posterior to the main incision. A long-arm cast is applied with the elbow flexed 60 to 90 degrees and the forearm in neutral or slight pronation. The cast and pins are removed in 3 weeks if there is adequate healing on x-rays. Early active motion is started at that time. If necessary, pin removal can be delayed 1 to 2 weeks to allow further healing in older children.

Technique of Open Reduction and Internal Fixation of Lateral Humeral Condylar Fractures

The elbow is exposed through a 5- to 6-cm lateral approach, placing two thirds of the incision above the joint and one third distal (Fig. 15-11). In the interval between the brachioradialis and the triceps, the dissection is carried down to the lateral humeral condyle. The joint's anterior surfaces are exposed by separating the fibers of the common extensor muscle mass. Soft tissue detachment is limited to only that necessary to expose the fragment, the fracture, and the joint; the posterior soft tissues are left intact. Retracting the antecubital structures exposes the anterior joint surface. The trochlea and the more medial entry point of the condylar fracture are inspected. The displacement and the size of the fragment are always greater than is apparent on the x-rays because much of the fragment is cartilaginous. The fragment usually is rotated as well as displaced. The joint is irrigated to remove blood clots and debris, the articular surface and the metaphyseal fragment are reduced accurately, and the reduction is confirmed by observing the articular surface,

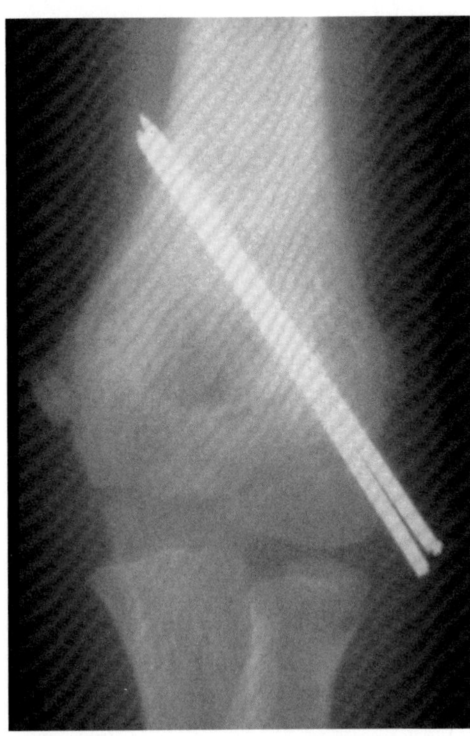

FIGURE 15-10 Fixation of lateral condylar fracture with two smooth K-wires, crossing just medial to the condylar fragment.

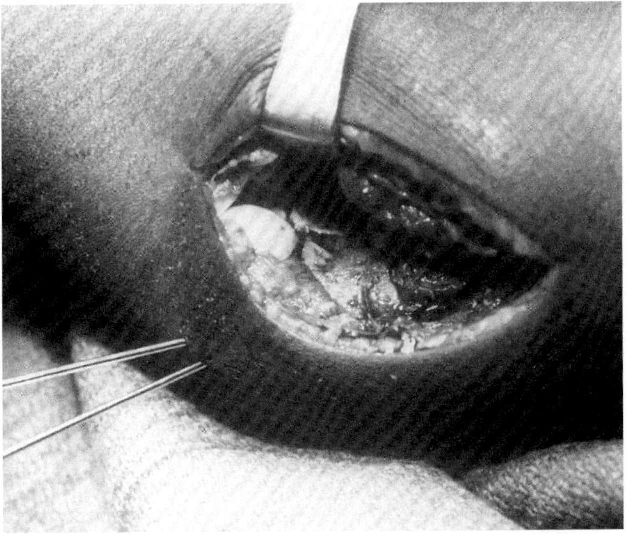

FIGURE 15-11 Lateral approach for open reduction and internal fixation of a lateral humeral condylar fracture of the left elbow. The approach is made through the brachioradialis–triceps interval; an anterior retractor is used to expose the joint surfaces, and the fracture is reduced and pinned percutaneously posterior to the incision.

particularly at the trochlea. The position is held with a small tenaculum, bone holder, or towel clip. When a large metaphyseal fragment is present, two smooth K-wires are inserted across it into the medial portion of the metaphysis. When the epiphyseal portion is small, as is more common, two smooth K-wires are inserted through the condyle, across the physis, and into the humeral metaphysis, penetrating the medial cortex of the humerus. The wires are directed 45 to 60 degrees; the reduction and the position of the internal fixation are checked by AP and lateral x-rays before closing the wound. The ends of the wires are cut off beneath the skin but are left long enough to allow easy removal. The arm is placed in a posterior plaster splint with the elbow flexed 60 to 90 degrees.

The splint is worn for 2 to 3 weeks after surgery. The pins can be removed at 3 weeks if union is progressing. Gentle active motion of the elbow is then usually resumed and continued until full range of motion returns.

Delayed Union and Nonunion

If sophisticated surgical treatment is unavailable, these fractures may go untreated or unrecognized for a prolonged period. Even in modern medical settings, elbow injuries may be treated as "sprains," and the diagnosis of a displaced lateral condylar fracture is not made. Thus, patients often present months or even years later with a nonunited or malunited fracture fragment.

Delayed Union

Delayed union, in contrast to nonunion or malunion, occurs in a fracture in which the fracture fragments are in satisfactory position but union of the lateral condylar fragment to the metaphysis is delayed. Various reasons have been suggested for delayed union of lateral condylar fractures. Flynn and Richards (52) speculated that it was caused by poor circulation to the metaphyseal fragment. Hardacre et al (39) believed that bathing the fracture site by articular fluid inhibited fibrin formation and subsequent callus formation. It is most likely that a combination of these two factors, in addition to the constant tension forces exerted by the muscle arising from the condylar fragment, is responsible for delayed union.

This complication is most common in patients treated nonoperatively. The symptoms and clinical examination determine the aggressiveness of treatment. The fragment is usually stable during clinical examination, the elbow is nontender, and the range of elbow motion increases progressively. On x-rays, the fragment's position remains unchanged. With time, these fractures usually heal (Fig. 15-12). Lateral spur formation or cubitus varus is relatively common with these fractures. The need for further treatment depends on the presence of significant symptoms or further displacement that may disrupt the joint surface and cause functional impairment. If neither of these conditions is present, the x-ray persistence of the fracture line requires only follow-up observation. If there is any question as to the integrity of the joint surface, an MRI may help determine any loss of continuity and the need for surgical treatment as a nonunion rather than a simple delayed union.

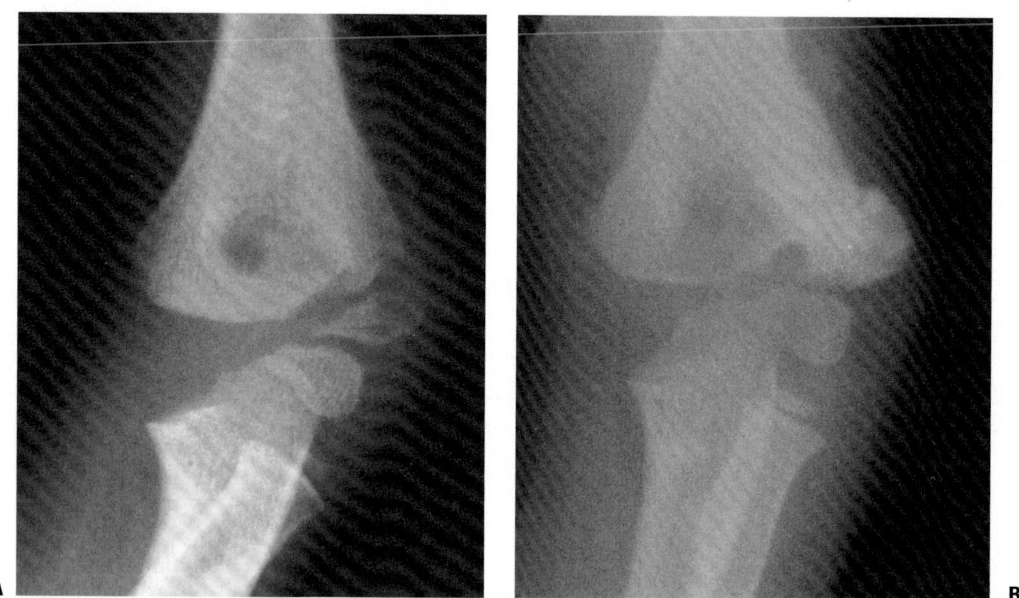

FIGURE 15-12 Delayed union and cubitus varus. **A.** Stage III lateral condylar fracture in a 7-year-old boy was treated in a cast. **B.** Seven months later, delayed union with malunion of the fracture and cubitus varus deformity were present.

Flynn and Richards (52) recommended long-term immobilization for minimally displaced fractures with delayed union. They found that 70% of minimally displaced fractures had united by 12 weeks. Jeffrey (40) recommended screw fixation with bone grafting. Hardacre et al (39), however, found that minimally displaced fractures with delayed union ultimately united if there was no significant displacement of the condylar fragment.

Controversy exists as to whether elbow function can be improved by a late open reduction and internal fixation of the fracture fragment. Delayed open reduction has been complicated by osteonecrosis and further loss of elbow motion. Speed and Macey (32) were among the first investigators to question whether patients treated with late surgery did better than those not treated. In patients with malunion who were treated late, they found a high incidence of poor results due to "epiphyseal changes" that probably represented osteonecrosis. There have been many subsequent reports of osteonecrosis occurring after late open reduction. The high incidence of osteonecrosis of the fragment is believed to be due to the extensive soft tissue dissection necessary to replace the fragment (Fig. 15-13). Böhler (35), on the other hand, had good results in his patients with delayed treatment. He avoided extensive soft tissue dissection by approaching the fragment transarticularly after performing an osteotomy of the olecranon.

The key to preventing osteonecrosis is to recognize the course of the blood supply to the lateral condyle. Only a small portion of the condyle is extra-articular. In his studies, Haraldsson (53) found that the vessels that supply the lateral condylar epiphysis penetrate the condyle in a small posterior nonarticular area (Fig. 15-14).

Jakob and Fowles (18) reported that patients treated later than 3 weeks after the fracture did no better than those who received no treatment at all. They found that early callus and fibrous tissue made it extremely difficult to obtain a satisfactory open reduction without performing considerable soft tissue dissection. All their patients treated after 3 weeks lost range of motion (at least 34 degrees on average), and osteonecrosis, premature physeal closure, as well as valgus deformity were common. In patients who received no treatment, valgus deformity due to nonunion and malunion was frequent, but no osteonecrosis of the lateral condylar epiphysis occurred. These investigators recommended that no open reduction should be performed for fractures older than 3 weeks, but that early ulnar nerve transposition should be performed to eliminate the possibility of late ulnar nerve symptoms that occur with cubitus valgus deformity after nonunion. Dhillon et al (54) and Zionts and Stolz (55) also reported that osteonecrosis was frequent after late open reduction and recommended no treatment for these fractures.

Nonunion

In 1932, Cooper (56) drew attention to the development of nonunion after lateral humeral condylar fractures when he described his findings in two cadaver specimens. He pointed out that there was absolutely no bony continuity between the distal humerus and the condylar fragment. True nonunion with significant deformity is rare because it usually is the result of a nontreated displaced fracture of the lateral condylar physis (37,41).

True nonunion occurs in patients with progressive displacement of the fragment. The mobile fragment can be palpated, or the patient has weakness or pain in the elbow. According to

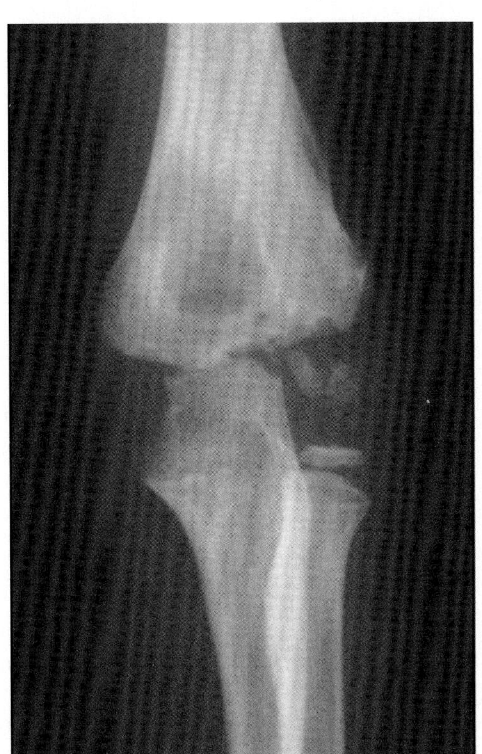

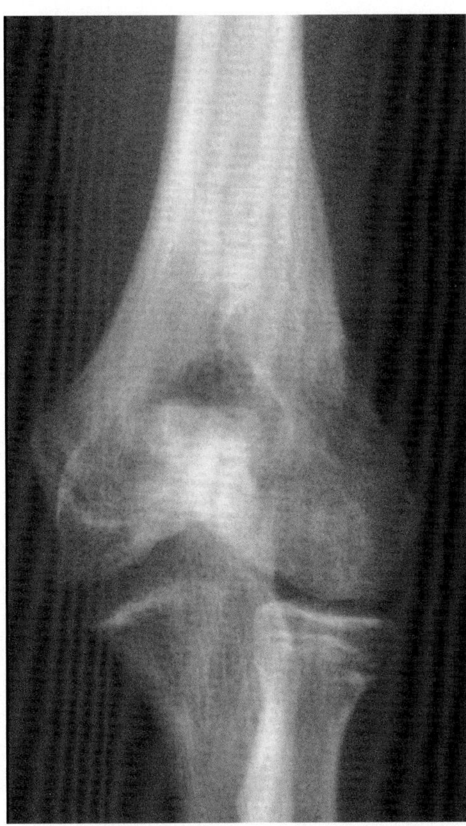

FIGURE 15-13 Osteonecrosis of the lateral condyle after lateral condylar fracture in a 10-year-old boy. AP **(A)** and lateral **(B)** x-rays.

the criteria of Flynn et al (57), if the fracture has not united by 12 weeks, it is classified as a nonunion.

Nonunion can occur with or without angular deformity. Many patients with nonunions and minimal fragment displacement have no angulation and remain relatively asymptomatic for normal activities (Fig. 15-14). Others have weakness or symptoms when the arm is used for high-performance activities. Because they are not significantly displaced, these fractures can often be stabilized with minimal extra-articular dissection using a combination of screw fixation and a laterally placed bone graft.

Nonunion with subsequent fragment displacement is more common after unstable fractures with stage II and III displacement. If the fragment becomes free, it tends to migrate proximally with a subsequent valgus elbow deformity. Nonunion can lead to a cubitus valgus deformity, which in turn, is associated with the development of a tardy ulnar nerve palsy.

Nonunion seems to occur when the distal fragment is displaced enough to allow the condylar fragment's cartilaginous articular surface to oppose the bony surface of the humeral metaphysis. In such a situation, union is impossible. Flynn and Richards (52) reported successful treatment of nonunion 9 months to 3 years after fracture and strongly advised early surgery for established nonunion when the condylar fragment is in "good position" in a child with open physes. Papandrea and Waters (58) recommended stable internal fixation with percutaneously placed pins or cannulated screws for early (less than 12 weeks), minimally displaced nonunions. For late displaced nonunions, they recommended staged procedures: ulnar nerve transposition and bone grafting and fixation in situ of the lateral condyle followed by osteotomy to correct angulation once the nonunion is healed and elbow range of motion is regained.

The most common sequela of nonunion with displacement is the development of a progressive cubitus valgus deformity. The fragment migrates both proximally and laterally, giving not only an angular deformity but also lateral translocation of the proximal radius and ulna (Fig. 15-15). Milch (14) noted that lateral translocation is not as likely to develop in the more lateral type of these fractures (Milch type I) because the lateral crista of the trochlea is intact (Fig. 15-16).

Surgical treatment of the nonunion deformity of the lateral condylar fragment is difficult and requires correcting two problems. First, articular cartilage may be opposing the distal humeral metaphysis, and union seldom can be obtained without mobilizing the fragments and applying an internal compressive device. The second problem is correcting the angular deformity (Fig. 15-17).

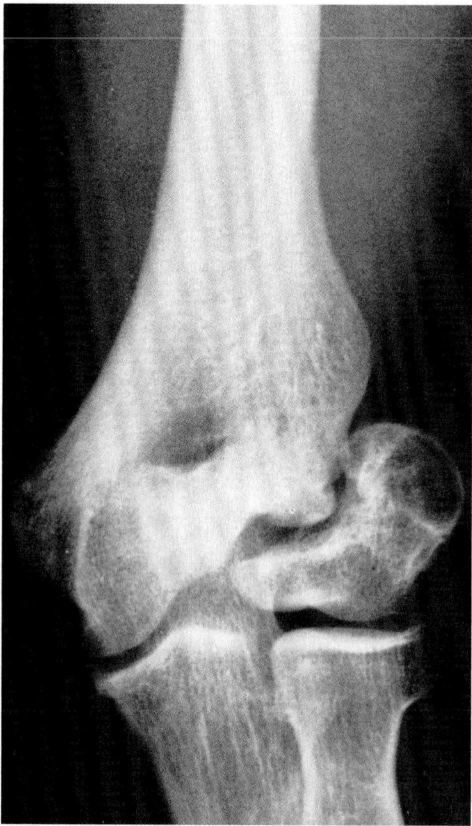

FIGURE 15-14 Asymptomatic nonunion of a lateral condyle in a 19-year-old military recruit. Because the patient had a completely normal and asymptomatic range of motion in his nondominant extremity, operative stabilization was not thought to be necessary.

Shimada et al (59) reported excellent or good results in 15 of 16 patients at an average follow-up of 11 years after osteosynthesis for nonunion of fractures of the lateral humeral condyle. The one patient with a poor result had evidence of osteonecrosis of the fragment. The average interval between injury and osteosynthesis was 5 years (range, 5 months to 10 years). To prevent progression of cubitus valgus deformity and subsequent ulnar nerve dysfunction, Shimada et al (59) recommended osteosynthesis for nonunion of lateral humeral condylar fractures in children because union is easily achieved, the range of motion is maintained, ulnar nerve function usually returns, and remodeling of the articular surfaces can be expected. They noted that bone grafting is essential to bridge the defect, to obtain congruity of the joint, and to promote union; damage to the blood supply should be avoided to prevent osteonecrosis.

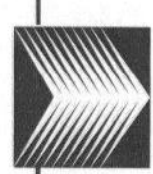

AUTHORS' PREFERRED TREATMENT

We distinguish between fractures seen late (more than 7 to 14 days after injury) and established nonunions (usually from 3 months to several years after injury). If we believe that we can obtain fracture union without loss of elbow motion and avoid osteonecrosis of the lateral condyle, then we recommend surgery for selected patients.

Treating an established nonunion of a lateral humeral condylar fracture poses a difficult dilemma. If no treatment is rendered, a progressive cubitus valgus deformity may occur with growth. Patients are usually asymptomatic except for those with high-demand athletic or labor activities. A mild flexion contracture of the elbow is present, but the cubitus valgus deformity is more cosmetic than functional. The danger in this approach is failure to recognize and treat early a tardy ulnar nerve palsy. If surgery is performed for an established nonunion, the potential risks of osteonecrosis and loss of elbow motion must be carefully considered.

We believe the criteria outlined by Flynn et al (52,57) are helpful in determining if surgical treatment is appropriate for an established nonunion:

1. A large metaphyseal fragment
2. Displacement of less than 1 cm from the joint surface
3. An open, viable lateral condylar physis

It is also helpful to distinguish between three distinct clinical situations. First, for an established nonunion with a large metaphyseal fragment, minimal migration, and an open lateral condylar physis, we recommend modified open reduction, screw fixation, and a lateral extra-articular iliac crest bone graft. This technique is markedly different from the surgical treatment of an acute lateral condylar fracture. The metaphyseal fragment of the lateral condyle and the distal humeral metaphysis are exposed, but no attempt is made to realign the articular surface. Intra-articular dissection should be avoided to help prevent any further loss of elbow motion. The metaphyseal fragments are debrided by gently removing any interposed fibrous tissue. The lateral condylar fragment can usually be moved distally a small distance. The metaphyseal fragments are firmly apposed, and a cancellous or cortical screw is used to fix the fragments with interfragmentary compression. Iliac crest bone graft can be placed between the metaphyseal fragments and laterally. The elbow is immobilized in 80 to 90 degrees of flexion for 3 to 4 weeks (Fig. 15-18).

Second, in patients with a nonunion who have cosmetic concerns but no functional complaints, treatment is similar to that for cubitus varus deformity after a supracondylar humeral fracture. If the patient and family desire, a supracondylar osteotomy can be performed (60). Rigid internal fixation should be used to allow early motion. Late osteosynthesis of the lateral condyle is rarely indicated in an adolescent or young adult with high functional demands and symptoms of instability.

Third, patients with asymptomatic nonunion, cubitus valgus deformity, and symptomatic tardy ulnar nerve palsy should be treated with anterior transposition of the ulnar nerve.

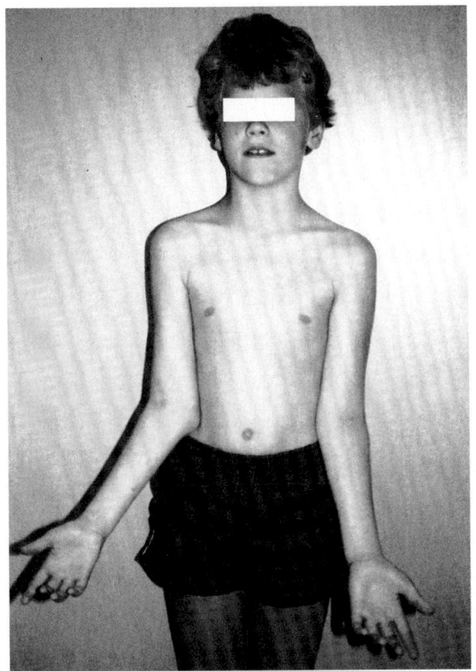

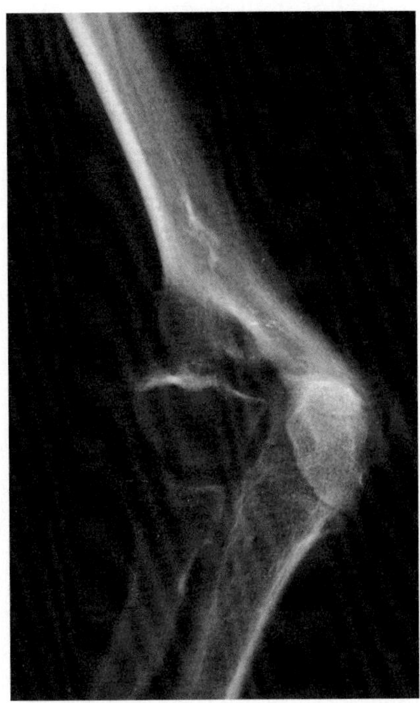

FIGURE 15-15 **A.** A 10-year-old boy with cubitus valgus resulting from a fracture of the lateral condylar physis with nonunion. **B.** Nonunion with cubitus valgus. X-ray showing both angulation and translocation secondary to nonunion of the condylar fragment.

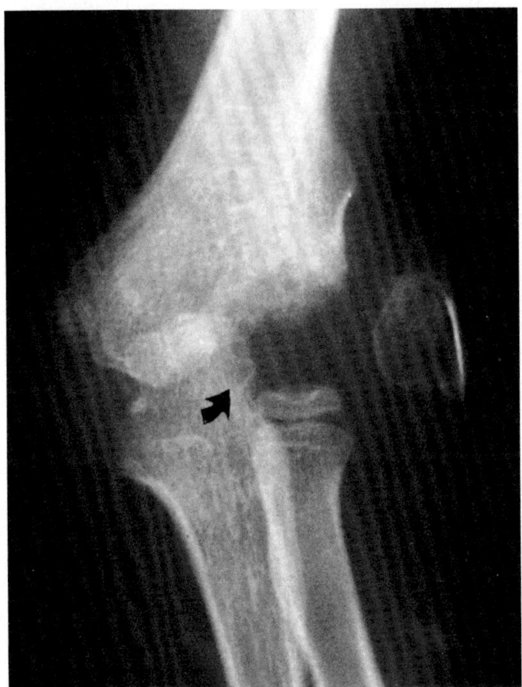

FIGURE 15-16 Nonunion without translocation. Milch type I fracture pattern. Despite nonunion, elbow stability was maintained because the lateral crista of the trochlea had remained intact (*arrow*). Valgus angulation also developed.

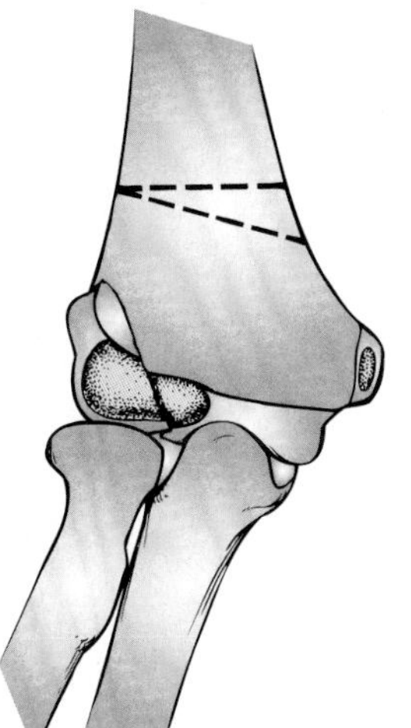

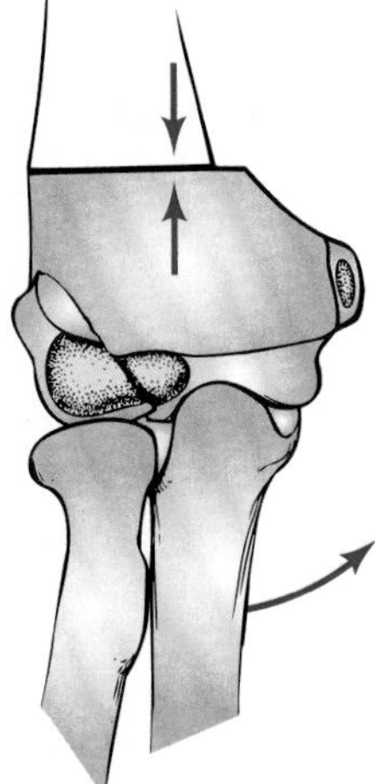

FIGURE 15-17 In the Milch type I fracture pattern, there is only an angular deformity that can be easily corrected with a closing wedge osteotomy. (Modified and reprinted with permission from Milch HE. Fractures and fracture–dislocations of the humeral condyles. *J Trauma* 1964;4:592–607.)

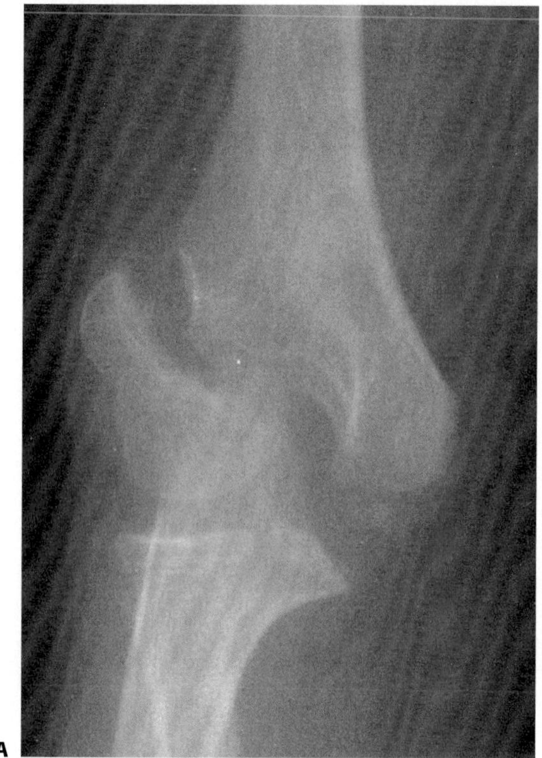

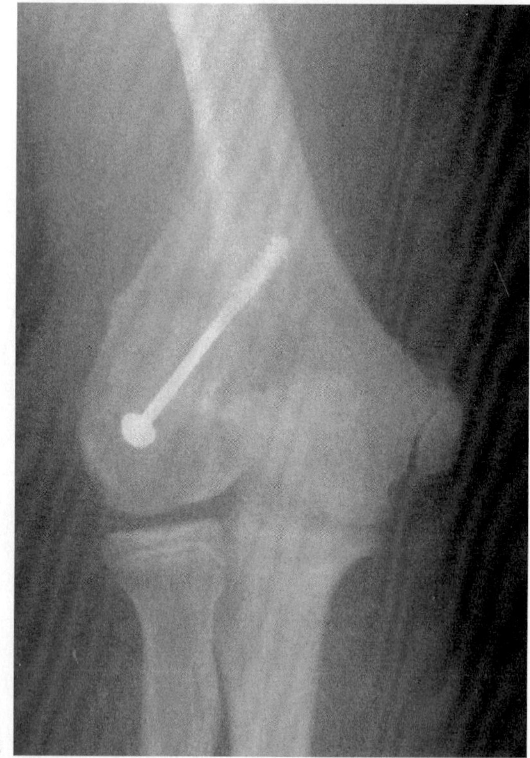

FIGURE 15-18 **A.** Established nonunion with a large metaphyseal fragment. **B.** After fixation with a cancellous screw and bone grafting of the metaphyseal fragment.

Complications

If an adequate reduction is obtained promptly and maintained with solid fixation, results are uniformly good. In supracondylar fractures, an incomplete reduction may result in a cosmetic deformity, but functional results are generally good. In displaced fractures of the lateral condylar physis, a marginal reduction can result in both cosmetic deformities and functional loss of motion (13). The complications that affect the outcome can be classified as either biologic or technical. Biologic problems occur as a result of the healing process, even if a perfect reduction is obtained. These problems include spur formation with pseudocubitus varus or a true cubitus varus. The technical problems usually arise from management errors and result in nonunion or malunion with or without valgus angulation and osteonecrosis. Other technical problems can arise from the injury itself, including neurologic injuries and myositis ossificans.

Lateral Spur Formation

Lateral condylar spur formation is one of the most common deformities after a fracture involving the lateral condylar physis. Cotton (15) believed that it is caused by coronal rotation of the distal fragment, which tends to displace laterally the flap of periosteum associated with the distal fragment. This periosteum then produces new bone formation in the form of a spur.

The spur occurs after both nonoperative and operative treatment. After nonoperative treatment, it results from the minimal displacement of the metaphyseal fragment and usually has a smooth outline. In patients with no real change in carrying angle, the lateral prominence of the spur may produce an appearance of mild cubitus varus (pseudovarus). In patients in whom a true cubitus varus develops, the presence of the lateral spur accentuates the varus alignment (Fig. 15-19A,B). The spur that occurs after operative treatment has a more irregular outline and is usually the result of hypertrophic bone formation from extensive dissection at the time of open reduction and internal fixation. During open reduction, care should be taken to limit the aggressiveness of the dissection and to carefully replace the lateral periosteal flap of the metaphyseal fragment.

Before treatment of lateral condylar fractures, the parents may be told that either lateral overgrowth with mild cubitus varus or lateral spur may develop, regardless of the treatment method. They should be told that this mild deformity is usually not of cosmetic or functional significance.

Cubitus Varus

Reviews of lateral condylar fractures show that a surprising number heal with some residual cubitus varus angulation (9,41,61–65). In some series, the incidence of cubitus varus is as high as 40% (61,64), and the deformity seems to be as frequent after operative treatment as after nonoperative treatment (63,64). Skak et al (66) reported visible varus deformities in six and valgus deformities in three of 28 children with displaced lateral condylar fractures. All patients with a valgus tilt of the joint surface were younger than 9 years of age at the time of injury. These investigators concluded that reduced growth potential at the trochlear groove is a regular complication of Milch type III fractures. The exact cause is not completely understood. In some instances, it is probably a combination of both an inadequate reduction and growth stimulation of the lateral condylar physis from the fracture insult (Fig. 15-20) (64).

The cubitus varus deformity is rarely severe enough to cause concern or require further treatment. This is probably because it is a pure coronal varus angulation and does not have the horizontal anterior rotation of the lateral condyle along with the sagittal extension that makes the cubitus varus that occurs after supracondylar fractures such an unacceptable deformity. Some investigators have noted that children with cubitus varus deformities have pain, decreased range of motion, epicondylitis, and problems with sports such as sidearm pitching, swimming, judo, and pushups. Davids et al (67) reported lateral condylar fractures in six children with pre-existing cubitus varus deformities from previous elbow fractures, usually supracondylar humeral fractures. They concluded that posttraumatic cubitus varus deformity may predispose a child to subsequent lateral condylar fracture and should be viewed as more than just a cosmetic deformity. They recommended valgus supracondylar osteotomy of the distal humerus.

Cubitus Valgus

Cubitus valgus is much less common after united lateral condylar fractures than cubitus varus. It has rarely been reported to result from premature epiphysiodesis of the lateral condylar physis (19). As with cubitus varus, it is usually minimal and is rarely of clinical or functional significance. The more difficult type of cubitus valgus associated with nonunions was discussed in the preceding section on nonunions.

Growth Disturbance: Fishtail Deformity

Two types of "fishtail deformity" of the distal humerus may occur. The first, a sharp-angled wedge, commonly occurs after fractures of the lateral condyle (Fig. 15-21). It is believed that this type of malformation is caused by persistence of a gap between the lateral condylar physis ossification center and the medial ossification of the trochlea (19,44). Because of this gap, the lateral crista of the trochlea may be underdeveloped, which may represent a small "bony bar" in the distal humeral physis (9). Despite some reports of loss of elbow motion with this type of fishtail deformity (19), most investigators (20,34,54,61) have not found this type of x-ray deformity to produce any functional deficiency. Nwakama et al (68) reported four patients (average age, 5 years) with fishtail deformities accompanied by premature closure of a portion of the distal humeral physis with resultant deformity, length retardation, decreased elbow motion, and functional impairment. Kim et al (69) reviewed the records of 18 children in whom trochlear deformities developed after distal humeral fractures (12 transcondylar or transphyseal, five supracondylar, one lateral condylar) and found that 17 of the 18

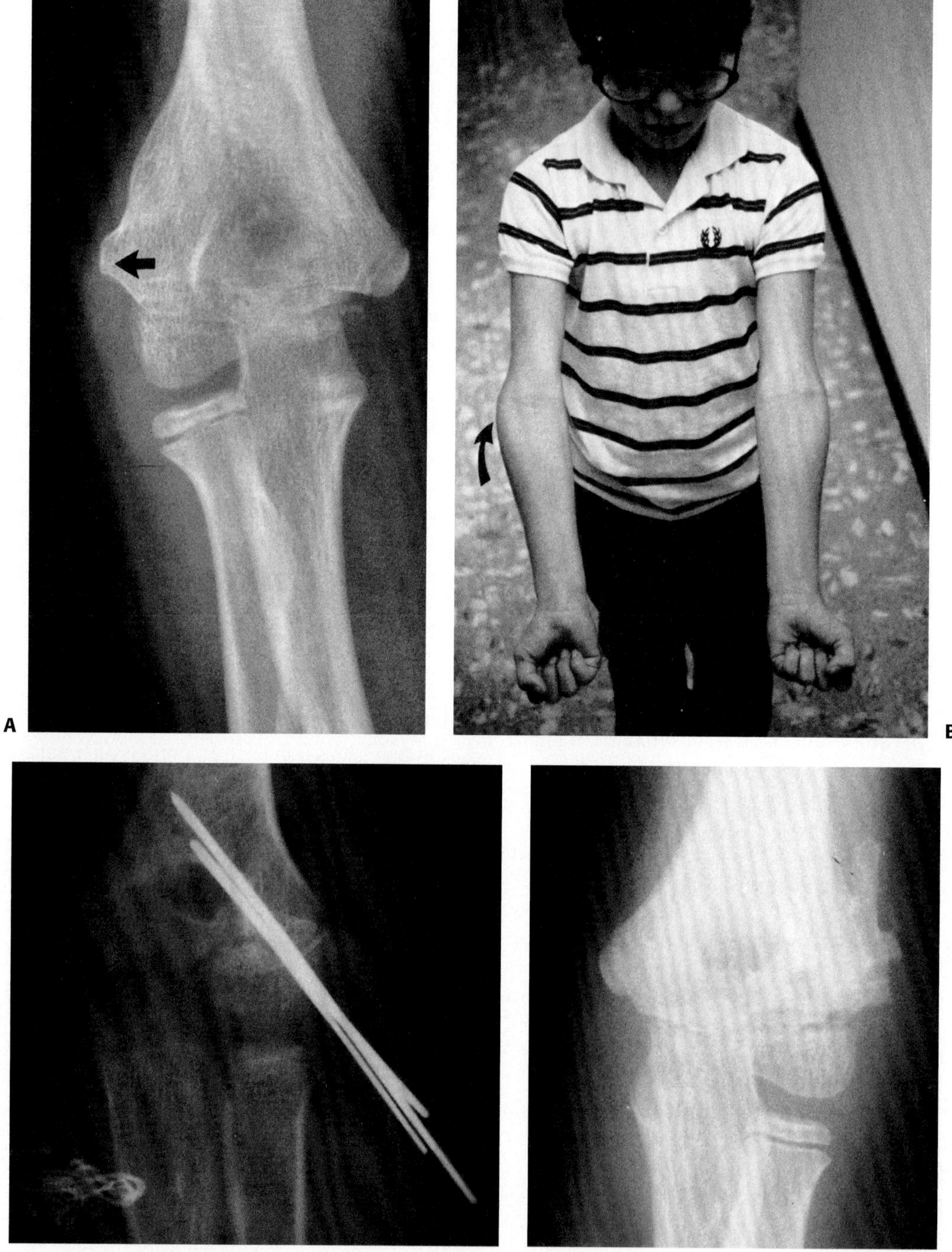

FIGURE 15-19 Spur formation. **A.** Follow-up x-ray of a boy whose lateral condylar fracture was treated nonoperatively. The periosteal flap produced a spur on the lateral aspect of the metaphysis (*arrow*). This fracture healed with a mild varus angulation as well. **B.** Clinically, the spur accentuated the lateral prominence (*arrow*) of the elbow, which in turn accentuated the mild valgus angulation. **C.** Considerable soft tissue dissection was performed in the process of open reduction of this lateral condylar fracture. **D.** At 2 months postsurgery, there is a large irregular spur formation secondary to periosteal new bone formation from the extensive dissection. (From Wilkins KE. Residuals of elbow fractures. *Orthop Clin N Am* 1990;21:289–312; with permission.)

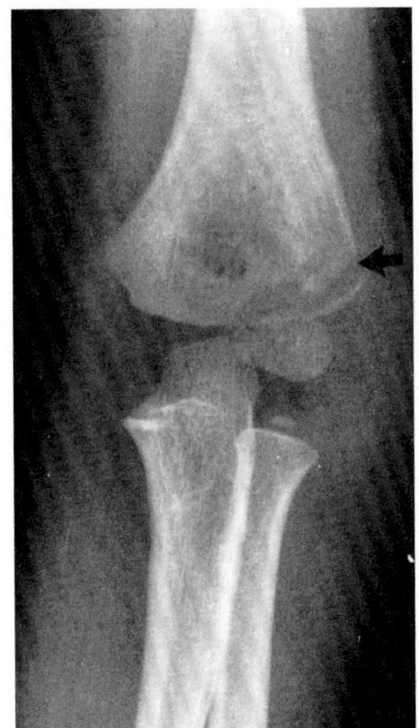

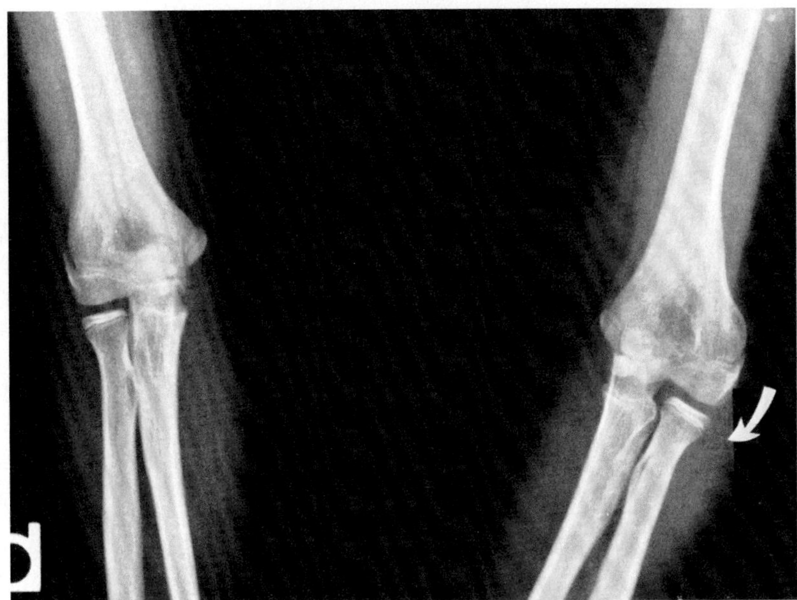

FIGURE 15-20 True varus. **A.** The injury film with a minimally displaced fracture (*arrow*). This 5-year-old child was treated with simple immobilization until the fracture was healed. **B.** Five years later, the patient had a persistent cubitus varus (*arrow*) that remained clinically apparent. The uninjured right elbow's carrying angle measured 5 degrees of valgus; the injured elbow had 10 degrees of varus. (From Wilkins KE. Residuals of elbow trauma in children. *Orthop Clin N Am* 1990;21:289–312, with permission.)

had cubitus varus deformities (varus angulation from 2 to 18 degrees). Bony defects in the medial and central trochlea were evident on x-rays as early as 1 month after injury (average, 3.4 months). At intermediate follow-up, eight of 10 patients evaluated had no progression of their deformities, and none of the five patients seen at long-term follow-up (more than 10 years) had progression.

The second type of fishtail deformity is a gentler, smooth curve. It is usually believed to be associated with osteonecrosis of the lateral part of the medial crista of the trochlea (62). The mechanisms of the development of this type of deformity are discussed in the section on osteonecrosis of the trochlea.

Neurologic Complications

The neurologic complications can be divided into two categories: acute nerve problems at the time of the injury and delayed neuropathy involving the ulnar nerve (the so-called tardy ulnar nerve palsy).

Acute Nerve Injuries

Reports of acute nerve injuries associated with this injury are rare. Smith and Joyce (43) reported two patients with posterior interosseous nerve injury after open reductions of the lateral condylar fragment, both of whom recovered spontaneously. McDonnell and Wilson (41) reported a case of transient radial nerve paralysis after an acute injury.

Friedman and Smith (70) reported a delayed radial nerve laceration from the tip of the screw that was used to stabilize a lateral condylar fracture 26 years earlier. This occurred when the patient sustained a hyperextension injury to the elbow.

Tardy Ulnar Nerve Palsy

Tardy ulnar nerve palsy as a late complication of fractures of the lateral condylar physis is well known, especially after the development of cubitus valgus from malunion or nonunion of fractures of the lateral condylar physis (71). The symptoms are usually gradual in onset. Motor loss occurs first, with sensory changes developing somewhat later (71). In Gay and Love's series (71) of 100 patients, the average interval of onset was 22 years.

Various treatment methods have been advocated, ranging from anterior transposition of the ulnar nerve (originally the most commonly used procedure) to simple relief of the cubital tunnel. We prefer simple subcutaneous anterior transposition of the nerve.

Physeal Arrest

Physeal arrest may be manifest by no more than premature fusion of the various secondary ossification centers to each other, with little or no deformity. Such a situation occurs much later than the original fracture. This phenomenon probably occurs because the fracture stimulates the ossification centers to

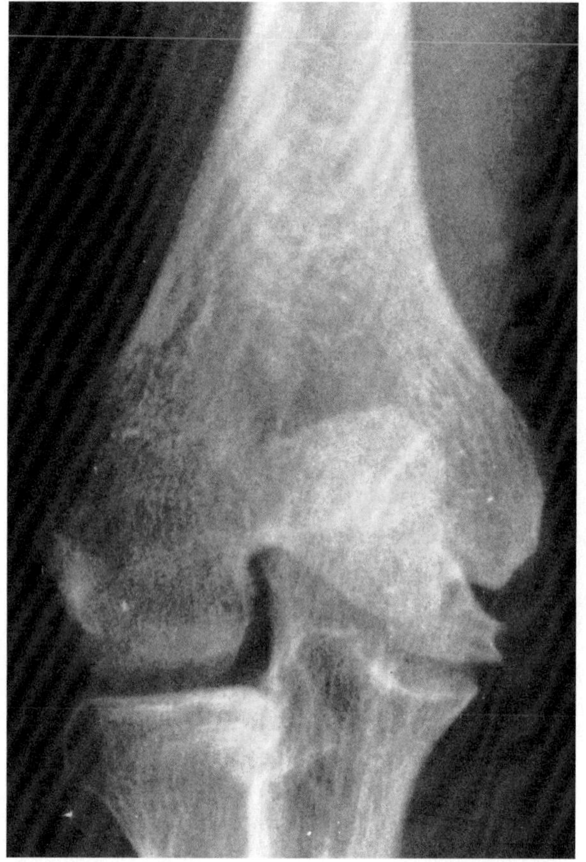

FIGURE 15-21 An angular "fishtail" deformity that persisted in this 14-year-old boy after operative treatment of a lateral condylar fracture 6 years previously.

grow more rapidly, and thus they reach maturity sooner; it is rarely caused by inadvertent dissection in the lateral condylar physis. Because only 20% of humeral growth occurs in the distal physis, physeal arrest seldom causes any significant angular or length deformities.

Malunion

The fragment rarely unites in an undesirable position. Cubitus valgus has been reported to occur as a result of malunion of the fracture fragments (19). Malunion of a Milch type I fracture pattern can result in the development of a bifid lateral condyle (Fig. 15-22). No reliable operative treatment has been described to re-establish the congruity of the articular surfaces in condylar malunions, and they are probably best left untreated. We have seen several patients with malunions in which the lateral condyle rotates in the coronal plane, with subsequent cubitus varus deformity.

Osteonecrosis

Osteonecrosis of the condylar fragment may be iatrogenic and is most commonly associated with the extensive dissection necessary to effect a late reduction or from loss of the blood supply at the time of injury (18,39,41). Wilson (44), however, described partial osteonecrosis in an essentially nondisplaced fracture of the lateral condylar physis that had an x-ray appearance and clinical course similar to those of osteochondritis dissecans. Osteonecrosis is rare in fractures of the lateral condylar physis that receive little or no initial treatment and result in nonunion (18,24).

Overly vigorous dissection of fresh fractures can result in osteonecrosis of either the lateral condylar ossification center (61,72) or, rarely, the metaphyseal portion of the fragment, leading to nonunion (Fig. 15-23). If the fracture unites, osteonecrosis of the lateral condyle reossifies over many years, much like Legg-Calvé-Perthes disease in the hip. Any residual deformity is usually related to loss of motion.

Ipsilateral Injuries

Fractures of the lateral condyle have been associated with elbow dislocations (35), ulnar shaft fractures (10,73), and fractures of the medial epicondyle. Often, an elbow dislocation is misdiagnosed in a patient with a lateral condylar fracture. Loss of the lateral crista can make the elbow unstable and allow the proximal radius or ulna to translocate laterally. This is a part of a normal pathologic condition associated with completely displaced lateral condylar fractures. In a true elbow dislocation, the proximal radius and ulna are displaced not only medially or laterally but also proximally (Fig. 15-24).

Fractures of the Capitellum

Fractures of the capitellum involve only the true articular surface of the lateral condyle. This includes, in some instances, the articular surface of the lateral crista of the trochlea. Generally, this fragment comes from the anterior portion of the distal articular surface. In adults, these fractures are not uncommon, but they are rare in children. In their review of 2,000 elbow fractures in children, Marion and Faysse (74) found only one fracture of the capitellum. Since then, this fracture has been frequently reported in older adolescents (48,74–77). Marion and Faysse (74) pointed out that verified fractures of the capitellum have not been described in children under 12 years of age. There have been two reports (78,79), however, of so-called anterior sleeve fractures of the lateral condyles, both in 8-year-olds (Fig. 15-25). These fractures involved a good portion of the anterior articular surface, although technically they could not be classified as pure capitellar fractures because they contained nonarticular epicondylar and metaphyseal portions in the fragment. This fracture is often difficult to diagnose because there is little ossified tissue. It is composed mainly of pure articular surface from the capitellum and essentially nonossified cartilage from the secondary ossification center of the lateral condyle.

Classification

Two fracture patterns have been described. The first is the more common Hahn-Steinthal type (80), which usually contains a

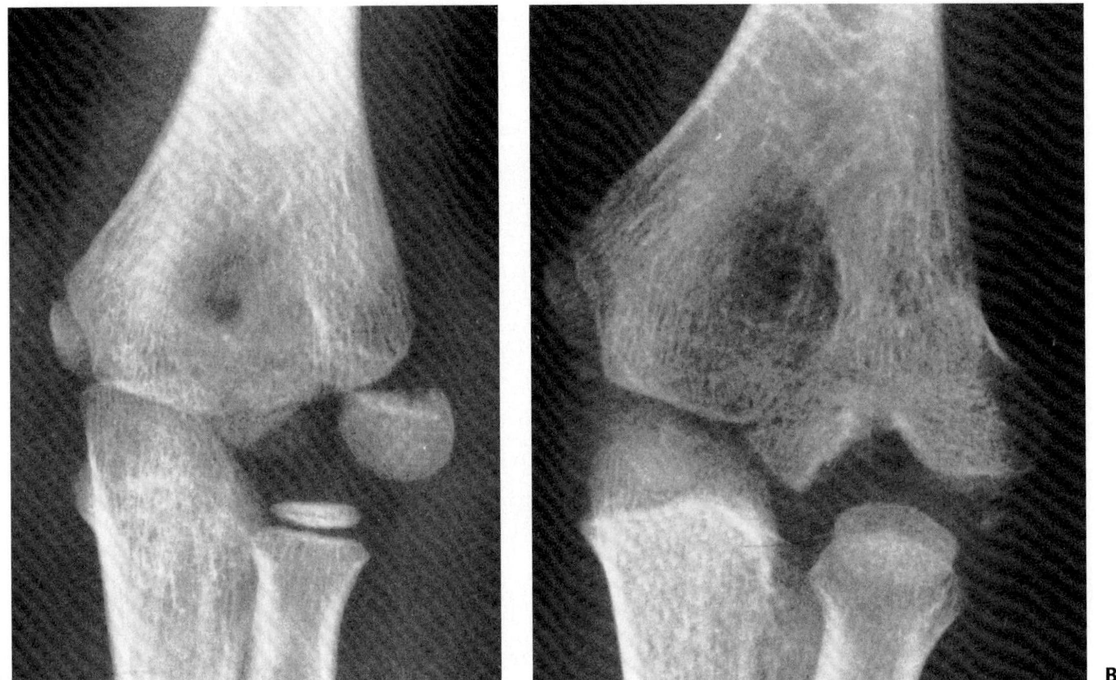

FIGURE 15-22 **A.** Injury film of a 7-year-old who sustained a Milch type I lateral condylar fracture. This patient was treated with cast immobilization alone. **B.** X-ray taken 2 years later showed complete fusion of the condylar epiphysis to the metaphysis, with the development of a "bifid" condyle.

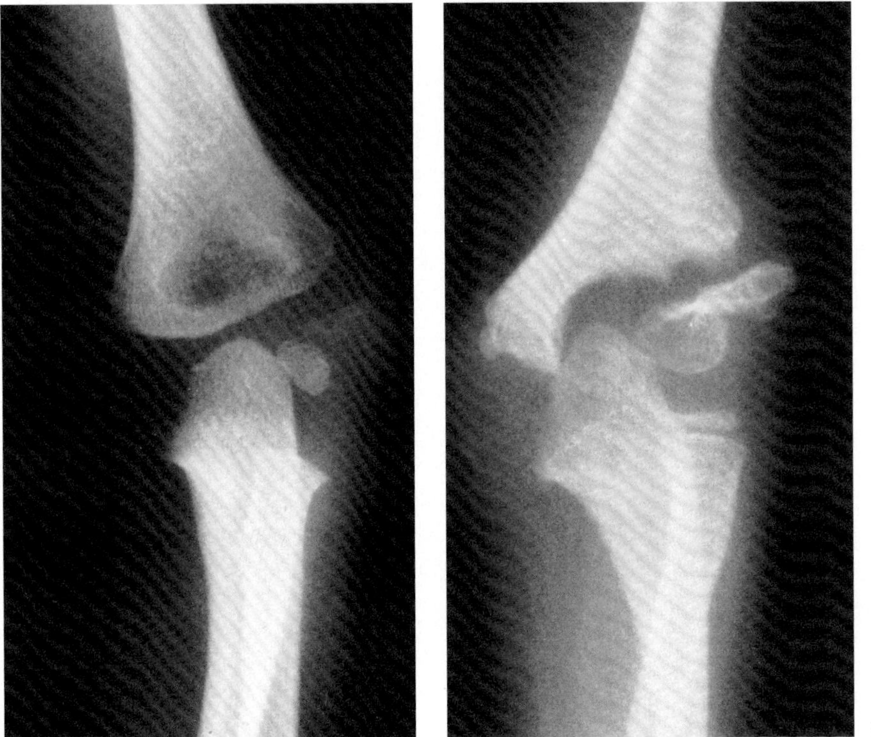

FIGURE 15-23 Osteonecrosis and nonunion developed in this child after of extensive dissection and difficulty in obtaining a primary open reduction. **A.** Injury film. **B.** Two years later, there was extensive bone loss in the metaphysis and a nonunion of the condyle.

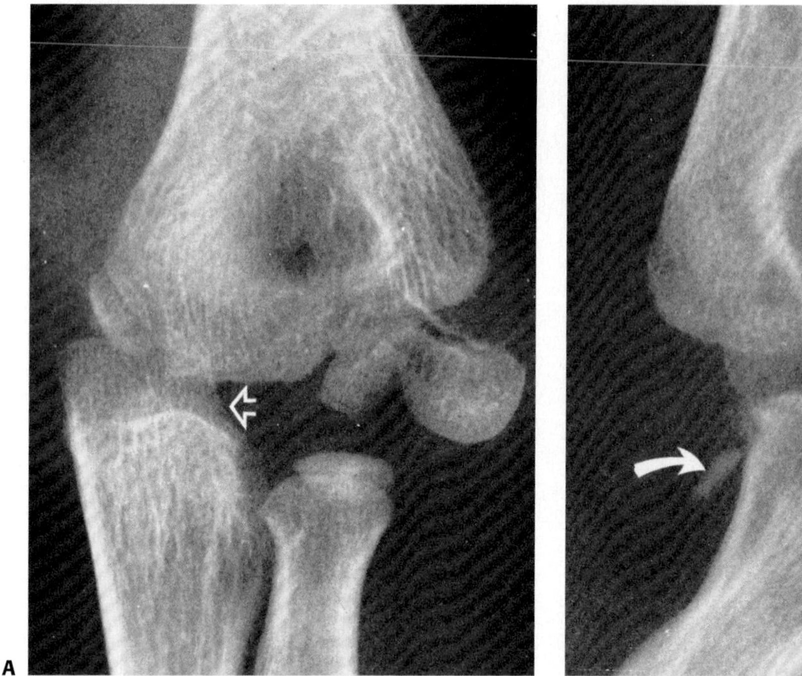

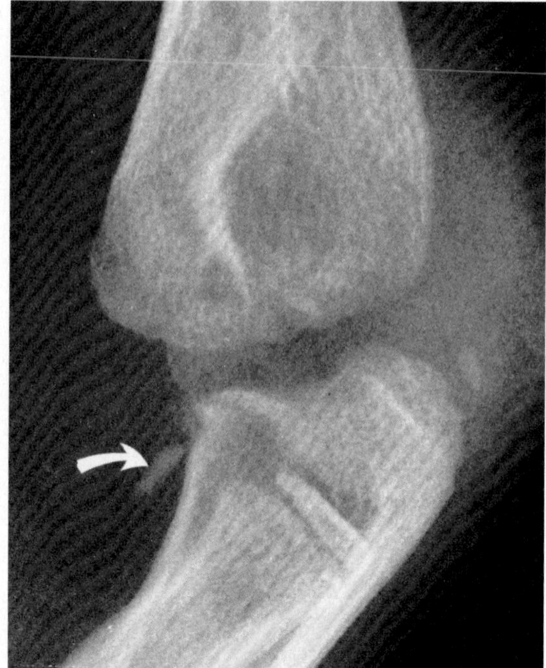

FIGURE 15-24 Ipsilateral injury. **A.** AP x-ray of an 8-year-old boy with a true posteromedial elbow dislocation (*open arrow*) and a Milch type I lateral condylar fracture. **B.** A small fracture of the coronoid process of the ulna (*closed arrow*) confirms the elbow dislocation's primary nature on the lateral x-ray.

rather large portion of cancellous bone of the lateral condyle. The lateral crista of the trochlea is often also included (Fig. 15-26). The second, or Kocher-Lorenz, type is more of a pure articular fracture with little if any subchondral bone attached and may represent a piece of articular cartilage from an underlying osteochondritis dissecans. This type of fracture is rare in children (78).

Mechanism of Injury

The most commonly accepted mechanism is that the anterior articular surface of the lateral condyle is sheared off by the radial head (75). The presence of cubitus recurvatum or cubitus valgus seems to predispose the elbow to this fracture pattern.

Diagnosis

Often, swelling is minimal, and the presence of the fragment restricts flexion. If the fragment is large, it may be readily apparent on a lateral x-ray (Fig. 15-27). On an AP x-ray, however, the fragment may be obliterated by the overlying distal metaphysis (Fig. 15-26). If the fragment is small, oblique views may be necessary to show the fragment. In younger children, arthrography or MRI may be required to diagnose this rare fracture. Letts et al (81) recommended computed tomography to help delineate the fracture type.

Associated Injuries

Because the mechanism is postulated to be a pushing off of the capitellum by the radial head, it stands to reason that there may be an associated radial head or neck fracture (76). In Palmer's (77) large series, including both children and adults, 31% had associated injuries of the proximal radius.

Treatment

Excising the fragment and open reduction and reattachment are the two most common forms of treatment. Closed reduction is not likely to be successful.

Excision of the Fragment

Through an open arthrotomy, the fragment can be either excised or reattached. Most investigators (74,75) favor excision because of its simplicity. In addition, motion and rehabilitation can be initiated early. Fowles and Kassab (75) reported good results after excision and noted that the earlier the fragment was excised, the better the results were. Even when large fragments were excised, joint instability did not appear to be a problem. In patients in whom treatment is delayed, although the results are not as good as when treatment is provided immediately after injury, improvement in function can be expected, even with late excision.

Reattachment of the Fragment

If the fragments are reattached, the fracture's stability is provided by wires or screws inserted through the lateral condyle's posterior surface. The major problems with reattachment are associated with osteonecrosis of the reattached fragment. Letts et

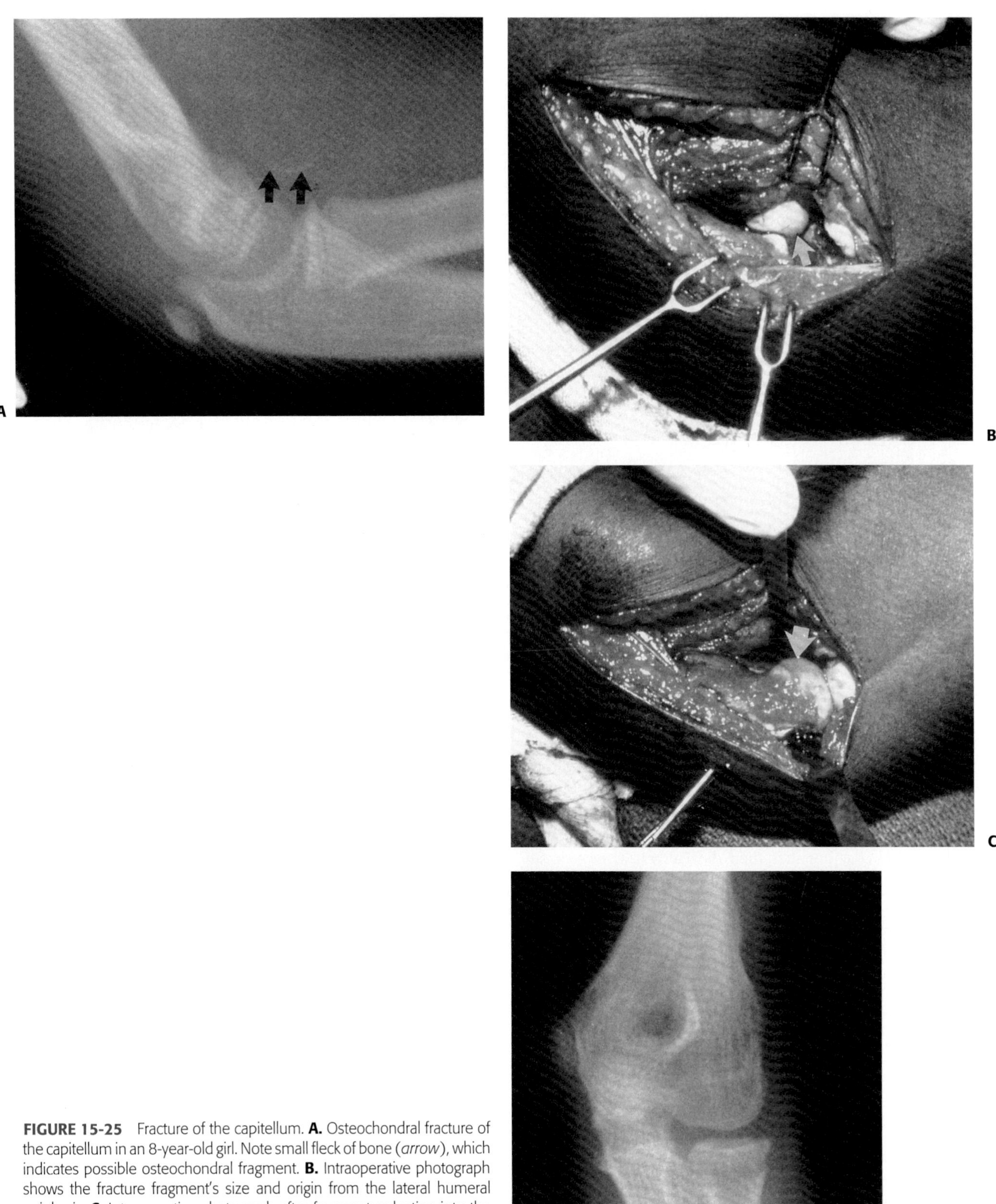

FIGURE 15-25 Fracture of the capitellum. **A.** Osteochondral fracture of the capitellum in an 8-year-old girl. Note small fleck of bone (*arrow*), which indicates possible osteochondral fragment. **B.** Intraoperative photograph shows the fracture fragment's size and origin from the lateral humeral epiphysis. **C.** Intraoperative photograph after fragment reduction into the bed of the capitellum. **D.** Healed fracture with articular congruity, restoration of cartilage space, and no osteonecrosis. (From Drvaric DM, Rooks MD. Case report. Anterior sleeve fracture of the capitellum. *J Orthop Trauma* 1990;4:188, with permission.)

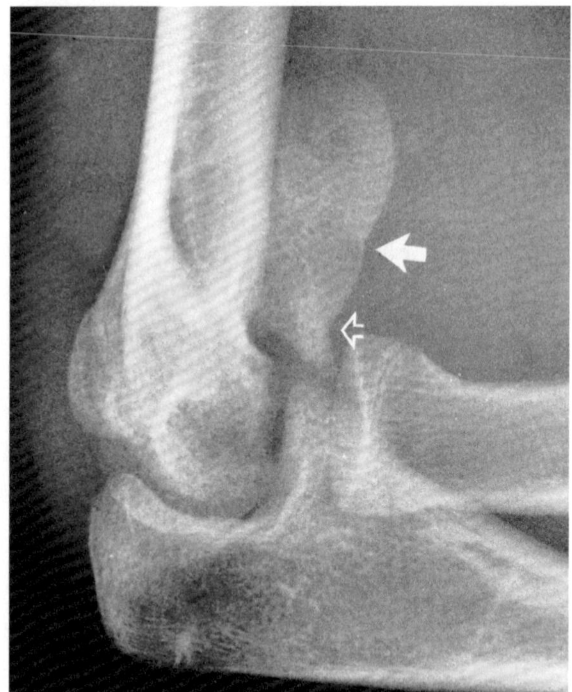
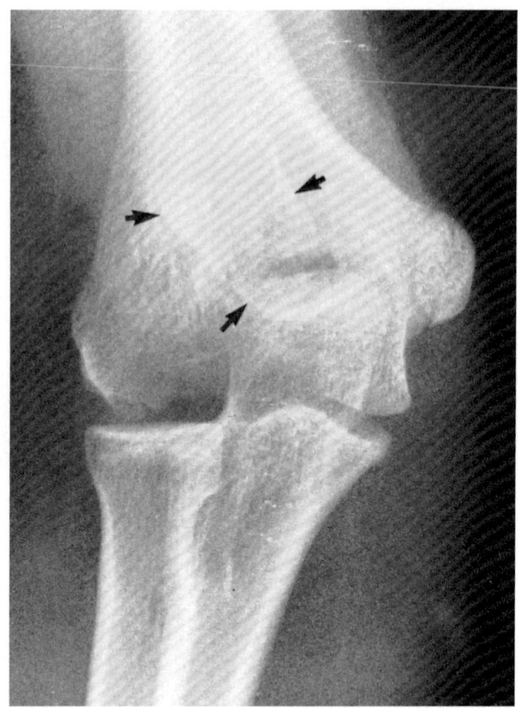

FIGURE 15-26 Fracture of the capitellum in a 13-year-old girl. **A.** Injury film, lateral view, shows the large capitellar fragment lying anterior and proximal to the distal humerus. Both the radiocapitellar (*solid arrow*) and trochlear grooves (*open arrow*) are seen in the fragment. **B.** In the AP view, only a faint outline of the fragment is seen (*arrows*).

al (81) reported satisfactory results with fixation of five capitellar fractures using K-wires (three fractures), Herbert screws (one fracture), and a cannulated screw (one fracture). In a biomechanical cadaver study, Elkowitz et al (82) demonstrated that Acutrac compression screws provided more stable fixation of simulated capitellar fractures than did Herbert screws. In an earlier study (83), they determined that fixation with posteroanteriorly directed cancellous lag screws was significantly more stable than fixation with anteroposteriorly directed lag screws; however, anteroposteriorly directed Acutrac compression screws provided significantly more stable fixation than the posteroanteriorly directed lag screws. An advantage of screw fixation is that it may not require later removal.

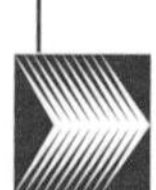

AUTHORS' PREFERRED TREATMENT

If the fragment is large, if the fracture is acute, and if an anatomic reduction can be achieved with a minimum of open manipulation or dissection, then we prefer to reattach it with two small cannulated screws inserted from posterior to anterior through a lateral approach. Enough bone must be present in the capitellar fragment to engage the screw threads, and if possible, countersink the heads of the screws (Fig. 15-27). If the fracture is old, if there is any comminution of the fragment, or if there is little bone in which to engage the screw threads, we believe the appropriate treatment is to simply excise the fragment and start early motion.

Complications

The major complication is osteonecrosis of the fragment. This, of course, occurs only in fractures in which the capitellar fragment is retained. Posttraumatic degenerative arthritis can occur whether the fragments are excised or retained. Many patients who are treated either operatively or nonoperatively can expect to lose some range of motion, but this loss is not always of functional or cosmetic significance. It is important to emphasize to the parents before the onset of treatment that complications can occur regardless of the treatment method.

Fractures Involving the Medial Condylar Physis

Fractures involving the medial condylar physis have two components. The intra-articular component involves, in some manner, the trochlear articular surface. The extra-articular portion includes the medial metaphysis and medial epicondyle. Because the fracture line extends into the articular surface of the trochlea, these often are called *trochlear fractures*. For purposes of description in this chapter, fractures of the trochlea are those that include only the articular surface.

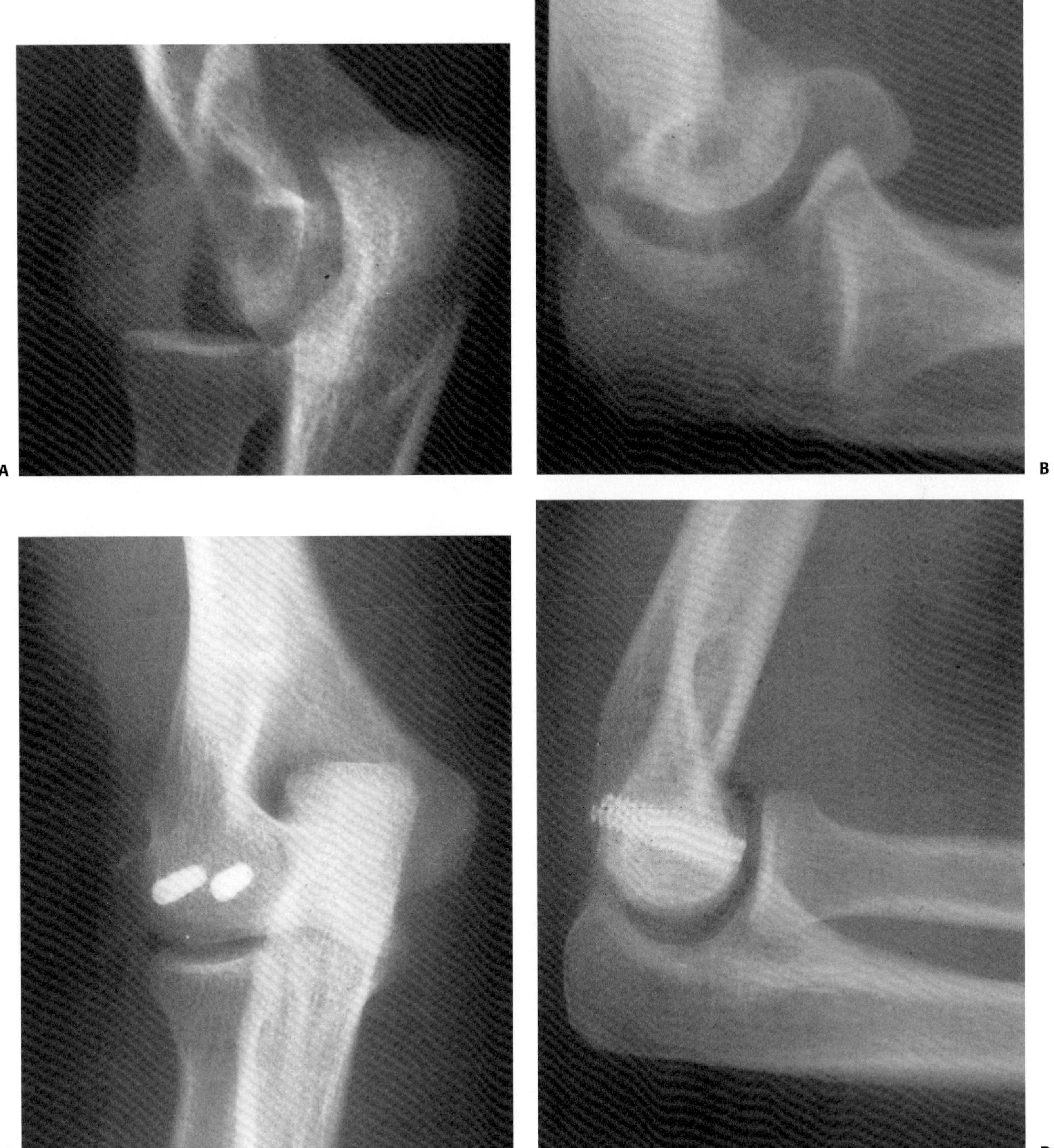

FIGURE 15-27 **A,B.** Fracture of the capitellum in a 14-year-old boy. **C,D.** After open reduction and fixation with two small cannulated screws through a lateral approach.

Incidence

Fractures involving the medial condylar physis are rare in skeletally immature children, accounting for less than 1% of fractures involving the distal humerus (84).

Many of the large series of elbow fractures in the literature and early fracture texts do not mention these fractures as a separate entity. Blount (85) described only one such fracture in his classic text. In Faysse and Marion's (86) review of more than 2,000 fractures of the distal humerus in children, only 10 fractures involved the medial condylar physis. Although it has been reported in a child as young as 2 years of age (87), this fracture pattern is generally considered to occur during later childhood.

Most series (86,88) show medial condylar fractures occurring somewhat later than lateral condylar fractures. A review of 38 patients in nine series (49,86–94) in which the specific ages were given showed that 37 patients were in the age range of 8 to 14 years. Thus, this fracture seems to occur after the ossification centers of the medial condylar epiphysis begin to appear. This fracture can occur as early as 6 months of age, however, before any ossification of the distal humerus has appeared (95,96), making the diagnosis extremely difficult.

Surgical Anatomy and Pathology

Fractures of the medial condylar physis involve both intra- and extra-articular components. They behave as Salter-Harris type IV physeal injuries, but not enough fractures have been described to show whether the fracture line courses through the secondary ossification center of the medial condylar epiphysis or whether it enters the common physeal line separating the lateral condylar ossification center from the medial condylar ossification center. This common physeal line terminates in the notch of the trochlea. The trochlea's lateral crista is ossified from the lateral condylar epiphysis. Only the medial crista is ossified by the secondary ossification centers of the medial condylar epiphysis. We believe that this fracture is a "mirror image" of the lateral condylar physeal injury and thus has characteristics of Salter-Harris type IV physeal injuries (Fig. 15-28). The deformity that develops if the fracture is untreated is nonunion, similar to that after lateral condylar physeal fracture, rather than physeal fusion, as occurs after a typical Salter-Harris type IV injury. The resultant deformity is cubitus varus instead of the cubitus valgus deformity that occurs with nonunion of the lateral condyle.

Characteristically, the metaphyseal fragment includes the intact medial epicondyle along with the common flexor origin of the muscles of the forearm. These flexor muscles cause the loosened fragment to rotate so that the fracture surface is facing anteriorly and medially and the articular surface is facing posteriorly and laterally (Fig. 15-29) (87,89). Rotation of the fragment is especially accentuated when the elbow is extended. Chacha (89) also noted that often the lateral aspect of the common flexor origin and the anterior capsule of the joint were torn and the fracture surface could usually be reached through this anterior opening into the joint.

The blood supply to the medial epicondyle and medial metaphysis courses extra-articularly along with the medial flexor muscle groups. The blood supply to the lateral ossification center of the medial crista of the trochlea, however, must traverse the surface of the medial condylar physis. If the fracture line disrupts these small intra-articular vessels, disruption and subsequent circulation loss to the lateral portion of the medial crista can result, leading to the development of a fishtail deformity.

Mechanism of Injury

Two separate mechanisms can produce physeal fractures of the medial condyle. Ashurst's (87) patients described falling directly

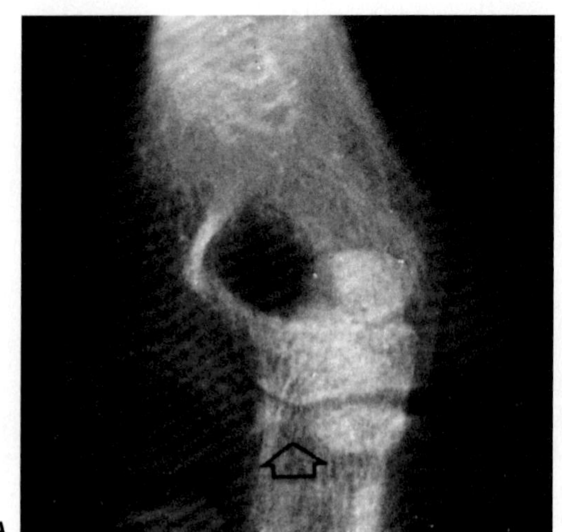

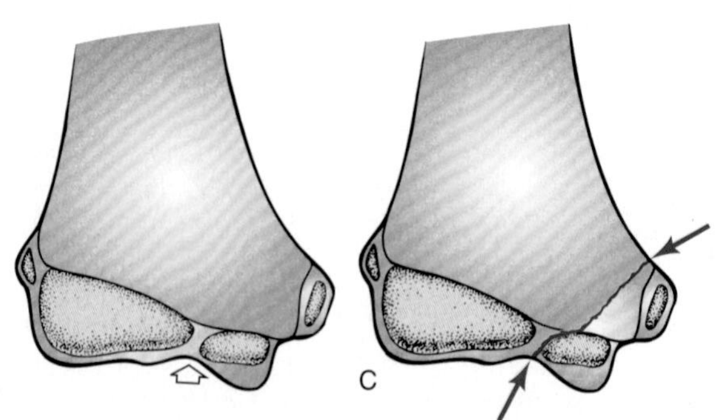

FIGURE 15-28 **A.** The AP x-ray of a 9-year-old boy demonstrates the location of the ossification centers. A common physeal line (*arrow*) separates the medial and lateral condylar physes. **B.** Relationship of the ossification centers to the articular surface. The common physis terminates in the trochlear notch (*arrow*). **C.** Location of the usual fracture line involving the medial condylar physis (*arrows*).

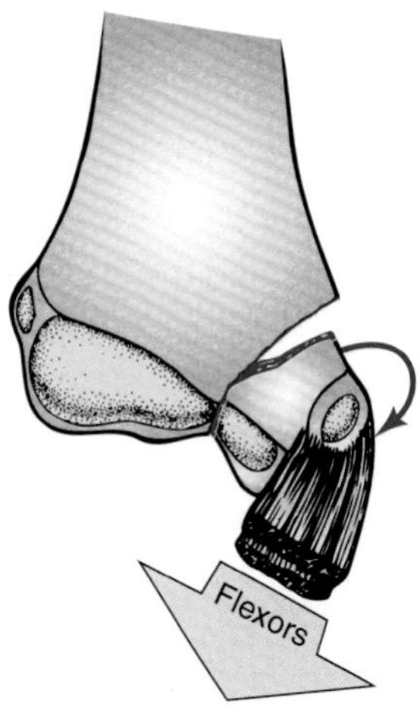

FIGURE 15-29 Displacement of the medial condyle. The pull of the forearm flexor muscles rotates the fragment so that the fracture surface is facing anteromedially and the articular surface is posterolateral. (Modified and reprinted with permission from Chacha PB. Fractures of the medial condyle of the humerus with rotational displacement. *J Bone Joint Surg [Am]* 1970;52:1453–1458.)

on the point of the flexed elbow. This mechanism was also implicated in other reports (89,93,95,97). In this mechanism, it is speculated that the semilunar notch's sharp edge of the olecranon splits the trochlea directly (Fig. 15-30A). In three more recent series (91,98,99), many patients sustained this injury when they fell on their outstretched arms. The theory is that this is an avulsion injury caused by a valgus strain at the elbow (Fig. 15-30B). Fowles and Kassab (99) reported a patient with a concomitant valgus greenstick fracture of the olecranon associated with a fracture of the medial condylar physis. They believed this fracture provided further evidence that this was a valgus avulsion type of injury.

Once the fragment becomes disassociated from the distal humerus, the forearm flexor muscles produce a sagittal anterior rotation of the fragment.

Classification

Classification, as with fractures of the lateral condylar physis, is based on the fracture line's location and the degree of the fracture's displacement.

Location of the Fracture Line

Milch (100) classified fractures of the medial condylar physis in adults into two types. In type I fractures, the fracture line traverses the apex of the trochlea. In type II fractures, it traverses the capitulotrochlear groove. He believed that the origin of the fracture line depended on whether the radial head, as in type II, or the semilunar notch of the olecranon, as in type I, served as the impinging force for the abduction injury. Both fracture patterns occur in children (Fig. 15-31), but type I fractures seem to be more common because the common physeal line, which serves as a point of weakness, ends in the apex of the trochlea.

Displacement of the Fracture

Kilfoyle (101) described three fracture displacement patterns that can be helpful in determining appropriate treatment (Fig. 15-32). In type I, the fracture line in the medial condylar metaphysis extends down to the physis. He noted that some of these might represent incomplete supracondylar fractures. Unless there is a greenstick crushing of the medial supracondylar column, these fractures are usually of no clinical significance. In type II, the fracture line extends into the medial condylar physis. The intra-articular portion, as it is in preosseous cartilage, is often not recognized. In this second type, the medial condylar fragment usually remains undisplaced. In type III, the condylar fragment is both rotated and displaced.

Bensahel et al (95) and Papavasiliou et al (88) found that type III displacement fractures, which accounted for only 25%, were more likely to occur in older adolescents, and type I fractures were more common in younger children. These studies also confirmed the correlation between the type of displacement and the treatment method.

Medial condylar physeal fractures have been reported in association with greenstick fractures of the olecranon and with true posterolateral elbow dislocations (Fig. 15-33) (95,102). Some investigators (95,96) found that child abuse was more common in their younger patients with these fractures than with other elbow fractures.

Diagnosis

Clinically and on x-rays, a fracture of the medial condylar physis is most often confused with a fracture of the medial epicondyle (103). In both types of intra- and extra-articular fractures, swelling is concentrated medially, and there may be valgus instability of the elbow joint. In a true intra-articular fracture, however, there is varus instability as well. Such is usually not the case with an isolated extra-articular fracture of the medial epicondyle. Ulnar nerve paresthesia may be present with both types of fractures.

In older children with a large metaphyseal fragment, involvement of the entire condyle is usually obvious on x-rays; in younger children, in whom only the epicondyle is ossified, fracture of the medial condylar physis may be erroneously diagnosed as an isolated fracture of the medial epicondyle (Fig. 15-34) (49,90,99).

In differentiating these two fractures, it is helpful to remember that medial epicondylar fractures are often associated with elbow dislocations, usually posterolateral, and that elbow dislocations are rare before ossification of the medial condylar epiphysis begins. With medial condylar physeal fractures, the elbow tends to subluxate posteromedially (90) due to the loss of trochlear stability.

Any metaphyseal ossification with the epicondylar fragment suggests the presence of an intra-articular fracture of the medial

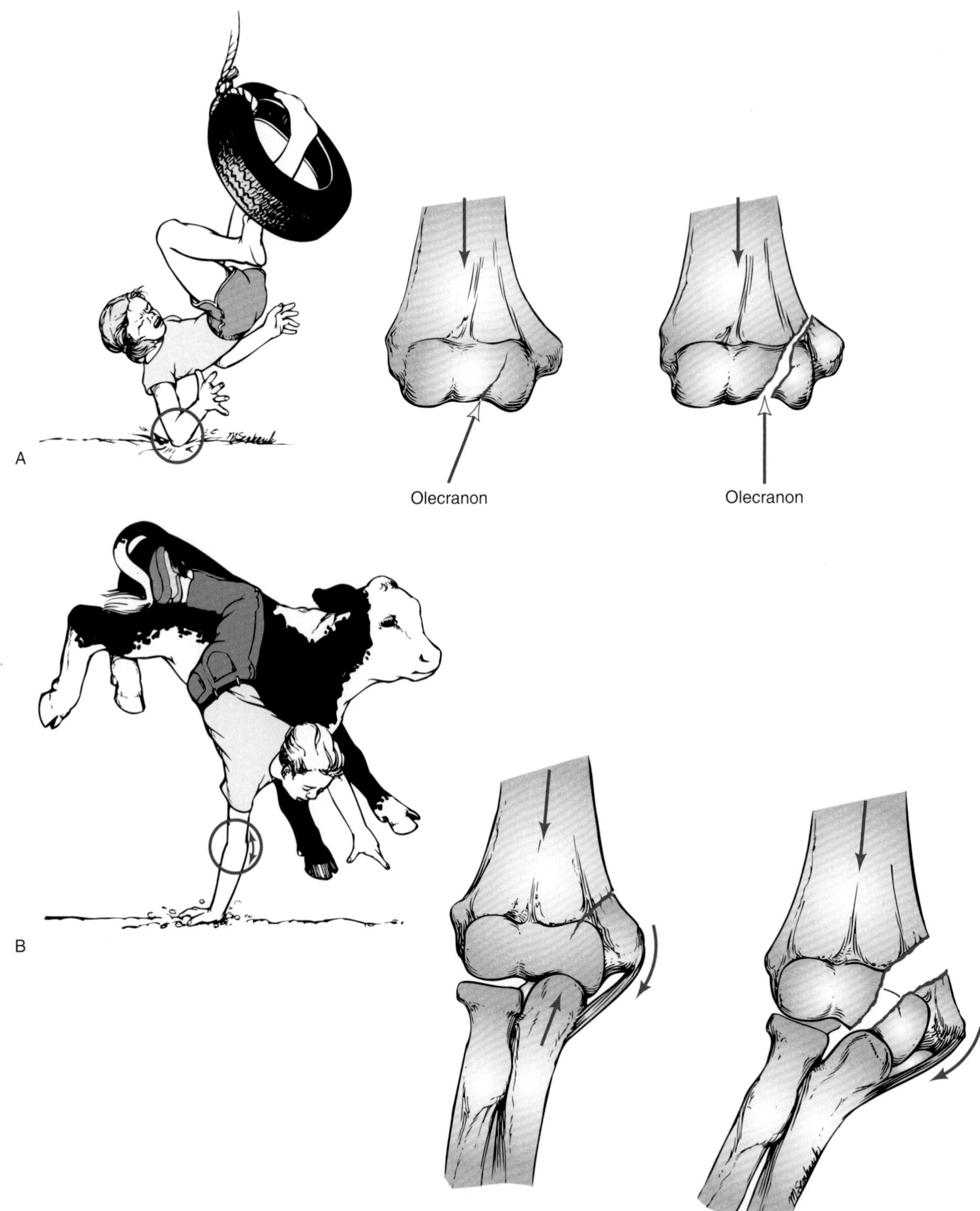

FIGURE 15-30 Medial condylar fracture mechanisms of injury. **A.** A direct force applied to the posterior aspect of the elbow causes the olecranon's sharp articular margin to wedge the medial condyle from the distal humerus. **B.** Falling on the outstretched arm with the elbow extended and the wrist dorsiflexed causes the medial condyle to be avulsed by both ligamentous and muscular forces.

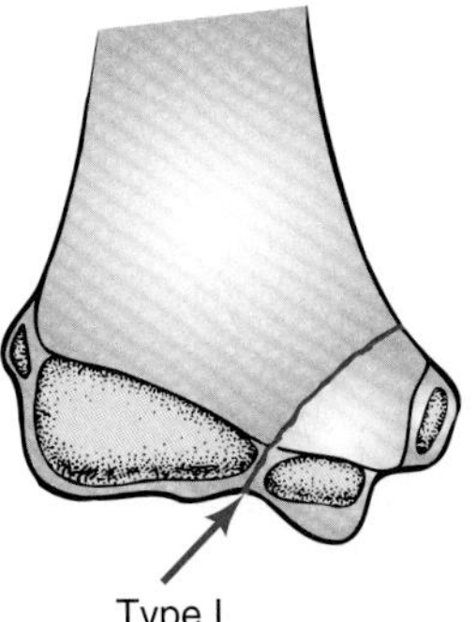

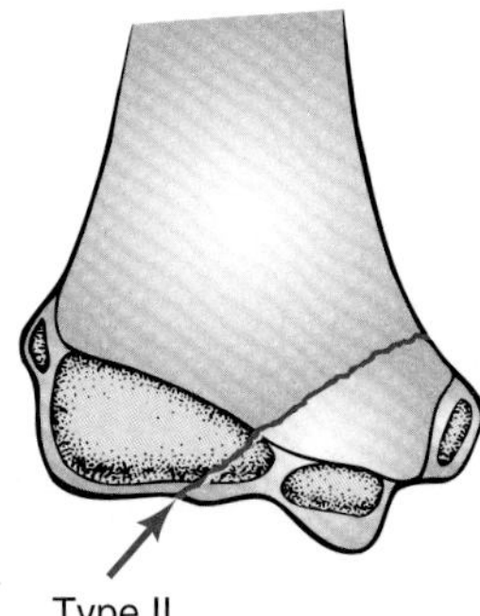

FIGURE 15-31 Medial condylar fracture patterns. In the Milch type I injury, the fracture line terminates in the trochlear notch (left, *arrow*). In the Milch type II injury, the fracture line terminates more laterally in the capitulotrochlear groove (right, *arrow*). (Modified and reprinted with permission from Milch H. Fractures and fracture–dislocations of the humeral condyles. *J Trauma* 1964;4:592–607.)

condyle and is an indication for further evaluation. Often, the medial condyle and the medial epicondyle are markedly displaced as a unit. A positive fat pad sign indicates that the injury has entered the elbow joint and a fracture of the medial condyle is likely (97,104). Isolated fractures of the medial epicondyle are extra-articular and usually do not have positive fat pad signs.

If the true location of the fracture line is questionable in a child younger than 8 to 10 years of age with significant medial elbow ecchymosis, arthrography or MRI of the elbow should be performed.

Treatment

For displaced fractures, open reduction with internal fixation is the most often used treatment method (88,91,93,95,98,99, 101,105). The fracture fragment can be approached by a posteromedial incision that allows good exposure of both the fracture site and the ulnar nerve. Fixation is easily achieved with smooth K-wires (Fig. 15-33) or with screws in older adolescents. Two wires are necessary because of the sagittal rotation forces exerted on the fracture fragment by the common flexor muscles. El Ghawabi (91) reported frequent delayed union and nonunion in fractures that were not rigidly stabilized.

In Kilfoyle's displacement types I and II fracture patterns, enough residual internal stability is usually present to allow the fracture to be simply immobilized in a cast or posterior splint (86,88,91,95,101). As with fractures of the lateral condylar physis, union may be slow. In fractures treated promptly, results have been satisfactory (49,89,99). Because there usually is more displacement in older children, the results in this age group are not as satisfactory as those in younger children, who tend to have relatively nondisplaced fractures (95).

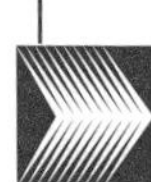

AUTHORS' PREFERRED TREATMENT

We generally treat type I nondisplaced fractures with simple observation and a posterior splint. Follow-up x-rays at weekly intervals are taken to ensure there is no late displacement. When there is good callus at the metaphyseal portion of the fracture line by 3 to 4 weeks, the splint is removed and early active motion is initiated. We continue to follow the patient until there is a full range of motion and obliteration of the fracture line.

Types II and III displaced fractures must be reduced and stabilized. This is usually difficult to do by closed methods because the swelling associated with this injury makes it hard to accurately identify the landmarks for pin placement. We proceed with an open reduction through a medial approach with identification and protection of the ulnar nerve. The posterior surface of the condylar fragment and the medial aspect of the medial crista of the trochlea should be avoided in the dissection because these are the blood supply sources to the ossific nuclei of the trochlea. Fixation with two parallel pins should be in the metaphyseal segment if possible (Fig. 15-35). Cannulated screw fixation can be used in adolescents near skeletal maturity.

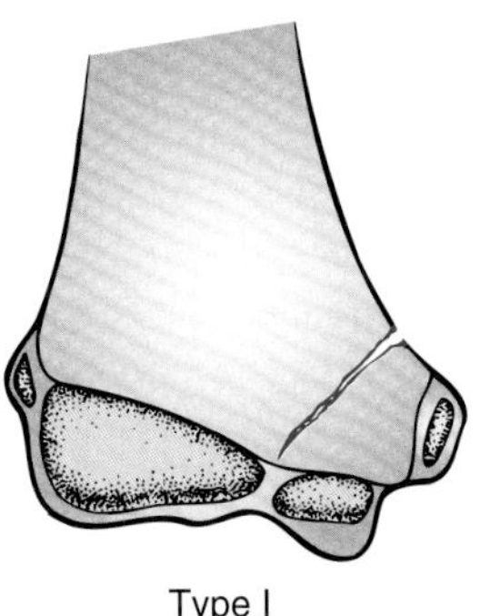

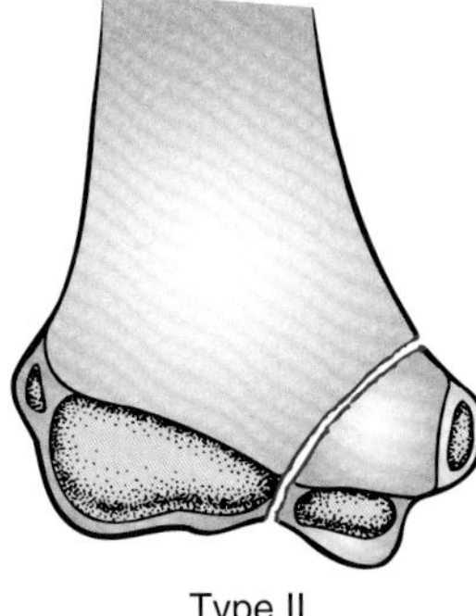

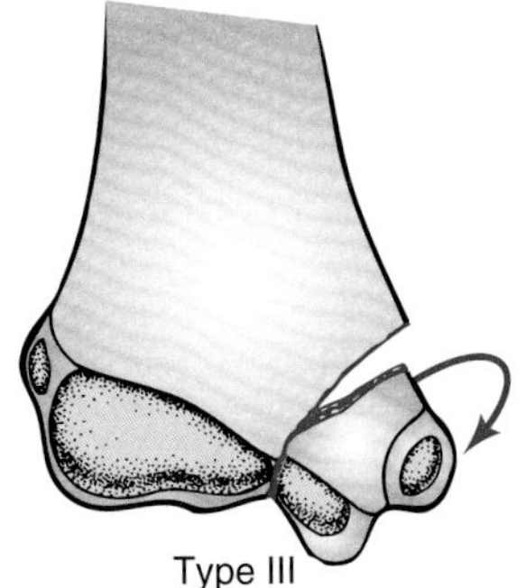

FIGURE 15-32 Kilfoyle classification of displacement patterns. (Modified and reprinted with permission from Kilfoyle RM. Fractures of the medial condyle and epicondyle of the elbow in children. *Clin Orthop* 1965;41: 43–50.)

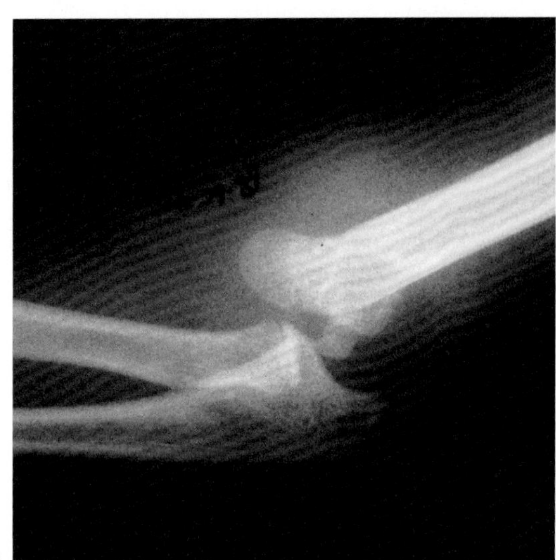

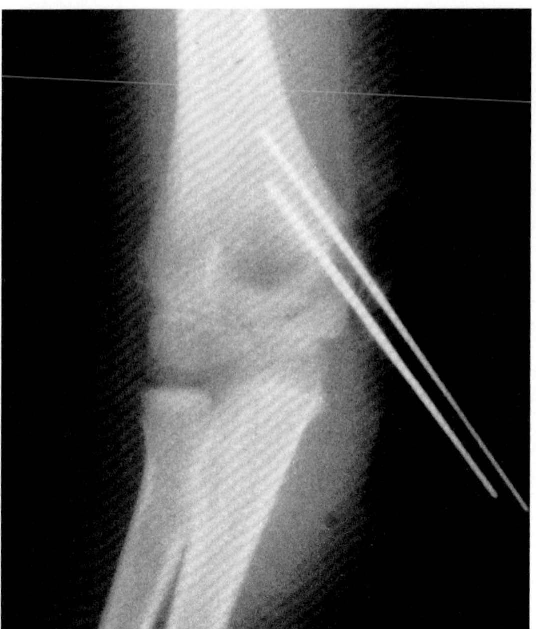

FIGURE 15-33 **A.** Injury film of a 10-year-old girl who sustained a type III displaced fracture of the medial condyle associated with a posterolateral elbow dislocation. **B.** After open reduction and K-wire fixation through an anteromedial approach. (Courtesy of Elizabeth A. Szalay, MD.)

Complications

The major complication is failure to make the proper diagnosis. This is especially true in younger children, in whom a medial condylar fracture can be confused with a displaced fracture of the medial epicondyle (Fig. 15-34). When the diagnosis is a real possibility, especially in a child with no ossification of the trochlea, examination with anesthesia, arthrography, or MRI may be helpful. Leet, Young, and Hoffer (106) reported complications after 33% of 21 medial condylar fractures, including osteonecrosis of the trochlea, nonunion, and loss of reduction. Untreated displaced fractures usually result in nonunion with cubitus varus deformity (Fig. 15-36) (94,99). We have seen one nonunion after a fracture of the medial condyle. Delayed union has been reported in patients treated with insecure fixation or simply placed in a cast (91,101).

Some disturbance of the vascular supply to the medial condylar fragment may occur during open reduction and internal fixation or at the time of initial injury. Several investigators have reported subsequent avascular changes in the medial crista of the trochlea (88,91,99,101). Hanspal (92) reviewed Cothay's original patient (90) 18 years after delayed open reduction and found that despite some minimal loss of motion, the patient was asymptomatic. X-rays, however, showed changes compatible with osteonecrosis of the medial condyle.

Both cubitus varus and valgus deformities have been reported in patients whose fractures united uneventfully. The valgus deformity appears to be caused by secondary stimulation or overgrowth of the medial condylar fragment. Some simple stimulation of the medial epicondyle's prominence may also produce the false appearance of a cubitus valgus deformity. Cubitus varus appears to result from decreased growth of the trochlea, possibly caused by a vascular insult. Principles for treating nonunion of lateral condylar fractures are generally applicable to nonunions of the medial condyle (Fig. 15-37).

El Ghawabi (91) described one partial ulnar neuropathy occurring after this type of injury. The neuropathy almost completely recovered after anterior transposition of the ulnar nerve.

Fractures of the Trochlea

Osteochondral fractures involving only the articular portion of the trochlea are extremely rare in skeletally immature children; only one such fracture has been reported in the English-language literature. Grant and Miller (107) reported a 13-year-old boy who had a posterolateral dislocation of the elbow with marked valgus instability and fractures of the medial epicondyle and radial neck. When the elbow was explored to secure the epicondyle, a large osteochondral fragment from the medial crista of the trochlea was found lying between the two articular surfaces. The fragment was replaced and fixed, and a satisfactory result was obtained, although the presence of the fragment was not detected preoperatively.

In an older child who sustains an elbow dislocation and in whom there is some widening of the joint after reduction, an intra-articular fracture of the trochlea or capitellum should be suspected. Arthrography, MRI, or computed tomography-arthrography, should be used for confirmation.

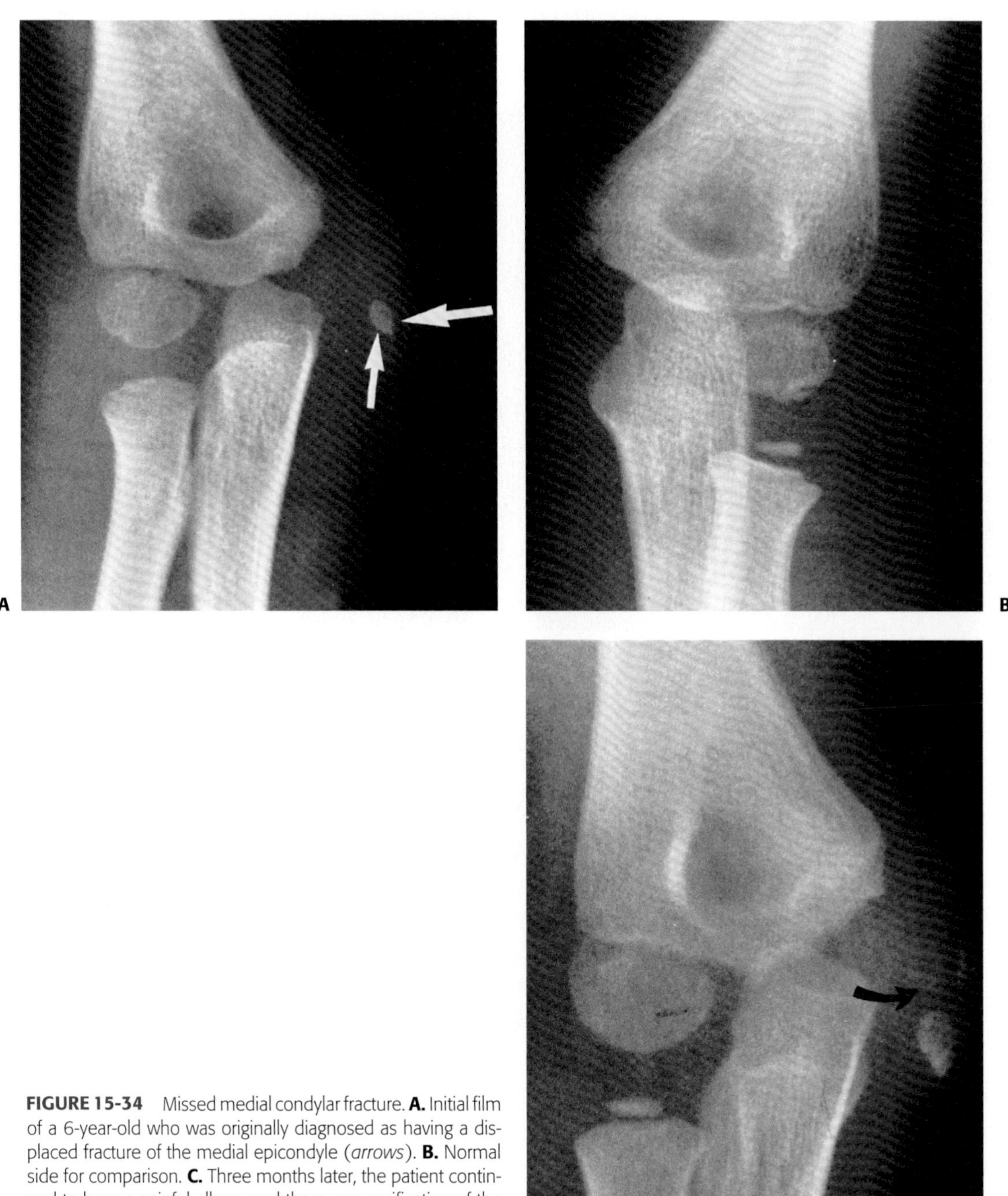

FIGURE 15-34 Missed medial condylar fracture. **A.** Initial film of a 6-year-old who was originally diagnosed as having a displaced fracture of the medial epicondyle (*arrows*). **B.** Normal side for comparison. **C.** Three months later, the patient continued to have a painful elbow, and there was ossification of the metaphysis (*arrow*) adjacent to the epicondyle.

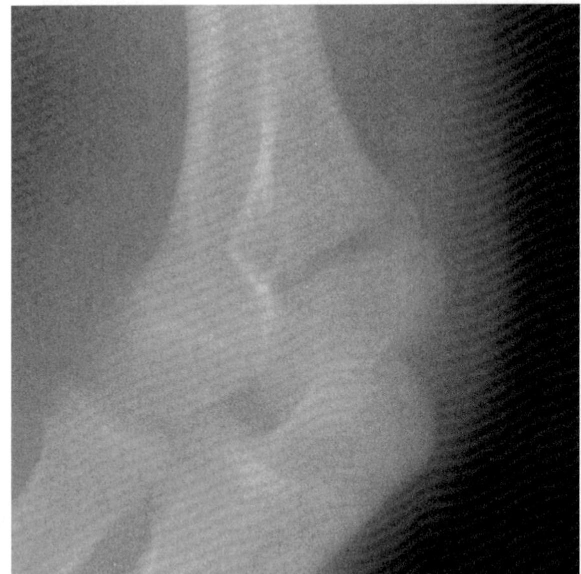

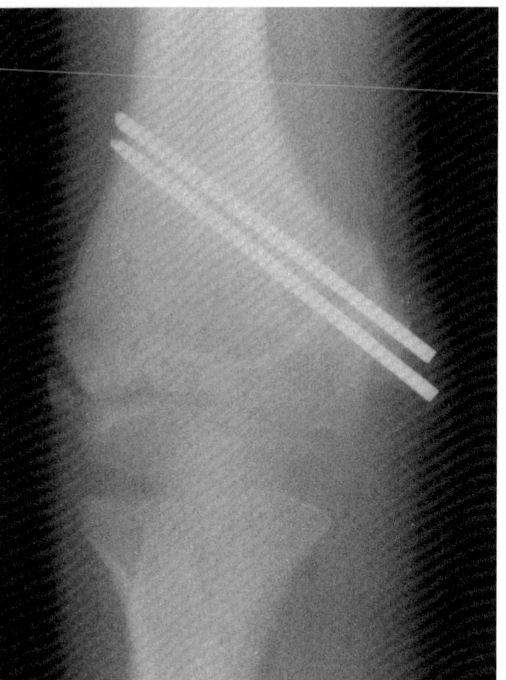

FIGURE 15-35 **A.** Stage II fracture of the medial condyle in a 10-year-old girl. **B.** After open reduction and Kirschner wire fixation through a medial approach.

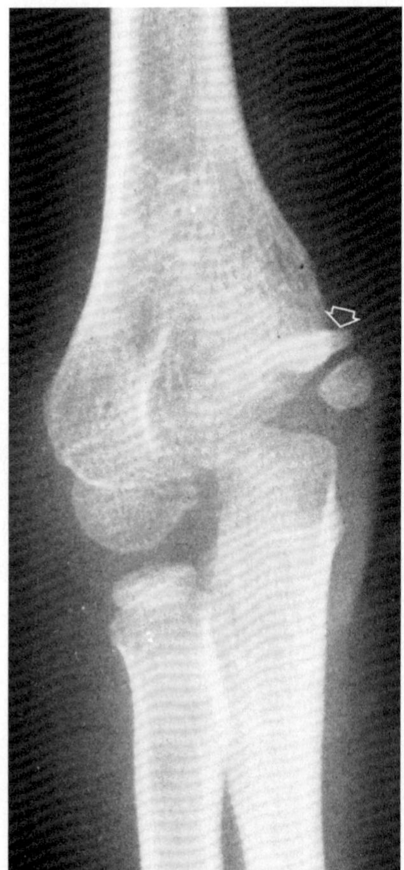

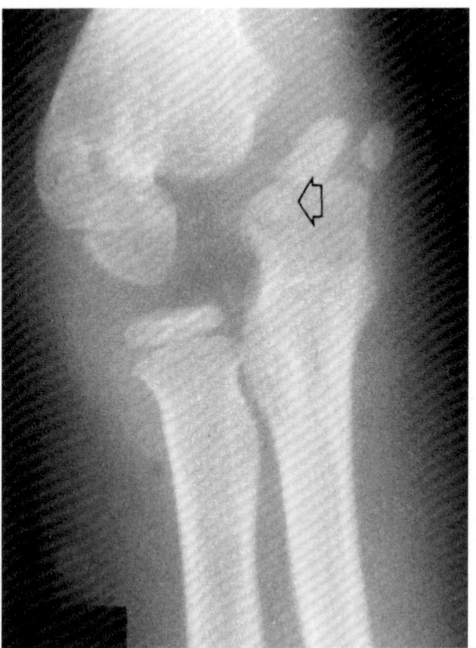

FIGURE 15-36 Nonunion in addition to cubitus varus deformity. **A.** Original film of a 5-year-old girl who sustained an injury 1 year previously. The metaphyseal fragment (*arrow*) is attached to the medial epicondyle. **B.** Film taken 2 years later. Some ossification has developed in the medial condylar epiphysis (*arrow*). (Courtesy of Roy N. Davis, MD.)

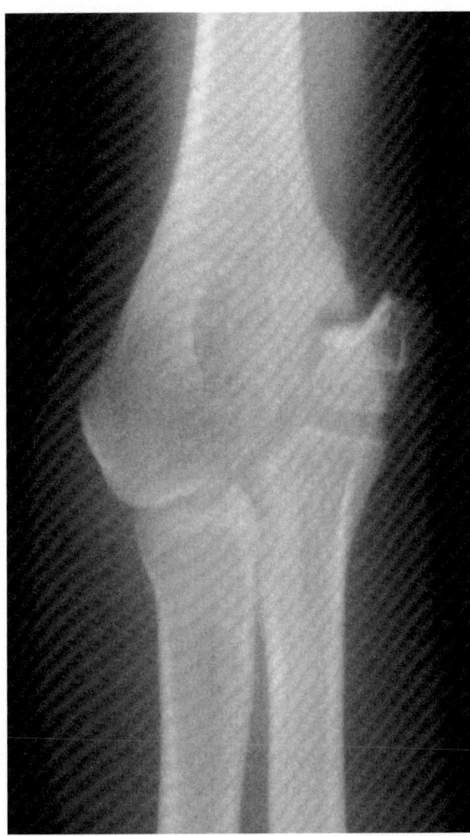

FIGURE 15-37 Nonunion of a medial condylar fracture in a 10-year-old girl. Note medial subluxation of the radius and ulna.

Fractures Involving the Entire Distal Humeral Physis

Incidence

From 1960 to 1978, many individual patients were reported (108–111). Once the presence of this injury became recognized, larger series appeared. Seven separate series reported a total of 45 fractures (84,112–117), and Abe et al (118) reported a series of 21 fractures. Originally thought to be a rare injury, it appears that fractures involving the entire distal humeral physis occur frequently in children. The major problem is the initial recognition of this injury.

Surgical Anatomy

The distal humeral epiphysis extends across to include the secondary ossification of the medial epicondyle until about 6 to 7 years of age in girls and 8 to 9 years in boys. Thus, fractures involving the entire physeal line include the medial epicondyle up to this age. In older children, only the lateral and medial condylar physeal lines are included.

Most fractures involving the entire distal humeral physis occur before the age of 6 or 7. The younger the child is, the greater the volume of the distal humerus that is occupied by the distal epiphysis will be. As the humerus matures, the physeal

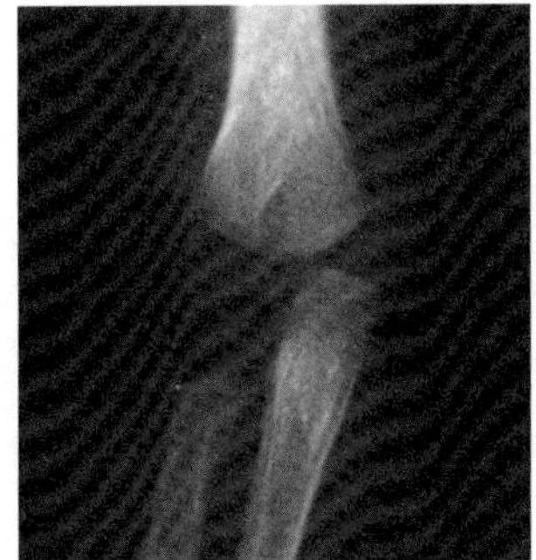

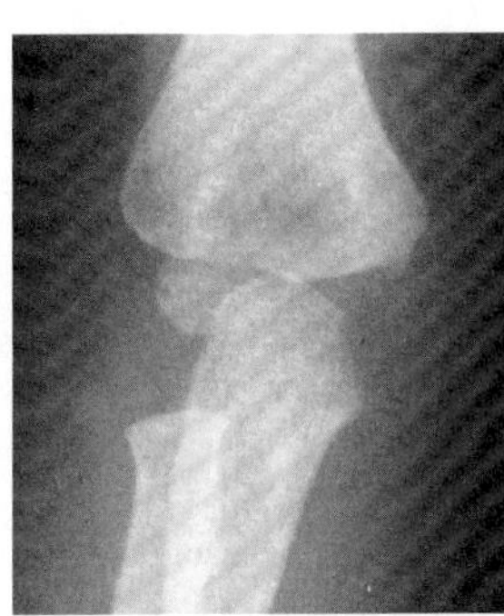

FIGURE 15-38 **A.** At 5 months of age, the metaphysis has advanced only to the supracondylar ridges. **B.** By 4 years of age, the edge of the metaphysis has advanced well into the area of the epicondyles.

line progresses more distally, with a central V forming between the medial and lateral condylar physes (Fig. 15-38). Ashhurst (87) believed that this V-shaped configuration of the physeal line helps protect the more mature distal humerus from physeal fractures.

Because fractures coursing along the distal humeral physis traverse the anatomic centers of the condyles, they are the pediatric counterparts of the adult bicondylar fracture. Because the fracture is distal, the fracture surfaces are broader than those proximally through the supracondylar fractures. This broader surface area of the fracture line may help prevent tilting of the distal fragment. Because the fracture lines do not involve the articular surface, development of joint incongruity with resultant loss of elbow motion is unlikely if malunion occurs.

Finally, part of the blood supply to the medial crista of the trochlea courses directly through the physis. The blood supply to this area is vulnerable to injury, which may cause osteonecrosis in this part of the trochlea.

Because the physeal line is more proximal in young infants, it is nearer the center of the olecranon fossa (Fig. 15-38). A hyperextension injury in this age group is more likely to result in a physeal separation than a bony supracondylar fracture (119).

Mechanism of Injury

The exact mechanism of this injury is unknown and probably varies with the age group involved. A few consistent factors are evident.

First, many fractures of the entire distal humeral physis have occurred as birth injuries associated with difficult deliveries (110,112,120–122). Siffert (110) noted that the clinical appearance of these injured elbows at the time of delivery was not especially impressive. There was only moderate swelling and some crepitus.

Second, DeLee et al (84) noted a high incidence of confirmed or suspected child abuse in their very young patients. Other reports (112,113,123) have confirmed the frequency of child abuse in infants and young children with these fractures.

Bright (124) showed that a physis is more likely to fail with rotary shear forces than with pure bending or tension forces.

Young infants have some residual flexion contractures of the elbow from intrauterine positioning; this prevents the hyperextension injury that results in supracondylar elbow fractures in older children. Rotary forces on the elbow, which can be caused by child abuse or birth trauma in young infants, are probably more responsible for this injury than hyperextension or varus or valgus forces, which produce other fracture patterns in older children.

Abe et al (118) reported 21 children, ranging in age from 1 to 11 years (average, 5 years), with fracture separations of the distal humeral epiphysis, all of which were sustained in falls.

Classification

DeLee et al (84) classified fractures of the entire distal humeral physis into three groups based on the degree of ossification of the lateral condylar epiphysis (Fig. 15-39). Group A fractures occur in infants up to 12 months of age, before the secondary ossification center of the lateral condylar epiphysis appears (Fig. 15-39A,B). They are usually Salter-Harris type I physeal injuries. This injury is often not diagnosed due to the lack of an ossification center in the lateral condylar epiphysis. Group B fractures occur most often in children 12 months to 3 years of age in whom there is definite ossification of the lateral condylar epiphysis (Fig. 15-39C). Although there may be a small flake of metaphyseal bone, this is also essentially a type I Salter-Harris physeal injury. Group C fractures occur in older children, from 3 to 7 years of age and result in a large metaphyseal fragment that is most commonly lateral but can be medial or posterior (Fig. 15-39D,E).

These fractures are almost always extension-type injuries with the distal epiphyseal fragment posterior to the metaphysis. A rare flexion type of injury can occur in which the epiphyseal fragment is displaced anteriorly (121). Stricker et al (125) reported a coronal plane transcondylar (Salter-Harris type IV) fracture in a 3-year-old child that was initially diagnosed as a fracture of the lateral humeral condyle. No growth disturbance was evident 3 years after open reduction and pin fixation.

Clinical Signs and Symptoms

In an infant less than 18 months of age, whose elbow is swollen secondary to trauma or suspected trauma, a fracture involving the entire distal humeral physis should be considered. In a young infant or newborn, swelling may be minimal with little crepitus. Poland (126) described the crepitus as "muffled" crepitus because the fracture ends are covered with softer cartilage than the firm osseous tissue in other fractures about the elbow. The relationship between the epicondyles and the olecranon is maintained. Because of the large, wide fracture surfaces, there are fewer tendencies for tilting with distal fragment rotation, and the angular deformity is less severe than that with supracondylar fractures. Often in older children, the elbow is so swollen that a clinical assessment of the bony landmarks is impossible, and x-ray evaluation must provide confirmation of the diagnosis (Fig. 15-39A,B).

X-Ray Findings

X-ray diagnosis can be difficult, especially if the ossification center of the lateral condyle is not visible in an infant. The only relationship that can be determined is that of the primary ossification centers of the distal humerus to the proximal radius and ulna. The proximal radius and ulna maintain an anatomic relationship to each other but are displaced posteriorly and medially in relation to the distal humerus. This posteromedial relationship is diagnostic. Although theoretically, the distal fragment can be displaced in any direction, with rare exceptions (121) most fractures reported have been displaced posteromedially. Comparison views of the opposite uninjured elbow may be helpful to determine the presence of posteromedial displacement (Fig. 15-39A,B).

Once the lateral condylar epiphysis becomes ossified, displacement of the entire distal epiphysis is much more obvious. The anatomic relationship of the lateral condylar epiphysis with the radial head is maintained, even though the distal humeral epiphysis is displaced posterior and medial in relation to the metaphysis of the humerus (Fig. 15-39C,D).

Because they have a large metaphyseal fragment, type C fractures may be confused with either a low supracondylar fracture or a fracture of the lateral condylar physis. The key diagnostic point is the smooth outline of the distal metaphysis in fractures involving the total distal physis. With supracondylar fractures, the distal portion of the distal fragment has a more irregular border.

Differentiation from a fracture of the lateral condylar physis and the rare elbow dislocation in an infant can be made on x-ray. With a displaced fracture of the lateral condylar physis, the relationship between the lateral condylar epiphysis and the proximal radius is usually disrupted (Fig. 15-8B). If the lateral crista of the trochlea is involved, the proximal radius and ulna may be displaced posterolaterally.

Elbow dislocations are rare in the peak age group for fractures of the entire distal humeral physis. With elbow dislocations, the displacement of the proximal radius and ulna is almost always posterolateral, and the relationship between the proximal radius and lateral condylar epiphysis is disrupted.

If differentiation of this injury from an intra-articular fracture is uncertain, arthrography or MRI may be helpful (Fig. 15-5) (112,116,120,127).

In neonates and infants in whom ossification has not begun, ultrasonography can be used to outline the epiphysis of the humerus (128). Comparison with the opposite uninjured humeral epiphysis may help determine the presence of a separation.

If the diagnosis is delayed, new periosteal bone forms around the distal humerus, and the whole epiphysis may remain displaced posteriorly and medially (Fig. 15-40).

Treatment

Treatment is first directed toward prompt injury recognition. Because this damage may be associated with child abuse, the parents may delay seeking treatment.

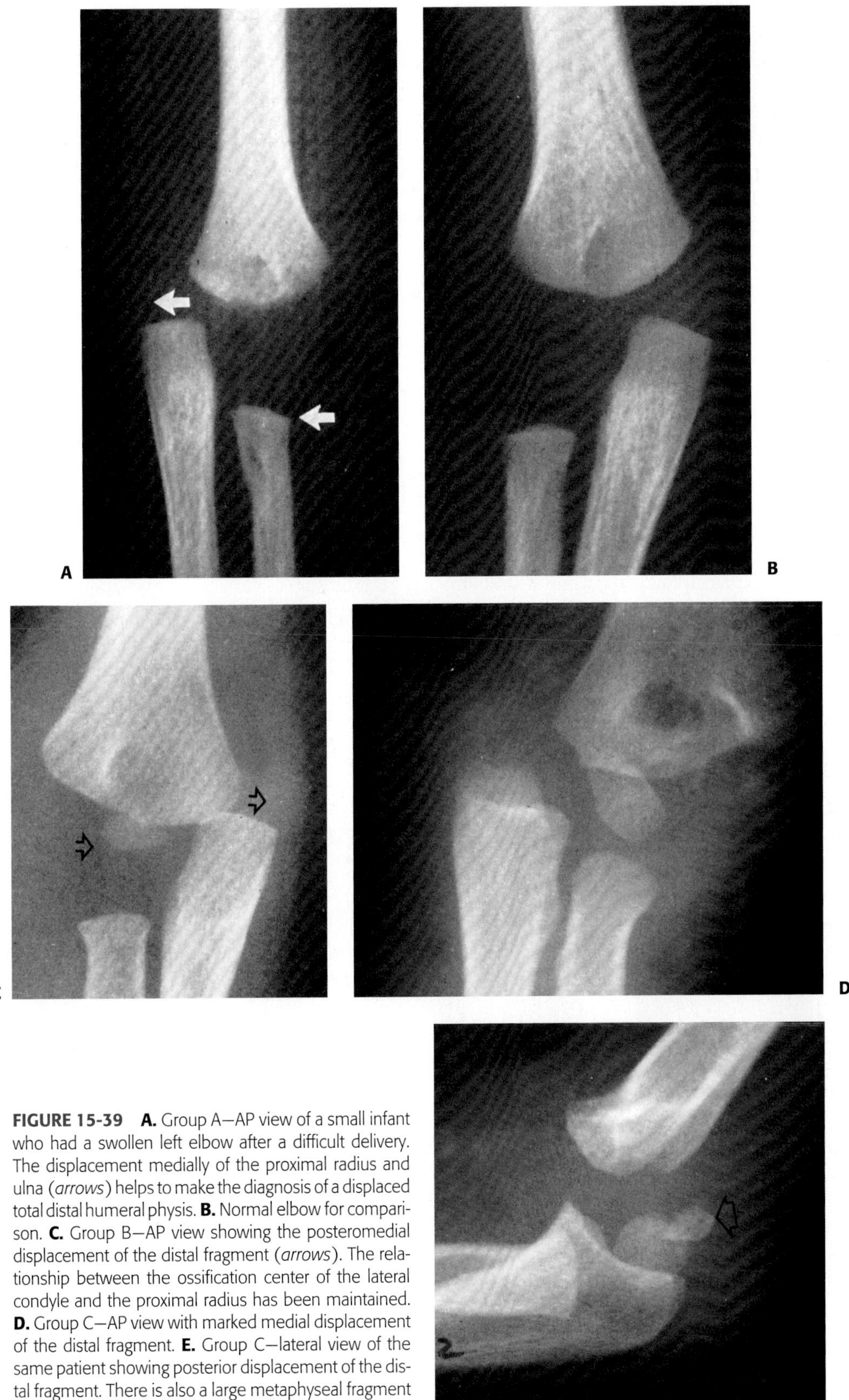

FIGURE 15-39 **A.** Group A—AP view of a small infant who had a swollen left elbow after a difficult delivery. The displacement medially of the proximal radius and ulna (*arrows*) helps to make the diagnosis of a displaced total distal humeral physis. **B.** Normal elbow for comparison. **C.** Group B—AP view showing the posteromedial displacement of the distal fragment (*arrows*). The relationship between the ossification center of the lateral condyle and the proximal radius has been maintained. **D.** Group C—AP view with marked medial displacement of the distal fragment. **E.** Group C—lateral view of the same patient showing posterior displacement of the distal fragment. There is also a large metaphyseal fragment associated with the distal fragment (*arrow*).

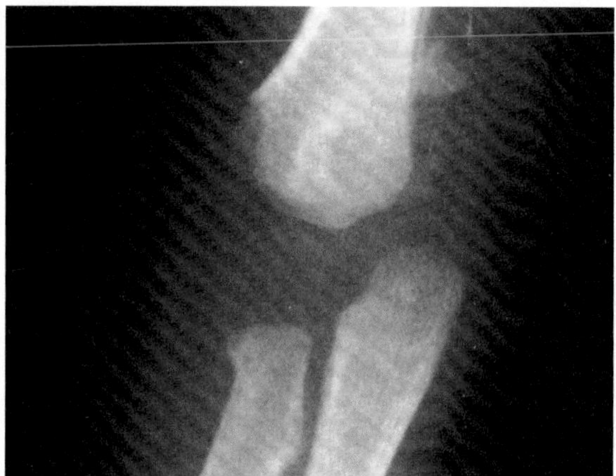

FIGURE 15-40 The true nature of this injury as involving the entire distal humeral physis was not appreciated until periosteal new bone became visible 3 weeks after injury.

De Jager and Hoffman (113) reported 12 fracture separations of the distal humeral epiphysis, three of which were initially diagnosed as fractures of the lateral condyle and one as an elbow dislocation. Due to the frequency of cubitus varus after this injury in young children, they recommended closed reduction and percutaneous pinning in children younger than 2 years of age so that the carrying angle can be evaluated immediately after reduction and corrected if necessary.

Several investigators have reported open reduction, usually performed owing to misdiagnosis as a displaced fracture of the lateral humeral condyle (109,112,114,123). Mizuno et al (116), however, recommended primary open reduction because of his poor results with closed reduction. They approached the fracture posteriorly by removing the triceps insertion from the olecranon with a small piece of cartilage.

If the fracture is old (more than 5 to 6 days) and the epiphysis is no longer mobile, manipulation should not be attempted, and the elbow should be splinted for comfort. Many essentially untreated fractures remodel completely without any residual deformity if the distal fragment is only medially translocated and not tilted (Fig. 15-41).

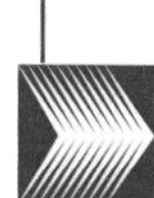

AUTHORS' PREFERRED TREATMENT

We usually first attempt a manipulative closed reduction of fresh fractures. The elbow is initially manipulated into extension to correct the medial displacement, and then the fragment is stabilized by flexing the elbow and pronating the forearm. The distal epiphysis is more securely held with the elbow flexed and the forearm pronated. When the fore-

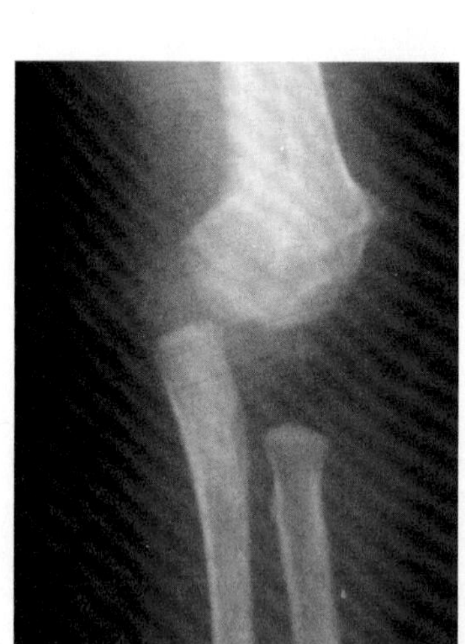

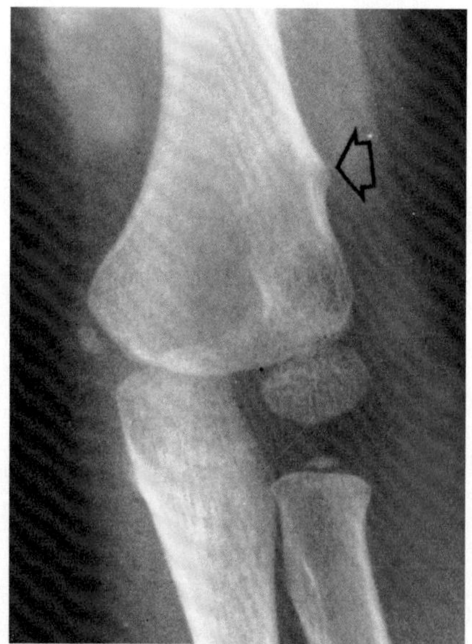

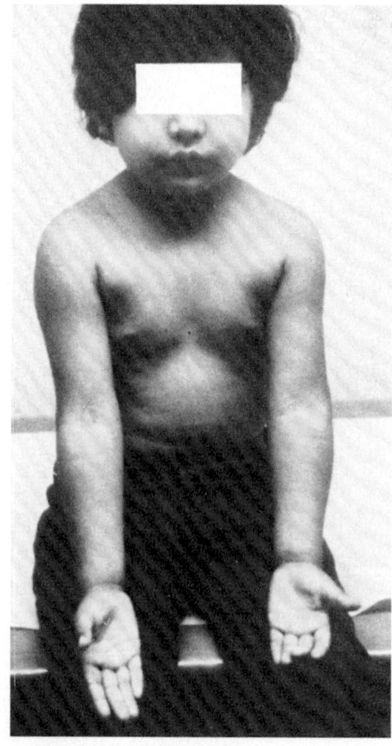

FIGURE 15-41 Remodeling of untreated fractures. **A.** AP view of a 2-year-old who had an unrecognized and untreated fracture of the distal humeral physis. The medial translocation is apparent. There was no varus or valgus tilting. **B.** Four years later, there had been almost complete remodeling of the distal humerus. A small supracondylar prominence (*arrow*) remains as a scar from the original injury. **C.** Clinical appearance 4 years after injury shows no difference in elbow alignment.

arm is supinated with the elbow flexed, the distal fragment tends to displace medially. This displacement is usually a pure medial horizontal translocation without mediolateral coronal tilting.

In neonates and very small infants in whom general anesthesia or percutaneous pin fixation may be difficult, we typically simply immobilize the extremity in 90 degrees of flexion with the forearm pronated. The extremity is then externally stabilized with a figure-of-eight splint.

In most older infants and young children, external immobilization is usually not dependable in maintaining the reduction. As a rule, in these patients, we perform the manipulation with the patient under general anesthesia and secure the fragment with two lateral pins (Fig. 15-42). Due to the swelling and immaturity of the distal humerus, the medial epicondyle is difficult to define as a distinct landmark, making it risky to attempt the percutaneous placement of a medial pin. If a medial pin is necessary for stable fracture fixation, a small medial incision can be made to allow direct observation of the medial epicondyle. In small infants and young children with minimal ossification of the epiphyseal fragment, an intraoperative arthrogram may be obtained to help determine the quality of the reduction.

The cast or splint and pins are removed in 3 weeks to allow active elbow motion to resume. The patient is then followed until full motion is regained and until there is x-ray evidence of normal physeal and epiphyseal growth. Usually, 3 weeks of immobilization is sufficient.

If treatment is delayed more than 3 to 5 days and if the epiphysis is not freely movable, the elbow is simply immobilized in a splint or cast. It is probably better to treat any resulting deformity later with a supracondylar osteotomy rather than risk the complication of physeal injury or osteonecrosis of the epiphysis by performing a delayed open

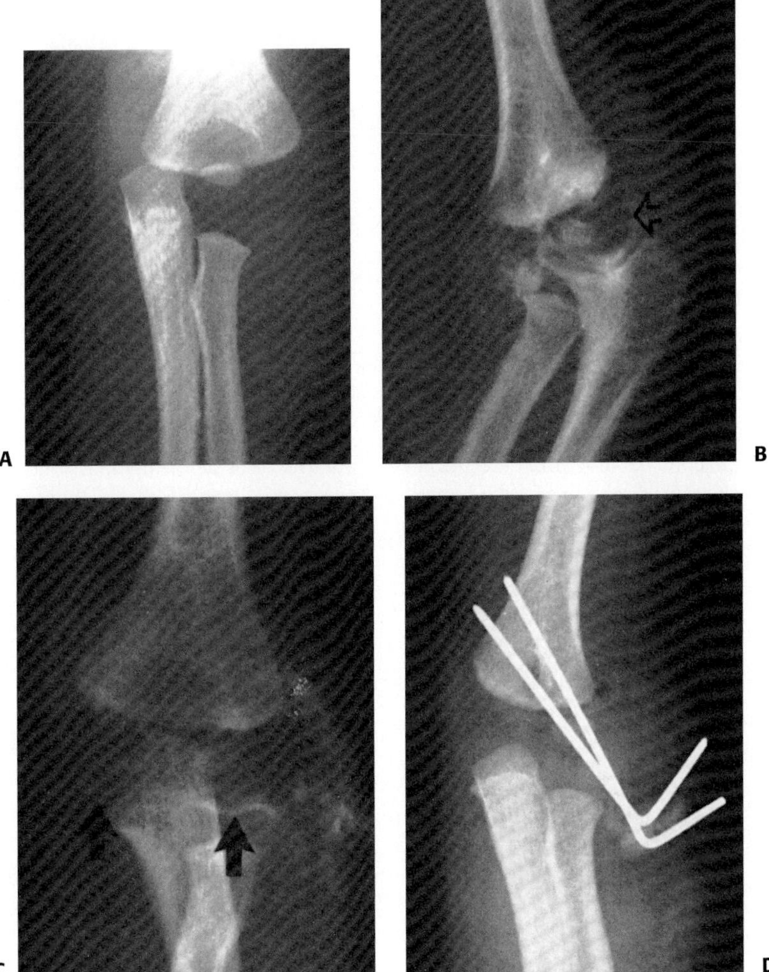

FIGURE 15-42 **A.** Injury film of a 20-month-old showing medial displacement of the distal fragment. **B,C.** The medial and posterior displacement of the condylar fragment (*arrow*) is better defined after an arthrogram. **D.** Fixation is achieved by two lateral pins placed percutaneously.

reduction. Only occasionally does an untreated patient have a deformity severe enough to require surgical correction at a later date. Because the articular surface is intact, complete functional recovery can usually be expected.

Child Abuse

Complications

Child abuse should always be considered in children with this injury, especially a type A fracture pattern, unless it occurs at birth. A young infant is unlikely to incur this type of injury spontaneously from the usual falls that occur during the first year of life. Of the 16 fractures reported by DeLee et al (84), six resulted from documented or highly suspected child abuse, all in children younger than 2 years of age.

Neurovascular Injuries

Neurovascular injuries, either transient or permanent, are rare with this fracture, probably because the fracture fragments are covered with physeal cartilage and do not have sharp edges as do other fractures in this area. In addition, the fracture fragments are usually not markedly displaced.

Nonunion

Only one nonunion after this fracture has been reported; it occurred in a patient seen 3 months after the initial injury (116). Because of the extreme vascularity and propensity for osteogenesis in this area, union is rapid even in patients who receive essentially no treatment.

Malunion

Significant cubitus varus deformity is common after this injury (Fig. 15-43) (114,118). Because the fracture surfaces are wider with this injury than with supracondylar fractures, the distal fragment tends to tilt less, which seems to account for the lower incidence of cubitus varus after this injury than after untreated supracondylar fractures (Fig. 15-43); however, reduction and percutaneous pinning are recommended for acute fractures with displacement.

Osteonecrosis

Osteonecrosis of the epiphysis of the lateral condyle or the trochlear epiphysis has rarely been reported after fractures of the entire distal humeral physis. Yoo et al (129) reported eight patients with osteonecrosis of the trochlea after fracture separations of the distal end of the humerus. Six of the eight fractures were diagnosed initially as medial condylar fractures, lateral condylar fractures, or traumatic elbow dislocation. All eight patients had rapid dissolution of the trochlea within 3 to 6 weeks after injury, followed by the development of a medial or central condylar fishtail defect. We have noted osteonecrosis of the trochlea after three fractures of the entire humeral physis, two of which were inadequately reduced and one of which was anatomically reduced by closed methods (Fig. 15-44). All three had marked displacement of the distal epiphyseal fragment. In one, the osteonecrosis of the trochlea produced a secondary cubitus varus deformity that continued to progress with growth and a significant loss of elbow motion. The etiology of this complication was discussed in the section on osteonecrosis of the trochlea.

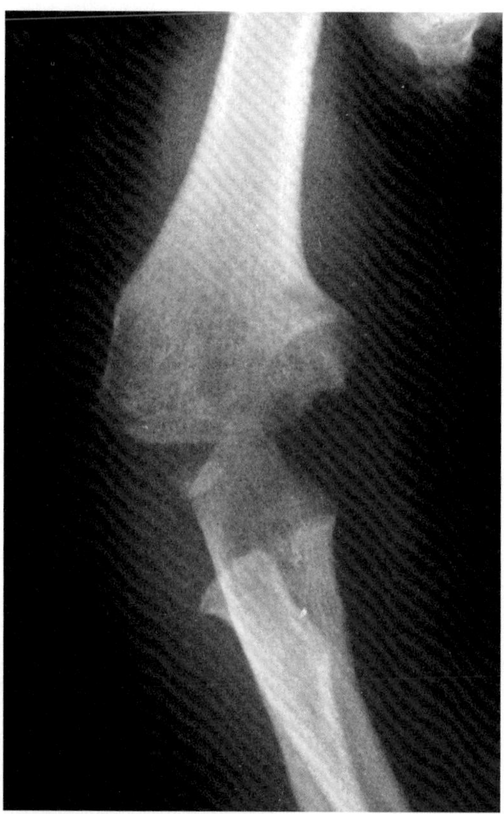

FIGURE 15-43 An AP view of a residual cubitus varus in a 2-year-old 6 months after physeal fracture of the distal humerus. This patient was treated initially with simple immobilization.

APOPHYSEAL INJURIES OF THE DISTAL HUMERUS

Fractures Involving the Medial Epicondylar Apophysis

In the early 1900s, it was recognized that this fracture was often associated with elbow dislocation, and the apophyseal fragment could become entrapped within the joint (130). Much of the discussion during that era centered on the manipulative techniques used to extract the fragment from the joint. In recent years, the proponents of uniform nonoperative management (131–133) have outnumbered the proponents of uniform operative management (134). In the interval since the third edition of this volume, little has been written about the treatment of

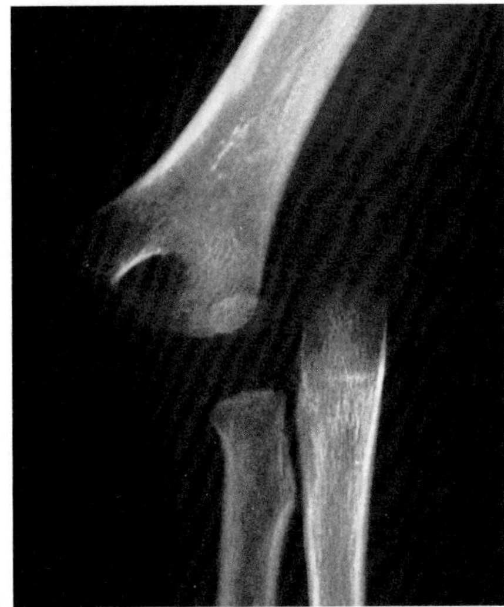
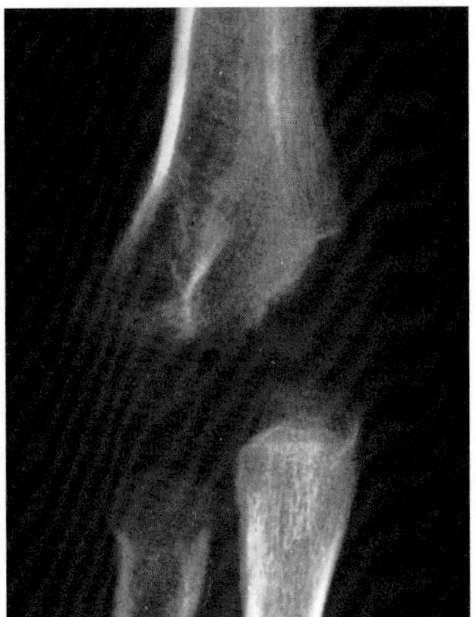

FIGURE 15-44 Osteonecrosis. **A.** Injury film in a 5-year-old with marked displacement of the distal epiphysis. Closed reduction was followed by lateral pin fixation. **B.** Nevertheless, x-rays taken 14 months later showed early evidence of osteonecrosis of the medial condyle. (Courtesy of Salvador J. Mendez, MD.)

this injury; most of the focus has been on the increased recognition of this injury occurring during sports (135–137).

Incidence

Fractures involving the medial epicondylar apophysis constitute approximately 14.1% of fractures involving the distal humerus and 11.5% of all fractures in the elbow region (138–140).

Fractures involving the epicondylar apophysis have a later peak age, similar to fractures involving the medial condylar physis. The youngest reported patient with this injury was 3.9 years (140). In the large series of fractures of the medial epicondylar apophysis, most occurred between ages 9 and 14, and the peak age incidence was 11 to 12 years (132–134,138, 141–144). Fractures of the epicondylar apophysis affect boys by a ratio of almost 4 to 1. In six large series in the literature, boys constituted 79% of the patients (130,133,141,145–147).

Association With Elbow Dislocation

The reported incidence of association with dislocation of the elbow has varied from as low as 30% to as high as 55% in many of the reported series (133,138). Two bilateral injuries associated with bilateral elbow dislocations have been reported (139,148). Both patients sustained their injuries while participating in gymnastics.

In summary, the peak age for fractures of the epicondylar apophysis is 9 to 12 years. The injury occurs in boys four times more often than in girls. About 50% of such injuries are associated with elbow dislocations. In at least 15% to 18% of patients, the fragment is incarcerated in the joint (Table 15-1).

Ossification

Surgical Anatomy

The medial epicondyle is a traction apophysis, so the term *apophysis* rather than *physis* is used throughout the description of this injury. The forces across its physis are tension rather than the compressive forces present across the condylar physes of the distal humerus. Because it is an apophysis, it does not contribute to the distal humerus' overall length.

In the early ossification process, the medial epicondylar apophysis is part of the entire distal humeral epiphysis. With growth and maturity, it becomes separated from the entire distal humeral epiphysis by intervening metaphyseal bone. In younger children, when there is a separation of the distal humeral epiphysis, the medial epicondylar apophysis is included as part of the distal fragment.

Posteromedial Location.

The medial epicondylar apophysis actually arises from the posterior surface of the medial distal humeral metaphysis. As was mentioned in Chapter 14, this posterior location is important when percutaneous pin fixation is used. Likewise, this posterior position affects the image of the apophysis on x-rays (Fig. 15-45).

TABLE 15-1 Fractures of the Medial Epicondylar Apophysis: Incidence

Overall incidence: Fractures of the distal humerus, 14.1%
Overall incidence: Fractures of the elbow region, 11.5%
Age: peak, 11–12 years
Sex: males, 79% (4 : 1, male : female)
Association with elbow dislocation: Approximately 50% (15% to 18% of these involve incarceration of the epicondylar apophysis)

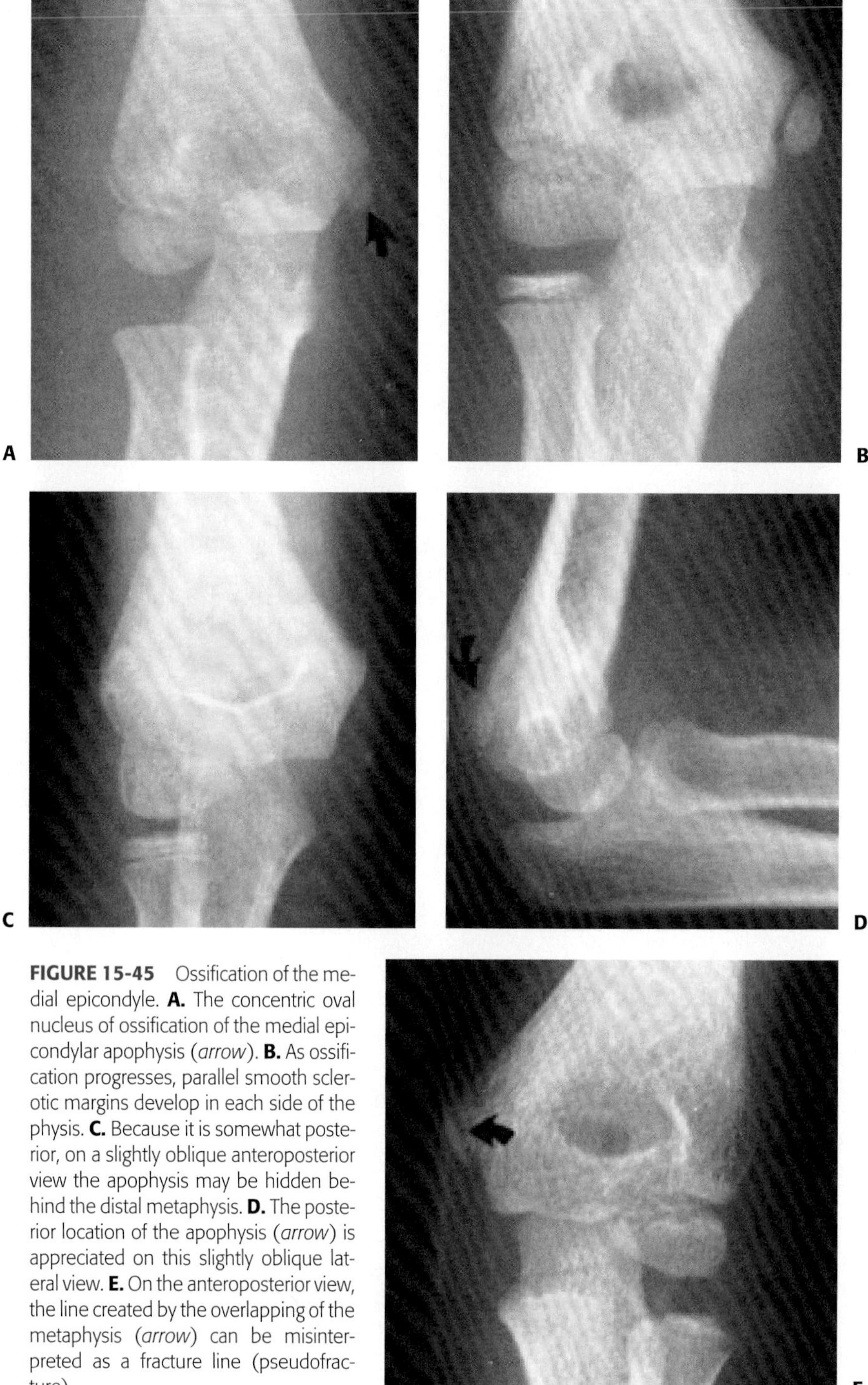

FIGURE 15-45 Ossification of the medial epicondyle. **A.** The concentric oval nucleus of ossification of the medial epicondylar apophysis (*arrow*). **B.** As ossification progresses, parallel smooth sclerotic margins develop in each side of the physis. **C.** Because it is somewhat posterior, on a slightly oblique anteroposterior view the apophysis may be hidden behind the distal metaphysis. **D.** The posterior location of the apophysis (*arrow*) is appreciated on this slightly oblique lateral view. **E.** On the anteroposterior view, the line created by the overlapping of the metaphysis (*arrow*) can be misinterpreted as a fracture line (pseudofracture).

Ossification Sequence. Silberstein et al (149) described various unique aspects of the ossification process of the medial epicondylar apophysis. The following discussion is paraphrased from their work.

Ossification begins from 4 to 6 years of age, with fusion occurring at about 15 years of age. It is the last secondary ossification center to fuse with the distal humeral metaphysis. The ossification center starts as a small eccentric oval nucleus (Fig. 15-45A). As it matures, parallel sclerotic margins develop along both sides of the physis (Fig. 15-45B). There may be some irregularity of the ossification process, which gives the ossific nucleus a fragmented appearance. This fragmentation may be falsely interpreted as a fracture.

Because the apophysis is posteromedial, the ossification center may be difficult to see on an AP x-ray, especially if the elbow is slightly oblique (Fig. 15-45C). The posterior position of the apophysis is best appreciated on a lateral x-ray. If the elbow is slightly oblique, the epicondyle's outline may be better appreciated (Fig. 15-45D). Because of this posterior location on AP x-rays, the distal medial metaphyseal border may overlap the ossific nucleus of the apophysis. This overlapping may appear as a lucent line that can be misinterpreted as a fracture (Fig. 15-45E).

Soft Tissue Attachments

Flexor Mass

The flexor mass, which includes the origin of the flexor carpi radialis, flexor carpi ulnaris, flexor digitorum superficialis, and palmaris longus and part of the pronator teres, originates from the anterior aspect of the apophysis (Fig. 15-46) (149). Part of the flexor carpi ulnaris also originates on the posterior aspect of the epicondyle.

Capsule. In younger children, some of the capsule's origin extends up to the physeal line of the epicondyle. In older children and adolescents, as the epicondyle migrates more proximally, the capsule is attached only to the medial crista of the trochlea (87). Thus, in younger children, a fracture line involving the medial epicondylar apophysis can enter the joint because part of the capsule is attached to the epicondylar fragment. In older children, however, if there is a pure avulsion force on the epicondyle, the capsule may remain attached to the trochlea's outer border. In this age group, the fracture may be totally extra-articular.

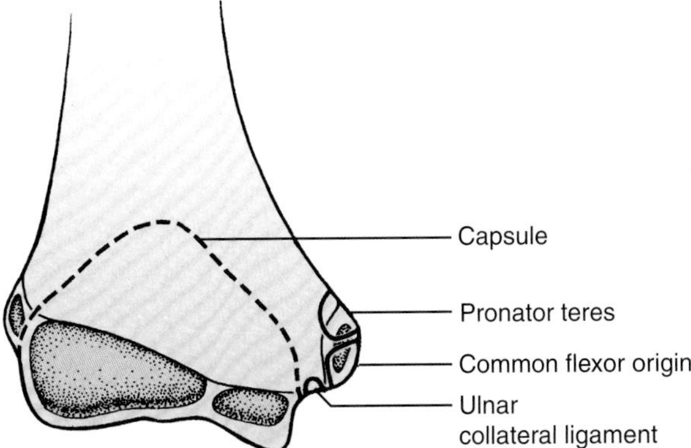

FIGURE 15-46 Soft-tissue attachments. The AP view of the distal humerus demonstrates the relationship of the apophysis to the origins of the medial forearm muscles. The origin of the ulnar collateral ligament lies outside the elbow capsule. The margin of the capsule is outlined by the dotted line.

Ligamentous Structures

The two major medial collateral ligaments originate from this apophysis. The ulnar collateral ligament is composed of three separate bands (Fig. 15-47) (150). Woods and Tullos (150) pointed out that the major stabilizing ligamentous structure in the elbow is the anterior band of the ulnar collateral ligament. The band's anterior portion is taut in extension, and the posterior fibers are taut in flexion. The fibers of the posterior band of the ulnar collateral ligament are relaxed in extension and are taut in flexion (Fig. 15-47). Thus, this posterior band provides stability only in flexion. Because the radial collateral ligaments do not attach directly to the ulna or radius, but instead attach to the orbicular ligament, they provide only minimal stability to the elbow joint.

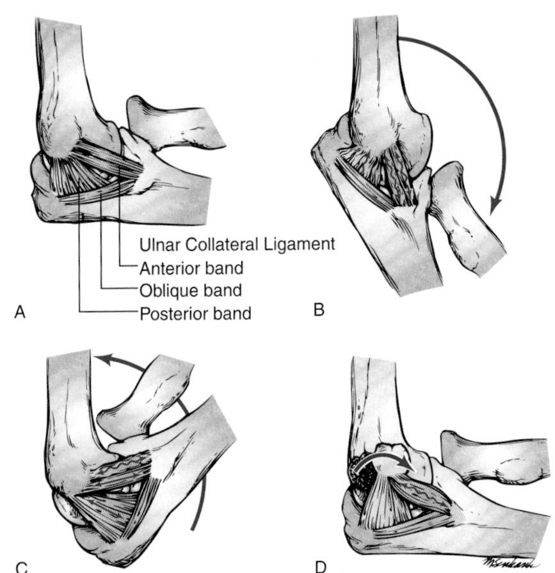

FIGURE 15-47 Ligamentous structures. **A.** The ulnar collateral ligament is divided into anterior, posterior, and oblique bands. **B.** On extension, the anterior fibers of the anterior band are taut. The posterior fibers of the anterior band and the entire posterior band are loose in this position. **C.** In flexion, the posterior fibers of the anterior bands and posterior band become taut. The anterior fibers of the anterior band become loose. **D.** When the epicondyle is rotated anteriorly, the entire anterior band can become loose. (From Woods WG, Tullos HS. Elbow instability and medial epicondyle fractures. *Am J Sports Med* 1977;5:23–30, with permission.)

Mechanism of Injury

Injuries to the medial epicondylar apophysis most commonly occur as acute injuries in which a distinct event produces a partial or a complete separation of the apophyseal fragment. Three theories have been proposed about the mechanism of acute medial epicondylar apophyseal injuries: a direct blow, avulsion mechanisms, and association with elbow dislocation (Table 15-2).

Direct Blow

Stimson (28) speculated that this type of injury could occur as a result of a direct blow on the posterior aspect of the epicondyle. Among more recent investigators, however, only Watson-Jones (151) described this injury as being associated with a direct blow to the posterior medial aspect of the elbow.

In rare patients in whom the fragment is produced by a direct blow to the joint's medial aspect, the medial epicondylar fragment is often fragmented (Fig. 15-48). In these injuries, there may also be more superficial ecchymosis in the skin.

Avulsion Mechanisms

Various investigators have suggested that some of these injuries are due to a pure avulsion of the epicondyle by the flexor muscles of the forearm (142,152). This muscle avulsion force can occur in combination with a valgus stress in which the elbow is locked in extension, or as a pure musculature contraction that may occur with the elbow partially flexed.

Avulsion and Extension (Valgus Stress)

Smith (143) proposed that when a child falls on his outstretched upper extremity with the elbow in extension, the wrist and fingers are often hyperextended as well, placing an added tension force on the epicondyle by the forearm flexor muscles (Fig. 15-49). The normal valgus carrying angle tends to accentuate these avulsion forces when the elbow is in extension. Many

TABLE 15-2 Fractures of Medial Condylar Apophysis: Mechanism of Injury

Acute injuries
Direct blow
Avulsion mechanisms
Avulsion in elbow extension (valgus stress)
Avulsion with elbow flexed (pure muscle forces)
Associated with elbow dislocation
Chronic tension stress injuries

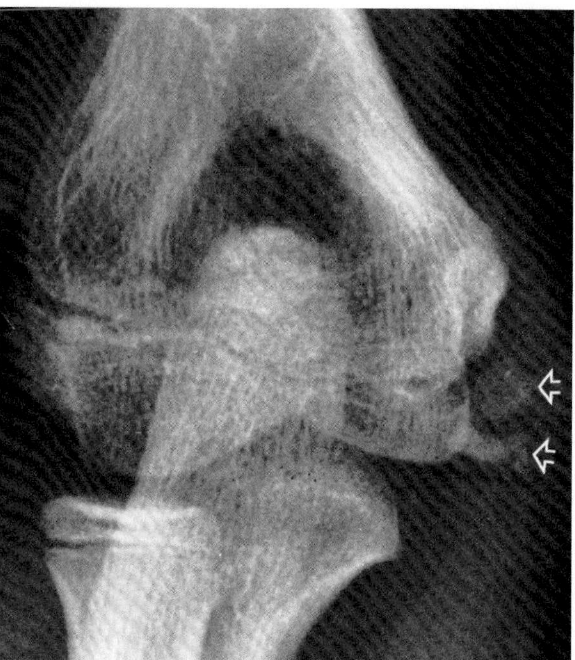

FIGURE 15-48 Direct fragmentation. The fragmented appearance of the medial epicondyle (*arrows*) in a 13-year-old who sustained a direct blow to the medial aspect of the elbow. (From Wilkins KE. Fractures of the medial epicondyle in children. *Instr Course Lect* 1991;40:1–8; with permission.)

proponents of this theory point to the other associated elbow fractures that have been seen with this injury as evidence to confirm that a valgus force is applied across the elbow at the time of the injury. These associated injuries include radial neck fractures with valgus angulation and greenstick valgus fractures of the olecranon (142).

Isolated Muscle Avulsions

Isolated avulsion can also occur in adolescents with the simple act of throwing a baseball. In this instance, the sudden contracture of the forearm flexor muscles may be sufficient to cause the epicondyle to fail (Fig. 15-50). The literature has reflected a high incidence of medial epicondylar apophyseal avulsions occurring with arm wrestling in patients near skeletal maturity (136,137). The largest series, reported by Nyska et al (137) from Israel, involved 8 boys 13 to 15 years of age, all of whom were treated conservatively with good results.

Associated With Elbow Dislocations

The final mechanism proposed is that this injury is associated with elbow dislocation in which the ulnar collateral ligament provides the avulsion force. If the elbow is dislocated when the patient is initially seen, there is no doubt that this is a major factor in the cause of this fracture. The question of whether this fracture is caused by an occult or partial elbow dislocation that

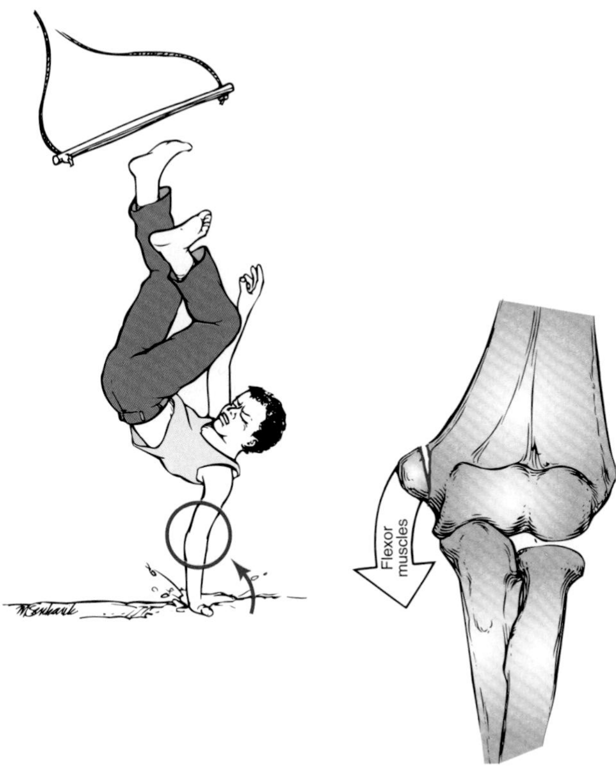

FIGURE 15-49 Hyperextension forces. When a person falls on the outstretched upper extremity, the wrist and fingers are forced into hyperextension (*solid arrow*), which places tension on the forearm flexor muscles. This sudden tension along with the normal valgus carrying angle tends to place a strong avulsion force on the medial epicondyle (*open arrow*).

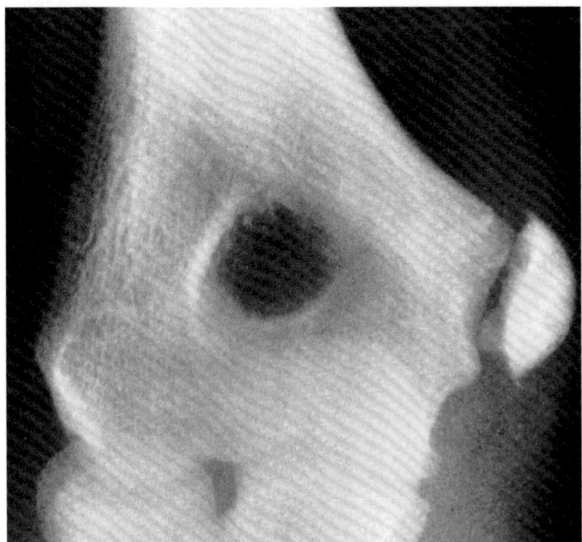

FIGURE 15-50 Muscle avulsion. Isolated avulsion of the medial epicondyle occurred suddenly in this 14-year-old Little League pitcher after throwing a curve ball. (From Wilkins KE. Fracture of the medial epicondyle in children. *Instr Course Lect* 1991;40:1–8; with permission.)

has reduced spontaneously is often raised. Some investigators (138,139,141) have noticed calcification development in the lateral collateral ligaments and adjacent lateral periosteum after fracture. They believed this calcification was evidence that this ligament had been stretched during the process of elbow dislocation. Marion and Faysse (145) found that most elbow dislocations associated with this injury were posterolateral, but some pure lateral, posterior, and posteromedial dislocations were also observed.

The question arises as to whether incarceration of the epicondylar fragment into the joint can occur without a dislocation. Patrick (152) believed that when an extreme valgus stress was applied to the joint, a vacuum was created within the joint that "sucked in" the avulsed epicondylar fragment.

It appears that any of these mechanisms can produce an acute apophyseal injury of the distal humerus. The direct blow mechanism appears to occur only rarely. Many of these injuries may be associated with an elbow dislocation that may or may not have reduced spontaneously.

Acute Fractures

Usually, the epicondyle is displaced distally. Avulsion generally involves only the apophysis, but a small flake of metaphyseal bone is occasionally attached to the apophyseal fragment. The fracture line rarely passes through the apophysis, and only part of the apophysis is avulsed (149). Although these partial avulsions may appear as only minor injuries, the partial fragment can be incarcerated within the joint just as easily as the full apophysis (Fig. 15-51).

Chronic Incarceration

When the fragment becomes incarcerated into the joint, the raw bone surface may become adherent to the coronoid process of the ulna (147). In late cases, this union of the fragment to the coronoid process may make extraction difficult. A universal finding when the fragment is incarcerated within the joint is a thick fascial band that binds the ulnar nerve to the underlying muscle (87,152). The constriction that this band creates is believed to be responsible for either the immediate or late dysfunction of the ulnar nerve.

Associated Injuries

Other elbow fractures that can be associated with this injury include fracture of the radial neck, olecranon, or coronoid process. If the epicondyle fragment is only rotated on its axis, the anterior band of the ulnar collateral ligament can become lax. This laxity can produce some medial elbow instability during extension (150).

Classification

The various classifications proposed for this injury (138,145) are similar. We have combined them to form a comprehensive

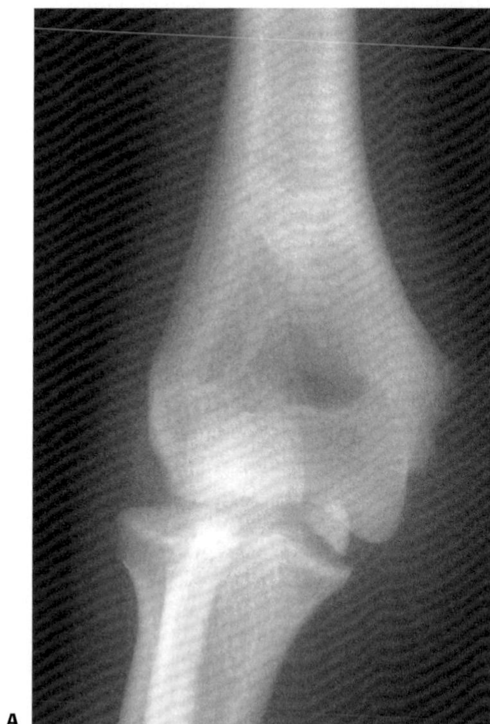

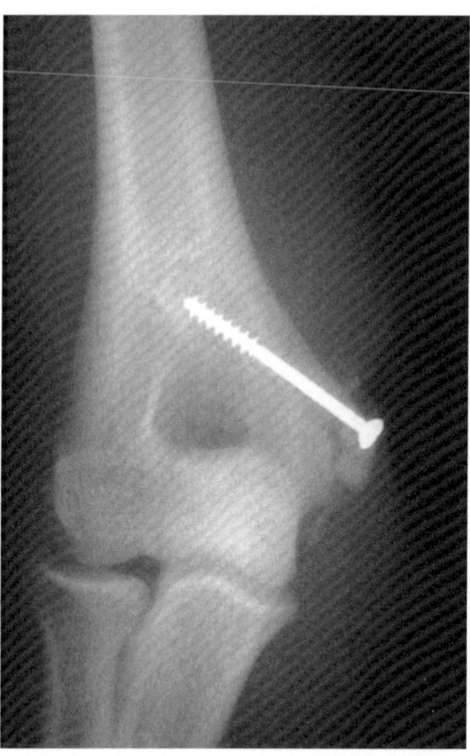

FIGURE 15-51 **A.** Entrapment of fracture fragment in medial epicondylar fracture with posterolateral elbow dislocation. **B.** After fragment extraction, open reduction, and screw fixation.

classification (Table 15-3) that can be useful in determining the proper treatment method. In the discussion of this classification, the clinical and x-ray findings are delineated for each type of fracture pattern. Initially, we have separated these injuries into two primary categories based on whether the injuries are acute or chronic.

Acute Injuries

Undisplaced or Minimally Displaced Fractures. In undisplaced fractures, the physeal line remains intact. The clinical manifestations usually consist only of swelling and local tenderness over the medial epicondyle. Crepitus and motion of the epicondyle are usually not present. On x-ray, the smoothness of the physeal line's edge remains intact. Although there may be some loss of soft tissue planes medially on the x-ray, displacement of the elbow fat pads may not be present because the pathology is extra-articular (153).

Minimally displaced fractures usually result from a stronger avulsion force, so there is often more soft tissue swelling. Palpating the fragment may elicit crepitus because the increased displacement allows motion of the fragment. On x-ray, there is a loss of parallelism of the smooth sclerotic margins of the physis (Fig. 15-52) (149). The radiolucency in the area of the apophyseal line is usually increased in width.

TABLE 15-3 **Fractures of the Medial Epicondyle Apophysis: Classification**

Acute injuries
Undisplaced or minimally displaced
Displaced fractures
Incarcerated fractures (without elbow dislocation)
Incarcerated fractures (with elbow dislocation)
Chronic tension (stress) injuries

Significantly Displaced Fractures. In significantly displaced fractures, there is no question as to whether the fragment is displaced, as it may be palpable and freely movable. Because it is displaced a considerable distance from the distal humerus, crepitus between the fragments may not be present. There may have been an elbow dislocation that reduced spontaneously or by manipulation. On the other hand, there may have been no documentation of the original dislocation. On x-ray, the long axis of the epicondylar epiphysis is rotated medially (Fig. 15-53). The displacement usually exceeds 5 mm, but the fragment remains proximal to the true joint surface. This fragment may contain a metaphyseal fragment.

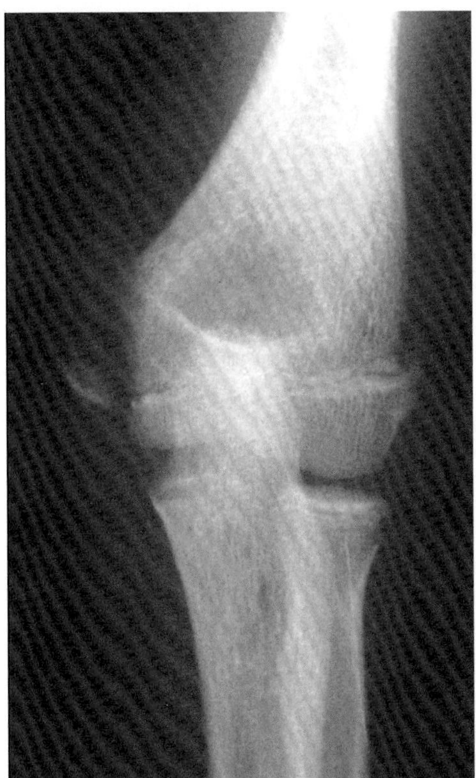

FIGURE 15-52 AP x-ray shows loss of normal smooth margins of the physis after type II medial epicondylar fracture.

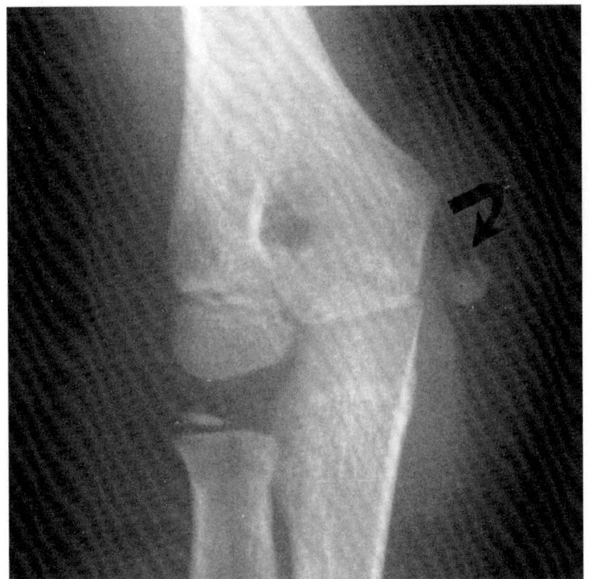

FIGURE 15-53 Type III displaced medial epicondylar fracture. AP view of an elbow in which the epicondyle (*arrow*) is significantly displaced both distally and medially. In addition, the fragment is rotated medially.

Entrapment of the Epicondylar Fragment Into the Joint

Without Elbow Dislocation. In many instances, the elbow appears reduced. The key clinical finding is a block to motion, especially extension. The epicondylar fragment is usually between the joint surfaces of the trochlea and the semilunar notch of the olecranon. On x-ray, any time the fragment appears at the level of the joint, it must be considered to be totally or partially within the elbow joint until proven otherwise (152). If the x-ray is examined carefully, the elbow is usually still found to be incompletely reduced. Due to an impingement of the fragment within the joint, a good AP view may be difficult to obtain caused by the inability to extend the elbow fully. If the fracture is old and if the fragment is fused to the coronoid process, widening of the medial joint space may be the only clue that the fragment is lying in the joint. The epicondylar ossification center may become fragmented and mistaken for the fragmented appearance of the medial crista of the trochlea (140,147). Absence of the apophyseal center on x-ray may be further confirmatory evidence that the fragment is within the joint. Comparison x-rays of the opposite elbow may be necessary to delineate the true pathology.

With Elbow Dislocation. Even if the elbow is dislocated, the fragment can still lie within the joint and prevent reduction. Recognition of this fragment as being within the joint before a manipulation should alert the physician of the possible need for open reduction. There should be adequate relaxation during the manipulative process. An initial manipulation to extract the fragment from the elbow joint may need to be accomplished before a satisfactory closed reduction of the elbow joint can be obtained (Fig. 15-54).

Fractures Through the Epicondylar Apophysis

Fractures through the body of the epicondyle can result from either a direct blow or avulsion of only part of the apophysis. In either case, the fragments may or may not be displaced. The normal lucent line formed by the overlying metaphyseal border should not be confused with this injury. Although described by Silberstein et al (149), this intrafragment fracture is a rare presentation.

Clinical Findings

Valgus Stress Test. Because many of the clinical diagnostic points have been discussed in the previous section on the classification of this injury, much of the emphasis in this section is on the determination of elbow instability. Because the ulnar collateral ligament's anterior oblique band may be attached to the medial epicondylar apophysis, the elbow may exhibit some instability after injury. To evaluate the elbow's medial stability, Woods and Tullos (150) and Schwab et al (155) advocated a simple valgus stress test. This test is performed with the patient supine and the arm abducted 90 degrees. The shoulder and arm are externally rotated 90 degrees. The elbow must be flexed at least 15 degrees to eliminate the stabilizing force of the olecra-

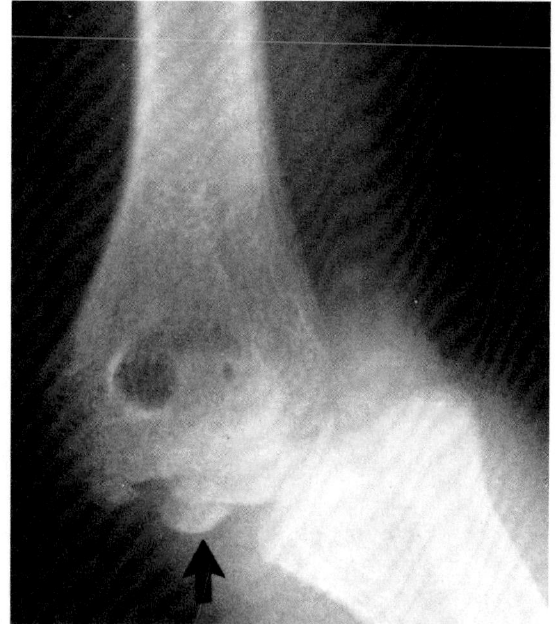

A

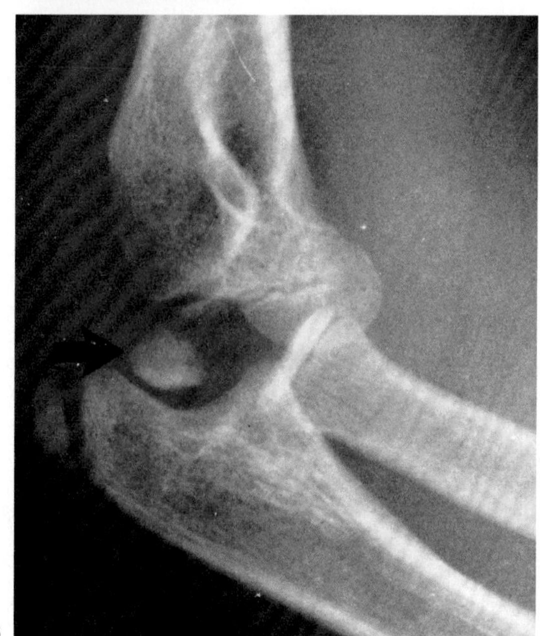

B

FIGURE 15-54 Dislocation with incarceration. **A.** AP view showing a posterolateral elbow dislocation. The presence of the medial epicondyle within the elbow joint (*arrow*) prevented a closed reduction. **B.** The lateral view of the same elbow demonstrates the fragment (*arrow*) between the humerus and olecranon.

non. If the elbow is unstable, simple gravity forces will open the medial side. A small additional weight or sedation may be necessary to acquire an accurate assessment of the medial stability with this test.

Evaluating the Ulnar Nerve. The function of the ulnar nerve must be carefully assessed. It is especially wise to document the presence or absence of an ulnar nerve injury before instituting therapy.

X-Ray Findings

Widening or irregularity of the apophyseal line may be the only clue in fractures that are only slightly displaced or nondisplaced. If the fragment is significantly displaced, the x-ray diagnosis is usually obvious. If the fragment is totally incarcerated in the joint, however, it may be hidden by the overlying ulnar or distal humerus. The clue here is the total absence of the epicondyle from its normal position just medial and posterior to the medial metaphysis.

Potter (31) suggested that properly performed MRI might disclose acute or chronic injury to the medial epicondylar apophysis. Recommended pulse sequences for evaluating the apophysis include fat-suppressed gradient echo imaging. On MRI, increased signal intensity and abnormal widening of the medial epicondylar physis are seen, typically with surrounding soft tissue edema.

Fractures of the medial epicondyle, even if displaced, may not produce positive fat pad signs (149,153). If the fracture is only minimally displaced and if it is the result of an avulsion injury, there may be no effusion because all the injured tissues remain extra-articular. In fractures associated with elbow dislocation, there is rupture of the capsule, so its ability to confine the hemarthrosis is lost. In minimally displaced fractures of the medial epicondyle with significant hemarthrosis, the evaluation must be especially thorough to ensure that an unrecognized fracture involving the medial condylar physis or an associated elbow dislocation is not present.

Differential Diagnosis

The major injury to differentiate involves the medial condylar physis. This is especially true if the secondary ossification centers are not present (see the earlier section on Fractures Involving the Medial Condylar Physis). If there is a significant hemarthrosis or a significant piece of metaphyseal bone accompanying the medial epicondylar fragment, arthrography or MRI may be indicated to determine if there is an intra-articular component to the fracture (Fig. 15-55).

Treatment

Areas of General Agreement

There seems to be universal agreement as to the proper method of treating fractures that are undisplaced or only minimally displaced. These first two types are easily treated with simple immobilization for comfort. Some investigators have recommended initiation of motion early to prevent stiffness, which is the most common complication of this injury (139,143). Likewise, if the fragment is incarcerated in the joint, the accepted treatment is to extract the fragment from the joint by manipulation or surgical intervention.

The controversy seems to be in determining the proper treatment method for patients with significant displacement (fragment displacement more than 5 mm).

Nonoperative Management. In reports in which only one method (i.e., operative or nonoperative) of treatment of all displaced fractures was used, results tend to support that method. The best argument for surgical management comes from Hines et al (134) whose practice was to surgically repair all fractures displaced more than 2 mm. They found that 96% of their patients had good to excellent results. Bad results were attributed mainly to technical errors. Josefsson and Danielsson (131) obtained equal results and treated all of these injuries nonoperatively. Although more than 60% of their patients demonstrated nonunion on x-ray, these investigators had an equal number of good results at a mean follow-up of 11 years. Other reports in the literature (132,133,154) also demonstrated the overall good results with nonoperative management.

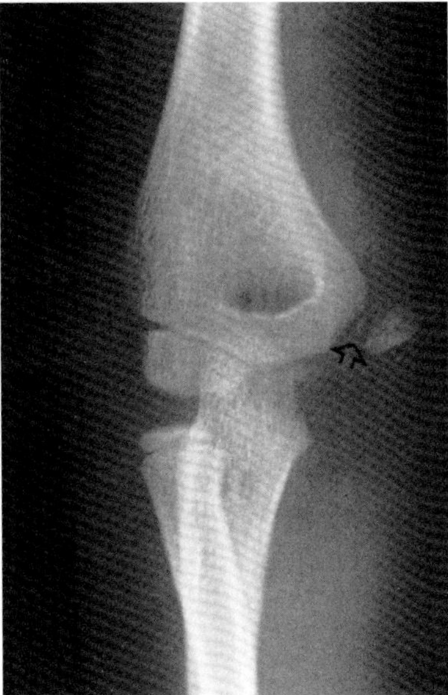

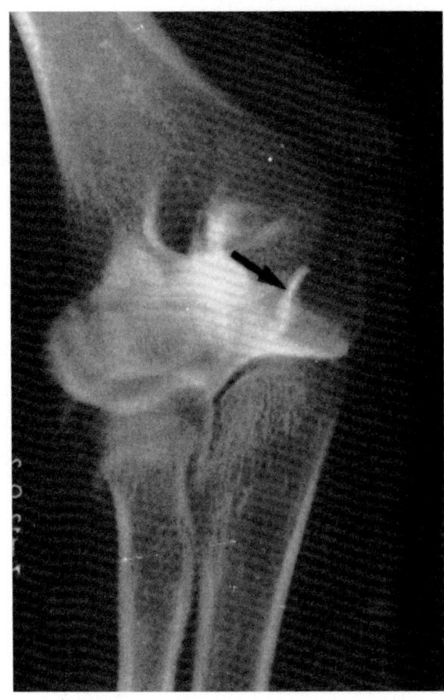

FIGURE 15-55 Intra-articular extension. **A.** Injury film in a 7-year-old girl who was initially suspected of having only a fracture of the medial epicondyle. In addition to moderate displacement, there was a significant metaphyseal fragment (*arrow*). **B.** An arthrogram revealed intra-articular components (*arrow*), which defined this injury instead as a fracture involving the medial condylar physis. (Courtesy of Carl McGarey, MD.)

The best comparison of operative and nonoperative treatment results comes from reports in which both methods were used in the same institution. Bede et al (138) had superior results in patients treated nonoperatively compared with those treated operatively. This same superiority of nonoperative management has been found in subsequent reports as well (133,139,141).

The results of fractures associated with a documented elbow dislocation are poorer (138,141) for patients treated operatively and nonoperatively. Fowles et al (141) reported that surgical intervention only added to the original trauma produced by the dislocation, increasing the residual loss of motion.

Indications for Operative Intervention. The indications for operative intervention in acute injuries are divided into two categories: absolute and relative. The single absolute indication is incarceration of the epicondylar fragment within the joint. The relative indications include ulnar nerve dysfunction and a need for elbow stability.

Incarceration in the Joint—Absolute. If the fragment is found in the joint acutely, it must be removed. There are proponents and techniques of both nonoperative and operative extraction of the fragment.

Nonoperative Extraction. Various methods of extracting the fragment by nonoperative methods have been proposed. The success rate of extracting the fragment successfully from the joint by manipulation alone is only about 40% (152). All the nonoperative methods require either heavy sedation or light general anesthesia.

Roberts' Manipulative Technique. The manipulative technique most commonly used is the method popularized by Roberts (148,156). It involves placing a valgus stress on the elbow while supinating the forearm and simultaneously dorsiflexing the wrist and fingers to place the forearm muscles on stretch; theoretically, this maneuver should extract the fragment from the joint. To be effective, this procedure should be carried out within the first 24 hours after injury.

Operative Extraction. Failure to extract the fragment by manipulative techniques is an indication to proceed with open surgical extraction. Once open extraction and reduction have been performed, many methods have been advocated to stabilize the fragment, including screw fixation or sutures in the comminuted fracture. Excision has also been advocated, especially if the fragment is comminuted.

Incarceration Discovered Late. Fowles et al (157) challenged the opinion that surgery is detrimental in patients with late incarceration, and the idea remains controversial. In their patients in whom the fragment was surgically extracted an average of 14 weeks after injury, 80% more elbow motion was regained. In addition, the patients' preoperative pain was relieved, and the ulnar dysfunction resolved. On a long-term basis, intra-articular retention of the fragment may not be all that disabling. Rosendahl (147) reported an 8-year follow-up of a fragment retained within the joint. The epicondyle had fused to the semilunar surface of the ulna, producing a large bony prominence clinically. There was only minor loss of elbow motion, with little functional disability.

Ulnar Nerve Dysfunction—Relative. Ulnar nerve dysfunction is a relative indication for operative intervention. If there are mild-to-moderate ulnar nerve symptoms at the time of the injury, there is usually no need to explore the nerve, because most of these mild symptoms resolve spontaneously (139,158). If the dysfunction is complete, then the ulnar nerve is probably wrapped around the fragment and should be explored surgically. One of the original fears was that the fracture fragment's raw surface would create scar tissue around or adjacent to the nerve and cause continued dysfunction. Thus, it was originally recommended that the ulnar nerve should be transposed at the time of open reduction (151). Subsequent reports have not found this step to be necessary (159).

There is some question as to whether delayed ulnar nerve symptoms can even occur after fractures of the epicondyle that are not associated with elbow dislocation. In a review of more than 100 patients with uncomplicated fractures involving the medial epicondylar apophysis, Patrick (152) could not find any instance in which a delayed ulnar neuritis developed. He found some patients with late ulnar neuritis after fractures that were associated with elbow dislocation. Bernstein et al (139) found that their patients with initial ulnar nerve symptoms all did well when treated nonoperatively. Thus, the original fear of delayed ulnar nerve dysfunction has been dispelled.

Joint Stability—Relative. Woods and Tullos (150) suggested that even minor forms of valgus instability after elbow injuries involving the medial epicondylar apophysis can cause significant disability in athletes. This condition is especially true in athletes who must have a stable upper extremity, such as baseball pitchers, gymnasts, or wrestlers. In younger adolescents (younger than 14 years of age), the anterior band of the ulnar collateral ligament often displaces with the apophyseal fragment. In older individuals (15 years or older), large fragments may be avulsed without a ligamentous injury. Rather than depending on arbitrary measurements of fracture displacement, Woods and Tullos (150) recommended using the gravity valgus stress test to determine the presence or absence of valgus instability. They believed that demonstration of a significant valgus instability, using this simple gravity test, was an indication for surgical intervention in patients who require a stable elbow for their athletic activities. Pimpalnerkar et al (105) also suggested

TABLE 15-4 Authors' Preferred Treatment

Nonoperative treatment

- Nondisplaced, minimally displaced
  - Significantly displaced in patients with low-demand upper-extremity function

Operative treatment Indications

- Absolute: Irreducible incarcerated fragment in the elbow joint
- Relative: Ulnar nerve dysfunction
- Relative: Patient with high-demand upper extremity-function

that clinical evidence of instability, as shown by gravity valgus stress testing, is an indication for operative fixation.

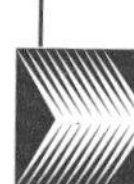

AUTHORS' PREFERRED TREATMENT

We use the classification scheme (Table 15-3) as a rough guide to treatment. We also strongly consider the expected activity of the involved extremity in deciding on nonoperative or operative treatment (Table 15-4).

For most uncomplicated fractures, regardless of the number of millimeters of displacement, we prefer nonoperative management (Fig. 15-56), including fractures associated with elbow dislocations. The parents are warned that no matter which type of treatment is provided, some loss of elbow extension may occur. They should be reassured, however, that this loss of motion, if it does occur, is not usually of any functional or cosmetic significance. The elbow is immobilized initially with a removable posterior splint, used mainly for comfort and some support.

Because stiffness is the most common complication of this injury, we promote early active motion. The patient is encouraged to remove the splint and start active motion as soon as 3 to 4 days after injury. The splint is exchanged for a sling as soon as the patient feels he or she no longer needs it for support. The same instructions apply to the sling: it is also discarded when it is no longer needed. This regimen of early motion is also used in fractures associated with a documented dislocation. Redislocation after elbow dislocation is rare, but elbow stiffness is common, so it is more important to initiate motion as soon as possible after reduction of the elbow. Due to the greater amount of soft-tissue injury associated with an elbow dislocation, the patient may not feel comfortable initiating early motion until about 5 to 7 days after reduction.

Physical therapy should be used only if voluntary active motion is difficult to obtain. The therapist should emphasize

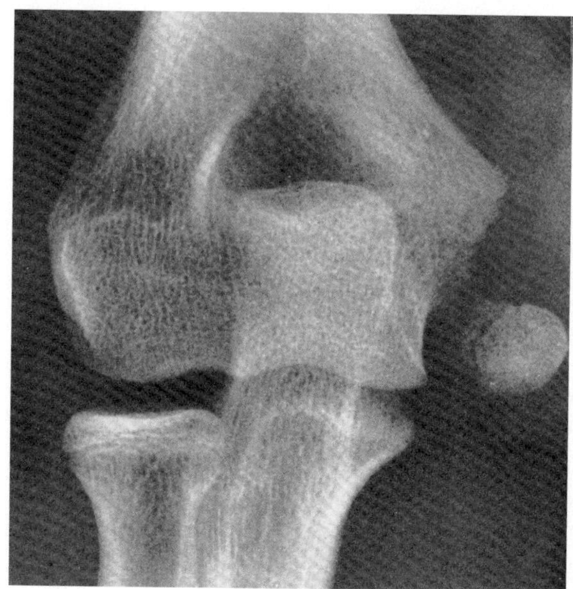

A

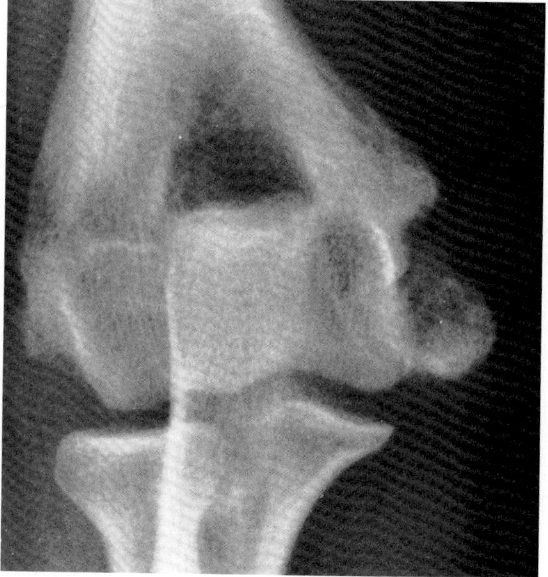

B

FIGURE 15-56 Nonoperative management. **A.** Postreduction film of a 13-year-old girl who sustained a displaced medial epicondyle following an acute elbow dislocation in her nondominant extremity. She was treated nonoperatively. **B.** One year later, the fragment has remained distally displaced with an apparent fibrous union. The patient, however, had a full painless range of elbow motion. (From Wilkins KE. Fractures of the medial epicondyle in children. *Instr Course Lect* 1991;40:1–8; with permission.)

modalities designed to decrease swelling and pain and reestablish strength. Range of motion should be achieved only by active means, not by passive stretching.

Operative Indications

Our indications for operative intervention are basically twofold. First and foremost are fractures in which the fragments cannot be extracted by manipulative means from within the elbow joint. Second, we stabilize the epicondyles operatively in patients whose expected high-level physical activity requires a stable elbow. We realize, however, that it is difficult to predict the athletic potential of a young child.

Acute Incarceration in the Joint.

If the elbow is reduced and if the ulnar nerve is intact, we use Roberts' manipulative technique (156) to attempt to extract the fragment before reduction. If this technique fails to remove the fragment, or if there is any ulnar nerve dysfunction, we proceed directly with an open procedure. The fragment is then extracted under direct vision just before reducing the elbow dislocation. If the elbow is reduced and if the fragment is incarcerated, we avoid the initial manipulation and proceed directly with an open extraction. We usually stabilize these fractures with a single cannulated screw rather than wires or pins, which allows almost immediate motion.

Follow-up is essentially the same as after closed treatment. Active motion is initiated 5 to 10 days postoperatively.

Prevention of Valgus Instability.

Currently, our most common indication for operative intervention is to ensure a stable elbow in patients participating in high-demand activities with their upper extremity (Fig. 15-57). This usually involves the dominant extremity of baseball pitchers, tennis players, or football quarterbacks. In wrestlers and gymnasts, the stability of the nondominant extremity also must be considered, which is best achieved with operative fixation.

We have not found the valgus stress test to be helpful in deciding on the need for operative stabilization of an athlete's medial epicondyle. Almost all of these patients with any significant displacement have a positive valgus stress test. Our decision is based primarily on the patient's need to have a very stable elbow for his or her athletic or work activity.

Fixation must be stable enough to allow early motion. Pins provide stability but do not allow early motion. Fortunately, most patients are mature enough so that the fragment can be secured with a cannulated screw.

Operative Technique

Our operative technique involves a direct medial approach to the fracture site. We make a longitudinal incision just anterior to the medial epicondyle. The fragment is usually displaced

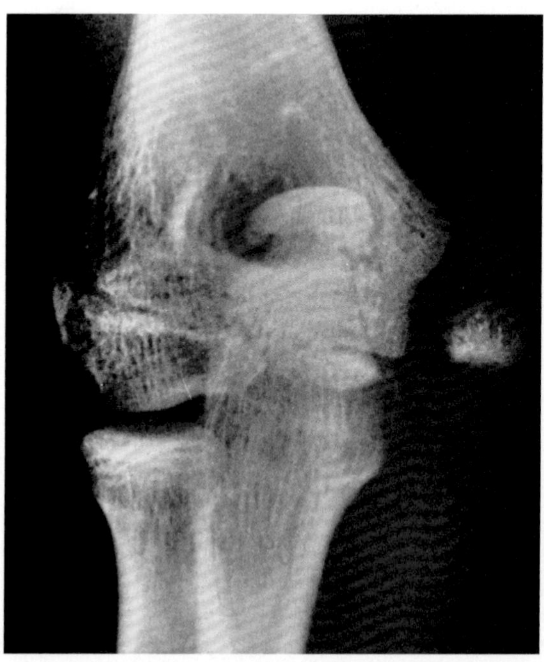
A

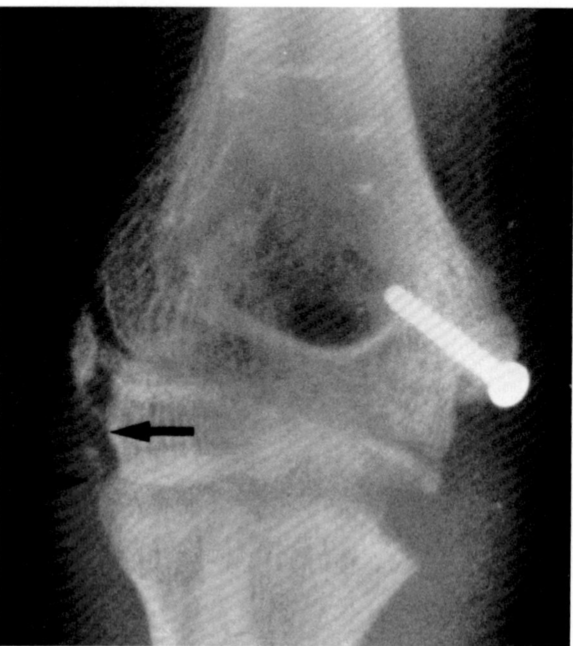
B

FIGURE 15-57 Operative stabilization. **A.** Injury film in a 12-year-old gymnast. Although this was a nondominant extremity, it was thought that both elbows needed stability. **B.** X-rays taken 4 weeks postoperatively show stabilization of the fragment with a single screw. There was also calcification of the lateral ligaments (*arrows*), confirming that the elbow was probably originally dislocated as well. (From Wilkins KE. Fractures of the medial epicondyle in children. *Instr Course Lect* 1991;40:1–8; with permission.)

distally and anteriorly. The periosteum is removed from the fracture site, and the clot is extracted by irrigation. It is important to identify and protect the ulnar nerve, but a complete dissection of the nerve is usually unnecessary. A small towel clip is used to reduce the fracture while the elbow is flexed and the forearm is pronated. Again, the medial epicondyle is normally situated posteriorly. The fragment is reduced and stabilized temporarily with one or two small K-wires. The final fixation is achieved using a screw, either partially threaded and overdrilled in the epicondylar fragment to compress it against the metaphysis or a cannulated 4.0-mm screw. After removal of the K-wires, the elbow is checked to ensure valgus stability and re-establishment of a full range of motion. After the surgical incision is closed, the extremity is placed in a long-arm cast, which is bivalved at 5 to 10 days, and active motion is initiated.

Fragmented Apophysis

If the epicondyle is fragmented and if there is a need to achieve elbow stability, an ASIF spike washer can be used to secure the multiple pieces to the metaphysis. If the washer is used, a second procedure may be necessary to remove the spike washer once the epicondyle is securely united to the metaphysis. If removal is impossible, we simply excise the fragments and reattach the ligament to the bone and periosteum at the base of the epicondylar defect.

Complications

Although much has been written about fractures involving the medial epicondylar apophysis, few complications are attributed to the fracture itself. The major complications that result in loss of function are failure to recognize incarceration in the joint and ulnar or medial nerve dysfunction. Most of the other complications are minor and result in only minimal functional or cosmetic sequelae (Table 15-5).

TABLE 15-5 Fractures of the Medial Epicondylar Apophysis: Complications

Major
Failure to recognize incarceration in the elbow
Ulnar nerve dysfunction
Minor
Loss of elbow extension
Myositis ossificans
Calcification of the collateral ligaments
Loss of motion
Cosmetic effects
Nonunion in the high-performance athlete

Major Complications

Failure to Recognize Incarceration. Failure to recognize incarceration of the epicondylar fragment into the joint can result in significant loss of elbow motion, especially if it remains incarcerated for any length of time. The management for late incarceration was detailed in the previous section on treatment.

Ulnar Nerve Dysfunction. The other major complication associated with this injury is the development of ulnar nerve dysfunction. The incidence of ulnar nerve dysfunction varies from 10% to 16% (138,145). If the fragment is entrapped in the joint, the incidence of ulnar nerve dysfunction may be as high as 50% (138,148).

The incidence of delayed ulnar nerve neuritis is low. More profound ulnar nerve injury has been reported after manipulative procedures (152). Thus, in patients with fragments incarcerated in the joint, manipulation may not be the procedure of choice if a primary ulnar nerve dysfunction is present. Patients in whom the fragment was left incarcerated in the joint for a significant time have experienced poor recovery of the primary ulnar nerve injury (145).

Dysfunction. Although the ulnar nerve is the major nerve injured, the median nerve may be trapped between a bony fragment and the distal humerus (58). It is speculated that the nerve can be entrapped between the apophyseal fragment and the distal humerus at the time of the original injury. This type of injury is described in greater detail in the section on complications of elbow dislocations.

Minor Complications

Other complications are minimal. Nonunion of the fragment with the distal metaphysis occurs in up to 50% of fractures with significant displacement (138). This appears to be more of an x-ray problem than a functional problem.

Another common problem is loss of the final degrees of elbow extension. A loss of 5% to 10% can be expected to develop in about 20% of these fractures. Little functional deficit is attributed to this loss of elbow dysfunction. Prolonged immobilization seems to be the key factor in loss of elbow extension. Again, it is important to emphasize before treatment is begun that loss of motion is common after this injury, regardless of the treatment method used.

Myositis ossificans is a rare occurrence following vigorous and repeated manipulation to extract the fragment from the joint. As with many other elbow injuries, myositis may be a result of the treatment rather than the injury itself. Myositis ossificans must be differentiated from ectopic calcification of the collateral ligaments, which involves only the ligamentous structures. This condition may occur after repeated injuries to

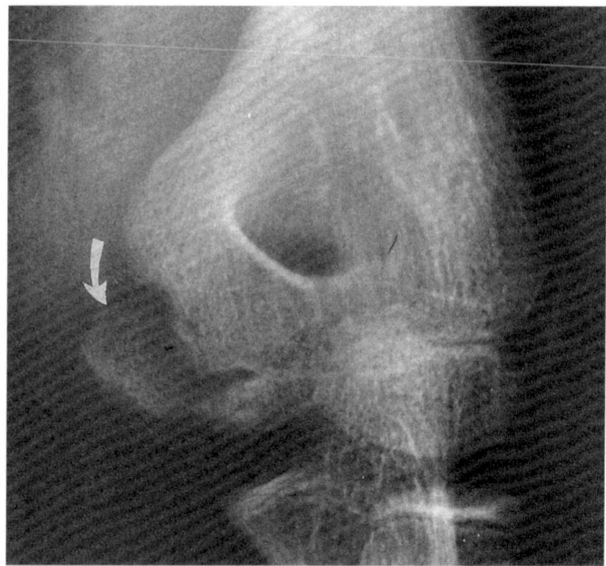

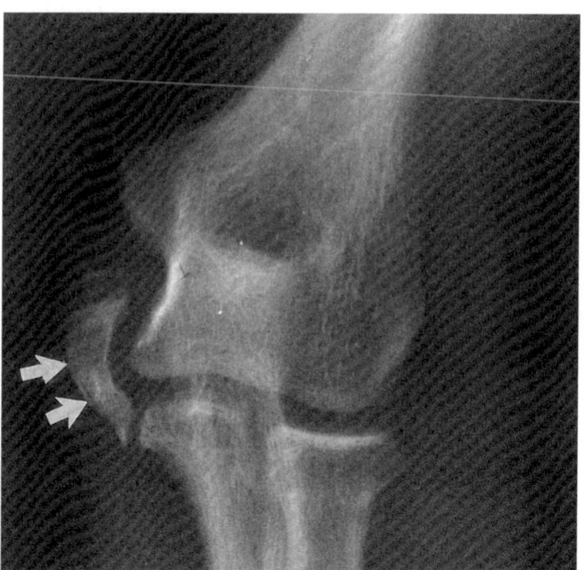

FIGURE 15-58 Heterotopic calcification. **A.** Injury to an 11-year-old who had moderate displacement of the medial epicondyle (*arrow*). **B.** One year later, she had considerable calcification of the ulnar collateral ligament (*arrows*). Other than mild instability with valgus stress, the patient had full range of motion and was asymptomatic. (Courtesy of Mark R. Christofersen, MD.)

the epicondyle and ligamentous structures (Fig. 15-58). Often, this calcified ligament is asymptomatic and does not seem to create functional disability. The cosmetic effects are minimal. In some patients, an accentuation of the epicondyle's medial prominence creates a false appearance of an increased carrying angle of the elbow. In his extensive review, Smith (143) recognized only a slight decrease in the carrying angle in two patients.

Nonunion in a high-performance athlete may be difficult to treat. One of the authors has treated a high-performance adolescent baseball pitcher who had to stop pitching after nonoperative management of a medial epicondylar fracture. The patient had developed a fibrous nonunion (Fig. 15-59). Attempts to establish union surgically were unsuccessful. The patient continued playing baseball, but had to change to another position.

Fractures Involving the Lateral Epicondylar Apophysis

Incidence

Fracture of the lateral epicondylar apophysis is a rare injury, with only a few isolated injuries described, mostly in textbooks.

Anatomic Considerations

Because the presence of this apophysis is often misinterpreted as a small chip fracture, a thorough understanding of the anatomy and ossification process is essential for evaluating injuries in this area.

Late Ossification

The lateral epicondylar apophysis is present for a considerable period but does not become ossified until the second decade. The best discussion of the anatomy of the ossification process

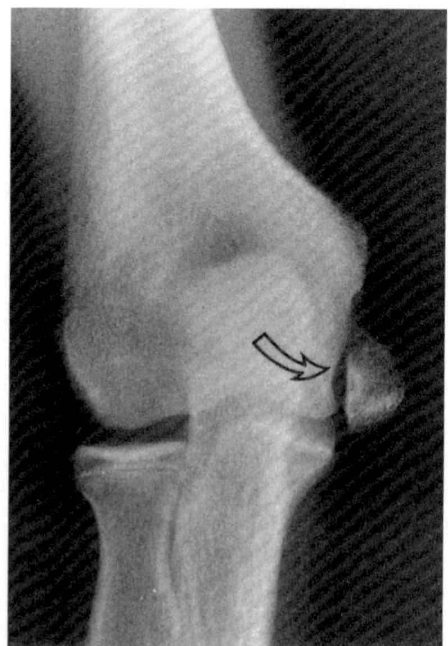

FIGURE 15-59 Nonunion in an athlete. This 15-year-old baseball pitcher had an untreated medial epicondyle fracture 1 year before this x-ray. He developed a fibrous union, but the epicondyle was shifted distally (*arrow*). His elbow was unstable enough to prevent him from pitching.

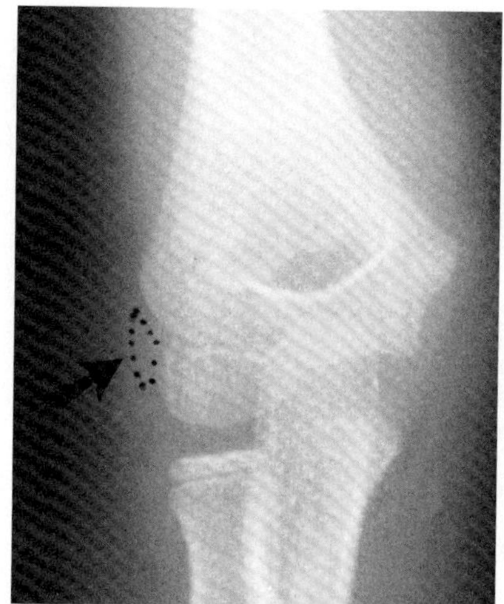

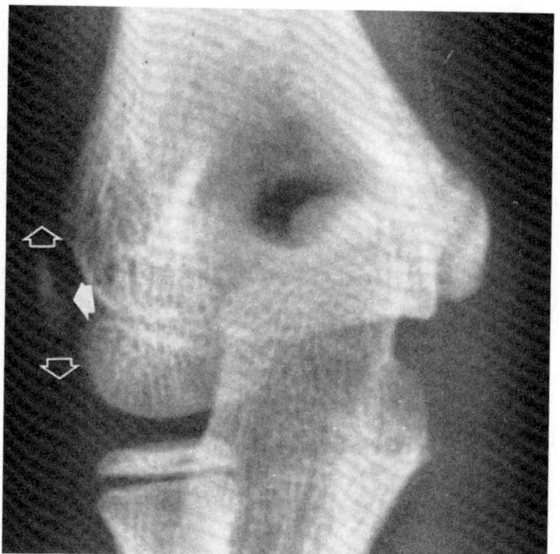

FIGURE 15-60 Lateral epicondylar apophysis. **A.** The cartilaginous apophysis occupies the wedge-shaped defect at the margin of the lateral condyle and metaphysis (*arrow*). The dotted line shows the margin of the cartilaginous apophysis. **B.** Ossification of the apophysis begins at the central portion of the wedge defect (*solid arrow*) and progresses both proximally and distally (*open arrows*) to form a triangular center.

is in a report by Silberstein et al (160), and much of the following discussion is paraphrased from their work. Just before ossification of the apophysis, the ossification margin of the lateral supracondylar ridge of the distal metaphysis curves abruptly medially toward the lateral condylar physis (Fig. 15-60). This process causes the osseous borders on the lateral aspect of the distal humerus to take the shape of the number 3. The central wedge of this defect contains the cartilaginous lateral epicondylar apophysis, which begins to ossify around 10 to 11 years of age. Ossification begins at the level of the lateral condylar physeal line and proceeds proximally and distally to form a triangle, with the apex directed toward the physeal line. The shape of the epicondylar apophyseal ossification center may also be in the form of a long sliver of bone with an irregular ossification pattern.

Silberstein et al (160) noted that the fracture line involving the lateral condylar physis often involves the proximal physeal line of the lateral epicondylar apophysis. Thus, this apophysis is almost always included with the lateral condylar fragment.

Mechanism of Injury

In adults, the most common etiology is that of a direct blow to the lateral side of the elbow. In children, because the forearm extensor muscles originate from this area, it is believed that avulsion forces from these muscles can be responsible for some of these injuries. Hasner and Husby (161) suggested that the fracture line's location in relation to the origins of the various extensor muscles determines the degree of displacement that can occur (Fig. 15-61). If the proximal part of the fracture line lies between the origin of the common extensors and the extensor carpi radialis longus, there is usually little displacement. If the fracture lines enter the area of origin of the extensor carpi radialis longus, then considerable displacement can occur.

X-Ray Findings

Because the ossification process starts on the external surface of the apophysis and proceeds centrally, the ossification center often appears separated from the lateral metaphysis and lateral condylar epiphysis. This natural separation can be confused with an avulsion fracture. The key to determining true separation is looking beyond the osseous tissues for the presence of associated soft tissue swelling (Fig. 15-62). If the ossification center lies distal to the osteochondral border of the lateral condylar epiphysis, it should be considered displaced (Fig. 15-63).

Treatment

Unless the fragment is incarcerated within the joint (162), treatment usually consists of simple immobilization for comfort. Al-

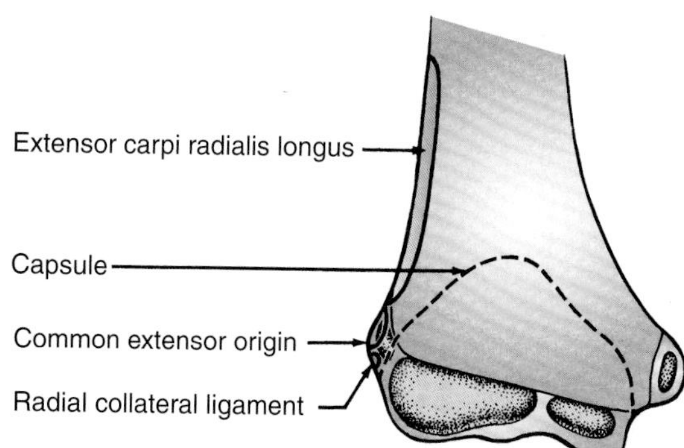

FIGURE 15-61 Soft tissue attachments. The origins of the forearm and wrist extensor muscles, radial collateral ligament, and outline of the capsule are shown in relation to the lateral epicondylar apophysis. (From Hasner E, Husby J. Fracture of the epicondyle and condyle of humerus. *Acta Chir Scand* 1951;101:195–202; with permission.)

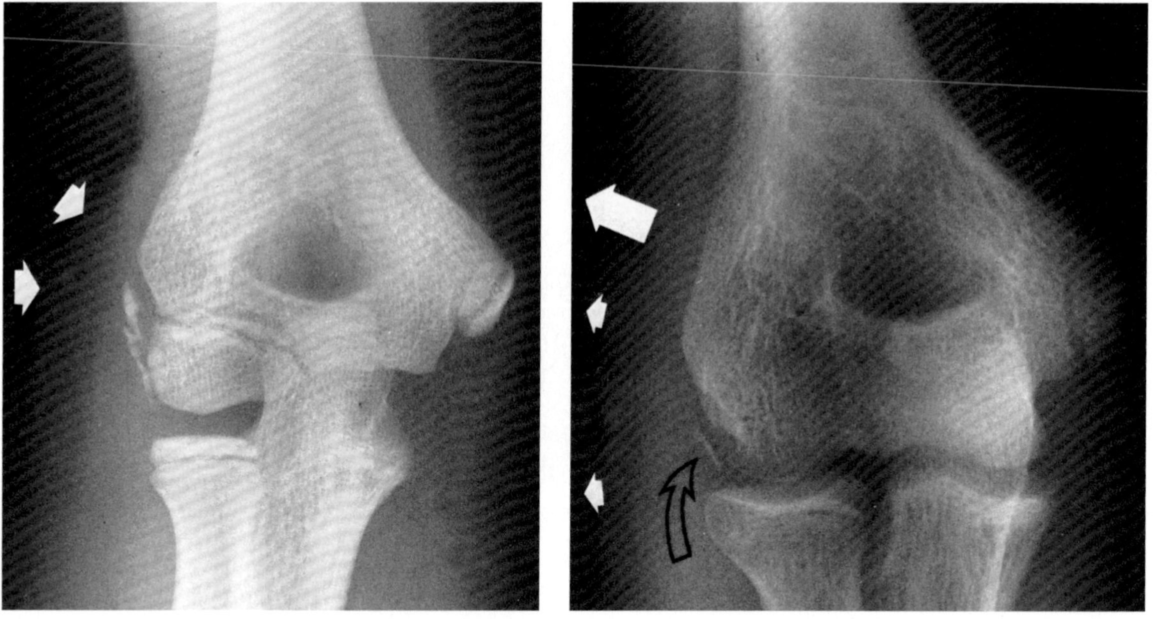

FIGURE 15-62 Lateral swelling. **A.** Soft tissue swelling in the area of the lateral epicondylar apophysis (*arrows*) suggests an undisplaced fracture involving the apophysis. The fragmentation of the apophysis is caused by irregular ossification. **B.** A small avulsion of the lateral epicondyle (*open arrow*) in an adolescent who is almost skeletally mature. There was considerable soft tissue swelling in this area (*solid arrows*).

though nonunion of the fragment can occur, this x-ray finding usually does not affect elbow function.

Complications

Only one rare major complication has been described with fractures involving the lateral epicondylar apophysis: entrapment of the fragment, either within the elbow joint (162) or between the capitellum and the radial head (163).

Fractures Involving the Olecranon Apophysis

Fractures involving the olecranon apophysis are believed to be caused by avulsion forces on the proximal ulna that occur with

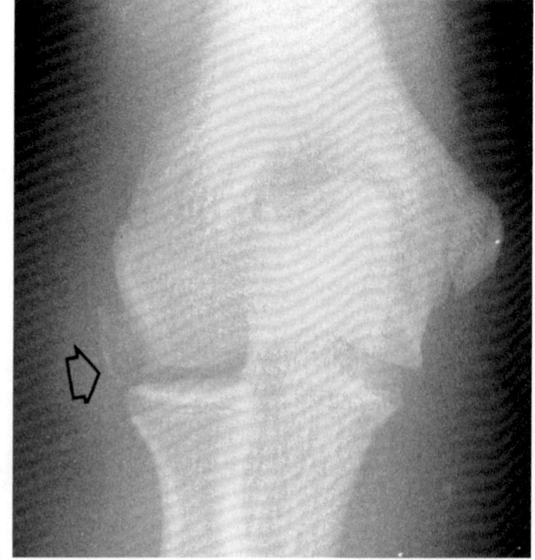

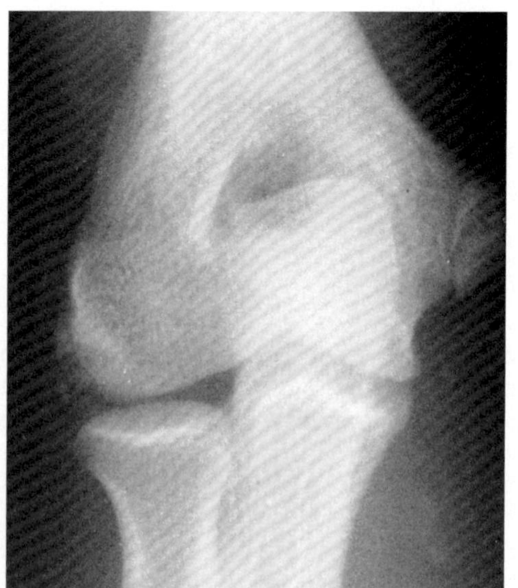

FIGURE 15-63 Avulsion injury. **A.** Avulsion of a portion of the lateral epicondyle in an adolescent (*arrow*). The fragment is at the level of the joint. Most of the epicondyle has fused to the condyle. **B.** The appearance 9 months later shows fragmentation and partial union of the fragment. (Courtesy of R. Chandrasekharan, MD.)

the elbow flexed (164). This injury is rare in normal children because an avulsion force generated through the expansion of the triceps tendon inserting on the metaphysis distal to the physis usually results in a fracture through the more distal metaphysis. Bracq (165) noted that fractures of the olecranon apophysis appeared to occur more often in children with osteogenesis imperfecta (OI), and several reports since that time have confirmed his observation (164,166–169). Why children with OI may be predisposed to this injury is unknown. Zionts and Moon (164) suggested that a combination of weakness of the subchondral bone adjacent to the physis of the proximal olecranon and increased laxity of the triceps expansion might make the olecranon apophysis more vulnerable to injury in children with OI. Because OI was not recognized in half of their patients, they suggested that OI should be considered in any child who has an isolated, displaced fracture of the olecranon apophysis, especially when the injury results from relatively minor trauma.

Undisplaced fractures can be treated with cast immobilization. Operative treatment is usually recommended for displaced fractures of the olecranon apophysis in all children, although the amount of "acceptable" displacement ranges from 3 mm to 5 mm. Fixation is with two smooth intramedullary K-wires and a tension band of either stainless-steel wire or absorbable suture. Problems with the K-wires backing out and re-fracture after hardware removal have been reported in children with OI (164,167,170,171); Gwynne-Jones (167) suggested that retaining the hardware or using nonabsorbable sutures might decrease the risk of re-fracture.

Reports in the literature indicate that approximately 70% of children with OI who sustain an olecranon apophyseal fracture later have a fracture of the contralateral olecranon apophysis; the mean time to second fracture reported by Gwynne-Jones (167) was 7 months and by Zionts and Moon (164). Parents should be advised of this possibility and the child's high-risk activities should be avoided.

Chronic Tension Stress Injuries (Little League Elbow)

This chronic injury is related to overuse in skeletally immature baseball pitchers. Brogdon and Crow described the original x-ray findings in 1960 (172). Later, Adams (173) demonstrated that the x-ray changes were due to excessive throwing and emphasized the need for preventive programs. This injury is thought to be due to excessive tension on the medial epicondyle with secondary tendinitis. There can also be a repeated compression on the lateral condyle, producing an osteochondritis.

Studies have shown that as long as the rules outlined by the Little League are followed (i.e., two innings per game, six innings per week), the incidence of these chronic tension stress injuries is fairly low (146). Most of the problems arise when overzealous parents and coaches require excessive pitching preseason and at home between practices. Albright (154) found a greater incidence in pitchers who had improper pitching techniques. The spectrum of these chronic injuries is outlined in Table 15-6.

TABLE 15-6 Spectrum of Chronic Tension Stress Injuries of Medial Epicondylar Apophysis

Stress fracture of the epicondylar physis
Calcification of the ulnar collateral ligaments
Hypertrophy of the medial epicondyle
Acceleration of growth maturity with generalized synovitis and stiffness
Osteochondritis of the lateral condyle

In chronic tension stress injuries (Little League Elbow Syndrome), the history is usually quite characteristic. It is found in young baseball pitchers who are throwing an excessive number of pitches or who are just starting to throw curve pitches (146). Clinically, this syndrome is manifested by a decrease in elbow extension. Medial epicondylar pain is accentuated by a valgus stress to the elbow in extension. There is usually significant local tenderness and swelling over the medial epicondyle.

On x-rays, the density of the bone of the distal humerus is increased due to the chronicity of the stress. The physeal line is irregular and widened. If the stress has been going on for a prolonged period, there may be hypertrophy of the distal humerus with accelerated bone growth. The bone age of the elbow is greater than the patient's chronologic age (Fig. 15-64).

We use a multifaceted approach that involves educating the parents, coaches, and player. Once symptoms develop, all pitching activity must cease until the epicondyle and adjacent flexor muscle origins become nontender. In addition, local and systemic measures to decrease the inflammatory response are used. Once the initial pain and inflammation have decreased, a program of forearm and arm muscle strengthening is initiated. The pitching technique is also examined to see if any corrections need to be made. Once strength has been re-established in the muscles in the upper extremity and motion has been fully re-established, the patient is gradually returned to pitching with careful monitoring of the number of innings and pitches within a specified time period.

OSTEONECROSIS OF THE TROCHLEA

Three theories have been proposed to account for the posttraumatic changes that occur in the distal humerus after fractures in the vicinity of the trochlea: malunion, partial growth arrest, and vascular injury. The most common form follows some type of elbow trauma. In some cases, the trauma is occult or poorly

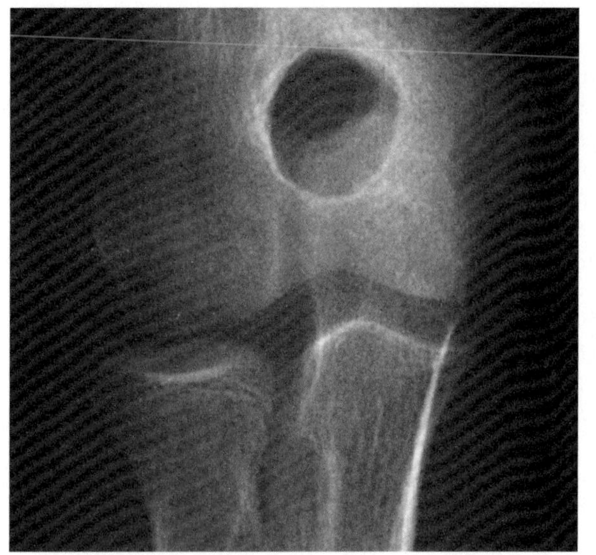
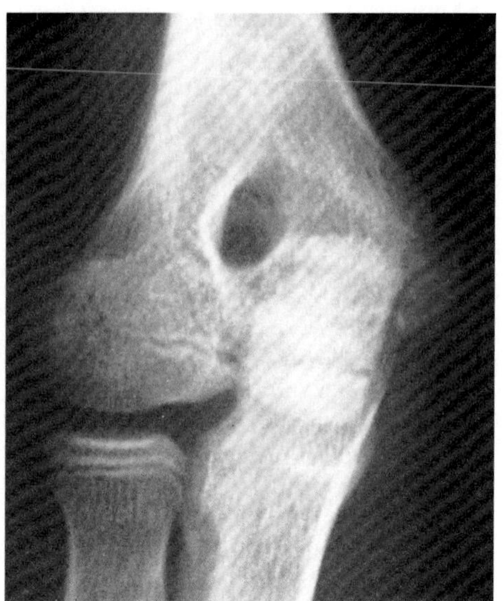

FIGURE 15-64 Chronic tension stress. **A.** AP view of a 13-year-old pitcher with chronic pain and significant loss of elbow motion. The bone age is around 15 years. **B.** Same view of the opposite elbow with a bone age of 13 years.

defined (174,175–179). This form results in a spectrum from simply a small defect of the trochlea (fishtail deformity) to complete destruction of the medial aspect of the distal humerus with a progressive varus deformity, decreased range of motion, and associated instability of the elbow. Because it is seldom reported in the literature, the exact incidence is unknown. Toniolo and Wilkins (180) reported a series of 30 cases collected over the past 20 years from various sources and suggested that osteonecrosis of the trochlea is probably one of the most unrecognized sequela of injuries to the distal humerus.

Vascular Anatomy

In Haraldsson's classic studies (181,182) of the blood supply of the distal humerus, he demonstrated that the medial crista of the trochlea had two separate blood supply sources (Fig. 15-65). Neither has anastomoses with each other or with the other metaphyseal vessels. In the young infant, the vessels are small and lie on the surface of the perichondrium.

The lateral vessels supply the trochlea's apex and the lateral aspect of the medial crista. These vessels cross the physis to enter the posterior aspect of the lateral trochlear ossification center. Their terminal branches lie just under the articular surface. Thus, they are particularly vulnerable to injury when the fracture line occurs through this area, as is typical in fractures of the medial condylar physis, lateral condyle, or a T-condylar fracture. By the same token, a fracture in the supracondylar area in which the fracture line is very distal, or a total distal humeral physeal displacement can also disrupt the lateral trochlear epiphyseal vessels as they course along the surface of the metaphysis or at their entrance into the physeal plate.

Another set of vessels enters medially through the nonarticulating surface of the trochlea. This set of vessels supplies the most medial aspect of the medial crista or the medial portion of the trochlear epiphysis. As shown in Haraldsson's (181,182) studies, there appear to be no anastomoses between these two sets of vessels supplying the trochlear epiphysis.

Ossification centers need blood supply for their appearance and development. Before these centers appear, the vessels are more superficial and less well defined. It is speculated that a lesion in these immature vessels in children leads only to a delay in the appearance of the centers. In older children, where there is already a well-defined ossification center, disruption produces a true bony osteonecrosis of one or both of the trochlea's ossification centers. This can result in a partial or total absence of further epiphyseal ossification, leading to hypoplasia of the central or whole medial aspect of the trochlea.

Patterns of Osteonecrosis

Osteonecrosis of the trochlea can appear as either a central defect (type A) or total hypoplasia manifest by complete absence of the trochlea (type B), depending on the extent of the vascular injury.

Type A—Fishtail Deformity

In the type A deformity, only the lateral portion of the medial crista or apex of the trochlea becomes involved in the necrotic process, which produces the typical fishtail deformity (Fig. 15-66). This more common pattern of necrosis seems to occur with very distal supracondylar fractures or with fractures involving the lateral condylar physis.

Type B—Malignant Varus Deformity

The type B deformity involves osteonecrosis of the entire trochlea and sometimes part of the metaphysis (Fig. 15-67).

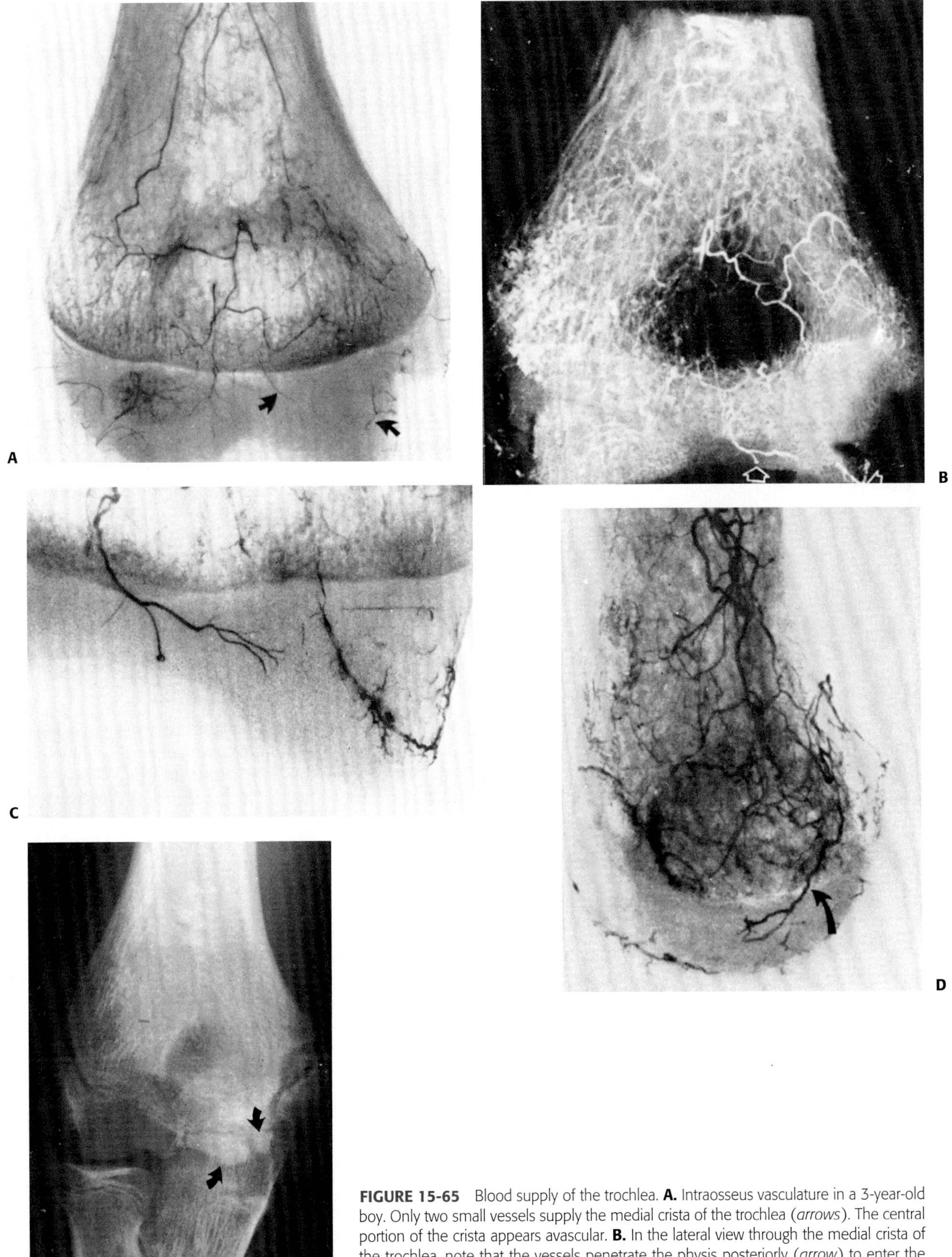

FIGURE 15-65 Blood supply of the trochlea. **A.** Intraosseus vasculature in a 3-year-old boy. Only two small vessels supply the medial crista of the trochlea (*arrows*). The central portion of the crista appears avascular. **B.** In the lateral view through the medial crista of the trochlea, note that the vessels penetrate the physis posteriorly (*arrow*) to enter the epiphyseal cartilage. (From Haraldsson S. On osteochondritis deformans juvenilis capituli humeri. *Acta Orthop Scand* 1959;38, with permission.)

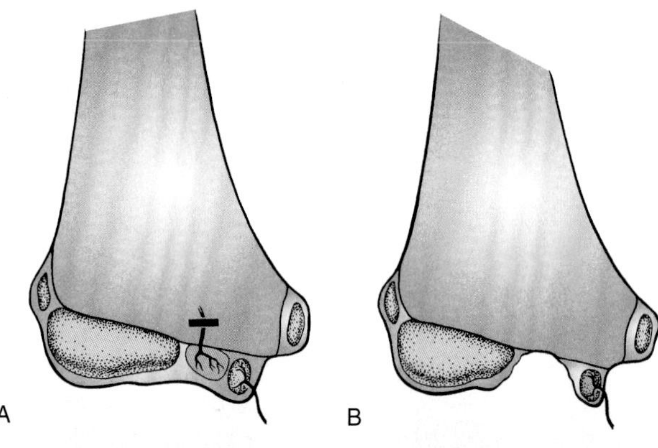

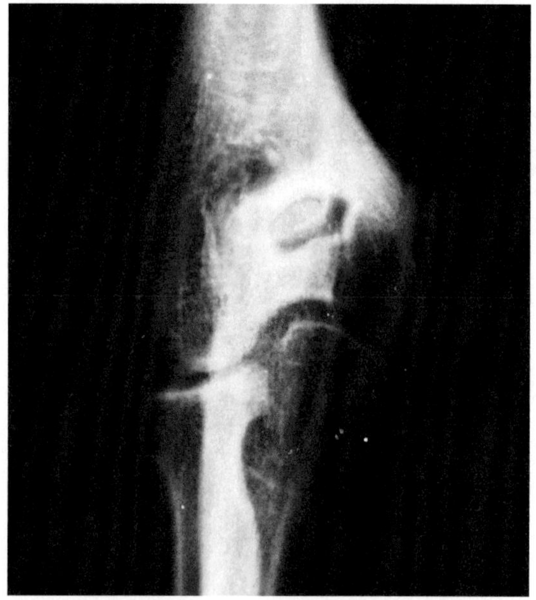

FIGURE 15-66 Fishtail deformity. **A,B.** Type A deformity. Osteonecrosis of only the lateral ossification center creates a defect in the trochlear groove's apex. **C.** The typical fishtail deformity is seen in an x-ray of a 14-year-old boy who sustained an undisplaced distal supracondylar fracture 5 years previously.

This type of necrosis has occurred as a sequela of fractures involving the entire distal humeral physis or fractures of the medial condylar physis (183) and can lead to a cubitus varus deformity in which the angulation progresses as the child matures.

The clinical signs and symptoms differ considerably between the two patterns of necrosis.

Patients who have the type A or fishtail deformity usually do not develop any angular deformities. The severity of the fishtail deformity is related to the degree of necrosis and seems to dictate the severity of the symptoms. In children who have a pattern of total osteonecrosis of the trochlea, including part of the nonarticular surface, a progressive varus deformity usually develops. Because the total medial trochlear surface is disrupted, significant loss of range of motion also develops. These deformities usually worsen cosmetically and functionally as the child matures. Early degenerative joint disease with a loss of range of motion is the most common sequela in severe cases.

Some children with osteonecrosis of the trochlea develop late-onset ulnar neuropathy (184–187), thought to be due to a multiplicity of factors, including joint malalignment, abnormal position of the ulnar nerve and triceps tendon, loss of protection by a deep ulnar groove, and the acute angle of entrance of the two heads of the flexor carpi ulnaris.

Treatment

Because the osteonecrosis of the trochlea is a direct consequence of trauma to the vessels at the time of injury, there is no effective prevention or treatment of the primary necrosis. Treatment is aimed at only the sequelae of the osteonecrosis of the trochlea. If a loss of range of motion is due to a significant disruption of the articular surface itself, there does not appear to be any good operative or nonoperative method that significantly improves elbow function. If the osteonecrosis of the trochlea has resulted in a varus deformity of the elbow, this deformity can be corrected by a supracondylar osteotomy with ulnar nerve transposition. The correction of the carrying angle is mostly cosmetic, with little functional improvement. Surgical treatment carries the risk of increased stiffness to the already limited elbow.

T-CONDYLAR FRACTURES

In T-condylar fractures, the fracture line originates in the central groove of the trochlea and courses proximal to the olecranon and the coronoid fossae, where it divides and separates the medial and lateral bony columns of the distal humerus. If the proximal fracture lines are oblique, the fracture may be termed *Y-condylar*. This injury is rare in skeletally immature children.

Incidence

The early modern literature reflects only reports by Blount (85) and Zimmerman (188), who each described a case in an 11-year-old patient. The average age of patients reported in three major series (189–191) was 12.6 years. Thus, Maylahn and Fahey (192), who reported six patients near skeletal maturity, were accurate when they said, "the fractures [T-condylar] take on the characteristics of an adult fracture and should be treated as such."

The actual incidence in younger children is certainly low, but it may be underdiagnosed because it is often confused with other fractures, such as those involving the lateral condylar physis or total distal physis. Special imaging studies such as arthrograms or MRI may be necessary to demonstrate the intracondylar aspect in young children. The combination of an increased awareness of the possibility of this injury and a more aggressive diagnostic approach may result in more cases being uncovered in this younger age group.

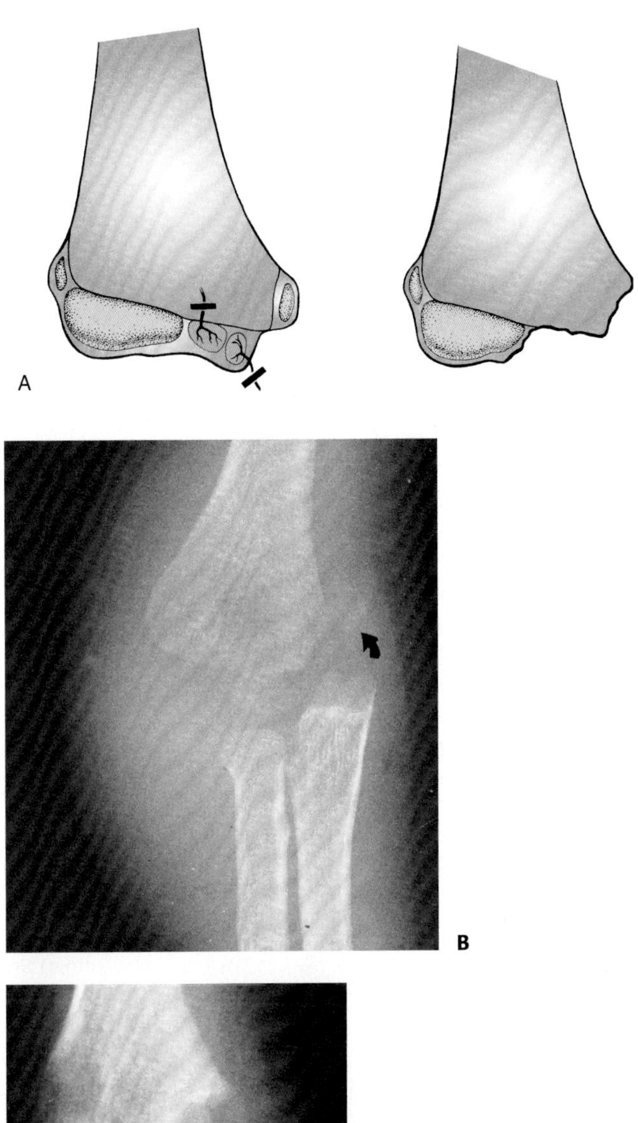

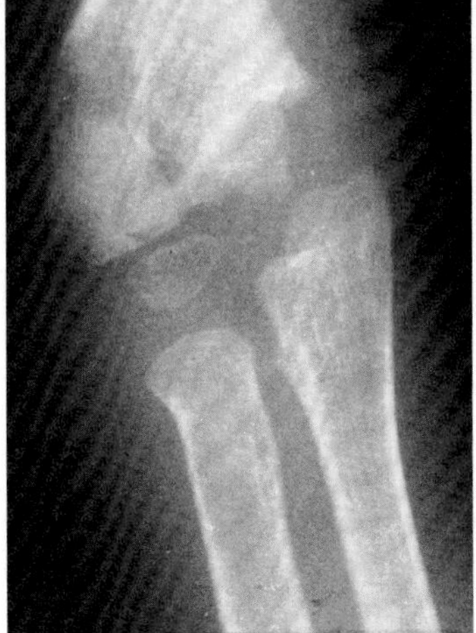

FIGURE 15-67 Osteonecrosis of the entire trochlea. **A.** In this type B deformity,. loss of blood supply from both the medial and lateral vessels results in osteonecrosis of the entire medial crista along with a portion of the metaphysis. **B.** X-ray of a 4-year-old boy who sustained a type II physeal fracture involving the entire distal humeral physis. In this injury film, there is a large metaphyseal fragment on the medial side (*arrow*). **C.** As shown by the appearance 5 months later, a mild varus deformity present is due to an incomplete reduction. The ossification in the medial metaphyseal fragment has disappeared.

Mechanism of Injury

The primary mechanism of this injury is the direct wedge effect of the articular surface of the olecranon on the distal end of the humerus. The sharp edge of the semilunar notch or coronoid process acts as a wedge to break the trochlea and split the condyles, which in turn separates the two columns of the distal humerus. Flexion and extension types of injuries have been described.

The most common mechanism producing a flexion injury is a direct blow to the posterior aspect of the elbow, usually when the child falls directly on the flexed elbow. This flexion mechanism in young children contributes to its rarity because most upper-extremity injuries in children have a component of elbow hyperextension. In these flexion injuries, the wedge effect is produced at the apex of the trochlea by the central portion of the trochlear notch. In these flexion injuries, the condylar fragments usually lie anterior to the shaft (Fig. 15-68A,B).

A T-condylar fracture may be caused by a fall on the outstretched arm with the elbow in only slight flexion. This extension mechanism has been suggested by patients in their description of the dynamics of the fall, and indirectly by the position of the distal fragments in relation to the diaphyses of the humerus—in other words, lying posterior (Fig. 15-68C,D). In the extension type of injury, the coronoid portion of the semilunar notch produces the wedge effect.

It has been suggested that contraction of the elbow flexor and extensor muscles may play a role in the displacement pattern of this fracture. Because of their origins on the epicondyles, they accentuate both the separation in the coronal plane and the forward displacement in the sagittal plane. This displacement pattern is often evident on the injury films (Fig. 15-68C,D).

Fracture Patterns

The fracture pattern in adolescents is similar to that in adults. The condylar fragments are often separated, with the articular surface completely disrupted. In addition to separation of the condylar fragments by the force of the original injury, the muscles that originate on these condylar fragments rotate them in both the coronal and sagittal planes (Fig. 15-68C,D). In the sagittal plane, the position of the condylar fragments in relation to the humeral shaft and metaphysis can either be anterior (flexor mechanism; Fig. 15-68B) or posterior (extension mechanism; Fig. 15-68D).

In skeletally immature patients, the central portions of the condylar fragments are usually separated, but the articular surface may remain intact because of its large cartilage component (Fig. 15-69) (191). Thus, the disruption and displacement are primarily in the osseous supracondylar area. The elasticity of the cartilage of the distal end of the humerus often protects the articular surface from being completely disrupted.

Classification

Various classifications (189,193) for adult T-condylar fractures have been proposed, but there are problems with applying these classifications to children's injuries. For example, the number of children with this fracture is so small that no clinician can include all types of fracture patterns in his or her own experience. In addition, there is no useful classification for younger patients, in whom the unossified intact articular cartilage is not visible on x-ray. Toniolo and Wilkins (194) proposed a simple classification based on the degree of displacement and comminution of the fracture fragments. Type I fractures are minimally displaced (Fig. 15-70A,B). Type II fractures are displaced but do not have comminution of the metaphyseal fragments (Fig. 15-70C). Type III fractures are displaced fractures with comminution of the metaphyseal fragments (Fig. 15-70D,E).

In a child, the integrity of the articular surface may be difficult to determine without using arthrography or MRI. Because the initial integrity of the articular surface may not be that important to the prognosis, this factor was not believed to significantly contribute to a general classification scheme.

In adolescents aged 12 years or older, classification and treatment are as those in adults (see Chapter 28, Fractures and Dislocations in Adults).

Diagnosis

Clinically, these fractures are most often confused with extension-type supracondylar fractures. The extended position of the elbow, along with the massive swelling, is almost identical to that of the displaced extension type of supracondylar fracture.

Plain x-rays are the cornerstone to the diagnosis. In older children, the differentiation must be made from that of a comminuted supracondylar fracture. Sometimes the diagnosis is not obvious until the fragments have been partially reduced, which allows the vertical fracture lines splitting the trochlea to become more evident. In younger children, the diagnosis is much more difficult because the articular surface is not visible. In addition, because of its rarity, the possibility of a T-condylar fracture may not be considered in this age group.

The diagnosis must exclude common fracture patterns of either the isolated lateral or medial condyles and complete separation of the distal humeral physis. In these latter fractures, an important sign is the presence of a medial or lateral Thurston-Holland fragment in the metaphysis (195). The key differential for the T-condylar fracture is the presence of a vertical fracture line extending down to the apex of the trochlea.

If the diagnosis is suspected after a careful evaluation of the static x-ray films, it can be confirmed with varus or valgus stress films made while the patient is under general anesthesia (195). The use of contrast medium in the form of an arthrogram also is helpful.

Treatment

Because of the rarity of this injury, treatment recommendations cannot be based on multiple case experiences. Most of the experience has been based on isolated cases or small series (189–191,195). Regardless of the treatment method, certain basic principles must be considered in dealing with these frac-

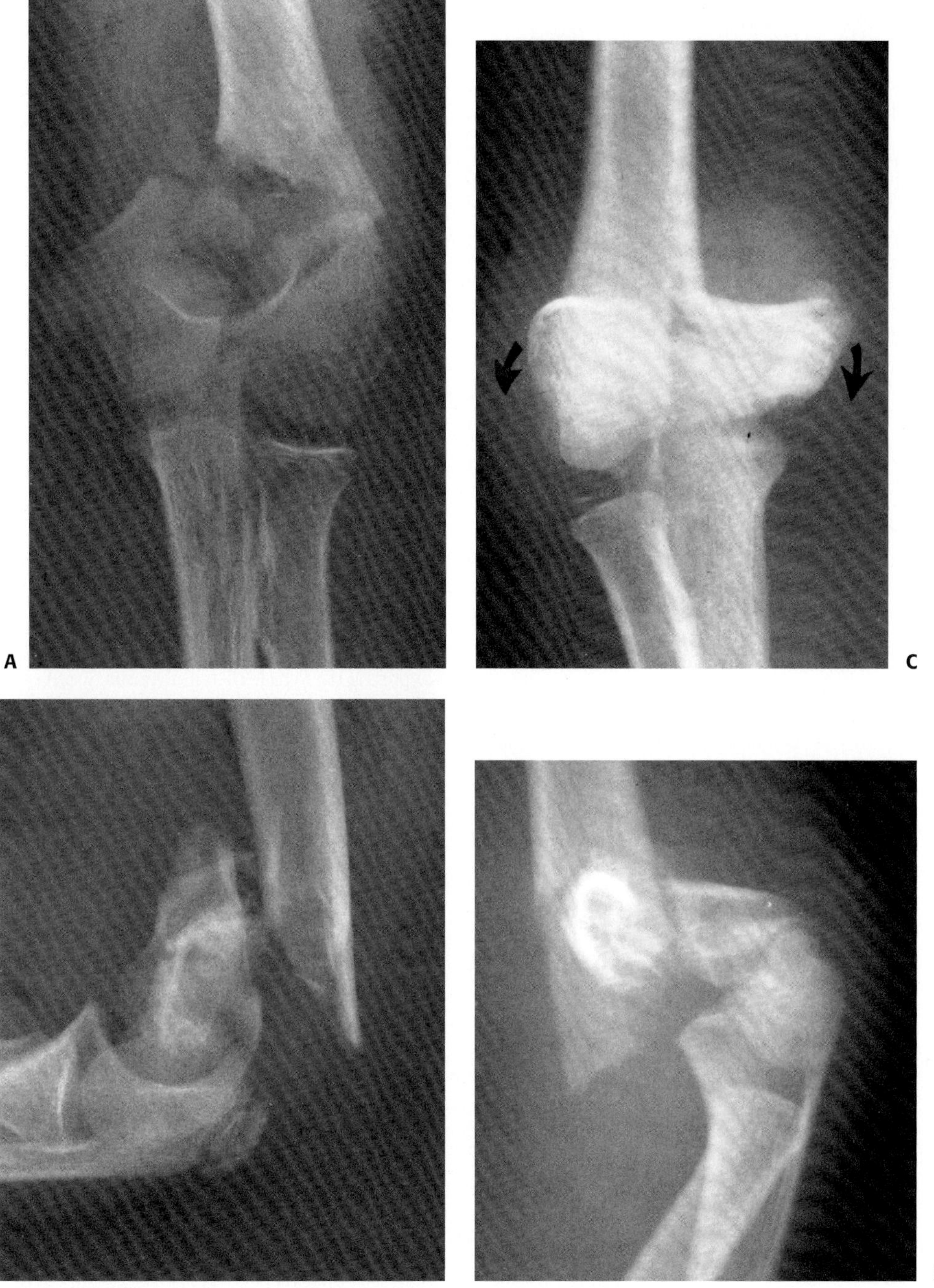

FIGURE 15-68 Mechanism patterns. **A,B.** The more common flexion pattern in which the condylar fragments are situated anterior to the distal shaft. **C,D.** An extensor pattern in which the condylar fragments are situated posterior to the distal shaft. The muscle origins on the respective condyles cause them to diverge in the coronal plane (*arrows*) and flex in the sagittal plane.

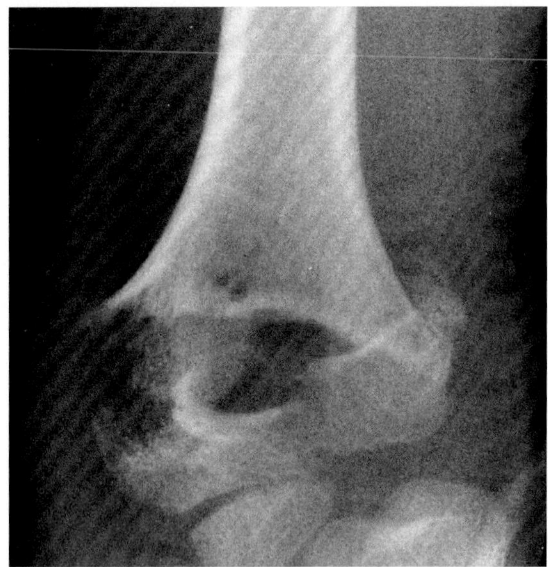

FIGURE 15-69 Intact articular surface. In this T-condylar fracture in a 7-year-old boy, the thick articular cartilage remains essentially intact, preventing separation of the condylar fragments. This fracture was secured with simple percutaneous pins.

tures. A treatment plan must be individualized for the specific fracture and the surgeon's level of expertise and experience. The following principles must be considered in planning a treatment method:

1. Elbow articular mobility depends on articular congruity, correct alignment of the axis of motion, and debris- and bone-free fossae.
2. The stability depends on the integrity of the lateral and medial supracondylar columns.
3. The T-condylar fracture is an articular fracture, so the first goal is to restore and stabilize the joint surface.
4. Closed methods alone usually cannot produce an acceptable result because of the muscle forces applied to the fragments.
5. Most patients are adolescents with minimal potential for bone remodeling.
6. Although surgical reduction may produce an acceptable reduction on x-ray, it may add to the already extensive damage to soft tissues; this in turn can contribute to postoperative stiffness.

The literature reflects good results with surgical management. Zimmerman (188) advocated establishing an anatomic reduction with internal fixation so that early motion could facilitate a more rapid rehabilitation. In the two young children described by Beghin et al (195), operative intervention was necessary to achieve a satisfactory reduction. A review of three series (189–191) supports surgical management: 29 of the 31 elbows in these combined series were treated operatively. The investigators of these series maintained that open reduction and internal fixation was the best way to restore the articular surface's integrity and stabilize the fracture sufficiently to allow early mobilization. All but one of the patients in this combined series who were treated surgically had good or very good results at follow-up.

Kanellopoulus and Yiannakopoulos (196) described closed reduction of the intra-articular component, with fixation by partially threaded pins for interfragmentary compression. Two elastic titanium intramedullary nails were used for stabilizing the supracondylar component. T-condylar fractures in two adolescents healed without complications after using this technique. Both patients returned to sports with full elbow range of motion at 6 weeks after surgery.

The surgical approach most widely accepted is the posterior longitudinal splitting of the triceps without an osteotomy of the olecranon. This approach gives adequate exposure of the fracture and the articular surface and does not seem to produce any loss of strength from splitting the triceps (190). Although one reported patient had x-ray evidence of osteonecrosis of the trochlea (191), another had a nonunion (190), and many had some loss of range of motion, none of these surgically treated patients demonstrated any significant loss of elbow function or discomfort.

Bryan and Morrey (197) described a triceps-sparing approach in which the extensor mechanism is reflected laterally, exposing the whole distal humerus. Remia et al (198) evaluated triceps function and elbow motion in nine patients with T-condylar fractures treated with open reduction through a triceps-sparing approach and compared them to those reported after a triceps-splitting approach. No statistically significant differences were found in function or range or motion.

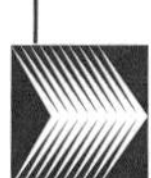

AUTHORS' PREFERRED TREATMENT

Because this fracture is rare in children, there is no standard recommended treatment. Our suggestions are based on a combination of our clinical experience and the experience of others in a few series (189–191). Our first consideration in these fractures is to re-establish the integrity of the articular surface to maintain the congruity of the joint. Usually, this cannot be achieved adequately by closed methods, so we proceed with an open surgical technique. We have found the simple classification into three types based on the degree of displacement or comminution to be helpful in guiding the aggressiveness of our treatment.

Type I (Undisplaced or Minimally Displaced)

In type I injuries, there is little displacement of the bony supracondylar columns. In children, the periosteum is often intact and can provide some intrinsic stability. In addition, the thicker articular and epiphyseal cartilage in skeletally immature children may still be intact, even if the bony epiphysis appears severed by a vertical fracture line. Because of this condition, we have found two methods to be successful for these types of fractures.

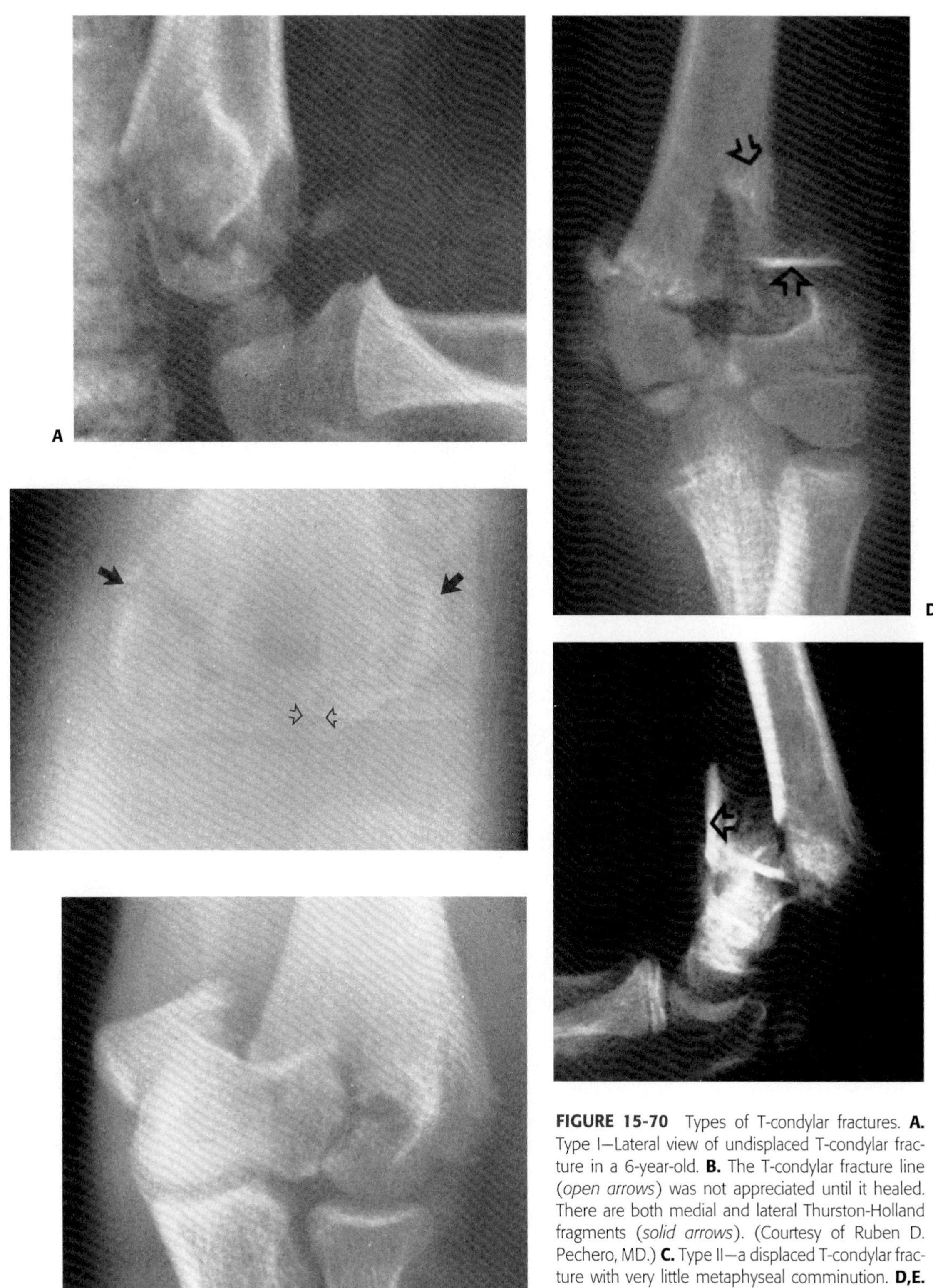

FIGURE 15-70 Types of T-condylar fractures. **A.** Type I—Lateral view of undisplaced T-condylar fracture in a 6-year-old. **B.** The T-condylar fracture line (*open arrows*) was not appreciated until it healed. There are both medial and lateral Thurston-Holland fragments (*solid arrows*). (Courtesy of Ruben D. Pechero, MD.) **C.** Type II—a displaced T-condylar fracture with very little metaphyseal comminution. **D,E.** Type III—two views of a markedly comminuted T-condylar fracture with multiple displaced fragments (*arrows*) in a 12-year-old.

Closed Reduction—Percutaneous Pin Fixation. These fractures require minimal manipulation under general anesthesia and x-ray control to re-establish the supracondylar columns. If there is anterior or posterior rotation in the sagittal plane of the metaphyseal portion of the column, a pin placed into that column can be used as a "joy stick" to manipulate the fragment into a satisfactory position. Once a satisfactory reduction is achieved, the pin can then be advanced across the fracture site for fixation. These fractures usually require multiple pins placed percutaneously, such as those used in comminuted supracondylar fractures (Fig. 15-71). Because of the rapid healing, the pins can be removed at 3 weeks to allow early active motion.

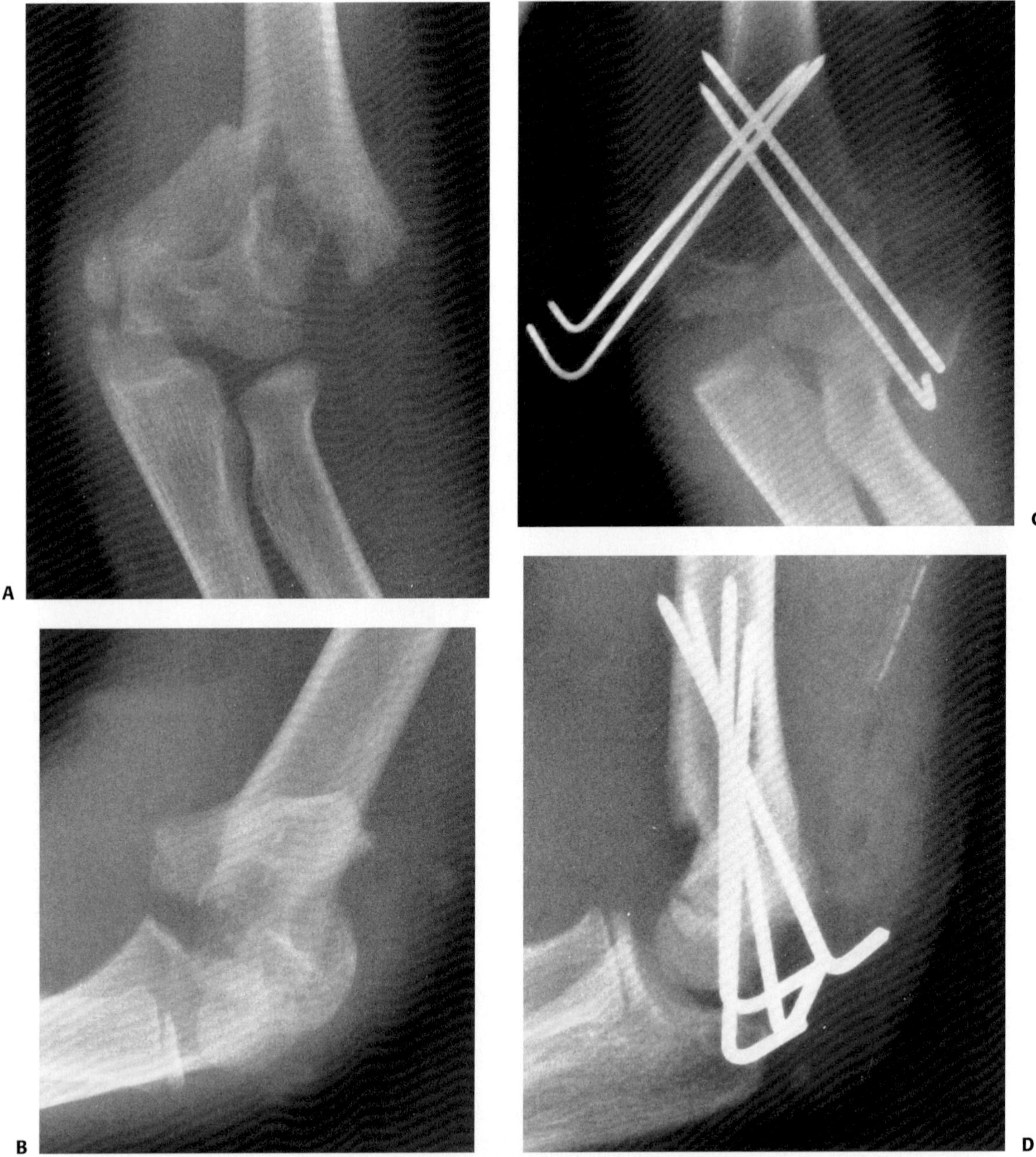

FIGURE 15-71 Closed reduction and pin fixation. **A,B.** Two views of a type II T-condylar fracture in a 15-year-old. **C,D.** Because an anatomic reduction was achieved by manipulative closed reduction, it was secured with simple multiple pin fixation placed percutaneously. The articular surface was minimally displaced. The pins were removed at 3 weeks. At this age, healing was rapid enough to pull the pins at 3 weeks to allow active motion. Ultimately, the patient was deficient only 10 degrees from achieving full extension.

Traction. If the articular cartilage is intact, it may close as a hinge with traction. The rotational displacement of the condyles created by the origins of the forearm muscles can be neutralized with olecranon traction, in which the elbow is suspended at 90 degrees of flexion. There is usually adequate stability from the callus around the fracture site at 2 to 3 weeks to discontinue the traction. The elbow is then immobilized in a hinged cast brace for an additional 2 to 3 weeks. This immobilization allows the initiation of protected active motion. With the present emphasis on short hospitalization, however, we find that skeletal traction is less acceptable for both social and financial reasons. Skeletal traction may be the only acceptable method of treatment in patients seen on a delayed basis with extensive skin abrasions, severe soft tissue injury, or gross comminution, in which cast application or other operative interventions might carry a high risk of infection.

Type II (Displaced Without Comminution)

Open Reduction and Internal Fixation. If there is wide separation of the condylar fragments with marked disruption of the articular surface, stability and articular congruity can be established only with an open surgical procedure. We prefer the Bryan-Morrey posterior triceps-sparing approach (197). The patient is placed prone on the operating table with the arm supported on a pillow and the forearm hanging down off the edge of the operating table. This position provides the best approach for direct observation of the posterior surface of the distal humerus. Olecranon osteotomy is reserved for severely comminuted articular fractures in adolescents.

Reconstruction of the Articular Surface. Our first priority is to re-establish the integrity of the articular fragments—in other words, to convert it to a supracondylar fracture (Fig. 15-72A–C). The olecranon and coronoid fossae must be cleared of bony fragments or debris to eliminate the chance of bony impingement with their respective processes. The best way to stabilize the condyles is with a screw passed transversely through the center of the axis of rotation in such a manner as to apply transverse compression. This stabilization method may require a small temporary secondary transverse pin proximal to the screw to prevent rotation of the fragments as the guide hole is drilled or when the compression screw is being applied. This pin can be removed after the fragments are secured.

Stabilization of the Supracondylar Columns. Once the condylar and articular integrity has been re-established, the distal fragments must be secured to the proximal fragment by stabilizing the supracondylar fragment columns. The decision here is how important it is to initiate early motion. In a younger child with rapid bony healing, pin fixation is often satisfactory; the pins can be removed in 3 weeks to start protected motion. In an older adolescent nearer to skeletal maturity, we prefer fixation—usually plates or screws—that allows early motion (Figs. 15-72E,F and 15-73). Before applying the plates, the su-

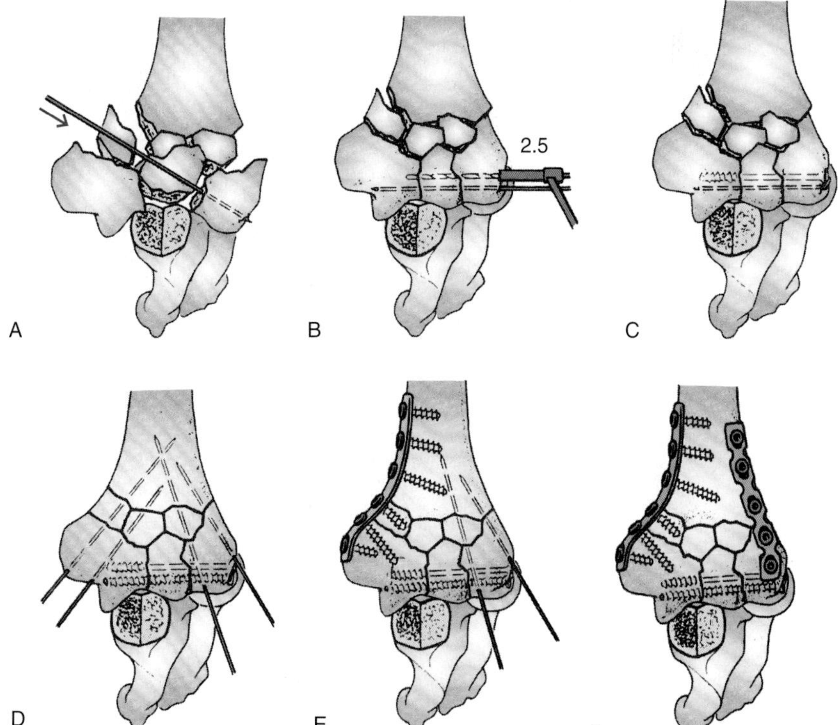

FIGURE 15-72 Sequence of distal humerus reconstruction. **A–C.** First, the articular portions are reassembled with provisional K-wire fixation, followed by screw fixation. **D.** K-wires can then also be used to provide temporary fixation of the distal humerus. **E.** A one-third tubular plate is attached to the medial side. **F.** A 3.5 pelvic reconstruction plate was attached to the posterolateral border. (From Heim U, Pfeiffer KM. *Internal fixation of small fractures,* 3rd ed. Berlin: Springer-Verlag, 1988; with permission.)

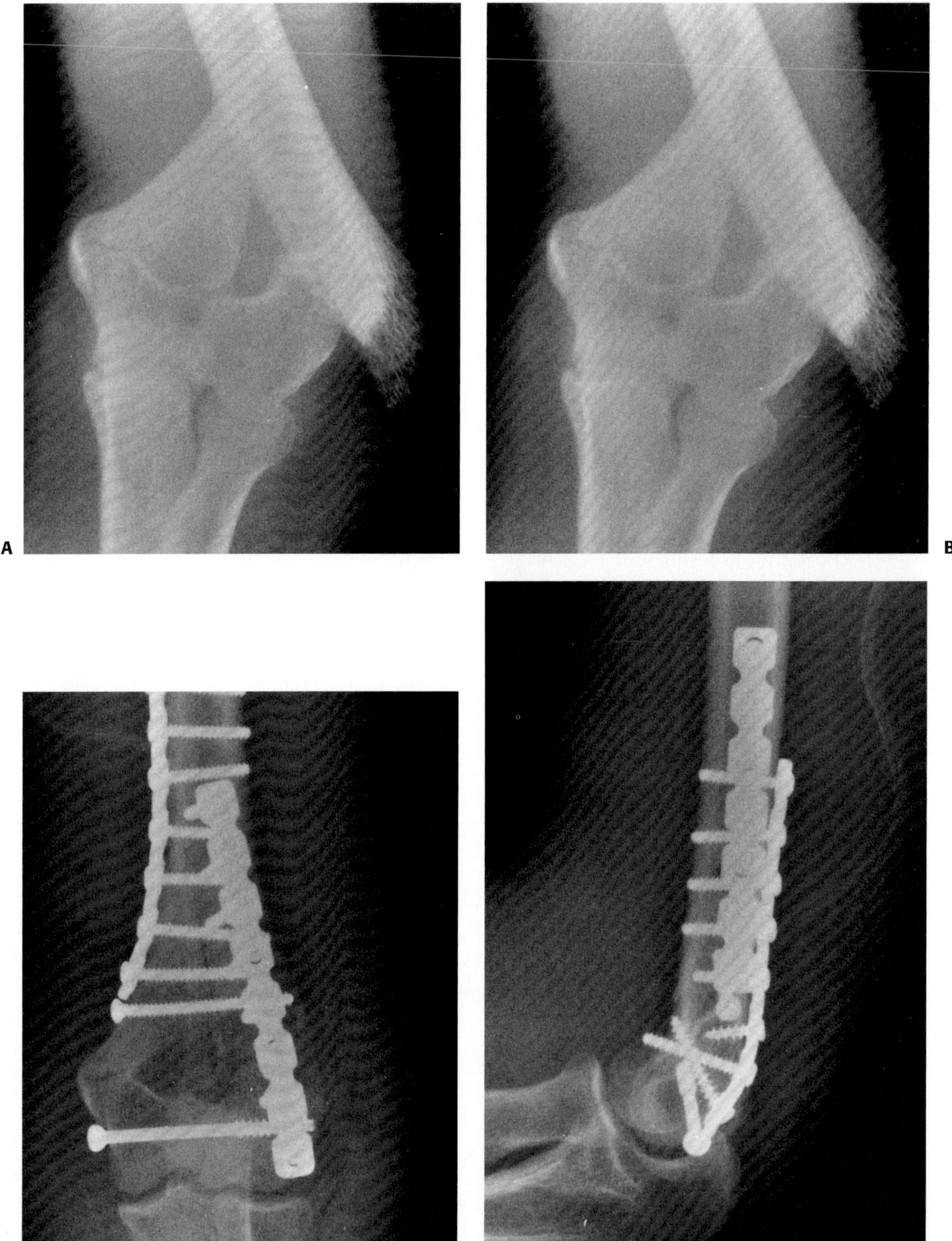

FIGURE 15-73 T. condylar numeral fractures with plate and screw fixation. **A,B.** Injury films of a type II flexion pattern in a 16-year-old boy. **C,D.** Articular integrity was first restored with a transcondylar compression screw. The condyles were secured to the metaphysis and distal shaft using pelvic reconstruction plates placed at 90 degrees to each other.

pracondylar columns can be stabilized temporarily with pin fixation (Fig. 15-73D).

Principles of Plate Fixation. The plates must be strong; thin semitubular plates are inadequate and may break (199). The reinforced malleable reconstructive type of plates used for fixation of pelvic fractures provide very secure fixation. A J-type of plate can also provide rigid fixation when used to stabilize the lateral column (200). It is best to place the plates at 90 degrees to each other, which provides for a more stable construct (201–203).

In most adolescents, this is essentially an adult type of fracture pattern. The reader is therefore referred to *Fractures in Adults* for a more detailed description of the various techniques used in treating adults with this type of fracture.

Postoperative Care

If plate fixation is used, we place the extremity in a supporting posterior splint for 5 to 7 days to allow the soft tissue swelling to decrease and the incisions to heal. At this time, active flexion and extension are initiated and the arm is protected with a removable cast brace.

Type III (Displaced With Comminution)

Limited Open Reduction Followed by Traction. Sometimes the supracondylar columns are too fragmented to allow adequate fixation. In such cases, we have found that in children the best initial treatment method involves re-establishing the articular surface and joint congruity with a limited open reduction. The separated condyles are secured with a transverse screw providing compression through the axis of rotation. This procedure can usually be done with minimal soft tissue dissection. Once this is stabilized, the supracondylar columns are then re-established by placing the extremity in olecranon traction and allowing them to reconstitute with callus formation. Traction must be maintained until there appears to be good osseous tissue formed in the supracondylar areas. While in traction, motion can be initiated. This technique can also be used in patients seen late with contaminated soft tissue abrasions or severe soft tissue problems. In selected patients, such as an adolescent with severe bone loss, plating followed by bone grafting may be indicated.

Complications

It is important to emphasize to the parents initially that this is a serious fracture. Because of the considerable soft tissue injury and the involvement of the articular surface of the distal humerus, stiffness and loss of motion of the elbow can be expected regardless of the treatment mode (189,191,192). In adolescents, failure to provide solid internal fixation that facilitates early motion (i.e., using only pin fixation) can result in a satisfactory x-ray appearance but considerable dysfunction due to residual loss of elbow motion.

Although neurovascular complications have not been mentioned in the few cases reported in the literature, the incidence is probably about equal to that of supracondylar fractures. Because these fractures occur late in the growth process, partial or total growth arrest due to internal fixation is not thought to be a major complication. Likewise, because these are older children, little remodeling can be expected. Nonunion (190), osteonecrosis of the trochlea (191), and failure of internal fixation have also been reported as complications.

REFERENCES

1. Peterson CA, Peterson HA. Analysis of the incidence of injuries to the epiphyseal growth plate. *J Trauma* 1972;12:273–279.
2. Fowles JV, Kassab MT. Displaced fracture of medial humeral condyle in children. *J Bone Joint Surg* 1980;62:1159–1163.
3. Hardacre JA, Nahigian SH, Froimson AI, et al. Fracture of the lateral condyle of humerus in children. *J Bone Joint Surg* 1971;53:1983–2095.
4. Houshian S, Mehdi B, Larsen MS. The epidemiology of elbow fracture in children: analysis of 355 fractures, with special reference to supracondylar humerus fractures. *J Orthop Sci* 2001;6:312–315.
5. Landin LA, Danielsson LG. Elbow fractures in children. An epidemiological analysis of 589 cases. *Acta Orthop Scand* 1986;57:309–312.
6. DeLee JC, Wilkins KE, Rogers LF, et al. Fracture separation of the distal humeral epiphysis. *J Bone Joint Surg* 1980;67:46–51.
7. Moucha CS, Mason DE. Distal humeral epiphyseal separation. *Am J Orthop* 2003;32: 497–500.
8. Griffith JF, Roebuck DJ, Cheng JC, et al. Acute elbow trauma in children: spectrum of injury revealed by MR imaging not apparent on radiographs. *Am J Roentgenol* 2001; 176:53–50.
9. Herring JA. Lateral condylar fracture of the elbow. *J Pediatr Orthop* 1986;6:724–727.
10. Menkowitz M, Flynn JM. Floating elbow in an infant. *Orthopedics* 2002;25:185–186.
11. Ippolito E, Tudisco C, Farsetti P, et al. Fracture of the humeral condyles in children: 49 cases evaluated after 18–45 years. *Acta Orthop Scand* 1996;67:173–178.
12. Smith FM. An 84-year follow-up on a patient with ununited fracture of the lateral condyle of humerus. *J Bone Joint Surg* 1973;55:378–380.
13. Stans AA, Maritz NG, O'Driscoll SW, Morrey BF. Operative treatment of elbow contracture in patients twenty-one years of age or younger. *J Bone Joint Surg (Am)* 2002; 84A:382–387.
14. Milch H. Fractures and fracture dislocations of humeral condyles. *J Trauma* 1964;4: 592–607.
15. Cotton FJ. Elbow fractures in children. *Ann Surg* 1902;35:75–104.
16. Salter RB, Harris WR. Injuries involving the epiphyseal plate. *J Bone Joint Surg* 1963; 45:587–632.
17. Mirsky EC, Karas EH, Weiner LS. Lateral condyle fractures in children: evaluation of classification and treatment. *J Orthop Trauma* 1997;11:117–120.
18. Jakob R, Fowles JV. Observations concerning fractures of the lateral humeral condyles in children. *J Bone Joint Surg* 1975;40:430–436.
19. Wadsworth TG. Premature epiphyseal fusion after injury of capitulum. *J Bone Joint Surg* 1964;46:46–49.
20. Badelon O, Bensahel H, Mazda K, et al. Lateral humeral condylar fractures in children: a report of 47 cases. J Pediatr Orthop 1988;8:31–34.
21. Major NM, Crawford ST. Elbow effusions in trauma in adults and children: is there an occult fracture? *Am J Roentgenol* 2002;178:413–418.
22. Petit P, Sapin C, Henry G, et al. Rate of abnormal osteoarticular radiographic findings in pediatric patients. *Am J Roentgenol* 2001;176:987–990.
23. Horn BD, Herman MJ, Crisci K, et al. Fractures of the lateral humeral condyle: role of the cartilage hinge in fracture stability. *J Pediatr Orthop* 2002;22:8–11.
24. Wilson PD. Fracture of the lateral condyle of humerus in children. *J Bone Joint Surg* 1936;18:299–316.
25. Conner A, Smith MGH. Displaced fracture of lateral humeral condyle in children. *J Bone Joint Surg* 1970;52:460–464.
26. Rovinsky D, Ferguson C, Younis A, et al. Pediatric elbow dislocations associated with a Milch type I lateral condyle fracture of the humerus. *J Orthop Trauma* 1999;13: 458–460.
27. Heyl JH. Fractures of the external condyle of the humerus in children. *Ann Surg* 1935; 101:1069–1077.
28. Stimson LA. *A practical treatise on fractures and dislocations*. Philadelphia: Lea Brothers & Co., 1900.
29. Finnbogason T, Karlsson G, Lindberg L, et al. Nondisplaced and minimally displaced fractures of the lateral humeral condyle in children: a prospective radiographic investigation of fracture stability. *J Pediatr Orthop* 1995;15:422–425.
30. Kamegaya M, Shinohara Y, Kurokawa M, et al. Assessment of stability in children's minimally displaced lateral humeral condyle fracture by magnetic resonance imaging. *J Pediatr Orthop* 1999;19:570–572.

31. Potter HG. Imaging of posttraumatic and soft tissue dysfunction of the elbow. *Clin Orthop* 2000;370:9–18.
32. Speed JS, Macey HB. Fracture of humeral condyles in children. *J Bone Joint Surg* 1933; 15:903–919.
33. Bast SC, Hoffer MM, Aval S. Nonoperative treatment for minimally and nondisplaced lateral humeral condyle fractures in children. *J Pediatr Orthop* 1998;18:448–450.
34. Beaty JH, Wood AB. Fractures of the lateral humeral condyle in children. Presented at the Annual Meeting of the American Academy of Orthopedic Surgeons, Las Vegas, 1985.
35. Böhler L. *The treatment of fractures*, vol. 1. New York: Grune & Strattion, 1956.
36. Mintzer CM, Water PM, Brown DJ, et al. Percutaneous pinning in the treatment of displaced lateral condyle fractures. *J Pediatr Orthop* 1994;14:462–465.
37. Blount WP, Schalz I, Cassidy RH. Fractures of the elbow in children. *JAMA* 1951;146: 699–704.
38. Editorial. Fractures of the lateral condyle of the humerus in children. *Injury* 1985;16: 363.
39. Hardacre JA, Nahigian SH, Froimson AI, et al. Fractures of the lateral condyle of the humerus in children. *J Bone Joint Surg* 1971;53:1083–1095.
40. Jeffrey CC. Nonunion of epiphysis of the lateral condyle of the humerus. *J Bone Joint Surg* 1958;40:396–405.
41. McDonnell DP, Wilson JC. Fracture of the lower end of the humerus in children. *J Bone Joint Surg* 1948;30:347–358.
42. Morin B, Fassier F, Poitras B, et al. Resultats du traitement chirurgical precoce des fractures du condyle humeral externe chez l'enfant. *Rev Chir Orthop* 1988;74:129–131.
43. Smith FM, Joyce JJ. Fracture of lateral condyle of humerus in children. *Am J Surg* 1954; 87:322–329.
44. Wilson JN. Fracture of external condyle of humerus in children. *Br J Surg* 1936;18: 299–316.
45. Zeir FG. Lateral condylar fracture and its many complications. *Orthop Rev* 1981;10: 49–55.
46. Launay F, Leet AI, Jacopin S, et al. Lateral humeral condyle fractures in children: a comparison of two approaches to treatment. *J Pediatr Orthop* 2004;24:385–391.
47. Fontanetta P, Mackenzie DA, Rosman M. Missed, maluniting, and malunited fractures of the lateral humeral condyle in children. *J Trauma* 1978;18:329–335.
48. Yuan Zhang M, Chun Bo Z, Tai Len Z, et al. Percutaneous probe reduction of frontal fractures of the humeral capitellum. *Clin Orthop* 1984;183:17–21.
49. Fahey JJ, O'Brien E. Fracture-separation of the medial humeral condyle in a child confused with fracture of the medial epicondyle. *J Bone Joint Surg (Am)* 1971;53: 1102–1104.
50. Sharma JC, Arora A, Mathur NC, et al. Lateral condylar fractures of the humerus in children: fixation with partially threaded 4.0 mm AO cancellous screws. *J Trauma* 1995;39:1129–1133.
51. Mohan N, Hunter JB, Colton CL. The posterolateral approach to the distal humerus for open reduction and internal fixation of fractures of the lateral condyle in children. *J Bone Joint Surg (Br)* 2000;82:643–645.
52. Flynn JC, Richards JF. Non union of minimally displaced fractures of the lateral condyle of humerus in children. *J Bone Joint Surg (Am)* 1971;53:1096–1101.
53. Haraldsson S. On osteochondrosis deformans juvenilis capituli humeri including investigation of intra osseous vasculature in distal humerus. *Acta Orthop Scand* 1959;(Suppl): 38.
54. Dhillon KS, Sengupta S, Singh BJ. Delayed management of fracture of the lateral humeral condyle in children. *Acta Orthop Scand* 1988;59:419–424.
55. Zionts LE, Stolz MR. Late fracture of the lateral condyle of the humerus. *Orthopedics* 1984;7:541–545.
56. Cooper AP. *A treatise on dislocations and fractures of the joints*. Boston: Lilly, Wait, Carter, and Hendee, 1932.
57. Flynn JC, Richards JF, Saltzman RI. Prevention and treatment of non union of slightly displaced fractures of the lateral humeral condyle in children. *J Bone Joint Surg (Am)* 1975;57:1087–1092.
58. Papandrea R, Waters PM. Posttraumatic reconstruction of the elbow in the pediatric patient. *Clin Orthop* 2000;370:115–126.
59. Shimada K, Masada K, Tada K, et al. Osteosynthesis for the treatment of non union of the lateral humeral condyle in children. *J Bone Joint Surg (Am)* 1997;79:232–238.
60. Masada K, Kawai H, Kawabata H, et al. Osteosynthesis for old, established non union of the lateral condyle of the humerus. *J Bone Joint Surg (Am)* 1990;72:32–40.
61. Foster DE, Sullivan JA, Gross RH. Lateral humeral condylar fractures in children. *J Pediatr Orthop* 1985;5:16–22.
62. Morrissy RT, Wilkins KE. Deformity following distal humeral fracture in childhood. *J Bone Joint Surg (Am)* 1984;66:557–562.
63. Rutherford AJ. Fractures of the lateral humeral condyle in children. *J Bone Joint Surg (Am)* 1985;67:851–856.
64. So YC, Fang D, Orth MC, et al. Varus deformity following lateral humeral condylar fracture in children. *J Pediatr Orthop* 1985;5:569–572.
65. Van Vugt AB, Severijnen RVSM, Festern C. Fractures of the lateral humeral condyle in children: late results. *Arch Orthop Trauma Surg* 1988;107:206–209.
66. Skak SV, Olsen SD, Smaabrekke A. Deformity after fracture of the lateral humeral condyle in children. *J Pediatr Orthop B* 2001;10:142–152.
67. Davids JR, Maguire MF, Mubarak SJ, et al. Lateral condylar fracture of the humerus following posttraumatic cubitus varus. *J Pediatr Orthop* 1994;14:466–470.
68. Nwakama AC, Peterson HA, Shaughnessy WJ. Fishtail deformity following fracture of the distal humerus in children: historical review, case presentations, discussion of etiology, and thoughts on treatment. *J Pediatr Orthop B* 2000;9:309–318.
69. Kim HT, Song MB, Conjares JN, Yoo CI. Trochlear deformity occurring after distal humeral fractures: magnetic resonance imagines and its natural progression. *J Pediatr Orthop* 2002;22:188–193.
70. Friedman RJ, Smith RJ. Radial nerve laceration twenty six years after screw fixation of a humeral fracture. *J Bone Joint Surg (Am)* 1984;66:959–960.
71. Gay JR, Love JG. Diagnosis and treatment of tardy paralysis of the ulnar nerve. *J Bone Joint Surg* 1947;29:1087–1097.
72. Papavasiliou VA, Beslikas TA. Fractures of the lateral humeral condyle in children: an analysis of 39 cases. *Injury* 1985;16:364–366.
73. Ravessoud FA. Lateral condylar fracture and ipsilateral ulnar shaft fracture: monteggia equivalent lesions? *J Pediatr Orthop* 1985;5:364–366.
74. Marion J, Faysse R. Fracture du capitellum. *Rev Chir Orthop* 1962;48:484–490.
75. Fowles JV, Kassab MT. Fracture of the capitulum humeri, treatment by excision. *J Bone Joint Surg (Am)* 1974;56:794.
76. Johansson J, Rosman M. Fracture of the capitulum humeri in children: a rare injury, often misdiagnosed. *Clin Orthop* 1980;146:157–160.
77. Palmer I. Open treatment of transcondylar T fracture of the humerus. *Acta Chir Scand* 1961;121:486–490.
78. Agins HJ, Marcus NW. Articular cartilage sleeve fracture of the lateral humeral condyle capitellum: a previously undescribed entity. *J Pediatr Orthop* 1984;4:620–622.
79. Drvaric DM, Rooks MD. Anterior sleeve fracture of the capitellum. *J Orthop Trauma* 1990;4:188–192.
80. Steinthal D. Die Isolirte Fraktur der Eminentia Capitata im Ellenbogengelenk. *Zentralbl F Chir* 1898;15:17–20.
81. Letts M, Rumball K, Bauermeister S, et al. Fractures of the capitellum in adolescents. *J Pediatr Orthop* 1997;17:313–318.
82. Elkowitz SJ, Kubiak EN, Polatsch D, et al. Comparison of two headless screw designs for fixation of capitellum fractures. *Bull Hosp Jt Dis* 2003;61:123–126.
83. Elkowitz SJ, Polatsch DB, Egol KA, et al. Capitellum fractures: a biomechanical evaluation of three fixation methods. *J Orthop Trauma* 2002;16:503–506.
84. DeLee JC, Wilkins KE, Rogers LF, et al. Fracture-separation of the distal humerus epiphysis. *J Bone Joint Surg* 1980;62:46–51.
85. Blount WP. *Fractures in children*. Baltimore: Williams & Wilkins, 1955.
86. Faysse R, Marion J. Fractures du condyle interne. *Rev Chir Orthop* 1962;48:473–477.
87. Ashurst APC. *An anatomical and surgical study of fractures of the lower end of the humerus*. Philadelphia: Lea & Febiger, 1910.
88. Papavasiliou V, Nenopoulos S, Venturis T. Fractures of the medial condyle of the humerus in childhood. *J Pediatr Orthop* 1987;7:421–423.
89. Chacha PB. Fractures of the medial condyle of the humerus with rotational displacement. *J Bone Joint Surg* 1970;52:1453–1458.
90. Cothay DM. Injury to the lower medial epiphysis of the humerus before development of the ossific centre. Report of a case. *J Bone Joint Surg (Br)* 1967;49:766–767.
91. El Ghawabi MH. Fracture of the medial condyle of the humerus. *J Bone Joint Surg (Am)* 1975;57:677–680.
92. Hanspal RS. Injury to the medial humeral condyle in a child reviewed after 18 years. Report of a case. *J Bone Joint Surg (Br)* 1985;67:638–639.
93. Potter CMC. Fracture-dislocation of the trochlea. *J Bone Joint Surg* 1954;36:248–251.
94. Varma BP, Srivastava TP. Fractures of the medial condyle of the humerus in children: a report of 4 cases including the late sequelae. *Injury* 1972;4:171–174.
95. Bensahel H, Csukonyi Z, Badelon O, et al. Fractures of the medial condyle of the humerus in children. *J Pediatr Orthop* 1986;6:430–433.
96. De Boeck H, Casteleyn PP, Opdecam P. Fracture of the medial humeral condyle. *J Bone Joint Surg (Am)* 1987;69:1442–1444.
97. Harrison RB, Keats TE, Frankel CJ, et al. Radiographic clues to fractures of the unossified medial humeral condyle in young children. *Skel Radiol* 1984;11:209–212.
98. Case SL, Hennrikus WL. Surgical treatment of displaced medial epicondyle fractures in adolescent athletes. *Am J Sports Med* 1997;25:682–686.
99. Fowles JV, Kassab MT. Displaced fractures of the medial humeral condyle in children. *J Bone Joint Surg* 1980;62:1159–1163.
100. Milch H. Fractures and fracture–dislocations of humeral condyles. *J Trauma* 1964;4: 592–607.
101. Kilfoyle RM. Fractures of the medial condyle and epicondyle of the elbow in children. *Clin Orthop* 1965;4143–4150.
102. Saraf SK, Tuli SM. Concomitant medial condyle fracture of the humerus in a childhood posterolateral dislocation of the elbow. *J Orthop Trauma* 1989;3:352–354.
103. Lee HH, Shen HC, Chang JH, et al. Operative treatment of displaced medial epicondyle fractures in children and adolescents. *J Shoulder Elbow Surg* 2005;14:178–185.
104. Skaggs DL, Mirzayan R. The posterior fat pad sign in association with occult fracture of the elbow in children. *J Bone Joint Surg (Am)* 1999;81:1429–1433.
105. Pimpalnerkar AL, Balasubramaniam G, Young SK, et al. Type four fractures of the medial epicondyle: a true indication for surgical intervention. *Injury* 1998;29:751–756.
106. Leet AI, Young C, Hoffer MM. Medial condyle fractures of the humerus in children. *J Pediatr Orthop* 2002;22:2–7.
107. Grant IR, Miller JH. Osteochondral fracture of the trochlea associated with fracture-dislocation of the elbow. *Injury* 1975;6:255–258.
108. Kaplan SS, Reckling FW. Fracture separation of lower humeral epiphysis with medial displacement. *J Bone Joint Surg* 1971;53:1105–1108.
109. Rogers LF, Rockwood CA. Separation of entire distal humeral epiphysis. *Radiology* 1973;106:393–399.
110. Siffert RS. Displacement of distal humeral epiphysis in newborn infant. *J Bone Joint Surg* 1963;45:165–169.
111. Sutherland DH. Displacement of the entire distal humeral epiphysis. *J Bone Joint Surg* 1974;56:206.
112. Akbarnia BA, Silberstein MJ, Rende RJ, et al. Arthrography in the diagnosis of fractures of the distal end of the humerus in infants. *J Bone Joint Surg (Am)* 1986;68:599–602.

113. de Jager LT, Hoffman EB. Fracture-separation of the distal humeral epiphysis. *J Bone Joint Surg (Br)* 1991;73B:143–146.
114. Holda ME, Manoli A, LaMont RL. Epiphyseal separation of the distal end of the humerus with medial displacement. *J Bone Joint Surg* 1980;62:52–57.
115. McIntyre WM, Wiley JJ, Charette RJ. Fracture–separation of the distal humeral epiphysis. *Clin Orthop* 1984;188:98–102.
116. Mizuno K, Hirohata K, Kashiwagi D. Fracture–separation of distal humeral epiphysis in young children. *J Bone Joint Surg* 1979;61:570–573.
117. Peiro A, Mut T, Aracil J, et al. Fracture–separation of the lower humeral epiphysis in young children. *Acta Orthop Scand* 1981;52:293–296.
118. Abe M, Ishizu T, Nagaoka T, et al. Epiphyseal separation of the distal end of the humeral epiphysis: a follow up note. *J Pediatr Orthop* 1995;15:426–434.
119. Dameron TB. Transverse fractures of distal humerus in children. *Instr Course Lect* 1981; 30:222–233.
120. Barrett WP, Almquist EA, Staheli LT. Fracture separation of the distal humeral physis in the newborn. *J Pediatr Orthop* 1984;4:617–619.
121. Berman JM, Weiner DS. Neonatal fracture separation of the distal humeral chondroepiphysis: a case report. *Orthopedics* 1980;3:875–879.
122. Downs DM, Wirth CR. Fracture of the distal humeral chondroepiphysis in the neonate. A case report. *Clin Orthop* 1982;169:155–158.
123. Willems B, Stuyck J, Hoogmartens M, et al. Fracture–separation of the distal humeral epiphysis. *Acta Orthop Belg* 1987;53:109–111.
124. Bright RW. Epiphyseal-plate cartilage. A biomechanical and histological analysis of failure modes. *J Bone Joint Surg (Am)* 1974;56:688–703.
125. Stricker SJ, Thomson JD, Kelly RA. Coronal plane transcondylar fracture of the humerus in a child. *Clin Orthop* 1993;292:306–309.
126. Poland J. *A practical treatise on traumatic separation of the epiphyses.* London: Smith, Elder & Co., 1898.
127. Hansen PE, Barnes DA, Tullos HS. Case report—arthrographic diagnosis of an injury pattern in the distal humerus of an infant. *J Pediatr Orthop* 1982;2:569–572.
128. Dias JJ, Lamont AC, Jones JM. Ultrasonic diagnosis of neonatal separation of the distal humeral epiphysis. *J Bone Joint Surg (Br)* 1988;70:825–828.
129. Yoo CI, Suh JT, Suh KT, et al. Avascular necrosis after fracture–separation of the distal end of the humerus in children. *Orthopedics* 1992;15:959–963.
130. Walker HB. A case of dislocation of the elbow with separation of the internal epicondyle and displacement of the latter into the joint. *Br J Surg* 1928;15:667–679.
131. Josefsson PO, Danielsson LG. Epicondylar elbow fracture in children: 35 year follow up of 56 unreduced cases. *Acta Orthop Scand* 1986;57:311–313.
132. Papavasilou VA. Fracture–separation of the medial epicondylar epiphysis of the elbow joint. *Clin Orthop* 1982;171:172–174.
133. Wilson NIL, Ingran R, Rymaszewski L, et al. Treatment of fractures of the medial epicondyle of the humerus. *Injury* 1988;19:342–344.
134. Hines RF, Herndon WA, Evans JP. Operative treatment of medial epicondyle fractures in children. *Clin Orthop* 1987;221:170–174.
135. Lokiec F, Velkes S, Engel J. Avulsion of the medial epicondyle of the humerus in arm wrestlers: a report of five cases and a review of the literature. *Injury* 1991;22:69–70.
136. Low BY, Lim J. Fracture of humerus during arm wrestling: report of 5 cases. *Singapore Med J* 1991;32:47–49.
137. Nyska M, Peiser J, Lukiec F, et al. Avulsion fracture of the medial epicondyle caused by arm wrestling. *Am J Sports Med* 1992;20:347–350.
138. Bede WB, Lefebure AR, Rosmon MA. Fractures of the medial humeral epicondyle in children. *Can J Surg* 1975;18:137–142.
139. Bernstein SM, King JD, Sanderson RA. Fractures of the medial epicondyle of the humerus. *Contemp Orthop* 1981;637–641.
140. Chessare JW, Rogers LF, Whihte H, et al. Injuries of the medial epicondyl ossification center of the humerus. *Am J Roentgenol* 1977;129:49–55.
141. Fowles JV, Slimane N, Kassab MT. Elbow dislocation with avulsion of the medial humeral epicondyle. *J Bone Joint Surg (Br)* 1990;72B:102–104.
142. Kilfoyle RM. Fracture of the medial condyle and epicondyle of the elbow in children. *Clin Orthop* 1965;41:43–50.
143. Smith FM. Medial epicondyle injuries. *JAMA* 1950;142:396–402.
144. Murakami Y, Komiyama Y. Hypoplasia of the trochlea and the medial epicondyle of the humerus associated with ulnar neuropathy—report of two cases. *J Bone Joint Surg (Br)* 1978;60:223–225.
145. Marion J, Faysse R. Fractures de l'epitrochlea. *Rev Chir Orthop* 1962;48:447–469.
146. Frances R, Bunch T, Chandler B. Little league elbow: a decade later. *Phys Sports Med* 1978;88–94.
147. Rosendahl B. Displacement of the medial epicondyle into the elbow joint: the final result in a case where the fragment has not been removed. *Acta Orthop Scand* 1959; 28:212–219.
148. Fairbank HAT, Buxton JD. Displacement of the internal epicondyle into the elbow joint. *Lancet* 1934;2:218.
149. Silberstein JJ, Brodeur AE, Graviss ER, et al. Some vagaries of the medial epicondyle. *J Bone Joint Surg* 1981;63:524–528.
150. Woods GM, Tullos HB. Elbow stability and medial epicondyle fracture. *Am J Sports Med* 1977;5:23–30.
151. Watson-Jones R. Primary nerve lesions in injuries of the elbow and wrist. *J Bone Joint Surg* 1930;12:121–140.
152. Patrick J. Fracture of the medial epicondyle with displacement into the elbow joint. *J Bone Joint Surg* 1946;28:143–147.
153. Harrison RB, Keats TE, Frankel CJ, et al. Radiographic clues to fractures of the unossified medial humeral condyle in young children. *Skel Radiol* 1984;11:209–212.
154. Albright JA, Jokl P, Shaw R, Albright JP. Clinical studies of baseball players: correlation of injury to throwing arm with method of delivery. *Am J Sports Med* 1978;6:15–21.
155. Schwab GH, Bennett JB, Woods GW, et al. Biomechanics of elbow instability: the role of the medial collateral ligament. *Clin Orthop* 1980;146:42–52.
156. Roberts NW. Displacement of the internal epicondyle into the joint. *Lancet* 1934;2: 78–79.
157. Fowles JV, Kassab MT, Moula T. Untreated intra articular entrapment of the medial humeral epicondyle. *J Bone Joint Surg (Br)* 1984;60:562–565.
158. Dias JJ, Johnson GV, Hoskinson J, et al. Management of severely displaced medial epicondyle fractures. *J Orthop Trauma* 1987;1:59–62.
159. Tayob AA, Shively RA. Bilateral elbow dislocations with intra articular displacement of medial epicondyles. *J Trauma* 1980;20:332–335.
160. Silberstein JJ, Brodeur AE, Graviss ER. Some vagaries of the lateral epicondyle. *J Bone Joint Surg (Am)* 1982;64:444–448.
161. Hasner E, Husby J. Fracture of the epicondyle and condyle of the humerus. *Acta Chir Scand* 1951;101:195–205.
162. McLeod GG, Gray AJ, Turner MD. Elbow dislocation with intra articular entrapment of the lateral epicondyle. *J R Coll Surg Edinb* 1993;38:112–113.
163. Fowles JV, Kassab MT. Displaced fracture of the medial humeral condyle in children. *J Bone Joint Surg* 1980;62:1159–1163.
164. Zionts LE, Moon CN. Olecranon apophysis fractures in children with osteogenesis imperfecta revisited. *J Pediatr Orthop* 2002;22:745–750.
165. Bracq H. Fractures of the olecranon. *Rev Chir Orthop* 1987;73:469–471.
166. DiCesare PE, Sew-Hoy A, Krom W. Bilateral isolated fractures in an infant as presentation of osteogenesis imperfecta. *Orthopedics* 1992;15:741–743.
167. Gwynne-Jones DP. Displaced olecranon apophyseal fractures in children with osteogenesis imperfecta. *J Pediatr Orthop* 2005;25:154–157.
168. Kocher MS, Shapiro F. Osteogenesis imperfecta. *J Am Acad Orthop Surg* 1998;6: 225–236.
169. Stott NS, Zionts LE. Displaced fractures of the apophysis of the olecranon in children who have osteogenesis imperfecta. *J Bone Joint Surg (Am)* 1993;75:1026–1033.
170. Fabry J, De Smet L, Fabry G. Consequences of a fracture through a minimally ossified apophysis of the olecranon. *J Pediatr Orthop B* 2000;9:212–214.
171. Mudgal CS. Olecranon fracture in osteogenesis imperfecta: a case report. *Acta Orthop Belg* 1992;58:453–456.
172. Brogdon BJ, Crow NE. Little leaguer's elbow. *Am J Roentgenol* 1960;83:671–675.
173. Adams JE. Injury to the throwing arm. *Calif Med* 1965;102:127–132.
174. Beyer WF, Heppt P, Gluckert K, et al. Aseptic osteonecrosis of the humeral trochlea (Hegemann's disease). *Arch Orthop Trauma Surg* 1990;110:45–48.
175. Jakob R, Fowles JV, Rang M, et al. Observations concerning fractures of the lateral humeral condyle in children. *J Bone Joint Surg* 1975;57:430–436.
176. McDonnell DP, Wilson JC. Fractures of the lower end of the humerus in children. *J Bone Joint Surg* 1948;30:347–358.
177. Mead CA, Martin M. Aplasia of the trochlea—an original mutation. *J Bone Joint Surg (Am)* 1963;45:379–383.
178. Morrissey TT, Wilkins KE. Deformity following distal humeral fracture in childhood. *J Bone Joint Surg (Am)* 1984;66A:557–562.
179. Yoo CI, Kim YJ, Suh JT, et al. Orthopedic surgery in Korea. Avascular necrosis after fracture separation of the distal end of the humerus in children. *Orthopaedics* 1992; 15:959–963.
180. Toniolo RM, Wilkins KE. Avascular necrosis of the trochlea. Scientific Presentation at the 15th Annual Meeting of European Orthopaedic Society, April 13, 1996, Prague, Czech Republic.
181. Haraldsson S. The interosseous vasculature of the distal end of the humerus with special reference to capitulum. *Acta Orthop Scand* 1957;27:81–93.
182. Haraldsson S. Osteochondrosis deformans juvenilis capituli humeri including investigation of intraosseous vasculature in distal humerus. *Acta Orthop Scand* 1959;38(Suppl).
183. Varma BP, Srivastava TP. Fractures of the medial condyle of the humerus in children: a report of 4 cases including the late sequelae. *Injury* 1972;4:171–174.
184. Minami A, Sugawara J. Humeral trochlear hypoplasia secondary to epiphyseal injuries as a cause of ulnar nerve palsy. *Clin Orthop* 1988;221:225–230.
185. Royle SG, Burke D. Ulna neuropathy after elbow injury in children. *J Pediatr Orthop* 1990;10:495–496.
186. Tanabu S, Yamauchi T, Fukushima M. Hypoplasia of the trochlea of the humerus as a cause of ulnar nerve palsy. Report of two cases. *J Bone Joint Surg (Am)* 1985;67: 151–154.
187. Yngve DA. Distal humeral epiphyseal separation. *Orthopaedics* 1985;8:102.
188. Zimmerman H. Fractures of the elbow. In: Weber BG, Brunner C, Freuler F, eds. *Treatment of fractures in children and adolescents.* New York: Springer-Verlag, 1980.
189. Jarvis JG, D'Astous JL. The pediatric T supracondylar fracture. *J Pediatr Orthop* 1984; 4:697–699.
190. Kasser JR, Richards K, Millis M. The triceps dividing approach to open reduction of complex distal humerus fractures in adolescents: a cybex evaluation of triceps function and motion. *J Pediatr Orthop* 1990;10:93–96.
191. Papvasilious VA, Beslikas TA. T condylar fractures of the distal humeral condyles during childhood: an analysis of six cases. *J Pediatr Orthop* 1986;6:300–303.
192. Maylahn DJ, Fahey JJ. Fracture of the elbow in children. *JAMA* 1958;166:220–226.
193. Riseborough EJ, Radin EL. Intercondylar T fracture of the humerus in the adult. A comparison of operative and nonoperative treatment in 29 cases. *J Bone Joint Surg (Am)* 1969;51A:130–141.
194. Toniolo RM, Wilkins KE. Part VI: T-condylar fractures. Fractures and dislocations of the elbow region. In: Rockwood CA Jr, Wilkins KE, Beaty JH, eds. *Fractures in children*, 4th ed. Philadelphia: Lippincott-Raven, 1996.

195. Beghin JL, Bucholz RW, Wenger DR. Intercondylar fractures of the humerus in young children. *J Bone Joint Surg (Am)* 1982;64A:1083–1086.
196. Kanellopoulos AD, Yiannakopoulos CK. Closed reduction and percutaneous stabilization of pediatric T-condylar fractures of the humerus. *J Pediatr Orthop* 2004;24:13–16.
197. Bryan RS, Morrey BF. Extensive posterior exposure of the elbow. A triceps sparing approach. *Clin Orthop* 1982;166:188–192.
198. Remia LF, Richards K, Waters PM. The Bryan-Morrey triceps-sparing approach to open reduction of T-condylar humeral fractures in adolescents: cybex evaluation of triceps function and elbow motion. *J Pediatr Orthop* 2004;24:615–619.
199. Wildburger R, Mahring M, Hofer HP. Supraintercondylar fractures of the distal humerus: results of internal fixation. Review of two consecutive series. *J Orthop Trauma* 1991;5:299–305.
200. Schemitsch EH, Tencer AF, Henley MB. Biomechanical evaluation of methods of internal fixation of the distal humerus. *J Orthop Trauma* 1994;8:468–475.
201. Helfet DL, Hotchkiss RN. Internal fixation of the humerus: a biomechanical comparison of methods. *J Orthop Trauma* 1990;4:258–262.
202. Kirk P, Goulet JA, Freiberg A, et al. A biomechanical evaluation of fixation methods for fractures of the distal humerus. *Orthop Trans* 1990;14:674.
203. Sanders RA, Raney EM, Pipkin S. Operative treatment of bicondylar intraarticular fractures of the distal humerus, original research. *Orthopedics* 1992;15:159–163.

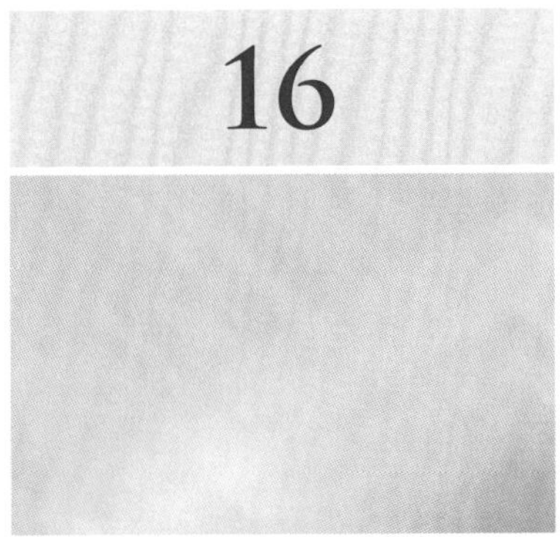

16

DISLOCATIONS OF THE ELBOW

Anthony A. Stans and Stephen D. Heinrich

Disruptions of the articular surfaces of the elbow represent a spectrum of injuries involving three separate articulations: the radiocapitellar, the ulnotrochlear, and the proximal radioulnar joints. Collectively they are common injuries, although the incidence of each subtype can vary widely.

SURGICAL AND APPLIED ANATOMY

Constraints about the elbow preventing dislocation can be considered either dynamic or static. Dynamic elbow stabilizers consist of elbow musculature, over which the patient has conscious control, and change depending on the degree of muscular contraction. Unlike the shoulder, dynamic stabilizers play a role of modest importance contributing to elbow stability. One indirect but important role of elbow musculature related to elbow stability is determining elbow position in space at the time of injury. In general, flexion and supination is a position of stability, while extension and pronation is a position of relative instability.

Static constraints can be further divided into osseous or ligamentous (Figs. 16-1, 16-2, and 16-3). The bone geometry of the

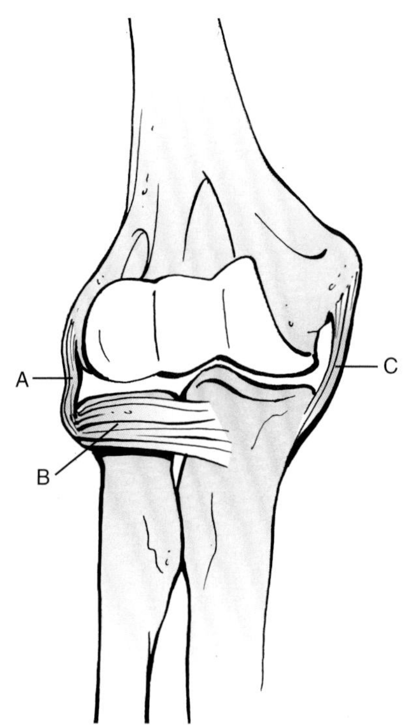

FIGURE 16-1 AP view of the elbow illustrates the bone and ligamentous structures that contribute to elbow stability. A, lateral collateral ligament; B, annular ligament; C, medial collateral ligament.

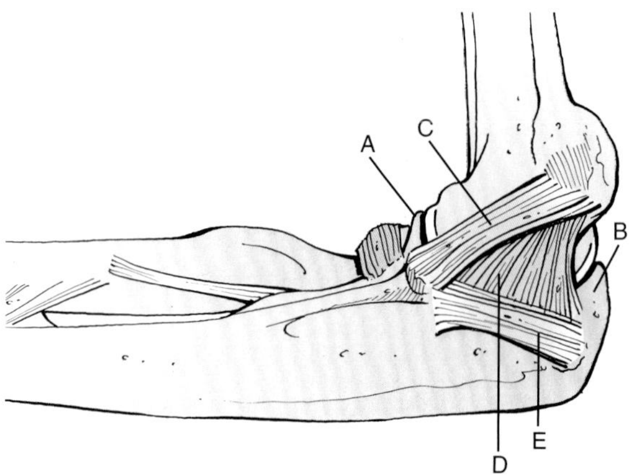

FIGURE 16-3 The medial elbow is stabilized by the hinge articulation between the proximal ulna and the humerus. Three components of the ulnar collateral ligament provide additional elbow stability. A, coronoid process; B, olecranon process; C, anterior oblique medial collateral ligament; D, posterior oblique medial collateral ligament; E, transverse medial collateral ligament.

elbow creates a relatively constrained hinge. The coronoid and olecranon form a semicircle of approximately 180 degrees into which the trochlea of the humerus securely articulates. The concave surface of the radial head matches the convex capitellum and provides stability to the lateral aspect of the elbow joint. The bone geometry of the medial and lateral aspects of the elbow complement each other, with the ulnohumeral articulation providing stability against medial/lateral or longitudinal translation and the radiocapitellar joint providing resistance to axial compression.

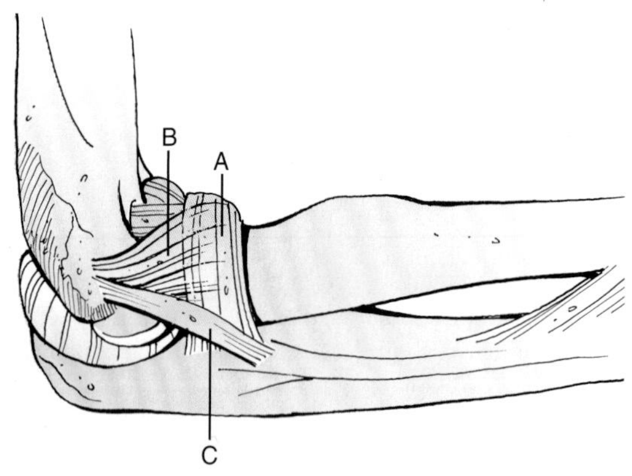

FIGURE 16-2 The annular ligament and lateral collateral ligament complex provides stability to the proximal radioulnar joint and radiocapitellar articulation. A, annular ligament; B, lateral collateral ligament insertion on annular ligament; C, lateral collateral ligament inserting on ulna.

Ligamentous constraints include the annular ligament, which encircles the radial neck and head, having its origin and insertion on the proximal ulna. Radial (lateral) collateral ligaments originate from the lateral epicondyle and insert into the annular ligament and the lateral aspect of the proximal ulna. The primary roles of the annular ligament and lateral collateral ligament complex are to provide stability to the proximal radiocapitellar and proximal radioulnar joints and to resist varus stress. The ulnar (medial) collateral ligament resists opening of the medial aspect of the elbow with valgus stress. Having its origin from the medial epicondyle, the medial collateral ligament has two primary components that contribute to elbow stability. The primary stabilizing segment courses from the medial epicondyle to the coronoid process. A fan-shaped posterior oblique ligament inserts on the olecranon and functions only in flexion. A small transverse ligament runs from olecranon to coronoid but has little functional importance.

CLASSIFICATION

Elbow dislocations are described by the relative position of the proximal radioulnar joint to the distal humerus: posterior, anterior, medial, or lateral. Posterior dislocations are further subdivided into posterolateral and posteromedial displacement.

Occasionally, the proximal radioulnar joint is disrupted. Most commonly, the radius and ulna diverge from each other in a mediolateral direction. Rarely, the radius and ulna translocate, with the radius medial and the ulna lateral.

Isolated dislocations of the radial head are uncommon and must be differentiated from congenital dislocations. Isolated dislocations of the proximal ulna are exceedingly rare and have not been reported in children.

Included in this chapter is a discussion of the commonly occurring subluxation of the radial head ("nursemaid's elbow"). This is not a true subluxation but rather a partial entrapment of the annular ligament in the radiocapitellar joint.

POSTERIOR ELBOW DISLOCATIONS

Principles of Management

Dislocations of the elbow joint are not common in children. Henrikson (1) studied 1,579 injuries about the elbow in skeletally immature patients in Gothenburg, Sweden, in 1966 and found only 45 dislocations, for an overall incidence of 3%. While the peak incidence of supracondylar fractures was in the first decade of life, pediatric elbow dislocations typically occurred in the second decade, usually between 13 and 14 years of age, when the physes begin to close. The same second-decade peak incidence was reported by Josefsson and Nilsson (2) in 1986. In their series, most elbow dislocations occurred in conjunction with sports activities.

Four series (3–6) have published data on elbow dislocations in both adults and children. There were 317 dislocations reported in the four series. One hundred fifty-seven occurred in children. All of these were posterior (posterior, posterolateral, or posteromedial) except for 10 lateral dislocations, 5 anterior dislocations, and 16 unclassified. Male gender and the left elbow were predominantly involved, and there was a high incidence of associated distal humerus, proximal radial, and proximal ulna fractures.

Carlioz and Abols (7) reported 58 elbow dislocations in children and adolescents, all posterior. The mean age at dislocation was 12 years (range 6 to 15 years). There were 41 boys (71%) and 35 left elbows (60%). Associated elbow fractures occurred in 37 children (64%).

Mechanism of Injury

The first stage in a posterior or posterolateral dislocation is a disruption of the ulnar collateral ligaments. This produces valgus instability. The force applied to the medial aspect of the elbow can produce an avulsion fracture of the medial epicondyle with its associated flexor muscle group. The proximal radius and ulna displace laterally, with the intact biceps tendon acting as the center of rotation for the displaced forearm (Fig. 16-4).

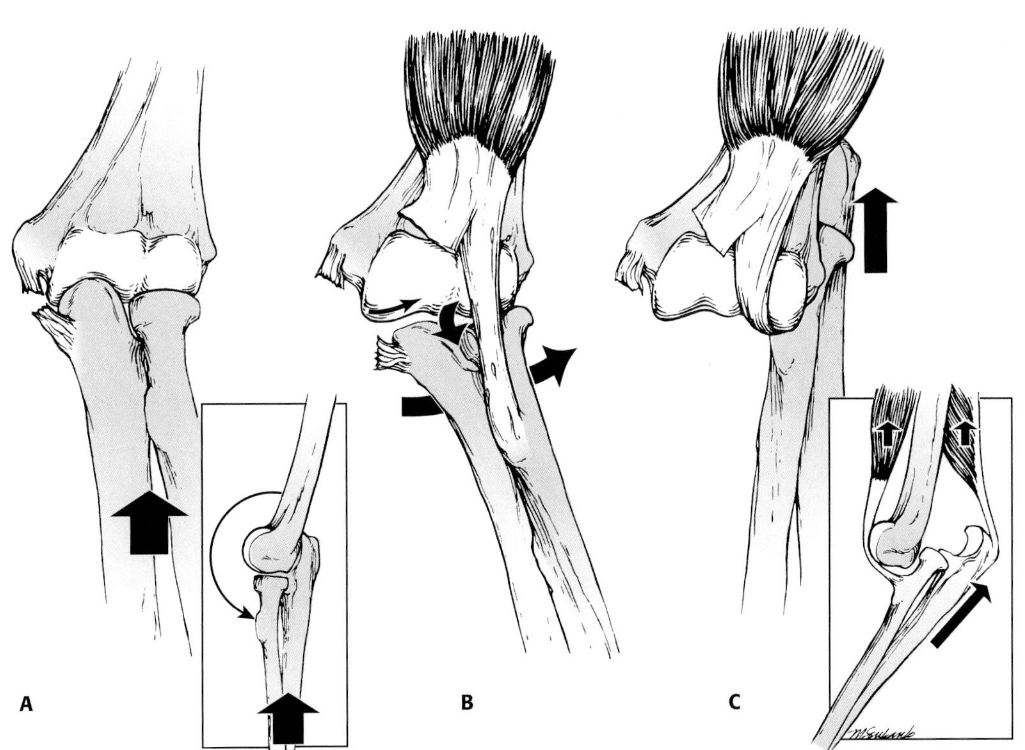

FIGURE 16-4 Mechanism of injury producing a posterior elbow dislocation. **A.** The elbow is forced into extension, which ruptures the medial collateral ligaments. The normal valgus alignment of the elbow accentuates the valgus force at the elbow. **B.** The lateral slope of the medial crista of the trochlea forces the proximal ulna posterolaterally (*small arrow*). The biceps tendon serves as a fulcrum for rotation (*medium arrow*), leading to valgus hinging (*large arrow*) of the forearm. **C.** The proximal ulna and radius are then impacted posteriorly and held against the distal articular surface by the contraction of the biceps and triceps (*arrows*).

The most commonly accepted mechanism of posterior elbow dislocation involves the application of both abduction and extension forces. However, there is controversy as to whether the elbow is initially hyperextended. Osborne and Cotterill (8) believed that initially the elbow was in slight flexion and that the lateral sloping surface of the medial crista of the trochlea served as a cam, converting the vertical thrust on the forearm to lateral rotation and valgus strain. Other investigators believe that there is first hyperextension of the elbow with rupture of the ulnar collateral ligaments (9,10). The elbow is then forced into moderate valgus (see Fig. 16-4). Posterior dislocations have been most commonly produced by initial hyperextension in cadaver studies (10,11). However, Sojbjerg et al (12), in a study of 10 cadaver elbows, produced posterior dislocations through a valgus and external rotation force in on a semiflexed elbow. Dislocation could not be produced with a varus and internal rotation force. O'Driscoll et al (13) found similar results in their study on 13 fresh autopsy specimens.

Soft Tissue Injury

Posterior dislocations normally produce moderate soft tissue injury and can be associated with neurovascular injuries and concomitant fractures (Fig. 16-5). The anterior capsule fails in tension, opening the joint cavity. Radial head displacement strips the capsule from the posterolateral aspect of the lateral condyle with the adjacent periosteum. Because of the large amount of cartilage on the posterolateral aspect of the lateral condyle, the posterior capsule may not reattach firmly with healing. This lack of a strong reattachment is believed to be a major factor in recurrent elbow dislocations (8).

Medially, the ulnar collateral ligament complex is disrupted either by an avulsion of the medial epicondyle or a direct tear of the ligament (10,12). Cromack (14) found that with medial epicondylar fractures, the origins of the ulnar collateral ligaments and the medial forearm flexor muscles remain as a unit, along with most of the pronator teres, which is stripped from its humeral origin proximal to the epicondyle. These structures are then displaced posterior to the medial aspect of the distal humerus. The ulnar collateral ligaments and the muscular origins of the common flexor muscles tear if the epicondyle remains attached to the humerus. With posterolateral displacement of the forearm, the medial aspect of the distal humerus dissects the intermuscular space between the pronator teres posteriorly and the brachialis anteriorly. The brachialis, because it

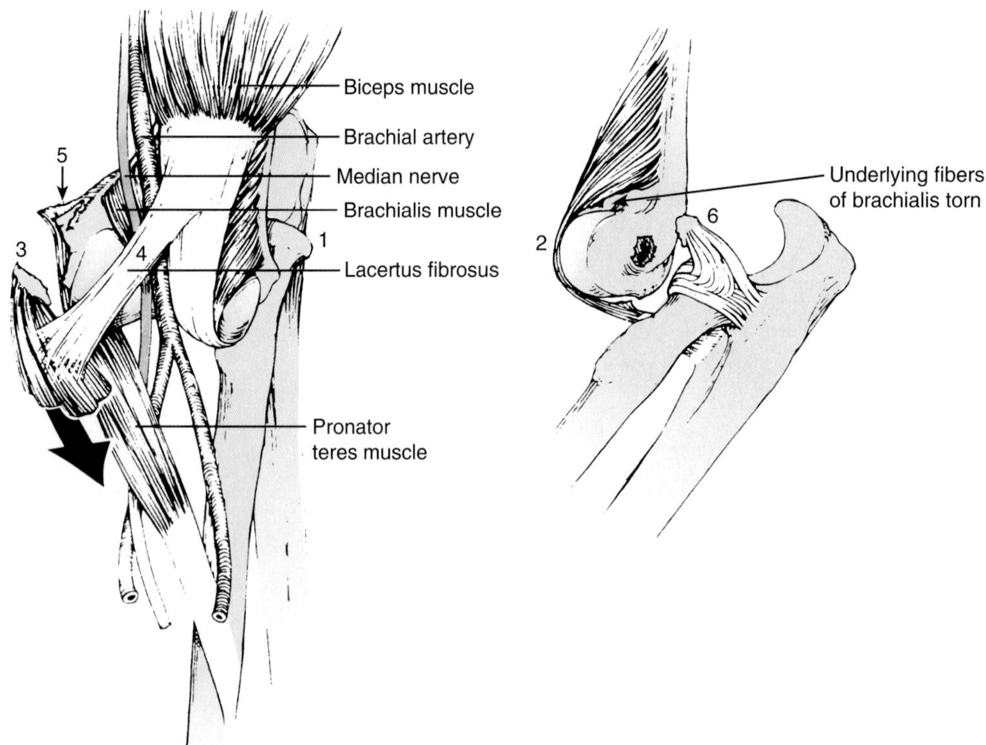

FIGURE 16-5 Injuries associated with elbow dislocation. *1:* The radial head and olecranon are displaced posterolaterally. *2:* The brachialis muscle is stretched across the articular surface of the distal humerus. *3:* The origins of the medial forearm flexion muscles are either torn or avulsed with the medial epicondyle from the medial condyle. *4:* The median nerve and brachial artery are stretched across the medial condyle and held firmly by the lacertus fibrosus. *5:* The medial condyle lies in the subcutaneous tissue between the brachialis anteriorly and the pronator teres posteriorly. *6:* The lateral (radial) collateral ligaments often avulse a piece of cartilage or bone from the lateral condyle.

has little distal tendon, is easily ruptured. The rent in the anterior capsule usually is in this same area.

The structure most commonly torn on the lateral aspect of the elbow is the annular ligament (12). On rare occasions, the lateral collateral ligament either avulses a small osteochondral fragment from the lateral epicondyle or tears completely within its substance.

Neurovascular Injuries

When the elbow is dislocated, the medial aspect of the distal humerus lies subcutaneously between the pronator teres posteriorly and the brachialis anteriorly. The median nerve and brachial artery lie directly over the distal humerus in the subcutaneous tissues. In a cadaver and clinical study by Louis et al (15), there was a consistent pattern of disruption of the anastomosis between the inferior ulnar collateral artery and the anterior ulnar recurrent artery. If the main brachial arterial trunk is also compromised, the loss of this collateral system can result in the loss of circulation to the forearm and hand.

The ulnar nerve also is at risk in posterior elbow dislocation because of its position posterior to the medial epicondyle.

Associated Fractures

Concomitant fractures occur in over half of posterior elbow dislocations (3–6). Fractures involving the medial epicondyle, radial head and neck, and coronoid process are most common. Fractures involving the lateral epicondyle, lateral condyle, olecranon, capitellum, and trochlea occur less frequently. In the 58 dislocations reported by Carlioz and Abols (7), there were 24 fractures involving the medial aspect of the elbow, 6 fractures from the lateral region, 2 with fractures from both regions, 2 coronoid process fractures, and 3 radial neck fractures.

Signs and Symptoms

Posterior elbow dislocation must be differentiated from extension-type supracondylar fracture of the distal humerus. With both injuries, the elbow is held semiflexed, and swelling may be considerable. Swelling usually is less with a dislocation than with a type III supracondylar humerus fracture. Crepitus is usually absent in children with a dislocation. The forearm appears shortened. The prominence produced by the distal humeral articular surface is more distal and is palpable as a blunt articular surface. The tip of the olecranon is displaced posteriorly and proximally so that its triangular relationship with the epicondyles is lost. The skin may have a dimpled appearance over the olecranon fossa. If the dislocation is posterolateral, the radial head also may be prominent and easily palpable in the subcutaneous tissues.

Radiographic and Other Imaging

Anteroposterior (AP) and lateral x-rays usually are diagnostic of a posterior elbow dislocation. There is a greater superimposition of the distal humerus on the proximal radius and ulna in the AP view. The radial head may be proximally and laterally displaced, or it may be directly behind the middistal humerus, depending on whether the dislocation is posterolateral, posterior, or posteromedial (Fig. 16-6). The normal

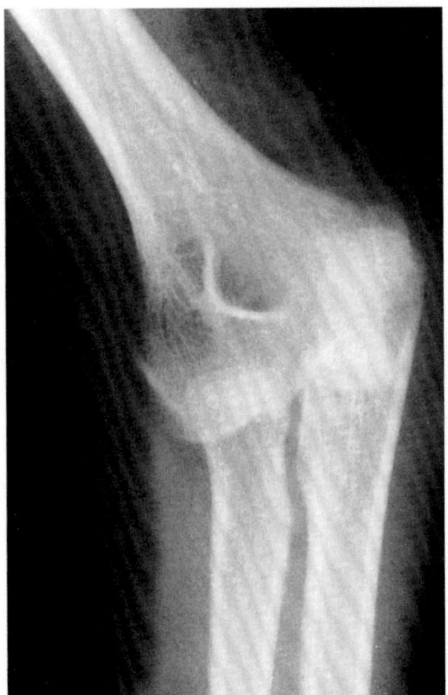

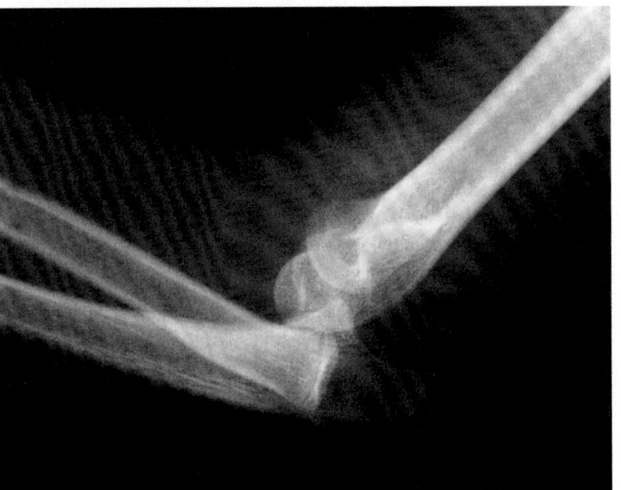

FIGURE 16-6 Radiographic findings. **A.** AP x-ray. The radial head is superimposed behind the distal humerus. There is increased cubitus valgus. The medial epicondyle has not been avulsed. **B.** Lateral x-ray showing that the proximal radius and ulna are both displaced posteriorly to the distal humerus.

valgus angulation between the forearm and the arm is usually increased. On the lateral view, the coronoid process lies posterior to the condyles. The x-rays must be examined closely for associated fractures.

Treatment Options

Closed Reduction

In the combined series (3–6) of 317 dislocations, only two cases (3) could not be reduced by closed methods. In the Carlioz and Abols series (7), two dislocations reduced spontaneously and closed reduction was successful in 50 cases but failed in 6 cases (10%). Josefsson et al (16) reported that all 25 dislocations without associated fractures were successfully reduced.

Progressive elbow swelling secondary to the soft tissue injury associated with an elbow dislocation makes it imperative that the joint be promptly reduced. Royle (6) found that dislocations reduced soon after the injury had better outcomes than those in which reduction was delayed.

All methods of closed reduction must overcome the deforming muscle forces so that the coronoid process and the radial head can slip past the distal end of the humerus. The forearm is hypersupinated to dislodge the coronoid process and radial head from their position behind the distal humerus before the reducing forces are applied. The reducing forces are applied in two major directions (Fig. 16-7). The first reducing force must be along the long axis of the humerus to overcome the contractions of the biceps and brachialis anteriorly and the triceps posteriorly. Once these forces are neutralized, the proximal ulna and radius must be passed from posterior to anterior. This requires a second force along the long axis of the forearm. This may require that the elbow be extended or even hyperextended to lever the coronoid process past the distal humerus.

Some investigators (17,18) have strongly advised against initial hyperextension before reduction forces area applied to the elbow. Loomis (17) showed that when the coronoid process is locked against the posterior aspect of the humerus and the elbow is extended, the force applied is magnified by as much as five times in the anterior muscles because of the increased leverage. This places a marked strain on the injured anterior capsule and the brachialis muscle (Fig. 16-8). By contrast, when the distal force is applied to the proximal forearm with the elbow flexed, the force exerted against the muscles across the elbow is equal to the distracting force.

Osborne and Cotterill (8) suggested that the best way to dislodge the coronoid process and the radial head from the distal humerus is to hypersupinate the forearm and then apply traction along the forearm with the elbow flexed. Others (19,20) have warned that in posterolateral dislocations, the lateral dis-

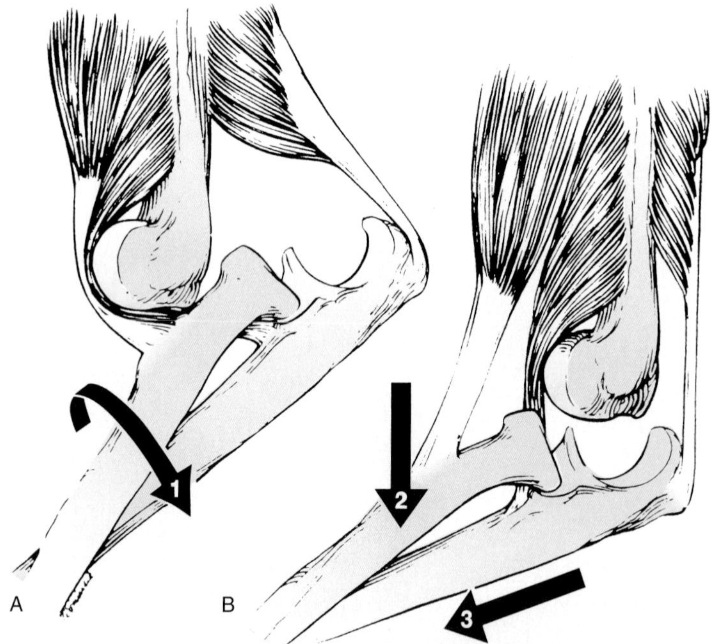

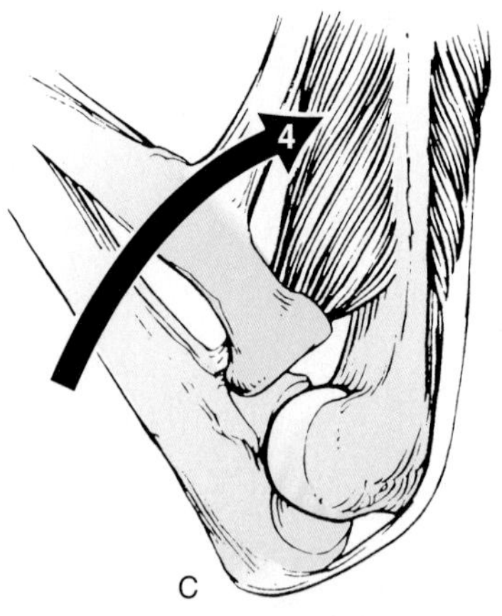

FIGURE 16-7 Forces required to reduce posterior elbow dislocations. **A.** The forearm is hypersupinated (*arrow 1*) to unlock the radial head. **B.** Simultaneous forces are applied to the proximal forearm along the axis of the humerus (*arrow 2*) and distally along the axis of the forearm (*arrow 3*). **C.** The elbow is then flexed (*arrow 4*) to stabilize the reduction once the coronoid is manipulated distal to the humerus.

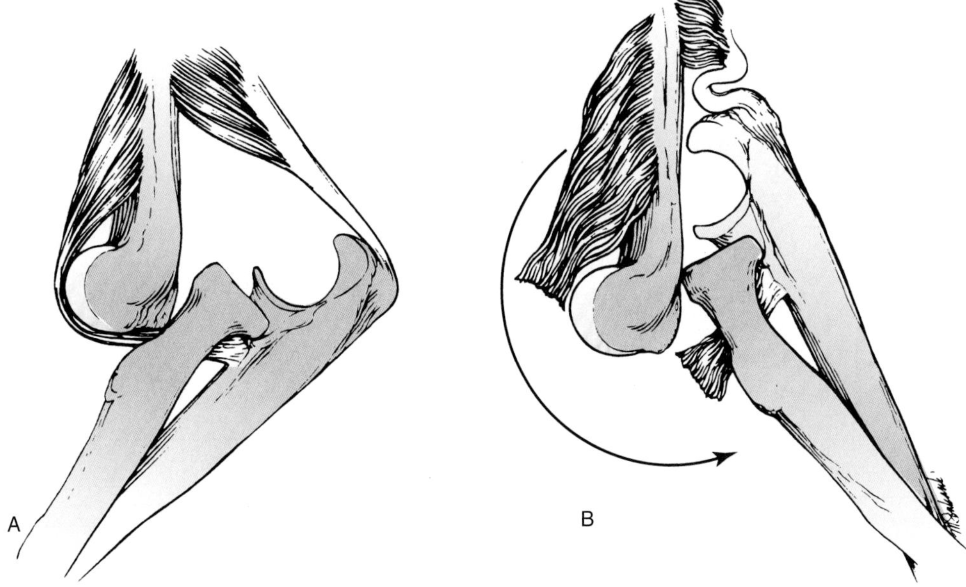

FIGURE 16-8 Hyperextension forces. **A.** The brachialis is stretched across the distal humerus. **B.** Hyperextending the elbow before it is reduced greatly increases the arc of motion and leverage placed across the brachialis. This can result in rupture of large portions of the muscle. (Reprinted from Loomis LK. Reduction and after-treatment of posterior dislocation of the elbow. *Am J Surg* 1944;63:56–60; with permission.)

placement of the proximal radius and ulna must first be corrected to prevent the median nerve from being entrapped or injured during reduction. Pronating the forearm during the reduction maneuver may also be a factor in entrapping the median nerve in the joint.

Although numerous reduction techniques have been advocated, they all have the common goal of applying the two major traction forces along the axes of the humerus and forearm. Each of these forces is resisted by its respective counterforce. There appears to be two main groups in the method of applying force to counteract the muscles of the arm: the "pullers" (Figs. 16-9, 16-10, and 16-11) (21–23) and the "pushers" (Fig. 16-12) (24–26). There also are combined unassisted pusher–puller techniques (27,28).

Postreduction Care. After reduction, the surgeon should determine and document the stability of the elbow. A concentric reduction must be documented in all cases. Some type of immobilization, usually a posterior splint, is advocated by most investigators after successful closed reduction. The standard period of immobilization recommended is usually three weeks (3,17,23,29), although some have advocated early motion (6,30,31). Ninety degrees of elbow flexion appears to be the standard position of immobilization. O'Driscoll et al (13) believed that if the elbow was stable to valgus stress with the forearm pronated, the anterior portion of the medial collateral ligament was intact and the patient could begin early motion.

Open Reduction

Indications for primary open reduction are an inability to obtain a concentric closed reduction, an open dislocation, and a displaced osteochondral fracture.

Inadequate Closed Reduction. Carlioz and Abols (7) reported that 19 of 58 posterior dislocations required open reduction. In 13, the reduction was stable and the surgery was for the treatment of displaced fractures. In six, open reduction of the joint was necessary: two each for an entrapped medial epicondyle, an ulnar osteochondral fragment, and a ligamentous fragment.

Adults with posterior elbow dislocations without concomitant fracture have no better function or stability following a primary ligamentous repair than those treated nonoperatively (32,33). The mean lack of elbow extension in both groups was 10 degrees. Similar results were reported by Josefsson et al (16) in 28 children and adolescents with simple posterior dislocations treated nonoperatively. However, Durig et al (34) recommended primary operative treatment of uncomplicated dislocations, because early surgery produced satisfactory functional results in all 10 of their patients. Cromak (14) reported full function in 14 children and adolescents treated by early operative repair.

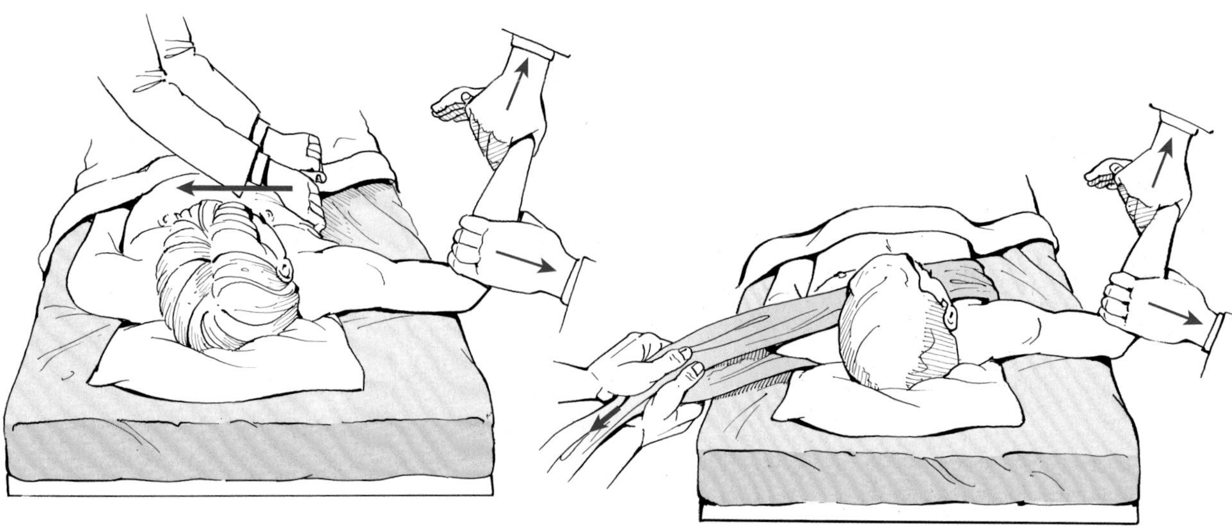

FIGURE 16-9 Reduction by "puller" techniques in a supine position. **A.** With the elbow flexed to almost 90 degrees, a force is applied to the anterior portion of the forearm with one hand while the other hand pulls distally along the forearm. A counterforce is applied to counteract the manipulating forces by direct stabilization of the patient by a second medical person. **B.** The counterforce is applied with a sheet around the chest in the ipsilateral axilla. (Redrawn from Parvin RW. Closed reduction of common shoulder and elbow dislocations without anesthesia. *Arch Surg* 1957;75:972–975; with permission. Copyright 1957, American Medical Association.)

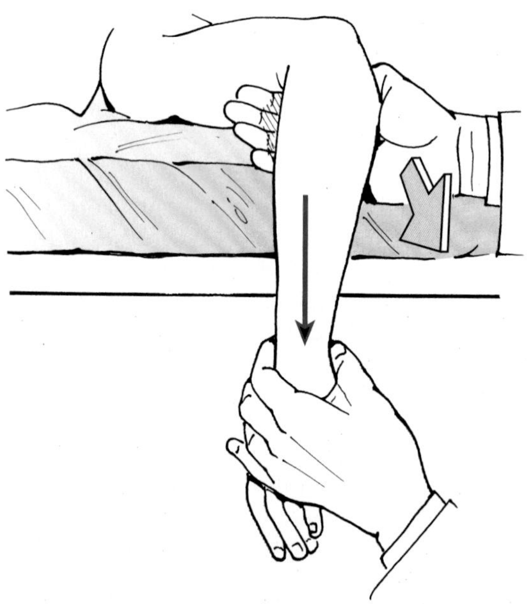

FIGURE 16-10 Reduction by "puller" technique in a prone position. The same forces are applied to the proximal portion of the anterior forearm and distal forearm as in the supine position. The table provides a counterforce against the anterior portion of the distal humerus when the patient is prone.

Open Posterior Dislocations. Open dislocations usually have a high incidence of arterial injuries (3,15,35,36). For this reason, operative intervention usually is necessary for debridement and evaluation of the brachial artery.

Associated Fractures. Children with an elbow dislocation can have an associated fracture of the coronoid, the olecranon (Fig. 16-13), or the medial epicondyle (Fig. 16-14). The presence of a concomitant displaced fracture is a common indication for surgical intervention (7,37,38). Surgery for associated fractures produced better results than nonoperative treatment in the series of Carlioz and Abols (7). Similar results were reported by Wheeler and Linscheid (38). Fowles et al (37), however, had poorer results in nine children with a concomitant medial epicondyle fracture stabilized surgically. They recommended surgery only for children in whom the medial epicondyle is entrapped in the joint (Fig. 16-15) or significantly displaced after closed reduction. Repair of an associated medial epicondylar fracture also may improve elbow stability in throwing athletes (10,31) when the injury is in the dominant arm.

Postoperative Care. Immobilization after surgery depends on the procedure performed. After open reduction, management is similar to that after satisfactory closed reduction. The length of immobilization for fractures usually is 3 to 5 weeks.

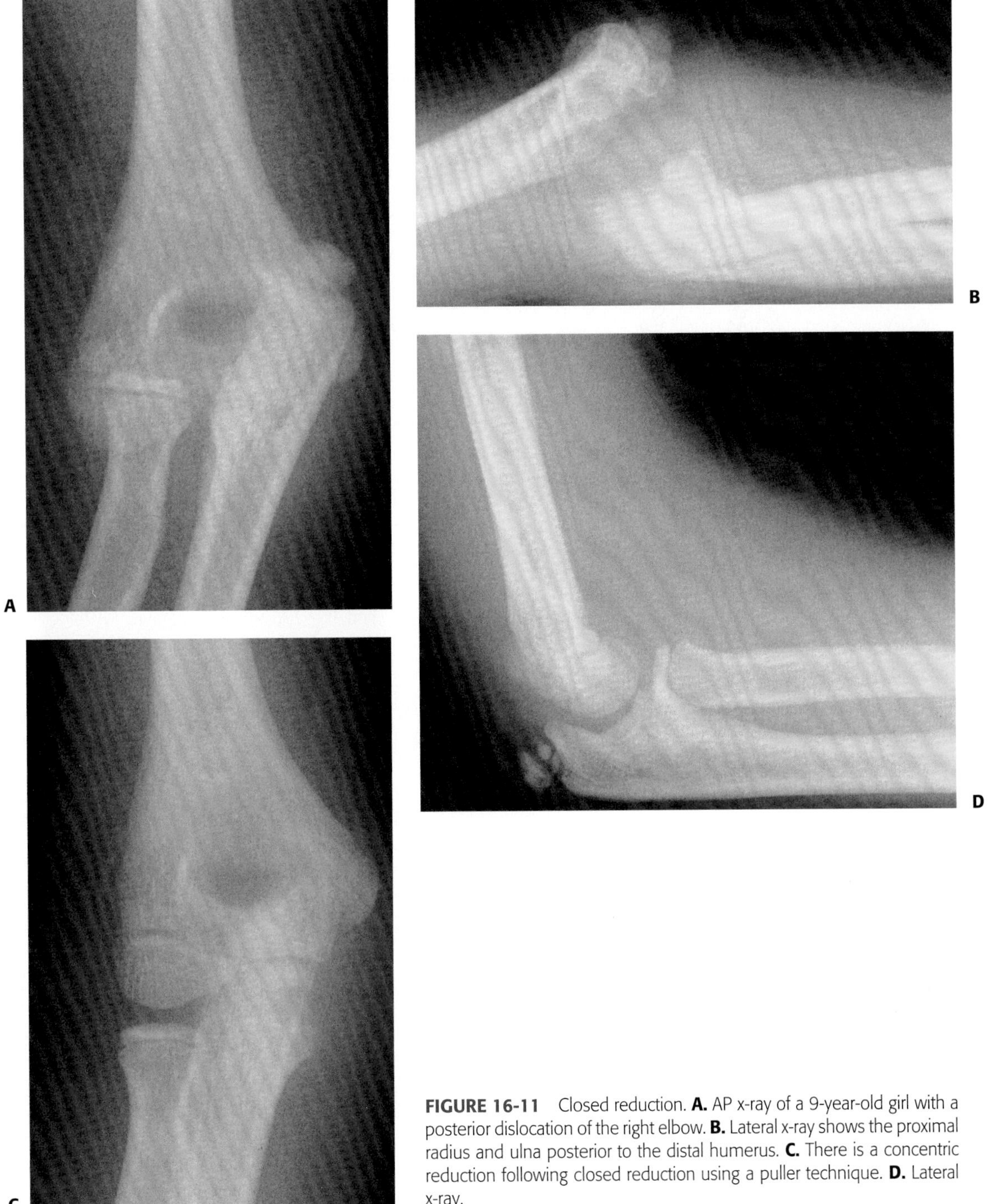

FIGURE 16-11 Closed reduction. **A.** AP x-ray of a 9-year-old girl with a posterior dislocation of the right elbow. **B.** Lateral x-ray shows the proximal radius and ulna posterior to the distal humerus. **C.** There is a concentric reduction following closed reduction using a puller technique. **D.** Lateral x-ray.

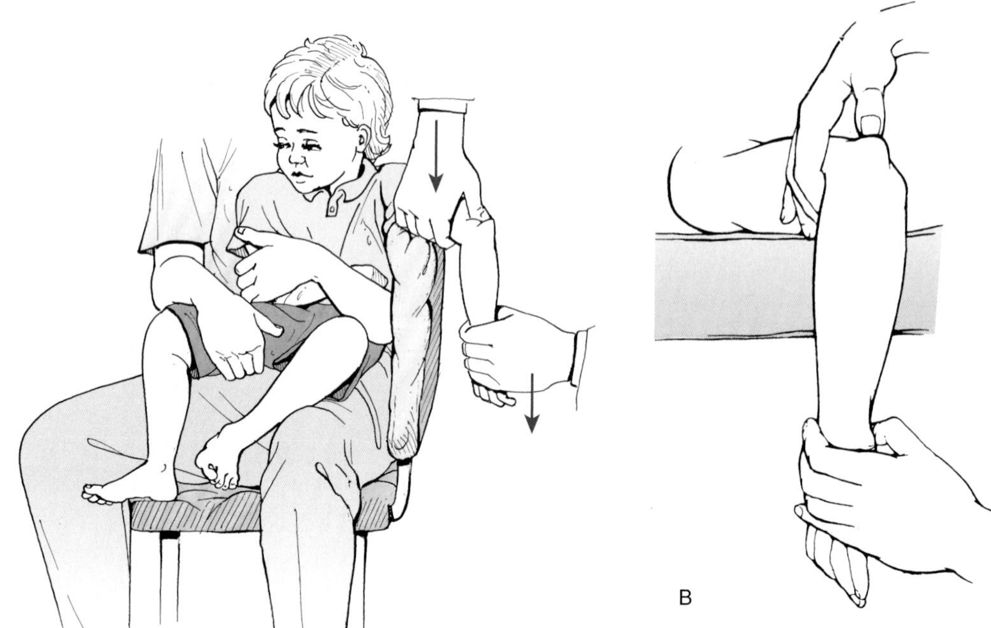

FIGURE 16-12 Reduction by "pusher" techniques. **A.** Lavine's method. The child is held by the parent while the elbow is draped over the edge of the chair. The olecranon is pushed distally past the humerus by the thumb of the physician while the other arm pulls distally along the axis of the forearm. **B.** Meyn's technique with patient lying prone on the table. (Redrawn from Meyn MA, Quigley TB. Reduction of posterior dislocation of the elbow by traction on the dangling arm. *Clin Orthop* 1974;103:106–107; with permission.)

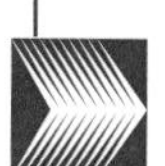

AUTHORS' PREFERRED TREATMENT

The "push-off" technique of reduction of an elbow dislocation is preferred in children 9 years of age or less. In this age group, the child often can be seated comfortably in the parent's lap (see Fig. 16-12). Hanging the arm over the back of a well-padded chair may provide some stabilization.

For the child 9 years of age and older, the puller technique advocated by Parvin (23) is used (see Figs. 16-9 and 16-10). The forearm must remain supinated during the process of reduction. Occasionally, it is necessary to hypersupinate the forearm to unlock the coronoid process and radial head before reduction. Closed reduction is done either with heavy sedation or general anesthesia. X-rays are obtained after the manipulation to assess the adequacy of the reduction (see Fig. 16-11). The elbow is immobilized in a posterior splint with the elbow flexed 90 degrees. If there is a question of persistent instability, the forearm is held in full supination. If the elbow is absolutely stable following reduction, the forearm may be immobilized in mid-pronation simply to allow the patient to be more functional in the splint.

Because the major complication of elbow dislocations is stiffness, the splint is removed after approximately 1 week and the patient begins intermittent active elbow motion. The patient can discard the splint and use a sling after 10 to 14 days. The emphasis is on early active motion to prevent the stiffness that often occurs after this injury. Before reduction, it is important to emphasize to the parents that there may be some loss of motion, especially extension, regardless of the treatment. This is usually not of functional or cosmetic significance.

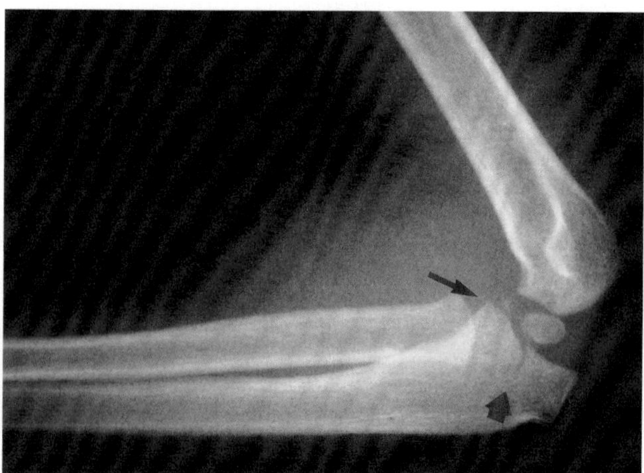

FIGURE 16-13 Lateral x-ray of a 4-year-old child who sustained an elbow dislocation with a concomitant olecranon fracture (*large arrow*) and a coronoid fracture (*small arrow*).

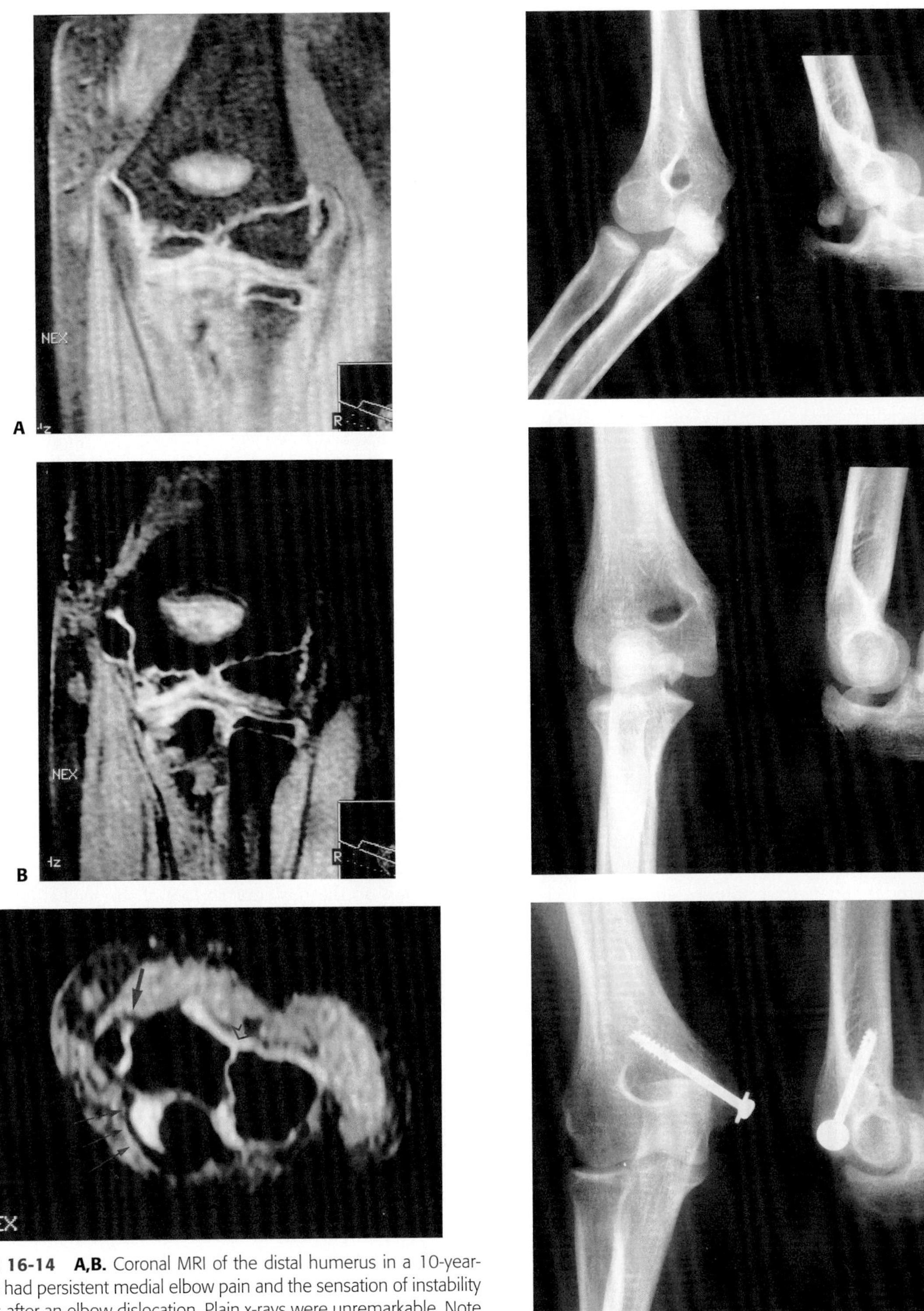

FIGURE 16-14 **A,B.** Coronal MRI of the distal humerus in a 10-year-old who had persistent medial elbow pain and the sensation of instability 4 weeks after an elbow dislocation. Plain x-rays were unremarkable. Note the joint effusion and the increase in signal intensity between the distal medial humerus and the medial epicondyle. Note the difference compared to the other distal humerus growth plates. **C.** An axial image shows widening and increased signal intensity in the medial epicondyle physis (*arrow*). There is an effusion posteriorly (*darts*). There is no disruption between the lateral condyle and the remaining portion of the distal humerus, as evidenced by a normal-appearing physis (*open arrow*). This patient was placed into a hinged elbow brace that limited extension for 3 weeks, with good results.

FIGURE 16-15 **A.** AP and lateral x-rays of a 14-year-old boy who sustained an elbow dislocation with an ipsilateral medial epicondyle fracture. **B.** Anterior and posterior x-rays after a closed reduction. Note the entrapment of the medial epicondyle in the joint. **C.** This patient was treated with an open reduction to extract the medial epicondyle from the joint and an internal fixation using a cannulated screw, which allowed rapid mobilization of his elbow.

A careful neurologic examination must be done before and after the reduction, with special attention to the median nerve. This same careful examination must be made at all follow-up evaluations.

Complications

Complications associated with posterior elbow dislocations can be divided into those occurring early and those occurring later. Early complications include neurologic and vascular injuries. Late complications include loss of motion, myositis ossificans, recurrent dislocations, radioulnar synostosis, and cubitus recurvatum. The special problems of chronic, unreduced dislocations are not considered complications of treatment.

Neurologic Injuries

In the combined series (3–6) of 317 patients, 32 patients (10%) had nerve symptoms after reduction. There was no breakdown as to the ages of the patients with the nerve injuries. Twenty-one patients had isolated ulnar nerve injuries and seven isolated median nerve injuries. In four patients both the median and ulnar nerves were involved. Most were transient paresthesias with rapid recovery. Only one patient failed to recover fully (3). Carlioz and Abols (7) reported no neurologic injuries with 58 dislocations in children and adolescents, although two children had transient ulnar nerve symptoms.

Ulnar Nerve Lesions. There is an increased incidence of ulnar nerve injuries associated with elbow dislocations (3,7,18, 39,40). There were 21 ulnar nerve injuries and 4 combined ulnar and median nerve injuries in the combined series (3–6). Watson-Jones (18) described 16 nerve lesions in 97 elbow dislocations, 12 of which involved the ulnar nerve; 9 of these were associated with a medial epicondylar fracture. Galbraith and McCullough (40) found six ulnar nerve injuries in 187 elbow dislocations. Four of these patients had medial epicondyle fractures and two had radial head fractures; all had posterior elbow dislocations. Linscheid and Wheeler (3) reported neurologic complications in 24 of 110 elbow dislocations, including 16 isolated ulnar nerve injuries and 4 injuries to both the ulnar and medial nerves. They recommended ulnar nerve transposition if ulnar nerve symptoms were present in a patient undergoing open reduction and internal fixation of a displaced medial epicondylar fracture. Cotton (39) reported 10 children with posterior dislocations associated with medial epicondylar fractures and ulnar nerve neuropathy. Except for the one patient described by Linscheid and Wheeler (3), these reported ulnar nerve injuries were transient and resolved completely.

Radial Nerve Lesions. Watson-Jones (18) is the only investigator to report a radial nerve injury associated with an elbow dislocation. He described two patients in whom the symptoms rapidly resolved after reduction.

Median Nerve Lesions. The most serious neurologic injury involves the median nerve, which can be damaged directly by the dislocation or can be entrapped within the joint. Median nerve injuries occur most commonly in children 5 to 12 years of age. There were seven median and four median/ulnar nerve injuries (3%) in the combined series (3–6).

Types of Median Nerve Entrapment. Fourrier et al (41) in 1977 delineated three types of medial nerve entrapment (Fig. 16-16).

Type 1. The child has an avulsion of the medial epicondyle or has a rupture of the medial muscles at their origin and the ulnar collateral ligaments (see Fig. 16-16A). This allows the median nerve, with or without the brachial artery, to displace posteriorly. The nerve is especially prone to being entrapped between the trochlea and the olecranon during the process of reduction if the lateral displacement of the proximal radius and ulna is not corrected before reduction. Hallett (42) showed in cadavers that pronation of the forearm while the elbow is hyperextended forces the median nerve posteriorly during the process of reduction, making it also vulnerable to entrapment. This type of entrapment has also been reported by other authors (19,20,41, 43–49). Delay in diagnosis is common. In some patients with an associated medial epicondyle fracture, the nerve can be so severely damaged after being entrapped that resection of the injured portion with reanastomosis is necessary (19,45,46). Good recovery of nerve function has been reported.

If the nerve has been entrapped for a considerable period, the Matev sign may be present on the x-rays (46). This represents a depression on the posterior surface of the medial epicondylar ridge where the nerve has been pressed against the bone (42–49). This groove is represented radiographically by two sclerotic lines parallel to the nerve (Fig. 16-17). This sign disappears when the pressure from the nerve has been released.

Type 2. The nerve is entrapped between the fracture surfaces of the medial epicondyle and the distal humerus (see Fig. 16-16B). The fracture heals and the nerve is surrounded by bone, forming a neo-foramen (47,49,50). This may or may not be visible radiographically. The medial epicondyle can be osteomized to free the nerve.

Type 3. The nerve is kinked and entrapped between the distal humerus and the olecranon (see Fig. 16-16C). Only three injuries of this type have been reported (43,51,52). Resection and reanastomosis resulted in return of good function over 6 to 24 months.

al-Qattan et al (53) described a fourth type of median nerve entrapment in a 14-year-old boy who had a posterior elbow dislocation with a medial epicondylar fracture. The median nerve was found entrapped in a healed medial epicondylar fracture (type 2) in an anterior-to-posterior direction 18 months after injury. The nerve then passed through the elbow joint

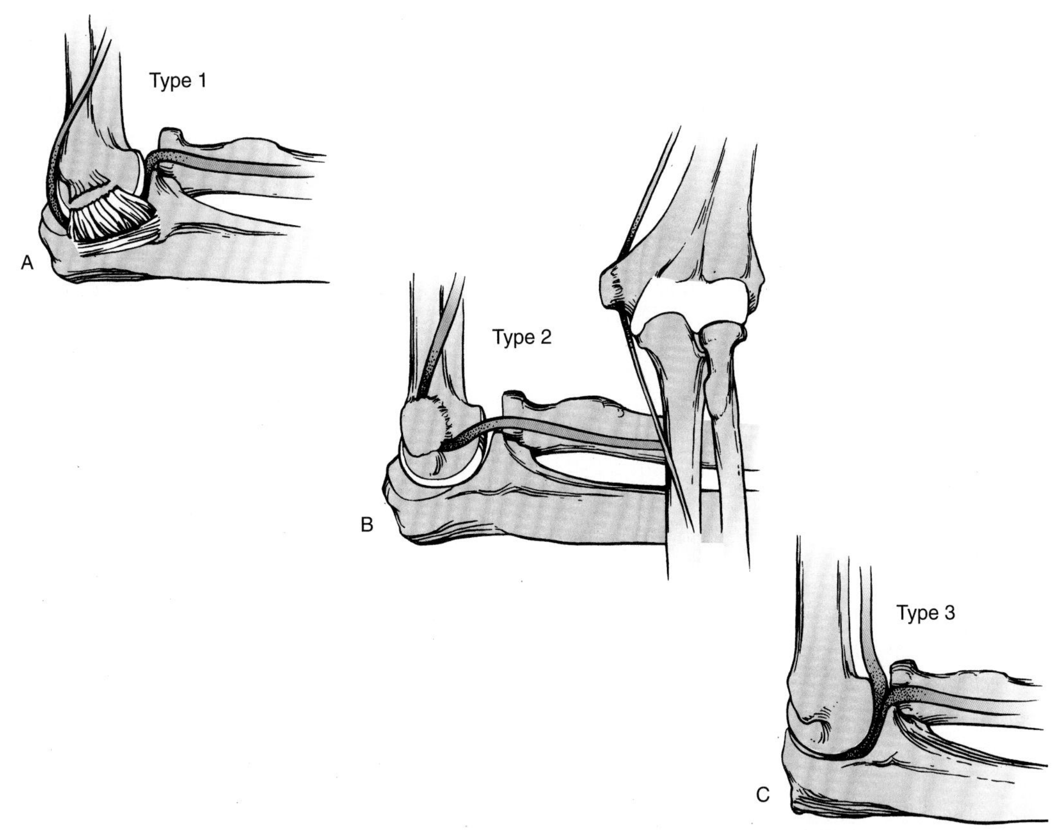

FIGURE 16-16 Median nerve entrapment. **A.** Type 1. Entrapment within the elbow joint with the median nerve coursing posterior to the distal humerus. **B.** Type 2. Entrapment of the nerve between the fracture surfaces of the medial epicondyle and the medial condyle. **C.** Type 3. Simple kinking of the nerve into the anterior portion of the elbow joint. (Redrawn from Hallett J. Entrapment of the median nerve after dislocation of the elbow. *J Bone Joint Surg [Br]* 1981;63:408–412; with permission.)

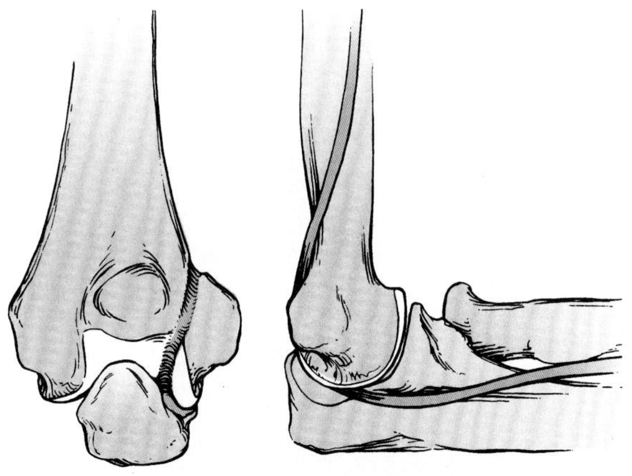

FIGURE 16-17 The Matev sign suggesting entrapment of the median nerve in the elbow joint and impingement of the nerve against the posterior surface of the medial condyle. This produces a depression with sclerotic margins. (Redrawn from Matev I. A radiographic sign of entrapment of the median nerve in the elbow joint after posterior dislocation. *J Bone Joint Surg [Br]* 1976;58:353–355; with permission.)

in a posterior-to-anterior direction (type 1). The nerve was so severely damaged that it had to be resected and repaired with sural nerve grafts.

The combination of an associated fracture of the medial epicondyle and significant median nerve dysfunction was cited by Rao and Crawford (48) as an absolute indication for surgical exploration of the nerve because of the frequency of median nerve entrapment with fractures of the medial epicondyle (types 1 and 2). MRI may be helpful in defining the course of the median nerve if entrapment is suspected. Once the entrapped nerve is removed from the joint, neurologic function typically improves even if the nerve appears seriously damaged. Resection and reanastomosis rarely are necessary.

Arterial Injuries

Arterial injuries are uncommon with posterior elbow dislocations in children and adolescents (15,35–37,54–59). Only eight vascular injuries (3%) were reported in the combined series (3–6). However, Carlioz and Abols (7) reported four patients with diminished radial pulses that resolved after reduction. Arterial injuries have been associated with open dislocations in which collateral circulation is disrupted (15,35,36,58). Usually the brachial artery is ruptured (15,35,36,55,56,60), but it also can be thrombosed (59) as well as entrapped in the elbow joint (54,57,59). Pearce (57) reported an entrapped radial artery in which there was a high bifurcation of the brachial artery.

When there is a complete rupture, there usually is evidence of severe ischemia distally. Unfortunately, the presence of good capillary circulation to the hand or a Doppler pulse at the wrist does not always mean the artery is intact (55,60). Arteriograms usually are not necessary because the arterial injury is at the site of the dislocation. Intravenous digital angiography has been used to confirm complete obstruction of the brachial artery if there is clinical evidence of distal ischemia (55).

Treatment usually consists of relocation of the elbow dislocation, which returns the displaced brachial vessels to their normal position (54,59), and operative repair of those that are ruptured or severely damaged. Ligation of the ends has been done, especially if there was good capillary circulation distally (35,36), but this may predispose to late ischemic changes such as claudication and cold sensitivity. Most investigators recommend direct arterial repair or a vein graft (15,55,56,58,60). Louis et al (15) recommended arterial repair because their cadaver studies showed that a posterior elbow dislocation usually disrupted the collateral circulation necessary to maintain distal blood flow.

Loss of Motion

Almost all patients with elbow dislocations lose some range of elbow motion (7,16,32,33,37). This loss is less in children than in adults (16) and is usually no more than 10 degrees of extension. This is rarely is of functional or cosmetic significance. However, this potential for loss of motion must be explained to the parents before reduction and may be an indication for a supervised rehabilitation program.

Myositis Ossificans versus Heterotopic Calcification

True myositis ossificans should be differentiated from heterotopic calcification, which is a dystrophic process. Myositis ossificans involves ossification within the muscle sheath that can lead to a significant loss of range of motion of the elbow. Disruption of the brachialis muscle is believed to be a contributory factor (17). Fortunately, myositis ossificans is rare in children (16,61). Although heterotopic calcification in the ligaments and capsule of the elbow is common (5,16), it rarely results in loss of elbow function (Fig. 16-18).

In Neviaser and Wickstrom's (4) series of 115 patients, 10 had radiographic evidence of myositis ossificans; all, however, were asymptomatic. Only Roberts (5) differentiated true myositis ossificans from heterotopic calcification. In his series of 60 elbow dislocations, only three patients had true myositis ossificans. Linscheid and Wheeler (3) noted that the incidence of some type of heterotopic calcification was 28%, which was most common around the condyles. Only in five patients was it anterior to the capsule (which probably represented true myositis ossificans in the brachialis muscle). Four of these patients had some decrease in elbow function. Josefsson et al (16) reported that 61% of 28 children with posterior dislocations had periarticular calcification, but this did not appear to be functionally significant.

Radioulnar Synostosis

In dislocations with an associated fracture of the radial neck, the incidence of a secondary proximal radioulnar synostosis is

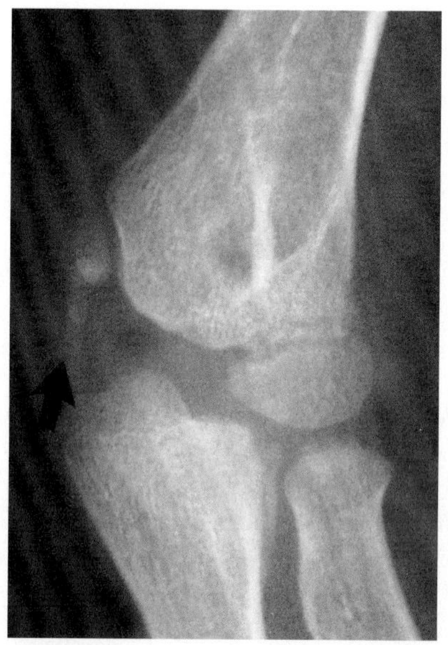

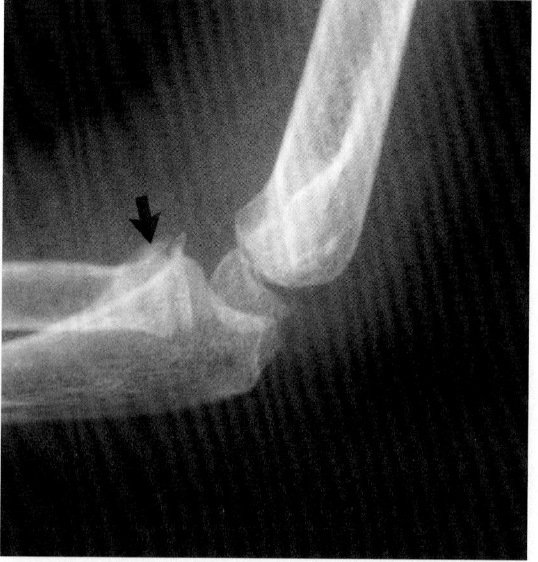

FIGURE 16-18 A. "Heterotopic calcification" of the ulnar collateral ligaments in an elbow that had been dislocated 2 months (*arrow*). **B.** Lateral view of the same elbow. Some "myositis" ossification has occurred where the brachialis inserts into the coronoid process (*arrow*).

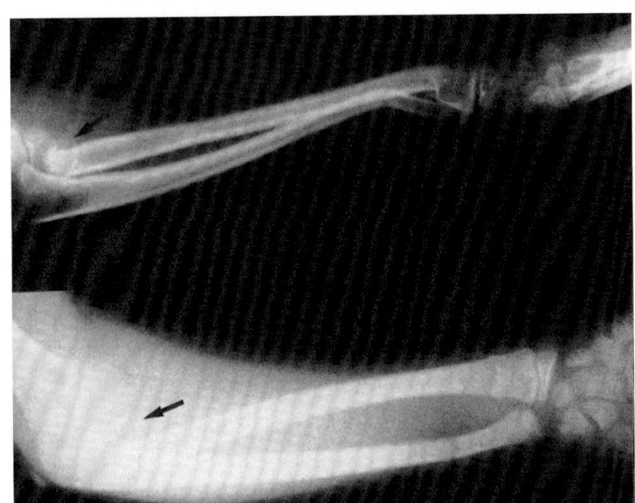

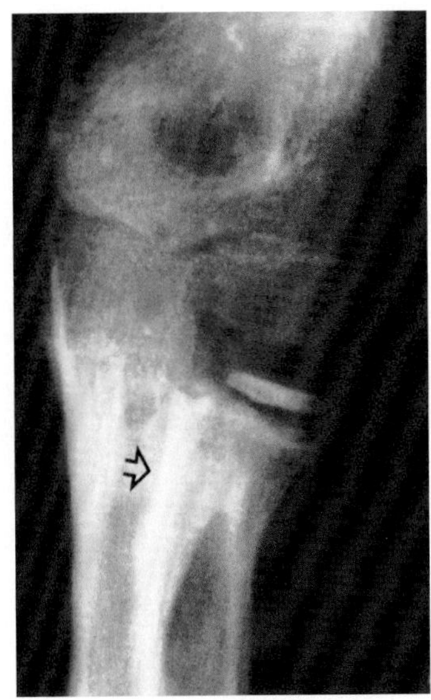

FIGURE 16-19 Radioulnar synostosis. **A.** Injury x-rays showing a posterolateral dislocation associated with a Salter-Harris type II proximal radius fracture (*arrow*). Open reduction of the proximal radial fracture was performed. **B.** Six months later, the patient developed a proximal radioulnar synostosis (*arrow*). (Courtesy of Ruben Pachero, MD.)

increased (Fig. 16-19). This can occur regardless of whether the radial neck fracture is treated operatively or nonoperatively (7,13,20). Carlioz and Abols (7) reported a synostosis in one of three patients with a posterior elbow dislocation associated with radial neck fracture.

Cubitus Recurvatum

Occasionally, a severe elbow dislocation results in significant tearing of the anterior capsule. As a result, after reduction, when all the stiffness created by the dislocation has subsided, the patient may have some hyperextension (cubitus recurvatum) of the elbow. This usually is minimally symptomatic.

Recurrent Posterior Dislocations

Recurrent posterior elbow dislocation is rare. In the combined series of dislocations, only two (0.1%) recurrent dislocations were reported (3–6). Although recurrent posterior elbow dislocations almost always involve adult patients (8,34,62–77), the initial dislocation has occurred before skeletal maturity. Approximately 80% of recurrent dislocations are in males. Three investigators have reported bilateral cases (66,71,78).

Mechanism of Injury

The pathology of recurrent dislocation involves collateral ligament deformation, capsular laxity, and bone defects.

Ligamentous and Capsular Laxity. Osborne and Cotterill (8) suggested that articular changes are secondary and that the primary defect is a failure of the posterolateral ligamentous and capsular structures to become reattached after reduction (Fig. 16-20). Posterior dislocations usually cause attenuation of the ulnar collateral ligaments, and this further contributes to the instability. With recurrent dislocations, the radial head impinges against the posterolateral margin of the capitellum, creating an osteochondral defect (Fig. 16-21).

Osborne and Cotterill (8) attributed the failure of the capsule to reattach to the presence of the large distal humerus articular cartilage surface area, which provides a poor surface for reattachment, and the presence of synovial fluid, which further inhibits healing. In addition to the defect in the capitellar articular surface, a similar defect develops in the anterior articular margin of the radial head. When these two defects oppose each other, recurrence of the dislocation is more likely. Subsequent studies have confirmed these findings in almost all recurrent dislocations, especially in children (34,63,72–74,76).

O'Driscoll et al (29) described posterolateral instability in five patients, including two children, in whom laxity of the ulnar part of the radial collateral ligament allowed a transitory rotary subluxation of the ulnohumeral joint and a secondary dislocation of the radiohumeral joint. Patients with posterolateral instability often describe a history of recurrent temporary dislocation of the elbow but when examined exhibit no unusual clinical findings.

The instability is diagnosed with a posterolateral rotary instability test. In some patients posterolateral rotary instability can be detected only with the patient completely relaxed under general anesthesia. This test is performed by holding the arm over the head while applying proximal axial compression plus a valgus and supination force to the forearm with the elbow flexed to 20 to 30 degrees (Fig. 16-22). O'Driscoll et al reported that surgical repair of the lax ulnar portion of the radial collateral ligament eliminated the posterolateral rotary instability (72).

Schwab et al (10) described treatment of the laxity of the

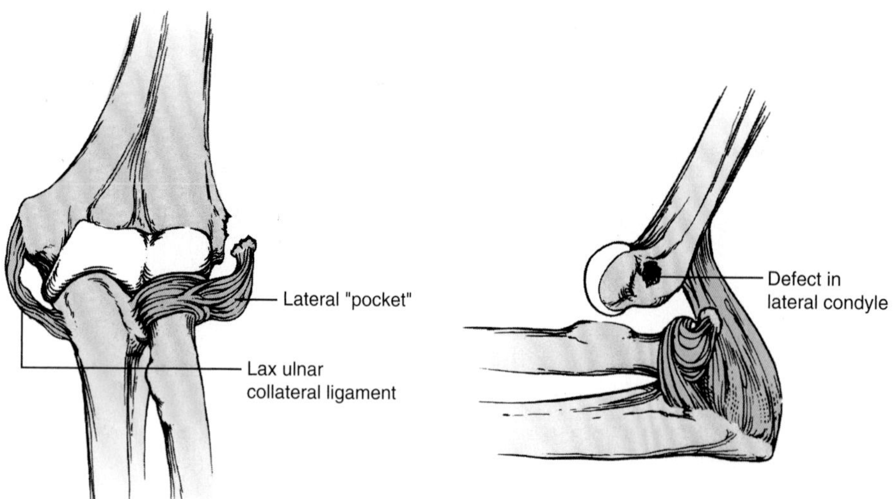

FIGURE 16-20 Pathology associated with recurrent elbow dislocations. The three components that allow the elbow to dislocate are a lax ulnar collateral ligament, a "pocket" in the radial collateral ligament, and a defect in the lateral condyle. (Reprinted from Osborne G, Cotterill P. Recurrent dislocation of the elbow. *J Bone Joint Surg [Br]* 1966;48: 340–346, with permission.)

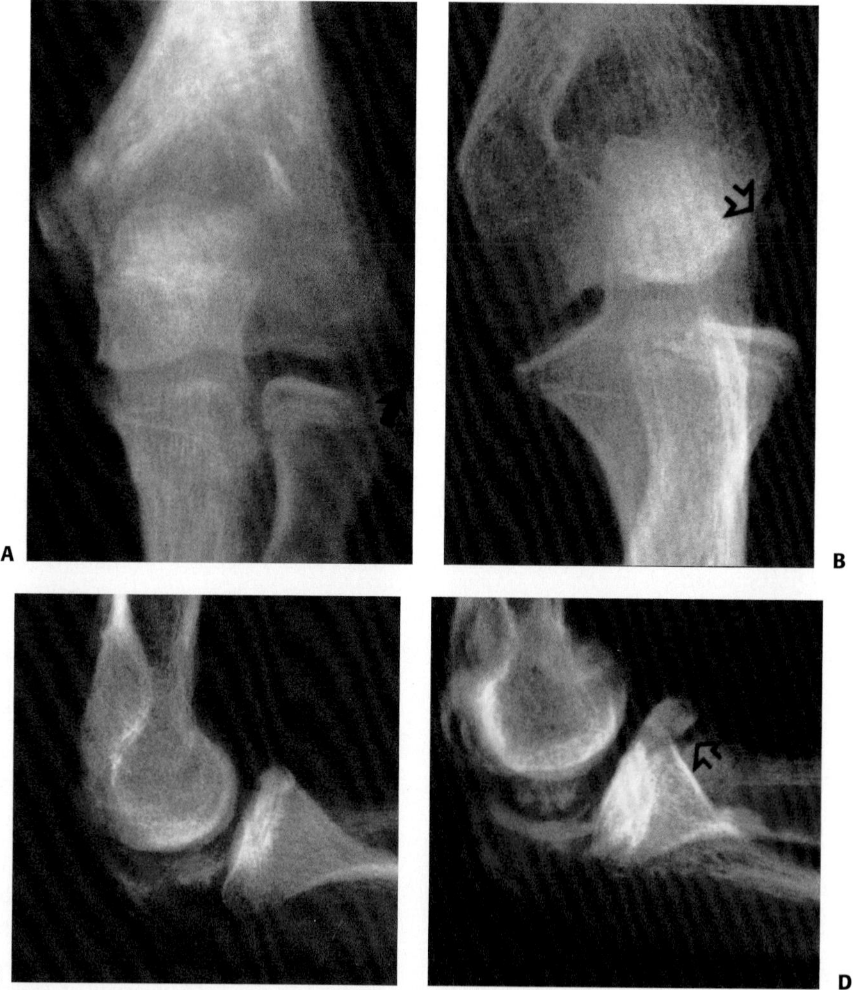

FIGURE 16-21 Radiographic changes associated with recurrent elbow dislocation. **A.** AP x-ray of a 13-year-old who had recurrent dislocations. An osteochondral fragment (*arrow*) is attached to the lateral ligament. **B.** An oblique x-ray shows the defect (*arrow*) in the posterolateral condylar surface. **C.** X-rays of an 11-year-old after his first dislocation. **D.** One year later, after recurrent dislocation and subluxations, blunting of the radial head has developed (*arrow*). (Courtesy of Marvin E. Mumme, MD.)

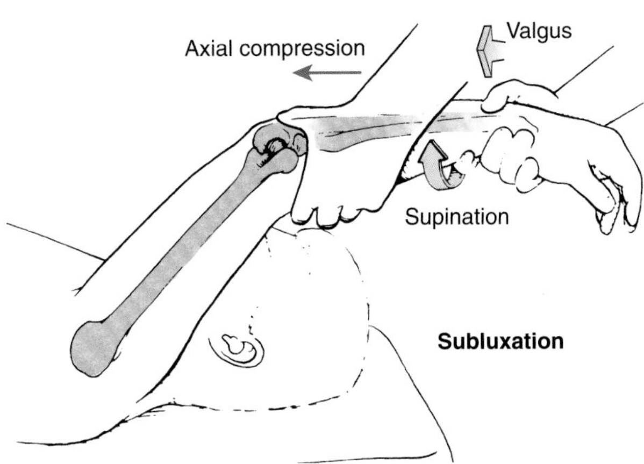

FIGURE 16-22 Posterolateral rotary instability is best demonstrated with the upper extremity over the head with the patient supine. The radial head can be subluxated or dislocated by applying a valgus and supination force to the forearm while proximal axial compression is applied along the forearm. (Reprinted from O'Driscoll SW, Bell DF, Morrey BF. Posterolateral rotary instability of the elbow. *J Bone Joint Surg [Am]* 1991;73:441, with permission.)

medial collateral ligament with advancement of the medial epicondyle proximally to tighten the medial collateral ligament.

Bone Defects. In addition to the previously described osteochondral defects in the capitellum and radial head, bone defects may include a shallow semilunar notch resulting from a coronoid fossa process fracture or multiple recurrent dislocations. Osteochondral fragments in the elbow joint also can contribute to instability.

Treatment Options

Nonoperative. There is only one report of successful nonsurgical management of recurrent elbow dislocations. Herring (64) used an orthosis that blocked the last 15 degrees of extension. After his patient wore this orthosis constantly for 2 years and with vigorous activities for another 6 months, there were no further dislocations, but the follow-up period was only 1 year. Beaty and Donati (79) emphasized that physical therapy and the use of an orthosis should be tried before surgery is considered.

Surgical Procedures. The treatment of recurrent posterior elbow dislocations is predominately surgical. Various surgical procedures have been described to correct bone and soft tissue abnormalities (Fig. 16-23).

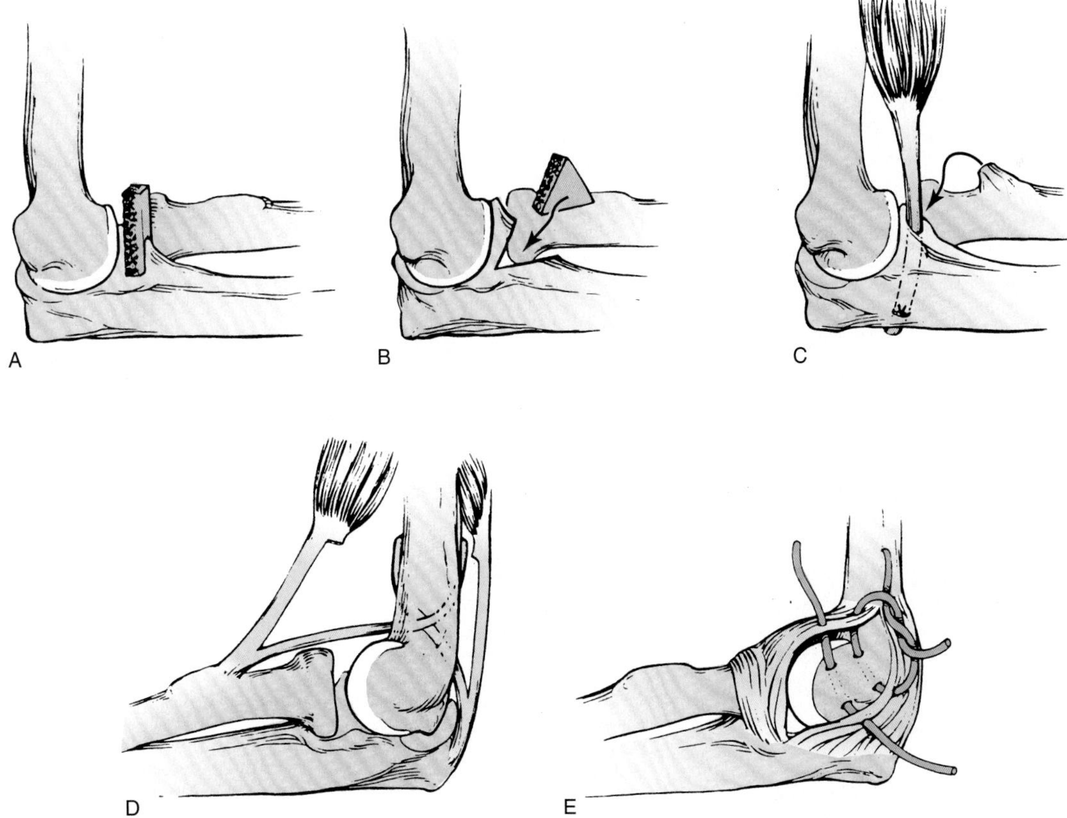

FIGURE 16-23 Surgical procedures for recurrent dislocation. **A.** Simple coronoid bone block. **B.** Open wedge coronoid osteotomy. **C.** Biceps tendon transfer to coronoid process. **D.** Cruciate ligament reconstruction. **E.** Lateral capsular reattachment of Osborne and Cotterill.

Bone Procedures. These are directed more toward correcting dysplasia of the semilunar notch of the olecranon. Milch (71) inserted a boomerang-shaped bone block. Others (62,70,75) found that a simple bone block was all that was necessary (see Fig. 16-23A). Mantle (69) increased the slope of the semilunar notch in two patients with an opening wedge osteotomy of the coronoid process (see Fig. 16-23B).

Schwab et al (10), believing the ulnar collateral ligament to be the mainstay of elbow stability, advocated tightening the medial side by osteotomizing the medial epicondyle and reattaching it proximally, but reported no results.

Soft Tissue Procedures. Reichenheim (78) and King (67) transferred the biceps tendon just distal to the coronoid process to reinforce it (see Fig. 16-23C). Kapel (66) developed a cruciate ligament reconstruction in which distally based strips of the biceps and triceps tendon were passed through the distal humerus (see Fig. 16-23D). Beaty and Donati (79) modified this technique by transferring a central slip of the triceps through the humerus posterior to anterior and attaching it to the proximal ulna.

The most widely accepted technique is that described by Osborne and Cotterill (8), in which the lateral capsule is reattached to the posterolateral aspect of the capitellum with sutures passing through holes drilled in the bone (see Fig. 16-23E). The joint should be inspected at surgery because osteocartilaginous loose bodies may be present (63,68,73). Since Osborne and Cotterill's (8) initial report of eight patients, successful use of this technique has been reported in numerous others (34,63,68,72–74,76). Zeier (77) and O'Driscoll et al (72) reinforced the lateral repair with strips of fascia lata, triceps fascia, or palmaris longus tendon. Malkawi (68) transferred the ulnar nerve and reinforced the medial repair in a patient with ulnar neuropathy.

Posttreatment Care

Postoperatively, especially after the repair described by Osborne and Cotterill (8), the arm is immobilized in a long-arm cast with the elbow flexed 90 degrees for approximately 4 weeks. Active range of motion exercises are then begun.

Complications

Major complications after correction of recurrent dislocations include loose osteocartilaginous fragments and destruction of the articular surface of the joint (Fig. 16-24), elbow stiffness, or recurrent instability.

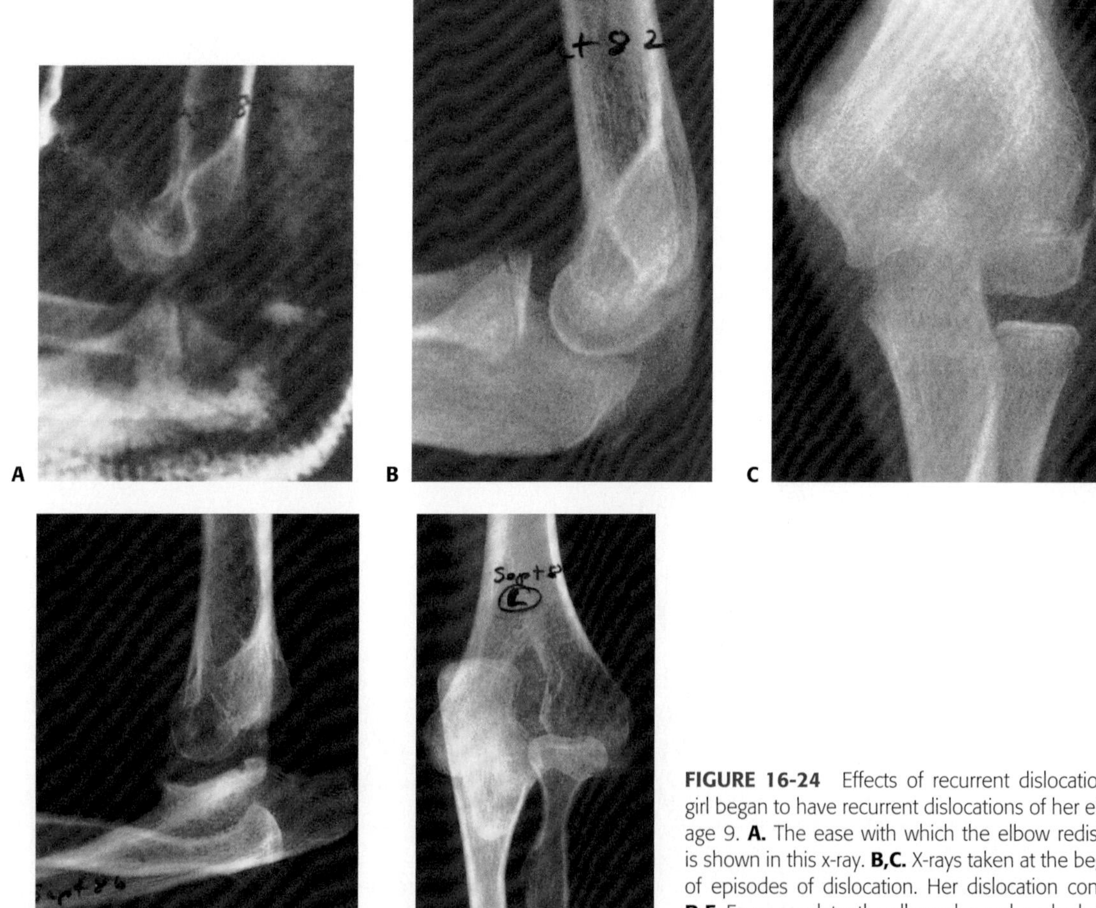

FIGURE 16-24 Effects of recurrent dislocation. This girl began to have recurrent dislocations of her elbow at age 9. **A.** The ease with which the elbow redislocates is shown in this x-ray. **B,C.** X-rays taken at the beginning of episodes of dislocation. Her dislocation continued. **D,E.** Four years later the elbow showed marked changes in its architecture. (Courtesy of David J. Mallams, MD.)

Unreduced Posterior Elbow Dislocations

Untreated posterior dislocations of the elbow in children are extremely rare in North America. Most reported series are from other countries (80–85).

Diagnosis

Children with untreated dislocations typically have pain and limited mid-range of motion (Fig. 16-25). Pathologically, there is subperiosteal new bone formation that produces a radiohumeral horn, myositis ossificans of the brachialis muscle, capsular contractures, shortening of the triceps muscle, contractures of the medial and lateral collateral ligaments, and tightening of the ulnar nerve (41,81,85). These factors have to be considered when planning treatment.

Treatment Options

Closed reduction of dislocations recognized within 3 weeks of injury may be possible (80,81). If this fails or if the dislocation is of longer duration, open reduction is necessary.

Surgical Procedures. Open reduction through a posterior approach, as described by Speed (86), involves lengthening of the triceps muscle and release or transposition of the ulnar nerve (81,84,85). Others have advocated posterolateral or medial and lateral incisions for better exposure (80,82). Satisfactory results usually can be obtained if a stable concentric reduction is achieved within 3 months of the initial dislocation (80,82). Results after surgical reconstruction decline thereafter but still may produce some improvement in function (81,84) (see Fig. 16-25). Fixation of the elbow joint to maintain reduction for 2 to 4 weeks followed by vigorous physical therapy has been recommended (81,84). Relatively large Kirschner wires or Steinmann pins may be used to stabilize the elbow and minimize the risk of intraarticular breakage.

Mahaisavariya et al (83) reported improved extension and better functional results in 34 patients with unreduced elbow dislocations 1 to 3 months after injury in whom the triceps tendon was not lengthened compared with 38 patients who had the triceps lengthened at surgery.

Congenital Elbow Dislocations

Chronic elbow dislocation may be congenital in origin. Altered anatomy and limited motion predispose these patients to injury. The key to differentiating a congenital from an acute traumatic elbow dislocation is examination of the radiographic architecture of the articulating surfaces. In a congenitally dislocated elbow, there is marked atrophy of the humeral condyles and the semilunar notch of the olecranon (Fig. 16-26). Unfortunately, these same changes can result from chronic recurrent dislocation after trauma, making the differentiation between congenital and chronic traumatic dislocation difficult. Certainly,

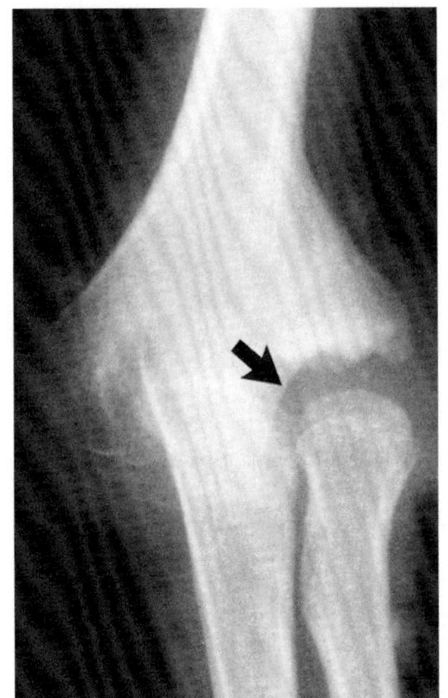

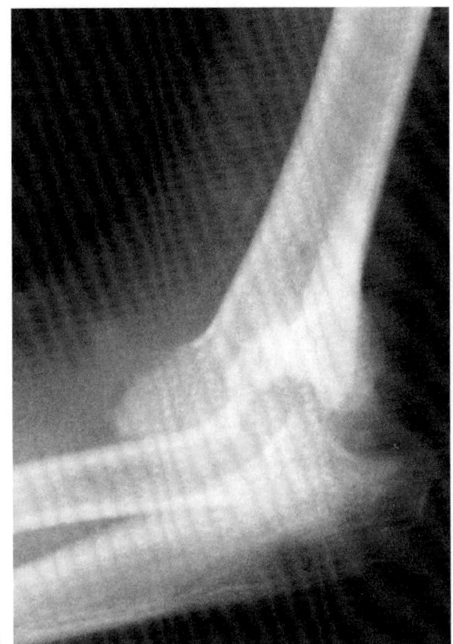

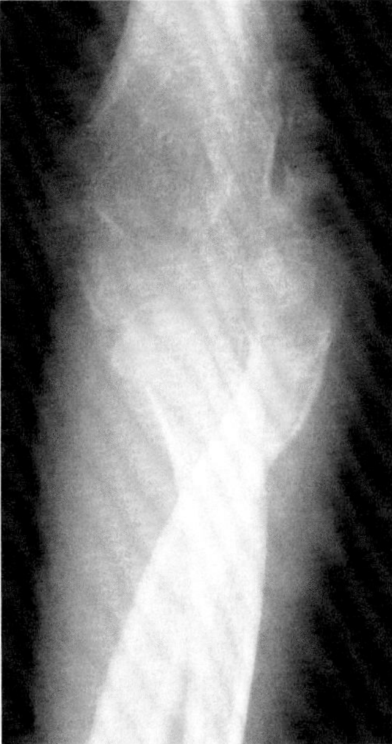

FIGURE 16-25 Unreduced dislocation. **A.** Preoperative AP x-ray. The elbow sustained an injury 3 years before surgery. Elbow motion was extremely limited and painful. The lateral supracondylar ridge had been eroded by the radial head (*arrow*). **B.** Lateral x-ray. The posterior position of the olecranon is apparent. **C.** AP x-ray 3 months postoperatively. Total elbow motion was 30 degrees, but there was less pain and more stability.

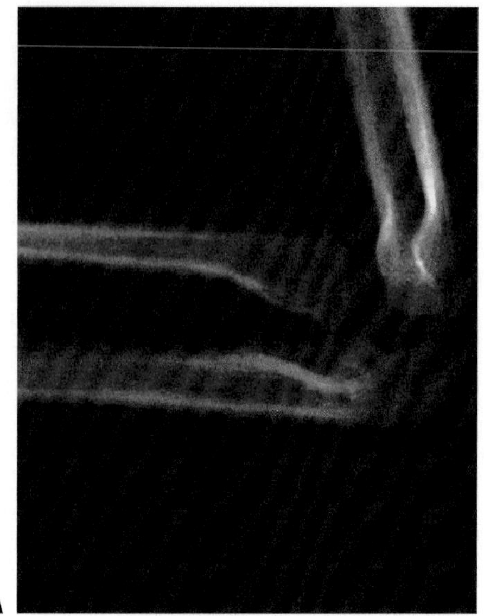

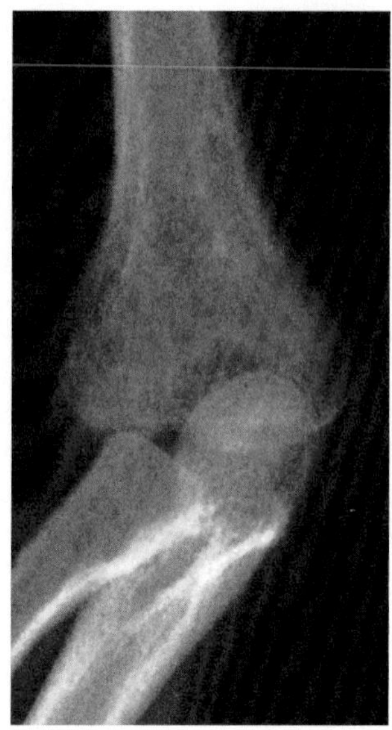

FIGURE 16-26 Lateral **(A)** and AP **(B)** x-rays of an elbow with congenital dislocation. The patient had sustained a minor injury. The fact that similar findings were seen in the opposite uninjured elbow confirms the congenital origin. (Courtesy of Earl A. Staple, MD.)

if other congenital anomalies are present or the child has an underlying syndrome, such as Ehlers-Danlos or Larsen's syndrome, the dislocation is likely to be congenital.

Posteromedial Dislocation

Posteromedial elbow dislocations are rare. One patient described by Wilkins et al (87) developed a recurrent dislocation. This 12-year-old boy had trochlear hypoplasia secondary to a very distal supracondylar fracture (Fig. 16-27). It was believed that hypoplasia of the trochlea contributed to the instability of the medial aspect of his elbow joint, predisposing him to recurrent dislocations. With time and continued follow-up, he subsequently became asymptomatic.

ANTERIOR ELBOW DISLOCATIONS

Principles of Management

Anterior elbow dislocations are rare. Of the 317 elbows in the combined series (3–6), only 5 were anterior, for an incidence of slightly over 1%. They are associated with an increased incidence of complications, such as brachial artery disruption and associated fractures, compared with posterior dislocations (88–93).

Mechanism of Injury

Anterior elbow dislocations usually are caused by a direct blow to the posterior aspect of the flexed elbow (89,93). Hyperextension of the elbow also has been implicated in one study (92). Twisting of the forearm on the elbow commonly occurs.

Signs and Symptoms

The elbow is in extension. There is a fullness in the antecubital fossa. Swelling usually is marked because of the soft tissue disruption associated with this type of dislocation. There is severe pain with attempted motion. A careful neurovascular examination is mandatory.

Radiographic and Other Imaging Studies

Routine AP and lateral x-rays are diagnostic. In most cases, the proximal radius and ulna dislocate in an anteromedial direction (Fig. 16-28). Associated fractures are common. In children, the triceps insertion may be avulsed from the olecranon with a small piece of cortical bone (93). This fragment usually reduced to the olecranon after reduction. Wilkerson (92) reported an anterior dislocation associated with a displaced olecranon fracture in a 7-year-old boy. Inoue and Horii (89) reported an 11-year-old girl with an anterior elbow dislocation with displaced fractures of the trochlea, capitellum, and lateral epicondyle. These were repaired with open reduction and internal fixation using Herbert bone screws.

Treatment Options

Closed Reduction

Reduction usually is accomplished by flexing the elbow and pushing the forearm proximally and downward at the same time (93). As with posterior dislocations, a force must first be applied longitudinally along the axis of the humerus with the elbow semiflexed to overcome the forces of the biceps and triceps. The longitudinal force along the axis of the forearm is directed toward the elbow (Fig. 16-29). To make reduction easier, the distal humerus can be forced in an anterior direction by pushing on the posterior aspect of the distal arm.

Surgical Procedures

Surgery usually is not required unless the dislocation is open, the brachial artery injury is present, or there is an associated

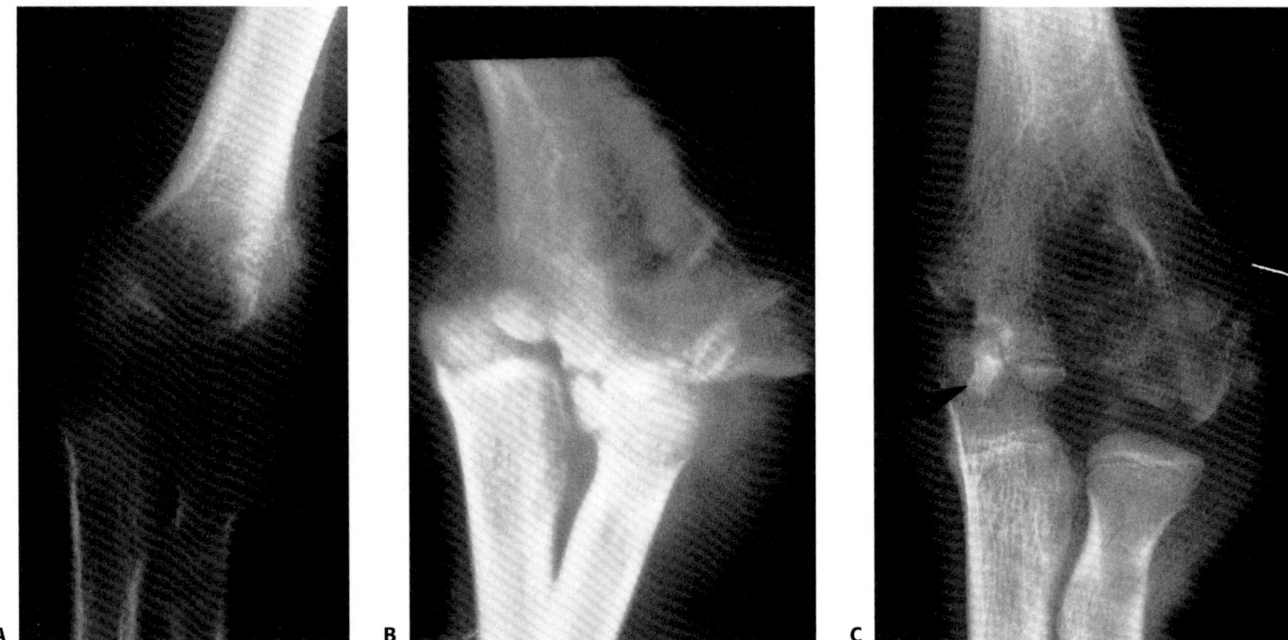

FIGURE 16-27 Posteromedial dislocation. **A.** At 6 years of age, this boy sustained what was thought to be a simple undisplaced but very distal supracondylar fracture. This x-ray taken 4 weeks after injury shows periosteal new bone formation along both supracondylar columns (*arrow*). **B.** Four years later, he began sustaining recurrent posteromedial dislocations. **C.** Reduction shows delayed development of the medial ossification center of the crista (*arrow*). It was thought that this hypoplastic trochlea contributed to his elbow instability. (Courtesy of Stephen A. Cord, MD.)

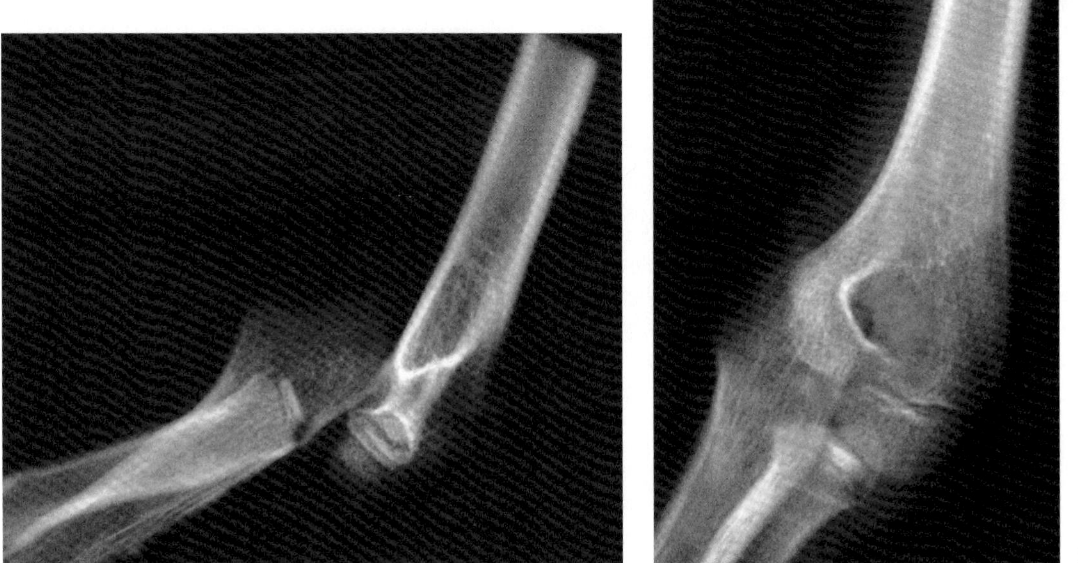

FIGURE 16-28 Anterior dislocation of the elbow. **A.** Initial AP x-ray. The olecranon lies anterior to the distal humerus. **B.** Initial lateral x-ray. The proximal ulna and radial head lie anteromedial, and the elbow carrying angle is in varus. (Courtesy of Hilario Trevino, MD.)

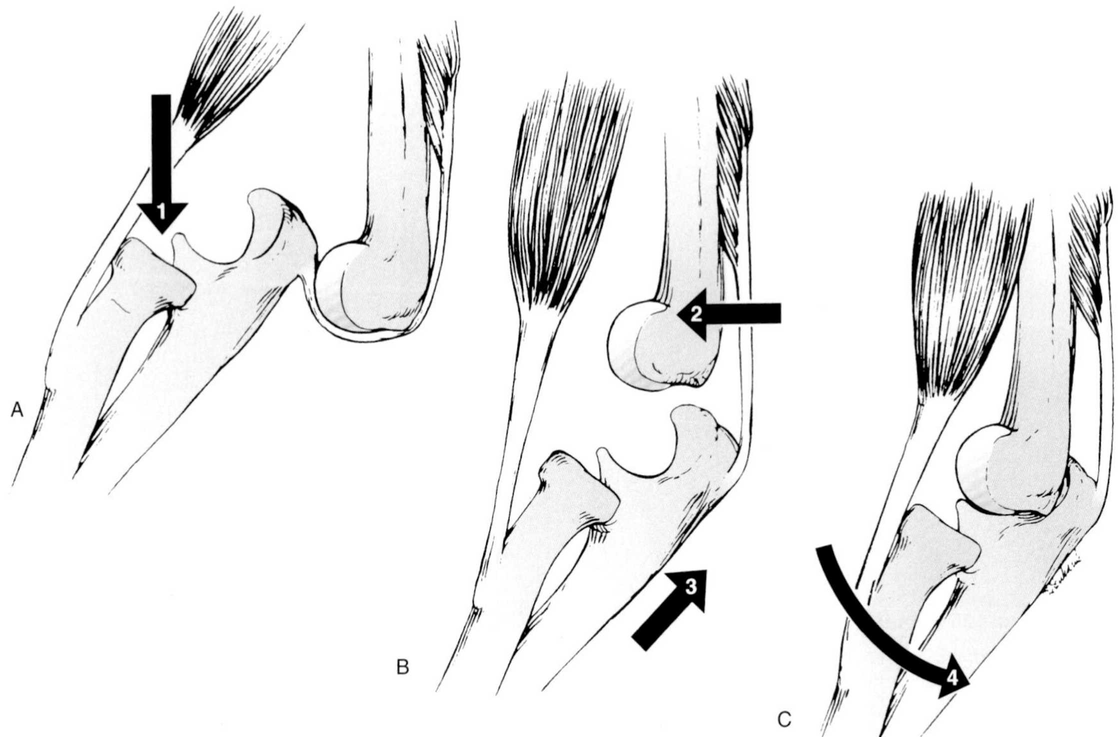

FIGURE 16-29 Reduction of anterior dislocation. **A.** With the elbow semiflexed, a longitudinal force is applied along the long axis of the humerus (*arrow 1*). Pulling distally on the forearm may be necessary to initially dislodge the olecranon. **B.** Once the olecranon is distal to the humerus, the distal humerus is pushed anteriorly (*arrow 2*) while a proximally directed force is applied along the long axis of the forearm (*arrow 3*). **C.** Finally, the elbow is immobilized in some extension (*arrow 4*).

fracture that does not realign satisfactorily after closed reduction. Open reduction and internal fixation of the fracture may then be necessary (89,92).

Postreduction Care

Because most anterior dislocations occur in flexion, the elbow should be immobilized in some extension for 2 to 3 weeks, followed by active range-of-motion exercises. Early motion after open reduction and internal fixation of an associated olecranon fracture usually can be allowed (89,92).

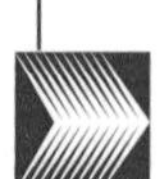

AUTHORS' PREFERRED TREATMENT

Closed reduction (see Fig. 16-29) is the initial procedure of choice. A distal force must be applied in line with and parallel to the long axis of the humerus first. Once the length has been reestablished, a posteriorly directed force along the axis of the forearm is applied until the elbow is reduced.

Complications

There appears to be an increased incidence of brachial artery rupture or thrombosis associated with anterior elbow dislocations (90,91). When present, prompt arterial repair is necessary.

MEDIAL AND LATERAL ELBOW DISLOCATIONS

These are rare dislocations. Lateral dislocations, either incomplete or complete, are more common than medial dislocations. There are no recent reports of medial dislocations in children.

Signs and Symptoms

In an incomplete lateral dislocation, the semilunar notch articulates with the capitellotrochlear groove and the radial head appears more prominent laterally. There is often good flexion and extension of the elbow, increasing the likelihood that a lateral dislocation will be overlooked. In a complete lateral dislocation, the olecranon is displaced lateral to the capitellum. This gives the elbow a markedly widened appearance.

Radiographic and Other Imaging Studies

AP x-rays of the elbow usually are diagnostic. On the lateral view the elbow may appear reduced.

Treatment Options

These rare dislocations are treated by closed reduction. A longitudinal force is applied along the axis of the humerus to distract the elbow, and then direct medial or lateral pressure (opposite the direction of the dislocation) is applied over the proximal forearm (Fig. 16-30).

DIVERGENT ELBOW DISLOCATION

Divergent dislocation represents a posterior elbow dislocation with disruption of the interosseous membrane between the

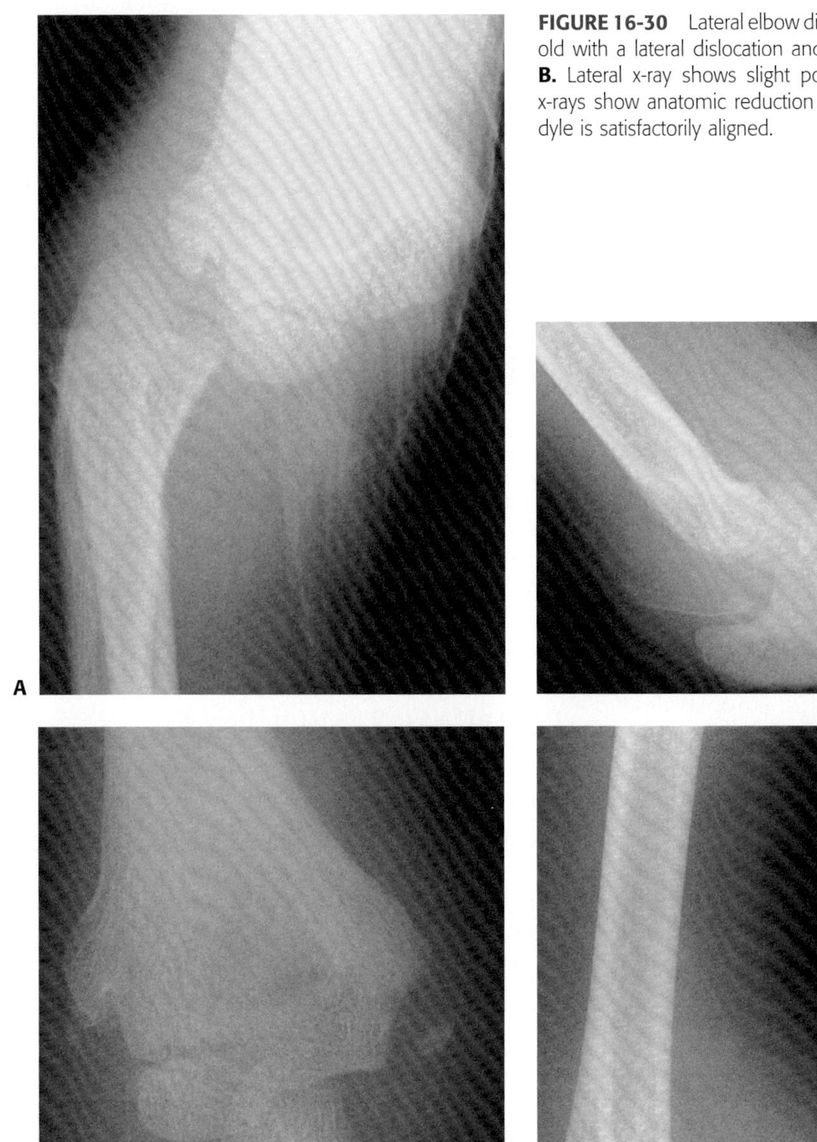

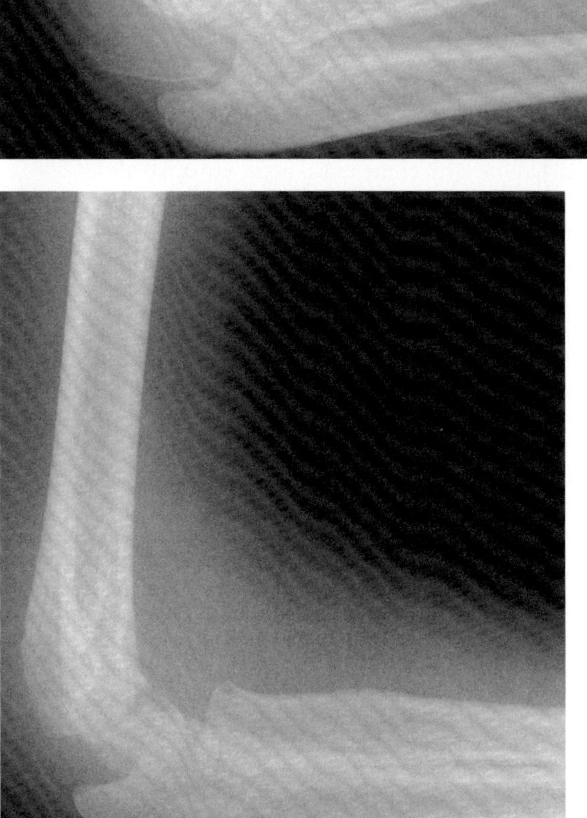

FIGURE 16-30 Lateral elbow dislocation. **A.** Initial AP x-ray in this 6-year-old with a lateral dislocation and displaced medial epicondyle fracture. **B.** Lateral x-ray shows slight posterior dislocation. **C,D.** Postreduction x-rays show anatomic reduction of the dislocation. The medial epicondyle is satisfactorily aligned.

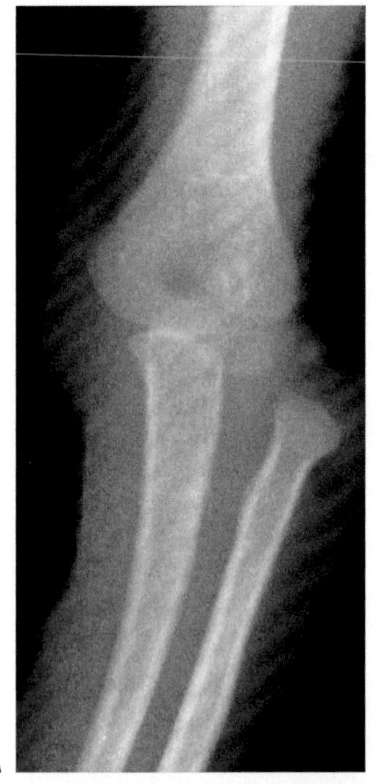

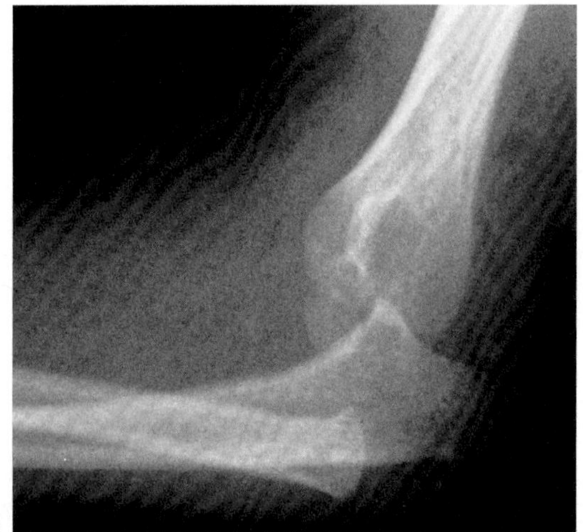

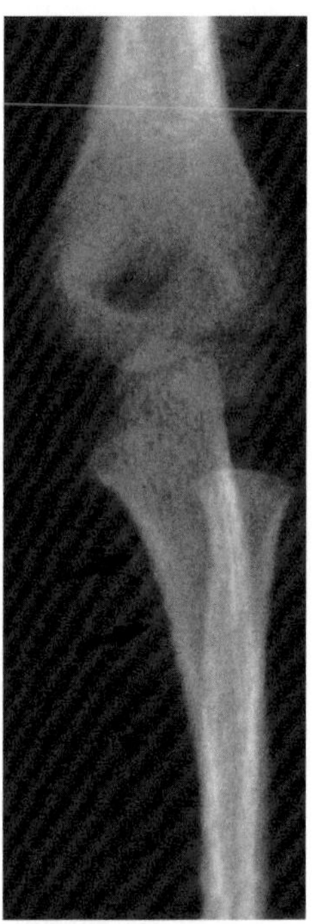

FIGURE 16-31 Medial-lateral divergent dislocation. **A.** AP view showing disruption of the proximal radioulnar joint with the radius lateral and the ulna medial. **B.** Lateral x-ray confirms that the radius and ulna are both posterior to the distal humerus. **C.** An x-ray taken 4 weeks after injury shows periosteal new bone formation (*arrows*), indicating where the soft tissues were extensively torn away from the proximal ulna.

proximal radius and ulna with the radial head displaced laterally and the proximal ulna medially (Fig. 16-31). These dislocations are extremely rare (29,94–103).

Divergent dislocations usually are caused by high-energy trauma. Associated fractures of the radial neck, proximal ulna, and coronoid process are common (95,97,103). It has been speculated that, in addition to the hyperextension of the elbow that produces the dislocation, a strong proximally directed force is applied parallel to the long axis of the forearm, disrupting the annular ligament and interosseous membrane and allowing the divergence of the proximal radius and ulna.

Treatment Options

Closed Reduction

Divergent dislocations are typically easily closed reduced under general anesthesia. Reduction is achieved by applying longitudinal traction with the elbow semiextended and at the same time compressing the proximal radius and ulna together.

Open Reduction

This is rarely indicated. There have been only two divergent dislocations reported that required open reduction (97,100). Closed reduction failed in one child (100), and the other had a displaced fracture of the proximal ulna (97).

Postreduction Care

After successful closed reduction, the elbow is immobilized in 90 degrees of flexion and the forearm in neutral for approximately 2 to 3 weeks. Active range-of-motion exercises are then begun. Most patients typically regain full elbow motion, including forearm pronation and supination.

PROXIMAL RADIOULNAR TRANSLOCATION

Principles of Management

Translocation of the proximal radius and ulna is extremely rare injury, with fewer than 10 cases reported in the English literature (95,104–109). Radioulnar translocation is commonly missed on the AP x-ray unless the proximal radius and ulna are noted to be completely reversed in relation to the distal humerus.

Mechanism of Injury

Translocations are believed to be caused by a fall onto the pronated hand with the elbow in full or nearly full extension, producing an axial force on the proximal radius. The anterior radial head dislocation occurs first, followed by the posterior dislocation of the olecranon. The radial head, depending on the degree of pronation, can be lodged in the coronoid fossa or dislocated posteriorly. As a consequence, fractures of the radial head, radial neck, or coronoid process may occur (95,104,105,109). Harvey reported a case in which the cause of radioulnar translocation may have been iatrogenic, the result of inappropriate technique used to reduce a posterior elbow dislocation (107).

Signs and Symptoms

Swelling and pain may obscure the initial examination, and minimal deformity may be apparent. Once pain has adequately been managed with analgesics, the most consistent finding on clinical examination is limited elbow range of motion, especially in supination.

Associated Injuries

Radial neck fracture is the most common fracture associated with proximal radioulnar translocation (104,105,108,109). Eklof also reported one patient who sustained a fracture of the tip of the coronoid (105). Proposed soft tissue injuries include radial collateral ligament, medial collateral ligament, annular ligament, and interosseous ligament injury (105,108). Isbister described transient ulnar nerve paresthesia, which resolved after reduction of the translocation (108). Osteonecrosis of the radial head was noted in one case after open reduction of proximal radioulnar translocation (107).

Rationale

There are no long-term follow-up reports of the natural history of untreated proximal radioulnar translocation, but in several of the reported cases a delay in diagnosis and treatment did occur. In each case, delayed treatment resulted in pain and limited motion until reduction of the elbow was achieved. Even after elbow relocation, initial delay in diagnosis resulted in a greater likelihood that elbow stiffness would persist (105,107). This information suggests that proximal radioulnar elbow translocation should be reduced promptly.

Diagnosis and Classification

The diagnosis of radioulnar translocation is frequently missed or delayed (105,106). Lack of supination is the most consistent physical examination finding. Elbow x-rays are often initially interpreted as normal; the carrying angle is often acceptable and the radius and ulna appear to align properly with the humerus. More careful inspection shows that the bones of the forearm are transposed, with the radius aligning with the trochlea and the ulna aligning with the capitellum. Remembering the constant rule that the radial head must align with the capitellum on all views can prevent missing this diagnosis.

Current Treatment Options

Nonoperative Treatment: Closed Reduction

Successful closed reduction of proximal radioulnar translocation has been reported (108,109). The patient must be completely relaxed under general anesthesia; sedation or regional anesthesia is unlikely to provide sufficient relaxation. With the elbow flexed approximately 90 degrees, longitudinal traction is applied to the elbow while the forearm is supinated (Fig. 16-32). If the radial head can be palpated, gentle anterior-directed pressure may help slide the radial head and neck over the coronoid process, allowing the proximal radius and ulna to resume their normal configuration. As always, just the right amount of force should be used; excessive force risks iatrogenic fracture to the proximal radius. Successful closed reduction should be confirmed radiographically and the elbow immobilized for approximately 3 weeks with the forearm supinated and the elbow flexed 90 to 100 degrees.

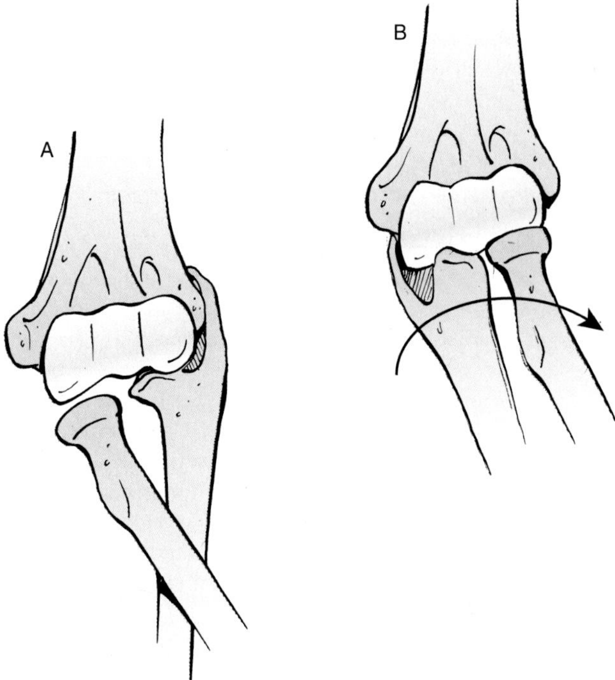

FIGURE 16-32 Proximal radioulnar translocation. **A.** Position of the proximal radius and ulna with a proximal radioulnar translocation. **B.** Closed reduction is rarely successful but may be attempted under general anesthesia using gentle longitudinal traction while supinating the forearm. (Redrawn from Harvey S, Tchelebi H. Proximal radio-ulnar translocation. *J Bone Joint Surg [Am]* 1979;61:447–449; with permission.)

Surgical Treatment: Open Reduction

Most reported radioulnar translocations have required open reduction (95,104–108). A lateral approach provides adequate exposure to the translocation and radial neck fracture if present. At surgery the radial head and neck is typically found trapped beneath the trochlea of the distal humerus. Elbow extension tightens the biceps tendon, making reduction more difficult. With the elbow flexed a Freer or Joker elevator may be placed beneath the radial head and neck, facilitating delivery over the coronoid process as the forearm is supinated. If present, the radial neck fracture may now be treated on its own merits. Internal fixation also may be necessary for an unstable displaced fracture.

Harvey and Tchelebi (107) used an osteotomy of the proximal ulna to expose and reduce the radius, which was complicated by a postoperative ulnar nerve paralysis that recovered completely over 2 months.

After successful closed or open reduction, the forearm is

immobilized for approximately 3 weeks with the forearm supinated and the elbow flexed 90 to 100 degrees, followed by an active elbow range-of-motion exercises.

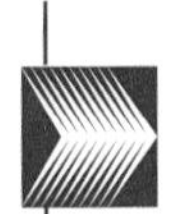

AUTHORS' PREFERRED TREATMENT: PROXIMAL RADIOULNAR TRANSLOCATION

Closed Versus Open Reduction

Within 24 hours of injury, before swelling and contracture impede reduction, the patient is brought to the operating room, where as little as possible but as much as necessary is done to obtain and maintain a stable reduction of the elbow. With the patient completely relaxed under general anesthesia and pharmacologic paralysis, closed reduction is attempted by applying longitudinal traction to the flexed elbow while the forearm is gently but firmly supinated. If the radial head can be palpated, gentle anterior-directed pressure may help slide the radial head and neck over the coronoid process, allowing the proximal radius and ulna to resume their normal configuration.

If closed reduction cannot be achieved, then open reduction is performed through a lateral approach as described above. Once closed or open reduction is achieved, stability of the elbow is assessed. The elbow is immobilized in the position of maximum stability, which typically involves flexion of 90 to 100 degrees and forearm supination. If the elbow remains unstable, radiocapitellar pin placement may be considered. A pin of adequate size must be selected and the elbow immobilized the entire time the pin is in place (typically 3 weeks) to avoid pin breakage. Annular ligament reconstruction or ulnar osteotomy has not been necessary but might be considered if a stable reduction cannot be achieved by other means.

Pearls and Pitfalls

Closed reduction should be performed under general anesthesia with complete paralysis to provide optimal conditions for success. Excessive force must be avoided to prevent iatrogenic radial neck fracture.

RADIAL HEAD DISLOCATION

Principles of Management

Isolated traumatic dislocation of the radial head is not common but not rare and is frequently missed on initial evaluation. Case reports (110–116) as well as small series have been reported (116–129).

The most common age for patients to sustain this injury is approximately 7 years, and the most common direction for radial head dislocation is anterior. Vesely (127) combined the experience of the members of the Association of Bone and Joint Surgeons to accumulate 17 dislocations; 13 were anterior, 3 were lateral, and 1 was posterior. Often patients with radial head dislocation have minimal pain and reasonable function but are most affected by increasing deformity and decreasing motion, therefore warranting treatment.

Mechanism of Injury

The most common mechanism of injury involves a fall onto an outstretched arm with the forearm pronated and the elbow near full extension, and often with additional varus strain applied to the elbow (119). Wiley et al (128) found in cadaver studies that anterior dislocations of the radial head could be produced only with great force. Dislocation required complete division of the anterior capsule and annular ligament, pronation, and application of an anterior force to the posterior aspect of the radial head. Tearing of the interosseous membrane sometimes occurred before the dislocation could be achieved.

Isolated radial head dislocations are variants of Monteggia lesions (118–121,130,131). (The mechanisms of injury of the various Monteggia lesions are discussed in Chapter 12.) Often, if the patient and the x-rays are carefully examined, an occult fracture of the olecranon or proximal ulna is discovered (120,122,132). The fracture may not be apparent until bowing of the proximal ulna or olecranon is noticed during the healing phase (118).

Lincoln and Mubarak (121) reviewed isolated anterior radial head dislocations in which there was no overt evidence of a fracture of the ulna. In each, there was subtle anterior bowing of the shaft of the ulna. They described this as the "ulnar bow sign." Normally the dorsal margin of the ulna is a straight line (Fig. 16-33). Based on their findings, they suggested that the

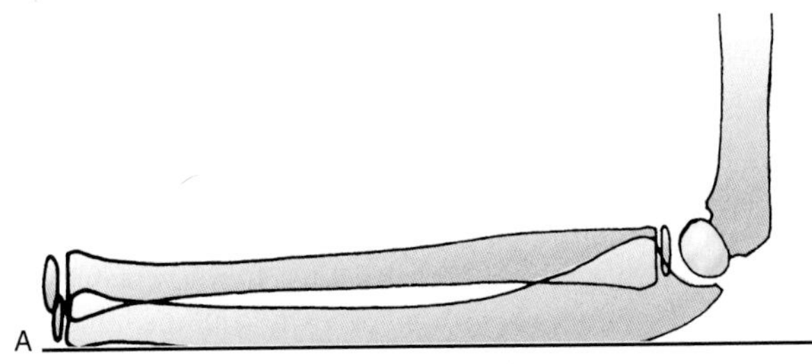

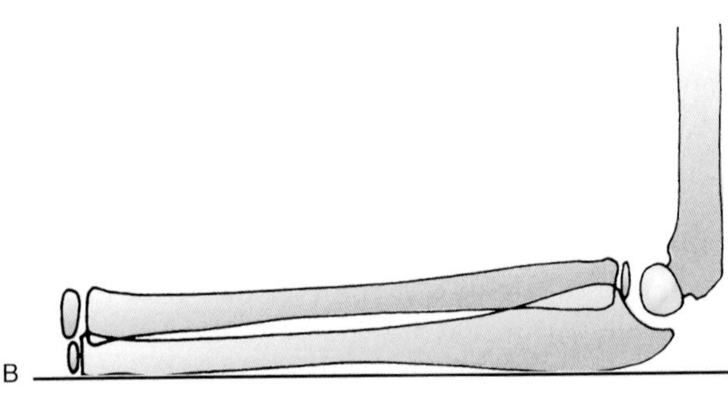

FIGURE 16-33 Ulnar bow sign. **A.** The normal posterior border of the ulna is represented by a straight line. **B.** In minimal type I Monteggia lesions, there is loss of this ulnar straight line with anterior bowing of the posterior border of the ulna and complete dislocation or partial subluxation of the radial head anteriorly. (Reprinted from Lincoln TL, Mubarak SH. "Isolated" traumatic radial-head dislocation. *J Pediatr Orthop* 1994;14: 455; with permission.)

term *isolated radial head dislocation* was a misnomer and that these be considered type I Monteggia injuries. The mechanism creating an isolated dislocation of the radial head appears to be the same as in Monteggia lesions (119–121,124,130).

Elbow hyperextension with the forearm fully supinated has also been proposed as a less common mechanism for radial head dislocation. Stanley reported a case in which an extreme degree of hyperextension was demonstrated in a 12-year-old with an isolated radial head dislocation (115). He believed ligamentous laxity contributed significantly to the etiology. Ligamentous laxity has not been mentioned by other investigators, but most radial head dislocations occur at approximately 7 years of age, when physiologic ligamentous laxity is at its peak.

Weisman et al recently described tardy displacement of traumatic radial head dislocation in two cases where the radial head was located on initial x-rays and dislocation occurred subsequently (133). The proposed explanation was that the radial head dislocated at the time of impact, spontaneously reduced by the time the first x-rays were obtained, and redislocated while the arm was in a cast. Careful radiographic assessment of the radiocapitellar joint using the radiocapitellar line is required in children with elbow and forearm injuries at presentation and when the cast is removed to detect delayed displacement of traumatic radial head dislocation. Delayed radial head dislocation as a late sequela of trauma has been described as well. Vocke-Hell et al reported five cases in which posttraumatic dysplasia of the distal humerus occurred, followed by secondary radial head overgrowth and dislocation (134).

Signs and Symptoms

After acute trauma the elbow is typically swollen, motion is limited, the radial head may or may not be palpable, and radial head dislocation may be impossible to distinguish clinically from other traumatic elbow injury. In a chronic dislocation, the radial head usually is palpable and there is a lack of full flexion and extension. Pronation often is full, while supination is limited (119). The carrying angle may be increased, resulting in visible deformity (135). Patients may also experience the sensation of instability or weakness when performing activities such as push-ups. Eventually the elbow may become painful as degenerative changes occur.

Associated Injuries

As noted above, plastic deformity of the ulna commonly accompanies apparent isolated radial head dislocation. Five of 22 patients treated by Horii et al had radial or ulnar nerve neuropraxia associated with radial head dislocation (136).

Rationale

Although there is consensus that an acute radial head dislocation should be reduced, there is controversy regarding reduction of a chronic radial head dislocation. Kadic and Bloem reported a case of minimal elbow dysfunction 32 years after a dislocation of a radial head that was not treated (137). On the other hand, Lloyd-Roberts and Bucknill reported a case of untreated radial head dislocation 50 years after injury in which the patient developed limited elbow motion from 80 to 100 degrees of flexion, restricted pronation and supination, and an unstable valgus deformity of 30 degrees (122).

Elbow joint stability depends on joint congruity, and reduction of the radial head is very important for normal elbow function. Chronic radial head dislocation may lead to increasing valgus deformity of the elbow with subsequent ulnar or radial nerve disfunction, restriction of flexion due to obstruction by the radial head, and consequent loss of function due to a combination of stiffness and instability. The longer the time interval between injury and radial head reduction, the greater symptoms patients are likely to experience and the more severe the pathologic changes preventing stable reduction (135). All considered, despite the risk of complications, relocation of the radial head is now recommended for most active patients as soon as possible to limit growth deformity and soft tissue contracture (136).

Diagnosis and Classification

Traumatic. As described above, the most common cause of radial head dislocation involves a fall onto an outstretched arm with the forearm pronated and the elbow near full extension, and often with additional varus strain applied to the elbow.

Congenital. It is important to be able to differentiate a congenital dislocation of the radial head that requires no treatment from an acute or chronic traumatically dislocated radial head that may benefit from treatment. Congenital dislocations are commonly bilateral, posterior, and associated with other anomalies, but some are idiopathic (138–142). Because of the lack of significant disability, the parents often are unaware that their child has a congenital radial head dislocation. If the child sustains an injury to the elbow with subsequent pain and swelling, accurate radiographic interpretation may be difficult.

Isolated traumatic dislocations of the radial head in newborns have been documented (110,111,114). This gives credence to the theory that some congenital dislocations may actually have a traumatic etiology that was unrecognized. Because most congenital dislocations are bilateral, it was initially thought that unilateral dislocations were probably traumatic in origin. Mardam-Bey and Ger (139) argued that if there were other congenital musculoskeletal abnormalities, if there was a positive family history of dislocated radial heads, or if the patient had bilateral dislocations, these were probably congenital in origin. Agnew and Davis (143) reported six patients with isolated unilateral dislocations in whom there had been no history of trauma and the presence of the dislocation had been recognized since early childhood. Thus, it may be difficult to determine definitively whether a long-standing unilateral radial head dislocation is congenital or traumatic in etiology.

There is also the question of congenital radial head subluxation. Southmayd and Ehrlich (144) reported three children with symptomatic subluxations of the radial head, two of whom had unilateral involvement. It was uncertain whether there was a relationship with congenital dislocation of the radial head. Similarly, Bell et al (145) reported congenital subluxations and dislocations of 34 elbows in 27 patients without other musculoskeletal anomalies; only 7 were bilateral.

Surgical reconstruction and relocation for congenital radial head dislocation remains controversial. For most patients with congenital radial head dislocation, their limited symptoms do not justify surgical relocation when considering the unpredictable results reported for this subgroup. However, there have been recent reports suggesting that surgical reconstruction may be indicated for select patients (146). Anterior radial head dislocation, unilateral dislocation, minimal dysplastic changes, and progressive elbow malalignment are factors that might influence the surgeon and family to consider relocation of a congenitally dislocated radial head. Interestingly, these same factors raise the question as to whether the dislocation is truly congenital or an early, undiagnosed traumatic dislocation.

Unusual Dislocation Patterns

Cubitus Varus. Cubitus varus after a supracondylar fracture of the distal humerus has been shown by Abe et al (147) to predispose to radial head dislocation. They described four dislocations that were chronic, recurrent, and precipitated by further injury. The radial head dislocated when the forearm was supinated and reduced when it was pronated. In addition to ligamentous repair, a supracondylar osteotomy was performed to correct the distal humerus deformity.

Osteochondritis Dissecans. Klekamp et al (148) reported seven older children and adolescents with osteochondritis dissecans of the capitellum who developed instability of the radial head: five subluxations and two posterolateral dislocations. Treatment was based on the presence of loose bodies and the characteristics of the osteochondral defect.

Birth Trauma. Birth trauma is an extremely rare mechanism of injury. Danielsson and Theander (111) reported an anterior dislocation, Schubert (114) an isolated anterolateral radial head dislocation, and Bayne and Rang (110) an anteromedial dislocation. Interestingly, all three infants were breech deliveries.

Imaging

Routine AP and lateral elbow x-rays typically show an isolated radial head dislocation, but distinguishing a traumatic from a congenital dislocation can be difficult. In a review of 50 patients with congenital dislocations of the radial head, Mardam-Bey and Ger (139) found the following radiographic characteristics in all their patients: relatively short ulna or long radius, hypoplastic or absent capitellum, partially defective trochlea, prominent medial epicondyle, dome-shaped radial head with long neck, and grooving of the distal humerus. Similar findings have been reported by McFarland (140) and Miura (141). Unfortunately, these same changes can be found in children with long-standing traumatic dislocations (Fig. 16-34) (118,138,149). When the radiographic findings described by Mardam-Bey and Ger (139) are seen, all that can be said with certainty is that the dislocation is long-standing.

Arthrograms have been advocated by Mizuno et al (123) in the differentiation of congenital and traumatic dislocations. Their differentiation was based on whether the radial head was intraarticular or extraarticular. If the radial head remained

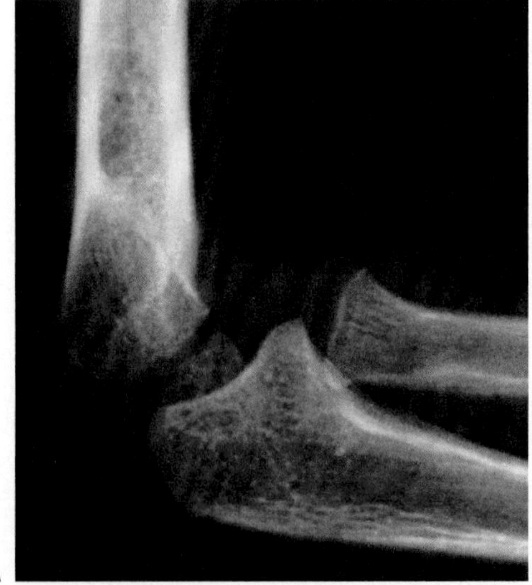
A

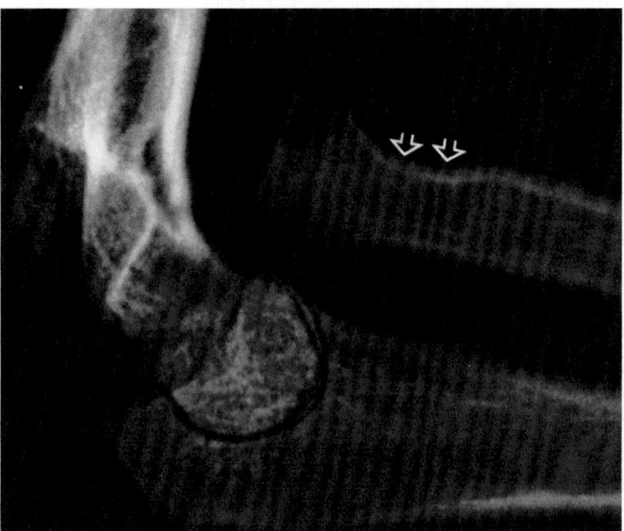
B

FIGURE 16-34 Progression of changes. **A.** Initial injury x-ray in a 5-year-old who sustained an acute minimally displaced anterior dislocation of the radial head. This dislocation was not appreciated initially. **B.** Three years later, the displacement had progressed and the radius had grown proximally. The radial neck also has become narrowed and elongated (*arrows*). These findings are similar to those described for a congenital dislocation of the radial head. (Courtesy of Charles T. Price, MD.)

within the intact but distended capsule, the dislocation was considered congenital. In 15 traumatic dislocations, the capsule was torn and the radial head was extraarticular.

Current Treatment Options

Nonoperative Treatment: Closed Reduction

A sound general philosophy to keep in mind when treating radial head dislocations is to do as little as possible but as much as necessary to obtain and maintain a stable reduction of the radiocapitellar joint. Most acute radial head dislocations can be satisfactorily treated by closed reduction and immobilization (116,119,126–129). With the patient adequately sedated or anesthetized, gentle longitudinal traction is applied while pressure is used to direct the radial head toward the radiocapitellar joint as the elbow is flexed and supinated. Once reduced, the elbow is examined while the patient is anesthetized to assess reduction stability. If the reduction is stable, the elbow is immobilized for 3 to 6 weeks in a safe position of greatest stability (116,119,126,127), most frequently with the elbow flexed 90 degrees or more and the forearm supinated (Fig. 16-35). Extreme flexion should be avoided to reduce the risk of neurovascular problems to the forearm; we recommend flexing the forearm just the right amount. Supination decreases the pull of the biceps muscle and creates tension in the interosseous membrane, which may contribute to radiocapitellar joint stability. Obtaining follow-up x-rays in the cast after 5 to 10 days is imperative to confirm that the radiocapitellar joint reduction is maintained in the cast. Closed reduction has not been successful when treatment is delayed greater than 3 weeks following injury.

Surgical Treatment

In the past it has been suggested that dislocations older than 1 month should be left alone and possibly treated by radial head excision if the elbow became symptomatic (126). More recently, it has been recognized that even chronic radial head dislocations can be significantly improved by surgical reconstruction. Therefore, if a stable reduction of a traumatic radial head dislocation cannot be achieved by closed means, open reduction should strongly be considered. The devil is in the details of determining for each patient the minimal intervention necessary to achieve a stable reduction, balancing the risk of recurrence against the increased surgical morbidity and complications.

Open Reduction. When closed reduction is unsuccessful, the orthopaedist must determine why a stable closed reduction cannot be achieved and with surgical treatment address all factors preventing stable reduction. Factors that may prevent stable radial head reduction include contracted and scarred annular ligament and joint capsule, loss of soft tissue stabilizers, angular deformity of the ulna, and relative ulnar shortening. In general, the longer time interval between dislocation and surgery, the more numerous and severe are the factors preventing radiocapitellar joint stability (146). A corollary is that the longer surgical relocation is delayed, the more extensive an operation may be necessary to achieve a successful result. Just how aggressive a procedure is necessary to ensure success is controversial and must be individualized for each patient, as is the question of whether there is a maximum acceptable time interval between dislocation and reconstructive surgery beyond which no surgery should be attempted.

Several authors recommend open reduction alone, without annular ligament repair, reconstruction, or osteotomy as an effective treatment for traumatic radial head dislocation (150–152). In De Boeck's series of four patients treated with open reduction, soft tissue debridement, and transcapitellar pinning, the average time from injury to surgery was 10 months, with a maximum of 21 months. Preoperative factors that may

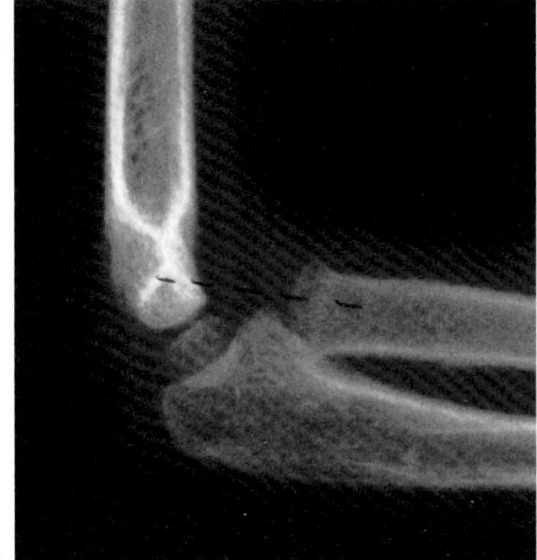

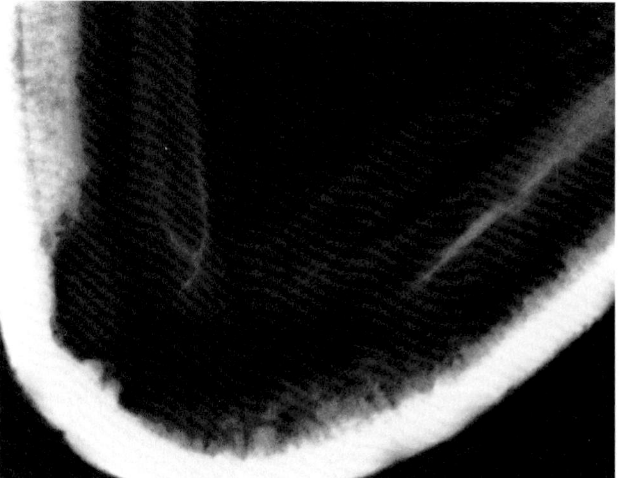

FIGURE 16-35 Closed reduction. **A.** Acute injury x-ray shows that the long axis of the radius (*dotted line*) passes proximal to the center of the capitellum, indicating a dislocation. **B.** After reduction, this relation has been reestablished and is maintained with the elbow immobilized in hyperflexion.

affect the outcome after surgery include increased carrying angle compared to the contralateral elbow, especially when associated with flexion contracture (146). It is unclear just how long after injury open reduction and pinning of radial head dislocation is effective, but in selected patients without significant associated forearm deformity this approach has been shown to be successful.

Annular Ligament Repair. There is little written about the results of annular ligament repair as a treatment for radial head dislocation. Cadaveric dissection and surgical treatment have shown that for radial head dislocation to occur, the annular ligament must tear or be avulsed from its ulnar attachment (128). For any hope of success, the annular ligament repair must be performed after acute injury because the ligament quickly contracts and becomes fibrous tissue interposed within the radiocapitellar joint.

Annular Ligament Reconstruction. For chronic radial head dislocations, more than open reduction and pinning is likely to be necessary to maintain a stable radiocapitellar joint. Bell Tawse popularized annular ligament reconstruction for the treatment of chronic radial head dislocation using a strip of triceps tendon, a technique that has subsequently been modified by others with good results (124,153–156). Seel and Peterson described an anatomic and physiologic annular ligament reconstruction method, reporting excellent results in patients treated as long as 7 years after traumatic dislocation (Figs. 16-36 and 16-37) (125). Their primary prerequisite for reconstruction was maintenance of a normal concave radial head articular surface, independent of the dislocation chronicity.

Ulnar Osteotomy. Ligament reconstruction alone may facilitate radial head stability when the alignment of the forearm is normal, but it is not sufficient when the forearm is malaligned (Fig. 16-38). In addition to open reduction and reconstruction of the annular ligament, osteotomy of the proximal ulna sometimes is necessary to achieve reduction of the radial head (117,118,124, 131,157). Bouyala et al (117) reported the use of this technique in 15 patients, including 9 with isolated dislocations of the radial head. There were no redislocations, and all had improved elbow motion. Their technique is essentially the same as that used for chronic Monteggia lesions (124,153–156).

McGuire and Myers (131) reported seven patients successfully treated with open reduction and ulnar osteotomy without annular ligament reconstruction. Since it is difficult to know the optimal position for the ulna, it is important to allow its position to be guided by the reduction of the radial head. Mc Guire and Myers contoured the ulnar plate until the radial head rotated against the capitellum during a full range of flexion, extension, pronation, and supination. All patients regained full elbow motion. It may be that correcting the ulnar deformity so as to redirect the radial head toward the capitellum is more important when trying to achieve radiocapitellar joint stability than annular ligament reconstruction. This is essentially what occurs when a Monteggia fracture is reduced closed. The annular ligament is torn but does not require reconstruction for stability.

In a chronic radial head dislocation, the ulna may be functionally short relative to the radius, and lengthening of the ulna may necessary to avoid excessive pressure on the radial head. Horii recommends an oblique osteotomy of the proximal ulna to facilitate lengthening (136). Iliac bone grafting of the osteot-

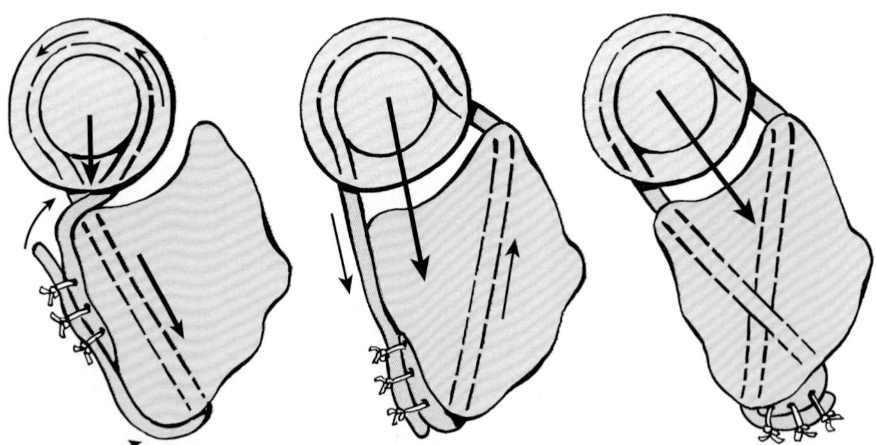

FIGURE 16-36 Drawings of transverse cuts of the proximal right radius and ulna (viewed from distally) at the level of the radial head. *Left:* Route of triceps tendon in Bell Tawse reconstruction. Direction of stability is posterior (*large arrow*). *Center:* Drill hole placed obliquely to exit the ulna at the site of medial annular ligament attachment. Direction of stability is posteromedial (*large arrow*). *Right:* Two drill holes exit the ulna at the sites of medial and lateral annular ligament attachments. Direction of stability is anatomic (*arrow*). (Reprinted from Seel MJ, Peterson HA. Management of chronic posttraumatic radial head dislocation in children. *J Pediatr Orthop* 1999;9:306–312, with permission.)

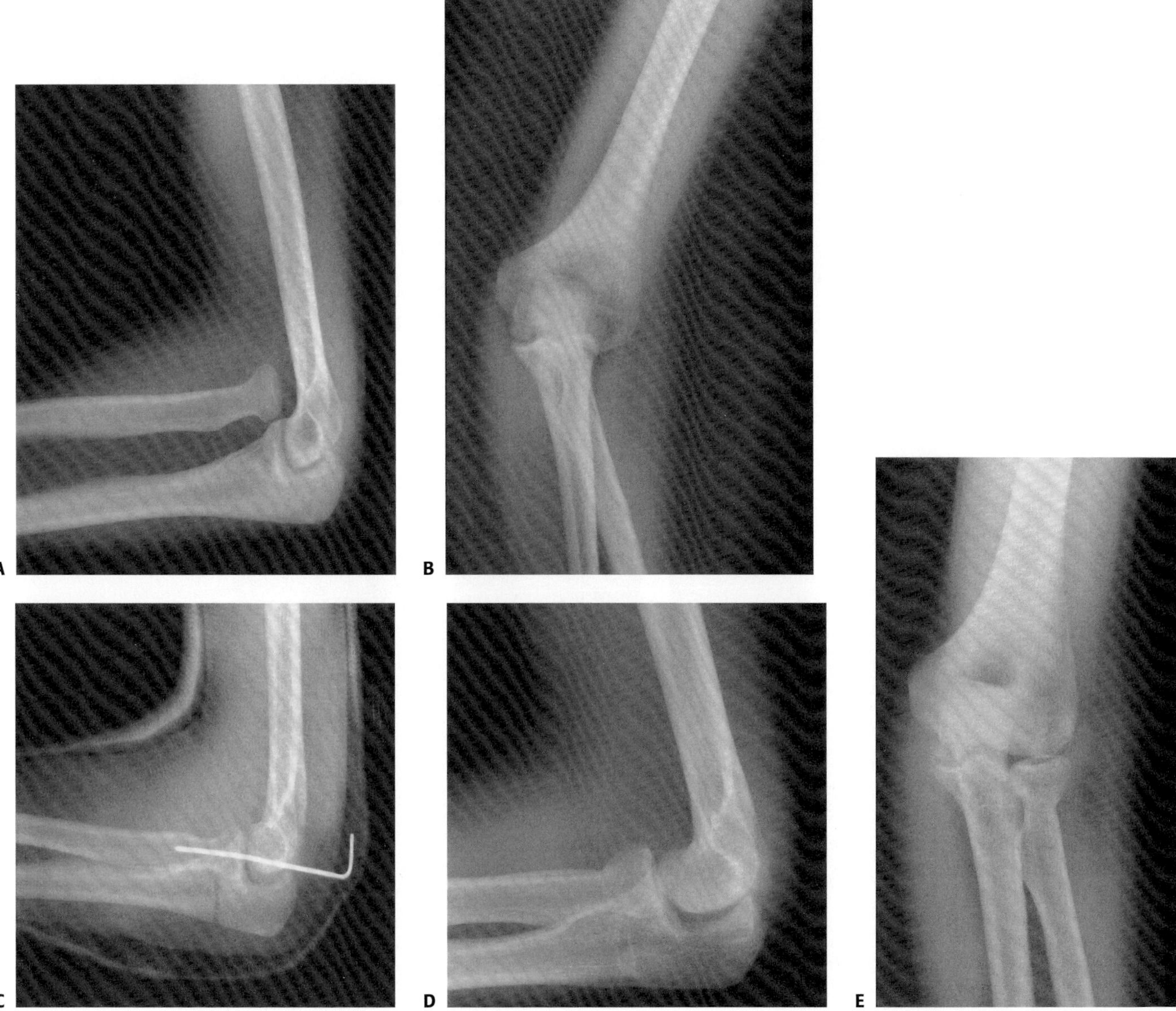

FIGURE 16-37 A,B. A 15-year-old boy had sustained a right elbow injury 5 years ago and presented with these x-rays, complaining of elbow stiffness and discomfort. **C.** Relocation of the radial head with reconstruction of the annular ligament as described by Seel and Peterson was performed. **D,E.** Two years postoperatively the patient has full, painless elbow motion.

omy was performed in some patients if necessary. Fixation of the ulnar osteotomy site with intramedullary Kirschner wires does not provide secure fixation of angular correction or lengthening osteotomy and has been associated with redislocation of the radial head. Rigid plate fixation preserves length and facilitates early elbow range of motion postoperatively. The osteotomy should be performed in the proximal ulnar metaphysis; osteotomy at the ulnar diaphysis middle of the ulnar shaft has been associated with a high incidence of treatment failure (136).

In type I Monteggia lesions, the shaft of the ulna is bowed anteriorly and the radial head is dislocated anteriorly. In type III Monteggia lesions, the proximal ulnar metaphysis or olecranon is bowed radially (laterally) and the radial head is dislocated anterolaterally. Late repair seems to be more successful when treating anterior dislocations than anterolateral dislocations (124).

Radial Osteotomy. Occasionally, when the radial head has been dislocated for a long time, there may be contracture of adjacent soft tissues, including the interosseous membrane and biceps tendon. This soft tissue contracture may cause significant proximal migration and overlap of the radius with the capi-

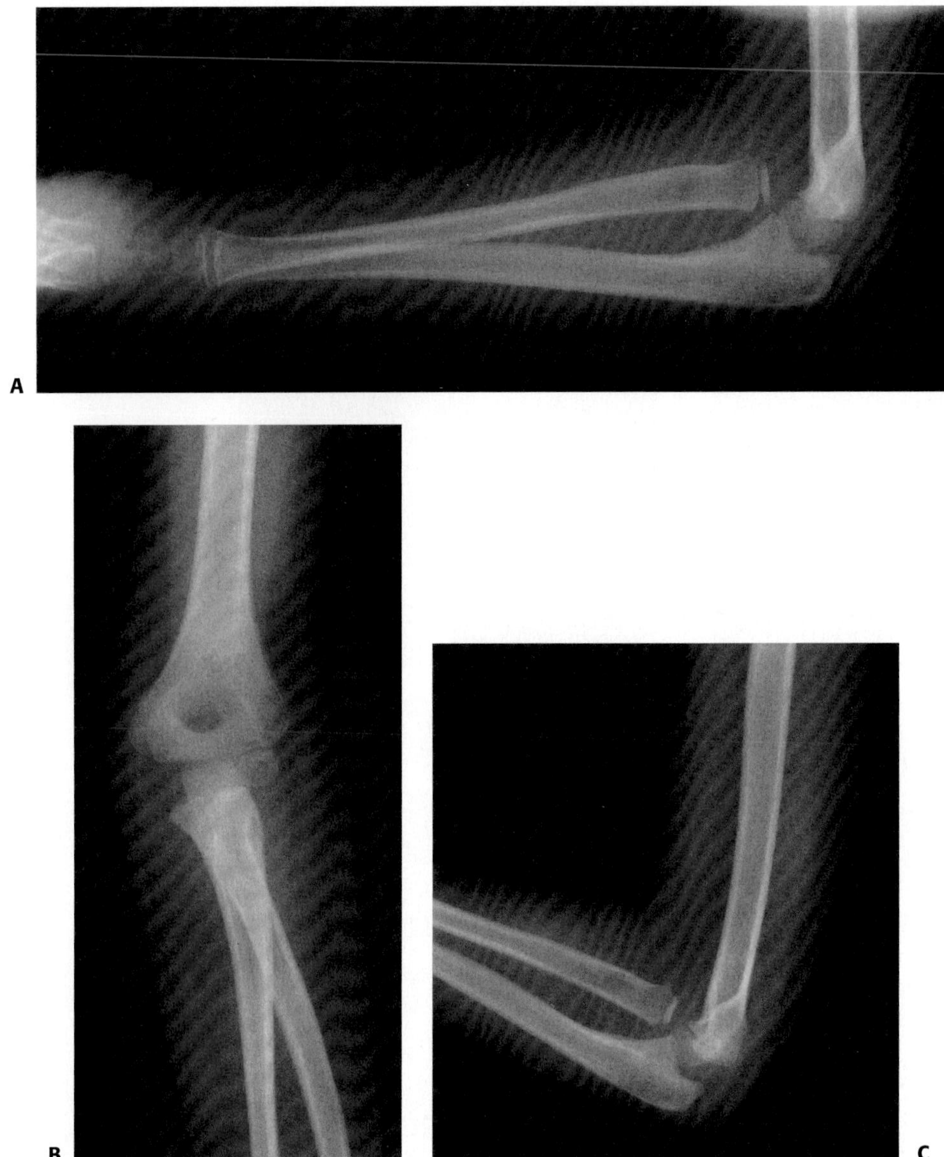

FIGURE 16-38 Missed radial head dislocation and anterior ulnar bow. **A,B.** This 7-year-old girl sustained an elbow injury on a trampoline. The radial head dislocation and ulnar bow were recognized 4 weeks after injury. Two unsuccessful surgical procedures were performed attempting to reduce the radial head. **C,D.** Four months after her injury the patient had a painful elbow with a 50-degree motion arc seen on maximum flexion and extension x-rays. (*continues*)

tellum, preventing radial head reduction. To address excessive radial length, a radial shaft shortening osteotomy can be performed through a separate midshaft incision, reducing the tension in the soft tissues and reducing pressure on the radial head (135). The amount of radial shortening corresponding to the length of radius protruding beyond the ulna coronoid process can be measured on preoperative x-rays to give the surgeon an estimate of the amount of radial shortening necessary. The final amount of shortening is determined by intraoperative assessment of radial head stability. Shortening of approximately 1.0 cm is often adequate to reduce compressive forces. A rotational adjustment to the radial osteotomy can be made if the radial head is severely deformed and associated radial neck angular deformity (exaggerated neck–shaft angle) is contributing to instability.

If the radial head dislocation is anterior and can be reduced

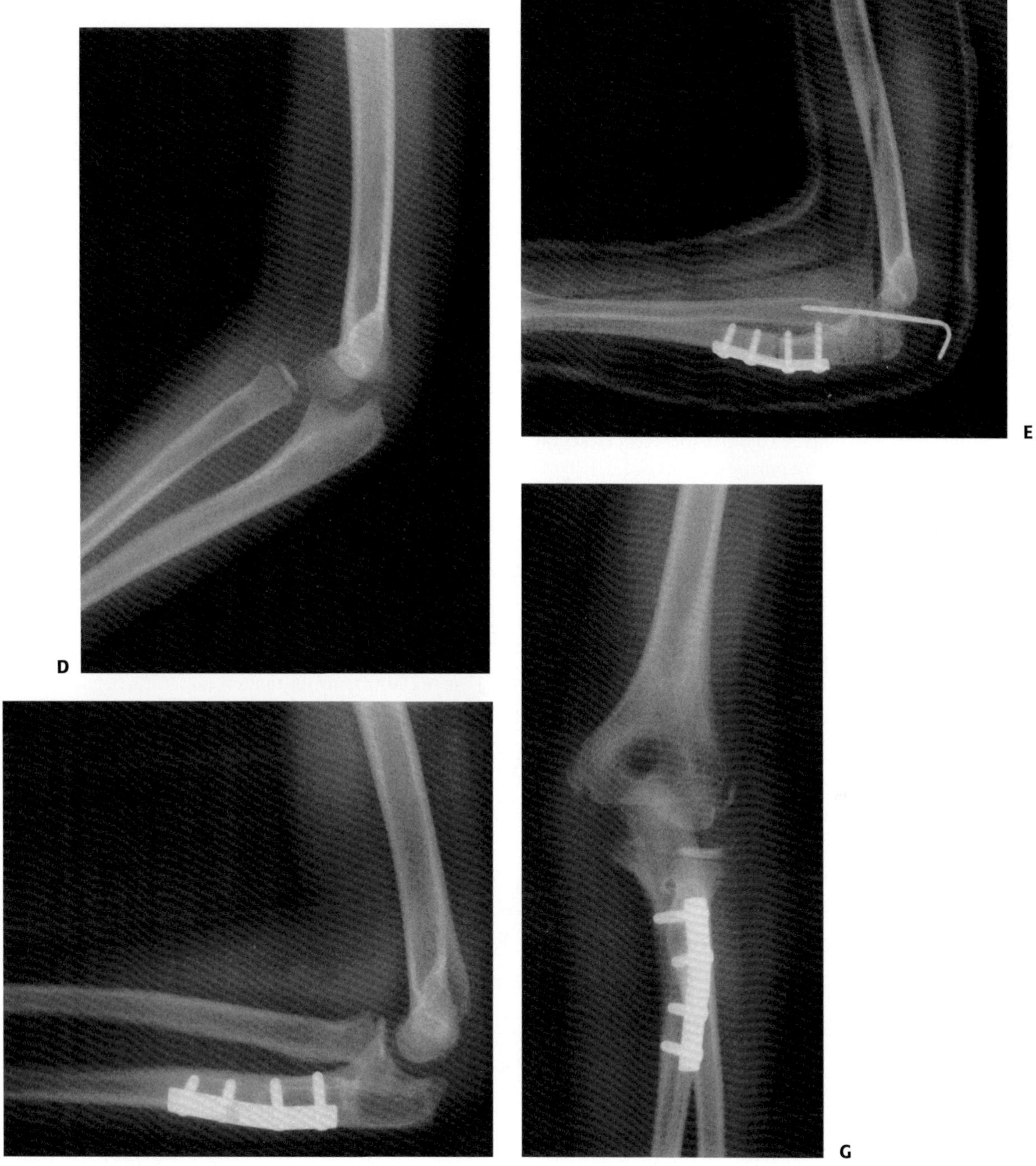

FIGURE 16-38 (*continued*) **E.** Excision of interposed soft tissue, reduction and pinning of radiocapitellar joint, and reconstruction of annular ligament as described by Seel and Peterson, with plating of proximal ulnar osteotomy in the position of maximal radial head stability, resulted in successful radial head reduction. **F,G.** X-rays at the time of plate removal 1 year later showed anatomic alignment of the radiocapitellar joint. Flexion-extension motion arc measured 130 degrees.

closed by manually supinating the forearm, Futami et al (112) achieved stability with a rotation osteotomy of the radius at midshaft. With the radial head reduced in maximum supination, the distal shaft segment was then rotated and fixed in pronation. This was thought to decrease the tension on the biceps, theorized to be one of the major deforming forces, but it may have the effect of reducing active supination.

Radial Head Excision. Results of radial head resection in children are unpredictable. Bell reported results of 10 patients under age 18 after radial head excision for chronic posterior radial head subluxation or dislocation and observed that 70% had lost motion in either the extension-flexion plane or the pronation-supination plane and that pain was relieved only in the short term (145). Lloyd-Roberts and Bucknill concurred that early excision poses problems of proximal radius migration, valgus deformity, and instability, recommending reconstruction for skeletally immature and symptomatic patients (122). In congenital as well as traumatic radial head dislocation, radial head excision may relieve pain and deformity but has not consistently improved elbow motion, as it does not address the soft tissue contractures that have developed over time (158,159).

In contrast, Hresko et al (160) reported significant improvement in motion in 27 elbows in 25 patients under 18 years of age who had radial head excision for a variety of conditions that caused a stiff, painful radiocapitellar joint.

Pros and Cons of Surgical Options for Radial Head Dislocation

Pros and cons of surgical options for radial head dislocation are summarized in Table 16-1.

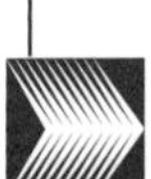

AUTHORS' PREFERRED TREATMENT

Acute Radial Head Dislocation

Most acute radial head dislocations can be treated by closed manipulation under sedation or general anesthesia. The key to maintaining the reduction is to immobilize the elbow in adequate flexion (at least 100 degrees) (see Fig. 16-35). The forearm is held in the position of maximum radial head stability, usually in supination.

Chronic Radial Head Dislocation

Open Reduction With Peterson Annular Ligament Reconstruction and Ulnar Osteotomy as Necessary. Our general philosophy is to do as little as possible but as much as necessary to obtain and maintain a stable reduction of the elbow. For posttraumatic dislocations greater than 3 weeks after injury, this almost always requires surgical treatment. We prefer open reduction and debridement of interposed soft tissue from the radiocapitellar joint, reconstruction of the annular ligament using a lateral strip of triceps tendon as described by Petersen (125), and proximal ulnar osteotomy if necessary (see Fig. 16-38). The radiocapitellar joint and proximal ulna are exposed through a Kocher approach to the elbow. The radiocapitellar joint can be stabilized with a Steinmann pin rather than a small-diameter Kirschner wire to decrease the risk of pin breakage. The elbow is immobilized for 3 to 5 weeks, after which the radiocapitellar pin is removed and active elbow range-of-motion exercise is begun.

Pearls and Pitfalls

The presence of ulnar deformity (Monteggia equivalent) must be detected and corrected for successful restoration of radiocapitellar joint stability.

TABLE 16-1 Pros and Cons of Surgical Options for Radial Head Dislocation

Operation	Pros	Cons
Annular ligament repair	Physiologic; attempts to restore injured normal anatomy	Injured ligament rapidly contracts, providing inadequate tissue for secure repair
Annular ligament reconstruction	Ample tissue available to achieve strong reconstruction	Additional exposure necessary to harvest tendon for reconstruction
Ulnar osteotomy	Restores normal anatomy; corrects angular deformity and relative shortening of ulna, which may be contributing to radial head instability	Slight increase in surgical exposure necessary
Radial osteotomy	Addresses relative excess radial length or malrotation	Nonphysiologic; requires second incision; may limit supination
Radial head excision	Quick; technically simple; acceptable solution for arthritic joint or joint where congruent reduction is not possible	Ablative; may lead to radial shortening, cubitus valgus, pain, and stiffness

Complications

Complications can occur with all of the reconstruction techniques, including open reduction, annular ligament reconstruction, ulnar osteotomy, and radial osteotomy. Rodgers et al (156) reported 14 complications in seven patients undergoing these procedures.

Annular Ligament Calcification

Dystrophic calcification of the capsule and annular ligament after reduction of radial head dislocations is common (113,122,126,132). It appears as a semilunar calcification surrounding the radial head and may become evident as early as 2 weeks after injury. In most patients, this calcification spontaneously resolves. This localized, well-defined calcification is not to be confused with the diffuse pattern of myositis ossificans after elbow injuries.

Recurrent Dislocation

Recurrent dislocation has been associated with failure to correct forearm malalignment, usually in the form of ulnar bowing or relative shortening, at the time of radial head relocation. Inadequate ulnar osteotomy fixation with intramedullary Kirschner wires has been associated with recurrent dislocation (136). The location of the ulnar osteotomy also appears to affect radial head stability, with diaphyseal osteotomy associated with redislocation. The ulnar osteotomy should be performed in the proximal metaphysis whenever possible.

Stiffness

Loss of motion is the most common complication after reduction of chronic radial head dislocation (136,146). Pronation and extension are the planes of motion most likely restricted, with supination and flexion also occasionally limited. Prolonged immobilization and lack of rigid fixation have been associated with postoperative stiffness (136).

Others

Radioulnar synostosis has been reported after chronic radial head relocation (146,161). Radial neck notching or narrowing has been noted radiographically but is of questionable significance (146,162). De Boeck reported a case of osteonecrosis of the radial neck and head after reduction and annular ligament reconstruction for chronic radial head dislocation (163).

PULLED ELBOW SYNDROME (NURSEMAID'S ELBOW)

Subluxation of the annular ligament, or pulled elbow syndrome, is a common elbow injury in young children (164–175). The term *nursemaid's elbow* and other synonyms have been used to describe this condition (176,177). The demographics associated with the subluxation of the radial head have been well described (164–175). The mean age at injury is usually 2 to 3 years, with the youngest reported patient 2 months of age. It rarely occurs after 7 years of age. Sixty percent to 65% of the children affected are girls, and the left elbow is involved in approximately 70%. It is difficult to determine the actual incidence because many subluxations are treated in primary care physicians' offices or resolve spontaneously before being seen by a physician.

Principles of Management

Mechanism of Injury

Longitudinal traction on the extended elbow is the usual mechanism of injury (Fig. 16-39). Cadaver studies have shown that longitudinal traction on the extended elbow can produce a partial slippage of the annular ligament over the head of the radius and into the radiocapitellar joint, sometimes tearing the subannular membrane. Displacement of the annular ligament occurs most easily with the forearm in pronation. In this position the lateral edge of the radial head, which opposes the main portion of the annular ligament, is narrow and round at its margin (171,178). In supination the lateral edge of the radial head is wider and more square at its margin, thereby restricting slippage. McRae (179) showed that forearm pronation maintains the displacement of the annular ligament.

Although the annular ligament slips proximally, it slips only partially over the radial head. This anatomic finding has been confirmed in numerous cadaver experiments (177–179). Salter and Zaltz (177) found that if the annular ligament slipped over the equator of the radial head, the maximum AP diameter, the ligament could not be reduced to its original position. The two reports of surgical exploration of this injury in the acute stage confirmed this observation (177,180). After 5 years of age, the distal attachments of the subannular membrane and annular ligament to the neck of the radius have strengthened sufficiently to prevent its tearing and subsequent displacement (177).

It was initially believed that the radial head diameter was less in children than in adults and this contributed to subluxation of the annular ligament. However, cadaver studies of infants, children, and adults have shown that the ratio of the head and neck diameters is essentially the same (177,181). Griffin (168) suggested that the lack of ossification of the proximal radial epiphysis in children less than 5 years of age made it more pliable, thereby facilitating slippage of the annular ligament.

Amir et al (164) performed a controlled study comparing 30 normal children with 100 who had pulled elbow syndrome. They found an increased incidence of hypermobility or ligamentous laxity among children with pulled elbows. Also, there was an increased incidence of hypermobility in one or both parents of the involved children compared with normals. It was these investigators' contention that hypermobility could be a factor predisposing children to this condition.

Thus, the most widely accepted mechanism is that the injury occurs when the forearm is pronated, the elbow is extended, and longitudinal traction is applied to the patient's wrist or hand (see Fig. 16-39) (174,178,179). Such an injury typically occurs when a young child is lifted or swung by the forearm or when

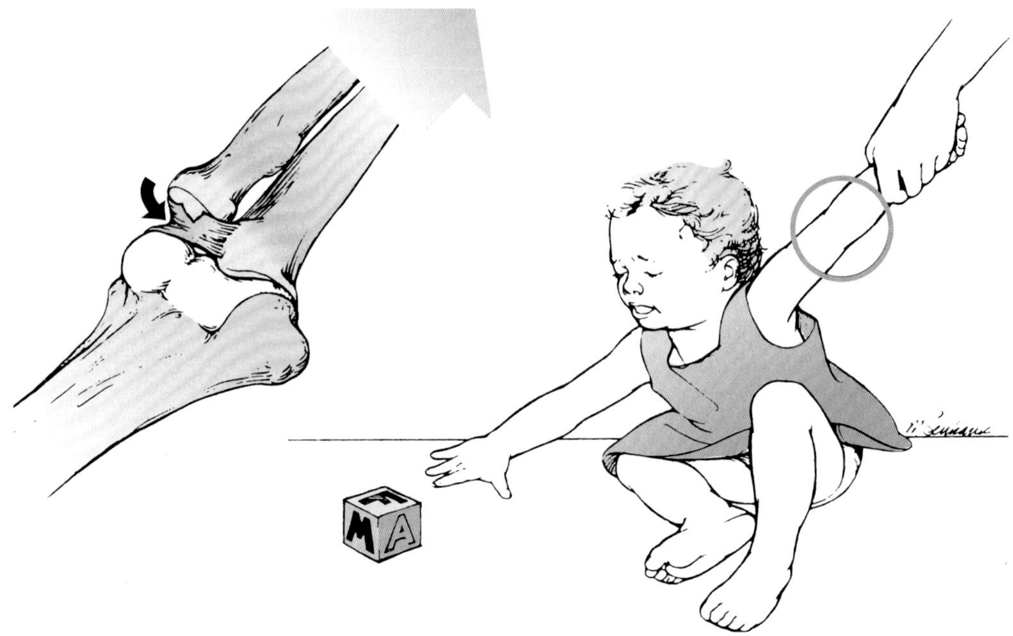

FIGURE 16-39 The injury most commonly occurs when a longitudinal pull is applied to the upper extremity. Usually the forearm is pronated. There may be a partial tear in the subannular membrane, allowing the annular ligament to subluxate into the radiocapitellar joint.

the child suddenly steps down from a step or off a curb while one of the parents is holding the hand or wrist.

Unusual Mechanisms. Newman (182) reported that five of six infants under 6 months of age with a pulled elbow sustained the injury when rolling over in bed with the extended elbow trapped under the body. It was believed that this maneuver, especially if the infant was given a quick push to turn over by an older sibling or a parent, provided enough longitudinal traction to displace the annular ligament proximally.

Signs and Symptoms

The history is critical in making the diagnosis. There almost always is an episode of a sudden longitudinal pull on the elbow of the young child. The initial pain usually subsides rapidly and the child does not appear to be in distress, except that he or she is reluctant to use the involved extremity. The upper extremity is typically held at the side with the forearm pronated. A limited painless arc of flexion and extension may be present. However, any attempt to supinate the forearm produces pain. Although there is no evidence of an elbow effusion, local tenderness may be present over the radial head and annular ligament. In some patients the pain is referred proximally to the shoulder or distally to the wrist (164,169).

Unfortunately, the classic history is not always present (166,172–174,183). In some studies 33% to 49% of patients had no clear history of a sudden longitudinal pull (174,183). There are several reasons why the history may not be characteristic: the parents are reluctant to give the true mechanism for fear they may be accused of child abuse, or the injury was not observed by a reliable adult witness. Often the child is crying and thus impossible to examine adequately until he or she has calmed down. In patients without a witnessed longitudinal traction injury, other causes, such as occult fracture or early septic arthritis, must be carefully ruled out.

Associated Injuries

As noted above, a few patients with pulled elbow syndrome may have a tear of the annular ligament instead of simple subluxation, which is of no apparent clinical significance. No other associated injuries have consistently been linked with pulled elbow syndrome.

Rationale

There are no reported cases of clinically significant sequelae following untreated pulled elbow syndrome. Patients with pulled elbow syndrome have limited painful elbow motion. The rationale for treatment is based on the goal of restoring full, painless elbow motion.

Diagnosis and Classification

There is essentially only one type of pulled elbow syndrome and therefore no commonly used classification system for this condition.

Imaging

Should x-rays be taken of every child before manipulation is attempted? If there is a classic history, the child is 5 years of age or younger, and the clinical findings strongly support the diagnosis, x-rays are not necessary (164,166,173,177,180). If, however, there is an atypical history or clinical examination, x-rays should be obtained before manipulation is attempted.

AP and lateral x-rays usually are normal (165–178,184), but subtle abnormalities may be present. Normally, the line down the center of the proximal radial shaft should pass through the center of the ossification center of the capitellum (radiocapitellar line) (184,185). Careful review of x-rays may demonstrate the radiocapitellar line to be lateral to the center of the capitellum in up to 25% of patients (184,185). To determine this subtle change requires a direct measurement on the x-ray. One problem is that these views often are taken with the forearm supinated and the subluxation is reduced when the technician places the forearm into supination to position it. Bretland (186) found that if the best x-ray that can be obtained is an oblique view with the forearm in pronation, pulled elbow syndrome is the likely diagnosis.

Arthrography. Matles and Eliopoulos (178) reported the use of arthrograms in some patients. Interposition of the annular ligament produces a defect between the radial head and the capitellum that is visible on arthrography (Fig. 16-40). Arthrography should be considered only in unusual circumstances when the diagnosis is in doubt, such as in the child who has persistent symptoms despite several attempts at closed reduction of the annular ligament.

Ultrasonography. When the diagnosis is not evident, ultrasonography may be helpful (171,187). The diagnosis is made by showing an increase in the echo-negative area between the articular surfaces of the capitellum and the radial head and increased radiocapitellar distance. Kosuwon et al (187) found that this distance is normally about 3.8 mm with the forearm pronated. With a subluxated radial head, this measured 7.2 mm. A difference of 3 mm between the normal and affected sides, therefore, suggests radial head subluxation.

Current Treatment Options

Nonoperative Treatment: Closed Reduction

Virtually all annular ligament subluxations are successfully treated by closed reduction. This is usually best done by forearm supination (166,168–176). Some have recommended that supination be performed with the elbow flexed, and others have found that supination alone with the elbow extended can effect a reduction. In many patients, a snapping sensation can be both heard and palpated when the annular ligament reduces (Fig. 16-41). Macias et al (176) reported in a randomized study that hyperpronation was more successful than supination. Reduction was successful in 40 of 41 patients (98%) in the hyperpronation group, compared with 38 of 44 patients (86%) in the supination group. They concluded that the hyperpronation technique was more successful, required fewer attempts, and was often successful when supination failed.

The value of immobilizing the elbow after reduction has been debated. Taha reported a decreased rate of recurrence during the 10 days after reduction if the elbow was splinted in a flexed supinated position for 2 days after reduction (188). Salter and Zaltz (177) recommended the use of a sling, mainly to prevent the elbow from being pulled a second time. Kohlhaas and Roeder (189) recommended a T-shirt technique for flexed elbow stabilization in very young children. This provided adequate immobilization without the use of a sling by pinning the sleeve of the long-sleeved T-shirt to the opposite chest. In general, after a successful closed reduction of a first-time annular ligament subluxation, immobilization of the extremity is not necessary if the child is comfortable and using the arm normally. After the reduction, it is important to explain to the parents the mechanism of injury and to emphasize the need to prevent longitudinal pulling on the upper extremities.

Surgical Treatment

Even if untreated, most annular ligament subluxations reduce spontaneously. There are no reported cases of long-term sequelae of untreated annular ligament subluxation. Therefore, open reduction is rarely if ever indicated for annular ligament subluxation. An indication for surgery might be the chronic symptomatic irreducible subluxation (180). In these cases, the annular ligament must be partially transected to achieve reduction.

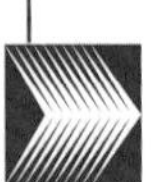

AUTHORS' PREFERRED TREATMENT

It is important to try to elicit a history of the child having had a longitudinal force applied across the extended elbow. The entire extremity is then carefully examined. Focal tenderness should be present directly over the radiocapitellar joint. If the history or physical examination is not entirely consistent with annular ligament subluxation, then x-rays of the upper extremity are obtained to assess for other injuries before manipulating the elbow.

Once the diagnosis of annular ligament subluxation is clearly established, manipulation is performed. First explain to the parents there will be a brief episode of pain, followed by significant relief of the symptoms. The patient usually is seated on the parent's lap. The patient's forearm is grasped with the elbow semiflexed while the thumb of the surgeon's opposite hand is placed over the lateral aspect of the elbow. The forearm is first supinated. If this fails to produce the characteristic snap of reduction, then the elbow is flexed maximally until the snap occurs (see Fig. 16-41). Just before reaching maximal flexion, there often is an increase in the resistance to flexion. At this point, a little extra pressure toward flexion must be applied, which usually produces the characteristic snap as the annular ligament suddenly returns to its normal position. If this fails, the hyperpronation technique of Macias et al (176) is used.

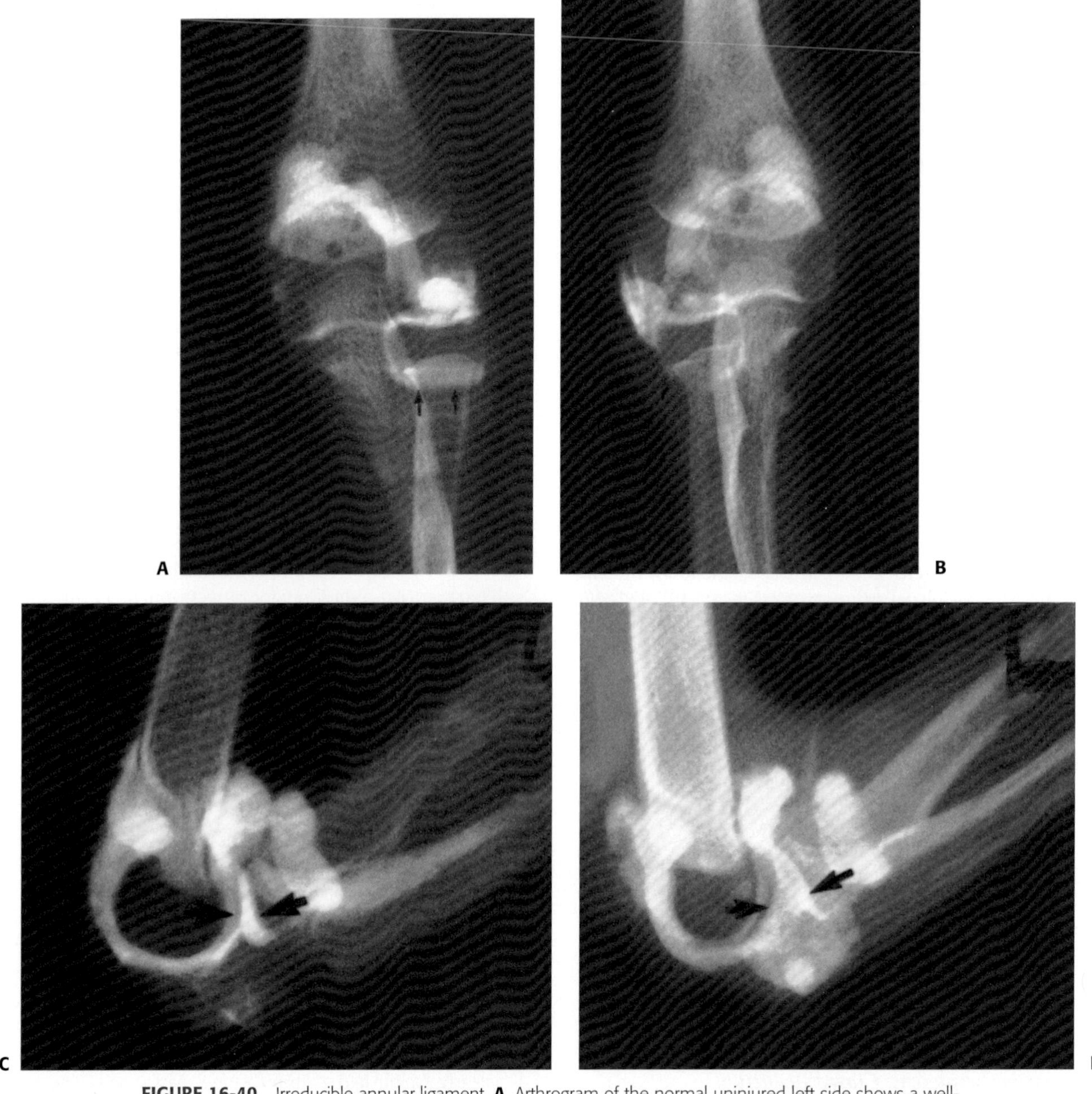

FIGURE 16-40 Irreducible annular ligament. **A.** Arthrogram of the normal uninjured left side shows a well-defined margin to the capsule and annular ligament at the radial neck (*arrows*). **B.** On the affected side, this margin has lost its sharp definition and the lateral aspect has migrated somewhat proximally. **C.** On the lateral x-ray of the normal elbow, the radial head articulates directly with the capitellum (*arrows*) when the elbow is fully flexed. **D.** On the injured side there is some limitation to full flexion. At surgery, the gap between the two articular surfaces (*arrows*) was filled with the interposed annular ligament. (Courtesy of Robert M. Campbell, Jr., MD.)

What should be done if a definite snap or pop is not felt or if the patient fails to use the extremity after manipulation? In a few patients, discomfort persists despite successful annular ligament reduction. If the subluxation has occurred more than 12 to 24 hours before the child is seen, there often is a mild secondary synovitis, and recovery may not be as dramatic. There also may be a small amount of blood in the elbow joint. Confirm that the initial diagnosis was correct. If they were not taken before the manipulation, x-rays should be obtained and the entire extremity carefully reexamined. If the x-rays are normal and the elbow can be fully flexed with free supination and pronation, the physician

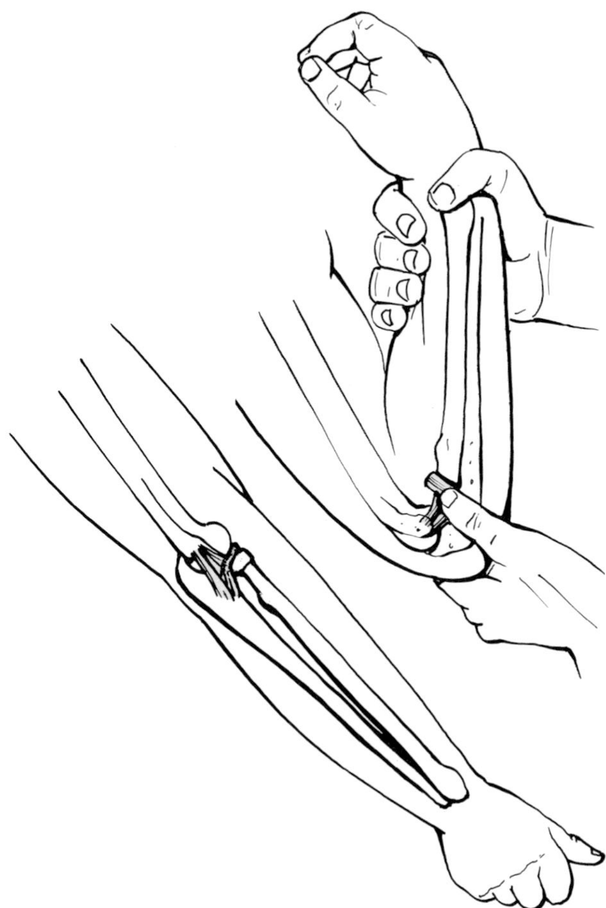

FIGURE 16-41 Reduction technique for "nursemaid's elbow." *Left:* The forearm is first supinated. *Right:* The elbow is then hyperflexed. The surgeon's thumb is placed laterally over the radial head to feel the characteristic snapping as the ligament is reduced.

can be assured that the subluxated annular ligament has been reduced. In this circumstance, the patient's arm may be placed in a splint or sling for a few days to a week and reexamined clinically and radiographically if needed.

Pitfalls and Pearls

Never assume that an unwitnessed fall has resulted in annular ligament subluxation. Such an injury mechanism is much more likely to result in a fracture (possibly occult) about the elbow.

Complications

There are no reports of long-term sequelae from unrecognized and unreduced subluxations. Almost all subluxations reduce spontaneously. The only problem seems to be discomfort to the patient until the annular ligament reduces.

Recurrent Subluxations. The reported incidence of recurrent subluxation has varied from 5% to 39% (166,168,169,172–175,190). Children 2 years of age or younger appear to be at greatest risk for recurrence (174,180). Recurrent subluxations usually respond to the same manipulative procedure as the initial injury. They eventually cease after 4 to 5 years, when the annular ligament strengthens. These recurrences do not lead to any long-term sequelae. If recurrent annular ligament subluxation significantly affects a patient's quality of life because of pain or limited activity, immobilization in an above-elbow cast with the forearm in supination or neutral position for 2 to 3 weeks is usually effective at preventing recurrence.

ACKNOWLEDGMENTS

We thank Kaye Wilkins and George Thompson for their contributions to this chapter. The information presented in this chapter is based on their efforts in previous editions.

REFERENCES

1. Henrikson B. Supracondylar fractures of the humerus in children. *Acta Chir Scand* 1966;(suppl)369:1–72.
2. Josefsson PO, Nilsson BE. Incidence of elbow dislocation. *Acta Orthop Scand* 1986;57:537–538.
3. Linscheid RL, Wheeler DK. Elbow dislocations. *JAMA* 1965;194:113–118.
4. Neviaser JS, Wickstrom JK. Dislocation of the elbow: a retrospective study of 115 patients. *South Med J* 1977;70:172–173.
5. Roberts PH. Dislocation of the elbow. *Br J Surg* 1969;56:806–815.
6. Royle SG. Posterior dislocation of the elbow. *Clin Orthop* 1991;269:201–204.
7. Carlioz H, Abols Y. Posterior dislocation of the elbow in children. *J Pediatr Orthop* 1984;4:8–12.
8. Osborne G, Cotterill P. Recurrent dislocation of the elbow. *J Bone Joint Surg [Br]* 1966;48:340–346.
9. Johnsson O. Capsular and ligament injuries of the elbow joint. A clinical and arthrographic study. *Acta Chir Scand* 1962;(suppl):287:50–65.
10. Schwab GH, Bennett JB, Woods GW, et al. A biomechanics of elbow instability: the role of the medial collateral ligament. *Clin Orthop* 1980;146:42–52.
11. Thomas TT. A contribution of the mechanism of fractures and dislocations in the elbow region. *Ann Surg* 1929;89:108–121.
12. Sojbjerg JO, Helmig P, Kjaersgaard-Andersen P. Dislocation of the elbow: an experimental study of the ligamentous injuries. *Orthopedics* 1987;12:461–463.
13. O'Driscoll SW, Morrey BF, Korinek S, et al. Elbow subluxation and dislocation. A spectrum of instability. *Clin Orthop* 1992;280:186–197.
14. Cromack PI. The mechanism and nature of the injury in dislocations of the elbow and a method of treatment. *Aust NZ J Surg* 1960;30:212–216.
15. Louis DS, Ricciardi JE, Spengler DM. Arterial injury: a complication of posterior elbow dislocation. A clinical and anatomical study. *J Bone Joint Surg [Am]* 1974;56:1631–1636.
16. Josefsson PO, Johnell O, Gentz CF. Long-term sequelae of simple dislocation of the elbow. *J Bone Joint Surg [Am]* 1984;66:927–930.
17. Loomis LK. Reeducation and after-treatment of posterior dislocation of the elbow. With special attention to the brachialis muscle and myositis ossificans. *Am J Surg* 1944;63:56–60.
18. Watson-Jones R. Primary nerve lesions in injuries of the elbow and wrist. *J Bone Joint Surg* 1930;12:121–140.
19. Boe S, Holst-Nielsen F. Intra-articular entrapment of the median nerve after dislocation of the elbow. *J Hand Surg [Br]* 1987;12:356–358.
20. Capo SR, Tito AV, Cuesta FJG, et al. Paralysies du nerf median consecutives a des fractures et luxations du conde. A propos d'une serie de douze cas. *Ann Chir* 1984;38:270–273.
21. Bhan S, Mehara AK. A method of closed reduction of posterior dislocation of the elbow. *Int Orthop* 1994;18:271–272.
22. Crosby EH. Dislocation of the elbow reduced by means of traction in four directions. *J Bone Joint Surg* 1936;18:1077.
23. Parvin RW. Closed reduction of common shoulder and elbow dislocations without anesthesia. *Arch Surg* 1957;75:972–975.
24. Lavine LS. A simple method of reducing dislocations of the elbow joint. *J Bone Joint Surg [Am]* 1953;35:785–786.
25. Meyn MA, Quigley TB. Reduction of posterior dislocation of the elbow by traction on the dangling arm. *Clin Orthop* 1974;103:106–108.
26. Minford EJ, Beattie TF. Hanging arm method for reduction of dislocated elbow. *J Emerg Med* 1993;11:161–162.

27. Hankin FM. Posterior dislocation of the elbow. A simplified method of closed reduction. *Clin Orthop* 1984;190:254–256.
28. Kumar A, Ahmed M. Technical tricks. Closed reduction of posterior dislocation of the elbow: a simple technique. *J Orthop Trauma* 1999;13:58–59.
29. Shankarappa YK, Tello E, Ferris BD. Transverse divergent dislocation of the elbow with ipsilateral distal radius epiphyseal injury in a seven-year-old. *Injury* 1998;29: 798–802.
30. Ross G, McDevitt ER, Chronister R, et al. Treatment of simple elbow dislocation using an immediate motion protocol. *Am J Sports Med* 1999;27:308–311.
31. Woods GW, Tullos HS. Elbow instability and medial epicondyle fracture. *Am J Sports Med* 1977;5:23–30.
32. Josefsson P, Gentz C-F, Johnell O, et al. Surgical versus nonsurgical treatment of ligamentous injuries following dislocations of the elbow joint. *Clin Orthop* 1987;214: 165–169.
33. Josefsson PO, Gentz C-F, Johnell O, et al. Surgical versus nonsurgical treatment of ligamentous injuries following dislocations of the elbow joint. A prospective randomized study. *J Bone Joint Surg [Am]* 1987;69:605–608.
34. Durig M, Gauer EF, Muller W. Die Operative Behandlung der Rezidivierenden und Traumatischen Luxation des Ellenbogengelenkes nach Osborne une Cotterill. *Arch Orthop Unfall Chir* 1976;86:141–156.
35. Henderson RS, Roberston IM. Open dislocation of the elbow with rupture of the brachial artery. *J Bone Joint Surg [Br]* 1952;34:636–637.
36. Kilburn P, Sweeney JG, Silk FF. Three cases of compound posterior dislocation of the elbow with rupture of the brachial artery. *J Bone Joint Surg [Br]* 1962;44:119–121.
37. Fowles JV, Slimane N, Kassab MT. Elbow dislocation with avulsion of the medial humeral epicondyle. *J Bone Joint Surg [Br]* 1990;72:102–104.
38. Wheeler DK, Linscheid RL. Fracture-dislocations of the elbow. *Clin Orthop* 1967;50: 95–106.
39. Cotton FJ. Elbow dislocation and ulnar nerve injury. *J Bone Joint Surg* 1929;11: 348–352.
40. Galbraith KA, McCullough CJ. Acute nerve injury as a complication of closed fractures or dislocations of the elbow. *Injury* 1979;11:159–164.
41. Fourrier P, Levai JP, Collin JP. Incarceration du nerf median au cours d'une luxation du coude. *Rev Chir Orthop* 1977;63:13–16.
42. Hallett H. Entrapment of the median nerve after dislocation of the elbow. A case report. *J Bone Joint Surg [Br]* 1981;63:408–412.
43. Ayala H, De Pablos J, Gonzalez J, et al. Entrapment of the median nerve after posterior dislocation of the elbow. *Microsurgery* 1983;4:251–220.
44. Danielsson LG. Median nerve entrapment and elbow dislocation. A case report. *Acta Orthop Scand* 1986;57:450–452.
45. Green NE. Case report. Entrapment of the median nerve following elbow dislocation. *J Pediatr Orthop* 1983;3:384–386.
46. Matev I. A radiological sign of entrapment of the median nerve in the elbow joint after posterior dislocation. A report of two cases. *J Bone Joint Surg [Br]* 1976;58:353–355.
47. Pritchett JW. Case report. Entrapment of the median nerve after dislocation of the elbow. *J Pediatr Orthop* 1984;4:752–753.
48. Rao SB, Crawford AH. Median nerve entrapment after dislocation of the elbow in children. A report of 2 cases and review of the literature. *Clin Orthop* 1995;312: 232–237.
49. Steiger RN, Larrick RB, Meyer TL. Median-nerve entrapment following elbow dislocation in children. A report of two cases. *J Bone Joint Surg [Am]* 1969;51:381–385.
50. Roaf R. Foramen in the humerus caused by the median nerve. *J Bone Joint Surg [Br]* 1957;39:748–749.
51. Pritchard DJ, Linscheid RL, Svien HJ. Intra-articular median nerve entrapment with dislocation of the elbow. *Clin Orthop* 1973;90:100–103.
52. Rana NA, Kenwright J, Taylor RG, et al. Complete lesion of the median nerve associated with dislocation of the elbow. *Acta Orthop Scand* 1974;45:365–369.
53. al-Qattan MM, Zuker RM, Weinberg MJ. Type 4 median nerve entrapment after elbow dislocation. *J Hand Surg [Br]* 1994;19:613–615.
54. Hennig K, Franke D. Posterior displacement of brachial artery following closed elbow dislocation. *J Trauma* 1980;20:96–98.
55. Hofammann KE III, Moneim MS, Omer GE, et al. Brachial artery disruption following closed posterior elbow dislocation in a child. A case report with review of the literature. *Clin Orthop* 1984;184:145–149.
56. Manouel M, Minkowitz B, Shimotsu G, et al. Brachial artery laceration with closed posterior elbow dislocation in an eight-year-old. *Clin Orthop* 1993;296:109–112.
57. Pearce MS. Radial artery entrapment. *Int Orthop* 1993;17:127–182.
58. Rubens MK, Auliciano PL. Open elbow dislocation with brachial artery disruption: case report and review of the literature. *Orthopaedics* 1986;9:539–542.
59. Wilmshurst AD, Millner PA, Batchelor AG. Brachial artery entrapment in closed elbow dislocation. *Injury* 1989;20:240–241.
60. Grimer RJ, Brooks S. Brachial artery damage accompanying closed posterior dislocation of the elbow. *J Bone Joint Surg [Br]* 1985;67:378–381.
61. Thompson HC, Garcia A. Myositis ossificans after elbow injuries. *Clin Orthop* 1967; 50:129–134.
62. Gosman JA. Recurrent dislocation of the ulna at the elbow. *J Bone Joint Surg* 1943;25: 44
63. Hassmann GC, Brunn F, Neer CS. Recurrent dislocation of the elbow. *J Bone Joint Surg [Am]* 1975;57:1080–1084.
64. Herring JA. Instructional case. Recurrent dislocation of the elbow. *J Pediatr Orthop* 1989;9:483–484.
65. Jacobs RL. Recurrent dislocation of the elbow joint. A case report and review of the literature. *Clin Orthop* 1971;74:151–154.
66. Kapel O. Operation for habitual dislocation of the elbow. *J Bone Joint Surg [Am]* 1951; 33:707–710.
67. King T. Recurrent dislocation of the elbow. *J Bone Joint Surg [Br]* 1953;35:50–54.
68. Malkawi H. Recurrent dislocation of the elbow accompanied by ulnar neuropathy. A case report and review of the literature. *Clin Orthop* 1981;161:270–274.
69. Mantle JA. Recurrent posterior dislocation of the elbow. *J Bone Joint Surg [Br]* 1966; 48:590.
70. McKeller Hall R. Recurrent posterior dislocation of the elbow joint in a boy. Report of a case. *J Bone Joint Surg [Br]* 1953;35:56.
71. Milch H. Bilateral recurrent dislocation of the ulna at the elbow. *J Bone Joint Surg* 1936; 18:777–780.
72. O'Driscoll SW, Bell DF, Morrey BF. Posterolateral rotatory instability of the elbow. *J Bone Joint Surg [Am]* 1991;73:440–446.
73. Symeonides PO, Paschaloglou C, Stavrou Z, et al. Recurrent dislocation of the elbow. Report of three cases. *J Bone Joint Surg [Am]* 1975;57:1084–1086.
74. Trias A, Comeau Y. Recurrent dislocation of the elbow in children. *Clin Orthop* 1974; 100:74–77.
75. Wainwright D. Recurrent dislocation of the elbow joint. *Proc R Soc Med* 1947;40: 880–886.
76. Witvoet J, Tayon B. La luxation recidivante du coude. A propos de 6 cas. *Rev Chir Orthop* 1974;60:485–495.
77. Zeier FG. Recurrent traumatic elbow dislocation. *Clin Orthop* 1982;169:211–214.
78. Reichenheim PP. Transplantation of the biceps tendon as a treatment for recurrent dislocation of the elbow. *Br J Surg* 1947;35:201–204.
79. Beaty JH, Donati NL. Recurrent dislocation of the elbow in a child. A case report and review of the literature. *J Pediatr Orthop* 1991;11:392–396.
80. Allende G, Freytes M. Old dislocation of the elbow. *J Bone Joint Surg* 1944;26:692–706.
81. Fowles JV, Kassab MT, Douik M. Untreated posterior dislocation of the elbow in children. *J Bone Joint Surg [Am]* 1984;66:921–926.
82. Krishnamoorthy S, Bose K, Wong KP. Treatment of old unreduced dislocation of the elbow. *Injury* 1976;8:39–42.
83. Mahaisavariya B, Laupattarakasem W, Supachutikul A, et al. Late reduction of dislocated elbow. Need triceps be lengthened? *J Bone Joint Surg [Br]* 1992;75:426–428.
84. Naidoo KS. Unreduced posterior dislocations of the elbow. *J Bone Joint Surg [Br]* 1982; 64:603–606.
85. Silva JF. Old dislocations of the elbow. *Ann R Coll Surg Engl* 1958;22:363–381.
86. Speed JS. An operation for unreduced posterior dislocation of the elbow. *South Med J* 1925;18:193–197.
87. Wilkins KE, Beaty JH, Chambers HG, et al. Fractures and dislocations of the elbow region. In: Rockwood CA, Green DP, Bucholz RW, et al., eds. *Rockwood and Green's fractures in adults*, 4th ed. Philadelphia: Lippincott-Raven, 1996:653–904.
88. Cohn I. Forward dislocation of both bones of the forearm at the elbow. Review of recorded cases and the literature with report of a case. *Surg Gynecol Obstet* 1922;35: 776–788.
89. Inoue G, Horii E. Case report. Combined shear fractures of the trochlea and capitellum associated with the anterior fracture–dislocation of the elbow. *J Orthop Trauma* 1992; 6:373–375.
90. Jackson JA. Simple anterior dislocation of the elbow joint with rupture of the brachial artery. Case report. *Am J Surg* 1940;47:479–486.
91. Spear HC, Jones JM. Rupture of the brachial artery accompanying dislocation of the elbow or supracondylar fracture. *J Bone Joint Surg [Am]* 1951;33:889–894.
92. Wilkerson RD. Anterior elbow dislocation associated with olecranon fractures. Review of the literature and case report. *Iowa Orthop J* 1993;13:223–225.
93. Winslow R. A case of complete anterior dislocation of both bones of the forearm at the elbow. *Surg Gynecol Obstet* 1913;16:570–571.
94. Andersen K, Mortensen AC, Gron P. Transverse divergent dislocation of the elbow. A report of two cases. *Acta Orthop Scand* 1985;56:442–443.
95. Carey RPL. Simultaneous dislocation of the elbow and the proximal radioulnar joint. *J Bone Joint Surg [Br]* 1984;66:254–256.
96. DeLee JC. Transverse divergent dislocation of the elbow in a child. Case report. *J Bone Joint Surg [Am]* 1981;63:322–323.
97. El Bardouni A, Mahfoud M, Ouadghiri M, et al. Divergent dislocation of the elbow. A case report. *Rev Chir Orthop* 1994;80:150–152.
98. Hemmadi SS, Trivedi JM. Divergent dislocation of the elbow in a child (a case report). *J Postgrad Med* 1991;37:221–222.
99. Holbrook JL, Green NE. Divergent pediatric elbow dislocation. A case report. *Clin Orthop* 1988;234:72–74.
100. McAuliffe TB, Williams D. Transverse divergent dislocation of the elbow. *Injury* 1988; 19:279–280.
101. Nakano A, Tanaka S, Hirofuji E, et al. Transverse divergent dislocation of the elbow in a six-year-old boy: case report. *J Trauma* 1992;32:118–119.
102. Sovio OM, Tredwell SJ. Case report. Divergent dislocation of the elbow in a child. *J Pediatr Orthop* 1986;6:96–97.
103. Vicente P, Orduna M. Transverse divergent dislocation of the elbow in a child. A case report. *Clin Orthop* 1993;294:312–313.
104. Carl A, Prada S, Teixeira K. Case report and review of the literature. Proximal radioulnar transposition in an elbow dislocation. *J Orthop Trauma* 1992;6:106–109.
105. Eklof O, Nybonde T, Karlsson G. Luxation of the elbow complicated by proximal radio-ulnar translocation. *Acta Radiol* 1990;31:145–146.
106. Gillingham BL, Wright JG. Convergent dislocation of the elbow. *Clin Orthop* 1997; 340:198–201.
107. Harvey S, Tchelebi H. Proximal radio-ulnar translocation. A case report. *J Bone Joint Surg [Am]* 1979;61:447–449.

108. Isbister ES. Proximal radioulnar translocation in association with posterior dislocation of the elbow. *Injury* 1991;22:479–482.
109. MacSween WA. Transposition of radius and ulna associated with dislocation of the elbow in a child. *Injury* 1978;10:314–316.
110. Bayne O, Rang M. Case report. Medial dislocation of the radial head following breech delivery. *J Pediatr Orthop* 1984;4:485–487.
111. Danielsson LG, Theander G. Traumatic dislocation of the radial head at birth. *Acta Radiol Diagn [Stockh]* 1981;22:279–382.
112. Futami T, Tsukamoto Y, Fujita T. Rotation osteotomy for dislocation of the radial head. Six cases followed for seven (three to ten) years. *Acta Orthop Scand* 1992;63:455–456.
113. Neviaser RJ, LeFevre GW. Irreducible isolated dislocation of the radial head. *Clin Orthop* 1971;80:72–74.
114. Schubert JJ. Dislocation of the radial head in the newborn infant. Case report and review of the literature. *J Bone Joint Surg [Am]* 1965;47:1019–1023.
115. Stanley D. Isolated traumatic anterior dislocation of the radial head: a mechanism of injury in children. *Injury* 1986;17:182–183.
116. Tait GR, Sulaiman SK. Isolated dislocation of the radial head: a report of two cases. *Injury* 1988;19:125–126.
117. Bouyala JM, Bollini G, Jacquemrier M, et al. Le traitement des luxations anciennes de la tete radial e chez l'enfant par l'osteotomie haute du cubitus. *Rev Chir Orthop* 1988; 74:173–182.
118. Bucknill TM. Anterior dislocation of the radial head in children. *Proc R Soc Med* 1977; 70:620–624.
119. Hudson DA, De Beer JDV. Isolated traumatic dislocation of the radial head in children. *J Bone Joint Surg [Br]* 1986;68:378–381.
120. Hume AC. Anterior dislocation of the head of the radius associated with undisplaced fracture of the olecranon in children. *J Bone Joint Surg [Br]* 1957;39:508–512.
121. Lincoln TL, Mubarak SJ. "Isolated" traumatic radial-head dislocation. *J Pediatr Orthop* 1994;14:454–457.
122. Lloyd-Roberts GC, Bucknill TM. Anterior dislocation of the radial head in children. Aetiology, natural history and management. *J Bone Joint Surg [Br]* 1977;59:402–407.
123. Mizuno K, Usui Y, Kohyama K, et al. Familial congenital unilateral anterior dislocation of the radial head: differentiation from traumatic dislocation by means of arthrography. A case report. *J Bone Joint Surg [Am]* 1991;73:1086–1089.
124. Oner FC, Diepstraten AFM. Treatment of chronic post-traumatic dislocation of the radial head in children. *J Bone Joint Surg [Br]* 1993;75:577–581.
125. Seel MJ, Peterson HA. Management of chronic posttraumatic radial head dislocation in children. *J Pediatr Orthop* 1999;19:306–312.
126. Stelling FH, Cote RH. Traumatic dislocation of head of radius in children. *JAMA* 1956; 160:732–736.
127. Vesely DG. Isolated traumatic dislocations of the radial head in children. *Clin Orthop* 1967;50:31–36.
128. Wiley JJ, Pegington J, Horwich JP. Traumatic dislocation of the radius at the elbow. *J Bone Joint Surg [Br]* 1974;56:501–507.
129. Wiley JJ, Loeher J, McIntyre W. Isolated dislocation of the radial head. *Orthop Rev* 1991;20:973–976.
130. Evans EM. Pronation injuries of the forearm with special reference to the anterior Monteggia fracture. *J Bone Joint Surg [Br]* 1949;31:578–588.
131. McGuire TP, Myers P. Ulnar osteotomy for missed Monteggia fractures. *J Bone Joint Surg [Br]* 1986;68:336.
132. Earwaker J. Posttraumatic calcification of the annular ligament of the radius. *Skel Radiol* 1992;21:149–154.
133. Weisman DS, Rang M, Cole WG. Tardy displacement of traumatic radial head dislocation in childhood. *J Pediatr Orthop* 1999;19:523–526.
134. Vocke-Hell AK, von Laer L, Slongo T, et al. Secondary radial head dislocation and dysplasia of the lateral condyle after elbow trauma in children. *J Pediatr Orthop* 2001; 21:319–323.
135. Kim HT, Conjares JN, Suh JT, et al. Chronic radial head dislocation in children, part 1: Pathologic changes preventing stable reduction and surgical correction. *J Pediatr Orthop* 2002;22:583–590.
136. Horii E, Nakamura R, Ioh S, et al. Surgical treatment for chronic radial head dislocation. *J Bone Joint Surg [Am]* 2002;84:1183–1188.
137. Kadic MA, Bloem RM. Traumatic isolated anterior dislocation of the radial head. A case with a 32–year follow-up. *Acta Orthop Scand* 1991;62:288–289.
138. Almquist EE, Gordon LH, Blue AI. Congenital dislocation of the head of the radius. *J Bone Joint Surg [Am]* 1969;51:1118–1127.
139. Mardam-Bey T, Ger E. Congenital radial head dislocation. *J Hand Surg* 1979;4: 316–320.
140. McFarland B. Congenital dislocation of the head of the radius. *Br J Surg* 1936;24: 41–49.
141. Miura T. Congenital dislocation of the radial head. *J Hand Surg* 1990;15:477–481.
142. Sachar K, Mih AD. Congenital radial head dislocations. *Hand Clin* 1998;14:39–47.
143. Agnew DK, Davis RJ. Congenital unilateral dislocation of the radial head. *J Pediatr Orthop* 1993;13:526–528.
144. Southmayd W, Ehrlich MG. Idiopathic subluxation of the radial head. *Clin Orthop* 1976;121:271–274.
145. Bell SN, Morrey BF, Bianco AJ. Chronic posterior subluxation and dislocation of the radial head. *J Bone Joint Surg [Am]* 1991;73:392–396.
146. Kim HT, Park BG, Suh JT, et al. Chronic radial head dislocation in children. part 2: results of open treatment and factors affecting final outcome. *J Pediatr Orthop* 2002; 22:591–597.
147. Abe M, Ishizu T, Nagaoka T, et al. Recurrent posterior dislocation of the head of the radius in post-traumatic cubitus varus. *J Bone Joint Surg [Br]* 1995;77:582–585.
148. Klekamp J, Green NE, Mencio GA. Osteochondritis dissecans as a cause of developmental dislocation of the radial head. *Clin Orthop* 1997;338:36–41.
149. Caravias DE. Some observations on congenital dislocation of the head of the radius. *J Bone Joint Surg [Br]* 1957;39:86–90.
150. De Boeck H. Treatment of chronic isolated radial head dislocation in children. *Clin Orthop* 2000;(380):215–219.
151. Devnani AS. Missed Monteggia fracture dislocation in children. *Injury* 1997;28: 131–133.
152. Hirayama T, Takemitsu Y, Yagihara K, et al. Operation for chronic dislocation of the radial head in children. *J Bone Joint Surg [Br]* 1987;69:639–642.
153. Bell Tawse AJS. The treatment of malunited anterior Monteggia fractures in children. *J Bone Joint Surg [Br]* 1965;47:718–723.
154. Best TN. Management of old unreduced Monteggia fracture dislocations of the elbow in children. *J Pediatr Orthop* 1994;14:193–199.
155. Cappellino A, Wolfe SW, Marsh JS. Use of a modified Bell Tawse procedure for chronic acquired dislocation of the radial head. *J Pediatr Orthop* 1998;18:410–414.
156. Rodgers WB, Waters PM, Hall JE. Chronic Monteggia lesions in children. Complications and results of reconstruction. *J Bone Joint Surg [Am]* 1996;78:1322–1329.
157. Kemnitz S, De Schrijver F, De Smet L. Radial head dislocation with plastic deformation of the ulna in children. A rare and frequently missed condition. *Acta Orthop* 2000;66: 359–362.
158. Kelly DW. Congenital dislocation of the radial head: Spectrum and natural history. *J Pediatr Orthop* 1981;1:295–298.
159. Wiley JJ, Loehr J, McIntyre W. Isolated dislocation of the radial head. *Orthop Rev* 1991; 20:973–976.
160. Hresko MT, Rosenburg BN, Pappas AM. Excision of the radial head in patients younger than 18 years. *J Pediatr Orthop* 1999;19:106–113.
161. Oner FC, Diepstraten AFM. Treatment of chronic post-traumatic dislocation of the radial head in children. *J Bone Joint Surg [Br]* 1993;75:577–581.
162. Fowles JV, Sliman N, Kassab MT. The Monteggia lesion in children: fracture of the ulna and dislocation of the radial head. *J Bone Joint Surg [Am]* 1983;65:1276–1283.
163. De Boeck H. Radial neck osteolysis after annular ligament reconstruction. A case report. *Clin Orthop* 1997;(342):94–98.
164. Amir D, Frankl U, Pogrund H. Pulled elbow and hypermobility of joints. *Clin Orthop* 1990;257:94–99.
165. Broadhurst BW, Buhr AJ. The pulled elbow. *Br Med J* 1959;1:1018–1019.
166. Choung W, Heinrich SD. Acute annular ligament interposition into the radiocapitellar joint in children (nursemaid's elbow). *J Pediatr Orthop* 1995;15:454–456.
167. Costigan PG. Subluxation of the annular ligament at the proximal radio-ulnar joint. *Alberta Med Bull* 1952;17:7–9.
168. Griffin ME. Review article. Subluxation of the head of the radius in children. *Pediatrics* 1955;15:103–106.
169. Illingsworth CM. Pulled elbow: a study of 100 patients. *Br Med J* 1975;2:672–674.
170. Jongschaap HCN, Youngson GG, Beattie TF. The epidemiology of radial head subluxation ("pulled elbow") in the Aberdeen City area. *Health Bull [Edinb]* 1990;48:58–61.
171. Magill HK, Aitken AP. Pulled elbow. *Surg Gynecol Obstet* 1954;98:753–756.
172. Piroth P, Gharib M. Die Traumatische Subluxation des Radiuskopfchens (Chassaignac). *Deutsch Med Wochenschr* 1976;101:1520–1523.
173. Quan L, Marcuse EK. The epidemiology and treatment of radial head subluxation. *Am J Dis Child* 1985;139:1194–1197.
174. Schunk JE. Radial head subluxation: epidemiology and treatment of 87 episodes. *Ann Emerg Med* 1990;19:1019–1023.
175. Snellman O. Subluxation of the head of the radius in children. *Acta Orthop Scand* 1959; 28:311–315.
176. Macias CG, Bothner J, Wiebe R. A comparison of supination/flexion to hyperpronation in the reduction of radial head subluxations. *Pediatrics* 1998;102:10.
177. Salter RB, Zaltz C. Anatomic investigations of the mechanism of injury and pathologic anatomy of pulled elbow in young children. *Clin Orthop* 1971;77:134–143.
178. Matles A, Eliopoulos K. Internal derangement of the elbow in children. *Int Surg* 1967; 48:259–263.
179. McRae R, Freeman PA. The lesion of pulled elbow. *J Bone Joint Surg [Br]* 1965;47:808.
180. Triantafyllou SJ, Wilson SC, Rychak J. Irreducible pulled elbow in a child. A case report. *Clin Orthop* 1992;284:153–155.
181. Ryan JR. The relationship of the radial head to radial neck diameters in fetuses and adults with reference to radial-head subluxation in children. *J Bone Joint Surg [Am]* 1969;51:781–783.
182. Newman J. "Nursemaid's elbow" in infants 6 months and under. *J Emerg Med* 1985; 2:403–404.
183. Sacchetti A, Ramoska EE, Glascow C. Nonclassic history in children with radial head subluxations. *J Emerg Med* 1990;8:151–153.
184. Snyder HS. Radiographic changes with radial head subluxation in children. *J Emerg Med* 1990;8:265–269.
185. Frumkin K. Nursemaid's elbow. A radiographic demonstration. *Ann Emerg Med* 1985; 14:690–693.
186. Bretland PM. Pulled elbow in childhood. *Br J Radiol* 1994;67:1176–1185.
187. Kosuwon W, Mahaisavariya B, Saengnipanthkul S, et al. Ultrasonography of pulled elbow. *J Bone Joint Surg [Br]* 1993;75:421–422.
188. Taha AM. The treatment of pulled elbow: a prospective randomized study. *Arch Orthop Trauma Surg* 2000;120:336–337.
189. Kohlhaas AR, Roeder J. Tee shirt management of nursemaid's elbow. *Am J Orthop* 1995; 24:74.
190. Teach SJ, Schutzman SA. Prospective study of recurrent radial head subluxation. *Arch Pediatr Adolesc Med* 1996;150:164–166.

17

PROXIMAL HUMERUS, SCAPULA, AND CLAVICLE

John F. Sarwark, Erik C. King, and Scott J. Luhmann

FRACTURES OF THE PROXIMAL HUMERUS

Fractures of the proximal humerus are relatively uncommon injuries of childhood, with an incidence of 1.2 to 4.4 per 1,000 per year (1–3), fewer than 5% of all pediatric fractures (2,4–7). Fractures in this region have enormous potential to heal and remodel, perhaps more so than anywhere else in the body, mainly due to the thick periosteum at the proximal humerus and the proximity to the physis. Thus, proximal humeral fractures in children can be expected to heal without significant residual functional or cosmetic deficits in most cases.

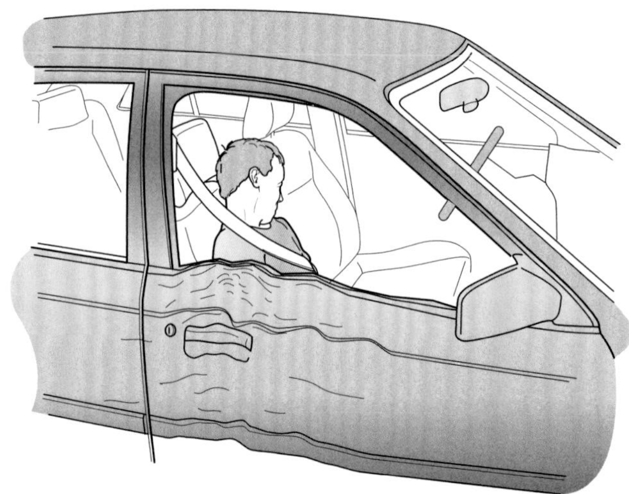

FIGURE 17-2 Motor vehicle crashes may result in proximal humeral fracture due to blunt trauma to the shoulder region.

Principles of Management

Mechanism of Injury

Fractures of the proximal humerus can be a common birth-related injury (8,9). As an infant is passing through the birth canal, the arm may be placed in a variety of abnormal positions that can result in a separation through the physis of the proximal humerus (8–14). These fractures are generally believed to result from hyperextension and/or rotation of the arm during the passage through the birth canal (Fig. 17-1) (8–14). As might be expected, obstetric proximal humeral fractures occur most frequently during vaginal deliveries of infants with larger size or breech presentation (9,15–17). Prenatal size and presentation, however, have not been accurate predictive factors for these fractures, because proximal humeral fractures can and do occur during vaginal deliveries of infants of all sizes and weights; hence, other infant and maternal factors play a role (15–17).

In older children, the predominant cause of fractures in the proximal humerus is trauma, both direct and indirect. In this age group, these fractures can involve the metaphysis, the physis, or both. The trauma can be a direct blow to the shoulder area, especially to the posterior aspect (10,18,19), or indirect, as in a fall onto an outstretched hand that transmits the force through the arm to the proximal humerus (17,20,21). Indirect trauma can result in forced or nonphysiologic positioning of the upper extremity, which in turn may cause a fracture of the proximal humerus. Specifically, six potential mechanisms of upper extremity positioning have been proposed to explain the resulting proximal humeral fractures: forced extension, forced flexion, forced extension with lateral or medial rotation, and forced flexion with lateral or medial rotation (22). Although trauma has been acknowledged as the most common mechanism of pediatric proximal humeral fractures, it is still controversial whether a fall or a direct blow is the more common etiology of the fracture.

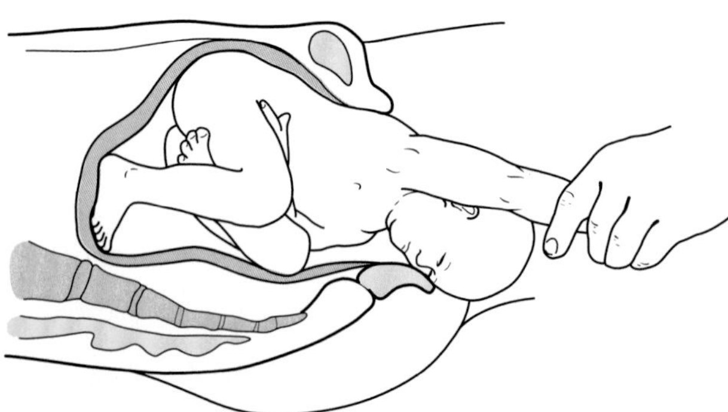

FIGURE 17-1 Hyperextension or rotation of the ipsilateral arm may result in a proximal humeral or physeal injury during birth.

Proximal humeral fractures are typically moderate- to higher-energy injuries and are frequently seen in motor vehicle crashes and sporting activities (Figs. 17-2 and 17-3) (23,24). Approximately 50% of shoulder girdle fractures in children have

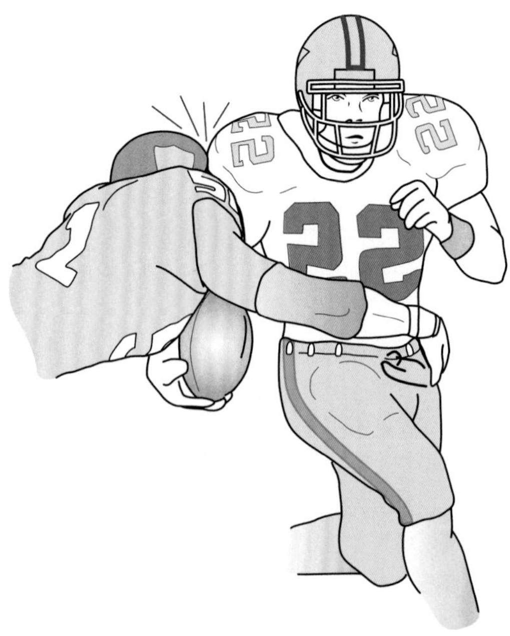

FIGURE 17-3 Blunt trauma from contact sports may result in fracture of the proximal humerus in children.

been reported to be associated with sports and play activities (25). Athletic activities associated with proximal humeral fractures include contact sports (football, hockey), horseback riding (fall from horses), gymnastics (upper extremity impact and weight bearing), and baseball (repetitive throwing) (6,26–29).

Less often, pediatric proximal humeral fractures result from other conditions such as malignant or benign tumors and pituitary gigantism (30–33). They also can be a complication of radiation therapy to the shoulder region (34). In addition, shoulder joint neuropathy secondary to Arnold-Chiari malformation, myelomeningocele, or syringomyelia has been implicated as an etiologic factor in proximal humeral fractures (23,35). An unknown percentage of pediatric proximal humeral fractures are part of the injuries associated with child abuse (Fig. 17-4) (36). Because no clear fracture pattern in the proximal humerus is suggestive of abuse, an index of suspicion must remain high when evaluating infants or young children with humeral fractures (37).

Signs and Symptoms

Clinical features of proximal humeral fractures in newborns may be subtle and not readily identified. For example, the infant may be irritable when handled by caregivers or when there is movement of the upper extremity. The infant may refuse to move the arm, giving the appearance of paralysis, called "pseudoparalysis." Infants exhibiting upper extremity paralysis also may be suffering from posterior humeral head dislocation (38).

Older children typically report a history consistent with a proximal humeral fracture: a traumatic injury with the immediate development of moderate to severe global shoulder pain exacerbated by motion of the arm. They often present with an obvious deformity, or fullness, in the anterior shoulder region, with the overall contour of the shoulder altered in comparison with the contralateral uninjured shoulder. The arm is internally rotated against the abdomen and the patient usually refuses to use the involved arm. Pain, swelling, and ecchymosis are invariably present to some degree.

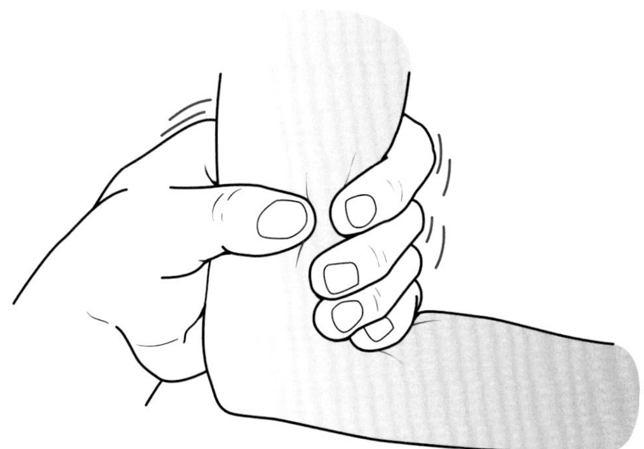

FIGURE 17-4 Although the exact mechanism of injury may vary in child abuse, fracture of the proximal humerus may result from twisting at the elbow or forearm.

The internally rotated position of the injured extremity is due to the pull of the pectoralis major muscle on the distal fragment. With posterior fracture dislocations, children demonstrate limited and extremely painful external rotation. Some children with fractures of the greater tuberosity have an unusual presentation of luxatio erecta where the involved shoulder is positioned in extreme abduction (39). This position reduces the displacement across the fracture as the greater tuberosity is pulled superiorly by the supraspinatus muscle. The elbow is typically flexed in luxatio erecta, allowing the hand to be near or above the head (39,40). Fractures of the lesser tuberosity affect the function of the inserting subscapularis muscle; hence, abduction and external rotation of the shoulder will be limited and painful (41–43).

Associated Injuries

In high-energy trauma, fractures of the proximal humerus may be associated with concomitant dislocations of the glenohumeral joint. The direction of the dislocation may be anterior, posterior, or inferior (36,39,40,44–47). Neurologic injury to the brachial plexus can result from fractures and fracture–dislocations of the proximal humerus (39,47–50). Typically these nerve deficits are transient, and full function typically returns in less than 6 months (51,52). Fractures of the proximal humerus in children also can be associated with other injuries, including rib fractures and pneumothorax (33).

Diagnosis and Classification

The proximal humeral epiphysis is not visible on plain x-rays until about 6 months of age (51–53), and plain x-rays are of limited value in evaluation of proximal humeral fractures in infants. On an anteroposterior (AP) x-ray, a change in the positional relationship between the proximal humeral metaphysis and the scapula and acromion often is visible. A comparison with the uninjured contralateral shoulder may reveal this alteration more clearly. A "vanishing epiphysis" sign also has been reported to describe posteriorly displaced physeal fractures of the proximal humerus (Fig. 17-5) (54,55). On an AP x-ray the epiphysis appears to vanish when it is displaced posteriorly. For complete evaluation of proximal humeral fractures in newborns and infants, ultrasonographic studies can be diagnostic and informative (56–59). Computed tomography (CT) also may be useful, especially for complex fractures with posterior dislocations (60). In addition to proximal humeral fractures, the differential diagnosis for such "paralysis" in infants includes brachial plexus injury, septic shoulder, and clavicular fractures.

For evaluation of proximal humeral fractures in older children, two x-rays in perpendicular views can be diagnostic (61). Ideally, a true AP view of the shoulder and an axillary lateral view provide the most information about the fracture. Because some lesser tuberosity fractures may be visible only on an axillary lateral view, this x-ray should be included whenever possible (62). Often, however, an axillary lateral view is difficult to

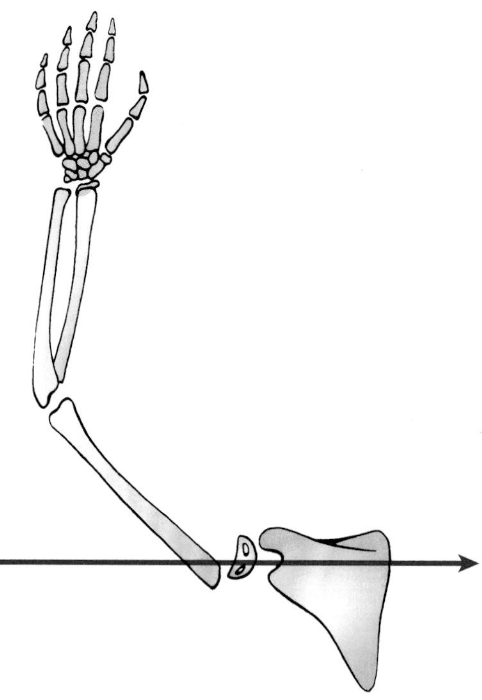

FIGURE 17-5 Vanishing epiphysis sign.

obtain in a child with an acutely fractured proximal humerus. In these instances, transthoracic axillary view or scapular-Y views can be obtained. In addition, an apical oblique view, an AP x-ray with the x-ray beam at 45 degrees of caudal tilt, also can provide significant information about the proximal humerus (63). In fact, some authors report that most shoulder trauma can be evaluated with AP and apical oblique x-rays and that a lateral view (axillary lateral or scapular-Y view) can be obtained if a humeral fracture is suspected (64).

When adequate x-rays cannot be obtained, CT is useful in evaluating proximal humeral fractures. CT may be especially useful in characterizing posterior fracture–dislocations (43,45). If the child continues to report shoulder pain despite negative radiographic and CT results, an occult fracture must be ruled out. For this purpose, magnetic resonance imaging (MRI) can be diagnostic, due to its ability to identify the intramedullary signal change of edema and the fracture plane (1,65,66). A bone scan may also be useful in equivocal cases. However, due to the normally increased radionuclide uptake at the physis of the proximal humerus, additional uptake due to a fracture may be difficult to interpret.

Fractures of the proximal humerus in the pediatric population are broadly categorized by their anatomic location. The fractures may involve the physis, the metaphysis, the lesser tuberosity, or the greater tuberosity. In addition, the degree of fracture deformity (angulation and translation) plays an important role in the overall treatment option. Other fracture characteristics that must be evaluated include the presence or absence of open fractures, concomitant glenohumeral dislocations, and fracture stability.

Fractures involving the physis are classified according to the Salter-Harris classification (Fig. 17-6) (67). Salter-Harris type I injuries with fractures through the physis occur mostly in patients under 5 years of age (10,68). After 11 years of age, most fractures of the proximal humerus are Salter-Harris type II injuries, with the fracture line exiting through the metaphysis (10,57,68,69), and they occasionally are associated with an additional anterolateral bony fragment (69). Salter-Harris type III injuries with the fracture line exiting through the epiphysis rarely occur in the proximal humerus of children (10,68) and have been reported with and without concomitant glenohumeral dislocation (44,45,70–72). Salter-Harris type IV injuries involving both the metaphysis and the epiphysis of the proximal humerus have not been reported in children.

Fractures of the metaphysis occur mostly in children 5 to 12 years of age (Fig. 17-7) and are categorized by their anatomic location and degree of displacement (10). This rather unexpected finding has been attributed to the rapid metaphyseal growth that occurs during this age, which in turn results in a relative structural weakness of the metaphysis (10). The anatomic location is described in relation to the major deforming forces in the region, namely the insertions of the pectoralis major and the deltoid muscles. Presence or absence of other fractures in the ipsilateral upper extremity also must be documented, because segmental fractures may require alternative treatments (73–75). Other isolated fractures of the proximal humerus may include the greater and the lesser tuberosities (39–42,76).

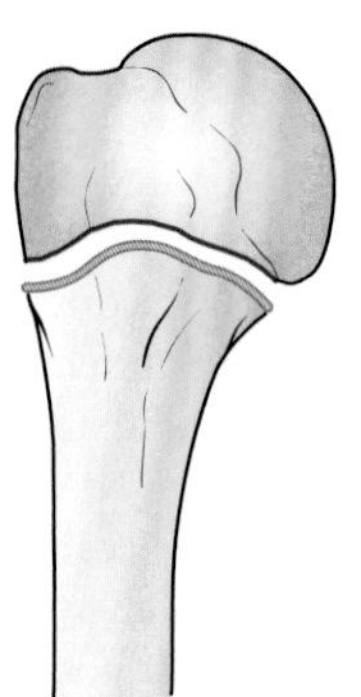

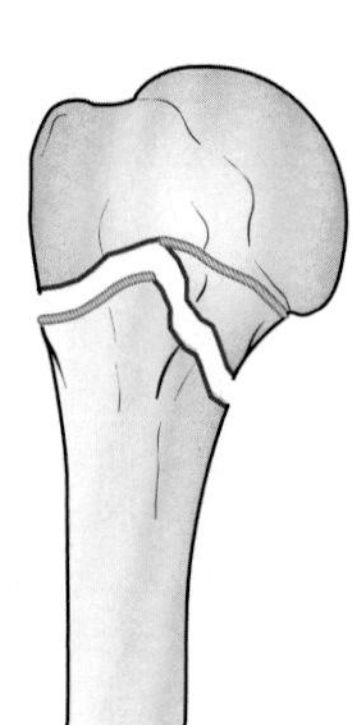

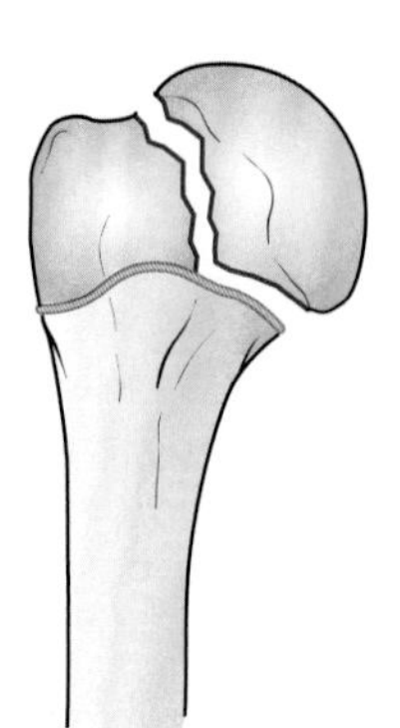

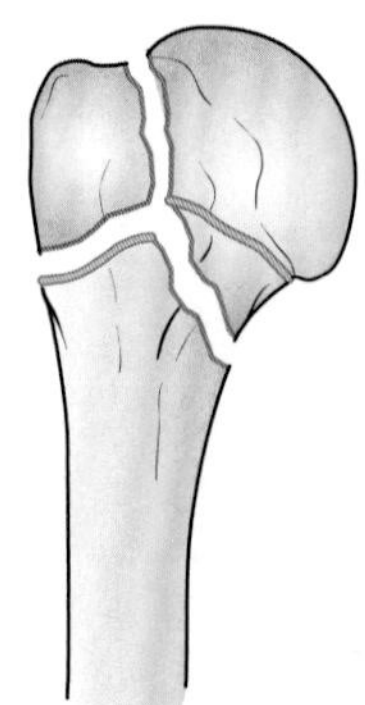

FIGURE 17-6 Physeal fractures of the proximal humerus. **A.** Salter-Harris I. **B.** Salter-Harris II. **C.** Salter-Harris III. **D.** Salter-Harris IV.

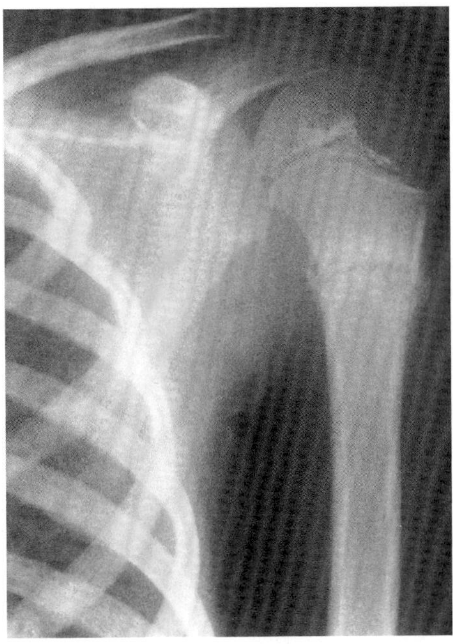

FIGURE 17-7 Healing undisplaced fracture of the proximal humerus in a 5-year-old child. Note the absence of a physeal injury.

The degree of displacement in proximal humerus fractures is classified with respect to the shaft diameter of the humerus (18). In grade I injuries, there is up to 5 mm of displacement. In grade II and III injuries, fractures are displaced by up to one third and two thirds of the humeral shaft diameter, respectively. Displacement of greater than two thirds of the shaft diameter is classified as a grade IV injury. In addition to degree of displacement, fractures in this region typically demonstrate concomitant angular deformities.

Surgical and Applied Anatomy

The proximal humeral ossification center cannot be seen on plain x-rays until about 6 months of age (51–53). In addition to the proximal humerus, both the greater and lesser tuberosities contain their own separate ossification centers. The ossification center for the greater tuberosity appears at around 1 to 3 years of age, while the ossification center for the lesser tuberosity takes form at 4 to 5 years of age (53,77). The two tuberosities typically coalesce between 5 and 7 years of age and subsequently fuse with the humeral head at 7 to 13 years of age (53,77).

The proximal physis of the humerus continues to be active well into the teenage years and is ultimately responsible for approximately 80% of the overall humeral growth (78–81). Interestingly, longitudinal growth at the proximal humeral physis changes during development, such that it is responsible for only 75% of humeral growth before age 2 but up to 90% of growth after age 11 (78–80). For girls, this growth continues until around 14 years of age, with subsequent fusion of the epiphysis to the shaft at 14 to 17 years of age (78,81,82). For boys, growth continues until about age 16, when closure of the physis begins (78–80).

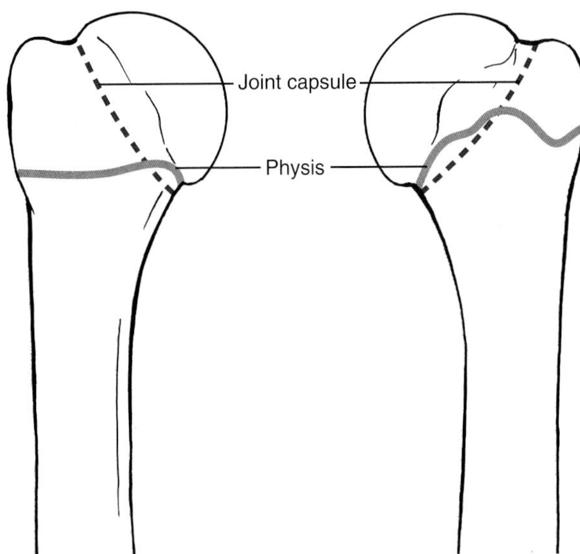

FIGURE 17-8 The anatomy of the proximal humerus.

For most boys, the proximal humeral physis is closed by about 18 years of age (82). The extracapsular location of the proximal humeral physis makes this structure susceptible to injury. Physeal fractures are thought to occur through the zone of hypertrophy and provisional calcification while relatively sparing the cells in the resting and proliferative zones (67). Salter-Harris type I or II fractures in children have high remodeling potential and rarely result in growth arrest (10,83).

The articular surface of the proximal humerus covers most of the medial aspect of the epiphysis as well as the proximal medial corner of the metaphysis (Fig. 17-8). The glenohumeral joint capsule surrounds the articular surface such that most of the medial epiphysis and the proximal medial corner of the metaphysis are intraarticular (Fig. 17-9). Conversely, a predom-

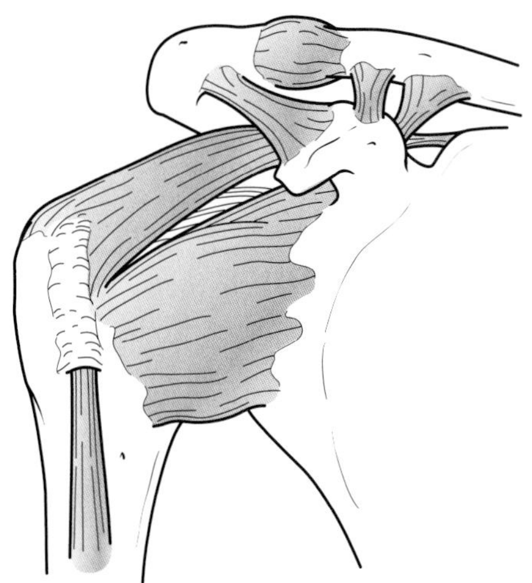

FIGURE 17-9 Glenohumeral joint capsule.

inant proportion of the physis is extracapsular and remains susceptible to injury. Most fractures of the pediatric proximal humerus involve the physis (10,68,69). The periosteum is quite strong in the posteromedial aspect of the proximal humerus, but the periosteum in the anterolateral aspect is relatively weak, occasionally allowing the fractured fragment to penetrate and prevent reduction (10).

The proximal humerus is the site of insertion for a number of different muscles that can influence the pattern of fracture displacement. These muscles and their attachments form early during development and are grossly similar to those of an adult shoulder by the time of birth. The four muscles of the rotator cuff insert onto the epiphysis. The subscapularis muscle inserts on the anterior aspect of the epiphysis on the lesser tuberosity, whereas the teres minor, the infraspinatus, and the supraspinatus muscles insert onto the superior and posterior aspect of the epiphysis near the greater tuberosity (Fig. 17-10). In addition to the rotator cuff muscles, the deltoid and pectoralis major muscles can also affect fracture displacement. The deltoid muscle attaches in the lateral aspect of the humeral shaft, whereas the pectoralis major muscle attaches to the anteromedial aspect of the metaphysis.

The muscular attachments to the proximal humerus contribute to the degree and the overall pattern of fracture displacement. With fractures of the physis (Salter-Harris types I, II, and III) and metaphyseal fractures proximal to the insertion of the pectoralis major muscle, the rotator cuff muscles displace the epiphysis into abduction, flexion, and slight external rotation. The distal fragment is displaced proximally by the deltoid muscle, whereas the pectoralis major muscle displaces the fragment anteriorly and medially. If the metaphyseal fracture occurs between the insertions of the deltoid and the pectoralis major muscles, the proximal fragment is adducted by the pull of the pectoralis major muscle, and the distal fragment is pulled proximally and abducted by the deltoid muscle. If the fracture occurs distal to the deltoid muscle insertion, the proximal fragment is abducted by the deltoid muscle and displaced anteriorly by the pectoralis major muscle. The distal fragment is pulled proximally and medially by the biceps and the triceps muscles (84).

The vascular supply to the proximal humerus arises from the axillary artery. Distal to the pectoralis minor muscle, three different arterial branches arise from the axillary artery before it becomes the brachial artery to supply the upper extremity. One of these branches is the subscapular artery, which runs with the subscapular nerve to supply the rotator cuff muscles. The remaining two branches, the anterior and the posterior humeral circumflex arteries, supply the proximal humerus. Most of the humeral head vascularity is from the arcuate artery, which in turn is from the ascending branch of the anterior humeral circumflex artery (85,86). The posterior humeral circumflex artery is a less dominant vascular supplier of the proximal humerus because it supplies a small portion of the greater tuberosity and posteroinferior portion of the humeral head (Fig. 17-11) (85).

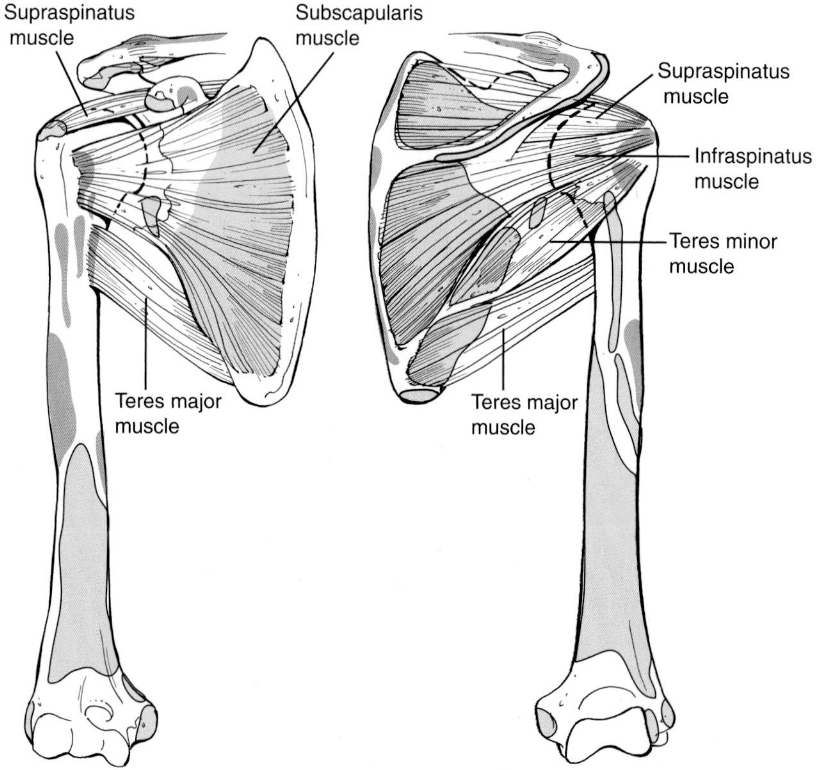

FIGURE 17-10 Origins and insertions of the cuff muscles in a child: subscapularis, teres minor, infraspinatus, and supraspinatus.

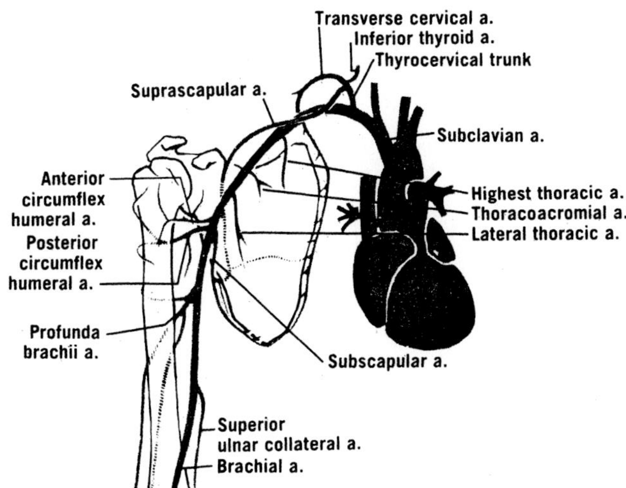

FIGURE 17-11 The arterial anatomy of the shoulder region.

The close proximity of the axillary nerve to the proximal humerus makes this neural structure susceptible to injury during fracture and fracture–dislocations of the proximal humerus (39,47,48). The axillary nerve is a branch of the posterior cord of the brachial plexus. It traverses the anterior aspect of the subscapularis muscle before passing inferior to the glenohumeral joint to the posterior aspect of the proximal humerus (Fig. 17-12). The axillary nerve provides innervation to the deltoid muscle as well as cutaneous sensation over the lateral aspect of the shoulder. Documentation of the normal motor and sensory function of this nerve at the initial evaluation and prior to treatment is essential.

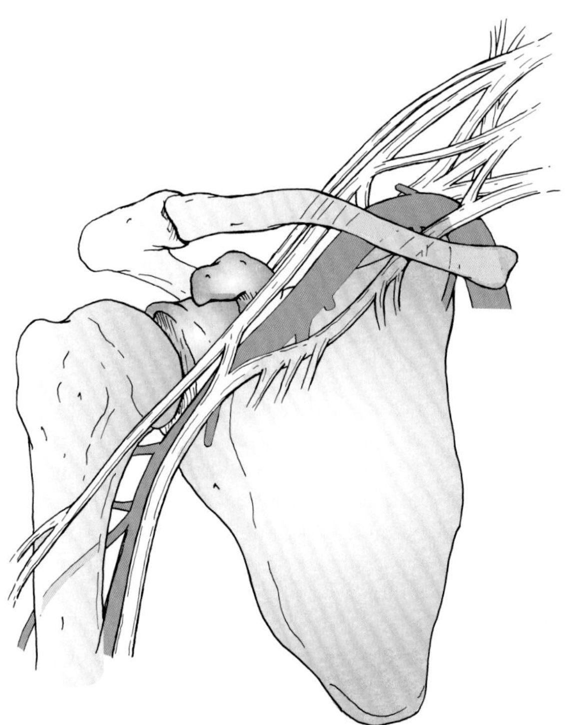

FIGURE 17-12 Relationship of the brachial plexus and artery to the proximal humerus and the scapula.

Current Treatment Options

Because of their tremendous potential for healing and remodeling, fractures of the proximal humerus in children infrequently require operative reduction and fixation (Table 17-1). This is especially true for obstetric proximal humeral fractures in infants. If needed, these fractures are amenable to gentle reduction with minimal anesthesia or sedation. If desired, the adequacy of the reduction can be evaluated via ultrasonography, but due to the incredible remodeling capability in this age group this is not routine. With or without anatomic reduction, the affected upper extremity should then be immobilized to the body by using a safety pin to attach the shirt sleeve to the shirt (33). Proximal humeral fractures in this age group heal quite rapidly, typically within 2 to 3 weeks, and result in no residual functional or cosmetic deficits (9,10,12,17,87,88).

Nondisplaced or minimally displaced proximal humeral fractures (Neer grades I and II) in older children and adolescents also should be treated nonoperatively. Initial management of these fractures involves sling-and-swathe immobilization (Fig. 17-13) followed by protected motion. Overall, nonoperative treatment provides excellent long-term results (10,39,89).

The remodeling potential of the fracture in young children is significant but decreases with the increasing age of the child; hence, the degree of acceptable displacement and angulation also changes with the age of the child. Generally, relative greater displacement and angulation can be accepted in younger children. For fractures in children under the age of 11, good to excellent long-term outcomes have been reported regardless of the fracture displacement (10,18,19,90). Various types of shoulder immobilization to maintain reduction have been advocated and include sling-and-swathe, thoracobrachial bandage (Velpeau), hanging arm cast, shoulder spica cast, salute position shoulder spica cast, and "Statue of Liberty" cast (10,12,18,89,90).

Grossly displaced or angulated proximal humeral fractures (Neer grades III and IV) in children over 11 are managed with fracture reduction and sometimes with specialized immobilization (10,18,90,91). Multiple maneuvers exist for the reduction of pediatric proximal humeral fractures. Most fractures can be reduced by applying longitudinal traction to the arm while positioning it in abduction, flexion, and external rotation. If this maneuver does not sufficiently reduce the fracture, better reduction can be obtained by moderate abduction, flexion to 90 degrees, and external rotation (18). Alternatively, the fracture can be reduced by direct manual manipulation of the fragments while the arm is placed in marked abduction (about 135 degrees), slight flexion (about 30 degrees), and longitudinal traction (17,21,88). Despite signifi-

TABLE 17-1 Interventions for Proximal Humerus Fractures

	Immobilization	Operative Reduction & Immobilization	Operative Reduction & Internal Fixation
Birth fractures	X		
Chronic slipped proximal humeral epiphysis	X		
Metaphyseal fractures	X	X	X
SH I before age 11 years	X	X	X
SH I after age 11 years	X		X

cant efforts, however, some fractures cannot be adequately reduced because of a barrier at the fracture site. Anatomic structures that can prevent reduction of proximal humeral fractures include the periosteum, the shoulder joint capsule, and the biceps tendon (87,92–96). In these situations, open reduction through a small deltopectoral incision is needed to remove the obstacles to reduction.

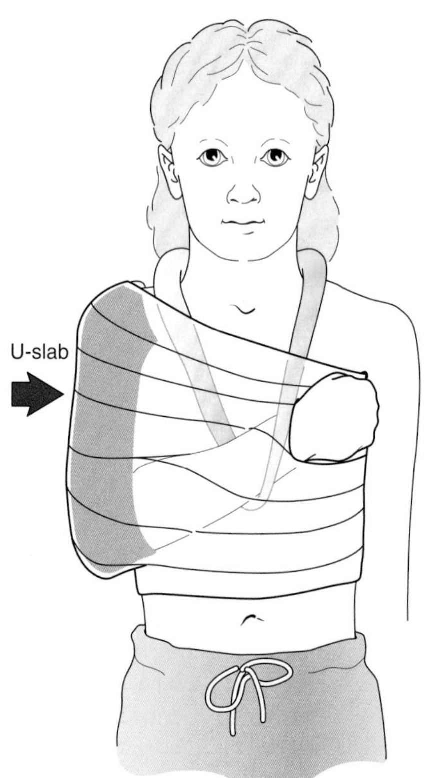

FIGURE 17-13 Sling-and-swathe for immobilization of proximal humeral fracture.

In children over 11 years old, some investigators recommend reducing selected Neer grade III and all grade IV fractures and immobilizing in salute-position shoulder spica casts (18). Other investigators suggest gentle reduction of Salter-Harris type I and II fractures with greater than 50% displacement, followed by immobilization with a thoracobrachial bandage (Velpeau) or shoulder spica cast (Fig. 17-14) (10). An acceptable reduction of proximal humeral fractures in children over 11 years of age has been proposed by some to be less than 50% displacement and 20 degrees of angulation (91). Traditional thinking has been that nonoperative treatment of pediatric proximal humeral fractures has produced good to excellent results in all age groups (10,18,90). Because of this, the reported indications for operative treatment of pediatric proximal humeral fractures have been limited to include open fractures, fractures associated with neurovascular injury, fractures associated with multiple trauma, displaced intraarticular fractures (i.e., Salter-Harris type III fractures), irreducible fractures, and significantly displaced fractures in older adolescents (4,23,68,71,95,97–102).

Interestingly, the cited literature that has been reported to support nonoperative treatment regimens for all patients actually supports this method for children less than 11 years of age and in fractures with no to minimal displacement (10,18,90). These classic references identified fractures in older children (11 years of age or older) and those with Neer grades III and IV displacements at increased risk for less-than-optimal outcome (10,18,90). Minimal remodeling, specifically angular correction, occurs in the older child and adolescent, which can lead to limitation of glenohumeral motion (abduction) and pain (10,90). Two issues exist in this fracture in children 11 years of age and older: achieving adequate reduction and maintaining the desired alignment during the healing process. Achieving acceptable fracture alignment can typically be accomplished with closed manipulation of the fracture and only infrequently requires an open reduction to remove

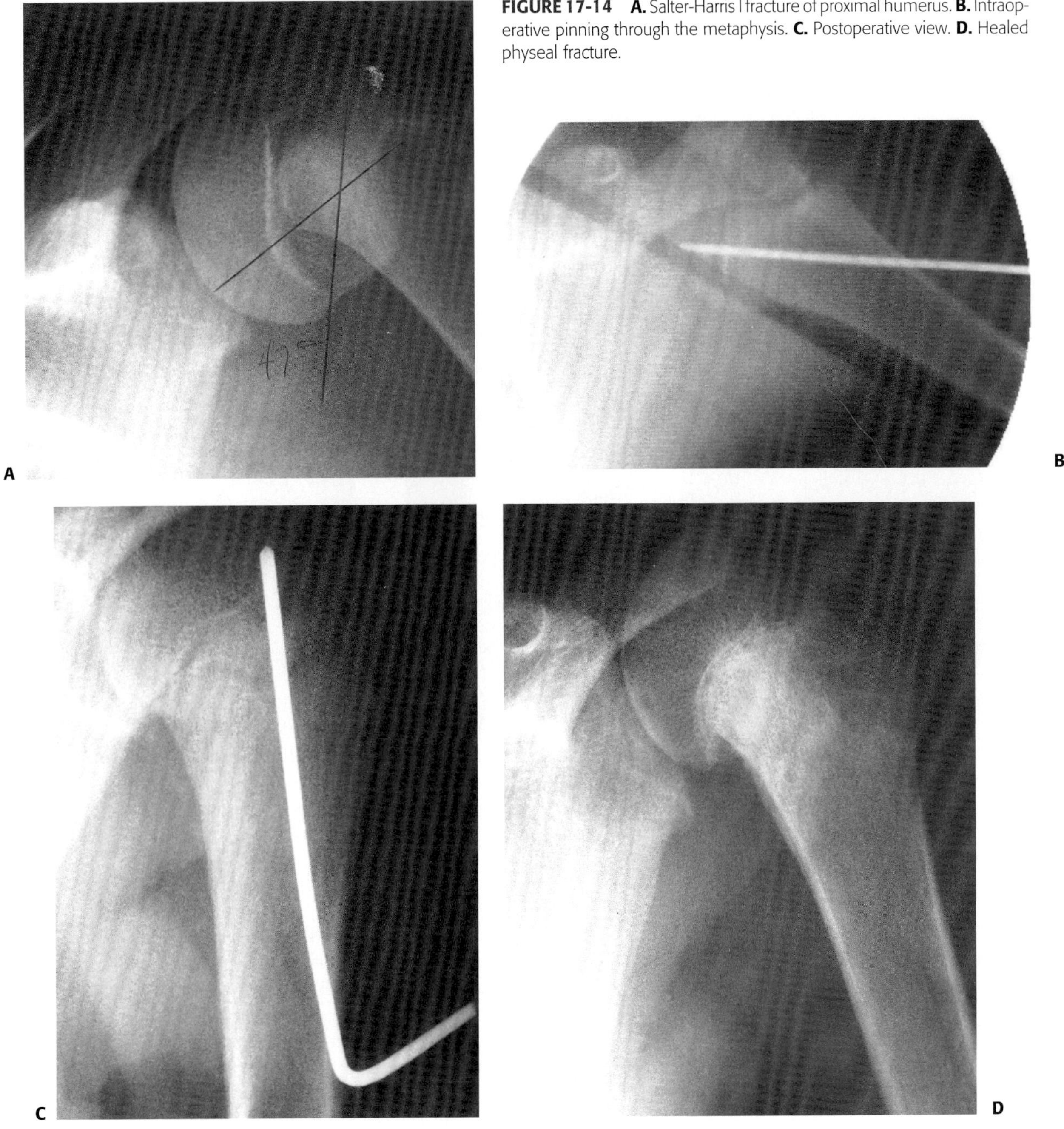

FIGURE 17-14 **A.** Salter-Harris I fracture of proximal humerus. **B.** Intraoperative pinning through the metaphysis. **C.** Postoperative view. **D.** Healed physeal fracture.

obstructions. Immobilization of the reduced fracture comes in two types: specialized casts or splints, or internal fixation. Various types of external immobilization have been reported to maintain reduction (10,12,18,89,90). Loss of reduction has been reported to be as high as 50% in one series in which only external immobilization was used (18). Internal fixation with cannulated screws or more commonly Kirschner wires (Fig. 17-15) can be used to stabilize the reduction, which obviates the need for cumbersome immobilization such as a Velpeau bandage or spica cast (23). Intramedullary fixation is also a viable option for stabilizing displaced proximal metaphyseal fractures (Fig. 17-16).

A stress fracture of the metaphysis or a slipped epiphysis can be produced by chronic or repetitive trauma, such as repetitive throwing, gymnastics with humeral weight bearing, and localized radiation therapy (26–29,34,103). Because of the tremen-

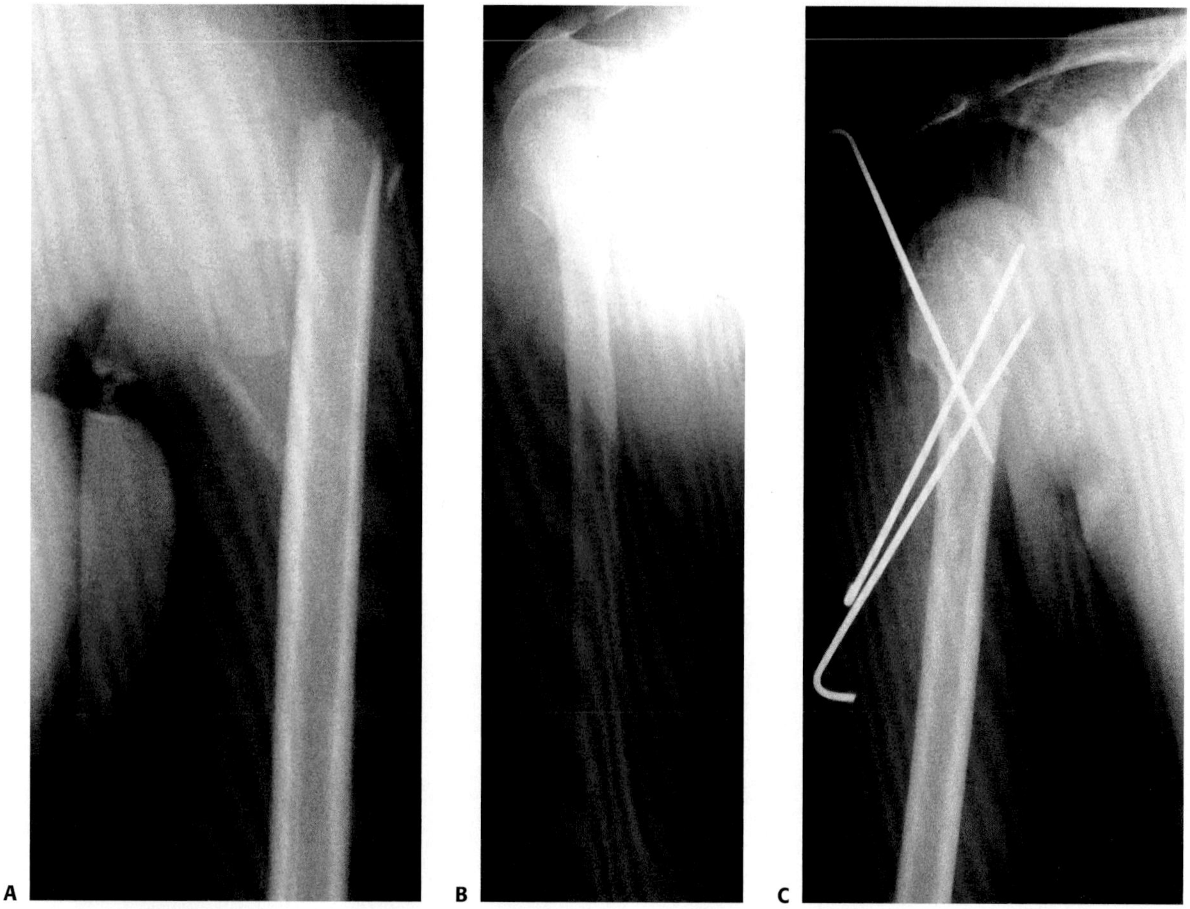

A B C

FIGURE 17-15 **A.** AP x-ray of displaced fracture of the proximal humerus metaphysis with shortening with apparent inferior subluxation of the humeral head with respect to the glenoid. **B.** Attempted axillary view. **C.** Intraoperative film status after percutaneous pinning. Note the apparent inferior subluxation while under general anesthesia.

dous healing and remodeling potential in the pediatric proximal humerus, these injuries can be successfully treated with conservative nonsurgical therapy.

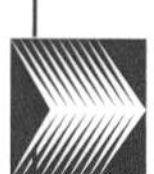

AUTHORS' PREFERRED TREATMENT

Surgical Procedure

Proximal humeral fractures that have significant displacement (Neer grades III and IV) and angulation in patients over 11 years of age are the fractures that typically undergo reduction to improve fracture alignment. General anesthesia is typically necessary for patient comfort and for adequate muscle relaxation due to the difficulties that can be encountered in obtaining and maintaining an acceptable reduction. A radiolucent operating table is optimal, but a regular operating room table can be used if the patient's torso is moved as far lateral as possible and supported by an additional piece of radiolucent Plexiglas. Adequate fluoroscopic imaging is essential for a successful intervention, and the fluoroscope is set up in the AP projection; it is not routinely moved during the procedure. A small towel bump is placed under the medial border of the ipsilateral scapula to elevate the shoulder away from the table to allow adequate circumferential access to the shoulder. The sterile preparation should be medial enough to allow the surgeon the option of performing a low deltopectoral or axillary approach to the shoulder should closed reduction be inadequate. Reduction is performed with longitudinal traction on the injured limb while the arm is placed in abduction, external rotation, and flexion to align the distal fragment with the epiphysis. Increasing the abduction (up to 90 degrees) and flexion (up to 90 degrees) of the distal fragment may be necessary to reduce the fracture. For fractures requiring operative reduction, percutaneous Kirschner wire stabilization is routinely used. The starting point for percutaneously placed implants is at the lateral cortex of the distal fragment, near the insertion of

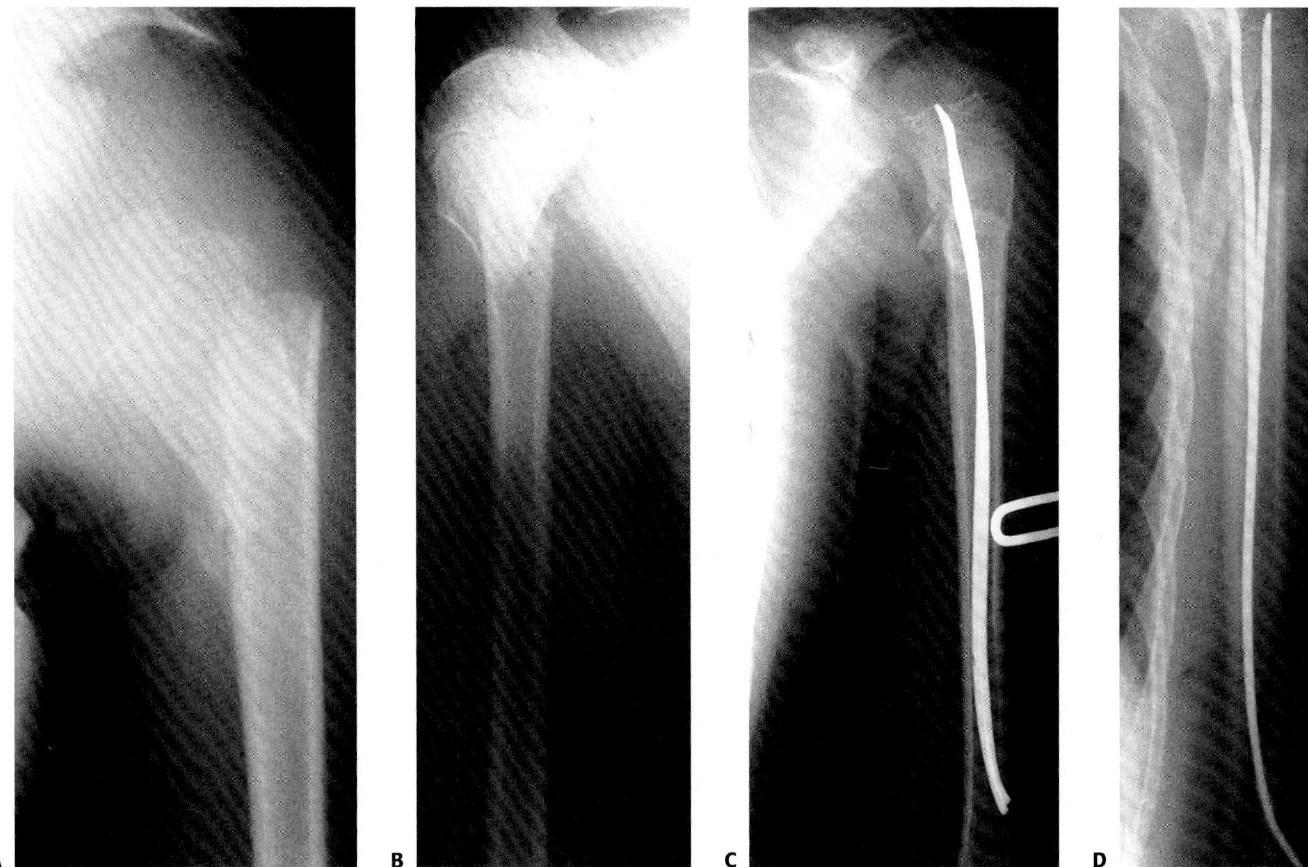

FIGURE 17-16 **A.** AP x-ray of displaced, shortened fracture of the proximal humerus. **B.** Axillary image of same. **C.** Intramedullary fixation using retrograde technique. Note the satisfactory restoration of alignment. **D.** Postoperative lateral view.

the deltoid muscle, and aimed obliquely into the humeral epiphysis. At least two pins (0.062 or 5/64 inches), and preferentially three pins, are used and typically allow adequate stabilization. The Kirschner wires may be cut beneath the level of the skin or may be left through the skin and protected with Jergen's balls. The arm is placed into a shoulder immobilizer, with the arm at the patient's side, while the patient is under general anesthesia. The implants can usually be removed as early as 4 weeks after surgery after documenting healing on x-ray.

Pearls and Pitfalls

- Most fractures of the proximal humeral physis are managed nonoperatively. This includes nondisplaced and most minimally to moderately displaced physeal injuries of the proximal humerus, which are treated with a shoulder sling or immobilizer. Range-of-motion exercises (pendulum) are initiated as soon as tolerated, and the immobilization is discontinued when healing is confirmed by x-rays and clinical examination. The great majority of metaphyseal fractures are also treated nonoperatively, with only a few requiring closed reduction. Because of the tremendous remodeling potential of metaphyseal fractures in children, up to 1 cm of displacement is acceptable if the fracture is in bayonet apposition.
- Due to the significant instability after reduction of displaced fractures involving the humeral epiphysis or metaphysis, we prefer to percutaneously pin these fractures, particularly those in children over 11 years of age (see Fig. 17-15). The rationale behind reduction and percutaneous pinning of proximal humeral physeal fractures is a more rapid return of normal active and passive range of motion, improved patient comfort, and easier care of the patient. There is a minimally increased, but acceptable, risk of infection. In our opinion, this approach is more acceptable than leaving the fracture unreduced and risking a decrease in shoulder range of motion with secondary shoulder pain. We prefer to place the pin percutaneously through the metaphyseal fragment up into the physis, similar conceptually to the pinning of a slipped capital femoral epiphysis in the hip (see Fig. 17-14). One drawback of Kirschner wire fixation is that if the wires are left under the skin, another general anesthetic is needed to remove the implants. In metaphyseal fractures, if the fracture is more distal, it may not be technically feasible to place a percutaneously placed Kirschner wire obliquely into the epiphysis. In this situation, intramedullary

fixation with flexible nails is an effective method (see Fig. 17-16). Occasionally a fracture is irreducible. In older children, open reduction is indicated. Generally the biceps is the offending structure. An anterior deltopectoral exposure is used.

- Fracture–dislocations of the shoulder require closed reduction of the glenohumeral joint dislocation with appropriate anesthesia. After reduction of the glenohumeral dislocation, radiographic confirmation of the reduction and reevaluation of the physeal or metaphyseal fracture is essential. If the dislocation does not concentrically reduce or the fracture is in unacceptable alignment, open reduction is generally done through a low anterior or axillary approach to the proximal humerus.
- Displaced fractures of the lesser tuberosity generally are treated with open reduction to restore the subscapularis tendon and anterior capsule. Lag screws or suture anchors are very useful in this region, particularly for injuries with small bony fragments. Fractures of the greater tuberosity generally are associated with acute dislocations of the shoulder and are typically treated nonoperatively after closed reduction of the shoulder dislocation. Rarely, after closed reduction of the shoulder dislocation, the greater tuberosity fracture reduction is unacceptable, and an open approach to repair the tuberosity fracture along with the rotator cuff is required.

Complications

Early Complications

Diagnosis of a proximal humeral fracture can be delayed in a child who is asymptomatic or minimally symptomatic. In children with multiple trauma, the diagnosis can be delayed due to the need to focus on more life- or limb-threatening problems and the absence of any dramatic limb malalignment. Even after the diagnosis of proximal humeral fracture is made, full evaluation and characterization of the fracture pattern can remain incomplete because of inadequate radiographic studies. A high index of suspicion, thorough physical examination, and insistence on high-quality x-rays must all be present to ensure prompt diagnosis and treatment of proximal humeral fractures.

Neurologic injury to the brachial plexus can result from fractures and fracture–dislocations of the proximal humerus (39,47–50). Most nerve deficits can be diagnosed immediately because the clinical signs are readily apparent. Rarely, however, nerve deficits from proximal humeral fractures can evolve slowly and delay the diagnosis (49). Typically, these nerve deficits are transient, and full function typically returns in less than 6 months (51,52). If the neurologic deficit persists longer than 3 months, further evaluation with electromyography is warranted. If no evidence of nerve recovery or regeneration is present, nerve exploration, repair, and grafting can be considered (48,104). Salvage operations for permanent nerve deficits include proximal humeral osteotomy and muscle or tendon transfers (105–109).

Fractures of the proximal humerus in children also can be associated with other injuries, including rib fractures and pneumothorax (33). In adults, these fractures have been associated with disruptions and thrombosis of the axillary vessels as well (110–113). Operative fixation of proximal humeral fractures with pins and wires has been associated with hardware migration, which can be fatal (114,115). Therefore, serial radiographic monitoring of the hardware after shoulder operations is essential.

Late Complications

Humerus varus after trauma is a rare complication that typically affects neonates and children under 5 years of age (116–120). Children with humerus varus have a significant decrease in the humeral neck–shaft angle and shortening of the upper extremity. Although shoulder abduction may be moderately limited, most children with humerus varus have only mild functional deficits and do not require surgical correction of the deformity (116–118,120). If, however, active abduction and flexion are severely limited, corrective osteotomy of the proximal humerus can produce good results (119,121).

Hypertrophic scarring can occur after surgical reduction of proximal humeral fractures. When the scarring is present in the anterior shoulder region after an anterior deltopectoral incision, the cosmetic deformity may be significant and psychologically damaging, especially for girls (93,122). Therefore, many investigators have argued for the more cosmetically appealing axillary or anterior axillary incision (123,124).

Limb length inequality after proximal humeral fractures occurs more frequently in children treated with surgical intervention than in those treated nonoperatively (10,83,125). This is likely due to the degree of damage to the physis at the time of injury and not iatrogenically induced due the surgical reduction. The inequality is not significantly affected by the quality of initial fracture reduction and may be more pronounced in older children (1 to 3 cm) (18,83). Despite this inequality, however, these children rarely develop any functional deficits to warrant surgical intervention. Full arrest of physeal growth after traumatic proximal humeral fractures is extremely uncommon (10). Although still quite rare, it does occur more frequently in children with pathologic fractures through unicameral bone cysts (126–128). If the functional or cosmetic deficit is significant, a limb-lengthening procedure may be of benefit for these children (129).

Osteonecrosis of the humeral head after proximal humeral fractures occurs frequently in adults but is rare in children (130,131). Even after acute disruption of the vascular supply to the proximal humeral epiphysis, subsequent remodeling and revascularization usually occur in children and lead to excellent clinical results (71). Similarly, glenohumeral subluxation after proximal humeral fractures is a rare complication in the pediatric population that typically results in good clinical outcomes (131). These children are best treated with a short period of immobilization followed by early physical therapy and rehabilitation (33).

Controversies and Future Directions

Little controversy exists in the treatment of minimally displaced fractures and fractures in children 11 years old and younger;

the main area of controversy is in the treatment of displaced fractures in the patient older than 11 years old. Two main areas of controversy are the amount of acceptable displacement (angulation and translation), and the optimal method of stabilization. The Neer classification is currently the most widely accepted method for the radiographic classification of proximal humeral fractures, but it has not been validated as a guide for treatment (18). This system defines the fractures based on the bony translation at the fracture site but does not integrate fracture angulation into the schema. Multiple published reports document a high percentage of good and excellent outcomes in Neer grade III and IV fractures (10,18,90,91). It is likely that fracture angulation, and not translation, is the more important factor in the overall outcome of these fractures. Unfortunately, due to the anatomy of the proximal humerus and epiphysis, plain radiographic assessment of fracture angulation can be very imprecise, especially in physeal fractures. This makes preoperative and postoperative analysis of the fracture alignment difficult, if not impossible. Further study into the role of fracture angulation, and the ability to quantify angulation, is likely to shed new light onto this topic by improving treatment algorithms and patient outcomes.

The classic treatment method for stabilization of the reduced proximal humerus fracture has been a specialized cast or splint designed to position the distal fracture fragment in alignment with the proximal fragment. Improvements in intraoperative imaging and equipment have permitted an evolution in pediatric fracture care to more widespread use of percutaneously placed Kirschner wires or cannulated screws. Both methods, external immobilization and internal fixation, have their advantages and disadvantages in proximal humerus fractures (Table 17-2), but direct comparison of the techniques has not been performed to date.

FRACTURES OF THE SCAPULA

Injury to the scapula is rare because it is well protected by multiple layers of muscle and other soft tissues. Due to this inherent protection, fractures and dislocations of the scapula are rare: only 1% of all fractures involve the scapula (132,133). However, when scapular injuries occur, they are almost certainly a result of high-energy trauma and may be associated with significant injuries to other major organ systems (134–136). Therefore, all children with apparently isolated scapular fractures should be meticulously evaluated on the secondary trauma survey for the presence of potentially life-threatening visceral injuries that require further intervention.

Principles of Management

Mechanism of Injury

Glenoid. Fractures of the glenoid typically occur in a fall onto an upper extremity. This is believed to drive the humeral head into the glenoid fossa, which in turn results in the fracture. Depending on the direction of the force, the fracture may injure the rim of the glenoid or the entire glenoid fossa. Less commonly, fractures may result from direct trauma to the glenoid.

Body of Scapula. Fractures to the body of the scapula occur via direct impact or avulsion mechanisms. The direct impact mechanism is typically of high energy and rarely is an isolated injury. As with all other high-energy injuries, child abuse must be excluded as a cause for scapular injury when no clear traumatic cause is evident (137). The avulsion-type fractures may occur at any of the several muscle attachments on the scapula.

TABLE 17-2 Treatment Pros and Cons: Proximal Humerus Fractures

	Pros	Cons
No reduction (sling or shoulder immobilizer)	1) No anesthesia/sedation 2) Sling/shoulder immobilizer well tolerated	1) No improvement of fracture alignment 2) Loss of shoulder range of motion
Reduction and external immobilization	1) Improves fracture alignment 2) No implant concerns (infection, migration, malposition, etc.) 3) No need for secondary anesthesia for implant removal	1) Need general anesthesia 2) Cumbersome cast/splint 3) No direct rigid fixation of fracture (potential for loss of reduction)
Reduction and internal fixation	1) Improves fracture alignment 2) Direct rigid fixation of fracture 3) Improved patient comfort (due to rigid fracture fixation) 4) No cumbersome cast or splint	1) Need general anesthesia 2) Minimal increased risk of infection 3) Implant concerns 4) Possible need for implant removal

Signs and Symptoms

Children with scapular fractures have significant pain and tenderness around the shoulder girdle and resist movement of the affected arm. Localized edema may obscure the overall shoulder contour, which may be more evident by comparison with the contralateral shoulder. The diagnosis of scapular fractures is frequently missed because of the attention required by more significant injuries.

Associated Injuries

Greater than 75% of patients with scapular fractures have associated injuries (135,138–140), many of which are life-threatening. In one reported series, the rate of death among patients with scapular fractures exceeded 14% (135).

Because of the proximity of the scapula to the axillary artery and the brachial plexus, fractures of the scapula often are associated with neurovascular injury (see Fig. 17-12) (135). The ipsilateral arm must be carefully examined to document arterial or neurologic deficits before the initiation of treatment. When injury to axillary or distal vasculature is suspected, an angiogram may be performed to examine the integrity of the vessels.

Scapular fractures also are associated with several life-threatening injuries, such as hemothorax, pneumothorax, cardiac contusions, as well as fractures of the spine, clavicle, rib, and humerus (134,135).

Diagnosis and Classification

Scapular fractures typically are discovered during the evaluation of the multiply injured patient. In the rare case where the scapular fracture is the initially identified fracture, a complete trauma evaluation should be undertaken for head, chest, abdominal, and retroperitoneal injuries. If suspicion is high, a general trauma evaluation may be requested. Conversely, scrutiny for fractures of the scapula should be included in the evaluation of the multiply traumatized child.

Imaging Studies. Most scapular injuries are identified initially on the AP chest x-ray from a trauma series. However, AP and lateral x-rays of the scapula will facilitate detection of fractures not evident on the AP chest view, as well as allowing better description of the fracture pattern. In addition to these, other special radiographic views can aid in fracture characterization. The Stryker notch view, for example, better reveals coracoid fractures, whereas the axillary lateral view is better suited to identify glenoid fractures. The axillary lateral view also is helpful in confirming the location of the humeral head with the glenoid. When available, CT with three-dimensional reconstruction provides the most detailed representation of scapular anatomy. In addition, CT is essential in characterizing intraarticular injuries of the glenoid.

In high-energy trauma, the AP chest x-ray should also be scrutinized for evidence of scapulothoracic dissociation. Scapulothoracic dissociation typically occurs in patients with massive, direct trauma to the chest or proximal upper extremity and is highly associated with ipsilateral neurovascular injury (141,142). This devastating injury should be suspected if the medial border of the scapula is displaced laterally, if there is a clavicular fracture with a large displacement, or if there is a complete acromioclavicular joint separation with large displacement (142,143).

Developmental variations in scapular anatomy may confuse radiographic interpretation. For example, os acromiale is commonly mistaken for an acute fracture. This variation occurs when the centers of ossification in the acromion fail to unite (144). Os acromiale is considered a normal variant, is present in 10% of normal shoulders, and is bilateral in 60% of affected individuals (143,145). Typically, os acromiale is located in the anterior and inferior aspect of the distal acromion and has a smooth and uniform appearance on x-rays. Occasionally os acromiale is symptomatic. If radiographic studies and clinical examination cannot distinguish between a fracture and a developmental variation, further evaluation with a bone scan may be clarify the diagnosis (141). Other variants in scapular anatomy include Sprengel's anomaly, absent acromion, bipartite or tripartite acromion, bipartite coracoid, and coracoid duplication (144,146–149).

Classification. Multiple classification systems for scapular fractures have been reported. Many are descriptive and based primarily on the anatomic location of fracture. Ada and Miller divided scapular fractures into categories of acromion, spine, coracoid, neck, glenoid, and body (138). In their series, fractures occurred most often in the body (35%), followed by the neck (27%); fractures of the coracoid were least common (7%). Thompson et al classified scapular fractures into three broad anatomic locations: fractures of the glenoid and the glenoid neck, fractures of the acromion and the coracoid, and fractures of the body (Fig. 17-17) (135). Other anatomic location–based scapular fracture classifications have been reported by Imatani and by Wilbur and Evans (136,139).

The classification described below is also based on the anatomic location of the fracture, with additional subclassifications based on multiple reported studies (see Fig. 17-17 and Table 17-3). However, most of these studies are not specific for pediatric scapular fractures, so application of this classification system and its supportive studies to pediatric scapular fractures should be individualized to each child. The fracture should be adequately evaluated for its anatomic location, displacement, comminution, and articular involvement. In addition, ipsilateral neurovascular status, the overall status of the patient, and other concomitant injuries should be fully characterized.

Fractures of the body and the spine of the scapula, which make up nearly 50% of all scapular fractures, are broadly categorized into those with and without displacement. Although an isolated fracture of the scapular neck is believed to be a stable bony construct, ipsilateral fractures to both the scapular neck and the clavicle may lead to disruption of the suspensory mechanism of the shoulder (132,150). Therefore, fractures of the scapular neck are categorized into those with and without concomitant injury to the clavicle. For similar considerations, fractures

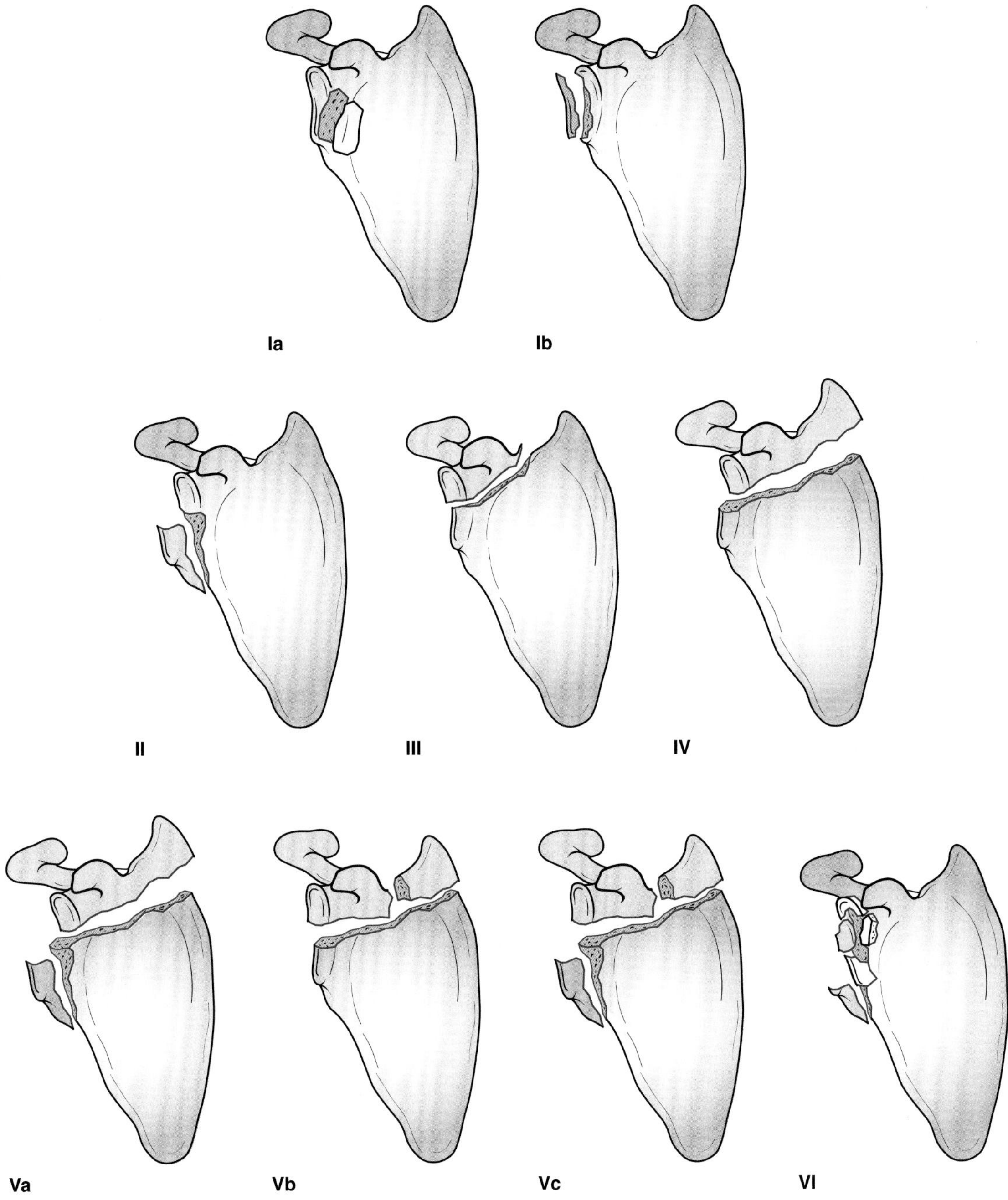

FIGURE 17-17 General classification of scapular/glenoid fractures.

of the coracoid process are categorized into those with and without concomitant injury to the acromioclavicular joint.

Fractures of the acromion are categorized into those with and without displacement. Displaced fractures are further subclassified based on the presence or absence of subacromial narrowing. Subacromial space narrowing may occur after inferior displacement of the acromion or after superior displacement of an ipsilateral glenoid fracture. When treated conservatively, these fracture patterns often lead to subacromial impingement in adults and result in decreased range of shoulder motion and increased shoulder pain (151). Although its applicability to acromial fractures in younger children is still debated, this finding significantly affects the treatment options for acromial fractures in older children.

Fractures of the glenoid typically occur when the humeral head is driven onto the glenoid fossa. Depending on the direction of the force applied to the humeral head, the fracture may involve the entire fossa or just the rim. If the entire fossa is

TABLE 17-3 Interventions for Scapular Fractures

	Immobilization	Operative Reduction & Immobilization	Operative Reduction & Internal Fixation
Body of scapula	X		
Acromion	X		X
Glenoid rim/fossa	X		X
Scapula-thoracic dissociation	X	X	

involved, the fracture line may then exit in multiple locations about the scapula. Hence, fractures of the glenoid are classified into five distinct groups based on their anatomic location and course of the fracture. This system was initially proposed by Ideberg and later expanded by Goss (Fig. 17-18) (152–154). Type I fractures are isolated glenoid rim fractures, with Ia involving the anterior rim and Ib involving the posterior rim. Type II, III, and IV fractures are glenoid fractures with fracture lines exiting through lateral, superior, and medial aspects of the scapula, respectively. Type V fractures are various combinations of type II, III, and IV fractures. Type Va, for example, is a combination of types II and IV. Type Vb is a combination of types III and IV, whereas type Vc is a combination of types II, III, and IV. Type VI fractures are comminuted fractures of the glenoid fossa. These various types of glenoid fractures are associated with distinct patterns of morbidity and treatment options.

Scapulothoracic dissociation occurs when all attachments or articulations between the thorax and the scapula are completely severed. When there is an ipsilateral neurovascular injury, it is sometimes referred to as a forequarter amputation. This is in contrast to scapulothoracic dislocation, where only the inferior scapulothoracic articulation is displaced (141). Although intrathoracic dissociations have been reported (155), scapulothoracic dissociations are typically laterally displaced. These injuries are categorized as open or closed with intact or compromised neurovascular status.

Surgical and Applied Anatomy

During development, the scapula forms in the first trimester of gestation. It first appears near the level of lower cervical spine, C4–C7, and then descends to its final position on the lateral aspect of the upper thorax during development. Most of the scapula is formed by intramembranous ossification. Numerous centers of ossification exist for the scapula: three for the body, two for the coracoid process, two to five for the acromion (144), and one for the glenoid. These ossification centers during childhood are often mistakenly identified as fractures. In some developmental anomalies, distinct ossification centers fail to fuse and persist into adulthood (147). These conditions are also frequently characterized as fractures. With few exceptions, however, a developmental variation and a fracture can be distinguished by clinical history, physical examination, and radiographic appearance.

The scapula is roughly triangular and has a complex three-dimensional structure. It is responsible for linking the upper extremity to the axial skeleton (Fig. 17-19) and contains attachments to 17 distinct muscles. The anterior aspect of the scapular body is a relatively flat surface, most of which is covered by the subscapularis muscle. The posterior aspect of the scapula is divided into two fossae by the scapular spine. These superior and inferior scapula fossae are mostly covered by the supraspinatus and the infraspinatus muscles, respectively. The anteromedial border of the scapular body provides attachment to the serratus anterior muscle. The posteromedial border contains the attachment sites of the levator scapulae, rhomboideus major and minor, and latissimus dorsi muscles. The omohyoid muscle attaches to the superior aspect of the scapular body, whereas the teres minor and major muscles and the triceps muscle attach to the lateral border. The scapular spine provides attachments to the trapezius and deltoid muscles, and the long head of the biceps muscle originates from the superior rim of the glenoid. Finally, the pectoralis minor muscle, as well as the conjoined tendon of the coracobrachialis and short head of the biceps muscles, attach to the coracoid process.

In addition to these muscle attachments, the scapula participates in the formation of both glenohumeral and acromioclavicular joints. The glenohumeral joint is stabilized by multiple dynamic and static forces about the joint, which are discussed separately. The acromioclavicular joint is stabilized in part by the presence of two coracoclavicular ligaments that position the distal clavicle immediately medial to the acromion. The two ligaments are the conoid and the trapezoid ligaments, with the conoid being the more medial of the two.

In close proximity to the scapula are a number of neurovascular structures that can be injured during a scapular fracture. Most notable are the brachial plexus and the axillary artery,

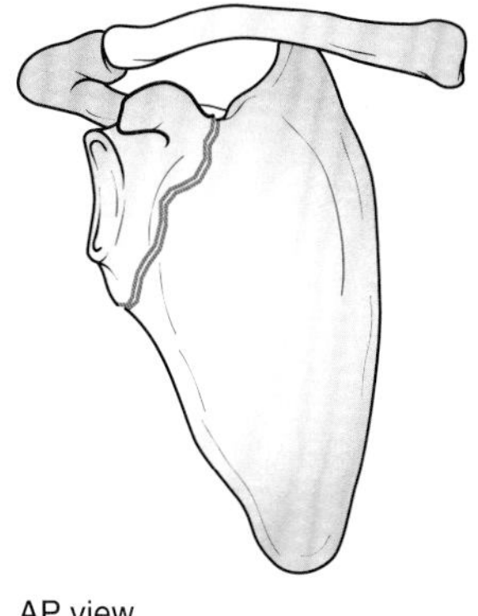

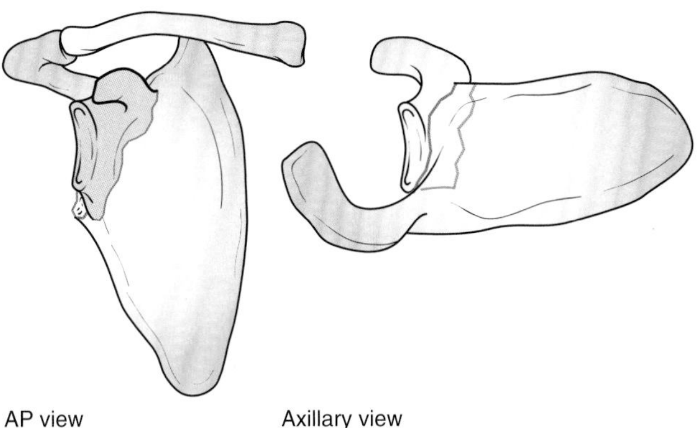

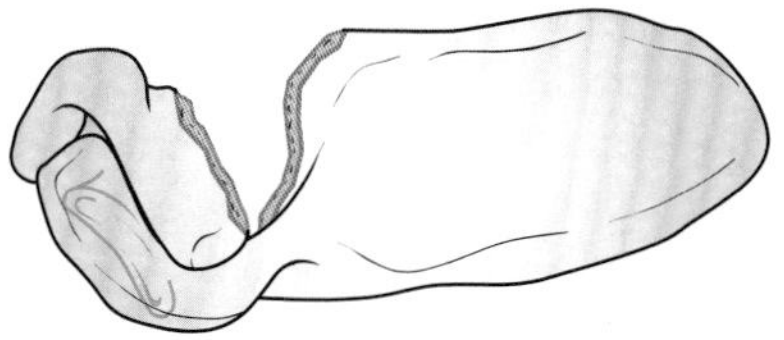

FIGURE 17-18 Classification of fractures of the glenoid neck.

which course across the anterosuperior aspect of the scapula. They are immediately posterior and inferior to the tip of the coracoid process. Medial to the base of the coracoid process is the scapular notch with the overlying transverse scapular ligament. The suprascapular nerve and artery pass under and over the ligament, respectively, in the scapular notch and are susceptible to injury with nearby fractures. The axillary nerve travels within an intermuscular interval immediately inferior to the glenoid and is also susceptible to injury with displaced fractures of the glenoid neck (156).

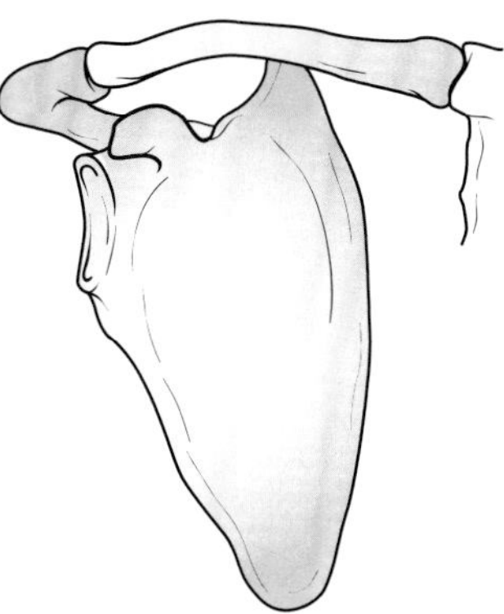

FIGURE 17-19 Relationship between the scapula, clavicle, and sternum.

A traumatic insult may cause fractures in multiple locations about the scapula, with one fracture influencing the stability of another. Goss proposed this and subsequently introduced the concept of a superior shoulder suspensory complex (SSSC) (132). The SSSC is a set of bony struts attached to a circular complex of structures at the lateral end of the scapula (Fig. 17-20). The superior and inferior bony struts are the middle clavicle and the lateral scapula body/spine, respectively. The circular complex is composed of the acromioclavicular ligament, acromion, glenoid process, coracoid process, coracoclavicular ligament, and distal clavicle. As a whole, the SSSC is responsible for linking the upper extremity to the axial skeleton. Traumatic injury to any single component of the SSSC may result in a minimally displaced fracture, because the inherent stability of the circular complex is still intact. However, when multiple structures of the circular complex are injured, a double disruption to the circle occurs. This, in turn, results in significant instability. Similarly, injury to one of the structures of the ring complex with a concomitant injury to a bony strut also may create an unstable construct. Goss proposed that the treatment decisions for scapular injuries should be based on the maintenance of SSSC integrity (132).

Current Treatment Options

There are few published studies to provide evidence-based recommendations regarding current treatment options for scapular fractures in children. Therefore, most of the following comments are inferred from studies of adult populations.

Isolated fractures of the scapular body do not affect the integrity of the SSSC. In addition, because of the numerous muscle attachments, fractures of the scapular body are quite stable and can be treated conservatively in most cases (see Table 17-3). Several studies have shown that conservative treatment of nondisplaced or minimally displaced scapular body fractures in adults is generally associated with excellent results. Based on these studies, similar treatment is recommended for equivalent fractures in the pediatric population (139,140,157,158). In adults, conservative treatment of scapular body fractures with

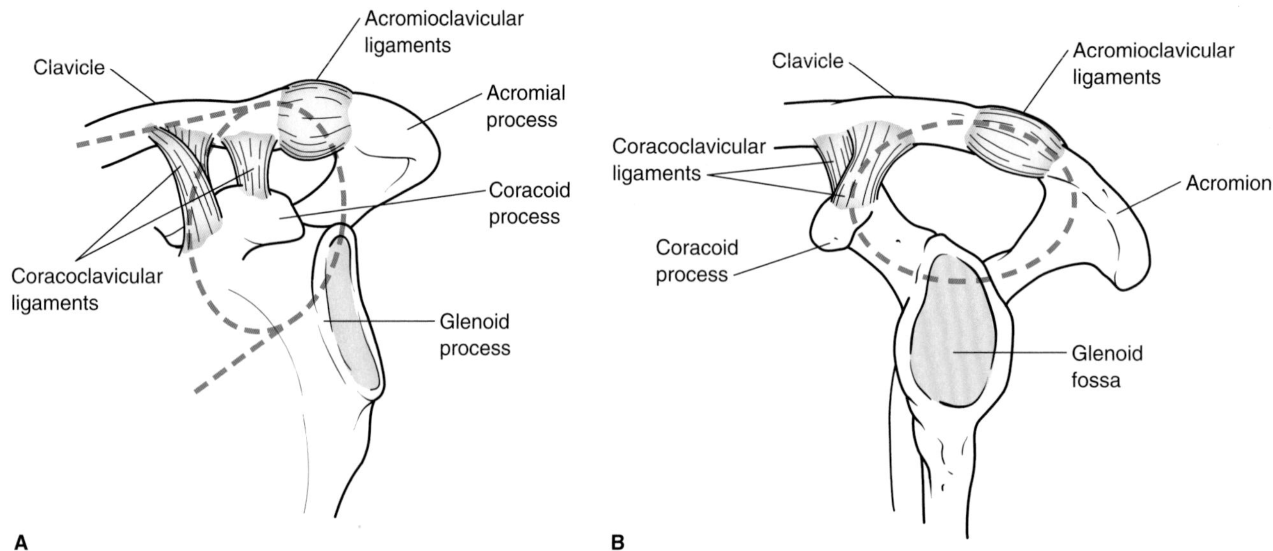

FIGURE 17-20 Superior shoulder suspensory complex. **A.** AP view of the bone–soft tissue ring and superior and inferior bone struts. **B.** Lateral view of the bone–soft tissue ring.

significant displacement of more than 10 mm, however, resulted in unfavorable outcomes (157). Since a comparable study of pediatric scapular body fractures has not yet been reported, we can only assume that widely displaced fractures in children would have a similarly poor long-term outcome. The threshold for acceptable displacement has not been described.

Nondisplaced or mildly displaced scapular neck fractures without concomitant injury to the clavicle can be treated conservatively (159). However, if there is also ipsilateral clavicular injury, surgical intervention generally is recommended to reestablish the SSSC (138,150,160,161). Whether open reduction and fixation of the clavicle is sufficient to stabilize the fracture (160) or whether the neck fracture also must be reduced in addition to the clavicle (150) is debatable. For patients in whom surgical intervention is not possible, external fixation or traction may be an acceptable option (162).

Fractures of the coracoid process typically occur at the base. Isolated fractures of the coracoid process usually are nondisplaced and can be treated conservatively with a sling and mobilization as tolerated. Displaced coracoid fractures occur with ipsilateral injury to the distal clavicle or the acromioclavicular joint. Most investigators favor open reduction and internal fixation of these fractures to restore the integrity of the SSSC (136,140,163). Displaced coracoid fractures near the suprascapular notch with injury to the suprascapular nerve also have been described, with some investigators advocating early exploration (164).

Isolated fractures of the acromion in children are typically nondisplaced. In adults, acromial fractures with subacromial narrowing are associated with subsequent development of subacromial impingement when treated nonsurgically (151). Therefore, most investigators recommend open reduction and internal fixation for displaced acromial fractures where the subacromial space has been compromised (151), or with another disruption in the SSSC (132).

Fractures of the glenoid neck typically are nondisplaced unless other elements of the SSSC are disrupted. These fractures generally have excellent outcomes with nonsurgical treatment. Significant displacement or angulation, however, may limit glenohumeral motion (157,162). In adults, glenoid neck fractures with more than 10 mm of displacement or 40 degrees of angulation result in poor outcomes when treated without surgical reduction (138). Therefore, it is reasonable to infer that pediatric glenoid neck fractures with significant displacement or angulation also require surgical intervention.

Treatment of glenoid rim fractures (types I and II) is based on the presence or absence of shoulder instability. Closed treatment of asymptomatic glenoid rim fractures rarely results in long-term morbidity (165). For glenoid rim fractures with resulting shoulder subluxation or instability, however, operative reduction and fixation are recommended to prevent permanent or recurrent dislocations (133,162,166). In adults, shoulder instability occurs when the fracture was displaced more than 10 mm or when the fracture involved more than either 25% of the anterior or 33% of the posterior aspects of the glenoid (162). Anterior and posterior approaches to the glenoid generally are recommended for open reduction and internal fixation of anterior and posterior rim fractures, respectively (132).

Nondisplaced glenoid fossa fractures (types III through VI) also can be successfully treated nonsurgically (132). Displaced fractures, on the other hand, are associated with significant morbidity (pain, stiffness, and limited range of motion) when treated without surgical reduction. Patients with intraarticular displacement greater than 5 mm should be considered for surgical reduction and fixation (162,167,168). In type IV glenoid fractures, where significant comminution is present, acceptable operative reduction and fixation may be difficult to achieve (132,154), and these fractures may be better treated with nonsurgical options (132,154). For open reduction and internal fixation of these fractures, a posterior approach generally provides the most acceptable exposure (132).

Initial treatment of scapulothoracic dissociations generally focuses on stabilization and repair of the neurovascular injury. If the axillary artery and the brachial plexus are not salvageable, an early amputation should be considered (142). Limb salvage is usually attempted if limb viability cannot be determined. Immediate exploration of the brachial plexus is warranted when a concomitant vascular injury requires an operative repair. If a vascular injury is not present, the brachial plexus need not be explored acutely. After a period of 4 to 6 weeks, the extent of the brachial plexus injury should be documented (physical examination, electromyography/nerve conduction velocity, MRI) prior to surgical reconstruction, such as nerve repair or musculotendinous transfer (132,142). Immediate operative stabilization of an ipsilateral clavicular fracture generally is necessary only if the bony instability compromises the integrity of the neurovascular structures.

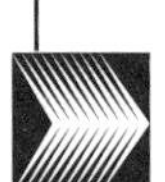

AUTHORS' PREFERRED TREATMENT

Once the patient is stabilized, the approach to the scapula or glenoid fractures can be undertaken more thoroughly. With rare exception, scapula fractures are treated without surgery. Fractures of the glenoid generally are treated with observation and follow-up, including physical therapy and rehabilitation. For the rare displaced glenoid intraarticular and highly displaced fractures, open reduction with internal fixation is recommended (169). This is generally performed via an anterior deltopectoral approach, but posterior approaches to the scapula and glenoid may be necessary depending on the fracture type.

Intrathoracic dislocation is rare. Most can be reduced by closed manipulative methods. In those associated with residual scapular deformity, an open approach may be required. With scapulothoracic disassociation, it is important to attend to the priorities of trauma care, including an appropriate and detailed neurovascular examination. Vascular consultation or evaluation may be required, given the potential for massive injury to the brachial artery or plexus. In these instances, early or late amputation should be considered.

Pearls and Pitfalls

- Suspect scapula fractures in patients with multiple trauma, and scrutinize the x-rays.
- Maintain a high index of suspicion for visceral injuries when a scapula body fracture presents as an isolated injury.
- Be aware of normal variants in scapular anatomy, such as os acromiale. Review x-rays of the contralateral scapula if necessary.
- Look for radiographic evidence of scapulothoracic dissociation.
- Most scapula fractures are managed without surgery.
- Highly displaced scapula body fractures and glenoid fossa fractures require open reduction and internal fixation.

Complications

Early Complications

Complications of scapular fractures are rare. The concomitant injuries frequently associated with scapular fractures were discussed throughout this section (135,139,140,143). Due to their proximity, the axillary and the suprascapular nerves may be injured in association with glenoid and coracoid fractures, respectively (156,164). In addition, the energy required to create scapular fractures likely results in other injuries, such as rib fractures, pneumothorax, and vascular avulsions. All or portions of the lower brachial plexus are susceptible to injury with scapulothoracic dissociations (141,142,149). This devastating injury also has been associated with the development of compartment syndrome in the upper arm (158). The presence of a complete brachial plexus avulsion is predictive of a poor functional outcome with a scapulothoracic dissociation (170).

Late Complications

Late complications associated with scapular fractures generally involve improper functioning of the upper extremity. Displaced fractures of the scapular body and spine, for example, infrequently result in upper extremity weakness and pain with movement (138). Similarly, fractures of the acromion can result in pain and decreased range of upper extremity motion secondary to subacromial impingement (151). Displaced intraarticular fractures of the glenoid are associated with glenohumeral subluxation or dislocation, as well as early progression of degenerative arthritis (132,133,162,166).

Symptomatic nonunion of scapula body fractures has been reported (171,172). Most problems related to injuries of the scapula are not necessarily related to treatment but are more often related to failure to accurately evaluate associated major systems injuries.

FRACTURES OF THE CLAVICLE

The clavicle has the important function of linking, as a strut, the axial skeleton to the upper extremity (see Fig. 17-19). Through its sternoclavicular and the acromioclavicular joints, the clavicle contributes to the overall motion of the upper extremity. The clavicle can protract and retract (173). It also rotates and elevates to contribute to shoulder abduction (173–175). In addition, the clavicle provides the attachment site for the two predominant mobilizers of the upper extremity: the pectoralis major and the deltoid muscles. The integrity of the clavicle, therefore, is crucial to the optimal functioning of the entire upper extremity.

As a result of two factors, the clavicle is one of the most frequently fractured bones in the body. First, the clavicle is subcutaneous throughout most its span, being situated on the anterosuperior aspect of the thorax. Second, nearly all of the forces imparted onto the upper extremity are transmitted through the clavicle to the trunk. The clavicle is the bone most commonly injured during labor and delivery, occurring in 0.5% of all deliveries and accounting for nearly 90% of all obstetrical fractures (176–179). In older children, clavicular fractures occur frequently, with the reported rates ranging between 8% and 15% of all pediatric fractures (180–182).

Principles of Management

Mechanism of Injury

The clavicle is the most common site of all obstetrical fractures, and clavicular fractures occur in 1% to 13% of all births (176–178,183–189). The incidence of obstetrical clavicle fractures is increased for larger-birthweight infants (176,179, 186,190). In addition, deliveries requiring the use of instruments or specialized obstetric maneuvers are more likely to result in clavicular fractures (176,185,186,190). Based on these findings, it has been postulated that fractures in these difficult deliveries result from lateral-to-medial pressure on the shoulders during passage through the narrow birth canal. However, despite the above trends, the majority of birth-related clavicular fractures occur in deliveries of average-birthweight infants who receive routine and otherwise uneventful obstetrical care. Thus, on the whole, obstetrical clavicle fractures are sometimes unavoidable consequences of vaginal deliveries for anatomic or physiologic reasons that may not be evident before or even after delivery.

The most common mechanism of clavicular fractures in children is a fall onto the shoulder (182,191,192). Other mechanisms include accidents where the traumatic insult is applied directly to the clavicle (192). Indirect applications of force, typically falling onto an outstretched hand, are much less likely to result in clavicular fractures (192). Clavicular fractures may also occur in children victimized by child abuse, but no pathognomonic pattern for isolated clavicular fractures resulting from child abuse has been described (193,194).

A significant amount of energy can be applied directly to the clavicle during athletic activities such as football or indirectly through athletic activities such as gymnastics. Most commonly, the direct mechanism is responsible for clavicle fractures, acromioclavicular joint injuries, or sternoclavicular joint injuries (180,182). A large proportion of these sports injuries may be preventable with the use of protective equipment and adequate padding (195). Although rare, stress fractures of the clavicle have been reported (174,196).

Signs and Symptoms

Clavicular fractures in newborns may be difficult to identify. The presence of generalized edema may prevent the palpation of normal clavicular margins (197). To minimize pain, newborns with clavicular fractures demonstrate pseudoparalysis of the affected arm, characterized by voluntary splinting or immobilization of the ipsilateral arm (198,199). Frequently this pseudoparalysis is mistaken for brachial plexus injury. To reduce the pull of the sternocleidomastoid muscle across the fracture site, affected infants turn their head toward the side of the fracture. In addition, infants with acute clavicular fractures typically exhibit an asymmetric Moro reflex (200,201). In the absence of radiographic confirmation, the diagnosis of clavicle fracture may be suspected and later confirmed after a mass is noticed in the affected clavicle. This mass represents a healing fracture callus that forms 7 to 10 days after the initial trauma. Often by this point the fracture is sufficiently stabilized by fracture callus that it causes little discomfort to the infant.

Diagnosis of clavicular fractures in older children is usually straightforward. Children have moderate to severe pain around the area of the fracture and voluntarily immobilize and stop using the affected arm. Tenderness, ecchymosis, and edema are invariably present; in fractures with large displacement, a bony prominence or deformity may be noted. Most children with clavicular fractures keep their heads turned to the side of the fracture to relax the sternocleidomastoid muscle (197).

Crepitus and instability may be detected over the affected joints in children with either acromioclavicular or sternoclavicular joint injuries. True dislocations of the acromioclavicular joint or the sternoclavicular joint are rare. Failure usually occurs at the physis before joint dislocation, and injuries to the medial and lateral end of the clavicle in children are commonly physeal fractures.

Associated Injuries

Atlantoaxial (C1-2) rotatory displacement (subluxation) and clavicular fracture occur together on rare occasions. Attributing acute torticollis entirely to the clavicular fracture may delay the diagnosis of atlantoaxial displacement, and delayed diagnosis of atlantoaxial displacement increases the risk of permanent atlantoaxial rotatory fixation (202,203). When present, the child's head will be laterally bent toward and rotated away from the fractured clavicle. The diagnosis of C1-2 subluxation is best confirmed by dynamic CT.

Posterior dislocations of the sternoclavicular joint or posterior displaced physeal separations of the medial clavicle are particular worrisome for associated injury or compression of the great vessels, the esophagus, or the trachea (204,205). Suspicion of these injuries is further increased in children who have difficulty speaking, breathing, or swallowing. Pulses in the ipsilateral upper extremity may be diminished or absent, and the neck veins may be distended. Obviously, any of these injuries associated with posterior sternoclavicular joint dislocations can be life-threatening, and precautionary diagnostic and treatment steps should be taken at the onset of treatment. If available, a thoracic or vascular surgeon should be consulted or notified prior to reduction attempts.

Diagnosis and Classification

Imaging Studies. An AP x-ray of the clavicle is the standard study with which a clavicular fracture is initially evaluated. In addition, ultrasonography is been a valuable supplement in establishing the diagnosis of clavicular fractures in neonates (206–208). Ultrasonography is particularly useful in detecting occult clavicular fractures as well as sternoclavicular joint dislocations in this young group (206,209). Bone healing may be detected on ultrasound 1 week before on x-rays.

For older children, other radiographic studies may be necessary to supplement the AP x-ray in evaluating the clavicular fracture. For fractures in the middle third of the clavicle, several views may be beneficial: the cephalad-directed views, the apical oblique view, and the apical lordotic view. The cephalad-directed views are helpful in illustrating the degree of fracture displacement. These views are taken with the x-ray beam 20 to 40 degrees cephalad to the clavicle (Fig. 17-21A). The apical oblique view is taken with the x-ray beam 45 degrees lateral to the axial axis of the body and 20 degrees cephalad to the clavicle. This view is better suited to identify fractures in the middle third of the clavicle, where significant curvature is present in the bone (210). The apical lordotic view is a perpendicular view of the AP x-ray. It is taken laterally with the shoulder abducted more than 130 degrees (see Fig. 17-21B). This degree of shoulder abduction, however, can cause significant discomfort in children with acute clavicular fractures. Therefore, this radiographic view may be better suited for evaluating the healing of the clavicular fracture rather than for the initial assessment of the fracture (211).

Fractures in the lateral aspect of the clavicle may require additional radiographic views for full assessment. In addition to the views mentioned above, an axillary lateral view is helpful in evaluating the fracture and its displacement. If the injury in this portion of the clavicle or the acromioclavicular joint is not obvious on the obtained x-rays, a radiographic stress view may provide more useful information. A radiographic stress view is an AP x-ray of the lateral clavicle with distraction on the ipsilateral upper extremity. Distraction can be achieved by asking the child to hold 5 to 10 pounds of weight with his or her hand or by simply having an assistant gently pull on the arm downward. The stress view may show subtle injuries to the distal clavicle or the acromioclavicular joint. If enhanced evaluation of the acromioclavicular joint is desired, a CT scan should be performed.

Additional radiographic views are usually necessary to characterize fractures of the medial third of the clavicle and sternoclavicular injuries. The "serendipity" view, where a broad x-ray beam with 40 degrees of cephalic tilt projects both clavicles on the same film, is helpful for evaluating fractures in this portion of the clavicle (Fig. 17-22) (212). By comparing with the uninjured contralateral side, the location of injury and the degree of displacement often can be determined. Currently, CT is highly effective for evaluating injuries in the medial third of the clavicle. CT provides detailed information about the morphology of the medial clavicle, the medial physis, the degree of displacement, and possible injury to the underlying intrathoracic structures (Fig. 17-23). Virtually every acute injury of the medial end of the clavicle should be evaluated with CT, and it also is useful for follow-up of chronic injuries. Nonetheless, the technique for serendipity views continues to be useful for intraoperative radiography.

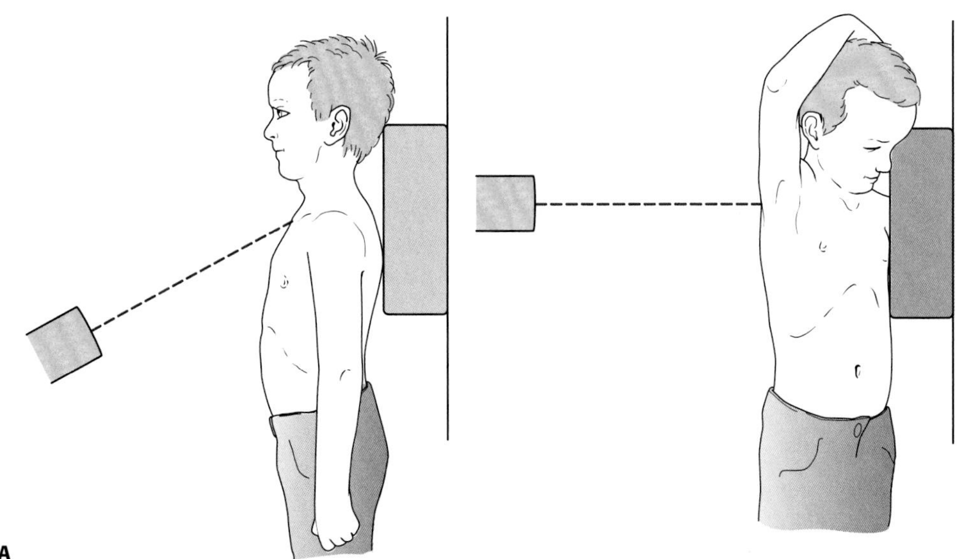

FIGURE 17-21 **A.** Cephalad-directed views. **B.** Apical lordotic view.

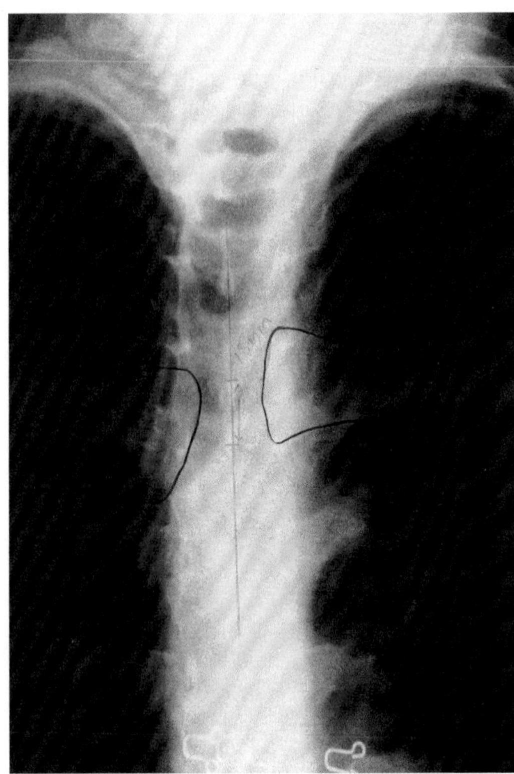

FIGURE 17-22 Serendipity view of the medial clavicle.

Classification. Because of differences in the mechanism and rate of injury, prognosis, and treatment options, clavicular fractures are broadly categorized by their anatomic location: medial third, middle third, and distal third (Fig. 17-24). Most clavicular fractures occur at the middle third, with the reported rates ranging from 76% to 85% (182,213). The second most common site of clavicular injury is the distal third, with the reported rates between 10% and 21% (182,213–215). Fractures in the medial third of the clavicle are relatively uncommon and represent only 3% to 5% of all clavicular fractures (182,215).

The widely used classification for clavicular fracture is based on the anatomic location of the fracture (216) (see Fig. 17-24). Type I fractures occur in the middle third of the clavicle and generally include all fractures lateral to the sternocleidomastoid muscle and medial to the coracoclavicular ligament. Type II fractures are in the distal clavicle, including and lateral to the coracoclavicular ligament. Type III fractures are medial to the sternocleidomastoid muscle. Type III fractures are relatively uncommon. Within this general framework, further classifications exist for injuries to the distal and medial ends of the clavicle.

Distal Clavicular Injuries. Distal clavicular injuries lateral to the coracoclavicular ligament and injuries to the acromioclavicular joint are categorized by a system proposed by Dameron and Rockwood (Fig. 17-25) (198). Although similar to the system for adult distal clavicular injuries, this classification system incorporates the observation that the distal clavicle displaces through a disruption in its periosteal sleeve rather than by true disruption of the coracoclavicular ligaments. Also, true acromioclavicular dislocations rarely occur in children. Most fractures in this region are either metaphyseal or physeal fractures (217,218). However, because distal clavicular epiphyseal ossification does not occur until age 18 or 19, these injuries may have the radiographic appearance of an acromioclavicular dislocation rather than a fracture (pseudodislocation) (217–219).

Type I acromial clavicular injuries are caused by low-energy trauma and are characterized by mild strains of the ligaments. No gross changes are seen on x-rays. Type II injury includes complete disruption of the acromioclavicular ligaments, with mild damage to the superolateral aspect of the periosteal sleeve. Mild instability of the distal clavicle results from this type of injury, and minimal widening of the acromioclavicular joint may be seen on an x-ray. In type III injury, complete disruption of the acromioclavicular ligaments occurs in addition to a large disruption in the periosteal sleeve. Noticeable superior displacement of the distal clavicle is seen on an AP x-ray, and the coracoid–clavicle interval is 25% to 100% greater than on the contralateral uninjured side (220,221). Similar soft tissue disruptions are seen in type IV injuries. The distal clavicle, however, is displaced posteriorly and is often embedded in the trapezius muscle (222). Minimal changes may be noted on an AP x-ray, and an axillary lateral x-ray may be required to identify the posterior clavicular displacement. Type V injuries are similar to type III injuries; the difference lies in the fact that the superior aspect of the periosteal sleeve is completely disrupted in type V injuries. This allows displacement of the distal clavicle into the subcutaneous tissues, occasionally splitting the deltoid and the trapezius muscles. On an AP x-ray, the coracoid–clavicle interval is more than 100% greater than on the contralateral uninjured side. In type VI injuries, the distal clavicle is displaced inferiorly, with its distal end located inferior to the coracoid process (223).

Medial Clavicular Injuries. The medial physis of the clavicle is the last physis in the body to close, and the fusion of this epiphysis to the shaft occurs as late as 23 to 25 years of age (224,225). The sternoclavicular ligaments attach primarily to the epiphysis, leaving the physis unprotected outside the capsule (194). Because of its unique anatomy, traumatic insults to the medial end of the clavicle in children typically result in fractures through the physis rather than dislocations through the sternoclavicular joint. Therefore, these injuries are categorized most appropriately in the Salter-Harris classification system (226). Most fractures at the medial end of the clavicle are Salter-Harris type I or II fractures. These fractures are further subdivided by the direction of the clavicular displacement, either anterior or posterior. Although anterior displacement of the clavicle occurs more frequently, more attention is given to fractures with posterior displacement due

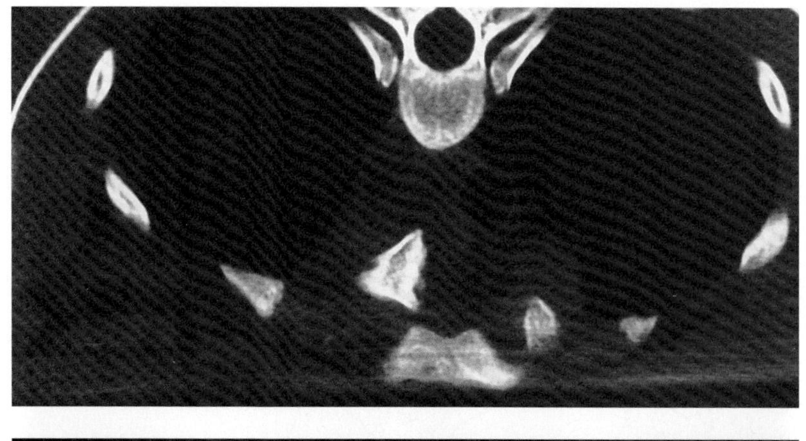

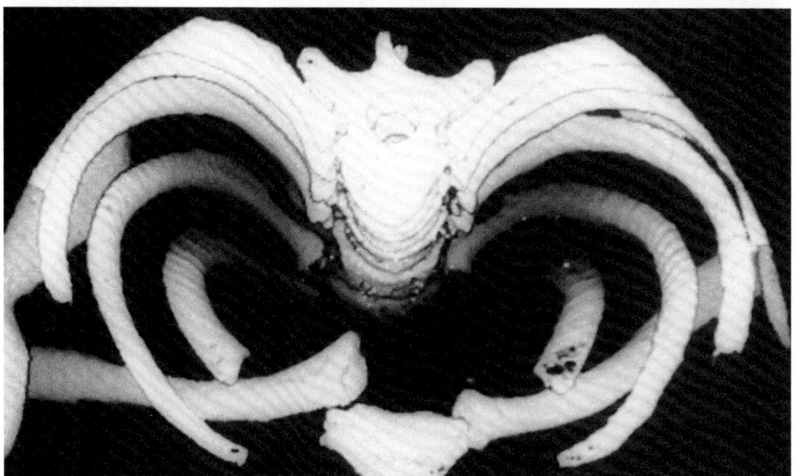

FIGURE 17-23 A. CT image of the clavicle showing posterior retrosternal dislocation of the medial end of the clavicle. **B.** Three-dimensional reconstruction of image shown in **A**.

to the possibility of concomitant mediastinal injuries requiring emergent intervention.

Surgical and Applied Anatomy

The clavicle is an S-shaped bone whose medial end is connected to the axial skeleton through the sternoclavicular joint. The medial two thirds of the bone is tubular, whereas the lateral end is flatter and is stabilized in its position by the two coracoclavicular ligaments. The clavicle appears early during embryonic development. By the 5th or 6th week of gestation, it begins ossification at two separate centers, medial and lateral (173,227,228). By the 7th or 8th week of gestation, its overall

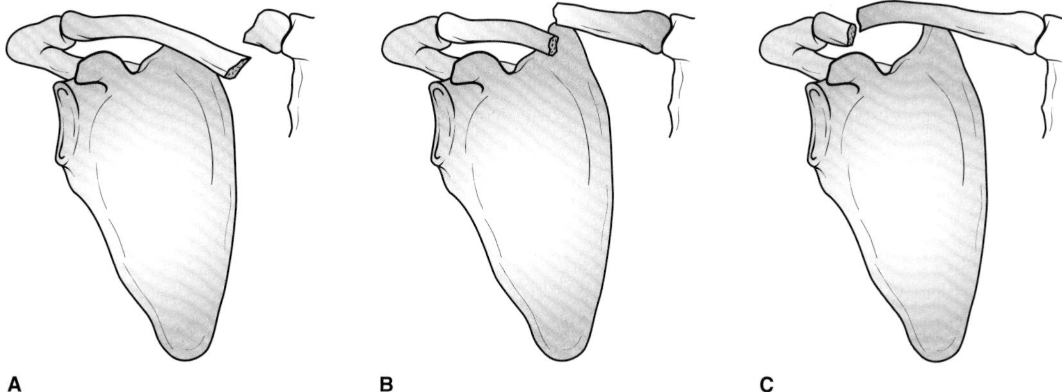

FIGURE 17-24 A. Fracture of the medial third of the clavicle. **B.** Fracture of the middle third of the clavicle. **C.** Fracture of the lateral third of the clavicle.

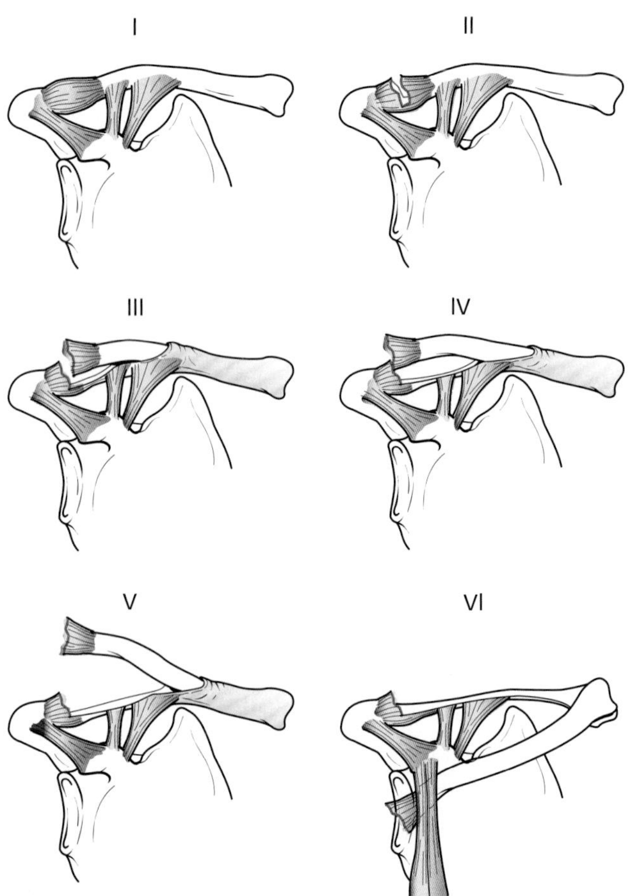

FIGURE 17-25 Dameron and Rockwood classification of distal/lateral fractures.

contour and shape are already formed (227). During childhood, approximately 80% of clavicular growth and longitudinal growth occur at the medial physis (229). Despite this early ossification and growth, complete growth of the clavicle does not occur until early adulthood. The lateral physis continues to proliferate until 18 to 19 years of age, and the medial physis does not close until 23 to 25 years of age (219,224,225).

The distal clavicle articulates with the scapula through the acromioclavicular joint, a joint that lacks inherent structural stability. It is held together in part by the acromioclavicular ligaments, which are relatively weak secondary stabilizers. The primary stabilizers of the joint are the two coracoclavicular ligaments, the conoid and the trapezoid, which place the lateral end of the clavicle immediately next to the acromion. Although the distal clavicle and the coracoid process usually do not articulate, a coracoclavicular joint has been reported in adults (230). In children, the distal clavicle and the acromion are surrounded by thick periosteum that forms a protective tube around the bony structures. The coracoclavicular ligaments are attached to the periosteum on the inferior surface of the distal clavicle. Because these ligament attachments are stronger than the periosteum, displacement of the distal clavicle occurs through a disruption in the periosteum rather than by detachment of the ligaments. In fact, displacement of the distal clavicle through this periosteum in children has been likened to having "a banana being peeled out of its skin." As mentioned above, the distal clavicular physis does not ossify until early adulthood (219). Therefore, fractures through the distal clavicular physis or metaphysis may be mistakenly identified as acromioclavicular joint dislocations.

Medially, the clavicle articulates with the sternum and the first rib through the sternoclavicular joint. Similar to the acromioclavicular joint, this joint also lacks inherent structural stability. It is held together by a series of strong ligaments, including the intraarticular disc ligament, the anterior and posterior capsular ligaments, the interclavicular ligament, and the costoclavicular ligament (231). In children, the medial physis of the clavicle is still open, and the capsular ligaments attach primarily to the epiphysis (224,225,231). Therefore, injuries to the medial clavicle typically result in physeal fractures with the epiphysis attached to the sternum.

The clavicle also serves as attachment sites for a number of different muscles. On its superior surface, the clavicular head of the sternocleidomastoid muscle is attached. On the posterior surface, the trapezius muscle is attached, whereas the pectoralis major and the deltoid muscles are attached on the anterior surface. Inferiorly, the clavicle provides attachment sites for the subclavius muscle as well as the clavipectoral fascia.

The clavicle provides protection for the subclavian vessels and the brachial plexus. These vital structures are located posterior to the clavicle, crossing the clavicle at the junction between the medial two thirds and lateral one third of the bone (see Fig. 17-12). Due to this close proximity, the neurovascular status of the ipsilateral upper extremity may be jeopardized in children with displaced clavicular shaft fractures. In addition, as discussed above, posterior dislocation of the sternoclavicular joint can lead to compression or injuries of the great vessels within the mediastinum. Therefore, the neurovascular status of the ipsilateral upper extremity must be documented before the initiation of treatment for any clavicular injury.

The clavicle contributes significantly to the overall motion and optimal function of the upper extremity. In the anterior to posterior direction, the clavicle can protract and retract approximately 35 degrees (173). Laterally, it can rotate and elevate to contribute approximately 30 degrees to shoulder abduction (173,175). The clavicle also provides the attachment sites for the major mobilizers of the upper arm, the pectoralis major and the deltoid muscles. Finally, together with the scapula, the distal clavicle forms the SSSC (described in the scapula section). As proposed by Goss, the SSSC provides a scaffold from which the upper extremity suspends and articulates in order to function (232).

Current Treatment Options

Treatment options are listed in Tables 17-4 and 17-5 as well as in the following text.

TABLE 17-4 Interventions for Clavicle Fractures

	Immobilization	Closed Reduction & Immobilization	Operative Reduction & Internal Fixation
Middle third	X		Rare
Distal third	X		Rare
Medial third	X		
SC dislocation, anterior		X	
SC dislocation, posterior		X—Emergency	Rare—see text

Middle-Third Fractures

Treatment of the obstetrical clavicle fracture is nonoperative. For most birth-related clavicular fractures, minimal or no treatment is required. If the infant appears to be in significant discomfort, the affected arm can be immobilized to the body for a short period of time, typically less than 2 weeks. Immobilization of the affected arm can be easily and effectively accomplished by using a safety pin to attach the long shirt sleeve to the shirt (233–235). The parents should be warned not to disturb the upper extremity by unnecessary excessive movements in the acute period. In addition, they should be informed that the infant will develop a noticeable mass over the fracture site that will typically resolve within 6 months (200).

Good to excellent results also can be expected from nonoperative treatment of most clavicle fractures in older children. A figure-of-eight splint is an acceptable method of nonoperative treatment and has been widely used with successful outcomes (200,236–238). It can be applied directly or after an attempt at closed reduction with retraction of the shoulders (239). In general, younger children do not require reduction of the fracture because their potential for remodeling is greater (239). A sling to support the weight of the arm is sufficient treatment in most cases.

The figure-of-eight splint, unfortunately, can be uncomfortable for some children. In addition, inappropriate use of the splint, on rare occasions, can lead to a number of complications, including edema, compression of the axillary vessels, and brachial plexopathy (237,240,241). Use of a sling, on the other hand, is typically well tolerated by children and is not associated with any of these complications. Treatment of both nondisplaced and displaced clavicular fractures with a sling has shown remarkably good results. In fact, in comparison with a figure-of-eight splint, treatment of clavicular fractures with a sling resulted in similar final outcomes (236,242,243). Therefore, it appears that nonoperative treatment of middle-third clavicular fractures with a simple sling can result in excellent outcomes without compromising the child's comfort.

Reported indications for operative treatment of middle-third

TABLE 17-5 Treatment Pros and Cons: Clavicle Fractures

	Pros	Cons
No reduction (sling or shoulder immobilizer)	1) No anesthesia/sedation 2) Sling/shoulder immobilizer well tolerated	1) No improvement of fracture alignment 2) Functional loss of shoulder range of motion (rare)
Reduction and internal fixation (rare)	1) Improves fracture alignment 2) Direct rigid fixation of fracture 3) Improved patient comfort (due to rigid fracture fixation) 4) No cumbersome cast or splint	1) General anesthesia 2) Minimal increased risk of infection 3) Significant implant concerns 4) Implant removal

clavicular fractures include severely displaced and irreducible fractures that threaten skin integrity, concomitant vascular injury requiring repair, irreducible compression of the subclavian vessels, compromise of the brachial plexus, and open fractures (244–248). In addition, as discussed separately in this chapter, concomitant displaced fractures in various regions of the scapula, including the acromion, the coracoid, and the scapular neck, may compromise the SSSC and require operative repair (232). For the rare surgical case, either plating or intramedullary fixation can be performed. Intramedullary stabilization with elastic nails is increasingly popular because it is a safe, minimally invasive procedure (249,250).

Distal-Third Fractures

Injuries to the distal clavicle in the pediatric population typically are pseudodislocations of the acromioclavicular joint, with fractures through the metaphysis or the physis (218,251). The acromioclavicular joint and the coracoclavicular ligaments usually are undamaged, and most of the periosteal sleeve is intact. Therefore, exceptional potential for growth and remodeling exists for these fractures, allowing successful nonoperative treatment for most injuries to the distal clavicle.

Most investigators agree that undisplaced or minimally displaced injuries of the distal clavicle (types I, II, and III) are treated without surgery (198,218,252–254). These injuries are managed with a sling or a figure-of-eight splint immobilization followed by early rehabilitation with range-of-motion exercises. Most children treated with nonoperative management have no significant long-term functional or cosmetic deficits.

The treatment of displaced types IV, V, and VI distal clavicle fractures remains controversial. Some investigators report that most children experience no functional deficits regardless of the method of treatment (252,253). Others report that distal clavicular injuries with either fixed or gross displacement should be treated with open reduction and internal fixation to prevent permanent deformity (198,217,218,220,253,255–257). One report suggested that although displaced distal clavicular injuries in children under 13 years of age may be amenable to nonoperative treatment, those in children over 13 years of age should be treated with open reduction and internal fixation (251).

Although no clear consensus exists for the treatment of grossly displaced distal clavicular fractures in children, as long as the integrity of the SSSC is maintained, it appears that neither nonoperative nor operative management results in long-term deficit in the normal function of the shoulder. Treatment options, therefore, should be individualized for each child and his or her family based on compliance as well as acceptance of the possible cosmetic deformity.

Medial-Third Clavicular Injuries

Most pediatric injuries in the medial clavicle are fractures through the physis. Similar to distal clavicular injuries, these fractures have vast potential for healing in an acceptable position, and subsequent remodeling and nonoperative management is appropriate.

Nondisplaced fractures of the medial physis do not require active intervention. Symptomatic treatment is all that is required for these stable fractures. In fact, nondisplaced fractures often are missed during initial examination and are only discovered after a mass or bump is noted over the medial clavicle. The parents should be warned that the mass is a healing callus surrounding the fracture and that it should remodel and disappear in 4 to 8 months.

Anterior displaced medial clavicular fractures and sternoclavicular dislocations can be safely reduced in the emergency department or operating room. Longitudinal traction is applied to the ipsilateral upper extremity while the shoulder is abducted to 90 degrees (235). Gentle posterior pressure also should be applied over the fracture to encourage reduction. After the reduction is accomplished, the clavicle should be immobilized with a figure-of-eight splint (235).

Posteriorly displaced medial clavicular fractures and sternoclavicular dislocations require immediate evaluation for the presence of concomitant injuries of the airway and/or great vessels. Minimally displaced fractures and dislocations can be treated without reduction. These mildly displaced injuries can be expected to remodel without significant residual deformity or pain. For fractures and dislocations with significant posterior displacement or those associated with compromise of the airway or great vessels, urgent reduction should be performed. Under general anesthesia, closed reduction is attempted, followed by open reduction if necessary. Before beginning closed reduction in the operating room, appropriate instruments should be prepared for a possible open reduction. It is advisable to notify a thoracic surgeon before beginning reduction maneuvers in case an associated airway or vascular injury becomes apparent.

Technique of Reduction. After induction of general anesthesia, a bolster is placed in the midline between the scapulae with the patient in the supine position. This positioning alone may cause reduction. Gentle longitudinal traction through the ipsilateral arm is then applied if necessary. If these reduction maneuvers are unsuccessful, direct reduction using a sterile towel clip is then attempted. After sterile preparation of the skin, the surgeon pierces the skin with the towel clip and grasps the medial end of the clavicle while an assistant applies longitudinal traction to the ipsilateral upper arm. The clavicle is then manipulated into a reduced position (235). If the above reduction techniques are unsuccessful or in the case of open injuries, open reduction is performed with the repair of the interposed ligaments.

Once these fractures or dislocations are reduced, they are often stable and require no internal fixation. If loss of reduction occurs intraoperatively, suture or wire stabilization can be performed for physeal fractures, or ligament repair for true sternoclavicular joint dislocations (258). A figure-of-eight harness is used for postoperative immobilization for 3 to 6 weeks, or until the injury is nontender. Internal fixation with metal implants is contraindicated because of the possibility of implant migration, with resulting fatal consequences (259).

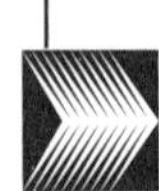

AUTHORS' PREFERRED TREATMENT

The approach to neonatal or birth injuries is one of diagnosis and reassurance and education of the parents. The family is told that a bump will develop over the fracture site and that the fracture will heal uneventfully. If the infant initially demonstrates discomfort with the fracture, the long arm sleeve of the infant's shirt can be pinned to the shirt for 7 to 10 days to provide adequate immobilization.

Older children who present to the emergency room generally have a significant level of pain and discomfort. We usually prefer a sling for relief of pain through immobilization. Occasionally, we use a figure-of-eight harness to provide retraction of the shoulder, to gain length at the level of the fracture, and to reduce pain. With the use of the figure-of-eight harness, it is important to inspect the skin on weekly follow-ups for 3 weeks to ensure that no unusual sharp bone fragments create any skin problems at the site of passage of the figure-of-eight harness over the fracture (Fig. 17-26). Despite this intervention, the parents are still informed that the fracture will take a couple of months to remodel and that there may be a bump for up to a year after the fracture.

Operative management of clavicular fractures is rarely indicated. The indications for surgery are fractures that have the potential to develop full-thickness skin loss over the apex of a fracture and fractures that cause clavicular impingement on either the brachial plexus or the subclavian vessels. Even with these fractures, gentle manipulation and closed reduction should be attempted. Open fractures also may be treated

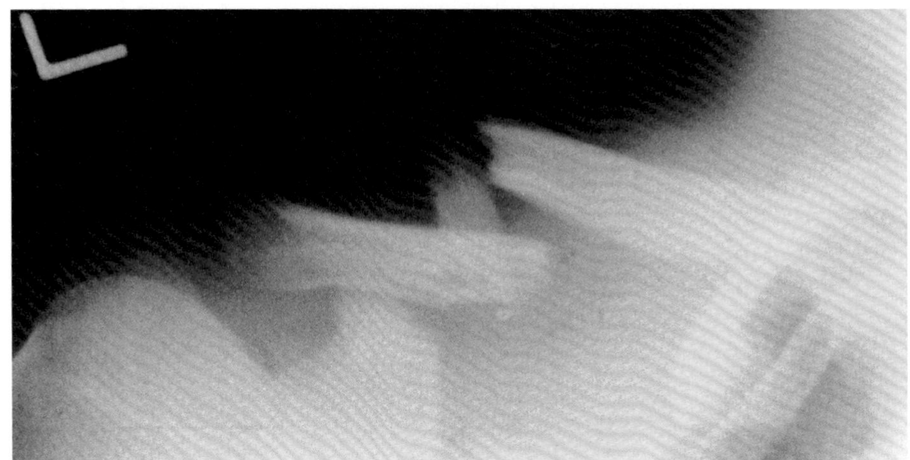
A

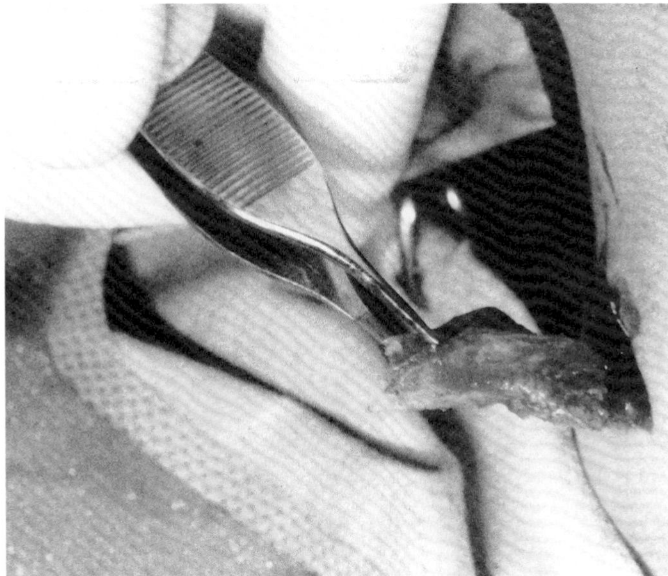
B

FIGURE 17-26 A. AP x-ray of comminuted clavicular fracture. **B.** Skin erosion over fracture fragment due to figure-of-eight splint.

with open surgery. If open repair is done, the fractured clavicle generally can be placed into the periosteal sleeve and the periosteal sleeve can be repaired over the fractured clavicle without the need for additional internal fixation.

Most fractures of the medial end of the clavicle are treated nonoperatively. A CT study is performed acutely on every posterior displaced fracture or dislocation, and on the majority of injuries with anterior displacement as well. If posterior displacement causes impingement of posterior vital structures, closed reduction is performed under general anesthesia in the operating room, followed by open reduction if closed techniques are unsuccessful. We use the open reduction techniques described above, and we perform suture repair in every case (203). Most injuries are stable in the reduced position. Postoperatively, we place the patient in a figure-of-eight harness for 3 to 6 weeks.

Anterior displacements of the medial end of the clavicle generally are associated with a physeal disruption and usually can be treated with closed reduction. Longitudinal traction is applied to the upper extremity with moderate abduction of the humerus, and general pressure is applied over the scapuloclavicular joint. Persistent instability of the scapuloclavicular joint is acceptable in anterior displacements because of the significant potential for remodeling in this area. After 2 to 4 weeks of immobilization, a program of progressive rehabilitation can begin.

Posterior dislocations of the medial end at the clavicle of the sternoclavicular joint may be either joint dislocations or associated with a physeal disruption. This injury may be acute and life-threatening. Most of these injuries can be treated successfully with closed reduction with general anesthesia and stand-by support of the cardiovascular service. The technique for the closed reduction is quite specific and involves the placement of a bolster in the midline along the level of the spine and spinous processes. Both humeri are adducted to the level of the chest, and anterior pressure is placed over the deltoid and humeral head toward the table with a downward pressure over both proximal humeri. This is generally sufficient to provide adequate retraction of the shoulder and restore the length of the clavicle at the level of the sternoclavicular joint. Further downward pressure to the level of the table provides a fulcrum force to reduce the medial end of the clavicle anteriorly into the sternoclavicular joint. A towel clip may be required to assist the reduction in difficult cases. When performed, the towel clip is placed subcutaneously and grasps the medial third of the clavicle to aid in the reduction process. Open reduction of the medial end of the sternoclavicular joint is indicated when closed reduction fails or results in an unstable retrosternal displacement. If the dislocation is unstable, generally repair of the capsule with a nonabsorbable suture through the capsule of the joint at the level of the sternum through holes drilled into the medial end of the clavicle is sufficient to provide anterior stability of the dislocation. Internal fixation is not recommended in this location.

Most injuries to the distal end of the clavicle in children and adolescents are treated nonoperatively. These fractures heal rapidly because of the early deposition of periosteal new bone and remodeling. Generally, patients can be treated with a sling and pain management with appropriate oral analgesics and ice to control swelling. Early range-of-motion therapy is recommended at approximately 10 days to 2 weeks. Clinical union is generally seen by 4 to 6 weeks.

For the rare type IV, V, or VI displaced distal clavicular injury, an open approach can be useful in replacing the distal clavicle in its periosteal sleeve, and repair of the periosteal sleeve may be sufficient to provide adequate fixation.

Pearls and Pitfalls

- Every newborn with a delivery-related clavicle fracture should be evaluated for concurrent brachial plexus palsy.
- Obtain a CT scan for posterior displaced medial clavicle fractures and posterior displaced sternoclavicular dislocations.
- When performing reduction of posterior displaced clavicles with a towel clip, grasp the clavicle in the central portion of the middle third. This enables better mobilization than grasping near the medial end.

Complications

Early Complications

Serious vascular injuries also have been described in association with clavicular fractures, including subclavian and axillary artery disruption, subclavian vessel compression, and arteriovenous fistula (244,260–263). In addition, displaced fractures of the medial clavicle may result in compression or injury of the great vessels within the mediastinum (204,205). Occasionally, these compressions can be relieved nonoperatively by reducing the fracture and eliminating the excessive pressure on the vessels (244,262). However, if nonoperative treatment does not alleviate the compression, operative reduction of the fracture and possible vascular repair may be required. Certainly, if the structural integrity of the vessels is compromised, operative repair by an experienced vascular or thoracic surgeon is necessary.

In addition to the compression of the great vessels, displaced medial clavicular fractures can result in compression of the trachea and esophagus, causing difficulty with the airway or with swallowing (204,205). Clavicular fractures resulting from severe trauma can be associated with pneumothorax (264,265). Rarely, a pneumothorax results from obstetrical clavicular fractures (266).

Neurologic deficits of the brachial plexus have been reported in association with clavicular fractures. Brachial plexus palsy may present early or late after the traumatic insult and occasionally requires operative reduction of the fracture (244,260, 267–269). Rarely, such nerve deficits can result from inappropriate use of the figure-of-eight splints (237,241). Although permanent nerve deficits have been reported, most brachial plexus injuries resolve spontaneously (269,270).

Failure to recognize and treat associated atlantoaxial rotatory displacement promptly can lead to fixed C1-2 deformity (203). Displacement recognized in the first 3 weeks of injury can be successfully treated without surgery. Fixed deformity can result if the diagnosis and treatment is delayed 6 weeks or longer. Once fixed deformity is established, limited cervical fusion will be necessary.

Late Complications

Implants and internal fixation devices for clavicular fractures have been associated with numerous complications, including hardware migration, infection, and nonunion (199,259,271–275). Although most of these complications can be adequately treated, some can have fatal results (259). Therefore, whenever possible, fixation of pediatric clavicular fractures should use minimal or no hardware.

Malunions are common after initial fracture healing, but most children experience no long-term deformities because of their tremendous potential for remodeling. Rare cases of clavicular reduplication and cleidoscapular synostosis have been reported (218,276). These unusual complications may require additional intervention.

Nonunions following traumatic clavicular fractures should be distinguished from congenital pseudarthrosis and pseudarthrosis secondary to other pathologic processes (214,273, 277–281). Operative indications for posttraumatic clavicle fracture pseudarthroses are unacceptable cosmetic deformity and pain (278,281–283). However, operative repair with grafting and internal fixation of the pseudarthroses can be associated with additional iatrogenic complications, such as pneumothorax, subclavian vessel damage, air embolism, and brachial plexus deficit (284).

Controversies and Future Directions

Whether internal fixation of clavicle fractures with titanium elastic nails (TEN) will take hold for severely displaced fractures remains to be seen. In any event, management of this fracture remains nonproblematic on the whole.

GLENOHUMERAL SUBLUXATION AND DISLOCATION

Dislocation of the glenohumeral joint in children is rare. None of the ancient writings of Hippocrates (460–375 B.C.), Galen (A.D. 131–201), and Paul of Aegena (A.D. 625–690) made specific mention of this injury in children (285). Most textbooks that address children's shoulder problems do not even discuss dislocations of the glenohumeral joint, and others merely touch on the subject (286–291). A review of the literature would suggest that glenohumeral dislocations in children less than 12 years of age are rare. Although several case reports have been presented, no large series of this entity are available (292–295). In Rowe's review of 500 dislocated shoulders (296), only 8 patients were under 10 years of age. In this same series, 99 patients were 10 to 20 years of age, but no details on skeletal maturity were given (296,297). Rockwood reported a series of 44 patients with shoulder dislocations, predominantly adolescents (285). Many articles have been published on adolescent patients without discussing their skeletal maturity (298–301). As the child reaches adolescence, the incidence of shoulder instability increases, but in the skeletally immature patient, this injury can still be considered rare. Marans et al (302) in 1992 presented a series of 21 patients with open physes from two major trauma centers.

Principles of Management

Mechanism of Injury

Traumatic Dislocations. Significant evidence of trauma should be present to assign patients to this group, whereas patients who dislocate with relatively minor trauma should be assigned to the atraumatic group. The vast majority of traumatic dislocations are anterior. The mechanism of injury is similar to that observed in the adult. Typically, a force applied to the outstretched hand forces the arm and shoulder into a maximally abducted, externally rotated position. At this point, the humeral head is levered out of the glenoid process anteriorly, with the head lodging against the anterior neck of the glenoid. This occurs commonly in contact sports, falls, fights, and motor vehicle accidents (303–305).

Posterior dislocations are rare. In reported series of all age groups, posterior dislocations represent only 2% to 4% of all traumatic dislocations. The history for posterior dislocations is one of violent trauma with the arm in a position of flexion, internal rotation, and adduction. This can occur in falls and in motor vehicle accidents as the arm braces the body against impact. The other common mechanisms that produce posterior dislocations include convulsions and electroshock. In these cases, the shoulder is dislocated posteriorly by the violent contraction of the shoulder internal rotators, which normally are stronger than the shoulder external rotators. The history of the mechanism of injury and a high index of suspicion are necessary to avoid missing a posterior dislocation (306–310).

In neonates, pseudodislocation of the shoulder can occur (311). This problem represents traumatic epiphyseal separation of the proximal humerus, which is certainly much more common than a true traumatic dislocation of the shoulder in this age group. Most true traumatic dislocations of the shoulder in the neonatal period occur in babies with underlying birth trauma to the brachial plexus or central nervous system.

Laskin and Sedlin (312) reported on a 3-month-old infant with Erb-Duchenne palsy who sustained a traumatic luxatio erecta of the shoulder during a planned shoulder manipulation. Posterior dislocation of the shoulder also can occur as a secondary traumatic phenomenon in unrecognized brachial plexus injuries of the upper trunk at delivery (313–316). Green and Wheelhouse (317) reported a dislocation in a 7.5-month-old infant that was secondary to a septic brain injury.

Atraumatic Dislocations. Atraumatic shoulder instability is more common in children and adolescents than previously reported. The child who presents with shoulder dislocation without a clear-cut significant history of trauma should arouse suspicion that atraumatic instability may be present. These patients have inherent joint laxity that allows the shoulder to be dislocated either voluntarily or involuntarily as the result of a minimally traumatic event (Fig. 17-27) (318). For example, throwing, hitting an overhead tennis shot, or pushing the body up when in bed would not constitute significant trauma. A high index of suspicion should be maintained with this kind of history. In the individual who dislocated voluntarily, conscious selective firing of muscles while antagonists are inhibited, combined with arm positioning, allows the shoulder to dislocate. A key to the diagnosis is that atraumatic instability, whether voluntary or involuntary, is not associated with much pain.

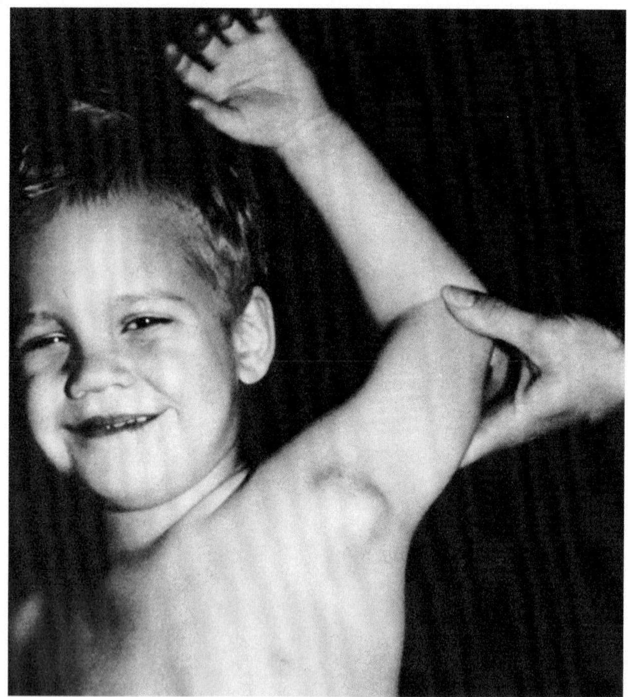
A

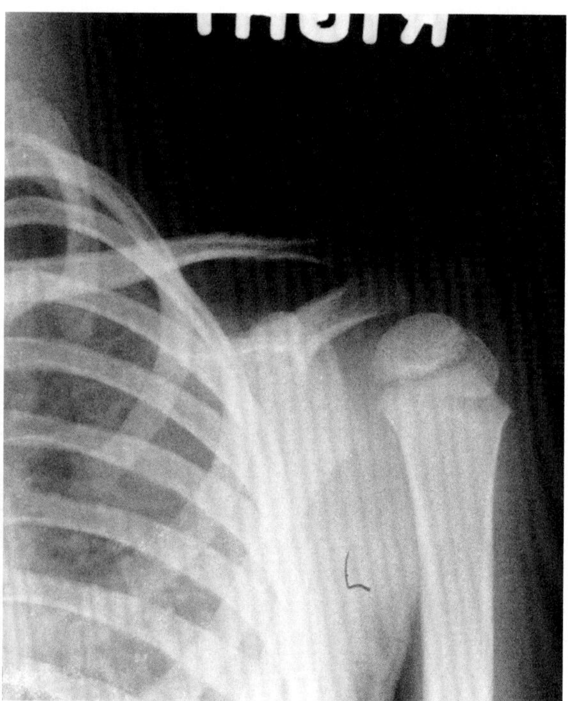
B

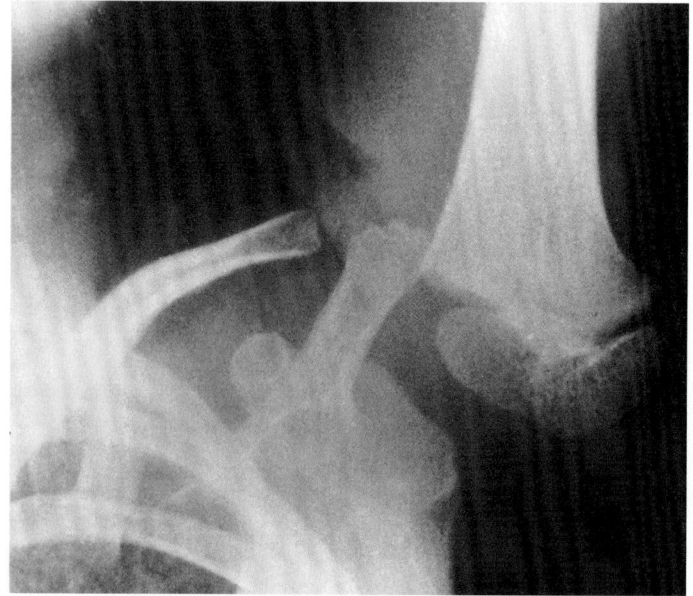
C

FIGURE 17-27 Congenital laxity of the left shoulder in a 4-year-old boy who is totally asymptomatic and has full range of motion of the left shoulder. **A.** With abduction and extension, the head subluxates anteriorly and inferiorly. **B.** An AP x-ray shows some lateral displacement of the humeral head. **C.** With overhead elevation, the humeral head is noted to displace anteriorly, laterally, and inferiorly. (Courtesy of Don Jones, MD.)

Even if reduction is necessary, the pain usually disappears rapidly. In most instances, spontaneous reduction occurs without manipulation (285).

Other causes of atraumatic shoulder instability, in addition to multidirectional joint laxity, include Ehlers-Danlos syndrome, congenital absence of the glenoid, deformities of the proximal end of the humerus, and emotional and psychiatric instability. True congenital dislocations of the shoulder are most commonly associated with developmental defects and multiple congenital abnormalities (319–323). Arthrogryposis, neglected septic arthritis, and neurologic defects also have been implicated in atraumatic dislocations in the young child (299,313, 315,317,324,325).

Signs and Symptoms

Traumatic Dislocations. The patient with a traumatic anterior dislocation presents with a painful, swollen shoulder. Obvious deformity is present with a prominent acromion and flattening of the contour of the lateral upper arm. The arm is often supported by the contralateral hand and held in an abducted and externally rotated position. Despite swelling, the humeral head can usually be palpated in a position anterior to the glenoid.

Careful examination of the neurologic and vascular status should be performed. The axillary nerve is the most commonly injured with anterior dislocation, and special attention to its function should be included in the physical examination (326). The sensory distribution of the axillary nerve is along the upper lateral arm, and motor innervation is to the deltoid and teres minor muscles. Light touch is adequate for sensory testing in the upper arm region. A convenient way to test deltoid function is to support the involved elbow in one of the examiner's hand while using the examiner's opposite hand to grab the muscle belly of the deltoid. The patient is asked to abduct the arm against resistance for about 1 inch so that deltoid firing is initiated. This examination confirms the status of the axillary nerve (Fig. 17-28).

In recurrent anterior dislocation or subluxation, the arm is well located with an overall normal appearance of the shoulder. The shoulder demonstrates a full range of motion, although the patient avoids the cocking position. The apprehension test with the arm abducted above 90 degrees is positive. A positive apprehension test, along with a suggestive history, is a very diagnostic physical sign for recurrent anterior instability.

For the much less common traumatic posterior dislocation, an affected patient presents with flattening of the anterior aspect of the shoulder and posterior fullness. The arm is held at the side with the forearm internally rotated across the chest. The patient resists any attempt at motion. Although difficult to elicit in the acute situation because of pain, hallmark findings of posterior dislocation are lack of shoulder external rotation and inability to supinate the forearm. It is advantageous to examine the shoulder with the patient seated so that the examiner can visualize the shoulders from above. From this perspective, posterior fullness and anterior flattening can be better visualized. As for anterior dislocations, the neurovascular status should be evaluated meticulously. A history of convulsion or electrical shock should raise the index of suspicion for posterior dislocation.

In neonates, traumatic separation of the upper humeral physis, the so-called pseudodislocation of the shoulder, can mimic an anterior dislocation. As is the case for true dislocations, the child is irritable and holds the affected arm abducted and exter-

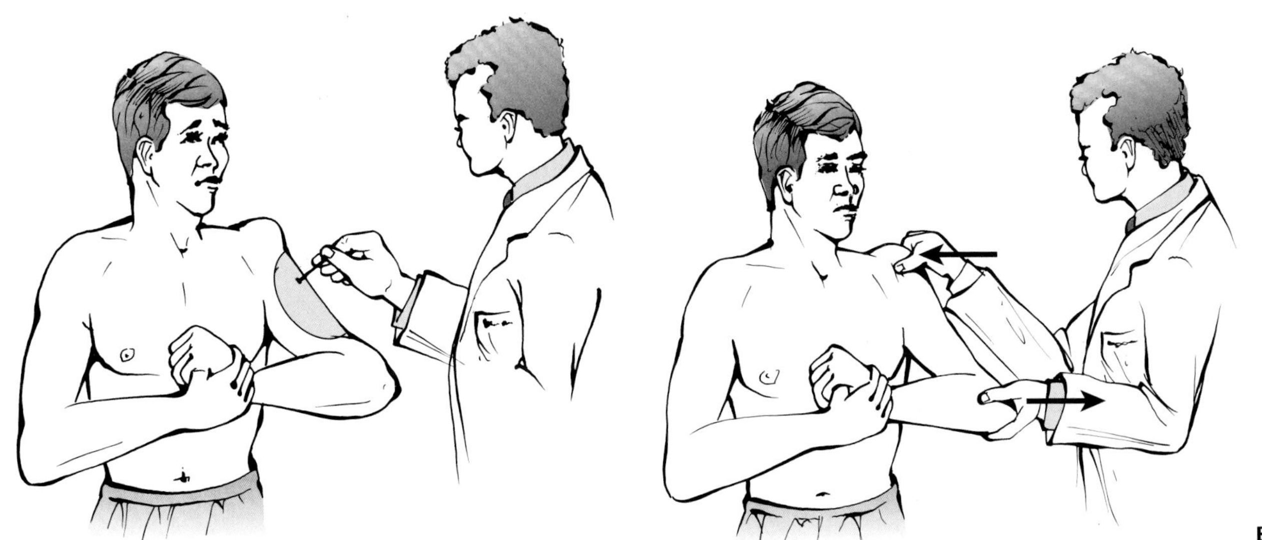

FIGURE 17-28 A. Sensory distribution for the axillary nerve important in anterior dislocation. **B.** Deltoid muscle can be tested in acute anterior dislocation by grabbing the muscle belly with the right hand while supporting the elbow with the left. The patient then can actively contract the deltoid by pushing the elbow against the examiner's hand while the examiner feels the muscle contraction.

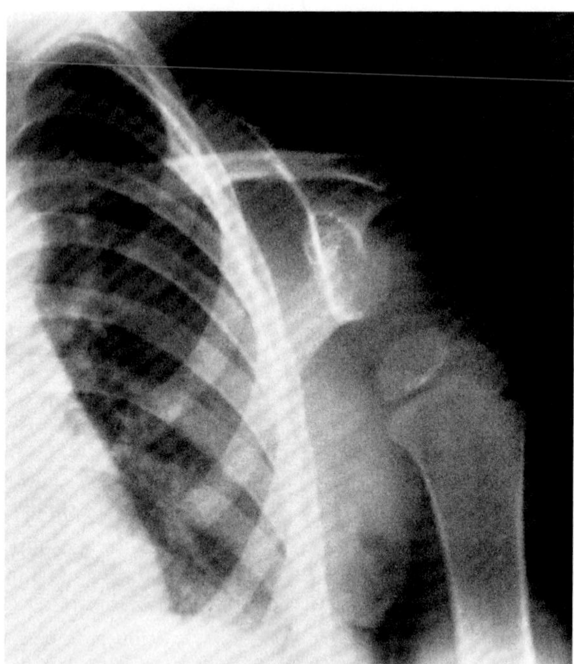

FIGURE 17-29 Dramatic demonstration of inferior subluxation of the glenohumeral joint in a patient with multidirectional instability. The clinical correlate is the sulcus sign.

nally rotated. There is resistance to any type of motion. Deformity in dislocation or pseudodislocation in the neonate is not apparent or subtle.

Atraumatic Dislocations. The most notable finding in patients with atraumatic shoulder instability is the relative lack of pain associated with the subluxation or dislocation (327–333). Even in cases of involuntary atraumatic dislocation, the minor pain associated with the dislocation itself subsides rapidly after reduction. Episodes of atraumatic subluxation and dislocation occur much more frequently than traumatic dislocations, and in almost all cases spontaneous reduction is the rule.

On clinical examination, multidirectional laxity or instability of the contralateral shoulder is usually present (285,298, 334,335). In addition, there is evidence of laxity of multiple joints (336). Characteristics of multiple joint laxity include hyperextension at the elbows, knees, and metacarpophalangeal joints. Not uncommonly, striae of the skin are present. Skin hyperelasticity is a noted characteristic of Ehlers-Danlos syndrome.

Multidirectional laxity of the shoulder is characterized by a positive sulcus sign and significant translation on an anterior and posterior drawer test. The sulcus sign is a dimpling of the skin below the acromion when manual longitudinal traction is applied to the arm (Fig. 17-29). This produces an inferior subluxation of the humeral head away from the acromion that enlarges the subacromial space and causes dimpling of the skin. The drawer or shift and load test is performed with the examiner seated behind the patient. The scapula is stabilized with one hand and forearm while the humeral head is manually translated anteriorly and posteriorly by the examiner's opposite hand (Fig. 17-30). Although some translation within the glenohumeral joint is expected in all patients, those with multidirectional laxity demonstrate translation of greater than 5 mm anteriorly and posteriorly from a neutral position.

In atraumatic dislocation, the shoulder often dislocates anteriorly, posteriorly, or inferiorly. The most common direction of dislocation in voluntary instability is posterior or inferior. The patient who can voluntarily dislocate the shoulder can force the humeral head posteriorly by contracting the anterior deltoid and internal rotators while inhibiting the antagonistic muscles

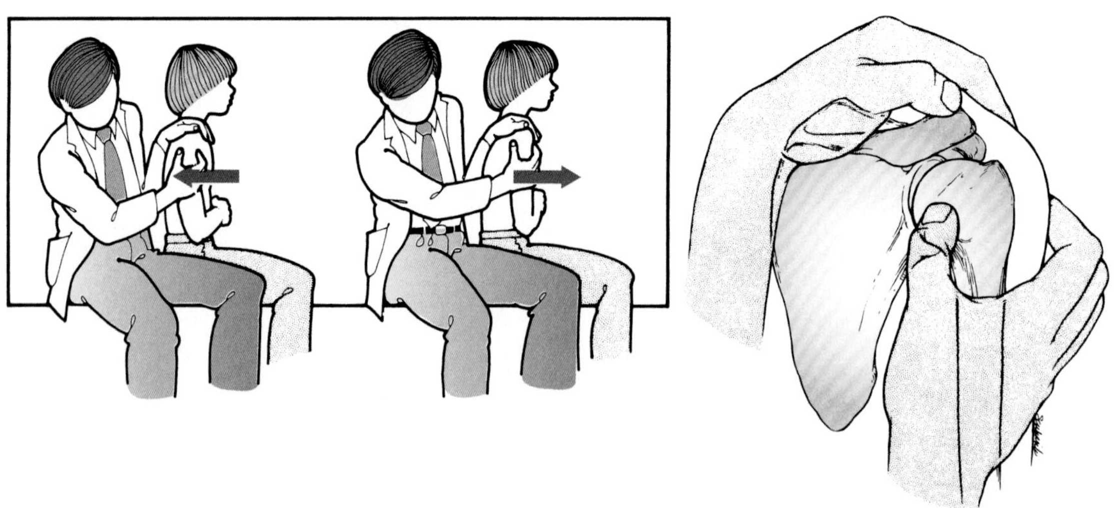

FIGURE 17-30 Drawer test. This technique is used to subluxate the shoulder manually both anteriorly and posteriorly to demonstrate multidirectional laxity.

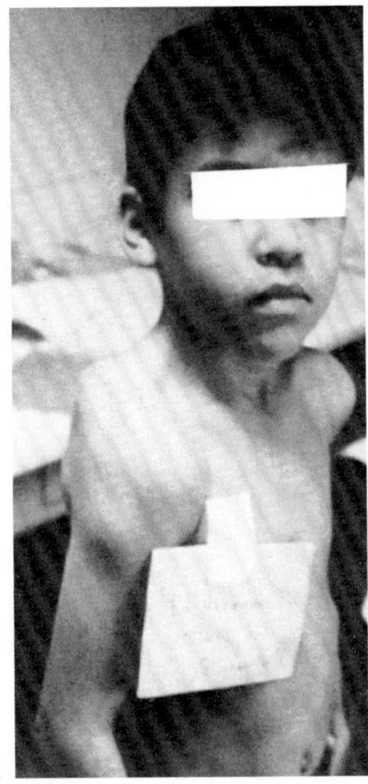
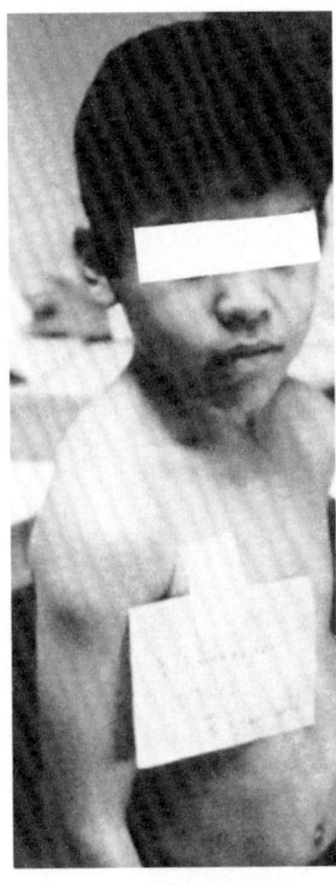

FIGURE 17-31 Voluntary anterior dislocation of the right shoulder in an 8-year-old boy. **A.** The patient voluntarily has dislocated the right shoulder anteriorly. **B.** The shoulder voluntarily reduced. The patient explained that he was taught to do this by an older brother who also had voluntary dislocation of the shoulders.

(Fig. 17-31). The elbow is positioned in horizontal adduction, and the head is dislocated. The arm can then be abducted, and the shoulder reduces, often with an audible clunk.

Associated Injuries

Although any of the nerves that traverse the axilla may be injured at the time of a shoulder dislocation, the axillary nerve is the most common associated nerve injury. Fortunately, most axillary nerve injuries associated with dislocations are neurapraxic and recover spontaneously with time and observation. In the event of complete axillary nerve palsy, significant disability can result due to the lack of deltoid function (326,337–341).

Vascular injuries are rare, but either the axillary artery or vein can be traumatized. Morrison and Egan (342) reported an axillary artery and a brachial plexus injury in a luxatio erecta dislocation in an 11-year-old child. The artery was rejoined with a vein graft and the brachial plexus injury fully recovered.

Diagnosis and Classification

Radiographic Studies. Children and adolescents with open growth plates have a low incidence of true traumatic dislocation of the shoulder. Traumatic lesions on plain x-rays are similar to those found in adults (Fig. 17-32). On the AP or internally rotated views of the proximal humerus, the Hill-Sachs compression lesion on the posterolateral aspect of the humeral head is commonly found. This injury to the proximal humerus occurs as the humeral head is impacted against the anterior rim of the glenoid during a dislocation (Fig. 17-33). Bony injury to the anterior glenoid rim can occur with dislocation as well. Injury to the glenoid ranges from small avulsion-type fractures to substantial bony fractures. Anterior glenoid rim injuries are best seen as a double density on the AP view of the shoulder or as a separate fragment on the axillary and West Point lateral views. The West Point lateral view projects the anteroinferior glenoid rim and most clearly shows this lesion when it is present. In traumatic posterior dislocation, the reverse Hill-Sachs lesion can be seen on the anterior part of the humeral head and in some cases will be seen in conjunction with fracture of the posterior rim of the glenoid.

In cases of traumatic subluxation of the shoulder in which the diagnosis may be unclear clinically, an arthrogram with CT scan can sometimes better delineate the extent of capsular stripping from the anterior glenoid rim. More recently, saline arthrograms and MRI have enhanced our ability to define the degree of injury to the labrum, capsule, and articular surfaces (335,343). CT scanning and MRI are useful for analyzing the significance of fractures of the glenoid rim (Figs. 17-34 and 17-35). In addition, the size of the reverse Hill-Sachs lesion of the humeral head in posterior dislocations is best analyzed with a CT scan (344,345).

With atraumatic dislocations in patients who do not have congenital or developmental defects, x-rays are usually normal. Among patients who do have congenital defects, the most common abnormality seen on x-rays is hypoplasia or aplasia of the glenoid. In patients with multidirectional laxity and atraumatic dislocation, stress x-rays can usually show instability in anterior, posterior, and inferior directions. The inferior component of multidirectional instability can be demonstrated by applying weights to the arm in an AP film. If laxity is present, this stress view will show the humeral head subluxating inferiorly in its relation to the glenoid (346).

Classification. The following scheme is useful for the classification of shoulder dislocation based on etiology:

1. Traumatic dislocations
    a. Primary trauma to the shoulder itself
    b. Secondary to birth trauma of the brachial plexus or central nervous system
2. Atraumatic dislocations—voluntary or involuntary
    a. Congenital abnormalities or deficiencies of bone or soft tissue
    b. Hereditary joint laxity problems, such as Ehlers-Danlos syndrome
    c. Developmental joint laxity problems
    d. Emotional and psychiatric disturbances

The above etiologic classification is commonly used in adults, but no consensus exists as to a classification scheme in children and adolescents.

Shoulder instability can be classified as to direction, degree,

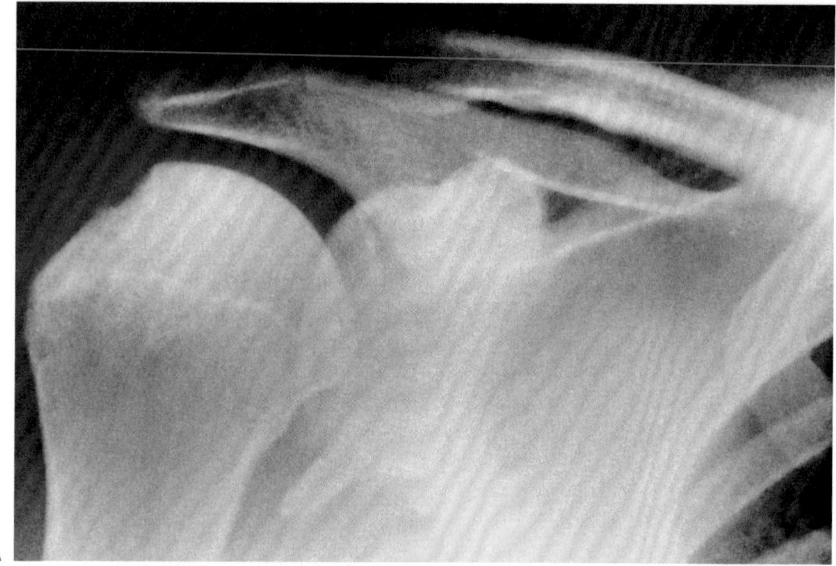

A

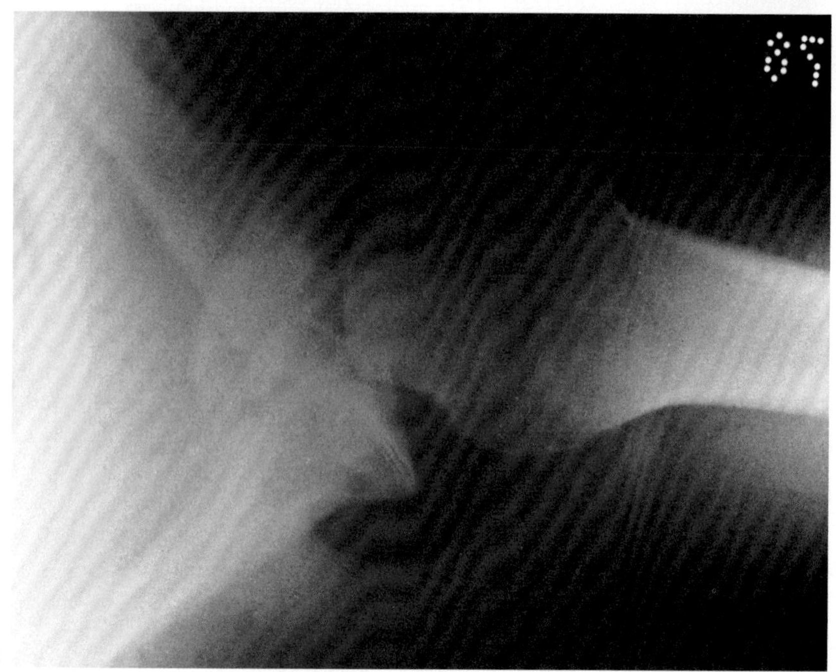

B

FIGURE 17-32 Traumatic anterior dislocation of the right shoulder in a 15-year-old boy. **A.** On the AP view, note the Hill-Sachs lesion as well as the anteroinferior bony fragment off the glenoid rim. **B.** Axillary x-ray made with the arm in 90 degrees of abduction demonstrates the anterior subluxation as well as the deficiency of the anterior glenoid rim.

and chronicity. Two basic schemes have been used to classify shoulder dislocations in children and adolescents. The more common of these is based on the direction or location of the dislocation. Although this scheme is useful in describing the clinical and radiographic features of the injury, it does not address the underlying pathology in children (285). Therefore, a second classification scheme describing the etiology of the dislocation is also useful when considering treatment options for this injury in children. This second system is similar to that used for adults but takes into account congenital and developmental problems unique to children. As discussed later in the section on treatment of this problem, accurate classification is important in selecting the appropriate conservative versus surgical options (347–349).

The directional classification has four categories: anterior, posterior, inferior (luxatio erecta), and multidirectional. As in adults, anterior dislocation in children is the most common, constituting at least 90% of glenohumeral dislocations (Fig. 17-36). Several isolated reports of posterior dislocation in children and adolescents have been documented, but posterior dislocation is rare in children, as in adults (293,350–352). Luxatio erecta or inferior locked dislocations are uncommon but have been reported in children (312,353,354). Multidirectional luxatio of the shoulder has been well described as a distinct clinical

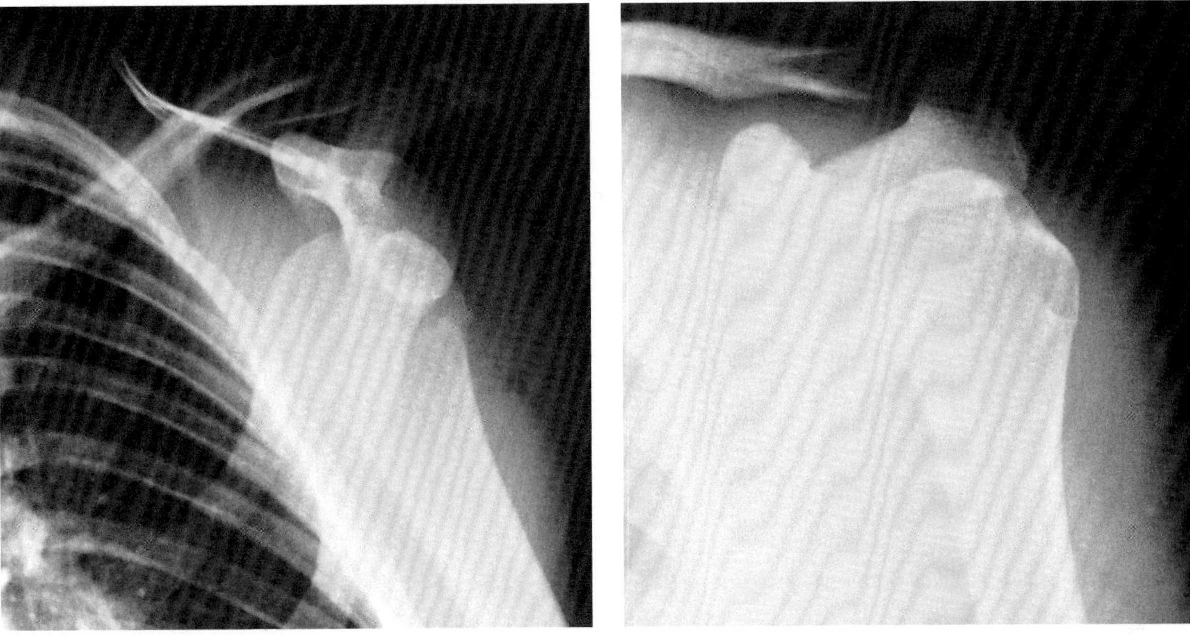

FIGURE 17-33 Anterior shoulder dislocation in a skeletally immature adolescent patient. **A.** AP x-ray shows the common appearance of an anterior dislocation of the shoulder. **B.** Postreduction AP x-ray of the shoulder shows a large posterolateral compression fracture of the humeral head or Hill-Sachs lesion.

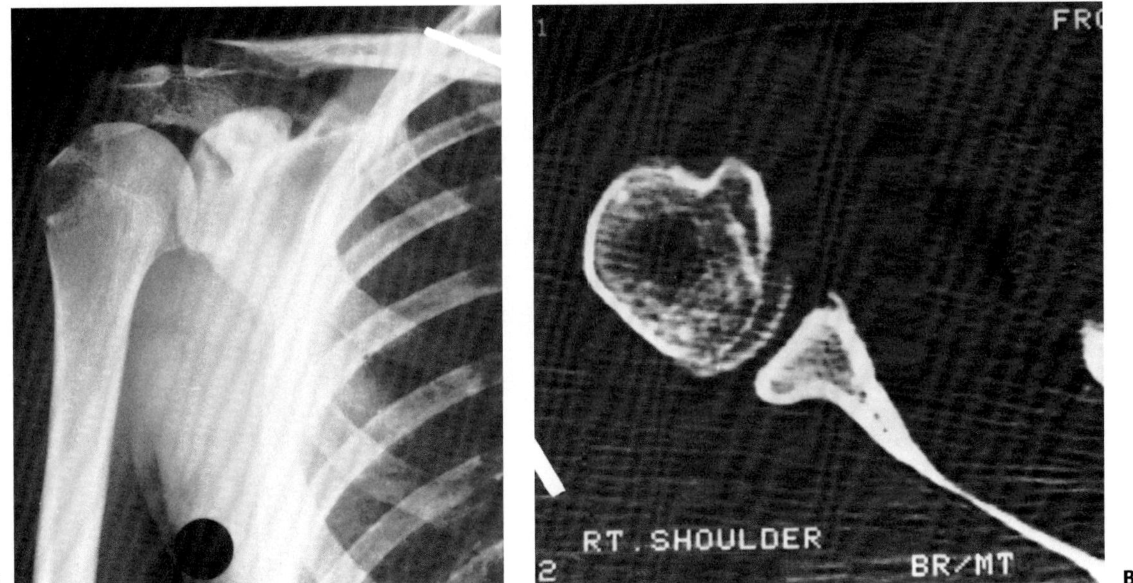

FIGURE 17-34 **A.** AP x-ray of a 14-year-old boy with recurrent anterior subluxation. Notice the presence of a Hill-Sachs compression fracture on the humeral head and a subtle double density at the anteroinferior glenoid rim. **B.** CT scan shows this to be an avulsion-type bony injury of the anterior glenoid.

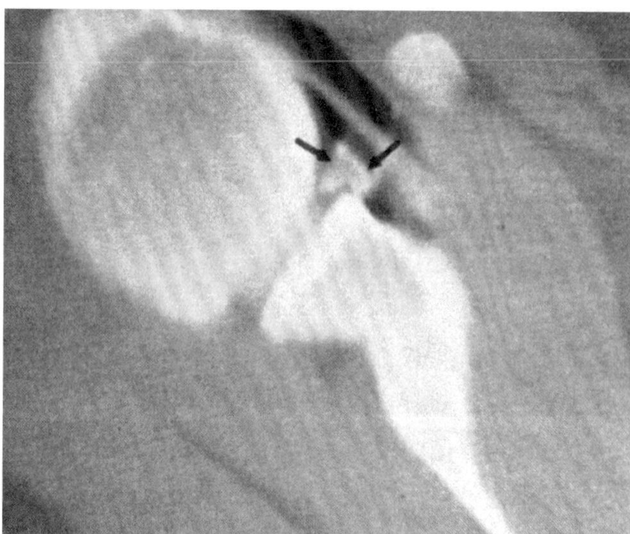

FIGURE 17-35 MRI in a patient with recurrent anterior instability of the shoulder. The *arrows* demonstrate a calcified bony Bankart's lesion.

entity by Burkhead and Rockwood (355), O'Driscoll and Evans (298), and Rockwood (285,335).

The degree of instability can be classified as a subluxation or a dislocation. A subluxation is an incomplete dislocation characterized by pain, a feeling of slipping, or a dead feeling in the arm. A complete dislocation of the humeral head out of the glenoid fossa is characterized by a displacement and locking of the head on the rim of the glenoid.

The chronicity of instability can be classified as acute, recurrent, or chronic. A single episode of instability can be described as an acute injury. As in the skeletally mature patient, an acute injury can lead to a recurrent instability, depending on the damage to the ligament and bony restraints of the joint. A chronic instability exists when an acute dislocation is not reduced, and it is usually associated with congenital dislocations.

Surgical and Applied Anatomy

Developmental anatomy is discussed previously in the section on fractures of the proximal humerus. The glenohumeral joint consists of the articulation between the large convex humeral head and the relatively flat glenoid fossa. Since there is very little bony constraint inherent to the glenohumeral joint, this joint is anatomically suited to accommodate the wide range of motion necessary to perform upper extremity function. The articular surface area and radius of curvature of the humeral head are about three times that of the relatively flat glenoid surface. Although the glenoid fossa is deepened by the labrum, the mismatch in the surface area and the radius of curvature explains the lack of joint stability.

The primary constraint for the glenohumeral joint is the capsular/ligamentous complex. The capsule on its inner surface is reinforced by thickened areas known as the anterior glenohumeral ligaments. This complex capsular/ligamentous structure must provide stability against abnormal translation while allowing a wide range of motion. With the arm abducted, the inferior capsule is highly redundant. The most important ligament is the anteroinferior glenohumeral ligament, located within the inferior redundant area. It is mechanically designed to tighten as the arm is abducted and externally rotated, much like the effect of wringing out a washcloth. This structure becomes the primary site of pathology in anterior shoulder instability, either when the anteroinferior glenohumeral ligament attachment to the glenoid and labrum is stripped from the anterior neck of the glenoid or as these ligaments are disrupted in substance (Fig. 17-37). Disruption of the capsular labral attachment is known as a Perthes or Bankart lesion.

The humeral attachment of the capsule of the glenohumeral joint is along the anatomic neck of the humerus except medially, where the attachment is more distal along the shaft. The physis, therefore, lies in an extracapsular position except on the medial side. As in most pediatric joint injuries, the strong capsular attachment to the epiphysis makes failure through the physis a much more common injury than true capsular/ligamentous injury (348,356,357). Therefore, fracture through the physis is more common than a dislocation in the skeletally immature patient.

The rotator cuff tendons consist of the subscapularis, supraspinatus, infraspinatus, and teres minor muscles. These muscle–tendon units surround the joint anteriorly, superiorly, and posteriorly. They serve an important function as dynamic secondary stabilizers of the joint by forming a force-couple with the large shoulder muscles (deltoid, pectoralis major, and latissimus dorsi). As the glenohumeral joint moves through its range of motion, the cuff provides a dynamic stabilizing effect, preventing excessive translation of the humeral head on the glenoid. This is important when addressing rehabilitation for the prevention of recurrent glenohumeral dislocation.

Current Treatment Options

Treatment options are listed in Table 17-6 as well as in the following text.

Traumatic Instability

The literature on the specific treatment of shoulder instability in children is limited (288,290,347,358). Most clinicians make the same treatment recommendations based on the sustained injury, regardless of the patient's age (303,359–363). The majority of treatment recommendations presented in this section are extrapolated from the adult and adolescent literature, as well as from the experience of Dameron and Rockwood (348).

Acute Dislocation

Patients with acute dislocations of the shoulder should undergo closed reduction by one of the standard techniques. For anterior dislocation, many reduction techniques have been described. Most clinicians prefer light sedation with intravenous or intramuscular injection. The traction/countertraction method is be-

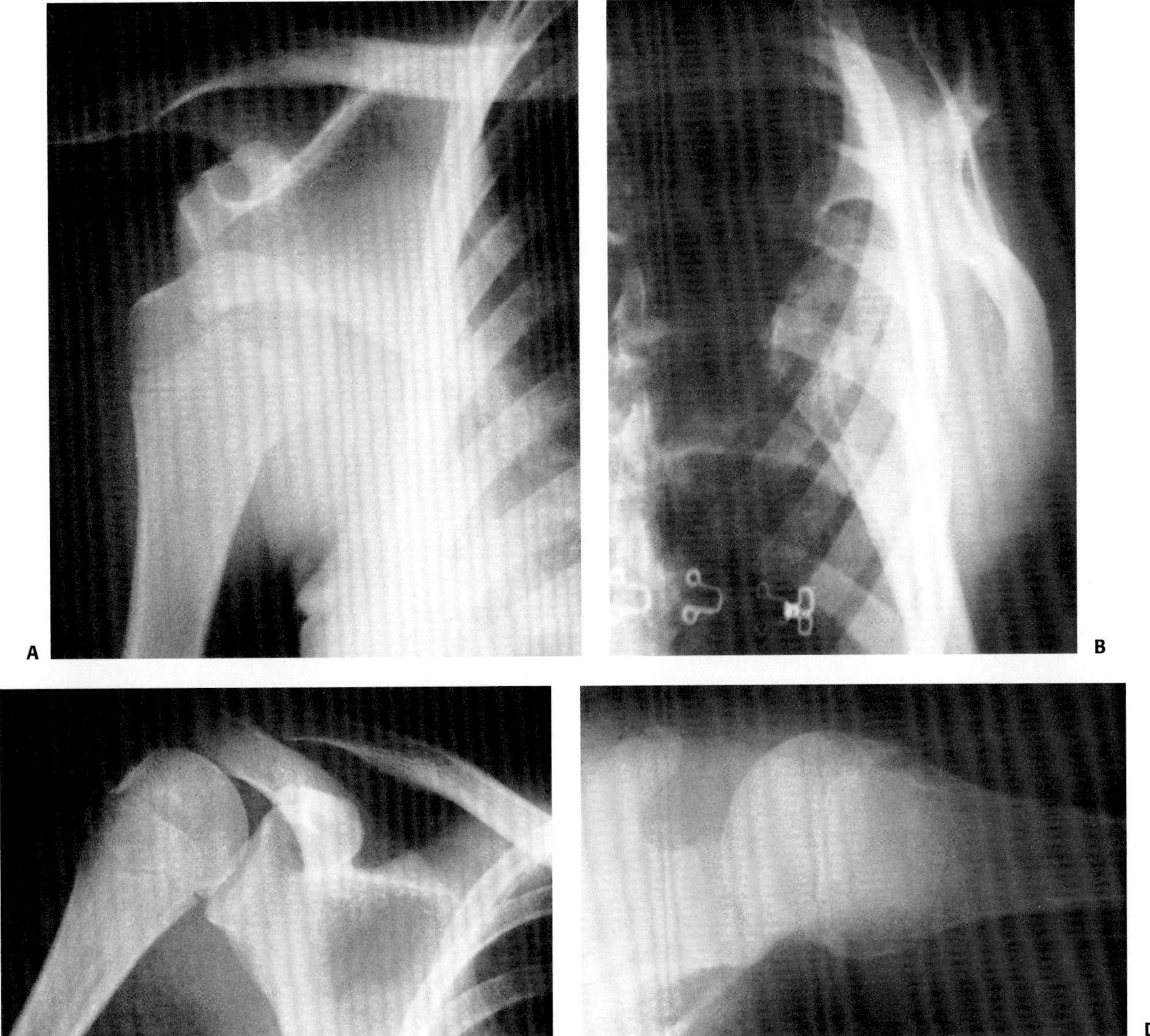

FIGURE 17-36 Anterior dislocation of the right shoulder in a 15-year-old girl. **A.** Note the typical subcoracoid position on the AP film. **B.** On a true scapular lateral film, note the anterior displacement of the humeral head. **C.** Postreduction film demonstrates a Hill-Sachs compression fracture in the posterolateral aspect of the humeral head. **D.** On the postreduction axillary film, note the posterolateral compression fracture of the humeral head.

lieved to be the most gentle. A bed sheet placed in the axilla of the affected shoulder passes above and below the patient so that countertraction can be applied to the body while longitudinal traction in line with the deformity is applied to the arm. Steady, continuous traction fatigues the muscles that lock the dislocation, and eventually reduction is accomplished by disimpacting the humerus from the glenoid.

The Stimson maneuver is equally effective. In this technique, the patient is placed prone on the examination table. A weight is applied to the affected arm. As the shoulder girdle muscles relax, reduction is achieved atraumatically (301). Another less-often-practiced technique is scapular manipulation. Kothari and Dronen (364) and McNamara (365) report that this latter technique is a safe, effective way to reduce glenohumeral dislocations.

Postreduction immobilization remains a subject for debate. The adult literature suggests that the period of immobilization may not be truly important in predicting recurrent dislocation. A sling or a sling-and-swathe with the arm internally rotated is the most common method of immobilization (360,366).

Closed reduction for acute posterior dislocations is somewhat similar to that for anterior dislocations. Traction–

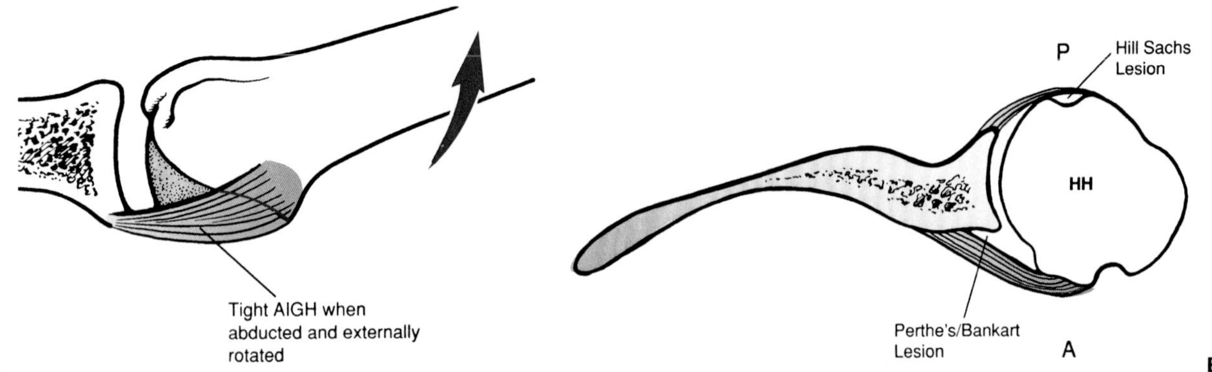

FIGURE 17-37 **A.** The tight anteroinferior glenohumeral ligament complex with the arm abducted and externally rotated. This ligament sling is the primary restraint against anterior instability of the shoulder. **B.** A cross-section in the transverse plane through the glenohumeral joint demonstrates the common lesions associated with anterior instability of the shoulder: Hill-Sachs lesion, Perthes-Bankart lesion, and redundant anteroinferior glenohumeral ligaments. *A*, anterior; *P*, posterior; *HH*, humeral head.

countertraction is the most effective method. Traction is applied in line with the deformity, and the humeral head is gently lifted back into its normal relationship with the glenoid. Most clinicians agree that immobilization should be with the arm in neutral rotation or slight external rotation at the shoulder. This may require the use of a spica cast or modified shoulder spica cast, as described by Dameron and Rockwood (348).

Recurrent Dislocation

The true incidence of recurrent dislocation after traumatic shoulder dislocation in children is understandably poorly defined, given the rarity of reports in the pediatric orthopaedic literature (321,367). In 1963, Rowe (297) reported a 100% incidence of recurrence in children 1 to 10 years of age with anterior dislocation. He also reported a 94% incidence of recurrence in adolescents and young adults (ages 11 to 20) (297). Elbaum et al (340) reported a recurrence rate of 71% in nine pediatric patients with traumatic anterior dislocations. The average age was 9 years. After reduction, they were immobilized for 3 weeks and then were treated with rehabilitation. However, Rockwood (285) reported a recurrence rate of only 50% in a series of adolescents and young adults 13.8 to 15.8 years of age. Hovelius et al (367) reported a 47% recurrence rate in patients less than 20 years of age. In a 10-year follow-up study, Hovelius et al (368) found that recurrent dislocation necessitating operative treatment had developed in 34% of shoulders in patients who were 12 to 22 years of age at the time of initial dislocation, compared with 28% in patients who were 23 to 29 and 9% in patients who were 30 to 40 years old. The type and duration of the initial treatment had no effect on the rate of recurrence. Vermeiren et al (369) reported a recurrence rate of 68% in patients younger than 20 years of age. They reported a better prognosis if the dislocation was associated with a fracture of the joint. Heck (292) reported a case of traumatic anterior dislocation in a 7-year-old boy who remained stable at a 5-year follow-up (Fig. 17-38). Endo et al (370) reported no recurrence in 2 patients, ages 3 and 9, with traumatic anterior dislocation. However, the follow-up was only 2 years in the 3-year-old and 1 year in the 9-year-old. Wagner and Lyne (295) reported an 80% recurrence rate in 10 patients with clearly

TABLE 17-6 Interventions for Glenohumeral Subluxation and Dislocation

	Closed Reduction & Immobilization	Closed Reduction & Early Reconstruction
Traumatic—acute, anterior	X	X (less common)
Traumatic—acute, posterior	X	
Atraumatic	X	
Atraumatic—multidirectional	X	X—with caution, see text

FIGURE 17-38 Traumatic anterior subluxation of the left shoulder in a 7-year-old boy. **A.** AP film of the left shoulder does not reveal any striking abnormality. **B.** An axillary film shows that the humeral head is subluxated away from the glenoid fossa. **C.** AP film of the left shoulder after manual reduction. (Courtesy of Charles C. Heck.)

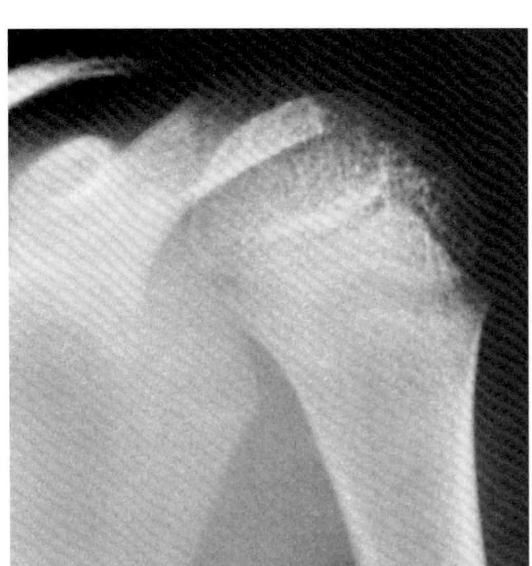

A

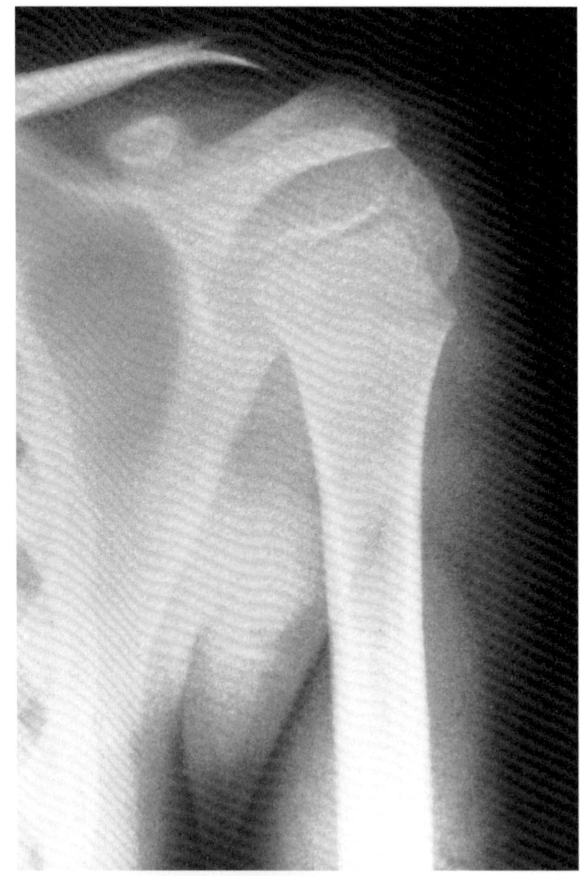

C

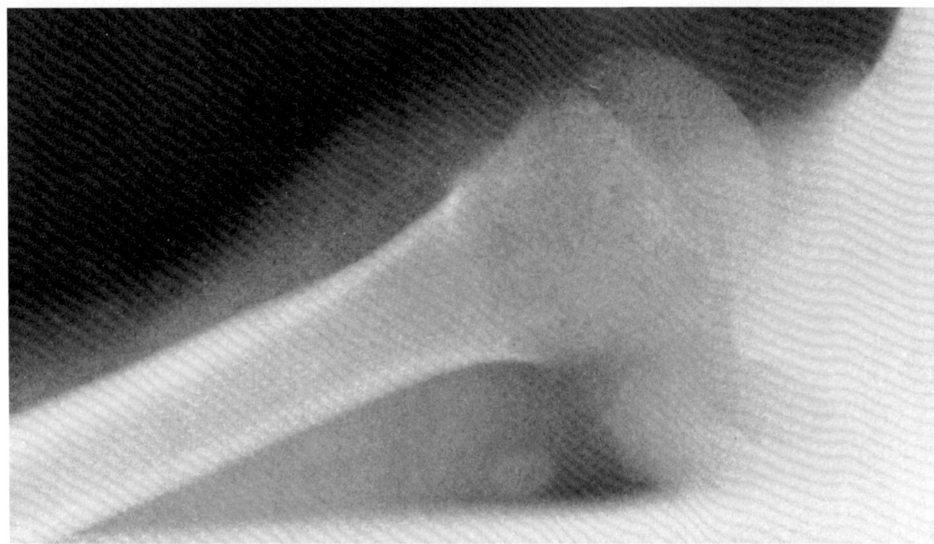

B

open proximal humeral epiphyses. Marans et al (302) reported the fate of traumatic anterior dislocations of the shoulder in 21 children (15 boys, 6 girls) in what may be the largest documented series to date. All the children had one or more documented anterior dislocations after the initial injury. Some of the children had been immobilized in a sling-and-swathe for 6 weeks. The literature reflects that the natural history of shoulder dislocations in adolescents and young adults demonstrates recurrence rates for dislocation of 50% to 90% despite the treatment program used after the initial dislocation.

Multiple surgical procedures have been described for the treatment of anterior shoulder instability. Once again, specific results for procedures such as the Putti-Platt, Bankart, and Magnuson-Stack have not been documented for children. Barry et al (361) described the effective use of the coracoid transfer for recurrent anterior instability in adolescents. Capsular procedures that specifically address the capsular pathology have been described by Neer and Foster (371), Jobe (372), and Rockwood et al (335), but results in children's dislocations were not documented. Goldberg et al (299) have reported on the use of arthroscopic techniques for capsular repair in adolescents.

Atraumatic Instability

Treatment of patients with atraumatic dislocations of the shoulder appears more difficult than treatment for true traumatic dislocations. Emphasis should be placed on careful diagnosis in these cases. Specific congenital bony or neurologic deficits should be recognized. The sequelae of Ehlers-Danlos syndrome or other collagen deficiency syndromes should be noted.

In patients with multidirectional laxity and voluntary or involuntary dislocations, a significant history of trauma is usually lacking. These patients have minimal pain associated with the dislocation and on clinical examination usually have other signs of multidirectional laxity of the opposite shoulder. Most of these dislocations reduce spontaneously and are associated with little pain. Rowe et al (332), Neer (336), and Burkhead and Rockwood (285,335,355) have described the use of a vigorous rehabilitation program involving strengthening of the rotator cuff as the treatment of choice for these patients. Most patients who do not have significant emotional and psychiatric problems are successful in improving their shoulder stability with such a program.

Most clinicians would agree that surgical intervention is considered only if a strict 6- to 12-month rehabilitation program fails. Routine shoulder reconstructions involving subscapularis shortening, including the Magnuson-Stack and Putti-Platt procedures, or "bone blocks" such as the Bristow are not sufficient for preventing future instability. Neer and Foster (371) described the inferior capsular shift reconstruction specifically for patients with multidirectional laxity of the shoulder with atraumatic instability. This procedure attempts to eliminate the overall capsular laxity and is used only after rehabilitation has failed. Huber and Gerber (373) reported on 25 consecutive children with 36 involved shoulders with voluntary subluxation of the shoulder. The children managed by "skillful neglect" had a satisfactory outcome, but only 50% of those treated with an operative procedure to prevent later degenerative arthritis had good results. They concluded that voluntary subluxation of the shoulder has a favorable result and that there is no indication for surgery with this problem in children.

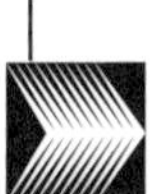

AUTHORS' PREFERRED TREATMENT

The initial challenge in managing shoulder dislocations in children is to establish whether the dislocation is traumatic or atraumatic in nature. A careful history of the mechanism of injury and physical examination designed to elicit evidence of multidirectional instability of the opposite shoulder, generalized joint laxity, or a congenital or developmental problem will facilitate this distinction. Care should be taken to identify the voluntary dislocator, who should be treated nonoperatively in all cases, with rare exceptions.

For all acute traumatic dislocations, gentle closed reduction with analgesia or anesthesia should be performed. Prereduction and postreduction x-rays are taken, and neurologic and vascular examinations are performed before and after reduction. We generally perform the traction–countertraction method under light sedation. For an anterior traumatic dislocation, we immobilize the shoulder in internal rotation for 4 weeks. For a posterior dislocation, we immobilize the shoulder for 4 weeks in a prefabricated commercially available splint or a modified spica cast with the shoulder in neutral rotation. After the 4 weeks of immobilization, we institute a rehabilitation program stressing rotator cuff strengthening.

The recurrence rate after a traumatic anterior dislocation is 50% or higher. Although we hesitate to intervene surgically after the initial dislocation, the patient and parents should be counseled regarding the high recurrence rate, in some cases even after compliance to rehabilitation program. With a second dislocation, the patient should be considered a recurrent dislocator, and surgical intervention should be considered. We use the capsular shift procedure as described by Rockwood (335). If present, the Bankart lesion is repaired anatomically to the anterior glenoid rim. Capsular shift is then performed to tighten the anteroinferior capsule.

A 6-month course of rehabilitation follows surgical intervention. For the first month, pendulum exercises and gentle elevation exercises are performed. The shoulder is protected in a sling, especially at night. The second and third months are used to regain range of motion, including protected external rotation. This procedure is designed to address the pathology without limiting motion. The fourth through sixth months are used for a progressive strengthening program, which includes strengthening of the rotator cuff and deltoid. At 6 months, the reconstruction is mature enough to release the child to a full activity level.

For atraumatic dislocation, reduction can be accomplished if necessary after an acute dislocation in a fashion similar to that described for traumatic dislocations. Again, attention should be focused on confirming the diagnosis of atraumatic dislocation. Patients with voluntary dislocation and their families should be counseled that the dislocations can be harmful to the joint and should be discouraged.

Patients with atraumatic instability should be treated with a vigorous rehabilitation program. Only in the face of recurrence after 6 to 12 months of supervised rehabilitation should surgical intervention be considered. Great care should be taken to exclude the voluntary dislocator as a surgical candidate. Psychiatric evaluation is instituted if necessary. A capsular procedure as described by Neer or the capsular shift technique described by Rockwood can be used to eliminate laxity of the joint capsule in a circumferential manner (285,335,336). Surgical management of the atraumatic dislocator is difficult and requires meticulous attention to detail during both the surgical procedure and the postoperative rehabilitation program.

Rehabilitation

The importance of an extensive rehabilitation program for instability about the shoulder for both traumatic and atraumatic problems is emphasized (348,360). Specific exercises are used to strengthen the rotator cuff and deltoid muscles. The scapular stabilizers are also strengthened. Three-inch wide strips of rubber (Thera-Bands) are used to strengthen the cuff and deltoid muscles; Theratubes are used later if necessary.

The amount of weight varies depending on the extent of the problem as well as the patient's age, size, and baseline strength. Exercises are performed four to six times a day. After basic strengthening has been accomplished, isokinetic exercises using the flexion/extension plane and the internal and external rotation plane are effective for maximizing endurance and strength in the shoulder girdle musculature.

Complications

Any of the neurologic or vascular injuries can occur at the time of dislocation or during relocation. Although rare, axillary or other nerve neuropraxia that does not spontaneously recover requires neurodiagnostic evaluation and possibly surgical reconstruction. Vascular injury should be evaluated immediately for repair.

Little information is available in the literature about the success or failure rates of surgical reconstruction of the shoulder for recurrent dislocation in children. As discussed, traumatic dislocation in a child or adolescent can progress to recurrent dislocation in 50% to 100% of cases. Rockwood et al have shown that more than 85% of atraumatic dislocators can be managed with a vigorous rehabilitation program and do not require surgery (285,335,355). Surgical treatment of these problems in children could be expected to have a success rate at least equal to that in adults. Greater than 90% success in stopping traumatic dislocations would be expected with surgical reconstruction (359,361,363).

Complications of surgical reconstruction of the shoulder include recurrent dislocation, recurrent subluxation, painfully restricted motion, problems with metal impingement or loosening about the shoulder, and neurologic injury. Perhaps the most common problem associated with the standard reconstructions about the shoulder that include subscapularis tendon-shortening procedures (Magnuson-Stack and Putti-Platt) is loss of external rotation. This loss in adults has been associated in some patients with a more rapid progression to glenohumeral arthritis (374,375).

Procedures that use metallic implants about the shoulder, including the Bristow and the DuToit stapling procedures, have been associated with complications of metal impingement on the humeral head or encroachment on the articular surface. Both problems can lead to pain and eventual arthritic change (286,334,376,377).

Controversies and Future Directions

The role of primary capsular repair (Bankart repair) for the acute first-time traumatic dislocator remains to be seen and played out in research of this injury. Initial indications seem to suggest that the procedure has value for the very active individual with a high likelihood of recurrent dislocation.

FRACTURES OF THE HUMERAL SHAFT

Fractures of the humeral shaft represent 10% or less of humerus fractures in children (378–380) and 2% to 5.4% of all children's fractures (378,381). They are most common in children under 3 and over 12 years of age (382). The incidence is greater in children with more severe trauma (383). The incidence is 12 to 30 per 100,000 per year (381,384,385). Birth injuries to the humerus have a reported incidence ranging from 0.035% to 0.34% (386,387).

Principles of Management

Mechanisms of Injury

Birth Injuries. Humeral fractures are more common in breech presentations and with macrosomic infants. The most difficult position is when the child's arms have gone above the head with maneuvers to bring the arm down after version and extraction (387).

Child Abuse. Humeral fractures in child abuse represent 61% of all new fractures and 12% of all fractures (388,389). Shaw et al (389), in a retrospective review of 34 humeral shaft fractures in children under 3 years of age, found that most occurred accidentally: only 6 were classified as caused by probable abuse. Child abuse must be part of the differential diagnosis in children with humeral diaphyseal fractures (390). The fractures may be spiral from a twisting injury or transverse from a direct blow.

Older Children. Older children sustain primarily transverse fractures from direct blows to the arm, frequently from falls, pedestrian/vehicle accidents, gunshot wounds, and machinery. Sports injuries are direct from contact sports or indirect from throwing. Throwing injuries occur as a stress injury from overuse or acutely during the throwing cycle from poor mechanics (391–401). A stress fracture also has been reported in an adolescent tennis player (402). Acute throwing fractures result from a sudden external rotation torque developed on the distal humerus with concomitant proximal internal rotation from the pectoralis major between the cocking and acceleration phases (403) as the shoulder external rotation and elbow flexion suddenly change to shoulder internal rotation and elbow extension. Humeral fractures may occur from arm wrestling in older adolescents (404–406). Many humeral fractures are pathologic through simple bone cysts or through dysplastic bones from osteogenesis imperfecta or fibrous dysplasia. Occasionally, pathologic fractures occur from benign or malignant tumors.

Signs and Symptoms

Evaluation of the Neonatal Shoulder

History. The infant who does not move the shoulder poses a diagnostic challenge. Establishing and evaluating a differential diagnosis is the first concern. By history, was the delivery normal? When was the problem noticed? Does the child move any part of the extremity? Was there a history of maternal gestational diabetes or of fetal macrosomia? Does the child nurse from each breast? A broad, useful differential diagnosis consists of clavicle fracture, proximal humeral physeal fracture, humeral shaft fracture, shoulder dislocation, brachial plexus palsy, septic shoulder, osteomyelitis, hemiplegia, and child abuse.

Examination. Initially, the child should be observed for spontaneous motion of the upper extremity. Is there any hand or elbow motion? Are there any areas of swelling, ecchymosis, or increased warmth? Does the child move the ipsilateral lower extremity? The clinician should carefully palpate each area of the upper extremity, starting with the clavicle and comparing it carefully with the opposite side for any change in soft tissue contour or tenderness. The upper arms and shoulders should then be examined, looking for any tenderness in the supraclavicular fossa. Lastly, the spine should be examined for tenderness or swelling.

Birth Fractures of the Humerus. In the newborn, a humeral fracture can simulate a brachial plexus palsy with pseudoparalysis and an asymmetric Moro reflex. The fracture site is tender and may have swelling or ecchymosis. The diagnosis is confirmed by plain radiography (387,407).

Older Children. In older children, the diagnosis is usually evident with pain, swelling, and unwillingness to move the arm. The arm is often supported by the opposite hand and is held tightly to the body (Fig. 17-39). It is essential to perform a complete neurologic and vascular examination of the extremity before any treatment except emergency splinting.

Children with torus or greenstick fractures may have localized tenderness but no deformity. In multiple-trauma victims, careful evaluation should be made of the arm because the diagnosis can be missed, especially if the patient is medically unstable (408). Humeral fractures should be sought in patients with massive upper extremity trauma.

Diagnosis and Classification

The simplest classification for humeral diaphyseal fractures describes the location (proximal third, middle third, or distal third, or the diaphyseal–metaphyseal junction), the pattern (spiral, short oblique, or transverse), the direction of displacement, and any tissue damage. Anatomically, the location is noted as proximal to the pectoralis major insertion, between the pectoralis

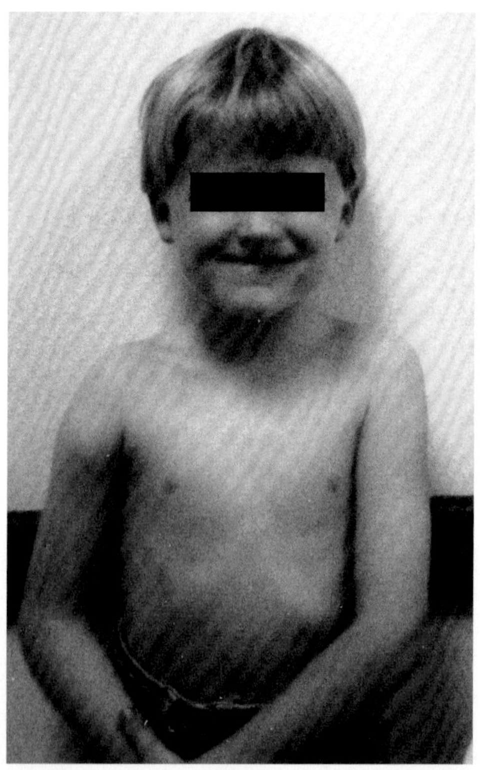

FIGURE 17-39 A young patient with a humeral shaft fracture, holding the arm tightly to his side.

major and deltoid insertions, below the deltoid insertion, or at the distal metaphyseal–diaphyseal junction (409). Humeral shaft fractures may be segmental, with fractures of the shaft and neck (410,411), or associated with shoulder dislocation (412,413). If they are associated with fractures of the ipsilateral forearm, they result in the so-called floating elbow (414,415).

The Association for the Study of Internal Fixation (AO-ASIF) has a classification for humeral shaft fractures (416,417), but it is not helpful in the evaluation and treatment of most children's humeral fractures, and like most classifications, it is subject to interobserver variability (418,419).

Imaging Studies. X-rays may be needed of the shoulder, clavicle, humerus, and cervical spine. Often the shoulder, clavicle, and humerus can be seen on a single AP view of both upper extremities and the chest. Ultrasonography can be used to identify a fracture of the clavicle or the proximal humeral epiphysis, a shoulder dislocation, or a shoulder effusion. A CT scan or arthrogram may be necessary. The radiographic findings for each fracture are discussed in the particular anatomic sections.

AP and lateral x-rays are sufficient and complete in most instances of humeral shaft fractures. In the occasional case where the diagnosis is suspect but not readily apparent on these views, oblique views may be useful.

Radiographic Findings. Birth fractures of the humerus are usually quite apparent on AP and lateral x-rays of the humerus. In older children, x-rays should be taken in both the AP and lateral planes to obtain two films perpendicular to each other. Most fractures are easily visualized on these x-rays. A true lateral view of the distal humerus is noted by superimposition of the posterior supracondylar ridges of the medial and lateral epicondyles (420,421). A supracondylar process of the humerus, when present, is best seen on an oblique x-ray showing the anterior medial aspect of the distal humerus.

Displaced fractures above the pectoralis major have marked abduction of the proximal fragment with external rotation by the rotator cuff attachment (409,422). The distal fragment is pulled proximally by the deltoid and medially by the pectoralis major. Displaced fractures between the pectoralis major and deltoid insertions show adduction of the proximal fragment from the pectoralis major and shortening by pull of the deltoid on the distal fragment. Fractures below the deltoid insertion have abduction of the long proximal fragment by the deltoid, but with shortening and medial displacement of the distal fragment by the pull of the biceps and triceps (409).

Pathologic bone may be evident (410,411). Simple bone cysts are a common cause of fractures. Periostitis or periosteal reaction of the humerus necessitates differentiating osteomyelitis or Ewing sarcoma from a stress fracture; every effort must be made to identify a cortical fissure using other imaging techniques (412–415).

Holstein and Lewis described a short oblique fracture of the distal third of the humerus with potential radial nerve palsy after closed reduction (416,417). This has been called the Holstein-Lewis fracture.

Surgical Applied Anatomy

Embryology and Development

The end of the embryonic period is marked by vascular invasion of the humerus at age 8 weeks. During the subsequent fetal period, the humerus resembles the adult bone in both form and muscular relationships (418–421). A bony collar is present very early with subsequent enchondral bone formation. The secondary ossification centers at the ends are not generally ossified radiographically until after birth (420,421).

Osseous

The proximal metaphysis of the humerus is wider than the thinner, triangular shaft. Distally, this flattens and widens to form the condylar region of the elbow. The deltoid inserts into a protuberance midway down the shaft known as the deltoid tuberosity. Distal to the tuberosity, the muscular spinal groove wraps posteriorly around the humerus. The groove gives origin to the uppermost fibers of the brachialis. The periosteum of the humeral diaphysis is thick and provides good remodeling potential (422,423). The main vascular foramen is at mid-shaft, but accessory foramina are common—most enter the anterior surface usually below the main foramen, but many are posterior (420,421,424).

Nerves

The radial nerve ordinarily lies close to the inferior lip of the spiral groove but not directly in it (425). The profunda artery either accompanies the radial nerve or passes in a second narrower grove. The nerve is protected from the humerus by a layer of either the triceps or the brachialis until the lower margin of the spiral groove near the lateral intermuscular septum (425). The ulnar nerve passes from anterior to posterior just distal to the humeral mid-shaft. A well-formed arcade and internal brachial ligament may hold the ulnar nerve (426). This ligament is always posterior to the medial intermuscular septum and subsequently joins the medial intermuscular septum proximal to the medial epicondyle. A few patients with a modified arcade have only superficial fibers of the triceps medial head passing superficial to the ulnar nerve and none deep to the nerve, making the nerve very close to the bone and vulnerable during a fracture (426).

Muscles

Several major muscle attachments occur throughout the metaphyseal and diaphyseal regions of the humerus. The pectoralis major muscle inserts laterally and distal to the bicipital grove along the anterior aspect of the humerus. The latissimus dorsi and teres major insert on the upper medial aspect of the humerus medial to the bicipital groove. The deltoid courses from the

TABLE 17-7 Interventions for Fractures of the Humeral Shaft and Distal Humeral Diaphyseal Fractures

	Nonoperative (sling/swathe; U plaster; hanging arm cast)	Functional Bracing	Operative Reduction & Internal Fixation
Birth fractures, humeral shaft	X		
Humeral shaft	X	X	
Distal humeral diaphyseal	X	X	Traction pin and traction (rare)

clavicle, acromion, and scapular spine to insert over a broad area of the deltoid tuberosity. The coracobrachialis arises from the coracoid process and inserts on the anterior medial aspect of the humerus at the junction of the middle and lower thirds. The brachialis originates from the anterior humerus about midway down the shaft. Knowledge of these muscles and their directions is essential to understand fracture displacement and treatment (422,427).

Current Treatment Options

Treatment options are listed in Tables 17-7 and 17-8 as well as in the following text.

Birth Injuries

Neonatal humeral shaft fractures heal and remodel quite well, with 40% to 50% remodeling within 2 years (Fig. 17-40) (428). Reported treatments include a sling-and-swathe (429) or a traction device using the von Rosen splint (430). The primary potential complication of birth injuries is an internal rotation deformity. Therefore, the fracture is best stabilized by splinting the arm in extension. If the parents will be moving the child, the splinted arm can be bound to the chest with a soft wrap. Children with arthrogryposis and brachial plexus palsies are prone to internal rotation contractures of the shoulder; these can be exacerbated if the birth fracture's rotation is not controlled.

Stress Fractures

Virtually all nondisplaced stress injuries heal well with temporary rest and immobilization (391,393,394,397,399,401–402, 431,432). They can displace if not treated (391). Displaced stress fractures should be treated like other humerus fractures.

TABLE 17-8 Treatment Pros and Cons: Fractures of the Humeral Shaft and Distal Humeral Diaphyseal Fractures

	Pros	Cons
No reduction (sling or shoulder immobilizer)	1) No anesthesia/sedation 2) Sling/shoulder immobilizer well tolerated	1) No improvement of fracture alignment 2) Loss of shoulder range of motion
Reduction and external immobilization	1) Improves fracture alignment 2) No implant concerns (infection, migration, malposition, etc) 3) No need for secondary anesthesia for implant removal	1) Need general anesthesia 2) Cumbersome cast/splint 3) No direct rigid fixation of fracture (potential for loss of reduction)
Reduction and internal fixation	1) Improves fracture alignment 2) Direct rigid fixation of fracture 3) Improved patient comfort (due to rigid fracture fixation) 4) No cumbersome cast or splint	1) Need general anesthesia 2) Minimal increased risk of infection 3) Implant concerns 4) Possible need for implant removal

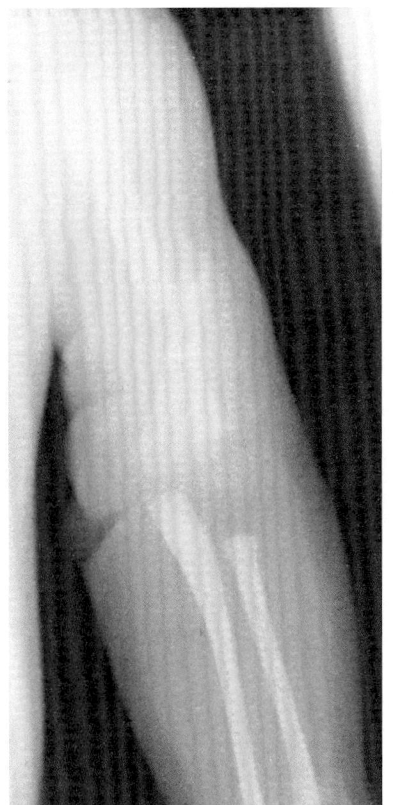

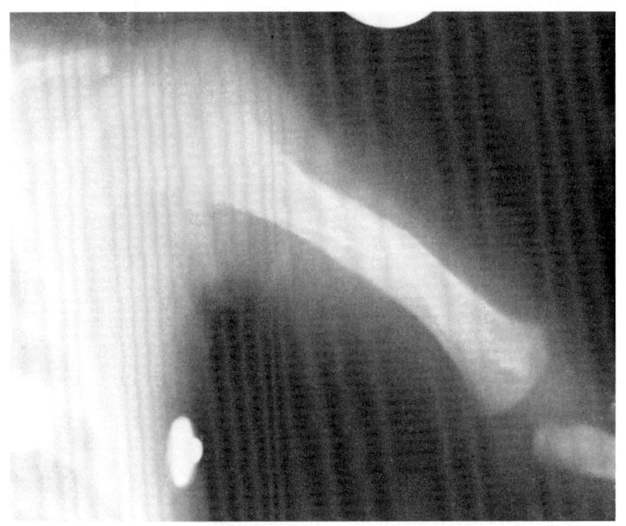

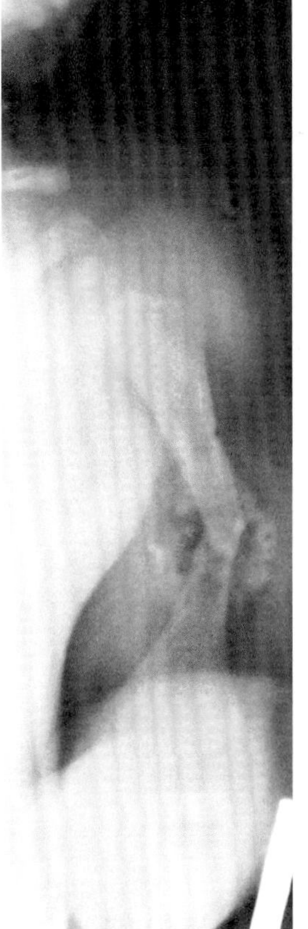

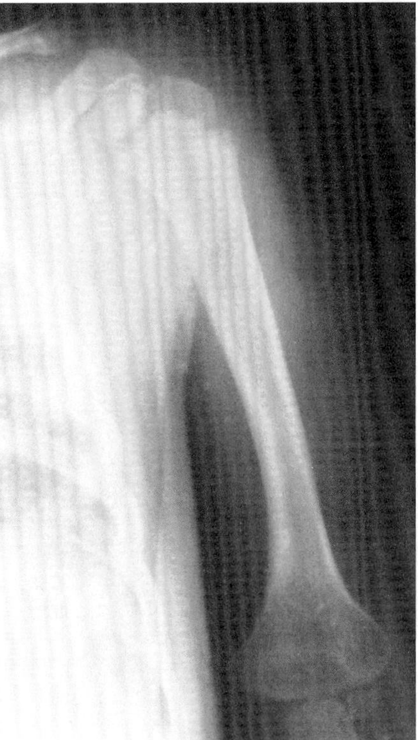

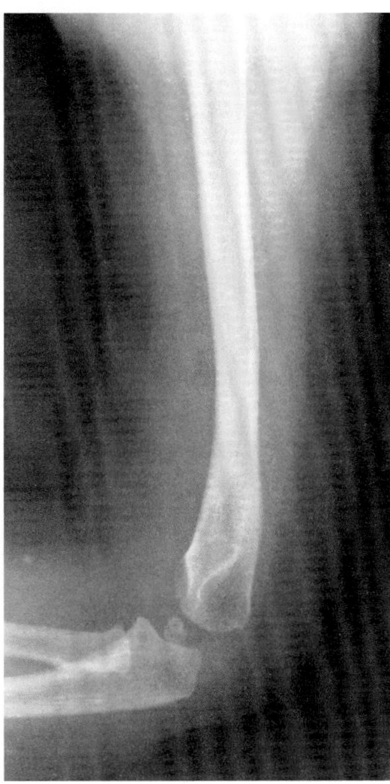

FIGURE 17-40 **A.** Fracture of the left humerus in a neonate that occurred during a difficult delivery. **B.** After 2 weeks of immobilization, clinical and radiographic union is evident, but with anterolateral angulation. **C.** At 2 months after injury, there is considerable remodeling. **D,E.** At 20 months, there is essentially complete remodeling of the fracture.

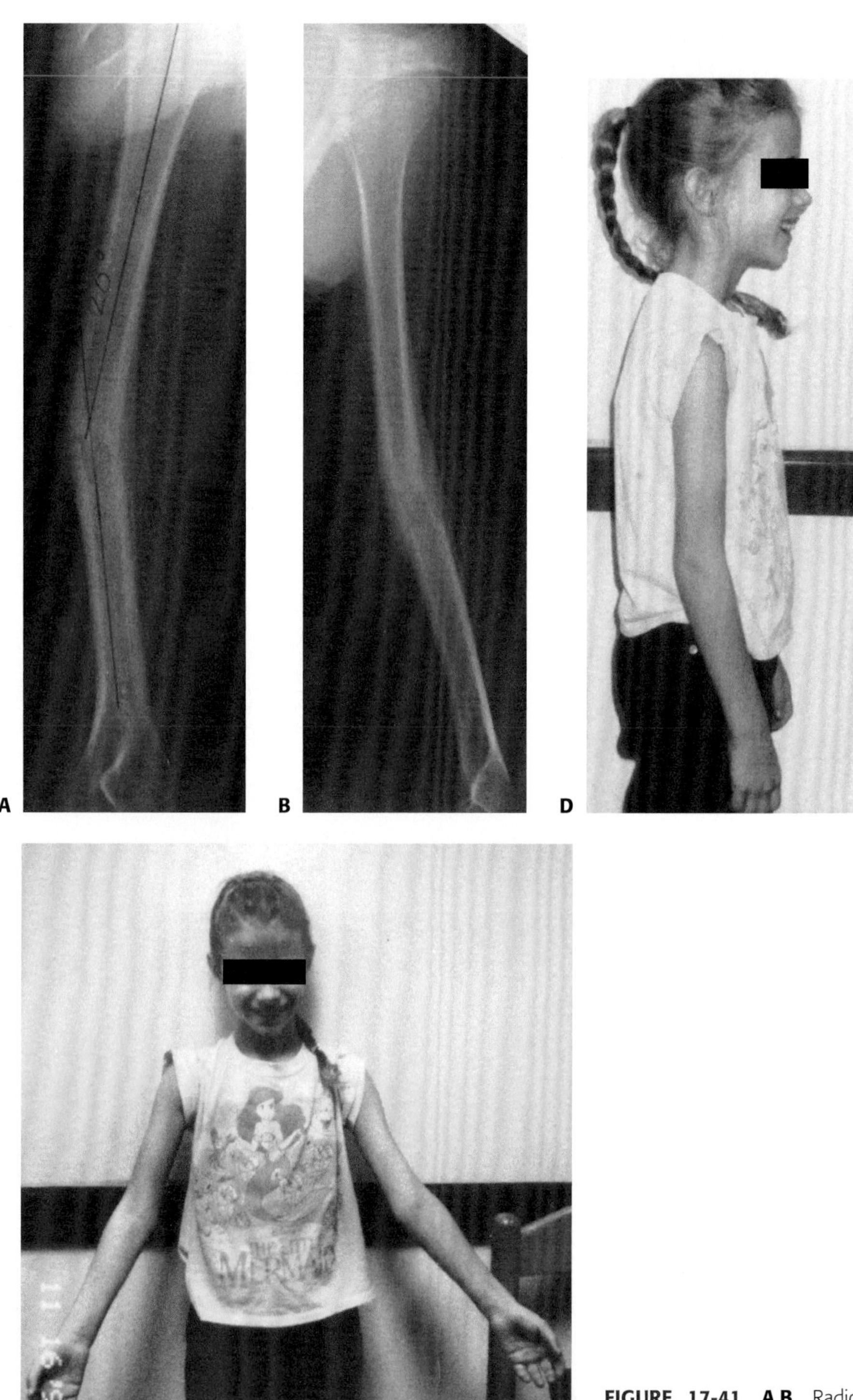

FIGURE 17-41 A,B. Radiographic appearance of a malunited humerus fracture showing 20 degrees of varus. **C,D.** The same patient with no deformity or disability, despite her thin extremities.

Acceptable Alignment

Because the humerus is not a weight-bearing bone, it does not require the precise mechanical alignment of the lower extremity. The marked mobility of the shoulder also allows some axial and rotational deviation without functional problems. Severe internal rotation contractures can cause difficulties in some overhead activities such as ball throwing and facial hygiene. Varus of 20 to 30 degrees is necessary before becoming clinically apparent (Fig. 17-41) (409,433,434). Anterior bowing may be apparent with 20 degrees of angulation (433). Functional impairment does not occur with 15 degrees or less of internal rotation deformity (409). Even adolescents can correct up to 30 degrees spontaneously (409). Beaty (382) gives guidelines based on the patient's age: children under 5 years of age tolerate 70 degrees angulation and total displacement, children 5 to 12 tolerate 40 to 70 degrees angulation, and children over 12 tolerate 40 degrees and 50% apposition. However, bayonet apposition is acceptable (435–237), with 1 to 2 cm of shortening well tolerated (Fig. 17-42). Clinical appearance is more important than radiographic alignment.

Nonoperative Treatment

Nonoperative treatment often increases internal rotation by 3 to 12 degrees at the expense of external rotation (409). This rarely is a functional problem. Nonoperative methods include a sling-and-swathe, the U plaster, a hanging arm cast, a thoracobrachial cast or dressing, a coaptation splint or functional bracing, and traction.

Sling-and-Swathe. The simplest form of treatment for fractures is a sling-and-swathe. It is sufficient for patients with minimally displaced greenstick and torus fractures (434,438). Although this treatment may yield good results in displaced fractures (439), it can be quite difficult to control anterior angulation (440) and may be uncomfortable.

U Plaster-Sugartong. Böhler (435) described a U plaster similar to the sugartong splint used on forearms. Plaster of appropriate width for the upper arm is formed from over the shoulder along the lateral aspect of the arm, underneath the olecranon, and along the medial aspect of the arm to the axilla. Cotton webbing is placed between the plaster and the skin, and the plaster is secured using a wrap (Fig. 17-43). Results have been quite good

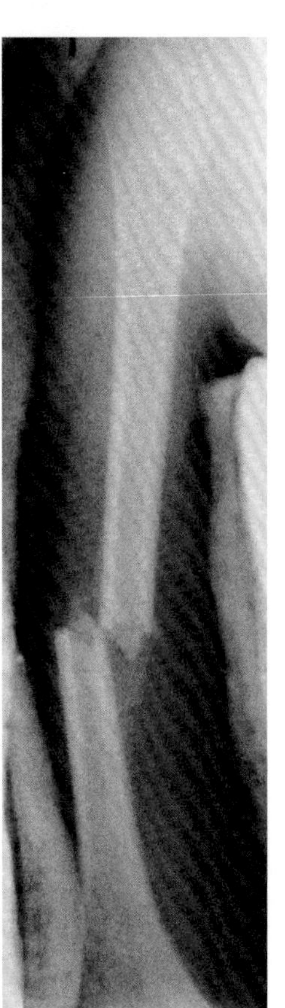

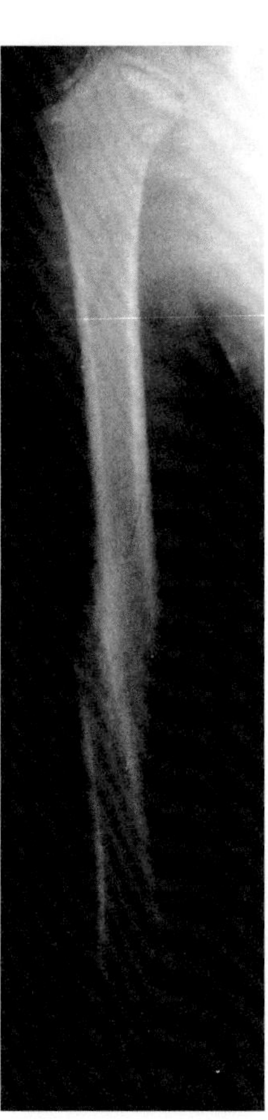

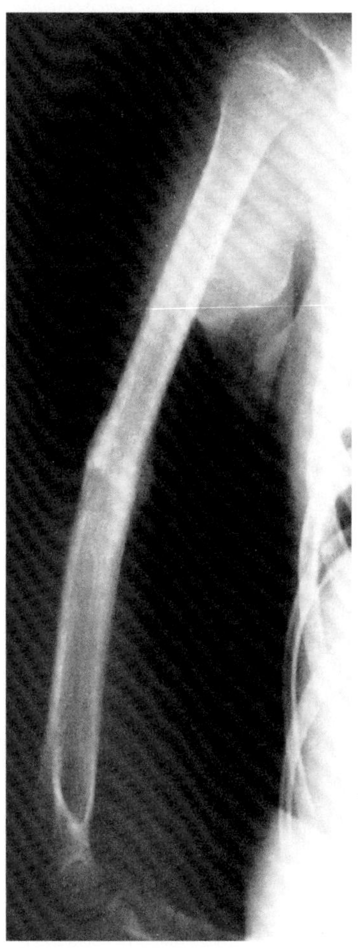

FIGURE 17-42 **A.** Humerus fracture allowed to heal in slight varus and bayonet apposition. **B,C.** The ultimate result, with essentially normal alignment.

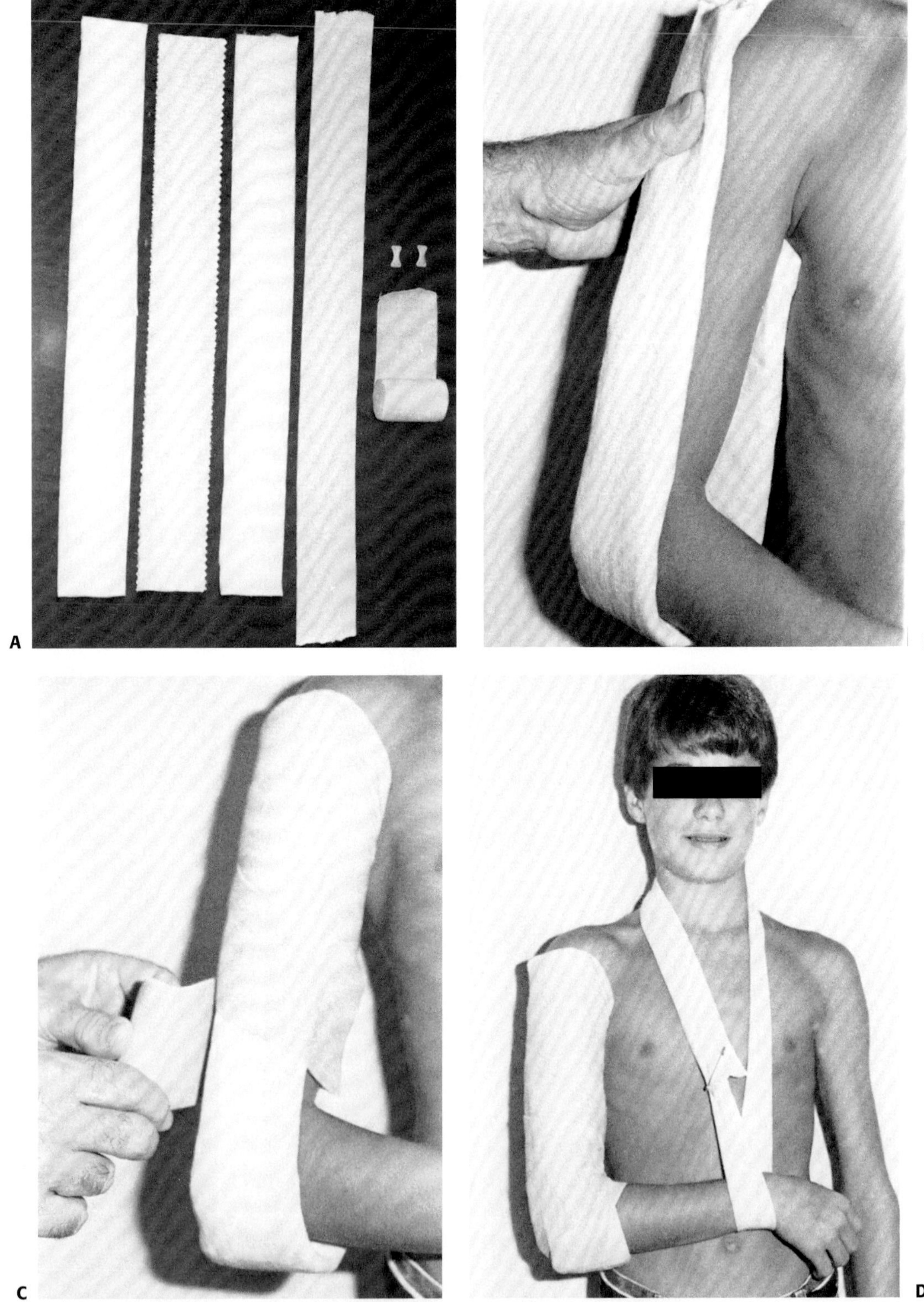

FIGURE 17-43 Coaptation splints with collar and cuff. **A.** The material used for a sugartong arm splint is two pieces of cast padding rolled out to the length of the plaster-of-paris splint and applied to each side of the splint after it is wet. The splint is then brought into the tubular stockinette of the same width but 4 inches longer than the splint. **B.** The plaster splint is applied to the arm from the axilla up to the tip of the acromion. **C.** As the plaster is setting, the splint is molded to the arm. An elastic bandage holds the splint in place. **D.** Stockinette is applied and attached to the wrist to form a collar-and-cuff sling.

(409), particularly in children (441). Holm (429) suggested applying benzoin before the cotton webbing and using a collar-and-cuff sling about the wrist. To prevent slippage, Shantharam (442) suggested applying the splint from the base of the neck, over the shoulder, and around to the axillary fold, with a strap securing the proximal end to the chest. The U plaster may not control alignment satisfactorily in more displaced fractures, which may require a thoracobrachial cast (429,434,436) or internal fixation. Böhler actually abandoned the immediate use of the U plaster for a thoracobrachial cast because of problems with early swelling (436,437).

Hanging Arm Cast. The hanging arm cast, described by Caldwell as a technique already in use (443), consists of a long-arm cast with a sling around the neck tied to the cast along the forearm. The weight of the cast and arm provides longitudinal traction. The position of the sling is modified to correct anterior or posterior angulation and varus or valgus. Rotation is difficult to control. Stewart and Hundley suggested not using it in children under age 12 because children cannot keep their arms in a dependent position during sleep and often keep the arm supported rather than hanging while awake (444). However, excellent results are reported in patients under age 10 (445). This is probably due to the marked remodeling and potential for good results regardless of treatment in children. Possible complications of the hanging cast include inferior shoulder subluxation (446), decreased external rotation (446), and shoulder stiffness (447), but these are rarely significant in children.

Thoracobrachial Immobilization. Severely unstable fractures uncontrollable in a hanging cast or U plaster may necessitate extending the cast to the chest as a thoracobrachial cast or splint (429,434,436,437,440). Various types of thoracobrachial dressings are often described as a Velpeau, but technically this is incorrect: Velpeau described a thoracobrachial bandage with acute elbow flexion. If a thoracobrachial cast or splint is used for a grossly unstable fracture, usually only a few degrees of abduction is necessary (429). Distal diaphyseal fractures rarely require extension to the chest.

Functional Bracing. Functional bracing, as described by Sarmiento (448), has been quite effective in adults (449–456). It may be difficult to use in children because size differences require a customized brace for each patient or a large supply of braces; however, modern thermoplastics can keep this economical (Fig. 17-44) (457). A prefabricated brace is placed on the initial visit if possible or on subsequent visits after placement of a U plaster or sling-and-swathe at the initial evaluation (458). The patient must be followed closely and the splint tightened as needed. It should not be used in bedridden patients because of loss of gravity support (449). Sarmiento (448,459,460) noted difficulty in controlling anterior angulation and indicated that patients should not lean on the elbow. The results in adults may be functionally superior to those of the U plaster (461).

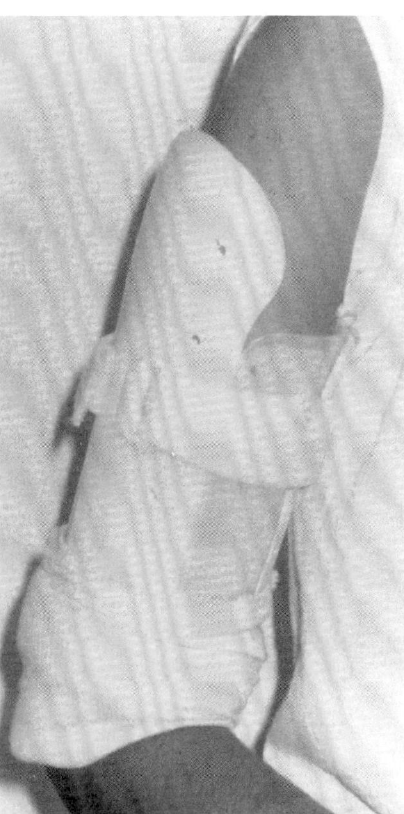

FIGURE 17-44 Light plastic functional braces are useful to maintain alignment and allow early restoration of motion, particularly in older children and adolescents.

Traction. Side-arm and overhead skin and skeletal forms of traction have been described (429,434,462,463). If olecranon skeletal traction is used, the AO method of an eye screw in the olecranon is less likely to produce ulnar nerve irritation than is a transolecranon pin (419,434). Excessive traction can lead to nonunion in adults (464) and elbow dislocation in children (465).

Operative Treatment

There are several surgical alternatives for humeral diaphyseal fractures: pinning, external fixation, intramedullary rodding, screw fixation, and compression plating. Biomechanically, interlocking rods are the stiffest in bending, and dynamic compression plating is stiffest in torsion. Flexible intramedullary rods are not as stiff as intact bone (466).

Open Reduction and Internal Reduction. Open reduction and internal reduction can be performed through either a posterior triceps-splitting approach, as advocated by the AO group (419,467), or through an anterior lateral approach between the brachialis and brachioradialis with extension proximally between the deltoid and pectoralis (468,469). The normal 4.5-mm dynamic compression plate does not provide adequate stability for the adult humerus shaft. The broad 4.5-mm dynamic compression plate is designed to allow compact screw placement without causing excessive stress on the humerus (419). At least six cortices of screw fixation proximal and distal to the fracture site are needed. With either the anterolateral or posterior approach, the lateral intermuscular septum should be split in the distal third to release the radial nerve's tether. Interfragmentary lag screws should be used when possible. The plate should be slipped underneath the radial nerve and vessels and some muscle placed between the plate and the nerve. Multiple screws in oblique fractures without a compression plate are unsatisfactory in adults (467) but may be sufficient in children. Extensively comminuted fractures should be grafted with autologous cancellous bone.

Generally, the results are good (468,470–474), and plating is particularly advocated in multiple-trauma patients to facilitate nursing care and management of other injuries (468). Potential complications include radial nerve palsy, infection, delayed union, nonunion, and failure of fixation (474).

Intramedullary Rodding. Several types of intramedullary rods are available. Currently, there are no indications for reamed intramedullary nailing in children because of potential proximal physeal damage and the small diaphyseal diameter. However, they may be used in older adolescents if the risk of physeal arrest is minimal and the canal has sufficient diameter (475). Reamed nailing has been reported in patients as young as 16 (476,477). The results are generally good (403,476,478–486), with a low risk of nonunion and infection (487).

Unreamed nails, such as Ender nails, Rush rods, or flexible titanium rods have been used primarily in adults. Nails or rods can be inserted via a posterior triceps-splitting approach through a hole just above the olecranon fossa. This can be useful for rapid management of fractures, including open fractures in patients with multiple trauma (392,488–491). Rods should not be inserted through the greater tuberosity in children (except under extenuating circumstances) because of the proximal humeral physis and the potential for shoulder impingement (492–494). Inserting these relatively large rods through the epicondyles results in a high incidence of nail back-out (491).

There are two techniques of using small, flexible, smooth wires. In the Hackethal technique (495), fluoroscopy is used with a tourniquet placed on the upper arm. A hole is made just proximal to the olecranon fossa using a triceps-splitting approach. Smooth, blunt-tipped Steinmann pins are placed up the canal of the humerus, progressively filling the canal with smaller and smaller pins as needed (Fig. 17-45). Results are generally good (496–502), although pin back-out can be a problem and care must be taken not to distract the fracture site. The rods should be bent 90 degrees at the cortical window (501). This technique may be useful for segmental and pathologic fractures (503).

The other technique consists of using small smooth rods or Steinmann pins placed through the epicondyles (504,505). The tips of the rods should be blunt and slightly bent. These are placed through the lateral epicondyle or through both the medial and lateral epicondyles. A hole is made in the epicondyle, and a blunt-tipped Steinmann pin is tapped up the diaphysis using a mallet or passed by hand, with a drill chuck holding the pin. The bend on the tip of the rods facilitates crossing the fracture site and manipulating the fracture reduction. A splint is necessary postoperatively. Alignment need be only within the tolerances for a closed reduction (Fig. 17-46).

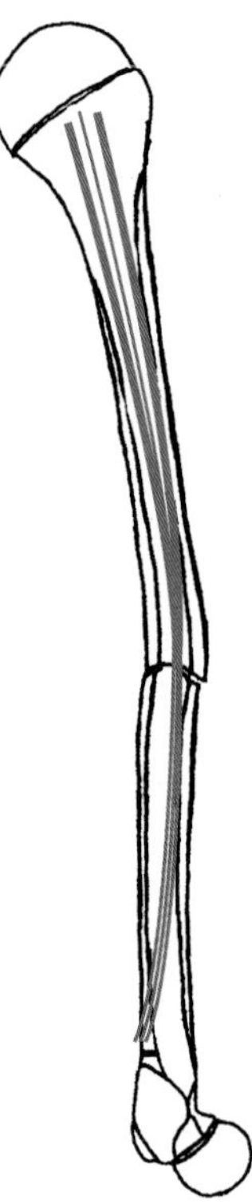

FIGURE 17-45 The Hackethal technique involves multiple smooth pins placed up the humeral shaft through a cortical window just above the olecranon fossa. The pins are placed until the canal is filled.

External Fixation. Both unilateral and multiplanar external fixation techniques are occasionally useful for humeral shaft fractures (462,506–508). External fixators are primarily useful for severe open fractures or as an alternative to internal fixation. In patients with open fractures, immediate external fixation with subsequent bone grafting yields good results (509,510). External fixation can be combined with internal fixation for immediate stability (511) for early rehabilitation. Severe open fractures with bone loss can be treated with primary shortening followed by callus distraction (512) to provide early soft tissue coverage and subsequent restoration of humeral length. Care must be taken during pin placement to avoid radial nerve injury. If screws are used, limited open screw placement can prevent this injury (509). Ring fixators may be useful for reconstructing the injured humerus (513–520).

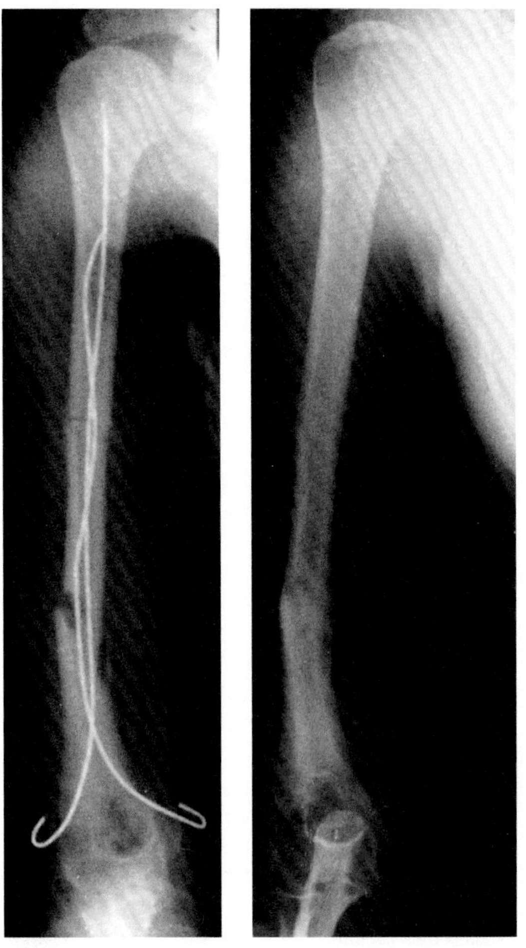

FIGURE 17-46 **A.** A segmental fracture difficult to align by nonoperative methods treated with two intramedullary smooth pins. **B.** Alignment need be only within the same tolerances as closed reduction.

Operative Versus Conservative Treatment

Because most humeral fractures are controllable nonoperatively, there are few surgical indications (521). Potential operative indications include open fractures, multiple trauma, bilateral injuries, arterial injuries, compartment syndromes, pathologic fractures, significant nerve injuries, inadequate closed reduction, and ipsilateral upper extremity injuries or paralysis.

Preadolescents can almost always be managed nonoperatively, except those with severe soft tissue injury. If fracture reduction cannot obtain less than 30 degrees varus and 20 degrees anterior angulation in older children and adolescents—or more importantly, if the arm appears deformed—alternatives such as internal fixation, intramedullary rodding, external fixation, a thoracobrachial cast, or traction should be considered. Inadequate closed reduction is most common in obese patients and in thin women with large breasts (467). However, obesity tends to hide the deformity of the fracture, and large breasts are seldom encountered in children.

Open fractures may require fixation. Small, stable grade 1 wounds can still be managed using coaptation splints or other closed methods. Unstable open fractures should be stabilized with internal or external fixation to protect soft tissues (467,490,522–525).

Multiple-trauma victims are often best treated with internal or external fixation for more rapid mobilization (382,392,468, 469,526,527). This is particularly true in patients with chest injuries, where thoracobrachial immobilization would compromise pulmonary care (490,524,526). Excellent results have been reported with external fixation (507,509,510,522), retrograde rodding using Ender nails or Rush rods (392), and internal fixation (468). In older adolescents, more rigid locked or unlocked intramedullary rodding can be used for patients requiring their upper extremities for mobility (469). However, this luxury does not exist for younger children.

Arterial injury and compartment syndromes requiring fasciotomy are potential indications for internal fixation (528–531). Continued fracture mobility can damage a vascular anastomosis (530–533), and fasciotomy can make the fracture less stable. Temporary vascular shunting before internal fixation allows the orthopaedist and the vascular surgeon to work under optimal conditions (534).

Most pathologic fractures in children, including those from malignancy (535), fibrous dysplasia (410,411,536), osteogenesis imperfecta, and simple bone cysts, can be treated nonoperatively. Simple bone cysts are discussed later in the section on proximal humerus fractures. A report of a 6-year-old with progressive ossifying fibrodysplasia suggests that internal fixation may prevent stiffness after fractures in this condition (537). In fractures secondary to malignancy, intramedullary rodding is necessary if extensive cortical loss causes instability (477,494,538–540). Spontaneous fracture in a severely brain-injured or unresponsive cerebral palsy patient is best treated nonoperatively (541).

Ipsilateral injuries, particularly fractures of the proximal or distal humerus and of the forearm, can be difficult to control. In adults with a floating elbow, internal fixation of the humeral fracture provides optimal results (392,542,543). This is also true for supracondylar humeral fractures in children but is not documented in diaphyseal fractures (414,415). The floating elbow is often associated with other organ system injuries; nerve injury occurs in up to 50% of these patients (544).

Humeral shaft fractures with ipsilateral brachial plexus palsies in adults heal best with open reduction and internal fixation (545). The same is true with spinal cord injuries (546). Functional bracing is precluded in these patients because the muscles do not function. Because of the excellent healing potential in children, they may be treated nonoperatively if satisfactory alignment can be maintained. Older adolescents should be treated like adults.

Radial Nerve Palsies

Radial nerve palsies with humeral shaft fractures have been reported in children (Fig. 17-47) (524,547). Primary radial nerve

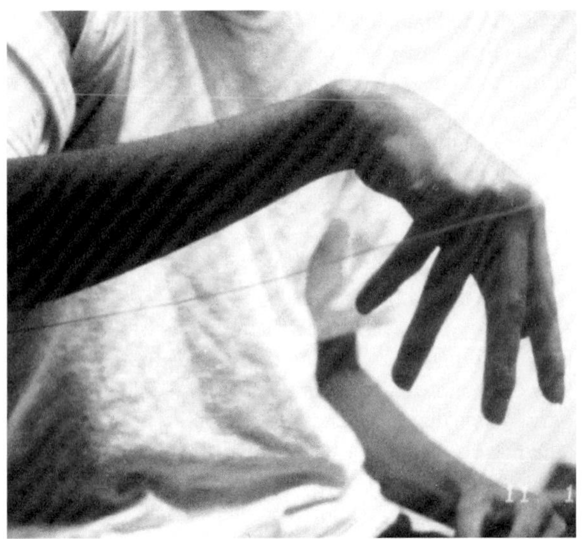

FIGURE 17-47 Radial nerve palsy secondary to a humeral shaft fracture from a low-velocity gunshot wound.

palsies occur at the time of the fracture; secondary radial nerve palsies occur after manipulation of the fracture. Many clinicians recommend exploration of primary (416,417,548–556) and secondary radial nerve palsies (381,382,409,550,553,554, 557,558). The incidence of concomitant radial nerve palsy with a humeral shaft fracture ranges from 2.4% to 20.6% (487,524,550,555,559–563) and has been reported in 4.4% of children's humeral shaft fractures (524). Most occur with middle and distal humeral shaft fractures, but they may occur with more proximal fractures as well (560). In explored primary radial nerve palsies, the incidence of complete nerve laceration is small (420,421,524,553,562,563). Commonly, the nerve is tented over the bone, trapped in the fracture site, or contused. The natural history is excellent, with recovery ranging from 78% to 100% (383,550,553,554,559,561–568). Therefore, many clinicians recommend observation rather than early exploration (383,550,553,554,559,561–563,567,568). Open fractures resulting in severe soft tissue injury requiring debridement should have the radial nerve explored and tagged (569) or preferably repaired (570). More severe open fractures should be stabilized using either intramedullary rodding or internal or external fixation to provide good soft tissue for radial nerve recovery. Early repair of the nerve provides the best anatomic results (571). Bostman et al (566) recommended exploration and internal fixation in patients with bayonet apposition because the abundant callus may endanger nerve recovery. The recommended waiting time before radial nerve exploration ranges from 8 weeks to 6 months (381,409,434,440,548,554, 557,560,561,564,567). Nerve grafting up to 18 months after the injury can provide good function (571,572). Seddon suggested a physiologic time of allowing 1 mm per day after the 1 to 2 months of Wallerian degeneration and nerve growth through the neuroma (573). Nerves grow 1 to 3 mm per day (573–575), and this rate has been used clinically with good success (569,576).

In secondary radial nerve palsies, the surgeon may feel compelled to explore the nerve because he or she "caused" the radial nerve injury. However, natural history studies of observed secondary radial nerve palsies show recovery rates of 80% to 100% with nonoperative treatment (550,566). Secondary palsies occurring after manipulation may be observed (456,559,562, 567,577). If the palsy occurs after a considerable time, the nerve is probably encased in callus and further investigation, including exploration, is warranted (578,579). Late presentation may result in an osseous foramen containing the nerve and requiring decompression (578).

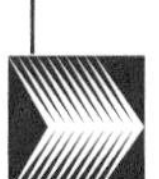

AUTHORS' PREFERRED TREATMENT

Birth fractures have a very good prognosis for full recovery. To prevent an internal rotation contracture, we place the arm in either a U plaster or a plaster coaptation splint with the palm facing anteriorly. A soft wrap holds the arm to the body so the child can be carried. The splint can be removed in 2 weeks. On healing, the radiographic angulation can be quite worrisome to the parents. We like to show them x-rays of other infants with marked remodeling, and we keep photographs handy for this purpose.

Most humeral diaphyseal fractures in children are treated nonoperatively. Torus fractures are treated with a commercial shoulder immobilizer or a sling. Greenstick fractures and displaced fractures in younger children are treated with a U plaster or a plaster coaptation splint; these are usually applied in the emergency department with mild sedation. We prefer general anesthesia if more manipulation is needed. A careful neurologic and vascular evaluation is performed before and after manipulation. We place a U plaster with Webril padding extending from over the deltoid, around the olecranon, and up to the axillary fold, and secure it with a gauze wrap followed by an elastic bandage. We have had similar results applying plaster coaptation splints on the medial and lateral aspects of the arm and rewrapping frequently with an elastic wrap. The patient is placed in a collar-and-cuff sling for forearm support. If alignment is unsatisfactory, a new splint is reapplied and molded.

In those rare fractures uncontrollable by closed means, we prefer smooth intramedullary rodding using two 2-mm rods placed retrograde through the epicondyles. For unstable fractures with extensive comminution, we prefer to use a unilateral external fixator, with small incisions made during screw placement to avoid the radial nerve. Open fractures are treated in a similar manner. Significant bone loss can be treated using bone transport techniques. We avoid plate fixation because it creates a stress riser, particularly in growing children. If a fracture occurs distal or proximal to the plate, it must be reexplored for plate removal, necessitating reexploration of the radial nerve and potential nerve damage. We observe both primary and early secondary radial nerve palsies, exploring them only after 1 to 2 months and growth of 1 mm per day if electromyography shows no return.

Rehabilitation

Patients treated with closed manipulation should be followed weekly for the first few weeks to ensure that alignment is maintained. The coaptation splint or long-arm cast should be replaced as needed. Patients with radial nerve palsies must be instructed in finger motion to keep the fingers supple and prevent contractures. Noncompliance requires formal hand therapy or a radial nerve outrigger. Stiffness of the shoulder and elbow is uncommon in children, but pendulum exercises are started at 3 to 4 weeks in older children and adolescents. Some form of immobilization is generally continued for 6 weeks. Patients should not return to contact sports until there is adequate healing, and the family should be cautioned that refracture may occur during the first 6 months after injury.

The prognosis for healing and remodeling of humeral shaft fractures in children is excellent. Internal rotation deformity is usually minimal, and the outlook for radial nerve palsies is good. Loss of shoulder motion may occur but is more common in older patients (434).

Complications

Early

Nerve Palsies. Radial nerve palsies were discussed previously. They also may occur immediately after operative treatment (580), or may be delayed and occur many years after internal fixation (581). Ulnar nerve paralysis has been reported from entrapment of the nerve in the fracture site (426). A few people have an abnormal arcade of Struthers in which only superficial fibers of the triceps medial head pass superficial to the ulnar nerve and none pass deep to the nerve, making the nerve extremely close to the bone and vulnerable to an abduction extension mechanism of fracture, which opens the anterior medial aspect of the humerus (426). In about 10% of the population, the median nerve crosses posterior to the brachial artery rather than anterior, placing it closer to the humerus. Median nerve palsy has been reported from an apex anterior mid-diaphyseal fracture (582). After an easy fracture reduction, the median nerve was caught in the fracture between the coracobrachialis and brachialis muscles, where the nerve crossed anteriorly. Anterior interosseous nerve palsies have not been reported in fractures above the supracondylar region.

Compartment Syndrome. The fascia of the upper arm is not as strong as it is in the lower arm, making compartment syndrome less common. Mubarak and Carroll (583) reported a dorsal forearm compartment syndrome in a 9-year-old boy with a humerus shaft fracture. Gupta and Sharma (584) described an adult with a triceps compartment syndrome from a middle-third minimally displaced fracture; this fracture did not disrupt the intercompartmental boundaries.

Vascular Injuries. Vascular injuries require a high index of suspicion and rapid treatment (580,585–587). The fracture should be stabilized sufficiently to prevent disruption of the vascular repair.

Infection. Infections have been reported in patients undergoing surgery. They have not been reported in closed fractures of the humerus in children, but have been reported in closed fractures elsewhere (588,589).

Late

Malunion. Malunion is uncommon in children's humeral diaphyseal fractures. Varus of 20 to 30 degrees can be accepted (see Fig. 17-41) (409,414,415,434,590), but anterior bowing of 20 degrees may be apparent (433). An internal rotation deformity of 15 degrees causes no functional impairment (409). Most patients under 6 years of age grow out of angular deformities (440). Children 6 to 13 years of age may not, although some remodeling is possible even in adolescents (440,591). Obese patients are more prone to malunion, but they also hide their deformity better (467). Green and Gibbs (594) noted that the deformity visible on the AP and lateral x-rays is generally not the maximum deformity, which is the vector sum of the two deformities. This can be appreciated by obtaining an x-ray perpendicular to the plane of the deformity, similar to the Stagnara view for scoliosis.

Nonunion. Primarily a problem in adults and occasionally in older adolescents, there are few reports of humeral nonunion in children—one in a child with progeria at age 4 (593), four in children with osteogenesis imperfecta (532), and three from severe trauma (534). In adults, numerous treatments have been used successfully. These include reamed nails (595) and modified flexible nails (596,597). However, the best results appear to be from ASIF techniques with the broad dynamic compression plate and autogenous bone grafting (416,417,598–602). Currently, treatment in children and adolescents must be extrapolated from adult treatment. In general, the atrophic ends of the nonunion are taken back to bleeding surfaces and apposed, a compression plate is applied with fixation of at least six cortical screws proximally and distally, and bone grafting is performed (601). The Ilizarov technique also reportedly produces good results (412,413,513,514,517–519). Electrical stimulation also has been used with success (603–608). Children with dysplastic bone, such as those with osteogenesis imperfecta, are best treated with intramedullary rodding and bone grafting (532).

Loss of Motion. Loss of shoulder and elbow motion is more common in older patients (440,609). The joint affected is usually the one closest to the fracture site.

Upper Extremity Limb Length Discrepancy. Overgrowth after humeral fracture occurs in about 81% of patients but is generally minimal (<1 cm) (438). Some generalized stimulus to the extremity is evident, with overgrowth of the carpals as well (610). In patients with limb length discrepancy of 3 cm or more at maturity, lengthening may be indicated (611,612). Unilateral or ring fixators may be used with Ilizarov's principles (514,515).

Other Complications. Uncommon complications include reflex sympathetic dystrophy (613) and fat embolism (614). Late refracture may occur from retained internal fixation (615).

DISTAL HUMERAL DIAPHYSEAL FRACTURES

Little has been written about distal humeral diaphyseal or metaphyseal–diaphyseal junction fractures, which are much less common than supracondylar humeral fractures. Fractures in this region should not be confused with supracondylar humeral fractures. The distal diaphysis is more triangular and the periosteum is thinner than in the supracondylar region (422,423), making these fractures generally less stable than supracondylar fractures. The cortical bone also heals more slowly than metaphyseal bone, requiring longer immobilization. The mobile wad, anconeus, and flexor pronator mass originate off the epicondyles; the biceps, brachialis, and triceps all insert distally. Therefore, forearm position greatly affects the fracture position. Because the brachial artery is tethered by the lacertus fibrosus, injury to the artery is more likely than with more proximal fractures.

Distal humeral diaphyseal–metaphyseal junction fractures may be caused by transverse or longitudinal loading, torsion, or moments generated by the forearm about the elbow. They are caused by direct blows and twisting more often than ulnar leverage in the olecranon fossa. The diagnosis, made on plain x-rays, must be differentiated from a supracondylar humerus fracture.

Diagnosis and Classification

Most distal humeral diaphyseal fractures are transverse, spiral, or short oblique. Occasionally, an oblique or spiral fracture extends distally toward or beyond the epicondyles (Fig. 17-48).

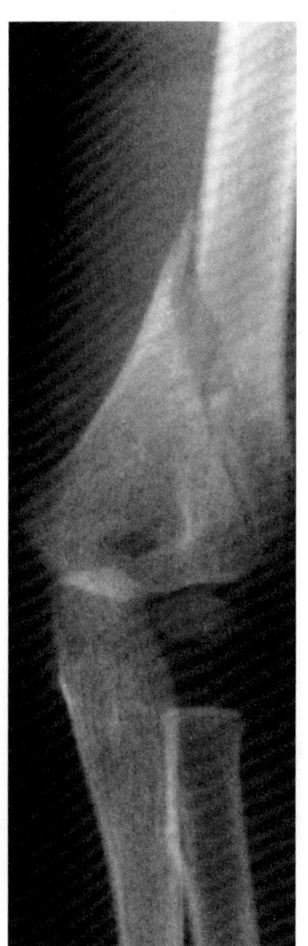
A

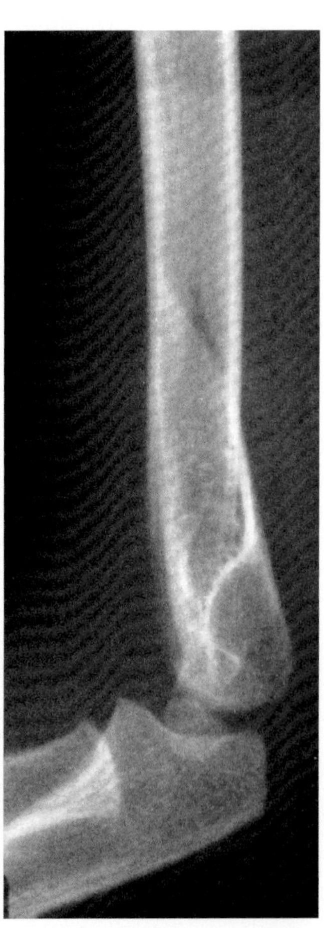
B

FIGURE 17-48 Distal humeral diaphyseal fracture extending to the epicondyles. This fracture was treated by casting with the forearm in pronation.

The description must include the direction of displacement, the neurologic and vascular status, and the degree of comminution. Medial column comminution predisposes to varus malunion.

Current Treatment Options

Nonoperative

Closed treatment usually is possible because acute flexion of the elbow, with potential vascular compromise, is not required to maintain reduction. These fractures tend toward varus malunion (Fig. 17-49) (616), which may be cosmetically unacceptable, particularly in more distal fractures. With 20% or less of humeral growth occurring distally (617–619), significant remodeling may not occur. Because of the proximity to the epicondyles with their muscular origins, supination and pronation affect fracture reduction. If one cortex is open, then the muscles originating on that side should be tightened to reduce the fracture (620). Because of the varus tendency, this is usually by pronation (435,437,531). However, this is best checked radiographically (Figs. 17-50 and 17-51).

Operative

Unstable fractures may require fixation (434,616) and possibly open reduction. Closed reduction and percutaneous pinning should be performed in a similar fashion to supracondylar humerus fractures. However, because the fracture is more proximal, it is difficult to get the pins into the diaphysis without crossing them at the fracture site (Fig. 17-52). Attempts should be made to pass the wires in intramedullary fashion up the lateral or medial and lateral columns separately to provide stability (Fig. 17-53) (434). This can be done by drilling the wires, but it is easier to create a starting site at the epicondyles and pass blunt-tipped wires up the columns. Holding the wires with a drill chuck helps, too. Because of the bony anatomy and the ulnar nerve, lateral wires are easier to place, particularly in younger children (Fig. 17-54). Alternatively, the fracture can be managed with skeletal traction until callus forms; then either a U plaster splint or a long-arm cast can be applied (Fig. 17-55). Brug et al reported the best results with flexible intramedullary rodding (616).

(text continues on page 761)

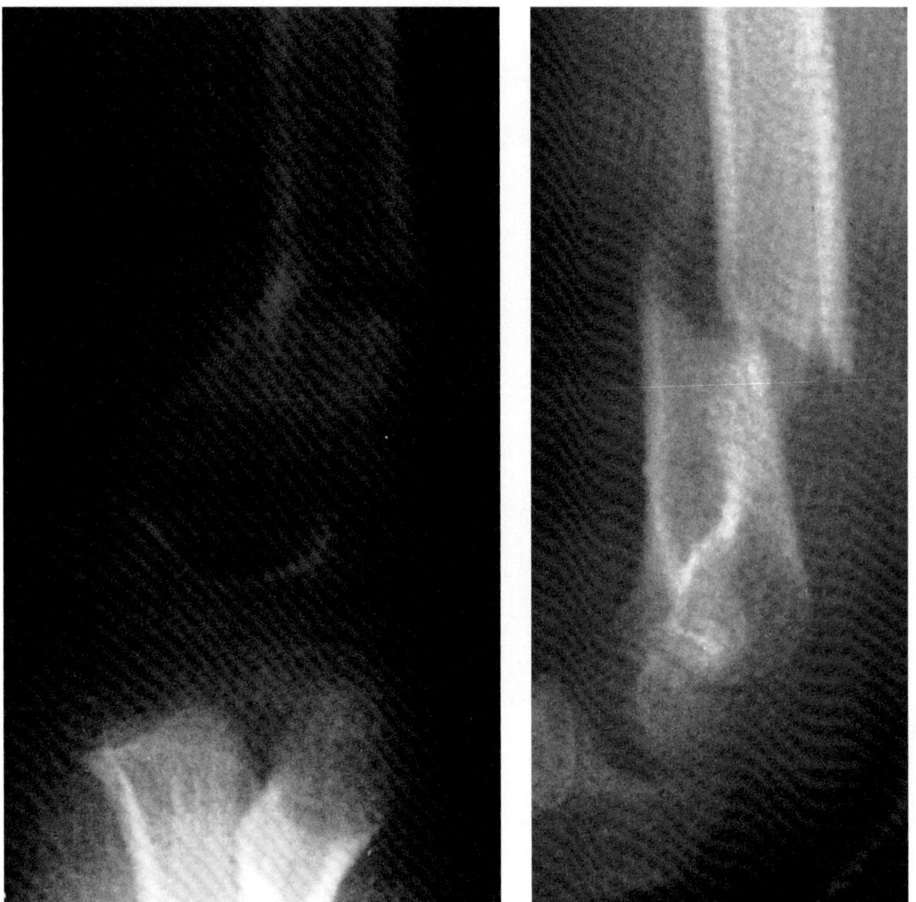

FIGURE 17-49 X-rays showing the tendency of distal humeral diaphyseal fractures toward varus malunion. This fracture required remanipulation.

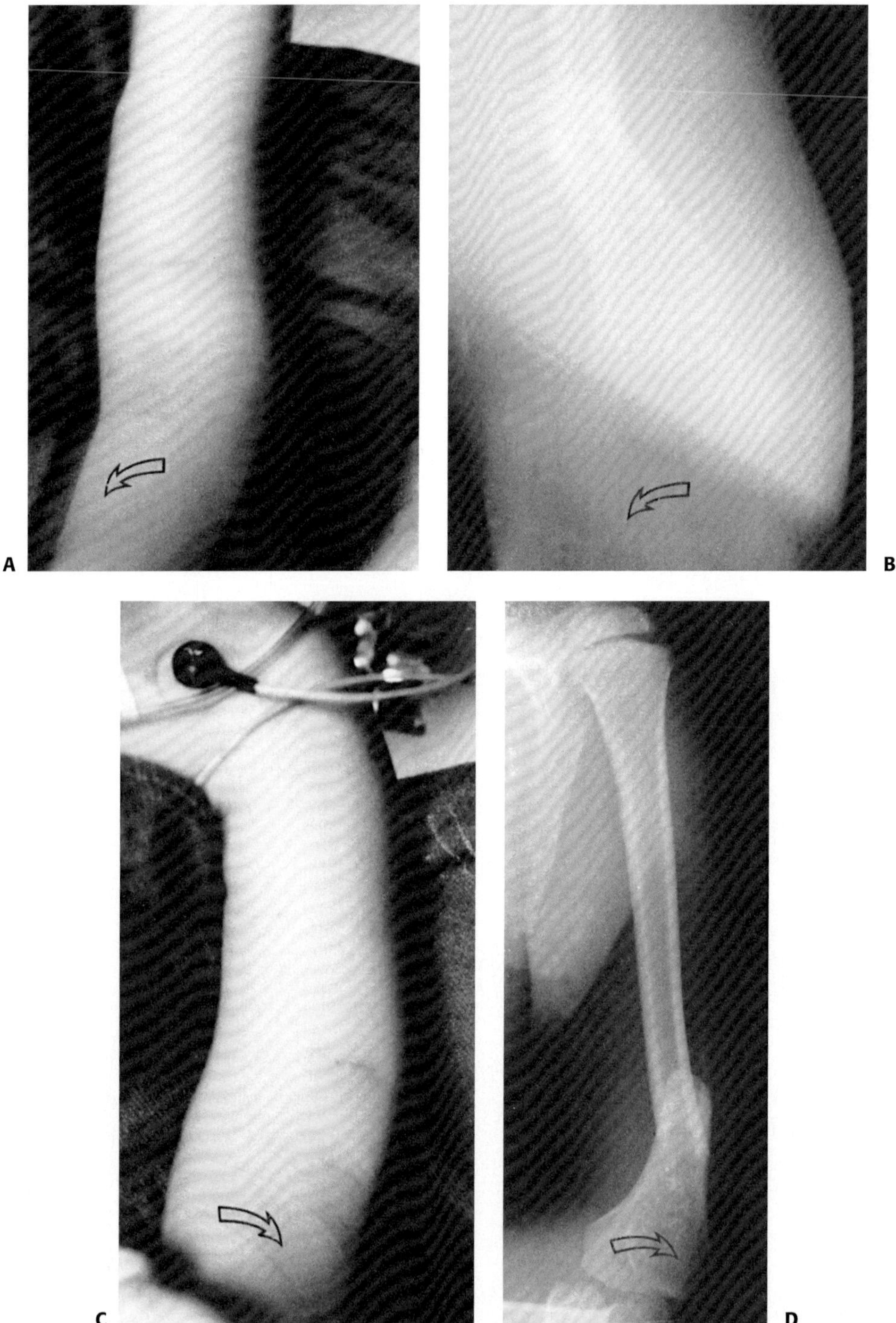

FIGURE 17-50 Influence of forearm rotation. Pronation **(A,B)** of the forearm produces a valgus angulation at the fracture site (*arrows*). Supination **(C,D)** creates a varus angulation (*arrows*).

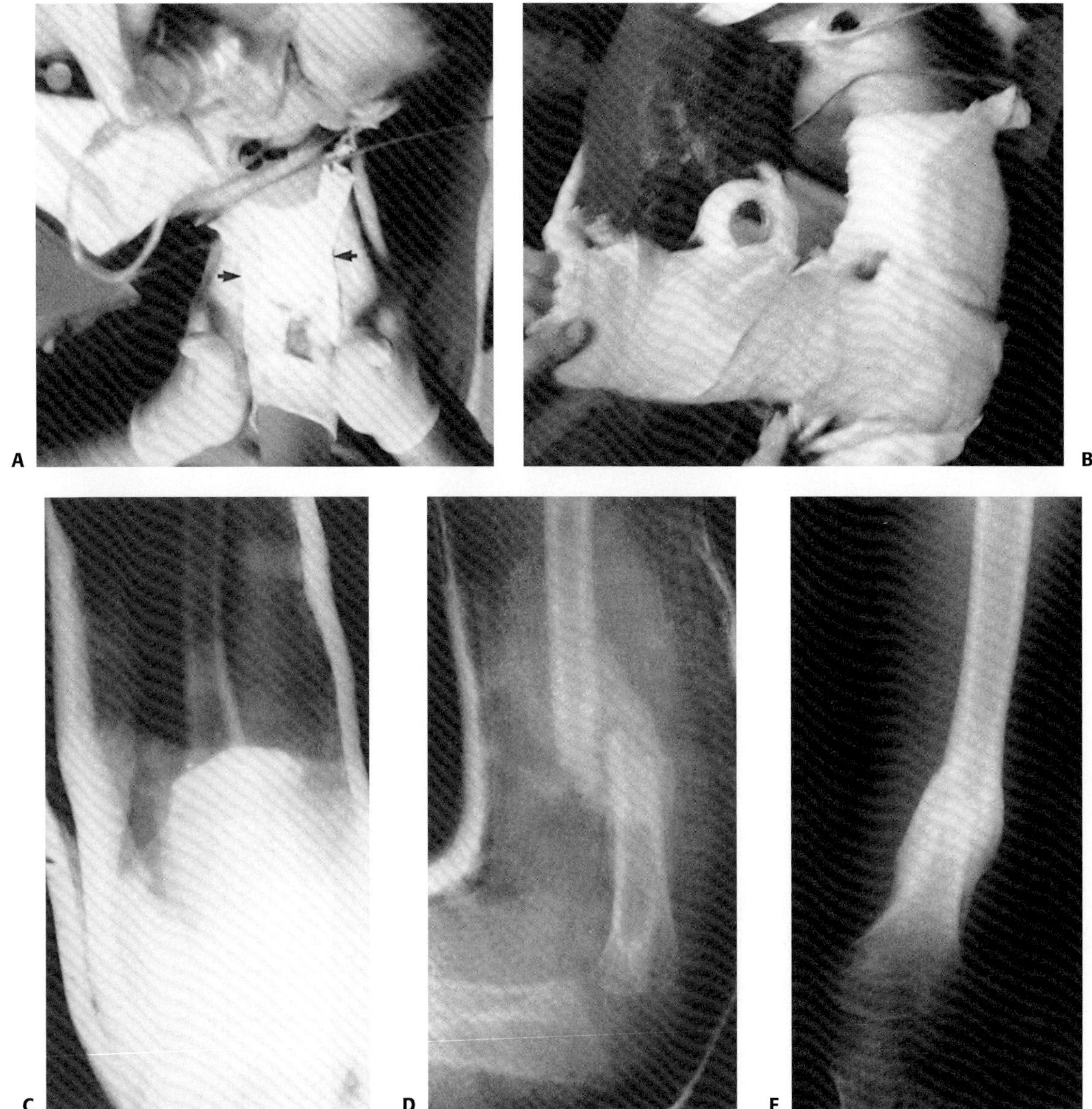

FIGURE 17-51 The same patient shown in Figure 17-50. **A.** The humeral coaptation splint is molded (*arrows*) with the forearm in neutral. **B.** A second forearm coaptation splint is added, and the extremity is suspended with a loop. **C.** X-rays show satisfactory linear alignment. **D,E.** The fracture healed in bayonet apposition but with satisfactory alignment.

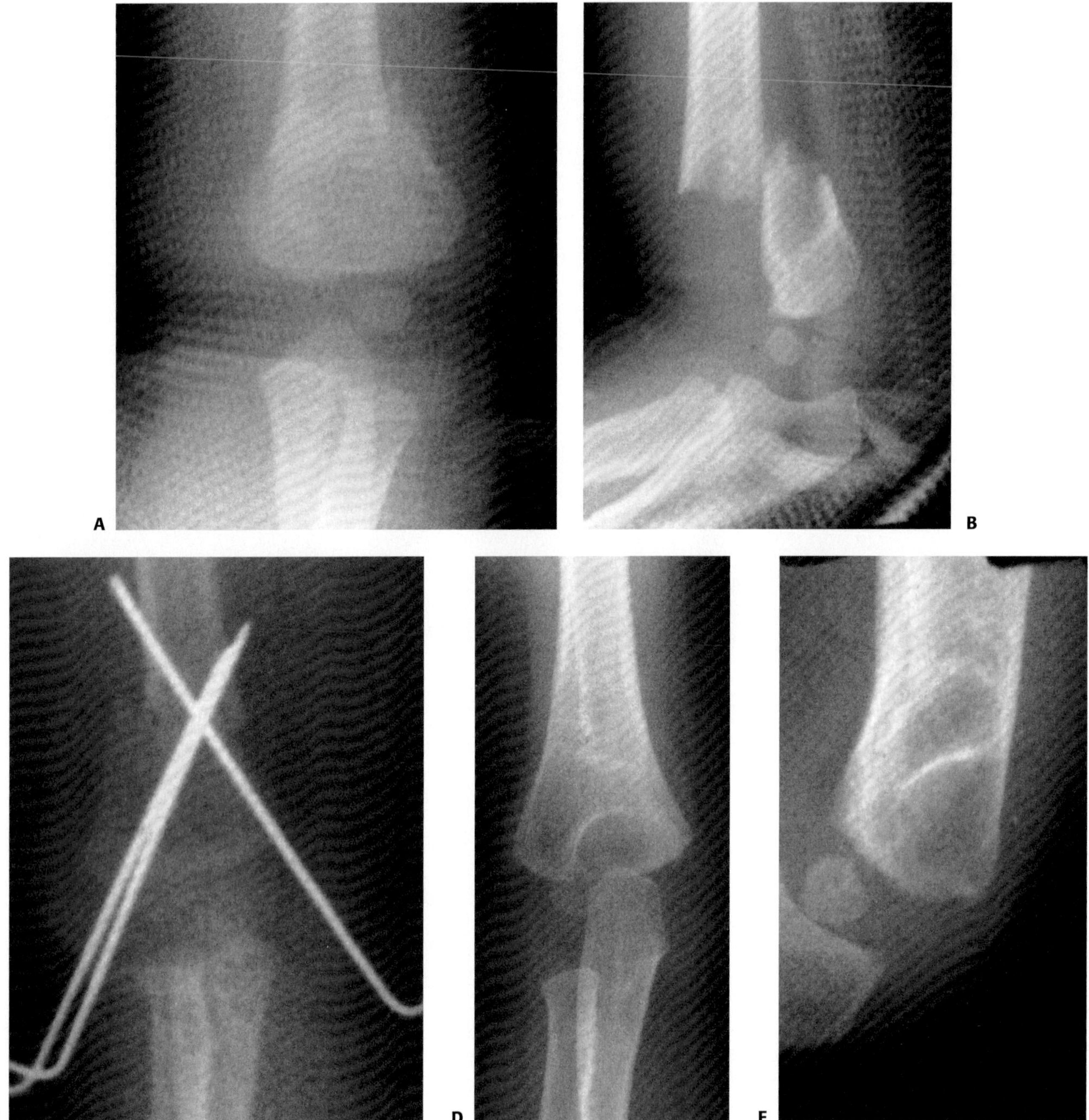

FIGURE 17-52 A,B. Distal humeral diaphyseal fracture in an 18-month-old treated with closed reduction and percutaneous pinning. **C.** The pins cross at the fracture site with decreased stability and some loss of position. **D,E.** The ultimate outcome was good.

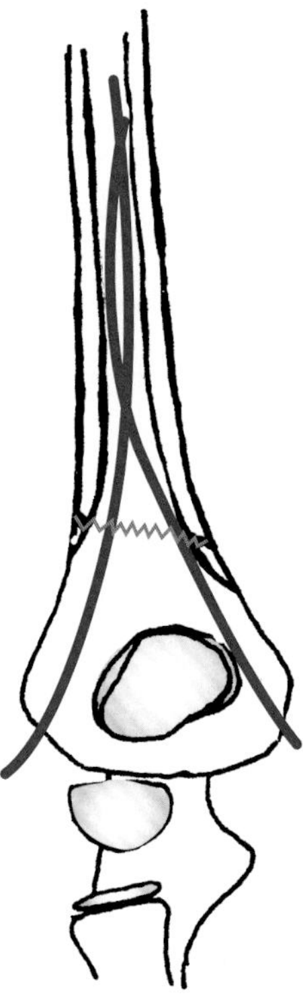

FIGURE 17-53 Ideally, pin fixation for distal humeral diaphyseal–metaphyseal junction fractures involves pins placed in intramedullary fashion up the medial and lateral columns.

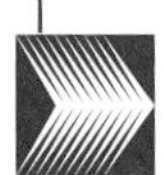

AUTHORS' PREFERRED TREATMENT

For distal humeral diaphyseal–metaphyseal junction fractures, we prefer closed treatment. Nondisplaced fractures are treated with a long-arm cast split to allow for swelling. A double sugartong splint is used if swelling is severe. We reduce displaced fractures under general anesthesia. Because supination and pronation of the forearm can affect the position, we use the image intensifier to determine the position best for maintaining the reduction; this is usually pronation. If the reduction obtained is unstable and cannot be held with a cast, we do not hesitate to treat it by percutaneous pinning, with small Steinmann pins placed through the medial and lateral epicondyles and up their respective columns, keeping the pins as divergent as possible at the fracture site or with lateral column pins. It is helpful to introduce them through the epicondyle and then tap rather than drill them up the column to prevent convergence at the fracture site. The pins are removed once good callus forms.

SUPRACONDYLAR PROCESS FRACTURES

Occasionally, a proboscis-like supracondylar process extends from a few centimeters above the medial epicondyle. The inci-

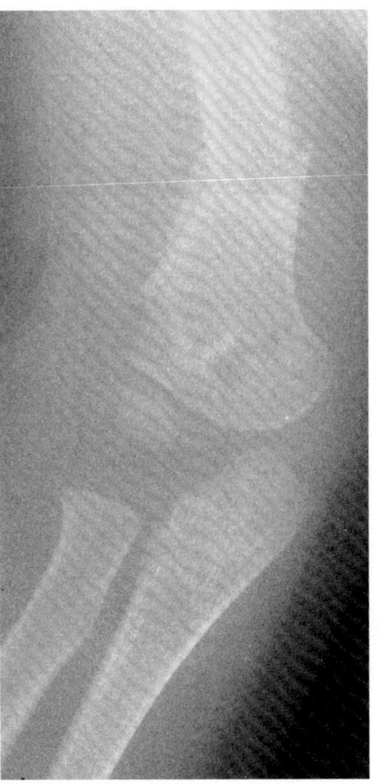

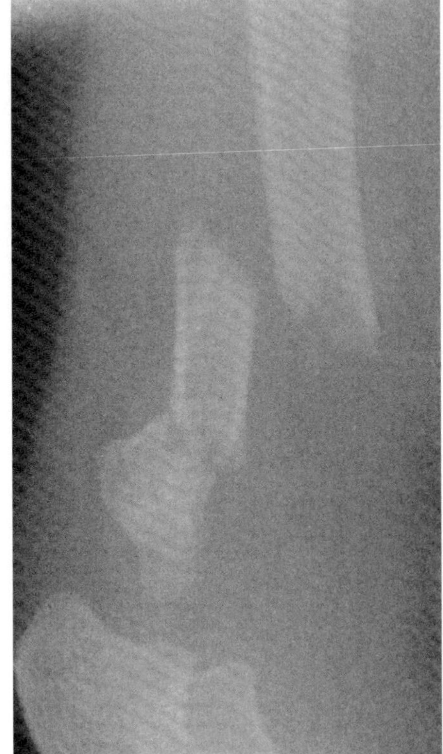

FIGURE 17-54 Segmental distal humeral diaphyseal and supracondylar fracture in a 4-year-old boy. **A,B.** Both fractures could not be controlled by closed means. *(continues)*

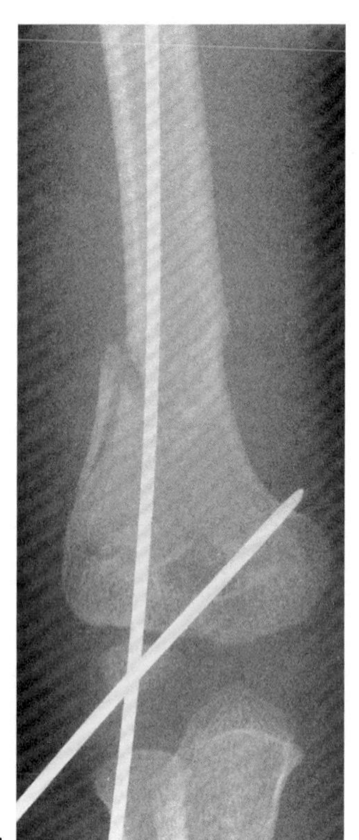
C

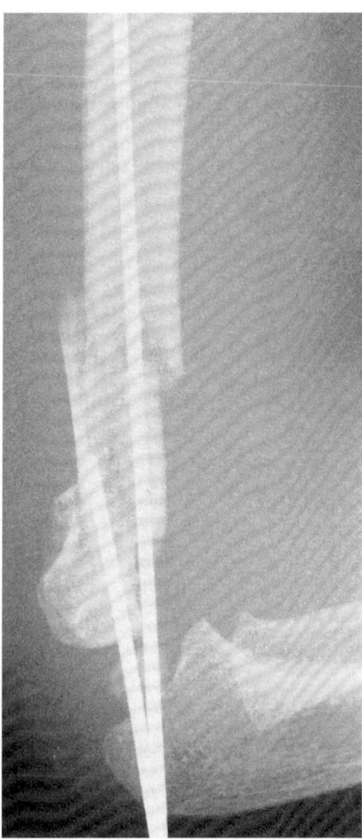
D

FIGURE 17-54 *(continued)* **C,D.** A lateral column pin acting as an internal splint is technically easier than medial column pins.

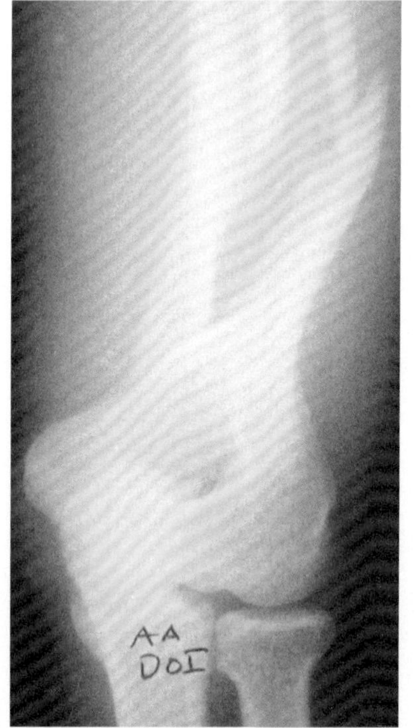

A

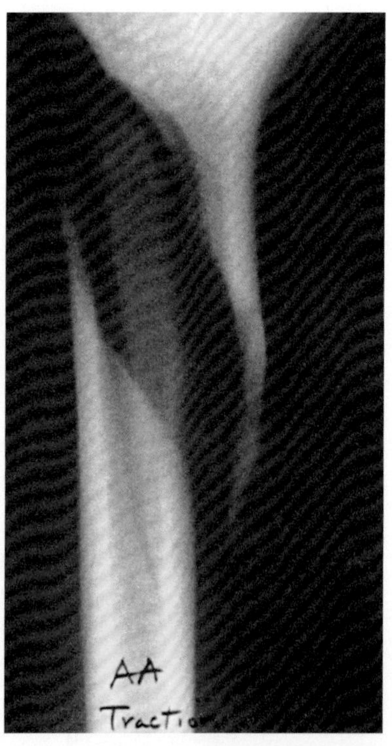

B

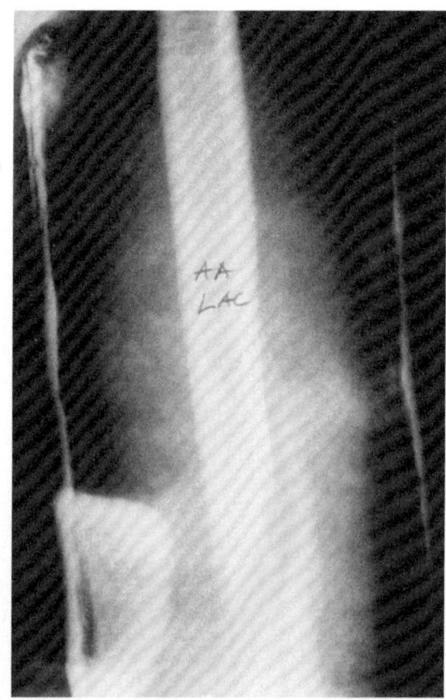

C

FIGURE 17-55 A comminuted distal humeral metaphyseal–diaphyseal fracture in a 14-year-old boy. Injury films **(A)** show multiple fragments in the metaphyseal–diaphyseal area. **B.** The patient was placed in traction for 2 weeks until callus appeared and then was transferred to a long-arm cast **(C)**.

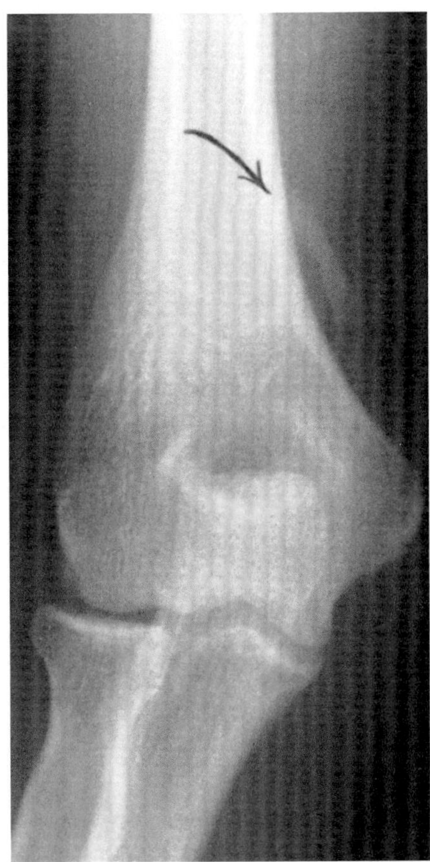

FIGURE 17-56 Radiographic appearance of a supracondylar process (*arrow*).

dence of this process ranges from 0.1% to 2.7%, with the lower percentages in blacks and the higher percentages in whites (621–623). The process extends obliquely downward and may be connected with the medial epicondyle by a tough fibrous band (507,621–624). Frequently, the foramen formed between the fibrous band and the humerus is traversed by the median nerve and the brachial artery. They may be entrapped by a fracture. Anomalous attachments of the coracobrachialis and the pronator teres may occur on the process (Fig. 17-56) (480,625).

Principles of Management

Supracondylar process fractures are the result of direct blows. There are no reports of avulsion from the anomalous muscle attachments.

Diagnosis and Classification

Supracondylar process fractures are classified as displaced or nondisplaced, with notation of median nerve or brachial artery compromise.

Current Treatment Options

Supracondylar process fractures have been reported in children (480) and usually are caused by direct blows to the distal humeral area. They may be quite painful and result in compression of the brachial artery or median nerve (480,621–625). The process is best seen on oblique views (623). If there are no symptoms of median nerve or brachial artery compression, they are treated by elevation, ice, and temporary immobilization for comfort. However, if a painful nonunion or neurovascular symptoms develop, the fragment should be excised (623). Fractures with neurologic signs or symptoms are treated by fragment excision and nerve and artery decompression.

REFERENCES

1. Berger PE, Ofstein RA, Jackson DW, et al. MRI demonstration of radiographically occult fractures: what have we been missing? *Radiographics* 1989;9:407–436.
2. Landin LA. Epidemiology of children's fractures. *J Pediatr Orthop* 1997;6:79–83.
3. Worlock P, Stower M. Fracture patterns in Nottingham children. *J Pediatr Orthop* 1986; 6:656–661.
4. Hohl JC. Fractures of the humerus in children. *Orthop Clin North Am* 1976;7:557–571.
5. Iqbal QM. Long-bone fractures among children in Malaysia. *Int Surg* 1974;59:410–415.
6. Landin LA. Fracture patterns in children: analysis of 8682 fractures with special reference to incidence, etiology and secular changes in Swedish urban populations. *Acta Orthop Scand Suppl* 1983;54:1–109.
7. Rose SH, Melton LJ 3rd, Morrey BF, et al. Epidemiologic features of humeral fractures. *Clin Orthop* 1982;168:24–30.
8. Lemperg R, Liliequest B. Dislocation of the proximal epiphysis of the humerus in newborns. *Acta Paediatr Scand* 1970;59:377–380.
9. Shulman BH, Terhune CB. Epiphyseal injuries in breech delivery. *Pediatrics* 1951;8: 693–700.
10. Dameron TB Jr, Reibel DB. Fractures involving the proximal humeral epiphyseal plate. *J Bone Joint Surg [Am]* 1969;51:289–297.
11. Gross SJ, Shime J, Farine D. Shoulder dystocia: predictors and outcome. *Am J Obstet Gynecol* 1987;156:334–336.
12. Haliburton RA, Barber JR, Fraser RL. Pseudodislocation: an unusual birth injury. *Can J Surg* 1967;10:455–462.
13. Harris BA. Shoulder dystocia. *Clin Obstet Gynecol* 1984;27:106–111.
14. Madsen TE. Fractures of the extremities in the newborn. *Acta Obstet Gynecol Scand* 1955;34:41.
15. Camus M, Lefebvre G, Veron P, et al. Obstetrical injuries of the newborn infant. Retrospective study apropos of 20,409 births. *J Gynecol Obstet Biol Reprod (Paris)* 1985;14: 1033–1043.
16. Gagnaire JC, Thoulon JM, Chappuis JP, et al. Injuries to the upper extremities in the new-born diagnosed at birth. *J Gynecol Obstet Biol Reprod (Paris)* 1975;4:245–254.
17. Jeffrey CC. Fracture separation of the upper humeral epiphysis. *Surg Gynecol Obstet* 1953;96:205–209.
18. Neer CS 2nd, Horowitz BS. Fractures of the proximal humeral epiphysial plate. *Clin Orthop* 1965;41:24–31.
19. Smith FM. Fracture–separation of the proximal humeral epiphysis: a study of cases seen at the Presbyterian Hospital, 1929–1953. *Am J Surg* 1956;91:627–635.
20. Aitken AP. End results of fractures of the proximal humeral epiphysis. *J Bone Joint Surg [Am]* 1936;18:1036–1041.
21. Bourdillan JF. Fracture–separation of the proximal epiphysis of the humerus. *J Bone Joint Surg [Br]* 1950;32:35–37.
22. Williams DJ. The mechanisms producing fracture-separation of the proximal humeral epiphysis. *J Bone Joint Surg [Br]* 1981;63:102–107.
23. Barber DB, Janus RB, Wade WH. Neuroarthropathy: an overuse injury of the shoulder in quadriplegia. *J Spinal Cord Med* 1996;19:9–11.
24. Kohler R, Trillaud JM. Fracture and fracture separation of the proximal humerus in children: report of 136 cases. *J Pediatr Orthop* 1983;3:326–332.
25. Nordqvist A, Petersson CJ. Incidence and causes of shoulder girdle injuries in an urban population. *J Shoulder Elbow Surg* 1995;4:107–112.
26. Dalldorf PG, Bryan WJ. Displaced Salter-Harris type I injury in a gymnast. A slipped capital humeral epiphysis? *Orthop Rev* 1994;23:538–541.
27. Lipscomb AB. Baseball pitching injuries in growing athletes. *J Sports Med* 1975;3: 25–34.
28. Tullos HS, Erwin WD, Woods GW, et al. Unusual lesions of the pitching arm. *Clin Orthop* 1972;88:169–182.
29. Tullos HS, Fain RH. Little League shoulder: rotational stress fracture of proximal epiphysis. *J Sports Med* 1974;2:152–153.
30. Ahn JI, Park JS. Pathological fractures secondary to unicameral bone cysts. *Int Orthop* 1994;18:20–22.
31. Kumar R, Cornah MS, Morris DL. Hydatid cyst—a rare cause of pathological fracture: a case report. *Injury* 1984;15:284–285.

32. Robin GC, Kedar SS. Separation of the upper humeral epiphysis in pituitary gigantism. *J Bone Joint Surg [Am]* 1962;44:189–192.
33. Sanders JO, Rockwood CA Jr, Curtis RJ. Fractures and dislocations of the humeral shaft and shoulder. In: Rockwood CA Jr, Wilkins KE, Beaty JH, eds. *Fractures in children.* Philadelphia: Lippincott-Raven, 1996:905–1021.
34. Edeiken BS, Libshitz HI, Cohen MA. Slipped proximal humeral epiphysis: a complication of radiotherapy to the shoulder in children. *Skel Radiol* 1982;9:123–125.
35. Lock TR, Aronson DD. Fractures in patients who have myelomeningocele. *J Bone Joint Surg [Am]* 1989;71:1153–1157.
36. Friedlander HL. Separation of the proximal humeral epiphysis: a case report. *Clin Orthop* 1964;35:163–170.
37. Shaw BA, Murphy KM, Shaw A, et al. Humerus shaft fractures in young children: accident or abuse? *J Pediatr Orthop* 1997;17:293–297.
38. Torode I, Donnan L. Posterior dislocation of the humeral head in association with obstetric paralysis. *J Pediatr Orthop* 1998;18:611–615.
39. Freundlich BD. Luxatio erecta. *J Trauma* 1983;23:434–436.
40. Kothari K, Bernstein RM, Griffiths JJ, et al. Luxatio erecta. *Skel Radiol* 1984;11:47–49.
41. Klasson SC, Vander Schilden JL, Park JP. Late effect of isolated avulsion fractures of the lesser tubercle of the humerus in children. Report of 2 cases. *J Bone Joint Surg [Am]* 1993;75:1691–1694.
42. Ross GJ, Love MB. Isolated avulsion fracture of the lesser tuberosity of the humerus: report of 2 cases. *Radiology* 1989;172:833–834.
43. Wadlington VR, Hendrix RW, Rogers LF. Computed tomography of posterior fracture–dislocations of the shoulder: case reports. *J Trauma* 1992;32:113–115.
44. Cohn BT, Froimson AI. Salter 3 fracture–dislocation of glenohumeral joint in a 10-year-old. *Orthop Rev* 1986;15:403–404.
45. Gregg-Smith SJ, White SH. Salter-Harris III fracture–dislocation of the proximal humeral epiphysis. *Injury* 1992;23:199–200.
46. Obremskey W, Routt ML Jr. Fracture–dislocation of the shoulder in a child: case report. *J Trauma* 1994;36:137–140.
47. Vastamaki M, Solonen KA. Posterior dislocation and fracture–dislocation of the shoulder. *Acta Orthop Scand* 1980;51:479–484.
48. Artico M, Salvati M, D'Andrea V, et al. Isolated lesion of the axillary nerve: surgical treatment and outcome in 12 cases. *Neurosurgery* 1991;29:697–700.
49. Drew SJ, Giddins GE, Birch R. A slowly evolving brachial plexus injury following a proximal humerus fractures in a child. *J Hand Surg [Br]* 1995;20:24–25.
50. Visser CPJ, Coene LN, Brand R, et al. Nerve lesions in proximal humeral fractures. *J Shoulder Elbow Surg* 2000;10:421–427.
51. Kuhns LR, Sherman MP, Poznanaski AK, et al. Humeral head and coracoid ossification in the newborn. *Radiology* 1973;107:145–149.
52. Jackson ST, Hoffer MM, Parrish N. Brachial plexus palsy in the newborn. *J Bone Joint Surg [Am]* 1988;70:1217–1220.
53. Ogden JA, Conlogue GJ, Jensen P. Radiology of postnatal skeletal development: the proximal humerus. *Skel Radiol* 1978;2:153–160.
54. Kleinman PK, Akins CM. The "vanishing" epiphysis: sign of Salter type I fracture of the proximal humerus in infancy. *Br J Radiol* 1982;55:865–867.
55. Scaglietti O. The obstetrical shoulder trauma. *Surg Gynecol Obstet* 1938;66:686.
56. Broker FHL, Burbach T. Ultrasonic diagnosis of separation of the proximal humeral epiphysis in the newborn. *J Bone Joint Surg [Am]* 1990;72:187–191.
57. Fisher NA, Newman B, Lloyd J, et al. Ultrasonographic evaluation of birth injury to the shoulder. *J Perinatol* 1995;15:398–400.
58. Howard CB, Shinwell E, Nyska M, et al. Ultrasound diagnosis of neonatal fracture separation of the upper humeral epiphysis. *J Bone Joint Surg [Br]* 1993;74:471–472.
59. van den Broek JA, Vegter J. Echography in the diagnosis of epiphysiolysis of the proximal humerus in a new-born infant. *Ned Tijdscr Geneeskd* 1988;132:1015–1017.
60. Troum S, Floyd WE 3rd, Waters PM. Posterior dislocation of the humeral head in infancy associated with obstetrical paralysis. A case report. *J Bone Joint Surg [Am]* 1993; 75:1370–1375.
61. Szalay EA, Rockwood CA Jr. Injuries of the shoulder and arm. *Emerg Med Clin North Am* 1984;2:279–294.
62. Howard FM, Shafer SJ. Injuries to the clavicle with neurovascular complications. A study of 14 cases. *J Bone Joint Surg [Am]* 1965;47:1335–1346.
63. Sloth C, Just SL. The apical oblique radiograph in examination of acute shoulder trauma. *Eur J Radiol* 1989;9:147–151.
64. Brems-Dalgaard E, Davidsen E, Sloth C. Radiographic examination of the acute shoulder. *Eur J Radiol* 1990;11:10–14.
65. Runkel M, Kreitner KF, Wenda K, et al. Nuclear magnetic tomography in shoulder dislocation. *Unfallchirurgie* 1993;96:124–128.
66. Tirman PF, Stauffer AE, Crues JV 3rd, et al. Saline magnetic resonance arthrogaphy in the evaluation of glenohumeral instability. *Arthroscopy* 1993;9:550–559.
67. Salter RB, Harris WR. Injuries involving epiphyseal plates. *J Bone Joint Surg [Am]* 1963; 45:587–622.
68. Peterson HA, Madhok R, Benson JT, et al. Physeal fractures: Part 1. Epidemiology in Olmsted County, Minnesota, 1979–1988. *J Pediatr Orthop* 1994;14:423–430.
69. Burgos-Flores J, Gonzales-Herranz P, Lopez-Mondejar JA, et al. Fractures of the proximal humeral epiphysis. *Int Orthop* 1993;17:16–19.
70. te Slaa RL, Nollen AJ. A Salter type 3 fracture of the proximal epiphysis of the humerus. *Injury* 1987;18:429–431.
71. Wang P Jr, Koval KJ, Lehman W, et al. Salter-Harris type III fracture–dislocation of the proximal humerus. *J Pediatr Orthop* 1997;6:219–222.
72. Wong-Chung J, O'Brien T. Salter Harris type III fracture of the proximal humeral physis. *Injury* 1988;19:453–454.
73. James P, Heinrich SD. Ipsilateral proximal metaphyseal and flexion supracondylar humerus fractures with an associated olecranon avulsion fracture. *Orthopedics* 1991;14: 713–716.
74. Macfarlane I, Mushayt K. Double closed fractures of the humerus in a child. A case report. *J Bone Joint Surg [Am]* 1990;72:443.
75. Olszewski W, Popinski M. Fractures of the neck and shaft of the humerus as a rare form of double fractures in children. *Chir Narzadow Ruchu Ortop Pol* 1974;39:121–123.
76. White GM, Riley LHJ. Isolated avulsion of the subscapularis insertion in a child. A case report. *J Bone Joint Surg [Am]* 1985;67:635–636.
77. Samilson RL. Congenital and developmental anomalies of the shoulder girdle. *Orthop Clin North Am* 1980;11:219–231.
78. Bortel DT, Pritchett JW. Straight-line graphs for the predictions of growth of the upper extremities. *J Bone Joint Surg [Am]* 1993;75:885–892.
79. Pritchett JW. Growth and predictions of growth in the upper extremity. *J Bone Joint Surg [Am]* 1988;70:520–525.
80. Pritchett JW. Growth plate activity in the upper extremity. *Clin Orthop* 1991;268: 235–242.
81. Stahl EJ, Karpman R. Normal growth and growth predictions in the upper extremity. *J Hand Surg [Am]* 1986;11:593–596.
82. Curtis RJJ, Dameron TB Jr, Rockwood CA Jr. *Fractures and dislocations of the shoulder in children,* 3rd ed. Philadelphia: JB Lippincott, 1991:829–919.
83. Baxter MP, Wiley JJ. Fractures of the proximal humeral epiphysis. Their influence on humeral growth. *J Bone Joint Surg [Br]* 1986;68:570–573.
84. Dameron TB Jr, Grubb SA. Humeral shaft fractures in adults. *South Med J* 1981;74: 1461–1467.
85. Gerber C, Schneeberger AC, Vinh TS. The arterial vascularization of the humeral head: an anatomical study. *J Bone Joint Surg [Am]* 1990;72:1486–1494.
86. Laing PG. The arterial supply of the adult humerus. *J Bone Joint Surg [Am]* 1956;38: 1105–1116.
87. Lentz W, Meuser P. The treatment of fractures of the proximal humerus. *Arch Orthop Trauma Surg* 1980;96:283–285.
88. Whitman RA. Treatment of epiphyseal displacement and fractures of the upper extremity of the humerus designed to assure deficit adjustment and fixation of the fragments. *Ann Surg* 1908;47:706–708.
89. Caldwell JA. Treatment of fractures in the Cincinnati General Hospital. *Ann Surg* 1933; 97:161.
90. Larsen CF, Kiaer T, Lindequist S. Fractures of the proximal humerus in children: 9-year follow-up of 64 unoperated on cases. *Acta Orthop Scand* 1990;61:255–257.
91. Sherk HH, Probst C. Fractures of the proximal humeral epiphysis. *Orthop Clin North Am* 1975;6:401–413.
92. Beaty JH. Fractures of the proximal humerus and shaft in children. *AAOS Instr Course Lect* 1992:369–372.
93. Fraser RL, Haliburton RA, Barber JR. Displaced epiphyseal fractures of the proximal humerus. *Can J Surg* 1967;10:427–430.
94. Jaberg H, Warner JJ, Jakob RP. Percutaneous stabilization of unstable fractures of the humerus. *J Bone Joint Surg [Am]* 1992;74:508–515.
95. Lee HG. Operative reduction of an unusual fracture of the upper epiphyseal plate of the humerus. *J Bone Joint Surg* 1944;26:401–404.
96. Visser JD, Rietberg M. Interposition of the tendon of the long head of biceps in fracture separation of the proximal humeral epiphysis. *Neth J Surg* 1980;32:12–15.
97. Curtis RJ Jr. Operative management of children's fracture of the shoulder region. *Orthop Clin North Am* 1990;21:315–324.
98. Loder RT. Pediatric polytrauma: orthopaedic care and hospital course. *J Orthop Trauma* 1987;1:48–54.
99. Markel DC, Donley BG, Blasier RB. Percutaneous intramedullary pinning of proximal humeral fractures. *Orthop Rev* 1994;23:667–671.
100. Müller ME, Allgöwer M, Schneider R, et al. *Manual of internal fixation. Techniques recommended by the AO-ASIF Group,* 3rd ed. Berlin: Springer-Verlag, 1991.
101. Sessa S, Lascombes P, Prevot J, et al. Centromedullary nailing in fractures of the upper end of the humerus in children and adolescents. *Chir Pediatr* 1990;31:43–46.
102. Stweart MJ, Hundley JM. Fractures of the humerus: a comparative study in methods of treatment. *J Bone Joint Surg [Am]* 1955;37:681–692.
103. Boyd KT, Batt ME. Stress fracture of the proximal humeral epiphysis in an elite junior badminton player. *Br J Sports Med* 1997;31:252–253.
104. Coene LN, Narakas AO. Operative management of lesions of the axillary nerve, isolated or combined with other nerve lesions. *Clin Neurol Neurosurg* 1992;94(suppl):64–66.
105. al Zahrani S. Modified rotational osteotomy of the humerus for Erb's palsy. *Int Orthop* 1993;17:202–204.
106. Covey DC, Riordan DC, Milstead ME, et al. Modification of the L'Episcopo procedure for brachial plexus birth palsies. *J Bone Joint Surg [Br]* 1992;74:897–901.
107. Hoffer MM, Phipps GJ. Closed reduction and tendon transfer for treatment of dislocations of the glenohumeral joint secondary to brachial plexus birth palsy. *J Bone Joint Surg [Am]* 1998;80:997–1001.
108. Kirkos JM, Papadopoulos IA. Late treatment of brachial plexus palsy secondary to birth injuries: rotational osteotomy of the proximal part of the humerus. *J Bone Joint Surg [Am]* 1998;80:1477–1483.
109. Phipps GJ, Hoffer MM. Latissimus dorsi and teres major transfer to rotator cuff for Erb's palsy. *J Shoulder Elbow Surg* 1995;4:124–129.
110. Linson MA. Axillary artery thrombosis after fracture of the humerus. A case report. *J Bone Joint Surg [Am]* 1980;62:1214–1215.
111. Seitz J, Valdes F, Kramer A. Acute ischemia of the upper extremity caused by axillary contused trauma. Report of 3 cases. *Rev Med Child* 1991;119:567–571.
112. Stromqvist B, Lidgren L, Norgren L, et al. Neurovascular injury complicating displaced proximal fractures of the humerus. *Injury* 1987;18:423–425.
113. Zuckerman JD, Flugstad DL, Teitz CC, et al. Axillary artery injury as a complication

of proximal humerus fractures. Two case reports and a review of the literature. *Clin Orthop* 1984;189:234–237.
114. Liebling G, Bartel HG. Unusual migration of a Kirschner wire following drill wire fixation of a subcapital humerus fracture. *Beitr Orthop Traumatol* 1987;34:585–587.
115. Lyons FA, Rockwood CA. Current concepts review. Migration of pins used in operations on the shoulder. *J Bone Joint Surg [Am]* 1990;72:1262–1267.
116. Ellefsen BK, Frierson MA, Raney EM, et al. Humerus varus: a complication of neonatal, infantile, and childhood injury and infection. *J Pediatr Orthop* 1994;14:479–486.
117. Langenskiöld A. Adolescent humerus varus. *Acta Chirurg Scand* 1953;105:353–363.
118. Lucas LS, Gill JH. Humerus varus following birth injury to the proximal humeral epiphysis. *J Bone Joint Surg* 1947;29:367–369.
119. Solonen KA, Vastamaki M. Osteotomy of the neck of the humerus for traumatic varus deformity. *Acta Orthop Scand* 1985;56:79–80.
120. Trueta J. *Studies of the development and decay of the human frame.* Philadelphia: WB Saunders, 1968.
121. Gill TJ, Waters P. Valgus osteotomy of the humeral neck: a technique for the treatment of humerus varus. *J Shoulder Elbow Surg* 1997;6:306–310.
122. Giebel G, Suren EG. Injuries of the proximal humeral epiphysis. Indications for surgical therapy and results. *Chirurgie* 1983;54:406–410.
123. Guibert L, Allouis M, Bourdelat D, et al. Fractures and slipped epiphysis of the proximal humerus in children. Place and methods of surgical treatment. *Chir Pediatr* 1983;24: 197–200.
124. Leslie JT, Ryan TJ. The anterior axillary incision to approach the shoulder joint. *J Bone Joint Surg [Am]* 1962;44:1193–1196.
125. Sakakida K. Clinical observations on the epiphysial separation of long bones. *Clin Orthop* 1964;34:119–141.
126. Herring JA, Peterson HA. Simple bone cyst with growth arrest. *J Pediatr Orthop* 1987; 7:231–235.
127. Moed BR, LaMont RL. Unicameral bone cyst complicated by growth retardation. *J Bone Joint Surg [Am]* 1982;64:1379–1381.
128. Norman A, Schiffman M. Simple bone cysts: factors of age dependency. *Radiology* 1977; 124:779–782.
129. Schopler SA, Lawrence JF, Johnson MK. Lengthening of the humerus for upper extremity limb length discrepancy. *J Pediatr Orthop* 1986;6:477–480.
130. Martin RP, Parsons DL. Avascular necrosis of the proximal humeral epiphysis after physeal fracture. A case report. *J Bone Joint Surg [Am]* 1997;79:760–762.
131. Yosipovitch Z, Goldberg I. Inferior subluxation of the humeral head after injury to the shoulder. A brief note. *J Bone Joint Surg [Am]* 1989;71:751–753.
132. Goss TP. Scapular fracture and dislocations: diagnosis and treatment. *J Am Acad Orthop Surg* 1995;3:22–33.
133. Hardegger FH, Simpson LA, Weber BG. The operative treatment of scapula fractures. *J Bone Joint Surg [Br]* 1984;66:725–731.
134. McGahan JP, Rab GT, Dublin A. Fractures of the scapula. *J Trauma* 1980;20:880–883.
135. Thompson DA, Flynn TC, Miller PW, et al. The significance of scapular fractures. *J Trauma* 1985;25:974–977.
136. Wilber MC, Evans EB. Fractures of the scapula: an analysis of forty cases and review of literature. *J Bone Joint Surg [Am]* 1977;59:358–362.
137. Kogutt MS, Swischuk LE, Fagan CJ. Patterns of injury and significance of uncommon fractures in the battered child syndrome. *Am J Roentgenol Radium Ther Nucl Med* 1974; 121:143–149.
138. Ada JR, Miller ME. Scapular fractures: analysis of 113 cases. *Clin Orthop* 1991;269: 174–180.
139. Imatani RJ. Fractures of the scapulae: a review of 53 fractures. *J Trauma* 1975;15: 473–478.
140. Rowe CR. Fractures of the scapula. *Surg Clin North Am* 1963;43:1565–1571.
141. Ebraheim NA, An HS, Jackson WT, et al. Scapulothoracic dissociation. *J Bone Joint Surg [Am]* 1988;70:428–432.
142. Oreck SL, Burgess A, Levine AM. Traumatic lateral displacement of the scapula: a radiographic sign of neurovascular disease. *J Bone Joint Surg [Am]* 1984;66:758–763.
143. Althausen P, Lee M, Finemeier C. Scapulothoracic dissociation: diagnosis and treatment. *Clin Orthop* 2003;416:237–244.
144. Chung SMK, Nissenbaum MM. Congenital and developmental defects of the shoulder. *Orthop Clin North Am* 1975;6:381–392.
145. Liberson F. Os acromiale? A contested anomaly. *J Joint Surg* 1937;19:683–689.
146. Kim SJ, Min BH. Congenital bilateral absence of the acromion: a case report. *Clin Orthop* 1994;300:117–119.
147. McClure JG, Raney RB. Anomalies of the scapula. *Clin Orthop* 1975;110:22–31.
148. Orrell KG, Bell DF. Structural abnormality of the clavicle associated with Sprengel's deformity: a case report. *Clin Orthop* 1990;258:157–159.
149. Samilson RL. Congenital and developmental anomalies of the shoulder girdle. *Orthop Clin North Am* 1980;11:219–231.
150. Leung KS, Lam TP. Open reduction and internal fixation of ipsilateral fractures of the scapular neck and clavicle. *J Bone Joint Surg [Am]* 1993;75:1015–1018.
151. Kuhn JE, Blasier RB, Carpenter JE. Fractures of the acromion process: a proposed classification system. *J Orthop Trauma* 1994;8:6–13.
152. Goss TP. Current concepts review: fractures of the glenoid cavity. *J Bone Joint Surg [Am]* 1992;72:299–305.
153. Ideberg R. Fractures of the scapula involving the glenoid fossa. In: Bateman JE, Walsh RD, eds. *Surgery of the shoulder.* Toronto: BC Decker, 1984:63–66.
154. Ideberg R. Unusual glenoid fractures. *Acta Orthop Scand* 1987;58:191–192.
155. Nettrour LF, Krufky EL, Mueller RE, Raycroft JF. Locked scapula: intrathoracic dislocation of the inferior angle. *J Bone Joint Surg [Am]* 1987;54:147–155.
156. McGahan JP, Rab GT. Fracture of the acromion associated with an axillary nerve deficit: a case report and review of the literature. *Clin Orthop* 1980;147:216–218.
157. Nordqvist A, Petersson C. Fracture of the body, neck, or spine of the scapula: a long-term follow-up study. *Clin Orthop* 1992;283:139–144.
158. Wippermann B, Schmidt U, Nerlich M. Results of treatment of compartment syndrome of the upper arm. *Unfallchirurgie* 1991;94:231–235.
159. Lindblom A, Leven H. Prognosis in fractures of body and neck of the scapula. *Acta Chir Scand* 1974;140:33–47.
160. Herscovici D Jr, Fiennes AG, Allgower M, et al. The floating shoulder: ipsilateral clavicle and scapular neck fractures. *J Bone Joint Surg [Br]* 1992;74:362–364.
161. Neer CS II. Fractures. In: *Shoulder reconstruction.* Philadelphia: WB Saunders, 1990: 412.
162. DePalma AF. *Surgery of the shoulder,* 3rd ed. Philadelphia: JB Lippincott, 1983.
163. Montgomery SP, Loyd RDL. Avulsion fracture of the coracoid epiphysis with acromioclavicular separation. *J Bone Joint Surg [Am]* 1977;59:963–965.
164. Neer CS II. Fractures about the shoulder. In: Wood CA, Green DP, ed. *Fractures.* Philadelphia: JB Lippincott, 1984:713–721.
165. Zravkovic D, Damholt VV. Comminuted and severely displaced fractures of the scapula. *Acta Orthop Scand* 1974;45:60–65.
166. Guttentag IJ, Rechtine GR. Fractures of the scapula: a review of the literature. *Orthop Rev* 1988;17:147–158.
167. Soslowsky LJ, Flatow EL, Bigliani LU, et al. Articular geometry of the glenohumeral joint. *Clin Orthop* 1992;285:181–190.
168. Lee S, Meinhard B, Schultz E, Toledano B. Open reduction and internal fixation of a glenoid fossa fracture in a child: a case report and rview of the literature. *J Orthop Trauma* 1997;11(6):452–454.
169. Cole P. Scapula fractures. *Orthop Clin North Am* 2002;33(1):1–18.
170. Zella B, Pape H, Gerich T, et al. Functional outcome following scapulothoracic dissociation. *J Bone Joint Surg [Am]* 2004;86:2–8.
171. Kaminsky S, Pierce V. Nonunion of a scapula body fracture in a high school football player. *Am J Orthop* 2002;31(8):456–457.
172. Ferraz I, Papadimitriou N, Sotreanos D. Scapular body nonunion: a case report. *J Shoulder Elbow Surg* 2002;11(1):98–100.
173. Moseley HF. The clavicle: its anatomy and function. *Clin Orthop* 1968;58:17–27.
174. Abbott A, Hannafin J. Stress fracture of the clavicle in a female lightweight rower. A case report and review of the literature. *Am J Sports Med* 2001;29(3):370–372.
175. Inman VT, Saunders JB, Abbott LC. Observations on the function of the shoulder joint. *J Bone Joint Surg* 1944;26:1–30.
176. Cohen AW, Otto SR. Obstetric clavicular fractures: a three year analysis. *J Reprod Med* 1980;25:119–122.
177. Farkas R, Levine S. X-ray incidence of fractured clavicle in vertex presentation. *Am J Obstet Gynecol* 1950;59:204–206.
178. Rubin A. Birth injuries: incidence, mechanisms, and end results. *Obstet Gynecol* 1964; 23:218–221.
179. Beall M, Ross M. Clavicel fracture in labor: risk factors and associated morbidities. *J Perinatol* 2001;21(8):513–515.
180. Landin LA. Fracture patterns in children: analysis of 8682 fractures with special reference to incidence, etiology, and secular changes in Swedish urban populations. *Acta Orthop Scand Suppl* 1983;54:1–109.
181. Lichtenberg RP. A study of 2532 fractures in children. *Am J Surg* 1954;87:330–338.
182. Nordqvist A, Petersson C. The incidence of fractures of the clavicle. *Clin Orthop* 1994; 300:127–132.
183. Camus M, Lefebvre G, Veron O, et al. Obstetrical injuries of the newborn infant: retrospective study apropos of 20409 births. *J Gynecol Obstet Biol Reprod (Paris)* 1985; 14:1033–1043.
184. Gilbert WM, Tchabo JG. Fractured clavicle in newborns. *Int Surg* 1988;73:123–125.
185. Gitch G, Schatten C. Incidence and potential factors in the genesis of birth injury induced clavicular fractures. *Zentralbl Gynakol* 1987;109:909–912.
186. Jelic A, Marin L, Pracny M, et al. Fractures of the clavicle in neonates. *Lijec Vjesn* 1992; 114:32–35.
187. Oppenheim WL, Davis A, Growdon WA, et al. Clavicle fractures in the newborn. *Clin Orthop* 1990;250:176–180.
188. Salonen IS, Uusitalo R. Birth injuries: incidence and predisposing factors. *Z Kinderchir* 1990;45:133–135.
189. Walle T, Hartikainen-Sorri A. Obstetric shoulder injury: associated risk factors, prediction, and prognosis. *Acta Obstet Gynecol Scand* 1993;72:450–454.
190. Levine MG, Holroyde J, Woods JR Jr, et al. Birth trauma: incidence and predisposing factors. *Obstet Gynecol* 1984;63:792–795.
191. Kreisinger V. Sur le traitement des fractures de la clavicule. *Rev Chir* 1927;65:396–407.
192. Stanley D, Trowbridge EA, Norris SH. The mechanism of clavicular fractures. A clinical and biomechanical analysis. *J Bone Joint Surg [Br]* 1988;70:461–464.
193. Herndon WA. Child abuse in a military population. *J Pediatr Orthop* 1983;3:73–76.
194. Kogutt MS, Swischuk LE, Fagan CJ. Patterns of injury and significance of uncommon fractures in the battered child syndrome. *Am J Roentgenol Radium Ther Nucl Med* 1974; 121:143–149.
195. Silloway KA, McLaughlin RE, Edlich RC, et al. Clavicular fractures and acromioclavicular joint dislocations in lacrosse: preventable injuries. *J Emerg Med* 1985;3:117–121.
196. Wu C, Chen Y. Stress fracture of the clavicle in a professional baseball player. *J Shoulder Elbow Surg* 1998;7(2):164–167.

197. Goddard NJ, Stabler J, Albert JS. Atlantoaxial rotatory fixation and fracture of the clavicle: an association and classification. *J Bone Joint Surg [Br]* 1990;72:72–75.
198. Dameron TB, Rockwood CA. Fractures and dislocations of the shoulder. In: Rockwood CA, Wilkins KE, King RE, eds. *Fractures in children.* Philadelphia: JB Lippincott, 1984: 624–653.
199. McCaughan JS Jr, Miller PR. Migration of Steinmann pin from shoulder to lung [Letter]. *JAMA* 1969;207:1917.
200. Post M. Current concepts in the treatment of fractures of the clavicle. *Clin Orthop* 1989; 245:89–101.
201. Sanford HN. The Moro reflex as a diagnostic aid in fracture of the clavicle in the newborn infant. *Am J Dis Child* 1931;41:1304–1306.
202. Abbott L, Lucas D. Function of the clavicle: its surgical significance. *Ann Surg* 1954; 140:583–599.
203. Bowen RE, Mah JY, Otsuka NY. Midshaft clavicle fractures associated with atlantoaxial rotatory displacement: a report of two cases. *J Orthop Trauma* 2003;17(6):444–447.
204. Gardner MA, Bidstrup BP. Intrathoracic great vessel injury resulting from blunt chest trauma associated with posterior dislocation of the sternoclavicular joint. *Aust N Z J Surg* 1983;53:427–430.
205. Worman LW, Leagus C. Intrathoracic injury following retrosternal dislocation of the clavicle. *J Trauma* 1967;7:416–423.
206. Graif M, Stahl-Kent V, Ben-Ami T, et al. Sonographic detection of occult bone fractures. *Pediatr Radiol* 1988;18:383–385.
207. Katz R, Landman J, Dulitzky F, et al. Fracture of the clavicle in the newborn. An ultrasound diagnosis. *J Ultrasound Med* 1988;7:21–23.
208. Kayser R, Mahlfeld K, Heyde C, Grasshoff H. Ultrasonographic imaging of fractures of the clavicle in newborn infants. *J Bone Joint Surg [Br]* 2003;85(1):115–116.
209. Pollock RC, Bankes MJ, Emery RJ. Diagnosis of retrosternal dislocation of the clavicle with ultrasound. *Injury* 1996;27:670–671.
210. Weinberg B, Seife B, Alonso P. The apical oblique view of the clavicle: its usefulness in neonatal and childhood trauma. *Skel Radiol* 1991;20:201–203.
211. Riemer BL, Butterfield SL, Daffner RH, et al. The abduction lordotic view of the clavicle: a new technique for radiographic visualization. *J Orthop Trauma* 1991;5:392–394.
212. Rockwood CA. Dislocations of the sternoclavicular joint. *AAOS Instr Course Lect* 1975; 24:144–159.
213. Miller DS, Boswick JA Jr. Lesions of the brachial plexus associated with fractures of the clavicle. *Clin Orthop* 1969;64:144–149.
214. Pyper JB. Nonunion of fractures of the clavicle. *Injury* 1978;9:268–270.
215. Rowe CR. An atlas of anatomy and treatment of midclavicular fractures. *Clin Orthop* 1968;58:29–42.
216. Al-Etani H, D'Astous J, Letts J, et al. Masked rotatory subluxation of the atlas associated with fracture of the clavicle: a clinical and biomechanical analysis. *J Bone Joint Surg [Am]* 1998;80:1477–1483.
217. Falstie-Jensen S, Mikkelsen P. Pseudodislocation of the acromioclavicular joint. *J Bone Joint Surg [Br]* 1982;64:368–369.
218. Ogden JA. Distal clavicular physeal injury. *Clin Orthop* 1984;188:68–73.
219. Todd TW, D'Errico J Jr. The clavicular epiphyses. *Am J Anat* 1928;41:25–50.
220. Browne JE, Stanley RF, Tullos HS, et al. Acromioclavicular joint dislocations: comparative results following operative treatment with and without primary distal clavisectomy. *Am J Sports Med* 1977;5:258–263.
221. Darrow JC, Smith JA, Lockwood RC. A new conservative method for the treatment of type III acromioclavicular separations. *Orthop Clin North Am* 1980;11:727–733.
222. Barber FA. Complete posterior acromioclavicular dislocation. *Orthopaedics* 1987;10: 493–496.
223. Gerber C, Rockwood CA. Subcoracoid dislocation of the lateral end of the clavicle. A report of three cases. *J Bone Joint Surg [Am]* 1987;69:924–927.
224. Jit I, Kulkarni M. Times of appearance and fusion of epiphysis at the medial end of the clavicle. *Ind J Med Res* 1976;64:773–782.
225. Owings-Webb PA. Epiphyseal union of the anterior iliac crest and medial clavicle in a modern multiracial sample of American males and females. *Am J Phys Anthropol* 1985; 68:457–466.
226. Salter RB, Harris WR. Injuries involving the epiphyseal plate. *J Bone Joint Surg [Am]* 1963;45:587–622.
227. Gardner E. The embryology of the clavicle. *Clin Orthop* 1968;58:9–16.
228. Ogata S, Uhthoff HK. The early development and ossification of the human clavicle. An embryologic study. *Acta Orthop Scand* 1990;61:330–334.
229. Ogden JA, Conlogue GJ, Bronson ML. Radiology of postnatal skeletal development. III. The clavicle. *Skel Radiol* 1979;4:196–203.
230. Kaur H, Jit I. Brief communication: coracoclavicular joint in northwest Indians. *Am J Phys Anthropol* 1991;85:457–460.
231. Bearn JG. Direct observations on the function of the capsule of the sternoclavicular support. *J Anat* 1967;101:159–170.
232. Goss TP. Scapular fracture and dislocations: diagnosis and treatment. *J Am Acad Orthop Surg* 1995;3:22–33.
233. Joseph PR, Rosenfeld W. Clavicular fractures in neonates. *Am J Dis Child* 1990;144: 165–167.
234. Madsen ET. Fractures of the extremities in the newborn. *Acta Obstet Gynecol Scand* 1955;34:41–74.
235. Sanders JO, Rockwood CA Jr, Curtis RJ. Fractures and dislocations of the humeral shaft and shoulder. In: Rockwood CA Jr, Wilkins KE, Beaty JH, eds. *Fractures in children.* Philadelphia: Lippincott-Raven, 1996:905–1021.
236. Jensen PO, Andersen K, Lauritzen J. Treatment of midclavicular fractures. A prospective randomized trial comparing treatment with a figure-of-eight dressing and a simple arm sling. *Ugeskr Laeger* 1985;147:1986–1988.
237. Mullick S. Treatment of mid-clavicular fractures. *Lancet* 1967:499.
238. Sankarankutty M, Turner BW. Fractures of the clavicle. *Injury* 1975;7:101–106.
239. Ogden JA. *Skeletal injury in the child,* 2nd ed. Philadelphia: WB Saunders, 1990.
240. Fowler AW. Treatment of fractured clavicle. *Lancet* 1968;1:46–47.
241. Leffert RD. Brachial plexus injuries. *N Engl J Med* 1974;291:1059–1067.
242. Andersen K, Jensen PO, Lauritzen J. Treatment of clavicular fractures. Figure-of-eight bandage versus a simple sling. *Acta Orthop Scand* 1987;58:71–74.
243. Stanley D, Norris SH. Recovery following fractures of the clavicle treated conservatively. *Injury* 1988;19:162–164.
244. Howard FM, Shafer SJ. Injuries to the clavicle with neurovascular complications: a study of fourteen cases. *J Bone Joint Surg [Am]* 1965;47:1335–1346.
245. Jablon M, Sutker A, Post M. Irreducible fracture of the middle third of the clavicle. Report of a case. *J Bone Joint Surg [Am]* 1979;61:296–298.
246. Mullaji AB, Jupiter JB. Low contact dynamic compression plating of the clavicle. *Injury* 1994;25:41–45.
247. Poigenfurst J, Rappold G, Fischer W. Plating of fresh clavicular fractures: results of 122 operations. *Injury* 1992;23:237–241.
248. Zenni EJ Jr, Krieg JK, Rosen MJ. Open reduction and internal fixation of clavicular fractures. *J Bone Joint Surg [Am]* 1981;63:147–151.
249. Kubiak R, Slongo T. Operative treatment of clavicle fractures in children: a review of 21 years. *J Pediatr Orthop* 2002;22(6):736–739.
250. Jubel A, Andermahr J, Schiffer G, et al. Elastic stable intramedullary nailing of midclavicular fractures with a titanium nail. *Clin Orthop* 2003;(408):279–285.
251. Eidman DK, Siff SJ, Tullos HS. Acromioclavicular lesions in children. *Am J Sports Med* 1981;9:150–154.
252. Black GH, McPherson JA, Reed MH. Traumatic pseudodislocation of the acromioclavicular joint in children. A 15-year review. *Am J Sports Med* 1991;19:644–646.
253. Havranek P. Injuries of distal clavicular physis in children. *J Pediatr Orthop* 1989;9: 213–215.
254. Rockwood CA Jr. The shoulder: facts, confusion, and myths. *Int Orthop* 1991;15: 401–405.
255. Bakalim G, Wilpulla E. Surgical or conservative treatment of total dislocation of the acromioclavicular joint. *Acta Chir Scand* 1975;141:43–47.
256. Dartoy C, Fenoll B, Hra B, et al. Epiphyseal fracture–avulsion of the distal extremity of the clavicle. *Ann Radiol (Paris)* 1993;36:125–128.
257. Roper BA, Levack B. The surgical treatment of acromioclavicular dislocations. *J Bone Joint Surg [Am]* 1982;69:1045–1051.
258. Waters P, Bae D, Kadiyala R. Short-term outcomes after surgical treatment of traumatic posterior sternoclavicular fracture-dislocations in children and adolescents. *J Pediatr Orthop* 2003;23(4):464–469.
259. Clark RL, Milgram JW, Yawn DH. Fatal aortic perforation and cardiac tamponade due to a Kirschner wire migrating from the right sternoclavicular joint. *South Med J* 1974; 67:316–318.
260. Bateman JE. Neurovascular syndromes related to the clavicle. *Clin Orthop* 1968;58: 75–82.
261. Jojart G, Nagy G. Ultrasonographic screening of neonatal adrenal apoplexy. *Int Urol Nephrol* 1992;24:591–596.
262. Mital MA, Aufranc OE. Venous occlusion following greenstick fracture of clavicle. *JAMA* 1968;206:1301–1302.
263. Tse DH, Slabaugh PB, Carlson PA. Injury to the axillary artery by a closed fracture of the clavicle. A case report. *J Bone Joint Surg [Am]* 1980;62:1372–1374.
264. Dugdale TW, Fulkerson JP. Pneumothorax complicating a closed fracture of the clavicle. A case report. *Clin Orthop* 1987;221:212–214.
265. Meeks RJ, Riebel GD. Isolated clavicle fracture with associated pneumothorax. A case report. *Am J Emerg Med* 1991;9:555–556.
266. Longo R, Ruggiero L. Left pneumothorax with subcutaneous emphysema secondary to left clavicular fracture and homolateral obstetrical paralysis of the arm. *Minerva Pediatr* 1982;34:273–276.
267. Della Santa D, Narakas A. Fractures of the clavicle and secondary lesions of the brachial plexus. *Z Unfallchir Versicherungsmed* 1992;85:58–65.
268. Della Santa D, Narakas A, Bonnard C. Late lesions of the brachial plexus after fracture of the clavicle. *Ann Chir Main Memb Super* 1991;10:531–540.
269. Jackson ST, Hoffer MM, Parrish N. Brachial plexus palsy in the newborn. *J Bone Joint Surg [Am]* 1988;70:1217–1220.
270. Jojart G, Zubek L, Toth G. Clavicle fractures in the newborn. *Orv Hetil* 1991;132: 2655–2657.
271. Fowler AW. Migration of a wire from the sternoclavicular joint to the pericardial cavity. *Injury* 1981;13:261–262.
272. Mazet R Jr. Migration of a Kirschner wire from the shoulder region into the lung: a report of 2 cases. *J Bone Joint Surg [Am]* 1943;25:477–483.
273. Nogi J, Heckman JD, Hakala M, et al. Nonunion of the clavicle in a child. A case report. *Clin Orthop* 1975;110:19–21.
274. Schwarz N, Hocker K. Osteosynthesis of irreducible fractures of the clavicle with 2.7-mm ASIF plates. *J Trauma* 1992;33:179–183.
275. Schwarz N, Leixnering M. Technique and results of clavicular medullary wiring. *Zentralbl Chir* 1986;111:640–647.
276. Qureshi AA, Kuo KN. Posttraumatic cleidoscapular synostosis following a fracture of the clavicle. *J Bone Joint Surg [Am]* 1999;81:256–258.
277. Brooks S. Bilateral congenital pseudarthrosis of the clavicles? Case report and review of the literature. *Br J Clin Pract* 1984;38:432–433.

278. Brunner C, Morger R. Congenital nonunion of the clavicle. *Pediatr Padol* 1981;16: 137–141.
279. O'Rourke IC, Middleton RWD. The place and efficacy of operative management of fractured clavicle. *Injury* 1975;6:236–240.
280. Wall JJ. Congenital pseudarthrosis of the clavicle. *J Bone Joint Surg [Am]* 1970;52: 1003–1009.
281. Wilkins RM, Johnston RM. Ununited fractures of the clavicle. *J Bone Joint Surg [Am]* 1983;65:773–778.
282. Boehme D, Curtis RJ, DeHaan JT, et al. Nonunion of fractures of the midshaft of the clavicle. Treatment with a modified Hagie intramedullary pin and autogenous bone grafting. *J Bone Joint Surg [Am]* 1991;73:1219–1226.
283. Manske DJ, Szabo RM. The operative treatment of midshaft clavicular nonunions. *J Bone Joint Surg [Am]* 1985;67:1367–1371.
284. Eskola A, Vainionpaa S, Myllynen P, et al. Surgery for ununited clavicular fracture. *Acta Orthop Scand* 1986;57:366–367.
285. Rockwood CA Jr. The shoulder: facts, confusions and myths. *Int Orthop* 1991;15: 401–405.
286. Blount WP. *Fractures in children.* Baltimore: Williams & Wilkins, 1955.
287. Pollen AG. *Fractures and dislocations in children.* Baltimore: Williams & Wilkins, 1973.
288. Rang M. *Children's fractures,* 2nd ed. Philadelphia: JB Lippincott, 1983.
289. Sharrard WJW. *Paediatric orthopaedics and fractures.* Oxford: Blackwell, 1971.
290. Tachdjian MO. *Paediatric orthopaedics.* Philadelphia: WB Saunders, 1990.
291. Weber BG, Brunner C, Freuler F. *Treatment of fractures in children and adolescents.* Berlin: Springer-Verlag, 1980:94–95.
292. Heck CC Jr. Anterior dislocation of the glenohumeral joint in a child. *J Trauma* 1981; 21:174–175.
293. Hernandez A, Drez D. Operative treatment of posterior shoulder dislocations by posterior glenoidplasty, capsulorrhaphy and infraspinatus advancement. *Am J Sports Med* 1986;14:187–191.
294. Lichtblau PO. Shoulder dislocation in the infant. Case report and discussion. *J Fla Med Assoc* 1977;64:313–320.
295. Wagner KT, Lyne ED. Adolescent traumatic dislocations of the shoulder with open epiphysis. *J Pediatr Orthop* 1983;3:61–62.
296. Rowe CR. Prognosis in dislocation of the shoulder. *J Bone Joint Surg [Am]* 1956;38: 957–977.
297. Rowe CR. Anterior dislocation of the shoulder: prognosis and treatment. *Surg Clin North Am* 1963;43:1609–1614.
298. O'Driscoll SW, Evans DC. Contralateral shoulder instability following anterior repair. An epidemiological investigation. *J Bone Joint Surg [Br]* 1991;73:941–946.
299. Goldberg BJ, Nirschl RP, McConnell JP, et al. Arthroscopic transglenoid suture capsulolabral repairs: preliminary results. *Am J Sports Med* 1993;21:656–665.
300. Matton D, Van Looy F, Geens S. Recurrent anterior dislocations of the shoulder joint treated by the Bristow-Latarjet procedure. *Acta Orthop Belg* 1992;58:16–22.
301. Montgomery WH 3rd, Jobe FW. Functional outcomes in athletes after modified anterior capsulolabral reconstruction. *Am J Sports Med* 1994;22:352–358.
302. Marans HJ, Angel KR, Schemitsch EH, et al. The fate of traumatic anterior dislocation of the shoulder in children. *J Bone Joint Surg [Am]* 1992;74:1242–1244.
303. Blazina ME, Satzman JS. Recurrent anterior subluxation of the shoulder in athletics—a distinct entity (proceedings). *J Bone Joint Surg [Am]* 1969;51:1037–1038.
304. Hovelius L. Anterior dislocation of the shoulder in teenagers and young adults. *J Bone Joint Surg [Am]* 1987;69A:393–399.
305. Morrey BF, Janes JM. Recurrent anterior dislocation of the shoulder. *J Bone Joint Surg [Am]* 1976;58:252–256.
306. Detenbeck LC. Posterior dislocations of the shoulder. *J Trauma* 1972;12:183–192.
307. Dimon JH III. Posterior dislocation and posterior fracture dislocation of the shoulder: a report of 25 cases. *South Med J* 1967;60:661–666.
308. Hawkins RJ, Koppert G, Johnston G. Recurrent posterior instability (subluxation) of the shoulder. *J Bone Joint Surg [Am]* 1984;66:169–174.
309. Norwood L, Terry GC. Shoulder posterior subluxation. *Am J Sports Med* 1984;12: 25–30.
310. Vastamaki M, Solonen KA. Posterior dislocation and fracture dislocation of the shoulder. *Acta Orthop Scand* 1980;51:479–484.
311. Haliburton RA, Barber JR, Fraser RL. Pseudodislocation: an unusual birth injury. *Can J Surg* 1967;10:455–462.
312. Laskin RS, Sedlin ED. Luxatio erecta in infancy. *Clin Orthop* 1971;80:126–129.
313. Babbitt DP, Cassidy RH. Obstetrical paralysis and dislocation of the shoulder in infancy. *J Bone Joint Surg [Am]* 1968;50:1447–1452.
314. Liebolt FL, Furey JG. Obstetrical paralysis with dislocation of the shoulder: a case report. *J Bone Joint Surg [Am]* 1953;35:227–230.
315. Wickstrom J. Birth injuries of the brachial plexus treatment defects in the shoulder. *Clin Orthop* 1962;23:187–196.
316. Wickstrom J, Haslam ET, Hutchinson RH. The surgical management of residual deformities of the shoulder following birth injuries of the brachial plexus. *J Bone Joint Surg [Am]* 1955;37:27–36.
317. Green NE, Wheelhouse WW. Anterior subglenoid dislocation of the shoulder in an infant following pneumococcal meningitis. *Clin Orthop* 1978;135:125–127.
318. Carter C, Sweetnam R. Recurrent dislocation of the patella and of the shoulder: their association with familial joint laxity. *J Bone Joint Surg [Br]* 1960;42:721–727.
319. Chung SMK, Nissenbaum MM. Congenital and development defects of the shoulder. *Orthop Clin North Am* 1975;6:381–392.
320. Cozen L. Congenital dislocation of the shoulder and other anomalies. *Arch Surg* 1937; 35:956–966.
321. Gartland JJ, Dowling JJ. Recurrent anterior dislocation of the shoulder joint. *Clin Orthop* 1954;3:86–91.
322. Grieg DM. On true congenital dislocation of the shoulder. *Edinb Med J* 1923;30: 157–175.
323. Pettersson H. Bilateral dysplasia of the neck of the scapula and associated anomalies. *Acta Radiol Diagn (Stockh)* 1981;22:81–84.
324. Heim M, Horoszowski H, Martinowitz U. Hemophilic arthropathy resulting in a locked shoulder. *Clin Orthop* 1986;202:169–172.
325. Stern WA. Arthrogryposis multiplex congenity. *JAMA* 1923;81:1507–1510.
326. Blom S, Dahlback LO. Nerve injuries in dislocations of the shoulder joint and fractures of the neck of the humerus. *Acta Chir Scand* 1970;136:461–466.
327. Davis AG. A conservative treatment for habitual dislocations of the shoulder. *JAMA* 1936;107:1012–1015.
328. Editorial. Voluntary dislocation of the shoulder. *Br Med J* 1973;4:505.
329. Keiser RP, Wilson CL. Bilateral recurrent dislocation of the shoulder (atraumatic) in a 13-year-old girl. *J Bone Joint Surg [Am]* 1961;43:553–554.
330. Lawhon SM, Peoples AB, MacEwen GD. Voluntary dislocation of the shoulder. *J Pediatr Orthop* 1982;2:590.
331. Magnuson PB, Stack JK. Bilateral habitual dislocation of the shoulders in twins: a familial tendency. *JAMA* 1940;114:2103.
332. Rowe CR, Pierce DS, Clark JG. Voluntary dislocation of the shoulder. *J Bone Joint Surg [Am]* 1973;55:445–459.
333. Shvartzman P, Guy N. Voluntary dislocation of shoulder. *Postgrad Med* 1988;84: 265–271.
334. O'Driscoll SW, Evans DC. Long-term results of staple capsulorrhaphy for anterior instability of the shoulder. *J Bone Joint Surg [Am]* 1993;75:249–258.
335. Rockwood CA, Matsen FA, Thomas SC. Anterior glenohumeral instability. In: Rockwood CA, Matsen FA, eds. *The shoulder.* Philadelphia: WB Saunders, 1990:592–598.
336. Neer CS II. Involuntary inferior and multidirectional instability of the shoulder: etiology, recognition, and treatment. *AAOS Instr Course Lect* 1985;34:232–238.
337. Barratta JB, Lim V, Mastromonaco E, et al. Axillary artery disruption secondary to anterior dislocation of the shoulder. *J Trauma* 1983;23:1009–1011.
338. Coene LN, Narakas AO. Operative management of lesions of the axillary nerve, isolated or combined with other nerve lesions. *Clin Neurol Neurosurg* 1992;94 (suppl):64–66.
339. Curr JF. Rupture of the axillary artery complicating dislocation of the shoulder: report of a case. *J Bone Joint Surg [Br]* 1970;52:313–317.
340. Elbaum R, Parent H, Zeller R, et al. Traumatic scapulohumeral dislocation in children and adolescents. Apropos of 9 patients. *Acta Orthop Belg* 1994;60:204–209.
341. Lucas GL, Peterson MD. Open anterior dislocation of the shoulder: case report. *J Trauma* 1977;17:883–884.
342. Morrison PD, Egan TJ. Axillary artery injury in erect dislocation of the shoulder (luxatio erecta): a case report. *J Ir Orthop* 1983;260–261.
343. Gudinchet F, Naggar L, Ginalski JM, et al. Magnetic resonance imaging of nontraumatic shoulder instability in children. *Skel Radiol* 1992;21:19–21.
344. Kummel BM. Arthrography in anterior capsular derangements of the shoulder. *Clin Orthop* 1972;83:170–176.
345. White SS, Blane CE, DiPietro MA, et al. Arthrography in evaluation of birth injuries of the shoulder. *J Can Assoc Radiol* 1987;38:113–115.
346. Jalovaara P, Myllyla V, Paivansalo M. Autotraction stress roentgenography for demonstration of anterior and inferior instability of the shoulder joint. *Clin Orthop* 1992;284: 136–143.
347. Asher MA. Dislocations of the upper extremity in children. *Orthop Clin North Am* 1976; 7:583–591.
348. Dameron TB, Rockwood CA. Fractures and dislocations of the shoulder. In: Rockwood CA, Wilkins KE, King RE, eds. *Fractures in children.* Philadelphia: JB Lippincott, 1984: 659–676.
349. Ogden JA. *Skeletal injury in the child.* Philadelphia: Lea & Febiger, 1982:227–228.
350. Boyd HB, Sisk TD. Recurrent posterior dislocation of the shoulder. *J Bone Joint Surg [Am]* 1972;54:779–786.
351. Foster WS, Ford TB, Drez D. Isolated posterior shoulder dislocation in a child. *Am J Sports Med* 1985;13:198–200.
352. May VR Jr. Posterior dislocation of the shoulder: habitual, traumatic and obstetrical. *Orthop Clin North Am* 1980;11:271–285.
353. Freundlich BD. Luxatio erecta. *J Trauma* 1983;23:434–436.
354. McNeil EL. Luxatio erecta [Letter]. *Ann Emerg Med* 1984;13:490–491.
355. Burkhead WZ Jr, Rockwood CA Jr. Treatment of instability of the shoulder with an exercise program. *J Bone Joint Surg [Am]* 1993;75:311–312.
356. Kleinman PK, Goss TP, Kanzaria PK, et al. Injuries of the glenoid labrum in athletic teenagers [Abstract]. *Pediatr Radiol* 1985;15:71.
357. Uhthoff HK, Piscopo M. Anterior capsular redundancy of the shoulder: congenital or traumatic? An embryological study. *J Bone Joint Surg [Br]* 1985;67:363–366.
358. Cleeman E, Flatow EL. Shoulder dislocations in the young patient. *Orthop Clin North Am* 2000;31:217–229.
359. Aamoth GM, O'Phelan EH. Recurrent anterior dislocation of the shoulder: a review of 40 athletes treated by subscapularis transfer (modified Magnuson-Stack procedure). *Am J Sports Med* 1977;5:188–190.
360. Aronen JG, Regan K. Decreasing the incidence of recurrence of first-time anterior shoulder dislocation with rehabilitation. *Am J Sports Med* 1984;12:283–291.

361. Barry TP, Lombardo SJ, Kerlan RK, et al. The coracoid transfer for recurrent anterior instability of the shoulder in adolescents. *J Bone Joint Surg [Am]* 1985;67:383–387.
362. DePalma AF, Silverstein CE. Results following a modified Magnuson procedure in recurrent dislocation of the shoulder. *Surg Clin North Am* 1963;43:1651–1653.
363. Karadimas J, Rentis G, Varouchas G. Repair of anterior dislocation of the shoulder using transfer of the subscapularis tendon. *J Bone Joint Surg [Am]* 1980;62:1147–1149.
364. Kothari RU, Dronen SC. Prospective evaluation of the scapular manipulation technique in reducing anterior shoulder dislocations. *Ann Emerg Med* 1992;21:1349–1352.
365. McNamara RM. Reduction of anterior shoulder dislocations by scapular manipulation. *Ann Emerg Med* 1993;22:1140–1144.
366. DePalma AF, Cooke AJ, Probhakar M. The role of the subscapularis in recurrent anterior dislocations of the shoulder. *Clin Orthop* 1967;54:35–49.
367. Hovelius L, Erikson GK, Fredin FH, et al. Recurrences after initial dislocation of the shoulder. *J Bone Joint Surg* 1983;65:343–349.
368. Hovelius L, Augustini BG, Fredin H, et al. Primary anterior dislocation of the shoulder in young patients: a ten-year prospective study. *J Bone Joint Surg [Am]* 1996;78: 1677–1684.
369. Vermeiren J, Handelberg F, Casteleyn PP, et al. The rate of recurrence of traumatic anterior dislocation of the shoulder. *Int Orthop* 1993;17:337–341.
370. Endo S, Kasai T, Fujii N, et al. Traumatic anterior dislocation of the shoulder in a child. *Arch Orthop Trauma Surg* 1993;112:201–202.
371. Neer CS II, Foster DR. Inferior capsular shift for involuntary inferior and multidirectional instability of the shoulder. *J Bone Joint Surg [Am]* 1980;62:897–908.
372. Lombardo SJ, Kerlan RK, Jobe FW, et al. The modified Bristow procedure for recurrent dislocation of the shoulder. *J Bone Joint Surg [Am]* 1976;58:256–261.
373. Huber H, Gerber C. Voluntary subluxation of the shoulder in children. A long-term follow-up study of 36 shoulders. *J Bone Joint Surg [Am]* 1994;76:118–122.
374. Hawkins RJ, Angelo RL. Glenohumeral osteoarthritis: acute complications of the Putti-Platt repair. *J Bone Joint Surg [Am]* 1990;72:1193–1197.
375. Lusard DA, Wirth MA, Wurtz D, et al. Loss of external rotation following anterior capsulorrhaphy of the shoulder. *J Bone Joint Surg [Am]* 1993;75:1185–1192.
376. Bach FR, O'Brien SJ, Warren RF, et al. An unusual neurological complication of the Bristow procedure: a case report. *J Bone Joint Surg [Am]* 1988;70:458–460.
377. Zuckerman JD, Matsen FA. Complications about the glenohumeral joint related to the use of screws and staples. *J Bone Joint Surg [Am]* 1984;66:175–180.
378. Cheng JC, Shen WY. Limb fracture pattern in different pediatric age groups: a study of 3350 children. *J Orthop Trauma* 1993;7:15–22.
379. Iqbal QM. Long-bone fractures among children in Malaysia. *Int Surg* 1974;59:410–415.
380. Lichtenberg RP. A study of 2532 fractures in children. *Am J Surg* 1954;87:330–338.
381. Webb LX, Green NE, Swiontkowski MF, eds. *Skeletal trauma in children.* Philadelphia: WB Saunders, 1993:257–281.
382. Beaty JH. Fractures of the proximal humerus and shaft in children. *AAOS Instr Course Lect* 1992;41:369–372.
383. Samardzic M, Grujicic D, Milinkovic ZB. Radial nerve lesions associated with fractures of the humeral shaft. *Injury* 1990;21:220–222.
384. Landin LA. Fracture patterns in children: analysis of 8682 fractures with special reference to incidence, etiology and secular changes in Swedish urban populations. *Acta Orthop Scand Suppl* 1983;54:1–109.
385. Worlock P, Stower M. Fracture patterns in Nottingham children. *J Pediatr Orthop* 1986; 6:656–661.
386. Camus M, Lefebvre G, Veron P, et al. Obstetrical injuries of the newborn infant. Retrospective study apropos of 20,409 births. *J Gynecol Obstet Biol Reprod (Paris)* 1985;14: 1033–1043.
387. Madsen TE. Fractures of the extremities in the newborn. *Acta Obstet Gynecol Scand* 1955;34:4.
388. Loder RT, Bookout C. Fracture patterns in battered children. *J Orthop Trauma* 1991; 5:428–433.
389. Shaw BA, Murphy KM, Shaw A, et al. Humerus shaft fractures in young children: accident or abuse? *J Pediatr Orthop* 1997;17:293–297.
390. O'Neill JA Jr, Meacham WF, Griffin JP, et al. Patterns of injury in the battered child syndrome. *J Trauma* 1973;13:332–339.
391. Allen ME. Stress fracture of the humerus: a case study. *Am J Sports Med* 1984;12: 244–245.
392. Brumback R, Bosse M, Poka A, et al. Intramedullary stabilization of humeral shaft fractures in patients with multiple trauma. *J Bone Joint Surg [Am]* 1986;68:960–970.
393. Garth WP Jr, Leberte MA, Cool TA. Recurrent fractures of the humerus in a baseball pitcher—a case report. *J Bone Joint Surg [Am]* 1988;70:305–306.
394. Gore RM, Rogers LF, Bowerman J, et al. Osseous manifestations of elbow stress associated with sports activities. *AJR Am J Roentgenol* 1980;134:971–977.
395. Gregersen HN. Fractures of the humerus from muscular violence. *Acta Orthop Scand* 1971;42:506–512.
396. Hennigan SP, Bush-Joseph CA, Kuo KN, et al. Throwing-induced humeral shaft fracture in skeletally immature adolescents. *Orthopedics* 1999;22:621–622.
397. Linn RM, Kerigshauser LA. Ball-thrower's fracture of the humerus—a case report. *Am J Sports Med* 1991;19:194–197.
398. Sprenger TR. Fracture of humerus from muscular violence: case report. *J Fla Med Assoc* 1985;72:101–103.
399. Sterling JC, Calvo RD, Holden SC. An unusual stress fracture in a multiple sport athlete. *Med Sci Sports Exerc* 1991;23:298–303.
400. Tullos HS, Erwin WD, Woods GW, et al. Unusual lesions of the pitching arm. *Clin Orthop* 1972;88:169–182.
401. Weseley MS, Barenfeld PA. Ball throwers' fracture of the humerus. *Clin Orthop* 1969; 64:153–156.
402. Rettig AC, Beltz HF. Stress fracture in the humerus in an adolescent tennis tournament player. *Am J Sports Med* 1985;13:55–58.
403. DiCicco JD, Mehlman CT, Urse JS. Fracture of the shaft of the humerus secondary to muscular violence. *J Orthop Trauma* 1993;7:90–93.
404. Bay BH, Sit KH, Lee ST. Mechanisms of humoral fractures in arm-wrestlers [Letter; Comment]. *Br J Clin Pract* 1992;46:98–99 and *Br J Clin Pract* 1993;47:279–280.
405. Low BY, Lim J. Fracture of humerus during arm-wrestling: report of 5 cases. *Singapore Med J* 1991;32:47–49.
406. Moon MS, Kim I, Han IH, et al. Arm-wrestler's injury: report of 7 cases. *Clin Orthop* 1980;147:219–221.
407. Howard NJ, Eloesser L. Treatment of fracture of the upper end of the humerus: an experimental and clinical study. *J Bone Joint Surg [Am]* 1934;16:1–29.
408. Langenberg R. Missed humeral fracture in multiple injury of the arm. *Zentralbl Chir* 1986;111:1536–1539.
409. Dameron TB Jr, Grubb SA. Humeral shaft fractures in adults. *South Med J* 1981;74: 1461–1467.
410. Thomas IH, Chow CW, Cole WG. Giant cell reparative granuloma of the humerus. *J Pediatr Orthop* 1988;8:596–598.
411. Stephenson RB, London MD, Harkan FM, et al. Fibrous dysplasia: an analysis of options for treatment. *J Bone Joint Surg [Am]* 1987;69:400–409.
412. Barquet A, Schimchak M, Carreras O, et al. Dislocation of the shoulder with fracture of the ipsilateral shaft of the humerus. *Injury* 1985;16:300–302.
413. Arrive L, Sellier N, Kalifa G, et al. Diagnostic difficulties of isolated symptomatic unilamellar periosteal appositions. Uncommon form of fatigue fracture in children. *J Radiol* 1988;69:351–356.
414. Stanitski CL, Micheli LJ. Simultaneous ipsilateral fractures of the arm and forearm in children. *Clin Orthop* 1980;153:218–222.
415. Bretagne MC, Mouton JN, Pierson M, et al. Periostitis or, rather, periosteal appositions in paediatrics. *J Radiol Electrol Med Nucl* 1977;58:119–123.
416. Müller ME, Allgöwer M, Schneider R, et al. *Manual of internal fixation. Techniques recommended by the AO-ASIF group,* 3rd ed. Berlin: Springer-Verlag, 1991.
417. Holstein A, Lewis GB. Fractures of the humerus with radial nerve paralysis. *J Bone Joint Surg [Am]* 1963;45:1382–1388.
418. Gardner E. Prenatal development of the human shoulder joint. *Surg Clin North Am* 1953;92:219–276.
419. Johnstone DJ, Radford WJ, Parnel EJ. Interobserver variation using the AO/ASIF classification of long-bone fractures. *Injury* 1993;24:163–165.
420. Gray DJ, Gardner E. The prenatal development of the human humerus. *Am J Anat* 1969;124:431–434.
421. Sonneveld GJ, Patka P, van Mourik JC, et al. Treatment of fractures of the shaft of the humerus accompanied by paralysis of the radial nerve. *Injury* 1987;18:404–406.
422. Curtis RJJ, Dameron TB Jr, Rockwood CA Jr, et al., eds. *Fractures in children,* 3rd ed. Philadelphia: JB Lippincott, 1991:829–919.
423. Dameron TB Jr. Transverse fractures of distal humerus in children. *AAOS Instr Course Lect* 1981;30:224–235.
424. Carroll SE. A study of the nutrient foramina of the humeral diaphysis. *J Bone Joint Surg [Br]* 1963;45:176–181.
425. Whitson RO. Relation of the radial nerve to the shaft of the humerus. *J Bone Joint Surg [Am]* 1954;36:85–88.
426. Kane E, Kaplan EB, Spinner M. Observations of the course of the ulnar nerve in the arm. *Ann Chir* 1973;27:487–496.
427. Hollingshead WH. *Anatomy for surgeons: the back and limbs.* New York: Harper & Row, 1982.
428. Bianco AJ, Schlein AP, Kruse RL, et al. Birth fractures. *Minn Med* 1972;55:471–474.
429. Holm CL. Management of humeral shaft fractures. Fundamental nonoperative technics. *Clin Orthop* 1970;71:132–139.
430. Astedt B. A method for the treatment of humerus fractures in the newborn using the S. von Rosen splint. *Acta Orthop Scand* 1969;40:234–236.
431. Devas MB. Stress fractures in athletes. *Proc R Soc Med* 1969;62:933–937.
432. Tullos HS, King JW. Lesions of the pitching arm in adolescents. *JAMA* 1972;220: 264–271.
433. Klenerman L. Fractures of the shaft of the humerus. *J Bone Joint Surg [Br]* 1966;48: 105–111.
434. Rang M. *Children's fractures,* 2nd ed. Philadelphia: JB Lippincott, 1983:154–151.
435. Böhler L. *The treatment of fractures.* New York: Grune & Stratton, 1956:618–694.
436. Böhler L. Conservative treatment of fresh closed fractures of the shaft of the humerus. *J Trauma* 1965;464.
437. Böhler L. *The treatment of fractures—supplement.* New York: Grune & Stratton, 1966.
438. Hedstrom O. Growth stimulation of long bones after fracture or similar trauma. A clinical and experimental study. *Acta Orthop Scand Suppl* 1969;122:1–134.
439. Spak I. Humeral shaft fractures. Treatment with a simple hand sling. *Acta Orthop Scand* 1978;49:234–239.
440. Hosner W. Fractures of the shaft of the humerus: an analysis of 100 consecutive cases. *Reconstr Surg Traumatol* 1974;14:38–64.
441. Koch G. Treatment of humeral fractures using the U splint. *Chirurgie* 1971;42:327–329.
442. Shantharam SS. Tips of the trade: 41. Modified coaptation splint for humeral shaft fractures. *Orthop Rev* 1991;20:1033–1039.
443. Caldwell JA. Treatment of fractures in the Cincinnati General Hospital. *Ann Surg* 1933; 97:16.

444. Stewart MJ, Hundley JM. Fractures of the humerus: a comparative study in methods of treatment. *J Bone Joint Surg [Am]* 1955;37:681–692.
445. Winfield JM, Miller H, LaFerte AD. Evaluation of the "hanging cast" as a method of treating fractures of the humerus. *Am J Surg* 1942;55:228–249.
446. Ciernik IF, Meier L, Hollinger A. Humeral mobility after treatment with hanging cast. *J Trauma* 1991;31:230–233.
447. Babin SR, Steinmetz A, Wuyts JL, et al. A reliable orthopedic technic in the treatment of humeral diaphyseal fractures in the adult: the hanging plaster. Report of a series of 74 cases. *J Chir (Paris)* 1978;115:653–658.
448. Sarmiento A, Kinman PB, Galvin EG, et al. Functional bracing of fractures of the shaft of the humerus. *J Bone Joint Surg [Am]* 1977;59:596–601.
449. Balfour GW, Mooney V, Ashby ME. Diaphyseal fractures of the humerus treated with a ready-made fracture brace. *J Bone Joint Surg [Am]* 1982;64:11–13.
450. Dufour O, Beaufils P, Ouaknine M, et al. Functional treatment of recent fractures of the humeral shaft using the Sarmiento method. *Rev Chir Orthop Reparatrice Appar Mot* 1989;75:292–300.
451. Galasko CS. The fate of simple bone cysts which fracture. *Clin Orthop* 1974;101: 302–304.
452. Hackstock H. Functional bracing of fractures. *Orthopadie* 1988;17:41–51.
453. Leung KS, Kwan M, Wong J, et al. Therapeutic functional bracing in upper limb fracture–dislocations. *J Orthop Trauma* 1999;2:308–313.
454. Michiels I, Broos P, Gruwez JA. The operative treatment of humeral shaft fractures. *Acta Chir Belg* 1986;86:147–152.
455. Naver L, Aalberg JR. Humeral shaft fractures treated with a ready-made fracture brace. *Arch Orthop Trauma Surg* 1986;106:20–22.
456. Peeters PM, Oostvogel HJ, Bongers KJ, van der Werken C. Early functional treatment of humerus shaft fractures by the Sarmiento method. *Aktuel Traumatol* 1987;17:150–152.
457. Bell CH. Construction of orthoplast splints for humeral shaft fractures. *Am J Occup Ther* 1979;33:114–115.
458. Zagorski JB, Latta LL, Zych GA, et al. Diaphyseal fractures of the humerus. treatment with prefabricated braces. *J Bone Joint Surg [Am]* 1988;70:607–610.
459. Sarmiento A. Functional fracture bracing: an update. *AAOS Instr Course Lect* 1987;36: 371–376.
460. Sarmiento A, Horowitch A, Aboulafia A, et al. Functional bracing for comminuted extra-articular fractures of the distal third of the humerus. *J Bone Joint Surg [Br]* 1990; 72:283–287.
461. Sharma VK, Jain AK, Gupta RK, et al. Nonoperative treatment of fractures of the humeral shaft: a comparative study. *J Indian Med Assoc* 1991;89:157–160.
462. Asche G. Use of external fixation in pediatric fractures. *Zentralbl Chir* 1986;111: 391–397.
463. Vichare NA. Fractures of the humeral shaft associated with multiple injuries. *Injury* 1974;5:279–282.
464. Hermichen HG, Pfister U, Weller S. Influence of the treatment of fractures on the development of pseudoarthroses of the humerus shaft. *Aktuel Traumatol* 1980;10: 137–142.
465. Heilbronner DM, Manoli A 2nd, Little RE. Elbow dislocation during overhead skeletal traction therapy: a case report. *Clin Orthop* 1981;154:185–187.
466. Henley MB, Monroe M, Tencer AF. Biomechanical comparison of methods of fixation of a midshaft osteotomy of the humerus. *J Orthop Trauma* 1991;5:14–20.
467. Rüedi T, Moshfegh A, Pfeiffer KM, et al. Fresh fractures of the shaft of the humerus—conservative or operative treatment? *Reconstr Surg Traumatol* 1974;14:65–74.
468. Bell MJ, Beauchamp CG, Kellam JK, et al. The results of plating humeral shaft fractures in patients with multiple injuries. The Sunnybrook experience. *J Bone Joint Surg [Br]* 1985;67:293–296.
469. Foster RJ, Dixon GL Jr, Bach AW, et al. Internal fixation of fractures and nonunions of the humeral shaft. Indications and results in a multicenter study. *J Bone Joint Surg [Am]* 1985;67:857–864.
470. Heim D, Herkert F, Hess P, et al. Can humerus shaft fractures be treated with osteosynthesis? *Helv Chir Acta* 1992;58:673–678.
471. Heim D, Herkert F, Hess P, et al. Surgical treatment of humeral shaft fractures—the Basel experience. *J Trauma* 1993;35:226–232.
472. Nast-Kolb D, Knoefel WT, Schweiberer L. The treatment of humeral shaft fractures. Results of a prospective AO multicenter study. *Unfallchirurgie* 1991;94:447–454.
473. Winker H, Vosberg W, Cyris A. Results of treatment of humerus shaft fractures. *Aktuel Traumatol* 1993;23(suppl):36–41.
474. Zinghi GF, Sabetta E, Bungaro P, et al. The role of osteosynthesis in the treatment of fractures of the humerus. *Ital J Orthop Traumatol* 1988;14:67–75.
475. Riemer BL, Foglesong ME, Burke CJ 3rd, et al. Complications of Seidel intramedullary nailing of narrow-diameter humeral diaphyseal fractures. *Orthopaedics* 1994;17:19–29.
476. Crolla RM, de Vries LS, Clevers GJ. Locked intramedullary nailing of humeral fractures. *Injury* 1993;24:403–406.
477. D'Ythurbide B, Augereau B, Asselineau A, et al. Closed intramedullary nailing of fractures of the shaft of the humerus. *Int Orthop* 1983;7:195–203.
478. Hall RF Jr. Closed intramedullary fixation of humeral shaft fractures. *AAOS Instr Course Lect* 1987;36:349–358.
479. Ingman AM, Waters DA. Locked intramedullary nailing of humeral shaft fractures. Implant design, surgical technique, and clinical results. *J Bone Joint Surg [Br]* 1994;76: 23–29.
480. Kolb LW, Moore RD. Fractures of the supracondylar process of the humerus. Report of 2 cases. *J Bone Joint Surg [Am]* 1967;49:532–534.
481. Marty B, Kach K, Candinas D, et al. Results of intramedullary nailing in humerus shaft fractures. *Helv Chir Acta* 1993;59:681–685.
482. Putz P, Lusi K, Baillon JM, Bremen J. The treatment of fractures of the humeral diaphysis with fasciculated intramedullary pins by the Hackethal method apropos of 194 cases. *Acta Orthop Belg* 1984;50:521–538.
483. Rommens PM, Vergruggen J, Broos PL. Retrograde locked nailing of humeral shaft fractures. *J Bone Joint Surg [Br]* 1995;77:84–89.
484. van der Ghinst M, De Geeter L, Thiry A. Treatment of collum and diaphyseal fractures of the humerus using Kirschner wire nailing. *Acta Chir Belg* 1972;(suppl 2):105–116.
485. Vander Griend RA, Ward EF, Tomasin J. Closed Kuntscher nailing of humeral shaft fractures. *J Trauma* 1985;25:1167–1169.
486. Zanasi R, Romano P, Rotolo F, et al. Intramedullary osteosynthesis: 3. Kuntscher nailing in the humerus. *Ital J Orthop Traumatol* 1990;16:311–322.
487. Babin SR, Graf P, Vidal P, et al. The risk of nonunion following closed-focus nailing and reaming. Results of 1059 interventions using the Kuntscher method. *Int Orthop* 1983;7:133–143.
488. Chapman MW. Closed intramedullary nailing of the humerus. *AAOS Instr Course Lect* 1983;32:324–328.
489. Confalonieri N, Simonatti R, Ramondetta V, et al. Intramedullary nailing with a rush pin in the treatment of diaphyseal humeral fractures. *Arch Putti Chir Organi Mov* 1990; 38:395–403.
490. DeLong WG Jr, Born CT, Marcelli E, et al. Ender nail fixation in long bone fractures: experience in a level I trauma center. *J Trauma* 1989;29:571–576.
491. Hall RFJ, Pankovich AM. Ender nailing of acute fractures of the humerus. A study of closed fixation by intramedullary nails without reaming. *J Bone Joint Surg [Am]* 1987; 69:558–567.
492. Mackay I. Closed Rush pinning of fractures of the humeral shaft. *Injury* 1984;16: 178–181.
493. Rose SH, Melton LJ 3rd, Morrey BF, et al. Epidemiologic features of humeral fractures. *Clin Orthop* 1982;168:24–30.
494. Stern PJ, Mattingly DA, Pomeroy DL, et al. Intramedullary fixation of humeral shaft fractures. *J Bone Joint Surg [Am]* 1984;66:639–646.
495. Hackethal KH. *Die Bundel-Nagelung.* Berlin: Springer-Verlag, 1961.
496. Champetier J, Brabant A, Charignon G, et al. Treatment of fractures of the humerus by intramedullary fixation. *J Chir (Paris)* 1975;109:75–82.
497. Destree C, Safary A. The treatment of fractures of the neck and diaphysis of the humerus by Hackethal's bundle nailing. *Acta Orthop Belg* 1979;45:666–677.
498. Durbin RA, Gottesman MJ, Saunders KC. Hackethal stacked nailing of humeral shaft fractures. Experience with 30 patients. *Clin Orthop* 1983;179:168–174.
499. Hennig F, Link W, Wofel R. Bundle nailing—an evaluation after 27 years. *Aktuel Traumatol* 1988;18:117–119.
500. Menger DM, Gauger JU, Schmitt-Koppler A. Experiences with cluster nailing of humeral shaft fractures. *Unfallchirurgie* 1985;11:70–75.
501. Peter RE, Hoffmeyer P, Henley MB. Treatment of humeral diaphyseal fractures with Hackethal stacked nailing: a report of 33 cases. *J Orthop Trauma* 1992;6:14–17.
502. Zifko B, Poigenfurst J. Treatment of unstable fractures of the proximal end of the humerus using elastic curved intramedullary wires. *Unfallchirurgie* 1987;13:72–81.
503. Link W, Herzog T, Hoffmann A. Bundle wire nailing in pathological upper arm fractures. *Zentralbl Chir* 1990;115:665–670.
504. Ligier JN, Metaizeau JP, Prevot J. Closed flexible medullary nailing in pediatric traumatology. *Chir Pediatr* 1983;24:383–385.
505. Metaizeau JP, Ligier JN. Surgical treatment of fractures of the long bones in children. Interference between osteosynthesis and the physiological processes of consolidation. Therapeutic indications. *J Chir (Paris)* 1984;121:527–537.
506. De Bastiani G, Aldegheri R, Renzi Brivio L. The treatment of fractures with a dynamic axial fixator. *J Bone Joint Surg [Br]* 1984;66:538–545.
507. Kamhin M, Michaelson M, Waisbrod H. The use of external skeletal fixation in the treatment of fractures of the humeral shaft. *Injury* 1978;9:245–248.
508. Kim NH, Hahn SB, Park HW, et al. The Orthofix external fixator for fractures of long bones. *Int Orthop* 1994;18:42–46.
509. Putnam MD, Walsh TM. External fixation for open fractures of the upper extremity. *Hand Clin* 1993;9:613–623.
510. Smith DK, Cooney WP. External fixation of high-energy upper extremity injuries. *J Orthop Trauma* 1990;4:7–18.
511. Costa P, Giancecchi F, Cavazzuti A. Internal and external fixation in complex diaphyseal and metaphyseal fractures of the humerus. *Ital J Orthop Traumatol* 1991;17:87–94.
512. Sales de Gauzy J, Vidal H, Cahuzac JP. Primary shortening followed by callus distraction for the treatment of a post-traumatic bone defect: case report. *J Trauma* 1993;34: 461–463.
513. Buachidze OS, Onoprienko GA, Shternberg AA, et al. Treatment of diaphyseal pseudarthrosis with transosseous osteosynthesis. *Vestn Khir Im I I Grek* 1977;119:84–87.
514. Cattaneo R, Catagni MA, Guerreschi F. Applications of the Ilizarov method in the humerus. Lengthenings and nonunions. *Hand Clin* 1993;9:729–739.
515. Cattaneo R, Villa A, Catagni MA, et al. Lengthening of the humerus using the Ilizarov technique. Description of the method and report of 43 cases. *Clin Orthop* 1990;250: 117–124.
516. Ciuccarelli C, Cervellati C, Montanari G, et al. The Ilizarov method for the treatment of nonunion in the humerus. *Chir Organi Mov* 1990;75:115–120.
517. Ilizarov GA. *Transosseous osteosynthesis.* Berlin: Springer-Verlag, 1992.
518. Ilizarov GA, Shevtsov VI. Bloodless compression–distraction osteosynthesis in the treatment of pseudarthroses of the humerus. *Voen Med Zh* 1974;27–31.
519. Shevtsov VI. Outcome of treatment of pseudarthroses of the humerus by methods of closed perosseous osteosynthesis by the Ilizarov technic. *Sov Med* 1977;75–79.
520. Shumada IV, Zhila IS, Rybachuk OI. Compression–distraction osteosynthesis in pseudarthroses of long tubular bones. *Vestn Khir Im I I Grek* 1976;116:90–94.
521. Beringer DC, Weiner DS, Noble JS, et al. Severely displaced proximal humeral epiphyseal fractures: a follow-up study. *J Pediatr Orthop* 1998;18:31–37.

522. Choong PF, Griffiths JD. External fixation of complex open humeral fractures. *Aust NZ J Surg* 1988;58:137–142.
523. Levin LS, Goldner RD, Urbaniak JR, et al. Management of severe musculoskeletal injuries of the upper extremity. *J Orthop Trauma* 1990;4:432–440.
524. Machan FG, Vinz H. Humeral shaft fracture in childhood. *Unfallchirurgie* 1993;19: 166–174.
525. Vinz H. Treatment of open fractures in children. *Zentralbl Chir* 1980;105:1483–1493.
526. Loder RT. Pediatric polytrauma: orthopaedic care and hospital course. *J Orthop Trauma* 1987;1:48–54.
527. Marcus RE, Mills MF, Thompson GH. Multiple injury in children. *J Bone Joint Surg [Am]* 1983;65:1290–1294.
528. Gainor BJ, Metzler M. Humeral shaft fracture with brachial artery injury. *Clin Orthop* 1986;204:154–161.
529. Pradhan DJ, Juanteguy JM, Wilder RJ, et al. Arterial injuries of the extremities associated with fractures. *Arch Surg* 1972;105:582–585.
530. Rich NM, Metz CW Jr, Hutton JE Jr, et al. Internal versus external fixation of fractures with concomitant vascular injuries in Vietnam. *J Trauma* 1971;11:463–473.
531. Smith RF, Szilagyi E, Elliott JP Jr. Fracture of long bones with arterial injury due to blunt trauma. Principles of management. *Arch Surg* 1969;99:315–324.
532. Gamble JG, Rinsky LA, Strudwick J, et al. Nonunion of fractures in children who have osteogenesis imperfecta. *J Bone Joint Surg [Am]* 1988;70:439–443.
533. McNamara JJ, Brief DK, Stremple JF, et al. Management of fractures with associated arterial injury in combat casualties. *J Trauma* 1973;13:17–19.
534. Chitwood WR Jr, Rankin JS, Bollinger RR, et al. Brachial artery reconstruction using the heparin-bonded Sundt shunt. *Surgery* 1981;89:355–358.
535. Rogalsky RJ, Black GR, Reed MH. Orthopaedic manifestations of leukemia. *J Bone Joint Surg [Am]* 1986;68:494–501.
536. Gibson MJ, Middlemiss JH. Fibrous dysplasia of bone. *Br J Radiol* 1971;44:1–13.
537. Nerubay J, Horoszowski H, Goodman RM. Fracture in progressive ossifying fibrodysplasia—a case report. *Acta Orthop Scand* 1987;58:289–291.
538. Colyer RA. Surgical stabilization of pathological neoplastic fractures. *Curr Probl Cancer* 1986;10:117–168.
539. Lewallen RP, Pritchard DJ, Sim FH. Treatment of pathologic fractures or impending fractures of the humerus with rush rods and methylmethacrylate. Experience with 55 cases in 54 patients, 1968–1977. *Clin Orthop* 1982;166:93–198.
540. Vail TP, Harrelson JM. Treatment of pathologic fracture of the humerus. *Clin Orthop* 1991;268:197–202.
541. Vastamaki M, Solonen KA. Posterior dislocation and fracture–dislocation of the shoulder. *Acta Orthop Scand* 1980;51:479–484.
542. Lange RH, Foster RJ. Skeletal management of humeral shaft fractures associated with forearm fractures. *Clin Orthop* 1985;195:173–177.
543. Rogers JF, Bennett JB, Tullos HS. Management of concomitant ipsilateral fractures of the humerus and forearm. *J Bone Joint Surg [Am]* 1984;66:552–556.
544. Pierce RO Jr, Hodurski DF. Fractures of the humerus, radius, and ulna in the same extremity. *J Trauma* 1979;19:182–185.
545. Brien WW, Gellman H, Becker V, et al. Management of fractures of the humerus in patients who have an injury of the ipsilateral brachial plexus. *J Bone Joint Surg [Am]* 1990;72:1208–1210.
546. Garland DE, Jones RC, Kunkle RW. Upper extremity fractures in the acute spinal cord injured patient. *Clin Orthop* 1988;233:110–115.
547. Chan D, Petricciuolo F, Maffulli N. Fracture of the humeral diaphysis with extreme rotation. *Acta Orthop Belg* 1991;57:427–429.
548. Alnot JY, Le Reun D. Traumatic lesions of the radial nerve of the arm. *Rev Chir Orthop Reparatrice Appar Mot* 1989;75:433–442.
549. Dabezies EJ, Banta CJ 2nd, Murphy CP, et al. Plate fixation of the humeral shaft for acute fractures, with and without radial nerve injuries. *J Orthop Trauma* 1992;6:10–13.
550. Garcia A, Maeck BH. Radial nerve injuries in fractures of the shaft of the humerus. *Am J Surg* 1960;99:625–627.
551. Kulenkampff HA, Rustemeier M. Clinical experiences in the treatment of humeral shaft fractures with the Sarmiento brace. *Unfallchirurgie* 1988;14:191–198.
552. Kwasny O, Maier R, Scharf W. The surgical treatment of humeral shaft fractures. *Aktuel Traumatol* 1990;20:87–92.
553. Packer JW, Foster RR, Garcia A, et al. The humeral fracture with radial nerve palsy: is exploration warranted? *Clin Orthop* 1972;88:34–38.
554. Postacchini F, Morace GB. Fractures of the humerus associated with paralysis of the radial nerve. *Ital J Orthop Traumatol* 1988;14:455–465.
555. Rommens PM, Vansteenkiste F, Stappaerts KH, et al. Indications, dangers and results of surgical treatment of humeral shaft fractures. *Unfallchirurgie* 1989;92:565–570.
556. Titze A. The operative treatment of fractures of the shaft of the humerus. *Reconstr Surg Traumatol* 1974;14:75–83.
557. Shaw JL, Sakellarides H. Radial nerve paralysis associated with fractures of the humerus. A review of 45 cases. *J Bone Joint Surg [Am]* 1967;49:899–902.
558. Vander Griend R, Tomasin J, Ward EF. Open reduction and internal fixation of humeral shaft fractures. Results using AO plating techniques. *J Bone Joint Surg [Am]* 1986;68: 430–433.
559. Bleeker WA, Nijsten MW, ten Duis HJ. Treatment of humeral shaft fractures related to associated injuries. A retrospective study of 237 patients. *Acta Orthop Scand* 1991; 62:148–153.
560. Mast JW, Spiegel PG, Harvey JP, et al. Fractures of the humeral shaft. A retrospective study of 240 adult fractures. *Clin Orthop* 1975;112:254–262.
561. Pollock FH, Drake D, Bovill EG, et al. Treatment of radial neuropathy associated with fractures of the humerus. *J Bone Joint Surg [Am]* 1981;63:239–243.
562. Shah JJ, Bhatti NA. Radial nerve paralysis associated with fractures of the humerus: a review of 62 cases. *Clin Orthop* 1983;172:171–176.
563. Vukadinovic S, Mikic Z, Lartey J. Humeral fractures complicated by radial nerve lesions. *Acta Chir Iugosl* 1981;28:211–217.
564. Amillo S, Barrios RH, Martinez-Peric R, et al. Surgical treatment of the radial nerve lesions associated with fractures of the humerus. *J Orthop Trauma* 1993;7:211–215.
565. Bostman O, Bakalim G, Vainionpaa S, et al. Immediate radial nerve palsy complicating fracture of the shaft of the humerus: when is early exploration justified? *Injury* 1985; 16:499–502.
566. Bostman O, Bakalim G, Vainionpaa S, et al. Radial palsy in shaft fracture of the humerus. *Acta Orthop Scand* 1986;57:316–319.
567. Di Filippo P, Mancini GB, Gillio A. Humeral fractures with paralysis of the radial nerve. *Arch Putti Chir Organi Mov* 1990;38:405–409.
568. Gjengedal E, Slungaard U. Treatment of humeral fractures with and without injury to the radial nerve—a follow-up study. *Tidsskr Nor Laegeforen* 1981;101:1746–1749.
569. Szalay EA, Rockwood CA. Fractures of the distal shaft of the humerus associated with radial nerve palsy. *Orthop Trans* 1982;6:455.
570. Foster RJ, Swiontkowski MF, Bach AW, et al. Radial nerve palsy caused by open humeral shaft fractures. *J Hand Surg [Am]* 1993;18:121–124.
571. Birch R, Bonney G, Payan J, et al. Symposium: peripheral nerve injuries. *J Bone Joint Surg [Br]* 1986;68:2–21.
572. Fisher TR, McGeorch CM. Severe injuries of the radial nerve treated by sural nerve grafting. *Injury* 1985;16:411–412.
573. Seddon HJ. Nerve lesions complicating certain closed bone injuries. *JAMA* 1947;135: 691–694.
574. Seddon HJ, Medawar PB, Smith H. Rate of regeneration of peripheral nerves in man. *J Physiol (Paris)* 1943;102:191–215.
575. Sunderland S. Rate of regeneration in human peripheral nerves. *Arch Neurol Psych* 1947;58:251–295.
576. Goodsell JO. The resilient radial nerve. *Mich Med* 1965;64:756–758.
577. Kwasny O, Maier R, Kutscha-Lissberg F, et al. Treatment procedure in humeral shaft fractures with primary or secondary radial nerve damage. *Unfallchirurgie* 1992;18: 168–173.
578. Duthie HL. Radial nerve in osseous tunnel at humeral fracture site diagnosed radiographically. *J Bone Joint Surg [Br]* 1957;39:746–747.
579. Stimson LA. *A practical treatise on fractures and dislocations,* 3rd ed. New York: Lea Brothers & Co, 1900.
580. de Mourgues G, Fischer LP, Gillet JP, et al. Recent fractures of the humeral diaphysis apropos of a continuous series of 200 cases, of which 107 were treated with a hanging cast alone. *Rev Chir Orthop Reparatrice Appar Mot* 1975;61:191–207.
581. Friedman RJ, Smith RJ. Radial nerve laceration 26 years after screw fixation of a humeral fracture—a case report. *J Bone Joint Surg [Am]* 1984;66:959–960.
582. Macnicol MF. Roentgenographic evidence of median-nerve entrapment in a greenstick humeral fracture. *J Bone Joint Surg [Am]* 1978;60:998–1000.
583. Mubarak SJ, Carroll NC. Volkmann's contracture in children: aetiology and prevention. *J Bone Joint Surg [Br]* 1979;61:285–293.
584. Gupta A, Sharma S. Volar compartment syndrome of the arm complicating a fracture of the humeral shaft—a case report. *Acta Orthop Scand* 1991;62:77–78.
585. Broyn T, Bie K. Peripheral arterial occlusion following traumatic intimal rupture. *Acta Chir Scand* 1966;131:167–170.
586. Makin GS, Howard JM, Green RL. Arterial injuries complicating fractures or dislocations: the necessity for a more aggressive approach. *Surgery* 1966;59:203–209.
587. McQuillan WM, Nolan B. Ischemia complicating injury. *J Bone Joint Surg [Am]* 1968; 50:482–492.
588. Canale ST, Puhl J, Watson FM, et al. Acute osteomyelitis following closed fractures. Report of 3 cases. *J Bone Joint Surg [Am]* 1975;57:415.
589. Watson FM, Whitesides TE Jr. Acute hematogenous osteomyelitis complicating closed fractures. *Clin Orthop* 1976;117:296–302.
590. Ellefsen BK, Frierson MA, Raney EM, et al. Humerus varus: a complication of neonatal, infantile, and childhood injury and infection. *J Pediatr Orthop* 1994;14:479–486.
591. Nonnemann HC. Limits of spontaneous correction of incorrectly healed fractures in adolescence. *Langenbecks Arch Chir* 1969;324:78–86.
592. Green SA, Gibbs P. The relationship of angulation to translation in fracture deformities. *J Bone Joint Surg [Am]* 1994;76:390–397.
593. Franklyn PP. Progeria in siblings. *Clin Radiol* 1976;27:327–333.
594. Lewallen RP, Peterson HA. Nonunion of long bone fractures in children: a review of 30 cases. *J Pediatr Orthop* 1985;5:135–142.
595. Christensen NO. Kuntscher intramedullary reaming and nail fixation for nonunion of the humerus. *Clin Orthop* 1976;116:222–225.
596. Gupta RC, Gaur SC, Tiwari RC, et al. Treatment of ununited fractures of the shaft of the humerus with bent nail. *Injury* 1985;16:276–280.
597. Pritchett JW. Delayed union of humeral shaft fractures treated by closed flexible intramedullary nailing. *J Bone Joint Surg [Br]* 1985;67:715–718.
598. Barquet A, Fernandez A, Luvizio J, et al. A combined therapeutic protocol for aseptic nonunion of the humeral shaft: a report of 25 cases. *J Trauma* 1989;29:95–98.
599. Chacha PB. Compression plating without bone grafts for delayed and nonunion of humeral shaft fractures. *Injury* 1973;5:283–290.
600. Fattah HA, Halawa EE, Shafy TH. Nonunion of the humeral shaft: a report on 25 cases. *Injury* 1982;14:255–262.
601. Healy WL, White GM, Mick CA, et al. Nonunion of the humeral shaft. *Clin Orthop* 1987;219:206–213.
602. Wright TW, Miller GJ, Vander Griend RA, et al. Reconstruction of the humerus with an intramedullary fibular graft. A clinical and biomechanical study. *J Bone Joint Surg [Br]* 1993;75:804–807.

603. Connolly JF. Selection, evaluation and indications for electrical stimulation of ununited fractures. *Clin Orthop* 1981;161:39–53.
604. Epps CH. Nonunion of the humerus. *AAOS Instr Course Lect* 1988;37:161–166.
605. Esterhai JL Jr, Brighton CT, Heppenstall RB, et al. Nonunion of the humerus. Clinical, roentgenographic, scintigraphic, and response characteristics to treatment with constant direct current stimulation of osteogenesis. *Clin Orthop* 1986;211:228–234.
606. Sedel L, Christel P, Duriez J, et al. Acceleration of repair of nonunions by electromagnetic fields. *Rev Chir Orthop Reparatrice Appar Mot* 1981;67:11–23.
607. Sedel L, Christel P, Duriez J, et al. Results of nonunions treatment by pulsed electromagnetic field stimulation. *Acta Orthop Scand Suppl* 1982;196:81–91.
608. Sturmer KM, Schmit-Neuerburg KP. Indications and clinical results of electromagnetically induced alternating current stimulation of poorly reacting pseudarthroses. *Unfallchirurgie* 1985;11:197–203.
609. Andre S, Feuilhade de Chauvin P, Camilleri A, et al. Recent fractures of the humeral diaphysis in adults—comparison of orthopedic and surgical treatment apropos of 252 cases. *Rev Chir Orthop Reparatrice Appar Mot* 1984;70:49–61.
610. Sattel W. Effect of dia- and pericondylar humeral fractures on the growth of the carpal bones in children. *Handchir Mikrochir Plast Chir* 1982;14:103–105.
611. Dal Monte A, Andrisano A, Manfrini M, et al. Humeral lengthening in hypoplasia of the upper limb. *J Pediatr Orthop* 1985;5:207.
612. Peterson HA. Surgical lengthening of the humerus: case report and review. *J Pediatr Orthop* 1989;9:596–601.
613. Fourastier J, Pialoux B, Bracq H, et al. Post-traumatic algodystrophy in children. *Chir Pediatr* 1986;27:313–317.
614. Kretzschmar HJ. Post-traumatic fat embolism in a 13-year-old girl. *Zentralbl Chir* 1970; 95:1223–1225.
615. Bransby-Zachary MA, MacDonald DA, Singh I, et al. Late fracture associated with retained internal fixation. *J Bone Joint Surg [Br]* 1989;71:539.
616. Brug E, Winckler S, Klein W. Distal diaphyseal fracture of the humerus. *Unfallchirurgie* 1994;97:74–77.
617. Bortel DT, Pritchett JW. Straight-line graphs for the predictions of growth of the upper extremities. *J Bone Joint Surg [Am]* 1993;75:885–892.
618. Pritchett JW. Growth and predictions of growth in the upper extremity. *J Bone Joint Surg [Am]* 1988;70:520–525.
619. Pritchett JW. Growth plate activity in the upper extremity. *Clin Orthop* 1991;268: 235–242.
620. Arnold JA, Nasca RJ, Nelson CL. Supracondylar fractures of the humerus. The role of dynamic factors in prevention of deformity. *J Bone Joint Surg [Am]* 1977;59:589–595.
621. Barnard BB, McCoy SM. The supracondyloid process of the humerus. *J Bone Joint Surg [Am]* 1946;28:845–850.
622. Lund HJ. Fracture of the supracondyloid process of the humerus. Report of a case. *J Bone Joint Surg [Am]* 1930;12:925–928.
623. Newman A. The supracondylar process and its fracture. *Am J Roentgenol Radium Ther Nucl Med* 1969;105:844–849.
624. Casadei R, Ferraro A, Ferruzzi A, et al. Supracondylar process of the humerus: four cases. *Chir Organi Mov* 1990;75:265–277.
625. Haagedoorn EL. Fracture of the supracondylar humeral process. *Ned Tijdschr Geneeskd* 1968;112:313–316.

SECTION

THREE

SPINE

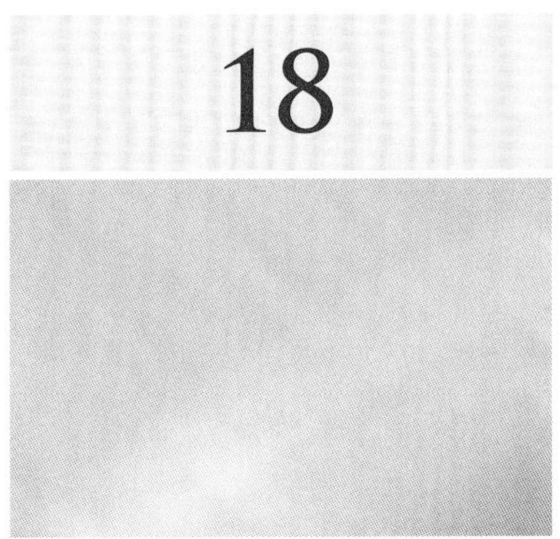

CERVICAL SPINE INJURIES IN CHILDREN

William C. Warner, Jr and Daniel J. Hedequist

Cervical spine fractures in children are rare, accounting for only 1% of pediatric fractures and 2% of all spinal injuries (1–11). The incidence is estimated to be 7.41 in 100,000 per year (12); however, that may be misleading because some injuries are not detected or are detected only at autopsy. Aufdermaur (13) examined the autopsied spines of 12 juveniles who had spinal injuries. All 12 had cartilage endplates that were separated from the vertebral bodies in the zone of columnar and calcified cartilage, similar to a Salter I fracture, although clinically and by x-ray a fracture was suggested in only 1 patient. Only x-rays at autopsy showed the disruption, represented by a small gap or apparent widening of the intervertebral space (13).

Cervical spine injuries in children younger than 8 years of age occur in the lower cervical spine, while older children and adolescents tend to have fractures involving either the upper or lower cervical spine (14). The upper cervical spine in children is more prone to injury because of the anatomic and biomechanical properties of the immature spine. The immature spine is hypermobile because of ligamentous laxity, and the facet joints are oriented in a more horizontal position; both of these properties predispose children to more forward translation. Younger children also have a relatively large head compared to the body, which changes the fulcrum of motion of the upper cervical spine. All of the factors predispose younger children to injuries of the upper cervical spine; with age, the anatomic changes lead to an increased prevalence of lower cervical spine injuries.

The mechanism of injury in pediatric patients also is age-related. Infants with cervical spine injuries should be evaluated for abuse (15). In children up to 9 years of age, the most common mechanism of injury is related to motor vehicle accidents; the second most common mechanism in this age group is falls (16,17). In older children and adolescents, the most common mechanism of cervical spine injuries is sporting activities, followed by motor vehicle accidents (16,18).

Cervical spine injuries associated with neurologic deficits are infrequent in children, and when incomplete there tends to be a better prognosis for recovery in children than in adults (19,20). Complete neurologic deficits, regardless of patient age, tend to have a poor prognosis for any recovery and may be indicative of the severity and magnitude of injury (21–24). Death from cervical spine injuries tends to be related to the level of injury and the associated injuries. Higher cervical spine injuries (i.e., atlanto-occipital dislocation) in younger children are associated with the highest mortality rate (25,26). Children with significant cervical spine injuries also may have associated severe head injuries, leading to an increase in mortality. In a study of 61 pediatric deaths related to spinal cord injuries, 89% of fatalities occurred at the scene, and most were related to high cervical cord injuries in patients who had sustained multiple injuries (27).

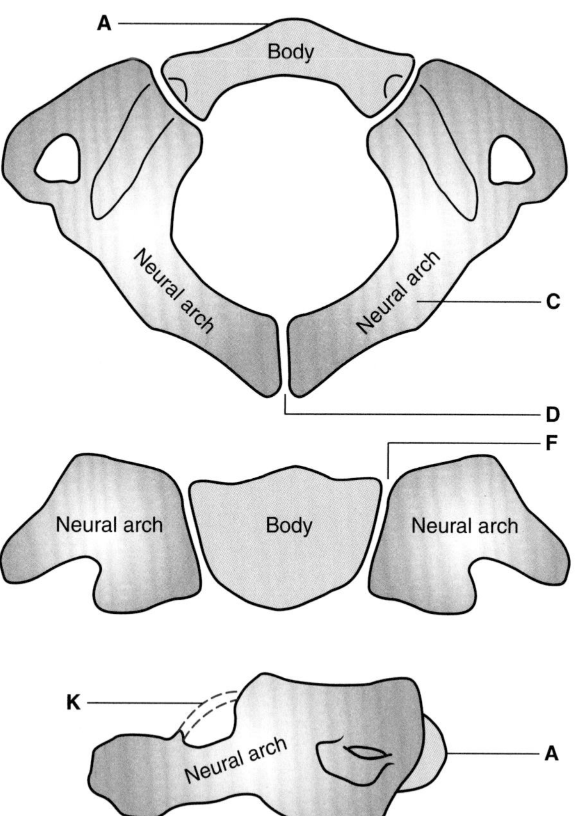

FIGURE 18-1 Diagram of C1 (atlas). The body (*A*) is not ossified at birth, and its ossification center appears during the first year of life. The body may fail to develop, and forward extension of neural arches (*C*) may take its place. Neural arches appear bilaterally about the 7th week (*D*), and the most anterior portion of the superior articulating surface usually is formed by the body. The synchondrosis of the spinous processes unites by the third year. Union rarely is preceded by the appearance of the secondary center within the synchondrosis. Neurocentral synchondrosis (*F*) fuses about the seventh year. The ligament surrounding the superior vertebral notch (*K*) may ossify, especially in later life. (Reprinted from Bailey DK. Normal cervical spine in infants and children. *Radiology* 1952;59:713–714; with permission.)

ANATOMY

Understanding the normal growth and development of the cervical spine is essential when treating a child with a suspected cervical spine injury. This will allow the physician to differentiate normal physes or synchondroses from pathologic fractures or ligamentous disruptions and will alert the physician to any possible congenital anomalies that may be mistaken for a fracture.

Upper Cervical Spine

At birth the atlas is composed of three ossification centers, one for the body and one for each of the neural arches (Fig. 18-1). The ossification center for the anterior arch is present in approximately 20% of individuals at birth, appearing in the remainder during the first year of life. Occasionally, the anterior arch is bifid, and the body may be formed from two centers or may fail to completely appear. The posterior arches usually fuse by the age of 3 years; however, occasionally the posterior synchondrosis between the two fails to fuse, resulting in a bifid arch. The neurocentral synchondroses that link the neural arches to the body are best seen on an open-mouth odontoid view. These synchondroses close by 7 years of age and should not be mistaken for fractures (28). The canal of the atlas is large to allow for the amount of rotation that occurs at this joint as well as some forward translation (29). The vertebral arteries are about 2 cm from the midline and run in a groove on the superior surface of the atlas. This must be remembered during lateral dissection at the occipital cervical junction. Because the ring of C1 reaches about normal adult size by 4 years of age, arthrodesis after this time should not cause spinal canal stenosis.

The axis develops from at least four separate ossification

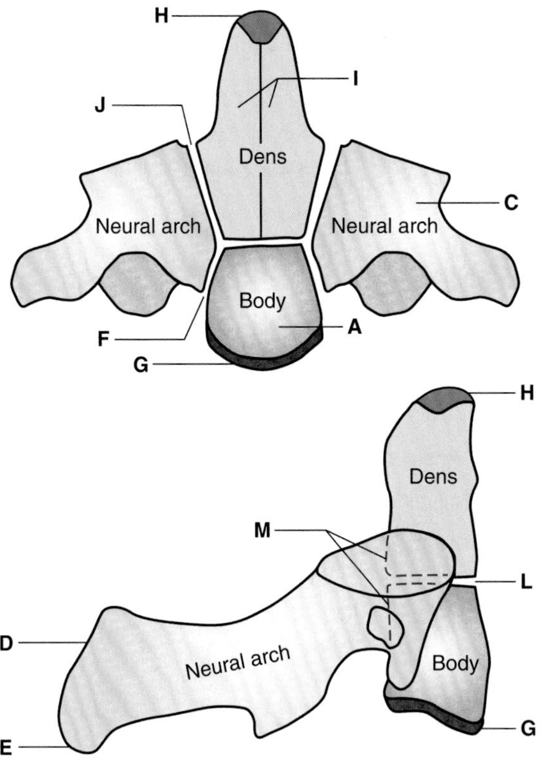

FIGURE 18-2 Diagram of C2 (axis). The body (*A*) in which one center (occasionally two) appears by the fifth fetal month. Neural arches (*C*) appear bilaterally by the seventh fetal month. Neural arches fuse (*D*) posteriorly by the second or third year. Bifid tip (*E*) of spinous process (occasionally a secondary center is present in each tip). Neurocentral synchondrosis (*F*) fuses at 3 to 6 years. The inferior epiphyseal ring (*G*) appears at puberty and fuses at about 25 years of age. The summit ossification center (*H*) for the odontoid appears at 3 to 6 years and fuses with the odontoid by 12 years. Odontoid (dens) (*I*). Two separate centers appear by the fifth fetal month and fuse with each other by the seventh fetal month. The synchondrosis between the odontoid and neural arch (*I*) fuses at 3 to 6 years. Synchondrosis between the odontoid and body (*L*) fuses at 3 to 6 years. Posterior surface of the body and odontoid (*M*). (Reprinted from Bailey DK. Normal cervical spine in infants and children. *Radiology* 1952;59:713–714; with permission.)

centers: one for the dens, one for the body, and two for the neural arches (Fig. 18-2). Between the odontoid and the body of the axis is a synchondrosis or vestigial disk space that often is mistaken for a fracture line. This synchondrosis runs well below the level of the articular processes of the axis and usually fuses at 6 to 7 years of age, although it may persist as a sclerotic line until 11 years of age (29). The most common odontoid fracture pattern in adults and adolescents is transverse and at the level of the articular processes. The normal synchondrosis should not be confused with this fracture; the synchondrosis is more cup-shaped and below the level of the articular processes. After 7 years of age, the synchondrosis should not be present on an open-mouth odontoid view; a fracture should be considered if a lucent line is present after this age. The neural arches of C2 fuse at 3 to 6 years of age; these are seen as vertical lucent lines on the open-mouth odontoid view. Occasionally, the tip of the odontoid is V-shaped (dens bicornum), or a small separate summit ossification center may be present at the tip of the odontoid (ossiculum terminale). An os odontoideum is believed to result from a history of unrecognized trauma. The differentiation between an os odontoideum and the synchondrosis of the body is relatively easy because of their relationships to the level of the C1-C2 facet (Fig. 18-3).

The arterial supply to the odontoid is derived from the vertebral and carotid arteries. The anterior and posterior ascending arteries arise from the vertebral artery at the level of C3 and ascend anterior and posterior to the odontoid, meeting superiorly to form an apical arcade. These arteries supply small penetrating branches to the body of the axis and the odontoid process. The internal carotid artery gives off cleft perforators that supply the superior portion of the odontoid. This arrangement of arteries and vessels is necessary for embryologic development and anatomic function of the odontoid. The synchondrosis prevents direct vascularization of the odontoid from C2, and vascularization from the blood supply of C1 is not possible because the synovial joint cavity surrounds the odontoid. The formation of an os odontoideum after cervical trauma may be related to this peculiar blood supply (Fig. 18-4).

Lower Cervical Spine

The third through seventh cervical vertebrae share a similar ossification pattern: a single ossification center for the vertebral body and an ossification center for each neural arch (Fig. 18-5). The neural arch fuses posteriorly between the second and third years, and the neurocentral synchondroses between the neural arches and the vertebral body fuse by 3 to 6 years of

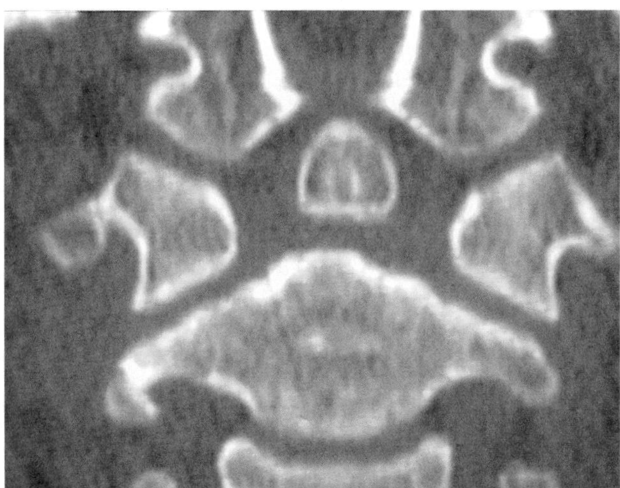

FIGURE 18-3 CT scan showing presence of an os odontoideum. Note the position of the os well above the C1-C2 facets. The scan also shows the vestigial scar of the synchondrosis between the dens and the body below the C1-C2 facet.

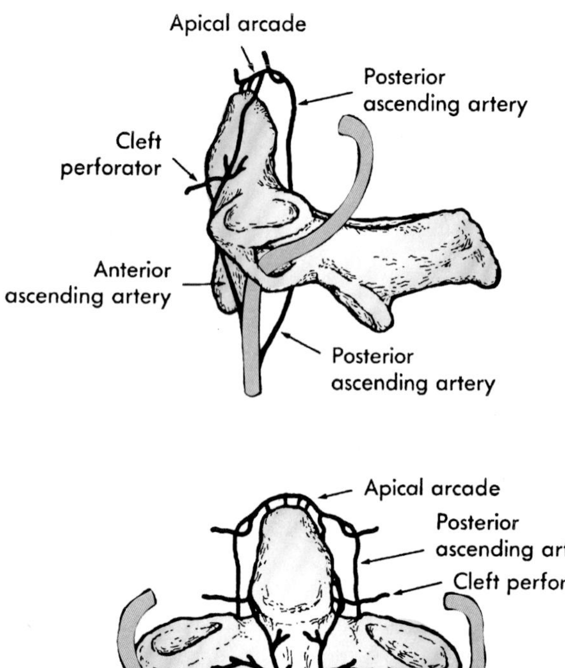

FIGURE 18-4 Blood supply to odontoid: posterior and anterior ascending arteries and apical arcade. (Reprinted from Schiff DC, Parke WW. The arterial supply of the odontoid process. *J Bone Joint Surg [Am]* 1973;55: 1450–1464; with permission.)

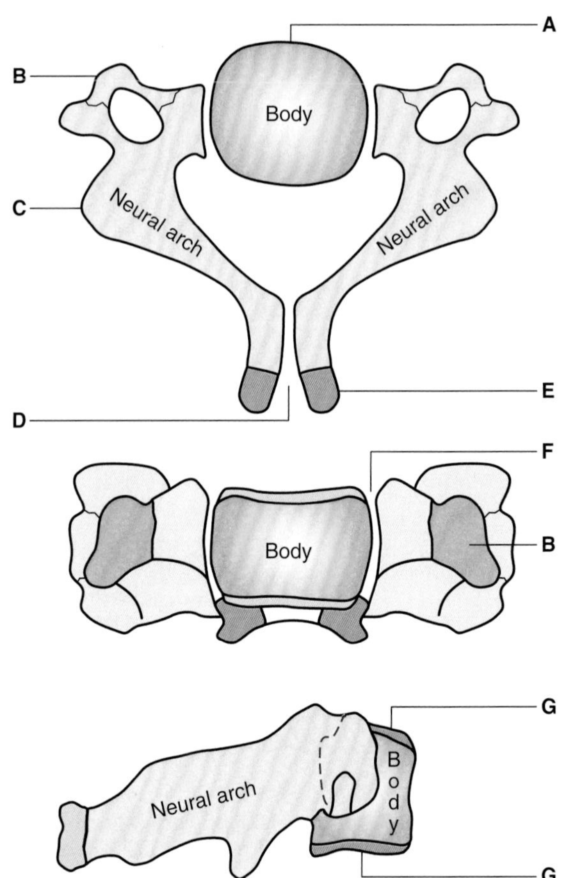

FIGURE 18-5 Diagram of typical cervical vertebrae, C3 to C7. The body (*A*) appears by the fifth fetal month. The anterior (costal) portion of the transverse process (*B*) may develop from a separate center that appears by the sixth fetal month and joins the arch by the sixth year. Neural arches (*C*) appear by the seventh to ninth fetal week. The synchondrosis between spinous processes (*D*) usually unites by the second or third year. Secondary centers for bifid spine (*E*) appear at puberty and unite with spinous process at 25 years. Neurocentral synchondrosis (*F*) fuses at 3 to 6 years. Superior and inferior epiphyseal rings (*G*) appear at puberty and unite with the body at about 25 years. The seventh cervical vertebra differs slightly because of a long, powerful, nonbifid spinous process. (Reprinted from Bailey DK. Normal cervical spine in infants and children. *Radiology* 1952;59:713–714; with permission.)

age. These vertebrae normally are wedge-shaped until 7 to 8 years of age (13,30,31). The vertebral bodies, neural arches, and pedicles enlarge by periosteal appositional growth, similar to that seen in long bones. By 8 to 10 years of age, a child's spine usually reaches near adult size and characteristics. There are five secondary ossification centers that can remain open until 25 years of age (30). These include one each for the spinous processes, transverse processes, and the ring apophyses about the vertebral endplates. These should not be confused with fractures.

The superior and inferior endplates are firmly bound to the adjacent disk. The junction between the vertebral body and the endplate is similar to a physis of a long bone. The vertebral body is analogous to the metaphysis and the endplate to the physis, where longitudinal growth occurs. The junction between the vertebral body and the endplate has been shown to be weaker than the adjacent vertebral body or disk, which can result in a fracture at the endplate in the area of columnar and calcified cartilage of the growth zone, similar to a Salter-Harris I fracture of a long bone (13). The inferior endplate may be more susceptible to this injury than the superior endplate because of the mechanical protection afforded by the developing uncinate processes (32).

The facet joints of the cervical spine change in orientation with age. The angle of the C1-C2 facet is 55 degrees in newborns and increases to 70 degrees at maturity. In the lower cervical spine, the angle of the facet joints is 30 degrees at birth and 60 to 70 degrees at maturity. This may explain why the pediatric cervical spine may be more susceptible to injury from the increased motion or translation allowed by the facet joint orientation.

Increased ligamentous laxity in young children allows a greater degree of spinal mobility than in adults. Flexion and extension of the spine at C2-C3 are 50% greater in children between the ages of 3 and 8 years than in adults. The level of the greatest mobility in the cervical spine descends with increasing age. Between 3 and 8 years of age the most mobile segment is C3-C4; from 9 to 11 years, C4-C5 is the most mobile segment, and from 12 to 15 years, C5-C6 is the most mobile segment (33,34). This explains the tendency for craniocervical injuries in the young children.

Several anomalies of the cervical spine may influence treatment recommendations. The atlas can fail to segment from the skull, a condition called occipitalization of the atlas, and can lead to narrowing of the foramen magnum, neurologic symptoms, and increased stresses to the atlantoaxial articulation, which often causes instability. Failure of fusion of the posterior arch of C1 is not uncommon and should be sought before any procedure that involves C1. Wedge-shaped vertebrae, bifid vertebrae, or a combination of these also can occur. Klippel-Feil syndrome consists of the classic triad of a short neck, low posterior hairline, and severe restriction of motion of the neck from fusion of the cervical vertebrae (35,36). Congenital fusion of the cervical spine may predispose a child to injury from trauma by concentrating stresses in the remaining mobile segments.

Hensinger et al (37) reported congenital anomalies of the odontoid, including aplasia (complete absence), hypoplasia (partial absence in which there is a stubby piece at the base of the odontoid located above the C1 articulation), and os odontoideum. Os odontoideum consists of a separate ossicle of the odontoid with no connection to the body of C2. The cause may be traumatic. These anomalies also may predispose a child to injury or instability.

HISTORY

Most cervical spine injuries in young children are the result of motor vehicle accidents, sporting injuries, or pedestrian injuries (38). Infants are at risk for cervical spine injuries during the obstetric period, as well as during early development because of their lack of head control; however, most cervical spine injuries in infants are spinal cord injury without radiologic abnormality (SCIWORA) and are related to child abuse (13). Younger children may sustain injuries to their neck from seemingly low-energy falls of less than 5 feet; however, most of their cervical spine injuries are sustained as a result of motor vehicle accidents (39,40). As children become adolescents the prevalence of sporting injuries increases, as does the prevalence of athletic-related SCIWORA (16,38). Regardless of the cause, an adequate history may be difficult to obtain at the initial evaluation, and repeat evaluations may be needed.

SYMPTOMS

The most common presenting symptom in patients with cervical spine injuries is pain localized to the cervical region. Other complaints, such as headache, inability to move the neck, subjective feelings of instability, and neurologic symptoms, all warrant complete evaluation. Infants may present with unexplained respiratory distress, motor weakness, or hypotonia, which warrant further evaluation. Patients with head and neck trauma, distracting injuries, or altered levels of consciousness are at high risk for a cervical spine injury and need to be thoroughly evaluated before obtaining cervical spine clearance (16). The presence of an occult cervical spine injury in an uncooperative or obtunded patient needs to be considered because of the frequency of SCIWORA in the pediatric population (9,10).

EVALUATION

The evaluation of any patient with a suspected cervical spine injury should begin with inspection. Head and neck trauma is associated with a high incidence of cervical spine injuries (13,33). Soft tissue abrasions or shoulder-harness marks on the neck from a seatbelt are clues to an underlying cervical spine injury (Fig. 18-6) (15,41,42). Unconscious patients should be treated as if they have a cervical spine injury until further evaluation proves otherwise. The next step in the evaluation is palpation of the cervical spine for tenderness, muscle spasm, and overall alignment. The most prominent levels should be the spinous processes at C2, C3, and C7. Anterior palpation should focus on the presence of tenderness or swelling. The entire spine should be palpated and thoroughly examined because 20% of patients with cervical spine injuries have other spinal fractures.

A thorough neurologic examination should be done, which can be difficult in pediatric patients. Strength, sensation, reflexes, and proprioception should be documented. In patients who are uncooperative because of age or altered mental status, repeat examinations are important; however, the initial neuro-

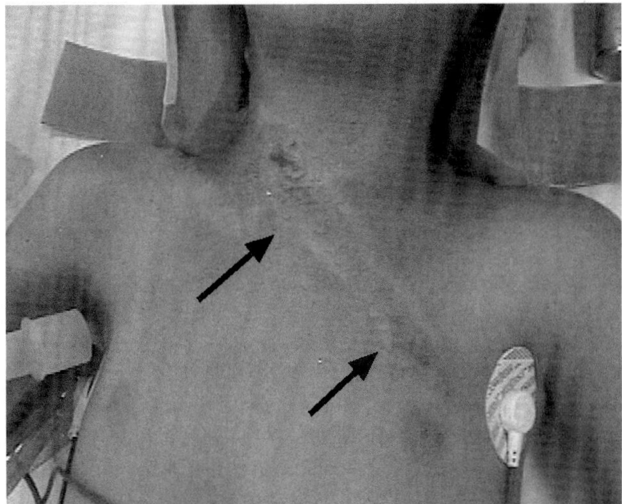

FIGURE 18-6 Clinical photograph of a patient with a cervical spine injury resulting from impact with the shoulder harness of a seat belt. Note location of skin contusions from the seat belt.

vascular examination should be documented even it if entails only gross movements of the extremities. The evaluation of rectal sphincter tone, bulbocavernosus reflex, and perianal sensation are important, especially in obtunded patients and patients with partial or complete neurologic injuries, regardless of age. Patients who are cooperative and awake can be asked to perform supervised flexion, extension, lateral rotation, and lateral tilt. Uncooperative or obtunded patients should not have any manipulation of the neck.

X-RAY EVALUATION

Plain X-Rays

Plain x-rays remain the standard for evaluating the cervical spine in children. There currently is no consensus regarding whether or not all pediatric trauma patients require cervical spine films. The presence of tenderness and a distracting injury are the most common clinical presentations of a cervical spine injury (43). While some studies have shown that plain x-rays are of low yield in patients without evidence of specific physical findings, the burden remains on the treating physician to clear the cervical spine (44–47). Clearly, patients with tenderness, distracting injuries, neurologic deficits, head and neck trauma, and altered levels of consciousness need to have a complete set of cervical spine x-rays. Initial x-rays should include an anteroposterior view, open-mouth odontoid view, and lateral view of the cervical spine. Patients who are deemed unstable in the emergency room and are not able to tolerate multiple x-rays should have a cross-table lateral view of the cervical spine until further x-rays can be taken. The false-negative rates for a single cross-table x-ray have been reported to be 23% to 26%, indicating that complete x-rays are necessary when the patient is stable (48,49).

Flexion and extension x-rays may further aid the evaluation of the cervical spine, but these views are unlikely to be abnormal when standard views show no abnormalities. These views are helpful, however, in ruling out acute ligamentous injury (50). We recommend flexion and extension views in an alert patient with midline tenderness who has normal plain films of the cervical spine. These views must be taken only with a cooperative and alert child; they should not be used in obtunded or uncooperative patients, nor should they be done by manually placing the child in a position of flexion and extension.

Evaluation of cervical spine x-rays should proceed with a knowledge of the anatomic ossification centers and variations that occur in children. Each vertebral level should be systematically evaluated, as should the overall alignment of the cervical spine with respect to the anterior and posterior aspects of the vertebral bodies, the spinolaminar line, and the interspinous distances. The absence of cervical lordosis, an increase in the prevertebral soft tissue space, and subluxation of C2 on C3 are all anatomic variations that may be normal in children (28). Ossification centers also may be confused with fractures, most commonly in evaluation of the dens. The presence of a synchondrosis at the base of the odontoid can be distinguished from a fracture based on the age of the patient and the location of synchondrosis well below the facet joints. Knowledge of these normal variants is useful in evaluating plain x-rays of the cervical spine in children (Table 18-1).

X-Ray Evaluation of Specific Areas of the Spine

Atlanto-Occipital Junction

The atlanto-occipital interval remains the most difficult to assess for abnormalities, partly because of the difficulty in obtaining quality x-rays and partly because of the lack of discrete and reproducible landmarks. The distance between the occipital condyles and the facet joints of the atlas should be less than 5 mm; any distance of more than this suggests an atlanto-occipital disruption (34,51). The foramen magnum and its relationship to the atlas also are useful in detecting injuries of the atlanto-occipital region. The anterior cortical margin of the foramen magnum is termed the basion, while the posterior cortical margin of the foramen magnum is termed the opisthion. The distance between the basion and the tip of the dens should be less

TABLE 18-1 Normal Ossification Centers and Anomalies Frequently Confused with Injury

Avulsion fracture
- Apical ossification center of the odontoid
- Secondary ossification centers at the tips of the transverse and spinous processes

Fracture
- Persistence of the synchondrosis at the base of the odontoid
- Apparent anterior wedging of a young child's vertebral body
- Normal posterior angulation of the odontoid seen in 4% of normal children

Instability
- Pseudosubluxation of C2-C3
- Incomplete ossification, especially of the odontoid process, with apparent superior subluxation of the anterior arch of C1
- Absence of the ossification center of the anterior arch of C1 in the first year of life may suggest posterior displacement of C1 on the odontoid
- Increase in the atlanto–dens interval of up to 4.5 mm

Miscellaneous
- Physiologic variations in the width of the prevertebral soft tissue due to crying misinterpreted as swelling due to edema or hemorrhage
- Overlying structures such as ears, braided hair, teeth, or hyoid bone. Plastic rivets used in modern emergency cervical immobilization collars can simulate fracture line.
- Horizontally placed facets in the younger child, creating the illusion of a pillar fracture
- Congenital anomalies such as os odontoideum, spina bifida, and congenital fusion or hemivertebrae

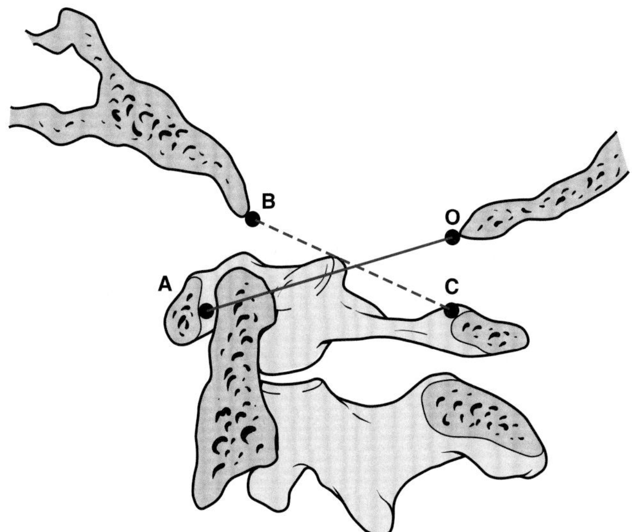

FIGURE 18-7 The Powers ratio is determined by drawing a line from the basion (*B*) to the posterior arch of the atlas (*C*) and a second line from the opisthion (*O*) to the anterior arch of the atlas (*A*). The length of the line BC is divided by the length of the line OA, producing the Powers ratio. (Reprinted from Lebwohl NH, Eismont FJ. Cervical spine injuries in children. In: Weinstein SL, ed. *The pediatric spine: principles and practice.* New York: Raven, 1994; with permission.)

than 12 mm as measured on a lateral x-ray (52). The Powers ratio (Fig. 18-7) is used to assess the position of the skull base relative to the atlas and is another way of evaluating the atlanto-occipital region. To determine this ratio, a line is drawn from the basion to the anterior cortex of the posterior arch of C1, and this distance is divided by the distance of a line drawn from the opisthion to the posterior cortex of the anterior arch of C1. The value should be between 0.7 and 1; a higher value indicates anterior subluxation of the atlanto-occipital joint and a lower value indicates a posterior subluxation. The problem lies in the fact that the basion is not always visible on plain x-rays. The Wackenheim line, which is drawn along the posterior aspect of the clivus, probably is the most easily identified line to determine disruption of the atlanto-occipital joint. If the line does not intersect the tip of the odontoid tangentially and if this line is displaced anteriorly or posteriorly, disruption or increased laxity about the atlanto-occipital joint should be suspected.

Atlantoaxial Joint

The atlanto–dens interval (ADI) and the space available for the spinal canal (SAC) are two useful measurements for evaluation of the atlantoaxial joint (Fig. 18-8). The ADI in a child is considered normal up to 4.5 mm, partly because the unossified cartilage of the odontoid, which is not seen on plain films, gives an apparent increase in the interval. At the level of the atlantoaxial joint, the space taken up is broken into Steel's rule of thirds: one third is taken up by the odontoid, one third by

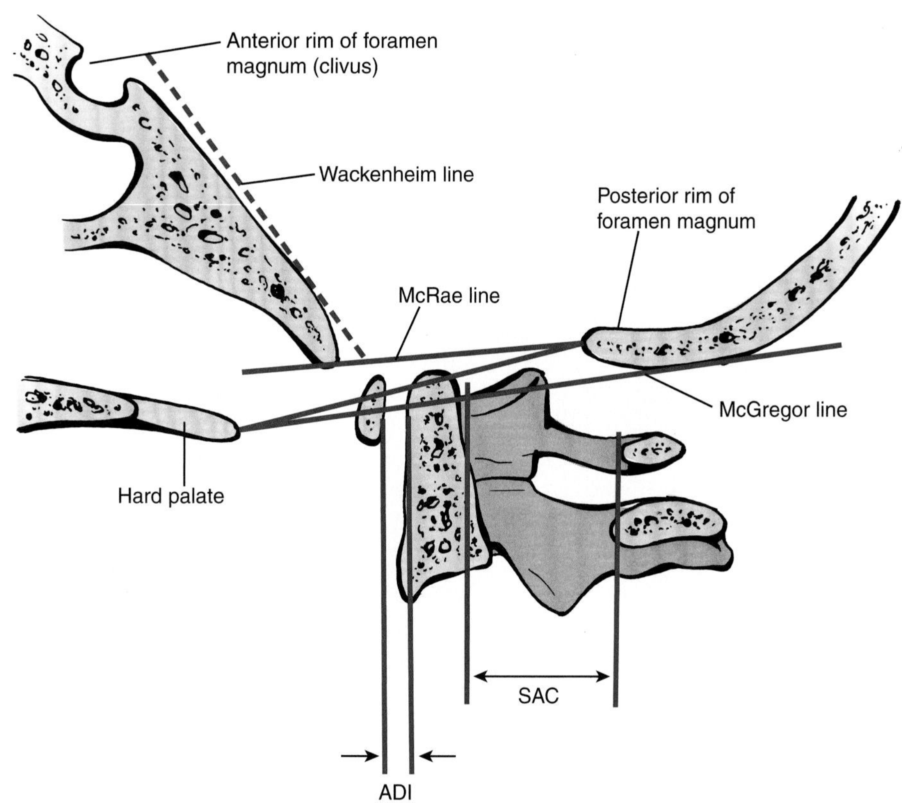

FIGURE 18-8 The atlantodens interval (ADI) and the space available for cord (SAC) are used in determining atlantoaxial instability. The Wackenheim clivus-canal line is used to determine atlantooccipital injury, while the McRae and McGregor lines are used in the measurement of basilar impression. (Reprinted from Copley LA, Dormans JP. Cervical spine disorders in infants and children. *J Am Acad Orthop Surg* 1998;6:204–214; with permission.)

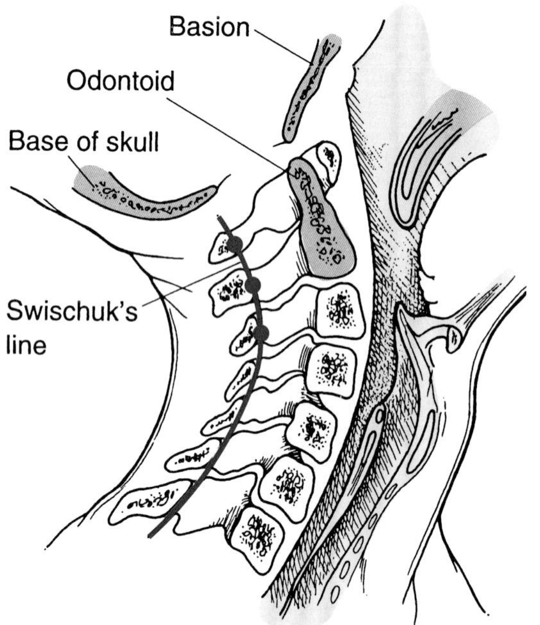

FIGURE 18-9 The spinolaminar line (Swischuk line) is used to determine the presence of pseudosubluxation of C2 on C3. (Reprinted from Copley LA, Dormans JP. Cervical spine disorders in infants and children. *J Am Acad Orthop Surg* 1998;6:201–214; with permission.)

the spinal cord, and one third is space available for the cord. These intervals also are easily measured on flexion and extension views and are helpful in determining instability. In children, extension views give the appearance of subluxation of the anterior portion of the atlas over the unossified dens, but this represents a pseudosubluxation and not instability (29,53).

Upper Cervical Spine

Anterior displacement of one vertebral body on another may or may not indicate a true bony or ligamentous injury. Displacement of less than 3 mm at one level is a common anatomic variant in children at the levels of C2-C3 and C3-C4. This displacement is seen on flexion x-rays and reduces in extension. The posterior line of Swischuk (54) has been described to differentiate pathologic subluxation from normal anatomic variation; this line is drawn from the anterior cortex of the spinous process of C1 to the spinous process of C3 (Fig. 18-9). The anterior cortex of the spinous process of C2 should lie within 3 mm of this line; if the distance is more than this, a true subluxation should be suspected (Fig. 18-10). Widening of the spinous processes between C1 and C2 of more than 10 mm also is indicative of a ligamentous injury and should be evaluated by further imaging studies (55).

Lower Cervical Spine

Lateral x-rays of the cervical spine should be evaluated for overall alignment as well as at each level. The overall alignment can be evaluated by the continuous lines formed by the line adjoining the spinous processes, the spinolaminar line, and the lines adjoining the posterior and anterior vertebral bodies (Fig. 18-11). These lines should all be smooth and continuous with

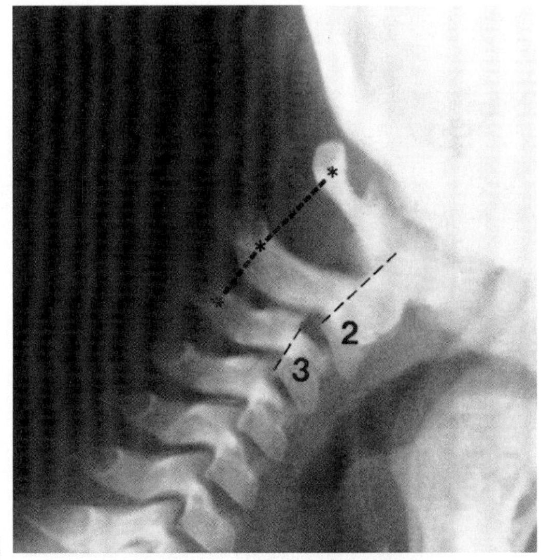

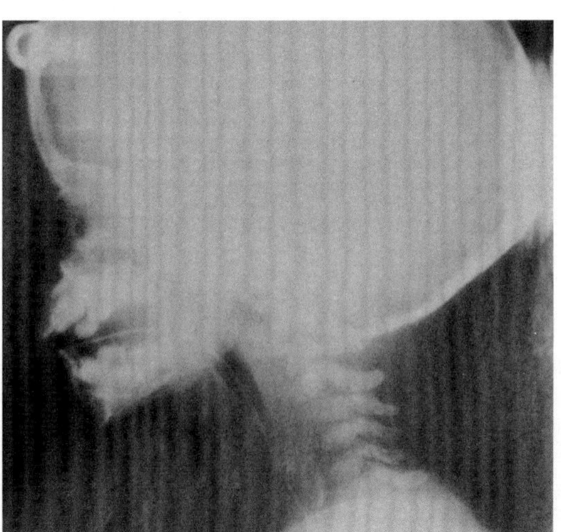

FIGURE 18-10 **A.** Pseudosubluxation of C2 on C3. **B.** True subluxation. In flexion the posterior element of C2 should normally align itself with the posterior elements C1 and C3. The relationship of the body of C2 with the body of C3 gives the appearance of subluxation; however, the alignment of the posterior elements of C1-C3 confirms pseudosubluxation.

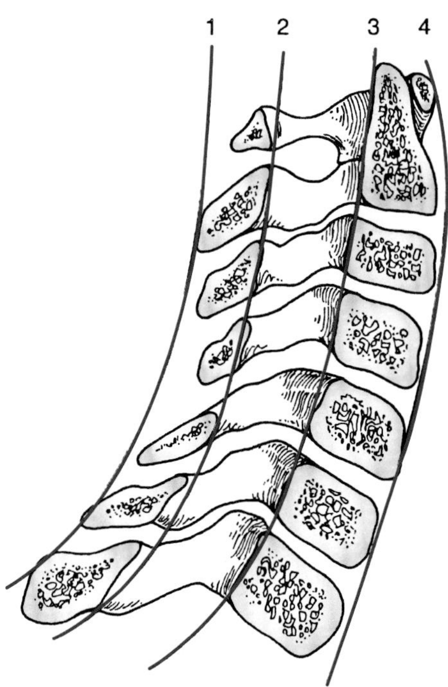

FIGURE 18-11 Normal relationships in the lateral cervical spine: *1,* spinous processes; *2,* spinolaminar line; *3,* posterior vertebral body line; *4,* anterior vertebral body line. (Reprinted from Copley LA, Dormans JP. Cervical spine disorders in infants and children. *J Am Acad Orthop Surg* 1998; 6:204–214; with permission.)

no evidence of vertebral translation at any level. Loss of normal cervical lordosis may be normal in children, but there should be no associated translation at any level (56). The interspinous distance at each level should be evaluated and should be no more than 1.5 times the distance at adjacent levels; if this ratio is greater, an injury should be suspected. There are calculated norms for the interspinous distances in children, and any value greater than two standard deviations above normal is indicative of a ligamentous injury (57). The measurement of soft tissue spaces is important in evaluating any evidence of swelling or hemorrhage, which may be associated with an occult injury. The normal retropharyngeal soft tissue space should be less than 6 mm at C3 and less than 14 mm at C6. These spaces may be increased in children without an injury who are crying at the time of the x-ray, because the attachment of the pharynx to the hyoid bone results in its forward displacement with crying, producing an apparent increase in the width of these spaces. These x-rays must be taken with the patient quiet and repeated if there is any doubt.

Special Imaging Studies

Most cervical spine injuries in children are detected by plain x-rays (1). Most ligamentous injuries can be identified on flexion and extension views of the cervical spine in a cooperative and alert patient. The roles of computed tomography (CT) scanning and magnetic resonance imaging (MRI) continue to evolve in the evaluation of trauma patients.

When CT scanning is used in children, a few salient points should be kept in mind. First, the proportion of a child's head to his or her body is greater than that of an adult, so care must be taken not to position the head in flexion to obtain the scan. Inadvertent flexion may potentiate any occult fracture not seen on plain films. Second, the radiation doses for CT scanning are significantly higher than for plain x-rays. CT protocols for children should be used to limit the amount of radiation that the head and neck receive during scanning of the cervical spine. While axial views are standard, coronal and sagittal reformatted images and three-dimensional reconstruction views provide improved anatomic details of the spine and can be obtained without any additional radiation to the patient (58). In patients with head injuries, CT scanning of the cervical spine can be done at the time of CT scanning of the head to reduce the number of plain films that may be required to document that there is not a neck injury (59). However, plain x-rays remain the standard for initial evaluation of the pediatric cervical spine; CT scanning as an initial imaging study is associated with an increase in radiation with no demonstrable benefit over plain films (60).

MRI has become increasingly useful in evaluating pediatric patients with suspected cervical spine injuries (Fig. 18-12), especially for ruling out ligamentous injuries in patients who cannot cooperate with flexion and extension views (61). The advantages of an early MRI are the ability to allow mobilization if no injury is present and the early detection of an unrecognized spinal fracture to allow proper treatment. MRI also is useful in

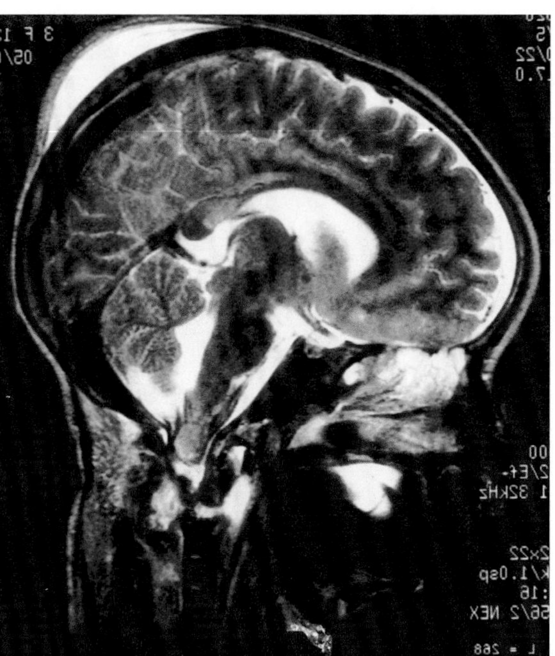

FIGURE 18-12 MRI depicts injury to the cervical cord and upper cervical spine.

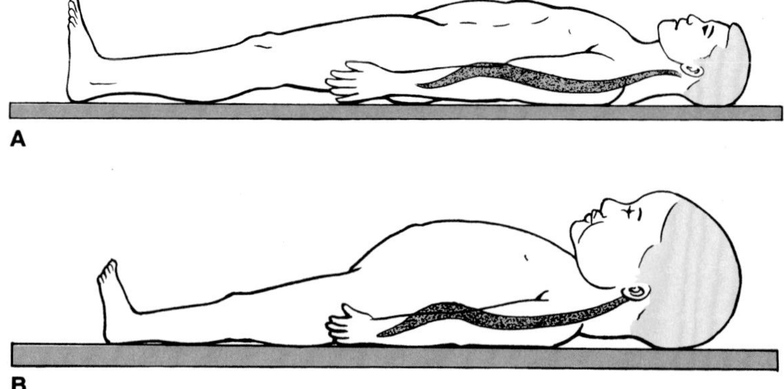

FIGURE 18-13 **A.** Adult immobilized on a standard backboard. **B.** Young child on a standard backboard. The relatively large head forces the neck into a kyphotic position. (Reprinted from Herzenberg JE, Hensinger RN, Dedrick DK, et al. Emergency transport and positioning of young children who have an injury of the cervical spine: the standard backboard may be hazardous. *J Bone Joint Surg [Am]* 1989;71:15–22; with permission.)

evaluating patients with SCIWORA. MR angiography has replaced standard arteriography for evaluation of the vertebral arteries in patients with upper cervical spine injuries who have suspected arterial injuries (62). MRI also remains the best imaging modality for evaluating injuries of the intervertebral disks and is especially useful to detect disk herniation in adolescent patients with facet joint injuries that may require operative reduction.

INITIAL MANAGEMENT OF CERVICAL SPINE INJURIES

The initial management of any child suspected of having a cervical spine injury starts with immobilization in the field. Extraction from an automobile or transport to the hospital may cause damage to the spinal cord in a child with an unstable cervical spine injury if care is not taken to properly immobilize the neck. The immobilization device should allow access to the patient's oropharynx and anterior neck if intubation or tracheostomy becomes necessary. The device should allow splintage of the head and neck to the thorax to minimize further movement.

The use of backboards in pediatric trauma patients deserves special attention because of the anatomic differences between children and adults. Compared to adults, children have a disproportionately larger head with respect to the body. This anatomic relationship causes a child's cervical spine to be placed in flexion if immobilization is done on a standard backboard. Herzenberg et al (63) reported 10 children under the age of 7 years whose cervical spines had anterior angulation or translation on x-ray when they were placed on a standard backboard. The use of a backboard with a recess so that the head can be lowered into it to obtain a neutral position of the cervical spine is one way to avoid unnecessary flexion. Another is a split-mattress technique in which the body is supported by two mattresses and the head is supported by one mattress, allowing the cervical spine to assume a neutral position. Children younger than 8 years of age should be immobilized on a backboard using one of these techniques (Figs. 18-13 and 18-14) (64).

Cervical collars supplement backboards for immobilization in the trauma setting. While soft collars tend to be more comfortable and cause less soft tissue irritation, rigid collars are preferred for patients with acute injuries because they provide better immobilization. Even rigid collars may allow up to 17 degrees of flexion, 19 degrees of extension, 4 degrees of rotation, and 6 degrees of lateral motion (65,66). Supplemental sandbags

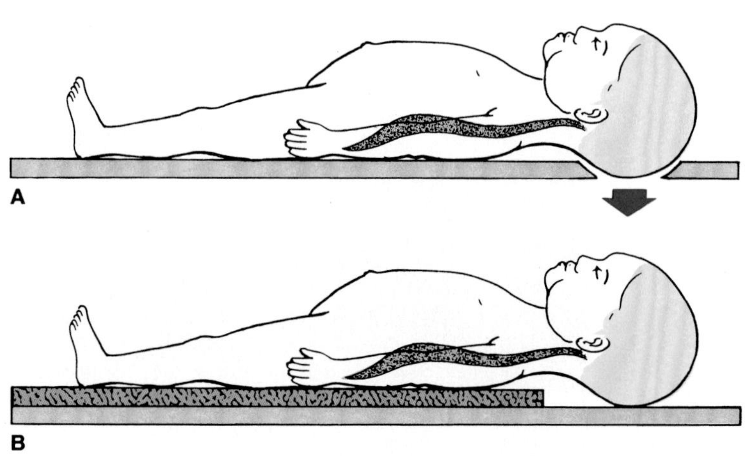

FIGURE 18-14 **A.** Young child on a modified backboard that has a cutout to the recess of the occiput, obtaining better supine cervical alignment. **B.** Young child on modified backboard that has a double-mattress pad to raise the chest, obtaining better supine cervical alignment. (Reprinted from Herzenberg JE, Hensinger RN, Dedrick DK, et al. Emergency transport and positioning of young children who have an injury of the cervical spine: the standard backboard may be hazardous. *J Bone Joint Surg [Am]* 1989;71:15–22; with permission.)

and taping on either side of the head are recommended in all children and have been shown to limit the amount of spinal motion to 3 degrees in any plane (39).

Further displacement of an unstable cervical injury may occur if resuscitation is required. The placement of pediatric patients on an appropriate board with the neck in a neutral position makes recognition of some fractures difficult because positional reduction may have occurred, especially with ligamentous injuries or endplate fractures. An apparently normal lateral x-ray in a patient with altered mental status or multiple injuries does not rule out a cervical spine injury. A study of four patients with unstable cervical spine injuries who had attempted resuscitation in the emergency department showed that axial traction actually increased the deformity (32). Any manipulation of the cervical spine, even during intubation, must be done with caution and with the assumption that the patient has an unstable cervical spine injury until proven otherwise.

Immobilization of the cervical spine may continue after the emergency setting if there is an injury that requires treatment. Specific injuries and their treatment are described later in this chapter. Further immobilization of some cervical spine injuries requires a cervical collar. A rigid collar can be used for immobilization if it is an appropriately fitting device with more padding than a standard cervical collar placed in the emergency department. More unstable or significant injuries can be treated with a custom orthosis, a Minerva cast, or a halo device. An advantage of custom devices is the ability to use lightweight thermoplastic materials that can be molded better to each patient's anatomy and can be extended to the thorax (Fig. 18-15). These devices must be properly applied for effective immobilization, and skin breakdown, especially over the chin region, needs to be carefully monitored. Minerva casts tend to provide more immobilization than thermoplastic devices, but their use is not as common and their application requires attention to detail.

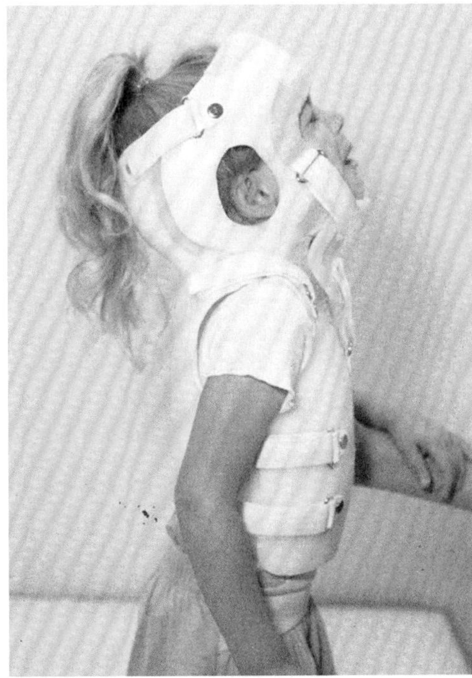

FIGURE 18-15 Custom-made cervicothoracic brace used to treat a C2 fracture that reduced in extension.

A halo device can be used for the treatment of cervical spine injuries even in children as young as 1 year old. The halo can be used as either a ring alone to apply traction or with a vest for definitive immobilization of an unstable cervical spine injury. The complication rate related to the use of a halo in one series of patients was 68%; however, all patients were able to wear the halo until fracture healing occurred or arthrodesis (67). The most common complications in this series were superficial pin track infection and pin loosening. Other complications that occur less frequently include dural penetration, supraorbital nerve injury, unsightly pin scars, and deep infection (67,68). Prefabricated halo vests are used in adults and are easily fitted to older adolescents. Because of the age and size ranges of children, however, a custom vest or even a cast vest may be needed. Prefabricated vests are available in sizes for infants, toddlers, and children, with measurements based on the circumference of the chest at the xiphoid process. Improper fitting of a vest may allow unwanted movement of the neck despite the halo, and any size mismatch requires a custom vest or cast vest (Fig. 18-16).

The fabrication of a halo for any patient needs to consider both the size of the ring and the size of the vest. Prefabricated rings and prefabricated vests are available for even for the smallest of patients and are based on circumferential measurements at the crown and at the xiphoid process. If the size of the patient or the anatomy of the patient does not fit within these standard sizes, the fabrication of a custom halo may be necessary. Mu-

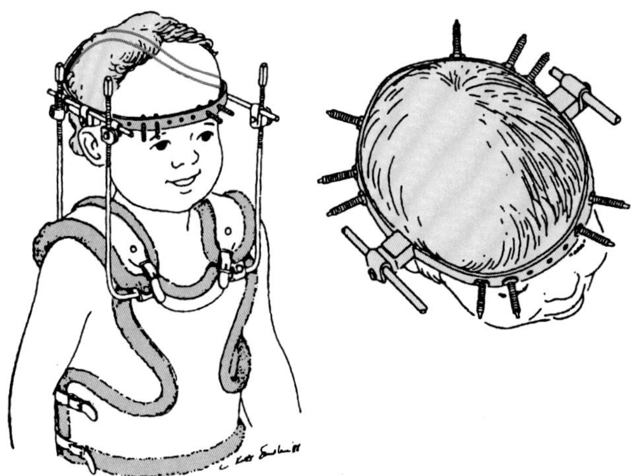

FIGURE 18-16 **A.** Custom halo vest and superstructure. **B.** In the multiple-pin, low-torque technique, 10 pins are used for an infant halo ring attachment. Usually, four pins are placed anteriorly, avoiding the temporal region, and the remaining six pins are placed in the occipital area. (Reprinted from Mubarak SJ, Camp JF, Fuletich W, et al. Halo application in the infant. *J Pediatr Orthop* 1989;9:612–613; with permission.)

barak et al (69) recommended the following steps in the fabrication of a custom halo for a child: (a) The size and configuration of the head are obtained with the use of the flexible lead wire placed around the head, (b) the halo ring is fabricated by constructing a ring 2 cm larger in diameter than the wire model, (c) a plaster mold of the trunk is obtained for the manufacture of a custom bivalved polypropylene vest, and (d) linear measurements are made to ensure appropriate length of the superstructure.

The placement of pins into an immature skull deserves special attention because of the dangers of inadvertent skull penetration with a pin. CT scanning before halo application aids in determining bone structure and skull thickness. It also aids in determining whether or not cranial suture interdigitation is complete and if the fontanels are closed. The thickness of the skull varies greatly up to 6 years of age and is not similar to that of adults until the age of 16 years (47). Garfin et al (70) evaluated the pediatric cranium by CT and determined that the skull is thickest anterolaterally and posterolaterally, making these the optimal sites for pin placement.

The number of pins used for placement of a ring and the insertion torques used in younger children also deserve special mention. The placement of pins at the torque pressures used in adults will lead to penetration during insertion (47). Pins should be inserted at torques of 2 to 4 inch-pounds; however, the variability and reliability of pressures found with various torque wrenches during cadaver testing are great, and each pin must be inserted cautiously (71). The use of 8 to 12 pins inserted at lower torque pressures aids in obtaining a stable ring with less chance of inadvertent penetration (Fig. 18-17). The insertion of each pin perpendicular to the skull also improves the pin–bone interface and the overall strength of the construct (72). We have had success using halo vests even in children younger than 2 years of age by using multiple pins inserted to finger-tightness rather than relying on torque wrenches.

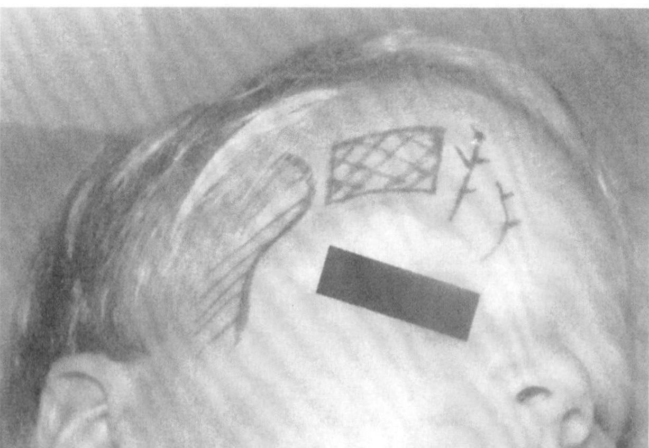

FIGURE 18-17 Shaded area represents the "safe zone" for pin placement, avoiding the supraorbital and supratrochlear nerves anteriorly and the temporalis posteriorly. (Reprinted from Crawford H. Traction. In: Weinstein SL, ed. *Pediatric spine surgery*, 2nd ed. Philadelphia: Lippincott Williams & Wilkins, 2001; with permission.)

Technique of Halo Application

A halo can be applied in older children and adolescents with a local anesthetic; however, in most younger children a general anesthetic should be used. The patient is positioned on the operating table in a position that prevents unwanted flexion of the neck and maintains the proper relationship of the head and neck with the trunk. The area of skin in the region of pin insertion is cleaned with antiseptic solution and appropriate areas are shaved as needed for pin placement posteriorly. The ring is placed while an assistant holds the patient's head; it should be placed just below the greatest circumference of the skull, which corresponds to just above the eyebrows anteriorly and 1 cm above the tips of the earlobes laterally. We recommend injection of local anesthetic into the skin and periosteum through the ring holes in which the pins will be placed. The pins are placed with sterile technique.

To optimize pin placement, a few points should be kept in mind. The thickest area of the skull is anterolaterally and posterolaterally, and pins inserted at right angles to the bone have greater force distribution and strength (70,72). Anterior pins should be placed to avoid the anterior position of the supraorbital and supratrochlear nerves (Fig. 18-18). Placement of the anterior pins too far laterally will lead to penetration of the temporalis muscle, which can lead to pain with mastication and talking, as well as early pin loosening. The optimal position for the anterior pins is in the anterolateral skull, just above the lateral two thirds of the orbit and just below the greatest circumference of the skull. The posterior pins are best placed posterolaterally directly diagonal from the anterior pins. We also recommend placing the pins to finger-tightness originally and tightening two directly opposing pins simultaneously. During placement of the pins, meticulous attention should be paid to the position of the ring in order to have a circumferential fit on the patient's skull and to avoid any pressure of the ring on the scalp, especially posteriorly.

The number of pins used and the torque pressures applied vary according to the age of the patient. In infants and younger children, we recommend the placement of multiple pins (8 to 12) tightened to finger-tightness or 2 to 4 inch-pounds to avoid unwanted skull penetration. In older children, six to eight pins are used and tightened to 4 inch-pounds. In general, in adolescents four to eight pins can be tightened with a standard torque wrench to 6 to 8 inch-pounds. Once the pins are tightened, they must be fastened to the ring by the appropriate lock nuts or set screws. The halo vest and superstructure are then applied, with care to maintain the position of the head and neck. Appropriate positioning of the head and neck can be done by adjusting the superstructure (see Fig. 18-18).

Daily pin care should consist of hydrogen peroxide/saline cleaning at the pin–skin interface. Retightening of pins at 48 hours should be avoided in infants and children to prevent skull penetration; however, in adolescents the pins can be retightened

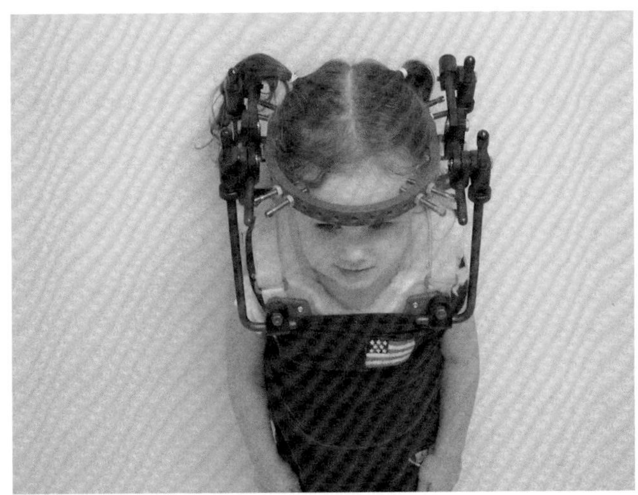

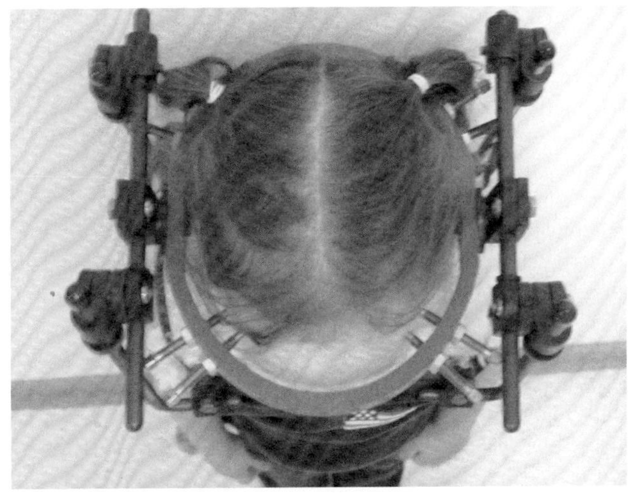

FIGURE 18-18 Child immobilized in a halo for C1-C2 rotary subluxation. Note the position of the anterior pins, as well as the placement of the posterior pins at 180 degrees opposite the anterior pins.

at 48 hours with a standard torque wrench. Local erythema or drainage may occur about the pins and can be managed with oral antibiotics and continued pin site care. If significant loosening occurs or the infection is more serious, the pin or pins should be removed. Occasionally, a dural puncture occurs during pin insertion or during the course of treatment. This necessitates pin removal and prophylactic antibiotics until the tear heals, usually at 4 to 5 days.

SPINAL CORD INJURY WITHOUT RADIOGRAPHIC ABNORMALITIES

Spinal cord injury without radiographic abnormalities (SCIWORA), a syndrome first brought to the attention of the medical community by Pang and Wilberger (9), is unique to children. This condition is defined as a spinal cord injury in a patient with no visible fracture or dislocation on plain x-rays, tomograms, or CT scans.

A complete or incomplete spinal cord lesion may be present, and the injury usually results from severe flexion or distraction of the cervical spine. SCIWORA is believed to occur because the spinal column (vertebrae and disk space) in children is more elastic than the spinal cord and can undergo considerable deformation without being disrupted (73,74). The spinal column can elongate up to 2 inches without disruption, whereas the spinal cord ruptures with only a quarter-inch of elongation.

SCIWORA also may represent an ischemic injury in some patients, although most are believed to be due to a distraction-type injury in which the spinal cord has not tolerated the degree of distraction but the bony ligamentous elements have not failed. Aufdermaur suggested another possibility (13): a fracture through a pediatric vertebral endplate reduces spontaneously (much like a Salter I fracture), giving a normal x-ray appearance, although the initial displacement could have caused spinal cord injury.

SCIWORA abnormalities are more common in children under 8 years of age than in older children (9,10,56,75), perhaps because of predisposing factors such as cervical spine hypermobility, ligamentous laxity, and an immature vascular supply to the spinal cord. The reported incidence of this condition varies from 7% to 66% of patients with cervical spine injuries (9,14,76).

Delayed onset of neurologic symptoms has been reported in as many as 52% of patients in some series (9,77). Pang and Pollock reported 15 patients who had delayed paralysis after their injuries (14). Nine had transient warning signs such as paresthesia or subjective paralysis. In all patients with delayed onset of paralysis, the spine had not been immobilized after the initial trauma, and all were neurologically normal before the second event. This underlines the importance of diligent immobilization of a suspected spinal cord injury in a child. Approximately half of the young children with SCIWORA in reported series had complete spinal cord injuries, whereas the older children usually had incomplete neurologic deficit injuries that involved the subaxial cervical spine (13,77–79).

Careful x-ray evaluation is helpful in the workup of these patients, but MRI will show a spinal cord lesion that often is some distance from the vertebral column injury. As many as 5% to 10% of children with spinal cord injuries have normal x-ray results (3,80).

SPINAL CORD INJURY IN CHILDREN

Spinal cord injuries are still rare in children. Rang reviewed spinal injuries at the Toronto Hospital for Sick Children over 15 years and found that children constituted a small percentage of the patients with acquired quadriplegia or paraplegia (81). He found that paraplegia was three times more common than quadriplegia. When a spinal cord injury is suspected, the neurologic examination must be complete and meticulous and may take several examinations of sensory and motor function. If an acute spinal cord injury is documented by examination, the administration of methylprednisolone within the first 8 hours after injury has been shown to improve the chances of neurologic recovery (82–85). Methylprednisolone in the treatment of acute spinal cord injuries has been shown to improve motor and sensory recovery when evaluated 6 weeks and 6 months after injury (84); however, this positive effect on neurologic recovery is limited to those treated within the first 8 hours of injury. The initial loading dose of methylprednisolone is 30 mg/kg body weight. If the loading dose is given within 3 hours after injury, then a maintenance infusion of 5.4 mg/kg is given for 24 hours after injury. If the loading dose is given between 3 and 8 hours after injury, then a maintenance infusion of 5.4 mg/kg is given for 48 hours after injury. Methylprednisolone decreases edema, has an anti-inflammatory effect, and protects the cell membranes from scavenging oxygen free radicals (82–85).

In several series (82–85) there was a slight increase in the incidence of wound infections but no significant increase in gastrointestinal bleeding. All of these studies involved patients 13 years or older, so no documentation of the efficacy in young children exists. A combination of methylprednisolone and GM1 ganglioside is being studied for its possible beneficial effect on an injured spinal cord (86–89). GM1 is a complex acid-like lipid found at high levels in the cell membrane of the central nervous system that is thought to have a neuroprotective and neurofunctional restorative potential. Early studies have shown that patients given both drugs had improved recovery over those who had received just methylprednisolone.

Once spinal cord injury is documented, routine care includes prophylaxis for stress ulcers, routine skin care to prevent pressure sores, and initial Foley catheterization followed by intermittent catheterization and a bowel training program. With incomplete lesions, children have a better chance than adults for useful recovery. Hadley et al (3) noted that 89% of pediatric patients with incomplete spinal cord lesions improved, whereas only 20% of patients with complete injuries had evidence of significant recovery. Laminectomy has not been shown to be beneficial and can actually be harmful (90,91) because it increases instability in the cervical spine; for example, it can cause a swan-neck deformity or progressive kyphotic deformity (92,93). The risk of spinal deformity after spinal cord injury has been investigated by several researchers (22,92,94–97). Mayfield et al (92) found that patients who had a spinal cord injury before their growth spurt all developed spinal deformities, 80% of which were progressive. Ninety-three percent developed scoliosis, 57% kyphosis, and 18% lordosis. Sixty-one percent of these patients required spinal arthrodesis for stabilization of their curves. Orthotic management usually is unsuccessful, but in some patients it delays the age at which arthrodesis is necessary. Lower extremity deformities also may occur, such as subluxations and dislocations about the hip. Pelvic obliquity can be a significant problem and may result in pressure sores and difficulty in seating in a wheelchair.

NEONATAL INJURY

Spinal column injury and spinal cord injury can occur during birth, especially during a breech delivery (98,99). Injuries associated with breech delivery usually are in the lower cervical spine or upper thoracic spine and are thought to result from traction, whereas injuries associated with cephalic delivery usually occur in the upper cervical spine and are thought to result from rotation. It is unclear whether cesarean section reduces spinal injury in neonates (100); however, Bresnan and Abroms (101) noted that neck hyperextension in utero (star-gazing fetus) in breech presentations is likely to result in an estimated 25% incidence of spinal cord injury with vaginal delivery and can be prevented by delivering by cesarean section.

Distraction-type injuries to the upper cervical spine have been reported in infants in forward-facing car seats. Because infants have poor head control and muscular development, if they are placed in a forward-facing car seat and a sudden deceleration occurs, the head continues forward while the remainder of the body is strapped in the car seat, resulting in a distraction-type injury (102,103).

Neuromuscular control of the cervical spine in neonates and infants is underdeveloped, and a normal infant cannot adequately support his or her head until about 3 months of age. Infants, therefore, cannot protect their spines against excessive forces that may occur during delivery or during the months after birth. Skeletal injuries from obstetric trauma are probably underreported because the infantile spine is largely cartilaginous and difficult to evaluate with x-rays, especially if the injury is through the cartilage or cartilage–bone interface (13). A cervical spine lesion should be considered in an infant who is floppy at birth, especially after a difficult delivery. Flaccid paralysis with areflexia usually is followed by a typical pattern of hyperreflexia once spinal cord shock is over. Brachial plexus palsies also warrant cervical spine x-rays. MRI can sometimes be helpful in this diagnosis.

Shulman et al (104) found atlanto-occipital and axial dislocations at autopsy, and Tawbin (99) found a 10% incidence of brain and spinal injuries at autopsy.

Treatment of neonatal cervical spine injuries is nonoperative and should consist of careful realignment and positioning of the child on a bed with neck support or a custom cervical thoracic orthosis. Healing of bony injuries usually is rapid and complete (11).

Caffey (28) in 1974 and Swischuk (105) in 1969 described a child abuse syndrome called the shaken infant syndrome. Children have weak and immature neck musculature and cannot support their heads when they are subjected to whiplash stresses. Intercranial and interocular hemorrhages can occur. This injury can result in death or cerebral injury with retardation and permanent visual and hearing defects. Fractures of the spinal column and spinal cord injuries can occur during violent shaking of a child. Swischuk reported a spinal cord injury in a 2-year-old that was the result of violent shaking that produced a cervical fracture dislocation that spontaneously reduced (105).

TABLE 18-2 Anderson and Montesano Classification of Occipital Condylar Fractures

Type	Description	Biomechanics
I	Impaction	Results from axial loading; ipsilateral alar ligament may be compromised, but stability is maintained by contralateral alar ligament and tectorial membrane.
II	Skull base extension	Extends from occipital bone via condyle to enter foramen magnum; stability is maintained by intact alar ligaments and tectorial membrane.
III	Avulsion	Mediated via alar ligament tension; associated disruption of tectorial membrane and contralateral alar ligament may cause instability.

(Modified from Hanson JA, Deliganis AV, Baxter AB, et al. Radiologic and clinical spectrum of occipital condyle fractures: retrospective review of 107 consecutive patients in 95 patients. *AJR Am J Roentgenol* 2002;178:1261–1268.)

OCCIPITAL CONDYLAR FRACTURE

Occipital condylar fractures are rare, and their diagnosis requires a high index of suspicion (106,107). CT with multiplanar reconstruction usually is necessary to establish the diagnosis. Tuli et al (108) recommended that a CT scan be obtained in the following circumstances: presence of lower cranial nerve deficits, associated head injury or basal skull fracture, or persistent neck pain despite normal x-rays. Reports of associated cranial nerve deficits vary from 53% to 31% of patients with occipital condylar fractures (1,79,108). Anderson and Montesano (1) described three types of occipital condylar fractures (Table 18-2, Fig. 18-19): type I, impaction fracture; type II, basilar skull fracture extending into the condyle; and type III, avulsion fractures. An avulsion fracture is the only type of occipital condylar fracture that is unstable. Type I injuries are the result of axial compression with a component of ipsilateral flexion. Type II injuries are basilar skull fractures that extend to involve the occipital condyle and usually are caused by a direct blow. Type III injuries are avulsion fractures of the inferomedial portion of the condyle that is attached to the alar ligament. Types I and II occipital condylar fractures usually are stable and can be treated with a cervical orthosis. Type III or avulsion fractures can be unstable and may require halo immobilization or occipitocervical arthrodesis (109).

TABLE 18-3 Tuli et al's Classification of Occipital Condylar Fractures

Type	Description	Biomechanics
1	Nondisplaced	Stable
2A	Displaced*	Stable; no x-ray, CT, or MRI evidence of occipitoatlantoaxial instability of ligamentous disruption
2B	Displaced*	Unstable; positive x-ray, CT, or MRI evidence of occipitoatlantoaxial instability or ligamentous disruption

* At least 2 mm of osseous separation.
(Modified from Hanson JA, Deliganis AV, Baxter AB, et al. Radiologic and clinical spectrum of occipital condyle fractures: retrospective review of 107 consecutive patients in 95 patients. *AJR Am J Roentgenol* 2002;178:1261–1268.)

Tuli et al (108) also classified occipital condylar fractures based on displacement and stability of the occiput/C1-C2 complex (Table 18-3). In their classification, type 1 fractures are nondisplaced and type 2 are displaced. They further subdivided type 2 fractures into type 2A, displaced but stable, and type

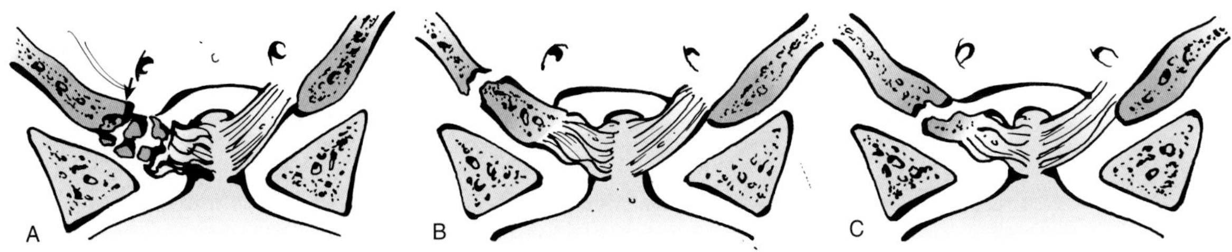

FIGURE 18-19 Classification of occipital condylar fractures according to Anderson and Monsanto. **A.** Type I fractures can occur with axial loading. **B.** Type II fractures are extensions of basilar cranial fractures. **C.** Type III fractures can result from an avulsion of the condyle during rotation, lateral bending, or a combination of mechanisms. (Reprinted from Hadley MN. Occipital condyle fractures. *Neurosurgery* 2002;50[Suppl]: S114–S119; with permission.)

2B, displaced and unstable. Most occipital condylar fractures can be treated with a cervical orthosis, but unstable fractures may need halo immobilization or occipital cervical fusion.

ATLANTO-OCCIPITAL INSTABILITY

Atlanto-occipital dislocation was once thought to be a rare fatal injury found only at the time of autopsy (Fig. 18-20) (13,82, 104,110,111). This injury is now being recognized more often, and children are surviving (67,112–114). This increase in the survival rate may be due to increased awareness and improved emergency care with resuscitation and spinal immobilization by emergency personnel. Atlanto-occipital dislocation occurs in sudden deceleration accidents, such as motor vehicle or pedestrian–vehicle accidents. The head is thrown forward, and this can cause sudden craniovertebral separation.

The atlanto-occipital joint is a condylar joint that has little inherent bony stability. Stability is provided by the ligaments about the joint. The primary stabilizers are the paired alar ligaments, the articular capsule, and the tectorial membrane (a continuation of the posterior longitudinal ligament). In children, this articulation is not as well formed as in adults and it is less cup-shaped. Therefore, there is less resistance to translational forces (13,52,104,110,111,115).

Diagnosis may be difficult because atlanto-occipital dislocation is a ligamentous injury. Although patients with this injury have a history of trauma, some may have no neurologic findings. Others, however, may have symptoms such as cranial nerve injury, vomiting, headache, torticollis, or motor or sensory deficits (111,113,116–119). Brain stem symptoms, such as ataxia and vertigo, may be caused by vertebrobasilar vascular insufficiency. Unexplained weakness or difficulty in weaning off a ventilator after a closed head injury may be a sign of this injury.

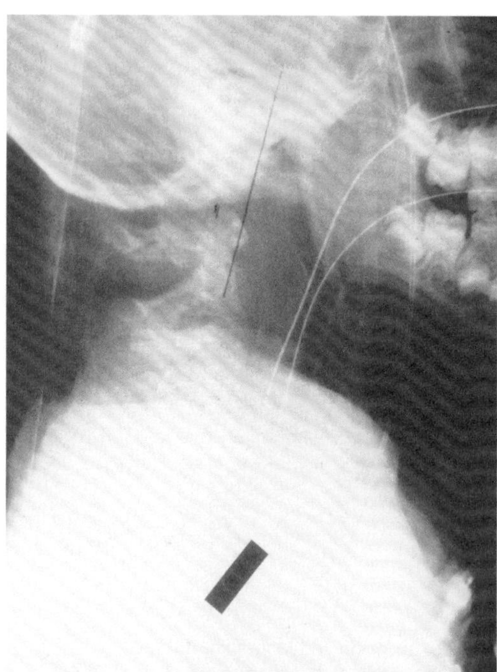

FIGURE 18-20 Patient with atlanto-occipital dislocation. Note the forward displacement of the Wackenheim line and the significant anterior soft tissue swelling.

The treating physician must have a high index of suspicion in children with closed head injuries or associated facial trauma and must be aware of the x-ray findings associated with atlanto-occipital dislocation. A significant amount of anterior soft tissue swelling usually can be seen on a lateral cervical spine x-ray. This increased anterior soft tissue swelling should be a warning sign that an atlanto-occipital dislocation may have occurred.

X-ray findings that aid in the diagnosis of atlanto-occipital dislocation are the Wackenheim line, Powers ratio, dens–basion interval, and occipital condylar distance. The Wackenheim line is drawn along the clivus and should intersect tangentially the tip of the odontoid. A shift anterior or posterior of this line represents either an anterior or posterior displacement of the occiput on the atlas (Fig. 18-21). This line is probably the most helpful because it is reproducible and easy to identify on a lateral x-ray. The Powers ratio (see Fig. 18-7) is determined by drawing a line from the basion to the posterior arch of the atlas (BC) and a second line from the opisthion to the anterior arch of the atlas (OA). The length of line BC is divided by the length of the line OA, producing the Powers ratio. A ratio of more than 1.0 is diagnostic of anterior atlanto-occipital dislocation. A ratio of less than 0.7 is diagnostic of posterior atlanto-occipital dislocation. Values between 1.0 and 0.7 are considered normal. Another x-ray measurement is the dens–basion interval. If the interval measures more than 1.2 cm, then disruption of the atlanto-occipital joint has occurred (52,120). Donahue et al (51) described an occipital condylar facet distance of more than 5 mm from the occipital condyle to the C1 facet as indicative of atlanto-occipital injury. They recommended measuring this distance from five reference points along the occipital condyle and the C1 facet (Fig. 18-22).

MRI is useful in diagnosing atlanto-occipital dislocation by showing soft tissue edema around the tectorial membranes and lateral masses and ligament injury or disruption (121).

Operative Treatment

Because atlanto-occipital dislocation is a ligamentous injury, nonoperative treatment usually is unsuccessful. Although Farley et al (122) reported successful stabilization in a halo, Georgopoulos et al (123) found persistent atlanto-occipital instability after halo immobilization. Immobilization in a halo should be used with caution: if the vest or cast portion is not fitted properly, displacement can increase (Fig. 18-23) because the head is fixed in the halo but movement occurs because of inadequate immobilization of the trunk in the brace or cast. Traction should be avoided because it can cause distraction of the skull from the atlas. Surgical stabilization is the recommended treatment (124). Posterior arthrodesis can be performed in situ, with wire fixation or fixation with a contoured Luque rod and wires (125–127). If the C1-C2 articulation is stable, arthrodesis should be only from the occiput to C1 so that C1-C2 motion is preserved (128). Some researchers have expressed reservations about the chance of obtaining fusion in the narrow atlanto-occipital interval and have

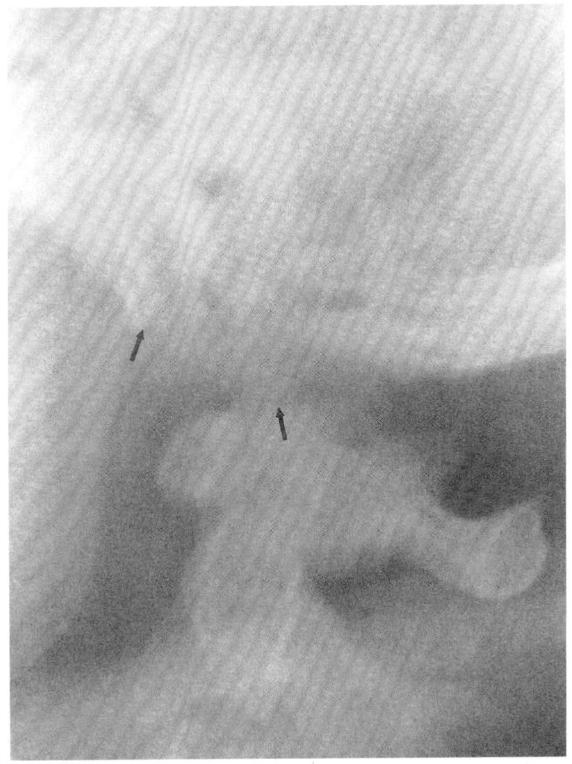

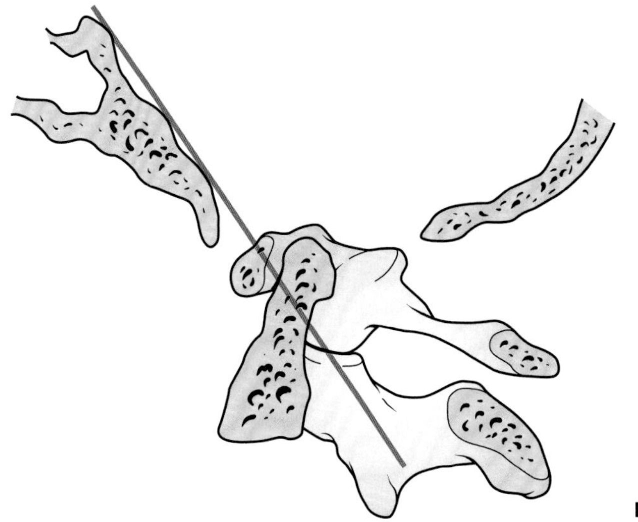

FIGURE 18-21 Craniovertebral dislocation. **A.** Lateral view shows extensive soft tissue swelling. The distance between the basion and the dens is 2.4 cm (*arrows*) (normal is <1 cm). **B.** Line drawing shows the abnormal relationship between the occiput and the upper cervical spine. (Reprinted from El-Khoury GY, Kathol MH. Radiographic evaluation of cervical trauma. *Semin Spine Surg* 1991;3:3–23; with permission.)

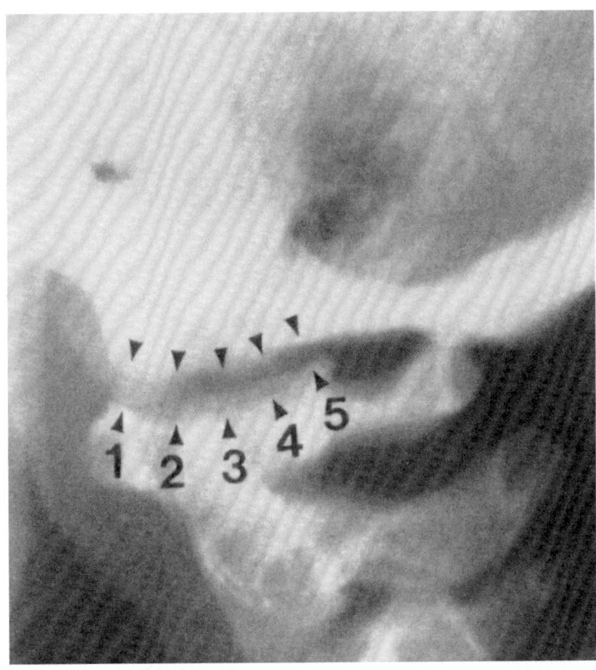

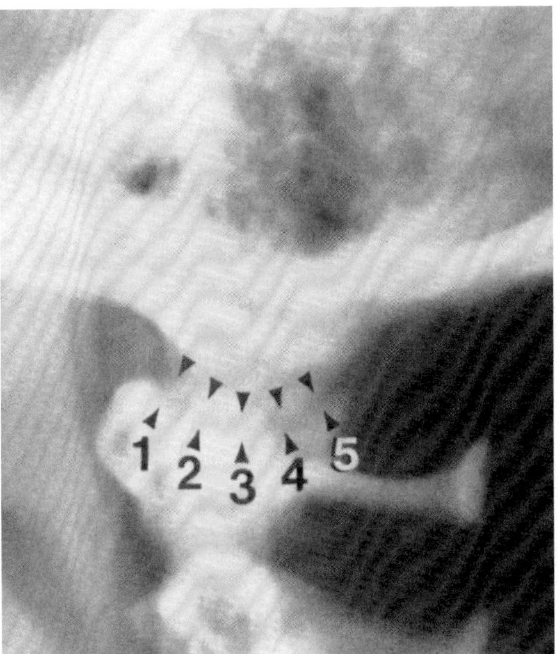

FIGURE 18-22 Atlanto-occipital joint measurement points 1 through 5 demonstrated on a normal cross-table lateral skull x-ray in an 8-year-old **(A)** and a 14-year-old **(B)**. (Reprinted from Kaufman RA, Carroll CD, Buncher CR. Atlantooccipital junction: standards for measurement in normal children. *AJNR Am J Neuroradiol* 1987;8:995–999; with permission.)

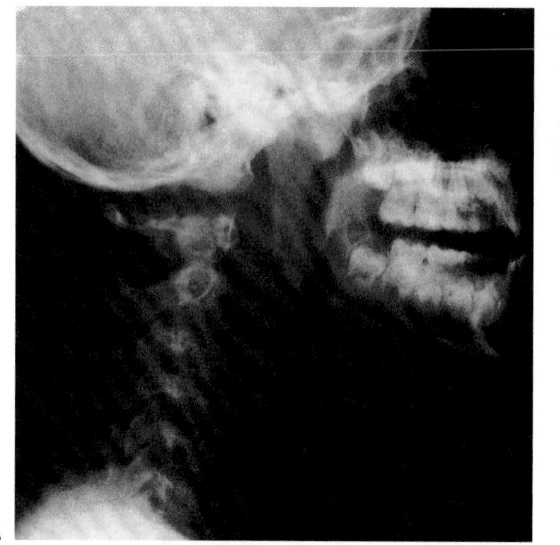

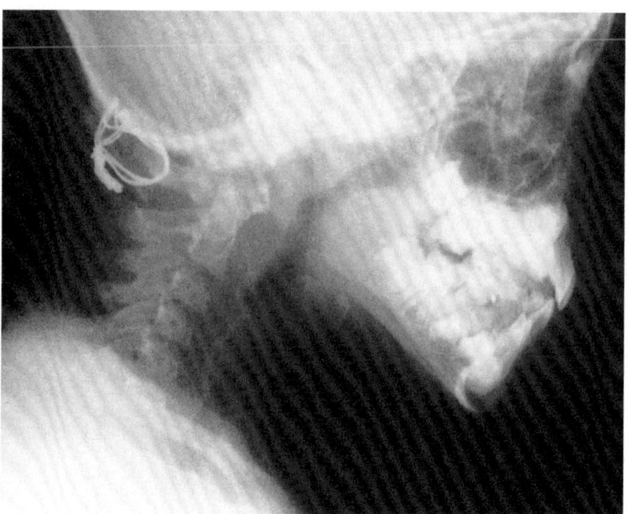

FIGURE 18-23 **A.** Lateral x-ray of a patient with atlanto-occipital dislocation. Note the increase in the facet condylar distance. **B.** Lateral x-ray after occipital C1 arthrodesis.

recommended arthrodesis from the occiput to C2. If stability of the C1-C2 articulation is questionable, arthrodesis should extend to C2 (129). Acute hydrocephalus can occur after this injury or in the early postoperative period because of changes in cerebrospinal fluid flow at the cranial cervical junction.

For a patient who presents very late with an unreduced dislocation, an in situ arthrodesis is recommended. DiBenedetto and Lee (130) recommended arthrodesis in situ with a suboccipital craniectomy to relieve posterior impingement.

Instability at the atlanto-occipital joint is increased in patients with Down syndrome as well as in those with a high cervical arthrodesis below the axis. These patients may be at risk of developing chronic instability patterns and are at higher risk of having instability after trauma.

Occiput to C2 Arthrodesis

Arthrodesis Without Internal Fixation. In younger children in whom the posterior elements are absent at C1 or separation is extensive in the bifid part of C1 posteriorly, posterior cervical arthrodesis from the occiput to C2 with iliac crest bone graft is performed using a periosteal flap from the occiput to provide an osteogenic tissue layer for the bone graft (Fig. 18-24) (131).

A halo is applied after the patient is anesthetized, endotracheal intubation is obtained, and all anesthesia lines are in place. For younger children, 8 to 12 pins with lower-pressure torque are used in the halo (see Fig. 18-17); in older children, 4 pins can be used.

An x-ray is obtained to evaluate the position of the head and cervical spine in the prone position with the halo in place. The

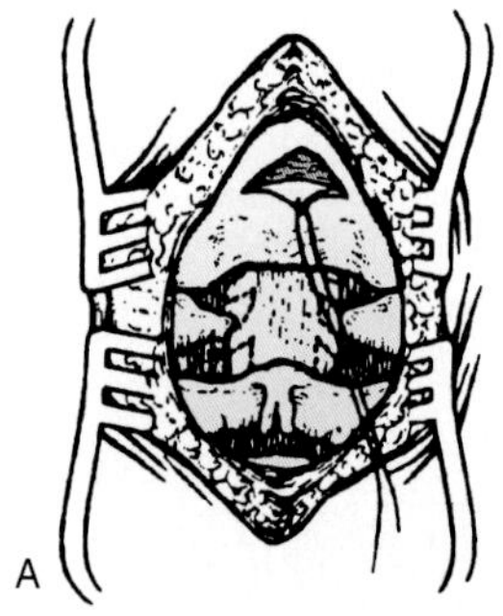

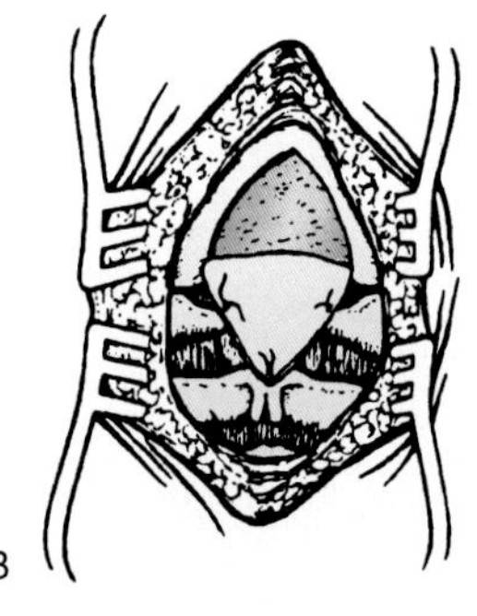

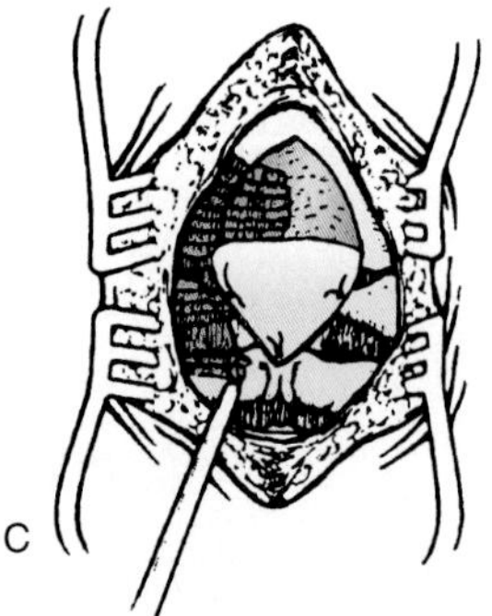

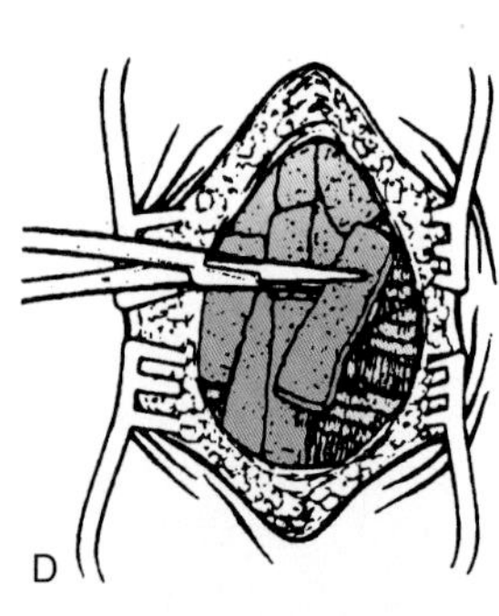

FIGURE 18-24 Technique of occipitocervical arthrodesis used when the posterior arch of C1 is absent. **A.** Exposure of the occiput, atlas, and axis. **B.** Reflection of periosteal flap to cover defect in atlas. **C.** Decortication of exposed vertebral elements. **D.** Placement of autogenous cancellous iliac bone grafts. (Redrawn from Koop SE, Winter RB, Lonstein JE. The surgical treatment of instability of the upper part of the cervical spine in children and adolescents. *J Bone Joint Surg [Am]* 1984;66:403; with permission.)

x-ray also aids in identifying landmarks and levels, although once the skin incision is made, the occiput and spinous processes can be palpated.

A straight posterior incision is made from the occiput to about C3, with care not to expose below C2 to avoid extension of the fusion to lower levels. An epinephrine and lidocaine solution is injected into the cutaneous and subcutaneous tissues to help control local skin and subcutaneous bleeding. The incision is deepened in the midline to the spinous processes of C2. Once identified, the level of the posterior elements of C1 or the dura is more easily found.

After C2 is identified, subperiosteal dissection is carried proximally. Extraperiosteal dissection is used to approach the occiput (see Fig. 18-24A). The dura is not completely exposed; if possible, any fat or ligamentous tissue present is left intact. The interspinous ligaments also should be left intact.

The occipital periosteum is mobilized by making a triangular incision directly on the posterior skull, with the apex posteriorly and the broad base over the foramen magnum region. A flap of 3 or 4 cm at the base can be created. With subperiosteal elevation, the periosteum can be reflected from the occiput to the spinous processes of C2 (see Fig. 18-24B). The apex of the flap is sutured to the spinous process of C2 and is attached laterally to any posterior elements that are present at C1 or other lateral soft tissues. After the periosteum is secured to the bone and any rudimentary C1 ring is exposed subperiosteally, a power bur is used to decorticate the occiput and any exposed portions of C1 and C2 (see Fig. 18-24C).

Iliac crest bone graft is harvested, and struts of iliac bone are placed across the area on the periosteal flap (see Fig. 18-24D). No internal fixation is used other than sutures to secure the periosteum. The wound is closed in a routine fashion, and a body jacket or cast is applied and attached to the halo. The halo cast is worn until x-rays show adequate posterior arthrodesis, usually in 8 to 12 weeks.

Arthrodesis With Triple-Wire Fixation. In older adolescents in whom the posterior elements of C1 and C2 are intact, a triple-wire technique, as described by Wertheim and Bohlman (132), can be used (Fig. 18-25). The wires are passed through the

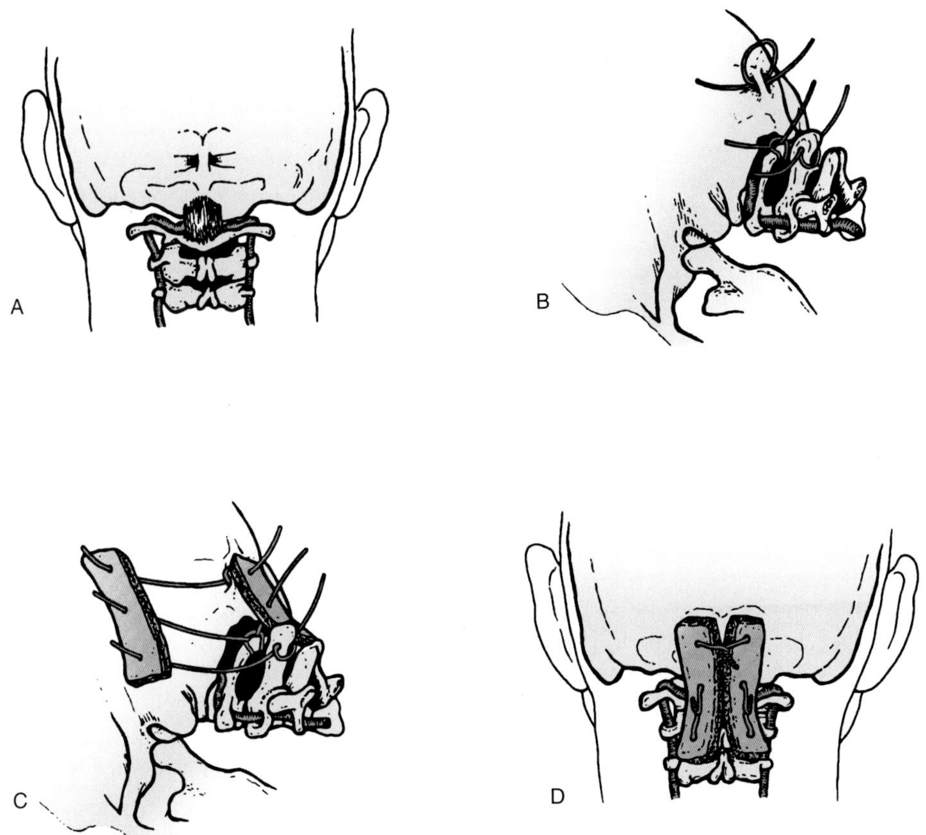

FIGURE 18-25 Technique of occipitocervical arthrodesis used in older adolescents with intact posterior elements of C1 and C2. **A.** A bur is used to create a ridge in the external occipital protuberance, and then a hole is made in the ridge. **B.** Wires are passed through the outer table of the occiput, under the arch of the atlas, and through the spinous process of the axis. **C.** Corticocancellous bone grafts are placed on the wires. **D.** Wires are tightened to secure grafts in place. (Redrawn from Wertheim SB, Bohlman HH. Occipitocervical fusion: indications, technique, and long-term results. *J Bone Joint Surg [Am]* 1987;69:833; with permission.)

outer table of the skull at the occipital protuberance. Because the transverse and superior sagittal sinuses are cephalad to the protuberance, they are not endangered by wire passage.

Stability of the spine is obtained preoperatively with cranial skeletal traction with the patient on a turning frame or cerebellar head rest. The patient is placed prone, and a lateral x-ray is obtained to document proper alignment. The subcutaneous tissues are injected with an epinephrine solution (1:500,000). A midline incision is made extending from the external occipital protuberance to the spine of the third cervical vertebra. The paraspinous muscles are sharply dissected subperiosteally with a scalpel, and a periosteal elevator is used to expose the occiput and cervical laminae, with special care to stay in the midline to avoid the paramedian venous plexus. At a point 2 cm above the rim of the foramen magnum, a high-speed diamond bur is used to create a trough on either side of the protuberance, making a ridge in the center (see Fig. 18-25A). A towel clip is used to make a hole in this ridge through only the outer table of bone. A 20-gauge wire is looped through the hole and around the ridge; then another 20-gauge wire is looped around the arch of the atlas. A third wire is passed through a hole drilled in the base of the spinous process of the axis and around this structure, giving three separate wires to secure the bone grafts on each side of the spine (see Fig. 18-25B).

A thick, slightly curved graft of corticocancellous bone of premeasured length and width is removed from the posterior iliac crest. The graft is divided horizontally into two pieces, and three holes are drilled into each graft (see Fig. 18-25C). The occiput is decorticated and the grafts are anchored in place with the wires on both sides of the spine (see Fig. 18-25D). Additional cancellous bone is packed around and between the two grafts. The wound is closed in layers over suction drains.

Either a rigid cervical orthosis or a halo cast is worn for 6 to 15 weeks, followed by a soft collar that is worn for an additional 6 weeks.

Occipitocervical Arthrodesis

The positioning of the patient and the procedure are done with the patient under general anesthesia and with monitoring of the somatosensory evoked potentials (Fig. 18-26). A halo ring is applied initially with the patient supine. Subsequently, the patient is carefully placed in the prone position, the halo is secured to the operating table with a halo-positioning device, and the alignment of the occiput and the cervical spine is confirmed with a lateral x-ray. The midline is exposed from the occiput to the second or third cervical vertebra. Particular care is taken to limit the lateral dissection to avoid damaging the vertebral arteries (133).

In patients who need decompression because of cervical stenosis or for removal of a tumor, the arch of the first or second cervical vertebra (or both) is removed, with or without removal of a portion of the occipital bone to enlarge the foramen magnum.

Four holes, aligned transversely, with two on each side of the midline, are made with a high-speed drill through both

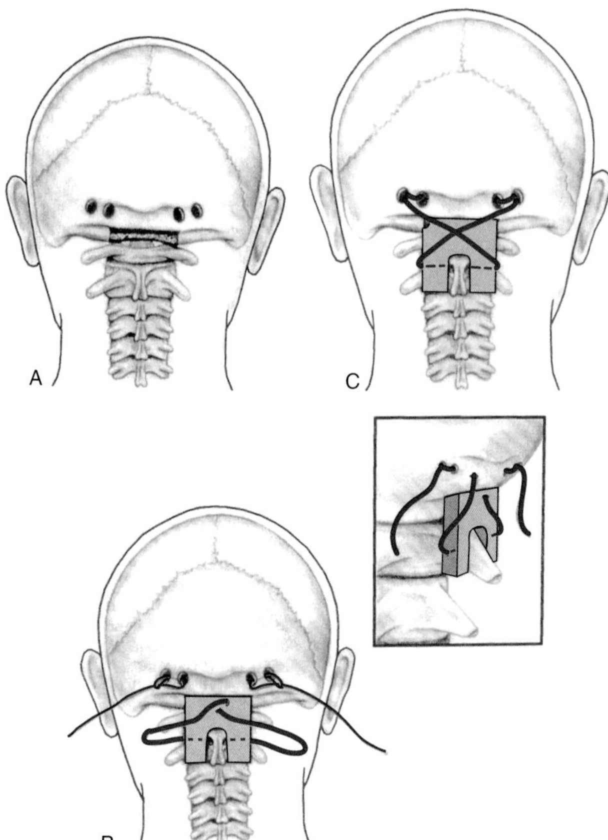

FIGURE 18-26 Occipitocervical arthrodesis. **A.** Four bur holes are placed into the occiput in transverse alignment, with two on each side of the midline, leaving a 1-cm osseous bridge between the two holes of each pair. A trough is fashioned into the base of the occiput. **B.** 16- or 18-gauge Luque wires are passed through the bur holes and looped on themselves. Wisconsin button wires are passed through the base of the spinous process of either the second or third cervical vertebra. The graft is positioned into the occipital trough and spinous process of the cervical vertebra at the caudal extent of the arthrodesis. The graft is locked into place by the precise contouring of the bone. **C.** The wires are crossed, twisted, and cut. The extension of the cervical spine can be controlled by positioning of the head with the halo frame, by adjustment of the size and shape of the bone graft, and to a lesser extent by tightening of the wires. (Reprinted from Dormans JP, Drummond DS, Sutton LN, et al. Occipitocervical arthrodesis in children. *J Bone Joint Surg [Am]* 1995;77:1234–1240; with permission.)

cortices of the occiput, leaving a 1-cm osseous bridge between the two holes of each pair. The holes are placed caudal to the transverse sinuses. A trough is fashioned into the base of the occiput to accept the cephalad end of the bone graft. A corticocancellous graft is obtained from the iliac crest and is shaped into a rectangle, with a notch created in the inferior base to fit around the spinous process of the second or third cervical vertebra. The caudal extent of the intended arthrodesis (the second or third cervical vertebra) is determined by the presence or absence of a previous laminectomy, congenital anomalies, or the level of the instability. On each side, a looped 16- or 18-gauge Luque wire is passed through the bur holes and looped on itself. Wisconsin button wires (Zimmer, Warsaw, IN) are passed through the base of the spinous process of either the second or the third cervical vertebra. The wire that is going into the left arm of the graft is passed through the spinous process from right to left. The graft is placed into the occipital trough superiorly and about the spinous process of the vertebra that is to be at the caudal level of the arthrodesis (the second or third cervical vertebrae). The graft is precisely contoured so that it fits securely into the occipital trough and around the inferior spinous process before the wires are tightened. The wires are subsequently crossed, twisted, and cut. An intraoperative x-ray is made at this point to assess the position of the graft and the wires as well as the alignment of the occiput and the cephalad cervical vertebrae. Extension of the cervical spine can be controlled by positioning of the head with the halo frame, by adjustment of the size and shape of the graft, and to a lesser extent by appropriate tightening of the wires.

Atlanto-Occipital Arthrodesis

Although most patients with atlanto-occipital dislocations are treated with fusion from the occiput to C2 or lower, Sponseller and Cass (128) described occiput–C1 fusion in two children with atlanto-occipital arthrodesis who had complete or near-complete neurologic preservation. Their rationale was that rotation would be preserved by sparing the C1-C2 articulation from fusion and that less stress would be concentrated on the lower cervical spine by fusing one level instead of two. In both of their patients, stable fusion was obtained and neurologic status was maintained.

Before surgery, x-rays and CT scans should be reviewed to be sure a bifid or hypoplastic C1 arch is not present. The positioning of the patient and the procedure are done with the patient under general anesthesia and with monitoring of the somatosensory evoked potentials. The procedure is done with the patient immobilized in a halo vest. The base of the skull to the ring of C1 is exposed and the periosteum of the skull is elevated so that it forms a flap from the foramen magnum located posteriorly-superiorly. The ring of C1 is carefully exposed, with care taken not to dissect more than 1 cm to either side of the midline to protect the vertebral arteries. Care also is taken not to expose any portion of C2 to prevent bridging of the fusion. The dissection of C1 should be done gently. A trough for the iliac crest bone graft is made in the occiput at a level directly cranial to the ring of C1. This trough is unicortical only and extends the width of the exposed portion of C1. Superior to this, two holes are drilled through the occiput as close to the trough as possible to avoid an anteriorly translating vector on the skull when tightening it down to C1. One 22-gauge wire is passed through the holes and another is placed around the ring of C1. The periosteal flap is turned down to bridge the occiput–C1 interval. A small, rectangular, bicortical, iliac crest bone graft approximately 1.5 cm wide and 1 cm high is shaped to fit the trough in the occiput; the graft is contoured to fit the individual patient's occiput–C1 interval. The inferior surface of the bone graft is contoured to fit snugly around the ring of C1 to keep it from migrating anteriorly into the epidural space. Two holes are drilled directly above the distal end of the graft, and the wire around C1 is passed through these holes, forming two distal strands; the wire passed through the occiput forms two proximal strands. These are twisted together and sequentially tightened to apply slight compression to the bone graft. This keeps the graft in the occipital trough and prevents migration into the canal by the occiput. Additional cancellous bone is added to any available space.

The halo vest is kept in place for 6 to 8 weeks in a young child and for as long as 12 weeks in an older child or adolescent. Union is confirmed by a coned, lateral x-ray of the posterior occiput–C1 interval and by flexion-extension lateral views. A rigid cervical collar is used for an additional 2 to 4 weeks to protect the fusion and support the patient's cervical muscles while motion is regained.

Occipitocervical Arthrodesis With Contoured Rod and Segmental Wire

Occipitocervical arthrodesis using a contoured rod and segmental wire has the advantage of achieving immediate stability of the occipitocervical junction (Fig. 18-27), which allows the patient to be immobilized in a cervical collar after surgery, avoiding the need for halo immobilization.

The base of the occiput and the spinous processes of the upper cervical vertebrae are approached through a longitudinal midline incision, which extends deep within the relatively avascular intermuscular septum. The entire field is exposed subperiosteally. A template of the intended shape of the stainless steel rod is made with the appropriate length of Luque wire. Two bur holes are made on each side, about 2 cm lateral to the midline and 2.5 cm above the foramen magnum. Care should be taken to avoid the transverse and sigmoid sinus when making these bur holes. At least 10 mm of intact cortical bone should be left between the bur holes to ensure solid fixation. Luque wires or Songer cables are passed in an extradural plane through the two bur holes on each side of the midline. The wires or cables are passed sublaminar in the upper cervical spine. The rod is bent to match the template; this usually will have a head–neck angle of about 135 degrees and slight cervical lordosis. A Bend Meister (Sofamor/Danek, Memphis, TN) may be helpful in bending the rod. The wires or cables are secured to the rod. The spine and occiput are decorticated and autogenous cancellous bone grafting is performed.

FRACTURES OF THE ATLAS

Fracture of the ring of C1 (Jefferson fracture) is caused by an axial load applied to the head and is not a common injury in children (129,134–139). The force is transmitted through the occipital condyles to the lateral masses of C1, causing a disruption in the ring of C1, usually in two places, with fractures

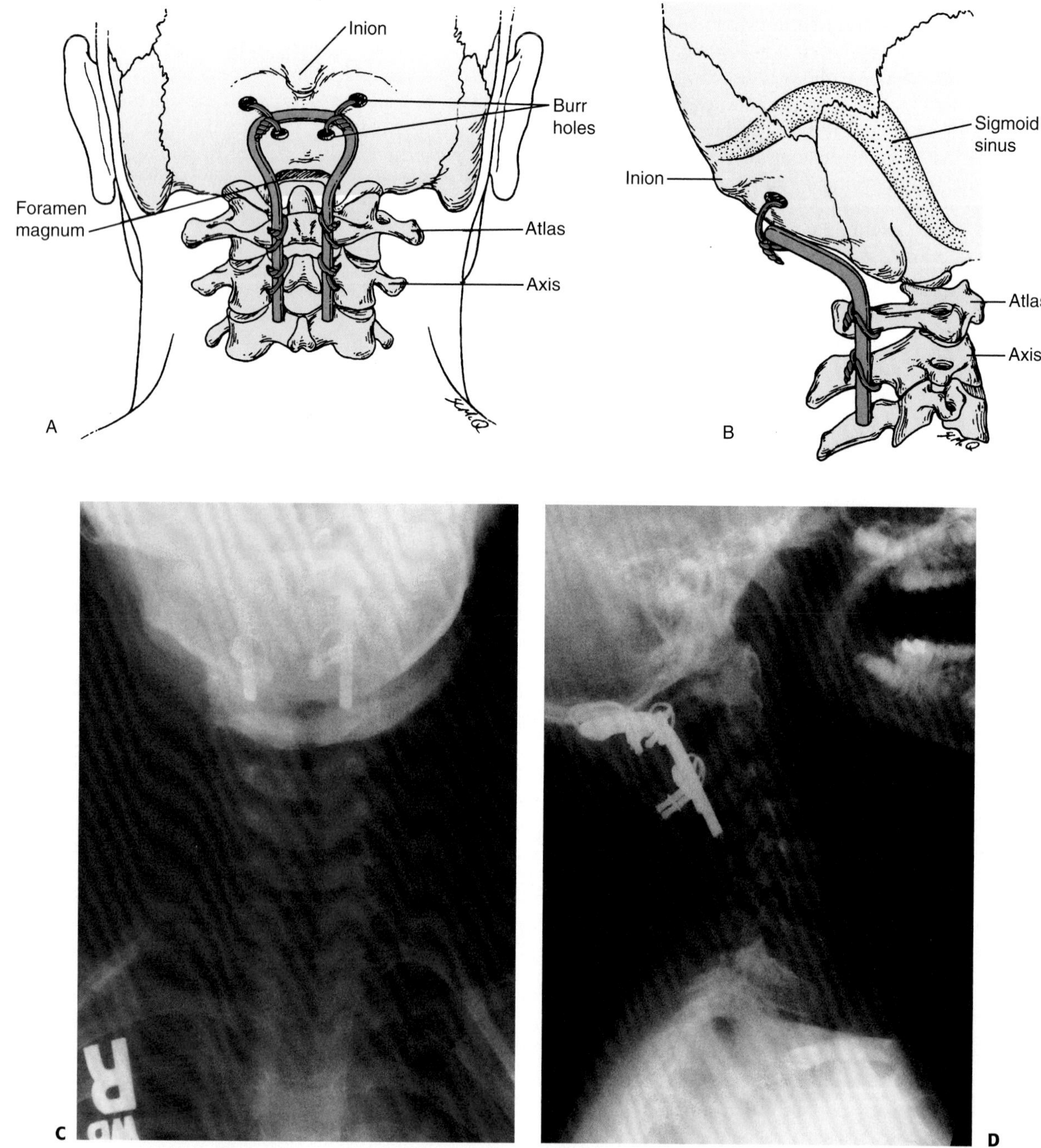

FIGURE 18-27 Occipitocervical arthrodesis using a contoured rod and segmental wire or cable fixation. (**A** and **B** reprinted from Warner WC. Pediatric cervical spine. In: Canale ST, ed. *Campbell's operative orthopaedics.* St. Louis: Mosby Year Book, 1998; with permission.)

occurring in both the anterior and posterior rings. In children an isolated single fracture of the ring can occur with the remaining fracture hinging on a synchondrosis. This is an important distinction in children because often fractures occur through a normal synchondrosis and there can be plastic deformation of the ring. This distinction can be seen on plain x-rays, with fractures appearing through what appears to be normal physes. As the lateral masses separate, the transverse ligament may be ruptured or avulsed, resulting in C1 and C2 instability (137). If the two lateral masses are widened more than 7 mm beyond the borders of the axis on an anteroposterior x-ray, then an injury to the transverse ligament is presumed. Injury to the

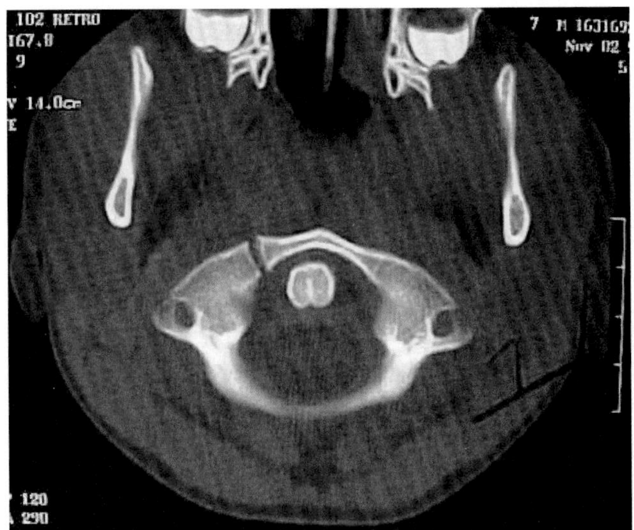

FIGURE 18-28 X-ray of an atlas fracture.

transverse ligament may be from a rupture of the ligament or an avulsion of the ligament attachment to C1. Jefferson fractures may be evident on plain x-rays, but CT scans are superior at showing this injury. CT scans also can be used to follow the progress of healing.

Treatment consists of immobilization in an orthosis (rigid collar or sternal occipital mandibular immobilizer [SOMI]), Minerva cast, or halo brace. If there is excessive widening (>7 mm), halo traction followed by halo brace or cast immobilization is recommended. Surgery rarely is necessary to stabilize these fractures (Fig. 18-28).

ATLANTOAXIAL INJURIES

Odontoid Fractures

Odontoid fractures are one of the most common fractures of the cervical spine in children (133), occurring at an average age of 4 years (140–142). The unique feature of odontoid fractures in children is that the fracture most commonly occurs through the synchondrosis of C2 distally at the base of the odontoid. This synchondrosis is a cartilage line at the base of the odontoid and looks like a physeal or Salter I injury.

A fracture of the odontoid usually is associated with head trauma from a motor vehicle accident or a fall from a height, although it also can occur after trivial head trauma. X-rays should be obtained in any child complaining of neck pain. Clinically, children with odontoid fractures complain of neck pain and resist attempts to extend the neck. Odent et al (143) reported that 8 of 15 odontoid fractures in children were the result of motor vehicle accidents, with the child fastened in a forward-facing seat. The sudden deceleration of the body as it is strapped into the car seat while the head continues to travel forward causes this fracture.

Most odontoid injuries are anteriorly displaced and usually have an intact anterior periosteal sleeve that provides some stability to the fracture when immobilized in extension and allows excellent healing of the fracture (144–147). Growth disturbances are uncommon after this type of fracture. This synchondrosis normally closes at about 3 to 6 years of age and adds little to the longitudinal growth of C2.

Most often the diagnosis can be ascertained by viewing the plain x-rays. Anteroposterior views usually appear normal, and the diagnosis must be made from lateral views because displacement of the odontoid usually occurs anteriorly. Plain x-rays sometimes can be misleading when the fracture occurs through the synchondrosis and has spontaneously reduced. When this occurs the fracture has the appearance of a nondisplaced Salter I fracture. CT scans with three-dimensional reconstruction views may be needed to fully delineate the injury (148). MRI also may be useful in nondisplaced fractures by detecting edema around the injured area, indicating that a fracture may have occurred. Dynamic flexion and extension views to demonstrate instability may be obtained in a cooperative child if a nondisplaced fracture is suspected. These studies should be done only in a cooperative child and under the direct supervision of the treating physician.

Odontoid fractures in children generally heal uneventfully and rarely have complications. Neurologic deficits rarely have been reported after this injury (143,149). Odent et al (143) described neurologic injuries in 8 of 15 patients, although most were stretch injuries to the spinal cord at the cervical thoracic junction and not at the level of the odontoid fracture.

Treatment of odontoid fractures is by closed reduction (usually extension or slight hyperextension of the neck), although complete reduction of the translation is not necessary. At least 50% apposition should be obtained to provide adequate cervical alignment, and then the patient should be immobilized in a Minerva or halo cast or custom orthosis. This fracture will heal in about 6 to 8 weeks. After bony healing, stability should be documented by flexion/extension lateral radiographs. Once the Minerva cast or halo is removed, a soft collar is worn for 1 to 2 weeks. If an adequate reduction cannot be obtained by recumbency and hyperextension, then a head halter or halo traction is needed. Rarely, manipulation under general anesthesia is needed for irreducible fractures (Fig. 18-29). Surgery with internal fixation rarely has been reported due to the good results that are achieved with conservative treatment in children (49,150–152).

Os Odontoideum

Os odontoideum consists of a round ossicle that is separated from the axis by a transverse gap, which leaves the apical segment without support. Fielding et al (153–157) suggested that this was an unrecognized fracture at the base of the odontoid. Some studies have documented normal x-rays of the dens with abnormal x-rays after trivial trauma. This can be explained by a distraction force being applied by the alar ligaments, which

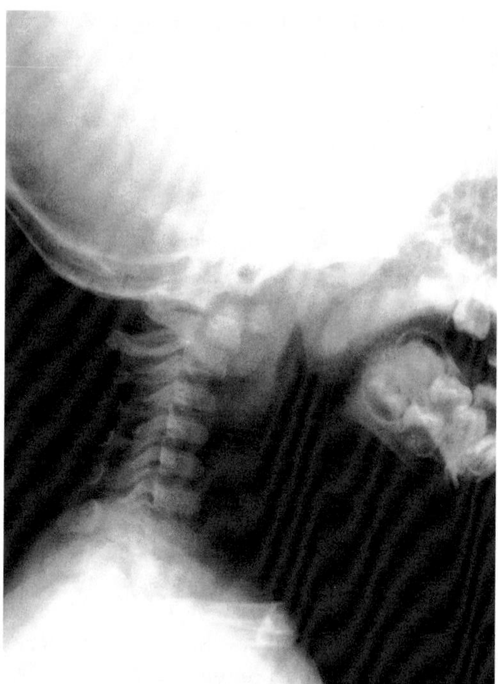

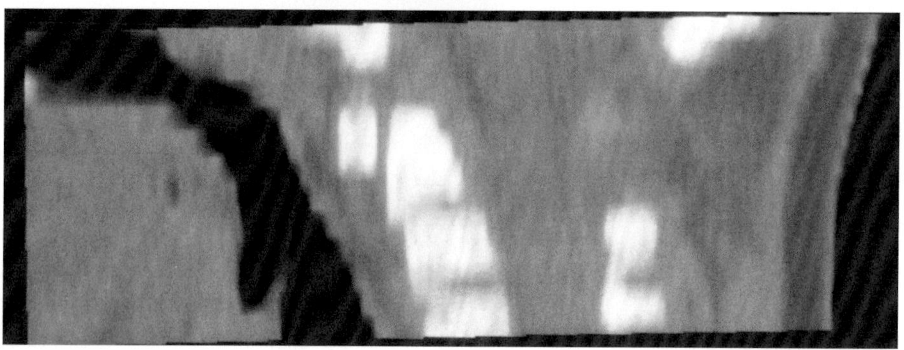

FIGURE 18-29 Lateral x-ray and CT reconstruction view of odontoid fracture through the synchondrosis of C2. Note the anterior displacement.

pulls the tip of the fractured odontoid away from the base and produces a nonunion (158–164). Other authors believe this to be of congenital origin because of its association with other congenital anomalies and syndromes (165–167).

The presentation of an os odontoideum can be variable. Signs and symptoms can range from a minor to a frank compressive myelopathy or vertebral artery compression. Presenting symptoms may be neck pain, torticollis, or headaches caused by local irritation of the atlantoaxial joint. Neurologic symptoms can be transient or episodic after trauma to complete myelopathy caused by cord compression (168). Symptoms may consist of weakness and loss of balance with upper motor neuron signs, although upper motor neuron signs may be completely absent. Proprioceptive and sphincter dysfunctions also are common.

Os odontoideum usually can be diagnosed on routine cervical spine x-rays, which include an open-mouth odontoid view (Fig. 18-30). Lateral flexion and extension views should be obtained to determine if any instability is present. With os odontoideum there is a space between the body of the axis and a bony ossicle. The free ossicle of the os odontoideum usually is half the size of a normal odontoid and is oval or round, with smooth sclerotic borders. The space differs from that of an acute fracture, in which the space is thin and irregular instead of wide and smooth. The amount of instability should be documented on lateral flexion and extension plain x-rays that allow measurement of both the anterior and posterior displacement of the atlas on the axis. Because the ossicle is fixed to the anterior arch of C1 and moves with the anterior arch of C1 both in flexion and extension, measurement of the relationship of C1 to the free ossicle is of little value because they move as a unit. A more meaningful measurement is made by projecting lines superiorly from the body of the axis to a line projected inferiorly from the posterior border of the anterior arch of the atlas. This gives more information as to the stability of C1-C2. Another measurement that is very helpful is space available for the cord, which

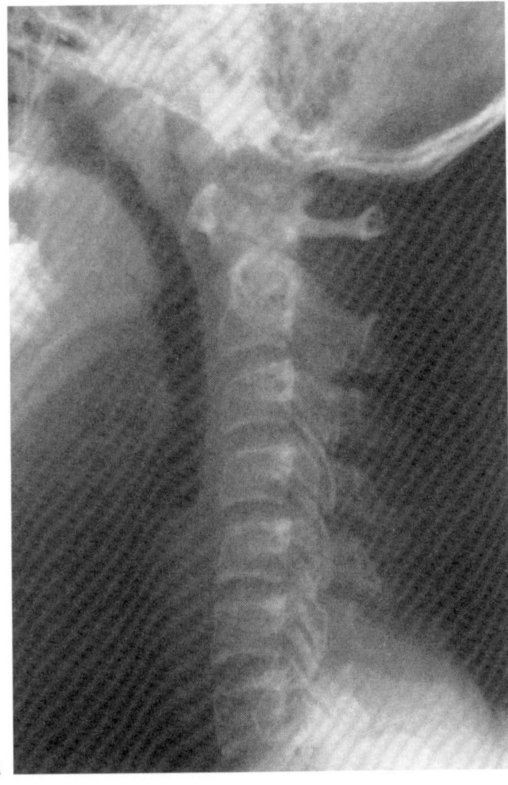

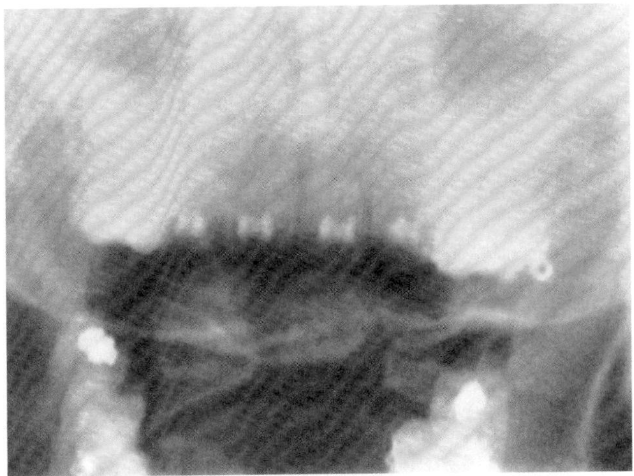

FIGURE 18-30 Lateral x-ray **(A)** and open-mouth odontoid x-ray **(B)** showing os odontoideum. (Reprinted from Warner WC. Pediatric cervical spine. In: Canale ST, ed. *Campbell's operative orthopaedics.* St. Louis: Mosby Year Book, 1999:2817; with permission.)

is the distance from the back of the dens to the anterior border of the posterior arch of C1.

Recommended treatment is posterior arthrodesis of C1 to C2. Before arthrodesis is attempted, the integrity of the arch of C1 must be documented by CT scan. Incomplete development of the posterior arch of C1 is uncommon but has been reported to occur with increased frequency in patients with os odontoideum. This may necessitate an occiput to C2 arthrodesis for stability. If a C1-C2 arthrodesis is done, one must be careful not to overreduce the odontoid and cause posterior translation. Care also must be taken in positioning the neck at the time of arthrodesis and when tightening the wires if a Gallie or Brooks arthrodesis is performed to prevent posterior translation (Figs. 18-31 and 18-32). Brockmeyer et al (169) and Wang et al (170) both reported good results with transarticular screw fixation and fusion in the treatment of children with os odontoideum. Wang et al reported the use of this technique in children as young as 3 years of age.

Traumatic Ligamentous Disruption

The transverse ligament is the primary stabilizer of an intact odontoid against forward displacement. Secondary stabilizers consist of the apical and alar ligaments, which arise from the tip of the odontoid and pass to the base of the skull. These also stabilize the atlanto-occipital joint indirectly (133). The normal distance from the anterior cortex of the dens to the posterior cortex of the anterior ring of C1 is 3 mm in adults and 4.5 mm in children. In children if the distance is more than 4.5 mm, disruption of the transverse ligament is presumed. The spinal canal at C1 is large compared with other cervical segments and accommodates a large degree of rotation and some degree of pathologic displacement without compromising the spinal cord. Steel expressed this as a rule of thirds: the spinal canal at C1

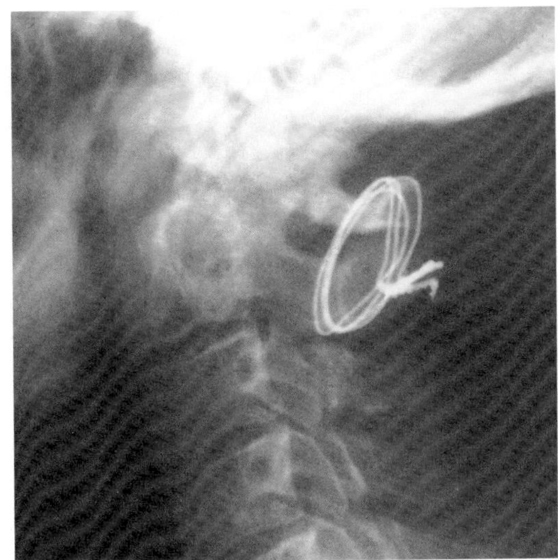

FIGURE 18-31 Posterior translation of atlas after C1-C2 posterior arthrodesis.

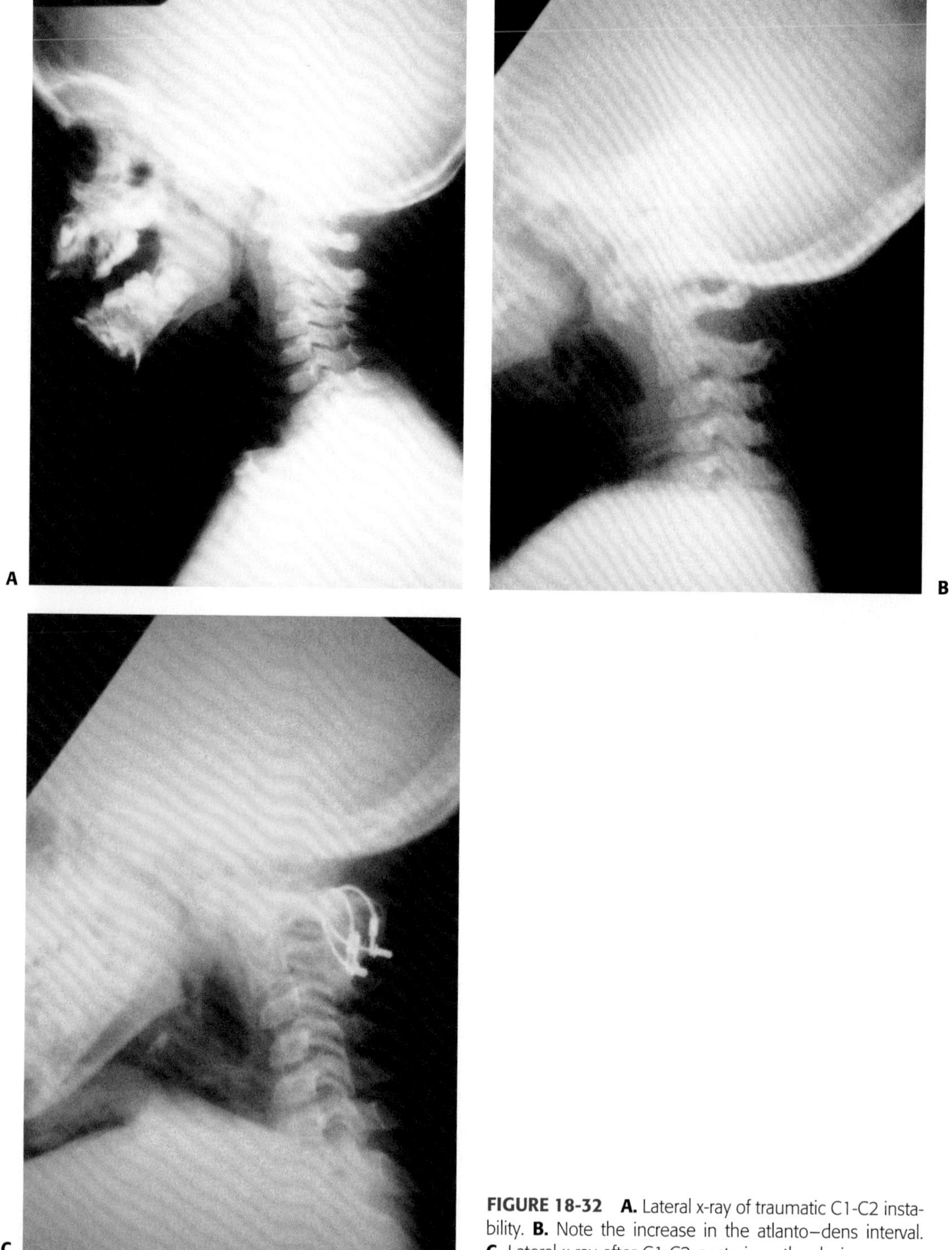

FIGURE 18-32 **A.** Lateral x-ray of traumatic C1-C2 instability. **B.** Note the increase in the atlanto–dens interval. **C.** Lateral x-ray after C1-C2 posterior arthrodesis.

is occupied equally by the spinal cord, odontoid, and a free space, which provides a buffer zone to prevent neurologic injury. Steel found that anterior displacement of the atlas that exceeds a distance equal to the width of the odontoid may place the spinal cord at risk (171).

Acute rupture of the transverse ligament is rare and reportedly occurs in fewer than 10% of pediatric cervical spine injuries (12,172). However, avulsion of the attachment of the transverse ligament to C1 may occur instead of rupture of the transverse ligament.

A patient with disruption of the transverse ligament usually has a history of cervical spine trauma and complains of neck pain, often with notable muscle spasms. Diagnosis is confirmed on lateral x-rays that show an increased atlanto–dens interval. An active flexion view may be required to show instability in cooperative patients with unexplained neck pain or neurologic findings. CT scans are useful to demonstrate avulsion of the transverse ligament from its origins to the bony ring of C1.

Although rarely used, conservative treatment of acute transverse ligament injuries has been reported. For acute injuries, reduction in extension is recommended, followed by surgical stabilization of C1 and C2 and immobilization for 8 to 12 weeks in a Minerva cast, a halo brace, or a cervical orthosis. Flexion and extension views should be obtained after stabilization to document stability.

OPERATIVE TREATMENT

Atlantoaxial Arthrodesis

Technique of Brooks and Jenkins. The supine patient is intubated in the supine position while still on a stretcher and is then placed prone on the operating table, with the head supported by traction; the head–thorax relationship is maintained at all times during turning (16) (Fig. 18-33). A lateral cervical spine x-ray is obtained to ensure proper alignment before surgery. The skin is prepared and draped in a sterile fashion and a solution of epinephrine (1:500,000) is injected intradermally to aid hemostasis.

C1 and C2 are exposed through a midline incision. With an aneurysm needle, a Mersiline suture is passed from cephalad to caudad on each side of the midline under the arch of the atlas and then beneath the lamina of C2. These serve as guides to introduce two doubled 20-gauge wires. The size of the wire used varies depending on the size and age of the patient. Two full-thickness bone grafts approximately 1.25 × 3.5 cm are harvested from the iliac crest and beveled so that the apex of the graft fits in the interval between the arch of the atlas and the lamina of the axis. Notches are fashioned in the upper and lower cortical surfaces to hold the circumferential wires and prevent them from slipping. The doubled wires are tightened over the graft and twisted on each side. The wound is irrigated and closed in layers over suction drains.

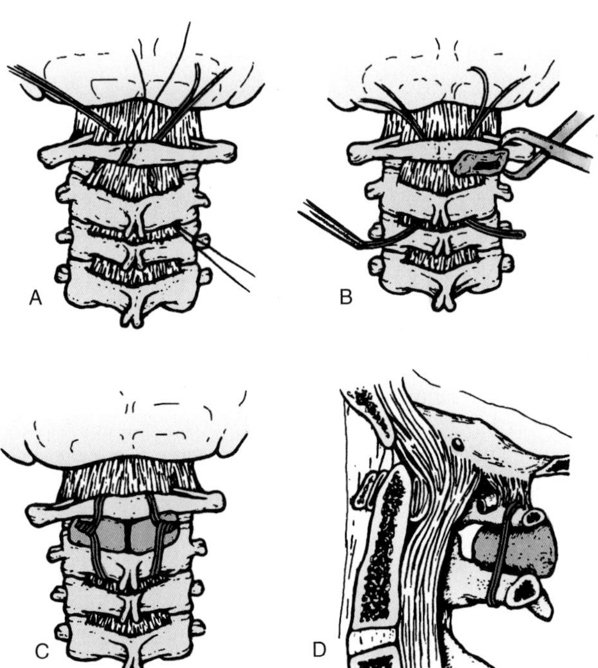

FIGURE 18-33 Technique of atlantoaxial arthrodesis (Brooks-Jenkins). **A.** Wires are inserted under the atlas and axis. **B.** Full-thickness bone grafts from the iliac crest are placed between the arch of the atlas and the lamina of the axis. **C,D.** The wires are tightened over the graft and twisted on each side. (Redrawn from Brooks AL, Jenkins EB. Atlantoaxial arthrodesis by the wedge compression method. *J Bone Joint Surg [Am]* 1978;60: 279; with permission.)

Technique of Gallie. The supine patient is intubated while on a stretcher (173) (Fig. 18-34). The prone patient then is placed on the operating table with the head supported by traction, maintaining the head–thorax relationship during turning. A lateral cervical spine x-ray is obtained to ensure proper alignment before surgery. The skin is prepared and draped in a sterile fashion, and a solution of epinephrine (1:500,000) is injected intradermally to aid hemostasis.

A midline incision is made from the lower occiput to the level of the lower end of the fusion, extending deeply within the relatively avascular midline structures, the intermuscular septum, or ligamentum nuchae. Care should be taken not to expose any more than the area to be fused to decrease the chance of spontaneous extension of the fusion. By subperiosteal dissection, the posterior arch of the atlas and the lamina of C2 are exposed. The muscular and ligamentous attachments from C2 are removed with a curet. Care should be taken to dissect laterally along the atlas to prevent injury to the vertebral arteries and vertebral venous plexus that lie on the superior aspect of the ring of C1, less than 2 cm lateral to the midline. The upper

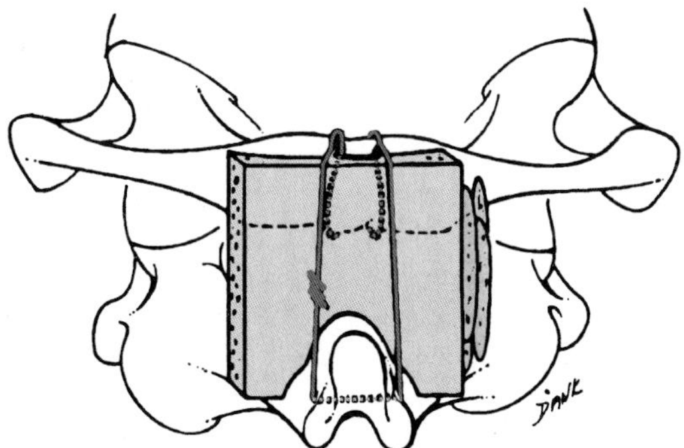

FIGURE 18-34 Wires are passed under the lamina of the atlas and through the spine of the axis and tied over the graft. This method is used most frequently. (Reprinted from Fielding JW, Hawkins RJ, Ratzan SA. Spine fusion for atlanto-axial instability. *J Bone Joint Surg [Am]* 1976;58: 400; with permission.)

surface of C1 is exposed no farther laterally than 1.5 cm from the midline in adults and 1 cm in children. Decortication of C1 and C2 generally is not necessary. From below, a wire loop of appropriate size is passed upward under the arch of the atlas either directly or with the aid of a Mersiline suture. The Mersiline suture can be passed with an aneurysm needle. The free ends of the wire are passed through the loop, grasping the arch of C1 in the loop.

A corticocancellous graft is taken from the iliac crest and placed against the lamina of C2 and the arch of C1 beneath the wire. One end of the wire is passed through the spinous process of C2, and the wire is twisted on itself to secure the graft in place. The wound is irrigated and closed in layers with suction drainage tubes.

Posterior C1-C2 Transarticular Screw Fixation. Preoperative evaluation must include flexion and extension x-rays to determine whether reduction is possible (127). CT of the craniocervical region with parasagittal reconstructions through the region of the axis pars interarticularis is necessary to determine the position of the vertebral artery; an aberrant position makes the procedure impossible.

The patient is positioned prone in traction with mild neck flexion. The foramen magnum and the upper four cervical vertebrae are exposed beyond the lateral facets, and the skin is prepared to the upper thoracic region to allow for the angle of drilling. The spinous processes and the lamina and facets from C1 to C3 are exposed. The ligamentum flavum is removed between C1 and C2 and the C2 nerve is exposed and elevated. The facet joint between C1 and C2 is identified. Venous bleeding from the venous plexus around C2 is controlled with judicious bipolar cauterization and packing. The C2 pars interarticularis is identified, and satisfactory alignment of the atlas and axis is confirmed.

A bone awl or a drill is used to penetrate the posterior cortical bone of C2 at the inferior facet 3 to 4 mm from the medial edge of the facet joint. The trajectory is marked out toward the dorsal cortical aspect of the anterior arch of C1. The drill is placed 10 degrees to the vertical, pointing medially to come through the C2 pars interarticularis. In the sagittal orientation, the trajectory is slightly medial to the vertical. The length of the screw and the screw path should be measured with CT reconstructions before the procedure. Guide wire insertion is monitored with fluoroscopy, and the guide wire must pass through the C1-C2 facet joint. As the wire traverses the joint space, the atlantoaxial articulation becomes rigid and fixed. A new stiffness can be felt in the guide wire and the tap that follows. If angulation is not possible for guide wire placement with the extent of exposure, a percutaneous technique is used.

The cannulated drill is passed over the guide wire and advanced with a pneumatic drill. The guide wire is secured beyond the pneumatic drill to prevent advancement into the parapharyngeal soft tissues. A guide wire of the same length as the screw length determined with preoperative CT is passed through the cannula, and the difference between the primary guide wire and the second guide wire is measured to confirm ideal screw length.

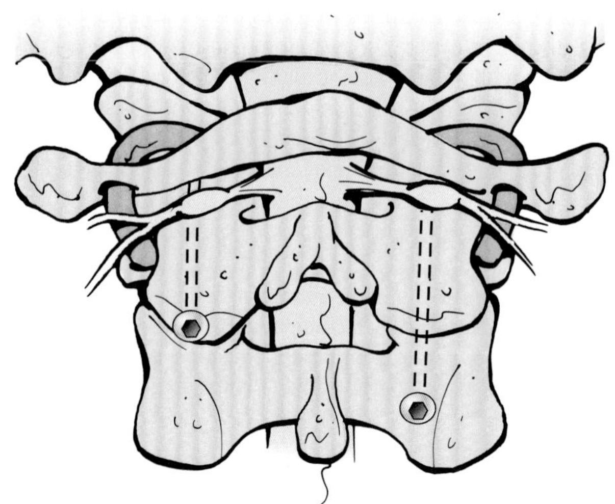

FIGURE 18-35 Position of vertebral arteries and position of screws across atlantoaxial joint. (Reprinted from Menezes AH. Surgical approaches to the craniocervical junction. In: Weinstein SL, ed. *Pediatric spine surgery*, 2nd ed. Philadelphia: Lippincott Williams & Wilkins, 2001.)

Opposite-side drilling is done before screw placement so that each guide wire can be identified with lateral fluoroscopy. When both guide wires are in satisfactory position, each screw is advanced over the guide wire and its purchase obtained into the lateral mass of the atlas (Fig. 18-35). The screw head should be flush against the bone, but the screws should not be overtightened to avoid shearing of the cortex of the pars interarticularis and facet.

Interlaminar bone fusion must be done after placement of the bilateral or unilateral screw. If the vertebral artery or vein has been injured, drilling must not be done on the opposite side. Because injury to one vertebral artery probably will not cause neurologic deficit, it is important not to proceed on the opposite side if injury has occurred.

Posterior C1-C2 Transarticular Screw Fixation. Preoperative CT scans are reviewed to confirm that the vertebral artery is not in an aberrant position and that the C1-C2 anatomy is suitable for transarticular screw placement (170). The patient is placed prone with the head held in a Mayfield skull clamp. The neck is manually flexed under fluoroscopic guidance to realign the atlas and axis. A routine posterior midline incision is used to expose the posterior aspect of C1 and C2. The C2 inferior facet is used as the landmark for screw entry: the entry point is 2 mm lateral to the medial edge and 2 mm above the inferior border of the C2 facet. The drill trajectory is angled medially 5 to 10 degrees. On the lateral fluoroscopic x-ray, the drill trajectory is adjusted toward the posterior cortex of the anterior arch of C1. After tapping, a 3.5-mm lag screw is placed across the C1-C2 joint. Another screw is then placed in exactly the same way on the other side. A bone graft is harvested from either the iliac crest or occipital bone. Multistranded titanium cable is passed under the lamina of C1. The bone graft is contoured and placed between the lamina of C1 and C2 and the wire looped around the spinal process of C2 is tightened and fixed. Care is taken not to overtighten the cable to avoid its cutting through the C1 lamina. The C1-C2 joint can be roughened with a curet and cancellous bone placed to enhance fusion. The fusion surfaces on the C1 and C2 lamina should be decorticated with a drill before the bone graft is placed.

Patients are immobilized in a hard cervical collar only; no halo or Minerva cast is used postoperatively.

Atlantoaxial Instability Associated With Congenital Anomalies and Syndromes

Although acute atlantoaxial instability in children is rare, chronic atlantoaxial instability occurs in certain conditions such as juvenile rheumatoid arthritis, Reiter syndrome, Down syndrome, and Larsen syndrome. Bone dysplasia—such as Morquio polysaccharidosis, spondyloepiphyseal dysplasia, and Kniest syndrome—also may be associated with atlantoaxial instability, as well as os odontoideum, Klippel-Feil syndrome, and occipitalization of the atlas (80,174–179).

Certain cranial facial malformations have high incidences of associated anomalies of the cervical spine, such as Apert syndrome, hemifacial microsomy, and Goldenhar syndrome (180). Treatment recommendations are individualized based on the natural history of the disorder and future risk to the patient. Although there is little literature on cervical spine instability in each of these syndromes, there has been considerable interest in the incidence and treatment of atlantoaxial instability in children with Down syndrome (181–186).

Some Down syndrome patients have C1-C2 instability of more than 5 mm. The Committee on Sports Medicine of the American Academy of Pediatrics issued a policy statement in 1984 (181) asserting that Down syndrome patients with 5 to 6 mm of instability should be restricted from participating in sports that carry a risk of stress to the head and neck. In 1995, the AAP retired this recommendation and issued the following statement (109): "From the available scientific evidence, it is reasonable to conclude that lateral plain radiographs of the cervical spine are of potential but unproven value in detecting patients at risk for developing spinal cord injury during sports participation." Current opinion is that in asymptomatic children, yearly examinations to detect any neurologic symptoms or signs of myelopathy are more predictive of progressive myelopathy or neurologic injury than are screening x-rays (182). Evaluation of lateral cervical spine x-rays in full flexion and full extension is still required before participation in sports considered by the Special Olympics to have potential risk: certain activities that axially load the head in flexion, such as gymnastics, diving, and soccer (187). Davidson (182) found that neurologic signs were more predictive of impending dislocation than the x-ray criteria. Studies have shown that by adolescence, the frequency of atlantoaxial instability approaches 10% to 30% (109,174,184,188,189). It also appears that 12% (174) to 16% (183) of children with Down syndrome who have instability develop neurologic signs and symptoms.

Surgical stabilization is indicated for patients with translation of more than 10 mm. In patients with less than 10 mm of translation and a neurologic deficit or history of neurologic symptoms, surgical stabilization also may be indicated. Once surgical stabilization is needed, the treating physician must understand the increased risk of complications (i.e., pseudarthrosis) in this patient population. Segal et al (188) reported a high complication rate after posterior arthrodesis of the cervical spine in patients with Down syndrome. Six of 10 patients developed resorption of the bone graft and associated pseudarthrosis. Other complications in this patient population after attempted posterior arthrodesis were wound infection, dehiscence of the operative site, instability of adjacent motion segments, and neurologic sequelae (180).

Atlantoaxial Rotatory Subluxation

Atlantoaxial rotatory subluxation is a common cause of childhood torticollis. This condition is known by several names, such as rotatory dislocation, rotatory displacement, rotatory subluxation, and rotatory fixation. Atlantoaxial rotatory subluxation probably is the most accepted term used, except for long-standing cases (3 months), which are called rotatory fixation.

A significant amount of motion occurs at the atlantoaxial joint; half of the rotation of the cervical spine occurs there. Through this range of motion at the C1-C2 articulation, some children develop atlantoaxial rotatory subluxation. The two most common causes are trauma and infection; the most common cause is an upper respiratory infection (Grisel syndrome) (190). Subluxation also can occur after a retropharyngeal abscess, tonsillectomy, pharyngoplasty, or trivial trauma. There is free blood flow between the veins and lymphatics draining the pharynx and the periodontoid plexus (75). Any inflammation of these structures can lead to attenuation of the synovial capsule or transverse ligament or both, with resulting instability. Another potential etiologic factor is the shape of the superior facets of the axis in children. Kawabe et al (191) showed that the facets are smaller and more steeply inclined in children than in adults. A meniscus-like synovial fold was found between C1 and C2 that could prohibit reduction after displacement has occurred.

Classification

Fielding and Hawkins (155) classified atlantoaxial rotatory displacements into four types based on the direction and degree of rotation and translation (Fig. 18-36). Type 1 is a unilateral facet subluxation with an intact transverse ligament. This is the most common and benign type. Type 2 is a unilateral facet subluxation with anterior displacement of 3 to 5 mm. The unilateral anterior displacement of one of the lateral masses may indicate an incompetent transverse ligament with potential instability. Type 3 is bilateral anterior facet displacement with more than 5 mm of anterior displacement. This type is associated with deficiencies of the transverse and secondary ligaments, which can result in significant narrowing of the space available

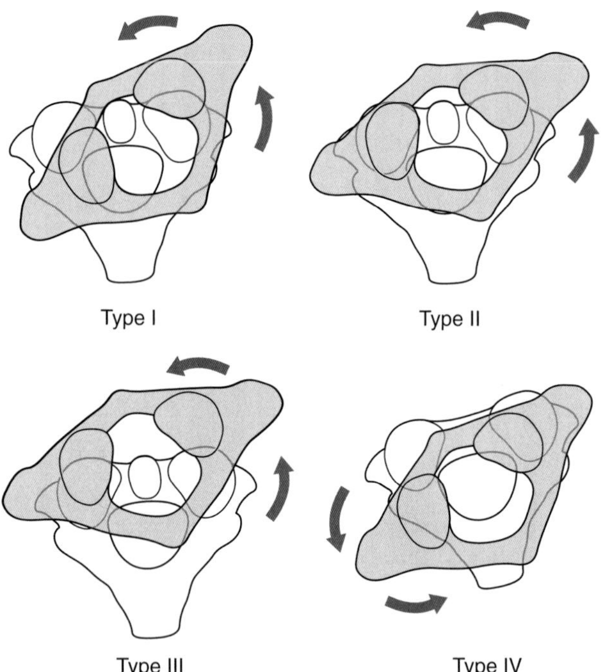

FIGURE 18-36 Classification of rotary displacement. (Reprinted from Fielding JW, Hawkins RJ. Atlantoaxial rotary fixation. *J Bone Joint Surg [Am]* 1977;59:37; with permission.)

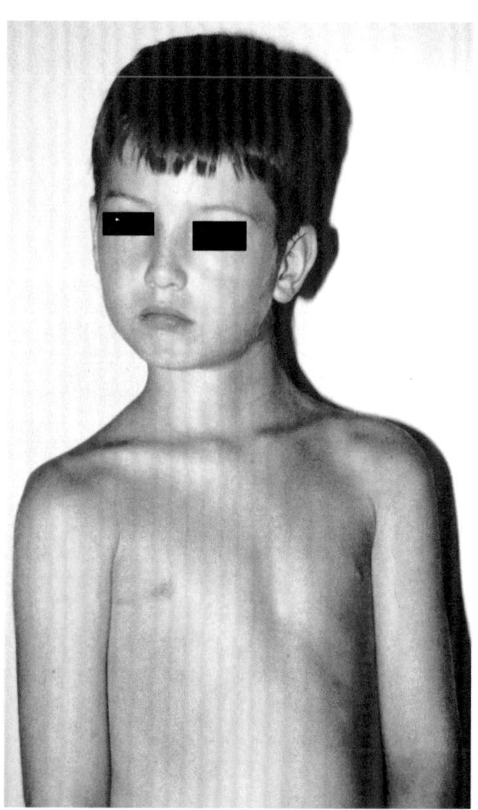

FIGURE 18-37 Child with rotary subluxation of C1 on C2. Note the direction of head tilt and rotation of the neck.

for the cord at the atlantoaxial level. Type 4 is an unusual type in which the atlas is displaced posteriorly. This usually is associated with a deficient dens. Although types 3 and 4 are rare, neurologic involvement may be present or instantaneous death can occur. Both types must be managed with great care.

Signs and Symptoms

Clinical findings include neck pain, headache, and a cock-robin position of rotating to one side as well as lateral flexion to the other (Fig. 18-37). When rotatory subluxation is acute, the child resists attempts to move the head and has pain with any attempts at correction. Usually the child is able to make the deformity worse but cannot correct it. Associated muscle spasms of the sternocleidomastoid muscle occur predominantly on the side of the long sternocleidomastoid muscle in an attempt to correct the deformity. If the deformity becomes fixed, the pain subsides but the torticollis and the decreased range of motion will persist (155). If rotatory fixation has been present for a long time in a small child, plagiocephaly is sometimes noted. Neurologic abnormalities are extremely rare, although a few cases have been reported.

X-Ray Findings

Adequate x-rays may be difficult to obtain because of the associated torticollis and difficulty in positioning the head and neck. Anteroposterior and open-mouth odontoid views should be taken with the shoulders flat and the head in as neutral a position as possible (192). Lateral masses that have rotated forward appear wider and closer to the midline, whereas the opposite lateral mass appears narrower and farther away from the midline on this view. One of the facet joints may be obscured because of apparent overlapping. The distance between the lateral mass and the dens also will be asymmetric. On the lateral view, the lateral facet appears anterior and usually appears wedge-shaped instead of the normal oval shape. The posterior arches of the atlas may fail to superimpose because of head tilt, giving the appearance of fusion of C1 to the occiput (occipitalization). Flexion and extension lateral views are recommended to exclude instability.

Cineradiography has been used for the evaluation of atlantoaxial rotatory subluxation (153,157,193). This technique is limited in the acute stage because pain restricts the motion necessary for a satisfactory study. With atlantoaxial rotatory fixation, cineradiography may be helpful in confirming the diagnosis by showing that the atlas and axis are rotating as a unit. However, this technique requires high radiation exposure and generally has been replaced by CT scanning (140,144,157, 194,195). CT should be performed with the head and body positioned as close to neutral as possible. This will show a superimposition of C1 on C2 in a rotated position and will allow the degree and amount of malrotation to be quantified. Some researchers have recommended dynamic CT scans taken with the patient looking to the right and the left to diagnose rotatory fixation (196). Three-dimensional CT scans also are helpful in identifying rotatory subluxation (146). MRI demonstrates more soft tissue detail, such as associated spinal cord compression and underlying vertebral or soft tissue infections (Fig. 18-38) (197).

Differential Diagnoses

Differential diagnoses include torticollis caused by ophthalmologic problems, sternocleidomastoid tightness from muscular torticollis, brain stem or posterior fossa tumors or abnormalities, congenital vertebral anomalies, and infections of the vertebral column.

Treatment

Treatment depends on the duration of the symptoms (196). Many patients probably never receive medical treatment, because symptoms may be mild and the subluxation may reduce spontaneously over a few days before medical attention is sought. If rotatory subluxation has been present for a week or less, a soft collar, anti-inflammatory medication, and an exercise program are indicated. If this fails to produce improvement and the symptoms persist for more than a week, head halter traction should be initiated. This can be done either at home or in the hospital, depending on the social situation and the severity of symptoms. Muscle relaxants and analgesics also may be needed. Phillips and Hensinger (196) found that if rotatory subluxation

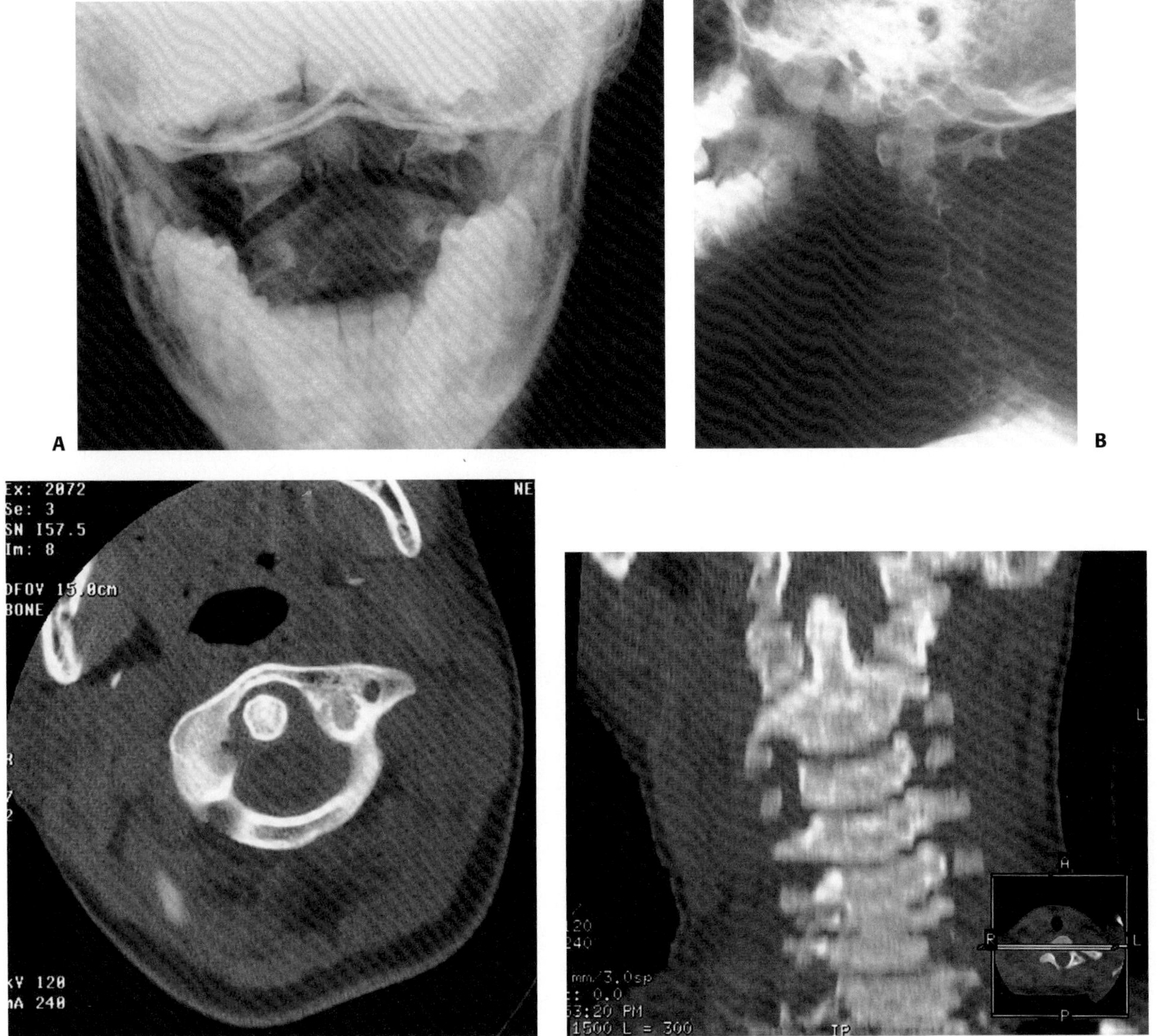

FIGURE 18-38 A,B. Odontoid view and lateral cervical spine x-ray of rotary subluxation of C1 on C2. **C.** Note the asymmetry on the open-mouth odontoid view. **D.** CT and CT reconstruction documenting rotary subluxation.

was present for less than 1 month, head halter traction and bed rest were usually sufficient to relieve symptoms. If the subluxation has been present for longer than a month, successful reduction is not very likely (116). However, halo traction can still be used to try to reduce the subluxation. The halo allows increased traction weight to be applied without interfering with opening of the jaw or causing skin pressure on the mandible. While the traction is being applied, active rotation to the right and left should be encouraged. Once the atlantoaxial rotatory subluxation has been reduced, motion has been restored, and the reduction is documented by CT scan, the patient is maintained in a halo vest for 6 weeks. If reduction cannot be maintained, posterior atlantoaxial arthrodesis is recommended. Even though internal rotation and alignment of the atlas and axis may not be restored, successful fusion should result in the appearance of normal head alignment by relieving the muscle spasms that occurred in response to the malrotation. Posterior arthrodesis also is recommended if any signs of instability or neurologic deficits secondary to the subluxation are present, if the deformity has been present for more than 3 months, or if conservative treatment of 6 weeks of immobilization has failed.

Hangman's Fracture

Bilateral spondylolisthesis of C2, or hangman's fractures, also may occur in children (197). The mechanism of injury is forced hyperextension. Most reports of this injury have been in children under the age of 2 years (195,198–204). This injury probably occurs more frequently in this age group because of the disproportionately large head, poor muscle control, and hypermobility. The possibility of child abuse also must be considered. Patients present with neck pain and resist any movement of the head and neck. There should be a positive history of trauma (Fig. 18-39).

X-rays reveal a lucency anterior to the pedicles of the axis, usually with some forward subluxation of C2 on C3. One must be sure this is a fracture and not a persistent synchondrosis of the axis. Several authors (205–208) have reported similar cases of persistent synchondrosis of the axis. CT scans showed the defect to be at the level of the neurocentral chondrosis. Later films showed ossification within the synchondrosis gap.

Treatment should be symptomatic with immobilization in a Minerva cast, halo, or cervical orthosis for 8 to 12 weeks. Traction is not needed to reduce this fracture and may even produce potentially dangerous distraction. Pizzutillo et al (195) reported that four of five patients healed with immobilization. If union does not occur, posterior arthrodesis or anterior arthrodesis can be performed to stabilize this fracture.

SUBAXIAL INJURIES

Fractures and dislocations involving C3 through C7 are rare in children and infants (90,209–211) and usually occur in teenagers or older children. Lower cervical spine injuries in children as opposed to those in adults can occur through the cartilaginous endplate (130). The endplate may break completely through the cartilaginous portion (Salter type I) or may exit through the bony edge (Salter type II). Usually the inferior endplate fractures because of the protective effect of the uncinate processes of the superior endplate (13).

Posterior Ligamentous Disruption

Posterior ligamentous disruption can occur with a flexion or distraction injury to the cervical spine. The patient usually has point tenderness at the injury site and complains of neck pain. Initial x-rays may be normal except for loss of normal cervical lordosis. This may be a normal finding in young children but should be evaluated for possible ligamentous injury in an adolescent. Widening of the posterior interspinous distance is suggestive of this injury. MRI may be helpful in documenting ligamentous damage.

With posterior ligamentous disruption, gradual displace-

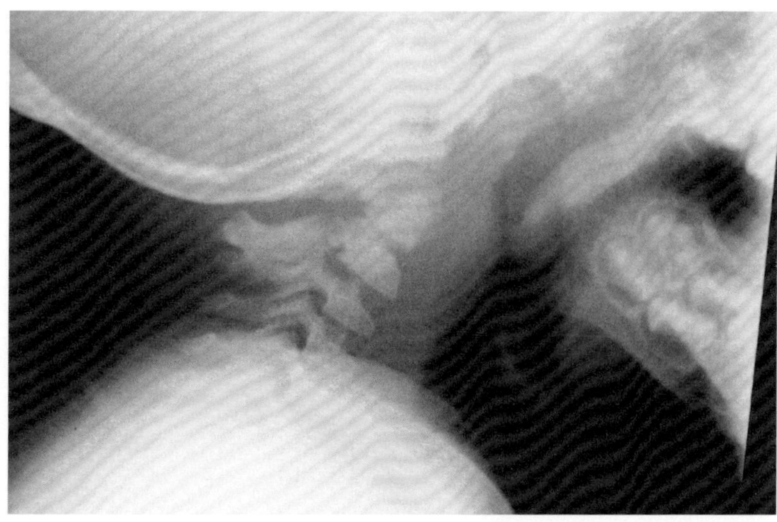

FIGURE 18-39 Lateral x-ray of patient with traumatic C2 spondylolisthesis (hangman's fracture).

ment of one segment on the other can occur, and secondary adaptive changes in the growing spine may make reduction difficult. Posterior ligamentous injuries should be protected with an extension orthosis, and patients should be followed closely for the development of instability. If signs of instability are present, then a posterior arthrodesis should be performed.

Compression Fractures

Compression fractures, the most common fractures of the subaxial spine in children, are caused by flexion and axial loading that results in loss of vertebral body height. This can be detected on a lateral x-ray. Because the vertebral disks in children are more resilient than the vertebral bodies, the bone is more likely to be injured. Compression fractures are stable injuries and heal in children in 3 to 6 weeks. Many compression fractures may be overlooked because of the normal wedge shape of the vertebral bodies in young children. Immobilization in a cervical collar is recommended for 3 to 6 weeks. Flexion and extension films to confirm stability should be obtained 2 to 4 weeks after injury. In children under 8 years of age, the vertebral body may reconstitute itself with growth, although Schwarz et al (212) reported that kyphosis of more than 20 degrees may not correct with growth. Associated injuries can include anterior teardrop, laminar, and spinous process fractures.

Unilateral and Bilateral Facet Dislocations

Unilateral facet dislocations and bilateral facet dislocations are the second most common injuries in the subaxial spine in children. Most occur in adolescents and are similar to adult injuries. The diagnosis usually can be made on anteroposterior and lateral x-rays. In children the so-called perched facet is a true dislocation. The cartilaginous components are overlapped and locked. On the x-ray, the facet appears perched because the overlapped cartilage cannot be seen. Unilateral facet dislocation is treated with traction and reduction. If reduction cannot be easily obtained, open reduction and arthrodesis are indicated. Complete bilateral facet dislocation, although rare, is more unstable and has a higher incidence of neurologic deficit (Fig. 18-40). Treatment consists of reduction and stabilization with a posterior arthrodesis.

Burst Fractures

Although rare, burst fractures can occur in children. These injuries are caused by an axial load. X-ray evaluation should consist of anteroposterior and lateral views. CT scans aid in detecting any spinal canal compromise from retropulsed fracture fragments and occult laminar fractures. If no neurologic deficit or significant canal compromise is present, then treatment consists of traction followed by halo immobilization. Anterior arthrodesis rarely is recommended in pediatric patients, except in a patient with a burst fracture and significant canal compromise (213). Anterior arthrodesis destroys the anterior growth potential; as posterior growth continues, a kyphotic deformity may occur (Fig. 18-41). In older children and adolescents, anterior instrumentation can be used for stabilization.

Spondylolysis and Spondylolisthesis

Spondylolysis and spondylolisthesis of C2 through C6 have been reported. These injuries can occur from either a hyperextension or flexion axial loading injury. Associated anterosuperior avulsion or compression fractures of the vertebral body may occur. The diagnosis usually is made on plain x-rays that show a fracture line through the pedicles. Oblique views may be necessary to better identify the fracture line. CT scanning may be useful in differentiating an acute fracture from a normal synchondrosis. Treatment consists of immobilization in a cervical orthosis or halo brace. Surgical stabilization is recommended only for truly unstable fractures or nonunions. Neurologic involvement is rare.

Operative Treatment

Posterior Arthrodesis

General anesthesia is administered with the patient supine (Fig. 18-42). The patient is turned prone on the operating table, with care taken to maintain traction and proper alignment of the head and neck. The head may be positioned in a head rest or maintained in skeletal traction. X-rays are obtained to confirm adequate alignment of the vertebrae and to localize the vertebrae to be exposed. Extension of the fusion mass can occur when extra vertebrae or spinous processes are exposed in the cervical spine. A midline incision is made over the chosen spinous processes, and the spinous process and lamina are exposed subperiosteally to the facet joints. If the spinous process is large enough, a hole is made in the base of the spinous process with a towel clip or Lewin clamp. An 18-gauge wire is passed through this hole, looped over the spinous process, and passed through the hole again. A similar hole is made in the base of the spinous process of the inferior vertebra to be fused, and the wire is passed through this vertebra. The wire is then passed through this hole, looped under the inferior aspect of the spinous process, and then passed back through the same hole. The wire is tightened and corticocancellous bone grafts are placed along the exposed lamina and spinous processes. The wound is closed in layers. If the spinous process is too small to pass wires, then an in situ arthrodesis can be performed and external immobilization used.

Hall et al (214) used a 16-gauge wire and threaded Kirschner wires. The threaded Kirschner wires are passed through the bases of the spinous processes of the vertebrae to be fused. This is followed by a figure-of-eight wiring with a 16-gauge wire (Fig. 18-43). After tightening the wire about the Kirschner wires, strips of corticocancellous and cancellous bone are packed over the posterior arches of the vertebrae to be fused.

In older children and adolescents, lateral mass plates or screw-and-rod systems can be used in the lower cervical spine. The instrumentation should be of appropriate size to match the size of the child's cervical spine.

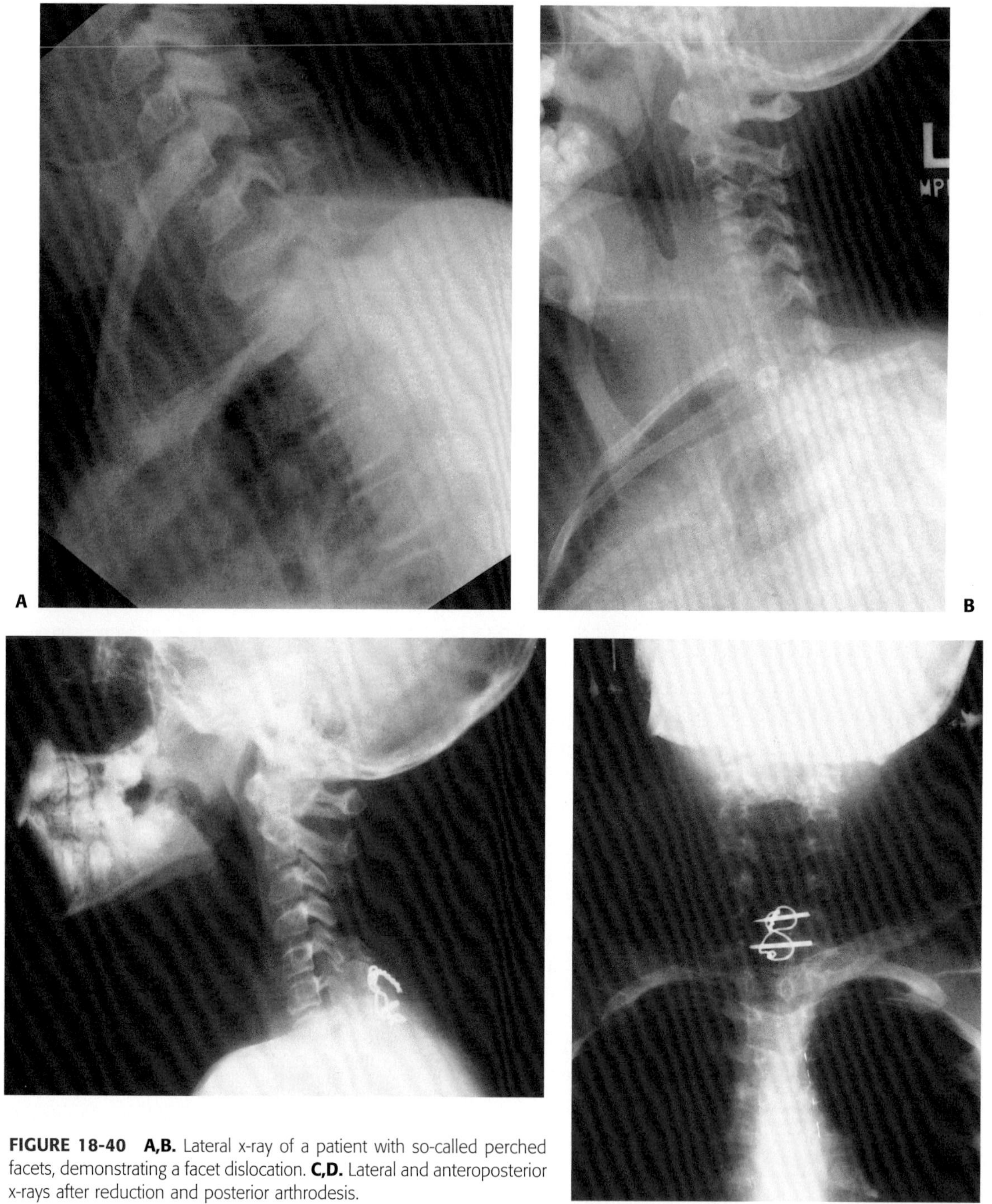

FIGURE 18-40 A,B. Lateral x-ray of a patient with so-called perched facets, demonstrating a facet dislocation. **C,D.** Lateral and anteroposterior x-rays after reduction and posterior arthrodesis.

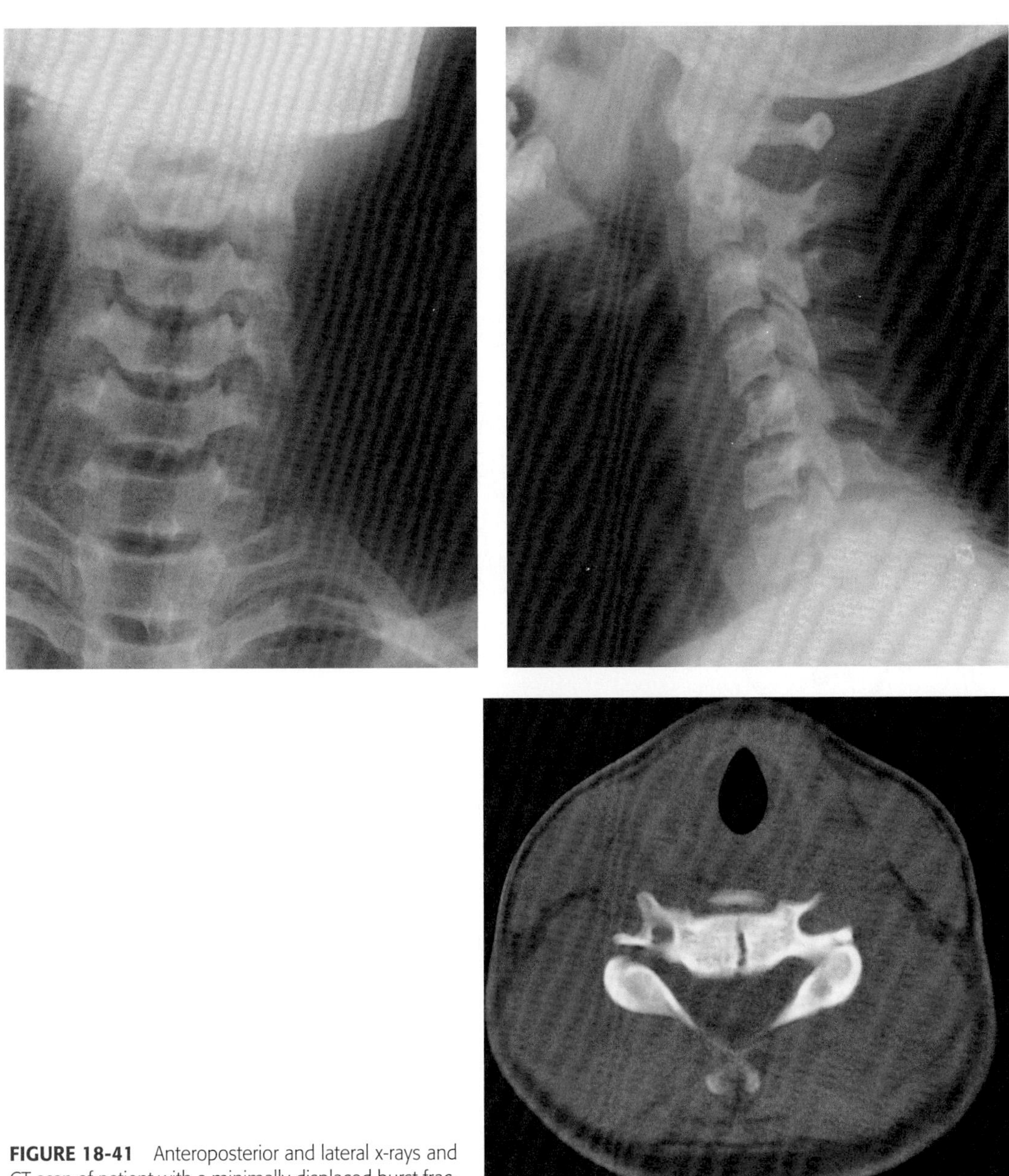

FIGURE 18-41 Anteroposterior and lateral x-rays and CT scan of patient with a minimally displaced burst fracture of C5.

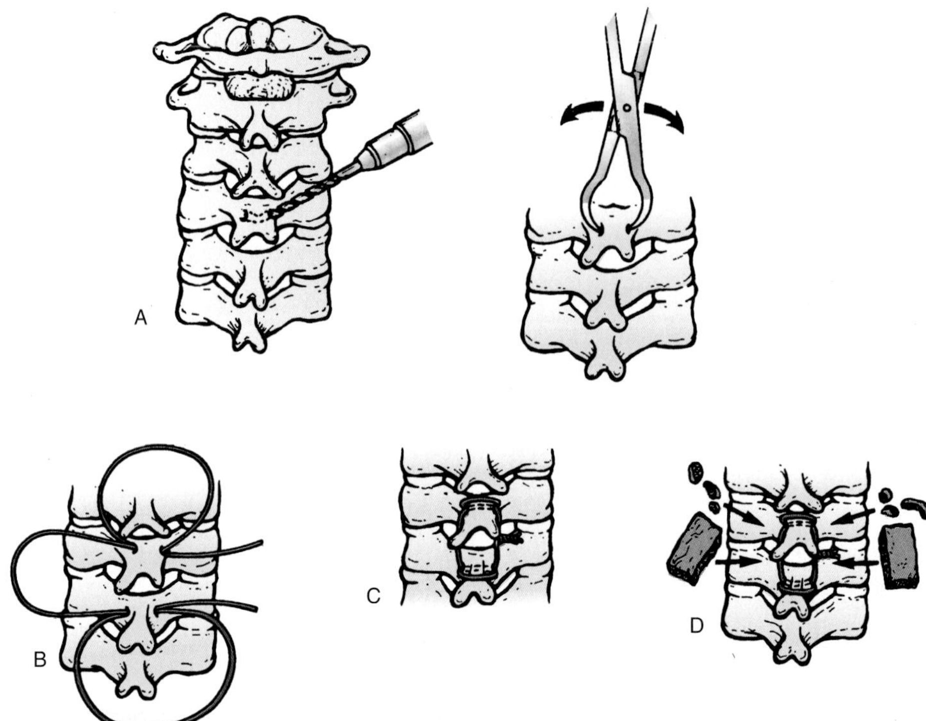

FIGURE 18-42 Technique of posterior arthrodesis in subaxial spine levels C3-C7. **A.** A hole is made in the spinous process of the vertebrae to be fused. **B.** An 18-gauge wire is passed through both holes and around the spinous processes. **C.** The wire is tightened. **D.** Corticocancellous bone grafts are placed. (Redrawn from Murphy MJ, Southwick WO. Posterior approaches and fusions. In: Cervical Spine Research Society. *The cervical spine.* Philadelphia: JB Lippincott, 1983; with permission.)

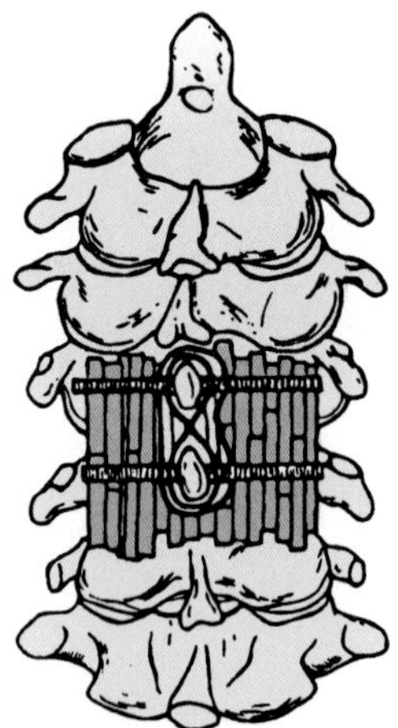

FIGURE 18-43 Alternative fixation method for posterior arthrodesis of C3-C7. A 16-gauge wire is placed in a figure-of-eight pattern around two threaded Kirschner wires passed through the bases of the spinous processes of the vertebrae to be fused. (Reprinted from Hall JE, Simmons ED, Danylchuk K, et al. Instability of the cervical spine and neurological involvement in Klippel-Feil syndrome: a case report. *J Bone Joint Surg [Am]* 1990;72:460; with permission.)

Posterior Arthrodesis With Lateral Mass Screw Fixation

Several techniques of lateral mass screw fixation for the lower cervical spine have been described. They differ primarily in the entry points for the screws and in the trajectory of screw placement, which yield different exit points (215,216).

Roy-Camille Technique. The entry point for the screw is at the center of the rectangular posterior face of the lateral mass or can be measured 5 mm medial to the lateral edge and midway between the facet joints (Fig. 18-44A). The drill is directed perpendicular to the posterior wall of the vertebral body with a 10-degree lateral angle (see Fig. 18-44B). This trajectory establishes an exit point slightly lateral to the vertebral artery and below the exiting nerve root. The lateral mass depth from C3 to C6 ranges from 6 to 14 mm in men (average 8.7 mm) and 6 to 11 mm in women (average 7.9 mm). An adjustable drill guide set to a depth of 10 to 12 mm is used to prevent penetration beyond the anterior cortex. The depth can be gradually and safely increased if local anatomy permits. If the additional 20% of pullout strength with bicortical fixation is desired, the exit point should be at the junction of the lateral mass and the transverse process. Lateral fluoroscopic imaging makes it easier to choose the optimal trajectory and avoid penetration of the subjacent facet joint (see Fig. 18-

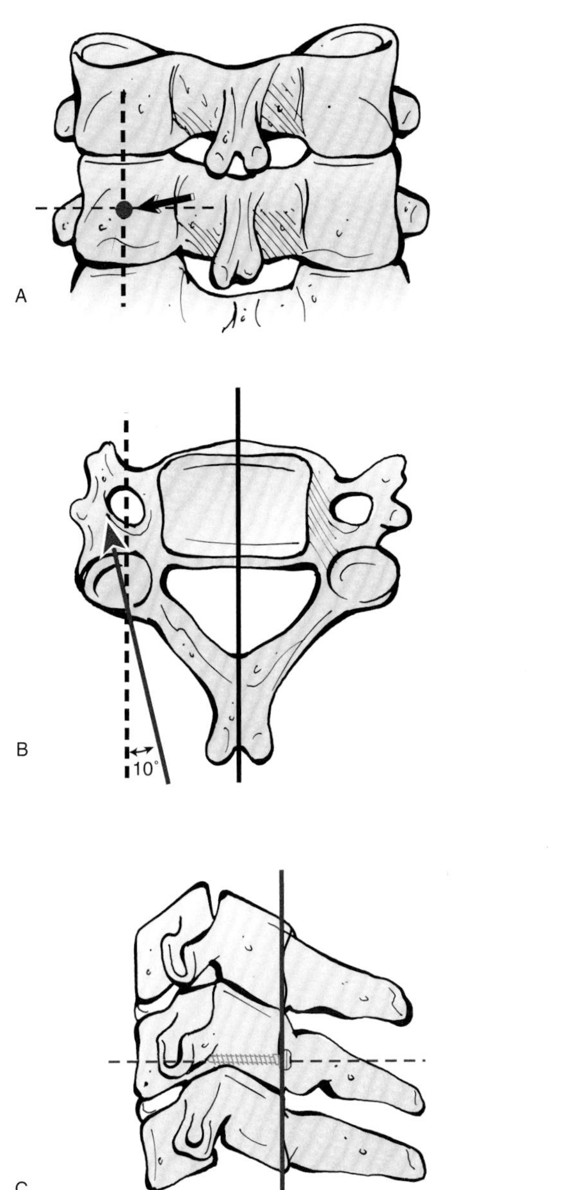

FIGURE 18-44 Roy-Camille technique of lateral mass screw insertion. **A.** Entry point for screw insertion. **B.** Drill is directed perpendicular to posterior wall of vertebral body with a 10-degree lateral angle. **C.** Final screw position. (Reprinted from Heller JG, Jeffords P. Internal fixation of the cervical spine. Posterior instrumentation of the lower cervical spine. In: Frymoyer JW, Wiesel SW, eds. *The adult and pediatric spine*, 3rd ed. Philadelphia: Lippincott Williams & Wilkins, 2004; with permission.)

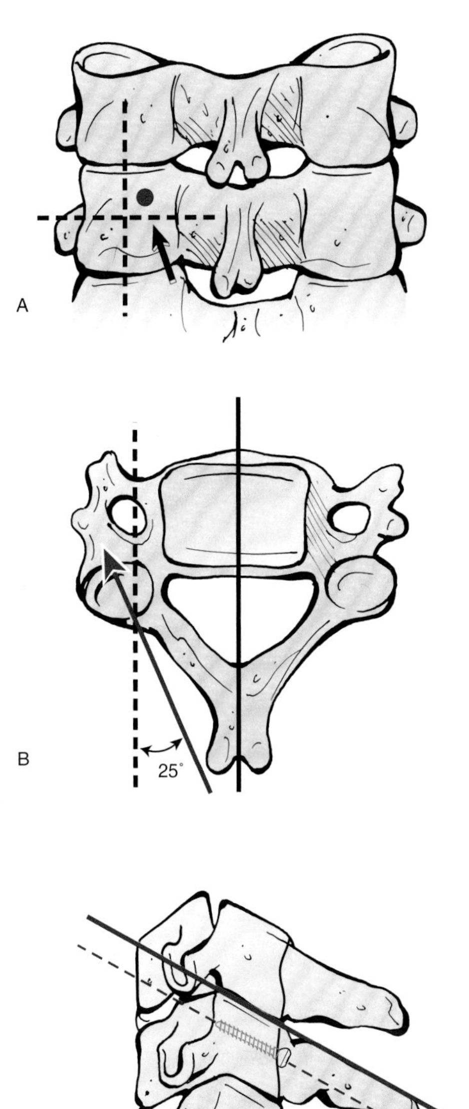

FIGURE 18-45 Magerl technique of lateral mass screw insertion. **A.** Entry point for screw insertion. **B.** Drill is directed at a 25-degree lateral angle. **C.** Final screw position. (Reprinted from Heller JG, Jeffords P. Internal fixation of the cervical spine. Posterior instrumentation of the lower cervical spine. In: Frymoyer JW, Wiesel SW, eds. *The adult and pediatric spine*, 3rd ed. Philadelphia: Lippincott Williams & Wilkins, 2004; with permission.)

44C), which is especially important at the caudal level of fixation because this joint should be included in the fusion.

Magerl Technique. The entry point for the screw is 1 mm medial and rostral (proximal) to the center point of the posterior surface of the lateral mass (Fig. 18-45A). It is oriented at a 45- to 60-degree rostral angle, parallel to the adjacent facet joint articular surface, and at a 25-degree lateral angle (see Fig. 18-45B). This trajectory establishes an exit point lateral to the vertebral artery and above the exiting nerve root while engaging the lateral portion of the ventral cortex of the superior articular facet (see Fig. 18-45C). The proper trajectory for this technique is more difficult to achieve that in the Roy-Camille technique. The prominence of the thorax can impede proper alignment of the drill and guide, risking injury to the nerve root if the second cortex is penetrated. The depth of penetration at this angle is approximately 18 mm, compared to 14 mm with the Roy-Camille technique, which has some implications for purchase strength and mode of screw failure.

REFERENCES

1. Anderson PA, Montesano PX. Morphology and treatment of occipital condyle fractures. *Spine* 1988;13:731–736.
2. Anderson JM, Schutt AH. Spinal injury in children: a review of 156 cases seen from 1950 through 1978. *Mayo Clin Proc* 1980;55:499–504.
3. Hadley MN, Zabramski JM, Browner CM, et al. Pediatric spinal trauma: review of 122 cases of spinal cord vertebral column injuries. *J Neurosurg* 1988;68:18–24.
4. Haffner DL, Hoffer MM, Wiedebusch R. Etiology of children's spinal injuries at Rancho Los Amigos. *Spine* 1993;18:679–684.
5. Herzenberg JE, Hensinger RN. Pediatric cervical spine injuries. *Trauma Q* 1989;5: 73–81.
6. Hubbard DD. Injuries of the spine in children and adolescents. *Clin Orthop* 1974;100: 56–65.
7. Kewalramani LS, Kraus JF, Sterling HM. Acute spinal-cord lesions in a pediatric population: epidemiological and clinical features. *Paraplegia* 1980;18:206–219.
8. Lebwohl NH, Eismont FJ. Cervical spine injuries in children. In: Weinstein SL, ed. *The pediatric spine: principles and practice.* Philadelphia: Lippincott Williams & Wilkins, 2001.
9. Pang D, Wilberger JE. Spinal cord injury without radiologic abnormalities in children. *J Neurosurg* 1982;57:114–129.
10. Ruge JR, Sinson GP, McLone DG, et al. Pediatric spinal injury: the very young. *J Neurosurg* 1988;68:25–30.
11. Stauffer ES, Mazur JM. Cervical spine injuries in children. *Pediatr Ann* 1982;11: 502–511.
12. McGrory BJ, Klassen RA, Chao EY, et al. Acute fracture and dislocations of the cervical spine in children and adolescents. *J Bone Joint Surg [Am]* 1993;75:988–995.
13. Aufdermaur M. Spinal injuries in juveniles: necropsy findings in twelve cases. *J Bone Joint Surg [Br]* 1974;56:513–519.
14. Pang D, Pollack IF. Spinal cord injury without radiologic abnormality in children: the SCIWORA syndrome. *J Trauma* 1989;29:654–664.
15. Ghatan S, Ellenbogen RG. Pediatric spine and spinal cord injury after inflicted trauma. *Neurosurg Clin North Am* 2002;13:227–233.
16. Brooks AL, Jenkins EB. Atlantoaxial arthrodesis by the wedge compression method. *J Bone Joint Surg [Am]* 1978;60:279–290.
17. Zuckerbraun BS, Morrison K, Baines B, et al. Effect of age on cervical spine injuries in children after motor vehicle collisions: effectiveness of restraint devices. *J Pediatr Surg* 2004;39:483–486.
18. Torg B, Das M. Trampoline and minitrampoline injuries to the cervical spine. *Clin Sports Med* 1985;4:45–60.
19. Birney TJ, Hanley EN. Traumatic cervical spine injuries in childhood and adolescence. *Spine* 1989;14:1277–1282.
20. Evans DL, Bethem D. Cervical spine injuries in children. *J Pediatr Orthop* 1989;9: 563–568.
21. Eleraky MA, Theodore N, Adams M, et al. Pediatric cervical spine injuries: report of 102 cases and review of the literature. *J Neurosurg* 2000;92(1 Suppl):12–17.
22. Kilfoyle RM, Foley JJ, Norton PL. Spine and pelvic deformity in childhood and adolescent paraplegia. *J Bone Joint Surg [Am]* 1965;47:659–682.
23. Nitecki S, Moir CR. Predictive factors of the outcome of traumatic cervical spine fracture in children. *J Pediatr Surg* 1994;29:1409–1411.
24. Patel JC, Tepas JJ III, Mollitt DL, Pieper P. Pediatric cervical spine injuries: defining the disease. *J Pediatr Surg* 2001;36:373–376.
25. Orenstein JB, Klein BL, Gotschall CS, et al. Age and outcome in pediatric cervical spine injury: 11-year experience. *Pediatr Emerg Care* 1994;10:132–137.
26. Orenstein JB, Klein BL, Oschensclager DW. Delayed diagnosis of pediatric cervical spine injury. *Pediatrics* 1992;89:1185–1188.
27. Hamilton MG, Myles ST. Pediatric spinal injury. Review of 61 deaths. *J Neurosurg* 1988; 77:705–708.
28. Caffey J. The whiplash shaken infant syndrome. *Pediatrics* 1974;54:396–403.
29. Cattell HS, Filtzer DL. Pseudosubluxation and other normal variations in the cervical spine in children. *J Bone Joint Surg [Am]* 1965;47:1295–1309.
30. Lawson JP, Ogden JA, Bucholz RW, et al. Physeal injuries of the cervical spine. *J Pediatr Orthop* 1987;7:428–435.
31. Rachesky I, Boyce WT, Duncan B, et al. Clinical prediction of cervical spine injuries in children: radiographic abnormalities. *Am J Dis Child* 1987;141:199–201.
32. Bohn D, Armstrong D, Becker L, et al. Cervical spine injuries in children. *J Trauma* 1990;30:463–469.
33. Committee on Pediatric Orthopaedics. Trauma of the Cervical Spine. Position Statement, American Academy of Orthopaedic Surgeons, 1990.
34. Pennecot GF, Gouraud D, Hardy JR, et al. Roentgenographical study of the stability of the cervical spine in children. *J Pediatr Orthop* 1984;4:346–352.
35. Hensinger RN, Lang JE, MacEwen GD. Klippel-Feil syndrome: a constellation of associated anomalies. *J Bone Joint Surg [Am]* 1974;56:1246–1252.
36. Klippel M, Feil A. Anomalies de la collone vertebrale par absence des vertebres cervicales; avec cage thoraque remontant jusqu'ala bas du crane. *Bull Soc Anat Paris* 1912; 87:185.
37. Hensinger RN, Fielding JW, Hawkins RJ. Congenital anomalies of the odontoid process. *Orthop Clin North Am* 1978;9:901–912.
38. Kokoska ER, Keller MS, Rallo MC, Weber TR. Characteristics of pediatric cervical spine injuries. *J Pediatr Surg* 2001;36:100–105.
39. Huerta C, Griffith R, Joyce SM. Cervical spine stabilization in pediatric patients. Evaluation of current techniques. *Ann Emerg Med* 1987;16:1121–1126.
40. Schwartz GR, Wright SW, Fein JA, et al. Pediatric cervical spine injury sustained in falls from low heights. *Ann Emerg Med* 1997;30:249–252.
41. Fuchs S, Barthel MJ, Flannery AM, et al. Cervical spine fractures sustained by young children in forward-facing car seats. *Pediatrics* 1989;84:348–354.
42. Hoy GA, Cole WG. The paediatric cervical seat belt syndrome. *Injury* 1993;24: 297–299.
43. Viccellio P, Simon H, Pressman BD, et al. A prospective multicenter study of cervical spine injury in children. *Pediatrics* 2001;108:E20.
44. Anderson LD, Smith BL, DeToree J, et al. The role of polytomography in the diagnosis and treatment of cervical spine injuries. *Clin Orthop Rel Res* 1982;165:64–68.
45. Dietrich AM, Ginn-Pease ME, Bartkowski HM, et al. Pediatric cervical spine fractures: predominately subtle presentation. *J Pediatr Surg* 1991;26:995–1000.
46. Lally KP, Senak M, Hardin WD, et al. Utility of the cervical spine radiograph in pediatric trauma. *Am J Surg* 1989;158:540–542.
47. Letts M, Kaylor D, Gouw G. A biomechanical study of halo fixation in children. *J Bone Joint Surg [Br]* 1987;70:277–279.
48. Bachulis BL, Long WB, Hynes GD, et al. Clinical indications for cervical spine radiographs in the traumatized patient. *Am J Surg* 1987;153:473–477.
49. Shaffer MA, Doris PE. Limitation of the cross-table lateral view in detecting cervical spine injuries: a retrospective review. *Ann Emerg Med* 1981;10:508–513.
50. Ralston ME, Chung K, Barnes PD, et al. Role of flexion-extension radiographs in blunt pediatric cervical spine injury. *Acad Emerg Med* 2001;8:237–245.
51. Donahue D, Muhlbauer M, Kaufman R, et al. Childhood survival of atlanto-occipital dislocation: underdiagnosis, recognition, treatment, and review of the literature. *Pediatr Neurosurg* 1994;21:105–111.
52. Bulas DI, Fitz CR, Johnson DL. Traumatic atlanto-occipital dislocation in children. *Radiology* 1993;188:155–158.
53. de Beer JD, Hoffman EB, Kieck CF. Traumatic atlantoaxial subluxation in children. *J Pediatr Orthop* 1990;10:397–400.
54. Swischuk EH Jr, Rowe ML. The upper cervical spine in health and disease. *Pediatrics* 1952;10:567–572.
55. Allington JJ, Zembo M, Nadell J, Bowen JR. C1-C2 posterior soft tissue injuries with neurologic impairment in children. *J Pediatr Orthop* 1990;10:596–601.
56. Walsh JW, Stevens DB, Young AB. Traumatic paraplegia in children without contiguous spinal fracture or dislocation. *Neurosurgery* 1983;12:439–445.
57. Kuhns LR, Strouse PJ. Cervical spine standards for flexion radiograph interspinous distance ratios in children. *Acta Radiol* 2000;7:615–619.
58. Hedequist DJ, Emans JB. The correlation of preoperative three-dimensional computed tomography reconstructions with operative findings in congenital scoliosis. *Spine* 2003; 28:2531–2534.
59. Keenan HT, Hollingshead MC, Chung CJ, et al. Using CT of the cervical spine for early evaluation of pediatric patients with head trauma. *AJR Am J Roentgenol* 2001;177: 1405–1409.
60. Adlegais KM, Grossman DC, Langer SG, et al. Use of helical computed tomography for imaging the pediatric cervical spine. *Acad Emerg Med* 2004;11:228–236.
61. Flynn JM, Closkey RF, Mahboubi S, et al. Role of magnetic resonance imaging in the assessment of pediatric cervical spine injuries. *J Pediatr Orthop* 2002;22:573–577.
62. Parbhoo AH, Govender S, Corr P. Vertebral artery injury in cervical spine trauma. *Injury* 2001;32:565–568.
63. Herzenberg JE, Hensinger RN, Dedrick DK, et al. Emergency transport and positioning of young children who have an injury of the cervical spine: the standard backboard may be hazardous. *J Bone Joint Surg [Am]* 1989;71:15–22.
64. Nypaver M, Treloar D. Neutral cervical spine positioning in children. *Ann Emerg Med* 1994;23:208–211.
65. Curran C, Dietrich AM, Bowman MJ, et al. Pediatric cervical-spine immobilization: achieving neutral position? *J Trauma* 1995;39:729–732.
66. Millington PJ, Ellingsen JM, Hauswirth BE, et al. Thermoplastic Minerva body jacket—a practical alternative to current methods of cervical spine stabilization. *Phys Ther* 1987; 67:223–225.
67. Dormans JP, Criscitiello AA, Drummond DS, et al. Complications in children managed with immobilization in a halo vest. *J Bone Joint Surg [Am]* 1995;77:1370–1373.
68. Baum JA, Hanley EN Jr, Pullekines J. Comparison of halo complications in adults and children. *Spine* 1989;14:251–252.
69. Mubarak SJ, Camp JF, Vueltich W, et al. Halo application in the infant. *J Pediatr Orthop* 1989;9:612–614.
70. Garfin SR, Roux R, Botte MJ, et al. Skull osteology as it affects halo pin placement in children. *J Pediatr Orthop* 1986;6:434–436.
71. Copley LA, Dormans JP, Pepe MD, et al. Accuracy and reliability of torque wrenches used for halo application in children. *J Bone Joint Surg [Am]* 2003;85:2199–2204.
72. Copley LA, Pepe MD, Tan V, et al. A comparison of various angles of halo pin insertion in an immature skull model. *Spine* 1999;24:1777–17800.
73. Burke DC. Spinal cord trauma in children. *Paraplegia* 1971;9:1–14.
74. Taylor AR. The mechanism of injury to the spinal cord in the neck without damage to the vertebral column. *J Bone Joint Surg [Br]* 1951;33:453–547.

75. Parke WW, Rothman RH, Brown MD. The pharyngovertebral veins: an anatomical rationale for Grisel's syndrome. *J Bone Joint Surg [Am]* 1984;66:568–574.
76. Yngve DA, Harris WP, Herndon WA, et al. Spinal cord injury without osseous spine fracture. *J Pediatr Orthop* 1988;8:153–159.
77. Menezes AH, Ryken JC. Craniovertebral junction abnormalities. In: Weinstein SL, ed. *The pediatric spine: principles and practice.* New York: Raven, 1994.
78. Annis JA, Finlay DB, Allen MJ, et al. A review of cervical-spine radiographs in casualty patients. *Br J Radiol* 1987;60:1059–1061.
79. Hanson JA, Deliganis AV, Baxter AB, et al. Radiologic and clinical spectrum of occipital condyle fractures: retrospective review of 107 consecutive fractures in 95 patients. *AJR Am J Roentgenol* 2002;178:1261–1268.
80. Hensinger RN, DeVito PD, Ragsdale CG. Changes in the cervical spine in juvenile rheumatoid arthritis. *J Bone Joint Surg [Am]* 1986;68:189–198.
81. Ranjith RK, Mullett JH, Burke TE. Hangman's fracture cause by suspected child abuse. A case report. *J Pediatr Orthop B* 2002;11:329–332.
82. Bracken MB. Treatment of acute spinal cord injury with methylprednisolone: results of a multi-center randomized clinical trial. *J Neurotrauma* 1991;8(suppl 1):47–50.
83. Bracken MB. Pharmacological treatment of acute spinal cord injury: current status and future projects. *J Emerg Med* 1993;11(suppl 1):43–48.
84. Bracken MB, Shepard MJ, Collins WF, et al. A randomized controlled trial of methylprednisolone or naloxone in the treatment of acute spinal cord injury: results of the Second National Spinal Cord Injury Study. *N Engl J Med* 1990;322:1405–1411.
85. Bracken MB, Shepard MJ, Collins WF, et al. Methylprednisolone and naloxone treatment after acute spinal cord injury: one-year follow-up data. Results of the Second National Acute Spinal Cord Injury Study. *J Neurosurg* 1992;76:23–31.
86. Geisler FH, Dorsey FC, Coleman WP. Recovery of motor function after spinal cord injury—a randomized, placebo-controlled trial with GM-1 ganglioside [erratum]. *N Engl J Med* 1991;325:1669–1670.
87. Geisler FH, Dorsey FC, Coleman WP. Recovery of motor function after spinal cord injury—a randomized, placebo-controlled trial with GM-1 ganglioside. *N Engl J Med* 1991;324:1829–1838.
88. Geisler FH, Dorsey FC, Coleman WP. GM-1 ganglioside in human spinal cord injury. *J Neurotrauma* 1992;9(suppl 1):407–416.
89. Geisler FH, Dorsey FC, Coleman WP. Past and current clinical studies with GM-1 ganglioside in acute spinal cord injury. *Rev Ann Emerg Med* 1993;22:1041–1047.
90. Sherk HH, Schut L, Lane J. Fractures and dislocations of the cervical spine in children. *Orthop Clin North Am* 1976;7:593–604.
91. Yasuoko F, Peterson H, MacCarty C. Incidence of spinal column deformity after multiple level laminectomy in children and adults. *J Neurosurg* 1982;57:441–445.
92. Mayfield JK, Erkkila JC, Winter RB. Spine deformities subsequent to acquired childhood spinal cord injury. *Orthop Trans* 1979;3:281–282.
93. Sim F, Svien H, Bickel W, et al. Swan neck deformity following extensive cervical laminectomy. *J Bone Joint Surg [Am]* 1974;56:564–580.
94. Banniza von Bazan UK, Paeslack V. Scoliotic growth in children with acquired paraplegia. *Paraplegia* 1977;15:65–73.
95. Bedbrook GM. Correction of scoliosis due to paraplegia sustained in pediatric age group. *Paraplegia* 1977;15:90–96.
96. Burke DC. Traumatic spinal paralysis in children. *Paraplegia* 1971;9:268–276.
97. Farley FA, Hensinger RN, Herzenberg JE. Cervical spinal cord injury in children. *J Spinal Disord* 1992;5:410–416.
98. Norman MG, Wedderburn LC. Fetal spinal cord injury with cephalic delivery. *Obstet Gynecol* 1973;42:355–358.
99. Tawbin A. CNS damage in the human fetus and newborn infant. *Am J Dis Child* 1951; 33:543–547.
100. Maekawa K, Masaki T, Kokubun Y. Fetal spinal cord injury secondary to hyperextension of the neck: no effect of caesarean section. *Dev Med Child Neurol* 1976;18:228–232.
101. Bresnan MJ, Abroms IF. Neonatal spinal cord transection secondary to intrauterine hyperextension of neck in breech presentation. *J Pediatr* 1974;84:734–737.
102. Conry BG, Hall CM. Cervical spine fractures and rear car seat restraints. *Arch Dis Child* 1987;62:1267–1268.
103. Givens T, Polley KA, Smith GF, Hardin WD Jr. Pediatric cervical spine injury: a three-year experience. *J Trauma* 1996;41:310–314.
104. Shulman ST, Madden JD, Esterly JR, et al. Transection of the spinal cord. A rare obstetrical complication of cephalic delivery. *Arch Dis Child* 1971;46:291–294.
105. Swischuk LE. Spine and spinal cord trauma in the battered child syndrome. *Radiology* 1969;92:733–738.
106. Momjian S, Dehdashti AR, Kehrli P, et al. Occipital condyle fractures in children: case report and review of the literature. *Pediatr Neurosurg* 2003;38:265–270.
107. Noble ER, Smoker WRK. The forgotten condyle: the appearance, morphology, and classification of occipital condyle fractures. *AJNR Am J Neuroradiol* 1996;17:507–513.
108. Tuli S, Tator CH, Fehlings MG, Mackay M. Occipital condyle fractures. *Neurosurgery* 1997;41:368–377.
109. American Academy of Pediatrics Committee on Sports Medicine and Fitness. Atlantoaxial instability in Down syndrome: subject review. *Pediatrics* 1995;96(1 pt 1):151–154.
110. Bohlman HH. Acute fractures and dislocations of the cervical spine. *J Bone Joint Surg [Am]* 1969;61:1119–1142.
111. Bucholz RW, Burkhead WZ. The pathological anatomy of fatal atlanto-occipital dislocations. *J Bone Joint Surg [Am]* 1979;61:248–250.
112. Evarts CM. Traumatic occipito-atlanto dislocation. *J Bone Joint Surg [Am]* 1970;52: 1653–1660.
113. Papadopoulos SM, Dickman CA, Sonntag VKH, et al. Traumatic atlantooccipital dislocation with survival. *Neurosurgery* 1991;28:574–579.
114. Sponseller PD, Herzenberg JE. Cervical spine injuries in children. In: *The cervical spine.* Philadelphia: Lippincott-Raven, 1998:357–371.
115. Bernini EP, Elefante R, Smaltino F, Tedeschi G. Angiographic study on the vertebral artery in cases of deformities of the occipitocervical joint. *AJR Am J Roentgenol* 1969; 107:526–529.
116. Burkus JK, Deponte RJ. Chronic atlantoaxial rotatory fixation: correction by cervical traction, manipulation, and branching. *J Pediatr Orthop* 1986;6:631–635.
117. Collato PM, Demuth WW, Schwentker EP, et al. Traumatic atlanto-occipital dislocation. *J Bone Joint Surg [Am]* 1986;68:1106–1109.
118. Harmanli O, Kaufman Y. Traumatic atlanto-occipital dislocation with survival. *Surg Neurol* 1993;39:324–330.
119. Hosono N, Yonenbou K, Kazuyoshi K, et al. Traumatic anterior atlanto-occipital dislocation. *Spine* 1993;18:786–790.
120. Powers B, Milber MD, Kramer RS, et al. Traumatic anterior occipital dislocation. *Neurosurgery* 1979;4:12–17.
121. Bundschumb CV, Allen JB, Ross M, et al. Magnetic resonance imaging of suspected atlanto-occipital dislocation. *Spine* 1992;17:245–248.
122. Farley FA, Graziano GP, Hensinger RN. Traumatic atlanto-occipital dislocation in a child. *Spine* 1992;17:1539–1541.
123. Georgopoulos G, Pizzutillo PD, Lee MS. Occipito-atlanto instability in children. A report of five cases and review of the literature. *J Bone Joint Surg [Am]* 1987;69:429–436.
124. Lynch JM, Meza MP, Pollack IF, et al. Direct injury to the cervical spine of a child by a lap-shoulder belt resulting in quadriplegia: case report. *J Trauma* 1996;41:747–749.
125. Arlet V, Aebi M. Anterior and posterior cervical spine fusion and instrumentation. In: Weinstein SL, ed. *Pediatric spine surgery*, 2nd ed. Philadelphia: Lippincott Williams & Wilkins, 2001.
126. Heller JG, Jeffords P. Internal fixation of the cervical spine. C. Posterior instrumentation of the lower cervical spine. In: Frymoyer JW, Wiesel SW, eds. *The adult and pediatric spine.* Philadelphia: Lippincott Williams & Wilkins, 2004.
127. Menezes AH. Surgical approaches to the craniocervical junction. In: Weinstein LD, ed. *Pediatric spine surgery*, 2nd ed. Philadelphia: Lippincott Williams & Wilkins, 2001.
128. Sponseller PD, Cass J. Atlanto-occipital arthrodesis for instability with neurologic preservation. *Spine* 1997;22:344–347.
129. Judd DB, Liem LK, Petermann G. Pediatric atlas fracture: a case of fracture through a synchondrosis and review of the literature. *Neurosurgery* 2000;46:991–995.
130. DiBenedetto T, Lee CK. Traumatic atlanto-occipital instability: a case report with follow-up and a new diagnostic technique. *Spine* 1990;15:595–597.
131. Koop SE, Winter RB, Lonstein JE. The surgical treatment of instability of the upper part of the cervical spine in children and adolescents. *J Bone Joint Surg [Am]* 1984;66: 403–411.
132. Wertheim SB, Bohlman HH. Occipitocervical fusion: indications, technique, and long-term results. *J Bone Joint Surg [Am]* 1987;69:833–836.
133. Grantham SA, Dick HM, Thompson RC, Stinchfield FE. Occipitocervical arthrodesis. *Clin Orthop* 1969;65:118–129.
134. Bivins HG, Ford S, Bezmalinovic Z, et al. The effect of axial traction during orotracheal intubation of the trauma victim with an unstable cervical spine. *Ann Emerg Med* 1988; 17:25–29.
135. Jefferson G. Fracture of the atlas vertebra: report of four cases and a review of those previously recorded. *Br J Surg* 1919–1920;7:407–422.
136. Marlin AE, Gayle RW, Lee JF. Jefferson fractures in children. *J Neurosurg* 1983;58: 277–279.
137. Mikawa Y, Watanabe R, Yamano Y, et al. Fractures through a synchondrosis of the anterior arch of the atlas. *J Bone Joint Surg [Br]* 1987;69:483.
138. Richards PG. Stable fractures of the atlas and axis in children. *J Neurol Neurosurg Psychiatry* 1984;47:781–783.
139. Tolo VT, Weiland AJ. Unsuspected atlas fractures and instability associated with oropharyngeal injury: case report. *J Trauma* 1979;19:278–280.
140. Dvorak J, Panjabi M, Gerber M, et al. CT-functional diagnostics of the rotatory instability of the cervical spine: 1. An experimental study on cadavers. *Spine* 1987;12:197–205.
141. Griffiths SC. Fracture of the odontoid process in children. *J Pediatr Surg* 1972;7: 680–683.
142. Seimon LP. Fracture of the odontoid process in young children. *J Bone Joint Surg [Am]* 1977;59:943–948.
143. Odent T, Langlais J, Glorion C, et al. Fractures of the odontoid process: a report of 15 cases in children younger than 6 years. *J Pediatr Orthop* 1999;19:51–54.
144. Apple JS, Kirks DR, Merten DF, et al. Cervical spine fractures and dislocations in children. *Pediatr Radiol* 1987;17:45–49.
145. Ries MD, Ray S. Posterior displacement of an odontoid fracture in a child. *Spine* 1986; 11:1043–1044.
146. Scapinelli R. Three-dimensional computed tomography in infantile atlantoaxial rotatory fixation. *J Bone Joint Surg [Br]* 1994;76:367–370.
147. Shaw BA, Murphy KM. Displaced odontoid fracture in a 9-month-old child. *Am J Emerg Med* 1999;1:73–75.
148. Sherburn EW, Day RA, Kaufman BA, et al. Subdental synchondrosis fracture in children: the value of 3-dimensional computerized tomography. *Pediatr Neurosurg* 1996; 25:256–259.
149. Stevens JM, Chong WK, Barber C, et al. A new appraisal of abnormalities of the odontoid process associated with atlantoaxial subluxation and neurological disability. *Brain* 1994;117:133–148.
150. Godard J, Hadji M, Raul JS. Odontoid fractures in the child with neurologic injury. Direct osteosynthesis with a cortico-spongious screw and literature review. *Childs Nerv Syst* 1997;13:105–107.

151. Price E. Fractured odontoid process with anterior dislocation. *J Bone Joint Surg [Br]* 1960;42:410–413.
152. Schippers N, Königs D, Hassler W, et al. Typical and atypical fractures of the odontoid process in young children. Report of two cases and a review of the literature. *Acta Neurochir (Wien)* 1996;138:524–530.
153. Fielding JW. Cineroentgenography of the normal cervical spine. *J Bone Joint Surg [Am]* 1957;39:1280–1288.
154. Fielding JW, Griffin PP. Os odontoideum: an acquired lesion. *J Bone Joint Surg [Am]* 1974;56:187–190.
155. Fielding JW, Hawkins RJ. Atlanto-axial rotary fixation (fixed rotary subluxation of the atlanto-axial joint). *J Bone Joint Surg [Am]* 1977;59:37–44.
156. Fielding JW, Hensinger RN, Hawkins RJ. Os odontoideum. *J Bone Joint Surg [Am]* 1980; 62:376–383.
157. Fielding JW, Stillwell WT, Chynn KY, et al. Use of computed tomography for the diagnosis of atlanto-axial rotatory fixation. *J Bone Joint Surg [Am]* 1978;60:1102–1104.
158. Hawkins RJ, Fielding JW, Thompson WJ. Os odontoideum: congenital or acquired. *J Bone Joint Surg [Am]* 1976;58:413.
159. Hukda S, Ora H, Okabe N, Tazima K. Traumatic atlantoaxial dislocation causing os odontoideum in infants. *Spine* 1980;5:207–210.
160. Kuhns LR, Loder RT, Farley FA, et al. Nuchal cord changes in children with os odontoideum: evidence for associated trauma. *J Pediatr Orthop* 1998;18:815–819.
161. Ricciardi JE, Kaufer H, Louis DS. Acquired os odontoideum following acute ligament injury. *J Bone Joint Surg [Am]* 1976;58:410–412.
162. Schuler TC, Kurz L, Thompson E, et al. Natural history of os odontoideum. *J Pediatr Orthop* 1991;11:222–225.
163. Stillwell WT, Fielding W. Acquired os odontoideum. *Clin Orthop* 1978;135:71–73.
164. Verska JM, Anderson PA. Os odontoideum. A case report of one identical twin. *Spine* 1997;22:706–709.
165. Giannestras NJ, Mayfield FH, Maurer J. Congenital absence of the odontoid process. *J Bone Joint Surg [Am]* 1964;46:839–843.
166. Sherk HH, Dawoud S. Congenital os odontoideum with Klippel-Feil anomaly and fatal atlanto-axial instability. *Spine* 1981;6:42–45.
167. Wollin DG. The os odontoideum. *J Bone Joint Surg [Am]* 1971;45:1459–1471.
168. Dyck P. Os odontoideum in children: neurological manifestations and surgical management. *Neurosurgery* 1978;2:93–99.
169. Brockmeyer DL, York JE, Apfelbaum RI. Anatomic suitability of C1-2 transarticular screw placement in pediatric patients. *J Neurosurg* 2000;92(Suppl 1):7–11.
170. Wang J, Vokshoor A, Kim S, et al. Pediatric atlantoaxial instability: management with screw fixation. *Pediatr Neurosurg* 1999;30:70–78.
171. Steel HH. Anatomical and mechanical consideration of the atlanto-axial articulation. *J Bone Joint Surg [Am]* 1968;50:1481–1482.
172. Lui T-N, Lee S-T, Wong C-W, et al. C1-C2 fracture-dislocations in children and adolescents. *J Trauma* 1996;40:408–411.
173. Gallie WE. Fractures and dislocations of the cervical spine. *Am J Surg* 1939;46: 495–499.
174. Burke SW, French HG, Roberts JM, et al. Chronic atlantoaxial instability in Down syndrome. *J Bone Joint Surg [Am]* 1985;67:1356–1360.
175. Dawson EG, Smith L. Atlanto-axial subluxation in children due to vertebral anomalies. *J Bone Joint Surg [Am]* 1979;61:582–587.
176. Hammerschlag W, Ziv I, Wald U, et al. Cervical instability in an achondroplastic infant. *J Pediatr Orthop* 1988;8:481–484.
177. Kobori M, Takahashi H, Mikawa Y. Atlanto-axial dislocation in Down's syndrome: report of two cases requiring surgical correction. *Spine* 1986;11:195–200.
178. Kransdorf MJ, Wherle PA, Moser RP Jr. Atlantoaxial subluxation in Reiter's syndrome. *Spine* 1988;13:12–14.
179. Miz GS, Engler GL. Atlanto-axial subluxation in Larsen's syndrome: a case report. *Spine* 1987;12:411–412.
180. Sherk HH, Whitaker LA, Pasquariello PS. Fascial malformations and spinal anomalies: a predictable relationship. *Spine* 1982;7:526–531.
181. Committee on Sports Medicine. Atlantoaxial instability in Down syndrome. *Pediatrics* 1984;74:152–154.
182. Davidson RG. Atlantoaxial instability in individuals with Down syndrome: a fresh look at the evidence. *Pediatrics* 1988;81:857–865.
183. Pueschel SM. Atlantoaxial subluxation in Down syndrome. *Lancet* 1983;1:980.
184. Pueschel SM, Scolia FH. Atlantoaxial instability in individuals with Down syndrome: epidemiologic, radiographic, and clinical studies. *Pediatrics* 1987;4:555–560.
185. Van Dyke DC, Gahagan CA. Down syndrome: cervical spine abnormalities and problems. *Clin Pediatr* 1988;27:415–418.
186. Wind WM, Schwend RM, Larson J. Sports for the physically challenged child. *J Am Acad Orthop Surg* 2004;12:126–137.
187. Special Olympics Bulletin. *Participation by individuals with DS who suffer from atlantoaxial dislocation.* Washington, DC: Special Olympics, 1983.
188. Segal LS, Drummond DS, Zanotti RM, et al. Complications of posterior arthrodesis of the cervical spine in patients who have Down syndrome. *J Bone Joint Surg [Am]* 1991; 73:1547–1560.
189. Windell J, Burke SW. Sports participation of children with Down syndrome. *Orthop Clin North Am* 2003;34:439–443.
190. Wetzel FT, Larocca H. Grisel's syndrome. A review. *Clin Orthop* 1989;240:141–152.
191. Kawabe N, Hirotoni H, Tanaka O. Pathomechanism of atlanto-axial rotatory fixation in children. *J Pediatr Orthop* 1989;9:569–574.
192. Maheshwaran S, Sgouros S, Jeyapalan K, et al. Imaging of childhood torticollis due to atlanto-axial rotatory fixation. *Childs Nerv Syst* 1995;11:667–671.
193. Hohl M, Baker HR. The atlanto-axial joint: roentgenographic and anatomical study of normal and abnormal motion. *J Bone Joint Surg [Am]* 1964;46:1739–1752.
194. Geehr RB, Rothman SLG, Kier EL. The role of computed tomography in the evaluation of upper cervical spine pathology. *Comput Tomogr* 1978;2:79–97.
195. Pizzutillo PD, Rocha EF, D'Astous J, et al. Bilateral fractures of the pedicle of the second cervical vertebra in the young child. *J Bone Joint Surg [Am]* 1986;68:892–896.
196. Phillips WA, Hensinger RN. The management of rotatory atlanto-axial subluxation in children. *J Bone Joint Surg [Am]* 1989;71:664–668.
197. Roche CJ, O'Malley M, Dorgan JC, Carty HM. A pictorial review of atlanto-axial rotatory fixation: key points for the radiology. *Clin Radiol* 2001;56:947–958.
198. Fardon DF, Fielding JW. Defects of the pedicle and spondylolisthesis of the second cervical vertebra. *J Bone Joint Surg [Br]* 1981;63:526–528.
199. Francis WR, Fielding JW, Hawkins RJ, et al. Traumatic spondylolisthesis of the axis. *J Bone Joint Surg [Br]* 1981;63:313–318.
200. Howard AW, Letts RM. Cervical spondylolysis in children: is it posttraumatic? *J Pediatr Orthop* 2000;20:677–681.
201. Kleinman PK, Shelton YA. Hangman's fracture in an abused infant: imaging. *Pediatr Radiol* 1997;27:776–777.
202. Parisi M, Lieberson R, Shatsky S. Hangman's fracture or primary spondylolysis: a patient and a brief review. *Pediatr Radiol* 1991;21:367–368.
203. Reinges MHT, Mayfrank L, Royhde V, et al. Surgically treated traumatic synchondrotic disruption of the odontoid process in a 15-month-old girl. *Childs Nerv Syst* 1998;14: 85–87.
204. Ruff SJ, Taylor TKF. Hangman's fracture in an infant. *J Bone Joint Surg [Br]* 1986;68: 702–703.
205. Matthews LS, Vetter LW, Tolo VT. Cervical anomaly stimulating hangman's fracture in a child. *J Bone Joint Surg [Am]* 1982;64:299–300.
206. Nordstrom REA, Lahdenrants TV, Kaitila II, et al. Familial spondylolisthesis of the axis is vertebra. *J Bone Joint Surg [Br]* 1986;68:704–706.
207. Smith T, Skinner SR, Shonnard NH. Persistent synchondrosis of the second cervical vertebra simulating a hangman's fracture in a child. *J Bone Joint Surg [Am]* 1993;75: 1228–1230.
208. Williams JP III, Baker DH, Miller WA. CT appearance of congenital defect resembling the hangman's fracture. *Pediatr Radiol* 1999;29:549–550.
209. Finch GD, Barnes MJ. Major cervical spine injuries in children and adolescents. *J Pediatr Orthop* 1998;18:811–814.
210. Jones ET, Hensinger RN. Cervical spine injuries in children. *Contemp Orthop* 1982;5: 17–23.
211. McClain RF, Clark CR, El-Khoury GY. C6–7 dislocation in a neurologically intact neonate: a case report. *Spine* 1989;14:125–126.
212. Schwarz N, Genelin F, Schwarz AF. Post-traumatic cervical kyphosis in children cannot be prevented by nonoperative methods. *Injury* 1994;25:173–175.
213. Shacked I, Ram Z, Hadani M. The anterior cervical approach for traumatic injuries to the cervical spine. *Clin Orthop* 1993;292:144–150.
214. Hall JE, Denis F, Murray J. Exposure of the upper cervical spine for spinal decompression by a mandible and tongue-splitting approach. Case report. *J Bone Joint Surg [Am]* 1977;59:121–125.
215. Magerl F, Seeman P. Stable posterior fusion of the atlas and axis by transarticular screw fixation. In: Kehr P, Weidner A, eds. *Cervical spine* Vienna: Springer-Verlag, 1985.
216. Roy-Camille R, Saillant G, Mazel C. Internal fixation of the unstable cervical spine by posterior osteosynthesis with plates and screws. In: Sherk HH, ed. *The cervical spine*, 2nd ed. Philadelphia: JB Lippincott, 1989.

THORACOLUMBAR SPINE FRACTURES

Peter O. Newton

Fractures of the thoracic and lumbar spine in pediatric patients are relatively uncommon compared to those in adults (1,2). Although cervical spine injuries outnumber thoracic and lumbar spinal column injuries, fractures of the thoracolumbar region certainly are not rare. The mechanisms of injury vary with age (3,4), while the classification of these injury patterns follows adult spine fracture guidelines: compression, burst, flexion–distraction, and fracture–dislocations. The treatment principles are based on the mechanism of injury and the "stability" of the fractures.

Clarifying the stability of any fracture can be challenging, and controversy remains as to how to establish which fractures require surgical stabilization. The status of the neurologic system is an important variable in treatment (5,6). In addition, other associated injuries are common (7), particularly with flexion–distraction ("lap belt") injuries (8–12). Understanding the mechanism of injury, the neurologic status, and the associated injuries will allow the treating surgeon to make logical decisions about the treatment approach to a child with a thoracolumbar spinal injury.

PRINCIPLES OF MANAGEMENT

Mechanism of Injury

One of the most important aspects of treating thoracolumbar spinal fractures is understanding the details of how the injury occurred. This is a basic element of the history, which must be sought in detail. In general, the mechanism of injury correlates with the age of the patient (4). Just as with other fractures in infants and young children, spinal trauma should generate concern about nonaccidental causes (13–15). Levin et al reported seven unstable thoracolumbar spinal fractures in abused children (16).

Motor vehicle accidents may be the most common cause of spinal column injury in all age groups (7). The type of seatbelt restraint has clear implications in the mechanism of force transferred to the spine, with the lap belt injury a common cause of both intra-abdominal and spinal injury (9–11,17,18). Addition of a shoulder strap or child seat with full frontal harness limits flexion with frontal impact injuries and protects the spine (and other parts of the body) from injury. The lap belt has been long known to create hyperflexion of the trunk over the belt, with the spine pinching the intra-abdominal organs anteriorly. The point of flexion is anterior to the spine, which causes anterior compression combined with posterior column distraction (Fig. 19-1).

Falls from a height generally result in axial loading of the spine, which may result in a "burst" fracture or wedge compression fracture, depending on the degree of flexion of the trunk at the time of impact. These fracture patterns are possible with any mechanism associated with axial compression and can occur with motor vehicle accidents and sporting injuries as well (4). Compression of the vertebra with the trunk flexed creates the greatest forces in the anterior aspect of the vertebra, usually causing anterior column wedging. This is in contrast to compression with the trunk extended, which loads the vertebral body more symmetrically, often causing the fracture to collapse with radial expansion or "bursting." Displacement of the posterior vertebral body fragments into the spinal canal may cause injury or compression of the neurologic elements (spinal cord or cauda equina) (19).

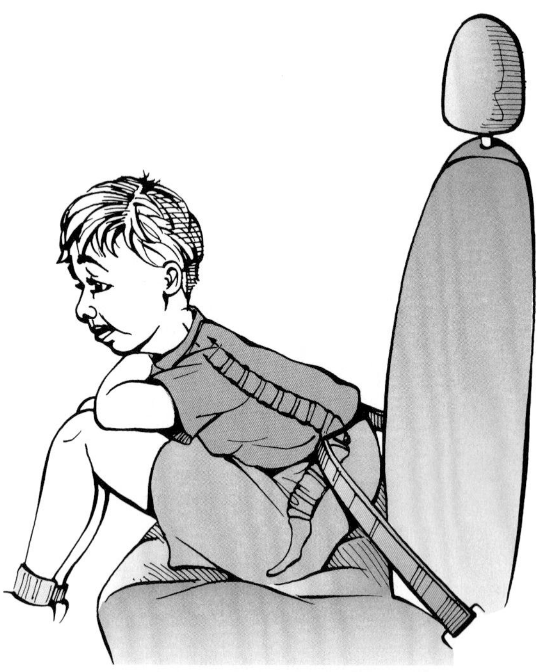

FIGURE 19-1 A lap belt in a child may create a point of rotation about which the spine may become flexed with an abrupt stop. This is a common mechanism for creating both intra-abdominal and flexion–distraction spinal injuries.

If the magnitude of injury sustained seems out of proportion to the force applied, diminished bone quality should be considered. Osteoporotic insufficiency fractures, common in the elderly, are rare in children, but several disease states may predispose to these fractures. Steroids, common in the management of many pediatric diseases, often lead to osteoporosis when taken chronically (20). In addition, primary lesions of bone, such as Langerhans histiocytosis, often affect the thoracic vertebrae (21,22). Other tumors and infections should be considered when nontraumatic compression fractures are identified (23,24).

Signs and Symptoms

Careful evaluation of a patient with a possible spinal injury begins as with any serious trauma victim. The ABCs of resuscitation are performed while maintaining cervical and thoracolumbar spinal precautions. Spinal injuries are frequent in the setting of major trauma (motor vehicle accidents and falls). After the cardiorespiratory systems are stabilized, symptoms of pain, numbness, and tingling should be sought if the patient is old enough and alert enough to cooperate. Pain in the back often is not appreciated when other distracting injuries exist and the patient is immobilized on a backboard. Examination of the back must not be forgotten and is performed by logrolling the patient. Visual inspection and palpation identify areas of swelling, deformity, ecchymosis, or tenderness that may provide a clue to the presence of a spinal injury.

Neurologic examination provides information on the integrity of the spinal cord. The age of the patient may limit the thoroughness of this assessment, but some indication of sensory and motor function should be sought. In patients with spinal cord deficits, detailed examinations of the strength of each muscle group, sensory levels, and rectal tone need to be compared over time, and the importance of the documentation cannot be overemphasized. The prognosis for recovery is significantly better if the spinal cord injury is incomplete (25–27). The status of neurologic function over time may lead to important treatment decisions regarding the need for and timing of surgical intervention. A progressive neurologic deficit warrants immediate surgical attention, while an improving status may suggest a less urgent approach.

Associated Injuries

Just as the mechanism of injury should raise suspicion of a particular injury (e.g., lap belt injury and flexion–distraction lumbar fracture pattern), the presence of one injury should raise suspicion of a concomitant associated injury. First, any spinal fracture should be considered a significant risk factor for a spinal fracture at another level. The traumatic force required to create one fracture often is enough to cause one or more additional fractures at other locations. Similarly, a cervical injury frequently is associated with closed head injury.

The lap belt mechanism of injury is well known to create flexion–distraction injuries of the spine and also is associated with intra-abdominal injury (9). Compressed between the seat belt and the spinal column, the aorta, intestinal viscera, and abdominal wall musculature are at risk for laceration. Ecchymosis on the anterior abdomen suggests intra-abdominal injury that warrants further evaluation with laparoscopy, laparotomy, or additional imaging by CT (7,17). A high index of suspicion is required, since any missed injuries may be life-threatening (10).

Associated injury to the spinal cord has obvious significance and may be present with many fracture patterns. Disruption of the stability of the spinal column or bony intrusion into the spinal canal may result in compromised neurologic function. All patients with a spinal column fractures or dislocations require a careful neurologic examination. Similarly, patients with traumatic neurologic deficits require careful evaluation of the spinal column integrity. A subset of patients present with spinal cord injury without radiographic abnormality (28,29). This scenario has been termed SCIWORA and is much more common in children than adults. It is thought that the flexibility of the immature spine allows spinal column segmental displacements great enough to lead to spinal cord injury without mechanically disrupting the bony or ligamentous elements (29). Although these injuries may not be visible on plain x-rays, nearly all of these patients will have some evidence of soft tissue injury of the spine on more sensitive MRI studies (30). SCIWORA is less relevant in the era of routine advanced imaging, which is always obtained in patients with spinal cord injury (31).

Rationale of Treatment

The goals of treatment for all spinal injuries are to maximize the potential for recovery of spinal cord function if a spinal cord injury is present and to provide skeletal stability to the spinal column to protect against future spinal cord injury. These two goals may be analyzed separately when both instability and spinal cord injury exist. Optimizing return of any lost spinal cord function is paramount, and the potential for recovery of spinal cord function in general is greater in children than in adults (6,27).

Spinal cord injuries in children have substantial potential for recovery. In a recent study from a major metropolitan trauma center, complete spinal cord injuries were associated with fatal injuries in one third and no neurologic recovery in one third, while most of the remaining third made improvements that ultimately allowed functional ambulation. Less surprisingly, nearly all patients with incomplete spinal cord injury made some improvement over time (27). This ability to recover, even from complete injuries, has led some to suggest more aggressive attempts at spinal cord decompression in the early course of treatment (32,33), while others have suggested a period of "spinal cord rest" with observation (34). There is certainly no controlled series of patients treated by both approaches to support either hypothesis. The data do, however, suggest a more optimistic view regarding the potential recovery of traumatic spinal cord injuries in children than in adults.

Assessment of the structural integrity of the spinal column is mandatory in all patients because the functional capacity of the vertebral elements to protect the spinal cord will continue to be required. This evaluation can be done with functional x-rays, such as flexion–extension views (much more common in the cervical spine), or with an MRI evaluation of associated soft tissue injuries that may coexist with more obvious bony fractures. Several methods of estimating spinal column stability have been proposed, including the three-column concept of Denis (35). Based on division into anterior, middle, and posterior columns, injuries to two and certainly three of these sagittal columns may be associated with an unstable injury pattern. Plain radiography with a CT scan is appropriate for evaluating the bony elements. An MRI often is required to evaluate the disc and ligamentous injuries (31,36,37). MRI is extremely sensitive and, given the brightness of edema fluid on T2-weighted images, may be overinterpreted. A recent study correlating MRI and intraoperative surgical findings, however, found high levels of both sensitivity and specificity in the MRI evaluation of posterior soft tissue injuries (Fig. 19-2) (38).

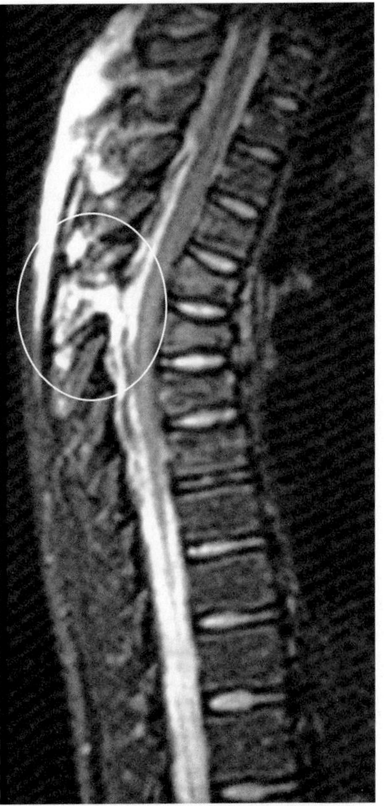

FIGURE 19-2 This sagittal MRI shows markedly increased signal in the posterior ligamentous complex. Anteriorly loss of height at the vertebra can be visualized, suggesting a three-column spinal injury.

The final treatment goal is a stable spinal column, which often requires surgical treatment for unstable fracture patterns. In contrast, most stable injuries can be managed nonoperatively. An associated spinal cord injury or a substantial associated deformity may alter the treatment approach of an otherwise mechanically stable injury. The presence of a complete spinal cord injury in a child younger than 10 years of age also may affect treatment strategies: the incidence of paralytic spinal deformity (scoliosis) is nearly 100% in such cases (39,40), and a long instrumented fusion will likely be required at some point. Depending on the fracture pattern and the age of the patient, it may be prudent to include much of the thoracic and lumbar spine in the initial instrumented fusion (41).

Classification

There are several methods of classifying thoracolumbar fractures (Holdsworth—two column, Denis—three column [35], McCormack—load sharing [42], Gertzbein—comprehensive [43]), each with proclaimed advantages. Designed primarily for adult spinal fracture patterns, the Denis classification seems to suffice for the categorization of most pediatric thoracolumbar injuries (44). Based on theories of stability related to the three-column biomechanical concept of the spine (anterior, middle, posterior columns), the Denis classification in its simplest form includes compression, burst, flexion–distraction, and fracture–dislocations (Fig. 19-3).

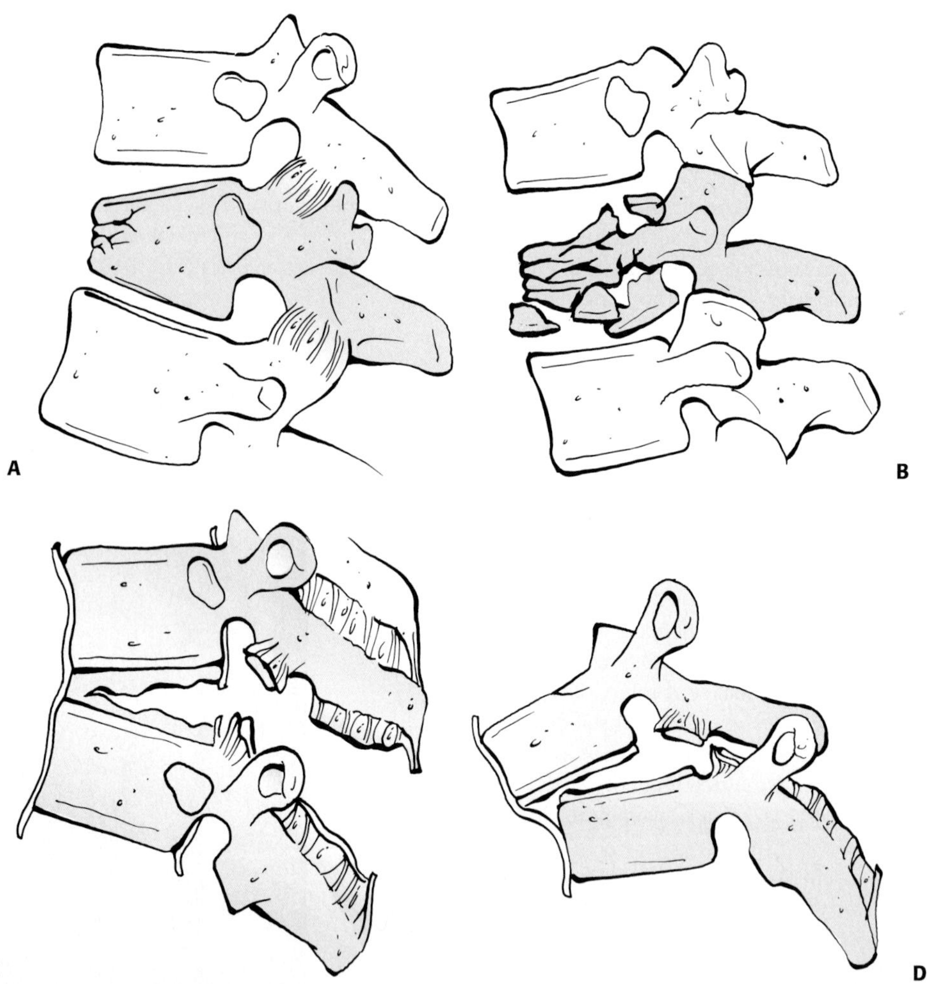

FIGURE 19-3 Denis classification of thoracolumbar fractures. **A.** Compression fracture results in mild wedging of the vertebra, primarily involving the anterior aspects of the vertebral body. The posterior vertebral height and posterior cortex remain intact. **B.** Burst fracture involves both the anterior and middle columns, with loss of height throughout the vertebral body. There may be substantial retropulsion of the posterior aspect of the vertebra into the spinal canal. In addition, posterior vertebral fractures and/or ligamentous injury may occur. **C.** Flexion–distraction injuries occur commonly after the seatbelt injury mechanism results in posterior distraction with disruption of the ligaments and bony elements of the posterior column, commonly extending into the anterior columns with or without compression of the most anterior aspects of the vertebra. **D.** Fracture–dislocations are complex injuries that involve marked translation of one vertebra on another, with frequently associated spinal cord injury as a result of translations through the spinal canal.

Compression fractures are the most common thoracolumbar spinal fracture pattern (45,46). The vertebral body loses height anteriorly compared to the posterior wall. Axial load with flexion is the common mechanism. Depending on the degree and direction of flexion, the wedging may be in the coronal or sagittal plane (Fig. 19-4). The percentage of lost height defines the severity of compression fractures, which rarely have an associated neurologic deficit. However, compression fractures often are associated with similar or occasionally more severe fractures at adjacent or distant levels. Contiguous compression fractures, each of a modest degree, may result in a substantial kyphotic deformity. Because the causes of these injuries, such as falls, are fairly common, it may be necessary to determine whether a wedged vertebra seen radiographically represents an acute compression fracture, a sequela of Scheuermann's kyphosis, or a remote injury. Clinical examination is certainly relevant, because acute injuries generally are painful; however, MRI or bone scanning can confirm an acute fracture based on signal changes and increased isotope uptake.

Burst fractures likely represent a more severe form of compression fracture that extends posteriorly in the vertebral body to include the posterior wall (middle column). Axial compression is the primary mechanism, although posterior ligamentous injury and posterior element fractures also may occur. Laminar fractures have been known to entrap the dural contents. Burst fractures are most common in the lower thoracic and upper lumbar levels. Associated neurologic injury is related to the severity of injury (greater injury index scores correlate with greater frequency of spinal cord injury [34]) and the degree of spinal canal encroachment by retropulsed bony fragments (19). Spinal cord injury at the thoracolumbar junction may result in conus medullaris syndrome or cauda equina syndrome. Careful examination of the perineal area is required to identify these spinal lesions.

Flexion–distraction injuries are especially relevant to the pediatric population because classic lap belt injuries are more frequent in back-seat passengers, particularly when a shoulder strap is lacking. Motor vehicle accidents are the primary cause of this injury. The lap belt, which restrains the pelvis in adults, may ride up onto the abdomen in children. Chance and later Smith described how with a frontal impact, the weight of the torso is driven forward, flexing over the restraining belt. The axis of rotation in front of the spine results in distractive forces in the posterior elements, with variable degrees of anterior vertebral compression. This three-column injury generally is unstable. The disruption of the posterior elements may occur entirely through the bony (Chance) or ligamentous (Smith) elements, although often the fracture propagates through both soft and hard tissues.

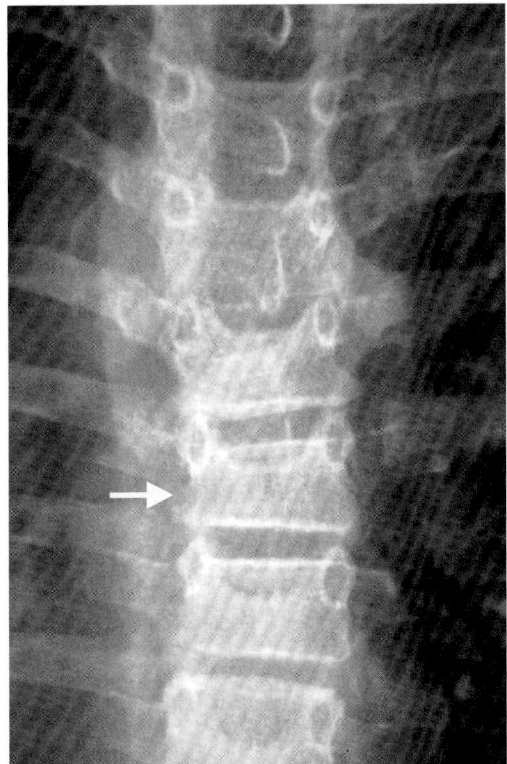

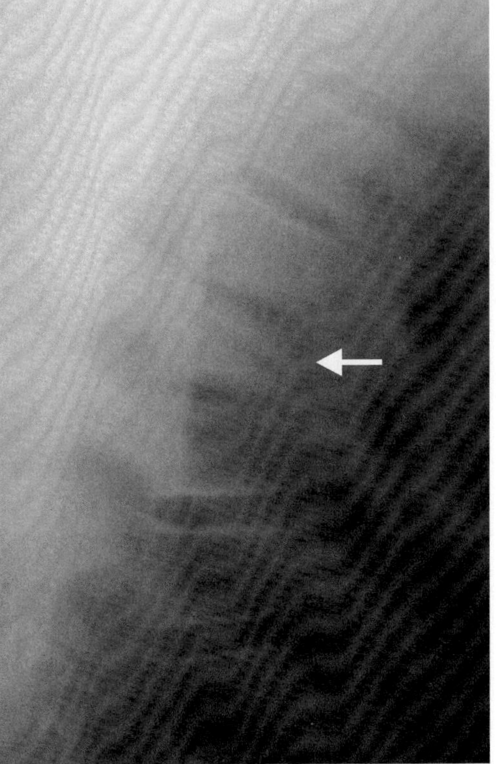

FIGURE 19-4 Compression fractures. **A.** This PA view shows wedging in the coronal plane. **B.** The more commonly recognized compression fractures involve wedging primarily in the sagittal plane, with loss of anterior vertebral height.

The injury is most obvious on lateral x-rays; however, if no fracture exists, widening of the intraspinous distance may be the only finding on an AP x-ray. Standard transverse plain CT imaging also may miss this injury, because the plane of injury lies within the plane of imaging. One classic finding in ligamentous flexion–distraction injuries is the "empty facet" sign. When the inferior articular process of the superior vertebra is no longer in contact with the superior articular process of the inferior vertebra, the facet appears empty in the transverse CT image (47). Sagittal reconstructions are most revealing, and MRI provides information about the integrity of the posterior ligamentous complex. Identification of a purely intravertebral flexion–distraction fracture is important, because this may alter the treatment to that for a severe ligamentous injury.

Fracture–dislocations of the spinal column result from complex severe loading mechanisms. These are by definition unstable injuries, with a component of shearing or rotational displacement. Of special concern in the pediatric population is the documentation of this injury pattern in young patients exposed to nonaccidental trauma (13,14).

Injury patterns specific to the pediatric population that do not fit the Denis classification include apophyseal avulsion fractures and the phenomenon described as SCIWORA (spinal cord injury without radiographic abnormality). Apophyseal injuries, typically of the lumbar spine, occur in adolescents as a result of trauma. The mechanism is thought to be related to flexion with a portion of the posterior corner of the vertebral body (ring apophysis) fracturing and displacing posteriorly into the spinal canal. Symptoms may mimic disc herniation, although the offending structure is bone and cartilage rather than disc material (Fig. 19-5) (48,49).

The concept of SCIWORA was popularized by Pang and Wilberger (28), who noted a series of patients with traumatic spinal cord injuries that were not evident on plain x-rays or tomograms. Several mechanisms to explain these findings have been proposed, including spinal cord stretch and vascular disruption or infarction. MRI studies have confirmed patterns of both cord edema and hemorrhage (30). Important additional information about SCIWORA includes the finding that some patients had a delayed onset of neurologic deficits. Transient neurologic symptoms were persistent in many who later developed lasting deficits. Additionally, younger patients (less than 8 years old) had more severe neurologic involvement (28,29,50).

Radiographic Evaluation

After a careful clinical examination, plain x-rays often are required. An alert, cooperative patient without pain or tenderness in the back can be cleared without x-rays. However, any patients with a significant mechanism (motor vehicle accident or fall of more than 10 feet) or associated injury (major long bone fracture, cervical or head injury) require thoracolumbar spine x-rays if they have spinal tenderness or are obtunded. Initial films should include AP and lateral views of the thoracic and lumbar spine.

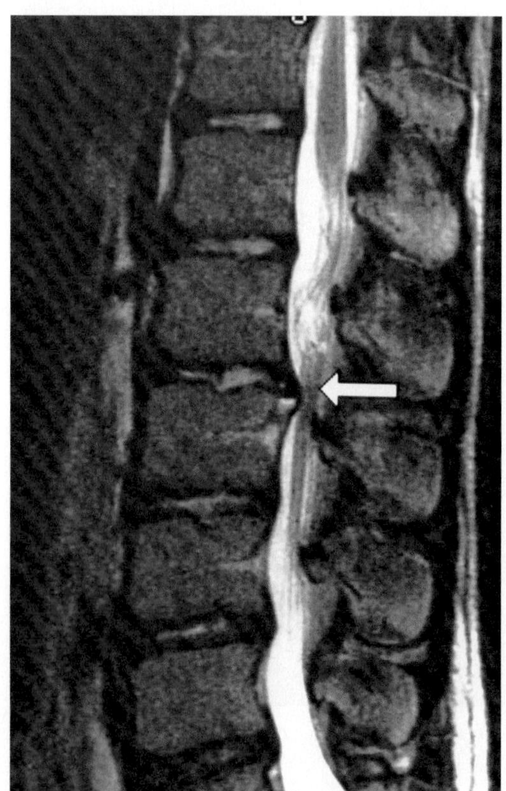

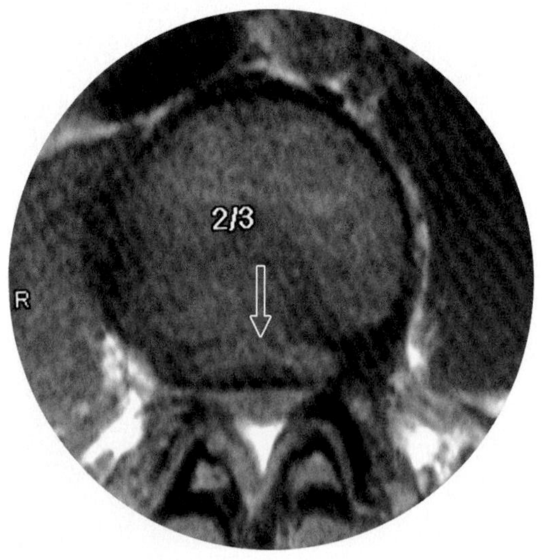

FIGURE 19-5 Ring apophyseal avulsion injuries. **A.** This lateral MRI image shows displacement of the ring apophysis, which functionally acts as a disc herniation. This, however, represents largely a bony and cartilaginous fragment, which results in neural element compression. **B.** Transverse image shows canal stenosis associated with this injury.

Plain x-rays often show relatively subtle findings. On AP x-rays, soft tissue shadows may be widened by paravertebral hematoma. The bony anatomy is examined for loss of height of the vertebral body as compared to adjacent levels. Similar comparisons can be made with regard to pedicle width and interspinous spacing. The lateral x-rays give important information about the sagittal plane: anterior vertebral wedging or collapse, posterior element distraction or fracture. Careful scrutiny of the plain x-rays is always prudent, but in reality CT scanning is nearly always used to clarify any suspected fractures.

CT is now a standard component of the evaluation of most trauma patients. Multidetector scanners allow rapid assessment with axial, coronal, and sagittal images for patients with abnormalities on plain x-rays. The axial images are best for evaluating the integrity of the spinal canal in patients with burst fractures, while the sagittal views demonstrate vertebral body compression as well as posterior element distraction or fracture. In addition, although major dislocations are easily seen on plain x-rays, CT scanning provides information about the space left in the spinal canal for the neurologic elements.

MRI is the modality of choice for evaluating the discs, spinal cord, and posterior ligamentous structures (31,38,51). Although more difficult to obtain in a multiply injured patient, this study is mandatory in patients with neurologic deficits to assess the potential cause of cord dysfunction. MRI can distinguish areas of spinal cord hemorrhage and edema. Assessment of the posterior ligamentous complex is critical in differentiating stable from unstable burst fractures as well as compression fractures from flexion–distraction injuries. Although subject to overinterpretation, MRI has been shown to correlate well with intraoperative findings of the structural integrity of posterior soft tissues (38).

APPLIED ANATOMY

The thoracic spine and the lumbar spine link the upper and lower extremities through the torso. The 12 thoracic and 5 lumbar vertebrae are joined by intravertebral discs and strong ligaments, both anteriorly and posteriorly. The bony architecture of the vertebra varies, with the smaller thoracic vertebra having a more shingled, overlapping configuration compared to the lumbar segments. The thoracic facets are oriented in the coronal plane, while those in the lumbar spine lie nearly in the sagittal plane (Fig. 19-6).

Mobility is less in the thoracic spine because of the adjacent and linked rib cage and the smaller intervertebral discs. The ribs make important connections with the vertebra, with the rib head articulating across a given disc space. This is in contrast to the relatively mobile lumbar segments, which have thick intervertebral discs that permit substantial flexion–extension, lateral bending, and axial rotation. The junction between the stiffer thoracic spine and the flexible lumbar spine is a region of frequent injury.

Ligamentous components include the anterior and posterior longitudinal ligaments, facet capsules, ligamentum flavum, and interspinous and supraspinous ligaments. Together these structures limit motion between vertebrae to protect the neurologic elements. The anterior longitudinal ligament rarely is disrupted in flexion injuries but may be rendered incompetent by extension loading or severe fracture–dislocation. Flexion is the primary mechanism of injury to the posterior ligaments (supraspinous and interspinous, facet capsule, ligamentum flavum). The healing capacity of the completely torn posterior ligamentous complex is limited; bony fractures are more likely to heal with stability.

The neural anatomy varies over the length of the thoracolumbar spine. The space within the canal is largest in the lumbar spine. The spinal cord traverses the entirety of the thoracic spine and typically terminates as the conus medullaris at the L1 or L2 level. Cauda equina occupies the dural tube below this level, and injuries below L1 generally are less likely to lead to permanent neurologic deficit. This is not to say that compression at this level cannot be serious, and careful examination of the perineum for sensation as well as rectal tone is important in the evaluation of potential conus medullaris and cauda equina syndromes.

CURRENT TREAMENT OPTIONS

Compression Fractures

Anterior vertebral body compression is the fracture pattern most likely to occur in the thoracic spine secondary to axial compression and flexion loading. The anterior aspect of the vertebral body is involved, but the posterior wall of the vertebral body is intact. The degree of wedging is variable, as is the loss of anterior height. These are nearly always stable injuries, although examination of the posterior soft tissues is required to rule out any more severe flexion–distraction injury, and a CT scan is required to rule out a burst fracture (Fig. 19-7).

Isolated fractures without neurologic involvement are the most common thoracolumbar fracture pattern and can nearly always be treated in an extension orthosis, such as a Jewitt brace. Immobilization with a brace that limits flexion provides pain relief and reduces further loading of the fracture. Most fractures heal in 4 to 6 weeks without significant additional collapse; however, in the first several weeks after injury x-rays should be obtained to monitor sagittal alignment. Long-term studies have suggested modest remodeling capacity of compression fractures in children (52,53). Asymmetric growth at the endplates seems to allow some correction in the wedged alignment over time in immature patients. Long-term results of compression fractures have been generally favorable, although fractures of the endplates are associated with later disc degeneration (54).

If the kyphosis associated with a fracture is initially greater than 40 degrees or markedly alters the local sagittal alignment, surgical treatment may be considered. This is most frequent with multiple adjacent compression fractures that create unacceptable kyphosis. The preferred surgical treatment of such patients generally is a posterior compression instrumentation con-

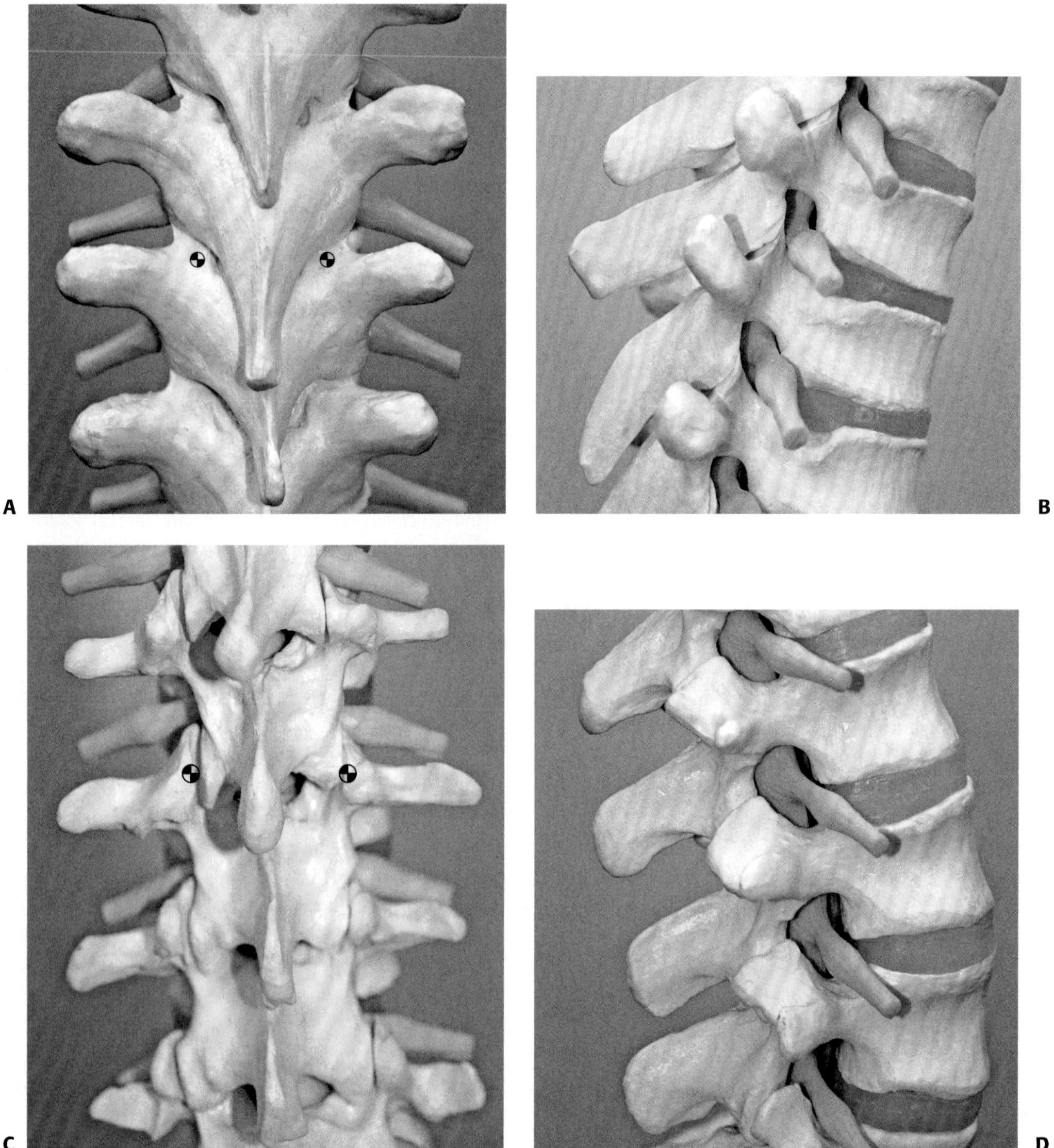

FIGURE 19-6 **A,B.** Thoracic spine posterior and lateral views show the overlapping lamina and spinous processes present in this region. The *circles* mark the location of the thoracic pedicles, which may be important in surgical reconstruction. **C,D.** Lumbar spine posterior and lateral projections show the differences in lumbar spine anatomy. Again, the *circles* mark locations of the lumbar pedicles relative to the facets and transverse processes.

struct that spans one or two levels above and below the affected vertebrae. Anterior surgical treatment is rarely required. The intact posterior vertebral wall provides a fulcrum to achieve kyphosis correction. The method of posterior fixation may be either hooks or pedicle screws. A posterior fusion over the instrumented segments ensures a lasting stable correction.

Osteoporosis from a variety of etiologies may affect children and adolescents to a degree that predisposes them to insufficiency fractures, most often compression fractures (Fig. 19-8). Multiple levels are more common in this setting, and problematic kyphosis may develop. Differentiating new from old fractures can be difficult if serial x-rays are not available. Use of a thoracic lumbar sacral orthosis for longer than is typical for simple compression fracture healing may be necessary to prevent progressive kyphosis, though treating the primary cause of the osteopenia is critical to maintaining normal alignment. An endocrinologic evaluation and an assessment of bone density by DEXA are advised.

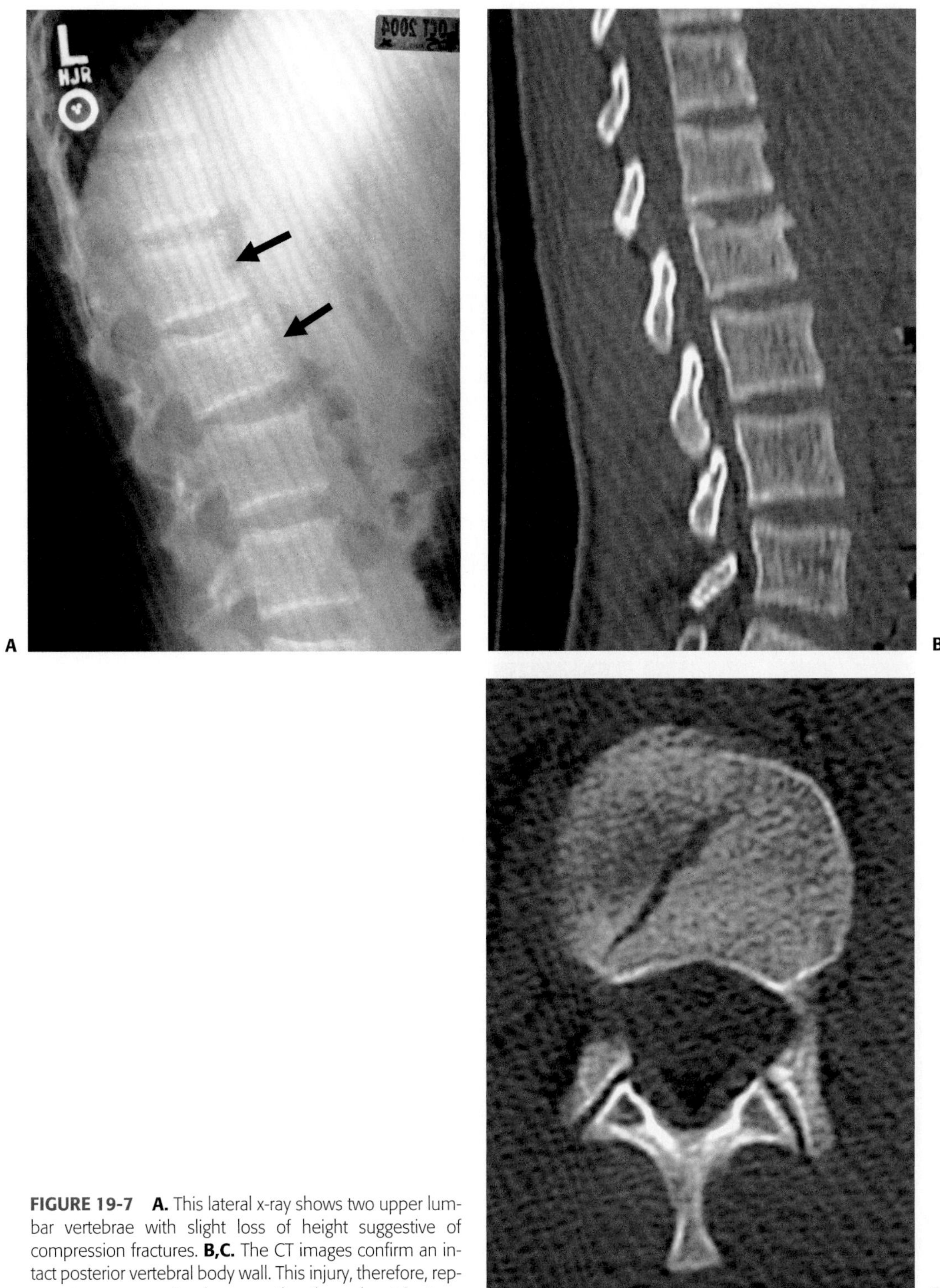

FIGURE 19-7 A. This lateral x-ray shows two upper lumbar vertebrae with slight loss of height suggestive of compression fractures. **B,C.** The CT images confirm an intact posterior vertebral body wall. This injury, therefore, represents a compression fracture rather than a burst fracture.

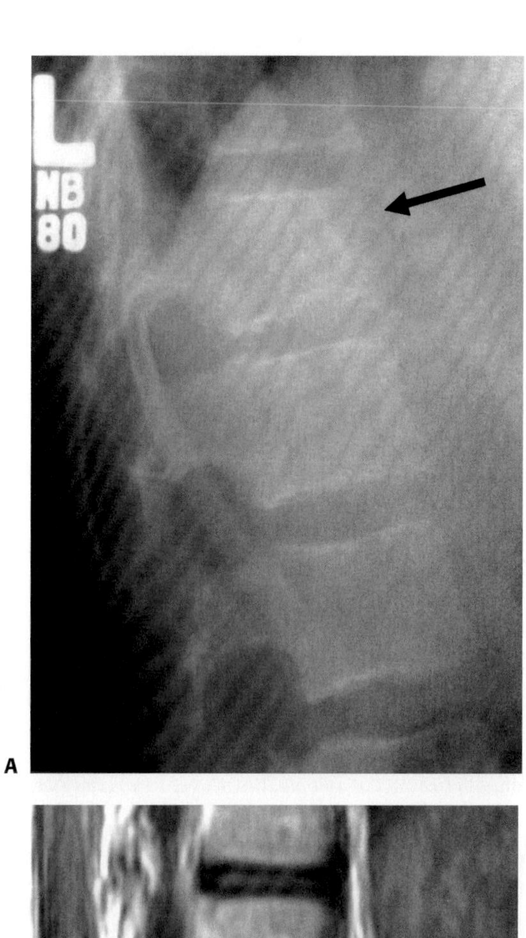

A

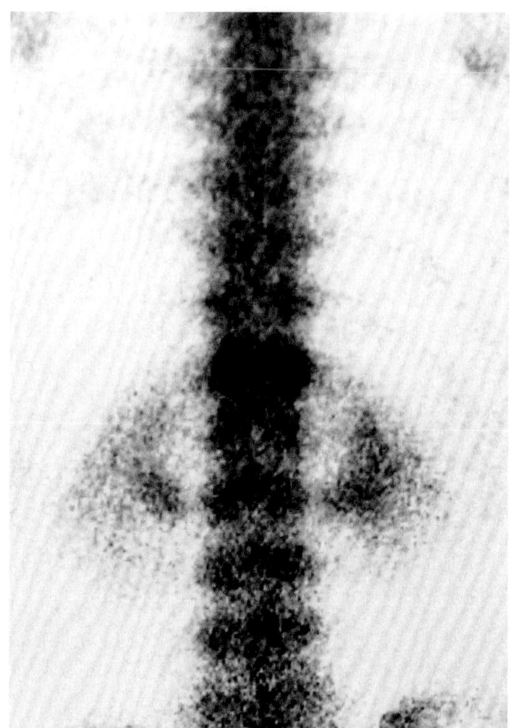
B

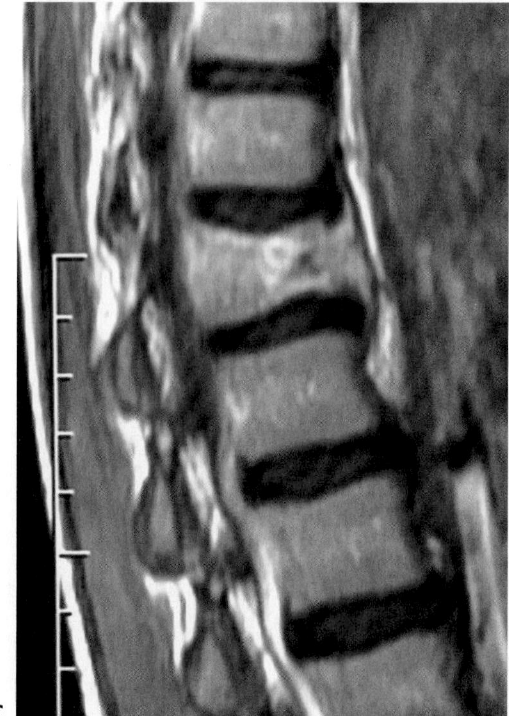
C

FIGURE 19-8 **A.** Lateral x-ray shows what appears to be a routine compression fracture. The patient did not have a significant history of trauma; however, pain was present and a bone scan was obtained to further evaluate this site. **B.** The bone scan shows markedly increased uptake, confirming an acute process and prompting additional study. **C.** An MRI shows loss of height and a lesion within the anterior aspect of the vertebral body, later confirmed to be an infectious process.

Burst Fractures

Axial compression injuries that are more severe and extend into the posterior wall of the vertebral body are called *burst fractures*. The treatment and classification of this fracture pattern are some of the more controversial areas of spinal trauma management. Some burst fractures can be easily managed nonoperatively in a brace, but others collapse further, resulting in increased deformity unless surgically stabilized. Defining the characteristics of stable and unstable burst fractures has been attempted by several authors (35,42,43). An additional compounding variable in the treatment algorithm is that concurrent spinal cord injury is more common than in compression fractures.

Assuming an intact neurologic system, defining stable and unstable burst fractures has been attempted based on the degree of comminution, loss of vertebral height, kyphotic wedging, and integrity of the posterior ligamentous complex. A load-sharing classification system assigns points based on comminution, fragment apposition, and kyphosis (42). Although the Denis classification suggests that all burst fractures are unstable because of at least two-column involvement, it is clear that often the addition of a third-column injury (posterior ligamentous complex) is required to result in an unstable condition. Some advocate differentiating stable and unstable burst fractures solely on the integrity of the posterior ligamentous complex (55,56). When a burst fracture is deemed stable, it must be done so on a presumptive basis. Treatment is then based on an extension molded cast or thoracic lumbar sacral orthosis, with the goal of allowing an upright position and ambulation (57). Frequent x-rays and neurologic follow-up are necessary to identify early failures. Depending on the age of the patient and the severity of the fracture, immobilization is suggested for 2 to 4 months.

Studies of immature patients treated for burst fractures are uncommon (44), but much of the literature about burst fractures in adults provides valuable information about the outcomes to expect following nonoperative treatment. Most of these fractures in adults heal with little change in kyphosis and function and minimal if any residual pain (58). It is reasonable to expect adolescents to heal at least as well, and probably faster. The controversy over operative and nonoperative treatment was addressed by Wood et al in a prospective, randomized study of patients with burst fractures who were neurologically intact, with a normal posterior ligamentous complex (55). The radiologic and functional outcomes were not substantially different, and these authors concluded that nonoperative treatment should be considered when the posterior ligamentous complex and neurologic function are intact. Functional outcome does not appear to correlate with the degree of spinal kyphosis, although long-term studies of scoliosis treatment do suggest that an alteration of sagittal alignment may be detrimental (flat back syndrome) in the long term.

Even some patients with injuries to the posterior ligamentous complex have been successfully treated nonoperatively (59); however, these three-column injuries often are operatively stabilized. When surgical treatment is selected, either an anterior or posterior approach can be used, although this also remains controversial. Anterior stabilization generally involves discectomy and strut grafting that spans the fractured vertebra. Stabilization with a plate or dual-rod system is appropriate. Posterior options include pedicle screw fixation one level above and below the fractured vertebra. The decision to use an anterior or posterior approach for the surgical treatment of a burst fracture is largely dictated by surgeon preference and to some degree the features of the fracture. Posterior approaches are familiar to all surgeons and can easily be extended over many levels. The spinal cord can be decompressed by indirect or direct methods. Restoration of the sagittal alignment frequently leads to spontaneous repositioning of the posteriorly displaced vertebral body fracture fragments. If additional reduction of posterior wall fragments is required, direct fracture reduction can be accomplished with posterolateral or transpedicular decompression (32). This also allows additional anterior column bone grafting, which may add structural integrity and speed fracture healing.

The anterior approach allows direct canal decompression through corpectomy of the fractured vertebra. Structural strut grafting restores the integrity of the anterior column. With this graft, a load-sharing anterior plate or rod system completes the reconstruction. This approach deals most directly with the pathology, which in a burst fractures lies within the anterior and middle vertebral columns (Fig. 19-9).

Flexion–Distraction Injuries (Chance Fractures)

The treatment of flexion–distraction injuries is dictated by the particular injury pattern and the associated abdominal injuries. In general, these fractures are reduced by an extension moment that can be maintained with either a cast or internal fixation. A hyperextension cast is ideal for younger patients (less than approximately 10 years) with a primary bony injury pattern who did not have significant intra-abdominal injuries. As described above, the posterior disruption may pass through ligaments or joint capsules in a purely soft tissue plane or may traverse an entirely bony path. The distinction is important, since bony fractures have the potential for primary bony union, while severe ligamentous injuries are less likely to heal with lasting stability without surgical intervention. As such, the greater the degree of ligamentous and facet disruption, the more likely the need for stabilization with an arthrodesis of the injured motion segment. Options for internal fixation include posterior wiring in young children (supplemented with a cast) and segmental fixation in a primarily compressive mode (Fig. 19-10).

Fracture–Dislocations

These highly unstable injuries nearly always require surgical stabilization. When the spinal cord function remains intact, instrumented fusion gives the greatest chance for maintaining cord function. On the other hand, if a complete spinal cord injury has occurred, internal fixation will aid in the rehabilitation process, allowing early transfers and upright sitting. At

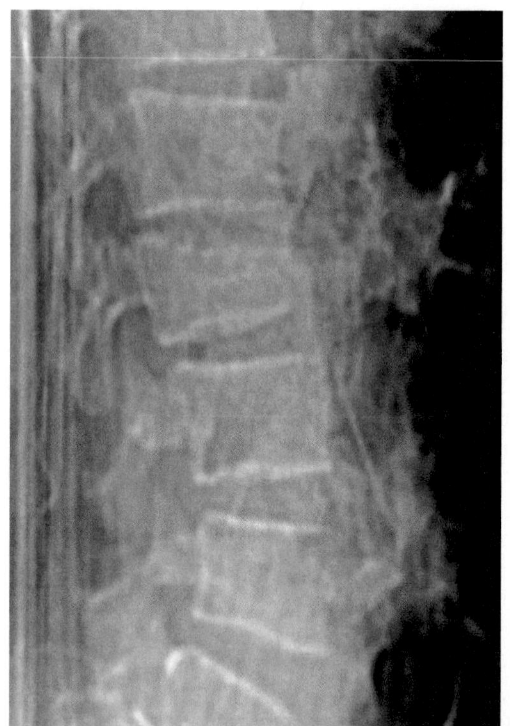

FIGURE 19-9 Burst fracture. **A.** This teenager presented with loss of vertebral body height associated with a motorcycle accident after jumping more than 20 feet. His neurologic examination was intact. **B.** CT scan confirmed a burst fracture component with very little retropulsion into the spinal canal. This appeared to be a stable injury and was initially managed with an orthosis. There was poor compliance with the orthosis and further collapse. **C,D.** Given the lack of compliance and progressive kyphosis, the patient underwent anterior reconstruction using iliac crest strut graft and plating.

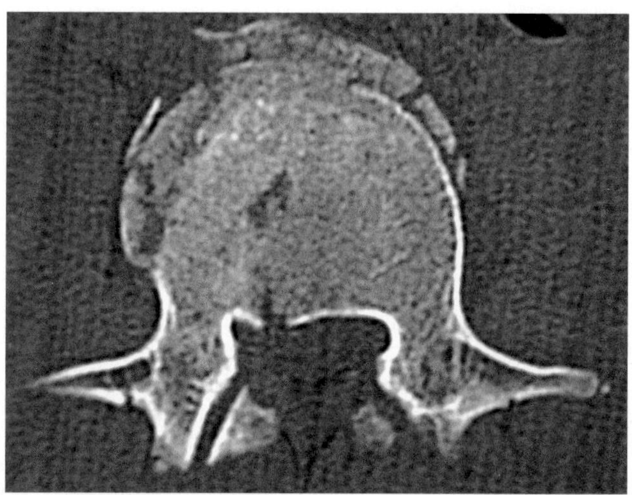

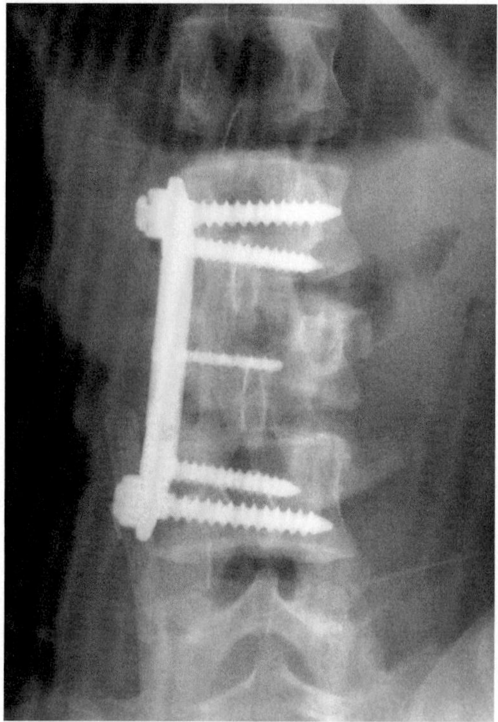

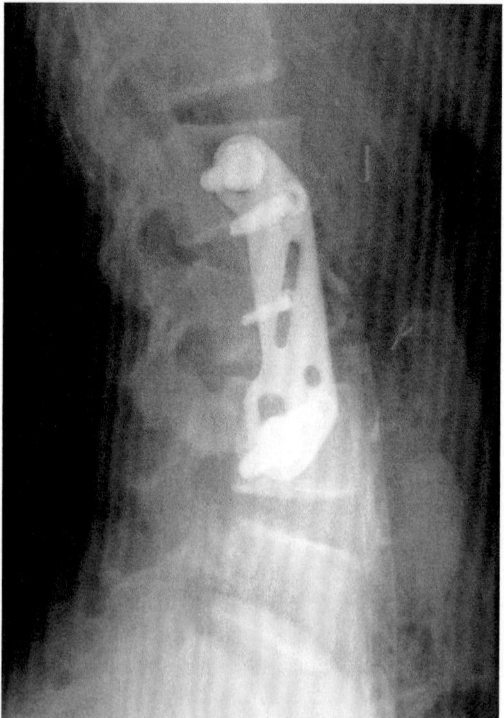

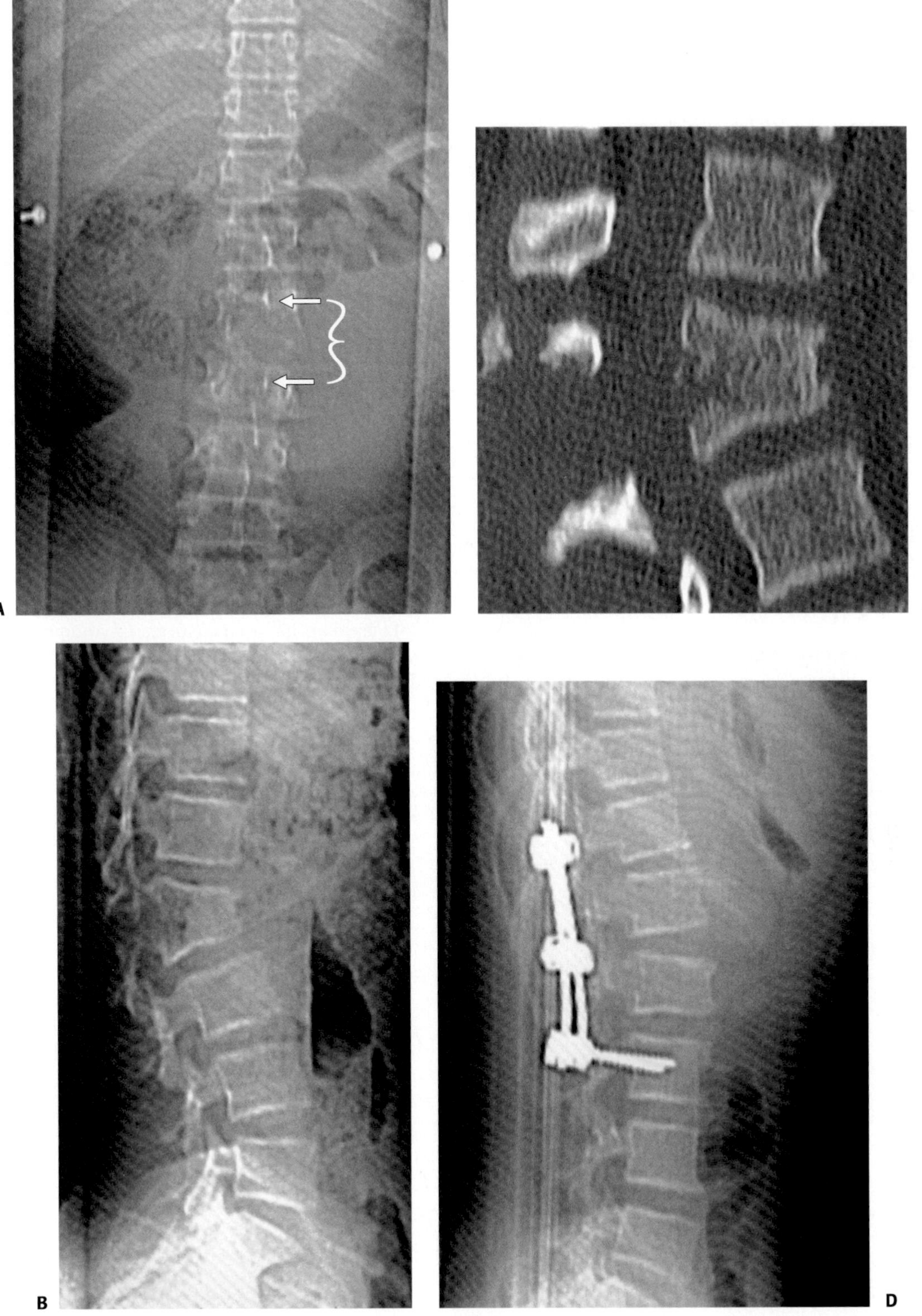

FIGURE 19-10 Flexion–distraction injury. **A,B.** Plain x-rays after a restrained back-seat passenger presented after a motor vehicle accident. The wedging of L2 with posterior distraction is visible on the lateral x-ray. The intraspinous widening is noted on the AP x-ray as well (*arrows*). **C.** Sagittal CT images confirm the injury pattern. **D.** Lateral x-rays after reconstruction with posterior spinal instrumentation.

least two levels above and below the level of injury should be instrumented to ensure restoration of stability. In patients younger than 10 years of age with a spinal cord injury, a longer fusion may be considered to reduce the incidence and severity of subsequent paralytic scoliosis. Those injured after the adolescent growth spurt are at low risk for late deformity if the fracture is well aligned at the time of initial fixation (Fig. 19-11).

Pearls and Pitfalls

- Make liberal use of advanced imaging, especially CT scanning.
- Understanding the mechanics of the injury allows a rationale treatment plan to be developed.
- Always seek to identify additional levels of spinal injury when one is discovered.
- Document the neurologic examination precisely and repeat it often.
- Watch for associated injuries, both musculoskeletal and others.
- Don't let MRI or CT findings replace a careful examination of the back.
- Not recognizing a changing neurologic status may limit the ability to intervene early and prevent permanent sequelae.

CONTROVERSIES

Several areas of controversy remain with regard to the management of acute spinal cord injury associated with thoracolumbar fractures. These include both nonoperative and operative methods of treatment. Investigations into the benefits of steroids in mitigating the effects of the secondary phase of spinal cord injury that follows the acute trauma have been mixed, although clinical trials have suggested benefit in specific instances.

Spinal cord injury that results from direct trauma may acutely disrupt the neural tissue, possibly with compression from fracture fragments or displacement. Once the initial injury occurs, biochemical cascades are set into motion that result in further injury of spinal cord tissue. Experimental studies have suggested that steroids administered early in the postinjury period can limit these detrimental secondary effects. Randomized clinical trails of methylprednisolone administration after acute spinal cord injury have been completed (60,61), and current recommendations for steroid use depend on the timing of administration relative to the occurrence of the injury. If the time lapse is less than 3 hours, a bolus of 30 mg/kg methylprednisolone is followed by an hourly infusion of 5.4 mg/kg for 24 hours. If the lapse between injury and treatment is 3 to 8 hours, an infusion of the same dose is continued for 48 hours. More importantly, if more than 8 hours have passed since the spinal cord injury, no steroids are recommended (61).

The benefit of steroids with regard to functional levels of recovery has been questioned, and in all studies of high-dose steroid use there has been an increased complication rate. Infection is the most consistent complication, with both pneumonia and sepsis occurring. Steroids are known to depress the immune

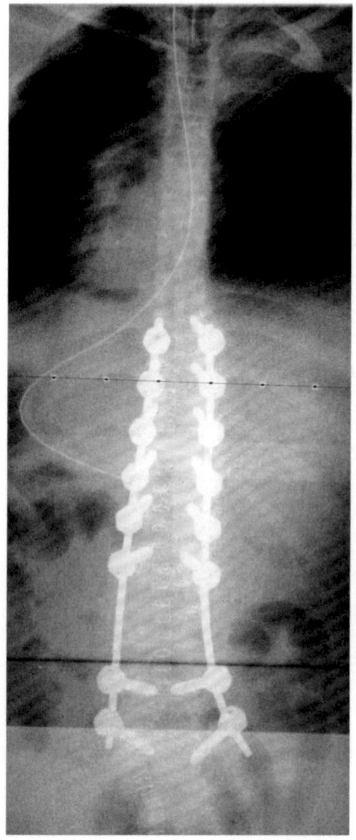

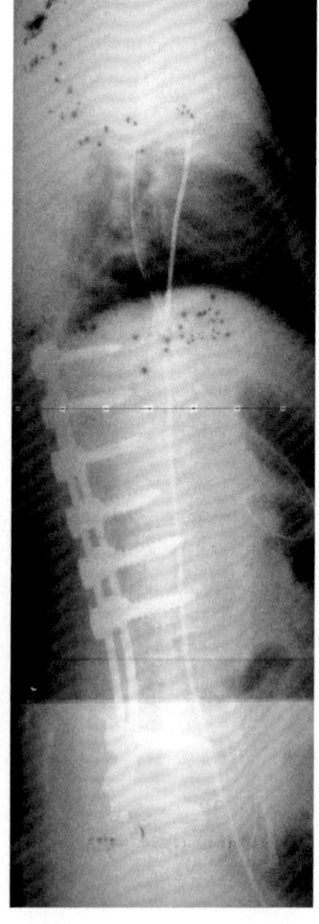

FIGURE 19-11 PA and lateral x-rays show reconstruction after a lower thoracic level complete spinal cord injury associated with fracture–dislocation in the lumbar spine combined with a burst fracture in the lower thoracic spine. Given the complete paraplegia present, a relatively long instrumentation construct was selected to provide stable foundation in this skeletally immature patient with paraplegia. Four years after surgery the patient has no evidence of progressive spinal deformity; however, there is certainly some risk remaining of developing pelvic obliquity and upper thoracic deformity, given the paraplegia.

response (62). These issues have resulted in an inconsistent adoption of the National Acute Spinal Cord Injury Study's recommendations.

The timing of and need for spinal decompression in patients with spinal cord injuries also remain debated. Traditional teaching suggests no benefit to decompression when a complete spinal cord injury exists. Experimentally, early decompression of an incomplete spinal cord injury appears to be beneficial, but it may be impossible to determine early on whether a patient has an incomplete injury masked by spinal shock. Spinal shock may last for 24 hours, leaving a patient with incomplete spinal cord injury completely unresponsive with regard to spinal cord function. The data to suggest a benefit to early decompression are largely experimental; however, one clinical study (33) reported a benefit. In a series of 91 pediatric patients, 66 with immediate decompression were compared with 25 in whom decompression was delayed. Improvement of at least one Frankel grade occurred in half of the early decompression patients compared to one quarter of those with delayed decompression.

In pediatric patients, it is difficult to argue against spinal cord decompression if the MRI documents persistent compression in a patient with a spinal cord injury. Children have substantial potential for recovery, and reducing pressure on the neural elements may be important in maximizing functional recovery. There is little controversy if spinal cord function is deteriorating and a compressive lesion is identified. This is an emergency that warrants decompression by either an anterior or posterior approach. Realignment of the spinal column and removal of fragments from the canal are required. The exact surgical approach depends on the location of the offending structures and the nature of the instability.

There certainly is room for vast improvements in our treatment of spinal cord injuries. Research into the mechanisms of secondary injury pathways as well as means of regeneration continues. Achieving bony stability remains relatively straightforward by instrumentation and fusion, although which injuries require surgery remain to be fully defined.

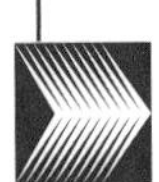

AUTHOR'S PREFERRED TREATMENT

Compression Fractures

Nearly all cases are managed nonoperatively in an off-the-shelf Jewitt brace. Occasionally a fracture is too proximal for such an orthosis and an extension to the chin/occiput is required. In cases with a fracture proximal to approximately T6, a Minerva brace is used. Compression fractures with greater than 50% loss of anterior vertebral height are considered for either a closed reduction in an extension molded body cast or surgical correction with posterior instrumentation. The determination of which of these two approaches to undertake is based on a discussion with the family and the associated injuries. Compression fractures associated with neurologic injury are managed surgically.

Burst Fractures

My preferred approach to neurologically intact patients with a burst fracture favors a nonoperative approach in light of recent studies. If the neurologic status is normal and the posterior soft tissues are intact, a thoracic lumbar sacral orthosis or cast is used for 3 months. A cast is used when local kyphosis is greater than 20 degrees, and the cast is placed in a hyperextension position in an attempt to restore sagittal alignment. If the posterior soft tissues are disrupted (and neurologically intact), then posterior surgical stabilization is preferred. An anterior decompression is used in cases of spinal cord injury if canal compromise is greater than 50%.

Flexion–Distraction Injuries

My treatment of Chance fractures is based on two findings: associated abdominal injuries and the presence of a ligamentous component to the fracture. If either exists, surgical treatment is the preferred approach. Casting in extension is appropriate for fractures that traverse an entirely bony plane without intra-abdominal pathology. A thigh is incorporated into the cast for greater control of lumbar lordosis. Surgical treatment is by a posterior approach and includes only the involved vertebrae. Monosegmental pedicle screw fixation generally is preferred.

Fracture–Dislocation

Posterior surgery is the treatment of choice for all cases of fracture–dislocation with or without neurologic injury. The timing of such intervention depends on the associated injuries and the ability of the patient to tolerate surgical intervention; however, stabilization as early as conveniently possible is preferred. Spinal cord injury nearly always complicates the management of these injuries, and a deteriorating neurological examination makes surgical treatment of the spine an emergency that is undertaken as quickly as possible.

Steroid Treatment

Despite the controversies, I continue to follow the recommendations of the Third National Acute Spinal Cord Injury Study and prescribe methylprednisolone if it can be given within 8 hours of the time of injury. I am skeptical that this provides significant benefit, but I believe this remains the current medical and legal standard.

REFERENCES

An asterisk denotes a Level I evidence-based reference.

1. Haffner DL, Hoffer MM, Wiedebusch R. Etiology of children's spinal injuries at Rancho Los Amigos. *Spine* 1993;18:679–684.

2. Roche C, Carty H. Spine trauma in children. *Pediatr Radiol* 2001;31:677–700.
3. Ruge JR, Sinson GP, McLeon DG, et al. Pediatric spinal injury: the very young. *Neurosurgery* 1988;68:25–30.
4. Cirak B, Ziegfeld S, Knight VM, et al. Spinal injuries in children. *Pediatr Surg* 2004;39: 607–612.
5. Augutis M, Levi R. Pediatric spinal cord injury in Sweden: incidence, etiology and outcome. *Spinal Cord* 2003;41:328–336.
6. Garcia RA, Gaebler-Spira D, Sisung C, et al. Functional improvement after pediatric spinal cord injury. *Am J Phys Med Rehabil* 2002;81:458–463.
7. Beaunoyer M, St-Vil D, Lallier M, et al. Abdominal injuries associated with thoracolumbar fractures after motor vehicle collision. *Pediatr Surg* 2001;36:760–762.
8. Mann DC, Dodds JA. Spinal injuries in 57 patients 17 years or younger. *Orthopedics* 1993;16:159–164.
9. Reid AB, Letts RM, Black GB. Pediatric Chance fractures: association with intraabdominal injuries and seatbelt use. *Trauma* 1990;30:384–391.
10. Letts M, Davidson D, Fleuriau-Chateau P, et al. Seat belt fracture with late development of an enterocolic fistula in a child. A case report. *Spine* 1999;24:1151–1155.
11. Griffet J, Bastiani-Griffet F, El-Hayek T, et al. Management of seatbelt syndrome in children. Gravity of 2-point seatbelt. *Eur J Pediatr Surg* 2002;12:63–66.
12. Inaba K, Kirkpatrick AW, Finkelstein J, et al. Blunt abdominal aortic trauma in association with thoracolumbar spine fractures. *Injury* 2001;32:201–207.
13. Kleinman PK, Marks SC. Vertebral body fractures in child abuse. Radiologic–histopathologic correlates. *Invest Radiol* 1992;27:715–722.
14. Diamond P, Hansen CM, Christofersen MR. Child abuse presenting as a thoracolumbar spinal fracture dislocation: a case report. *Pediatr Emerg Care* 1994;10:83–86.
15. Carrion WV, Dormans JP, Drummond DS, et al. Circumferential growth plate fracture of the thoracolumbar spine from child abuse. *J Pediatr Orthop* 1996;16:210–214.
16. Levin TL, Berdon WE, Cassell I, et al. Thoracolumbar fracture with listhesis—an uncommon manifestation of child abuse. *Pediatr Radiol* 2003;33:305–310.
17. Sivit CJ, Taylor GA, Newman KD, et al. Safety-belt injuries in children with lap-belt ecchymosis: CT findings in 61 patients. *AJR Am J Roentgenol* 1991;157:111–114.
18. Rumball K, Jarvis J. Seatbelt injuries of the spine in young children. *J Bone Joint Surg [Br]* 1992;74:571–574.
19. Hashimoto T, Kanada K, Abumi K. Relationship between traumatic spinal canal stenosis and neurologic deficits in thoracolumbar burst fractures. *Spine* 1988;13:1268–1272.
20. Varonos S, Ansell BM, Reeve J. Vertebral collapse in juvenile chronic arthritis: its relationship with glucocorticoid therapy. *Calcif Tissue Int* 1987;41:75–78.
21. Baghaie M, Gillet P, Dondelinger RF, et al. Vertebra plana: benign or malignant lesion? *Pediatr Radiol* 1996;26:431–433.
22. Garg S, Mehta S, Dormans JP. Langerhans cell histiocytosis of the spine in children. Long-term follow-up. *J Bone Joint Surg [Am]* 2004;86:1740–1750.
23. Ribeiro RC, Pui CH, Schell MJ. Vertebral compression fracture as a presenting feature of acute lymphoblastic leukemia in children. *Cancer* 1988;61:589–592.
24. Meehan PL, Viroslav S, Jr. Vertebral collapse in childhood leukemia. *J Pediatr Orthop* 1995;15:592–595.
25. Catz A, Thaleisnik M, Fishel B, et al. Recovery of neurologic function after spinal cord injury in Israel. *Spine* 2002;27.
26. Hadley MN, Zabramski JM, Browner CM, et al. Pediatric spinal trauma. Review of 122 cases of spinal cord and vertebral column injuries. *Neurosurg Clin North Am* 1988;68: 18–24.
27. Wang MY, Hoh DJ, Leary SP, et al. High rates of neurological improvement following severe traumatic pediatric spinal cord injury. *Spine* 2004;29:1493–1497.
28. Pang D, Wilberger JE. Spinal cord injury without radiographic abnormalities in children. *Neurosurgery* 1982;57:114–129.
29. Pang D, Pollack IF. Spinal cord injury without radiographic abnormality in children—the SCIWORA syndrome. *Trauma* 1989;29:654–664.
30. Grabb PA, Pang D. Magnetic resonance imaging in the evaluation of spinal cord injury without radiographic abnormality in children. *Neurosurgery* 1994;35:406–414.
31. Kerslake RW, Jaspan T, Worthington BS. Magnetic resonance imaging of spinal trauma. *Br J Radiol* 1991;64:386–402.
32. Gambardella G, Coman TC, Zaccone C, et al. Posterolateral approach in the treatment of unstable vertebral body fractures of the thoracic–lumbar junction with incomplete spinal cord injury in the paediatric age group. *Childs Nerv Syst* 2003;19:35–41.
33. Papadopoulos SM, Selden NR, Quint DJ, et al. Immediate spinal cord decompression for cervical spinal cord injury: feasibility and outcome. *Trauma* 2002;52:323–332.
34. Limb D, Shaw DL, Dickson RA. Neurological injury in thoracolumbar burst fractures. *J Bone Joint Surg [Br]* 1995;77:774–777.
35. Denis F. The three-column spine and its significance in the classification of acute thoracolumbar spinal injuries. *Spine* 1983;8:817–831.
36. Smith AD, Koreska J, Moseley CF. Progression of scoliosis in Duchenne muscular dystrophy. *J Bone Joint Surg [Am]* 1989;71:1066–1074.
37. Green RA, Saifuddin A. Whole spine MRI in the assessment of acute vertebral body trauma. *Skeletal Radiol* 2004;33:129–135.
38. Lee HM, Kim HS, Kim DJ, et al. Reliability of magnetic resonance imaging in detecting posterior ligament complex injury in thoracolumbar spinal fractures. *Spine* 2000;25: 2079–2084.
39. Parisini P, DiSilvestre M, Greggi T. Treatment of spinal fractures in children and adolescents: long-term results in 44 patients. *Spine* 2002;27:1989–1994.
40. Lancourt JE, Dickson JH, Carter RE. Paralytic spinal deformity following traumatic spinal cord injury in children and adolescents. *J Bone Joint Surg [Am]* 1981;63:47–53.
41. Mayfield JK, Erkkila JC, Winter RB. Spine deformity subsequent to acquired childhood spinal cord injury. *J Bone Joint Surg [Am]* 1981;63:1401–1411.
42. McCormack T, Karaikovic E, Gaines RW. The load sharing classification of spine fractures. *Spine* 1994;19:1741–1744.
43. Gertzbein SD, Court-Brown CM. Rationale for the management of flexion–distraction injuries of the thoracolumbar spine based on a new classification. *J Spinal Disord* 1989; 2:176–183.
44. Lalonde F, Letts M, Yang YP, et al. An analysis of burst fractures of the spine in adolescents. *Am J Orthop* 2001;30:115–120.
45. Carreon LY, Glassman SD, Campbell MJ. Pediatric spine fractures: a review of 137 hospital admissions. *J Spinal Disord* 2004;17:477–482.
46. Holmes JF, Miller PQ, Panacek EA, et al. Epidemiology of thoracolumbar spine injury in blunt trauma. *Acad Emerg Med* 2001;8:866–872.
47. Gellad FE, Levine AM, Joslyn JN, et al. Pure thoracolumbar facet dislocation: clinical features and CT appearance. *Radiology* 1986;161:505–508.
48. Epstein NE, Epstein JA. Limbus lumbar vertebral fractures in 27 adolescents and adults. *Spine* 1991;16:962–966.
49. Dietemann JL, Runge M, Badoz A, et al. Radiology of posterior lumbar apophyseal ring fractures: report of 13 cases. *Neuroradiology* 1988;30:337–344.
50. Bosch PP, Vogt MT, Ward WT. Pediatric spinal cord injury without radiographic abnormality (SCIWORA): the absence of occult instability and lack of indication for bracing. *Spine* 2002;27:2788–2800.
51. Sledge JB, Allred D, Hyman J. Use of magnetic resonance imaging in evaluating injuries to the pediatric thoracolumbar spine. *J Pediatr Orthop* 2001;21:288–293.
52. Mangus KK, Anders M, Ralph H, et al. A modeling capacity of vertebral fractures exists during growth: an up to 47-year follow-up. *Spine* 2003;28:2087–2092.
53. Pouliquen JC, Kassis B, Glorion C, et al. Vertebral growth after thoracic or lumbar fracture of the spine in children. *J Pediatr Orthop* 1997;17:115–120.
54. Kerttula LI, Serlo WS, Tervonen OA, et al. Posttraumatic findings of the spine after earlier vertebral fracture in young patients: clinical and MRI study. *Spine* 2000;25:1104–1108.
*55. Wood K, Butterman G, Mehbod A, et al. Operative compared with nonoperative treatment of a thoracolumbar burst fracture without neurological deficit. *J Bone Joint Surg [Br]* 2003;85:773–781.
56. Shen WJ, Liu TJ, Shen YS. Nonoperative treatment versus posterior fixation for thoracolumbar junction burst fractures without neurologic deficit. *Spine* 2001;26:1038–1045.
57. Shen WJ, Shen YS. Nonsurgical treatment of three-column thoracolumbar junction burst fractures without neurologic deficit. *Spine* 1999;24:412–415.
58. Weinstein JN, Collalto P, Lehmann TR. Thoracolumbar "burst" fractures treated conservatively: a long-term follow-up. *Spine* 1988;13:33–38.
59. Chow GH, Nelson BJ, Beghard JS, et al. Functional outcome of thoracolumbar burst fractures managed with hyperextension casting or bracing and early mobilization. *Spine* 1996;21:2170–2175.
*60. Bracken MB. Methylprednisolone in the management of acute spinal cord injuries. *Med J Aust* 1990;153:368.
*61. Bracken MB, Shepard MJ, Holford TR, et al. Administration of methylprednisolone for 24 or 48 hours or tirilazad mesylate for 48 hours in the treatment of acute spinal cord injury. Results of the Third National Acute Spinal Cord Injury Randomized Controlled Trial. *JAMA* 1997;277:1597–1604.
62. Galandiuk S, Raque G, Appel S, et al. The two-edged sword of large-dose steroids for spinal cord trauma. *Ann Surg* 1993;218:419–425.

SECTION FOUR

LOWER EXTREMITY

FRACTURES OF THE PELVIS

Roger F. Widmann

Pelvic fractures comprise less than 0.2% of all pediatric fractures (1,2), but pelvic fractures constitute between 1% and 5% of admissions to level 1 pediatric trauma centers (3–7). The most important aspect of treatment of these fractures is the appreciation of the high-energy mechanism of injury and the associated injuries to other systems including the neurovascular structures, abdominal viscera, genitourinary system, musculoskeletal system, and central nervous system. Injuries to the pelvis and spine are associated with the longest hospital stays and the most admissions to the intensive care unit, and the highest rates of mortality in patients with multiple injuries (8,9). When a pelvic fracture is identified in a child, it is an indication that the child may have other significant life-threatening injuries to soft-tissues including but not limited to the abdominal and genitourinary system. The mortality rate in children with pelvic fractures was between 2.4% and 14.8% in recent large series from level 1 pediatric trauma centers (3–7,10–16). Central nervous system head injury was cited as the most common cause of death in two recent large single-institution retrospective studies of pediatric pelvic fractures (4,14). Other causes of death include multiorgan failure and visceral injuries (4,7,10,14). In children, hemorrhage from pelvic fracture-related vascular injury was the cause of death in only 0.3% compared with 3.4% in adults (7).

PRINCIPLES OF MANAGEMENT

Mechanisms of Injury

Between 75% and 95% of pelvic fractures in children result from motor vehicle-related accidents (3,4,10–15,17–19). In the largest consecutive series of pediatric pelvic fractures from a single urban level 1 trauma center, the most common mechanism of injury was pedestrian struck by a motor vehicle (60%), followed by passenger in a motor vehicle (22%), and falls (13%) (14). Sporting activities account for between 4% and 11% of pelvic fractures in other series (13,15). Child abuse is a rare cause of pelvic fracture, but isolated fracture of the pelvis may be the only skeletal manifestation of child abuse (20). X-rays of the pelvis should be included in any skeletal survey for child abuse (21). Avulsion injuries most commonly occur secondary to athletic injuries, especially soccer, gymnastics, and track.

Signs and Symptoms

The evaluation of a child with a suspected or documented pelvic fracture begins with a thorough history and physical examination. The associated injuries including closed head injury, and chest, abdomen, and genitourinary injury take precedence over the pelvic fracture in terms of diagnosis, stabilization, and operative intervention. The examination of the pelvic area begins with a visual inspection. Areas of contusion, abrasion, laceration, ecchymosis, or hematoma, especially in the perineal and pelvic areas, should be recorded.

Pelvic landmarks including the anterior superior iliac spine, crest of the ilium, sacroiliac joints, and symphysis pubis should be palpated. Exerting posterior pressure on the anterior superior iliac crest produces pain at the fracture site as the pelvic ring is opened. Compressing the pelvic ring at the iliac crest from lateral to medial also causes pain, and crepitation may be felt if a pelvic fracture is present. Pressure downward on the symphysis pubis and posteriorly on the sacroiliac joints causes pain and motion if there is a fracture in the pelvic ring. The range of motion of the extremities, especially at the hip joint, should be determined. Careful examination of the head, neck, and spine should be performed to assess for spinal injury and closed head injury. A complete neurovascular examination including peripheral pulses should be part of the initial survey. Rectal examination and careful genitourinary evaluation must also be performed as part of the primary evaluation.

Associated Injuries

Because most pelvic fractures in children result from high-energy trauma, multisystem injuries are commonly present. Between 58% and 87% of pelvic fractures have at least one and often several associated injuries (4,6,13,14,22). Of the 57 consecutive children with pelvic fractures reported by Grisoni et al (6), 58% had one or more other body area injuries in addition to the pelvic fracture including nonpelvic fractures (49%), neurologic injury (26%), significant hemorrhage requiring transfusion (21%), abdominal injury (14%), thoracic injury (7%), and genitourinary injury (4%). The incidence of associated injuries increases with the severity of the pelvic fracture. Bond et al (3) noted that the location and number of pelvic fractures were strongly associated with the probability of abdominal injury: <1% for isolated pubic fractures, 15% for iliac or sacral fractures, and 60% for multiple fractures of the pelvic ring. The data of Grisoni et al did not support this finding, and their study found no association between multiple pelvic fractures and associated abdominal injuries (6). Almost all authors agree that the outcome of patients with pelvic fractures is largely determined by the associated injuries rather than the pelvic fracture itself (3,4,6,7,9,10,13,14,16,22).

The incidence of head injury in association with pelvic fracture is between 9% and 48% in recent retrospective studies (3,4,6,10–14,23). Rieger and Brug (13) reported the highest incidence of head injuries in 48% of the 54 patients in their series, ranging from mild concussion to brain death. The two largest single institution studies of pediatric pelvic fractures reported closed head injuries in 39% (4) and 44% of patients (14). The correlation of pelvic fractures with head injury has been noted by others as well (15). Brain injury merits the highest priority because it is the leading cause of death in patients with pelvic fracture.

Because children's bones have a lower modulus of elasticity, they deform more and absorb more energy that adult bones before fracture (24). In addition, there is greater elasticity in the sacroiliac joints and symphysis pubis in children, and greater energy is required to cause a fracture in an immature pelvis than in an adult pelvis (14). Thus, the presence of a pelvic fracture in a child is a marker of severe injury that should alert the clinician to search actively for other injuries including abdominal, genitourinary, neurologic, and other fractures (4). Although children with high-energy pelvic fractures often require blood transfusions, exsanguination is rarely the primary cause of death in children with pelvic fractures. In three recent studies, each with between 57 and 166 patients, the incidence of transfusion was between 20% and 30% (4–6). In none of these studies did children die of an exsanguinating pelvic fracture or associated vascular injury. Direct vascular injury with marked superior displacement of the hemipelvis can injure the superior and inferior gluteal arteries at the sciatic notch. Other studies on pelvic fractures in children have documented retroperitoneal hemorrhage secondary to injury of primary branches of the iliac artery in relationship to a grossly disrupted sacroiliac joint in children (10,18). Children are thought to have lower incidence of exsanguinating hemorrhage compared with adults because of a more effective vasoconstrictive response in younger patients with nonatherosclerotic blood vessels (7). Only McIntyre et al's (10) study of pelvic fractures in children correlated the risk of life-threatening hemorrhage to pelvic fracture complexity. In children with unstable fracture patterns or uncontrolled hypotension with ongoing transfusion requirements, external fixation, angiography, and selective embolization may be indicated.

Hematuria is noted on initial urinalysis in 14% to 52% of children with pelvic fractures (4,12,25). The incidence of significant lower urinary tract injuries including bladder rupture or urethral tear has been between 4% and 15% in recent retrospective studies (3,11–13,19,26). The two largest single-center retrospective studies of pediatric pelvic fractures by Silber et al (14) and Tarman et al (25) reported a 1% incidence of lower urinary tract injury in association with pelvic fracture. Although controversial, most authors agree that microhematuria can be followed expectantly, whereas patients with gross hematuria or significant local findings on physical examination should undergo formal urologic assessment. This should include imaging with abdominopelvic computed tomography (CT), retrograde urography, and cystography (25). Pediatric patients should also be carefully screened for the presence of vaginal and/or rectal lacerations because the incidence of these injuries is between 2% and 18% in children with pelvic fractures (11,19,25,27), and early detection and repair or diversion may prevent late pelvic abscess formation (28). The overall incidence of lower urinary tract injury (47%), vaginal laceration (33%), and rectal laceration (66%) is significantly increased in cases of open pelvic fractures (29). Some authors have correlated the presence of multiple pelvic fractures and anterior pelvic fractures with urogenital injury in children (3,9), but the largest series to address this issue found no association between pelvic fracture type or instability and urinary tract injury (25).

The incidence of abdominal injuries including solid organ injury and hollow viscus injury is between 14% and 21% in children with pelvic fractures (3–5,11,14). Rapid diagnosis of severe abdominal injury is important because abdominal injury ranks second to head injury as cause of death in children with pelvic fractures (4). The presence of extremity fractures in the presence of a pelvic fracture is associated with increased risk of abdominal injury (16). CT scan best demonstrates evidence of injury to solid organs, hollow viscera, and mesentery after blunt injury to the abdomen (4). The incidence of abdominal injury in association with pelvic fracture is similar in children (13.7%) and adults (16.7%) (5). Ultrasound and diagnostic peritoneal lavage may also be helpful in the diagnosis of intraabdominal injury and vascular injury.

Pelvic fractures with posterior displacement of the hemipelvis or iliac wing can damage the lumbosacral plexus as well as the sciatic nerve. The incidence of lumbosacral plexus injury is low, between 1% and 3% (9,19,22). Myelography with computed axial tomography or alternatively magnetic resonance imaging (MRI) is useful for the diagnosis of lumbosacral plexus injury or root avulsion. Complete neurologic examination of the extremities should be routine, and documentation of any neurologic deficit is essential. Surgical repair of nerve root avulsions is rarely performed, and deficits are usually permanent (30).

Fractures of other bones are present in 40% to 50% of children with pelvic fractures (4,6,10,13,14,22). The most frequently fractured bone is the femur followed by the tibia and fibula. Vazquez and Garcia (16), in a study of 79 children with pelvic fractures, found that the presence of any additional fracture was a significant indication that head or abdominal injury was also present and that transfusion would be required in the first 24 hours after injury. The patients with an additional fracture had twice the frequency of death, thorac injury, laparotomy, and other nonorthopaedic procedures compared with the group with pelvic fractures alone. Vazquez and Garcia (16) suggested that this easily identifiable risk factor can help identify patients who may benefit from early transfer to a regional pediatric trauma center.

Radiographic Studies and Other Imaging

Emergency assessment and stabilization of the child with pelvic trauma should be performed before obtaining survey x-rays because associated injuries account for most of the morbidity and mortality in patients with pelvic fractures. Once the patient is stabilized, pertinent x-rays should be ordered by the physician in charge. Scout views of the skull, cervical spine, chest, abdomen, pelvis, and long bones should be obtained quickly. If special views are necessary, then the physician ordering these films should be in attendance.

In a child with a pelvic fracture, unless there is a significant fracture-dislocation, multiple radiographic views can be deferred. A single anteroposterior x-ray may be sufficient to determine pelvic ring stability in the acute situation (31). The presence of sacroiliac displacement on the anteroposterior view indicates greater instability and the possibility of associated major hemorrhage. Two other views, the inlet and outlet views, are approximately at right angles to each other (31). The inlet view is obtained by directing the x-ray beam caudally at an angle of 60 degrees to the x-ray plate. The inlet view is best for the determination of posterior displacement of the pelvis. The outlet view is obtained by directing the x-ray beam in a cephalad direction at an angle of 45 degrees to the x-ray plate. The outlet view best demonstrates superior displacement of the posterior pelvis or superior or inferior displacement of the anterior portion of the pelvis (31). Internal and external rotation views help to determine fractures of the acetabulum. Comparison views of the contralateral apophysis may be helpful in evaluating avulsion fractures.

CT scanning helps determine the presence of fractures and any disruption or incongruity of the sacroiliac joint, sacrum, or acetabulum. Most authors agree that CT scanning is indicated if there is doubt about the diagnosis on plain x-ray or if operative intervention is planned (32). Some of the advantages of CT over plain x-rays include optimized imaging with CT reconstruction, as well as improved fracture definition, aid in decision making between conservative and operative treatment, and improved operative approaches (33). Others have noted that CT scans of the pelvis are more sensitive than plain x-rays in all anatomic areas including the iliac region, pubis, sacroiliac joint, hip, sacrum, and soft tissues (34). These authors note that pelvic x-rays may be superfluous in pediatric patients who will undergo pelvic CT scan for assessment of soft tissue injuries. MRI offers similar benefits, with the advantages over CT including better delineation of soft tissue injuries, absence of ionizing radiation, and improved imaging of posterior wall fractures in the setting of pediatric hip dislocations in which the posterior wall fragment is largely cartilaginous (35). Rarely, a radioisotope bone scan is useful for the diagnosis of nondisplaced pelvic fractures and in the identification of acute injuries in children and adults with head injuries or multiple-system injuries (31,36).

Classification

Quinby (18) and Rang (37) classified pelvic fractures in children into three categories: uncomplicated or mild fractures, fractures with visceral injury requiring surgical exploration, and fractures with immediate, massive hemorrhage often associated with multiple and severe pelvic fractures. This classification system emphasizes the importance of the associated soft tissue injuries, but does not account for the mechanism of injury or the prognosis of the pelvic fracture itself. Watts (38) classified pediatric pelvic fractures according to the severity of skeletal injury: (a) avulsion, caused by violent muscular contraction across the unfused apophysis; (b) fractures of the pelvic ring (secondary to crushing injuries), stable and unstable; and (c) acetabular fracture associated with hip dislocation.

Torode and Zieg (15) retrospectively reviewed 141 children with pelvic fractures and classified the injuries on the basis of the severity of the fractures as well as associated prognosis. Their classification does not include acetabular fractures (Fig. 20-1 and Table 20-1). The morbidity, mortality, and complications were greatest in the type IV group with segmental instability of the pelvis. Pennal et al (39) classified pelvic fractures according to the direction of force producing the injury: (a) anteroposterior compression, (b) lateral compression with or without rotation, and (c) vertical shear. This classification was modified and expanded by Tile et al (Table 20-2) (31). Burgess et al (40) further modified the Pennal system and incorporated subsets to the lateral compression and anteroposterior compression groups to quantify the amount of force applied to the pelvic ring. They also created a fourth category, combined mechanical injury, to include injuries resulting from combined forces that may not be strictly categorized according to the Pennal et al classification scheme.

The Tile classification has been incorporated into the Orthopaedic Trauma Association/AO classification, which is divided into bone segments, type, and groups (Table 20-3) (41). The Orthopaedic Trauma Association/AO system classifies pelvic fractures on the basis of stability versus instability, and surgical indications are based on the fracture types. Surgery is rarely

TABLE 20-1 Torode and Zieg Classification of Pelvic Fractures in Children

1. Avulsion fractures
2. Iliac wing fractures
   a. Separation of the iliac apophysis
   b. Fracture of the bony iliac wing
3. Simple ring fractures
   a. Fractures of the pubis and disruption of the pubic symphysis
   b. Fractures involving the acetabulum, without a concomitant ring fracture
4. Fractures producing an unstable segment (ring disruption fracture)
   a. "Straddle" fractures, characterized by bilateral inferior and superior pubic rami fractures
   b. Fractures involving the anterior pubic rami or pubic symphysis and the posterior elements (e.g., sacroiliac joint, sacral ala)
   c. Fractures that create an unstable segment between the anterior ring of the pelvis and the acetabulum

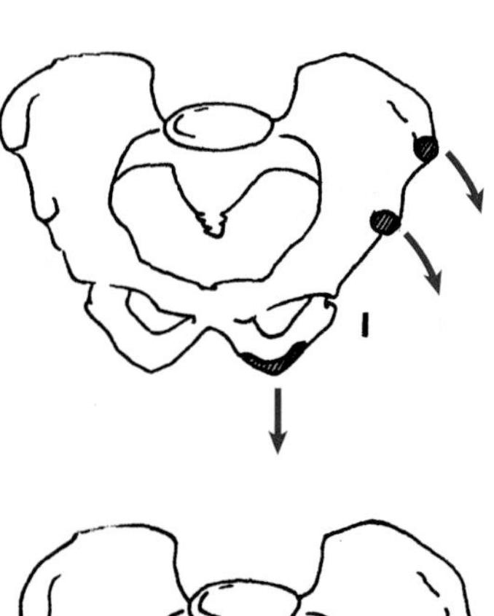

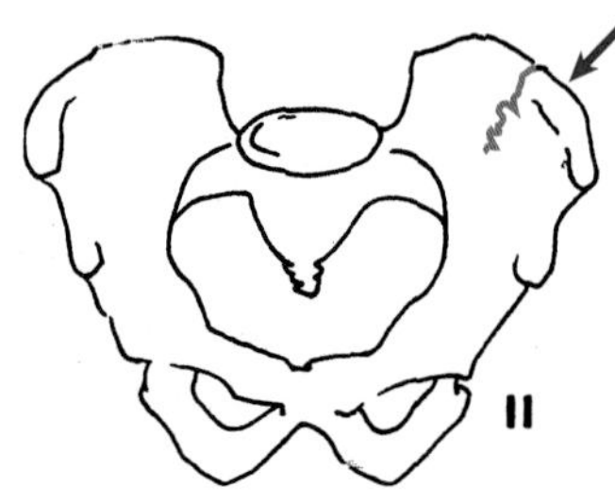

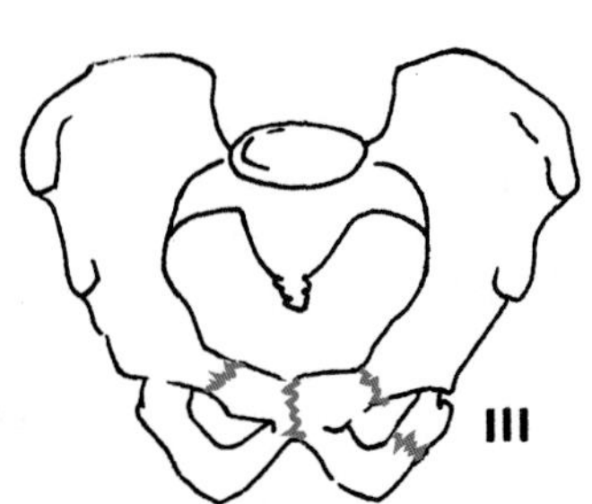

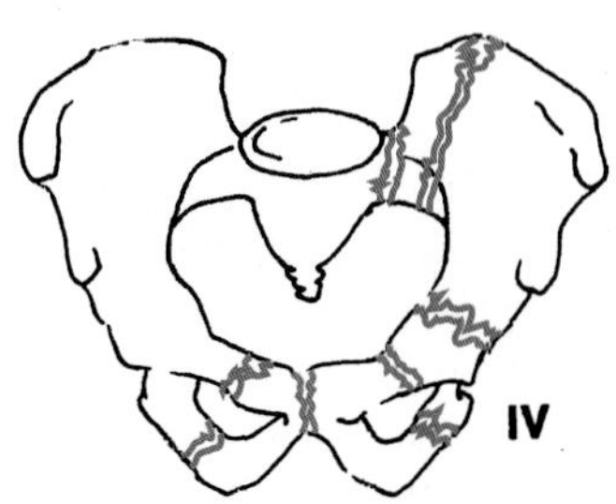

FIGURE 20-1 Torode and Zieg classification of pelvic fractures in children: type I, avulsion fractures; type II, iliac wing fractures; type III, simple ring fractures; type IV, ring disruption fractures.

TABLE 20-2 Tile and Pennal Classification of Pelvic Fractures

A. Stable fractures
- A1: Avulsion fractures
- A2: Undisplaced pelvic ring or iliac wing fractures
- A3: Transverse fractures of the sacrum and coccyx

B. Partially unstable fractures
- B1: Open-book fractures
- B2: Lateral compression injuries (includes triradiate injury)
- B3: Bilateral type B injuries

C. Unstable fractures of the pelvic ring
- C1: Unilateral fractures
    - C1-1: Fractures of the ilium
    - C1-2: Dislocation or fracture-dislocation of the sacroiliac joint
    - C1-3: Fractures of the sacrum
- C2: Bilateral fractures, one type B and one type C
- C3: Bilateral type C fractures

TABLE 20-3 AO/Association for the Study of Internal Fixation Classification of Pelvic Fractures

A. Stable fractures

B. Rotationally unstable fractures, vertically stable

C. Rotationally and vertically unstable fractures
- C1: Unilateral posterior arch disruption
    - C1-1 Iliac fracture
    - C1-2 Sacroiliac fracture-dislocation
    - C1-3 Sacral fracture
- C2: Bilateral posterior arch disruption, one side vertically unstable
- C3: Bilateral injury, both unstable

indicated for type A fractures, whereas anterior or posterior surgical stabilization or both may be indicated for types B and C. Numerous subtypes are included, and further details are described in the chapter on pelvic fractures in *Rockwood and Green's Fractures in Adults* (Volume 2, Chapter 35).

Silber and Flynn (42) reviewed x-rays of 133 children and adolescents with pelvic fractures and classified them into two groups: immature (Risser 0 and all physes open) and mature (closed triradiate cartilage). They suggested that in the immature group management should focus on the associated injuries because the pelvic fractures in this group rarely required surgical intervention; fractures in the mature group were best classified and treated according to adult pelvic fracture classification and management principles.

The multitude of classification systems makes the comparison of incidence, mechanism of injury, morbidity and mortality, and outcome difficult among studies using different systems. Although many recent studies of children's fractures use the Torode and Zieg (15) or Tile classifications or both, the basic classifications, (a) mature or immature pelvis and (b) stable or unstable fracture, are very useful information for making treatment decisions. Most pelvic fractures in children are stable injuries. Pelvic fractures in patients with closed triradiate cartilage should follow adult fracture classifications and treatment protocols (31,40,41).

APPLIED ANATOMY

There are several important anatomic differences between the pelvis of a child and that of an adult. First, a child's pelvis is more malleable because of the nature of the bone itself, the increased elasticity of the joints, and the ability of the more cartilaginous structures to absorb energy (43). Second, the elasticity of the joints may allow significant displacement and resultant fracture in only one area rather than the traditional concept of a mandatory "double break" in the ring for a displaced fracture (37,43). Third, avulsion fractures of an apophysis occur more often in children and adolescents than in adults because of the inherent weakness of cartilage compared with bone; fractures of the acetabulum into the triradiate cartilage also occur more often for the same reason (16,37). Fourth, fractures through physeal cartilage in children can ultimately cause growth arrest, leg-length discrepancy, and abnormal development (e.g., a fracture through the triradiate cartilage with resultant "bony bar" formation and ultimately a deficient and dysplastic acetabulum) (43).

Ossification Centers

The pelvis of a child consists of three primary ossification centers: the ilium, ischium, and pubis. The three centers meet at the triradiate cartilage and fuse at approximately 16 to 18 years of age (Fig. 20-2) (43). The pubis and ischium fuse inferiorly at the pubic rami at 6 or 7 years of age. Occasionally, at approximately the time of fusion of the ischium to the pubis, an asymptomatic mass, ischiopubic synchondrosis, is noted radiographically in this area. The child should be treated expectantly, and this should not be confused with a fracture of the pelvis.

The secondary centers of ossification include the iliac crest, ischial apophysis, anterior inferior iliac spine, pubic tubercle, angle of the pubis, ischial spine, and lateral wing of the sacrum. The iliac crest is first seen at 13 to 15 years and fuses at 15 to 17 years of age. The secondary ossification of the ischium is first seen at 15 to 17 years and fuses at 19 years of age, although fusion may be as late as 25 years of age. A center of ossification may be present at the anterior inferior iliac spine at approximately 14 years, fusing at 16 years of age (38,43). These second-

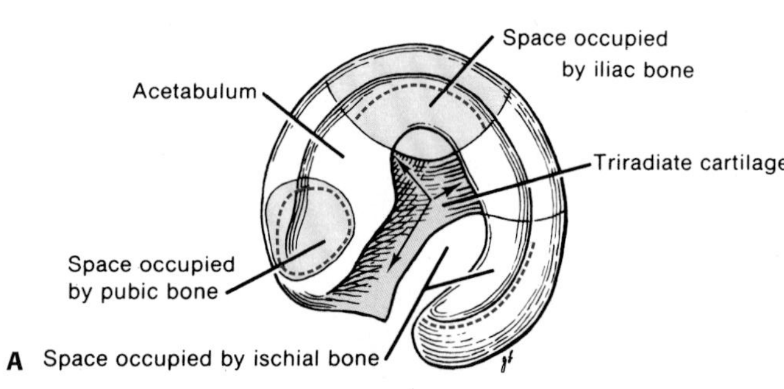

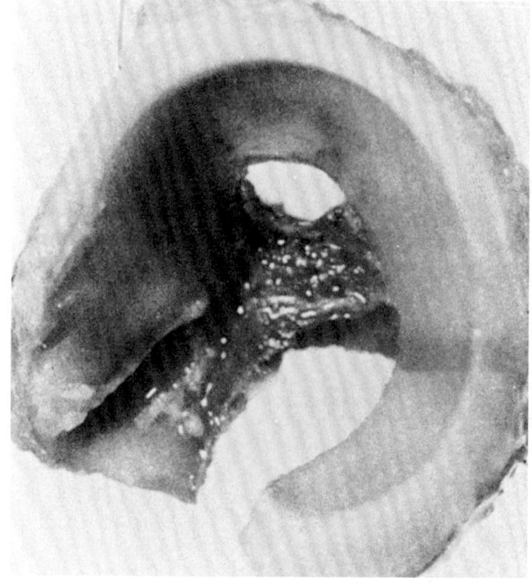

FIGURE 20-2 A. Triradiate-acetabular cartilage complex viewed from the lateral side, showing the sites occupied by the iliac, ischial, and pubic bones. **B.** Normal acetabular cartilage complex of a 1-day-old infant. The ilium, ischium, and pubis have been removed with a curet. The lateral view shows the cup-shaped acetabulum. (From Ponseti IV. Growth and development of the acetabulum in the normal child. Anatomical, histological, and roentgenographic studies. *J Bone Joint Surg Am* 1978;60(5): 575–585, with permission.)

ary centers of ossification and the age of appearance and fusion are described so they will not be confused with avulsion fractures.

The acetabulum contains the physes of the ilium, ischium, and pubis that merge to become the triradiate cartilage. Interstitial growth in the triradiate part of the cartilage complex causes the acetabulum to expand during growth and causes the pubis, ischium, and ilium to enlarge as well. The concavity of the acetabulum develops in response to the presence of a spherical head. The depth of the acetabulum increases during development as the result of interstitial growth in the acetabular cartilage, appositional growth of the periphery of this cartilage, and periosteal new bone formation at the acetabular margin (44). At puberty, three secondary centers of ossification appear in the hyaline cartilage surrounding the acetabular cavity. The *os acetabuli*, which is the epiphysis of the pubis, forms the anterior wall of the acetabulum. The epiphysis of the ilium, the *acetabular epiphysis* (38,44), forms a large part of the superior wall of the acetabulum. The small secondary center of the ischium is rarely seen. The os acetabuli, the largest part, starts to develop at approximately 8 years of age and forms a significant part of the anterior wall of the acetabulum; it unites with the pubis at approximately 18 years of age. The acetabular epiphysis develops in the iliac acetabular cartilage at approximately 8 years and fuses with the ilium at 18 years of age, forming a substantial part of the superior acetabular joint surface (Fig. 20-3). The *secondary center of the ischium*, the smallest of the three, develops in the ninth year, unites with the acetabulum at 17 years, and contributes very little to acetabular development. These secondary centers should not be confused with avulsion fractures or loose bodies in the hip joint.

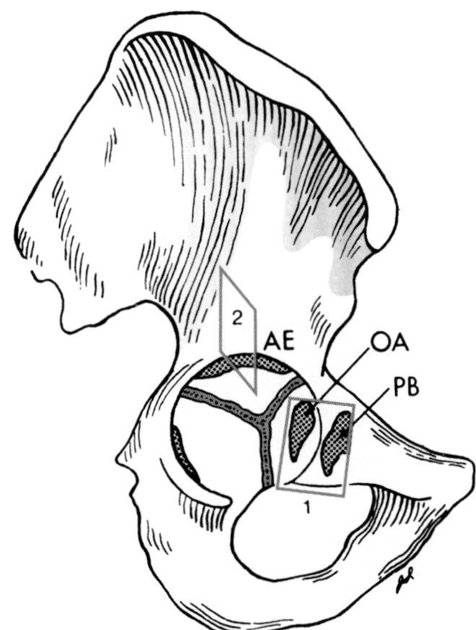

FIGURE 20-3 Right innominate bone of an adolescent. The os acetabuli (OA) is shown within the acetabular cartilage adjoining the pubic bone (PB); the acetabular epiphysis (AE), within the acetabular cartilage adjoining the iliac bone; and another small epiphysis (not labeled), within the acetabular cartilage adjoining the ischium (*left*). (From Ponseti IV. Growth and development of the acetabulum in the normal child. Anatomical, histological, and roentgenographic studies. *J Bone Joint Surg Am* 1978; 60(5):575–585; with permission.)

CURRENT TREATMENT OPTIONS: PELVIC FRACTURES

Avulsion Fractures

Avulsion fractures of the pelvis usually occur in adolescent athletes as a result of forceful contraction of the attached muscle while the athlete is actively engaged in activities such as kicking, running, or jumping (45–47). The incidence of avulsion fractures is most certainly underrepresented in large hospital-based clinical series because most of these injuries do not result in emergency department visits. The incidence in two large recent series was approximately 4% (12,13). Chronic repetitive traction on the developing iliac apophysis may result in an incomplete avulsion fracture or apophysitis without a history of acute trauma (48,49). The sartorius muscle attaches to the anterior superior iliac spine, the direct head of the rectus femoris attaches to the anterior inferior iliac spine, and the hamstrings and adductors attach to the ischial tuberosity.

Of the 268 pelvic avulsion fractures reported in the four largest series (Table 20-4) (45–47,50), 50% were ischial avulsions, 23% were avulsions of the anterior superior iliac spine, and 22% were avulsions of the anterior inferior iliac spine (Fig. 20-4). Avulsions of the lesser trochanter (3%) and iliac apophysis (2%) accounted for the rest.

Mechanism of Injury

The mechanism of injury is thought to be either sudden forceful concentric or eccentric contraction of large muscles, which have their insertion on the pelvic apophyses, or sudden passive lengthening while performing anteroposterior splits during

TABLE 20-4 Location of Pelvic Avulsion Fractures in Four Series (268 Fractures)*

Ischium	ASIS	AIIS	Lesser Trochanter	Iliac Apophysis
50%	23%	22%	3%	2%

* From Fernbach SK, Wilkinson RH. Avulsion injuries of the pelvis and proximal femur. *AJR Am J Roentgenol* 1981;137(3):581–584; Metzmaker JN, Pappas AM. Avulsion fractures of the pelvis. *Am J Sports Med* 1985;13(5):349–358; Rossi F, Dragoni S. Acute avulsion fractures of the pelvis in adolescent competitive athletes: prevalence, location and sports distribution of 203 cases collected. *Skeletal Radiol* 2001;30(3):127–131; and Sundar M, Carty H. Avulsion fractures of the pelvis in children: a report of 32 fractures and their outcome. *Skeletal Radiol* 1994;23(2):85–90; with permission.

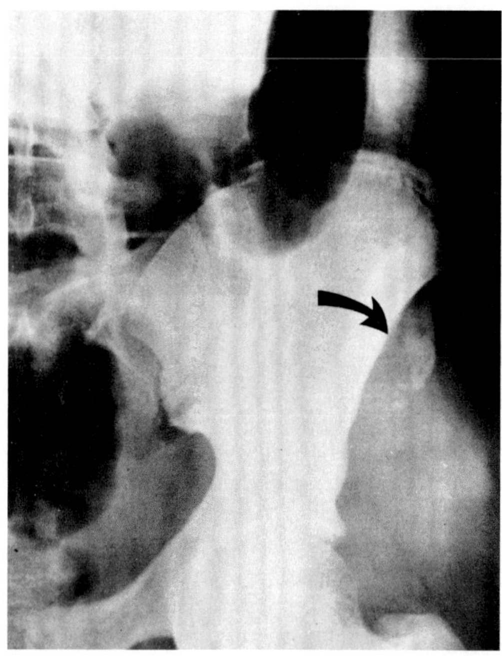

FIGURE 20-4 Displaced fracture of the anterosuperior iliac spine.

such activities as gymnastics or dance (46). The distribution of fracture patterns with respect to sporting activity reveals that gymnastics are responsible for the greatest number of acute ischial tuberosity avulsion fractures, whereas soccer is responsible for the greatest numbers of anterior superior and anterior inferior iliac spine avulsion fractures (47). Iliac apophysitis is most frequently associated with long distance running and thought to result from either repetitive muscular contraction and inflammation or subclinical stress fractures of the apophysis (49).

Diagnosis

Symptoms usually include localized swelling and tenderness about the site of the avulsion fracture. Motion is limited, and pain may be mild or marked. In patients with chronic avulsions caused by repetitive activity, pain and limitation of motion usually are gradually progressive. In patients with ischial avulsions, pain at the ischial tuberosity can be elicited by flexing the hip and extending the knee. In this position, if the hip is moved into abduction, more pain is elicited. Patients may also have pain while sitting or moving on the involved tuberosity.

In patients with anterior superior iliac spine avulsions, x-rays show slight displacement of the apophysis (Fig. 20-5). In patients with anterior inferior iliac spine avulsions, x-rays show minimal distal displacement of the fragment. Further displacement is probably prevented because this is a conjoined tendon, and the reflected head of the rectus femoris muscle is intact. Contralateral views can be obtained and compared to ensure that this fragment is not actually a secondary center of ossification, either the os acetabuli or acetabular epiphysis (Fig. 20-5). With ischial tuberosity avulsions, x-rays reveal a large fragment displaced distally compared with the opposite ischial tuberosity (Fig. 20-6). Significant displacement is resisted by the intact sacrotuberous ligament.

Because these avulsion fractures occur primarily through secondary centers of ossification before the center is fused with the pelvis, primarily in children ages 11 to 17 years (45,46,50), comparison views of the contralateral apophysis should be obtained to ensure that what appears to be an avulsion fracture is not in reality a normal adolescent variant. Later, exuberant callus formation can occasionally mimic a malignant neoplasm (51). Recognition of the initial fracture is important to avoid unnecessary evaluations such as CT, MRI, and radionuclide scans, and inappropriate biopsy.

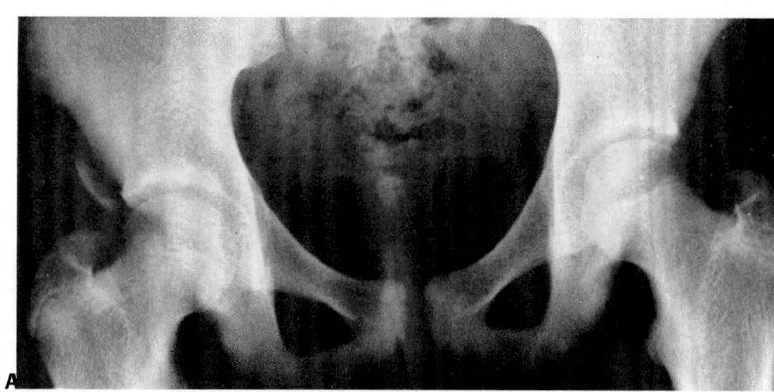

A

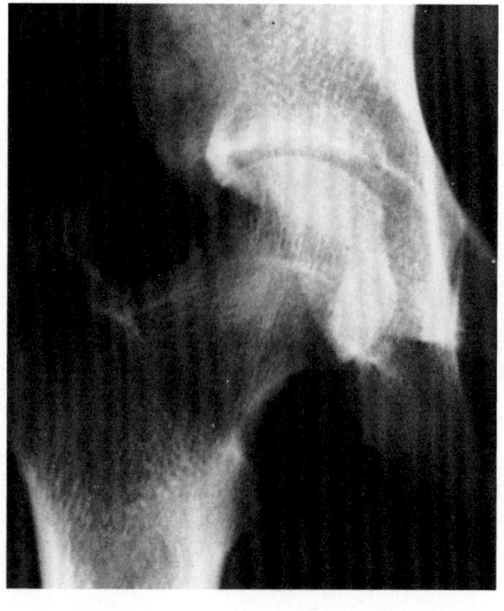

B

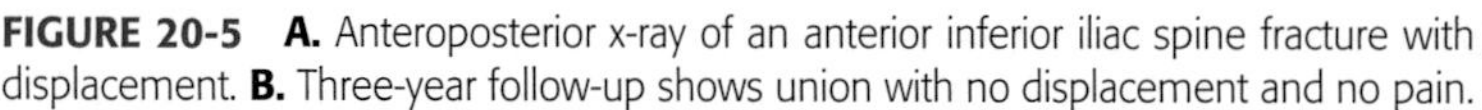

FIGURE 20-5 **A.** Anteroposterior x-ray of an anterior inferior iliac spine fracture with displacement. **B.** Three-year follow-up shows union with no displacement and no pain.

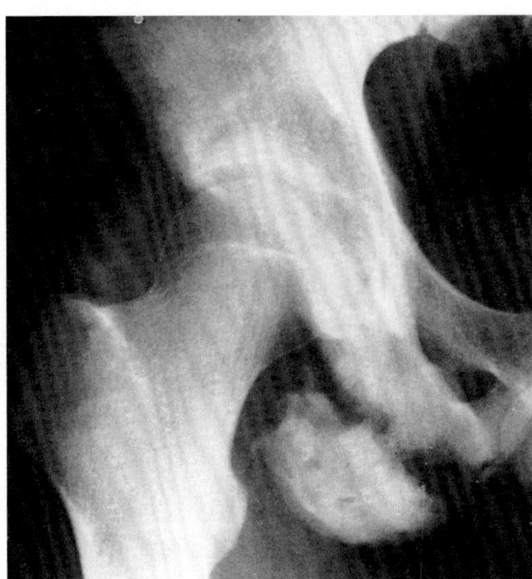

FIGURE 20-6 Large ischial tuberosity fracture.

Treatment and Prognosis

Most pelvic avulsion fractures in children do well with conservative nonoperative management including rest, partial weight bearing on crutches for 2 or more weeks, and extremity positioning to minimize muscle stretch. Two small series of adolescents with pelvic avulsion fractures treated conservatively concluded that nonsurgical treatment was successful in all patients, and all patients returned to preinjury activity levels (45,46). Others have suggested that conservative nonoperative treatment is associated with a significantly higher incidence of functional disability and inability to return to competitive athletic activity (Fig. 20-7) (50). On long-term follow-up of 12 patients with ischial avulsions, 8 reported significant reduction in athletic ability and 5 had persistent local symptoms (50). In the largest series published to date, only 3 of 198 competitive adolescent athletes with pelvic avulsion fractures were treated operatively (47). Anecdotally, long-term functional disability and inability to return to preinjury activity levels have been reported in the setting of conservatively managed ischial avulsion fractures (50,52). Controversy exists surrounding the acute management of ischial avulsion fractures, but most agree that excision of the ischial apophysis is indicated in the setting of chronic pain and disability. Some authors recommend open reduction and internal fixation of those rare acute pelvic avulsion fragments displaced more than 1 to 2 cm (53).

Fractures of the Pubis or Ischium

In children, pelvic rami fractures are usually caused by high-velocity trauma and have a significant number of associated injuries. Reed (12) reported that 45% of the pelvic fractures in children in his series were pubic rami fractures. Rieger and Brug (13) reported that 37% of their series of 54 pelvic fractures in children were "simple ring fractures," and McIntyre et al (10) reported that 40% of 57 pelvic fractures were "type I" (unilateral anterior) fractures. Silber et al (14) reported that 56% of pelvic fractures in their series of 166 consecutive pediatric pelvic fractures were simple ring fractures (excluding acetabular fractures) and were caused by motor vehicle versus pedestrian mechanism in 60%. Single ramus fractures are more common than multiple rami fractures, and the superior ramus is fractured more often than the inferior ramus (Fig. 20-8) (12).

In patients with isolated pubic ramus fractures, clinical examination reveals pain and possible crepitus at the fracture site; however, there should be little or no motion on deep palpation. CT scanning or inlet and outlet radiographic views are helpful in determining whether any other pelvic fractures are present. If there is significant displacement of the pubic rami, a second

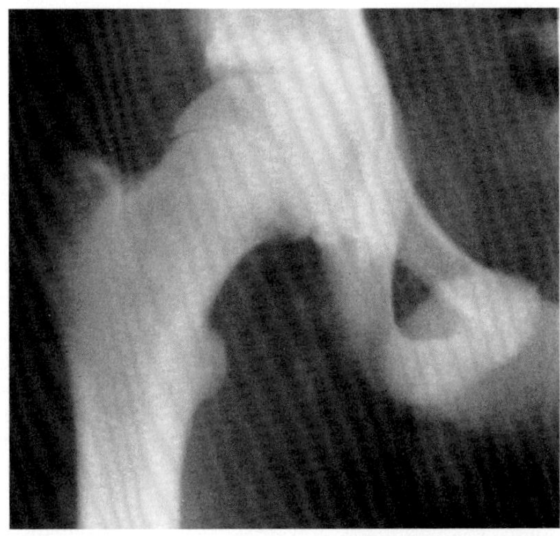

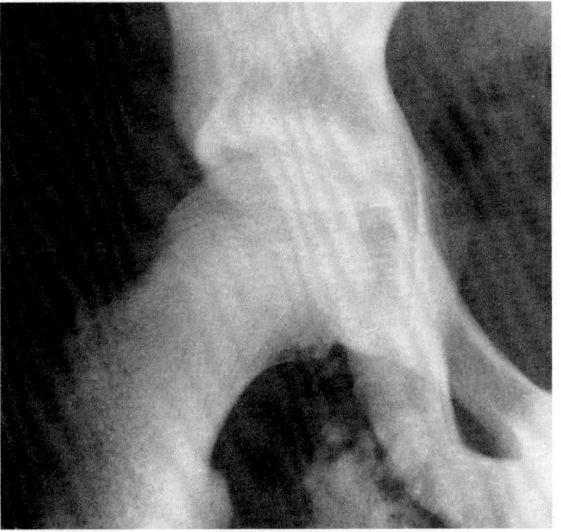

FIGURE 20-7 Ischial tuberosity fracture at time of fracture **(A)** and at 6-month follow-up **(B)**, showing abundant callus formation.

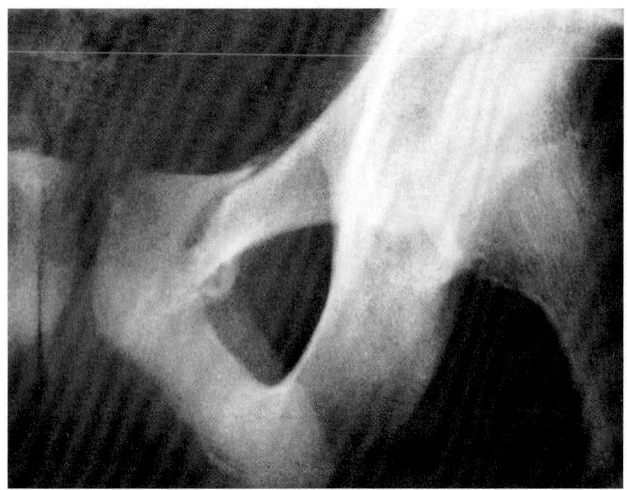

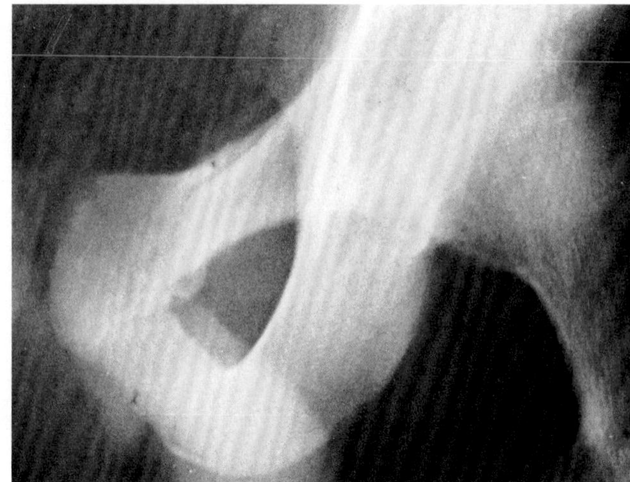

FIGURE 20-8 **A.** Stable superior pubic ramus fracture. The patient was allowed full weight bearing at 4 weeks postfracture. **B.** He was asymptomatic and x-ray showed early callus formation.

fracture through the pelvic ring should be suspected, although because of the plasticity of bone and elasticity of the symphysis and sacroiliac joints in children, more displacement can be expected than in adults with the same injury. Bed rest until pain subsides, followed by progressive weight bearing, usually is sufficient treatment.

Fractures of the Body of the Ischium

Fracture of the body of the ischium near the acetabulum is extremely rare in children. The fracture occurs from external force to the ischium, most commonly in a fall from a considerable height. The fracture usually is minimally displaced, and treatment consists of bed rest and progressive weight bearing (Fig. 20-9).

Stress Fractures of the Pubis or Ischium

Stress fractures are rare in small children, but they do occur in adolescents and young adults from chronic, repetitive stress to a bony area, and also occur during the last trimester of pregnancy. Stress fractures of the pubis are likewise uncommon, but a small

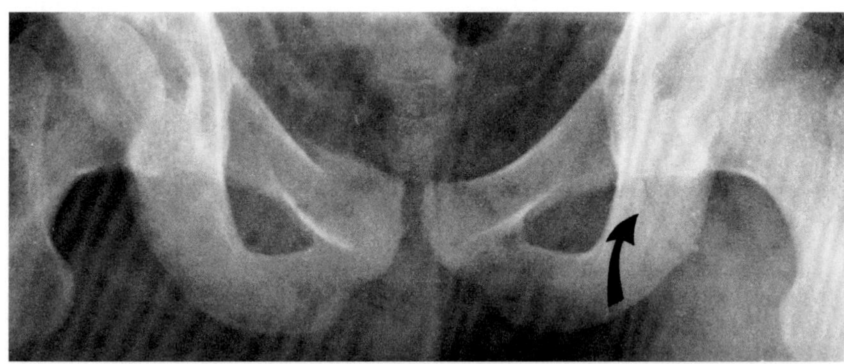

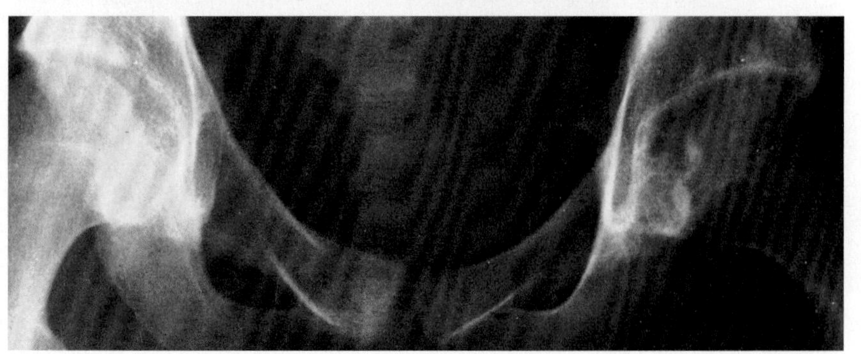

FIGURE 20-9 Nondisplaced fracture through the left ischium and contralateral pubic ramus fracture **(A)**. Follow-up x-ray shows mild displacement and incongruity of the acetabulum and complete healing of the superior pubic ramus fracture **(B)**. Either displacement of the fracture fragments or premature closure of the triradiate cartilage could have contributed to the incongruity of the femoral head in the acetabulum.

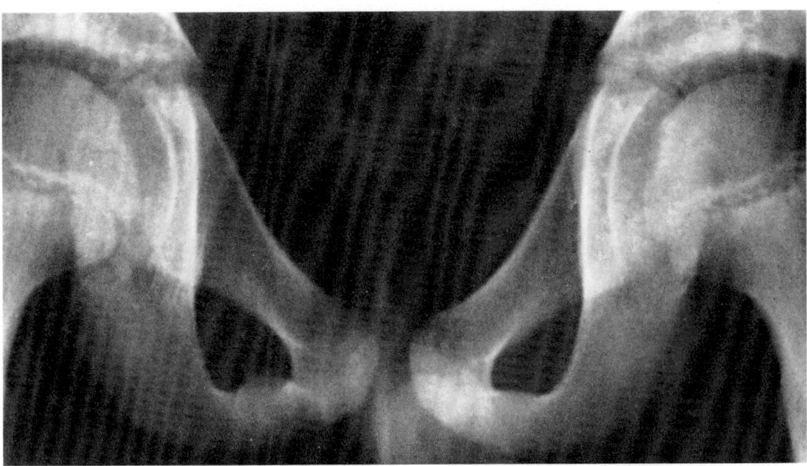

FIGURE 20-10 X-ray of the pelvis of a 9-year-old child. Although the differentiation could not be made between a fracture and fusion of the right ischiopubic ossification center at the time of the x-ray, the patient was asymptomatic and the mass was considered a variant of normal development.

series of stress fractures, primarily in the inferior pubic rami, has been reported. Chronic symptoms and pain increased by stress may be noted in the inferior pubic area. X-rays may show no evidence of fracture for as long as 4 to 6 weeks, and then only faint callus formation may be visible; however, imaging by MRI or a technetium bone scan may reveal increased uptake (36), indicating a stress fracture, 3 to 4 weeks before changes on x-ray. Treatment should consist of discontinuing the activity causing the repetitive stress, along with limited weight bearing on crutches for 4 to 6 weeks.

The ischiopubic synchondrosis usually closes between 4 and 8 years of age (54). X-rays of the ischiopubic junction are at best difficult to interpret and may be misinterpreted as a fracture. Caffey and Ross noted that bilateral fusion of the ischiopubic synchondrosis is complete in 6% of children at 4 years of age and in 83% of children at 12 years of age (55). Bilateral swelling of the synchondrosis was also noted in 47% of children at age 7 years. Irregular mineralization and swelling of the ischiopubic synchondrosis has been called ischiopubic osteochondrosis or van Neck disease (56). As noted above, the radiographic changes are common and usually asymptomatic. If this syndrome is noted in a child older than 10 years of age, a stress fracture may be suspected and treated as such (Fig. 20-10).

Fractures of the Wing of the Ilium (Duverney Fracture)

Direct trauma may cause a fracture of the wing of the ilium, but isolated iliac wing fractures are relatively rare. Reed (12) reported an incidence of 12% in children with fractures of the pelvis. Rieger and Brug (13) reported iliac wing fractures in only three (5.6%) of their patients, and McIntyre et al (10) reported only 7 (12%) in 57 fractures. However, this fracture often occurs in conjunction with other fractures of the pelvis, and thus the overall incidence of iliac wing fractures is probably significantly higher than the incidence of isolated iliac wing fractures.

Displacement of the fracture usually occurs laterally, but it can occur medially or proximally. Severe displacement is prevented by preservation of some of the attachments of the abdominal muscles and the hip abductors. Pain is located over the wing of the ilium, and motion at the fracture site may be noted. A painful Trendelenburg gait may be present because of spasm of the hip abductor muscles.

A fracture of the wing of the ilium may be overlooked on an underexposed x-ray of the pelvis where the ilium is poorly seen as a large area of radiolucency. Use of a "hot light" is helpful in making the diagnosis (Fig. 20-11).

Treatment of an iliac wing fracture usually is dictated by the associated injuries. Bed rest in a comfortable position, usually with the leg abducted, is all that is necessary for treatment of the fracture itself. This should be followed by partial weight bearing on crutches until the symptoms are completely re-

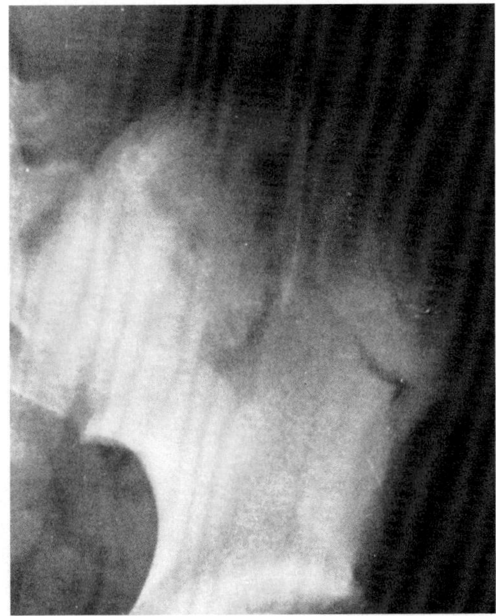

FIGURE 20-11 Minimally displaced fracture of the left iliac wing.

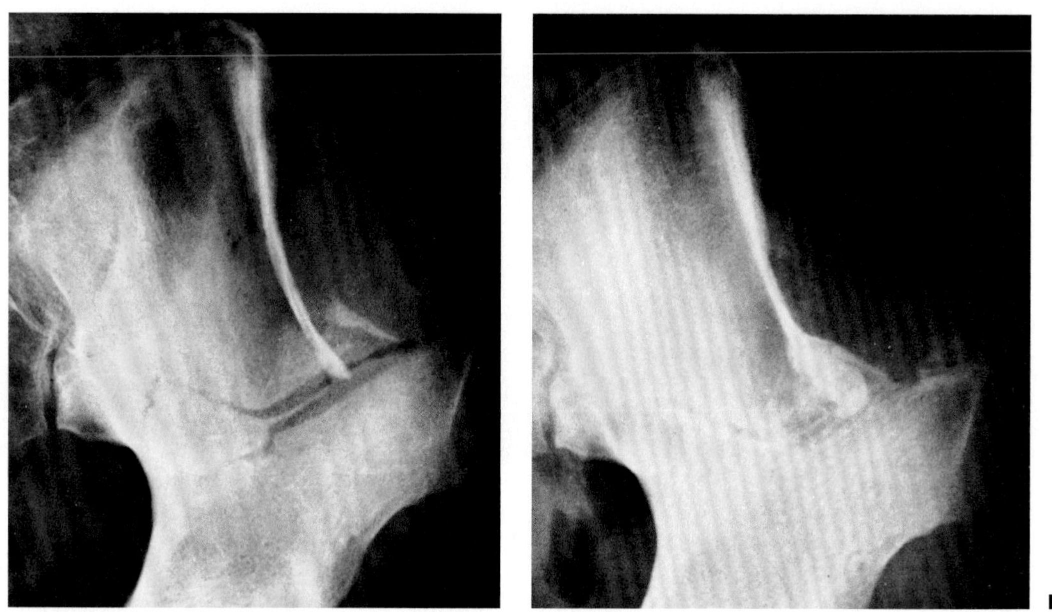

FIGURE 20-12 **A.** Severely comminuted fracture of the left iliac wing. **B.** X-ray at 3-month follow-up shows fracture healed with displacement, but the patient was asymptomatic.

solved. Regardless of the amount of comminution or displacement, these fractures usually unite without complications or sequelae (Fig. 20-12).

Fractures of the Sacrum

Sacral fractures constitute a small fraction of pelvic fractures reported in children. Rieger and Brug (13) reported two sacral fractures and seven sacroiliac fracture-dislocations in their 54 patients. Sacral fractures are probably more common than reported, but because they are obscured by the bony pelvis and the soft tissue shadows of the abdominal viscera, and because they are rarely displaced, they may be overlooked (Fig. 20-13). Nine of 166 patients (5.4%) with pelvic fractures in the series by Silber et al (14) had associated sacral fractures, none with

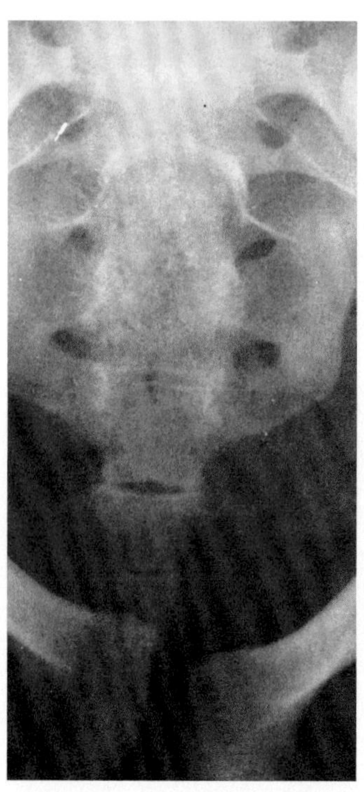

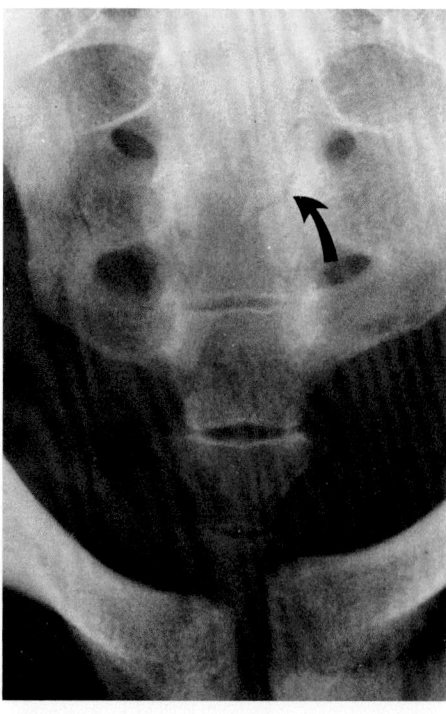

FIGURE 20-13 **A.** X-ray suggesting comminuted nondisplaced linear sacral fracture on the left. **B.** At 6-week follow-up, x-ray shows definite evidence of linear sacral fracture.

nerve root involvement. These fractures may be significant because they may damage the sacral nerves, resulting in loss of bowel and bladder function.

Sacral fractures are best diagnosed clinically. Pain and swelling may be present, usually over the lower part of the sacrum. Rectal examination elicits pain on palpation anterior to the sacrum. Occasionally, the fracture fragments may be felt. Repeated bimanual rectal examination with attempts at reduction should be avoided because a tear in the rectum may occur.

The fractures are difficult to see on x-rays. The fracture can be oblique, but most are transverse with minimal displacement and occur through a sacral foramen, which is the weakest part of the body of the sacrum. Minimal offset of the foramen or offset of the lateral edge of the body of the sacrum is an indication of sacral fracture. Lateral views are helpful only if there is anterior displacement, which is rare. A 35-degree caudad view of the pelvis may reveal a fracture of the body of the sacrum. CT scans and MRI scans are both helpful in the identification of sacral fractures missed on plain radiographic images (34,57,58). In one study comparing x-rays with CT scans in a consecutive series of 103 pediatric trauma patients with pelvic x-rays and pelvic CT scans, only three sacral fractures were identified with plain x-rays whereas nine sacral fractures were identified with CT (Fig. 20-14) (34).

Fractures of the Coccyx

Significant soft tissue injury to the coccyx makes it difficult to determine on x-rays whether a coccygeal fracture has occurred, especially in a child. However, historically, trauma to the coccyx is often refractory to treatment. For this reason, if clinical symptoms are sufficient, an injury to this area in a child should be considered a fracture regardless of whether a fracture can be seen on x-rays.

Coccygeal fractures are not included in most large series of fractures of the pelvis in adults and children, although the coccyx is part of the pelvis. The mechanism of injury is usually similar to that in adults: a direct fall onto the buttocks in the sitting position. These fractures rarely have associated injuries. Clinically, patients describe immediate, severe pain in the area of the coccyx. Pain on defecation may be present as well as pain on rectal examination. Because radiographic identification is difficult, the diagnosis should be made clinically by digital rectal examination. Exquisite pain may be elicited, and an abnormal mobility of the coccygeal fragments may be noted. Acute symptoms may abate in 1 to 2 weeks, but may persist on sitting for 4 weeks.

Lateral x-rays of the coccyx with the hips flexed maximally may reveal the fracture (Fig. 20-15). The coccyx may appear to be acutely angulated as a normal variant, and a fracture may not be seen, or the normal acute angulation may be falsely interpreted as a fracture or dislocation. CT and MRI scanning may be helpful in differentiating between physeal plates and fracture lines (59). Treatment consists of activity restriction and use of an inflated doughnut cushion with return to full activity in 4 to 6 weeks.

Fractures of the Two Ipsilateral Rami

Fractures of the ipsilateral superior and inferior pubic rami comprised 18% of pediatric pelvic fractures in the series of 120 pediatric pelvic fractures reviewed by Chia et al (4). Although these fractures are generally stable, they may be associated with increased incidence of associated injuries to abdominal viscera, especially the genitourinary system including bladder rupture (60). There is a high association as well with head injury, which correlates with the mechanism of injury, which is very often motor vehicle versus pedestrian (15).

Considerable force is necessary to cause this fracture pattern, and other associated fractures should be expected. A general

A
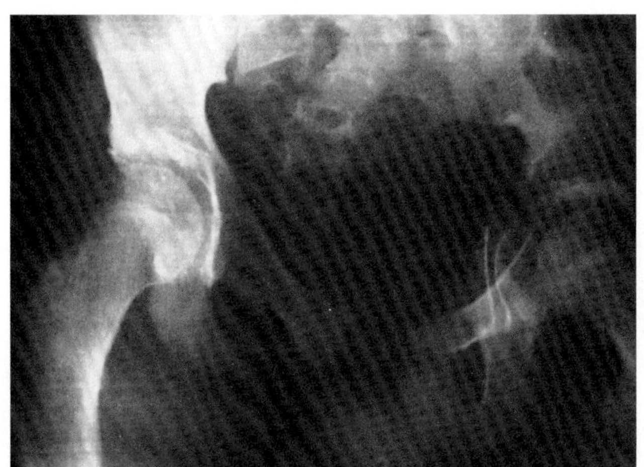
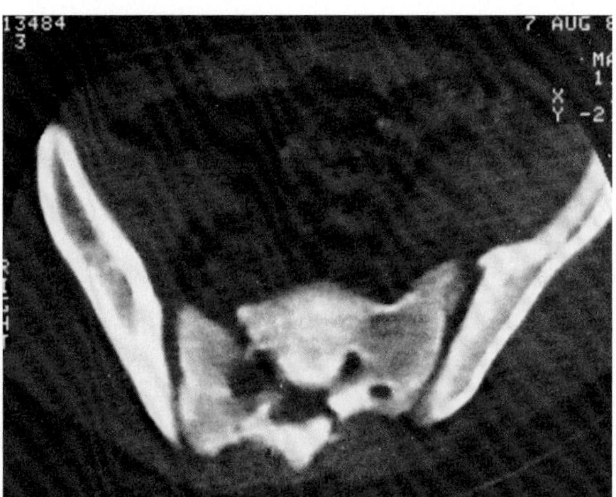

B

FIGURE 20-14 **A.** A 15-year-old boy with an obvious fracture of the left acetabulum and symphysis pubis diastasis, and a questionable ill-defined sacral fracture. **B.** CT scan reveals a comminuted displaced sacral fracture.

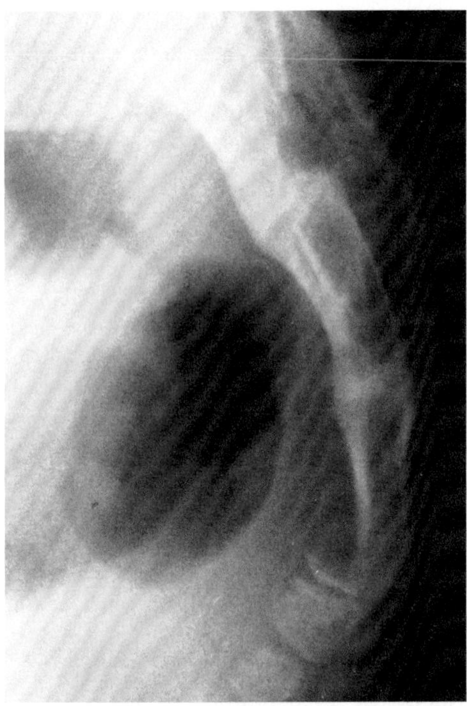

FIGURE 20-15 Lateral x-ray with the hips maximally flexed reveals displaced coccygeal fracture in a 14-year-old boy.

evaluation should be followed by examination of the pelvis and lower extremities, with special attention to abrasions, contusions, lacerations, and ecchymosis about the pelvis. Palpation reveals discomfort anteriorly, and crepitus at the fracture site may be noted.

Various methods of treatment have been advocated for adults. However, in children, the fracture almost always unites with adequate remodeling of even the most displaced fractures. For this reason, short-term bed rest followed by progressive weight bearing on the involved side is all that is necessary (Fig. 20-16).

Fractures Near or Subluxation of the Symphysis Pubis

Isolated injuries in the symphysis pubis area are rare, primarily because they usually occur in association with disruption of posterior structures such as the sacroiliac joint. Although significant force appears to be necessary to disrupt or fracture the symphysis pubis, isolated disruption of the symphysis pubis can occur (38). Usually, there is some normal elasticity at the symphysis in adults (0.5 mm in men, 1.5 mm in women), and there is probably even more in children, depending on maturity. In children and adolescents diastasis greater than or equal to 2.5 cm or rotational deformity greater than 15 degrees suggests significant instability and the need for reduction (61).

Clinically, exquisite pain is present anteriorly at the symphysis; the legs are externally rotated and often pain is worse in the supine position than in the side-lying position (38). Motion of the hips in flexion, abduction, external rotation, and extension is restricted and painful (fabere sign).

X-rays may reveal subluxation and widening of the symphysis, as if opening a book (62). Offset may be superior, inferior, anterior, or posterior (Fig. 20-17). Furthermore, a fracture near or into the symphysis may produce an equivalent subluxation of the symphysis pubis (Fig. 20-18). Because of the variable normal separation of the symphysis in children of different ages, the amount of traumatic separation may be difficult to evaluate. Watts (38) suggested x-rays with and without lateral compression of the pelvis. More than 1 cm of difference in the width of the symphysis pubis between the two views suggests a symphysis pubis separation. Radiographic evaluation should be performed to specifically exclude sacroiliac joint disruption and

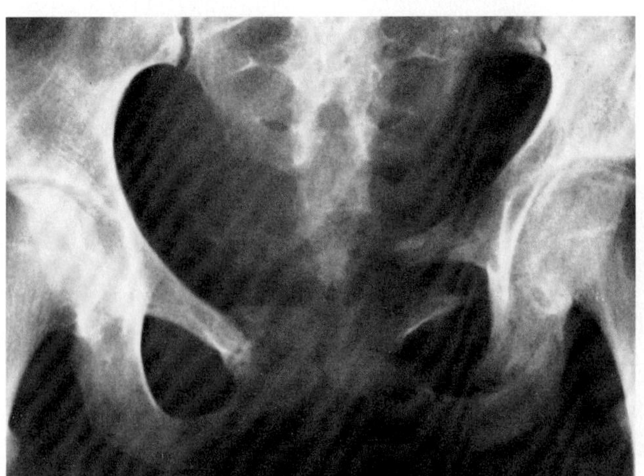

A

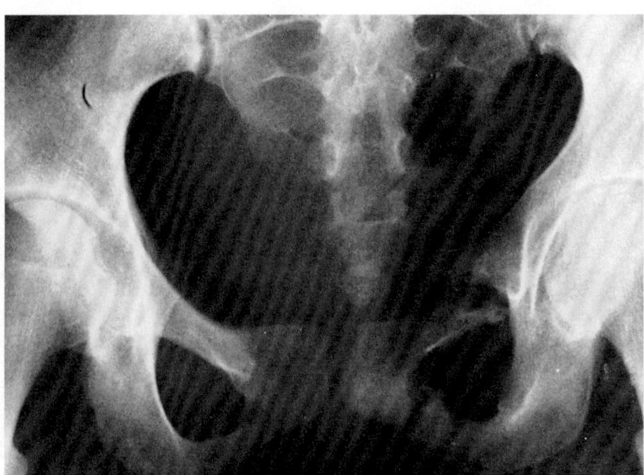

B

FIGURE 20-16 **A.** Ipsilateral left pubic rami fractures with a contralateral right superior ramus fracture. **B.** At 2-year follow-up, nonunion of the ipsilateral rami fractures is evident, but the patient is asymptomatic.

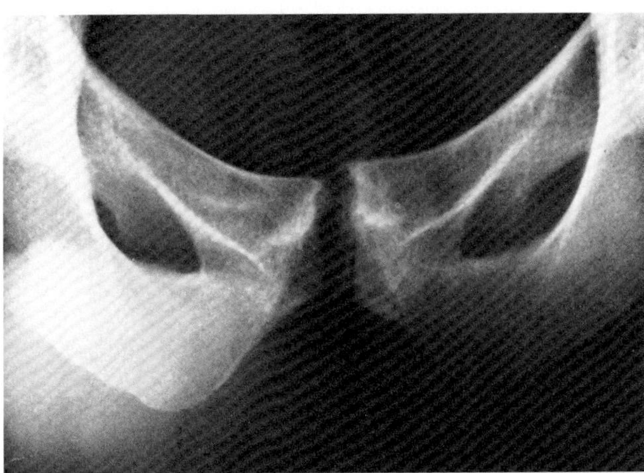

FIGURE 20-17 Mild symphysis pubis subluxation with superior displacement. At 4-year follow-up, the patient is asymptomatic.

triradiate cartilage fracture because both of these injuries may occur in association with symphysis pubis separation (43).

Treatment of isolated fractures or subluxations of the symphysis pubis should consist of bed rest, usually in a side-lying position, especially if other injuries are present. Unilateral Buck's traction may relieve pain, but it rarely improves alignment of the fracture or subluxation. Application of a spica cast in the lateral position with lateral compression may also reduce the displacement and decrease the length of hospitalization (38). External fixation with an anterior frame may provide immediate stability and allow early mobilization in displaced fractures or severe subluxation (63).

Fractures Near or Subluxation of the Sacroiliac Joint

Fractures near or subluxation of the sacroiliac joint are rare, isolated injuries, probably even less common than isolated fractures at the weaker symphysis pubis. More commonly, disruptions of the sacroiliac joint occur with fractures or dislocations of the anterior portion of the pelvis, causing an instability of the pelvis. Sacroiliac dislocations differ from those in adults in several ways. In children, fractures tend to be incomplete because of partial tearing of the anterior sacroiliac ligaments or epiphyseal iliac fracture adjacent to the joint (43). A subchondral fracture through structurally weak zones of physeal cartilage may leave the sacroiliac joint intact (64). Associated vascular and neurologic injuries may occur, and lumbosacral nerve root avulsions have been described in children with this fracture (30).

Subluxation of the sacroiliac joint should be suspected with high-velocity trauma and injury to the posterior aspect of the pelvis near the sacroiliac joint. In patients with these injuries, the fabere sign is markedly positive on the ipsilateral side (64,65). Comparison views of both sacroiliac joints should be carefully evaluated to determine any asymmetry of the wings of the ilium with increased separation at the sacroiliac joint (Fig. 20-19). Any offset of the distal articular surface of the sacrum and ilium on radiography is an indication of sacroiliac joint disruption. Oblique views for comparison of both sacroiliac joints often are beneficial. Because of the rarity of this subluxation or fracture, multiple views including inlet and outlet views, and axial CT scan may be necessary to ensure there is no anterior fracture (Fig. 20-20).

Bed rest and guarded weight bearing on crutches are probably all the treatment needed for isolated subluxations or fractures. Heeg and Klasen (65) reported sacroiliac joint dislocations in 18 children, 10 of whom had extensive degloving injuries of the posterior pelvis. Ten were treated nonoperatively, six with open reduction and internal fixation, one with open reduction but no internal fixation, and one with external fixation. Disabling long-term sequelae included occasional back pain in six, daily back pain in three, and incomplete neurologic recovery in six.

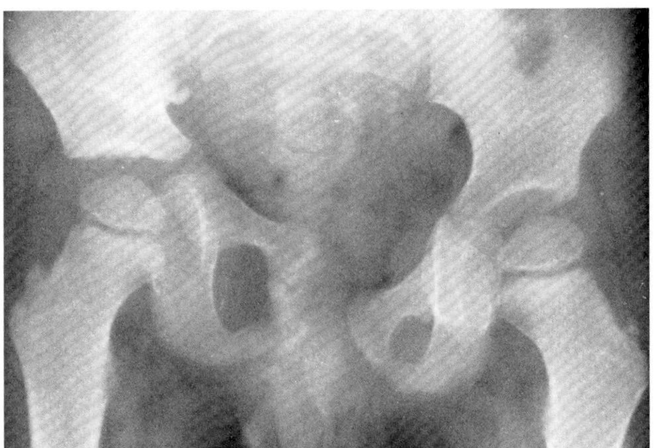

FIGURE 20-18 Fracture adjacent to the symphysis pubis with symphysis pubis separation.

Unstable Fracture Patterns

Unstable pelvic fracture combinations usually are of three types:

- Double vertical pubic rami fractures (straddle or floating fractures) or dislocations of the pubis that occur as an anterior double break in the pelvic ring anteriorly
- Double fractures in the pelvic ring anteriorly and posteriorly, through the bony pelvis, sacroiliac joint, or symphysis pubis (Malgaigne fractures)
- Multiple crushing injuries that produce at least two severely comminuted fractures in the pelvic ring

Bilateral Fractures of the Inferior and Superior Pubic Rami

Bilateral fractures of both the inferior and superior pubic rami (straddle fractures) cause a floating anterior arch of the pelvic

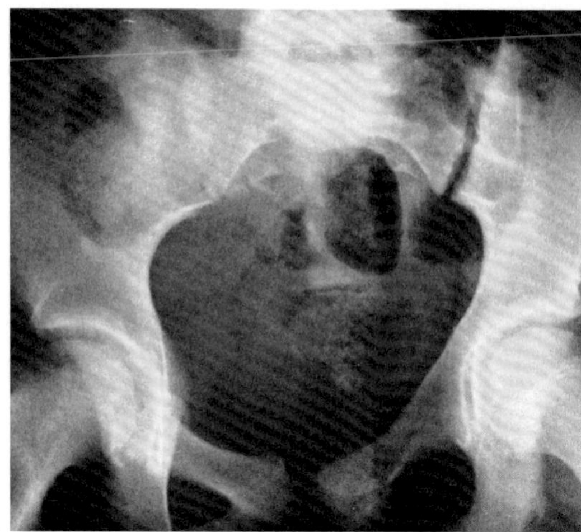

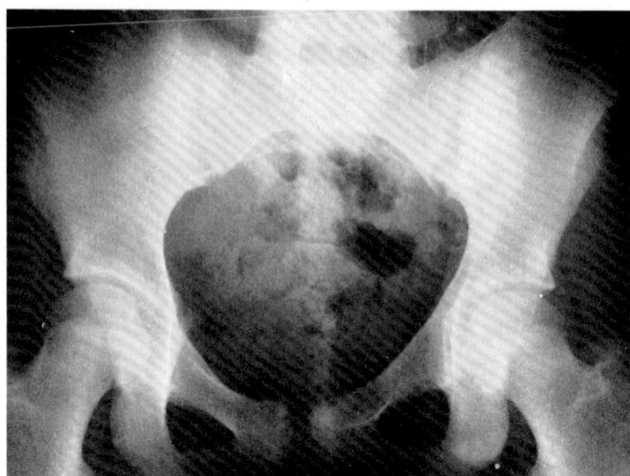

FIGURE 20-19 Separation of the left sacroiliac joint with asymmetry of the wings of the ilium. **A.** Careful scrutiny of the x-ray reveals contralateral pubic rami fractures. **B.** At 2-year follow-up, the sacroiliac joint is slightly wide, but the patient is asymptomatic.

ring that is inherently unstable (Fig. 20-21), as does dislocation of the symphysis pubis with fractures of both ipsilateral pubic rami. This fracture pattern frequently is associated with bladder or urethral disruption (43).

Bilateral fractures of the inferior and superior pubic rami can occur in a fall while straddling a hard object or by lateral compression on the pelvis. The floating fragment usually is displaced superiorly, being pulled in this direction by the rectus abdominis muscles (38). Radiographically, an inlet view most accurately determines the amount of true displacement of the floating fragment.

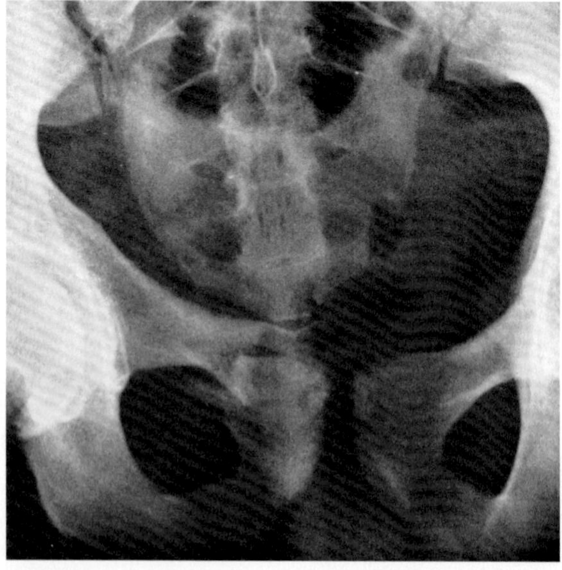

FIGURE 20-20 Fracture of the superior pubic ramus; occult fractures of the ipsilateral sacrum and the sacroiliac joint at the distal articular surface are also present.

In a child, regardless of the amount of displacement, the fracture should heal and remodeling can be expected. Because this fracture does not involve the weight-bearing portion of the pelvis, it does not cause leg-length discrepancy. Skeletal traction is unnecessary, and a pelvic sling is contraindicated because of the possibility that compression will cause medial displacement of the ilium (38,43).

Treatment should consist simply of supine bed rest in the semi-Fowler position with the hips flexed to relax the abdominal and adductor muscles. If the fracture was caused by lateral compression forces, the lateral decubitus position is contraindicated to avoid medial displacement of the ilium.

Complex Fracture Patterns

Fractures and dislocations of the posterior arch (posterior to the acetabulum) combined with anterior ipsilateral or contralateral fractures or dislocations of the anterior arch (Fig. 20-22) result in instability of the hemipelvis or acetabulum. These unstable fractures are associated with retroperitoneal and intraperitoneal bleeding. Bilateral anterior and posterior fractures are the most likely fracture pattern to cause severe hemorrhage. Initial treatment usually involves replacement of blood volume and stabilization of the child's overall condition before treatment of the pelvic fractures (9).

Three mechanisms of injury have been implicated in these fractures and fracture-dislocations: anteroposterior compression forces, lateral compression forces, and, with the hip fixed in extension and abduction, indirect forces transmitted proximally along the femoral shaft.

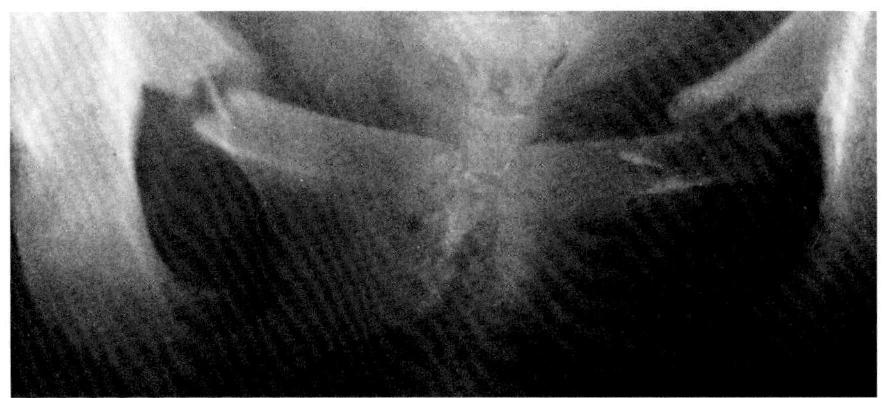

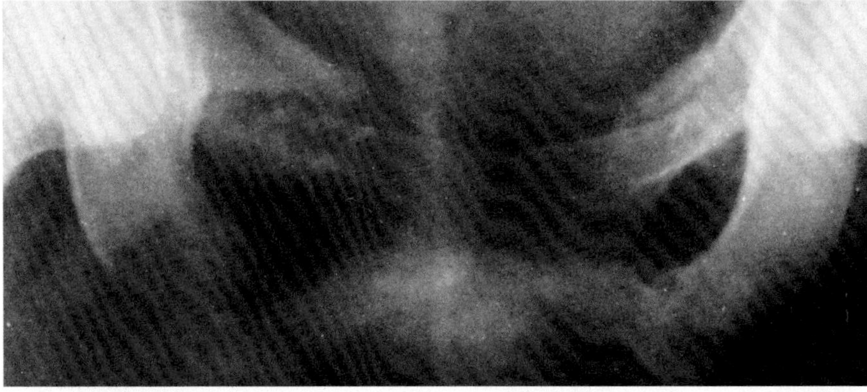

FIGURE 20-21 **A.** Classic example of a straddle fracture in a 16-year-old girl. **B.** At 6 weeks after injury, abundant callus formation is present and the fractures have healed.

Aside from the physical signs usually associated with pelvic fractures, leg-length discrepancy and asymmetry of the pelvis also may be present because of the displacement of the hemipelvis. If the measured distance from the umbilicus to the medial malleolus is unequal for the two extremities, and the distance from the anterior superior iliac spine to the medial malleolus is the same, pelvic obliquity or displacement is present rather than true leg-length discrepancy. Inlet and outlet x-rays and CT scan reveal the amount of pelvic displacement.

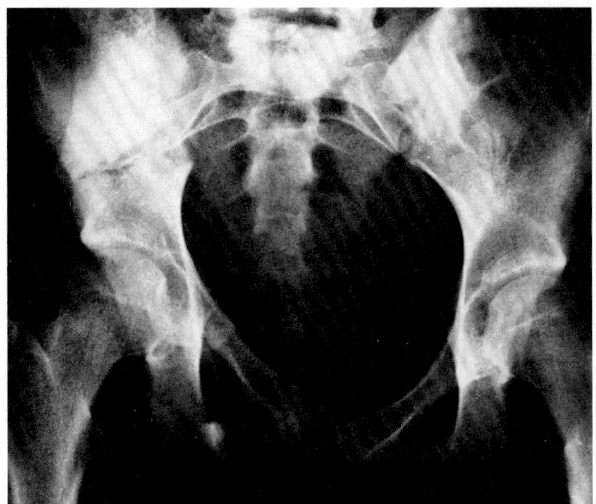

FIGURE 20-22 An unusual Malgaigne fracture; fracture extends through the ilium into the sacroiliac joint with ipsilateral pubic rami fractures.

Numerous treatment regimens have been successful, depending on the type of fracture and the amount of displacement. For fractures with minimal displacement, bed rest in the lateral recumbent position may be all that is necessary. If lateral displacement is severe, closed manipulation in the lateral decubitus position and spica casting can be used, as described in Chapter 35 in Volume 2 of this series. If the displacement is cephalad only, skeletal traction can be used in a small child. Occasionally, manipulation under anesthesia may be required. After successful manipulation of the fragments, traction on the involved side can be used to maintain the reduction. Open or percutaneous external fixation of the pelvis has been advocated to maintain accurate reduction of the fracture or dislocation, achieve earlier ambulation (toe-touch weight bearing), and decrease pain secondary to instability.

Schwarz et al (66), in a long-term (2–25 years) follow-up of 17 children with nonoperatively treated unstable pelvic fractures, reported moderate to severe pelvic asymmetry in eight patients (66). Measured leg length discrepancies between 2 and 5 cm were reported in five patients. These authors emphasized that reduction of the pelvic ring fractures should be as anatomic as possible because healing in malposition resulted in unsatisfactory results in half of the cases. Nierenberg et al (67), however, reported excellent or good results after conservative treatment of 20 unstable pelvic fractures in children despite radiographic evidence of deformity. They suggested that treatment guidelines for unstable pelvic fractures are not the same for children as for adults, and recommended that external or internal fixation should be used only when conservative methods fail. Silber and Flynn (42), in a retrospective review of 166 consecutive children with pelvic fractures, found that all four patients who required open reduction and internal fixation had a mature pelvis with a closed triradiate cartilage. These reviews suggest that younger children with an immature pelvis are unlikely to require operative intervention; however, treatment of children with unstable pelvic fractures and treatment of adolescents with a "mature" pelvis should follow adult pelvic fracture guidelines.

Operative treatment of pelvic fractures in children is not routinely recommended (68) because (a) exsanguinating hemorrhage is unusual in children, so operative pelvic stabilization to control bleeding rarely is necessary (11,68); (b) pseudarthrosis is rare in children and fixation is not necessary to promote healing; (c) the thick periosteum in children tends to help stabilize the fracture, so surgery usually is not necessary to obtain stability (12); (d) prolonged immobilization is not necessary for fracture healing (67); (e) significant remodeling may occur in skeletally immature patients (Fig. 20-23) (68); and (f) long-term morbidity after pelvic fracture is rare in children (6,11,69). Operative fixation may be indicated to facilitate wound treatment in open fractures, control hemorrhage during resuscitation, allow patient mobility and make nursing care easier, prevent deformity in severely displaced fractures that may not heal or adequately remodel, improve overall patient care in patients with polytrauma, minimize risk of growth disruption, or restore articular congruity.

Keshishyan et al (70) advocated external fixation of complex pelvic fractures, especially in children with polytrauma, and Gordon et al (61) suggested external fixation or open reduction and internal fixation in children older than 8 years of age because spica casting is poorly tolerated in older children. Stiletto et al (71) reported good results after open reduction and internal fixation of unstable pelvic fractures in two toddlers. AO small-fragment instrumentation was used in both. Large retrospective reviews of pediatric pelvic fractures suggest that conservative management is successful in patients with an immature pelvis, but operative management may be indicated for severely unstable or malaligned fractures or acetabular fractures (6,42).

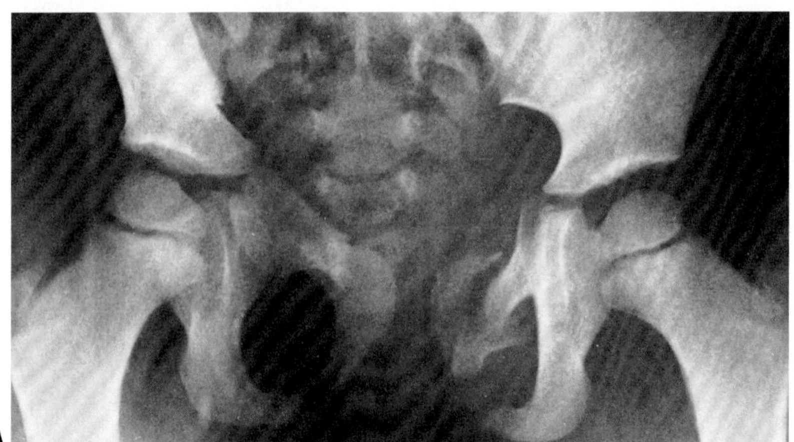

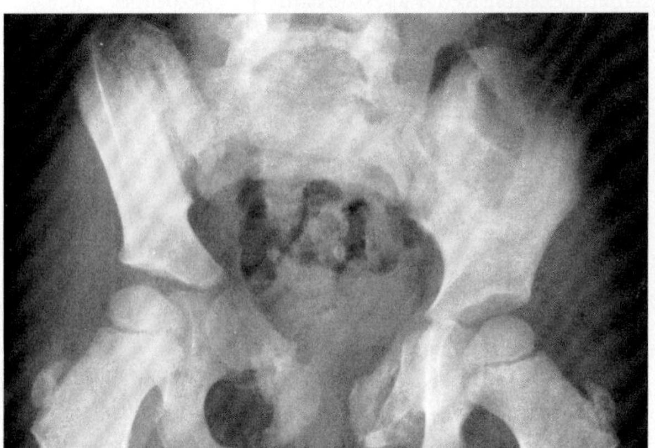

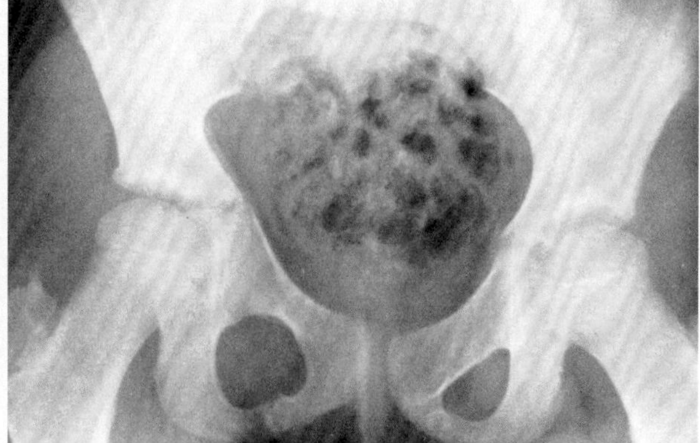

FIGURE 20-23 **A.** A 6-year-old child with a Malgaigne fracture with right sacroiliac joint displacement and multiple (four) pubic rami fractures. **B.** Four weeks after injury. **C.** At 5-year follow-up, complete remodeling is present.

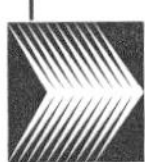

AUTHOR'S PREFERRED TREATMENT

Treatment is more likely to be conservative in children with an immature pelvis and operative in children with a mature pelvis or closed triradiate cartilage (42). For toddlers, we prefer to use bed rest and distal femoral traction on the displaced side of the hemipelvis. The younger the child, the more likely that traction will be adequate treatment and the pelvis will remodel. Open reduction and internal fixation rarely are required in a young child unless severe (>3 cm) displacement of the sacroiliac joint cannot be corrected with traction. Combining open reduction and internal fixation with external fixation may be necessary in a child older than 8 to 10 years of age with an unstable fracture and severe polytrauma (Fig. 20-24). The technical principles are identical to those used for unstable pelvic fractures in adults (see Chapter 35, Volume 2). In older adolescents, treatment should follow the guidelines for the treatment of adult fractures (see Chapter 35, Volume 2), including a combination of internal and external fixation for fracture stabilization and early mobilization.

Severe Multiple or Open Fractures

In patients with crushing injuries, distortion of the pelvis is severe and, in addition to multiple breaks in the pelvic ring, apparent or occult fractures of the sacrum may be present, with or without neurologic involvement. Massive hemorrhage, although common in adults with severe pelvic fractures (5), is much less common in children with pelvic fractures (42). Nevertheless, up to 20% of children with crushed open pelvic fractures in one series died within hours of admission secondary to uncontrolled hemorrhage (29). The overall need for blood transfusion in two large retrospective series including all types of pediatric pelvic fractures was between 21% and 33% (5,6). In the setting of hypovolemic shock, however, emergency measures outlined previously in this chapter may be necessary.

The patient should be stable without evidence of ongoing blood loss before operative intervention, either external fixation or open reduction. The rare patient may also require arterial embolization and placement of an inferior vena cava filter before operative intervention. It is important to recognize these severe pelvic fractures because mobile fracture fragments may penetrate viscera (e.g., the bladder or abdominal viscera), lacerate

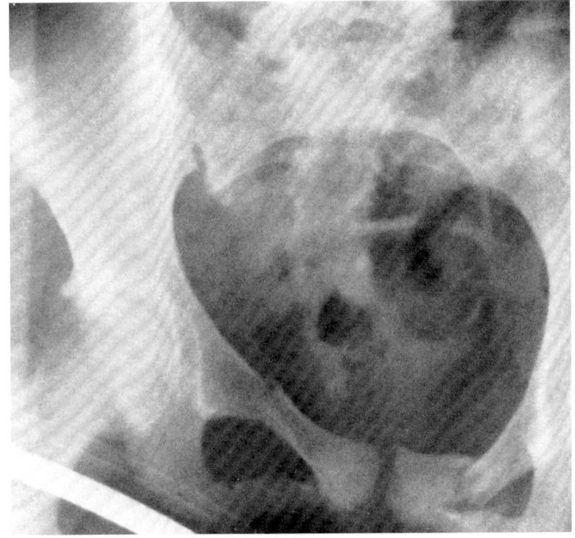

A

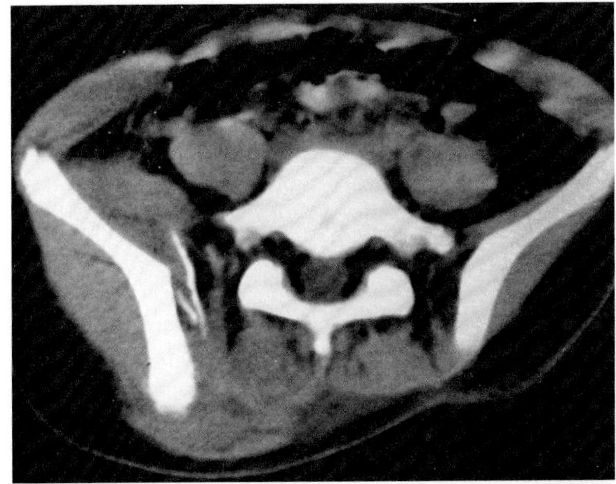

B

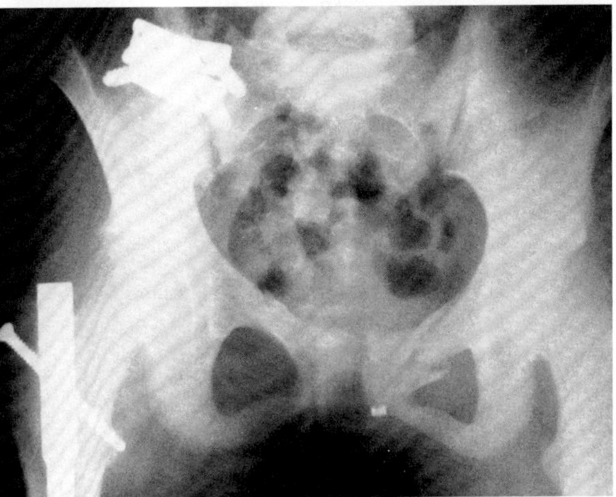

C

FIGURE 20-24 **A.** Multiple trauma in this 12-year-old child included three fractures of the pubic rami, disruption and fracture of the sacroiliac joint on the right, and a femoral shaft fracture on the right. **B.** Computed tomography (CT) shows fracture of the ilium and disruption of the sacroiliac joint. **C.** After open reduction and internal fixation of the sacroiliac joint and closed intramedullary nailing of the femoral shaft fracture. Note femoral nail inserted through the tip of the greater trochanter.

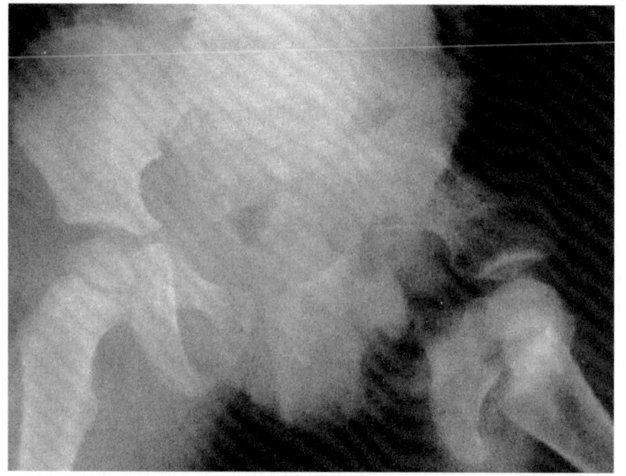
A

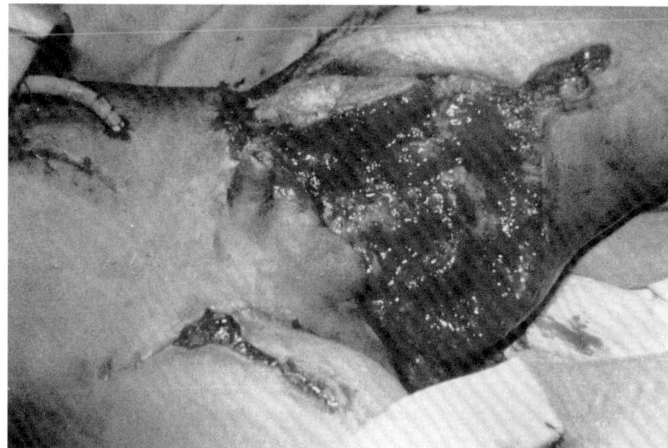
B

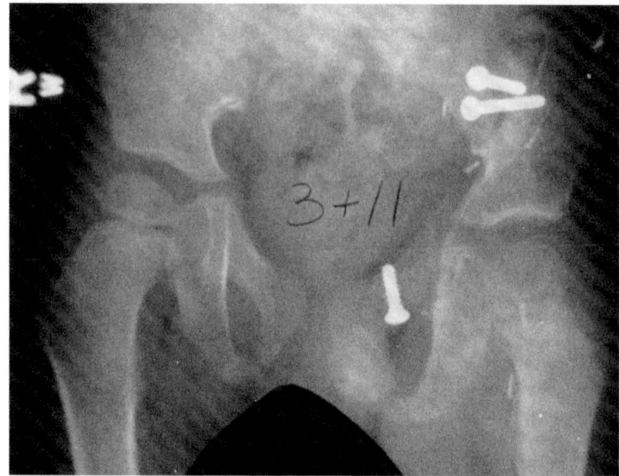

C

FIGURE 20-25 A,B. Complex open type IIIC pelvic fracture in a 3-year-old boy. Vascular (femoral artery and vein) and neurologic injuries were also present. Multiple debridements were required, as were colostomy and vesicostomy. The fractures of the wing of the ilium and pubic rami were fixed with small screws. **C.** One year after injury. (Courtesy of Dr. Gerry Clancy, Children's Hospital, Denver, CO.)

the abdominal vascular tree, or cause neurologic involvement (Fig. 20-25). Treatment of these acute soft-tissue injuries should take precedence over realignment of the pelvic architecture, although if possible during emergency surgery such as laparotomy, pelvic stabilization should be achieved quickly with a combination of internal and external fixation as needed while the patient is under general anesthesia. In particular, the application of an external fixator may decrease blood loss by stabilizing mobile, bleeding bone fragments, and decreasing the volume of the pelvis (31,62,63).

Open pelvic fractures are rare in children. Mosheiff et al (29) reported that 13% of 116 pediatric pelvic fractures seen over a 12-year period were open injuries. Fourteen of the 15 children were struck by motor vehicles, and one sustained a gunshot wound. Five children with stable fractures were treated nonoperatively, and 10 with unstable fractures were treated operatively: external fixation alone (eight patients), combined external fixation and internal fixation (three patients), and internal fixation alone (two patients). Three of the children died secondary to uncontrollable hemorrhage (two patients) and chest injury (one patient). Eleven of the 12 surviving children had deep wound infection or sepsis, and three had premature physeal closure. Mosheiff and colleagues (29) emphasized that the treatment of the soft tissue injuries depends on stabilization of the pelvis and that external fixation is often insufficient, and posterior internal fixation and stabilization are often necessary.

ACETABULAR FRACTURES

Acetabular fractures constitute only 6% to 17% of pediatric pelvic fractures, making them very uncommon (6,29,42). The mechanism of injury of acetabular fractures in children is similar to that in adults: The fracture occurs from a force transmitted through the femoral head. The position of the leg with respect to the pelvis and the location of the impact determine the fracture pattern; the magnitude of the force determines the severity of the fracture or fracture-dislocation. Patients with high-energy injuries usually have major associated injuries, whereas isolated acetabular fractures can occur from low-energy forces.

Classification

Watts (38) described four types of acetabular fractures in children: (a) small fragments that most often occur with dislocation of the hip, (b) linear fractures that occur in association with pelvic fractures without displacement and usually are stable, (c) linear fractures with hip joint instability, and (d) fractures secondary to central fracture-dislocation of the hip. More recently, however, acetabular fractures in both adults and children usually are classified by the system of Judet et al (72) and Letournel and Judet (73). A more comprehensive classification is based on the AO comprehensive fracture classification, which groups all fractures into A, B, and C types with increasing severity. Type A acetabular fractures involve a single wall or column; type B fractures involve both columns (transverse or T-types) and a portion of the dome remains attached to the intact ilium; and type C fractures involve both columns and separate the dome fragment from the axial skeleton by a fracture through the ilium. Both of these classification systems are discussed in more detail in Chapter 36, Volume 2 of this series.

Radiographic Evaluation

Anteroposterior and lateral views may not adequately show the amount of displacement of acetabular fragments after fracture. Inlet, outlet, and 45-degree oblique (Judet) views often are necessary to appreciate the amount of displacement. CT scanning can be used to determine the amount of acetabular displacement (Fig. 20-26) and whether any retained fragments in the acetabulum are preventing an accurate concentric reduction (74). Three-dimensional CT reconstructions can give an excellent view of the overall fracture pattern but often underestimate minimally displaced fractures, especially posterior acetabular wall fractures in children (Fig. 20-27) (35). Rubel et al (35) recommend MRI as an adjunctive imaging study for all pediatric acetabular fractures because MRI discloses the true size of largely cartilaginous posterior wall fragments in children.

Treatment

The aim of treatment for acetabular fractures in children is the same as for adults: to restore joint congruity and hip stability. Treatment guidelines in general follow those for adults. Bed rest or non–weight-bearing ambulation with crutches can be used for nondisplaced or minimally (≤1 mm) displaced fractures.

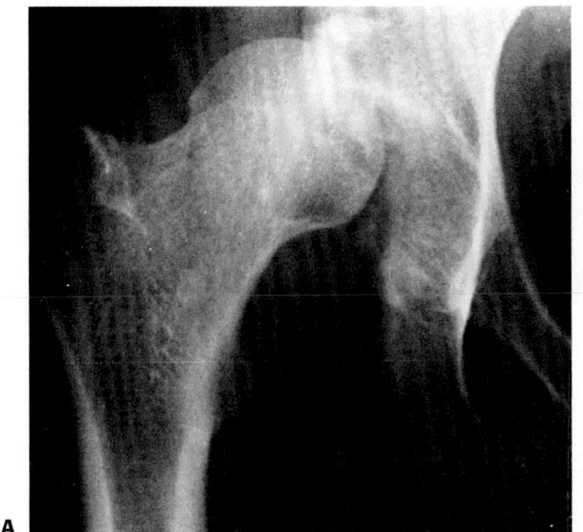
A

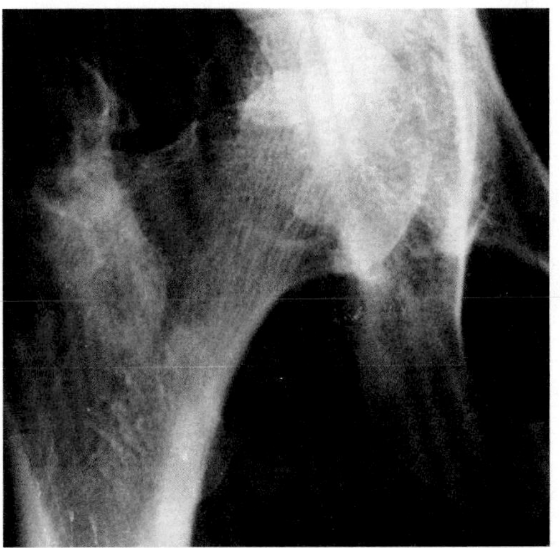
B

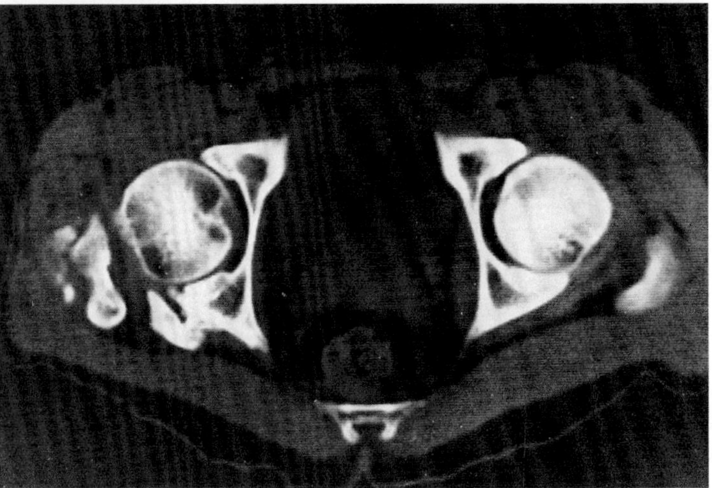
C

FIGURE 20-26 A. Traumatic dislocation with a small acetabular fragment. **B.** After reduction, a small fragment is visible, but it is not impeding hip congruity or function. **C.** At 12 weeks after injury, CT scan reveals that the fragment is from the posterior acetabulum, with mild displacement of the acetabulum posteriorly.

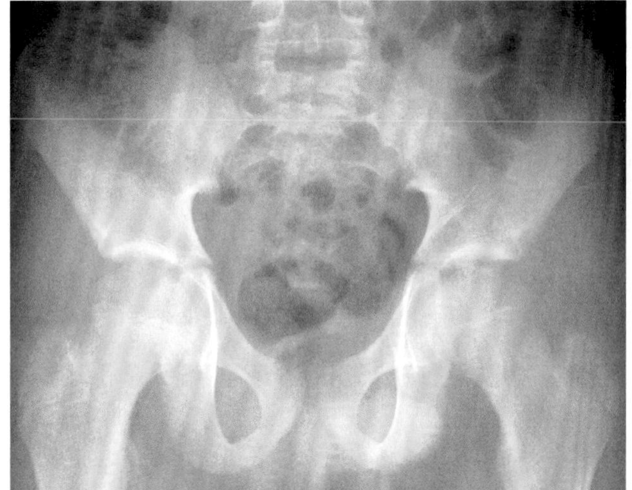

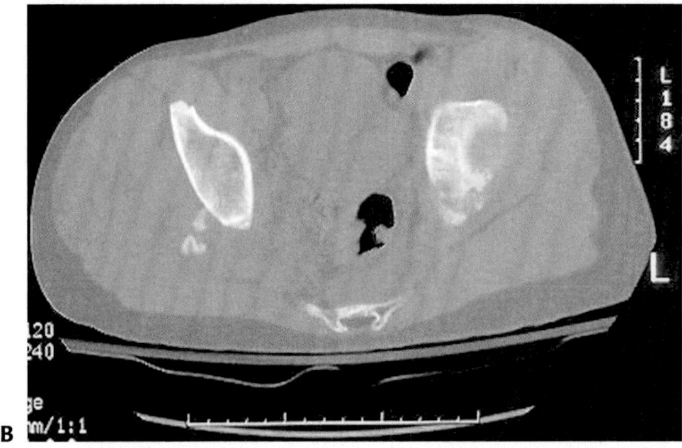

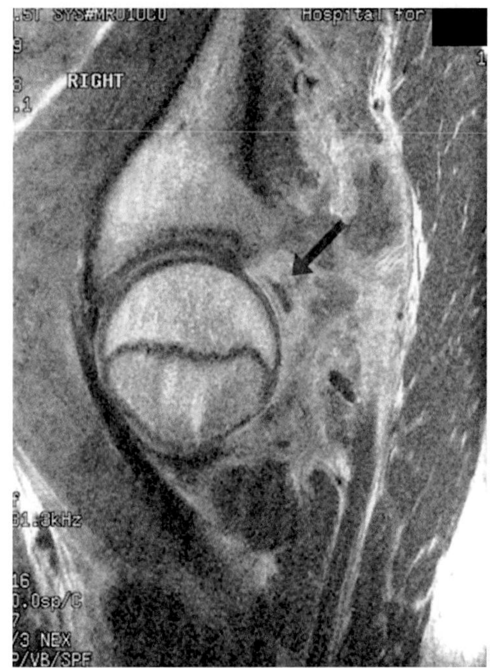

FIGURE 20-27 **A.** Postreduction x-ray of a left hip dislocation in a 12-year-old boy. **B.** CT scan demonstrates small ossified posterior wall fragments. **C.** Sagittal magnetic resonance imaging (MRI) demonstrates 90% posterior wall involvement with intraarticular step-off (*black arrow*). (Reproduced from Rubel IF, Kloen P, Potter HG, Helfet DL. MRI assessment of the posterior acetabular wall fracture in traumatic dislocation of the hip in children. *Pediatr Radiol* 2002;32(6):435–439, with permission.)

Because weight-bearing forces must not be transmitted across the fracture, crutch ambulation is appropriate only for older children who can be relied on to avoid putting weight on the injured limb. Non-weight bearing usually is continued for 6 to 8 weeks. In younger children, this may be shortened to 5 to 6 weeks, and in adolescents (>12 years of age), partial weight bearing should be continued for 3 to 4 more weeks. For fractures in which displacement can be reduced to less than 2 mm, skeletal traction with a traction pin in the distal femur can be used. Because traction must be maintained for 5 to 6 weeks, this option usually is not feasible in older children or adolescents.

Gordon et al (61) recommended accurate reduction and internal fixation of any displaced acetabular fracture in a child. They noted that the presence of incomplete fractures and plastic deformation may make accurate reduction difficult or impossible; they recommended that incomplete fractures be completed and that osteotomies of the pubis, ilium, or ischium be made if necessary for accurate reduction of the acetabulum. In children with open physes, all periacetabular metallic implants should be removed 6 to 18 months after surgery.

Improved outcomes with early (<24 hours) fixation of acetabular fractures in adults have been reported (75), and Gordon et al (61) noted that early fixation is especially important to prevent malunion in young patients in whom healing is rapid.

In addition, anatomic alignment of the triradiate cartilage should be obtained in children. Linear growth of the acetabulum occurs by interstitial growth in the triradiate part of the cartilage complex, causing the pubis, ischium, and ilium to enlarge. The depth of concavity of the acetabulum is in response to the presence of a spherical femoral head and increases during development as a result of interstitial growth in the acetabular cartilage. Cessation of growth of all or part of the triradiate cartilage occurring secondary to fracture may result in a dysplastic acetabulum.

Acetabular dysplasia secondary to growth arrest (bony bridge) of the triradiate cartilage has been reported after trauma to the acetabulum (Fig. 20-28). Heeg et al (76) reported acetabular deformity and subluxation of the hip in two of three patients with premature fusion of the triradiate cartilage. Peterson and Robertson (77) reported formation of a physeal osseous bar in a 7-year-old boy 2 years after fracture of the lateral portion of the superior ramus at the junction with the triradiate cartilage. After excision of the osseous bridge, the physis remained open. Although the injured physis closed earlier than the contralateral side, there was only a slight increase in the thickness of the

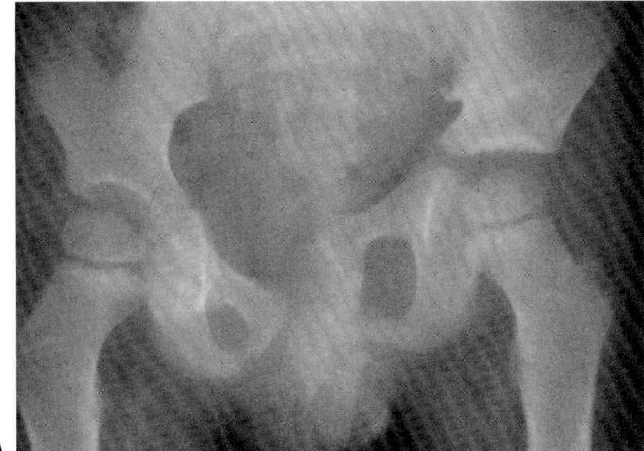

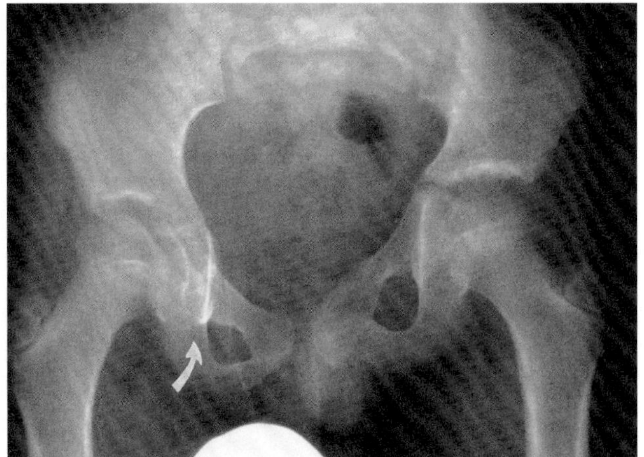

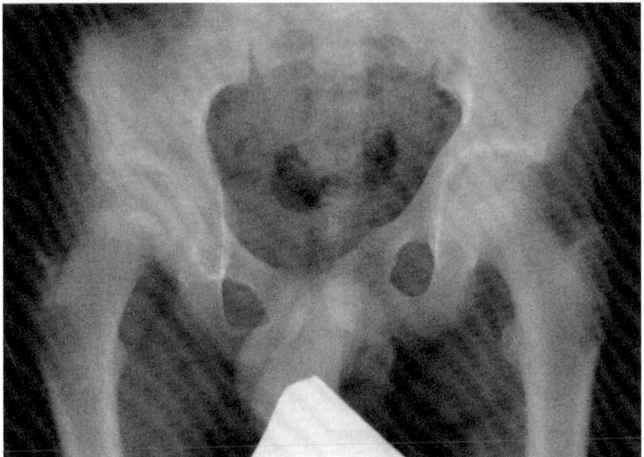

FIGURE 20-28 **A.** Fractures of the left superior and inferior pubic rami and the left ilium with injury to the right triradiate cartilage in a 5-year-old boy. **B.** Three years after injury, the pubic rami fractures are healed and remodeling has occurred, but acetabular dysplasia, widening of the "teardrop," and mild subluxation are evident in the right hip. **C.** At 15 years of age, the sequelae of the mild triradiate cartilage injury are still apparent, but he is not symptomatic.

acetabular wall and lateral displacement of the femoral head. Peterson and Robertson emphasized that early recognition and treatment are essential, before premature closure of the entire physis and development of permanent osseous deformity. The typical dysplastic changes seen after trauma to the triradiate cartilage differ significantly from developmental dysplasia and include both lateralization of the hip joint and acetabular retroversion (78).

Bucholz et al (79) noted two main patterns of physeal disturbance in nine patients with triradiate cartilage injury: a Salter-Harris type I or II injury, which had a favorable prognosis for continued normal acetabular growth, and a crush injury, which had a poor prognosis with premature closure of the triradiate cartilage caused by formation of a medial osseous bridge (Fig. 20-29). In either pattern, the prognosis depended on the child's age at the time of injury. In young children, especially those younger than 10 years of age, acetabular growth abnormality was common and resulted in a dysplastic acetabulum. By the time of skeletal maturity, disparate growth increased the incongruity of the hip joint and led to progressive subluxation. These authors found that acetabular reconstruction was frequently necessary to correct the gradual subluxation of the femoral head.

Surgical Treatment

The surgical treatment varies according to the pattern of the fracture and the direction of the displacement as determined on the preoperative x-rays and CT scans (61) (Table 20-5). Fractures of the posterior wall or posterior column can be approached through a Kocher-Langenbeck approach with the patient either in the lateral decubitus position (isolated posterior wall fracture) or supine (associated posterior column fracture). Anterior column injuries can be approached through an ilioinguinal approach. Some transverse fractures may require an extended iliofemoral approach (80). The extended lateral approaches, which include the extended iliofemoral and triradiate approaches, should be avoided as much as possible because of the risk of devascularization of the ilium and heterotopic bone formation (81).

The surgeon should be familiar with Judet et al's (72) treatise on the operative reduction of acetabular fractures and with Letournel and Judet's work before performing this surgery (73). For smaller children and smaller fragments, Watts (38) recommended threaded Kirschner wires for reduction. In larger children, cannulated screws may aid in reduction and provide secure fixation (Fig. 20-30). Small-fragment reconstruction plates,

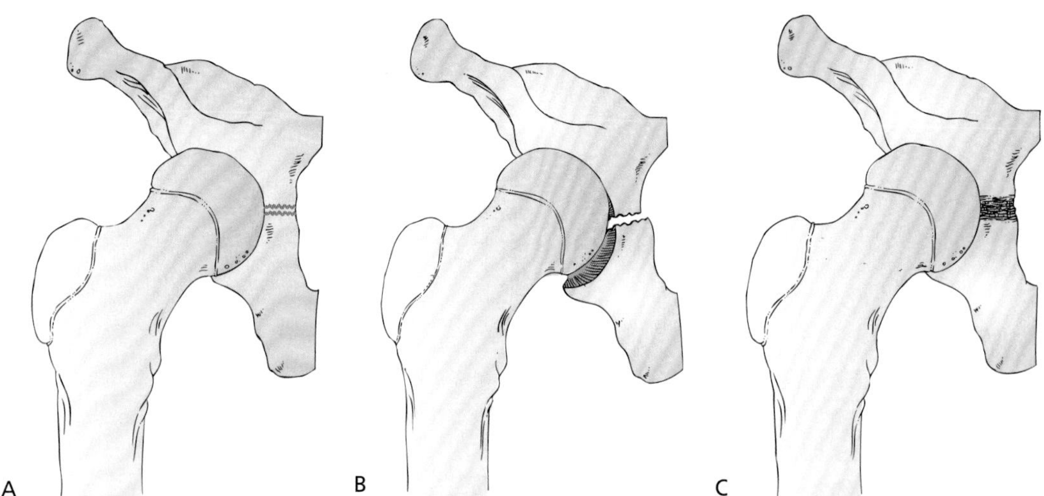

FIGURE 20-29 Types of triradiate cartilage fractures. **A.** Normal triradiate cartilage. **B.** Salter-Harris type I fracture. **C.** Salter-Harris type V (compression) fracture. (Redrawn from Scuderi G, Bronson MJ. Triradiate cartilage injury: report of two cases and review of the literature. *Clin Orthop* 1987;217:179–189, with permission.)

appropriately contoured, also can be used. Gordon et al (61) described the addition of a small (two- or three-hole) "hook plate" for small or comminuted fragments (Fig. 20-31). Because operative procedures about the hip may be necessary later, the hardware in a child may be removed in this situation.

Brown et al (82) described the use of CT image-guided fixation of acetabular fractures in 10 patients, including bilateral posterior wall fractures in a 14-year-old girl. They cite as advantages of image-guided surgery reduced operating time (~20% reduction), less extensive surgical dissection, reduced fluoroscopic time, and compatibility with traditional fixation techniques. Most important, it allows accurate and safe placement of screws and pins for acetabular fixation.

Postoperative Management

Small children can be immobilized in a spica cast for 6 weeks. If x-rays show adequate healing at that time, the cast is removed and free mobility is allowed. In an older child with stable fixation, crutches are used for protected weight bearing for 6 to 8 weeks. If x-rays show satisfactory healing, weight bearing is progressed as tolerated. Return to vigorous activities, especially competitive sports is delayed for at least 6 months.

TABLE 20-5 Surgical Exposure for Operative Fixation of Acetabular Fractures

Fracture Type	Exposure
Anterior column or wall	Ilioinguinal
Posterior column or wall	Kocher-Langenbeck
Transverse	Ilioinguinal (or extended lateral)
T-shaped	Ilioinguinal and Kocher-Langenbeck (or extended lateral)
Anterior column and posterior hemitransverse	Ilioinguinal
Both columns	Ilioinguinal (or extended lateral)

From Gordon RG, Karpik K, Hardy Sea. Techniques of operative reduction and fixation of pediatric and adolescent pelvic fractures. *Oper Tech Orthop* 1995;5:95–114; with permission.

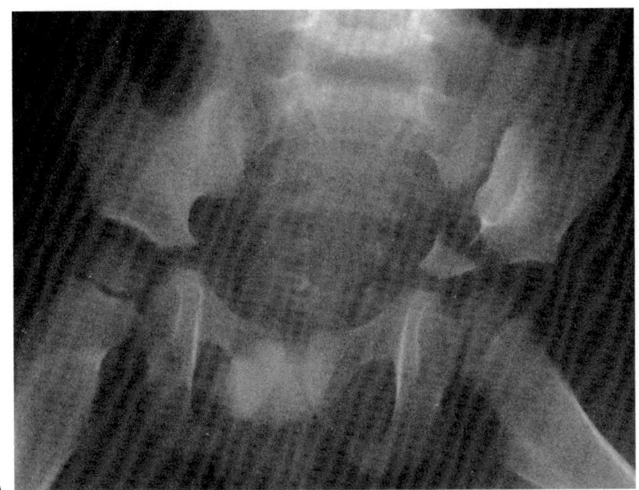

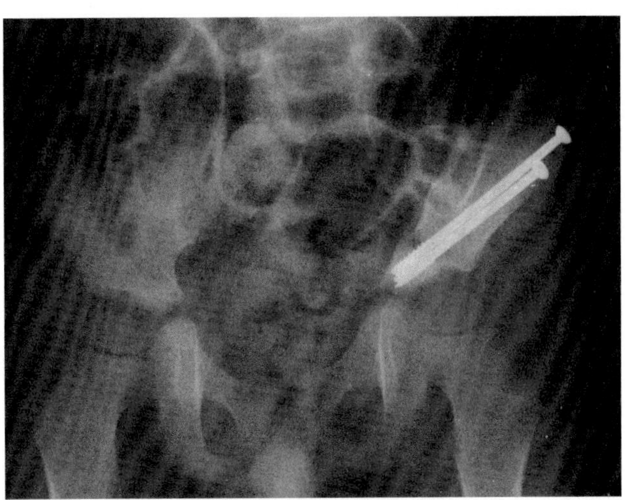

FIGURE 20-30 **A.** Fracture of the wing of the ilium with extension into the dome of the acetabulum in a 3-year-old boy. **B.** After reduction and fixation with two cannulated screws. (From Habacker TA, Heinrich SD, Dehne R. Fracture of the superior pelvic quadrant in a child. *J Pediatr Orthop* 1995;15(1):69–72; with permission.)

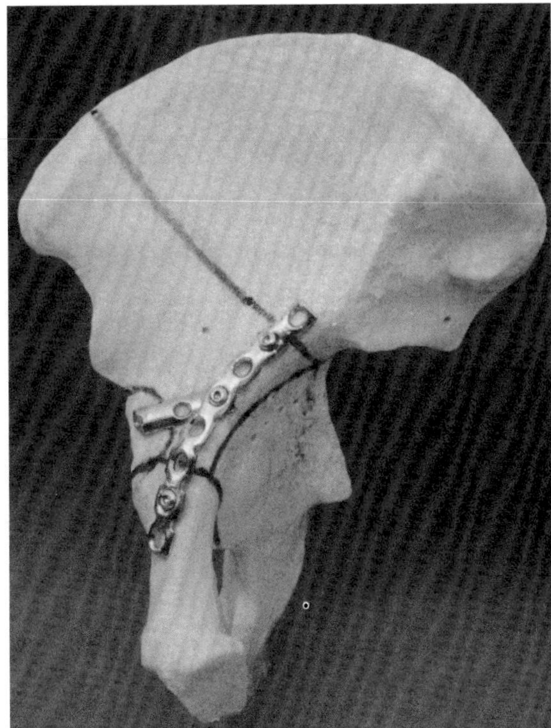

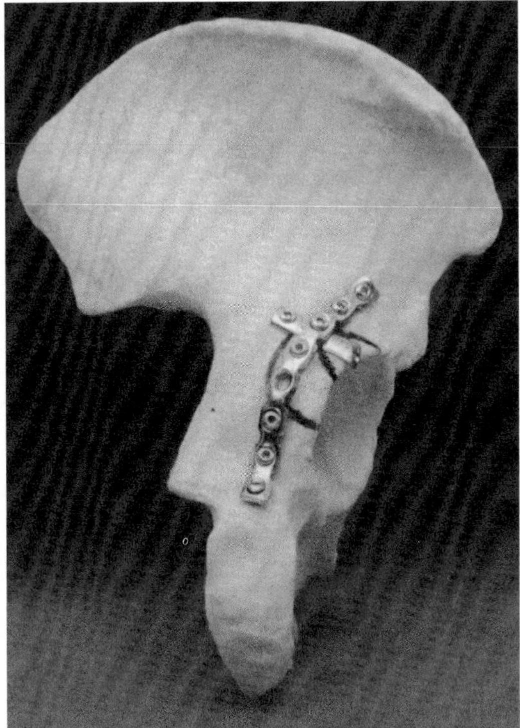

FIGURE 20-31 **A.** Anterior column plate and additional wall "hook" plate. **B.** Posterior wall buttress plate and hook plate. (From Gordon RG, Karpik K, Hardy SEA. Techniques of operative reduction and fixation of pediatric and adolescent pelvic fractures. *Oper Tech Orthop* 1995;5:95–114; with permission.)

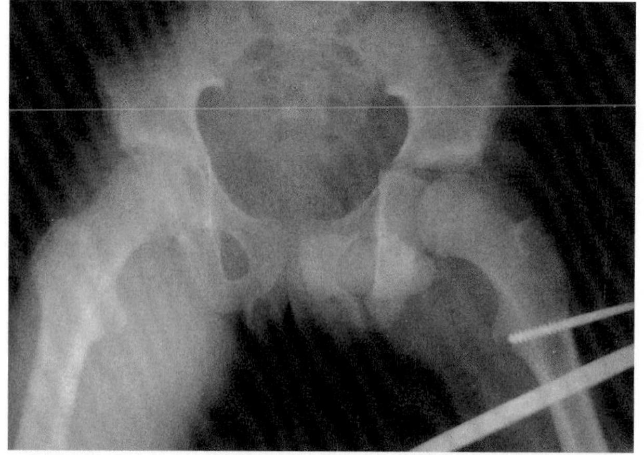

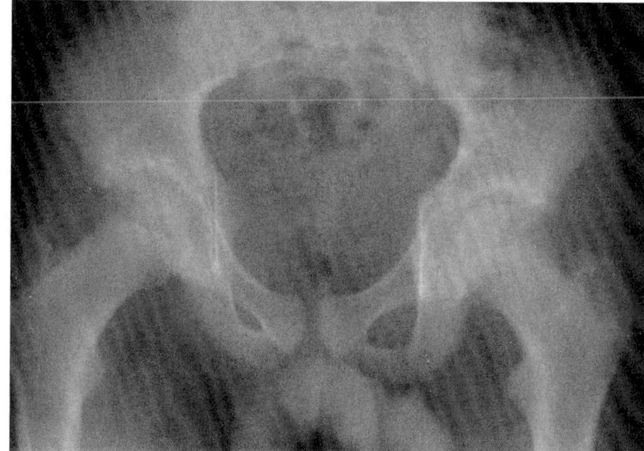

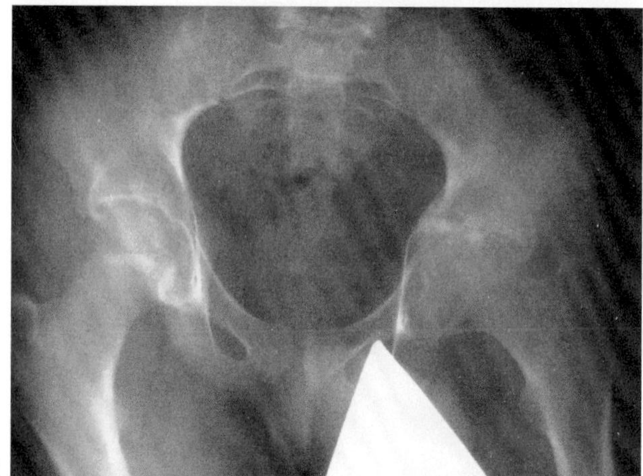

FIGURE 20-32 Central fracture-dislocation of the hip with injury to the triradiate cartilage in a 15-year-old boy. Note distraction and incongruous reduction. **A.** During skeletal traction after reduction of the hip dislocation. **B.** Six months after injury. **C.** Two years after injury, he has chondrolysis, mild osteonecrosis of the femoral head, and an ankylosed hip.

COMPLICATIONS

Because of the remodeling potential and rapid healing in young children, loss of reduction and malunion usually are not problems. Reported complications include premature triradiate cartilage closure, osteonecrosis, traumatic arthritis, sciatic nerve palsy, heterotopic myositis ossificans about the acetabulum and pelvis after acetabular fractures (Fig. 20-32), and pelvic asymmetry at long-term follow-up of female patients. Because this asymmetry may cause maternal dystocia during childbearing, pelvimetry is recommended before pregnancy. Rieger and Brug (13) reported one female patient who required cesarean section because of ossification of the symphysis pubis after nonoperative treatment of an open-book fracture. Schwarz et al (66) reported leg-length discrepancies of 1 to 5 cm in 10 of 17 patients after nonoperative treatment of unstable pelvic fractures; five had low back pain at long-term follow-up. Nine of 10 patients with lumbar scoliosis had low back pain.

REFERENCES

1. Worlock P, Stower M. Fracture patterns in Nottingham children. *J Pediatr Orthop* 1986;6(6):656–660.
2. Cheng JC, Ng BK, Ying SY, et al. A 10-year study of the changes in the pattern and treatment of 6,493 fractures. *J Pediatr Orthop* 1999;19(3):344–350.
3. Bond SJ, Gotschall CS, Eichelberger MR. Predictors of abdominal injury in children with pelvic fracture. *J Trauma* 1991;31(8):1169–1173.
4. Chia JP, Holland AJ, Little D, et al. Pelvic fractures and associated injuries in children. *J Trauma* 2004;56(1):83–88.
5. Demetriades D, Karaiskakis M, Velmahos GC, et al. Pelvic fractures in pediatric and adult trauma patients: are they different injuries? *J Trauma* 2003;54(6):1146–1151; discussion 1151.
6. Grisoni N, Connor S, Marsh E, et al. Pelvic fractures in a pediatric level I trauma center. *J Orthop Trauma* 2002;16(7):458–463.
7. Ismail N, Bellemare JF, Mollitt DL, et al. Death from pelvic fracture: children are different. *J Pediatr Surg* 1996;31(1):82–85.
8. Buckley SL, Gotschall C, Robertson W Jr, et al. The relationships of skeletal injuries with trauma score, injury severity score, length of hospital stay, hospital charges, and mortality in children admitted to a regional pediatric trauma center. *J Pediatr Orthop* 1994;14(4):449–453.
9. Tolo VT. Orthopaedic treatment of fractures of the long bones and pelvis in children who have multiple injuries. *Instr Course Lect* 2000;49:415–423.
10. McIntyre RC Jr, Bensard DD, Moore EE, et al. Pelvic fracture geometry predicts risk of life-threatening hemorrhage in children. *J Trauma* 1993;35(3):423–429.
11. Musemeche CA, Fischer RP, Cotler HB, et al. Selective management of pediatric pelvic fractures: a conservative approach. *J Pediatr Surg* 1987;22(6):538–540.
12. Reed MH. Pelvic fractures in children. *J Can Assoc Radiol* 1976;27(4):255–261.
13. Rieger H, Brug E. Fractures of the pelvis in children. *Clin Orthop* 1997;336:226–239.
14. Silber JS, Flynn JM, Koffler KM, et al. Analysis of the cause, classification, and associated injuries of 166 consecutive pediatric pelvic fractures. *J Pediatr Orthop* 2001;21(4):446–450.
15. Torode I, Zieg D. Pelvic fractures in children. *J Pediatr Orthop* 1985;5(1):76–84.
16. Vazquez WD, Garcia VF. Pediatric pelvic fractures combined with an additional skeletal injury is an indicator of significant injury. *Surg Gynecol Obstet* 1993;177(5):468–472.
17. Lane-O'Kelly A, Fogarty E, Dowling F. The pelvic fracture in childhood: a report supporting nonoperative management. *Injury* 1995;26(5):327–329.
18. Quinby WC Jr. Fractures of the pelvis and associated injuries in children. *J Pediatr Surg* 1966;1(4):353–364.
19. Reichard SA, Helikson MA, Shorter N, et al. Pelvic fractures in children—review of 120 patients with a new look at general management. *J Pediatr Surg* 1980;15(6):727–734.

20. Prendergast NC, deRoux SJ, Adsay NV. Non-accidental pediatric pelvic fracture: a case report. *Pediatr Radiol* 1998;28(5):344–346.
21. Ablin DS, Greenspan A, Reinhart MA. Pelvic injuries in child abuse. *Pediatr Radiol* 1992; 22(6):454–457.
22. Garvin KL, McCarthy RE, Barnes CL, et al. Pediatric pelvic ring fractures. *J Pediatr Orthop* 1990;10(5):577–582.
23. Tile M. Pelvic ring fractures: should they be fixed? *J Bone Joint Surg Br* 1988;70(1):1–12.
24. Currey JD, Butler G. The mechanical properties of bone tissue in children. *J Bone Joint Surg Am* 1975;57(6):810–814.
25. Tarman GJ, Kaplan GW, Lerman SL, et al. Lower genitourinary injury and pelvic fractures in pediatric patients. *Urology* 2002;59(1):123–126; discussion 126.
26. Landin LA. Epidemiology of children's fractures. *J Pediatr Orthop B* 1997;6(2):79–83.
27. Blount WP. *Fractures in Children*. Huntington, NY: Robert E. Krieger Publishing Company; 1977.
28. Niemi TA, Norton LW. Vaginal injuries in patients with pelvic fractures. *J Trauma* 1985; 25(6):547–551.
29. Mosheiff R, Suchar A, Porat S, et al. The "crushed open pelvis" in children. *Injury* 1999; 30(Suppl 2):B14–18.
30. Shaw BA, Holman M. Traumatic lumbosacral nerve root avulsions in a pediatric patient. *Orthopedics* 2003;26(1):89–90.
31. Tile M, Helfet DL, Kellam J, eds. *Fractures of the Pelvis and Acetabulum*. 3rd ed. Baltimore: Lippincott Williams & Wilkins; 2003.
32. Silber JS, Flynn JM, Katz MA, et al. Role of computed tomography in the classification and management of pediatric pelvic fractures. *J Pediatr Orthop* 2001;21(2):148–151.
33. Magid D, Fishman EK, Ney DR, et al. Acetabular and pelvic fractures in the pediatric patient: value of two- and three-dimensional imaging. *J Pediatr Orthop* 1992;12(5):621–625.
34. Guillamondegui OD, Mahboubi S, Stafford PW, et al. The utility of the pelvic radiograph in the assessment of pediatric pelvic fractures. *J Trauma* 2003;55(2):236–239; discussion 239–240.
35. Rubel IF, Kloen P, Potter HG, et al. MRI assessment of the posterior acetabular wall fracture in traumatic dislocation of the hip in children. *Pediatr Radiol* 2002;32(6): 435–439.
36. Heinrich SD, Gallagher D, Harris M, et al. Undiagnosed fractures in severely injured children and young adults. Identification with technetium imaging. *J Bone Joint Surg Am* 1994;76(4):561–572.
37. Rang M. *Children's Fractures*. 2nd ed. Philadelphia: J.B. Lippincott Company; 1983.
38. Watts HG. Fractures of the pelvis in children. *Orthop Clin North Am* 1976;7(3):615–624.
39. Pennal GF, Tile M, Waddell JP, et al. Pelvic disruption: assessment and classification. *Clin Orthop* 1980(151):12–21.
40. Burgess AR, Eastridge BJ, Young JW, et al. Pelvic ring disruptions: effective classification system and treatment protocols. *J Trauma* 1990;30(7):848–856.
41. Pohlemann T. Pelvic ring injuries: assessment and concepts of surgical management. In: Colton C, Dell'Oca A, Holz U, et al, eds. *AO Principles of Fracture Management*. New York: Thieme; 2000:391–439.
42. Silber JS, Flynn JM. Changing patterns of pediatric pelvic fractures with skeletal maturation: implications for classification and management. *J Pediatr Orthop* 2002;22(1):22–26.
43. Ogden JA. *Skeletal Injury in the Child*. 3rd ed. New York: Springer-Verlag; 2000.
44. Ponseti IV. Growth and development of the acetabulum in the normal child. Anatomical, histological, and roentgenographic studies. *J Bone Joint Surg Am* 1978;60(5):575–585.
45. Fernbach SK, Wilkinson RH. Avulsion injuries of the pelvis and proximal femur. *AJR Am J Roentgenol* 1981;137(3):581–584.
46. Metzmaker JN, Pappas AM. Avulsion fractures of the pelvis. *Am J Sports Med* 1985; 13(5):349–358.
47. Rossi F, Dragoni S. Acute avulsion fractures of the pelvis in adolescent competitive athletes: prevalence, location and sports distribution of 203 cases collected. *Skeletal Radiol* 2001;30(3):127–131.
48. Godshall RW, Hansen CA. Incomplete avulsion of a portion of the iliac epiphysis: an injury of young athletes. *J Bone Joint Surg Am* 1973;55(6):1301–1302.
49. Clancy WG Jr, Foltz AS. Iliac apophysitis and stress fractures in adolescent runners. *Am J Sports Med* 1976;4(5):214–218.
50. Sundar M, Carty H. Avulsion fractures of the pelvis in children: a report of 32 fractures and their outcome. *Skeletal Radiol* 1994;23(2):85–90.
51. Barnes ST, Hinds RB. Pseudotumor of the ischium. A late manifestation of avulsion of the ischial epiphysis. *J Bone Joint Surg Am* 1972;54(3):645–647.
52. Schlonsky J, Olix ML. Functional disability following avulsion fracture of the ischial epiphysis. Report of two cases. *J Bone Joint Surg Am* 1972;54(3):641–644.
53. Lynch SA, Renstrom PA. Groin injuries in sport: treatment strategies. *Sports Med* 1999; 28(2):137–144.
54. Keats TE, Anderson MW. *Atlas of Normal Roentgen Variants that May Simulate Disease*. St. Louis: Mosby; 2001:371.
55. Caffey J, Ross SE. The ischiopubic synchondrosis in healthy children: some normal roentgenologic findings. *Am J Roentgenol Radium Ther Nucl Med* 1956;76(3):488–494.
56. Kuhn JP, Slovis TL, Haller JA, eds. *Caffey's Pediatric Diagnostic Imaging*. Philadelphia: Mosby; 2004.
57. Grier D, Wardell S, Sarwark J, et al. Fatigue fractures of the sacrum in children: two case reports and a review of the literature. *Skeletal Radiol* 1993;22(7):515–518.
58. Shah MK, Stewart GW. Sacral stress fractures: an unusual cause of low back pain in an athlete. *Spine* 2002;27(4):E104–108.
59. Broome DR, Hayman LA, Herrick RC, et al. Postnatal maturation of the sacrum and coccyx: MR imaging, helical CT, and conventional radiography. *AJR Am J Roentgenol* 1998;170(4):1061–1066.
60. Dunn AW, Morris HD. Fractures and dislocations of the pelvis. *J Bone Joint Surg Am* 1968;50(8):1639–1648.
61. Gordon RG, Karpik K, Hardy Sea. Techniques of operative reduction and fixation of pediatric and adolescent pelvic fractures. *Oper Tech Orthop* 1995;5:95–114.
62. Tile M. Pelvic fractures: operative versus nonoperative treatment. *Orthop Clin North Am* 1980;11(3):423–464.
63. Alonso JE, Horowitz M. Use of the AO/ASIF external fixator in children. *J Pediatr Orthop* 1987;7(5):594–600.
64. Donoghue V, Daneman A, Krajbich I, et al. CT appearance of sacroiliac joint trauma in children. *J Comput Assist Tomogr* 1985;9(2):352–356.
65. Heeg M, Klasen HJ. Long-term outcome of sacroiliac disruptions in children. *J Pediatr Orthop* 1997;17(3):337–341.
66. Schwarz N, Posch E, Mayr J, et al. Long-term results of unstable pelvic ring fractures in children. *Injury* 1998;29(6):431–433.
67. Nierenberg G, Volpin G, Bialik Vea. Pelvic fractures in children: a follow-up in 20 children treated conservatively. *J Pediatr Orthop B* 1993;1:140–142.
68. Blasier RD, McAtee J, White R, et al. Disruption of the pelvic ring in pediatric patients. *Clin Orthop* 2000(376):87–95.
69. Junkins EP Jr, Nelson DS, Carroll KL, et al. A prospective evaluation of the clinical presentation of pediatric pelvic fractures. *J Trauma* 2001;51(1):64–68.
70. Keshishyan RA, Rozinov VM, Malakhov OA, et al. Pelvic polyfractures in children. Radiographic diagnosis and treatment. *Clin Orthop* 1995(320):28–33.
71. Stiletto RJ, Baacke M, Gotzen L. Comminuted pelvic ring disruption in toddlers: management of a rare injury. *J Trauma* 2000;48(1):161–164.
72. Judet R, Judet J, Letournel E. Fractures of the acetabulum: classification and surgical approaches for open reduction. Preliminary report. *J Bone Joint Surg Am* 1964;46: 1615–1646.
73. Letournel E, Judet R. *Fractures of the Acetabulum*. 2nd ed. New York: Springer-Verlag; 1993.
74. Canale ST, Manugian AH. Irreducible traumatic dislocations of the hip. *J Bone Joint Surg Am* 1979;61(1):7–14.
75. Plaisier BR, Meldon SW, Super DM, et al. Improved outcome after early fixation of acetabular fractures. *Injury* 2000;31(2):81–84.
76. Heeg M, Visser JD, Oostvogel HJ. Injuries of the acetabular triradiate cartilage and sacroiliac joint. *J Bone Joint Surg Br* 1988;70(1):34–37.
77. Peterson HA, Robertson RC. Premature partial closure of the triradiate cartilage treated with excision of a physical osseous bar. Case report with a fourteen-year follow-up. *J Bone Joint Surg Am* 1997;79(5):767–770.
78. Dora C, Zurbach J, Hersche O, Ganz R. Pathomorphologic characteristics of posttraumatic acetabular dysplasia. *J Orthop Trauma* 2000;14(7):483–489.
79. Bucholz RW, Ezaki M, Ogden JA. Injury to the acetabular triradiate physeal cartilage. *J Bone Joint Surg Am* 1982;64(4):600–609.
80. Crenshaw AH. Extensile acetabular approaches. In: Canale ST, ed. *Campbell's Operative Orthopaedics, 10th Edition*. Vol 1. St. Louis: Mosby; 2003:77–86.
81. Hall BB, Klassen RA, Ilstrup DM. Pelvic fractures in children: a long-term follow-up study. Unpublished.
82. Brown GA, Willis MC, Firoozbakhsh K, et al. Computed tomography image-guided surgery in complex acetabular fractures. *Clin Orthop* 2000(370):219–226.

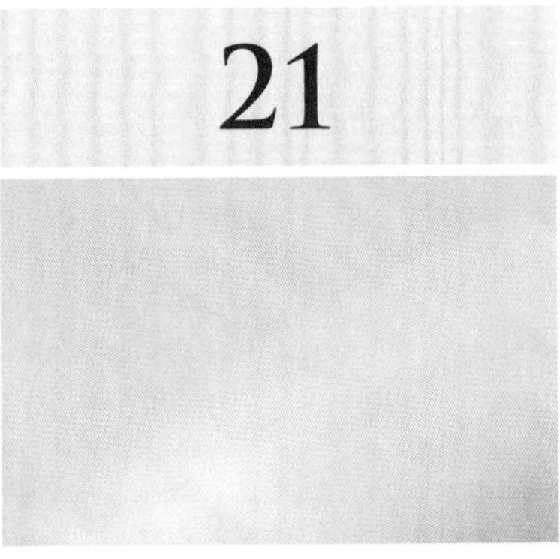

21

FRACTURES AND TRAUMATIC DISLOCATIONS OF THE HIP IN CHILDREN

R. Dale Blasier and Laurie O. Hughes

FRACTURES OF THE HIP

Fractures of the head and neck of the femur in children are exceedingly rare, accounting for fewer than 1% of all pediatric fractures (1). In comparison, the prevalence of fractures of the hip in children is less than 1% of that in adults. Therefore, most orthopaedic surgeons will treat only a few such fractures in a lifetime (2).

The pattern of fracture and thus the classification in children differ from those in adults. Because of the weak proximal femoral physis, a transphyseal separation can occur in children. Transcervical and cervicotrochanteric fractures have an extremely high risk for osteonecrosis (ON) and coxa vara compared with their adult counterparts. Intertrochanteric fractures are mechanically similar in both groups, although in children involvement of the greater trochanteric apophysis can result in premature closure.

The proximal femoral physis is at risk in hip fracture and has obvious implications for fracture care and prognosis. If the proximal physis is damaged, coxa vara or coxa breva may develop with further growth regardless of fracture alignment. Conversely, if the greater trochanteric apophysis fuses prematurely as a result of trauma, coxa valga may develop (3).

Although hip fractures in children can generally be expected to heal, their importance lies in the frequency and severity of complications, including ON, coxa vara, premature physeal closure, limb length discrepancy, and occasionally nonunion. Because the hip is developing in the growing child, deformities can progress with age.

Principles of Management

Mechanism of Injury

Hip fractures in children can be caused by axial loading, torsion, hyperabduction, or a direct blow to the hip. Almost all hip fractures in children are caused by severe, high-energy trauma. This is in marked contrast to hip fractures in the elderly, in whom minor torsional forces acting on osteoporotic bone cause most hip fractures. The proximal femur in children, except for the proximal femoral physis, is extremely strong, and high-energy forces, such as from motor vehicle accidents and high falls, are necessary to cause fracture (4).

Signs and Symptoms

Clinical examination usually reveals pain in the hip and a shortened, externally rotated extremity in a patient who cannot ambulate. An infant with a hip fracture holds the extremity flexed, abducted, and externally rotated. Pseudoparalysis, shortening, and a strong suspicion are the keys to diagnosis in this age group. With a nondisplaced or stress fracture of the femoral neck, the patient may be able to bear weight with a limp and may demonstrate hip or knee pain only with extremes of range of motion, especially internal rotation.

Associated Injuries

Because these fractures are caused by high-energy trauma, they frequently are accompanied by associated injuries that can affect the patient's overall functional outcome. Pape et al (5), in a series of 28 patients with a mean follow-up of 11 years, found favorable outcomes in types II, III, and IV fractures according to Ratliff's criteria (1). Poor functional outcomes were attributed to head trauma, amputation, or peripheral neurologic damage (5). In Mirdad's series (6) of 14 patients with hip fractures, all of which were caused by vehicular accidents or falls from heights, 12 patients had associated injuries including head injury, pelvic fracture, open femoral shaft fracture, subtrochanteric femoral fracture, facial injury, upper extremity and clavicle injuries, splenic injuries, perineal wounds, and retroperitoneal hematoma. Bagatur and Zorer (7) found five associated injuries in 4 of their 17 patients, including forearm, humeral, pelvic, and tibial fractures. All but 1 of the 17 fractures were caused by high-energy mechanisms (7).

Rationale for Management

Much of the early, classic literature on hip fractures in children documented the high rates of coxa vara, delayed union, and nonunion in patients treated without internal fixation (1,8). Canale and Bourland, noting that fractures treated by spica casting alone had a greater incidence of coxa vara, attributed their lower rate of coxa vara and nonunion to the use of internal fixation for all transcervical fractures (9). Subsequent authors have documented lower rates of ON, coxa vara, and nonunion in patients who were aggressively treated with anatomic open reduction and internal fixation within 24 hours of injury (5,7,10–12). Therefore, current management is directed at early, anatomic reduction of these fractures with stable internal fixation and supplemental external stabilization (casting), with the goal of minimizing devastating late complications.

Diagnosis

The diagnosis of hip fracture in a child is based on the history of high-energy trauma and the typical signs and symptoms of the shortened, externally rotated, and painful lower extremity.

A good-quality anteroposterior (AP) pelvic x-ray will provide a comparison view of the opposite hip if a displaced fracture is suspected. For the AP x-ray the leg should be held in extension and in as much internal rotation as possible without causing extreme pain to the patient. A cross-table lateral x-ray should be considered to avoid further displacement and unnecessary discomfort to the patient from an attempt at a frog-leg lateral view. Any break or offset of the bony trabeculae near Ward's triangle is evidence of a nondisplaced or impacted fracture.

Not all fractures can be detected on initial plain x-rays. Special studies may be required to reveal an occult fracture. A radioisotopic bone scan 48 hours after the onset of symptoms may show increased uptake at the fracture site. The typical magnetic resonance imaging (MRI) appearance of a fracture is a linear black line (low signal) on all sequences surrounded by a high-signal band of bone marrow edema and hemorrhage. The low signal represents trabecular impaction. MRI may detect an occult hip fracture within the first 24 hours after injury (13).

In a patient with posttraumatic hip pain without evidence of a fracture, other diagnoses must be considered, including synovitis, hemarthrosis, and infection. A complete blood count and evaluation of the erythrocyte sedimentation rate, C-reactive protein, and temperature are helpful. Ultrasonography can be used to detect fluid in the joint. If necessary, aspiration should be performed. A bloody aspirate establishes the diagnosis of fracture, whereas a serous or suppurative aspirate suggests synovitis or infection, respectively. In children under 5 years of age, developmental coxa vara can be confused with an old hip fracture (3).

Classification

Pediatric hip fractures generally are classified by the method of Delbet because its simplicity and uniformity allow accurate description and reporting of results of each fracture by type. Type I is a transepiphyseal separation, with (type IA) or without (type IB) dislocation of the femoral head from the acetabulum. Type II is a transcervical fracture. Type III is a cervicotrochanteric fracture. Type IV is an intertrochanteric fracture (Fig. 21-1) (14). Subtrochanteric fractures are not included in this classification and are discussed in Chapter 22.

Type I. Transphyseal fractures occur through the proximal femoral physis (Fig. 21-2). Such fractures are rare, constituting 8% of femoral neck fractures in children (2). True transphyseal fractures tend to occur in young children after high-energy trauma (9,15) and are different from unstable slipped capital femoral epiphysis of the preadolescent, which probably occurs as a result of a subtle endocrinopathy. In the absence of a history of significant trauma in a young child, battered child syndrome should be suspected (16). Rarely, this injury occurs during a difficult delivery or attempted closed reduction of a traumatic dislocation of the hip in adolescents (2). Approximately half of type I fractures are associated with a dislocation of the capital femoral epiphysis. In such cases, the outcome is dismal because

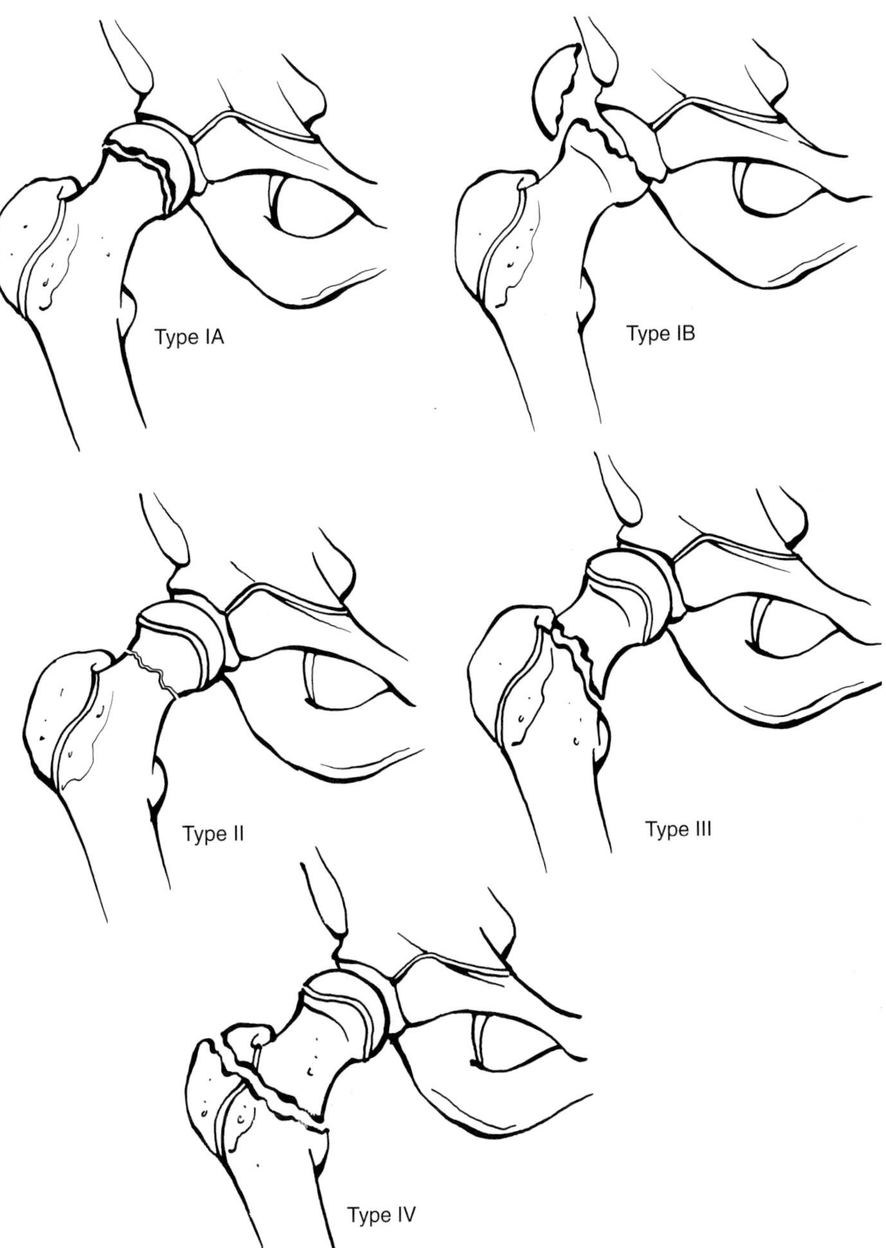

FIGURE 21-1 Delbet classification of hip fractures in children. *I,* transepiphyseal, with (IB) or without (IA) dislocation from the acetabulum; *II,* transcervical; *III,* cervicotrochanteric; and *IV,* intertrochanteric.

of ON and premature physeal closure in virtually 100% of patients (9,15).

Type I fractures in children under 2 or 3 years of age have a better prognosis than in older children. ON is unlikely, although coxa vara, coxa breva, and premature physeal closure can cause subsequent leg length discrepancy (17,18).

Type II. Transcervical fractures account for 46% of fractures of the head and neck of the femur in children (2). In three large series, 77% of all type II fractures were displaced (2). Nondisplaced fractures have a better prognosis and a lower rate of ON than displaced fractures, regardless of treatment (1,9). The risk of ON is thought by most investigators to be directly related to the initial displacement of the fracture, although a few have hypothesized an intraarticular hemarthrosis with tamponade (2,9) as the etiology of vascular impairment.

Type III. Cervicotrochanteric fractures are, by definition, located at or above the anterior intertrochanteric line and are the second most common type of hip fracture in children, representing about 34% of fractures (2). The incidence of ON is 20% to 30%, and, as in type II fractures, the risk of ON is directly related to the degree of displacement at the time of injury (2). Premature physeal closure occurs in 25% of patients and coxa

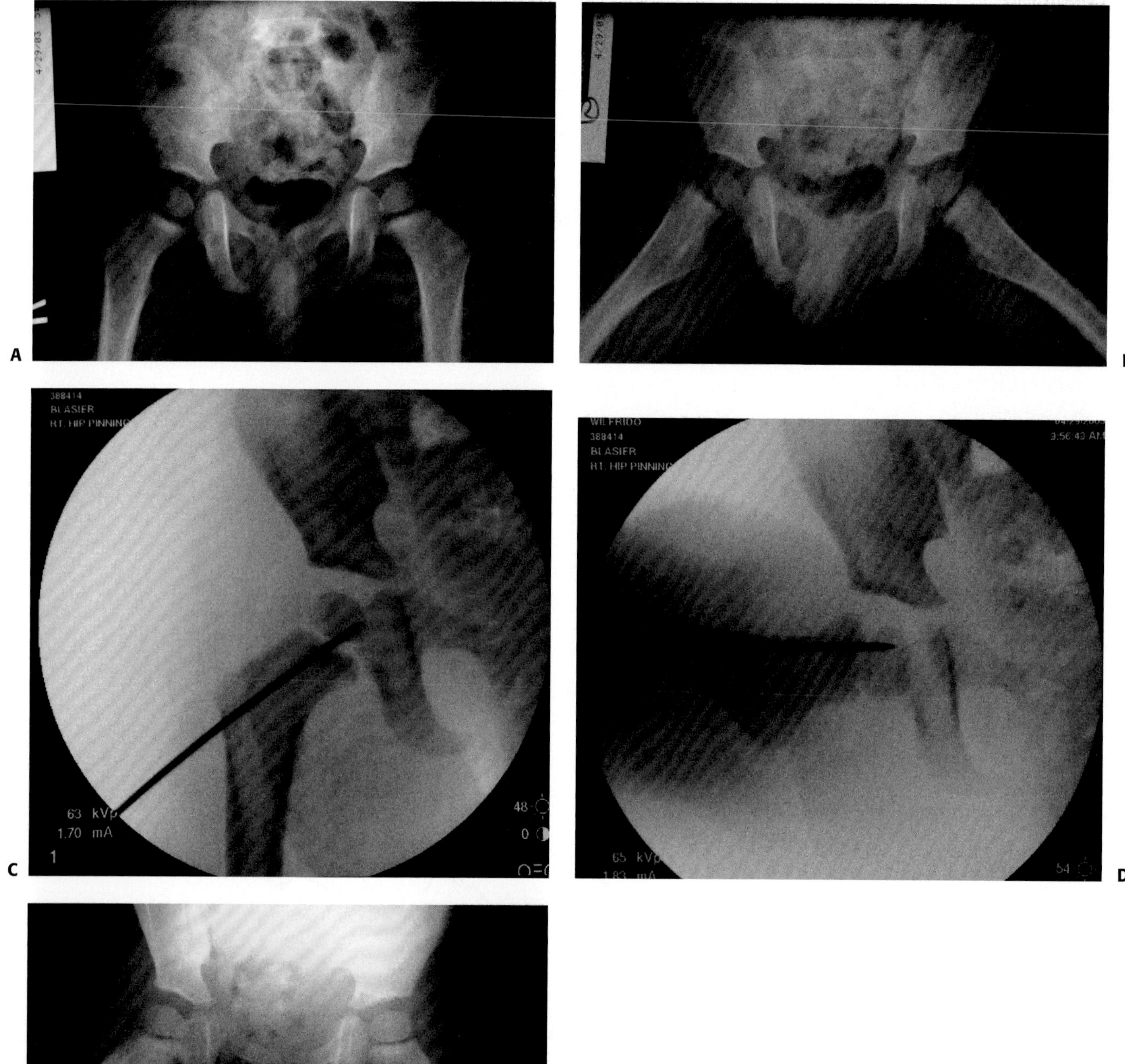

FIGURE 21-2 This 2-year-old boy fell on the trampoline and subsequently complained of right hip pain. **A.** AP x-rays were not grossly abnormal. **B.** Frog lateral x-ray revealed a Salter I epiphyseal separation. **C,D.** Closed reduction in the operating room was stabilized with a percutaneous pin. **E.** At 8 months he was asymptomatic and there was no evidence of ON.

vara in 14% (2). Displaced type III fractures are similar to type II fractures in regard to the development of complications. Nondisplaced type III fractures have a much lower complication rate than displaced fractures.

Type IV. Intertrochanteric fractures account for only 12% of fractures of the head and neck of the femur in children (2). This fracture has the lowest complication rate of all four types. Nonunion and ON after this fracture are rare. Coxa vara and premature physeal closure have occasionally been reported (1,2,8,9,19).

Unusual Fracture Patterns

Type I fracture in a neonate deserves special attention. This injury is exceedingly rare and, because the femoral head is not visible on plain x-rays, the index of suspicion must be high. The differential diagnosis includes septic arthritis and hip dislocation. Plain x-rays may be of assistance, but ultrasonography is useful if the diagnosis remains in doubt. Plain x-rays may show a high-riding proximal femoral metaphysis on the involved side, resembling a dislocation. Ultrasonography shows the cartilaginous head in the acetabulum with dissociation from the femoral shaft. The diagnosis can be missed if there is no history of trauma (such as in child abuse) or if there is an ipsilateral fracture of the femoral shaft (20).

Stress fractures are caused by repetitive injury and result in hip or knee pain and a limp. Pain associated with long-distance running, marching, or a recent increase in physical activity is suggestive of stress fracture. Close scrutiny of high-quality x-rays may identify sclerosis, cortical thickening, or new bone formation. Undisplaced fractures may appear as faint radiolucencies (Fig. 21-3).

An acute unstable slipped capital femoral epiphysis may be confused with an acute type I fracture of the proximal femur; however, a slipped capital femoral epiphysis is caused by an underlying abnormality of the physis and occurs after trivial trauma, usually in preadolescents, whereas type I fractures usually occur in young children.

Fracture after minor trauma suggests weakened bone. Intrinsic bone disease, tumors, cysts, and infections may weaken the bone. If the trauma is significant but the history is not consistent, nonaccidental trauma must always be considered (16,21).

It is easy to miss hip fractures that are overshadowed by more dramatic or painful injuries. X-rays of the proximal femur should be examined carefully in patients with femoral shaft fractures because ipsilateral fracture or dislocation of the hip is not unusual (20).

Surgical and Applied Anatomy

Ossification of the femur begins in the 7th fetal week (15). In early childhood, only a single proximal femoral physis exists (Fig. 21-4A,B). During the first year of life, the medial portion of this physis grows faster than the lateral, creating an elongated femoral neck by 1 year of age (see Fig. 21-4C). The capital femoral epiphysis begins to ossify at approximately 4 months in girls and 5 to 6 months in boys. The ossification center of

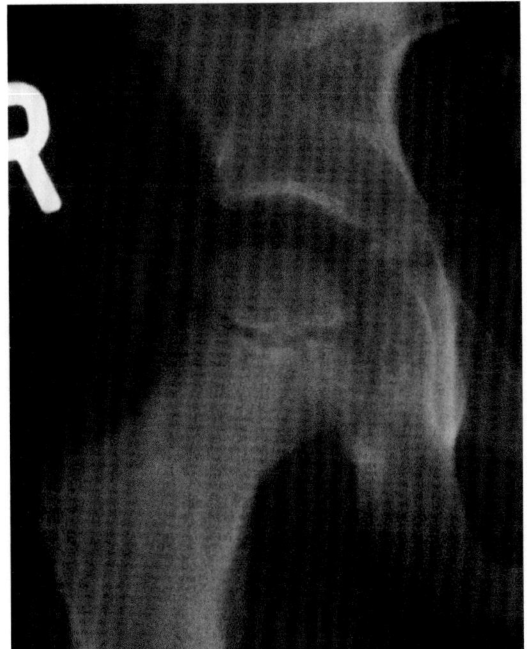

A

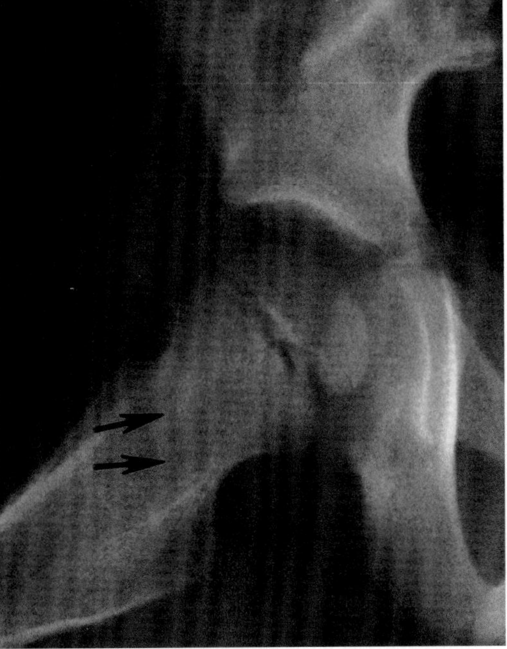

B

FIGURE 21-3 **A.** This 5-year-old boy jumped off his bunk bed and subsequently complained of right hip pain and limp. AP radiography yielded normal findings. **B.** Careful examination of the frog-leg lateral x-ray revealed a nondisplaced femoral neck fracture. Symptoms resolved after 4 weeks in a spica cast.

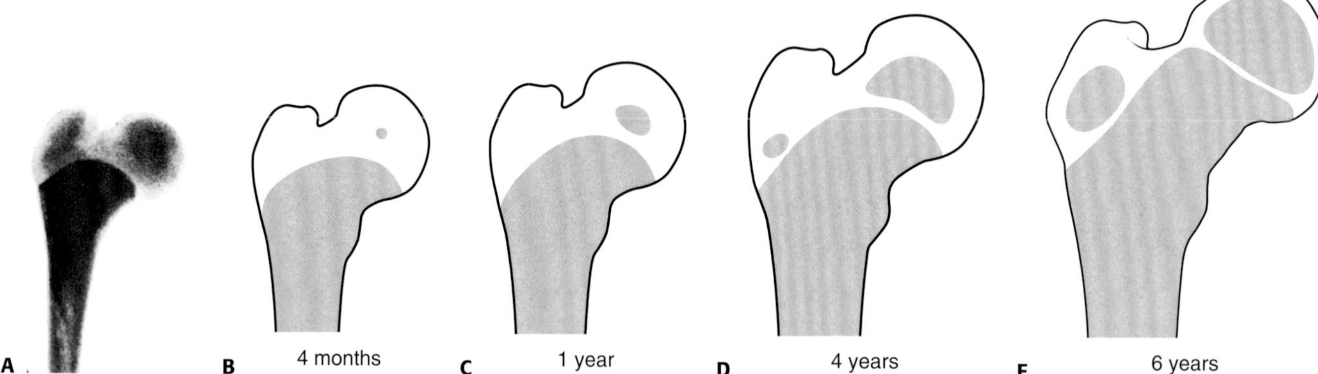

FIGURE 21-4 The transformation of the preplate to separate growth zones for the femoral head and greater trochanter. The diagram shows development of the epiphyseal nucleus in the proximal end of the femur. **A.** X-ray of the proximal end of the femur of a stillborn girl, weight 325 g. **B–E.** Drawings made on the basis of x-rays. (Reprinted from Edgren W. Coxa plana. A clinical and radiological investigation with particular reference to the importance of the metaphyseal changes for the final shape of the proximal part of the femur. *Acta Orthop Scand* 1965;84(suppl):24; with permission.)

the trochanteric apophysis appears at 4 years in boys and girls (2) (see Fig. 21-4D). The proximal femoral physis is responsible for the metaphyseal growth in the femoral neck, whereas the trochanteric apophysis contributes to the appositional growth of the greater trochanter and less to the metaphyseal growth of the femur (Fig. 21-5) (22). Fusion of the proximal femoral and trochanteric physes occurs at about the age of 14 in girls and 16 in boys (23). The confluence of the greater trochanteric physis with the capital femoral physis along the superior femoral neck (see Fig. 21-4E) and the unique vascular supply to the capital femoral epiphysis make the immature hip vulnerable to growth derangement and subsequent deformity after a fracture.

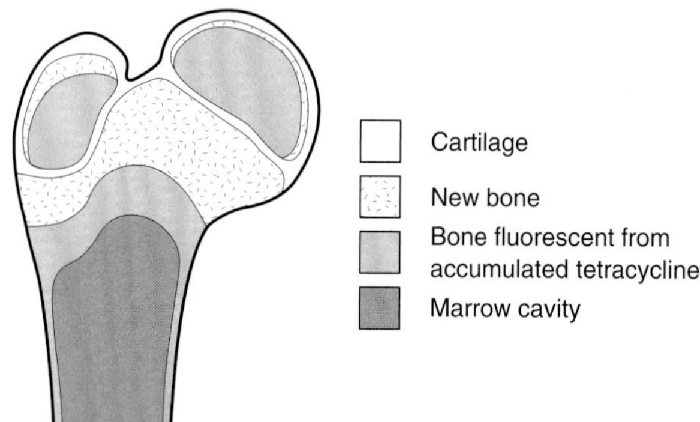

FIGURE 21-5 Drawing of a frontal section through the upper end of the femur of a 14-week-old pig injected 8 weeks previously with tetracycline (50 mg/kg). Diagram depicts the contribution of the capital femoral physis and greater trochanteric physis to new bone formation. (Reprinted from Edgren W. Coxa plana. A clinical and radiological investigation with particular reference to the importance of the metaphyseal changes for the final shape of the proximal part of the femur. *Acta Orthop Scand* 1965;84(suppl):24; with permission.)

Vascular Anatomy

Because of the frequency and sequelae of ON of the hip in children, the blood supply has been studied extensively (18,24–26). Postmortem injection and microangiographic studies have provided clues to the vascular changes with age. These observations are as follows:

1. The vessels of the ligamentum teres are of virtually no importance. They contribute little blood supply to the femoral head until age 8, and then only about 20% as an adult.
2. At birth, the branches of the medial and lateral circumflex arteries (metaphyseal vessels) traversing the femoral neck predominately supply the femoral head. These arteries gradually diminish in size as the cartilaginous physis develops and forms a barrier that prevents penetration of these vessels into the femoral head. This metaphyseal blood supply is virtually nonexistent by age 4.
3. When the metaphyseal vessels diminish, the lateral epiphyseal vessels predominate and the femoral head is primarily supplied by these vessels, which bypass the physeal barrier.
4. Ogden noted that the lateral epiphyseal vessels consist of two branches, the posterosuperior and posteroinferior branches of the medial circumflex artery (Fig. 21-6). At the level of the intertrochanteric groove, the medial circumflex artery branches into a retinacular arterial system (the posterosuperior and posteroinferior arteries). These arteries penetrate the capsule and traverse proximally (covered by the retinacular folds) along the neck of the femur to supply the femoral head peripherally and proximally to the physis.
5. Capsulotomy does not damage the blood supply to the femoral head, but violation of the intertrochanteric notch or the lateral ascending cervical vessels may render the head avascular.

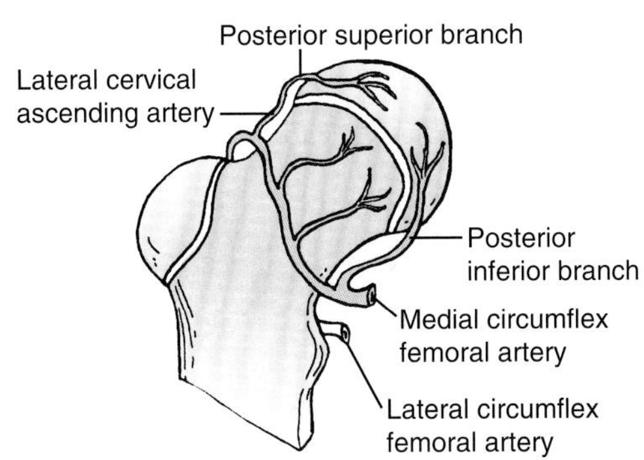

FIGURE 21-6 Arterial supply of the proximal femur. The capital femoral epiphysis and physis are supplied by the medial circumflex artery through two retinacular vessel systems: the posterosuperior and posteroinferior. The lateral circumflex artery supplies the greater trochanter and the lateral portion of the proximal femoral physis and a small area of the anteromedial metaphysis.

6. At about 3 to 4 years of age, the lateral posterosuperior vessels appear to predominate and supply the entire anterior lateral portion of the capital femoral epiphysis.
7. The posteroinferior and posterosuperior arteries persist throughout life and supply the femoral head.
8. The multiple small vessels of the young coalesce with age to a limited number of larger vessels. As a result, damage to a single vessel can have serious consequences; for example, occlusion of the posterosuperior branch of the medial circumflex artery can cause ON of the anterior lateral portion of the femoral head (3).

Soft Tissue Anatomy

The hip joint is enclosed by a thick fibrous capsule. Tense hemarthrosis after intracapsular fracture may tamponade the ascending cervical vessels and may have implications in the development of ON. The hip joint is surrounded on all sides by a protective cuff of musculature. Open hip fracture is rare. In the absence of associated hip dislocation, neurovascular injuries are rare after hip fracture and are more likely to occur during surgery.

The lateral femoral cutaneous nerve lies in the interval between the tensor and sartorius muscles and supplies sensation to the lateral thigh. This nerve must be identified and preserved during an anterolateral approach to the hip. The femoral neurovascular bundle is separated from the anterior hip joint by the iliopsoas. Thus, any retractor placed on the anterior acetabular rim should be carefully placed deep to the iliopsoas to protect the femoral bundle. Inferior and medial to the hip capsule, coursing from the deep femoral artery toward the posterior hip joint, is the medial femoral circumflex artery. Placement of a distal Hohmann retractor too deeply can tear this artery, and control of the bleeding may be difficult.

The sciatic nerve emerges from the sciatic notch beneath the piriformis and courses superficial to the external rotators and the quadratus medial to the greater trochanter.

Preferred Approaches

The Watson-Jones Approach. If open reduction is necessary, the Watson-Jones approach is the most useful and direct approach to the femoral neck. A lateral incision is made over the proximal femur, slightly anterior to the greater trochanter (Fig. 21-7A). The fascia lata is incised longitudinally (see Fig. 21-7B). The innervation of the tensor muscle by the superior gluteal nerve is 2 to 5 cm above the greater trochanter, and care should be taken not to damage this innervation. The tensor muscle is reflected anteriorly. The interval between the gluteus medius and the tensor muscles will be used (see Fig. 21-7C). The plane is developed between the muscles and the underlying hip capsule (see Fig. 21-7D). If necessary, the anteriormost fibers of the gluteus medius tendon can be detached from the trochanter for wider exposure. After clearing the anterior hip capsule, longitudinal capsulotomy is made along the anterosuperior femoral neck. A transverse incision can be added superiorly for wider exposure (see Fig. 21-7E). Once the hip fracture is reduced, wires can be passed perpendicular to the fracture along the femoral neck from the base of the greater trochanter.

The Smith-Peterson Approach. Alternatively, a bikini approach can be used through the Smith-Petersen interval (Fig. 21-8). Care should be taken to identify and protect the lateral femoral cutaneous nerve. The sartorius and rectus muscles can be detached to expose the hip capsule. Medial and inferior retractors should be carefully placed to avoid damage to the femoral neurovascular bundle and medial femoral circumflex artery, respectively. Care must be taken not to violate the intertrochanteric notch and the lateral ascending vessels. Because the lateral aspect of the greater trochanter is not exposed, wires must be passed percutaneously once the hip fracture is reduced.

Current Treatment Options

Type I

Fracture treatment is based on the age of the child and fracture stability after reduction. In toddlers under 2 years of age with nondisplaced or minimally displaced fractures, simple spica cast immobilization is likely to be successful. Because the fracture tends to displace into varus and external rotation, the limb should be casted in mild abduction and neutral rotation to prevent displacement. Displaced fractures in toddlers should be reduced closed by gentle traction, abduction, and internal rotation. If the fracture "locks on" and is stable, casting without fixation is indicated. If the fracture is not stable, it should be fixed with small smooth pins that access the femoral neck and cross the physis. If casting without fixation is done, repeat x-rays should be taken within days to look for displacement, because the likelihood of successful repeat reduction decreases rapidly with time and healing in a young child (Fig. 21-9).

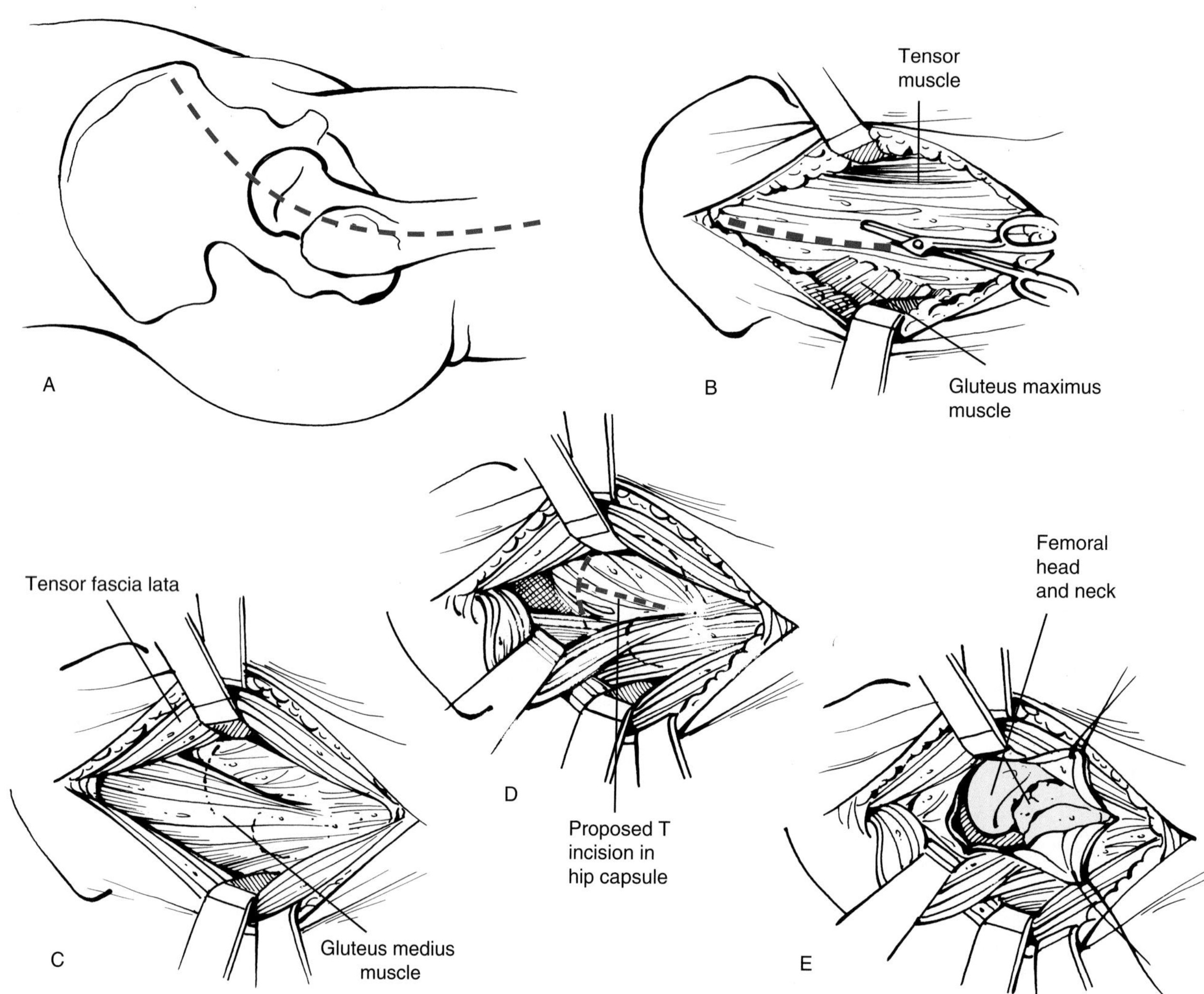

FIGURE 21-7 Watson-Jones lateral approach to the hip joint for open reduction of femoral neck fractures in children. **A.** Skin incision. **B.** Incision of the fascia lata between the tensor muscle (anterior) and gluteus maximus (posterior). **C.** Exposure of the interval between the gluteus medius and tensor fascia lata (retracted anteriorly). Development of the interval will reveal the underlying hip capsule. **D.** Exposure of hip capsule. **E.** Exposure of the femoral neck after T incision of the capsule.

Children older than 2 years should always have operative fixation even if the fracture is undisplaced because the complications of late displacement may be great. Smooth pins can be used in young children, but cannulated screws are better for older, larger children. Fixation should cross the physis into the capital femoral epiphysis. Irreducibility mandates an open reduction and internal fixation. Postoperative spica cast immobilization is mandatory in all but the oldest and most reliable adolescents. Fixation may be removed shortly after fracture healing to enable further growth in younger patients.

Closed reduction of type IB fracture–dislocations may be attempted, but immediate open reduction is necessary if a single attempt at closed reduction is unsuccessful. Internal fixation is mandatory. The surgical approach should be from the side to which the head is dislocated, generally posterolateral. Parents must be advised in advance about the risk of ON.

Type II and Type III

Displaced neck fractures should always be treated with anatomic reduction and stable internal fixation to minimize the risk of late complications. In two large series, the prevalences of coxa vara and nonunion were high in displaced transcervical

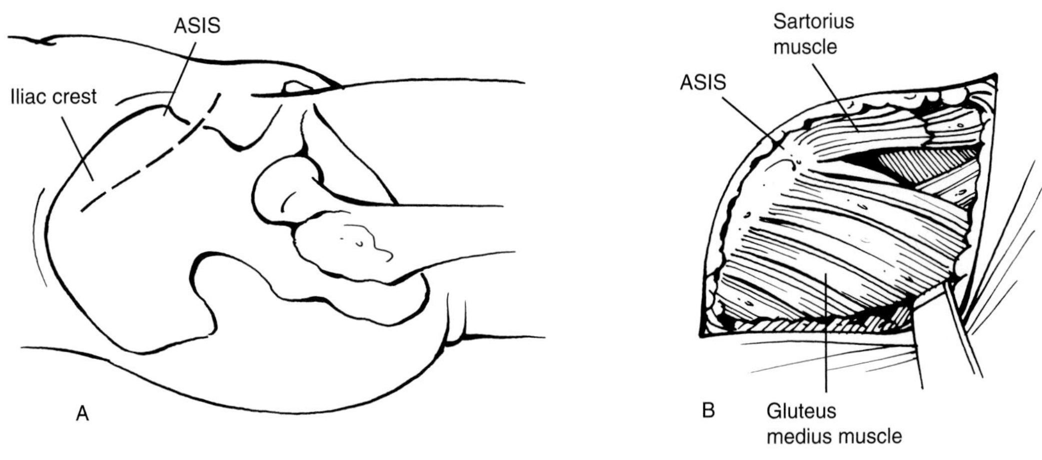

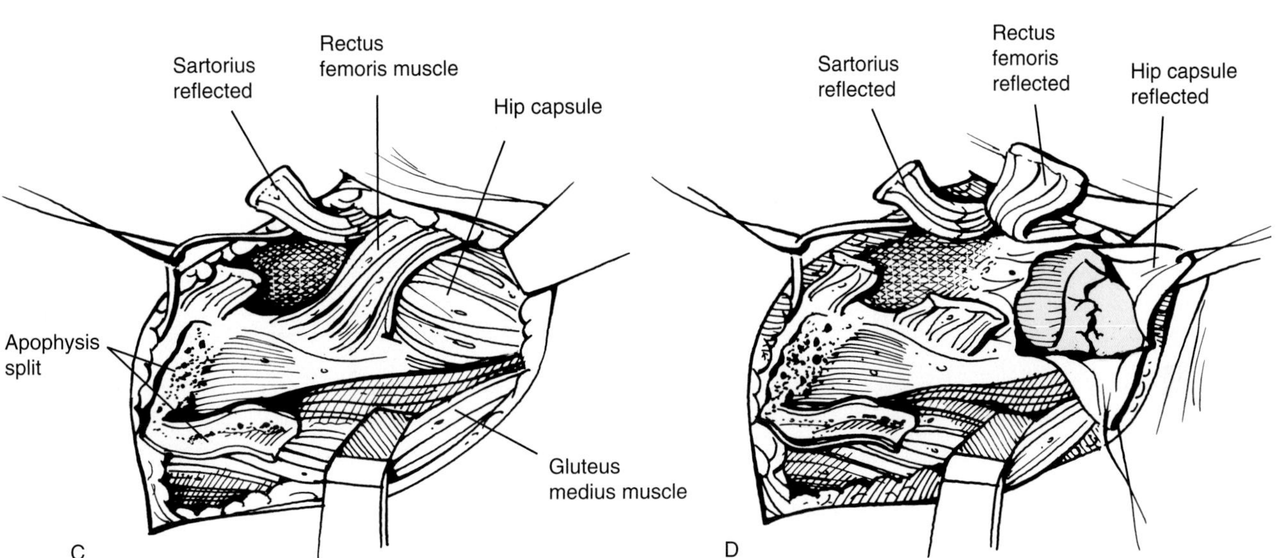

FIGURE 21-8 Smith-Petersen anterolateral approach to the hip joint. **A.** Skin incision. Incision is 1 cm below the iliac crest and extends just medial to the anterior superior iliac spine (ASIS). **B.** Skin is retracted, exposing the fascia overlying the ASIS. The interval between the sartorius and the tensor fascia lata is identifiable by palpation. **C.** The sartorius is detached from the ASIS. Splitting of the iliac crest apophysis and detachment of the rectus femoris (shown attached to anterior inferior iliac spine) will facilitate exposure of the hip capsule. **D.** The hip capsule is exposed. A T incision is made to reveal the femoral head and neck.

fractures treated with immobilization but without internal fixation (8,9). Much lower prevalences of these two complications have been documented in patients treated with anatomic closed or open reduction and internal fixation (9,10,12).

Internal fixation also is recommended by most investigators for nondisplaced transcervical fractures (2) because the risk of late displacement in such fractures far outweighs the risk of percutaneous screw fixation, especially in young children (27). Nondisplaced type II fractures in children under 5 years of age can be managed with spica casting and close follow-up (8,28), but fixation remains preferable. Even then, close follow-up is necessary to prevent varus displacement in the cast.

Gentle closed reduction of displaced fractures is accomplished with the use of longitudinal traction, abduction, and

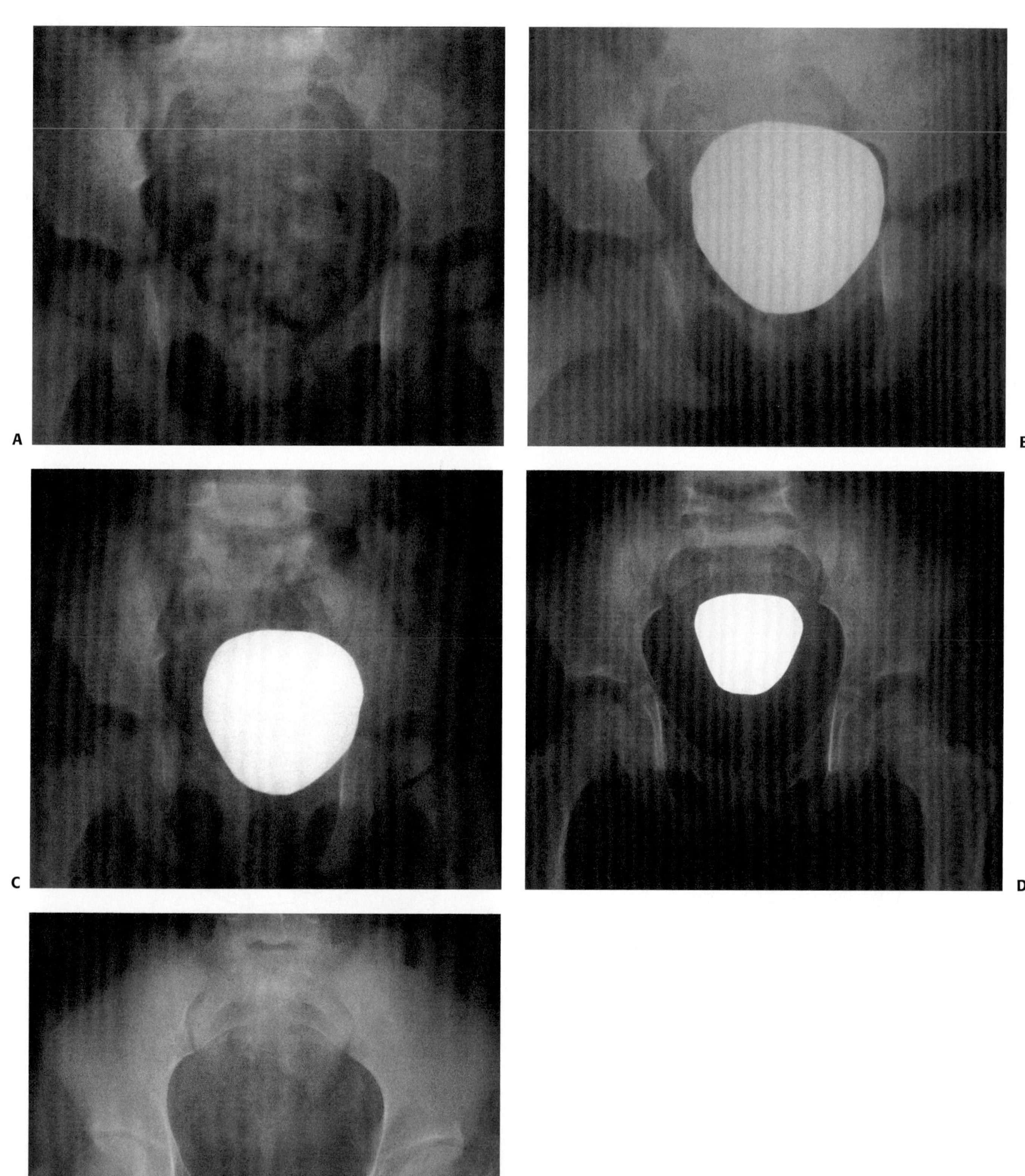

FIGURE 21-9 **A.** A 16-month-old boy with a type I fracture of the left hip. Note widening of the left femoral physis. **B.** Lateral x-ray at injury. Instability of the physis is apparent. **C.** AP x-ray after 1 month in a spica cast. **D.** At 2 years after the injury, the patient has mild coxa valga and coxa breva. **E.** At 10 years after the injury, coxa breva secondary to premature physeal closure is evident. Note the overgrowth of the greater trochanter.

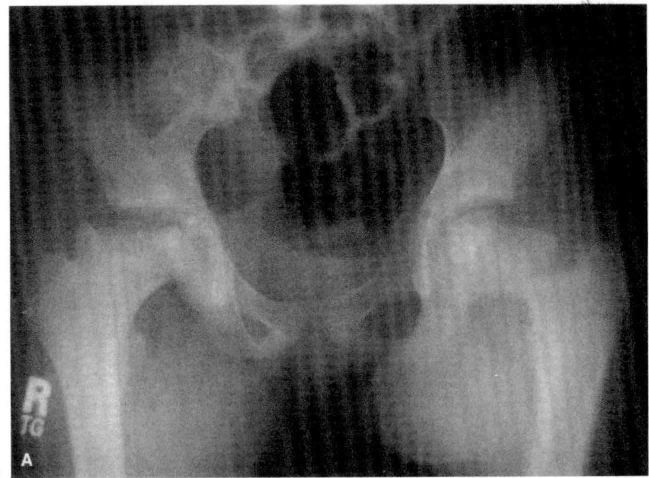

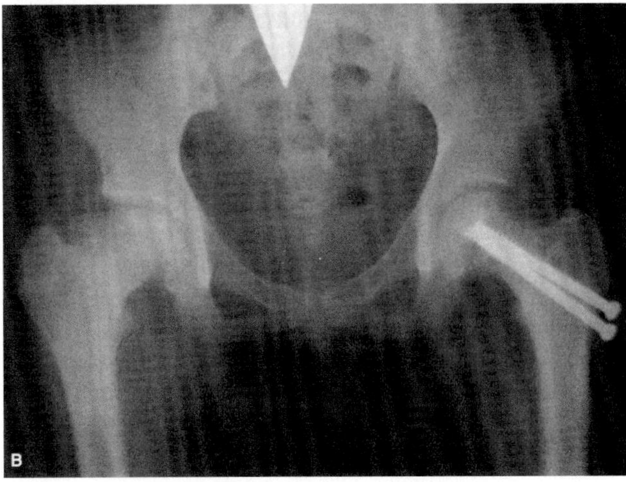

FIGURE 21-10 **A.** Pathologic type II fracture of left femoral neck in an 11-year-old girl with Gauchze disease and old osteonecrosis of the right hip. **B.** One year after open reduction and fixation with 40-mm cannulated hip screws.

internal rotation. Open reduction frequently is necessary for displaced fractures and should be done through a Watson-Jones surgical approach.

Internal fixation with cannulated screws is done through a small lateral incision. Three screws should be placed if possible. One screw should be placed low along the calcar and two above, spaced as widely as possible (27). Occasionally, the small size of the child's femoral neck will accommodate only two screws. Care should be taken to minimize drill holes in the subtrochanteric region because they increase the risk of subtrochanteric fracture. If possible, screws should be inserted short of the physis in type III fractures; however, if physeal penetration is necessary for purchase, it must be done (Figs. 21-10 and 21-11) (2,12). The risks of premature physeal closure and trochanteric overgrowth are much less than those of nonunion, pin breakage, and ON. Treatment of the fracture is the first priority, and any subsequent growth disturbance and leg length discrepancy are secondary.

Nondisplaced cervicotrochanteric fractures can be treated adequately in an abduction one-and-one-half spica cast with close follow-up (2). Displaced cervicotrochanteric fractures have been shown to have a complication rate similar to that for type II fractures and should be treated similarly. Fixation generally does not need to cross the physis in type III fractures.

In a more distal cervicotrochanteric fracture, especially in a child over 5 years of age, a pediatric hip compression screw can be used for more secure fixation. Consideration may be given to capsulotomy or aspiration of the joint to eliminate tense hemarthrosis at the time of surgery. Spica casting is routine, except in older reliable children (10). Hardware removal at 6 to 12 months after fracture union will avoid bony overgrowth of the hardware.

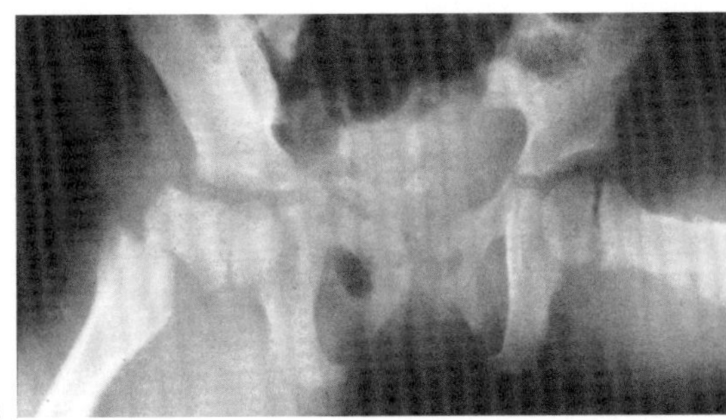

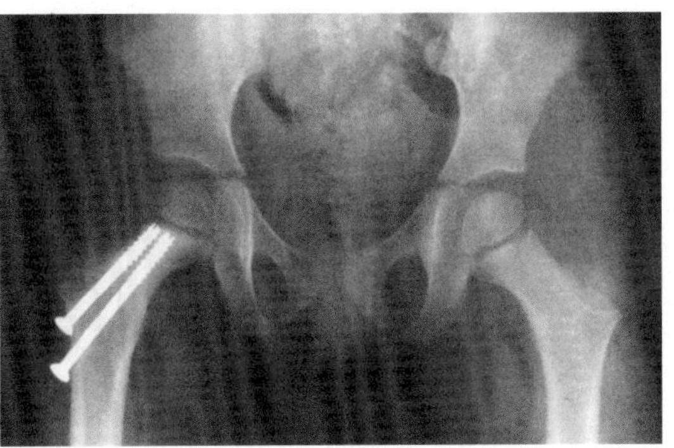

FIGURE 21-11 **A.** A boy age 4 years and 9 months sustained a type III femoral neck fracture in a motor vehicle accident. **B.** Three months after anatomic open reduction and internal fixation with two screws, sparing the physis.

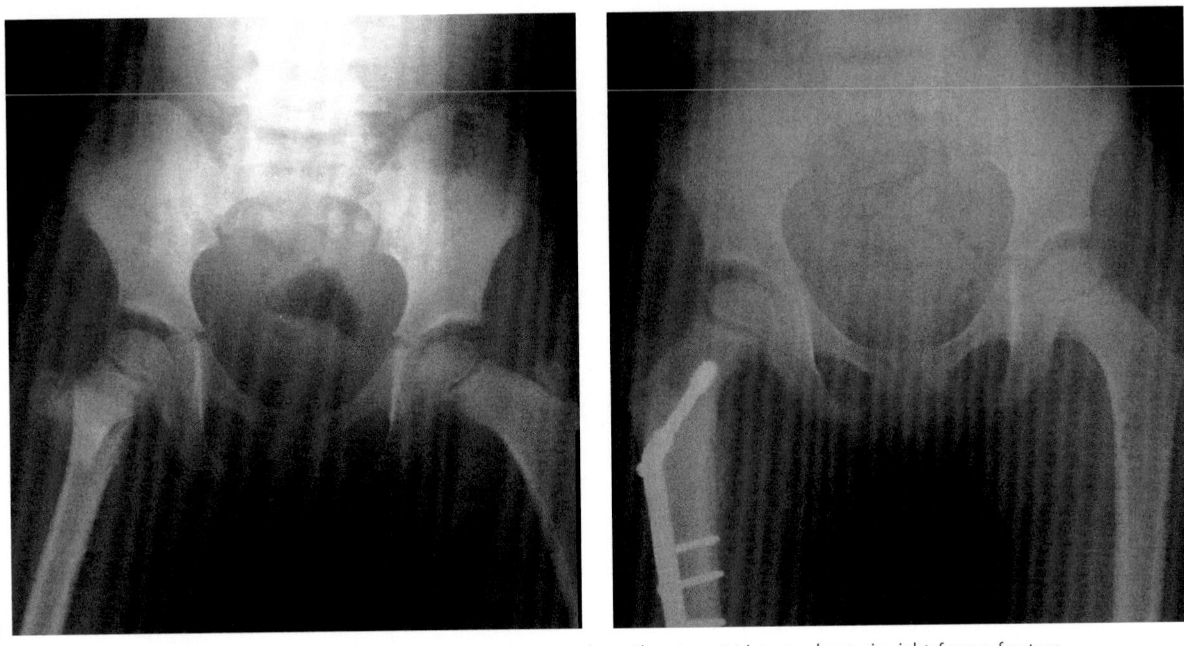

FIGURE 21-12 **A.** A girl age 3 years and 7 months with a type IV intertrochanteric right femur fracture. **B.** Three months after fixation with a pediatric sliding hip screw.

Type IV

Good results can be expected after closed treatment of most intertrochanteric fractures, regardless of displacement. Traction and spica cast immobilization are effective (2). Failure to maintain adequate reduction and polytrauma are indications for internal fixation. Children old enough to use crutches or those with multiple injuries can be treated with open reduction and internal fixation (Figs. 21-12 and 21-13). A pediatric hip screw provides the most rigid internal fixation for this purpose.

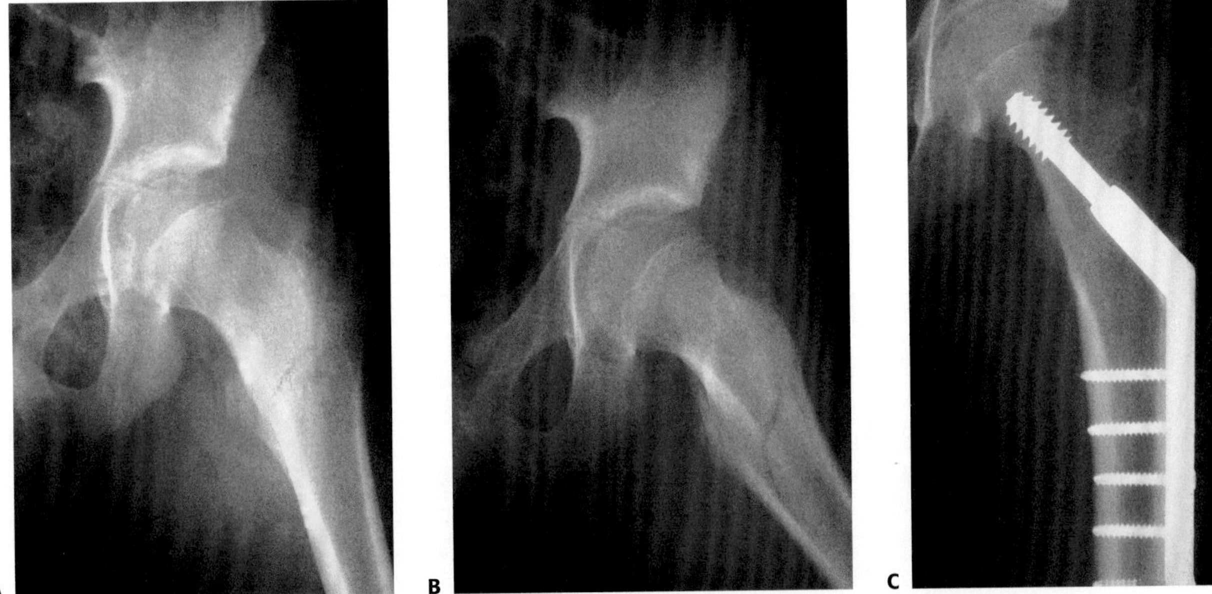

FIGURE 21-13 **A.** A 14-year-old boy who fell from a tree swing sustained this nondisplaced left intertrochanteric hip fracture. **B.** Lateral x-ray shows the long spiral fracture line. **C.** Three months after fixation with an adult sliding hip screw.

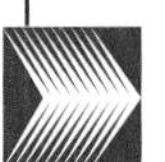

AUTHORS' PREFERRED TREATMENT

Type I

Truly undisplaced or minimally displaced fractures in toddlers up to age 2 should be treated in a spica cast without internal fixation. The limb should be casted in a position of abduction and neutral rotation to prevent displacement into varus. If the fracture requires reduction or moves significantly during reduction or casting maneuvers, then internal fixation is mandatory. Small, smooth Kirschner wires are inserted percutaneously to cross the physis. We recommend two or three wires. Wires should be cut off and bent below the skin for later retrieval under a brief general anesthetic at the time of spica cast removal. We do not recommend leaving the wires outside the skin. Frequent x-rays are necessary to check for migration of the pins into the joint space. A spica cast is always applied in this age group and should remain in place for at least 6 weeks (10).

Type I fractures in children older than 2 years should always have operative internal fixation, even if the fracture is anatomically reduced. While Kirschner wires are appropriate for small children, 4.0-mm cannulated screws crossing the physis should be used in older, larger children. If closed reduction is successful, a 4.5- to 5-cm lateral incision is made distal to the greater trochanter apophysis for insertion of pins or cannulated screws.

If gentle closed reduction cannot be achieved, a Watson-Jones approach is preferred for type IA fractures. For type IB fractures, the choice of approach is dictated by the position of the femoral epiphysis. If it is anterior or inferior, a Watson-Jones approach should be used. It is most commonly posterior, in which case a posterior approach should be selected.

Under direct vision, the fracture is reduced and guide wires are passed from the lateral aspect of the proximal femur up the neck perpendicular to the fracture. Because the femoral neck in children is denser and harder than the osteoporotic bone in elderly patients, predrilling and tapping are necessary before the insertion of screws.

Types II and III

Types II and III fractures should be fixed with 4.0-mm cannulated screws in small children up to age 8 years. After the age of 8 years, fixation with 6.5-mm cannulated screws is appropriate. Two or three screws should be used, depending on the size of the child's femoral neck. We prefer a Watson-Jones approach because it provides the most direct exposure of the femoral neck for fracture reduction. These fractures must be gently anatomically reduced under direct vision. Guide wires are then placed up the femoral neck perpendicular to the fracture. If possible, penetration of the physis should be avoided (10,11). However, in most unstable type II fractures, penetration of the physis may be necessary to achieve stability and avoid the complications associated with late displacement (2,12). Excellent fixation of type III fractures generally is possible without penetration of the physis. As in type I fractures, predrilling and tapping of the femoral neck are necessary to avoid displacement of the fracture while advancing the screws.

Type IV

Undisplaced type IV fractures in children younger than 3 years, or fractures in this age group in which a stable closed reduction can be achieved, can be treated without internal fixation with immobilization in a spica cast for 12 weeks. Frequent radiographic examination is necessary to assess for late displacement, particularly into varus. Displaced type IV fractures in all children over 3 years of age should be treated with internal fixation with a pediatric or juvenile compression hip screw. Closed reduction often is possible with a combination of traction and internal rotation of the limb. If open reduction is necessary, a Watson-Jones approach should be used.

Postoperative Fracture Care

Hip spica casting is used after internal fixation in all patients under 10 years of age. The cast should remain in place for 6 to 12 weeks depending on age. For children over 12 years of age, no postoperative cast is used and early ambulation with crutches is encouraged, as in adults. For children 10 to 12 years of age, the use of a postoperative cast depends on the stability of fracture fixation and the patient's compliance; if either is in doubt, a single hip spica cast is used. Formal rehabilitation usually is unnecessary unless there is a severe persistent limp, which may be due to abductor weakness. Stiffness rarely is a problem in the absence of ON.

Pearls and Pitfalls

- Table 21-1 summarizes the "pearls" of surgical stabilization of pediatric hip fractures, including recommended choices of implants for internal fixation.
- For young, small patients, the operation should be done on a radiolucent operating table rather than on a fracture table, which is more appropriate for older and larger adolescents.
- Because the femoral bone in children is harder than the osteoporotic bone in elderly patients, predrilling and pretapping are necessary for insertion of all screws.
- Multiple attempts at wire placement should be avoided because they result in empty holes in the subtrochanteric region of the femur. This predisposes to late subtrochanteric fracture below or at the level of the screw heads after removal of the spica cast.
- A hip spica cast must be used to supplement internal fixation in all patients who are younger than 10 years. For older patients, if the stability of the fracture is questionable or if the child's compliance is doubtful, the surgeon should not hesitate to apply a hip spica cast. The quality of reduction and the stability of the fixation have a direct impact on the occurrence of nonunion (1,8,10,12).

TABLE 21-1 Surgical Tips and Pearls for Hip Fractures in Children

Anterolateral approach
Age 0–3 yr: smooth pins, 5/64-inch or 3/32-inch
Age 3–8 yr: cannulated 4.0-mm screws
Age 8+ yr: 6.5- or 7.0-mm cannulated screws
Type IV fractures <8 yr: pediatric hip compression screw >8 yr: juvenile or adult hip compression screw
Always predrill and tap before inserting screws.
Avoid crossing physis if possible, but cross physis if necessary for stability.
Age <10 yr: hip spica for 6–12 wk.

- Growth of the femur and the contribution of the proximal femoral physis are important; however, this physeal contribution to growth is only 13% of the entire extremity, or 3 to 4 mm per year on average. Once the decision for internal fixation of a fracture of the head or neck of the femur is made, stable fixation of the fracture is a higher priority than preservation of the physis. If stability is questionable, the internal fixation device should extend into the femoral head for rigid, stable fixation, regardless of the type of fracture or the age of the child.

Complications

Osteonecrosis

ON is the most serious and frequent complication of hip fractures in children. Its overall prevalence is approximately 30%, based on nine series in the literature (2,11,29). It is the primary cause of poor results after fractures of the hip in children. The risk of ON is related to the extent of initial displacement of the fracture and to the damage to the blood supply at injury. The risk of ON is highest after displaced type IB, type II, and type III fractures (Fig. 21-14) (2). Cheng et al (11) and Flynn et al (10) both reported low rates of ON in their series of patients treated within 24 hours of injury with prompt reduction and internal fixation. They recommended an aggressive approach to early reduction and stabilization as a possible means of preventing this complication. Increased intraarticular pressure caused by fracture hematoma may be related to ON after intracapsular fracture, and evacuation of this hemarthrosis may decrease the ON rate (2,29,30). Aspirating the hematoma from the hip capsule may decrease the intracapsular pressure and increase blood flow to the femoral head (11,29) or may have no effect (2,5,31). If a child is going to have an anesthetic for treatment of a fracture, aspiration of the hematoma can easily be accomplished. Open reduction results in capsular evacuation at capsulotomy, or a small capsulotomy can be made if a straight lateral incision is used after unsuccessful closed reduction.

ON has been classified by Ratliff as follows: type I, involvement of the whole head; type II, partial involvement of the head; and type III, an area of necrosis from the fracture line to the physis (Fig. 21-15) (1). Type I is the most severe and most common form and has the poorest prognosis. Type I probably results from damage to all of the lateral epiphyseal vessels, type II from localized damage to one or more of the lateral epiphyseal vessels near their insertion into the anterolateral aspect of the femoral head, and type III from damage to the superior metaphyseal vessels. Type III is rare but has a good prognosis (1).

ON causes pain and limitation of motion. As early as 6 weeks after injury, plain x-rays may reveal decreased density of the femoral head with widening of the joint space. Fragmentation and collapse of the femoral head occur late. Technetium bone scanning with pinhole collimation may show decreased uptake in the involved femoral head early in the course of ON. With revascularization, changes may be variable. Signs and symptoms of ON usually develop within the first year after injury, but sometimes as late as 2 years (2,19). Patients should be followed with plain x-rays for at least 2 years after fracture to rule out late onset of ON. MRI reveals ON within a few days of injury (see the subsection on osteonecrosis under "Hip Dislocations in Children"). If MRI does not reveal ON within 6 weeks of injury, it is unlikely to develop. The long-term results of ON are poor in over 60% of patients (5,9,28,32). There is no clearly effective treatment for posttraumatic ON in children (2,19). Older children (more than 10 years of age) tend to have worse outcomes than younger children. Ongoing research includes the role of core decompression, vascularized fibular grafting (Fig. 21-16), and the trapdoor procedure. Results of the procedures in few reported patients must ultimately be compared with the natural healing of untreated ON. Remodeling can occur over many years and is more likely in younger children than in older ones. Degenerative arthritis in older children generally is irreversible. Valgus intertrochanteric osteotomy may improve coxa vara and leg length discrepancy if there is reasonable congruence in adduction of the hip preoperatively (Fig. 21-17).

Coxa Vara

The prevalence of coxa vara has been reported to be approximately 20% to 30% in nine series (2), although it is significantly lower in series in which internal fixation was used after reduction of displaced fractures (9). Coxa vara may be caused by malunion, ON, premature physeal closure, or a combination of these problems (Fig. 21-18). Severe coxa vara raises the greater trochanter in relation to the femoral head, causing shortening of the extremity and mechanical disadvantage of the abductors. The result is an abductor lurch. If the child is over 8 years of age, the neck–shaft angle is 110 degrees or less, and coxa vara has been persistent for more than 2 years, subtrochanteric valgus osteotomy may be considered to restore limb length and abductor strength (2).

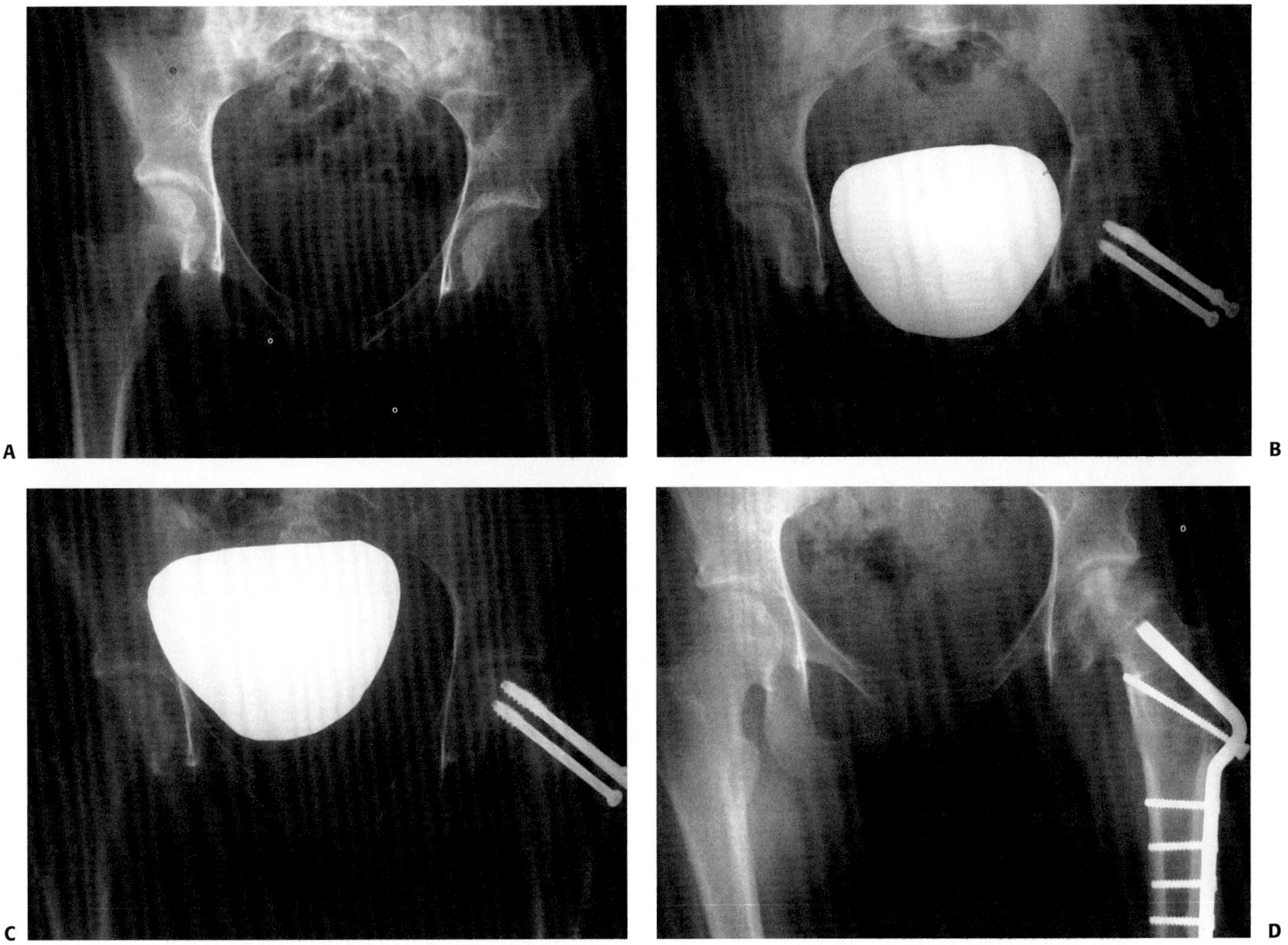

FIGURE 21-14 **A.** A 14-year-old girl with a type II fracture of the left femoral neck. **B.** After fixation with three cannulated screws. **C.** Seven months after injury. Osteonecrosis with collapse of the superolateral portion of the femoral head. **D.** After treatment with valgus osteotomy.

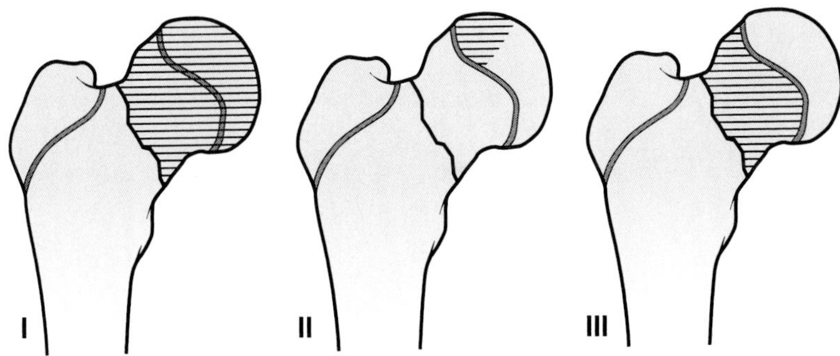

FIGURE 21-15 Three types of osteonecrosis. Type I, whole head; type II, partial head; and type III, femoral neck. (Reprinted from Ratliff AHC. Fractures of the neck of the femur in children. *J Bone Joint Surg [Br]* 1962;44:528; with permission.)

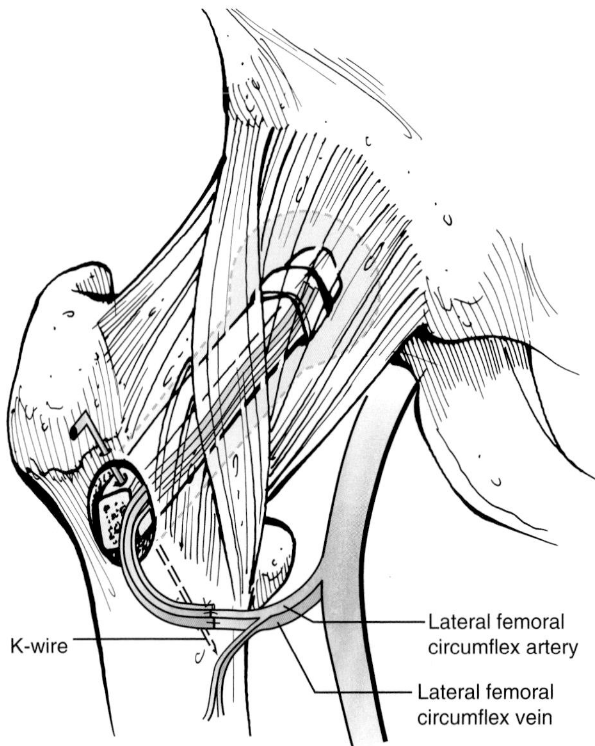

FIGURE 21-16 Vascularized fibular grafting for osteocrosis of the femoral head. (Redrawn after Aldridge JM III, Berend KR, Gunneson EE, et al. Free vascularized fibular grafting for the treatment of post collapse osteocrosis of the femoral head. *J Bone Joint Surg Ann* 2004;86:87–101; with permission.)

Premature Physeal Closure

Premature physeal closure has occurred after approximately 28% of fractures (2). The risk of premature physeal closure increases with penetration by fixation devices or when ON is present. It is most common in patients who have type II or III ON (see Fig. 21-18) (1,19).

The capital femoral physis contributes only 13% of the growth of the entire extremity and normally closes earlier than most of the other physes in the lower extremity. As a result, shortening due to premature physeal closure is not significant except in very young children (2,17). Treatment for leg length discrepancy is indicated only for significant discrepancy (2.5 cm or more projected at maturity) (2). Rarely, trochanteric epiphysiodesis may be used in progressive coxa vara.

Nonunion

Nonunion occurs infrequently, with an overall incidence of 7% of hip fractures in children (2). Nonunion is a complication of femoral neck fracture and is not generally seen after type I or type IV fractures. The primary cause of nonunion is failure to obtain or maintain an anatomic reduction (2,9). After femoral neck fracture in a child, pain should be gone and bridging new bone should be seen at the fracture site by 3 months after injury. A computed tomography (CT) scan may be helpful to look for bridging bone. If no or minimal healing is seen by 3 to 6 months, the diagnosis of nonunion is established. Nonunion should be treated operatively as soon as possible. Either rigid internal fixation or subtrochanteric valgus osteotomy should be performed to allow compression across the fracture (Fig. 21-19). Because the approach necessary for bone grafting is extensive, it should be reserved for persistent nonunion. Internal fixation should extend across the site of the nonunion, and spica cast immobili-

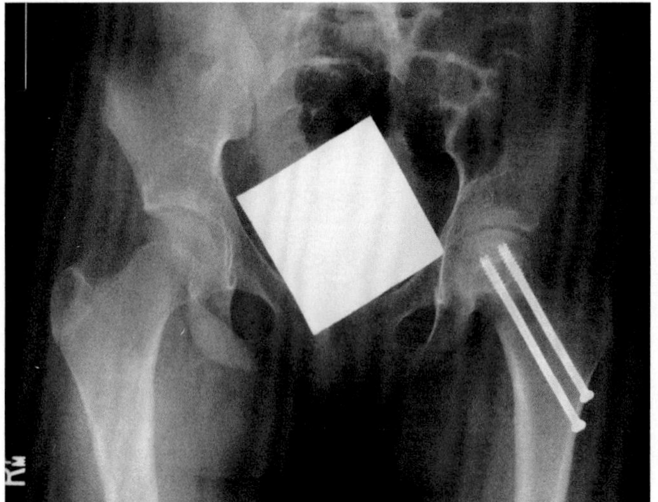

A

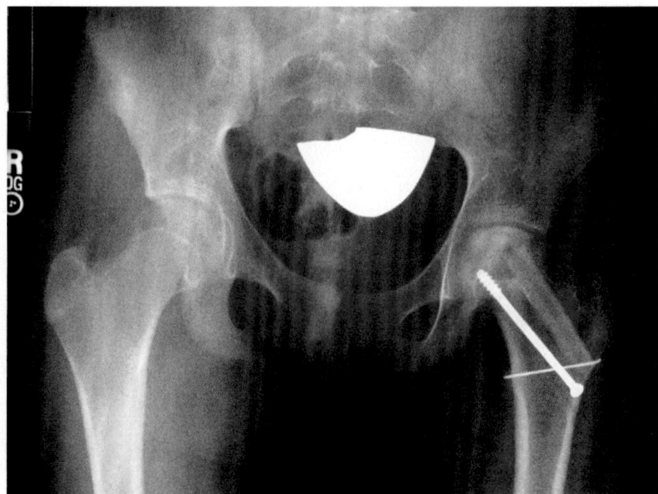

FIGURE 21-17 **A.** Osteonecrosis of the femoral head in an 11-year-old girl 6 months after type III femoral fracture. **B.** One year after vascularized fibular graft. (Courtesy of Dr. James Urbaniak.)

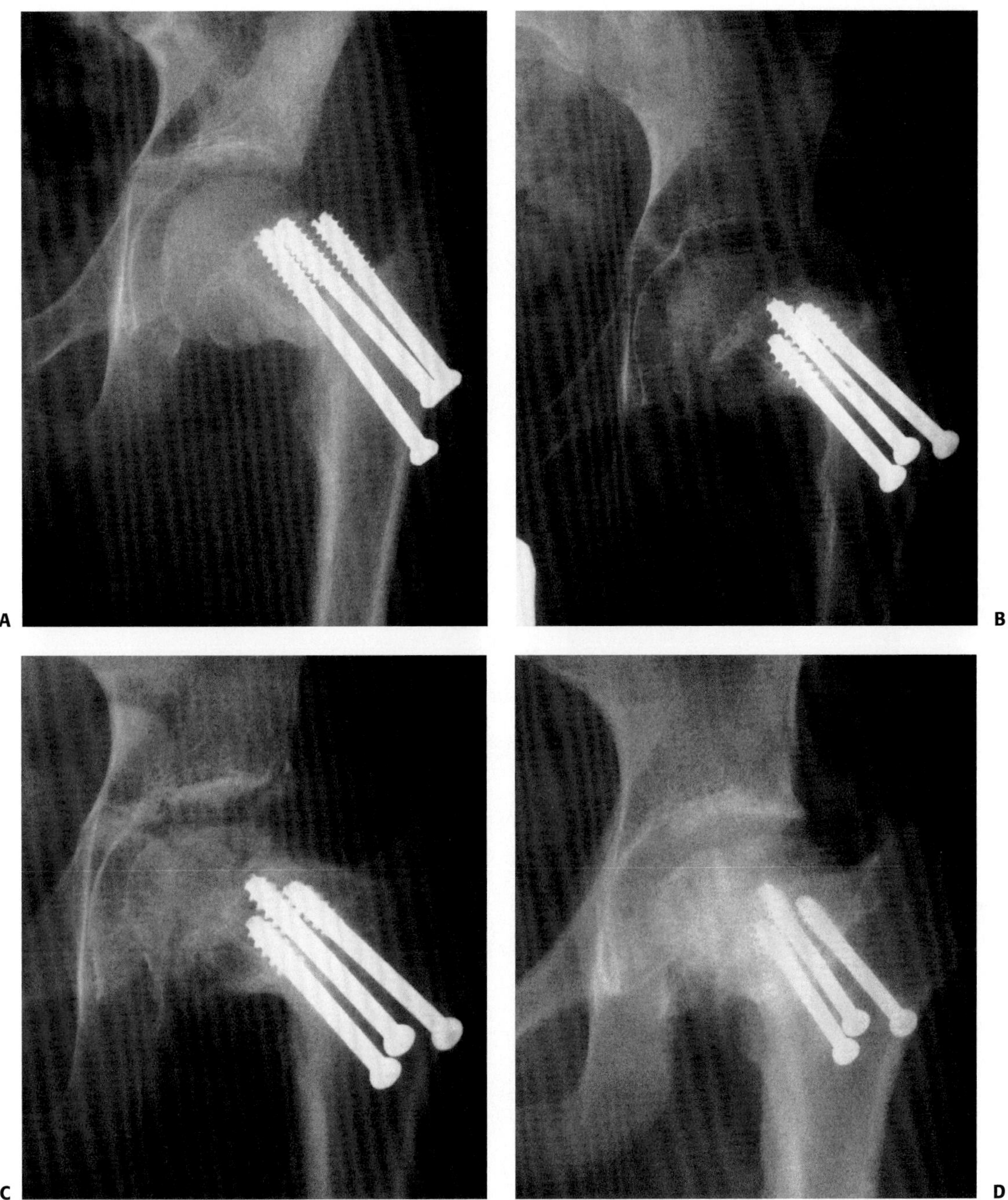

FIGURE 21-18 **A.** A 12-year-old boy with a type III left hip fracture. Poor pin placement and varus malposition are evident. **B.** The fracture united in mild varus after hardware revision. **C.** Fourteen months after injury. Collapse of the weight-bearing segment is evident (Ratliff type II ON). **D.** Six years after injury. Coxa breva and trochanteric overgrowth are seen secondary to ON, malunion, and premature physeal closure.

zation should be used in all but the most mature and cooperative adolescents.

Other Complications

Infection is uncommon after hip fractures in children. The reported incidence of 1% (1,8,9) is consistent with the expected infection rate in any closed fracture treated surgically with open reduction and internal fixation.

Chondrolysis is exceedingly rare and has been reported only in two series (7,32). Care must be taken to avoid persistent penetration of hardware into the joint, which can cause this condition.

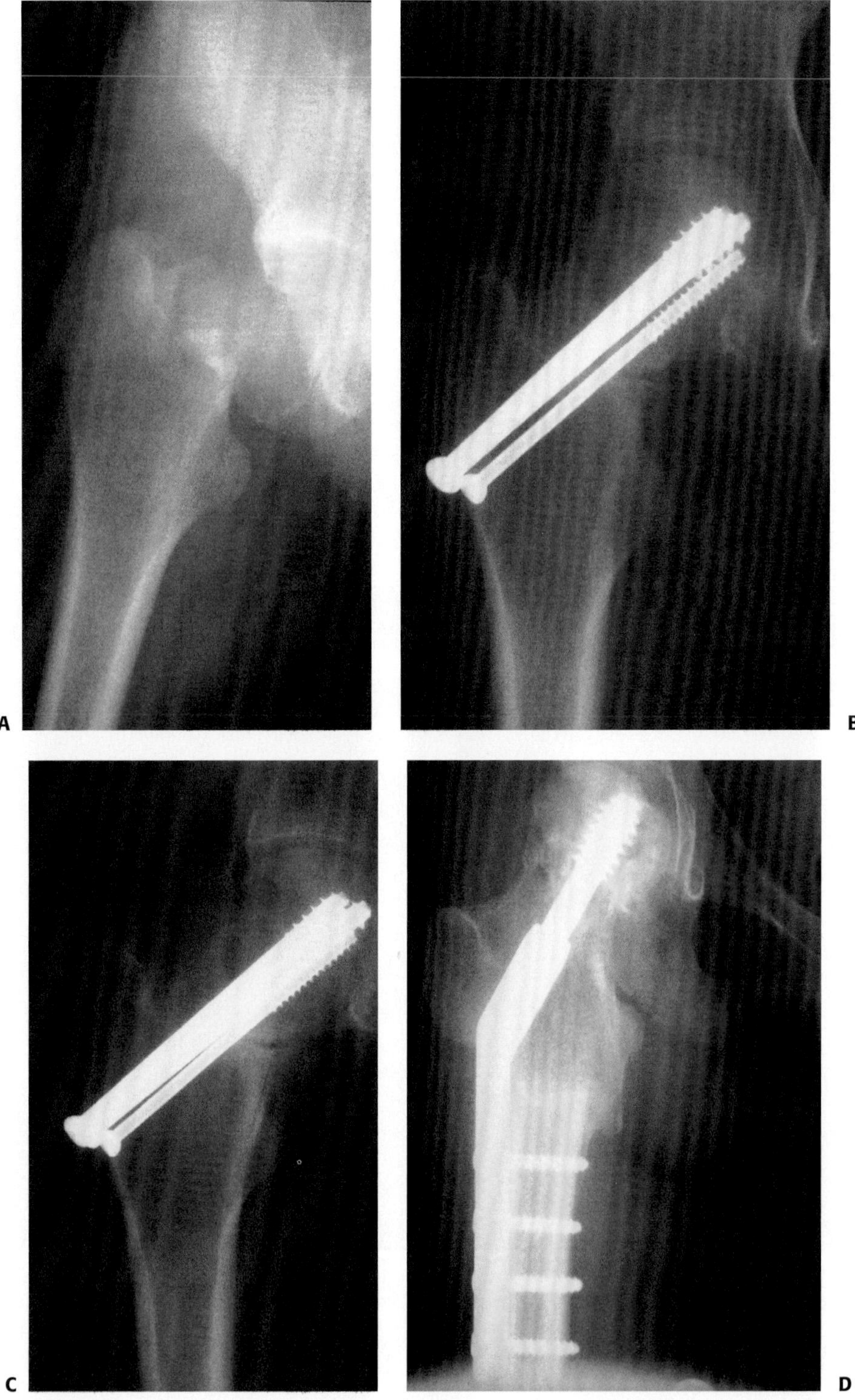

FIGURE 21-19 **A.** A 15-year-old girl with a markedly displaced type II femoral neck fracture. **B.** She underwent open reduction and internal fixation with two 7.3-mm cannulated screws and one 4.5-mm cannulated screw. Primary bone grafting of a large defect in the superior neck also was performed. **C.** X-ray at 5 months showing a persistent fracture line. **D.** Six weeks after valgus intertrochanteric osteotomy. The fracture is healing.

Stress Fractures

Stress fractures of the femoral neck are unusual in children: only 13 cases have been reported in the English-language literature. The rarity of such fractures underscores the need for a high index of suspicion when a child has unexplained hip pain, because early diagnosis and treatment are essential to avoid complete fracture with displacement.

Mechanism

Stress fractures of the femoral neck in children result from repetitive cyclic loading of the hip, such as that produced by a new or increased activity. A recent increase in the repetitive activity is highly suggestive of the diagnosis. Long-distance running, trampoline use, and scooter use are examples of such activities. Underlying metabolic disorders that weaken the bone may predispose to stress fracture. In adolescent female athletes, amenorrhea, anorexia nervosa, and osteoporosis have been implicated in the development of stress fractures of the femoral neck (33).

The usual presentation is that of progressive hip or groin pain with or without a limp. The pain may be perceived in the thigh or knee, and the pain may not be so severe as to preclude the offending activity. In the absence of displacement, examination typically reveals slight limitation of hip motion with increased pain, especially with internal rotation. Usually, plain x-rays reveal the fracture, but in the first 4 to 6 weeks after presentation, plain films may be negative. If there are no changes or only linear sclerosis, bone scan will help identify the fracture. MRI has been documented as a sensitive test for undisplaced fractures of the femoral neck because impaction of the bony trabeculae appears on both T1 and T2 images as a linear black signal (31). If a sclerotic lesion is seen on plain x-rays, the differential diagnosis should include osteoid osteoma, chronic sclerosing osteomyelitis, bone infarct, and osteosarcoma. Other causes of hip pain, including slipped capital femoral epiphysis, Legg-Calvé-Perthes disease, infection, avulsion injuries of the pelvis, and eosinophilic granuloma, should be considered. Stress fracture unrelieved by rest or treatment may progress with activity to complete fracture with displacement (34). For this reason, prompt diagnosis and treatment are important.

Classification

Devas classified femoral neck stress fractures into two types: compression fractures and tension fractures. The compression type appears as reactive bone formation on the inferior cortex without cortical disruption. This type rarely becomes completely displaced but may collapse into a mild varus deformity (35). Compression types have been reported to progress to complete fracture without early treatment (34). The tension type is a transverse fracture line appearing on the superior portion of the femoral neck (35). This type is inherently unstable because the fracture line is perpendicular to the lines of tension, and fractures heal best under compression. Tension stress fractures have not been reported in children but may occur in skeletally mature teenagers (34).

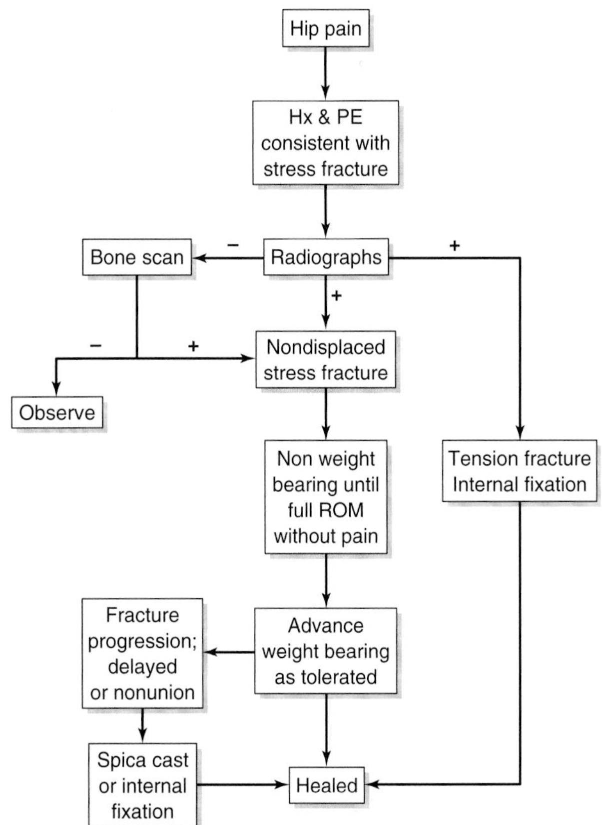

FIGURE 21-20 Treatment algorithm for hip pain in children and adolescents with a history and physical examination compatible with a stress fracture. (Reprinted from St. Pierre P, Staheli LT, Smith JB, et al. Femoral neck stress fractures in children and adolescents. *J Pediatr Orthop* 1995; 15:470–473.)

Treatment

Compression-type fractures generally can be treated with a period of non–weight bearing on crutches. Partial weight bearing can be allowed at 6 weeks and full weight bearing at 12 weeks if pain is resolved and there is radiographic evidence of healing. In small or uncooperative children, spica casting may be necessary. Displacement into varus, however minimal, mandates internal fixation. Tension fractures are at high risk for displacement and should be treated with in situ compression fixation using cannulated screws (Fig. 21-20).

Complications

Coxa vara is the most common complication of untreated compression-type fractures. Acute displacement of this type also has been described. Once displaced, the stress fracture is subject to all the complications of type II and type III displaced femoral neck fractures.

HIP DISLOCATIONS IN CHILDREN

Hip dislocations in children are relatively uncommon. They can occur in young children under age 5 as a result of seemingly trivial trauma (36–40). The child's acetabulum at that age is primarily soft pliable cartilage, and there is generalized ligamentous laxity that allows hip dislocation. Dislocations in older children usually require significant trauma because the acetabulum is bony and less resilient and the ligaments are stiffer (37–40). Most hip dislocations in children can be reduced easily and will heal satisfactorily (39,40), although the possibility of late problems exists (41). Difficulties after hip dislocation can include neurovascular injury, concomitant fracture, irreducibility, nonconcentric reduction, ON, coxa magna, arthritis, and recurrent dislocation.

Principles of Management

Mechanism of Injury

The mechanism of injury dictates the direction of hip dislocation. Posterior dislocations are the most common (36,40,41) and generally occur when a force is applied to the leg with the hip flexed. Anterior dislocations generally occur through a combination of external rotation and abduction.

Signs and Symptoms

The affected child has pain and inability to ambulate. Children sometimes feel the pain in the knee rather than in the hip (Fig. 21-21). The hallmark of the clinical diagnosis of dislocation of the hip is abnormal positioning of the limb, which is not seen in fracture of the femur. With posterior dislocation, the thigh tends to be flexed, adducted, and internally rotated. The greater trochanter is proximal to its normal position, and the femoral head often is palpable in the gluteal region. If the hip is dislocated anteriorly, the extremity generally is extended, abducted, and externally rotated.

Associated Injuries

Posterior dislocations of the femoral head can damage the sciatic nerve, and function of this nerve should be specifically tested after injury. Anterior dislocations can damage the femoral neurovascular bundle, and femoral nerve function and perfusion of the limb should be assessed. Fractures of the acetabulum, especially the posterior rim, are uncommon and especially rare in young children (42). Fractures of the femoral head or neck are rare. Tears of the capsule or acetabular labrum occur and prevent concentric reduction of the hip.

Diagnosis and Classification

Plain x-rays usually confirm the diagnosis. X-rays should be examined for fracture of the acetabular rim and proximal femur, which may be associated with dislocation. Ipsilateral femoral fracture has been described in a few patients (41). CT scanning is useful for evaluating the acetabulum and may be useful in localizing intraarticular bony fragments after reduction (43,44) (Fig. 21-22). The identification of nonbony fragments is difficult by CT without the use of concomitant arthrography (43). MRI is useful for evaluating soft tissues that may be interposed between the femoral head and acetabulum. MRI is especially helpful in nonconcentric reductions when the initial direction of dislocation is unknown. Soft tissue injury will dictate the surgical approach.

Spontaneous reduction may occur after hip dislocation (45–47), and the diagnosis will be missed if it is not considered. The presence of air in the hip joint, which may be detectable on CT scan of the pelvis, is evidence that a hip dislocation has occurred (48). Dislocation and spontaneous reduction with interposed tissue can occur and lead to late arthropathy if untreated (46). Widening of the joint space on plain x-rays suggests the diagnosis. In patients with hip pain, a history of trauma, and widening of the joint space, consideration should be given to MRI or arthrography to rule out dislocation with spontaneous relocation incarcerating soft tissue. If incarcerated soft tissues or osseous cartilage fragments are found, open reduction is required to obtain concentric reduction of the hip.

Hip dislocations in children generally are generally classified as anterior or posterior depending on where the femoral head lies after dislocation. Posterior dislocations are much more common than anterior dislocations and tend to occur as a result of an axial force on the femur applied toward the hip with the hip in flexion. Dashboard injury is a frequent cause. The limb assumes a position of shortening, internal rotation, and adduction (Fig. 21-23).

Anterior dislocations can occur superiorly or inferiorly and result from forced abduction and external rotation. In extension, the hip tends to dislocate anteriorly and superiorly. The limb appears shortened, the thigh is positioned in external rotation and extension, and the femoral head is palpable in the groin. If the hip dislocates with the leg flexed, the femoral head tends to dislocate inferiorly. The leg is held in abduction, external rotation, and flexion, and the femoral head is palpable near the obturator foramen (Fig. 21-24).

In very rare cases, the femoral head may dislocate inferiorly, a condition known as luxatio erecta femoris or infracotyloid dislocation. The hip is hyperflexed and the thigh rests upon the abdomen parallel to the long axis of the body. This condition is extremely rare but occurs more commonly in children than adults (42).

Fracture–dislocation of the hip involving the femoral head or the acetabulum is much more unusual in children than in adults. Older adolescents may sustain adult-type fracture–dislocations of the hip, and these are best classified by the methods of Thompson and Epstein and of Pipkin.

Habitual dislocation of the hip has been described in children. In this condition, the child can actually voluntarily dislocate the hip. Many factors may contribute to this ability, including generalized ligamentous laxity, excessive anteversion of the femur and acetabulum, coxa valga, and hyperlaxity disorders (49).

Surgical and Applied Anatomy

The hip joint is highly specialized. Although capable of bearing body weight, the hip still provides a tremendous range of

(text continues on page 23)

FIGURE 21-21 **A.** Not all children have severe pain with dislocation. An 8-year-old complained of pain and had difficulty walking after wrestling. Because of knee pain, a knee immobilizer was placed at an outside facility. **B.** The leg length discrepancy had gone unnoticed. **C.** The thigh was markedly shortened on the dislocated right side. **D.** Closed reduction was easily achieved under anesthesia. Thigh length was restored. She made an unremarkable recovery.

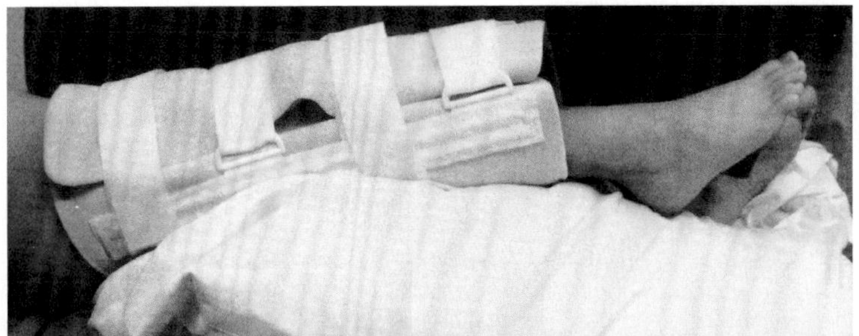
A

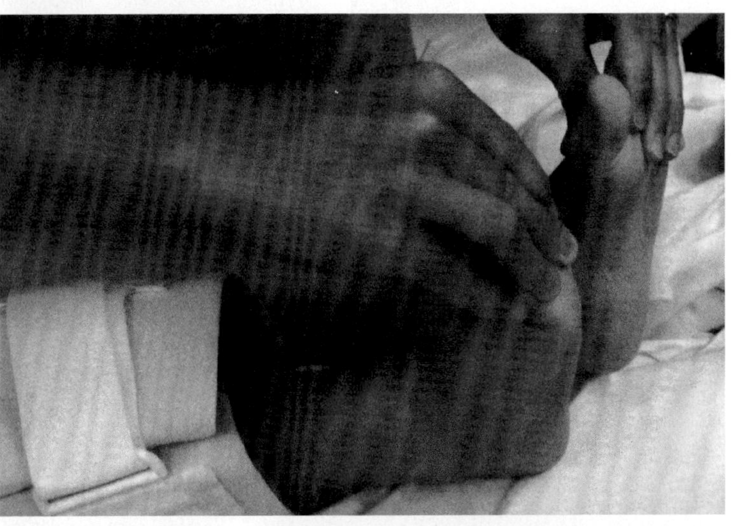
B

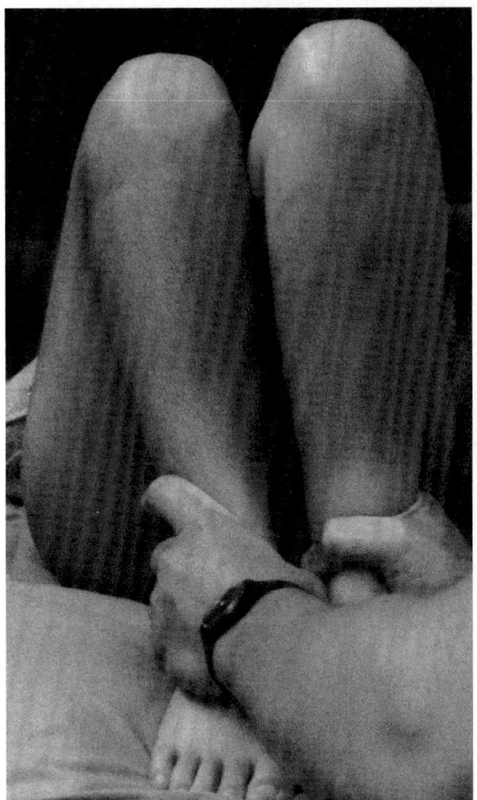
C

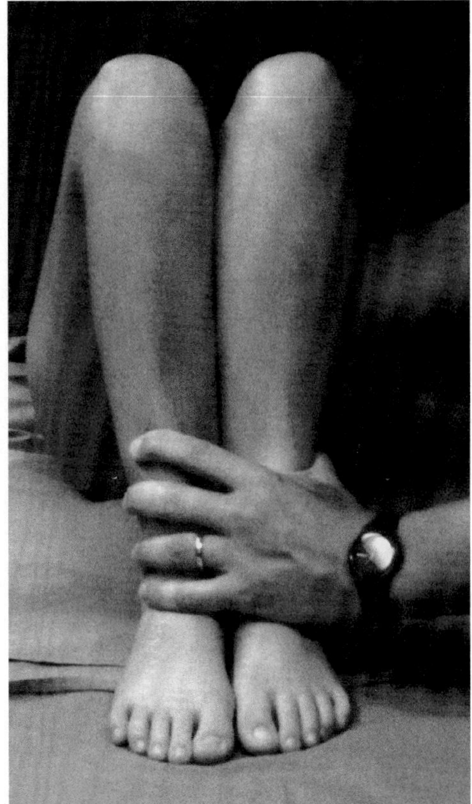
D

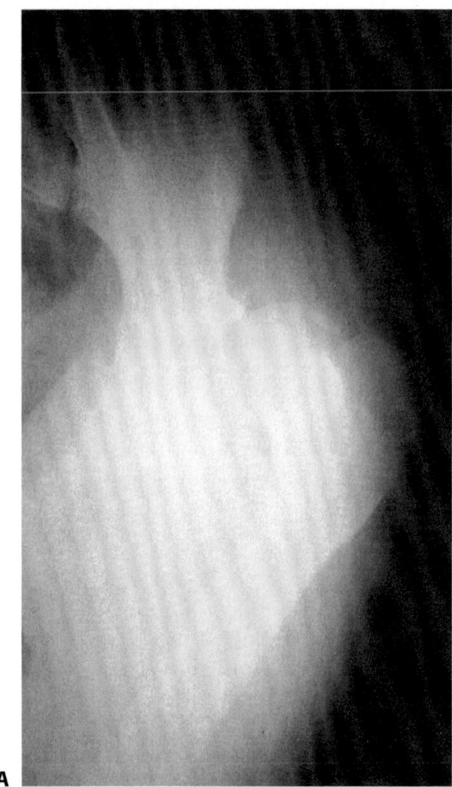

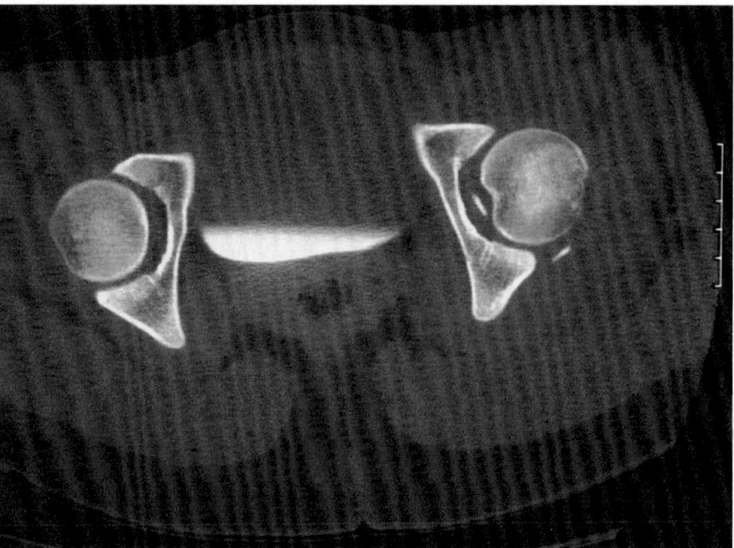

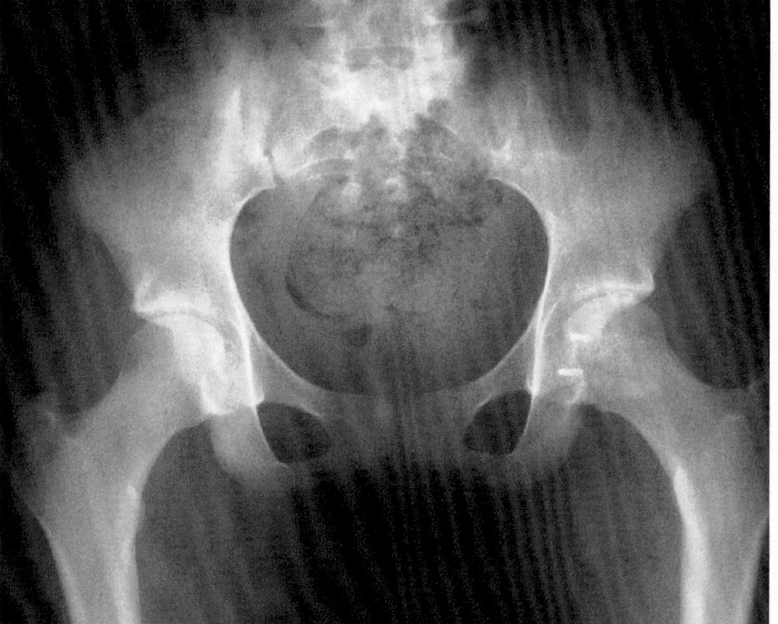

FIGURE 21-22 **A.** A girl age 13 years and 11 months sustained a left posterior hip dislocation in a motor vehicle accident. **B.** CT scan after reduction showed intraarticular bony fragments. **C.** At open reduction and capsulorrhaphy, the bony fragments were removed. Suture anchors were used to reattach capsule to bone. Ten months after injury, there is no sign of ON. Heterotopic ossification is seen.

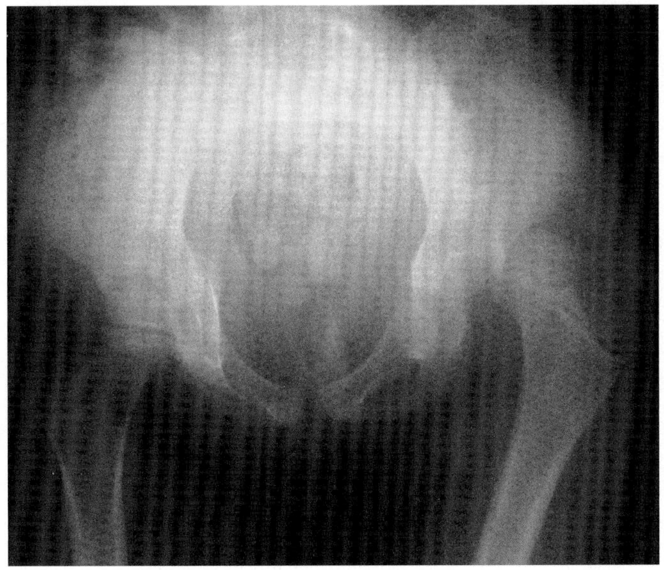

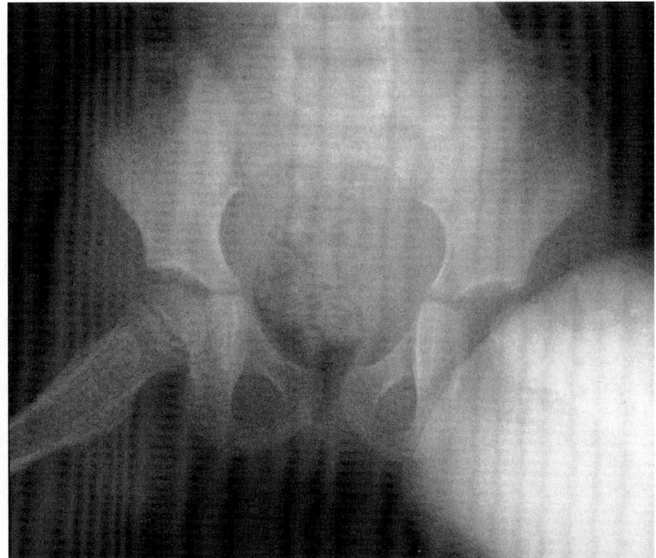

B

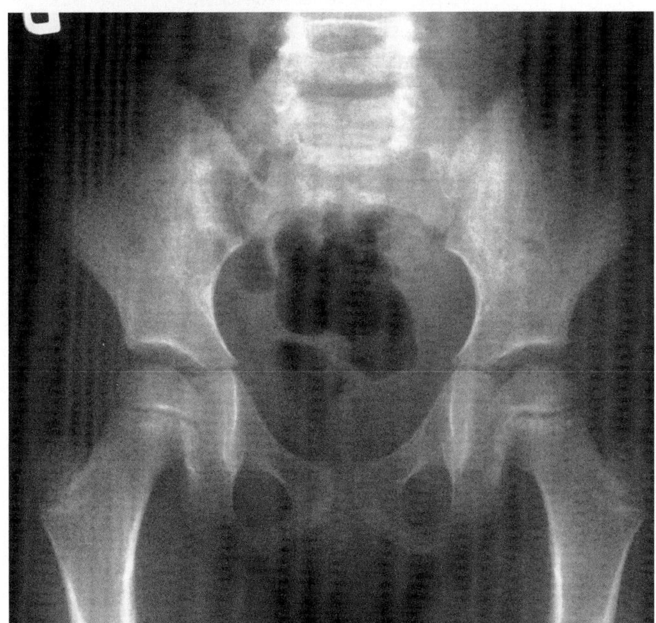

C

FIGURE 21-23 **A.** A girl age 4 years and 7 months presented with a posterior dislocation of the left hip. **B.** Frog-leg lateral x-ray at injury. **C.** Eight months after successful closed reduction, radiographic appearance is normal.

motion, surpassed only by the range of motion of the shoulder. The architecture of the hip joint is highly specialized and is centered on the spherical femoral head, which resides in the bony acetabulum. The relatively narrow femoral neck increases the range of motion possible at the hip joint in flexion, extension, abduction, and circumduction. A larger-diameter neck would impinge on the acetabular rim at extremes of motion.

Containment of the hip joint is ensured by several factors. The bony socket physically constrains the femoral head and is further deepened by the surrounding fibrocartilaginous acetabular labrum. In young children, the socket and labrum are largely cartilaginous and flexible. In older children, a larger proportion of the socket and rim is hard bone. Intimate contact between the cartilaginous surfaces of the round head and the socket, in the presence of joint fluid, provides a suction fit. In an intact joint, considerable force is required to disrupt this union. The strong fibrous joint capsule further contains the hip joint. The capsule is flexible enough to allow excellent range of motion but secure enough to maintain the hip reduced, except for extreme circumstances. The ligamentum teres does not provide any stability to the hip. The muscles that span the hip joint further provide active extrinsic stability by maintaining constant tension across the hip joint, which pushes the head into the acetabulum. These muscles, which provide the power

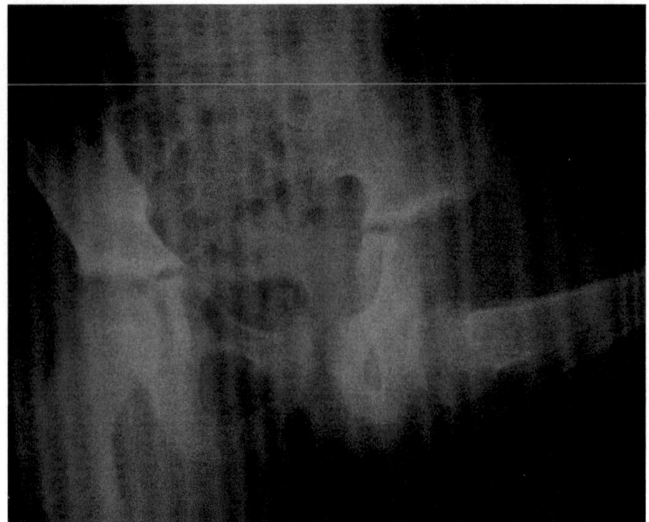

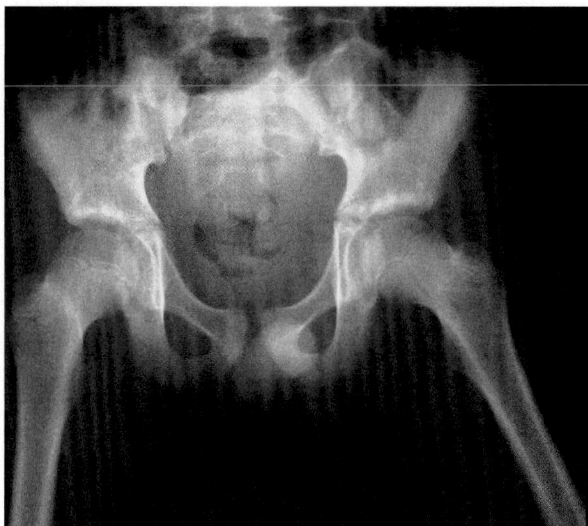

FIGURE 21-24 **A.** An 11-year-old girl sustained an anterior inferior dislocation of the hip. **B.** Immediate closed reduction was concentric.

for standing and locomotion, act around the fulcrum centered at the hip. Efficient transmission of muscle forces requires hip stability.

For the hip to dislocate, considerable force or mechanical advantage is required to overcome these restraints. The capsule must be torn or stretched. This will be deformed or disrupted at the time of dislocation. The ligamentum teres is likely to be torn, but this does not appear to result in any long-term sequelae.

Current Treatment Options

The immediate goal in the treatment of a dislocated hip is to obtain concentric reduction as soon as practical. Generally, closed reduction should be attempted initially. Successful closed reduction can be achieved with intravenous or intramuscular sedation in the emergency room in many patients (50). Complete muscle relaxation is required for others, and this is best provided in the operating room with a general anesthetic. Open reduction is indicated if closed reduction is unsuccessful or incomplete.

Several methods of closed reduction have been described. Stimson described a maneuver for reduction of posterior dislocation of the hip; it is also referred to as the gravity method of Stimson. In this method, the patient is placed prone with the lower limbs hanging over the edge of a table. Two persons are required to perform this maneuver. An assistant stabilizes the pelvis by applying pressure downward from above. The manipulator holds the affected knee and hip flexed 90 degrees and applies gentle downward pressure in an attempt to bring the posteriorly dislocated head over the posterior rim of the acetabulum and back into the socket. Gentle internal and external rotation may assist in the reduction.

Allis described a maneuver in which the patient is placed supine and the reducing surgeon stands above the patient. For this reason, either the patient must be placed on the floor or the surgeon must climb onto the operating table. The knee is flexed to relax the hamstrings. While an assistant stabilizes the pelvis, the surgeon applies longitudinal traction along the axis of the femur and gently manipulates the femoral head over the rim of the acetabulum and back into the socket.

Bigelow described a manipulative reduction in which the patient lies supine and an assistant provides downward pressure on the pelvis. The surgeon grasps the ipsilateral limb at the ankle with one hand, puts the opposite forearm behind the knee, and applies longitudinal traction in the axis of the femur. Internal rotation, adduction, and flexion of 90 degrees or more take the tension off the Y ligament and allow the surgeon to bring the femoral head to the level of the acetabulum, posteriorly. The femoral head is then levered into the acetabulum by abducting, externally rotating, and extending the hip. This is a more forceful maneuver than the others and may cause damage to the articular surfaces of hip or even fracture the femoral neck, so it should be used with great caution.

A technique called the reverse Bigelow maneuver can be used for anterior dislocation. In this technique, the hip is held in partial flexion and abduction. One of two reduction methods may be used. The first is a lifting method in which a firm jerk is applied to the thigh, which may result in reduction. If that fails, traction is applied in the line of the thigh and the hip is then sharply internally rotated, adducted, and extended. This manipulative method may result in reduction but also risks fracture of the femoral neck.

With any type of dislocation, traction along the axis of the thigh coupled with gentle manipulation of the hip often effects reduction after satisfactory relaxation of the surrounding muscles.

If satisfactory closed reduction cannot be obtained using reasonable measures, it is appropriate to proceed with open reduction to remove any obstructing soft tissues.

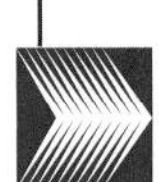

AUTHORS' PREFERRED TREATMENT

Expeditious closed reduction by applying traction in line with the femur and gently manipulating the femoral head back into the acetabulum is the first choice. Surgery is indicated for dislocations that are irreducible or nonconcentric.

Surgical Procedures

Open reduction of a posterior dislocation should be performed through a posterolateral approach. The patient is positioned in the lateral decubitus position with the dislocated side upward. The incision is centered on and just posterior to the greater trochanter and goes up into the buttock. Generally a straight incision can be made with the hip flexed approximately 90 degrees. Once the gluteal fascia lata is incised, the femoral head can be palpated beneath or within the substance of the gluteus maximus muscle. The fibers of the gluteus maximus can then be divided by blunt dissection, exposing the femoral head. The path of dislocation is followed through the short external rotator muscles and capsule down to the acetabulum. The sciatic nerve lies on the short external rotators and should be inspected. It may be necessary to detach the short external rotators to see inside the joint capsule.

Anterior dislocations should be approached through an anterior approach. This can be done through a bikini incision that uses the interval between the sartorius and the tensor fascia lata. The deep dissection follows the defect created by the femoral head down to the level of the acetabulum.

At the time of open reduction, the femoral head should be inspected for damage, scuffing, or fracturing. Before reduction, the acetabulum should be inspected and palpated for similar damage. Any intraarticular fragments should be removed. The labrum and capsule should be inspected for repairable tears. Labral fragments that cannot be securely replaced should be excised, but repair should be attempted. Frequently, the labrum or hip capsule is entrapped in the joint. The femoral head should be dislocated and any interposed soft tissue extracted. The labrum or capsule may be tied for ease in removal. Obstacles to reduction should be teased out of the way and the traumatic defect enlarged if necessary. The hip joint is then reduced under direct vision. X-rays should be taken to confirm concentric reduction. If the joint appears slightly widened, repeat investigation must rule out interposed tissue. Slight widening may be due to fluid in the hip joint, and this should settle out over the next few days. The capsule is repaired if possible. Closure is routine.

Open injuries should be treated with immediate irrigation and debridement. The surgical incision should incorporate and enlarge the traumatic wound. Inspection should proceed as detailed above. Capsular repair should be attempted if the hip joint is not contaminated. The wound should be left open or should be well drained to prevent invasive infection. As in all open fractures, intravenous antibiotics should be administered and repeat wound care performed as needed.

After reduction, treatment should be symptomatic. Generally a short period of recumbency, until the pain subsides, can be followed by return to ambulation with crutches if necessary (42). Bed rest, spica casting, skin traction, and non–weight bearing have not been proven to be beneficial (38,40,41). After open reduction with substantial capsulorrhaphy, immobilization or a spica cast may be indicated for 6 weeks to allow capsular healing. Return to full activities is encouraged.

Pearls and Pitfalls

- There are several pitfalls in the management of hip dislocations in children. It is always important to look for associated fractures. In older children, it is important to evaluate the posterior rim of the acetabulum after posterior dislocation to rule out fracture (Fig. 21-25). Relying on plain x-rays and CT may underestimate the extent of damage to the posterior wall of the acetabulum due to the incomplete ossification of the pediatric bone. MRI may be required to adequately assess the posterior wall of the acetabulum in children (51). Fractures at other sites in the femur must be considered. It is important to obtain x-rays that show the entire femur to rule out ipsilateral fracture. Fractures of the femoral head are distinctly unusual in children, but separation of the capital femoral epiphysis and femoral neck fracture have been reported in association with dislocation of the hip.
- Another pitfall is the possibility of spontaneous relocation of a dislocation of the hip. Failure to appreciate the presence of hip dislocation may lead to inadequate treatment. Traumatic hip subluxation occurs commonly in American football and may go undetected or may be treated as a sprain or strain if the diagnosis is not considered (45,47). Hip subluxation in football players may even result in ON without an overt hip dislocation (45). After dislocation and spontaneous reduction, soft tissue may become interposed in the hip joint. Chronic arthropathy may result. In a child with posttraumatic hip pain without obvious deformity, the possibility of dislocation–relocation must be considered. X-rays should be obtained to rule out joint space widening and undisplaced fracture.
- Another consideration after reduction of hip dislocations is interposed tissue. After reduction, hemarthrosis may initially cause the hip joint to appear slightly wide (50). With time, the hip should seat and the increased iliofemoral distance should subside (Fig. 21-26). If it fails to appear concentric after a few days, the possibility of interposed soft tissue must be considered (38,46,52,53).

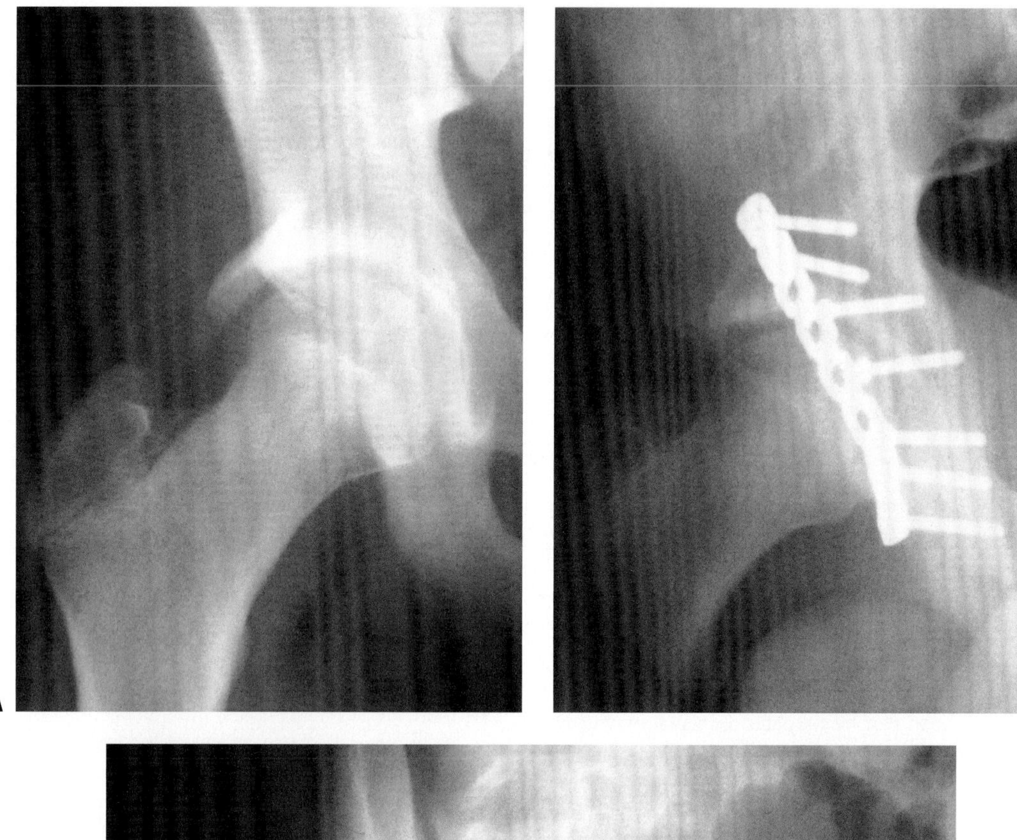

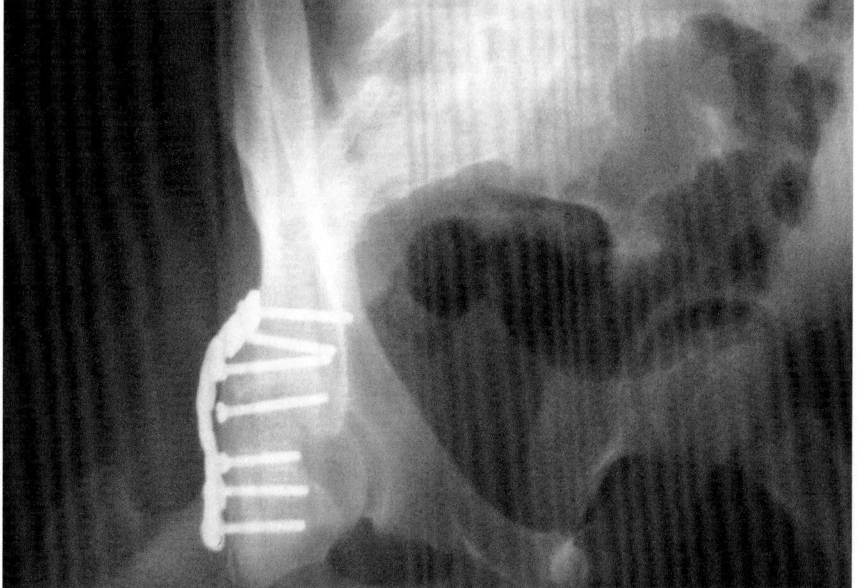

FIGURE 21-25 **A.** A 12-year-old boy was tackled from behind in football. The right hip was dislocated. Reduction was easily achieved, but the hip was unstable posteriorly as a result of fracture of the posterior rim of the acetabulum. **B.** The fracture and capsule were fixed via a posterior approach. **C.** Oblique view shows reconstitution of the posterior rim.

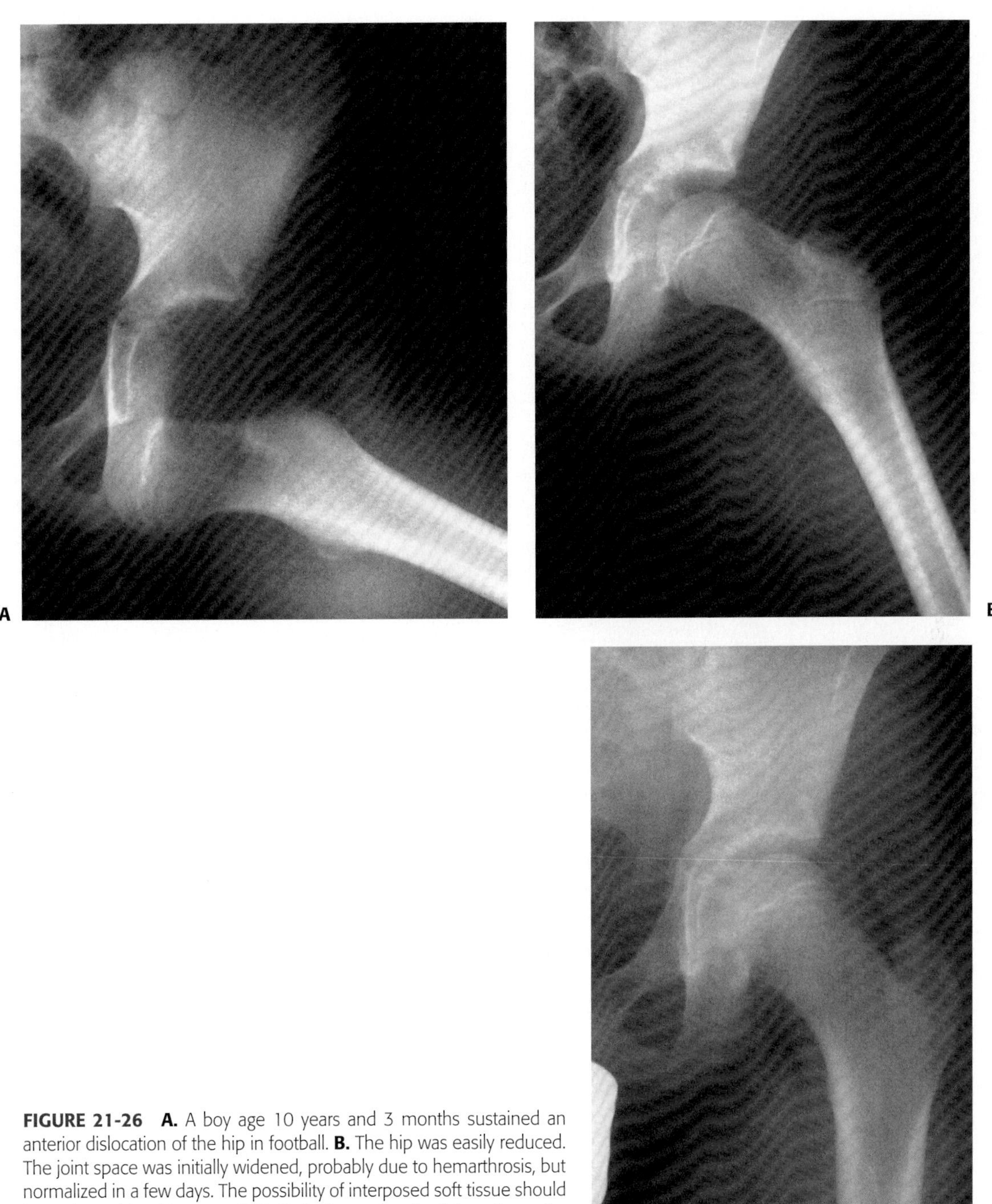

FIGURE 21-26 **A.** A boy age 10 years and 3 months sustained an anterior dislocation of the hip in football. **B.** The hip was easily reduced. The joint space was initially widened, probably due to hemarthrosis, but normalized in a few days. The possibility of interposed soft tissue should be evaluated by CT scan or MRI. **C.** At 4 months after injury, the radiographic appearance was normal.

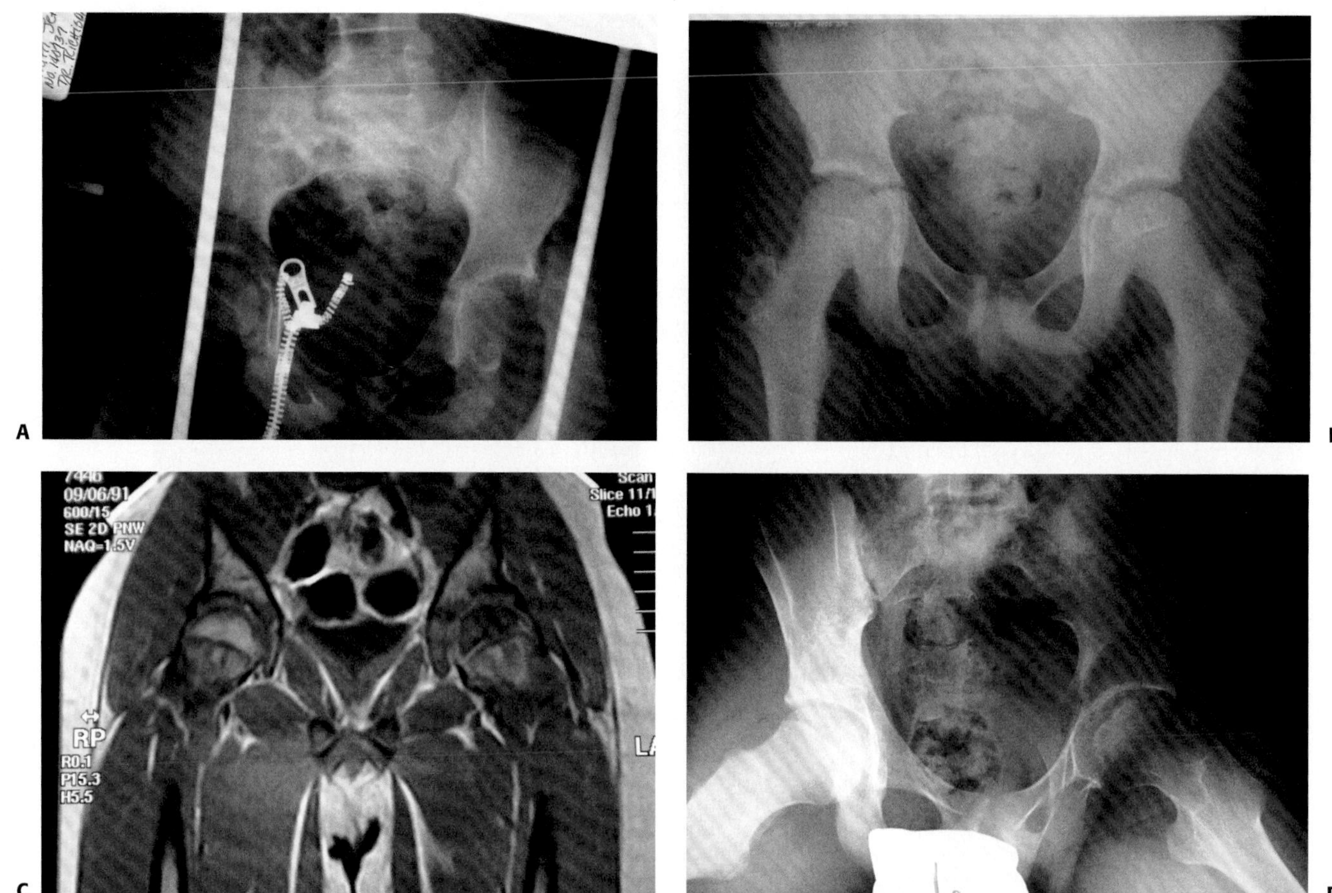

FIGURE 21-27 **A.** An 11-year-old boy dislocated his left hip while wrestling. **B.** The hip was easily reduced. **C.** After 5 months, hip pain led to an MRI, which shows ON of the capital femoral epiphysis. **D.** At 10 months after injury, there are typical changes of ON despite non–weight bearing.

Complications

Most hip dislocations in children resolve without sequelae. Complications are rare.

Vascular Injury

Impingement on the femoral neurovascular bundle has been described after anterior hip dislocation in children, and this may occur in 25% of patients (41). If there is femoral artery occlusion, the hip should be relocated as soon as possible to remove the offending pressure from the femoral vessels. If relocation of the hip fails to restore perfusion, immediate exploration of the femoral vessels is indicated.

Nerve Injury

The sciatic nerve may be damaged after a posterior dislocation of the hip in 2% to 13% of patients (40,41,54). Usually the nerve is directly compressed by the femoral head. The treatment is expedient relocation of the hip. Nerve function returns spontaneously in most patients (38,54). The nerve does not need to be explored unless open reduction is required for other reasons. If sciatic nerve function is shown to be intact and is lost during the reduction maneuver, the nerve should be explored to ensure that it has not displaced into the joint. Other nerves around the hip joint rarely are injured at dislocation. Treatment is generally expectant unless laceration or incarceration is suspected. If so, exploration is indicated.

Osteonecrosis

ON occurs in about 10% of hip dislocations in children (Fig. 21-27) (41,44,55). The most significant contribution to the blood supply to the superior portion of the femoral head is from the deep branch of the medial femoral circumflex artery, which terminates in two to four superior retinacular vessels. Experimental studies suggest that perfusion of the femoral head is interrupted by kinking or compression of extracapsular vessels, which explains why the incidence of ON is related to the period of time the hip is dislocated (56). This is why prompt relocation of the hip, especially within 24 hours, may decrease the incidence of this complication (37,44,41). The risk of ON probably is also related to the severity of initial trauma (41). If the force of hip dislocation is so strong as to disrupt the obturator externus muscle, the posterior ascending vessels may be torn (56). Increased intracapsular pressure as a result of hemarthrosis may have a role (50). The type of postreduction care has not been shown to influence the rate of ON.

Early technetium bone scanning detects ON as an area of decreased uptake. This is best seen on pinhole collimated images. After a few weeks, with the onset of revascularization and reossification, the uptake may appear normal or even increased.

MRI detects avascularity of the capital femoral epiphysis as loss of signal on T1-weighted images (57). Findings on T2-weighted images are abnormal but of variable signal intensity.

After hip dislocation, routine screening for ON by bone scan or MRI cannot be strongly recommended for several reasons. Even if a perfusion defect is detected, there is no known treatment that will reverse it. Secondly, MRI may be falsely negative if performed within a few days of injury (57). Furthermore, hips with abnormal bone scan and MRI weeks after injury may not develop symptomatic ON. In fact, a large proportion of perfusion defects seen on MRI spontaneously resolve after several months (57,58). Bone scanning to detect ON after hip dislocation is fraught with false-positive and false-negative results so cannot be considered to be a reliable predictor (44).

If hips are followed by serial x-rays for ON, it is recommended that they be studied for at least 2 years after dislocation, because radiographic changes may appear late (36). If MRI yields normal findings 4 to 6 weeks after injury, no further study is necessary because the risk of developing symptomatic ON is miniscule (57).

If ON develops, pain, loss of motion, and deformity of the femoral head are likely (Fig. 21-28) (59). ON in a young child resembles Perthes disease and may be treated like Perthes disease (59). Priorities are to maintain mobility and containment of the femoral head to maximize congruity after resolution. ON in older children should be treated as in adults and may require hip fusion, osteotomy, or reconstruction, as discussed following femoral neck fractures.

Recurrent Dislocation

Recurrence after traumatic hip dislocation is rare but occurs most frequently after posterior dislocation in children under 8 years of age (60,61) or in children with known hyperlaxity (Down syndrome, Ehlers-Danlos disease). The incidence is estimated at no more than 3% (39). At surgical exploration of these hips, recurrence has been found to result from either laxity or a defect in the capsule (60). Recurrence can be quite disabling and in the long term may result in damage to the articular surfaces due to scuffing. Arthrography is recommended to identify a capsular defect or redundancy (60). Prolonged spica casting (at least 3 months) may stop recurrence (62), but exploration with capsulorrhaphy is a more rapid and reliable solution (60–62). In older children, recurrent dislocation can occur as a result of a bony defect in the posterior rim of the acetabulum similar to that in adults and may require posterior acetabular reconstruction.

Habitual Dislocation

Habitual or voluntary dislocation of the hip usually is unrelated to trauma. Many factors may contribute to this ability, including generalized ligamentous laxity, excessive anteversion of the femur and acetabulum, and coxa valga. Initial management should include counseling the child to cease the activity (with or without psychiatric counseling) and observation. If episodes of dislocation persist, permanent changes such as secondary capsular laxity or osteocartilaginous deformation of the hip may occur. These changes may lead to pain, residual subluxation, or degenerative joint disease. Corrective surgery should be tailored to match the anatomic abnormality and may include capsular plication, periacetabular osteotomy, or osteotomy of the femur (49).

Chondrolysis

Chondrolysis has been reported after hip dislocation in up to 6% of children (38,39,55,63) and probably occurs as a result of articular damage at the time of dislocation. Chondrolysis cannot be reversed by medical means, and treatment should be symptomatic. Antiinflammatory medicines and weight-relieving devices should be used as needed. If the joint fails to reconstitute, fusion or reconstruction should be considered.

Coxa Magna

Coxa magna occasionally occurs after hip dislocation. The reported incidence ranges from 0% to 47% (39,55,63). It is believed to occur as a result of posttraumatic hyperemia (39). In most children, this condition is asymptomatic and does not require any treatment (39). There is no intervention that will prevent coxa magna.

Late Presentation

Not all hip dislocations in children cause severe or incapacitating symptoms. Ambulation may even be possible (see Fig. 21-19). As a result, treatment may be delayed or the diagnosis missed until shortening of the limb and contracture are well established, making reduction difficult. Prolonged heavy traction will sometimes effect reduction (64). Preoperative traction, extensive soft tissue release, or primary femoral shortening should be considered if open reduction is required. Open reduction will likely be difficult and will not always be successful. Even if the hip stays reduced, progressive arthropathy may lead to a stiff and painful hip. The likelihood of a good result decreases with the duration of dislocation.

Interposed Soft Tissue

Interposed tissues may cause nonconcentric reduction or result in complete failure of closed reduction. Muscle, bone, articular cartilage, and labrum have been implicated (37,38,47,52,53,65). CT arthrography or MRI provides information on obstacles to complete reduction and the direction of the initial dislocation (52,53). Open reduction generally is necessary to clear impeding tissues from the joint (38,39,52,53,65), even late

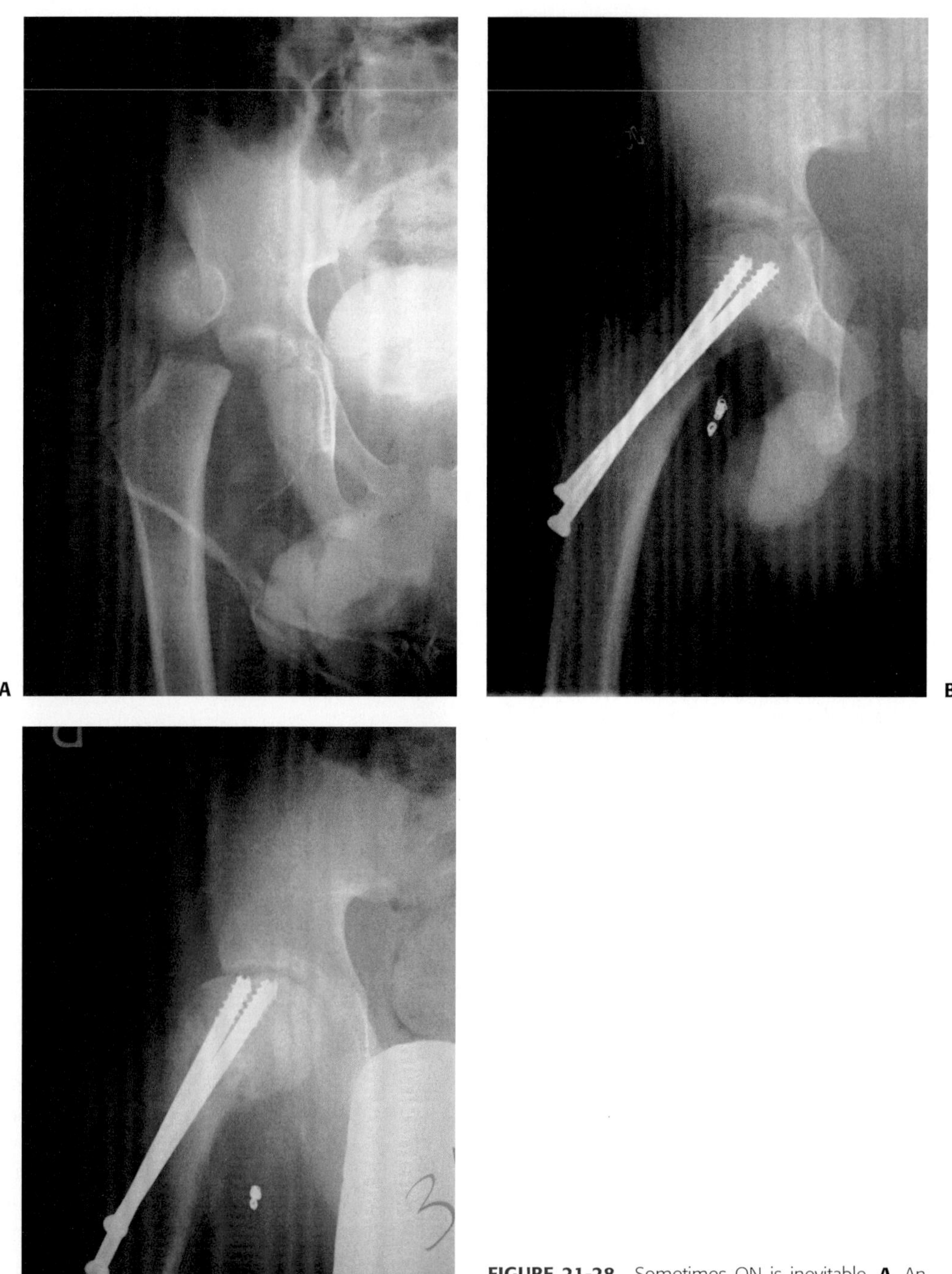

FIGURE 21-28 Sometimes ON is inevitable. **A.** An 11-year old boy struck by a car had a fracture–dislocation of the hip. **B.** Open reduction and internal fixation was successful. At surgery there was no soft tissue attached to the femoral head segment. **C.** At 7 months, ON was obvious.

(47). Untreated nonconcentric reduction may lead to permanent degenerative arthropathy (46).

REFERENCES

1. Ratliff AHC. Fractures of the neck of the femur in children. *J Bone Joint Surg [Br]* 1962; 44:528–542.
2. Hughes LO, Beaty JH. Current concepts review: fractures of the head and neck of the femur in children. *J Bone Joint Surg [Am]* 1994;76:283–292.
3. Canale ST, Beaty JH. Pelvic and hip fractures. In: Rockwood CA Jr, Wilkins KE, Beaty JH, eds. *Fractures in children,* 4th ed. Philadelphia: Lippincott-Raven, 1996:1109–1193.
4. Currey JD, Butler G. Mechanical properties of bone tissue in children. *J Bone Joint Surg [Am]* 1975;57:810–814.
5. Pape H, Krettek C, Friedrich A, et al. Long-term outcome in children with fractures of the proximal femur after high energy trauma. *J Trauma* 1999;46:58–64.
6. Mirdad T. Fractures of the neck of the femur in children: an experience at the Aseer Central Hospital, Abha, Saudi Arabia. *Injury Int J Care Injured* 2002;33:823–827.
7. Bagatur AE, Zorer G. Complications associated with surgically treated hip fractures in children. *J Pediatr Orthop B* 2002;11:219–228.
8. Lam SF. Fractures of the neck of the femur in children. *J Bone Joint Surg [Am]* 1971; 53:1165–1179.
9. Canale ST, Bourland WL. Fracture of the neck and intertrochanteric region of the femur in children. *J Bone Joint Surg [Am]* 1977;59:431–443.
10. Flynn JM, Wong KL, Yeh GL, et al. Displaced fractures of the hip in children: management by early operation and immobilization in a hip spica cast. *J Bone Joint Surg [Br]* 2002;84:108–112.
11. Cheng JCY, Tang N. Decompression and stable internal fixation of femoral neck fractures in children can affect the outcome. *J Pediatr Orthop* 1999;19:338–343.
12. Morsy HA. Complications of fracture of the neck of the femur in children. A long-term follow-up study. *Injury Int J Care Injured* 2001;32:45–51.
13. Ingari JV, Smith DK, Aufdemorte TB, et al. Anatomic significance of magnetic resonance imaging findings in hip fracture. *Clin Orthop Rel Res* 1996;332:209–214.
14. Colonna PC. Fracture of the neck of the femur. *J Bone Joint Surg [Am]* 1976;58:961–970.
15. Edgren W. Coxa plana. A clinical and radiological investigation with particular reference to the importance of the metaphyseal changes for the final shape of the proximal part of the femur. *Acta Orthop Scand Suppl* 1965;84:1–129.
16. Swischuk LE. Irritable infant and left lower extremity pain. *Pediatr Emerg Care* 1997; 13:147–148.
17. Jerre R, Karlsson J. Outcome after transphyseal hip fractures. *Acta Orthop Scand* 1997; 68:235–238.
18. Ogden JA. Changing patterns of proximal femoral vascularity. *J Bone Joint Surg [Am]* 1974;56:941–950.
19. Ratliff AHC. Complications after fractures of the femoral neck in children and their treatment. *J Bone Joint Surg [Br]* 1970;52:175.
20. Alho A. Concurrent ipsilateral fractures of the hip and femoral shaft. *Acta Orthop Scand* 1996;67:19–28.
21. Ashwood N, Wojcik AS. Traumatic separation of the upper femoral epiphysis in a 15-month-old girl: an unusual mechanism of injury. *Injury* 1995;26:695–696.
22. Langenskiold A, Salenius P. Epiphyseodesis of the greater trochanter. *Acta Orthop Scand* 1967;38:199–219.
23. Hansman CF. Appearance and fusion of ossification centers in the human skeleton. *AJR Am J Roentgenol* 1962;88:476–482.
24. Chung SMD. The arterial supply of the developing proximal end of the human femur in childhood. A report of six cases. *Ann Surg* 1928;88:902–907.
25. Trueta J. The normal vascular anatomy of the human femoral head during growth. *J Bone Joint Surg [Br]* 1957;39:358–393.
26. Trueta J, Morgan JD. The vascular contribution to osteogenesis. *J Bone Joint Surg [Br]* 1960;42:97–109.
27. Bray TJ. Femoral neck fracture fixation. *Clin Orthop Rel Res* 1997;339:20–31.
28. Davison BL, Weinstein SL. Hip fractures in children: a long-term follow-up study. *J Pediatr Orthop* 1992;12:355–358.
29. Ng GP, Cole WG. Effect of early hip decompression on the frequency of avascular necrosis in children with fractures of the neck of the femur. *Injury* 1996;27:419–421.
30. Soto-Hall R, Johnson LH, Johnson RA. Variations in the intra-articular pressure of the hip joint in injury and disease. *J Bone Joint Surg [Am]* 1964;46:509–516.
31. Maruenda JI, Barrios C, Gomar-Sancho F. Intracapsular hip pressure after femoral neck fracture. *Clin Orthop Rel Res* 1997;340:172–180.
32. Forlin E, Guille JT, Kumar SJ, et al. Transepiphyseal fractures of the neck of the femur in very young children. *J Pediatr Orthop* 1992;12:503–509.
33. Haddad FS, Bann S, Hill RA, et al. Displaced stress fracture of the femoral neck in an active amenorrhoeic adolescent. *Br J Sports Med* 1997;31:70–75.
34. St. Pierre P, Staheli LT, Smith JB, et al. Femoral neck stress fractures in children and adolescents. *J Pediatr Orthop* 1995;15:470–473.
35. Devas MB. Stress fractures of the femoral neck. *J Bone Joint Surg [Br]* 1965;47:728–738.
36. Barquet A. Traumatic hip dislocation in childhood. *Acta Orthop Scand* 1979;50:549–553.
37. Funk FJ. Traumatic dislocation of the hip in children. *J Bone Joint Surg [Am]* 1962;44: 1135–1145.
38. Hamilton PR, Broughton NS. Traumatic hip dislocation in childhood. *J Pediatr Orthop* 1989;18:691–694.
39. Offierski CM. Traumatic dislocation of the hip in children. *J Bone Joint Surg [Br]* 1981; 63:194–197.
40. Schlonsky J, Miller PR. Traumatic hip dislocations in children. *J Bone Joint Surg [Am]* 1973;55:1057–1063.
41. Scientific Research Committee of the Pennsylvania Orthopaedic Society. Traumatic dislocation of the hip in children. Final report. *J Bone Joint Surg [Am]* 1968;50:79–88.
42. Salisbury RD, Eastwood DM. Traumatic dislocation of the hip in children. *Clin Orthop Rel Res* 2000;377:106–111.
43. Hernandez RJ, Poznanski AK. CT evaluation of pediatric hip disorders. *Orthop Clin North Am* 1985;16:513–541.
44. Mehlman CT, Gregory WH, Crawford AH, et al. Traumatic hip dislocation in children. *Clin Orthop Rel Res* 2000;376:68–79.
45. Moorman CT, Warren RF, Hershman EB, et al. Traumatic posterior hip subluxation in American football. *J Bone Joint Surg [Am]* 2003;85:1190–1196.
46. Olsson O, Landin LA, Johansson A. Traumatic hip dislocation with spontaneous reduction and capsular interposition. *Acta Orthop Scand* 1994;65:476–479.
47. Price CT, Pyevich MT, Knapp DR, et al. Traumatic hip dislocation with spontaneous incomplete reduction: a diagnostic trap. *J Orthop Trauma* 2002;16:730–735.
48. Fairbairn KJ, Mulligan ME, Murphey MD, et al. Gas bubbles in the hip joint on CT: an indication of recent dislocation. *AJR Am J Roentgenol* 1996;166:472–473.
49. Song KS, Choi IH, Sohn YJ, et al. Habitual dislocation of the hip in children: a report of eight additional cases and literature review. *J Pediatr Orthop* 2003;23:178–183.
50. Rieger H, Pennig D, Klein W, Grunert J. Traumatic dislocation of the hip in young children. *Arch Orthop Trauma Surg* 1991;110:114–117.
51. Rubel IF, Kloen P, Potter HG, Helfet DL. MRI assessment of the posterior acetabular wall fracture in traumatic dislocation of the hip in children. *Pediatr Radiol* 2002;32: 435–439.
52. Gennari JM, Merrot T, Bergoin V, et al. X-ray transparency interpositions after reduction of traumatic dislocations of the hip in children. *Eur J Pediatr Surg* 1996;6:288–293.
53. Shea KP, Kalamachi A, Thompson GH. Acetabular epiphysis–labrum entrapment following traumatic anterior dislocation of the hip in children. *J Pediatr Orthop* 1986;6: 215–219.
54. Epstein HC. Traumatic dislocations of the hip. *Clin Orthop Rel Res* 1973;92:116–142.
55. Glass A, Powell HDW. Traumatic dislocation of the hip in children. An analysis of forty-seven patients. *J Bone Joint Surg [Br]* 1961;43:29–37.
56. Nötzli HP, Siebenrock KA, Hempfing A, et al. Perfusion of the femoral head during surgical dislocation of the hip. Monitoring by laser Doppler flowmetry. *J Bone Joint Surg [Br]* 2002;84:300–304.
57. Poggi JJ, Callaghan JJ, Spritzer CE, et al. Changes on magnetic resonance images after traumatic hip dislocation. *Clin Orthop Rel Res* 1995;319:249–259.
58. Godley DR, Williams RA. Traumatic dislocation of the hip in a child: usefulness of MRI. *Orthopedics* 1993;16:1145–1147.
59. Barquet A. Natural history of avascular necrosis following traumatic hip dislocation in childhood. A review of 145 cases. *Acta Orthop Scand* 1982;53:815–820.
60. Barquet A. Recurrent traumatic dislocation of the hip in childhood. *J Trauma* 1980;20: 1003–1006.
61. Gaul RW. Recurrent traumatic dislocation of the hip in children. *Clin Orthop Rel Res* 1973;90:107–109.
62. Wilchinsky ME, Pappas AM. Unusual complications in traumatic dislocation of the hip in children. *J Pediatr Orthop* 1985;5:534–539.
63. Hougard K, Thomsen PB. Traumatic hip dislocation in children. Follow-up of 13 cases. *Orthopedics* 1989;12:375–378.
64. Gupta RC, Shravat BP. Reduction of neglected traumatic dislocation of the hip by heavy traction. *J Bone Joint Surg [Am]* 1977;59:249–251.
65. Canale ST, Manugian AH. Irreducible traumatic dislocations of the hip. *J Bone Joint Surg [Am]* 1979;61:7–14.

22

FEMORAL SHAFT FRACTURES

James R. Kasser and James H. Beaty

Femoral shaft fractures, including subtrochanteric and supracondylar fractures, represent approximately 1.6% of all bony injuries in children. The male to female ratio of femoral fracture is 2.6:1 with a bimodal distribution (1–3). The first peak occurs in early childhood and the second in mid-adolescence. A review of the Maryland Hospital Discharge Database by Hinton et al (4) confirmed the bimodal distribution with peak incidences at 2 and 12 years of age. The annual rate of femoral shaft fracture in children was 1 per 5,000. In Switzerland, the incidence of pediatric femoral shaft fracture is 1 per 2,000 per year (5).

Although femoral shaft fractures are dramatic and disabling injuries, both to the patient and the family, most unite rapidly without significant complications or sequelae. Not many years ago, traction and casting were standard treatment for all femoral shaft fractures in children, and femoral fractures ranked high in duration of hospitalization for a single diagnosis (6). More recently, a variety of therapeutic alternatives, such as external fixation, compression or submuscular plating, and flexible or locked intramedullary nailing, have become available, decreasing impairment, increasing convenience, and decreasing cost of care. An increasingly aggressive approach to femoral shaft fractures appears to be continuing. It is important to note that treatment of "pediatric" femur fractures encompass the newborn to skeletally mature adolescent. Numerous treatment options are possible and should be tailored to each patient's case.

ANATOMY

Children's bone changes from primarily weak woven bone to stronger lamellar bone through remodeling during childhood (7). Strength also is increased by a change in geometry (Fig. 22-1). The increasing diameter and area of bone result in a markedly increased area moment of inertia, leading to marked increase in strength. This progressive increase in bone strength helps explain the bimodal distribution of femoral fractures. In early childhood, the femur is relatively weak and breaks under load conditions reached in normal play. In adolescence, high-velocity trauma is required to reach the stresses necessary for fracture.

MECHANISM OF INJURY

The etiology of femoral fractures in children varies with the age of the child. In children younger than walking age, up to 80% of femoral fractures may be caused by abuse (8–10); in children under 4 years of age, up to 30% of femoral fractures may be caused by abuse. Blakemore et al (11) reported that in 42 children 1 to 5 years of age who had femoral fractures, a history of fall was present in 34. Although the history was considered suspicious for intentional injury in 14 patients, only 1 patient had a documented abuse-related injury. Older children are unlikely to have a femoral shaft fracture caused by abuse, because their bone is sufficiently strong to tolerate forceful blows or is able to resist torque without fracture. In older children, femoral fractures are most likely to be caused by high-energy injuries, such as motor vehicle accidents, which account for over 90% of femoral fractures in this age-group (2,12,13). Gunshot wounds are an increasingly common cause of femoral fractures.

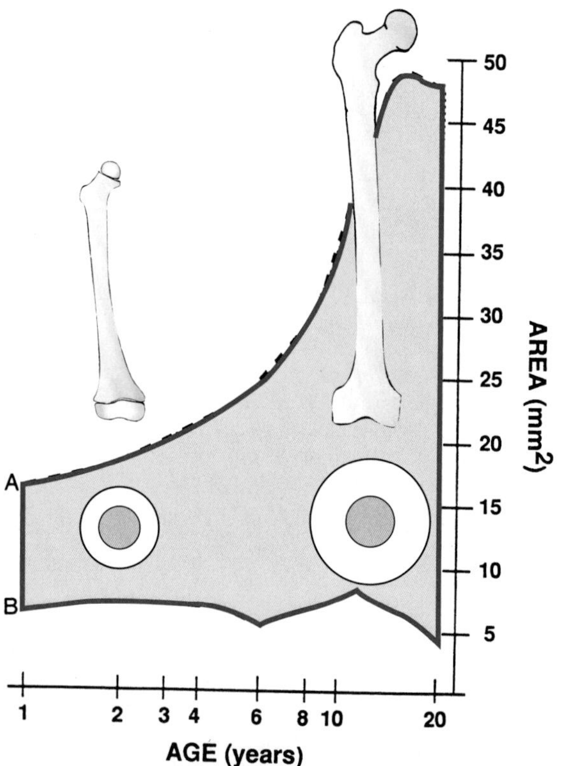

FIGURE 22-1 The shaded area represents cortical thickness by age-group. This rapid increase in cortical thickness may contribute to the diminishing incidence of femoral fractures during late childhood. (Redrawn from Netter FH. *The Ciba collection of medical illustrations.* Vol. 8. *Musculoskeletal System.* I. *Anatomy, Physiology, and Metabolic Disorders.* Summit, NJ: Ciba-Geigy; 1987; with permission.)

Pathologic femoral fractures are relatively rare in children, but they may occur because of generalized osteopenia in infants or young children with osteogenesis imperfecta. A femoral fracture in a young child with no history suggestive of abuse or significant trauma should suggest the possibility of osteogenesis imperfecta (14). Radiologic evaluation is often insufficient to diagnose osteogenesis imperfecta, and skin biopsy, collagen analysis, and bone biopsy may be required to make a definitive diagnosis. Generalized osteopenia also may accompany neurologic diseases, such as cerebral palsy or myelomeningocele, leading to fracture with minor trauma in osteopenic bone (1,15,16). Pathologic fractures may occur in patients with neoplasms, most often benign lesions such as nonossifying fibroma, aneurysmal bone cyst, unicameral cyst, or eosinophilic granuloma. Pathologic femoral fractures rarely occur in pediatric patients but one must always be looking for the subtle signs of primary lesions predisposing to fracture, such as mixed lytic-blastic areas disrupting trabecular architecture, break in the cortex and periosteal reaction in malignant lesions such as osteosarcoma, or better-defined sclerotic borders with an intact cortex seen in benign lesions such as nonossifying fibroma (Fig. 22-2).

Stress fractures may occur in any location in the femoral shaft (17–19). Most occur in adolescents involved in sports activity, such as football, lacrosse, and track. Although uncommon (4% of all stress fractures in children), femoral shaft or femoral neck stress fractures should be considered in a child with thigh pain because an unrecognized stress fracture may progress to a displaced femoral fracture. As the number of young children involved in athletics increases, stress fractures will become more frequent (20). Bilateral femoral stress fractures were reported in a rollerblade enthusiast, reflecting a departure from the traditional sports recognized as being related to this injury (21).

An unusual femoral fracture reported in infants is a greenstick fracture of the medial distal femoral metaphysis that occurs when the parent falls on a child who is straddling the parent's hip. It is important to recognize this fracture because it occurs in infants at an age when abuse is the leading cause of femoral fracture. The fracture is caused by bending of the femur, which produces a compression injury to the medial cortex. This injury

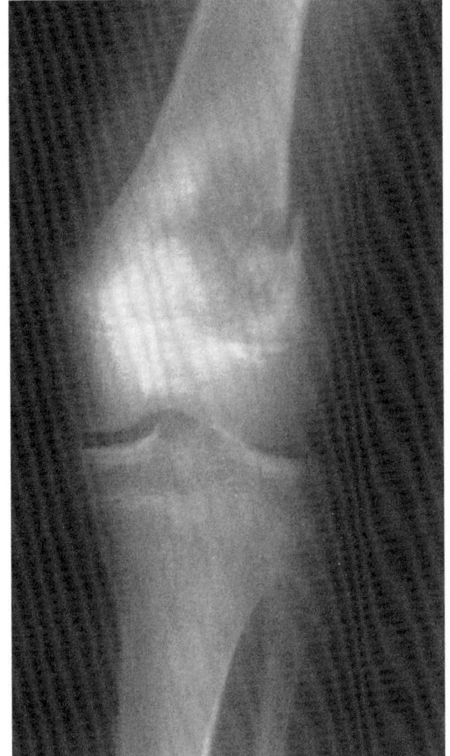

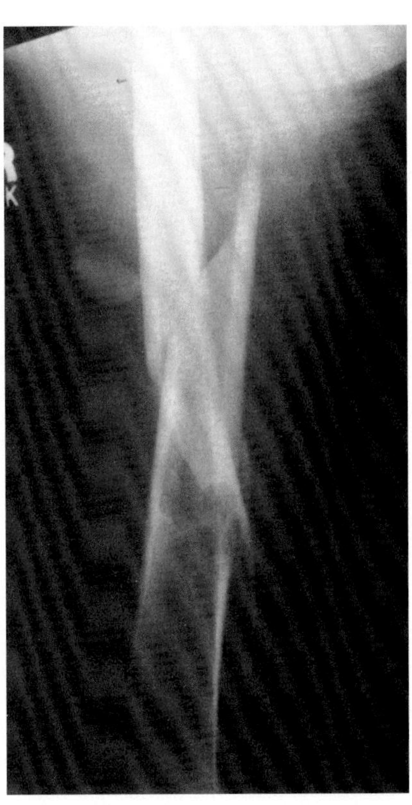

FIGURE 22-2 **A.** Femoral fracture through a poorly demarcated, mixed, osteoblastic, osteolytic lesion—an osteosarcoma. **B.** Sclerotic borders of this lesion in the distal femur are typical of a pathologic fracture through a nonossifying fibroma.

is not consistent with abuse and may confirm a parent's description of a fall as the cause.

DIAGNOSIS

Most patients with femoral shaft fractures are unable to walk and are in extreme pain with an obvious fracture. The diagnosis is more difficult in patients with multiple trauma or head injury and in nonambulatory, severely disabled children. A physical examination usually is sufficient to document the presence of a femoral fracture. Swelling, instability, crepitance, and tenderness usually are present. In patients lacking sensation (myelomeningocele), swelling and redness may simulate infection.

The entire child must be carefully examined. Hypotension rarely results from an isolated femoral fracture. Waddell's triad of femoral fracture, intra-abdominal or intrathoracic injury, and head injury are associated with high-velocity automobile injuries. Multiple trauma may necessitate rapid stabilization of femoral shaft fractures (13,22) to facilitate overall care. This is particularly true with head injury and vascular disruption.

The hemodynamic significance of femoral fracture has been studied by two groups (23,24). Hematocrit levels below 30% rarely occur without multisystem injury. A declining hematocrit should not be attributed to closed femoral fracture until other sources of blood loss have been eliminated (23,24).

X-RAY FINDINGS

X-ray evaluation should include the entire femur, including the hip and knee, because injury of the adjacent joints is common. Femoral shaft fractures may occur with intertrochanteric fractures of the hip, fractures of the femoral neck, and dislocation of the upper end of the femur (25,26). Distal femoral fractures may be associated with physeal injury about the knee, knee ligament injury, meniscal tears (27), and tibial fractures (28).

Plain x-rays generally are sufficient for making the diagnosis. Bone scanning and magnetic resonance imaging (MRI) occasionally may be helpful in the diagnosis of small buckle fractures in limping children or stress fractures in athletes, but usually are not necessary. Comminution or nondisplaced "butterfly" fragments, second fractures, joint dislocations, and pathologic lesions should be sought in every evaluation because such findings will alter therapy and ultimately affect outcome.

Roach and Hoschl (29) described diffuse uptake of radionuclide tracer throughout an entire femoral shaft in an 18-month-old child. This is significant because it demonstrates that the impact of a fracture on a bone of a young child is well beyond the isolated fracture obvious on plain x-ray. A similar finding has been shown in plastic deformation of the forearm in young children.

CLASSIFICATION

Femoral fractures are classified as (a) transverse, spiral, or oblique; (b) comminuted or noncomminuted; and (c) open or

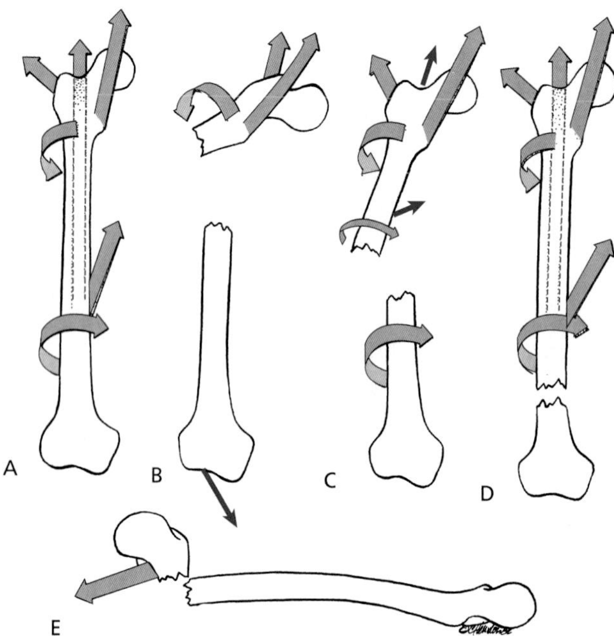

FIGURE 22-3 The relationship of fracture level and position of the proximal fragment. **A.** In the resting unfractured state, the position of the femur is relatively neutral because of balanced muscle pull. **B.** In proximal shaft fractures the proximal fragment assumes a position of flexion (iliopsoas), abduction (abductor muscle group), and lateral rotation (short external rotators). **C.** In mid-shaft fractures the effect is less extreme because there is compensation by the adductors and extensor attachments on the proximal fragment. **D.** Distal shaft fractures produce little alteration in the proximal fragment position because most muscles are attached to the same fragment, providing balance. **E.** Supracondylar fractures often assume a position of hyperextension of the distal fragment due to the pull of the gastrocnemius.

TABLE 22-1 Treatment Options for Femoral Shaft Fractures in Children and Adolescents

Age	Treatment
Birth to 24 mo	Pavlik harness (newborn to 6 mo) Immediate spica cast Traction → spica cast
24 mo to 5 yr	Immediate spica cast Traction → spica cast External fixation (rare) Flexible intramedullary rod (rare)
6–11 yr	Traction → spica cast Flexible intramedullary rod Compression plate External fixation
12 yr to maturity	Flexible intramedullary rod Compression plate Locked intramedullary rod External fixation

Treatment choices are influenced by polytrauma (vs. an isolated femoral shaft fracture) or open fractures with soft tissue trauma.

closed. Open fractures are classified according to Gustilo's system (6). The presence or absence of vascular and neurologic injury is documented and is part of the description of the fracture. The most common femoral fracture in children (over 50%) is a simple transverse, closed, noncomminuted injury.

The level of the fracture (Fig. 22-3) leads to characteristic displacement of the fragments based on the attached muscles. With subtrochanteric fractures, the proximal fragment lies in abduction, flexion, and external rotation. The pull of the gastrocnemius on the distal fragment in a supracondylar fracture produces an extension deformity (posterior angulation of the femoral shaft), which may make the femur difficult to align.

TREATMENT

Treatment of femoral shaft fractures in children is age dependent, with considerable overlap between age groups (Table 22-1). The child's size and age also must be considered, as well as the cause of the injury. Whether the femoral fracture is an isolated injury or part of polytrauma influences treatment choices. Economic concerns, the family's ability to care for a child in a spica cast or external fixator, and the advantages and disadvantages of any operative procedure also are important factors. In adolescents, the psychologic implications of treatment should be considered. Prolonged hospitalization alters the adolescent's self-image and interrupts social and educational development. The disadvantages of nonoperative treatment—time in traction or a cast, economic and social impact on the family—must be carefully weighed against the potential complications of a surgical procedure: infection, refracture after removal of fixation, neurologic injury, limb shortening or overgrowth, and osteonecrosis of the femoral head.

The comparative economics of nonoperative and operative treatment of femoral shaft fractures have been evaluated by several researchers, but no clear consensus has been reached. Reeves et al (30) reported that the cost of nonoperative treatment was 46% higher than that of operative treatment, even considering the necessity for a second surgical procedure for implant removal. Newton and Mubarak (31) analyzed the financial aspects of femoral shaft fracture treatment in 58 children and adolescents and determined that total charges were lowest for those treated with early spica casting and highest for those treated with skeletal traction or intramedullary nailing. Similarly, Coyte et al (32) found the cost of surgical treatment (external fixation) to exceed that of early spica casting in all cases. Stans and Morrissy (33), in evaluating the cost of treating femoral fractures in children 6 to 16 years of age, found that all surgical treatments cost approximately the same. This cost was three times that of early spica cast management and essentially equivalent to traction followed by spica cast. In all cost studies related to femoral fracture, the determinants of increased cost are (a) cost of fixation device, (b) cost of the operating room, and (c) cost of hospital days for recovery. Nork and Hoffinger (34) showed that hospital profit was highest in the traction group, despite charges being equivalent to the surgical group, because the actual hospital resources required were significantly less. In a study by Yandow et al (35) comparing cost of traction to immediate spica in young children, equivalent results occurred with 83% greater charges in the traction group. Wright (36) in an extensive review of the literature and meta-analysis concluded that immediate spica casting had a lower cost and lower malunion rate than traction. Hedin et al (37), in a cost analysis comparing three methods of treating femoral shaft fracture, found that the major determinant of cost was length of hospital stay. Certainly, cost is a factor, but it should not be the overriding consideration in discussions of treatment options with the family. In addition to monetary cost to the medical system, the social cost to the family of treatment choice is significant. This includes disruption of schedules, lost work, and time out of school.

Treatment Variation with Age

In infants, newborn to 6 months of age, femoral fractures usually are reasonably stable because of a thick periosteum. For stable proximal or mid-shaft femoral fractures, simple splinting or a Pavlik harness is all that is required. For unstable fractures in infancy, a simple splint can be tried, but usually the femur cannot be adequately treated in this manner. We have found that a Pavlik harness with a wrap around the thigh, as described by Wilkins, is beneficial. For femoral fractures with excessive shortening (>1 to 2 cm) or angulation (>30 degrees), spica casting may be required. Traction rarely is necessary in this age-group.

In children 6 months to 6 years of age, immediate or early spica casting is the treatment of choice for femoral fractures with less than 2 cm of initial shortening (Fig. 22-4). Femoral fractures with more than 2 cm of initial shortening or marked instability and fractures that cannot be reduced with immediate spica casting require 3 to 10 days of skin or skeletal traction. Skeletal stabilization by external fixation generally is reserved for children with open fractures or multiple trauma. Intramedullary rodding is used in children with metabolic bone disease that predisposes to fracture or after multiple fractures, such as in osteogenesis imperfecta. Larger children in whom reduction cannot be maintained with a spica cast occasionally may benefit from flexible intramedullary rodding or traction.

Treatment of femoral fractures in children 6 to 11 years of age is highly controversial. For stable, minimally displaced fractures, immediate spica casting usually produces satisfactory results; however, in large children with unstable comminuted fractures, traction followed by application of a cast brace or spica cast may be necessary. Because of the cost and the social

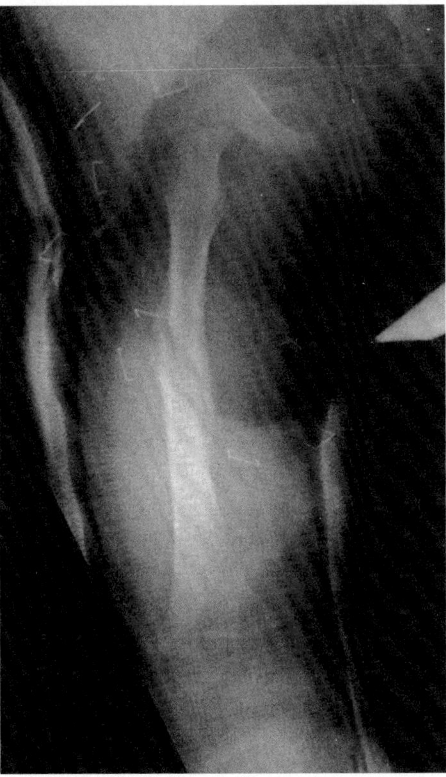
A

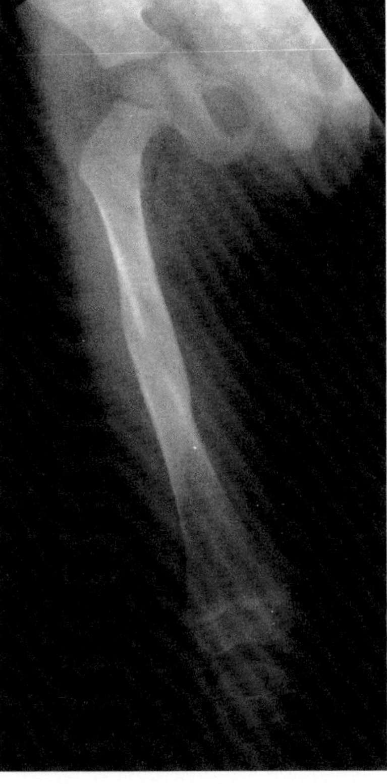
B

FIGURE 22-4 **A.** Three weeks after immediate spica casting of isolated femoral shaft fracture in 3-year-old child. **B.** Three months after injury, fracture is healed in good position.

problems that may accompany management of a child in a spica cast, enthusiasm for skeletal fixation has increased in recent years. Skeletal fixation frequently is used in children with multiple trauma, head injury, vascular compromise, floating knee injuries, or multiple fractures. Treatment options should be discussed with the parents before choosing the method of fracture fixation, even for isolated fractures.

Enthusiasm for treatment that decreases hospital stay has led to the use of external fixation and flexible intramedullary nails in children 6 years of age through adolescence. Compression plating has been reintroduced as a technique with low risks and significant benefit in the management of pediatric femoral fractures. As plating implants have evolved and imaging improved, subcutaneous bridge plating has become an increasingly popular treatment alternative. In older adolescents, antegrade rodding has been recommended as a standard procedure, but the recognized risks of osteonecrosis and growth disturbance have led to limited use of this as a standard technique. Using a greater trochanteric approach appears to offer a significant margin of safety over traditional piriformis insertion for an antegrade rod. Retrograde femoral rodding is another alternative to consider in older children near skeletal maturity with comminuted femoral fractures and an open proximal femoral physis.

Pavlik Harness

Morris et al (38) reported a group of 8 birth-related femoral fractures in 55,296 live births. Twin pregnancies, breech presentation, and prematurity were associated with this injury. The typical fracture is a spiral fracture of the proximal femur with flexion of the proximal fragment. In a newborn with a femoral fracture, one is faced with a very small child, a thick periosteum, and a remarkable remodeling potential. Stannard et al (39) popularized the use of the Pavlik harness for the treatment of this fracture. This treatment is ideal for a proximal or mid-shaft femoral fracture that occurs as a birth-related injury. In a newborn infant in whom a femoral fracture is noted in the intensive care unit or nursery, simple padding or immobilization of the femoral with a soft splint can be tried. For a stable fracture, this approach may be sufficient and will allow intravenous access to the feet if needed. If the fracture remains angulated, a Pavlik harness can be applied with the hip in moderate flexion and abduction. This often helps align the distal fragment with the proximal fragment (Fig. 22-5). Reduction can be aided by a wrap around the thigh if greater stability is needed. The reduction is easily evaluated in the sagittal plane with a lateral x-ray, but evaluation of angulation in the coronal plane (varus-valgus) is more difficult because of hyperflexion. Stannard et al (39) reported acceptable alignment in all patients with less than 1 cm of shortening. Morris et al (38) showed that all treatments, including traction, spica cast, and Pavlik harness, are effective and resulted in satisfactory outcome in all patients regardless of treatment.

In fractures occurring in infancy, management may include evaluation for underlying metabolic bone abnormality or abuse. Once these have been ruled out, a stable fracture should be managed using a simple splint. Unstable fractures should be managed using a Pavlik harness and a small wrap around the thigh, with immediate spica or traction reserved for the rare fracture that cannot be managed with simpler means because of failure to align the fracture or excessive shortening greater than 2 cm.

Immediate Spica Casting

Immediate spica casting, popularized by Irani et al (40) and Staheli et al (41), is indicated for isolated femoral shaft fractures in children under 6 years of age unless (a) shortening of more than 2 cm is present, (b) massive swelling of the thigh is noted, or (c) associated injuries are present. Its primary advantages are simplicity, low cost, and generally good results based on leg length equality, healing time, and motion (42,43).

Hughes et al (94) evaluated 23 children ranging in age from 2 through 10 years who had femoral fractures treated with immediate spica casting to determine the impact of treatment on the patients and their families. The greatest problems encountered by the family in caring for a child in a spica cast were transportation, cast intolerance by the child, and keeping the child clean. Although most children did not attend school while in the cast, no child was required to repeat a grade and no permanent psychologic effects were reported by the parents. The researchers found that overall treatment in a spica cast was much easier for families of preschool children than for those with school-age children. Kocher (45) in a similar study using a validated questionnaire for assessing the impact of medical conditions on families demonstrated unexpectedly high effect similar to that experienced with diseases such as leukemia. Considering this, assistance that facilitates care would be welcome by families, and efforts should be made at the time of discharge to help families cope with the burden of a child in a spica cast.

Illgen et al (46), in a series of 114 isolated femoral fractures in children under 6 years of age, found that 90 degree/90 degree (90/90) spica casting was successful in 86% without cast change or wedging, based on tolerance of shortening less than 1.5 cm and angulation less than 10 degrees. Of the 20 patients requiring spica change, only 2 healed with unacceptable position (>2 cm of leg length discrepancy). One of these overgrew by 1.5 cm, and the other was lost to follow-up. Illgen et al used an immediate spica regardless of initial shortening and placed the child in traction only if unacceptable shortening occurred. Shortening requiring spica cast change was associated with a knee flexion angle of less than 50 degrees. Similar excellent results have been reported by Czertak and Hennrikus (47) using the 90/90 spica cast. Infante et al (43) expanded the indications for spica casts to children up to age 10 and up to 100 pounds. Although exact selection criteria were not stated, it is clear that this technique can be applied beyond traditional accepted age and size limitations in selected cases. Ferguson and Nicol (42) conducted a prospective study of early spica casting in children less than 10 years of age including 101 fractures in a 30-month period. Only

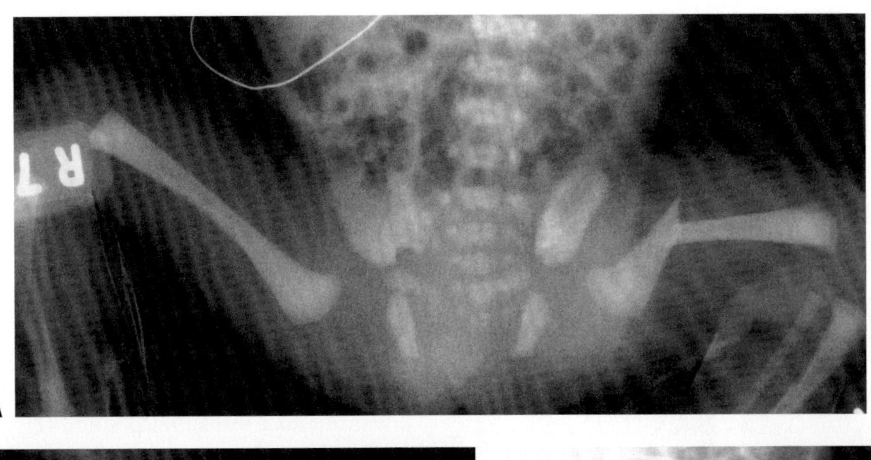

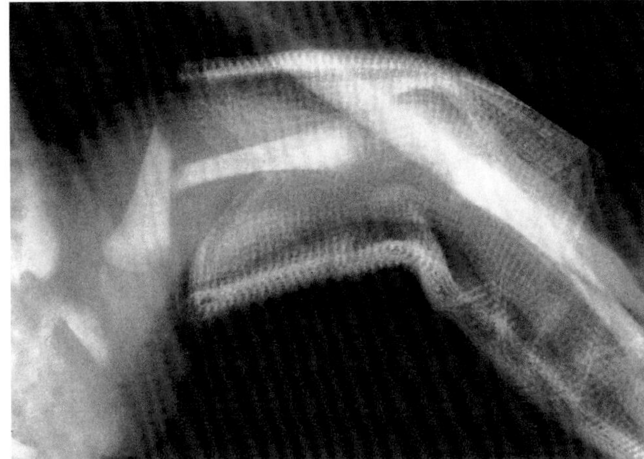

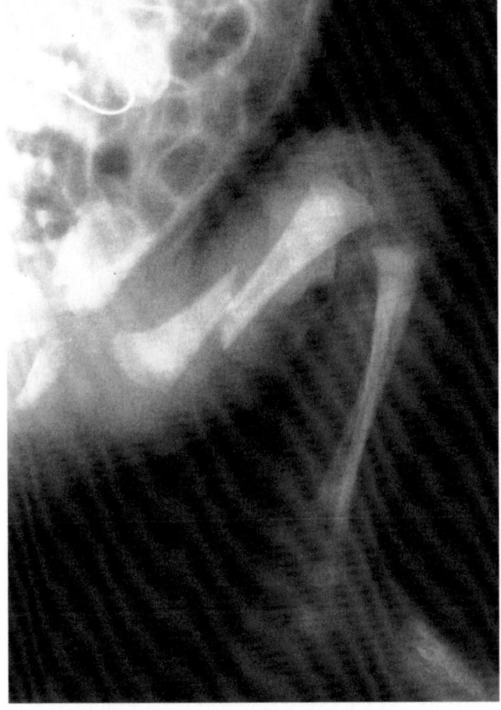

FIGURE 22-5 **A.** This infant had a birth-related left femoral fracture. **B.** An anteroposterior splint was used but ended at the fracture site, only increasing the angulation. **C.** A Pavlik harness reduced the fracture by flexing the distal fragment.

four spicas had to be removed for unacceptable position. Age greater than 7 years was a variable predictive of a higher risk of failure of this technique to achieve satisfactory alignment.

Thompson et al (48) described the telescope test in which patients were examined with fluoroscopy at the time of reduction and casting. If more than 3 cm of shortening could be demonstrated with gentle axial compression, traction was used rather than immediate spica casting. By using the telescope test, these researchers decreased unacceptable results (>2.5 cm of shortening) from 18% to 5%.

Martinez et al (49) reported excessive shortening and angular deformity in 26 of 51 patients after immediate spica casting, especially in comminuted fractures. Although shortening and angulation can occur in a spica cast, excessive deformity can be detected with weekly x-ray and clinical evaluations during the first 2 to 3 weeks after injury. Minimal shortening is acceptable but should not exceed 2 cm (Fig. 22-6). This is best measured on a lateral x-ray taken through the cast. If follow-up x-rays reveal significant varus (>10 degrees) or anterior angulation (>30 degrees), the cast may be wedged. However, Weiss et al (50) noted that wedging of 90/90 spica casts can cause peroneal nerve palsy, especially during correction of valgus angulation. For unacceptable position, the fracture can be manipulated and a new cast applied, or the cast can be removed and the patient placed in traction to regain or maintain length (Fig. 22-7). Angular deformity of up to 15 degrees in the coronal plane and up to 30 degrees in the sagittal plane may be acceptable, depending on the patient's age (Table 22-2). Finally, if shortening exceeds 2 cm, traction or an external fixator can be used.

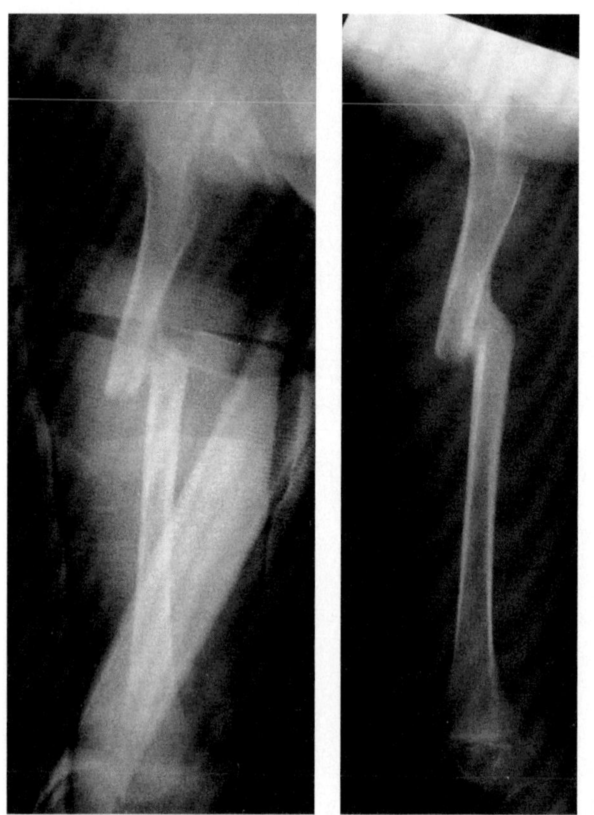

FIGURE 22-6 **A.** Immediate spica casting of isolated femoral shaft fracture in an 8-year-old child; shortening on initial x-ray was 2 cm. **B.** Four months after injury, shortening of 2 cm is seen with this healed fracture.

Shortening and angulation occur most often in fractures associated with polytrauma and those with loss of the periosteal sleeve (1,12) Fry et al (1) found that 50% (12 of 23) of closed femoral shaft fractures caused by high-energy trauma in children under 10 years of age required repeat reduction or other treatment to correct excessive shortening or angulation that occurred after initial reduction; only 8% (2 of 24) of low-energy fractures required repeat closed reduction. Wright (36) showed that limb length discrepancy and angular deformity are lower in spica treatment than with traction treatment. The lower cost of spica management is an added reason to pursue this method of management.

The position of the hips and knees in the spica cast is controversial. Spica cast application with the hip and knee extended and the bottom of the foot cut out to prevent excessive shortening has been described (51). Varying the amounts of hip and knee flexion in the spica cast based on the position of the fracture also has been recommended: the more proximal the fracture, the more flexed the hip should be (41).

An alternative to the standard hip-knee extended spica is the 90/90 spica cast or the sitting spica cast (52,53). A sitting spica cast (Fig. 22-8), with the hips and knees set in about 90 degrees of flexion, is the easiest and perhaps the most effective cast for femoral fractures in preschool-aged children, unless the fracture cannot be maintained in this position. The child is placed in a sitting position with the legs abducted about 30 degrees on either side. The synthetic material used for the cast gives it sufficient strength so that no bar is required between the legs. This not only allows the child to be carried on the parent's hip but also aids in toiletry needs, making bedpans unnecessary. Also, the child can sit upright during the day and can attend school in a wheelchair.

Spica Cast Application: Technique

The child is taken to the operating room or plaster room, where anesthesia or sedation is administered. A short leg cast is applied with the foot in neutral position (Fig. 22-9A). Extra padding and a felt pad are placed in the area of the popliteal fossa. The cast is then extended to a long leg cast with the knee held in 90 degrees of flexion (Fig. 22-9B). Be sure not to flex the knee after padding because this may predispose to vascular obstruction by producing a lump of cast material in the popliteal fossa. Because most diaphyseal fractures tend to fall into varus angulation while in a spica cast, a valgus mold is necessary (Fig. 22-9C). The patient is then placed on a spica table, supporting the weight of the legs with manual traction, and the remainder of the cast is applied with the hips in 90 degrees of flexion and 30 degrees of abduction, holding the fracture out to length (Fig. 22-9D). It is mandatory that excessive traction not be applied because compartment syndromes and skin sloughs have been reported, presumably secondary to overzealous traction and poor cast technique. Applying a long leg cast in one piece may be a technique that prevents a transition from short to long cast, which may cause problems. The leg should be placed in 15 degrees of external rotation to align the distal fragment with the external rotation of the proximal fragment. After the spica cast is in place, anteroposterior (AP) and lateral x-rays are obtained to ensure that length and angular and rotational alignment are maintained. Frick et al (54) reported two cases of compartment syndrome with immediate spica treatment in a position of 90 degrees of knee flexion and believed that increased knee flexion contributed to this problem. Caution about the position of the knee and cast padding are critical in avoiding this complication. We found that knee flexion greater than 60 degrees improved maintenance of length and reduction (46). However, if one applies excessive traction to maintain length, the risk of compartment syndrome is unacceptably high. Less traction, less knee flexion, and accepting a bit more shortening is a reasonable compromise. We observe all patients for 24 hours after spica application to be sure that neurovascular compromise and compartment syndrome are not present.

Gortex liners can be used to decrease the skin problems of diaper rash and superficial infection. This has been beneficial and has justified the cost of a Gortex liner. If angulation of more than acceptable limits occurs, the cast should be changed, with manipulation in the operating room. Casts can be wedged for less than 15 degrees of angulation. If shortening of more than 2 cm is documented, the child should be treated with cast change,

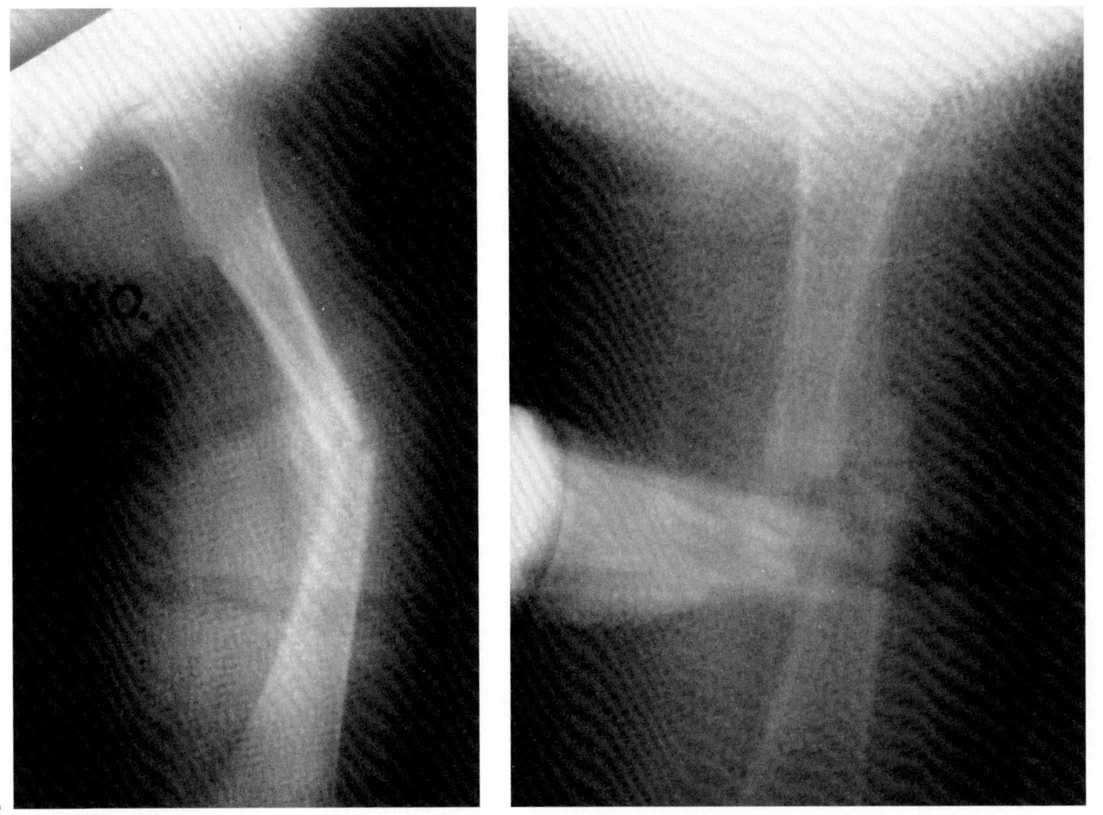

FIGURE 22-7 **A.** Unacceptable position of fracture in spica cast in a 2-year-old child. **B.** With manipulation, application of a new spica cast, and cast wedging, this angulation is corrected.

traction, or conversion to external fixation with lengthening for late detection. When conversion to external fixation is required, we recommend osteoclasis at the time of the application of the external fixator, with slow lengthening over a period of several weeks (1 mm per day) to reestablish acceptable length (Fig. 22-10).

Generally, the spica cast is worn for 4 to 8 weeks, depending on the age of the child and the severity of the soft tissue damage accompanying the fracture. After the cast has been removed, management should include skin care in young children and crutch-assisted or walker-assisted ambulation in older children. Ambulation is accomplished with weight bearing as tolerated. Stiff knees and weak hamstrings and quadriceps should be identified after the child begins to walk, and a physical therapy program should be started if needed. Long-term follow-up for leg length evaluation, range of motion, and quadriceps weakness should be maintained.

TABLE 22-2 **Acceptable Angulation**

Age	Varus/Valgus (degrees)	Anterior/ Posterior (degrees)	Shortening (mm)
Birth to 2 yr	30	30	15
2–5 yr	15	20	20
6–10 yr	10	15	15
11 yr to maturity	5	10	10

Traction and Casting

Since as early as the 18th century, traction has been used for management of femoral fractures. The French used the Hippocratic method of traction and coaptation splinting in extension. The English, influenced by Pott (55), treated patients on their sides with the hip and knee flexed. In 1861, Buck (56) introduced simple horizontal traction. Vertical overhead traction with the hip flexed 90 degrees and the knee straight was introduced by Bryant in 1873 (57,58), but this often resulted in vascular insufficiency (Fig. 22-11) (59), and it is now rarely used for treatment of femoral fractures, except occasionally in infants under 2 years of age and weighing less than 20 pounds. However, even in this infantile age-group, split Russell's traction (60) or immediate spica casting is preferable. Modified Bryant's

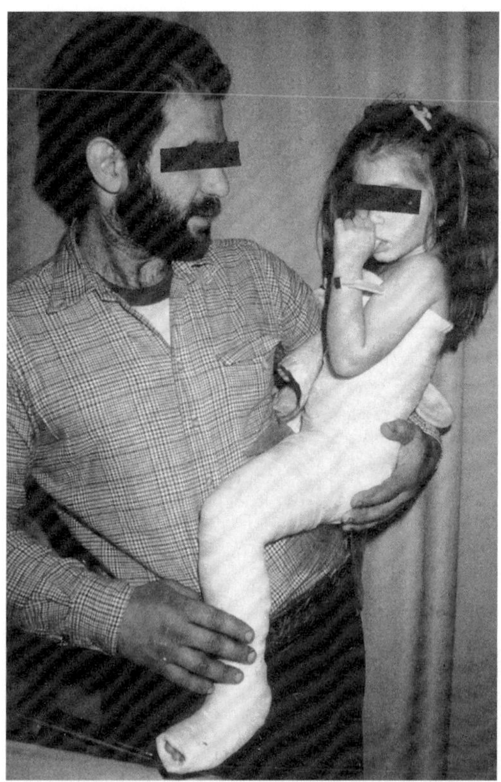

FIGURE 22-8 A 90 degree/90 degree spica cast allows a small child to be carried on the parent's hip. The child can be placed in a sitting position in a chair or on the toilet in this type of cast.

traction, in which the knee is flexed 45 degrees, increases the safety of overhead skin traction (61). Gallows traction also has been used (62).

The indications for skin or skeletal traction include (a) unstable femoral fracture in a child under 6 years of age with more than 2 to 3 cm of shortening, (b) femoral fracture that fails to maintain proper length and alignment in a spica cast in a child under 6 years of age, and (c) femoral fracture in a child 6 to 11 years of age, without multiple fractures, head trauma, or severe soft tissue or vascular injuries, who is able to cooperate with a period of bed rest and spica cast immobilization and whose family prefers no surgery. The limit of skin traction is the interface between skin and tape or skin and foam traction boot. Skin complications, such as slough and blistering, usually occur when more than 5 pounds of traction is applied. When more than 5 pounds of traction is required, or simply for ease in patient management, skeletal traction can be used to maintain alignment (63). Casas et al (64) studied a group of 41 patients between the ages of 4 and 10 years treated with skin traction followed by spica casting. Spica casts were applied at an average of 20.7 days. No leg length difference nor deformity resulted. In this situation hospital length of stay was not thought to be a reason to reject this conservative yet clearly effective method of management. Abandonment of traction and casting in the child less than 10 in many centers is in reaction to cost and convenience, not because of negative clinical outcome in children.

Skeletal traction also can be used in adolescents with comminuted proximal femoral shaft and intertrochanteric fractures in whom secure fixation cannot be obtained without risk of vascular compromise to the proximal femur. In general, however, skeletal traction is not recommended for children 12 years of age or older because of significant incidences of shortening and angular malunion.

The distal femur is the location of choice for a traction pin (63,65,66). Although proximal tibial traction pins have been recommended by some clinicians (67), growth arrest in the proximal tibial physis and subsequent recurvatum deformity have been associated with their use (Fig. 22-12). Also, knee ligament and meniscal injuries that sometimes accompany femoral fractures are aggravated by the chronic pull of traction across the knee. The rare indication for a tibial traction pin is a child in whom fracture configuration or skin problems prevent placement of a femoral traction wire and in whom no knee injury is present.

In a group of 45 patients with femoral fractures, Stanitski et al (68) calculated the radiation dose received by the patient while in traction. The average dose before casting was 0.699 rad. Although this is a significant radiation exposure, it was not excessive compared to that received by patients managed with other methods of treatment, particularly when intraoperative exposures are considered. However, radiation exposure during treatment must be considered.

Traction Pin Insertion: Technique

After preparation of the thigh circumferentially from the knee to the mid-thigh, the limb is draped in a sterile manner. The knee is held in the position in which it will remain during traction; that is, if 90/90 traction is being used, the traction pin should be inserted with the knee bent 90 degrees (Fig. 22-13A). The patient should be sedated and the wound treated with a local anesthetic, or general anesthesia should be given before the traction pin is inserted (Fig. 22-13B). The location of pin insertion is one finger breadth above the patella with the knee extended or just above the flare of the distal femur (Fig. 22-13C). A small puncture wound is made over the medial side of the femur (Fig. 22-13D). A medial-to-lateral approach is used so that the traction pin does not migrate into the area of the femoral artery that runs through Hunter's canal on the medial side of the femur. A traction pin between 3/32 inch and 3/16 inch is chosen depending on the size of the child. The pin is placed parallel to the joint surface (63) to help maintain alignment while in traction. After the pin protrudes through the lateral cortex of the femur, a small incision is made over the tip of the pin. The pin is then driven far enough through the skin to allow fixation with a traction bow (Fig. 22-13F). If 90/90 traction is used, a short leg cast is placed with a ring through its mid-portion to support the leg. Alternatively, a sling to sup-

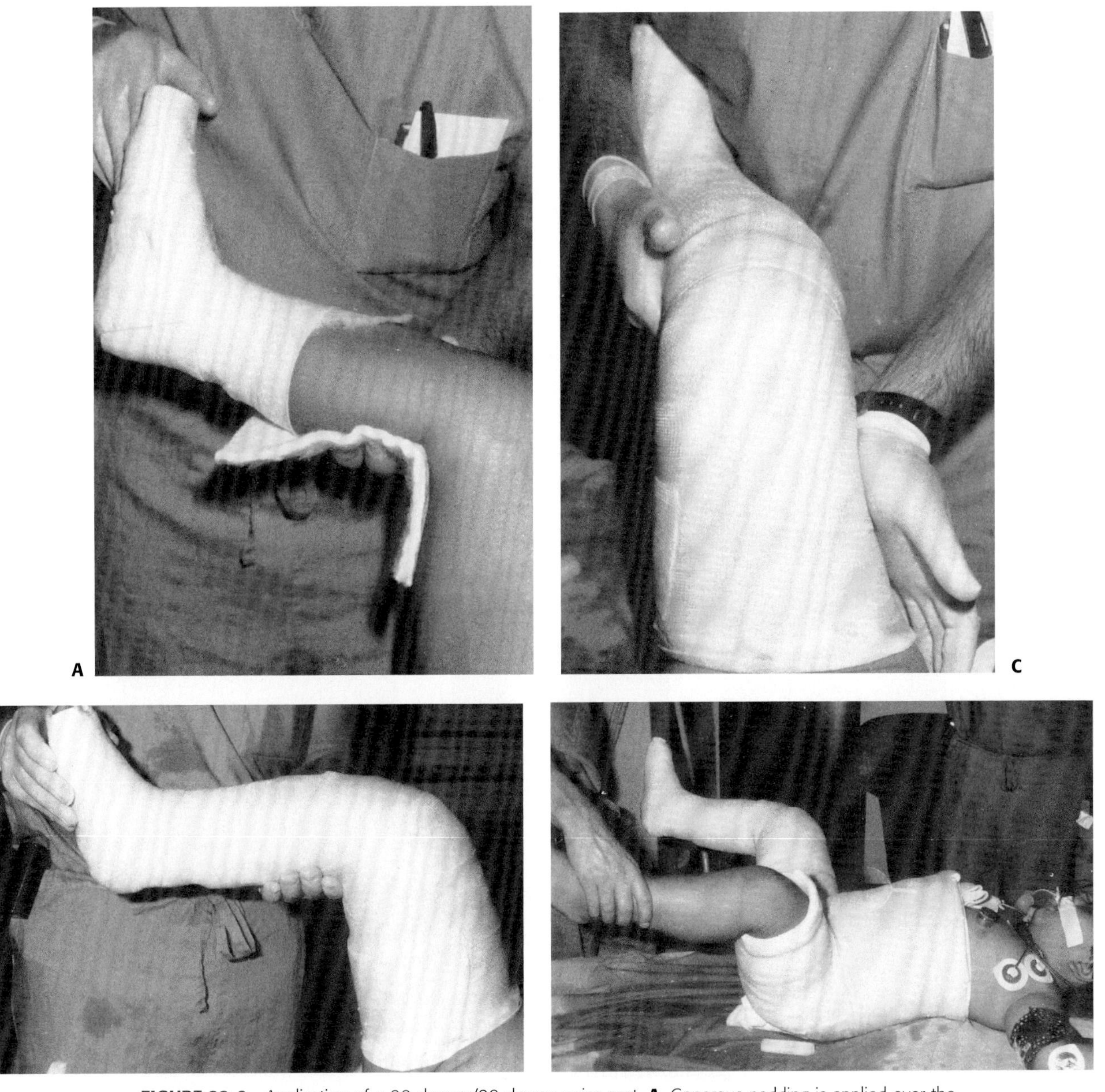

FIGURE 22-9 Application of a 90 degree/90 degree spica cast. **A.** Generous padding is applied over the foot, and a pad is placed on the popliteal fossa to prevent injury to the peroneal nerve and popliteal vessels. **B.** A long leg cast is applied with the knee flexed 90 degrees. **C.** A mold is placed over the apex of the fracture, generally correcting a varus deformity into slight valgus. **D.** Using a standard spica table, a 11/2 spica cast is applied with the hip flexed 90 degrees and abducted 30 degrees.

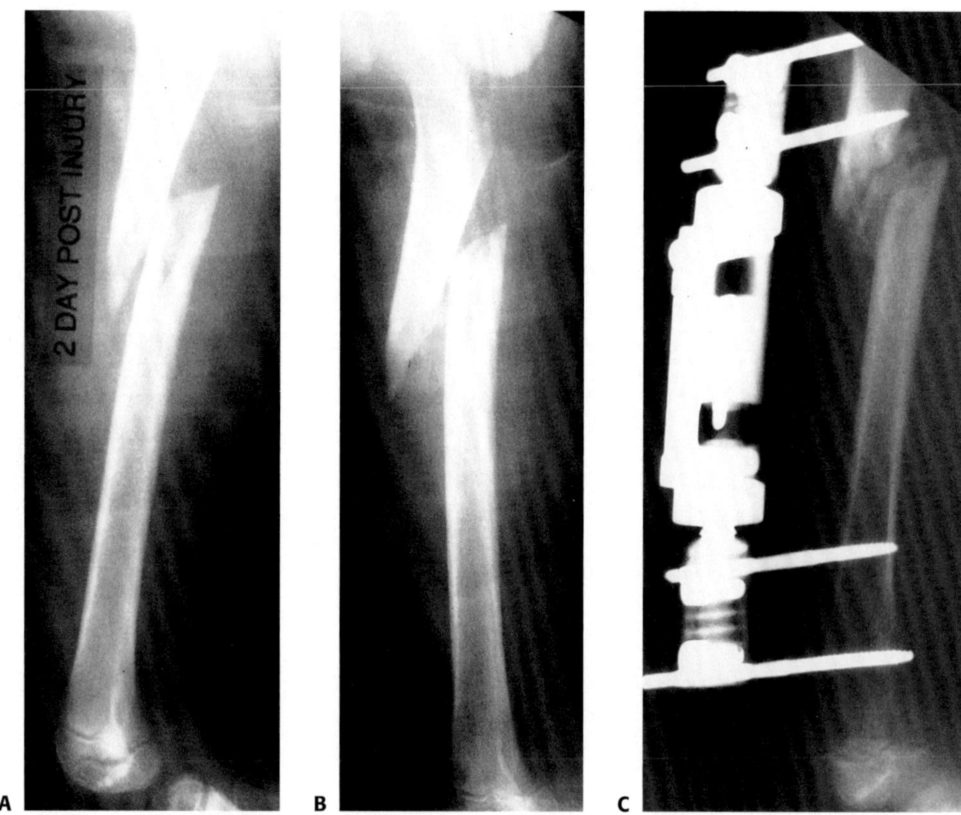

FIGURE 22-10 **A.** This 8-year-old child with a femoral fracture was treated with an immediate spica cast. **B.** After 3 weeks of immobilization, unacceptable shortening (2.2 cm) was noted. **C.** Closed osteoclysis and lengthening with an external fixation device solved the problem, with length achieved by callus distraction.

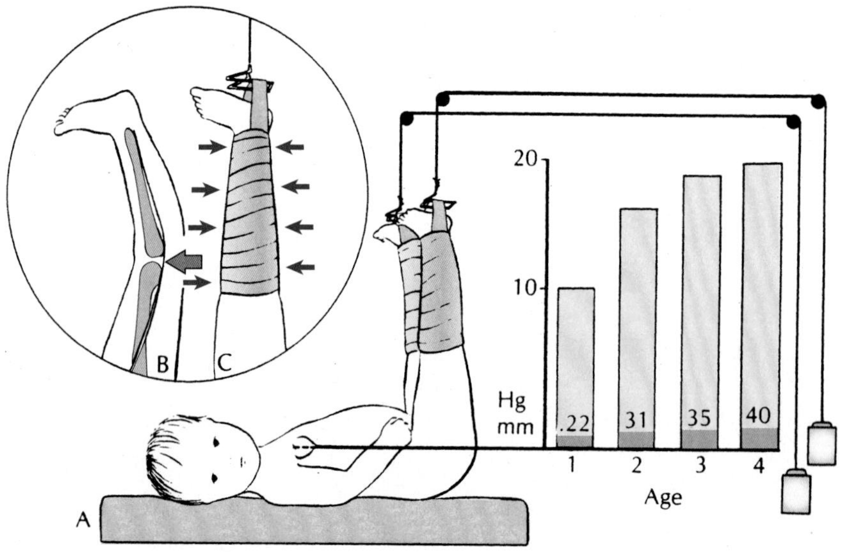

FIGURE 22-11 Adverse effect on limb circulation by overhead traction as detailed by Nicholson. **A.** Incremental increase in hydrostatic pressure necessary for limb perfusion due to increasing limb length. **B.** Hyperextension of the knee occurs if the infant moves to the foot of the bed, stretching the popliteal artery. **C.** Extrinsic compression of wrapping to maintain traction tapes aggravates the problem. Any or all of these factors contribute to the risk of overhead traction. (Redrawn from Nicholson J, Foster R, Heath R. Bryant's traction: a provocative cause of circulatory complications. *JAMA* 1955;157:4118; with permission.)

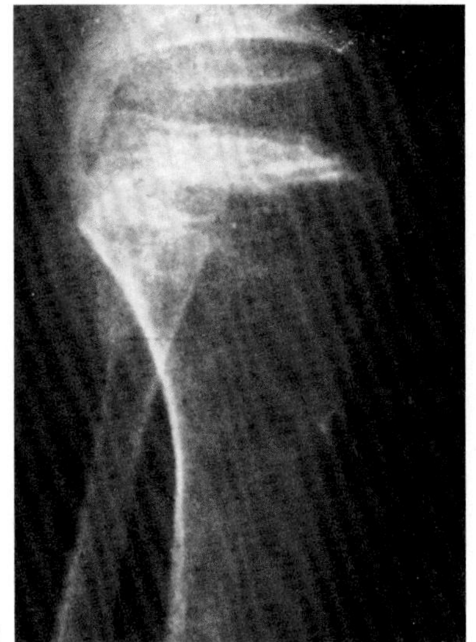
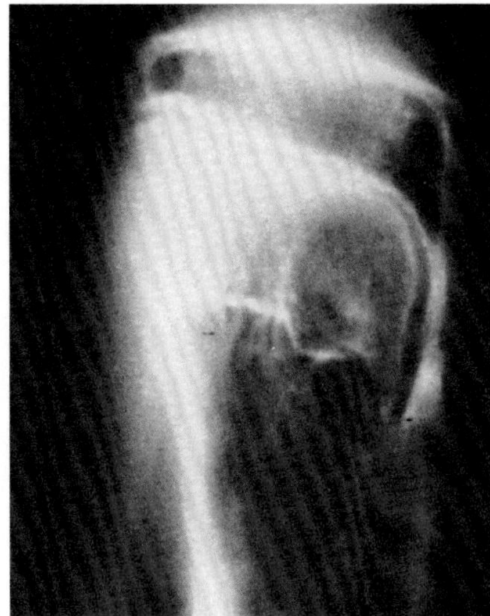
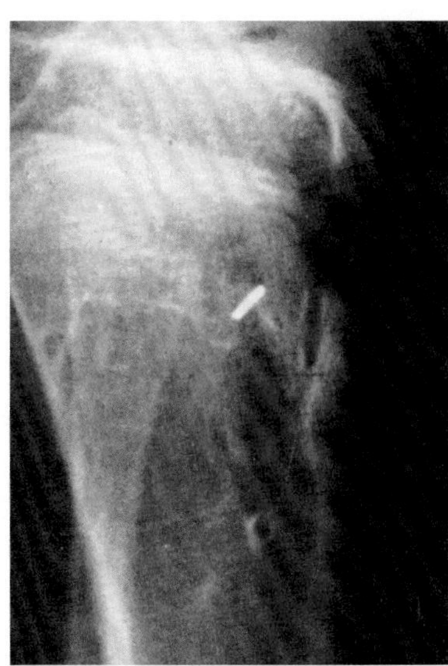

FIGURE 22-12 Tibial epiphyseal injury in association with tibial pin traction treatment for a femoral fracture. A 14-year-old boy sustained a femoral fracture that was treated by tibial skeletal traction. Two years later the fracture was well healed but 2.5 cm short. A recurvatum deformity of the same side was apparent. **A.** An apparent fusion of the tibial tubercle. **B.** The bridge was confirmed by tomography. **C.** Bridge resection was performed with free fat interposition. A marker was placed to facilitate subsequent evaluation of growth. A tibial pin, if used, should be inserted posterior to the anterior aspect of the tibial tubercle.

port the calf may be used. If a sling is used, heel cord stretching should be performed while the patient is in traction.

After the skeletal traction pin has been placed in the distal femur, traction is applied in a 90/90 position (the hip and knee flexed 90 degrees) (Fig. 22-14) or in an oblique position (the hip flexed 20 to 60 degrees). If the oblique position is chosen, a Thomas splint or sling is necessary to support the leg. The fracture may be allowed to begin healing in traction, and x-rays should be obtained once or twice a week to monitor alignment and length. In a child under 10 years of age, the ideal fracture position in traction should be less than 1 cm of shortening and slight valgus alignment to counteract the tendency to angulate into varus in the cast and the eventual overgrowth that may occur (average 0.9 cm). If this method is used for adolescents (11 years or older), normal length should be maintained.

Technique Tips. Threaded pins, although more difficult to remove, are preferable to smooth pins because of their secure fixation within the bone without side-to-side movement; however, they have a slightly higher incidence of skin interface complications.

Aronson et al (63) found that obliquely placed femoral traction pins were associated with an increased incidence of varus or valgus angulation. Pins for skeletal traction should be placed parallel to the axis of the knee joint or the articular surface, and in children over 11 years of age the fracture should be reduced without shortening.

Postoperative Care

Prolonged traction of 3 weeks or more followed by knee immobilization in a spica cast is well tolerated by young children. In children over 12 years of age or in children weighing over 100 pounds, maintaining the knee in 90 degrees of flexion for a prolonged period may lead to knee stiffness and a difficult period of rehabilitation (67).

Alternatives for treatment after traction application include (a) a 2- to 3-week period of traction until callus formation is apparent and the fracture is stable before pin removal and application of a spica cast or cast brace (51,56,69–71), (b) early incorporation of a traction pin into a spica cast; and (c) incorporation of a traction pin into a cast brace with intermittent traction to maintain length until callus formation is present (72). Each of these methods has advantages, costs, and risks, and a clear "best method" cannot be identified, and the interest in surgical treatment in this age group has decreased interest in these options.

Results of Traction and Casting

In a study by Gross et al (72), 72 children with femoral fractures were treated with early cast brace/traction management. In this technique, a traction pin is placed in the distal femur and then incorporated in a cast brace. The traction pin is left long enough to be used for maintaining traction while the patient is in the cast brace or traction is applied directly to the cast. The patient is allowed to ambulate in the cast brace starting 3 days after application. X-rays are taken of the fracture in the cast brace to document that excessive shortening is not occurring. The patient then is returned to traction in the cast brace until satisfactory callus is present to prevent shortening or angular deformity with weight-bearing. The technique was not effective in older adolescents with mid-shaft fractures but achieved excel-

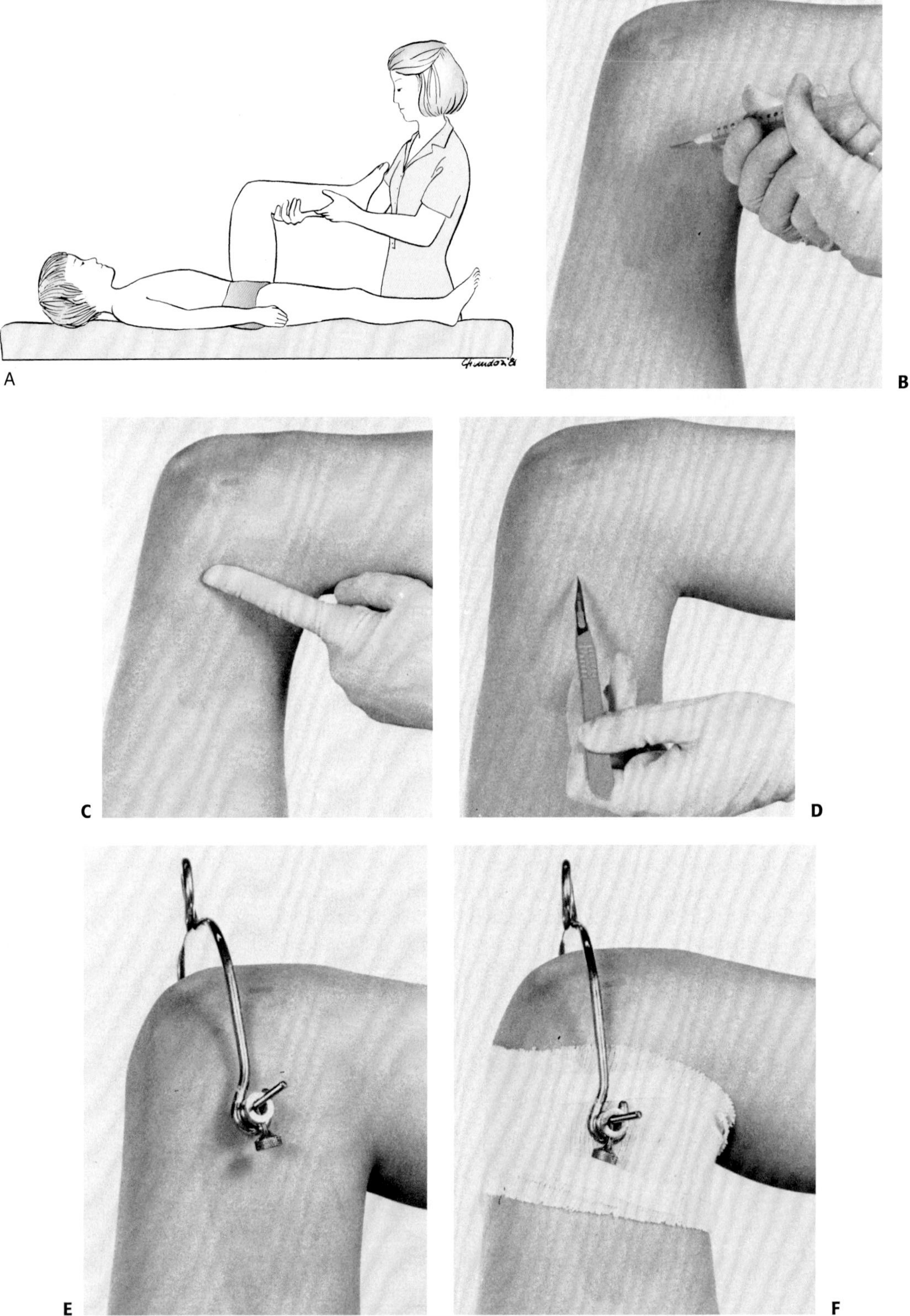

FIGURE 22-13 Insertion of femoral skeletal traction pin. **A.** The limb is held in the 90 degree/90 degree position by an assistant. **B.** A site just superior to the adductor tubercle is surgically prepared, both medially and laterally. **C.** Local anesthesia is applied in the skin and periosteum on both sides of the limb. **D.** The skin is penetrated with a scalpel. **E.** A threaded Steinmann pin is introduced at the level 1 cm proximal to the adductor tubercle. **F.** Dressing and traction bow in place.

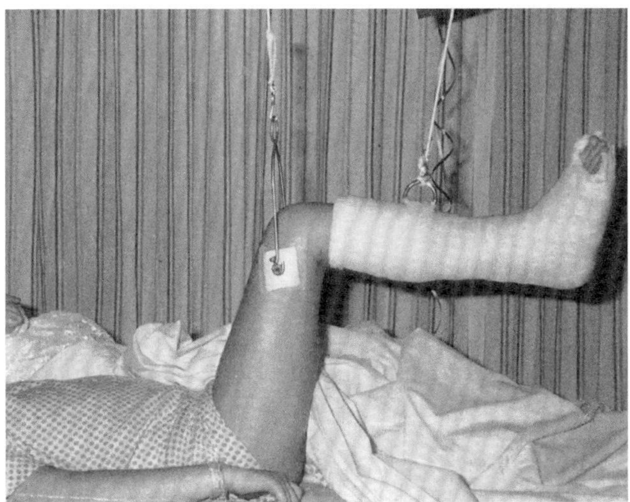

FIGURE 22-14 In 90 degree/90 degree traction, a femoral pin is used and the lower leg and foot are supported with a short leg cast or a sling.

lent results in children 5 to 12 years of age. The average hospital stay was 17 days.

Complications of Traction and Casting

Comparative studies and retrospective reviews have demonstrated unsatisfactory results in a small, yet significant, percentage of patients treated with skeletal traction (30,67,73,74). It is clear that traction remains an acceptable method of treatment of femoral shaft fractures in children under 12 years of age, but surgical methods are easier or more convenient with similar outcome.

External Fixation

External fixation of femoral shaft fractures offers a fast convenient method to align and stabilize the fractured femur. It is the method of choice when severe soft tissue injury is present and may be considered in any patient where traditional closed methods of management are not appropriate (14). In head-injured or multiply injured patients and those with open fractures, external fixation offers an excellent method of management. Wagner was an early advocate of monolateral frame fixation and developed an external fixation and lengthening device. Aronson and Tursky (75) in 1987 reported their early experience with 44 femoral fractures treated with primary external fixation and early weight-bearing. Most patients returned to school by 4 weeks after fracture and had full knee motion by 6 weeks after the fixator was removed. In this early study, end-on alignment was the goal and overgrowth was minimal. Following early enthusiasm for the use of external devices, the 1990s saw some waning interest in their use because of complications with pin track infections, scarring, delayed union, and refracture. With other methods of skeletal fixation such as flexible intramedullary rodding, the use of external fixation devices for primary treatment of femoral fractures has declined. However, there remain advocates for external fixation and devices have improved with corresponding improvement in outcome.

Hedin et al (76) reported a series of 98 fractures in 96 children between the ages of 3 and 15 years treated with monolateral external fixation devices, with generally good outcome in two nearby Swedish hospitals. The refracture rate after fixator removal was only 2% but three femurs slowly deformed at the fracture site, requiring corrective osteotomy. Therefore, the major complication rate was nearly 6%. Superficial infection was common, but deep infection did not occur. Their conclusion was that this was an effective method of fracture management that was easy to learn and apply.

Bar-On et al (77) compared external fixation with flexible intramedullary rodding in a prospective randomized study. They found that the early postoperative course was similar but that the time to return to school and to resume full activity was less with intramedullary fixation. Muscle strength was better in the flexible intramedullary fixation group at 14 months after fracture. Parental satisfaction was also significantly better in the flexible intramedullary rodding group. Bar-On et al (77) recommended that external fixation be reserved for open or severely comminuted fractures.

Fixator Design

The design of external fixator frames is important in determining the end result. In general, circular fixation devices are rarely, if ever, indicated for femoral fractures. External fixation should be performed using a monolateral or cantilever system. The monolateral devices are of two types. The AO system, in which pins can be placed at any point along a bar, with a special clamp holding the pins at a variable angle to the bar, has been in common use (Fig. 22-15). The advantage of this system is that the stability of fixation is increased if the two pins on each side of the fracture are spread widely, with one pin close to the fracture and one quite distant from it. A second longitudinal rod can be added to this system to increase its rigidity. A second type of external fixation system has pin clamps at the end of a telescopic tube. The pin clamps provide easy application, but the stability of the fixation device is decreased because the pins are widely separated from the fracture. The pin clamps may be constrained to rotation only (Wagner) or attached with a universal joint to the barrel of the device (Orthofix, EBI) (Fig. 22-16). The telescoping barrel provides lengthening or dynamization, and the universal joints provide adjustment. Sola et al (78) found that results were improved significantly by adding an auxiliary pin to the standard Orthofix type frame, providing better fixation near the fracture site. They reviewed 38 fractures in 37 children 5 to 18 years of age. Six of 22 femurs treated without auxiliary pins required remanipulation for loss of reduction, whereas only 1 of the 16 frames with an auxiliary pin required remanipulation. Although these researchers provided auxiliary pin fixation by attaching a pin to the barrel of the external fixator with methylmethacrylate, other methods of intermediate pin fixation are available at this time.

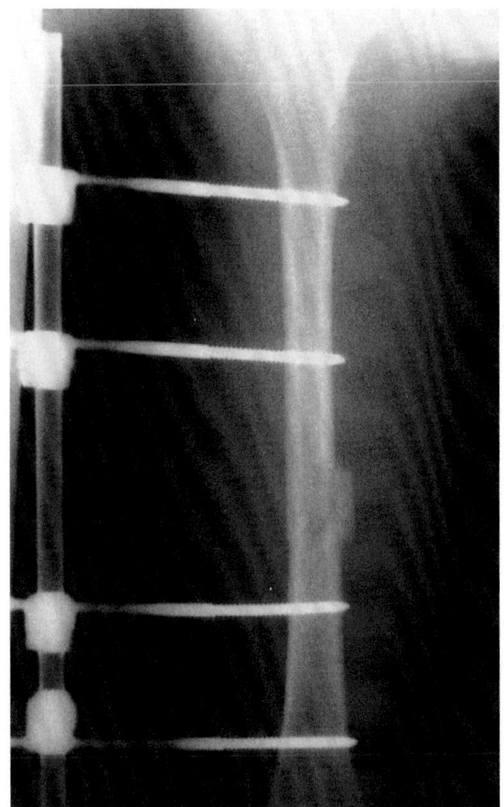

FIGURE 22-15 Application of AO external fixator. The most proximal and distal pins are placed a few centimeters from the fracture site to improve frame stability.

Variation of external fixation devices allow for varying amounts of "dynamization." Dynamization refers to the amount of motion allowed by a given frame or construct. A fracture can be dynamized before frame removal to increase strength of healing callus. Excessive rigidity is thought to relate to poor bone healing and strength. Domb et al (79) compared static to dynamic external fixation in pediatric femoral fractures. Average time to early callus formation was similar, and the average time to complete healing was 70.1 days in the dynamic group versus 63.1 days in the static group. The assumption that less rigid frames decrease fracture rate remains unproven.

Pins are more closely clustered and placed farther from the fracture site, and the frame itself is placed more laterally away from the femur, which should not be anatomically reduced.

A technical development in external fixation has been the use of hydroxyapatite-coated pins. The pin–bone interface was a problem with loosening in some devices. The strength of the pin–bone interface with hydroxyapatite-coated pins appears to be somewhat better, although large series with this device have not yet been reported.

The ease and speed with which an external fixation device can be applied makes it ideal for management of a polytrauma victim who cannot tolerate extended anesthesia. Nowotarski et al (80), in a review of 1,507 femoral fractures at a trauma center, found 59 (4%) that were managed with external fixation followed by intramedullary rodding. The average time to rodding was 7 days, and the infection rate was 1.7%, or 1 patient. They concluded that emergent external fixation followed by early intramedullary rodding was safe.

Frame Application: Technique

Preoperative planning is mandatory. Fracture lines indicative of comminution must be recognized. There must be length available between the trochanteric and the distal femoral physes for the device chosen.

After appropriate anesthesia, the leg is prepared and the patient is placed on a radiolucent table or a fracture table, depending on the preference of the surgeon and the size of the child. Either the fracture table or fluoroscopic table works well. We make the decision based on the size of the patient and the ease with which reduction can be obtained, as well as the available assistance. In general, a fracture table facilitates reduction and application of the external fixator.

First we try to reduce the fracture both in length and alignment. If the fracture is open, it should be irrigated and debrided before application of the external fixation device. With the fracture maximally aligned, fixation is begun. The minimal and maximal length constraints characteristic of all external fixation systems must be kept in mind. The angular adjustment intrinsic to the fixation device needs to be determined. If a universal joint at the end of the device only allows for 15 degrees of angular correction, one cannot expect 40 degrees of adjustment after application of the device. Rotation in general is constrained with all external fixation systems once the first pins are placed. That is, if parallel pins are placed with the fracture in 40 degrees of malrotation, a 40-degree malalignment will exist. Rotational correction must be obtained before placing the pins in the proximal and distal shafts of the femur.

Application of the fixator is similar no matter what device is chosen (Fig. 22-17). One pin is placed proximally in the shaft, and another pin is placed distally perpendicular to the long axis of the shaft. Alignment is always to the long axis of the shaft rather than to the joint surface. Rotation should be checked before the second pin is placed because it constrains rotation but not angulation or length. After pins are correctly placed, all fixation nuts are secured and sterile dressings are applied to pins.

Technique Tips. Pin sizes vary with manufacturers, as do drill sizes. In general the pins are placed through predrilled holes to avoid thermal necrosis of bone. Sharp drills should be used. The manufacturer's recommendation for drill and screw sizes should be checked before starting the procedure. Some self-drilling and self-tapping pins are available. At least two pins should be placed proximally and two distally. An intermediate or auxiliary pin may be beneficial.

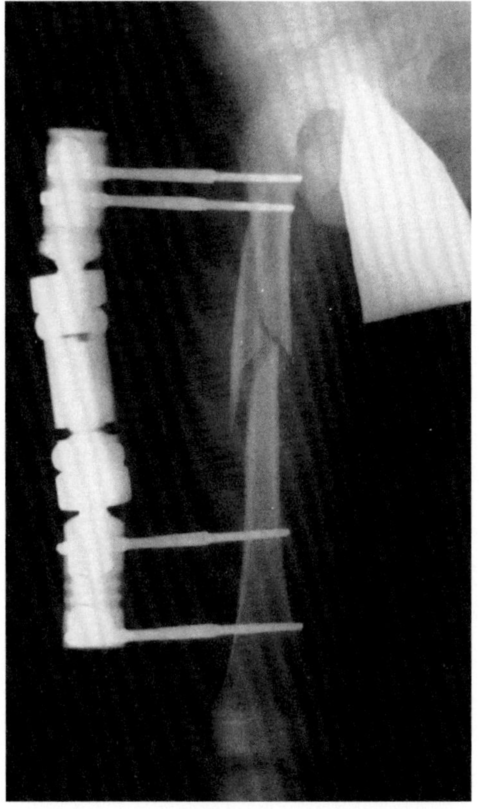

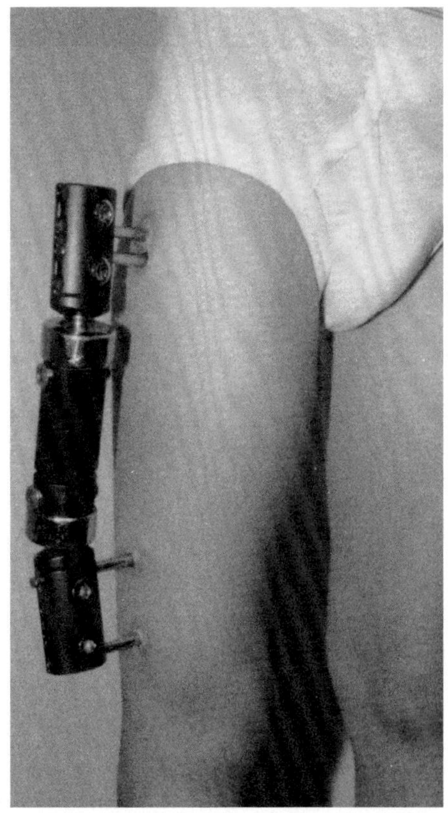

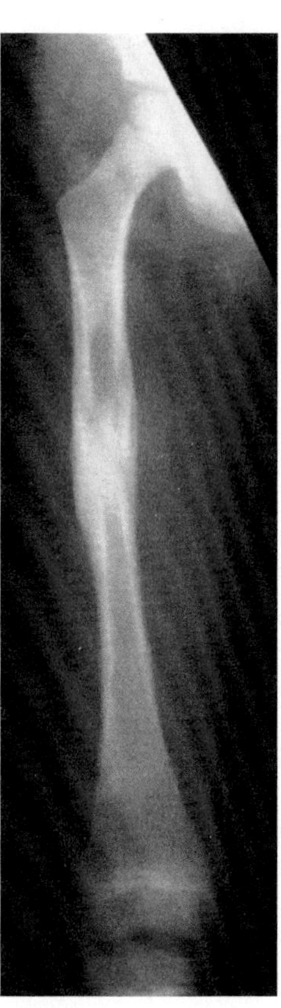

FIGURE 22-16 **A.** Two weeks after unilateral external fixation of a comminuted femoral shaft fracture in an 8-year-old child. **B.** Clinical photograph of external fixator in place. **C.** Four months after fracture, immediately after removal of the external fixator, fracture has healed in good position.

Postoperative Care. Pin site care is critical, and avoiding tension at the skin–pin interface is beneficial. Large pin sites are cleaned with peroxide daily. Showering is allowed once the wound is stable and there is no communication between the pin and the fracture hematoma. Antibiotics are used liberally because pin site infections are common and easily resolved with antibiotic treatment, usually cephalosporin. The external fixation device remains until the fracture is healed. Dynamization is performed before removal, allowing the bone to be stressed to full body weight. The device should not be removed until three or four cortices demonstrate bridging bone continuous on AP and lateral x-rays, typically 3 to 4 months after injury.

Complications of External Fixation

The most common complication of external fixation is pin track infection, which has been reported to occur in up to 72% of patients (81). This complication generally is mild and easily treated with oral antibiotics and local pin site care. Sola et al (78) reported a decreased number of pin track infections after changing their pin care protocol from cleansing with peroxide to simply having the patient shower daily. Superficial infections should be treated aggressively with pin track releases and antibiotics. Deep infections are rare, but if present, drainage and antibiotic therapy are mandatory. Any skin tenting over the pins should be released at the time of application or at follow-up.

In a study of complications of external fixators for femoral fractures, Gregory et al (82) reported a 30% major complication rate and a high minor complication rate. Among the major complications were five refractures or fractures through pin sites. Skaggs et al (83) reviewed the use of external fixation devices for femoral fractures and found a 12% rate of secondary fractures in 66 patients. Multivariate linear regression analysis showed no correlation between the incidence of refracture and the fracture pattern, percentage of bone contact after fixator application, type of external fixator used, or dynamization of the fracture. A statistically significant association was found between the number of cortices demonstrating bridging callus on both the AP and lateral views at the time of fixator removal and refracture. Fractures with fewer than three cortices with bridging callus had a 33% risk of refracture, whereas those with three or four cortices showing bridging callus had only a 4% rate of refracture. Other reports in the literature with smaller numbers, but still substantial experience, document refracture rates as high as 21.6% with more significant complications (81,83–88).

In 1997, in a follow-up of the original article by Aronson and Tursky (75), Blasier et al (89) reported 139 femoral fractures

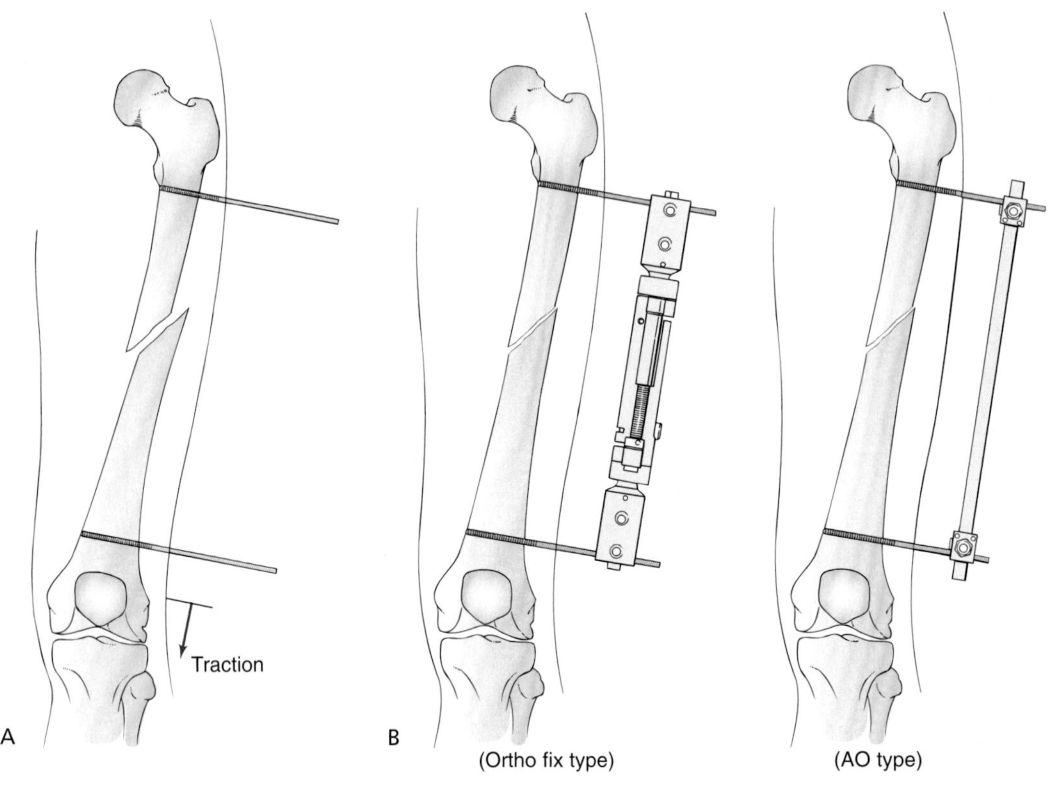

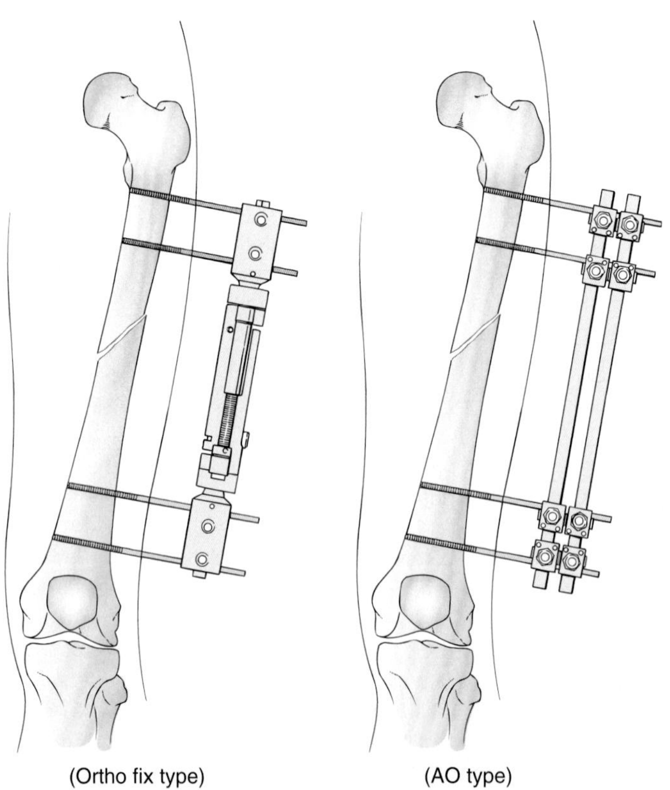

FIGURE 22-17 Technique of external fixation. **A.** With traction applied and provisional reduction of the fracture obtained, the proximal and distal pins are placed perpendicular to the long axis of the bone, being certain that rotational alignment is satisfactory. **B.** Provisional fixation is obtained by attaching the external fixation device with single pins in place. **C.** The second pin is added proximal and distal, providing secure fixation.

treated with external fixation between 1984 and 1993. The average age at treatment was 8.9 years, and the average time to healing was 11.4 weeks. Only 18 patients had definitive x-ray follow-up, with 15 patients demonstrating overgrowth averaging 8.7 mm. In the series of Blasier et al, pin track infection was common and there was a 2% incidence of fracture after removal of the device. El Hayek et al (90) demonstrated the benefit of modern techniques of external fixation in a series of 28 external fixators in fracture treatment in 21 children. Despite the complications, patients and treating physicians have found wound care and ability to lengthen through the fracture to be of great benefit with this technique.

Although joint stiffness has been noted in older patients treated with external fixation, it is relatively uncommon in children with femoral fractures unless major soft tissue injury is present (91).

Intramedullary Fixation

Since the introduction of intramedullary fixation of femoral fractures, enthusiasm for this form of internal fixation has varied but generally increased. Although various techniques have been described over the years, the modifications introduced by Winquist et al (92) and Ligier et al (93) were significant. In the 1970s, Winquist et al (92) developed techniques for closed intramedullary rodding and indirect methods of fixation with reamed and locked fixation devices. In the 1970s and 1980s, Ligier et al (93) introduced a dual flexible rod system that provided internal fixation of fractures with an indirect reduction method leading to less fracture stability but accelerated healing.

By the late 1980s, techniques of antegrade rodding had been refined, and enthusiasm grew for using this procedure in younger patients. The publication by Ligier et al (93) in 1988 of a group of patients treated with flexible intramedullary rodding seemed contrary to the tendencies toward more rigid and more secure fixation. With reports of osteonecrosis of the proximal femur by Beaty et al (94) beginning in the early 1990s, flexible rodding (either antegrade or retrograde) for femoral fractures has grown in favor over locked intramedullary nails. The relative safety of the technique combined with its simplicity have led to its greater acceptance. Comparative studies by Reeves et al (30) and Kirby et al (74), as well as retrospective reviews of traction and casting, suggest that femoral fractures in adolescents are better treated with intramedullary fixation (72–74,84,92,93,95–100) than with traditional traction and

TABLE 22-3 Results of Treatment of Femoral Shaft Fractures in Adolescents

Series	No. of Patients	Average Age (Range) in Years	Treatment	Results and Complications (n)
Kirby et al.	13	12 + 7 (10 + 11–15 + 6)	Traction + cast	Short > 2.5 cm (2) Significant residual angulation (4)
	12	12 + 0 (10 – 10–15 + 7)	Intramedullary nailing	No overgrowth No significant residual angulation
Ziv et al.	17	8 + 3 (6–12)	Intramedullary nailing (9 Rush pins, 9 Kuntscher nails)	No leg length discrepancy > 1 cm Change in AID 0.5–1 cm = 3 with Kuntscher nails
Reeves et al.	41	12 + 4 (9 + 9–16 + 4)	Traction + cast	Delayed union (4) Malunion (5) Growth disturbance (4) Psychotic episodes (2)
	49	14 + 11 (11–16 + 10)	Intramedullary nailing	No infection, nonunion, or malunion
Beaty et al.	30	12 + 3 (10–15)	Intramedullary nailing	Overgrowth >2.5 cm (2) AVN femoral head (1)
Aronson et al.	42	9 + 7 (2 + 5–17 + 8)	External fixation	8.5% Pin infection 10% Cast or reapplication
Ligier	123	10 (5–16)	Flexible IM rods	1 infection 13 wound ulcerations 2 LLD > 2 cm
Mazda	34	9.5 (6–17)	Flexible IM rods	1.0 to 1.5 cm overgrowth (3) 1.0 to 15° malalignment (2)

casting (Table 22-3). The development of trochanteric nail systems sparing the piriformis insertion point may bring antegrade rigid nailing back to the forefront of adolescent fracture care, but a cautious approach must be adopted.

Flexible Intramedullary Rod Fixation

Flexible intramedullary nailing of pediatric femoral fractures either with stainless steel (Ender) or titanium (Nancy) rods can be performed either antegrade or retrograde. The benefit of elastic internal fixation is that a healthy environment for fracture healing with some motion leads to increased callus formation. Properly used, flexible intramedullary rods provide sufficient stability in the fracture so that a cast is not needed, but they lack the rigidity of an external fixation device, which inhibits fracture healing. This lack of rigidity and inability to lock the flexible rods may predispose to deformity either with angular or axial deviation in unstable fractures. The lack of rigidity also may create an environment in which muscle spasm and postoperative pain become more of a problem than with traditional rigid intramedullary fixation devices.

Elastic nailing of femoral fractures carries with it a few controversies: (a) straight versus bent rods, (b) titanium versus steel, (c) immobilization versus no immobilization postoperatively, and (d) antegrade versus retrograde insertion.

Mechanical testing of femoral fracture fixation systems showed that the greatest rigidity is provided by an external fixation device and the least by flexible intramedullary rodding (101). Stainless-steel rods are stronger than titanium in bending tests. Stainless-steel rods have greater intrinsic strength and therefore are not as dependent on the opposing bend technique. Lee et al (101) analyzed a group of synthetic fractured femurs instrumented with Enders rods and determined that there was sufficient axial and torsional stiffness to allow "touch down weight-bearing" despite fracture type. Gwyn et al (102) similarly showed that 4-mm titanium rods impart satisfactory torsional stability regardless of fracture pattern. Flexible rods may be placed retrograde in a double "C" configuration or antegrade in a "C" and "S" manner through a single proximal lateral entry point. Frick et al (103) found there to be greater stiffness and resistance to torsional deformation with the retrograde double C pattern than with the antegrade C and S configuration. Surprisingly Kiely (104) showed that whether rods were straight, bent in a C pattern, or combined C and S pattern, similar mechanical properties were obtained when tested in four-point bending and torsion.

Bourdelet (105) compared retrograde and antegrade (ascending and descending) flexible intramedullary rodding in a group of 73 femoral fractures. Treatment was not randomized, but the subtrochanteric insertion site was preferred because there were fewer knee symptoms and earlier patient independence with the antegrade insertion technique. The insertion site used by Bourdelet was just below the level of the trochanter proximally with a standard medial and lateral distal insertion site. An antegrade transtrochanteric approach was recommended by Carey and Galpin (106), who reported excellent results in 25 patients without growth arrest of the upper femur and no osteonecrosis. Satisfactory alignment and fracture healing were obtained in all patients.

Retrograde intramedullary rodding with Ender rods or titanium rods has been reported by Ligier et al (93), Mann et al (107), Heinrich et al (108), Herscovici et al (109), and others (106,110,111). Heinrich et al (108) recommended a 3.5-mm Ender nail in children 6 to 10 years of age and a 4.0-mm nail in children over 10 years of age. Ligier and Metaizeau (93) used titanium rods ranging from 3 to 4 mm inserted primarily in a retrograde fashion. Heinrich et al (109) recommended flexible intramedullary nails for fixation of diaphyseal femoral fractures in children with multiple system injury, head injury, spasticity, or multiple long bone fractures. After early success in this selected group of patients, they expanded the use of flexible intramedullary rods to include isolated fractures in any patient over 6 years of age with a femoral fracture and parents willing to accept the risk of the surgical treatment. External immobilization with casts was rapidly discontinued in their series.

In 56 patients with femoral fractures stabilized with flexible titanium rods, Flynn et al (112) reported 4 with angular malalignment of more than 10 degrees. These angular deviations tended to occur in fractures toward the end of the bone rather than in diaphyseal fractures. Narayanan et al (113), in looking at complications in a group of 79 fractured femurs over 5 years, found irritation at the insertion site in 41, malunion in 8, refracture in 2, and superficial wound infection in 2. They suggested that these rates of complication could be reduced by leaving the rod ends straight tight against the metaphysis and always using matched-diameter rods. Luhmann et al (114) reported 21 complications in 43 patients with titanium flexible nails. Most of the problems were minor, but a hypertrophic nonunion and a septic joint occurred in their group. They suggested that problems could be minimized by using the largest nail possible and leaving only 2.5 cm out of the femoral cortex.

There is no series comparing titanium to stainless-steel rods in a randomized fashion, but both types of rods have high success rates when judged by rates of malunion, which are less than 5% in most series. Gregory et al (86) compared the use of flexible rods (Ender) with rigid antegrade nailing and found that both techniques produced satisfactory outcomes but flexible rods required much less operative and fluoroscopy time with similar patient satisfaction and outcome.

Fixation with Flexible Intramedullary Rods: Technique

Preoperative Planning. Patients in whom this method of fixation is appropriate are those between the ages of 5 and 16 years with noncomminuted femoral fractures. With unstable femoral fracture patterns, considerable experience is required to achieve satisfactory outcome with flexible intramedullary nailing. Postoperative cast immobilization or postoperative use of an external support device to supplement the internal flexible rod has been of value in unstable fractures.

In evaluating the x-ray, fracture lines that propagate beyond the obvious fracture should be noted (Fig. 22-18). Involvement of the distal metaphyseal region is a relative contraindication

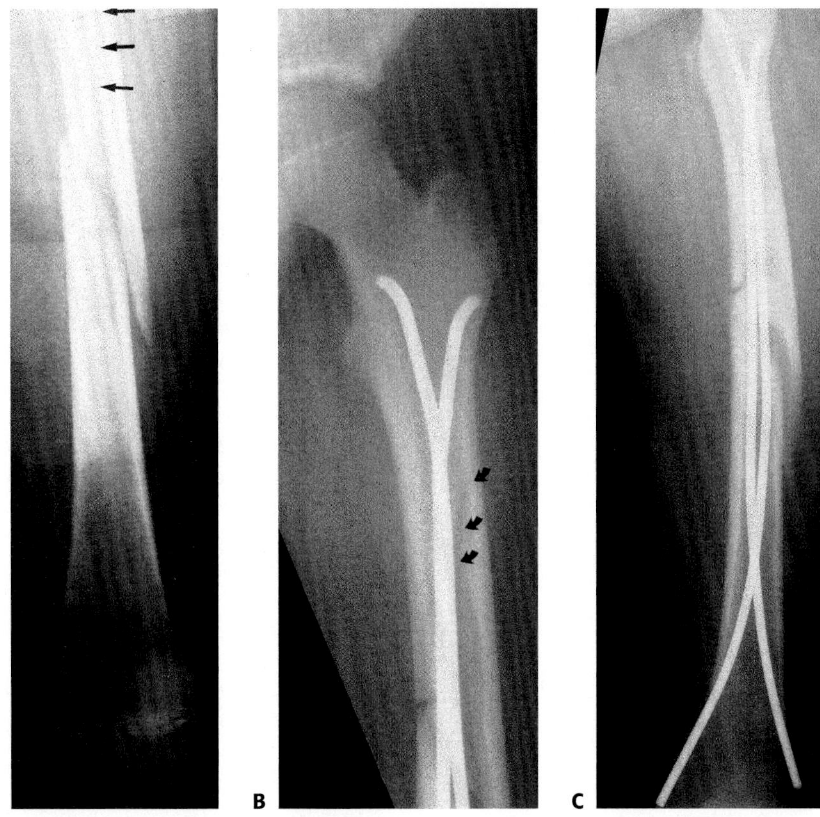

FIGURE 22-18 **A.** The initial anteroposterior x-ray of this 8-year-old child shows an oblique femoral fracture, but there is also a nondisplaced butterfly fragment (*arrows*). **B.** Flexible rods may be used in such a case, being careful not to displace the fragment and **(C)** burying the rods deep in the proximal femoral metaphysis to provide satisfactory fixation.

to this technique. The width of the canal is measured at the narrowest point in the diaphysis on both the AP and lateral views (Fig. 22-19), and this number is divided by 2. This represents the maximal diameter rod that can be used, and generally a rod 0.5 mm smaller than this radius should be used. Therefore, if the medullary canal measures 8 mm, a 3.5-mm rod probably should be used, filling approximately 80% of the canal diameter.

The procedure can be performed on a fracture table or fluoroscopy table, but reduction must be documented with fluoroscopy before insertion of the rods. The procedure is described with the use of a fracture table, but in small children (<80 pounds), we find this easier to do without a fracture table. The procedure described is with titanium elastic rods, but other devices are available and can be used with slight variations in procedure.

Rod Bending. The distance from the top of the inserted rod to the level of the fracture site is measured, and a gentle 30-degree bend is placed in the nail with the apex at what will be the level of the fracture. Next the rod tip is bent to facilitate placement, and to allow the rod to "bounce off" the opposite cortex at the time of insertion. This also facilitates spreading of the rods in the proximal metaphysis, either in the femoral neck or in the greater trochanter. Some surgeons prefer to avoid the second bend at the level of the fracture and use these rods as straight rods, much as in traditional intramedullary fixation. Although not consistent with the recommendation of Lascombes, satisfactory results have been achieved with this technique, especially with the stronger stainless-steel rods. The rods used generally are 3.0 to 4.0 mm in diameter, depending on the size of the bone and the child. Two rods of the same size should always be used, and varying sizes should be avoided.

The technique of elastic fixation of femoral fractures as described by Ligier et al (93) requires that a bend be placed in the mid-portion of the rod at the level of the fracture site. This produces a spring effect (Fig. 22-20) that adds to the rigidity of the fracture fixation. The spread of the rods in opposite directions provides a "prestressed" fixation, which increases resistance to bending. The opposite bends of the two rods at the level of the fracture significantly increase resistance to varus and valgus stress, as well as torsion.

Retrograde Insertion. After the child is placed on the fracture table, the leg is prepared and draped with the thigh (hip to

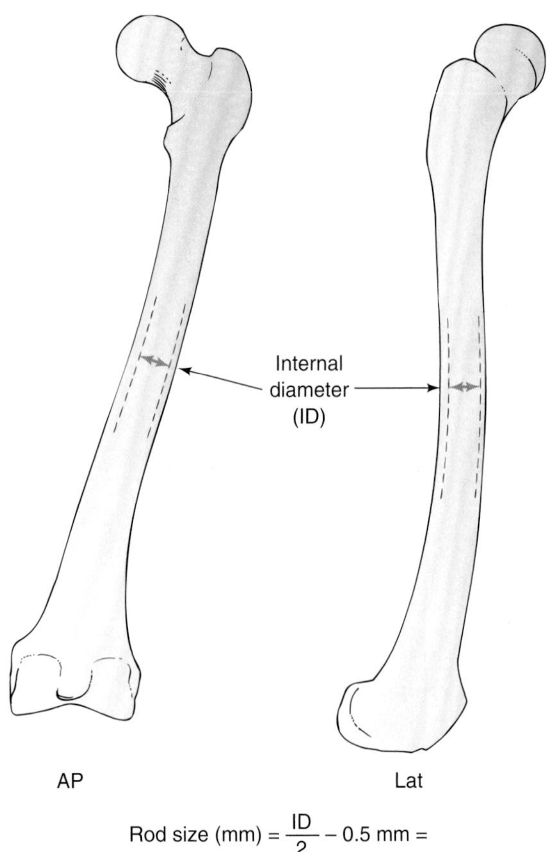

$$\text{Rod size (mm)} = \frac{ID}{2} - 0.5 \text{ mm} =$$

FIGURE 22-19 To determine the size of titanium flexible rods to be used, measure the diaphyseal internal diameter on both the anteroposterior and lateral views, divide by 2, and subtract 0.5 mm. Use the smaller of the number obtained from the anteroposterior and lateral views. AO rods range from 2.0 to 4.0 mm in diameter, in 0.5-mm increments.

knee) exposed (Fig. 22-21). The image intensifier is used to localize the placement of skin incisions by viewing the distal femur in the AP and lateral planes. Incisions are made on the medial and lateral side distal to the insertion site in the bone. The proximal end of the 3-cm incision should be at or just distal to the level of the insertion site, which is about 2.5 to 3 cm proximal to the distal femoral physis (Fig. 22-22). A 4.5-mm drill bit or awl is used to make a cortical hole in the bone. The distal femoral metaphysis is opened using a drill or awl at a point 2.5 cm proximal to the distal femoral physis. The drill is then inclined 10 degrees anteriorly and steeply angled in the frontal plane to facilitate passage of the nail through the dense pediatric metaphyseal bone.

Rods are inserted from the medial and lateral side and driven up to the level of the fracture. Upon insertion the rod glances off the cortex as it advances toward the fracture site. Both medial and lateral rods are inserted to the level of the fracture. At this point the fracture is reduced using longitudinal traction and a fracture reduction tool (Fig. 22-21B). This tool is radiolucent and holds the unstable femoral fracture in the appropriate position to allow fixation. After the first rod is driven across the fracture, approximately 2 to 3 cm, the second rod is driven across the fracture. The two rods then are driven into the proximal end of the femur, with one driven toward the femoral neck and the other toward the greater trochanter. When placing the second rod across the fracture site and rotating it, care must be taken not to wind one rod around the other. After the rods are driven across the fracture and before they are seated, fluoroscopy is used to confirm satisfactory reduction of the fracture and to ensure that the rods did not comminute the fracture as they were driven into the proximal fragment.

The rods are pulled back approximately 2 cm, the end of each rod is cut, and the rods are driven back securely into the femur. The end of the rod should lie adjacent to the bone of the metaphysis but should be at least 1 cm distal to the insertion hole to allow ease in later removal. Bending the rod ends should be avoided because it can cause a painful bursa over the rod end.

If the fracture is in the distal aspect of the femur, a proximal insertion site should be considered. The insertion site may be anterolateral just below the greater trochanter or through the lateral border of the trochanter. Through a skin incision at the level of the trochanter, two 4.5-mm holes are drilled into the metaphysis just below the apophysis and connected with a rongeur. The rods are inserted antegrade. The sizing of the rods and postoperative management are the same as in the retrograde technique.

Technique Tip. Mazda et al (115) emphasized that for insertion of titanium elastic nails, the nails have to be bent into an even curve over the entire length, and the summit of the curve must be at the level of the fracture or very close to it in comminuted fractures. The depth of curvature should be about three times the diameter of the femoral canal. Flynn et al (112) also stressed the importance of contouring both nails with similar gentle curvatures, choosing nails that are 40% of the narrowest diaphyseal diameter and using medial and lateral starting points that are at the same level in the metaphysis.

Postoperative Management. For unstable long oblique fractures or comminuted fractures, immobilization with a cast may be of benefit. To decrease knee pain and quadriceps spasm, we have found the use of a knee immobilizer to be beneficial in the early postoperative course. Physical therapy with touchdown weight-bearing should begin as soon as the patient is comfortable. Gentle knee exercises and quadriceps strengthening can be begun, but there should be no aggressive passive motion of the knee, which increases the motion at the fracture site and increases quadriceps spasm. Postoperative knee motion does return to normal, but this requires time. Full weight-bearing generally is tolerated by 6 weeks. Ozdemir et al (116) recommended the use of postoperative functional bracing, demonstrating effectiveness in a group of patients treated with elastic rodding. Such postoperative support may occasionally be required, but in most cases it appears not to be needed.

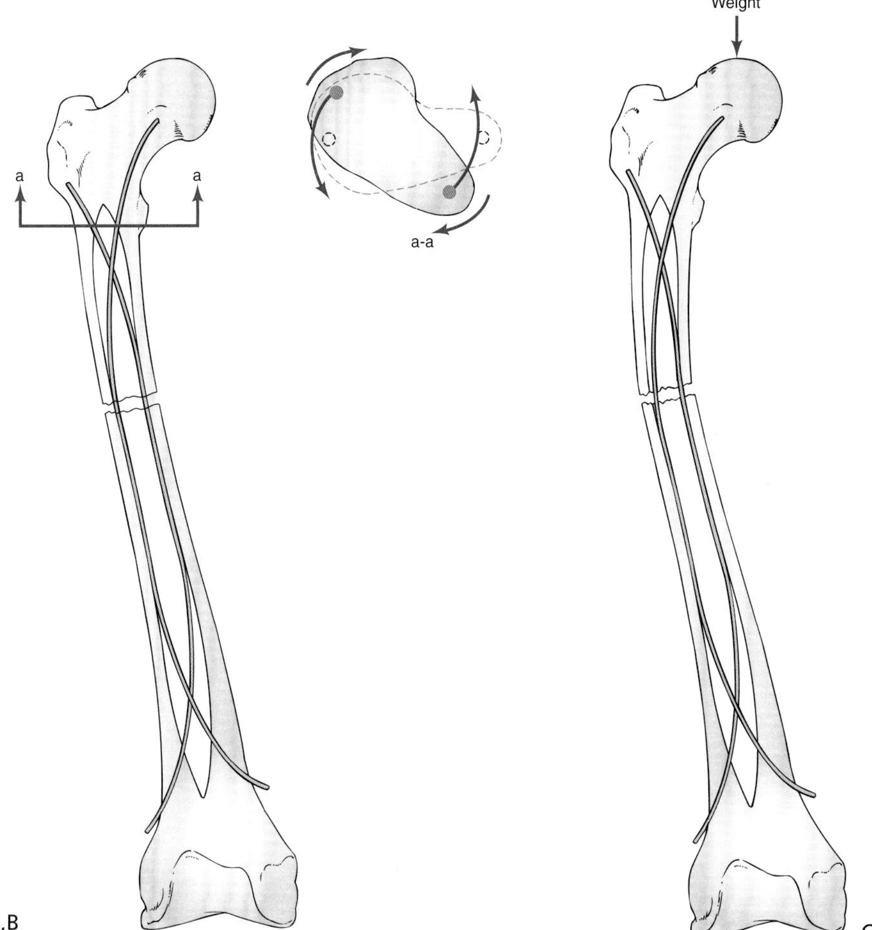

FIGURE 22-20 **A.** Stability from flexible rods comes from proper technique. **B.** Torsional stability results from divergence of the rods in the metaphysis. **C.** Resistance to sagittal and coronal bending results from spreading of the pre-bent rods through the diaphysis, as well as the size and material properties of the rods. Elastic rods return to their predetermined alignment when loaded unless plastic deformation occurs.

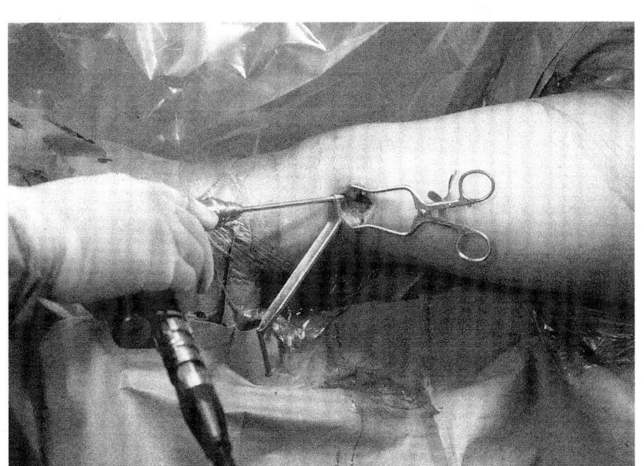

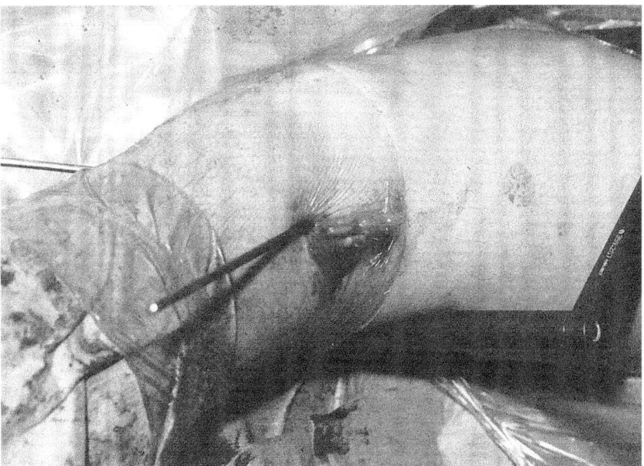

FIGURE 22-21 **A.** In children weighing more than 80 pounds, a fracture table can be used to provide traction and reduction of a femoral fracture. The leg is draped free, allowing medial and lateral rods to be placed. **B.** A radiolucent reduction bar may be beneficial to reduce angular deformity when passing the rods.

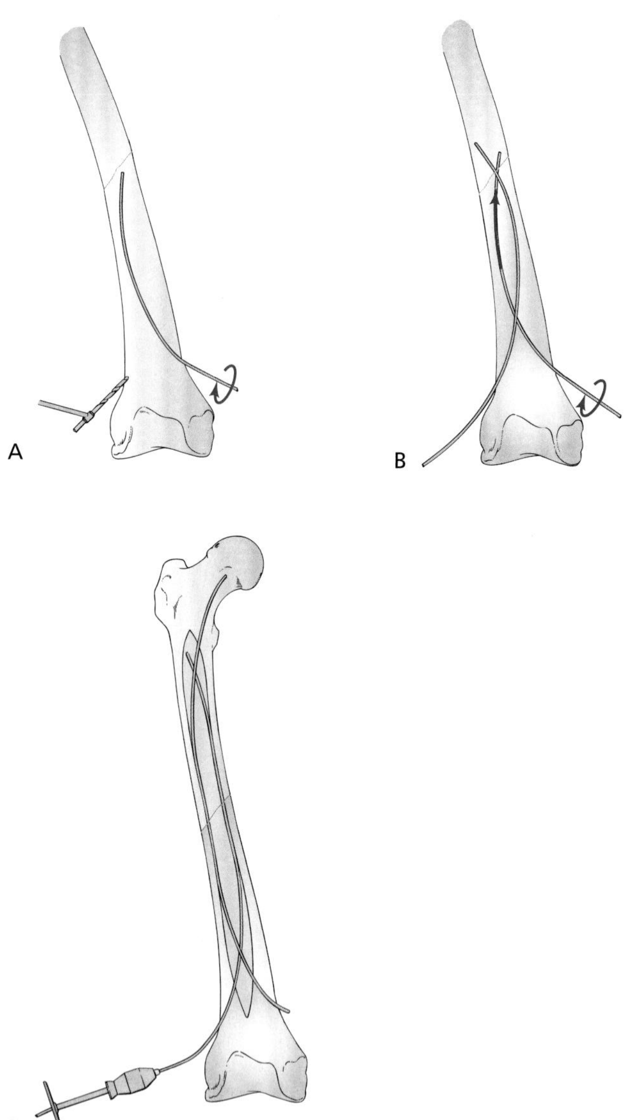

FIGURE 22-22 Retrograde insertion. **A.** The rods are inserted through a distal cortical hole 4.5 mm in diameter made either with a drill or an awl 2.5 cm above the physis. **B.** Rods are advanced to the level of the fracture site by rotating (reciprocally) or pounding with an inserter and mallet. The fracture is reduced, and one rod is driven across the fracture site 3 to 5 cm. **C.** Then the second rod is driven into the proximal fragment.

The rods can be removed 6 to 12 months after injury when the fracture is fully healed, usually as an outpatient procedure.

Complications of Flexible Intramedullary Nailing. Complications are relatively infrequent after flexible intramedullary nailing. In 351 fractures reported in 7 studies (77,93,106,114,115, 117,118), 1 nonunion, 1 infection, and no occurrence of osteonecrosis were reported. Approximately 12% of patients had malunions, most often mild varus deformities, and approximately 3% had clinically significant leg length discrepancies from either overgrowth or shortening. Mazda et al (115) pointed out a technique-related complication that occurred in 10 of their 34 patients: rods were left too long and caused painful bursae and limited knee flexion. All 10 patients had the nails removed 2 to 5 months after surgery. In a multicenter study that included 58 femoral fractures stabilized with titanium elastic nails, irritation of the soft tissue near the knee by the nail tip occurred in 4 patients (7%), leading to a deeper infection in 2 patients. This study also reported one refracture after premature nail removal, leading to a recommendation that nail removal be delayed until callus is solid around all cortices and the fracture line is no longer visible. Ozdemir et al (116) measured overgrowth with a scanogram and found that the average increase in length was 1.8 mm, suggesting that femoral overgrowth is not seen with this method of treatment.

Flynn et al (119) compared traction and spica cast with titanium elastic nails for treatment of femoral fractures in 83 consecutive school-aged children. The three unsatisfactory results were treated with traction followed by casting. The overall complication rate was 34% in the traction group and 21% in the elastic nail group. As in other studies the costs were similar in both arms of the study. The operative group returned to school sooner and overall had a quicker recovery form this injury.

After reviewing all available literature on this subject, it is clear that the complication rate rises with comminuted fractures in large patients, which has lead many to look at alternative techniques for management in such adolescents. These alternatives include trochanteric nailing and bridge plating.

Rigid Intramedullary Rod Fixation

Problems with angular malalignment and maintenance of length can be avoided with the use of rigid intramedullary fixation. Interlocking proximally and distally to maintain length and rotational alignment in unstable fractures, as in adults, appears to be of benefit to some adolescents (120–122). Beaty et al (94) reported the use of interlocking intramedullary nails for the treatment of 31 femoral shaft fractures in 30 patients 10 to 15 years of age. All fractures united, and the average leg length discrepancy was 0.51 cm. No angular or rotational malunions occurred. All nails were removed at an average of 14 months after injury; no refracture or femoral neck fracture occurred after nail removal. One case of osteonecrosis of the femoral head occurred, which was thought to be secondary to injury to the ascending cervical artery during nail insertion. A poll of the members of the Pediatric Orthopaedic Society disclosed 14 patients with osteonecrosis in approximately 1,600 femoral fractures. Despite the use of a "safe" transtrochanteric insertion site for antegrade femoral rodding, a case of osteonecrosis has been reported. Buford et al (123) showed in their MRI study of hips after antegrade rodding that subclinical osteonecrosis may be present. Antegrade rodding through the trochanter or the upper end of the femur appears to be associated with a risk of osteonecrosis in children with open physes, regardless of chronologic age.

Reamed antegrade nailing in children under 12 years of age is not recommended because of proximal femoral growth abnormalities (124), the risk of osteonecrosis of the femoral head (55,94,125,126), the size of the proximal femur, and the relative success of other treatment methods. However, Maruenda-Paulino et al (128) reported good results using 9-mm Kuntscher rods in children 7 to 12 years of age, and Beaty et al (94) reported the use of newer pediatric "intermediate" interlocking nails for femoral canals with diameters as small as 8 mm. In children 12 to 17 years of age, antegrade locked transtrochanteric fixation may occasionally be indicated for an unstable fracture in a large adolescent. Townsend and Hoffinger (128) and Momberger et al (129) published reviews of trochanteric nailing in adolescents with very good results. The combined series includes 82 patients age 10 to 17 + 6 years with no reported cases of osteonecrosis and no significant alteration in proximal femoral anatomy.

Open fractures in older adolescents can be effectively treated with intramedullary rodding, either as delayed or primary treatment, including those caused by gunshot wounds and high-velocity injuries (130,131). Antegrade intramedullary rod insertion maintains length, prevents angular malunion and nonunion, and allows the patient to be rapidly mobilized and discharged from the hospital. However, other techniques with fewer potential risks should be considered.

Retrograde rodding of the femur has become an accepted procedure in adults (Fig. 22-23) (132,133). In a large patient approaching skeletal maturity (bone age >16 years) but with an open proximal femoral physis and an unstable fracture pattern, one might consider this treatment as a way to avoid the risk of osteonecrosis yet stabilize the fracture. Growth from the distal femur will be less than 1 cm, so leg length inequality will not be a problem. Ricci et al (133) have shown that the complication rate with this technique compares favorably to that of antegrade nailing, with a higher rate of knee pain but a lower rate of hip pain. The malunion rate was slightly lower with retrograde rodding than with antegrade rodding of the femur.

Antegrade Transtrochanteric Intramedullary Nailing: Technique

The patient is placed either supine or in the lateral decubitus position on a fracture table. The upper end of the femur is approached through a 5-cm longitudinal incision proximal to the greater trochanter and in line with the femoral shaft by fluoroscopy. The skin incision can be precisely placed after localization on both the AP and lateral views. The gluteus maximus muscle is spread, and the gluteus medius muscle identified. The rod should be inserted just lateral to the tip of the trochanter. Posterior and medial dissection may place the vasculature of the proximal femur at risk. Identifying the piriformis fossa with vigorous dissection and placement of anterior and posterior retractors to the femoral neck also may cause injury to the lateral ascending cervical artery and must be avoided. Dissection should be limited to the lateral aspect of the greater trochanter, avoiding the piriformis fossa. This prevents dissection near the origin of the lateral ascending cervical artery medial to the piriformis fossa.

A threaded-tip guidewire is inserted into the proximal portion of the greater trochanter, followed by reaming with a 9-mm reamer. A ball-tip guidewire then can be inserted into the proximal femur. No dissection should be performed medial or posterior to the insertion site. The ball-tip guidewire is placed across the fracture site and into the distal fragment to a level just proximal to the distal femoral physis. Progressive reaming is performed before a reamed rod or a nonreamed rod is chosen. The smallest rod that maintains contact with the femoral cortices is used (generally 8 or 9 mm) and is locked proximally and distally. Only one distal locking screw is necessary, but two can be used (134). Rods that have an expanded proximal cross section should be avoided. The proximal end of the nail should be left slightly long (up to 1 cm) to make later removal easier. The rod chosen should be angled proximally and specifically designed for transtrochanteric insertion (Fig. 22-24).

Technique Tips. Dissection should be limited to the tip of the greater trochanter, without extending to the capsule or mid-portion of the femoral neck. Leaving the proximal end of the nail up to 1 cm long makes later removal easier.

Postoperative Management. Nails can be removed 9 to 18 months after radiographic union to prevent bony overgrowth over the proximal tip of the nail. Dynamization with removal of the proximal or distal screw generally is not necessary.

Complications of Locked Intramedullary Nailing. Although good results have been reported with this technique and patient satisfaction is high, problems with proximal femoral growth, osteonecrosis, and leg length discrepancy cannot be ignored.

In a series of intramedullary nailing of 31 fractures, Beaty et al (94) reported one patient with segmental osteonecrosis of the femoral head (Fig. 22-25), which was not seen on x-ray until 15 months after injury. Kaweblum et al (134) reported a patient with osteonecrosis of the proximal femoral epiphysis after a greater trochanteric fracture, suggesting that the blood supply to the proximal femur may have been compromised by vascular disruption at the level of the greater trochanter during rod insertion. Other researchers have reported single patients with osteonecrosis of the femoral head after intramedullary nailing (125,126,135). Chung (136) noted the absence of transphyseal vessels to the proximal femoral epiphysis and demonstrated that the singular lateral ascending cervical artery predominantly supplies blood to the capital femoral epiphysis (Fig. 22-26). He stated that all of the epiphyseal and metaphyseal branches of the lateral ascending cervical artery originate from a single stem that crosses the capsule at the trochanteric notch. Because the space between the trochanter and the femoral head is extremely narrow, this single artery is vulnerable to injury and appears to be so until skeletal maturity, regardless of chronologic age.

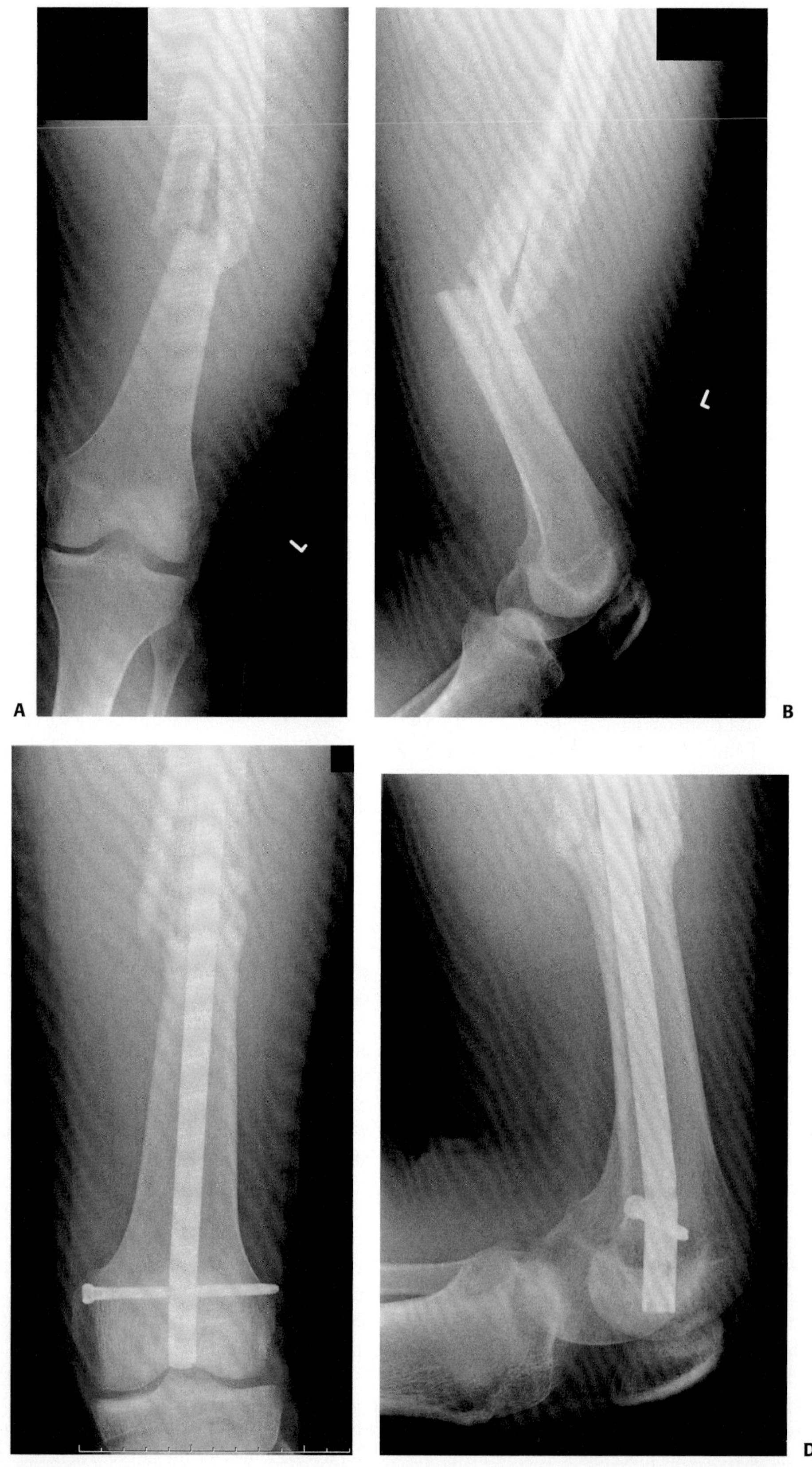

FIGURE 22-23 A,B. This 15-year-old with a comminuted femoral fracture was an ideal candidate for a retrograde locked rod to spare the proximal femur and the risk of osteonecrosis. **C,D.** The rod crosses the distal femoral physis and should only be used in children nearing the end of growth.

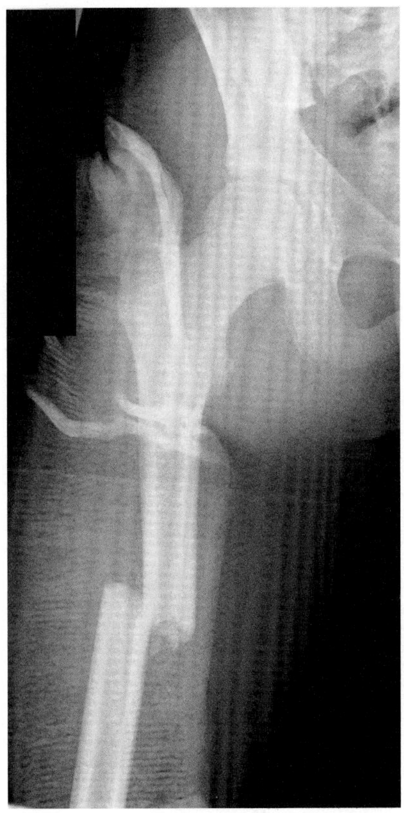

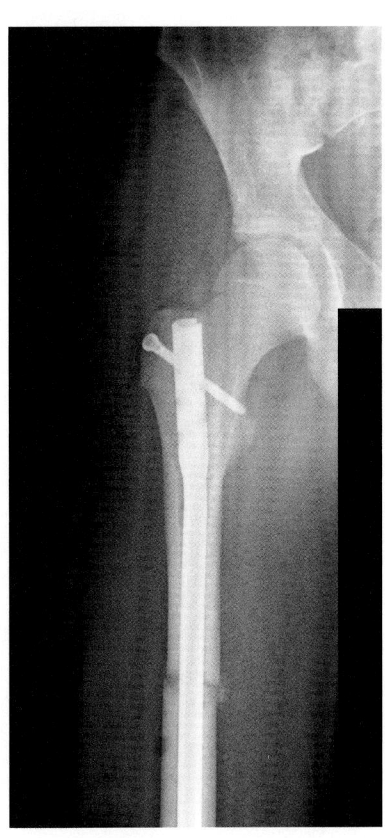

FIGURE 22-24 **A.** This 15-year-old patient had an open proximal femoral physis. He weighed 80 kg and represents an ideal indication for a trochanteric rod. **B.** The trochanteric insertion with a specifically designed trochanteric nail provides stable fixation and less risk of ostionecrosis.

Townsend and Hoffinger (128) reported no ostonecrosis in 34 patients in whom a trochanteric tip starting point was used. Simonian et al (137) in a long-term study of 52 children and adolescents with femoral fractures treated with plating and intramedullary rodding, found that excessive overgrowth was less common with nailing than with plating. Three patients had moderate valgus deformities of the hip and one had late arthrosis after intramedullary rodding despite using a transtrochanteric approach. Simonian et al (137) concluded that open physes were a contraindication to antegrade rodding even with a transtrochanteric approach. Thometz and Lamdan (126) also documented an association between osteonecrosis and antegrade rodding in an adolescent.

Growth abnormality in the proximal femur may occur with arrest of the greater trochanteric physis. Although most growth from the greater trochanter after 8 years of age is appositional, Raney et al (124) reported five patients who developed coxa valga and mild hip subluxation from trochanteric physeal arrest after antegrade nailing. These patients ranged in age from 9 to 13 years, suggesting that even in older children greater trochanteric physeal arrest occasionally can produce clinical problems. Beaty et al (94) reported two patients, boys age 13 years, with overgrowth of more than 2.5 cm that required epiphysiodesis because of leg length discrepancy. Gordon et al (97) in a study of the effect of trochanteric nailing on proximal femoral anatomy found no significant changes in the articulotrochanteric distance, the neck-shaft angle or the width of the femoral neck after trochanteric antegrade nailing. They also found no incidence of osteonecrosis.

The proximal femoral physis is a continuous cartilaginous plate between the greater trochanter and the proximal femur in young children. Interference with the physis may result in atrophy of the femoral neck, placing the child at a small risk for subsequent femoral neck fracture (137). Antegrade rodding with reaming of a large defect also may result in growth disturbance in the proximal femur as well as femoral neck fracture (Fig. 22-27). Beaty et al (94) reported no "thinning" of the femoral neck in their patients, which they attributed to an older patient group (10 to 15 years of age) and design changes in the femoral nail that allowed a decrease in the cross-sectional diameter of the proximal portion of the femoral rods.

Open Reduction and Internal Fixation with Plate and Screws

Ward et al (138), Kregor et al (139), Fyodorov et al (140), and Hansen (141) recommended this form of treatment in selected femoral fractures. Ward et al (138) reported the use of AO compression plates for the treatment of femoral shaft fractures in 25 children 6 to 16 years of age, 22 of whom had associated fractures or multisystem injuries. According to these investigators, plate fixation offers the advantages of anatomic reduction,

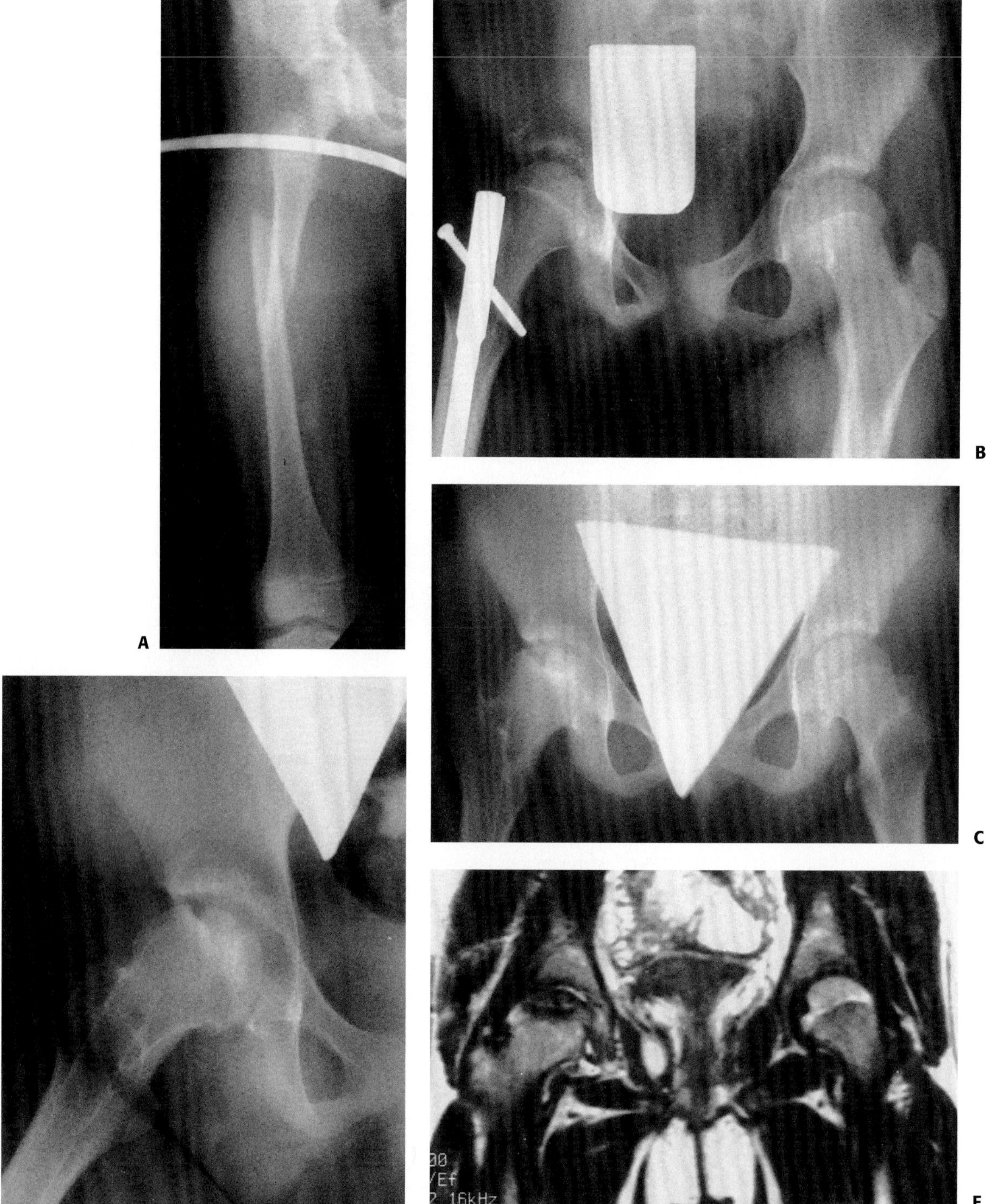

FIGURE 22-25 **A.** Isolated femoral shaft fracture in an 11 year old. **B.** After fixation with an intramedullary nail, femoral head appears normal. **C.** Eight months after injury, fracture is healed; note early signs of osteonecrosis of right femoral head. **D.** Fifteen months after injury, segmental osteonecrosis of the femoral head is evident on x-rays. **E.** Magnetic resonance image shows extent of osteonecrosis of right femoral head. (**D** reprinted from Beaty JH, Austin SM, Warner WC, et al. Interlocking intramedullary nailing of femoral-shaft fractures in adolescents: preliminary results and complications. *J Pediatr Orthop* 1994;14:178–183; with permission.)

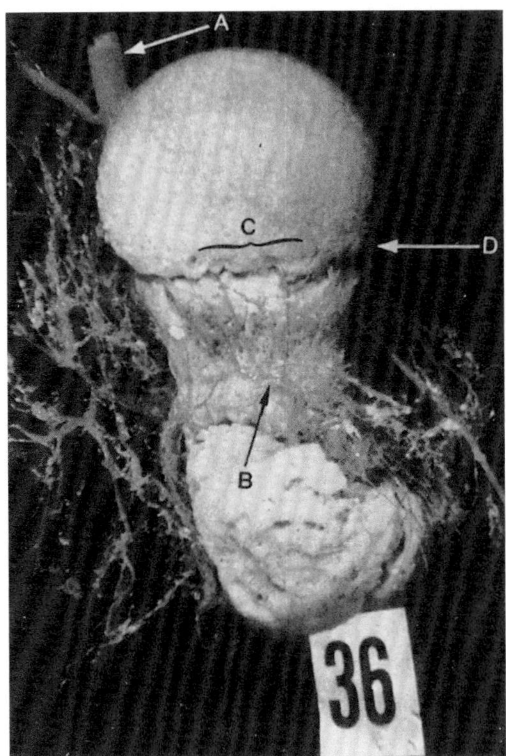

FIGURE 22-26 The single ascending cervical artery (*A*) is the predominant blood supply to the femoral head. The vessel is at risk during antegrade insertion of an intramedullary rod. (Reprinted from Chung S. The arterial supply of the developing proximal end of the femur. *J Bone Joint Surg Am* 1976;58:961; with permission.)

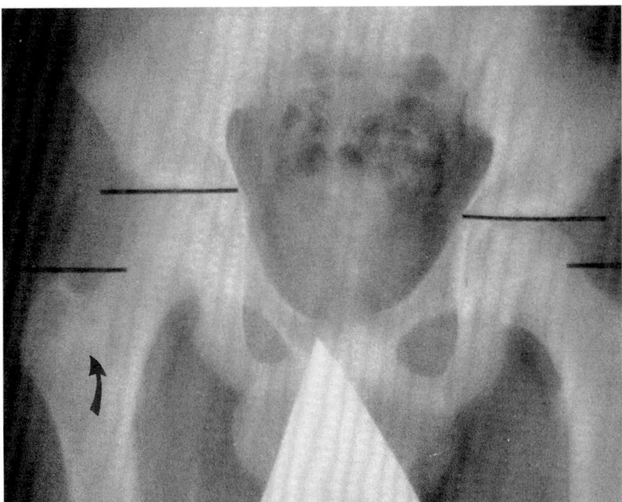

FIGURE 22-27 Fifteen-year-old boy 3 years after intramedullary nailing of the right femur. Articulotrochanteric distance increased by 1.5 cm; note partial trochanteric epiphysiodesis (*arrow*) with mild overgrowth of the femoral neck. (Reprinted from Beaty JH, Austin SM, Warner WC, et al. Interlocking intramedullary nailing of femoral-shaft fractures in adolescents: preliminary results and complications. *Pediatr Orthop* 1994;14: 178–183; with permission.)

ease of insertion, simplified nursing care, rapid mobilization without casting, and applicability to any size femoral shaft. Disadvantages of plate fixation include the long incision necessary and the risks of plate breakage and stress fracture after plate removal. They recommended plate fixation for children under 11 years of age with closed-head injuries or multiple trauma. All the patients reported by Kregor et al (139) had multiple trauma, and this form of treatment was selected to stabilize the femoral fracture quickly and mobilize the patient. Fyodorov et al (140) reviewed 21 patients in whom 4.5-mm DCP plates were used for fixation. Patients were kept non–weight-bearing on crutches for 8 weeks. There were two plate breakages requiring revision and one requiring spica casting to achieve healing.

Modern techniques of femoral plating (142) with maintenance of the periosteum may lead to greater acceptance of this method of management. Kanlic et al (98) reported a series of 51 patients using submuscular bridge plating with up to 10 year follow-up. Fifty-five percent had unstable fracture patterns. There were two significant complications: one plate breakage (3.5 mm) and one fracture after plate removal. Functional outcome was excellent with 8% significant leg length discrepancy. Rozbruch et al (142) described modern techniques of plate fixation popularized by the AO Association for the Study of Internal Fixation that include indirect reduction, biologic approaches to internal fixation, and greater use of blade plates and locked plates (Fig. 22-28).

Pathologic fractures, especially in the distal femoral metaphysis, create larger areas of bone loss that can be treated with open biopsy, plate fixation, and immediate bone grafting (Fig. 22-29).

Technique: Standard Compression Plating

In a sterile operating room environment after general anesthesia has been given, the patient is placed on a radiolucent operating table and the entire extremity is prepared and draped. The femur is approached laterally. The vastus lateralis is retracted anteriorly to expose the femur. Soft tissue attachments to the bone are preserved to the extent possible. Fragments are lagged into place and secured with a dynamic compression plate. A 4.5-mm or larger compression plate is used in children (Fig. 22-30). If the fracture is at either end of the bone, leaving insufficient bone for cortical fixation, fully threaded cancellous screws add to the stability of fixation and are preferable to either cortical or partially threaded cancellous screws. Both interfragmentary compression and dynamic compression techniques can be used to achieve stability and anatomic alignment.

Technique Tips. Soft tissue stripping should be limited, and three screws should be used proximal and distal to the fracture site.

Postoperative Management. Protected weight-bearing is progressed to weight-bearing to tolerance. Active range-of-motion exercise of the hip and knee is encouraged.

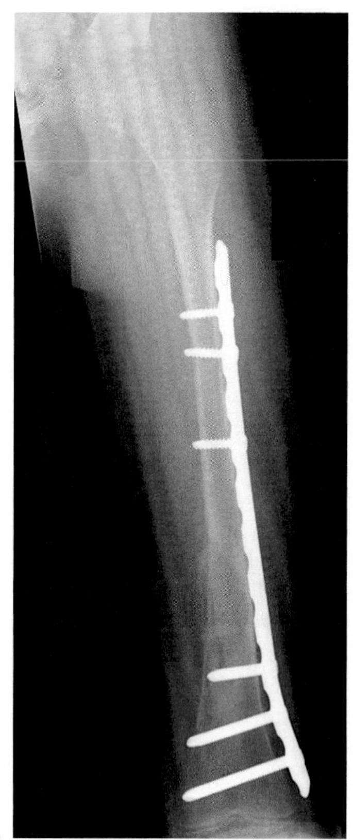

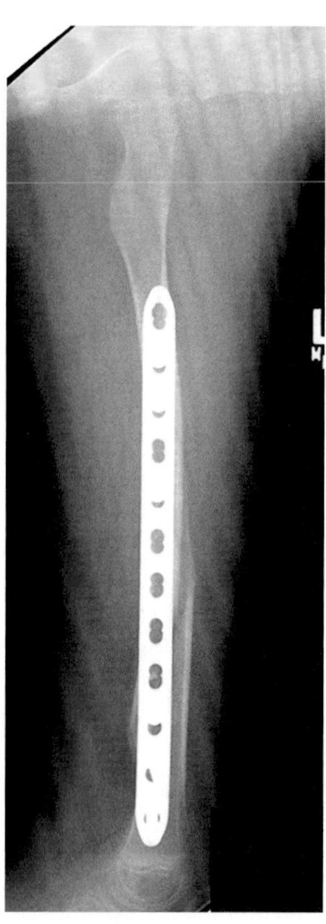

FIGURE 22-28 **A.** This child with an unstable femoral fracture in osteopenic bone was managed with a submuscular locking plate providing alignment and stability. **B.** The lateral bow of the femur may be partially preserved despite a straight plate.

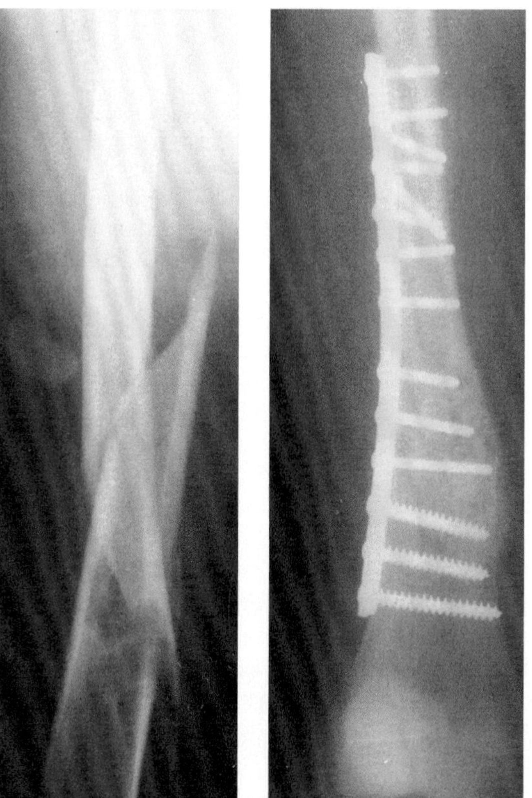

FIGURE 22-29 **A.** Pathologic fracture (nonossifying fibroma) of the femoral diaphysis. **B.** Plate fixation at the time of biopsy and bone grafting.

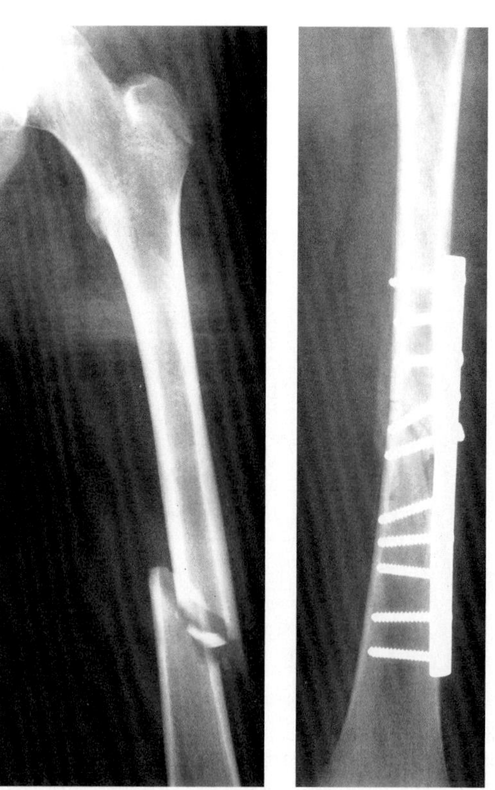

FIGURE 22-30 **A.** This oblique mid-shaft femoral fracture with some comminution in a 200-pound male occurred in an automobile accident. **B.** Stable fixation with plate and lag screw construction is highly successful and carries no risk of osteonecrosis.

Technique: Locked and Submuscular Plating

In selected cases in which there is limited bone for fixation between the fracture and the physes, locked plating techniques may be valuable. This technique provides greater stability by securing the plate with a fixed-angle screw in which the threads lock to the plate, as well as in the bone. This effectively converts the screw-plate to a fixed-angle blade plate device. In using this type of device, one should lock first, then compress, and finally lock the plate on the opposite side of the fracture. The locked plate can be used with an extensile exposure or with submuscular plating, but the latter is more difficult and should only be attempted when the technique is mastered.

Submuscular bridge plating is a technique (143) that has become more frequently used in adult orthopaedic trauma over the past few years. The technique is particularly applicable in children (Fig 22-31) with comminuted fractures, allowing for stable internal fixation with reduced blood loss and maintenance of vascularity to small fragments of bone, facilitating early healing. In the treatment of comminuted pediatric femoral fractures or unstable femoral fractures, there appears to be a role for bridge plating.

In this technique, a 4.5-mm narrow LC-DCP plate is used with minimal exposure. The plate is held to the bone using percutaneous screw technique with the plate positioned extraperiosteally and submuscularly. In certain situations, locked plating may be of value, but in the standard technique for bridge plating, locking is not necessary.

Preoperative x-rays of the contralateral femur are used to template a plate for fixation along the lateral side of the femur. A 4.5-mm narrow LC-DCP plate is used for several reasons. The plates are readily available. The width allows optimal contact with the shaft, and they are easy to contour. The length of the plate depends on the size of the femoral shaft and location of the fracture. Generally a 12- to 16-hole plate is used in order to have maximal spread of screws proximally and distally to achieve maximal stability. The plate is pre-bent to the contour of the femur, specifically recognizing the metaphyseal flare both proximally and distally. In general, we do not contour the plate to conform to the anterior bow of the femur. We do not use locking plates unless pathologic lesions, severe osteopenia, or severe comminution is present.

Technique: Submuscular Bridge Plating

The patient is placed supine on a radiolucent operating table with the leg free and traction held manually with either a traction pin and bow or simple distal skin traction. A 2-cm incision is made over the distal femur, just above the level of the physis. Exposure of the periosteum just below the vastus lateralis facilitates the submuscular passage of the plate. A Cobb elevator is used to dissect the plane between the periosteum and the vastus lateralis. The fracture site is not exposed, and, in general, a proximal incision is not required. The plate is inserted underneath the vastus lateralis, and the femoral shaft is held to length by traction. The plate is advanced slowly, allowing the surgeon

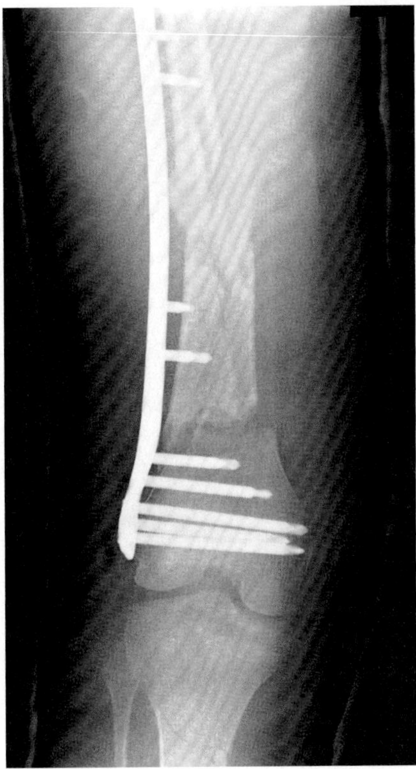

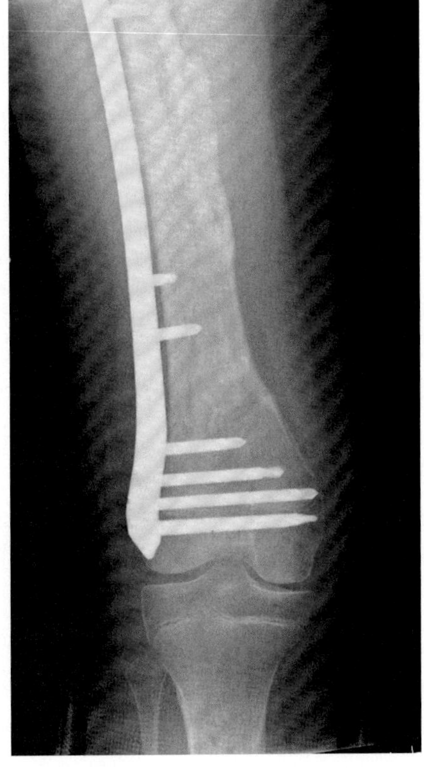

FIGURE 22-31 This 15-year-old boy had a comminuted distal femoral fracture stabilized with a locked plate **(A)** spanning the unstable segment, maintaining length and alignment. Blood supply was maintained to the healing fragments using a submuscular technique. Healing was uneventful **(B)**.

to feel the bone against the tip of the plate. Fluoroscopy is helpful in determining proper positioning of the plate. A bolster is placed under the thigh to help maintain sagittal alignment. Once the plate is in position and the femur is at length, a Kirschner wire is placed in the most proximal and most distal hole of the plate to maintain length (Fig. 22-32). Fluoroscopy is used to check the AP and lateral views and be sure the bone is at appropriate length at this point. A third Kirschner wire may be used to provide a more stable reduction of the femoral shaft. Although screws can be used to facilitate angular reduction to the plate, length must be achieved before the initiation of fixation.

The principles of external fixation are used in choosing sites for screw fixation. Greater spread of screws increases the stability of fracture fixation. We generally place one screw through the incision under direct visualization distally. The most proximal screw is then placed to fix length and provisionally improve alignment. Central screws are then placed, using a free-hand technique with the "perfect circle" alignment of the plate over the fracture fragments. Stab holes are made centrally for drill and screw insertion (Fig. 22-32). Rather than using a depth gauge directly, because the bone will be pulled to the plate, the depth gauge is placed over the thigh itself to measure appropriate length of the screw. When screws are inserted, a Vicryl tie is placed around the shank to avoid losing the screw during percutaneous placement. Self-tapping screws are required for this procedure. Six cortices are sought on either side of the fracture.

Following internal fixation, the patient requires only a simple dressing. At times, there is benefit to a knee immobilizer; however, in general, this is not required.

The postoperative management includes protected weight-bearing on crutches with no need for cast immobilization, as long as stable fixation is achieved. Early weight-bearing in some series of plate fixation has resulted in a low but significant incidence of plate breakage and nonunion. These complications should be decreased by a cautious period of postoperative management.

There are occasional cases in which there is sufficient osteopenia or comminution to require a locked plate to provide secure fixation. In using a locked plate submuscularly, a large enough incision must be used to be sure the bone is against the plate when it is locked. The articular fragment is fixed first to ensure that the angular relationship between the joint surface and the shaft is perfect.

Complications of Plate Fixation

Extensive dissection and periosteal stripping during plate application may lead to overgrowth. Overgrowth was not a significant problem in the series of Kregor et al (139), with an average increase in length of 0.9 cm (range 0.5 to 1.5 cm), but Ward et al (138) reported several patients with considerable overgrowth (approximately 1 inch), and Hansen (141) reported overgrowth of an inch in a 12-year-old boy, suggesting that overgrowth is possible in children over 10 years of age. Eren et al (144) re-

A 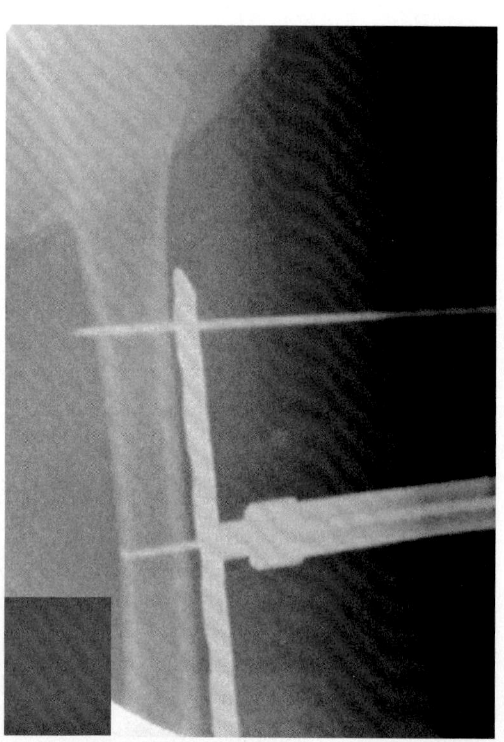

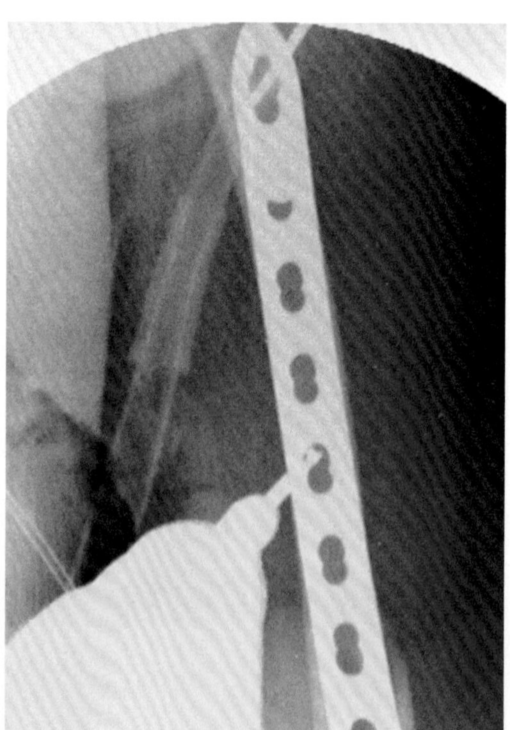 B

FIGURE 22-32 **A.** A Kirschner wire is inserted in the end holes of the plate to maintain length. **B.** Drill holes and screws are placed with fluoroscope imaging.

ported a series of 40 children age 4 to 10 years with significant lengthening on the operated side in 40% of patients averaging 1.2 cm (0.4 to 1.8 cm).

Fyodorov et al (140) reported hardware failure in 2 of 23 femoral shaft fractures treated with dynamic compression plating. One was treated with revision plating and the other with spica casting; both fractures healed uneventfully. No other complications were noted in their patients.

Refracture is rare at the end of the plate or through screw holes, and whether bone atrophy under a plate is caused by stress shielding or by avascularity of the cortex is unknown. Although still somewhat controversial, the plate and screws may be removed at 1 year after fracture to avoid fracture at the end of the plate.

Quadriceps strength after plate fixation appears not to be compromised (145), relative to intramedullary fixation or cast immobilization.

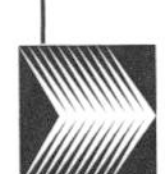

AUTHORS' PREFERRED TREATMENT

For stable femoral fractures in children under 6 months of age, we use a posterior splint or Pavlik harness. If the fracture is unstable, usually the proximal fragment is flexed and a Pavlik harness is the ideal device for reducing and holding the fracture. The use of a Pavlik harness requires an attentive and compliant caregiver. Traction with a spica cast occasionally is needed in this group. Abuse and metabolic bone disease must be considered in an infant with a femoral fracture.

In children 6 months to 6 years of age, an immediate spica cast with Gortex liner is almost always the treatment of choice. If length or alignment cannot be maintained in an immediate spica cast, traction followed by casting can be used. We usually use a distal femoral traction pin and place the child in a 90/90 or oblique position in the bed for traction. It is of note, however, that over 95% of young children with femoral fractures can be managed with immediate spicas with a low complication rate and low cost. In children with multiple trauma, either flexible intramedullary rodding or external fixation is chosen, based on the fracture anatomy and the soft tissue injury. Traction is very rarely used in the management of femoral fractures in this age group.

In children 6 to 12 years of age, flexible intramedullary rodding is frequently used, most often with retrograde insertion. External fixation is used for unstable fracture patterns, comminuted fractures, and fractures with severe soft tissue injury. Bridge plating offers significant advantage in this age group with unstable fracture patterns. Immediate spica casts may be used for the most stable fractures in this age group.

In children 12 years to maturity, we use flexible intramedullary rods as our treatment of choice. In a patient with an unstable fracture configuration, we would use either a submuscular bridge plate or a trochanteric antegrade rod, recognizing the potential significant risk of osteonecrosis of the femoral head. Locked plating is preferable for subtrochanteric and supracondylar fractures of the femur, whereas intramedullary nails are ideal for mid-shaft fractures. If antegrade rodding is chosen, a transtrochanteric approach is used. New methods are under development for fixation, using an infratrochanteric approach with a locked type of flexible rod. There is a limited role for retrograde locked intramedullary nailing in adolescents approaching skeletal maturity.

COMPLICATIONS OF FEMORAL SHAFT FRACTURES

Leg Length Discrepancy

The most common sequela after femoral shaft fractures in children is leg length discrepancy. The fractured femur may be initially short from overriding of the fragments at union; growth acceleration occurs to "make up" the difference, but often this acceleration continues and overgrowth occurs. The potential for growth stimulation from femoral fractures has long been recognized, but the exact cause of this phenomenon is still unknown. Growth acceleration has been attributed to age, sex, fracture type, fracture level, handedness, and the amount of overriding of the fracture fragments. Age seems to be the most constant factor, but fractures in the proximal third of the femur and oblique comminuted fractures also have been associated with relatively greater growth acceleration. According to Staheli (146) in patients over 10 years of age, shortening is more likely; in patients 2 to 10 years of age, overgrowth is more likely, especially if traction has been used.

Shortening

Because the average overgrowth after femoral fracture is approximately 1.5 cm, shortening of 2 to 3 cm in the cast is the maximal acceptable amount. The maximal acceptable shortening depends on the age of the child; for example, in a 6-year-old child, 2.5 cm may be acceptable, whereas only 1 to 2 cm should be accepted in a 14-year-old approaching skeletal maturity. In patients 2 to 10 years of age with more than 3 cm of shortening after immediate spica casting, the cast is removed, traction is reapplied until acceptable length is obtained, and then a new cast is applied. For early shortening of more than 3 cm in a patient 11 or 12 years old, a reinstitution of traction and reapplication of the cast also may be appropriate or surgical fixation. If, however, the shortening is unacceptable at 6 weeks after fracture, the decision must be made as to whether osteoclasis and distraction with external fixation is preferable to a later limb equalization procedure (lengthening or shortening). The trend is to correct the shortening immediately with external fixation if possible.

Overgrowth

Overgrowth after femoral fracture is common in children 2 to 10 years of age. The average overgrowth is 0.9 cm, with a range of 0.4 to 2.5 cm (147). Overgrowth occurs whether the fracture is short, at length, or overpulled in traction at the time of healing. In general, overgrowth occurs most rapidly during the first 2 years after fracture and to a much lesser degree for the next year or so (148).

Truesdell (149) first reported the phenomenon of overgrowth in 1921, and many researchers since have verified the existence of growth stimulation after fracture (150–159). The relationship of the location of the fracture to growth is somewhat controversial. Staheli (146) and Malkawi et al (158) reported that overgrowth was greatest if the fracture occurred in the proximal third of the femur, whereas Henry (159) stated that the most overgrowth occurred in fractures in the distal third of the femur. Other investigators have found no relationship between fracture location and growth stimulation (147, 157,160,161). The relationship between fracture type and overgrowth also is controversial. In general, most researchers believe that no specific relationship exists between fracture type and overgrowth, but some have reported overgrowth to be more frequent after spiral, oblique, and comminuted fractures associated with greater trauma.

Angular Deformity

Some degree of angular deformity is frequent after femoral shaft fractures in children, but this usually remodels with growth. Angular remodeling occurs at the site of fracture, with appositional new bone formation in the concavity of the long bone. Differential physeal growth also occurs in response to diaphyseal angular deformity. Wallace and Hoffman (162) stated that 74% of the remodeling that occurs is physeal, and appositional remodeling at the fracture site occurs to a much lesser degree. However, this appears to be somewhat age dependent. It is clear that angular remodeling occurs best in the direction of motion at the adjacent joint (162). That is, anterior and posterior remodeling in the femur occurs rapidly and with little residual deformity. In contrast, remodeling of a varus or valgus deformity occurs more slowly. The differential physeal growth in a varus or valgus direction in the distal femur causes compensatory deformity, which is usually insignificant. In severe varus bowing, however, a hypoplastic lateral condyle results, which may cause a distal femoral valgus deformity if the varus bow is corrected (Fig. 22-33).

Guidelines for acceptable alignment vary widely. The range of acceptable anterior and posterior angulation varies from 30 to 40 degrees in children up to 2 years of age, decreasing to 10 degrees in older children and adolescents (Fig. 22-34) (163). The range of acceptable varus and valgus angulation also becomes smaller with age. Varus angulation in infants and children should be between 10 and 15 degrees, although greater degrees of angulation may have a satisfactory outcome. Acceptable valgus angulation is 20 to 30 degrees in infants, 15 to 20 degrees in children up to 5 years of age, and 10 degrees in older children and adolescents. The muscle mass of the femur generally hides femoral deformity from direct observation. The acceptability of femoral deformity, in general, is a direct function of the degree of difficulty in changing the deformity and the appearance of the leg.

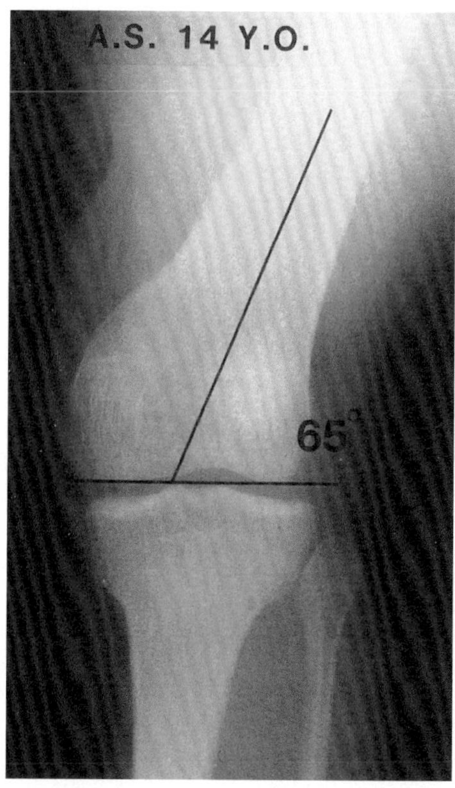

FIGURE 22-33 Long-standing varus deformity in the femoral shaft may lead to hypoplasia of the lateral condyle and a compensatory distal femoral valgus deformity after correction of the varus of the shaft.

Late development of genu recurvatum deformity of the proximal tibia after femoral shaft fracture has been most often reported as a complication of traction pin or wire placement through or near the anterior aspect of the proximal tibial physis, excessive traction, pin track infection, or prolonged cast immobilization (164). However, proximal tibial growth arrest may complicate femoral shaft fracture, presumably as a result of occult injury (165). Femoral pins are preferred for traction, but if tibial pins are required, the proximal anterior tibial physis must be avoided (166). Femoral traction pins should be placed one or two finger breadths proximal to the superior pole of the patella to avoid the distal femoral physis.

If significant angular deformity is present after fracture union, corrective osteotomy should be delayed for at least a year unless the deformity is severe enough to impair function. This will allow determination of remodeling potential before deciding that surgical correction is necessary. The ideal osteotomy corrects the deformity at the site of fracture. In juvenile patients, however, metaphyseal osteotomy of the proximal or distal femur may be necessary. In adolescents with mid-shaft deformities, diaphyseal osteotomy and fixation with an interlocking intramedullary nail are preferable.

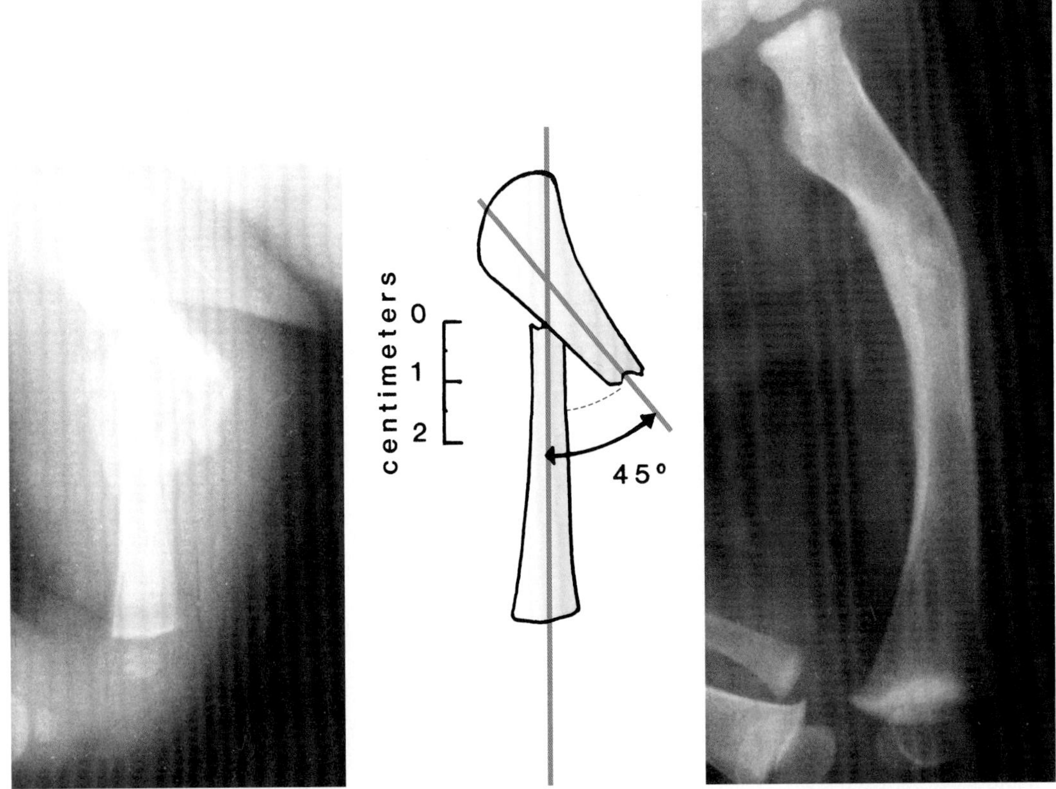

FIGURE 22-34 Remodeling potential of the femur during infancy. This infant sustained a femoral fracture during a breech delivery and was placed in a spica cast but with insufficient flexion of the hip. **Left.** At 3 weeks, union is evident with about 45 degrees of angulation in the sagittal plane and 1.5 cm of overriding. **Center.** Line drawing demonstrating true angulation. **Right.** Twelve months later the anterior angulation has reduced to a level such that it was not apparent to the family, and the shortening has reduced to less than 1 cm.

Rotational Deformity

According to Verbeek (167), rotational deformities of 10 degrees to more than 30 degrees occur in one third of children after conservative treatment of femoral shaft fractures. Malkawi et al (158) found asymptomatic rotational deformities of less than 10 degrees in two thirds of their 31 patients. Torsional deformity usually is expressed as increased femoral anteversion on the fractured side compared with the opposite side, as demonstrated by anteversion views; a difference of more than 10 degrees has been the criterion of significant deformity. However, Brouwer et al (168) challenged this criterion, citing differences of 0 to 15 degrees in a control group of 100 normal volunteers. The accuracy of measurements from plain x-rays also has been disputed, and Norbeck et al (169) suggested the use of computed tomographic (CT) scanning for greater accuracy.

Rotational remodeling in childhood femoral fractures is another controversy in the search for criteria on which to base therapeutic judgments. According to Davids (170) and Braten et al (171) up to 25 degrees of rotational malalignment at the time of healing of femoral fractures appears to be well tolerated in children. In their patients with more than 25 degrees of rotational malalignment, however, deformity caused clinical complaints. Davids (170) found no spontaneous correction in his study of malunions based on CT measurements, but the length of follow-up is insufficient to state that no rotational remodeling occurs. Brouwer et al (168) and others (167,172–174) reported slow rotational correction over time. Buchholz et al (175) documented 5 children with increased femoral anteversion of 10 degrees or more after fracture healing in children between 3 and 6 years old. In 3 of 5 children there was full correction of the rotational deformity but the oldest of the children failed to correct spontaneously.

Certainly, in older adolescents, no significant rotational remodeling will occur. In infants and juveniles, some rotational deformity can be accepted (176) because either true rotational remodeling occurs or functional adaptation allows resumption of normal gait. Up to 30 degrees of malrotation in the femur should result in no functional impairment unless there is preexisting rotational malalignment. The goal, however, should be to reduce a rotational deformity to 10 degrees, based on alignment of the proximal and distal femur radiographically, interpretation of skin and soft tissue envelope alignment, and correct positioning within a cast, based on the muscle pull on the proximal fragment. The distal fragment should be lined up with the position of the proximal fragment determined by the muscles inserted upon it (see Fig. 22-3).

Delayed Union

Delayed union of femoral shaft fractures is uncommon in children. The time to fracture union in most children is rapid and age dependent. In children under 5 years of age, healing usually occurs in 4 to 6 weeks. In children 5 to 10 years of age, fracture healing is somewhat slower, requiring 8 to 10 weeks. Throughout adolescence, the time to healing continues to lengthen. By the age of 15 years, the mean time to healing is about 13 weeks, with a range from 10 to 15 weeks (Fig. 22-35). The rate of healing also is related to soft tissue injury and type of treatment. Application of an external fixation device appears to delay callus formation and slow the rate of healing. In adults there is an association between nonunion and the use of NSAIDS after injury and delayed fracture healing (150), which is very significant. Perhaps in patients with risk factors for delayed healing avoidance of NSAIDS should be considered.

Bone grafting and internal fixation with either a compression plate or locked intramedullary nail is the usual treatment for delayed union in older children and adolescents. Delayed union of a femoral fracture treated with casting in a child 1 to 6 years of age is probably best treated by continuing cast immobilization until bridging callus forms or (rarely) by additional bone grafting.

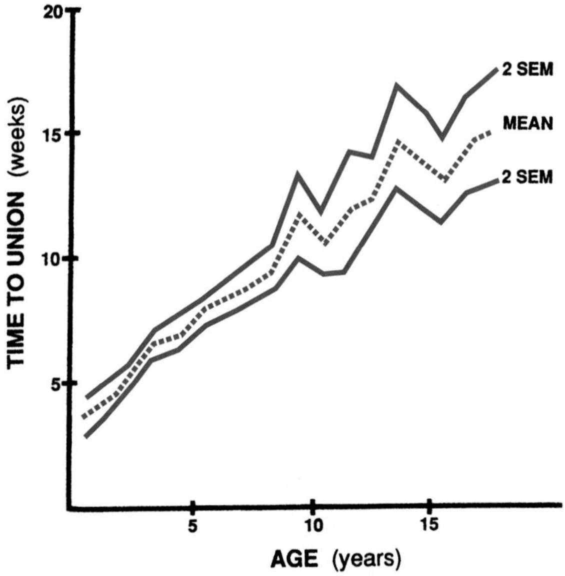

FIGURE 22-35 Time required for union of femoral shaft fractures in childhood and adolescence. (Redrawn from Skak SV, Jensen TT. Femoral shaft fracture in 265 children. *Acta Orthop Scand* 1988;59:704–707; with permission.)

Nonunion

Nonunions of pediatric femoral fractures are rare (177). They tend to occur in adolescents, in infected fractures, or in fractures with segmental bone loss or severe soft tissue loss. Most nonunions in children are of tibial fractures; femoral fractures account for only 15% of nonunions in children. Even in segmental fractures with bone loss, young children may have sufficient osteogenic potential to fill in a significant fracture gap (Fig. 22-36) (178). For the rare femoral shaft nonunion in a child 5 to 10 years of age, bone grafting and plate-and-screw fixation have been traditional treatment methods, but more recently insertion of an interlocking intramedullary nail and bone grafting have been preferred, especially in children over 10 to 12 years of age.

Robertson et al (179) reported the use of external fixators in 11 open femoral fractures. The time to union was delayed,

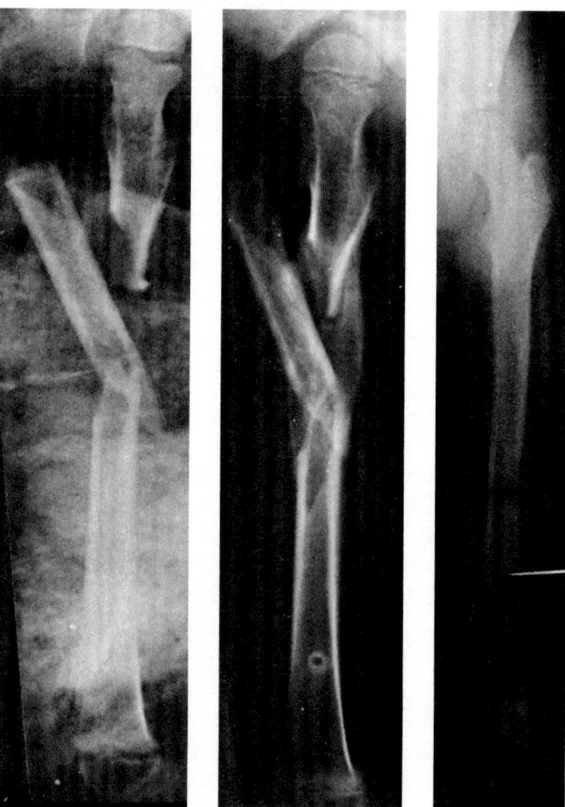

FIGURE 22-36 The effectiveness of remodeling of the femur in a child. **Left.** Comminuted fracture in an 8-year-old child managed with a femoral pin incorporated in a spica cast. The mid-fragment is markedly angulated. **Center.** Fracture after union 12 weeks later with filling in of the defect and early absorption of the protruding fragment. **Right.** Appearance at age 12 with only a minimal degree of irregularity of the upper femur remaining.

but a satisfactory outcome occurred without subsequent procedures. This supports the belief that the rates of delayed union and nonunion are low in pediatric femoral fractures, because open fractures would have the highest rates of delayed union.

Muscle Weakness

Weakness after femoral fracture has been described in the hip abductor musculature, quadriceps, and hamstrings, but persistent weakness in some or all of these muscle groups seldom causes a clinical problem. Hennrikus et al (180) found that quadriceps strength was decreased in 30% of his patients and 18% had a significant decrease demonstrated by a one-leg hop test. Thigh atrophy of 1 cm was present in 42% of patients. These deficits appeared to be primarily related to the degree of initial displacement of the fracture. Finsen et al (145) found hamstring and quadriceps deficits in patients with femoral shaft fractures treated with either rods or plates.

Damholt and Zdravkovic (181) documented quadriceps weakness in approximately one third of patients with femoral fractures, and Viljanto et al (182) reported that this weakness was present whether patients were treated operatively or nonoperatively. Biyani et al (183) found that hip abductor weakness was related to ipsilateral fracture magnitude, long intramedullary rods, and, to a lesser degree, heterotopic ossification from intramedullary rodding. Hedin and Larsson (184) found no significant weakness in any of 31 patients treated with external fixation for femoral fractures based on either Cybex testing or a one-leg hop test. He felt that the weakness seen in other studies may be related to prolonged immobilization.

Injury to the quadriceps muscle probably occurs at the time of femoral fracture, and long-term muscle deficits may persist in some patients regardless of treatment. Severe scarring and contracture of the quadriceps occasionally require quadricepsplasty (185).

Infection

Infection may rarely complicate a closed femoral shaft fracture, with hematogenous seeding of the hematoma and subsequent osteomyelitis. Fever is commonly associated with femoral fractures during the first week after injury (186), but persistent fever or fever that spikes exceedingly high may be an indication of infection.

Pin-track infections occasionally occur with the use of skeletal traction, but most are superficial infections that resolve with local wound care and antibiotic therapy. Occasionally, however, the infections may lead to osteomyelitis of the femoral metaphysis or a ring sequestrum that requires surgical debridement.

Neurovascular Injury

Nerve and vascular injuries are uncommon with femoral fractures in children (187–190). An estimated 1.3% of femoral fractures in children are accompanied by vascular injury (187–190) such as intimal tears, total disruptions, or injuries resulting in the formation of pseudoaneurysms (191). Vascular injury occurs most frequently with displaced Salter-Harris physeal fractures of the distal femur or distal metaphyseal fractures. If arteriography indicates that vascular repair is necessary after femoral shaft fracture, open reduction with internal fixation or external fixation of the fracture is recommended. Secondary limb ischemia also has been reported after the use of both skin and skeletal traction. Documentation of peripheral pulses at the time of presentation, as well as throughout treatment, is necessary.

Nerve abnormalities reported with femoral fractures in children include those caused by direct trauma to the sciatic or femoral nerve at the time of fracture and injuries to the peroneal nerve during treatment. Weiss et al (50) reported peroneal nerve palsies in 4 of 110 children with femoral fractures treated with early 90/90 hip spica casting. They recommended extending the initial short leg portion of the cast above the knee to decrease tension on the peroneal nerve.

Riew et al (192) reported 8 nerve palsies in 35 consecutive patients treated with locked intramedullary rodding. The nerve injuries were associated with delay in treatment, preoperative shortening, and boot traction. Resolution occurred in less than 1 week in 6 of 8 patients.

The natural history of peroneal nerve injury with femoral shaft fractures in children seems to be spontaneous correction. In infants, however, the development of an early contracture of the Achilles tendon is more likely. Because of the rapid growth in younger children, this contracture can develop quite early; if peroneal nerve injury is suspected, the extremity should be braced until the peroneal nerve recovers. If peroneal, femoral, or sciatic nerve deficit is present at initial evaluation of a closed fracture, no exploration is indicated. If a nerve deficit occurs during reduction or treatment, the nerve should be explored. Persistent nerve loss without recovery over a 4- to 6-month period is an indication for exploration.

Compartment Syndrome

Compartment syndromes of the thigh musculature are rare, but have been reported in patients with massive thigh swelling after femoral fracture and in patients treated with intramedullary rod fixation (193). If massive swelling of thigh musculature occurs and pain is out of proportion to that expected from a femoral fracture, compartment pressure measurements should be obtained and decompression by fasciotomy should be considered. It is probable that some patients with quadriceps fibrosis (161) and quadriceps weakness (47,194) after femoral fracture had intracompartmental pressure phenomenon. Mathews et al (195) reported two cases of compartment syndrome in the "well leg" occurring when the patient was positioned for femoral rodding in the hemilithotomy position. Vascular insufficiency related to Bryant's traction may produce signs of compartment syndrome with muscle ischemia (154). Janzing et al (102) reported the occurrence of compartment syndrome using skin traction for treatment of femoral fractures. Skin traction has been associated with compartment syndrome in the lower leg in both the fractured and nonfractured side. It is important to realize that in a traumatized limb, circumferential traction needs to be monitored closely and is contraindicated in the multiply injured or head-injured child.

SPECIAL FRACTURES OF THE FEMORAL SHAFT

Metaphyseal (Subtrochanteric and Supracondylar) Fractures

Subtrochanteric fractures in younger children can be treated in traction, followed by either a cast brace or single spica cast (Fig. 22-37) (197). Sponseller (personal communication) reported satisfactory results with conservative treatment of subtrochanteric fractures in children. Internal fixation with plate and screw devices also can produce satisfactory results (198). Intramedullary fixation of subtrochanteric fractures in children is generally not indicated. In adolescents, there is insufficient experience with this fracture to determine at what age intramedullary fixation with a reconstruction-type nail and an angled transfixion screw into the femoral neck is indicated. Antegrade intramedullary nail systems place significant holes in the upper femoral neck and should be avoided. Unlike subtrochanteric fractures in adults, nonunions are rare in children with any treatment method.

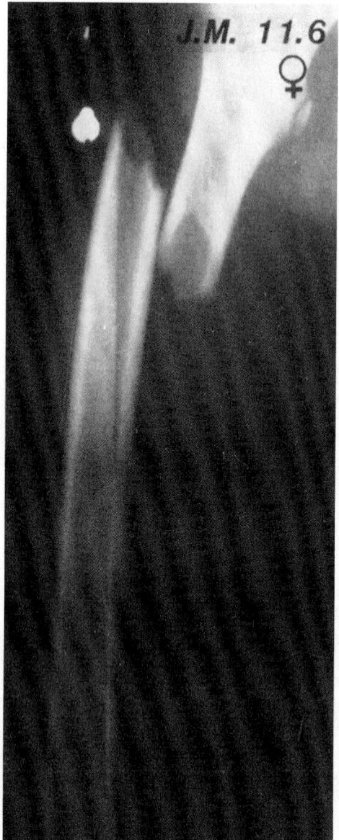

A

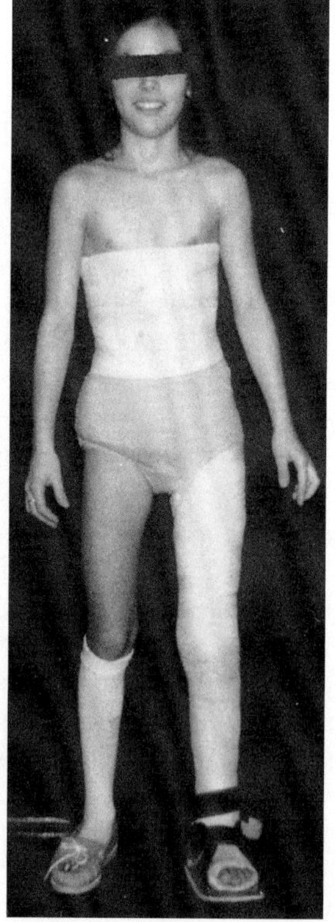

B

FIGURE 22-37 Subtrochanteric fractures **(A)** may be treated with traction followed by a one-legged ambulatory spica cast **(B)**.

With the admonition against intramedullary fixation in children with open physes combined with the fact that nonunions are rare, our recommendation is for traction followed by spica casting in young children up to approximately age 5 or 6, with plate and screw fixation in older children. The traction technique should be that of 90/90 traction in which the distal fragment is flexed to align with the proximal fragment and spica cast treatment may be either in an ambulatory one-legged spica cast or a flexed hip/flexed knee spica cast, depending on the fracture and healing. Ideally, locked plating will yield sufficient rigidity to maintain alignment despite having limited room for internal fixation. The method of plate and screw fixation may be either a straight plate with angled screws in the proximal fragment (Fig. 22-38) or hip screw configuration systems appropriately sized to a small child. Reconstruction intramedullary nailing is reserved for adolescents at skeletal maturity.

Supracondylar fractures represent as many as 12% of femoral shaft fractures (199) and are difficult to treat because the gastrocnemius muscle inserts just above the femoral condyles and pulls the distal fragment into a position of extension (200), making alignment difficult (see Fig. 22-3). The traditional methods of casting and single-pin traction may be satisfactory in young children (Fig. 22-39). If alignment cannot be achieved using these methods, however, open reduction with internal fixation or combined epiphyseal-metaphyseal traction can be used. Generally, internal fixation is preferable, either with locked plates (Fig. 22-40) and fully threaded cancellous screws if there is sufficient metaphyseal length to allow this or with crossed smooth K-wires transfixing the fracture from the epiphysis to the metaphysis, as described for distal femoral physeal separations (201). If there is sufficient metaphyseal length, antegrade flexible rods can be used. Pathologic fractures in this area are common, and a underlying lesion should always be sought.

Open Femoral Fractures

Open femoral fractures are uncommon in children because of the large soft tissue compartment around the femur. Proper wound care, debridement, stabilization, and antibiotic therapy are required to reduce the chance of infection (200). In a study by Hutchins et al (202), 70% of children with open femoral fractures had associated injuries and 90% were automobile related. The average time to healing was 17 weeks, and 50% of the Gustillo type III injuries developed osteomyelitis.

External fixation of open femoral shaft fractures simplifies wound care and allows early mobilization. The configuration of the external fixator is determined by the child's size and the fracture pattern. Generally, monolateral half-pin frames are satisfactory, but thin-wire circular frames may be necessary if bone loss is extensive. External fixation provides good fracture control, but, as always, family cooperation is required to manage pin and fixator care.

Plate fixation also allows early mobilization, as well as anatomic reduction of the femoral fracture. Wound care and treatment of other injuries are made easier in children with multiple

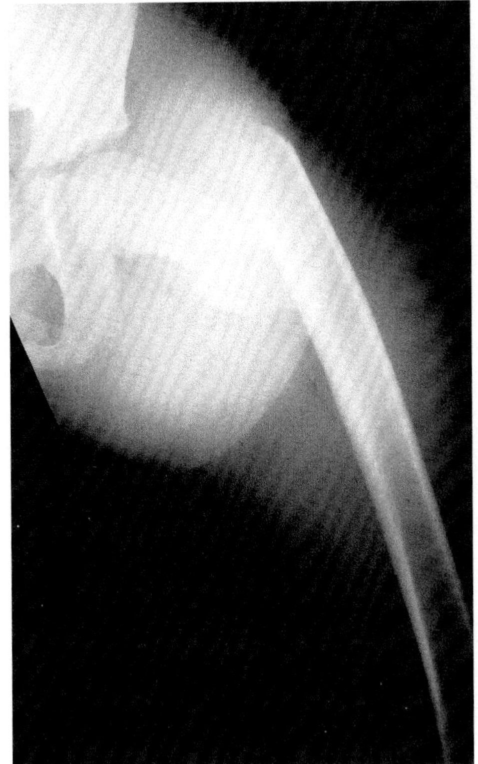

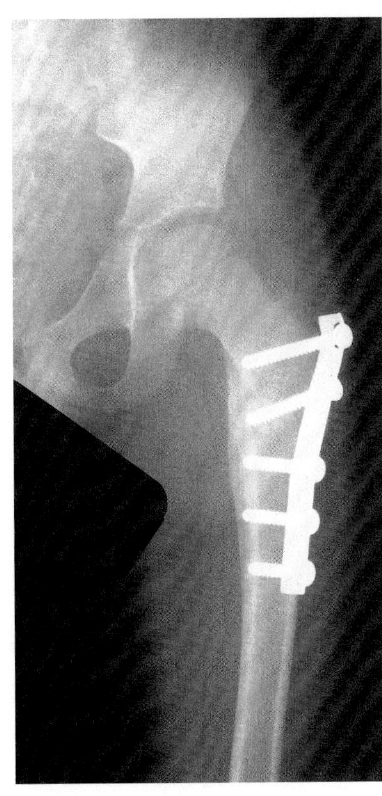

FIGURE 22-38 **A.** This 6-year-old boy sustained a subtrochanteric fracture of the femur. **B.** He was treated with plate and screw fixation supplemented with a spica cast.

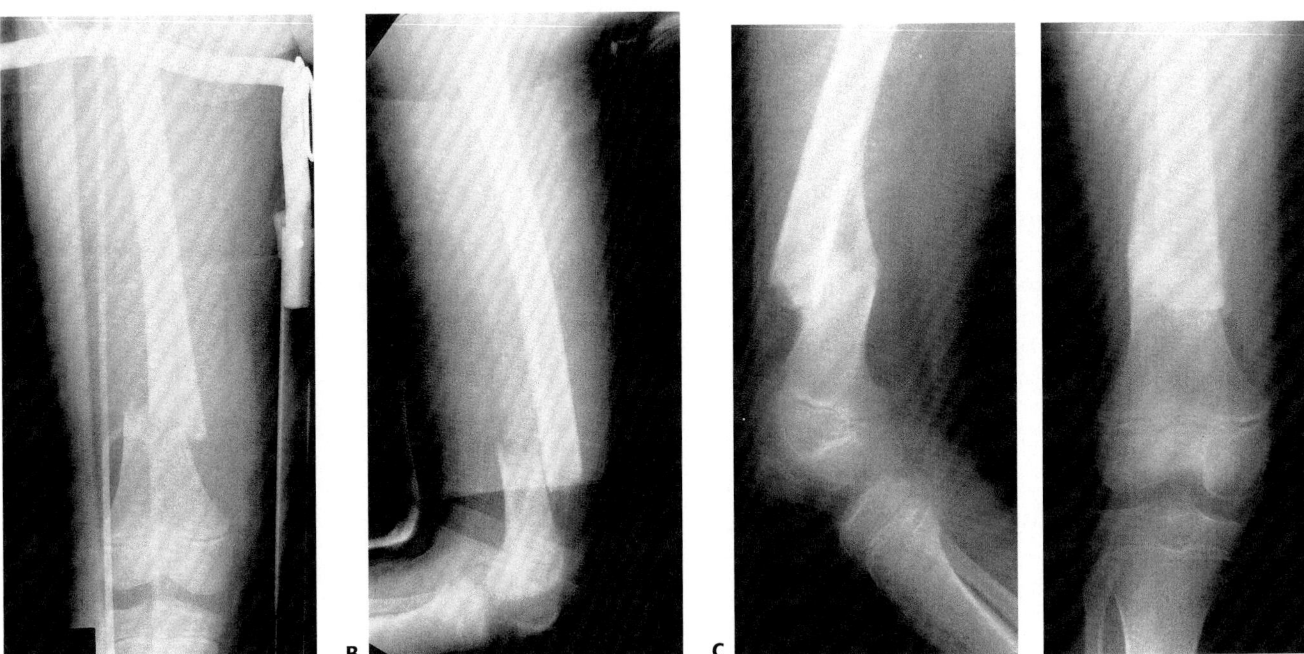

FIGURE 22-39 **A.** This 6-year-old patient sustained an unstable supracondylar fracture of the femur. **B.** The fracture was managed with immediate spica casting with the knee in 90 degrees of flexion, mandatory in such a case to prevent posterior angulation. **C.** Bayonet apposition is acceptable in a child this age.

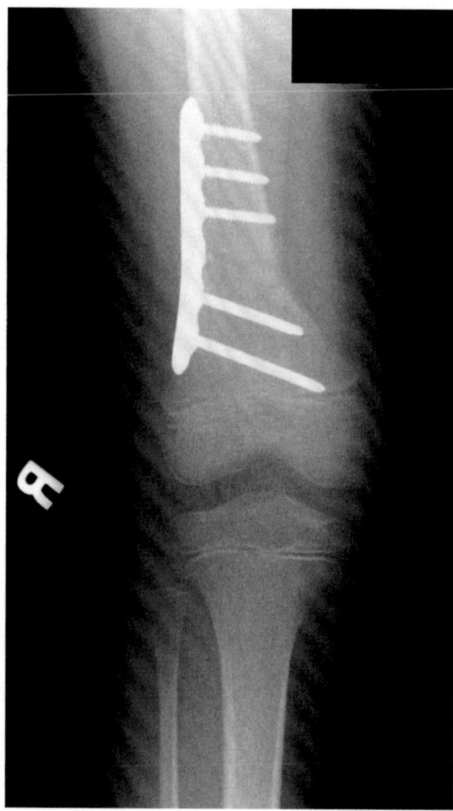

FIGURE 22-40 A locked plate provides stable fixation in small metaphyseal fractures, sparing the physis in unstable supracondylar fractures.

trauma. However, this is an invasive technique with the potential for infection and additional injury to the already traumatized soft tissues in the area of the fracture. In emergency situations, plate fixation or intramedullary fixation may be used for Gustillo-Anderson type I and II fractures; type III fractures in older adolescents are better suited for external fixation or intramedullary nailing. Plate breakage can occur if bone grafting is not used for severe medial cortex comminution.

In older adolescents, plating or flexible intramedullary nailing is especially useful. Closed nailing after irrigation and drainage of the fracture allows early mobilization and easy wound care in patients with Gustillo-Anderson type I, II, IIIA, and IIIB injuries, but the risk of osteonecrosis must be recognized.

Femoral Fractures in Patients with Metabolic or Neuromuscular Disorders

For patients with osteogenesis imperfecta who have potential for ambulation, surgical treatment with Rush, Bailey-Dubow, or Fassier rods (see Chapter 6) is recommended for repeated fractures or angular deformity. Cast immobilization is usually avoided in patients with myelomeningocele or cerebral palsy because of the frequency of osteoporosis and refracture in these patients. If possible, existing leg braces are modified for treatment of the femoral fracture. In nonambulatory patients, a simple pillow splint is used.

Floating Knee Injuries

These rare injuries occur when ipsilateral fractures of the femoral and tibial shafts leave the knee joint "floating" without distal or proximal bony attachments (Fig. 22-41A). They are high-velocity injuries, usually resulting from collision between a child pedestrian or cyclist and a motor vehicle. Most children with floating knee injuries have multiple trauma, including severe soft tissue damage, open fractures, and often head injuries.

In general, at least one of the fractures, usually the tibia, should be fixed. The femoral fracture can usually then be treated by the most appropriate option. If both fractures are open, external fixation of both the tibial and femoral fractures may be appropriate. If immediate mobilization is necessary, fixation of both fractures with external fixation, intramedullary nails, compression plates, or any combination of these may be indicated (Fig. 22-41B).

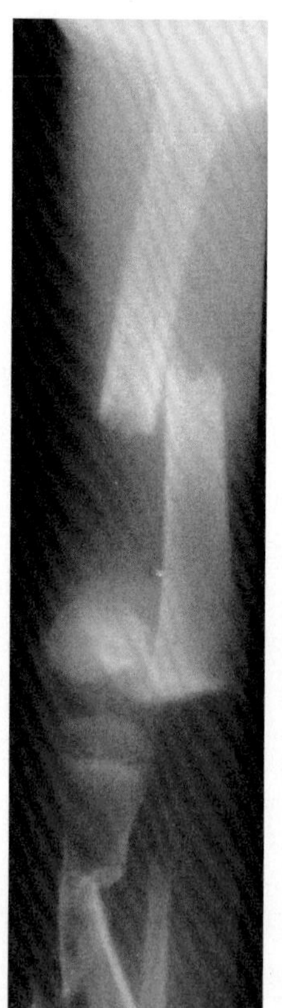
A

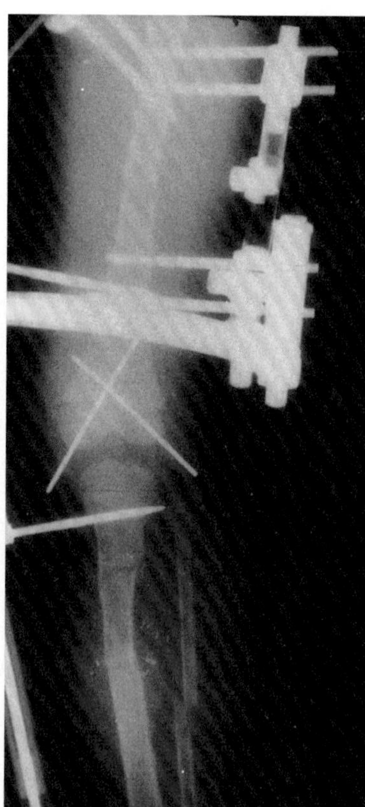
B

FIGURE 22-41 **A.** Floating knee injury in a 4-year-old girl: femoral shaft fracture, displaced physeal fracture of the distal femur, and open (type IIIB) proximal tibial fracture. **B.** After external fixation of femoral shaft fracture, closed reduction and percutaneous pinning of the distal femoral physeal fracture, and external fixation of the open tibial fracture; a free-flap was required for skin coverage.

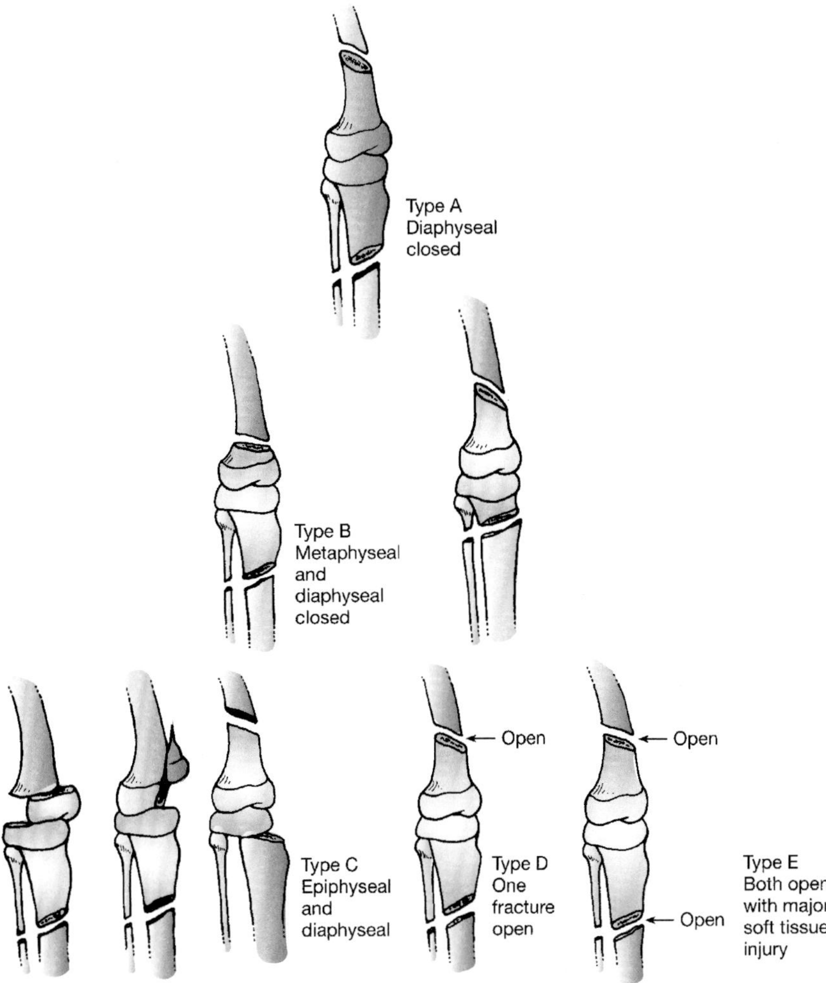

FIGURE 22-42 Classification of floating knee injuries in children. (Redrawn from Letts M, Vincent N, Gouw G. The "floating knee" in children. *J Bone Joint Surg Br* 1986;68:442; with permission.)

Letts et al (28) described five patterns of ipsilateral tibial and femoral fractures and made treatment recommendations based on those patterns (Fig. 22-42). Because of the high prevalence of complications after closed treatment, Bohn and Durbin (203) recommended open or closed reduction and internal fixation of the femoral fracture in older children. In children under 10 years of age, these investigators recommend 90/90 femoral pin traction for 4 weeks, followed by 1½ spica casting until fracture union. The tibial fracture was immobilized in a below-knee cast during the traction. Bohn and Durbin (203) listed four situations in which operative stabilization of the femoral fracture is indicated: (a) a child with severe head trauma with signs of posturing, (b) an adolescent near skeletal maturity, (c) a child with severe soft tissue injury, and (d) an inability to obtain acceptable closed reduction. Stabilization of the tibial fracture by external fixation is indicated if satisfactory closed reduction cannot be obtained or maintained and for open fractures with severe soft tissue injury, regardless of the age of the child. Arslan et al (204) evaluated the treatment of the "floating knee" in 29 consecutive cases, finding that those treated operatively had a shorter hospital stay, decreased time to weight-bearing, and fewer complications than those managed with splinting casting or traction. Arslan et al (204) demonstrated that open knee fracture rather than ligamentous injury was a risk factor for poor outcome and that angulation was a predictor of future compromise of function.

Letts et al (28) reported that maintaining adequate reduction by traction was difficult in children over 12 years of age and that complications were more frequent in children treated by traction alone. Complications in their patients treated by traction alone included pin track infection, osteomyelitis, limitation of knee motion, malunion, and leg length discrepancies of 1.5 cm or more. Bohn and Durbin (203) reported that of 19 patients with floating knee injuries, at long-term follow-up 11 had limb length discrepancy secondary to either overgrowth of the bone after the fracture or premature closure of the ipsilateral physis (7 patients), genu valgum associated with fracture of the proximal tibial metaphysis (3 patients), or physeal arrest (1 patient). Four patients had late diagnosis of ligamentous laxity of the knee that required operation. Other complications included peroneal nerve palsy, infection, nonunion, malunion, and refracture.

Fractures in the Head Trauma or Multiple Trauma Patient

In a study of 387 previously healthy children with femoral fractures, evaluated the effect of stabilization on pulmonary function. Patients with severe head trauma or cervical spine trauma are at greatest risk for pulmonary complications. Timing of treatment of femoral fractures appears to not affect the prevalence of pulmonary complications. Mendelson et al (205) similarly showed no effect of timing of femoral fixation on long-term outcome but early fracture fixation did decrease hospital stay without increasing the risk of central nervous system or pulmonary complications.

REFERENCES

1. Fry K, Hoffer MM, Brink J. Femoral shaft fractures in brain-injured children. *J Trauma* 1976;16:371–373.
2. Hedlund R, Lindgren U. The incidence of femoral shaft fractures in children and adolescents. *J Pediatr Orthop* 1986;6:47–50.
3. Landin LA. Fracture patterns in children: analysis of 8,682 fractures with special reference to incidence, etiology and secular changes in a Swedish urban population 1950–1979. *Acta Orthop Scand Supp* 1986;202:54.
4. Hinton RY, Lincoln A, Crockett MM, et al. Fractures of the femoral shaft in children: incidence, mechanisms, and sociodemographic risk factors. *J Bone Joint Surg Am* 1999; 81:5009.
5. Buess E, Kaelin A. One hundred pediatric femoral fracture: epidemiology, treatment attitudes, and early complications. *J Pediatr Orthop Br* 1998;7:186–192.
6. Henderson J, Goldacre MJ, Fairweather JM, et al. Conditions accounting for substantial time spent in hospital in children aged 1–14 years. *Arch Dis Child* 1992;67:83–86.
7. Schenk R. Basic histomorphology and physiology of skeletal growth. In: Weber B, Brunner C, Frueler F, eds. *Treatment of Fractures in Children and Adolescents*. New York: Springer-Verlag; 1980:3–19.
8. Beals RK, Tufts E. Fractured femur in infancy: the role of child abuse. *J Pediatr Orthop* 1983;3:583–586.
9. Gross RH, Stranger M. Causative factors responsible for femoral fractures in infants and young children. *J Pediatr Orthop* 1983;3:341–343.
10. Silverman FN. Radiological aspects of the battered child syndrome. In *The Battered Child*. Edited. University of Chicago Press; 1987:214–246.
11. Blakemore LC, Loder RT, Hensinger RN. Role of intentional abuse in children 1 to 5 years old with isolated femoral shaft fractures. *J Pediatr Orthop* 1996;16:585–588.
12. Daly KE, Calvert PT. Accidental femoral fracture in infants. *Injury* 1991;22:337–338.
13. Loder RT. Pediatric polytrauma: orthopaedic care and hospital course. *J Orthop Trauma* 1987;1:48–54.
14. Krettek C, Haas N, Walker J, et al. Treatment of femoral shaft fractures in children by external fixation. *Injury* 1991;22:263–266.
15. Katz JF. Spontaneous fractures in paraplegic children. *J Bone Joint Surg Am* 1953;35: 220–226.
16. Robin GC. Fractures in poliomyelitis in children. *J Bone Joint Surg Am* 1966;48: 1048–1054.
17. Burks RT, Sutherland DH. Stress fracture of the femoral shaft in children: report of two cases and discussion. *J Pediatr Orthop* 1984;4:614–616.
18. Johnson AW, Weiss CB Jr, Wheeler DL. Stress fractures of the femoral shaft in athletes: more common than expected—new clinical test. *Am J Sports Med* 1994;22:248–256.
19. Meaney JE, Carty H. Femoral stress fractures in children. *Skeletal Radiol* 1992;21: 173–176.
20. Brouwer KJ, Molenaar JC, van Linge B. Rotational deformities after femoral shaft fractures in childhood: a retrospective study 27–32 years after the accident. *Acta Orthop Scand* 1981;52:81–89.
21. Toren A, Goshen E, Katz M, et al. Bilateral femoral stress fractures in a child due to in-line (roller) skating. *Acta Paediatr* 1997;86:332–333.
22. Porat S, Milgrom, C, Nyska M, et al. Femoral fracture treatment in head-injured children: use of external fixation. *J Trauma* 1986;26:81–84.
23. Ciarallo L, Fleisher G. Femoral fractures: are children at risk for significant blood loss? *Pediatr Emerg Care* 1996;12:343–346.
24. Lynch JM, Gardner MJ, Gains B. Hemodynamic significance of pediatric femur fractures. *J Pediatr Surg* 1996;31:1358–1361.
25. Bennett FS, Zinar DM, Kilgus DJ. Ipsilateral hip and femoral shaft fractures. *Clin Orthop Relat Res* 1993;296:168–177.
26. Cannon SR, Pool CJ. Traumatic separation of the proximal femoral epiphysis and fracture of the mid-shaft of the ipsilateral femur in a child: a case report and review of the literature. *Injury* 1983;15:156–158.
27. Vangsness CT Jr, DeCampos J, Merritt PO, et al. Meniscal injury associated with femoral shaft fractures: an arthroscopic evaluation of incidence. *J Bone Joint Surg Br* 1993;75: 207–209.
28. Letts M, Vincent N, and Gouw G. The "floating knee" in children. *J Bone Joint Surg Br* 1986;68:442–446.
29. Roach J, Hoschl R. Diffuse femoral uptake on bone scan after fracture in an infant. *Q J Nucl Med* 1996;40:194–196.
30. Reeves RB, Ballard RI, Hughes JL. Internal fixation versus traction and casting of adolescent femoral shaft fractures. *J Pediatr Orthop* 1990;10:592–595.
31. Newton PO, Mubarak SJ. Financial aspects of femoral shaft fracture treatment in children and adolescents. *J Pediatr Orthop* 1994;14:508–512.
32. Coyte PC, Bronskill SE, Hirji ZZ, et al. Economic evaluation of 2 treatments for pediatric femoral shaft fractures. *Clin Orthop Relat Res* 1997;336:205–215.
33. Stans AA, Morrissy RT, Renwick SE. Femoral shaft fracture treatment in patients age 6 to 16 years. *J Pediatr Orthop* 1999;19:222–228.
34. Nork SE, Hoffinger SA. Skeletal traction versus external fixation for pediatric femoral shaft fractures: a comparison of hospital costs and charges. *J Orthop Trauma* 1998;12: 563–568.
35. Yandow SM, Archibeck MJ, Stevens PM, et al. Femoral-shaft fractures in children: a comparison of immediate casting and traction. *J Pediatr Orthop* 1999;19:55–59.
36. Wright JG. The treatment of femoral shaft fractures in children: a systematic overview and critical appraisal of the literature. *Can J Surg* 2000;43:180–189.
37. Hedin H, Borgquist L, Larsson S. A cost analysis of three methods of treating femoral shaft fractures in children: a comparison of traction in hospital, traction in hospital/home and external fixation. *Acta Orthop Scand* 2004;75:241–248.
38. Morris S, Cassidy N, Stephens M, et al. Birth-associated femoral fractures: incidence and outcome. *J Pediatr Orthop* 22:27–30.
39. Stannard JP, Christensen KP, Wilkins KE. Femur fractures in infants: a new therapeutic approach. *J Pediatr Orthop* 1995;15:461–466.
40. Irani RN, Nicholson JT, Chung SM. Long-term results in the treatment of femoral-shaft fractures in young children by immediate spica immobilization. *J Bone Joint Surg Am* 1976;58:945–951.
41. Staheli LT, Sheridan GW. Early spica cast management of femoral shaft fractures in young children: a technique utilizing bilateral fixed skin traction. *Clin Orthop Relat Res* 1977;126:162–166.
42. Ferguson J, Nicol RO. Early spica treatment of pediatric femoral shaft fractures. *J Pediatr Orthop* 2000;20:189–192.
43. Infante AF Jr, Albert MC, Jennings WB, et al. Immediate hip spica casting for femur fractures in pediatric patients: a review of 175 patients. *Clin Orthop Relat Res* 2000; 376:106–112.
44. Hughes BF, Sponseller PD, Thompson JD. Pediatric femur fractures: effects of spica cast treatment on family and community. *J Pediatr Orthop* 1995;15:457–460.
45. Kocher M. In: *American Academy of Orthopaedic Surgeons Specialty Day*. San Francisco, 2004.
46. Illgen R 2nd, Rodgers WB, Hresko MT, et al. Femur fractures in children: treatment with early sitting spica casting. *J Pediatr Orthop* 1998;18:481–487.
47. Czertak DJ, Hennrikus WL. The treatment of pediatric femur fractures with early 90-90 spica casting. *J Pediatr Orthop* 1999;19:229–232.
48. Thompson JD, Buehler KC, Sponseller PD, et al. Shortening in femoral shaft fractures in children treated with spica cast. *Clin Orthop Relat Res* 1997;338:74–78.
49. Maruenda-Paulino JI, Sanchis-Alfonso V, Gomar-Sancho F, et al. Kuntscher nailing of femoral shaft fractures in children and adolescents. *Int Orthop* 1993;17:158–161.
50. Weiss AP, Schenck RC Jr, Sponseller PD, et al. Peroneal nerve palsy after early cast application for femoral fractures in children. *J Pediatr Orthop* 1992;12:25–28.
51. McCullough N, Vinsant J, Sarmiento A. Functional fracture-bracing of long-bone fractures of the lower extremity in children. *J Bone Joint Surg Am* 1978;60:314.
52. McCarthy RE. A method for early spica cast application in treatment of pediatric femoral shaft fractures. *J Pediatr Orthop* 1986;6:89–91.
53. Miller ME, Bramlett KW, Kissell EU, et al. Improved treatment of femoral shaft fractures in children: the "pontoon" 90–90 spica cast. *Clin Orthop Relat Res* 1987;219:140–146.
54. Large TM, Frick SL. Compartment syndrome of the leg after treatment of a femoral fracture with an early sitting spica cast: a report of two cases. *J Bone Joint Surg Am* 2003;85:2207–2210.
55. Pott P. *Some Few General Remarks on Fractures and Dislocations*. Edited by Hawes L, Clarke E, Collins R. London, 1769.
56. Buck G. An improved method of treating fractures of the thigh illustrated by cases and a drawing. *Trans NY Acad Sci* 1861;2:232–250.
57. Bryant T. *The Practice of Surgery*. Edited, Philadelphia: HC Lea; 1873.
58. Cole WH. Results of treatment of fractured femurs in children with special reference to Bryant's overhead traction. *Arch Surg* 1922;5:702–716.
59. Nicholson JT, Foster RM, Heath RD. Bryant's traction: a provocative cause of circulatory complications. *J Am Med Assoc* 1955;157:415–418.
60. Russell RH. Theory and method in extension of the thigh. *Br Med J* 1921;2:637–639.
61. Ferry AM, Edgar MS Jr. Modified Bryant's traction. *J Bone Joint Surg Am* 1966;48: 533–536.
62. Holmes SJ, Sedgwick DM, Scobie WG. Domiciliary gallows traction for femoral shaft fractures in young children: feasibility, safety and advantages. *J Bone Joint Surg Br* 1983; 65:288–290.
63. Aronson DD, Singer RM, Higgins RF. Skeletal traction for fractures of the femoral shaft in children: a long-term study. *J Bone Joint Surg Am* 1987;69:1435–1439.
64. Casas J, Gonzalez-Moran G, Albinana J. Femoral fractures in children from 4 years to 10 years: conservative treatment. *J Pediatr Orthop Br* 2001;10:56–62.
65. Dencker H. Wire traction complications associated with treatment of femoral shaft fractures. *Acta Orthop Scand* 1964;35:158–163.
66. Ryan JR. 90–90 skeletal femoral traction for femoral shaft fractures in children. *J Trauma* 1981;21:46–48.
67. Humberger FW, Eyring EJ. Proximal tibial 90–90 traction in treatment of children with femoral-shaft fractures. *J Bone Joint Surg Am* 1969;51:499–504.

68. Stanitski CL, Monroe MT, Stanitski DF, et al. Radiation exposure during skeletal traction treatment of pediatric femoral fractures. *J Pediatr Orthop* 1998;18:271–272.
69. Connolly JF, Dehne E, Lafollette B. Closed reduction and early cast-brace ambulation in the treatment of femoral fractures. II. Results in one hundred and forty-three fractures. *J Bone Joint Surg Am* 1973;55:1581–1599.
70. Mital MA, Cashman WF. Fresh ambulatory approach to treatment of femoral shaft fractures in children: a comparison with traditional conservative methods. *J Bone Joint Surg Am* 1976;58:285.
71. Scott J, Wardlaw D, McLauchlan J. Cast bracing of femoral shaft fractures in children: a preliminary report. *J Pediatr Orthop* 1981;1:199–201.
72. Gross RH, Davidson R, Sullivan JA, et al. Cast brace management of the femoral shaft fracture in children and young adults. *J Pediatr Orthop* 1983;3:572–582.
73. Herndon WA, Mahnken RF, Yngve DA, et al. Management of femoral shaft fractures in the adolescent. *J Pediatr Orthop* 1989;9:29–32.
74. Kirby RM, Winquist RA, Hansen ST Jr. Femoral shaft fractures in adolescents: a comparison between traction plus cast treatment and closed intramedullary nailing. *J Pediatr Orthop* 1981;1:193–197.
75. Aronson J, Tursky RN. External fixation of femur fractures in children. *J Bone Joint Surg Am* 1987;69:1435–1439.
76. Hedin H, Hjorth K, Rehnberg L, et al. External fixation of displaced femoral shaft fractures in children: a consecutive study of 98 fractures. *J Orthop Trauma* 2003;17:250–256.
77. Bar-On E, Sagiv S, Porat S. External fixation or flexible intramedullary nailing for femoral shaft fractures in children: a prospective, randomised study. *J Bone Joint Surg Br* 1997;79:975–978.
78. Sola J, Schoenecker PL, Gordon JE. External fixation of femoral shaft fractures in children: enhanced stability with the use of an auxiliary pin. *J Pediatr Orthop* 1999;19:587–591.
79. Domb BG, Sponseller PD, Ain M, et al. Comparison of dynamic versus static external fixation for pediatric femur fractures. *J Pediatr Orthop* 2002;22:428–430.
80. Nowotarski PJ, Turen CH, Brumback RJ, et al. Conversion of external fixation to intramedullary nailing for fractures of the shaft of the femur in multiply injured patients. *J Bone Joint Surg Am* 2000;82:781–788.
81. Miner T, Carroll KL. Outcomes of external fixation of pediatric femoral shaft fractures. *J Pediatr Orthop* 2000;20:405–410.
82. Gregory P, Pevny T, Teague D. Early complications with external fixation of pediatric femoral shaft fractures. *J Orthop Trauma* 1996;10:191–198.
83. Simonian PT, Chapman JR, Selznick HS, et al. Iatrogenic fractures of the femoral neck during closed nailing of the femoral shaft. *J Bone Joint Surg Br* 1994;76:293–296.
84. Davis TJ, Topping RE, Blanco JS. External fixation of pediatric femoral fractures. *Clin Orthop Relat Res* 1995;318:191–198.
85. de Sanctis N, Gambardella A, Pempinello C, et al. The use of external fixators in femur fractures in children. *J Pediatr Orthop* 1996;16:613–620.
86. Gregory P, Sullivan JA, Herndon WA. Adolescent femoral shaft fractures: rigid versus flexible nails. *Orthopedics* 1995;18:645–649.
87. Hull JB, Sanderson PL, Rickman M, et al. External fixation of children's fractures: use of the Orthofix Dynamic Axial Fixator. *J Pediatr Orthop Br* 1997;6:203–206.
88. Probe R, Lindsey RW, Hadley NA, et al. Refracture of adolescent femoral shaft fractures: a complication of external fixation–report of two cases. *J Pediatr Orthop* 1993;13:102–105.
89. Blasier RD, Aronson J, Tursky EA. External fixation of pediatric femur fractures. *J Pediatr Orthop* 1997;17:342–346.
90. El Hayek T, Daher AA, Meouchy W, et al. External fixators in the treatment of fractures in children. *J Pediatr Orthop B* 2004;13:103–109.
91. Evanoff M, Strong ML, MacIntosh R. External fixation maintained until fracture consolidation in the skeletally immature. *J Pediatr Orthop* 1993;13:98–101.
92. Winquist RA, Hansen ST Jr, Clawson DK. Closed intramedullary nailing of femoral fractures: a report of five hundred and twenty cases. *J Bone Joint Surg Am* 1984;66:529–539.
93. Ligier JN, Metaizeau JP, Prevot J, et al. Elastic stable intramedullary nailing of femoral shaft fractures in children. *J Bone Joint Surg Br* 1988;70:74–77.
94. Beaty JH, Austin SM, Warner WC, et al. Interlocking intramedullary nailing of femoral-shaft fractures in adolescents: preliminary results and complications. *J Pediatr Orthop* 1994;14:178–183.
95. Cameron CD, Meek RN, Blachut PA, et al. Intramedullary nailing of the femoral shaft: a prospective, randomized study. *J Orthop Trauma* 1992;6:448–451.
96. Galpin RD, Willis RB, Sabano N. Intramedullary nailing of pediatric femoral fractures. *J Pediatr Orthop* 1994;14:184–189.
97. Gordon JE, Swenning TA, Burd TA, et al. Proximal femoral radiographic changes after lateral transtrochanteric intramedullary nail placement in children. *J Bone Joint Surg Am* 2003;85:1295–1301.
98. Kanlic EM, Anglen JO, Smith DG, et al. Advantages of submuscular bridge plating for complex pediatric femur fractures. *Clin Orthop Relat Res* 2004;426:244–251.
99. Timmerman LA, Rab GT. Intramedullary nailing of femoral shaft fractures in adolescents. *J Orthop Trauma* 1993;7:331–337.
100. Ziv I, Blackburn N, Rang M. Femoral intramedullary nailing in the growing child. *J Trauma* 1984;24:432–434.
101. Lee SS, Mahar AT, Newton PO. Ender nail fixation of pediatric femur fractures: a biomechanical analysis. *J Pediatr Orthop* 2001;21:442–445.
102. Gwyn DT, Olney BW, Dart BR, et al. Rotational control of various pediatric femur fractures stabilized with titanium elastic intramedullary nails. *J Pediatr Orthop* 2004;24:172–177.
103. Frick KB, Mahar AT, Lee SS, et al. Biomechanical analysis of antegrade and retrograde flexible intramedullary nail fixation of pediatric femoral fractures using a synthetic bone model. *J Pediatr Orthop* 2004;24:167–171.
104. Kiely N. Mechanical properties of different combinations of flexible nails in a model of a pediatric femoral fracture. *J Pediatr Orthop* 2002;224:424–427.
105. Bourdelat D. Fracture of the femoral shaft in children: advantages of the descending medullary nailing. *J Pediatr Orthop Br* 1996;5:110–114.
106. Carey TP, Galpin RD. Flexible intramedullary nail fixation of pediatric femoral fractures. *Clin Orthop Relat Res* 1996;332:110–118.
107. Mann DC, Weddington J, Davenport K. Closed Ender nailing of femoral shaft fractures in adolescents. *J Pediatr Orthop* 1986;6:651–655.
108. Heinrich SD, Drvaric D, Darr K, et al. Stabilization of pediatric diaphyseal femur fractures with flexible intramedullary nails (a technique paper). *J Orthop Trauma* 1992;6:452–459.
109. Herscovici D Jr, Scott DM, Behrens F, et al. The use of Ender nails in femoral shaft fractures: what are the remaining indications? *J Orthop Trauma* 1992;6:314–317.
110. Karaoglu S, Baktir A, Tuncel M, et al. Closed Ender nailing of adolescent femoral shaft fractures. *Injury* 1994;25:501–506.
111. McGraw JJ, Gregory SK. Ender nails: an alternative for intramedullary fixation of femoral shaft fractures in children and adolescents. *South Med J* 1997;90:694–696.
112. Flynn JM, Hresko T, Reynolds RA, et al. Titanium elastic nails for pediatric femur fractures: a multicenter study of early results with analysis of complications. *J Pediatr Orthop* 2001;21:4–8.
113. Narayanan UG, Hyman JE, Wainwright AM, et al. Complications of elastic stable intramedullary nail fixation of pediatric femoral fractures, and how to avoid them. *J Pediatr Orthop* 2004;24:363–369.
114. Luhmann SJ, Schootman M, Schoenecker PL, et al. Complications of titanium elastic nails for pediatric femoral shaft fractures. *J Pediatr Orthop* 2003;23:443–447.
115. Mazda K, Khairouni A, Pennecot GF, et al. Closed flexible intramedullary nailing of the femoral shaft fractures in children. *J Pediatr Orthop Br* 1997;6:198–202.
116. Ozdemir HM, Yensel U, Senaran H, et al. Immediate percutaneous intramedullary fixation and functional bracing for the treatment of pediatric femoral shaft fracture. *J Pediatr Orthop* 2003;23:453–457.
117. Fein LH, Pankovich AM, Spero CM, et al. Closed flexible intramedullary nailing of adolescent femoral shaft fractures. *J Orthop Trauma* 1989;3:133–141.
118. Heinrich SD, Drvaric DM, Darr K, et al. The operative stabilization of pediatric diaphyseal femur fractures with flexible intramedullary nails: a prospective analysis. *J Pediatr Orthop* 1994;14:501–507.
119. Flynn JM, Luedke LM, Ganley TJ, et al. Comparison of titanium elastic nails with traction and a spica cast to treat femoral fractures in children. *J Bone Joint Surg Am* 2004;86:770–777.
120. Benirschke SK, Melder I, Henley MB, et al. Closed interlocking nailing of femoral shaft fractures: assessment of technical complications and functional outcomes by comparison of a prospective database with retrospective review. *J Orthop Trauma* 1993;7:118–122.
121. Brumback RJ, Ellison TS, Poka A, et al. Intramedullary nailing of femoral shaft fractures. III. Long-term effects of static interlocking fixation. *J Bone Joint Surg Am* 1922;74:106–112.
122. Hajek PD, Bicknell HR Jr, Bronson WE, et al. The use of one compared with two distal screws in the treatment of femoral shaft fractures with interlocking intramedullary nailing: a clinical and biomechanical analysis. *J Bone Joint Surg Am* 1993;75:519–525.
123. Buford D Jr, Christensen K, Weatherall P. Intramedullary nailing of femoral fractures in adolescents. *Clin Orthop Relat Res* 1998;350:85–89.
124. Raney EM, Ogden JA, Grogan DP. Premature greater trochanteric epiphysiodesis secondary to intramedullary femoral rodding. *J Pediatr Orthop* 1993;13:516–520.
125. Mileski RA, Garvin KL, Huurman WW. Ostonecrosis of the femoral head after closed intramedullary shortening in an adolescent. *J Pediatr Orthop* 1995;15:24–26.
126. Thometz JG, Lamdan R. Osteonecrosis of the femoral head after intramedullary nailing of a fracture of the femoral shaft in an adolescent: a case report. *J Bone Joint Surg Am* 1995;77:1423–1426.
127. Maruenda-Paulino JI, Sanchis-Alfonso V, Gomar-Sancho F, et al. Kuntscher nailing of femoral shaft fractures in children and adolescents. *Int Orthop* 1993;17:158–161.
128. Townsend DR, Hoffinger S. Intramedullary nailing of femoral shaft fractures in children via the trochanter tip. *Clin Orthop Relat Res* 2000;376:113–118.
129. Momberger N, Stevens P, Smith J, et al. Intramedullary nailing of femoral fractures in adolescents. *J Pediatr Orthop* 2000;20:482–484.
130. Bergman M, Tornetta P, Kerina M, et al. Femur fractures caused by gunshots: treatment by immediate reamed intramedullary nailing. *J Trauma* 1993;34:783–785.
131. Tolo VT. External fixation in multiply injured children. *Orthop Clin North Am* 1990;21:393–400.
132. Ostrum RF, DiCicco J, Lakatos R, et al. Retrograde intramedullary nailing of femoral diaphyseal fractures. *J Orthop Trauma* 1998;12:464–468.
133. Ricci WM, Bellabarba C, Evanoff B, et al. Retrograde versus antegrade nailing of femoral shaft fractures. *J Orthop Trauma* 2001;15:161–169.
134. Kaweblum M, Lehman WB, Grant AD, et al. Osteonecrosis of the femoral head as sequela of fracture of the greater trochanter: a case report and review of the literature. *Clin Orthop Relat Res* 1993;294:193–195.
135. O'Malley DE, Mazur JM, Cummings RJ. Femoral head osteonecrosis associated with intramedullary nailing in an adolescent. *J Pediatr Orthop* 1995;15:21–23.
136. Chung SM. The arterial supply of the developing proximal end of the human femur. *J Bone Joint Surg Am* 1976;58:961–970.
137. Simonian PT, Chapman JR, Selznick HS, et al. Iatrogenic fractures of the femoral neck during closed nailing of the femoral shaft. *J Bone Joint Surg Br* 1994;76:293–296.

138. Ward WT, Levy J, Kaye A. Compression plating for child and adolescent femur fractures. *J Pediatr Orthop* 1992;12:626–632.
139. Kregor PJ, Song KM, Routt ML Jr, et al. Plate fixation of femoral shaft fractures in multiply injured children. *J Bone Joint Surg Am* 1993;75:1774–1780.
140. Fyodorov I, Sturm PF, Robertson WW Jr. Compression-plate fixation of femoral shaft fractures in children aged 8 to 12 years. *J Pediatr Orthop* 1999;19:578–581.
141. Hansen TB. Fractures of the femoral shaft in children treated with an AO-compression plate: report of 12 cases followed until adulthood. *Acta Orthop Scand* 1992;63:50–52.
142. Rozbruch SR, Muller U, Gautier E, et al. The evolution of femoral shaft plating technique. *Clin Orthop Relat Res* 1998;354:195–208.
143. Hedequist DJ, Sink E. Technical aspects of bridge plating for pediatric femur fractures. *J Orthop Trauma* 2005;19:276–279.
144. Eren OT, Kucukkaya M, Kockesen C, et al. Open reduction and plate fixation of femoral shaft fractures in children aged 4 to 10. *J Pediatr Orthop* 2003;23:190–193.
145. Finsen V, Harnes OB, Nesse O. Muscle function after plated and nailed femoral shaft fractures. *Injury* 1993;24:531–534.
146. Staheli LT. Femoral and tibial growth following femoral shaft fracture in childhood. *Clin Orthop Relat Res* 1967;55:159–163.
147. Shapiro F. Fractures of the femoral shaft in children: the overgrowth phenomenon. *Acta Orthop Scand* 1981;52:649–655.
148. Griffin PP, Green WT. Fractures of the shaft of the femur in children: treatment and results. *Orthop Clin North Am* 1972;3:213–224.
149. Truesdell ED. Inequality of lower extremity following fracture of the femoral shaft in childhood. *Ann Surg* 1921;74:606–612.
150. Aitken AP. Overgrowth of the femoral shaft following fracture in children. *Am J Surg* 1948;49:147–148.
151. Aitken AP, Blackett CW, Cincotti JJ. Overgrowth of the femoral shaft following fracture in childhood. *J Bone Joint Surg* 1939;21:334–338.
152. Anderson M, Green WT. Lengths of the femur and the tibia: norms derived from orthoroentgenograms of children from five years of age until epiphyseal closure. *Am J Dis Child* 1948;75:279–290.
153. Barfod BCJ. Fractures of the femoral shaft in children with special reference to subsequent overgrowth. *Acta Chir Scand* 1958;116:235–250.
154. Clark MW, D'Ambrosia RD, Roberts JM. Equinus contracture following Bryant's traction. *Orthopedics* 1978;1:311–312.
155. Cole WH. Compensatory lengthening of the femur in children after fracture. *Ann Surg* 1925;82:609–616.
156. Raney EM, Ogden JA, Grogan DP. Premature greater trochanteric epiphysiodesis secondary to intramedullary femoral rodding. *J Pediatr Orthop* 1993;13:516–520.
157. Edvardsen P, Syversen SM. Overgrowth of the femur after fracture of the shaft in childhood. *J Bone Joint Surg Br* 1976;58:339–342.
158. Malkawi H, Shannak A, Hadidi S. Remodeling after femoral shaft fractures in children treated by the modified Blount method. *J Pediatr Orthop* 1986;6:421–429.
159. Meals RA. Overgrowth of the femur following fractures in children: influence of handedness. *J Bone Joint Surg Am* 1979;61:381–384.
160. Henry AN. Overgrowth after femoral shaft fractures in children. *J Bone Joint Surg Br* 1963;45:222.
161. Reynolds DA. Growth changes in fractured long-bones: a study of 126 children. *J Bone Joint Surg Br* 1981;63:83–88.
162. Wallace ME, Hoffman EB. Remodelling of angular deformity after femoral shaft fractures in children. *J Bone Joint Surg Br* 1992;74:765–769.
163. MacEwen GD, Kasser JR, Heinrich SD. *Pediatric Fractures*. Edited. Baltimore: Williams & Wilkins; 1993:281.
164. Van Meter JW, Branick RI. Bilateral genu recurvatum after skeletal traction: a case report. *J Bone Joint Surg Am* 1980;62:837–839.
165. Hresko MT, Kasser JR. Physeal arrest about the knee associated with non-physeal fractures in the lower extremity. *J Bone Joint Surg Am* 1989;71:698–703.
166. Miller PR, Welch MC. The hazards of tibial pin replacement in 90–90 skeletal traction. *Clin Orthop Relat Res* 1978;135:97–100.
167. Verbeek H. Does rotational deformity following femur shaft fracture correct during growth. *Reconstr Surg Traumatol* 1979;17:77–81.
168. Brouwer KJ, Molenaar JC, van Linge B. Rotational deformites after femoral shaft fractures in childhood: a retrospective study 27–32 years after the accident. *Acta Orthop Scand* 1981;52:81–89.
169. Norbeck DE, Asselmeier M, Pinzor MS. Torsional malunion of a femur fracture: diagnosis and treatment. *Orthop Rev* 1990;19:625.
170. Davids JR. Rotational deformity and remodeling after fracture of the femur in children. *Clin Orthop Relat Res* 1994;302:27–35.
171. Braten M, Terjesen T, Rossvoll I. Torsional deformity after intramedullary nailing of femoral shaft fractures: measurement of anteversion angles in 110 patients. *J Bone Joint Surg Br* 1993;75:799–803.
172. Benum P, Ertresvag K, Hoiseth K. Torsion deformities after traction treatment of femoral fractures in children. *Acta Orthop Scand* 1979;50:87–91.
173. Hagglund G, Hansson LI, Norman O. Correction by growth of rotational deformity after femoral fracture in children. *Acta Orthop Scand* 1983;54:858–861.
174. Oberhammer J. Degree and frequency of rotational deformities after infant femoral fractures and their spontaneous correction. *Arch Orthop Trauma Surg* 1980;97:249–255.
175. Buchholz IM, Bolhuis HW, Broker FH, et al. Overgrowth and correction of rotational deformity in 12 femoral shaft fractures in 3–6-year-old children treated with an external fixator. *Acta Orthop Scand* 2002;73:170–174.
176. Ferry AM, Edgar MS Jr. Modified Bryant's traction. *J Bone Joint Surg Am* 1966;48:533–536.
177. Lewallen RP, Peterson HA. Nonunion of long bone fractures in children: a review of 30 cases. *J Pediatr Orthop* 1985;5:135–142.
178. Mesko JW, DeRosa GP, Lindseth RE. Segmental femur loss in children. *J Pediatr Orthop* 1985;5:471–474.
179. Robertson P, Karol LA, Rab GT. Open fractures of the tibia and femur in children. *J Pediatr Orthop* 1996;16:621–626.
180. Hennrikus WL, Kasser JR, Rand F, et al. The function of the quadriceps muscle after a fracture of the femur in patients who are less than seventeen years old. *J Bone Joint Surg Am* 1993;75:508–513.
181. Damholt B, Zdravkovic D. Quadriceps function following fractures of the femoral shaft in children. *Acta Orthop Scand* 1974;45:756.
182. Viljanto J, Kiviluoto H, Paananen M. Remodelling after femoral shaft fracture in children. *Acta Chir Scand* 1975;141:360–365.
183. Biyani A, Jones DA, Daniel CL. Assessment of hip abductor function in relation to peritrochanteric heterotopic ossification after closed femoral nailing. *Injury* 1993;24:97–100.
184. Hedin H, Larsson S. Muscle strength in children treated for displaced femoral fractures by external fixation: 31 patients compared with 31 matched controls. *Acta Orthop Scand* 2003;74:305–311.
185. Ikpeme JO. Quadricepsplasty following femoral shaft fractures. *Injury* 1993;24:104–108.
186. Staheli LT. Fever following trauma in childhood. *JAMA* 1967;199:503–504.
187. Connolly JF, Whittaker D, Williams E. Femoral and tibial fractures combined with injuries to the femoral or popliteal artery: a review of the literature and analysis of fourteen cases. *J Bone Joint Surg Am* 1971;53:56.
188. Dehne E, Kriz FK Jr. Slow arterial leak consequent to unrecognized arterial laceration: report of five cases. *J Bone Joint Surg Am* 1967;49:372–376.
189. Isaacson J, Louis DS, Costenbader JM. Arterial injury associated with closed femoral-shaft fracture: report of five cases. *J Bone Joint Surg Am* 1975;57:1147–1150.
190. Rosental JJ, Gaspar MR, Gjerdrum TC, et al. Vascular injuries associated with fractures of the femur. *Arch Surg* 1975;110:494–499.
191. Shah A, Ellis RD. False aneurysm complicating closed femoral fracture in a child. *Orthop Rev* 1993;22:1265–1267.
192. Riew KD, Sturm PF, Rosenbaum D, et al. Neurologic complications of pediatric femoral nailing. *J Pediatr Orthop* 1996;16:606–612.
193. Miller DS, Markin L, Grossman E. Ischemic fibrosis of the lower extremity in children. *Am J Surg* 1952;84:317–322.
194. Thomson SA, Mahoney LJ. Volkmann's ischaemic contracture and its relationship to fracture of the femur. *J Bone Joint Surg Br* 1951;33:336–347.
195. Mathews PV, Perry JJ, Murray PC. Compartment syndrome of the well leg as a result of the hemilithotomy position: a report of two cases and review of literature. *J Orthop Trauma* 2001;15:580–583.
196. Janzing H, Broos P, Rommens P. Compartment syndrome as a complication of skin traction in children with femoral fractures. *J Trauma* 1996;41:156–158.
197. DeLee JC, Clanton TO, Rockwood CA Jr. Closed treatment of subtrochanteric fractures of the femur in a modified cast-brace. *J Bone Joint Surg Am* 1981;63:773–779.
198. Ireland DC, Fisher RL. Subtrochanteric fractures of the femur in children. *Clin Orthop Relat Res* 1975;110:157–166.
199. Smith NC, Parker D, McNicol D. Supracondylar fractures of the femur in children. *J Pediatr Orthop* 2001;21:600–603.
200. Gustilo RB. Current concepts in the management of open fractures. *Instr Course Lect* 1987;36:359–366.
201. Shahcheraghi GH, Doroodchi HR. Supracondylar fracture of the femur: closed or open reduction? *J Trauma* 1993;24:499–502.
202. Hutchins CM, Sponseller, PD, Sturm P, et al. Open femur fractures in children: treatment, complications, and results. *J Pediatr Orthop* 2000;20:183–188.
203. Bohn WW, Durbin RA. Ipsilateral fractures of the femur and tibia in children and adolescents. *J Bone Joint Surg Am* 1991;73:429–439.
204. Arslan H, Kapukaya A, Kesemenli C,et al. Floating knee in children. *J Pediatr Orthop* 2003;23:458–463.
205. Mendelson SA, Dominick TS, Tyler-Kabara E, et al. Early versus late femoral fracture stabilization in multiply injured pediatric patients with closed head injury. *J Pediatr Orthop* 2001;21:594–599.

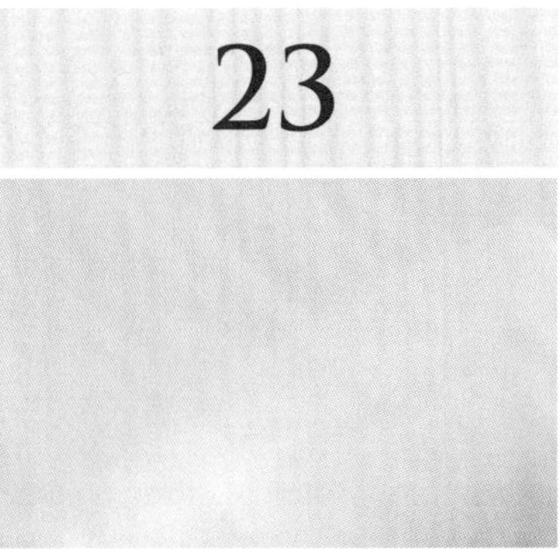

EXTRA-ARTICULAR INJURIES OF THE KNEE

David L. Skaggs

FRACTURES OF THE DISTAL FEMORAL EPIPHYSIS

Fractures involving the physes about the knee are particularly prone to complications and associated injuries and must be approached with care (Table 23-1). There is quite a significant risk of permanent injury to the physis, which may lead to growth disturbance and requires follow-up after fracture healing, and possibly future surgical treatment. In addition, associated injuries to nerves, vascular structures, ligaments, and the possibility of compartment syndrome require attention to detail in the evaluation and management of these fractures.

Principles of Management

Mechanism of Injury

Distal femoral physeal injuries account for 6% to 9% of all physeal injuries and far fewer than 1% of all fractures in children (1,2). In adults, ligaments usually fail before bone when a bending stress is applied across the knee joint. A common example of this is when an athlete with a planted foot is struck by an opponent on the lateral side of the knee, the valgus force may cause a failure of the medial collateral ligament (Fig. 23-1). In a skeletally mature individual, the medial collateral ligament and other soft-tissue structures are likely to fail as the knee falls into valgus (Fig. 23-2A). In an immature skeleton, the physis will fail in tension and the knee will fall into valgus though a Salter I or II fracture (Fig. 23-2B).

Both compression and distraction forces may occur simultaneously, in which case a Salter II fracture is more likely. On the tension side, the cartilaginous matrix of the physis is more

TABLE 23-1 Comparative Incidence of Epiphyseal Separations in the Lower Extremities

Location	Peterson[1]	Mann[2]
Proximal femur	1 (.5%)	4 (1%)
Distal femur	13 (6%)	29 (9%)
Proximal tibia	8 (4%)	12 (4%)
Distal tibia	104 (52%)	282 (86%)
Proximal fibula	1 (.5%)	
Distal fibula	68 (34%)	
Totals	195	327 (86%)

vulnerable to distraction, whereas on the compression side, the osseous metaphysis is more vulnerable to shear failure from compression (Fig. 23-3). A well-described mechanism of injury is forced hyperextension of the knee with posterior failure of the physis in tension. Pure compression injuries of the physis, also referred to as a Salter V injury, have been described, though are considered to be quite rare. A case of a 10-year-old girl with a Salter V injury has been reported in which a pure compression injury led to later valgus deformity of the knee, with tomograms indicating a fine mesh of bony beams passing through a continuous and apparently intact growth plate rather than one single bridge (3).

A series of 63 distal femoral physeal fractures in children aged 2 to 11 years were almost invariably caused by severe trauma, however those occurring in older children were usually secondary to less extensive trauma, most often sports injuries (4).

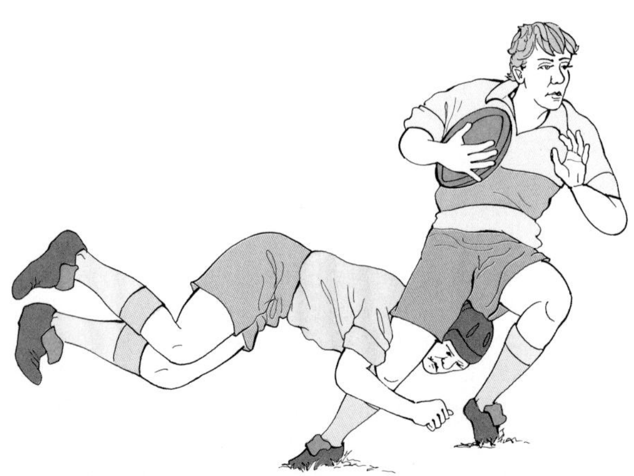

FIGURE 23-1 Valgus stress across the knee may cause a ligament injury or physeal separation.

One mechanism of injury deserving of special attention is an unrecognized physeal injury in association with nonphyseal fractures in the femur or tibia (5,6). For example, Navascues et al reports on six children who sustained distal femoral growth arrest after tibial shaft fractures (7).

Unusual mechanisms or underlying conditions, such as arthrogryposis, myelomeningocele, and lightening strike, may also cause distal femoral physeal injuries (8–11). Rodgers et al noted that physeal injuries in children with myelomeningocele may heal more slowly than metaphyseal fractures and may require splinting or casting for a longer period (10). Cases of epiphyseal separation of the distal femur have been reported in infants with breech delivery, even in cases of Caesarean section (12).

Signs and Symptoms

Physical Findings. The patient usually cannot walk or bear weight on the injured limb immediately after sustaining a displaced separation of the distal femoral epiphysis. Most often these injuries result from significant force, so malalignment of the limb, swelling, and/or ecchymosis make the diagnosis of a fracture likely from observation alone. Abrasion or laceration of the overlying soft tissues may be a clue to the mechanism of injury or to an open fracture. In Salter I and II fractures in which the periosteum may be intact on the compression side, more swelling may be noted on the opposite side which opened in tension.

Usually these children are in significant pain, and if the diagnosis of a fracture is suspected, it is probably kinder to perform x-rays before any manipulation. If muscle spasm can be relaxed, instability just above the knee joint may be felt. Crepitus sometimes may be absent if the periosteum is interposed between the metaphysis and the epiphysis. Abnormal laxity in a patient with negative x-rays may be caused by a nondisplaced physeal injury rather than by a ligamentous tear. At times there is a nondisplaced separation in which the patient may be able to walk. It sometimes is possible to localize tenderness to the level of the physis in cases of physeal fracture, which is at approximately the same level as the upper pole of the patella and the adductor tubercle, both of which can be used as reference points.

Extravasation of blood into the soft tissues of the distal thigh and popliteal fossa produces ecchymosis that may become apparent within 72 hours after injury.

Whenever a diagnosis of epiphyseal separation is suspected, careful neurovascular examination of the lower leg and foot should be done, including pulses, color, temperature, and motor and sensory status. The extremity may become cyanotic if venous return is impaired. The use of the Doppler may be helpful in evaluating circulation distal to the injury. Compartmental pressure recordings should be obtained if there are clinical findings of compartment syndrome.

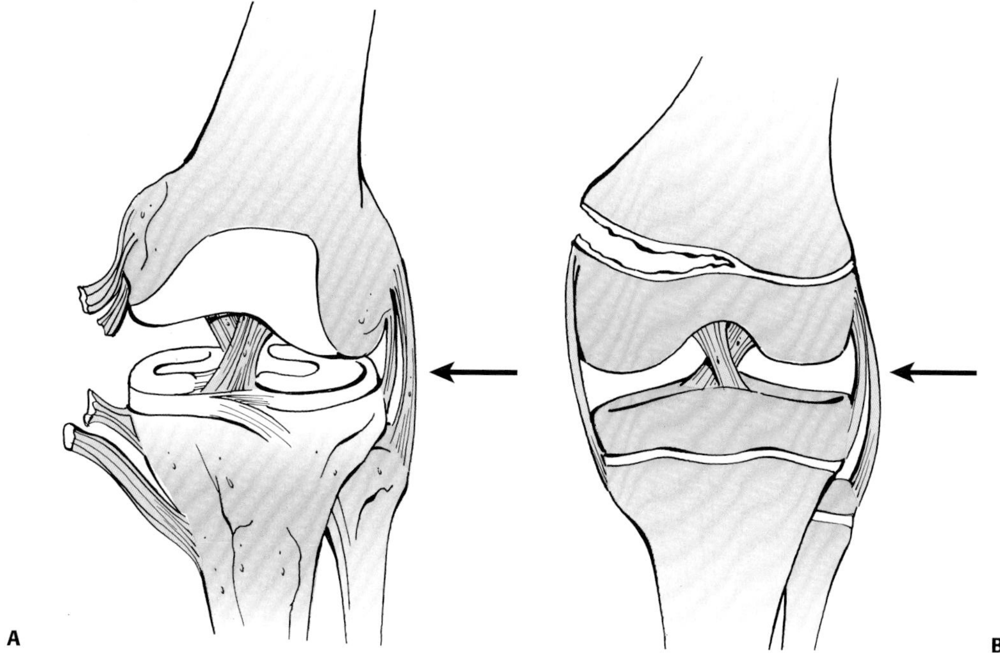

FIGURE 23-2 **A.** In skeletally mature patient with closed physis, tensile failure usually occurs across the ligament. **B.** In skeletally immature patient with open physis, failure usually occurs across the physis. (Reprinted with permission from Skaggs DL, Flynn JF. Trauma about the Knee, Tibia, and Foot. In Skaggs DL, Flynn JF, eds. *Staying out of Trouble in Pediatric Orthopaedics*. Philadelphia: Lippincott Williams & Wilkins, 2006.)

Direction of Displacement. Most commonly, displacement of the epiphysis occurs in the coronal plane, producing varus or valgus deformity. The protruding end of the metaphysis may be palpated through the distal portion of the vastus medialis with valgus injuries, or through the vastus lateralis with varus injuries.

With anterior displacement, the patella, riding forward on the femoral epiphysis, becomes extremely prominent. There is a palpable depression across the anterior thigh just proximal to the patella, and fullness in the popliteal fossa is produced by posterior displacement of the distal end of the metaphysis. Posterior protrusion of the metaphysis may put pressure on the popliteal artery, so that pulsations become palpable in the subcutaneous region of the popliteal fossa.

With posterior displacement of the distal femoral epiphysis, the distal end of the metaphysis is prominent on the anterior aspect of the distal thigh directly above the patella, and the epiphysis can be felt as a palpable fullness in the popliteal fossa. Whatever the direction of displacement, the patella and femoral condyles remain in line with the proximal tibia, a point useful in differentiating epiphyseal separation from dislocation of the knee.

Associated Injuries

Ligamentous Injuries. Symptomatic knee joint instability may persist after the epiphyseal separation has healed. This finding at follow-up implies concomitant injury to knee ligaments, often unappreciated at the time of initial management of the epiphyseal separation. Bertin and Goble found that 6 of 16 patients seen in follow-up for distal femoral physeal fractures had positive anterior drawer and Lachman tests; 1 patient had laxity to valgus stress (13). A 2002 review of 151 children with distal femoral physeal fractures found symptomatic knee ligamentous laxity in 12 patients (8%) (14). Brone and Wroble (15) reported three patients with Salter-Harris type III fractures of the femoral condyle associated with anterior cruciate ligament (ACL) tears, and found two more reported in the literature. All were near skeletal maturity. They emphasized the importance of early diagnosis of associated ligament injury. If there is no meniscal injury, a rehabilitation program is indicated initially. If there is a reparable meniscal tear, cruciate reconstruction at the time of meniscal repair after physeal healing may be indicated, depending on the patient's age and activity level.

Vascular Impairment. Vascular injuries are uncommon with this fracture, with many series not reporting any vascular injuries (4,14,16,17). Intimal tear and thrombosis in the popliteal artery may be caused by trauma from the distal end of the metaphysis when the epiphysis is displaced anteriorly with a hyperextension injury (18).

Arterial spasm or direct mechanical obstruction of the artery by the proximal fragment may be associated with displacement in the sagittal plane and resolve with fracture reduction. If vascular impingement occurs but is relieved by prompt reduction

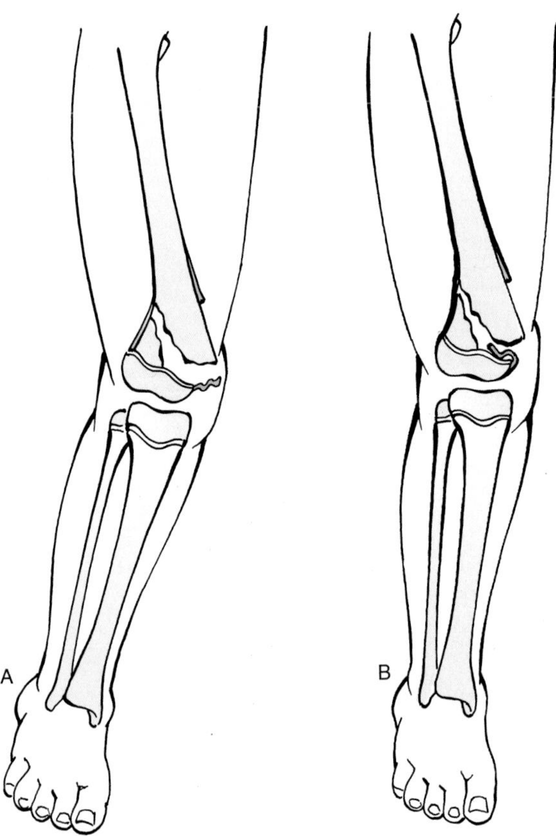

FIGURE 23-3 **A.** In a Salter-Harris type II fracture the side where the fracture occurred through the physis fails in tension, with disruption of the periosteum. The side of the fracture with the Thurston-Holland fragment failed in compression, with the periosteum usually intact. The intact periosteum can be used for fracture reduction. **B.** With fracture reduction, the periosteum may become interposed within the fracture site, preventing an anatomic reduction.

of the displaced epiphysis, the patient should be observed to rule out an intimal tear with thrombosis. If however, following fracture reduction and stabilization, the leg remains poorly perfused, arteriography and vascular consultation should be considered. If there is an associated fracture of the pelvis or femoral shaft, arteriography may be necessary to localize the vascular injury. In the cases of known vascular injury, as may occur in open fractures, vascular repair should be carried out following fracture stabilization and arteriography may not be indicated. Vascular impairment may develop slowly from increasing compartmental pressure. If the patient has inordinate persistent pain, with a cool and pale foot, a femoral arteriogram and compartment pressure measurement should be considered, even if peripheral pulses are present.

Whether vascular repair or fracture stabilization should be carried out first is open to debate (19,20). The vascular repair is at risk for avulsion during manipulation for fracture repair, if the vascular structures are repaired first. However, if there has been significant ischemia time, temporary re-vascularization of the artery with IV tubing should be considered prior to definitive fracture care to minimize the overall ischemia time (19).

Peroneal Nerve Injury. The peroneal nerve is the only nerve injured with any appreciable frequency in this type of fracture. It may be stretched by anterior or medial displacement of the epiphysis. It rarely requires treatment other than reduction of the separation. Resolution of peroneal neuropraxia may occur up to 6 months following fracture reduction (18,21). The exception to this is a transected nerve in association with an open injury, which may be treated with repair or grafting. Persistent neurologic deficit after 3 to 6 months warrants electromyographic examination. If the conduction time is prolonged and fibrillation or denervation is present in distal muscles, exploration and microneural reanastomosis or resection of any neuroma may be indicated.

Diagnosis and Classification

Separations of the distal femoral epiphysis have been classified according to the pattern of fracture, the direction of displacement, or the mechanism of injury (Table 23-2). The Salter-Harris classification (Fig. 23-4) (22) is useful for description and treatment planning. The direction and degree of displacement may help predict the type and severity of complications. Mechanisms of injury, as well as the implications of growth disturbance, vary with the patient's age.

Classification by Fracture Pattern. The Salter-Harris type I pattern is a separation through the distal femoral physis, without fracture through the adjacent epiphysis or metaphysis (Fig. 23-5). It occurs in newborns with birth injury and in adolescents, often as a nondisplaced separation. Either may go undetected. Sometimes the diagnosis is made only in retrospect, when subperiosteal new bone formation occurs along the adjacent metaphysis. If displacement is present, it is usually in the sagittal plane. Growth disturbance may occur after Salter-Harris type I distal femoral injuries, contrary to the usual expectations for Salter-Harris type I fractures in other locations.

The Salter-Harris type II pattern, characterized by an oblique extension of the fracture across one corner of the adjacent metaphysis, is the most common type of separation at the distal femur and usually occurs in adolescents (Fig. 23-6). The metaphyseal corner, which remains attached to the epiphysis, is called the Thurston-Holland fragment. The physeal separation occurs on the tension side, in which the physis is fractured. Displacement usually is toward the side of the metaphyseal fragment. The incidence of premature growth arrest, even with satisfactory reduction, is significant. If asymmetric growth follows a type II separation, the portion of the physis underneath the metaphyseal fracture usually is spared (Fig. 23-6). Therefore, if the metaphyseal fracture is medial, deformity is more likely to be valgus than varus.

A Salter-Harris type III injury consists of a partial separation of the physis, with a vertical fracture line extending from the physis down to the articular surface of the epiphysis (Fig. 23-7).

TABLE 23-2 Mechanism of Injury in Clinical Reviews of Separation of the Distal Femoral Epiphysis

	Neer[a]	Bassett[b]	Roberts[c]	Stephens[d]	Total
Sports injury	5	4	64	8	81 (49%)
Hit by automobile	9	8	15	10	42 (25%)
Falls	3	3	12	1	19 (12%)
Auto accident	–	3	5	1	9 (5%)
Other	4	7	4	–	15 (9%)

[a] Neer CS II. Separation of the lower femoral epiphyses. *Am J Surg* 1960;99:756–761.
[b] Bassett FH III, Goldner JL. Fractures involving the distal femoral epiphyseal growth line. *South Med J* 1962;55:545–557.
[c] Roberts JM. Fracture separation of the distal femoral epiphysis. *J Bone Joint Surg Am* 1973;55A:1324.
[d] Stephens DC, Louis DS, Louis E. Traumatic separation of the distal femoral epiphyseal cartilage plate. *J Bone Joint Surg Am* 1974;56:1383–1390.

The vertical fracture line is usually in line with the intercondylar notch. Salter-Harris type III injuries most often are caused by valgus stress in sports and usually involve the medial condyle. The fracture may be nondisplaced and detected only with a stress x-rays or magnetic resonance imaging (MRI) (23).

Salter-Harris type IV injuries of the distal femur are uncommon. A sagittal fracture line extends from the metaphyseal cortex down across the physis and enters the articular surface of the epiphysis. Even slight displacement of the fracture fragment may produce growth disturbance following formation of a bony bridge from the displaced epiphysis to the metaphysis. Therefore, anatomic reduction and internal fixation are advised. Figure 23-8 demonstrates that even minimally displaced fractures should be followed closely for growth plate injury.

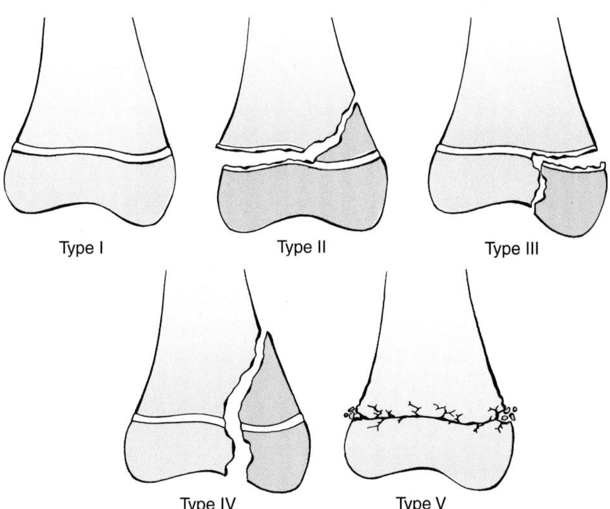

FIGURE 23-4 The Salter-Harris classification of fractures involving the distal femoral physis.

Salter-Harris type V injuries (without fracture) are rare. Most commonly, the diagnosis is made in retrospect at the time of evaluation for premature growth arrest and limb-length discrepancy or angular deformity (3).

Even less common is an avulsion injury to the edge of the physis. A small fragment, including a portion of the perichondrium and underlying bone, may be torn off when the proximal attachment of the collateral ligament is avulsed. This uncommon injury may also lead to localized premature growth arrest and progressive angular deformity (5). The bony bridge usually is small, localized, and surgically accessible, and excision is appropriate.

A triplane fracture infrequently occurs in the distal femur. Computed tomographic (CT) scans with three-dimensional (3D) modeling may be helpful in identifying and analyzing (24) this injury.

Classification by Displacement. Anterior displacement of the epiphysis results from hyperextension of the knee. The extension force on the distal femur is transmitted through the posterior capsule of the knee joint. The mechanism is similar to that of knee dislocations in adults. There is an increased risk of neurovascular injury. Posterior displacement of the epiphysis on the femur is uncommon. It has been reported in birth injuries and in older children struck on the front of the flexed knee. Reduction is obtained and maintained by extending the knee. Medial/lateral displacement currently is most common, usually with an associated fracture of the adjacent metaphysis (Salter-Harris type II).

Classification According to Age. Separations of the distal femoral epiphysis in infants may be associated with breech birth or

(text continues on page 8)

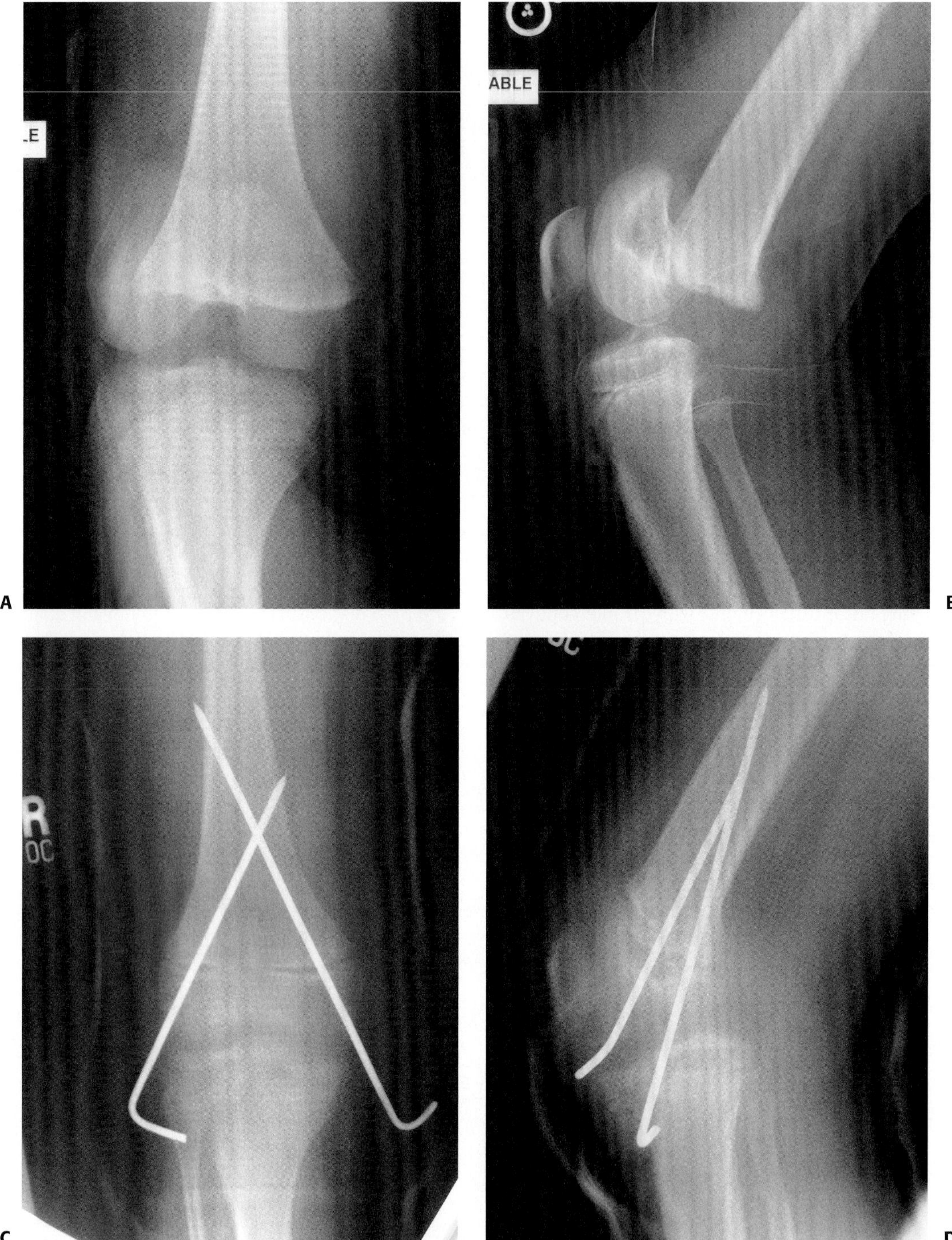

FIGURE 23-5 **A.** Salter-Harris type I fracture of the distal femur in an 8-year-old. **B.** Lateral view shows hyperextension. **C.** Fixation following closed reduction under general anesthesia. Note that pins are widely separated at the fracture site. **D.** Lateral view of fixation.

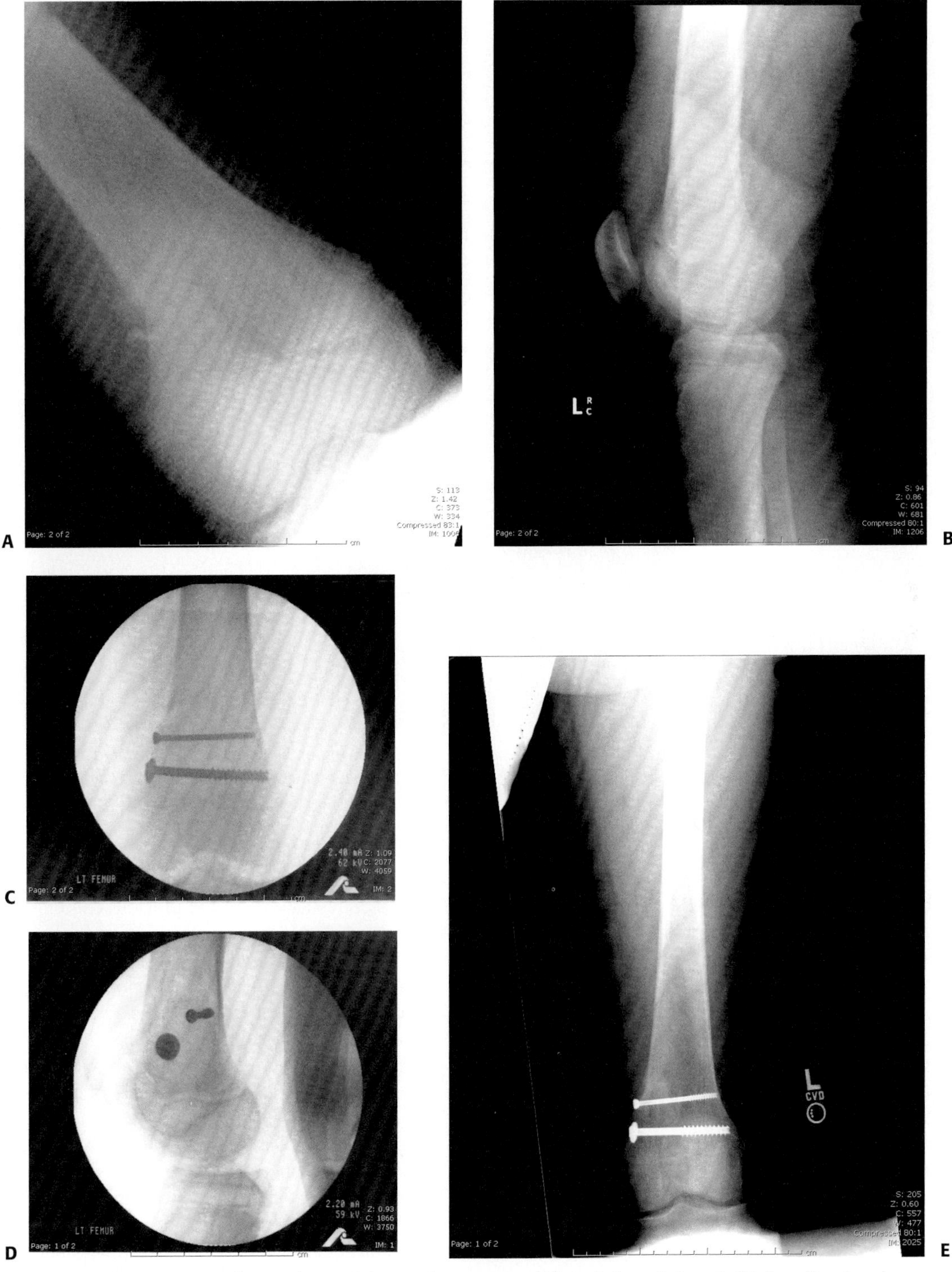

FIGURE 23-6 **A.** Salter-Harris type II fracture in a 12-year-old boy. **B.** Lateral view. **C.** AP view after closed reduction and fixation. Note that screws function in compression with threads across fracture line. **D.** Lateral view. **E.** Six months after injury this plain x-ray and clinical picture was suspicious of increased valgus. Note that x-ray is not centered on the distal physis, and thus the physis is difficult to visualize.

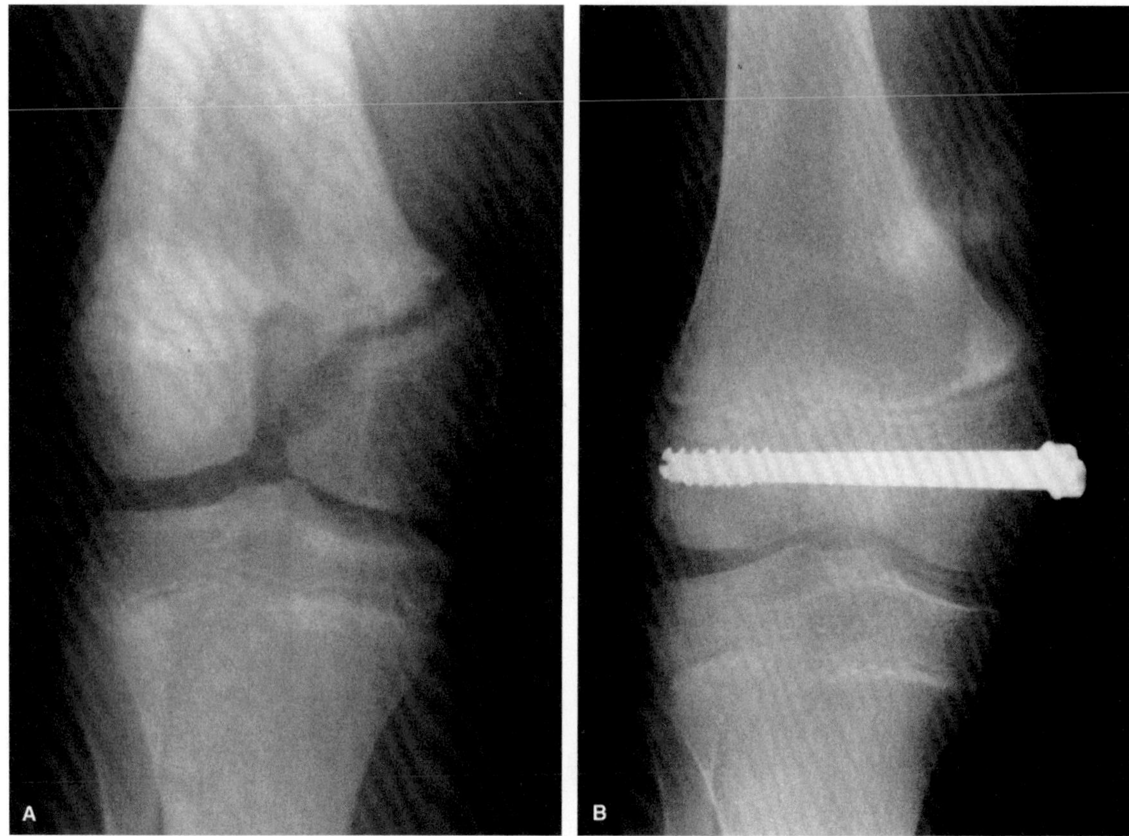

FIGURE 23-7 **A.** Salter-Harris type III fracture-separation of the distal femur. Note the vertical fracture line extending from the physis distally into the intercondylar notch with displacement. **B.** After reduction and fixation with two compression screws extending transversely across the epiphyseal fragments. Note closure and healing of the vertical fracture line in the epiphysis, with restoration of the articular surface.

child abuse (Fig. 23-9). Most are Salter-Harris type I injuries. Clinically differentiating between an epiphyseal separation and hematogenous osteomyelitis may be difficult. Ultrasonography or MRI (25) may be used to confirm fracture.

In most recent reviews, approximately two thirds of distal femoral epiphyseal separations occur in adolescents, often from contact sports (4,26). The most common patterns are Salter-Harris types I and II. The potential for growth disturbance is lowest in this group. Older children and preadolescents usually are injured in sports whereas younger children are often involved in high-energy accidents, such as a fall or being hit by a vehicle (4). Associated musculoskeletal and visceral injuries are common in the latter group.

Imaging

Because the physis normally is radiolucent, injury is diagnosed by displacement, widening, or adjacent bony disruption. However, a nondisplaced Salter-Harris type I or III fracture without separation can be easily overlooked (23). Oblique views of the distal femur may reveal an occult fracture through the epiphysis or metaphysis (Table 23-3).

It has been suggested in the previous edition of this text that stress views should be considered if multiple plain films are negative in a patient with an effusion or tenderness localized to the physis (Fig. 23-10). Another option is an MRI, which should be diagnostic in unclear cases. For many reasons timely MRI scans may have limited availability. Stress x-rays may be falsely negative if there is associated muscle spasm. (Please see Controversies section of this chapter for more discussion of stress views.)

Distal femoral physeal fractures have such a significant risk of growth disturbance, and may involve the articular surface of a weight-bearing joint. Thus, one should have a low threshold in ordering a CT scan to help determine if there is sufficient displacement to warrant surgical treatment and best visualize the fracture pattern.

A vertical fracture line extending from the articular surface of the distal femoral epiphysis into the radiolucent physis is usually diagnostic of a Salter-Harris type III fracture. The epiphyseal fracture line is often best seen on an anteroposterior view because it is oriented in the sagittal plane. The degree of displacement in this fracture pattern may be difficult to measure on plain films unless the radiographic projection is precisely in

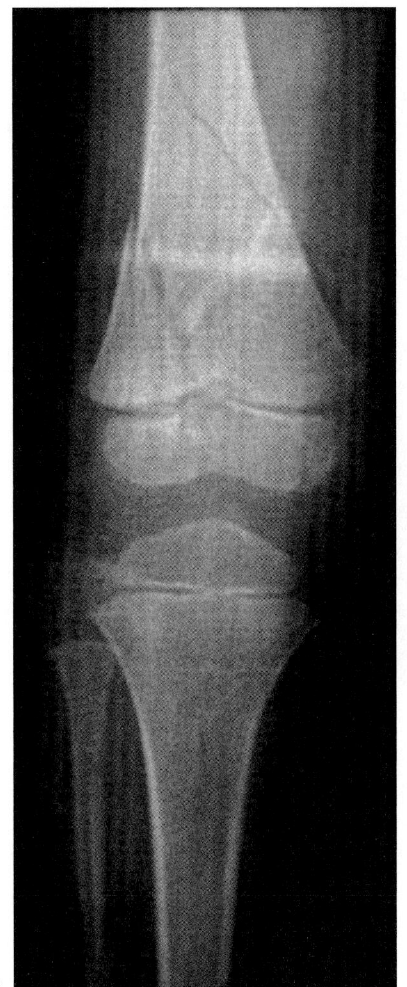
A

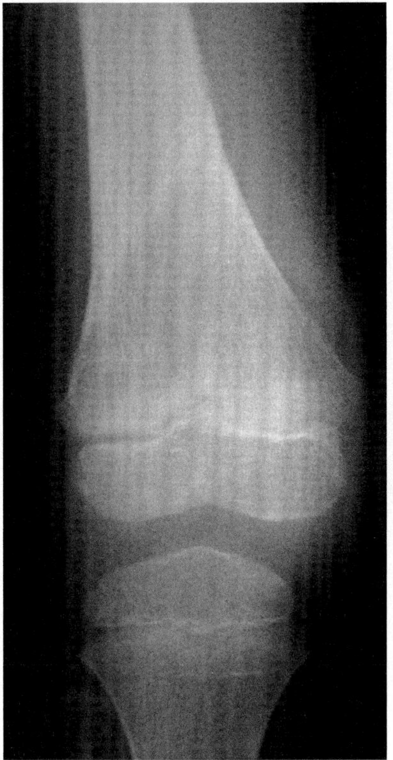
B

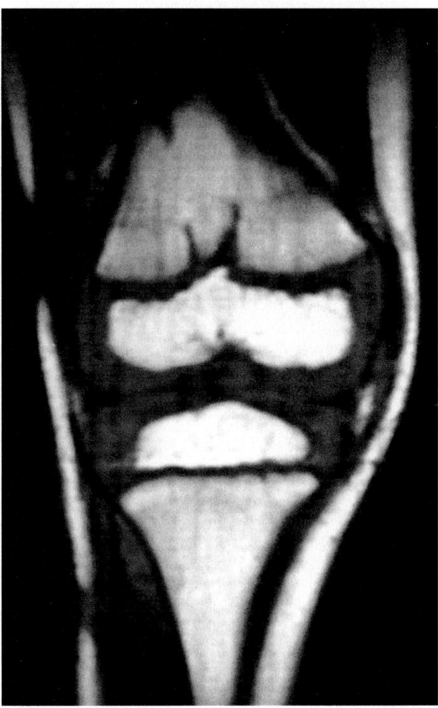
C

FIGURE 23-8 Five-year-old boy hit by car with Salter IV fracture of the distal femur.**A.** AP x-ray of a minimally displaced Salter IV fracture of the distal femur. **B.** AP x-ray of healed fracture. From this view it is difficult to tell if any injury to the physis has occurred, though a central growth arrest was suspected. **C** MRI shows that a central growth plate injury probably did occur, although this did not result in the formation of a bony bar or growth arrest. (Courtesy of Robert Kay, MD, Los Angeles, California.)

line with the plane of fracture. A fracture line extending from the epiphyseal surface across the physis and up through the metaphysis is characteristic of a Salter-Harris type IV injury. Even 1 to 2 mm of displacement is significant (27).

Anterior or posterior displacement of the epiphysis is best appreciated on the lateral projection. The anteriorly displaced epiphysis is usually tilted so that the distal articular surface faces anteriorly. The posteriorly displaced epiphysis is rotated so that the distal articular surface faces the popliteal fossa.

Separation of the distal femoral epiphysis in an infant is difficult to see on initial x-rays unless there is displacement because only the center of the epiphysis is ossified at birth. This ossicle should be in line with the axis of the femoral shaft on both anteroposterior and lateral views. Comparative views of the opposite knee may be helpful. MRI (25), ultrasonography, or arthrography of the knee may help to identify a separation of the relatively unossified femoral epiphysis.

When MRI is used to visualize the physis, fat-suppressed 3D spoiled gradient-recalled echo sequences have reportedly allowed best visualization (28). In a review of MRI scans in 315 children with traumatic knee injuries, physeal injuries of the distal femur was diagnosed in 7 patients and of the proximal tibial in 2 patients. Plain films available on 8 patients showed signs of fracture in 7 patients, but was only clearly delineated in one patient (29).

Surgical and Applied Anatomy

The epiphysis of the distal femur is the first epiphysis to ossify. From birth to skeletal maturity, the distal femoral physis con-

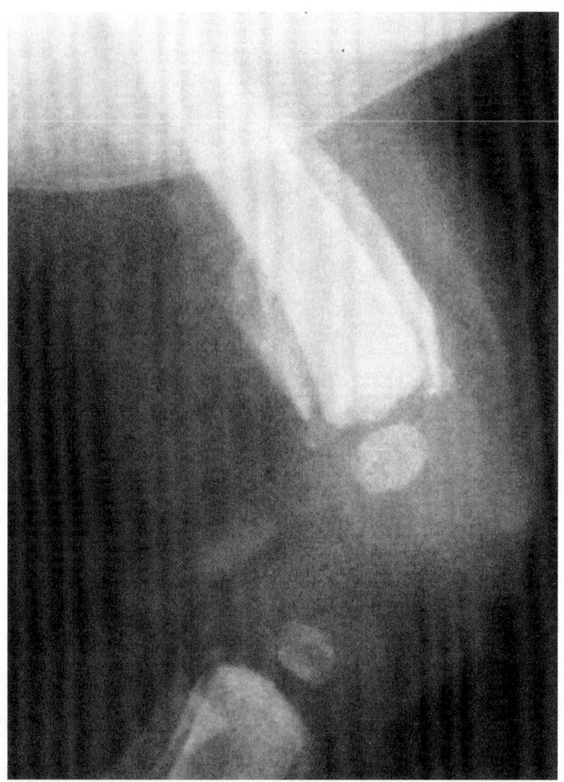

FIGURE 23-9 Lateral x-ray of a swollen knee in a 3-month-old girl who reportedly fell out of her crib 8 days earlier. Subperiosteal ossification along the distal femoral shaft indicates separation of the distal femoral epiphysis. Note evidence of fracture-separation of the proximal tibial epiphysis as well. Final diagnosis: abused child.

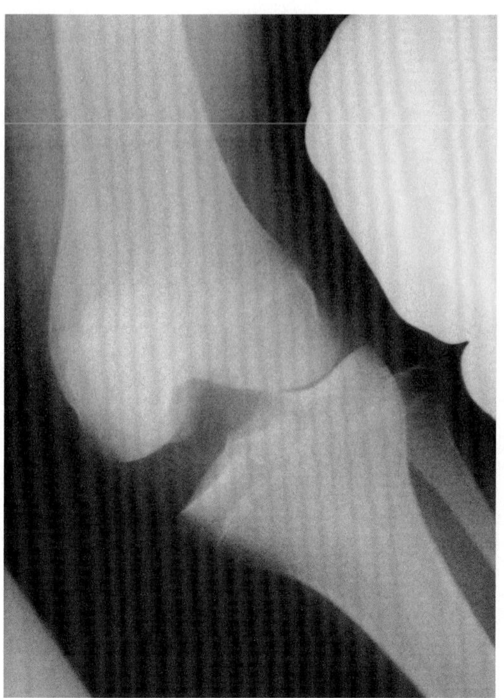

FIGURE 23-10 AP x-ray of the knee in an adolescent with a valgus stress view demonstrating opening of the medial joint space, with no osseous fracture. Thus, the diagnosis of a medial collateral ligament injury may be made.

TABLE 23-3 Imaging Studies in the Evaluation of Distal Femoral Physeal Fractures

Study	Indications	Limitations
Plain films	First study, often sufficient.	May miss nondisplaced Salter I or III fractures or underestimate fracture displacement.
CT scan	Best defines fracture pattern and amount of displacement. Useful in deciding if surgery is needed, and planning surgery.	Poor cartilage visualization. Less useful than MRI in evaluating for occult Salter I or III fracture.
MRI	Evaluation of occult Salter I or III fracture possible. Infants with little epiphyseal ossification.	Availability, cost, insurance company authorizations. Identifies associated soft-tissue injuries. Unclear that study changes initial treatment.
Stress views	Differentiate occult Salter fracture from ligament injury.	Painful, muscle spasm may not permit opening of fracture if patient awake. Unclear that study changes initial treatment.
Contralateral x-rays	Infants, or to assess physeal width	Usually not needed.

tributes 70% of the growth of the femur and 37% of the growth of the lower extremity. The annual rate of growth is approximately 3/8 in. or 9 to 10 mm. The growth rate slows at a mean skeletal age of 13 years in girls and 15 years in boys (30).

Bony Anatomy

Immediately above the medial border of the medial condyle, the metaphysis of the distal femur widens sharply to the adductor tubercle. In contrast, the metaphysis flares minimally on the lateral side to produce the lateral epicondyle. A line tangential to the distal surfaces of the two condyles (the joint line) is approximately horizontal in an upright stance. The longitudinal axis of the diaphysis of the femur inclines medially downward, with an angle of 9 degrees from vertical. The mechanical axis of the femur is formed by a line between the centers of the hip and knee joints (Fig. 23-11).

A large part of the surface of the distal femoral epiphysis is covered by cartilage for articulation with the proximal tibia and patella. The anterior or patellar surface has a shallow midline concavity to accommodate the longitudinal ridge on the undersurface of the patella. The distal or tibial surface of each condyle extends on either side of the intercondylar notch far around onto the posterior surface. Here, the articular cartilage nearly reaches the posterior margin of the physis.

There is a distinctly quadrupedal configuration of the distal femoral physis, undulating from side to side and front to back. The fact that the physis is not flat may help to resist shear and torsion. However, when subject to trauma significant enough to cause fracture, however, the epiphyseal ridges may grind against the metaphyseal projections and damage germinal cells. With a nonplaner physis, it is hypothesized that the fracture line may extend through multiple regions of the growth plate (4). Animal studies report that if a fracture line extends into the epiphyseal physeal border, there was a greater likelihood of subsequent physeal bar formation (31). Note that the clinical outcome of the distal femoral physis is quite different from the relatively planer distal radius physis in which growth plate disturbances are rare.

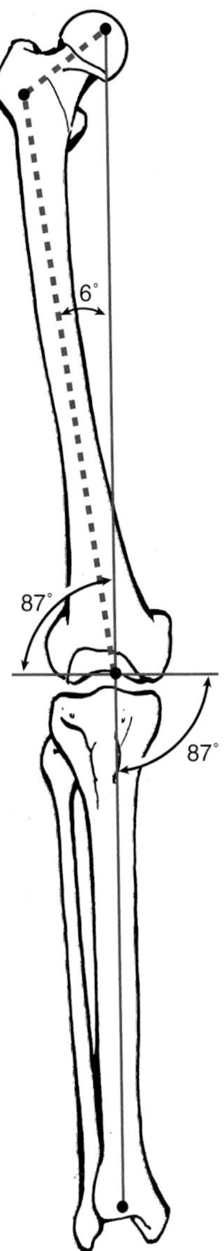

FIGURE 23-11 The mechanical and anatomic axis of the lower extremity. Note that the knee joint is in a mean of 3 degrees of valgus.

Soft-Tissue Anatomy

The distal femoral physis is completely extra-articular. Anteriorly and posteriorly, the synovial membrane and joint capsule of the knee attach to the femoral epiphysis close to the distal femoral physis. Anteriorly, the suprapatellar pouch balloons proximally over the anterior surface of the metaphysis. On the medial and lateral surfaces of the epiphysis, the proximal attachment of the synovium and capsule is below the physis and separated from the physis by the insertions of the collateral ligaments.

The strong posterior capsule, as well as all major supporting ligaments of the knee, is attached to the epiphysis of the femur distal to the physis. Both cruciate ligaments originate in the upward-sloping roof of the intercondylar notch distal to the physis. Compression and tension forces can be transmitted across the extended knee to the epiphysis of the femur by taut ligaments.

The medial and lateral head of the gastrocnemius originate from the distal femur, proximal to the joint capsule (32,33). Thus muscle pull would theoretically not seem to be as much of a factor as the pull of the ligaments in the initial displacement of the epiphysis at the time of injury.

Vascular Anatomy

The popliteal artery is separated from the posterior surface of the distal femur by only a thin layer of fat. Directly above the femoral condyles, the superior geniculate arteries pass medially and laterally to lie between the femoral metaphysis and the overlying muscles. As the popliteal artery continues distally, it lies on the posterior capsule of the knee joint between the femoral condyles. At this level, the middle geniculate artery branches directly forward to enter the posterior aspect of the distal femoral epiphysis. The popliteal artery and its branches are vulnerable to injury from the distal femoral metaphysis at the time of hyperextension injury. It is unlikely that the distal femoral epiphysis would be completely shorn of its blood supply because of the rich anastomosis supplied, in part, by the superior geniculate branches. Clinically osteonecrosis (ON) of the epiphysis is not a commonly recognized sequela of even severe fractures about the epiphysis.

Above the popliteal space, the sciatic nerve divides into the peroneal and tibial nerves. The peroneal nerve descends posteriorly between the biceps femoris muscle and the lateral head of the gastrocnemius muscle to a point just distal to the head of the fibula. Thus, there is interposed muscle protecting the nerve from the potentially sharp edges of a physeal fracture. The nerve is subject to stretch if the distal femoral epiphysis is tilted into varus or rotated medially.

Current Treatment Options

Rationale

The objectives of treatment of separation of the distal femoral epiphysis are to obtain and maintain satisfactory reduction, to regain a functional range of motion and strength, and to avoid further damage to the physis while addressing associated neurovascular injuries (34). Anatomic reduction of a displaced separation of the distal femoral epiphysis is desirable to maintain normal mechanical alignment of the limb, to help prevent growth disturbance, and minimize arthritis from joint incongruity.

In terms of remodeling, the closer the patient is to skeletal maturity, the greater the need for exact realignment. In contrast, in terms of future growth disturbance, skeletally immature children with growth remaining will develop significant deformity with a growth disturbance. Residual varus or valgus deformity after reduction remodels much less than remodeling in the plane of joint motion. The remodeling potential in infants is so great that considerable displacement can be accepted. Most infants can be treated by supportive traction or splinting, no matter how great the displacement.

Although growth may be adversely affected by the injury itself, further damage to the physis should be avoided during diagnostic stress x-rays, closed reduction, or open reduction. The use of general anesthesia decreases the forces across the physis.

At the time of initial evaluation and treatment planning, the short- and long-term problems and complications are explained to the patient and parents. The need for long-term follow-up is stressed from the beginning of treatment. The family is better able to accept the likelihood of growth disturbance, deformity, and need for further surgery is this is discussed at the initial consultation.

Closed Reduction and Immobilization

A nondisplaced separation is immobilized to prevent displacement and relieve pain. If there is tense effusion of the knee joint, aspiration under sterile precautions may be done for pain relief. A well-molded long leg cast is applied with the knee in approximately 15 degrees to 20 degrees of flexion with the intact periosteal hinge tightened. Thus, if the metaphyseal fragment of a nondisplaced Salter-Harris type II separation is on the lateral side of the metaphysis, the cast is applied with three-point molding into slight varus. Alternative methods of immobilization include a posterior splint, cylinder cast from high thigh to supramalleolar level, or a single hip spica cast. The more secure form of immobilization should be used if the patient is obese or of uncertain reliability. It must be stressed that there is a high chance of loss of reduction if a displaced fracture is reduced and not internally fixed (16). X-rays are made 1 week after immobilization to ensure that displacement has not occurred, and more frequently based on clinical suspicion of instability.

Closed reduction usually can be performed in older children up to 10 days after injury. Partial weight-bearing on crutches with touchdown gait may be started 2 to 3 weeks after injury. By 4 to 8 weeks after injury, depending on the x-rays, patient's age, and social situation, the cast is removed and may be converted to knee immobilizer for continued protection. Even with a nondisplaced fracture, growth inhibition may be caused by a compression force at the time of injury, and the patient should be followed for 12 to 24 months.

Series have reported rates of 43% to 70% of distal femoral fractures treated without internal fixation have displaced (16,36). Unless a fracture is truly nondisplaced and stable, immobilization without fixation is no longer the treatment of choice (26).

Closed Reduction and Fixation

A basic principle is that fixation devices should avoid crossing the physis if adequate fixation can be achieved. In Salter-Harris type III and IV separations, pins or screws may be placed transversely across the epiphysis. In Salter-Harris type II and IV separations, pins or screws are placed transversely across the metaphysis, engaging the triangular fragment if it is large enough (2 to 3 cm tall; Fig. 23-6B). Washers should be used with compression screws as the bone in the metaphysis and epiphysis is not cortical, and a screw head without a washer may migrate into the metaphysis.

If traversing the physis is unavoidable, smooth pins are used. Pins should be widely separated at the fracture site (Fig. 23-5C), which is generally easiest to achieve by crossing the pins proximal to the physis. Although it may not be possible to tell with 100% certainty if a subsequent growth disturbance arose from the injury or pins crossing the physis, clinical experience suggests smooth pins crossing a physis are exceeding unlikely to cause a growth disturbance. The treatment of supracondylar humerus fractures supports this belief. A rabbit model found a 2.5 mm drill hole (4% to 5% of the physeal area) across the distal femoral growth plate did not cause a growth disturbance

(37). In Salter I fractures, as well as Salter II fractures with small metaphyseal fragments crossing the physis may be necessary. It is important to obtain adequate fixation and avoid loss of reduction in the postoperative period.

The technique of closed reduction depends on the direction and degree of displacement of the epiphysis (Fig. 23-12A,B). General anesthesia often is helpful to decrease associated muscle spasm and diminish the risk of further injury to the physis. Joint aspiration may precede manipulation. Remember that the periosteum is usually intact on one side—the side of the metaphyseal fragment in a Salter II fracture, and the direction of displacement of the distal fragment in most Salter fractures. The first principal in reduction is do no harm to the physis. The maneuver should be 90% traction and 10% leverage. The first maneuver increases the deformity slightly with traction. The proximal edge of the displaced epiphysis can then be brought to the edge of the metaphysis on the same side of the periosteal tether. Reduction is then completed by realignment of the angular deformity. Grinding of the physeal cartilage against the metaphysis is thereby avoided. The sequence of events is to pull, tip, and close the separation.

Medial or Lateral Displacement. The patient is placed supine. The leg is grasped with the knee in extension and the hip in slight flexion. The thigh is fixed by an assistant. Moderate longitudinal traction is exerted by a handhold on the leg above the ankle. If the displacement of the epiphysis is medial, varus is increased gently and cautiously to avoid stretching the peroneal nerve. With one hand holding traction on the leg, the palm of the other hand is placed against the concave surface of the angulated distal femur. The epiphysis is pushed toward the metaphysis as the leg is realigned with the thigh. Once reduction is obtained, longitudinal traction is released. A long leg cast or hip spica cast is then applied, with the knee in slight flexion. External immobilization is continued for 5 to 6 weeks. Thereafter, the care is similar to that for a nondisplaced separation.

Anterior Displacement. Anterior displacement of the epiphysis can be reduced with the patient either supine or prone. With the patient supine, the hip is flexed approximately 60 degrees and the thigh is fixed by an assistant. Longitudinal traction is applied, with the knee in partial flexion. Posterior pressure on the epiphysis is exerted manually. With continuing traction on

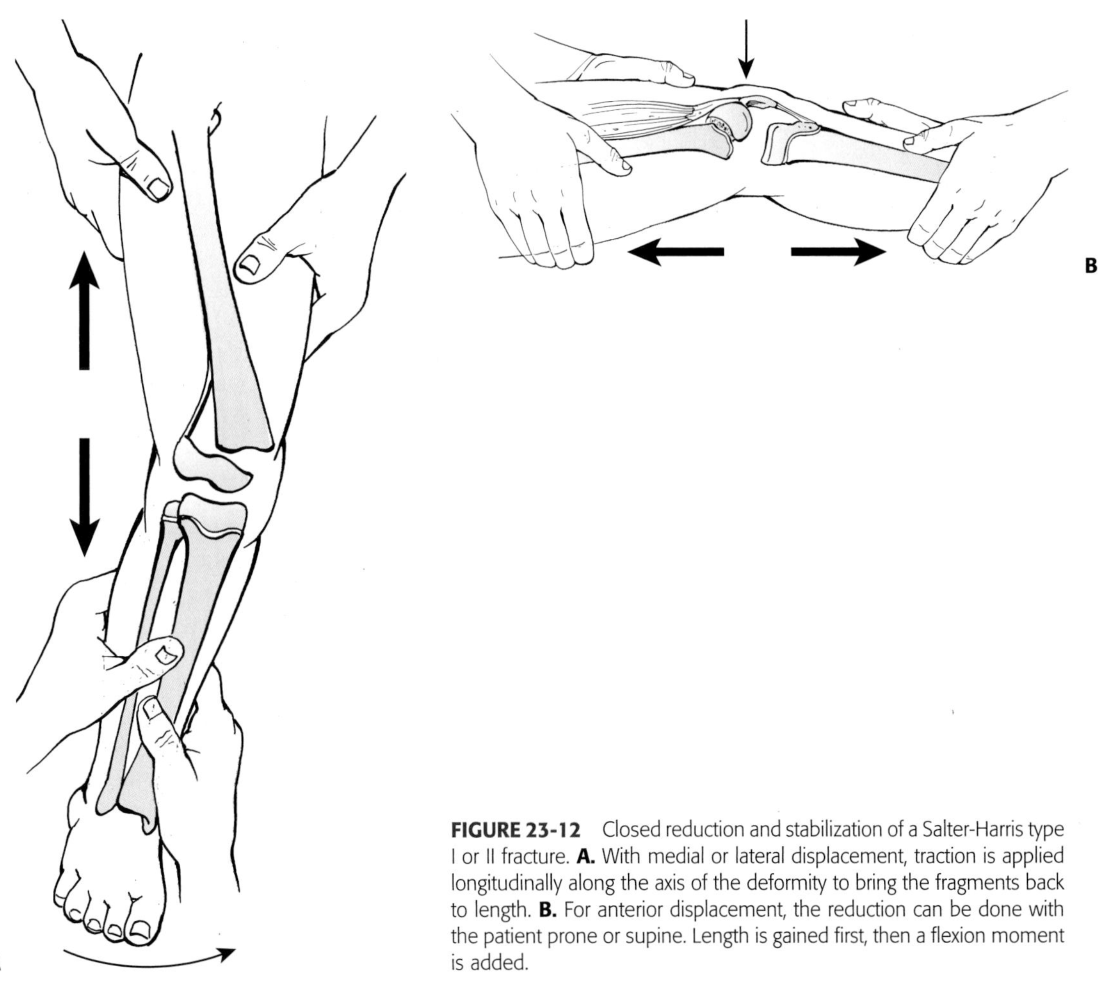

FIGURE 23-12 Closed reduction and stabilization of a Salter-Harris type I or II fracture. **A.** With medial or lateral displacement, traction is applied longitudinally along the axis of the deformity to bring the fragments back to length. **B.** For anterior displacement, the reduction can be done with the patient prone or supine. Length is gained first, then a flexion moment is added.

the leg, the knee is flexed 45 degrees to 90 degrees. Prone reduction requires fewer assistants. If the surgeon chooses to perform the reduction with the patient prone, traction is applied to the limb, an assistant pushes down on the posterior aspect of the proximal femur, and the knee is flexed further until approximately 110 degrees of flexion is reached. This sequence is similar to that for reduction of a supracondylar humerus fracture of the elbow.

After reduction of an anteriorly displaced epiphysis, it is important to check the pulses in the foot and ankle. Flexion of a swollen knee to beyond 90 degrees may compromise the popliteal vessels. If reduction is adequate, the knee may be immobilized in flexion by a long leg or hip spica cast. Griswold (38) noted difficulty regaining extension of the knee after prolonged immobilization in flexion. In addition, judgment of frontal plane alignment is difficult in the flexed knee. For these reason, pinning the knee in the reduced position, and casting in mild knee flexion of 20 degrees to 30 degrees may be preferable. If casting in flexion without fixation is chosen, it is important to increase the range of extension gradually during the 6-to-8-week period of immobilization with cast changes.

Posterior Displacement. To reduce posterior displacement of the distal femoral epiphysis, the patient is placed supine. The surgeon grasps the leg and exerts downward longitudinal traction while the knee is held partly flexed. Longitudinal traction is continued as the leg is brought up to extend the knee. An assistant pulls up directly under the distal femoral epiphysis with one hand and pushes down on the distal metaphysis of the femur with the other. Such flexion type injuries may be immobilized in extension (39).

Pin Fixation. The larger the metaphyseal fragment and the greater the displacement, the less stable the closed reduction. If the metaphyseal fragment is large enough, threaded pins or screws can be directed transversely across the metaphysis after reduction (Fig. 23-13; see also Fig. 23-6C). In the absence of a substantial metaphyseal fragment, smooth pins are directed through the side of each condyle to cross in the metaphysis proximal to the physis. The closer the pins are to crossing at the fracture site, the less stable they are. To make the pins cross at a point proximal to the fracture site, they should come in at a "high" angle, less than 45 degrees to the long axis of the femur. The pins may be cut off under the skin before application of the cast or left percutaneous. Infection is frequent if pins in this region are left out through the skin for greater than 4 to 6 weeks, and intra-articular pins may lead to a septic knee. The use of self-reinforced polyglycolic acid pins has been reported in fixation of distal femoral physeal fractures in a rabbit, with good healing and no growth disturbance at 28 weeks, though this short-term animal study can not necessarily be translated to use in humans (40).

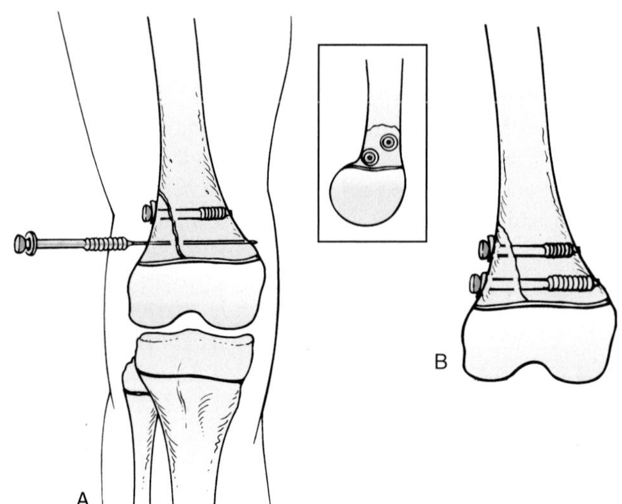

FIGURE 23-13 Screw fixation following closed or open reduction of Salter-Harris type II fracture with a large metaphyseal fragment. **A.** When using cannulated screws, place both guide wires before screw placement to avoid rotation of the fragment while drilling or inserting screw. Screw threads should be past the fracture site to enable compression. Washers help increase compression. Screws may be placed anterior and posterior to each other, which is particularly helpful when trying to fit multiple screws in a small metaphyseal fragment. **B.** This form of fixation is locally "rigid," but must be protected with long leg immobilization or long lever arm.

Open Reduction of Physeal Fractures

Open reduction is indicated for displaced Salter-Harris type III or IV fractures, for all other types in which satisfactory alignment cannot be obtained by closed means, open fractures, or when associated injuries mandate it (i.e., a "floating knee" or ligament injury). A tourniquet around the proximal thigh may be used for temporary hemostasis if it is placed proximally enough to avoid binding the thigh muscles under the inflated tourniquet. Although some fracture malalignment may be tolerated in Salter I and II injuries with subsequent remodeling (Fig 23-14), given the high rate of growth disturbance for these fractures, we do not recommend acceptance of clearly displaced fractures, and prefer open reduction in these instances.

How much of a "fracture gap" of a Salter II fracture is acceptable is open to debate. The simple presence of interposed periosteum is not an absolute indication for an open reduction. We know from animal studies that interposed periosteum in a Salter fracture, in the absence of intentional physeal ablation, does not lead to a growth disturbance. In these animals the periosteum was degraded or forced toward the metaphysis with normal growth. Only in animals where the physis was partially ablated did a physeal bar occur (41).

For a Salter-Harris type II separation in the coronal plane, a longitudinal incision opposite the metaphyseal fragment gives direct exposure of any obstacles to reduction and avoids disruption of the periosteal hinge. If the displacement is anterior, the procedure is done with the patient prone. After incision of the deep fascia dissection is continued, extending the plane of injury bluntly by spreading the muscle fibers to expose the end of the metaphysis. Irrigation and careful removal of clotted blood

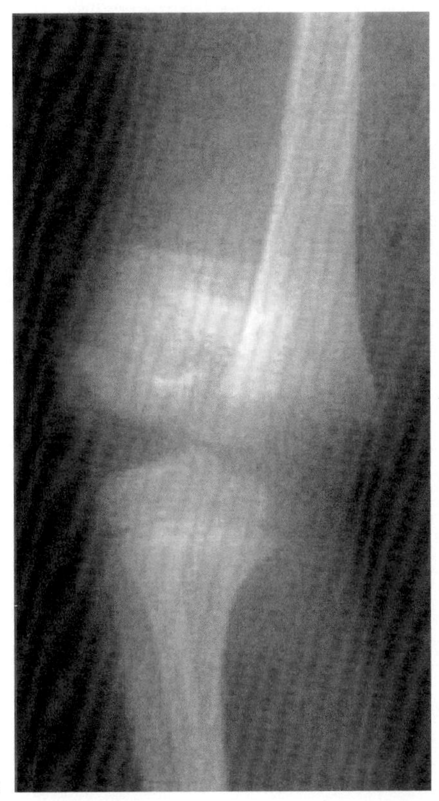
A

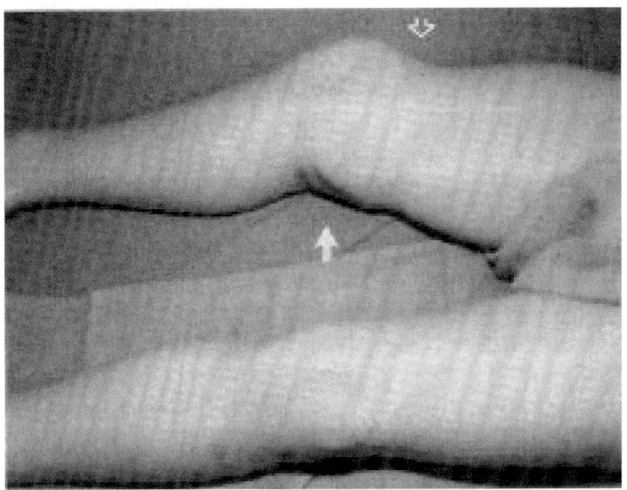
B

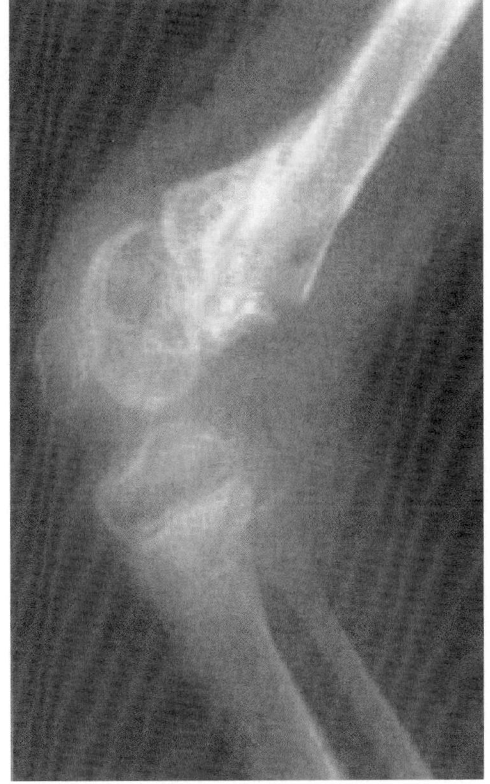
D

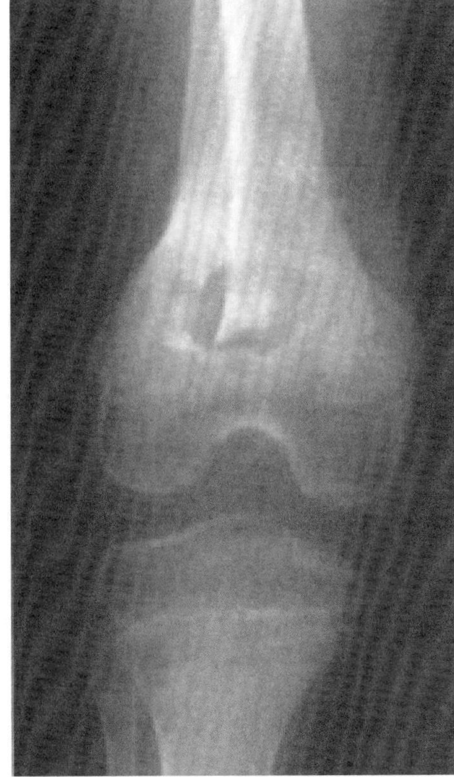
C

FIGURE 23-14 **A.** Completely displaced Salter-Harris type II fracture of the distal femur in a 6-year-old girl whose foot was on the back of the driver's headrest when the automobile in which she was riding was involved in an accident. **B.** Ecchymosis in the popliteal fossa and anterior displacement of the distal femur are evident. Clinical examination revealed absence of peroneal nerve function and a cold, pulseless foot. The fracture was irreducible by closed methods and required open reduction, internal fixation, and repair of a popliteal artery laceration. **C,D.** Incomplete reduction Salter II fracture in a 6-year-old girl with 25 degrees of posterior angulation and abundant callus formation. Further reduction should not be attempted at this point, as further injury to the physis is possible. *(continues)*

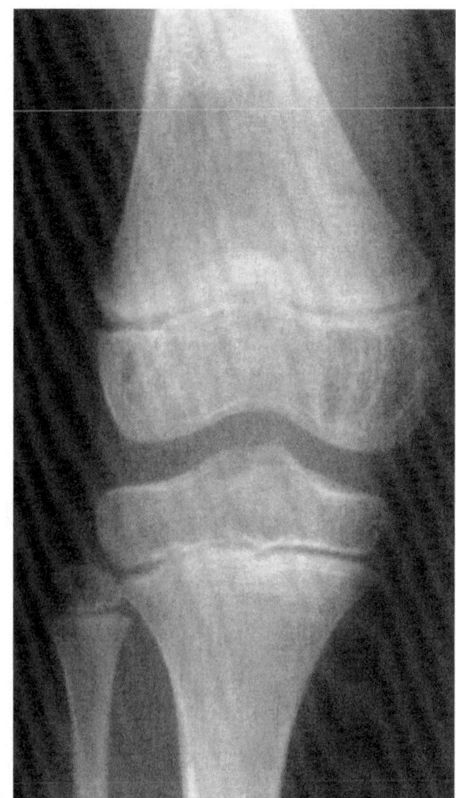

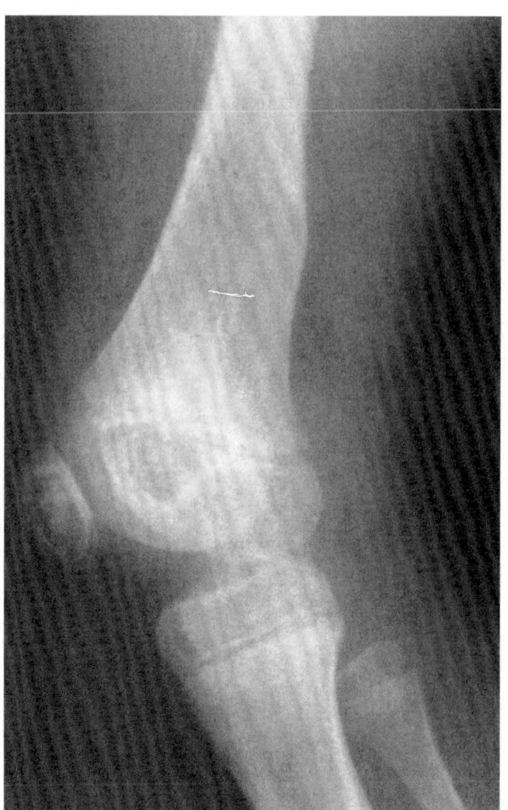

FIGURE 23-14 *(continued)* **E,F.** Four years later remodeling has occurred and no growth disturbance is noted. Results such as this cannot be relied upon, and early anatomic reduction is recommended.

permit better inspection of the separation. An interposed flap of periosteum may be identified between the epiphysis and metaphysis and removed. Special care is taken to avoid any additional damage to the physis. Once the muscle and periosteal flap are removed, reduction is carried out primarily with traction accompanied by gentle realignment. To avoid damage to the physis, instruments should not be placed in the physeal interval. Fixation should be performed as needed. After closure of the wound, a long leg or hip spica cast is applied.

For open reduction and internal fixation of a displaced Salter-Harris type III or IV separation, an anteromedial or anterolateral longitudinal incision is used (Fig. 23-15). In severely comminuted fractures an anterior incision may be used with a total knee replacement in mind for the future. The anterior physeal and articular margins of the fracture are exposed. Reduction is checked by noting the apposition of the articular surfaces, the physeal line anteriorly, and the fracture pattern (Fig. 23-15) and can be confirmed with fluoroscopy. The gastrocnemius has been reported as an obstacle to reduction in a Salter III fracture of the medial femoral epiphysis (42). Provisional stabilization is obtained with Kirschner guide wires. When reduction is accomplished, screws are directed transversely across the epiphysis in Salter-Harris type III separations or across the metaphysis and epiphysis in Salter-Harris type IV injuries (Figs. 23-15 and 23-16) If crossing the physis with fixation is unavoidable, smooth pins or wires should be used. After reduction and fixation are checked by intraoperative x-rays, the knee joint is thoroughly irrigated and inspected for other fractures and ligament disruption. After surgery, the reduction is protected by a long leg or hip spica cast. The use of indomethacin to reduce the incidence of growth disturbance in a rabbit distal femoral fracture model has been reported with equivocal results (43). Recommendation for this treatment in humans is premature.

If an associated collateral ligament injury is found, it can be repaired at the time of open reduction. Internal fixation is used to allow early mobilization and rehabilitation of both the physeal separation and the ligamentous injury.

If vascular repair is indicated, a posterior modified S-shaped incision or posteromedial incision is used to follow the course of the femoral artery. Care should be taken during incision because the vessel may be superficial beneath the skin, particularly in an anteriorly displaced fracture. The hamstring tendons may be "bowstrung" around the femoral metaphysis. The artery may be in spasm, occluded by intimal tear, or torn. After the vascular structures are identified, the fracture is reduced and

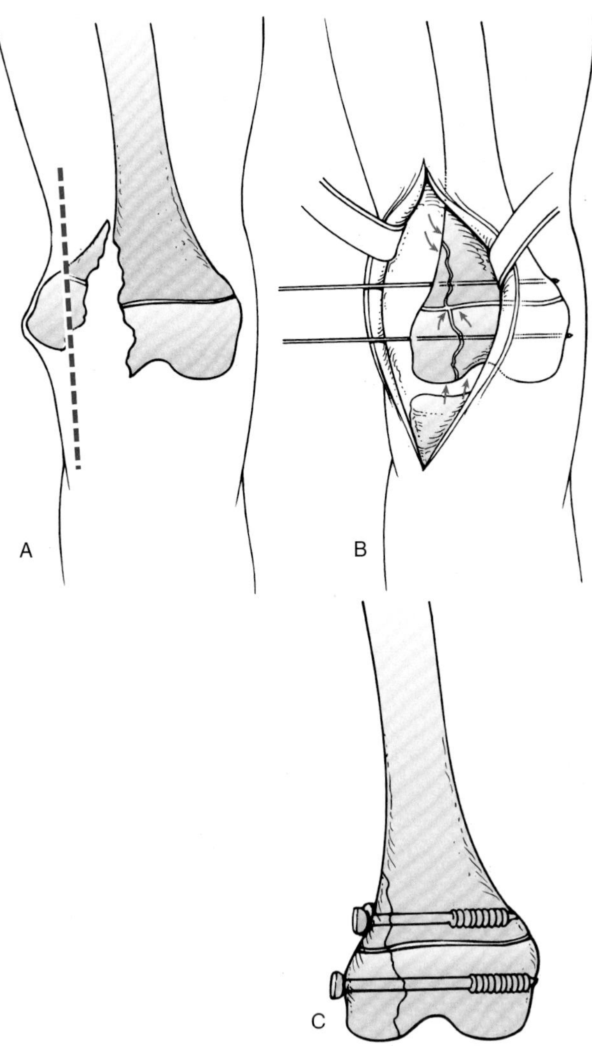

FIGURE 23-15 Open reduction of displaced lateral Salter-Harris type IV fracture of the distal femur. **A.** A longitudinal skin incision, cheating anteriorly if fracture severity raises concern of needing total knee replacement in future. **B.** Alignment of joint and physis are used to judge reduction. Guide wires for cannulated screws placed above and below physis, parallel to physis. **C.** Screws inserted in compression with washer on metaphyseal fragment. Washer optional in epiphyseal fragment if later prominence is of more concern than need for additional compression.

stabilized before vascular repair, except as noted above in the associated injuries section on vascular injury.

Open separations of the distal femoral epiphysis usually are caused by hyperextension, with anterior displacement of the epiphysis. A wound may be present in the popliteal fossa, overlying the posterior protruding end of the metaphysis. The patient is placed prone with the knee slightly flexed and the skin is thoroughly irrigated and debrided. The wound is enlarged to allow inspection of the contents of the popliteal fossa. Muscle or periosteum or both may be interposed in the fracture site. Because the patient is prone, reduction is obtained by bringing the leg up against downward pressure on the distal end of the femoral shaft, while maintaining longitudinal traction. Internal fixation is used to stabilize the fracture, especially if vascular or ligamentous repair is to be done. The knee immobilized in slight flexion with a long leg or hip spica cast.

External Fixation

In cases of significant soft-tissue injuries in which dressing changes or staged surgeries are planned, or in severely comminuted fractures, external fixation may be indicated. Because of the danger of secondary knee joint infection, external fixation is generally not indicated for most distal femoral physeal fractures (44).

Rigid Plate Fixation

Rigid plate fixation across the physis will stop all remaining growth. Thus, this option is reserved only for adolescents near the end of growth and/or children with severe injuries in which severe growth disturbance is believed to be inevitable. Growth remaining for an individual is difficult to predict, and family growth patterns and size should be carefully considered before taking this irreversible step (Table 23-4).

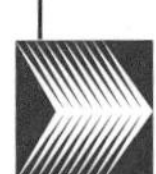

AUTHOR'S PREFERRED TREATMENT

Surgical Procedure

Nondisplaced Fractures. Truly nondisplaced fractures may be placed in a long leg cast for 6 weeks (Fig. 23-8). If there is any concern of fracture displacement, particularly in Salter type III and IV injuries a CT scan is obtained. The cast must be high on the thigh to avoid a large moment arm at the fracture, and short or obese children may require a hip spica cast. Weight-bearing is started in Salter I and II fractures at 2 to 3 weeks if there is no discomfort.

In the rare case of a nondisplaced distal femur fracture that cannot be differentiated from a collateral ligament injury on physical examination or x-rays, I place the patient in a knee immobilizer and reexamine in 10 to 14 days, including x-rays to look for periosteal new bone formation indicative of a healing facture.

Salter I and II Fractures. For displaced Salter I and II fractures, closed reduction and percutaneous fixation is performed under general anesthesia. In Salter I fractures, smooth pins, 2.0 to 3.2 mm in size is used in a cross pin configuration. Pins are bent to prevent migration, and the skin protected by sterile ¼ in. thick felt (Fig. 23-5). We attempt to maximally separate the pins at the fracture site for stability. In thin children, the pins may be brought out of the skin proximally to avoid the possibility of a pin infection leading to a septic knee.

In Salter II fractures, if the metaphyseal fragment is large enough, one or two cannulated cancellous screws are placed under compression using washers (Fig. 23-6). At least two guide

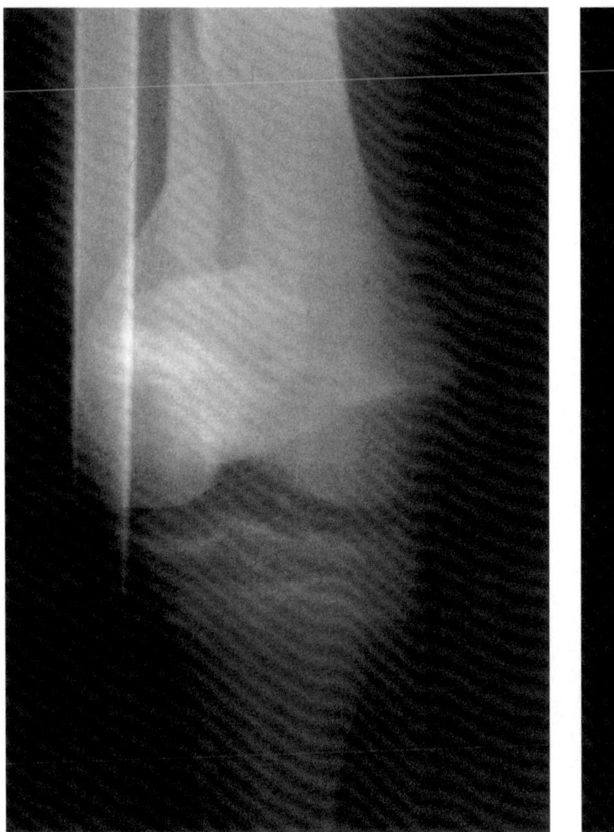

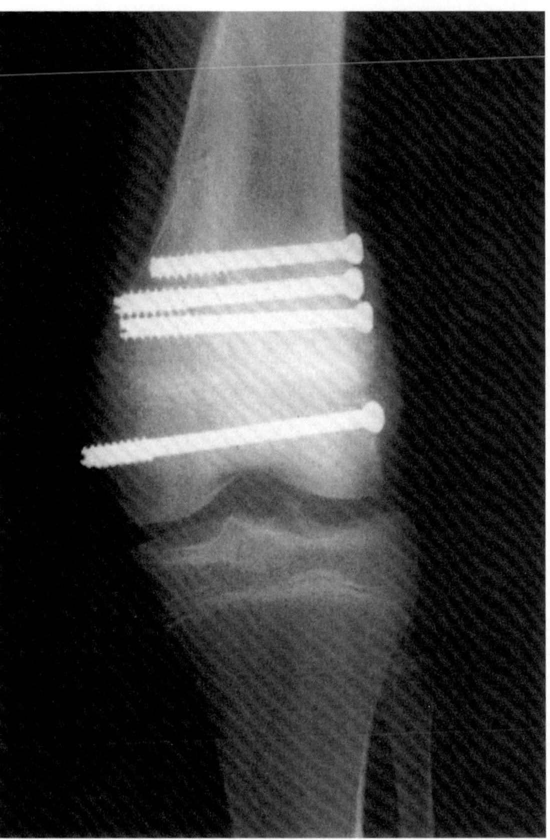

FIGURE 23-16 **A.** Comminuted Salter-Harris type IV fracture of the distal femur in a 14-year-old boy involved in a motor vehicle accident. **B.** Six months after open reduction and internal fixation with cannulated screws in the metaphysis and epiphysis.

TABLE 23-4 Methods of Treatment for Distal Femoral Physeal Fractures

Treatment	Pros	Cons	Indications
Closed reduction and immobilization	Avoids anesthesia	High risk of loss of reduction	Nondisplaced, stable fractures
Closed reduction and screw fixation	Minimal dissection	Only in reducible fractures	Reducible Salter II fractures Nondisplaced Salter III and IV
Closed reduction and smooth pinning	Minimal dissection	Pins may lead to joint infection or require later removal	Reducible Salter I fractures, and Salter II fractures with small metaphyseal fragment
Open reduction and screws and/or pins	Anatomic reduction	Stiffness	Nonreducible Salter I and II fractures, displaced Salter III and IV fractures
External fixation	Allows soft-tissue access	Pin site (joint) infection	Severe soft-tissue injury
Rigid plate crossing physis	Rigid fixation	Stops future growth	Rarely indicated Adolescents near the end of growth Severe injuries with severe growth disturbance inevitable

wires are placed before drilling and tapping to prevent rotation of the fragment. Different sized screws, such as a 7.3 mm screw in the bottom of the metaphyseal fragment and a 4.5 mm screw in the smaller upper portion, may be used. Titanium screws will improve the quality of MRI scans in the future of the growth plate if a physeal bar is suspected, but imaging with steel screws may be effective at visualizing the physis if they are sufficiently far from the physis (Fig. 23-6E).

In children younger than 10 years of age, as much as 20 degrees of posterior angulation is acceptable, but in patients closer to adolescence, we accept only minimal anteroposterior angulation and no more than 5 degrees of varus-valgus angulation. As long as alignment is acceptable, we accept a gap of up to 3 to 4 mm.

If the displacement is anterior, we perform the reduction with the patient supine. An assistant holds the thigh with the hip partly flexed over a bolster. The surgeon grasps the leg from behind the calf with one hand and pulls down in line with the thigh as he or she tries to tip and close the epiphysis against the metaphysis with the other hand. An above-the-knee cast is applied with the knee in 5 degrees to 10 degrees of flexion.

A long leg fiberglass cast is placed with the knee in 5 degrees to 10° of flexion, to allow for assessment of fracture reduction with postoperative imaging.

Salter III and IV Fractures. We prefer open anatomic reduction for all displaced type III and IV fractures to prevent the formation of a bony bar, which causes limb-length discrepancy and angular deformity. Preoperative CT scans are helpful in the diagnosis and preoperative planning for these fractures, and may identify unrecognized comminution that will influence fixation. In the truly nondisplaced type III fracture, percutaneous screw fixation is adequate. An anteromedial or anterolateral approach is performed based upon the location of the fracture. The fracture line, the physis, and the joint surface are observed to confirm anatomic reduction (Fig. 23-16). Cannulated screws are then inserted with either an open technique or percutaneously with the aid of image intensification, using the above principals (Fig. 23-15). Large osteochondral fragments may be fixed with headless screws (such as Herbert screws) in a subchondral position in the unusual instance where extra-articular fixation is not possible. Titanium screws will improve the quality of MRI scans in the future of the growth plate if a physeal bar is suspected. Every effort is made to achieve rigid fixation to allow early motion in about 6 weeks. A long leg fiberglass cast is placed with the knee in 5 degrees to 10 degrees of flexion.

Open fractures or fractures caused by massive penetrating trauma require meticulous debridement. We try to save and stabilize any viable fragments of epiphysis or articular surface, but totally free fragments are removed. Debridement is repeated as necessary, usually at 24 to 72 hours, and soft-tissue coverage is accomplished as soon as feasible.

Postreduction Care

Ambulation on crutches usually is possible within a few days. In children with percutaneous pins, signs and symptoms of infection should be explained to the parents and assessed at follow-up visits. At 1 week after reduction, the patient returns for x-rays taken through the cast. X-rays may be repeated at 2 and 3 weeks if loss of reduction is a concern (Fig. 23-17). Partial weight-bearing is started at 2 to 3 weeks for Salter I and II fractures. Pins may be removed at 3 to 4 weeks when there is early healing if there is any concern of infection. This may be done through a window in the cast. At 6 to 8 weeks after injury, if x-rays taken out of plaster show adequate healing, the cast is discontinued. Scanograms are often taken shortly following initial fracture care to identify a preexisting leg length discrepancy, because growth disturbances are common complications of the fracture. Many patients who underwent open reduction may benefit from physical therapy to increase range of motion and strength. At 6 months after injury, alignment, leg length, and gait are evaluated with comparative x-rays of the lower extremities. If alignment, leg length, and gait are within normal limits, the patient is dismissed from routine care but is counseled to return for evaluation of growth 12 and 24 months after injury.

Pearls and Pitfalls

- Reduction is 90% traction—10% leverage (Table 23-5).
- For screw fixation, use washers—do not hesitate to use 2 sizes of screws.
- The leg is a long, heavy lever arm. Protect your fixation with a cast that is high enough, or a single leg spica if the thigh is short and/or wide.
- Use fixation for any displaced fracture. Literature is clear that fractures without fixation often lose reduction.

Complications of fractures of the distal femoral epiphysis are listed in Table 23-6.

Complications

Recurrent Displacement

Separation of the distal femoral epiphysis may be quite unstable after reduction (26). In a series of 30 fractures, Thomson et al (16) showed 43% of fractures without internal fixation displaced, whereas no fractures with internal fixation displaced. Graham and Gross reported that 7 of 10 patients treated by closed means lost reduction (36).

The use of fixation in any fracture that requires reduction should minimize the risk of recurrent displacement. It is important to remember that the femur and tibia are a long lever arms with forces that may overcome almost any fixation about the knee (Fig. 23-17) The use of a knee immobilizer, long leg cast, or spica cast for patients with large thighs will further help minimize the risk of recurrent displacement.

Physeal Injury

Distal femoral physeal fractures are associated with high incidences of growth disturbance, resulting in asymmetry of length

(text continues on page 958)

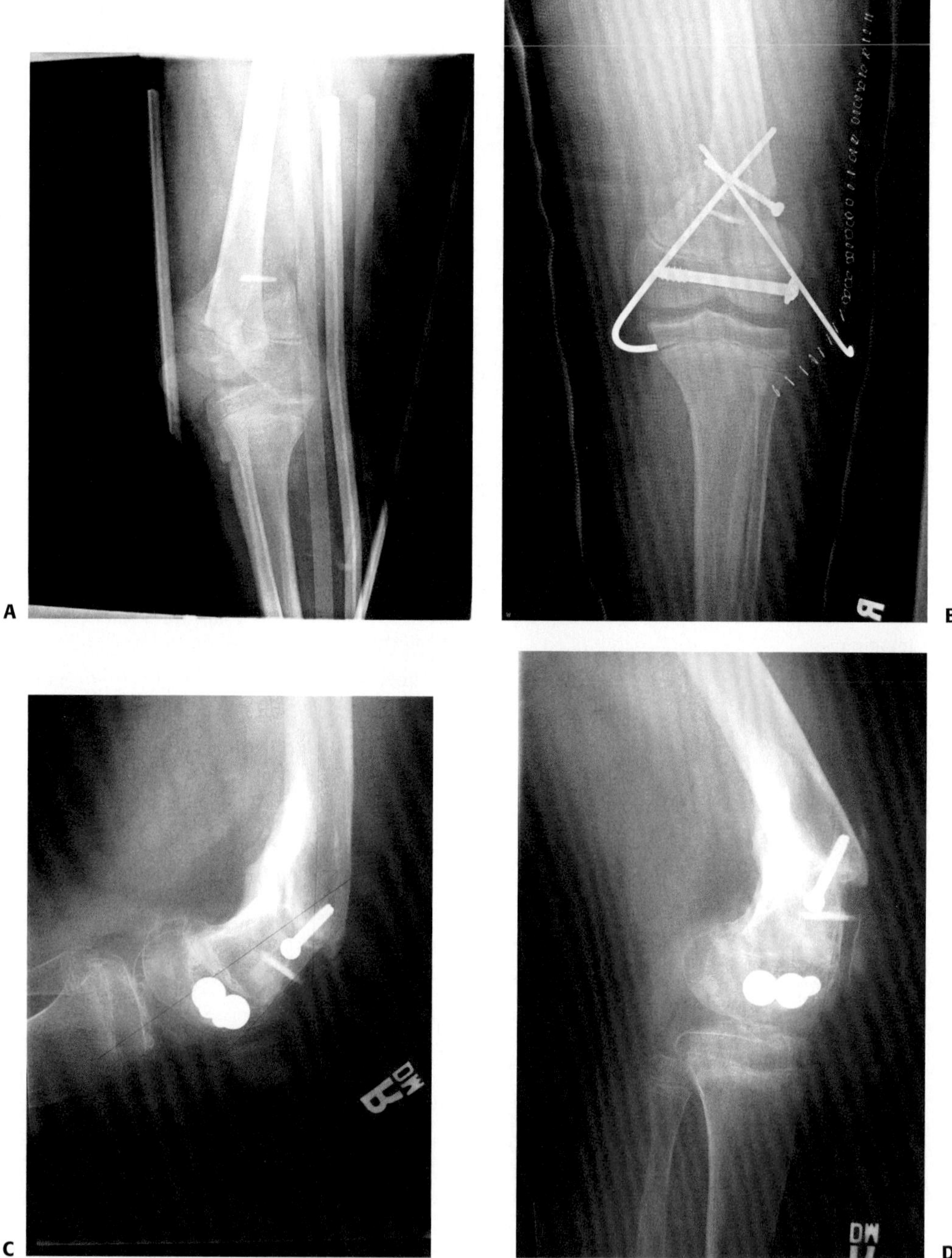

FIGURE 23-17 Thirteen-year-old boy with a "T" type fracture through the distal femoral physis and intercondylar notch. **A.** Preoperative x-rays. **B.** Reduction is not anatomic and fixation is inadequate. **C,D.** After fracture was believed to be healed, and child was being treated with physical therapy for a stiff knee, flexion and extension views reveal motion is through pseudoarthrosis, not through the knee joint. *(continues)*

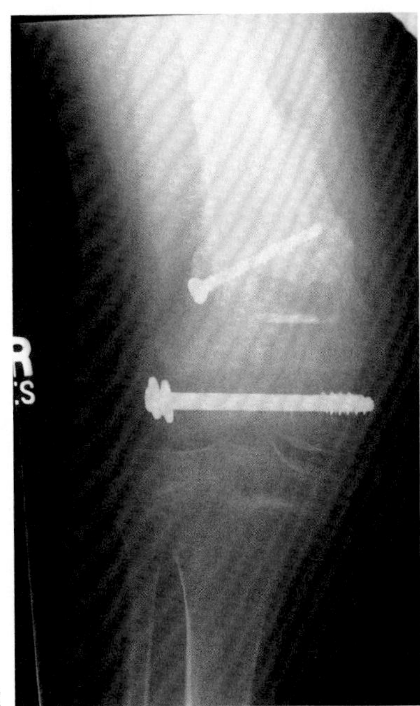

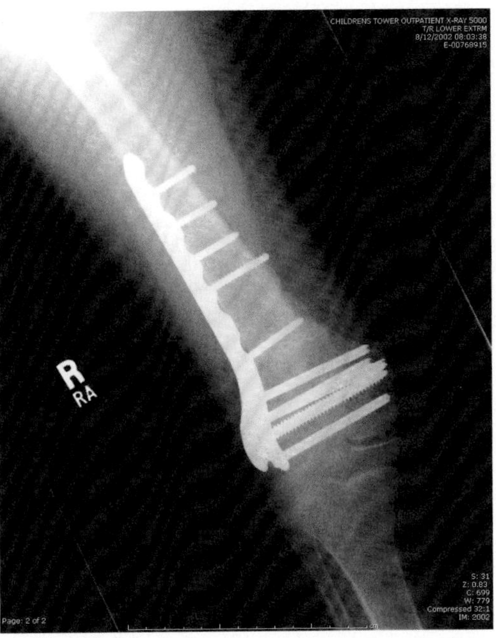

FIGURE 23-17 *(continued)* **E.** AP x-rays of the knee reveal growth plate closure. **F.** Subsequent ORIF with rigid fixation and contralateral epiphysiodesis of the distal femoral physis. Extensive knee release, continuous passive motion, and extensive physical therapy were performed. Two years following surgery the patient has a full range of knee motion and is playing basketball.

TABLE 23-5 Distal Femoral Physeal Fractures: Pitfalls and Prevention

Pitfall	Preventative Strategy
Missed diagnosis	Immobilize and reexamine if uncertain, or MRI Be cognizant of nondisplaced injury in unresponsive or multi-trauma patient
Redisplacement of fracture	High long leg cast or spica cast. X-rays at 1 week follow-up
Growth disturbance	Minimize trauma at reduction Follow-up at 6, 12, and possibly 24 months
Knee joint instability	Check ligaments when fracture stabilized or healed
Septic knee	When possible, avoid percutaneous pins through knee joint. Bury pins under skin, but this requires second procedure for removal. Frequent assessment and parental education on signs and symptoms of infection. Pull pins early, 3 to 6 weeks.
Peroneal nerve injury	Assess at time of injury Avoid excessive varus during reduction

TABLE 23-6 Complications of Fractures of the Distal Femoral Epiphysis

	No. Patients	Ligamentous Laxity	Compartment Syndrome	Angular Deformity	Shortening	Stiffness	Thigh Atrophy	Lost Reduction
Czitrom, 1981	41	0%		41%	14% clinical 68% radiographic	22%		
Riseborough, 1983*	66			25%	56%	23%		
Robert, 1988	41	18%		32%	36%	30%		20%
Thomson, 1995	30	2 associated ACL injuries		18%	47%	18%		20%
Eid, 2002	151	8% symptomatic 14% asymptomatic	1%	51%	38%	29%	28%	

* This series contains many patients referred after known complications so may not represent true incidence of complications in population.

or angulation, or both (4,14,16,17,26,34). Growth disturbance is caused by bony bridging resulting from direct physeal trauma or from lack of anatomic reduction of the physis. Several authors have shown that the likelihood of physeal disturbance is greater with significant (>50% of the width of the physis) initial displacement of the fracture (18,16). The complex contour of the physis makes it possible for shearing of the fracture line to occur across several zones of the physis at a microscopic level, even in fracture patterns that are typically considered to be benign, such as Salter-Harris type I and II injuries.

Physeal injury may be noted about 6 months following fracture healing on plain films taken centered on the physis by narrowing of the physis, or areas of osseous bridging. If Park-Harris growth lines are not parallel, their convergence points the area of growth arrest. The distance to these lines should be greater than the distance of the lines form the adjacent proximal tibial physis, which grows more slowly (34). An absence of Park-Harris lines suggests complete physeal closure as there is no growth. MRI can demonstrate transphyseal bridging or altered arrest lines in physeal fracture before they become manifest on x-rays (45). T2-gradient-recalled echo or proton-density sequences with fat suppression MRI has been recommended as the best MRI technique for diagnosis and follow-up of the growth plate (Fig. 23-18; see also Fig. 23-6) (46,47).

Physeal Injury with Progressive Angulation. Angular deformity following distal femoral physeal injury is reported in 18% to 51% of recent series (4,14,16,26). Progressive angulation after separation of the distal femoral epiphysis is usually caused by asymmetric growth (48) from either trauma to the physis at the initial injury (Salter-Harris type I or II) or physeal offset with bony bar formation after healing (49) (Salter-Harris type III or IV). Occasionally, progressive angulation follows nonphyseal fractures in which an associated Salter-Harris type V physeal injury presumably was not noted (3). The risk of significant angular disturbance is highest in patients with significant growth remaining. If the separation is a Salter-Harris type II

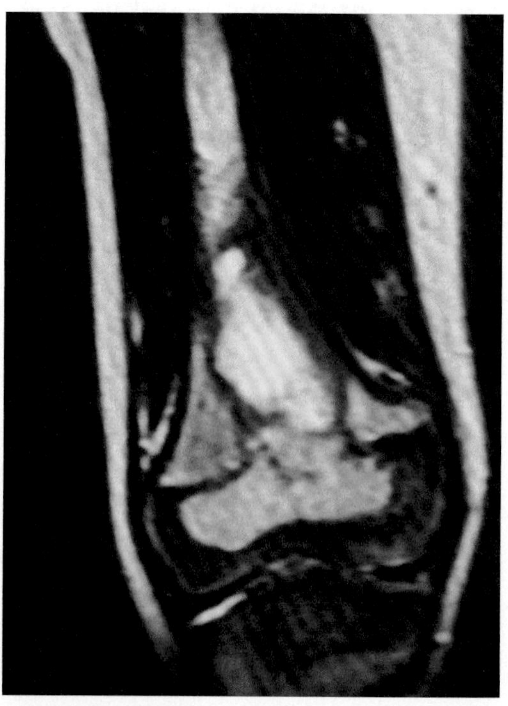

FIGURE 23-18 MRI of the distal femur demonstrating a central physeal bar following a Salter II fracture.

injury, the physis distal to the triangular metaphyseal fragment usually is spared (Fig. 23-6). The localized area of growth inhibition occurs in that portion of the physis not protected by the metaphyseal fragment.

If a localized area of premature arrest constitutes less than 25% to 50% of the total area of the physis and if at least 2 years of growth remain, excision of the bony bridge has been recommended (17,50–52). The bridge can be accurately defined by MRI as discussed above. Helical CT scans have been recommended to create a map of the injured physis (24,53). Kasser recommends that simultaneous corrective osteotomy should be performed when the angular deformity exceeds 20° (50).

The technique of excision is well described by Peterson (48,52). A peripheral bridge can be approached directly. A central bridge is approached through a metaphyseal window. The area of union between the epiphysis and the metaphysis is carefully removed with a curette and power bur. The defect is filled with an interposition material such as fat, cartilage, elastomer, or methylmethacrylate, though the superiority of one over the other is unclear (50). It is critically important to excise the osseous bridge in its entirety, which can be verified by seeing healthy growth plate at all edges of the bar resection. A dental mirror or arthroscope can be useful to visualize the growth plate following resection of a central bar.

Langenskiold reported on a series of 35 patients undergoing boney bridge resection and fat graft interposition, of which 18 were for the distal femur. Five patients required a secondary procedure, and 7 had questionable benefit (52). Hasler and Foster warn that despite a standardized operative technique and appropriate patient selection for physeal bar resection (a bar size less than 50% of the physis, and a prospective growth period greater than 2 years) failure may result. In their series of 22 patients with bar resections with interposition of autologous fat, 14 patients had only fair or poor results. Limited growth because of poor function of the remaining physis and secondary tethers (incomplete resection or recurrence of the bar) may prevent reestablishment of growth or lead to its premature cessation (54). Calcification of the provisional zone of the metaphysis shown by MRI indicates poor viability of the physis and has been associated with failure of bar resection (55).

It has been the author's experience that physeal resection about the distal femur has a high rate of failure, and one should consider epiphysiodesis, and even contralateral epiphysiodesis in older children. Robert suggests surgical epiphysiodesis at the time of fracture treatment in adolescents aged 15 years or over as a reasonable possibility (26).

Hemiepiphysiodesis may be considered in maturing adolescents with progressive varus or valgus angulation associated with a central bony bridge with some remaining growth medially or laterally. Enough growth may remain in the segment of physis between the bony bridge and the perimeter on the same side to correct the deformity. Because of the physeal bar, this procedure is unpredictable and must be followed closely postoperatively to assess for failure. If hemiepiphysiodesis is used to correct angular deformity, timely epiphysiodesis of the opposite limb may be required to prevent significant limb-length discrepancy.

If the patient is approaching skeletal maturity, corrective osteotomy is the preferred treatment. Opening-wedge osteotomy is applicable for correction when the angular deformity is 25° or less and the limb-length discrepancy is, or will be, 25 mm or less at maturity. This technique is described and illustrated by Scheffer and Peterson (56). An osteotomy is made at the supracondylar level, parallel to the articular surface of the condyles. The hinge of the osteotomy should be in metaphyseal bone, which is better able to deform plastically than is cortical bone. Usually no more than 15 degrees of correction can be obtained without cracking the hinge. The distal fragment is then tilted to place the articular surface in horizontal alignment. A triangular fragment of bone graft is inserted in the opening. The graft and correction may be internally fixed and the leg immobilized.

An alternative method of fixation for an opening-wedge osteotomy or for lengthening and angular correction of the distal femur is external fixation. The Ilizarov or similar constructs are useful because the amount of lengthening or angulation can be adjusted postoperatively, and significant angulation and length deformities can be corrected (57).

Physeal Injury with Leg-Length Discrepancy. Progressive leg-length discrepancy may follow a separation of the distal femoral epiphysis if premature arrest of the physis occurs. If the patient is within 2 years of skeletal maturity at the time of injury, the shortening probably will be insignificant. If there are more than 2 years from the time of injury to skeletal maturity, the leg-length discrepancy may progress at a rate of 1 cm (3/8 in.) per year (Fig. 23-17).

Sometimes the growth disturbance is not a discrete bar but a partial physeal slowing. The progression of leg-length discrepancy is best followed by serial examinations. Every 6 months, a scanogram and bone age are obtained and the clinical discrepancy is measured. The leg lengths can be plotted on the Moseley straight-line graph. After three sequential scanograms over a period of 12 to 18 months, discrepancy at skeletal maturity can be estimated by extrapolation according to the rate of growth of each limb.

Although limb length discrepancy is a frequently reported complication of distal femoral physeal fractures (4,14,16,26), in most cases the amount of discrepancy is not clinically significant (39). Management of the limb length discrepancy is well described (58,59).

Stiffness

Limitation of knee motion after separation of the distal femoral epiphysis may be caused by intra-articular adhesions, capsular contracture, or muscular contracture. This should be treated with active and active-assistive range-of-motion exercises. Following prolonged immobilization and osteoporosis, periarticular fractures from overzealous manipulation for knee contracture has been reported (60). Drop-out casts and dynamic braces may be of benefit in recalcitrant cases. For patients with stiff knees in whom conservative treatment has failed, surgical release of contractures and adhesions, followed by continuous passive motion, may regain significant motion (27).

Controversies

Stress X-rays

Stanitski presents a cogent argument against the use of stress views to differentiate between a collateral ligament injury and a physeal fracture of the distal femur. He reports that this test may have been needed in the past, when the treatment of a collateral ligament injury was operative, and the treatment of a nondisplaced physeal fracture was immobilization. Stanitski argues the current initial treatment of both a collateral ligament injury and a nondisplaced femur fracture is immobilization, thus the need for an immediate diagnosis and stress views is no longer valid (61). Another option for early diagnosis is an MRI scan, however the additional use of health care resources may be difficult to justify as it will not have a significant change in the initial treatment.

FRACTURES OF THE PROXIMAL TIBIAL EPIPHYSIS

Principles of Management

In contrast to the distal femoral physis, the proximal tibial physis has intrinsic anatomic stability. On the lateral aspect, the proximal tibial epiphysis is buttressed by the upper end of the fibula. Anteriorly, the tubercle projects down from the epiphysis to overhang the adjacent metaphysis. The superficial portion of the medial collateral ligament (MCL) extends beyond the physis to insert into the upper metaphysis.

Because of this protection, separation of the proximal tibial epiphysis is relatively rare and requires significant force (see Table 23-1). The intimate proximity and tethering of the popliteal artery to the proximal tibia contribute to fairly frequent vascular injury. Mann and Rajmaira (2) reviewed 2,650 long bone fractures in children; 15 (0.6%) were physeal separations of the proximal tibia, mostly in adolescent boys.

Mechanism of Injury

The mechanism of injury is usually due to motor vehicle trauma, jumping, or a lawn mower accident. Hyperextension force is a common mechanism, with the metaphyseal fragment displacing posteriorly. Child abuse has been reported to cause a Salter II fracture (35). Separations of this epiphysis have occurred during passive manipulation of the lower limbs in infants with arthrogryposis (8).

Rarely, a flexion force can cause a Salter II or III fracture (62). This mechanism occurs in adolescents with closure of the physis posteriorly, resulting in genu recurvatum deformity. These fractures represent a transition between tibial tubercle fractures and tibial epiphyseal separations, in comparing the mechanism of injury and fracture anatomy.

Initially unrecognized trauma to the proximal tibial physis and subsequent growth arrest has been associated with lower extremity nonphyseal fractures. Six cases of premature proximal tibial physeal closure secondary to diaphyseal fractures of the tibia in adolescents between 12 and 15 years of age have been described, though only one patient went on to require surgical correction (7). Hresko and Kasser reported on four cases of proximal femur fractures in 10- to 12-year-olds that went on to have 20 degrees to 25 degrees of recurvatum from a proximal tibial growth disturbance (5).

Signs and Symptoms

Physical Examination. A patient with a separation of the proximal tibial epiphysis usually has a knee joint tense with hemarthrosis. Extension is limited because of hamstring spasm. Typically, tenderness is present over the proximal tibial physis 1 to 1.5 cm distal to the joint line.

If the proximal end of the metaphysis is displaced posteriorly, a concavity is seen and felt anteriorly at the level of the tibial tubercle. If the metaphysis is displaced medially, a valgus deformity is present. There may be tenderness or angulation of the proximal fibula as well. If the proximal end of the metaphysis protrudes under the subcutaneous tissues on the medial aspect of the knee, a tear of the distal end of the MCL should be suspected. Vascular status must be carefully documented including distal pulses, and warmth and color of extremity. Compartments should be assessed by palpation and passive and active ankle and toe motion documented in evaluation for compartment syndrome.

Pearls and Pitfalls

Welch and Wynne (63) described a nondisplaced separation of the proximal tibial epiphysis that was initially misdiagnosed as an isolated tear of the MCL because tenderness over the medial aspect of the proximal tibia was interpreted as evidence of an avulsed ligament. Operative exploration showed the distal attachment of the ligament was intact below the level of the physis. Stress x-rays revealed an epiphyseal separation.

Radiographic Findings

Nondisplaced separations may not be visible radiographically. An associated hemarthrosis may be manifested by an increased space between the patella and distal femur on a lateral x-ray. The x-rays are scanned for evidence of fracture lines extending proximally through the epiphysis or distally through the metaphysis. A small bony fragment at the periphery of the metaphysis may be the only clue to the diagnosis. Fracture lines may be visible only on oblique views. Stress x-rays in both coronal and sagittal planes may be helpful, but severe hyperextension of the knee is best avoided because of the possibility of injury to the popliteal vessels. In contrast to the distal femur, initial treatment of a minimally displaced tibial physeal injury usually includes hospital admission for observation and gentle elevation due to the high possibility of vascular damage and/or compartment syndrome. Thus differentiating a proximal tibial physeal fracture from a ligament injury should be attempted at time of presentation, and stress views may be warranted.

Most patients with separations of the proximal tibial epiphysis are adolescents in whom the secondary ossification of the tibial tubercle has appeared. A smooth, horizontal radiolucent line through the base of the tubercle should not be confused with an epiphyseal fracture. It may represent an incomplete fusion of the two secondary ossification centers: the tubercle ossicle and the main portion of the proximal tibial epiphysis.

CT scans may be helpful in determining the treatment of Salter-Harris type III and IV injuries.

Associated Injuries

Ligamentous Injuries. Internal derangement of the knee joint may occur with separation of the proximal tibial epiphysis, and may have been under recognized in earlier series. Concomitant avulsion of the tibial eminence also has been reported in 4 of 10 patients with type III and IV fractures in one series (64).

Vascular Injuries. The most serious injury associated with proximal tibia physeal fracture is vascular compromise. The popliteal artery is tethered by its major branches near the posterior surface of the proximal tibial epiphysis. The posterior tibial branch passes under the arching fibers of the soleus. The anterior tibial artery passes forward through an aperture above the proximal border of the interosseous membrane. A hyperextension injury that results in posterior displacement of the upper end of the metaphysis may stretch and tear the bound popliteal artery (Fig. 23-19).

Routine angiography is not mandatory because ischemia usually resolves with reduction, but motor function, pulses, warmth, and color should be checked frequently during the initial 48 to 72 hours. It is important to remember, that even a fracture that appears minimally displaced at presentation in an emergency department, may have had significantly more displacement at the time of injury, particularly in motor vehicle accidents (Fig. 23-20). Careful attention to evaluating and monitoring the arterial status is particularly warranted in proximal tibial physeal fractures.

Arterial insufficiency may result from either a tear in the popliteal artery at the time of epiphyseal separation or from a compartment syndrome. Delay in recognition results in delay of treatment, which is potentially catastrophic. Arteriography is not mandatory for isolated injuries but may be helpful if the vascular supply is questionable. Fracture fixation should be followed by arterial exploration (posterior or posteromedial approach) and repair or vein grafting. Compartment syndrome is treated by fasciotomy and delayed wound closure or skin grafting.

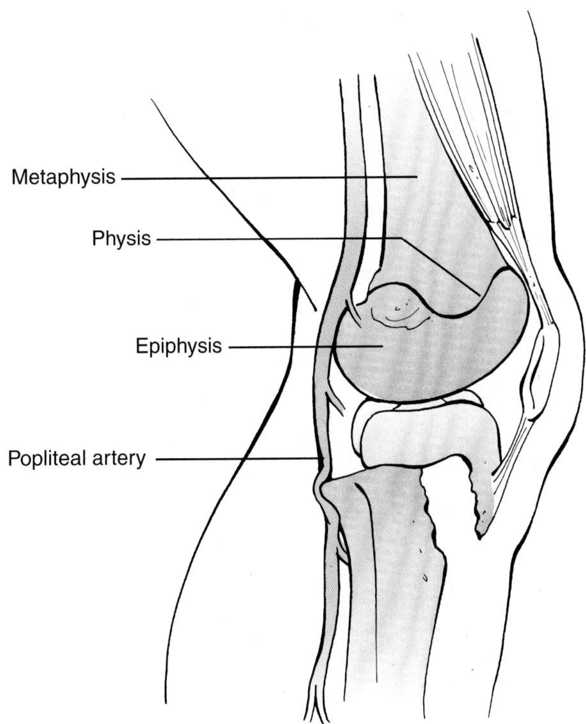

FIGURE 23-19 Posterior displacement of the epiphysis following fracture-separation at the time of injury can cause arterial injury. In addition, a posteriorly displaced fragment can cause persistent arterial occlusion by direct pressure. (Reprinted with permission from Skaggs DL, Flynn JF. Trauma about the Knee, Tibia, and Foot. In Skaggs DL, Flynn JF, eds. *Staying out of Trouble in Pediatric Orthopaedics*. Philadelphia: Lippincott Williams & Wilkins, 2006.)

Classification

Most separations of the proximal tibial epiphysis are Salter-Harris type I and II injuries (Tables 23-7 and 23-8). The frequency of Salter-Harris type III injuries may be skewed by the inclusion of displaced avulsion fractures of the tibial tubercle, and the incidence of Salter-Harris type IV injuries depends on whether open injuries to the knee (i.e., lawn mower) are included, as in the series by Burkhart and Peterson (65).

Fifty percent of Salter-Harris type I separations of the proximal tibia are nondisplaced. Stress x-rays may reveal widening on the medial or posterior aspect. If displaced, the metaphysis is medial or posterior relative to the epiphysis. Presumably, the overhanging tubercle prevents anterior displacement and the fibula prevents lateral displacement of the metaphysis. There may be an associated fracture of the proximal diaphysis of the fibula or a separation of the proximal fibular epiphysis.

Two thirds of Salter-Harris type II fracture–separations of the proximal tibial epiphysis are displaced. Displacement of the tibial metaphysis usually is medial (Fig. 23-21), and the associated metaphyseal fracture usually is lateral, resulting in valgus deformity. The proximal fibula also may be fractured.

Salter-Harris type III separations have a vertical fracture line

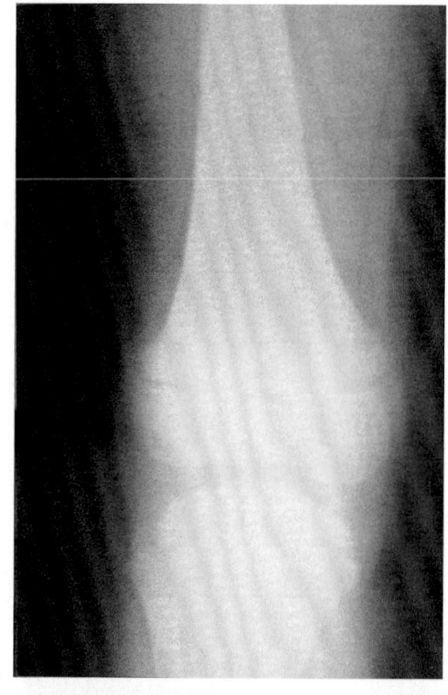

A

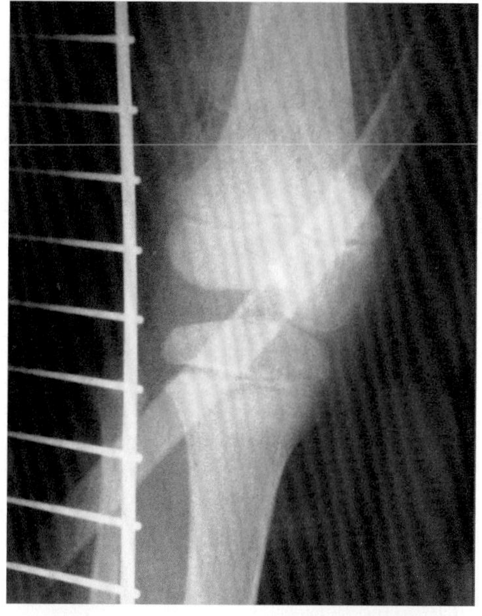

B

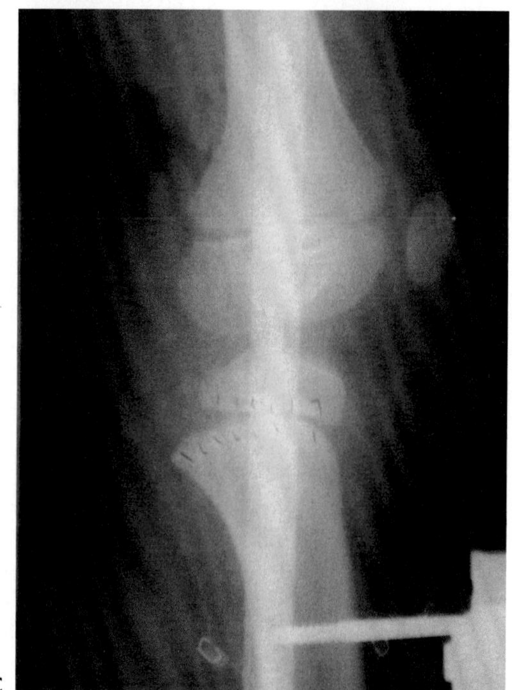

C

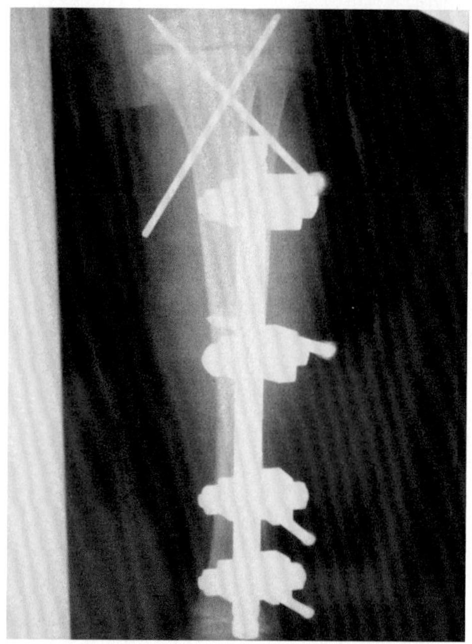

D

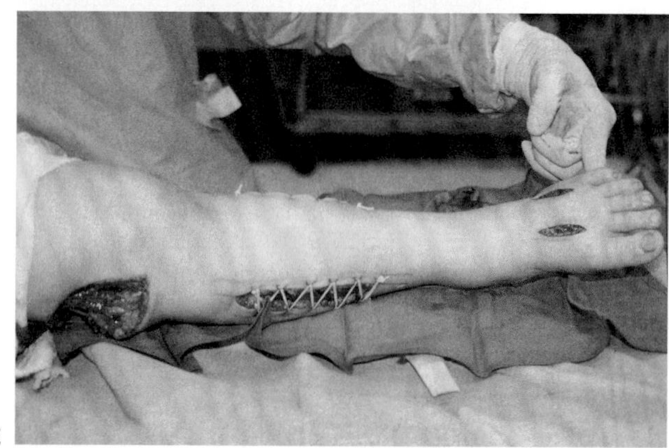

E

FIGURE 23-20 Child on back of bicycle struck by car sustained ipsilateral proximal femoral and tibial shaft fracture. **A,B.** Proximal tibial physeal fracture on initial x-rays were not appreciated. **C.** Following external fixation of the tibial diaphyseal fracture, a Salter-Harris type I fracture of the proximal tibial physeal is evident. **D.** Closed reduction and K-wire fixation were used to treat the proximal tibial physeal fracture. **E.** Compartment syndrome occurred, which is associated with proximal physeal fractures of the tibia. In this case, the contribution of concomitant injuries to the compartment syndrome is difficult to discern. (**A** and **E** reprinted with permission from Skaggs DL, Flynn JF. Trauma about the Knee, Tibia, and Foot. In Skaggs DL, Flynn JF, eds. *Staying out of trouble in pediatric orthopaedics*. Philadelphia: Lippincott Williams & Wilkins, 2006.)

TABLE 23-7 Classifications and Implications of Proximal Tibial Physeal Fractures

Classification	Implications
Mechanism of injury	
I. Hyperextension	Risk of vascular disturbance
II. Varus/valgus	Usually results from jumping; very near maturity
III. Flexion	See tibial tubercle fractures, type IV, in the next section
Salter-Harris pattern	
I	Fifty percent nondisplaced
II	Thirty percent nondisplaced
III	Associated collateral ligament injury possible
IV	Rare
V	Has been reported; diagnosis usually late

through the proximal epiphysis from the articular surface to the physis. There is some confusion in the literature as some series (66) include tibial tubercle avulsion fractures with proximal intra-articular extension as a type III proximal tibial physeal fracture. Most commonly, the lateral epiphysis is fractured, and the MCL frequently is torn. This lateral fragment may require internal fixation, and the MCL may require surgical repair. A coronal split fracture of the proximal tibia epiphysis through a partially closed physis has been described as well (67).

Salter-Harris type IV injuries can involve the medial or lateral tibial plateau. Salter-Harris type V injuries are rare but have been reported in the proximal tibia. Usually, the diagnosis is made in retrospect when progressive angulation or leg-length discrepancy is noted. A type V injury is rare but has been reported (68).

Proximal tibial fractures also can be classified by the direction of deformity (Fig. 23-22). The classic hyperextension type has an apex-posterior angulation and results from forced hyperextension. Varus and valgus types result from abduction or adduction forces. A flexion type injury, in which the fracture line begins along physis underlying the tibial tubercle and extends posterior along the proximal tibial physis may be considered either a proximal tibial physeal fracture, or an extension of a tibial tubercle fracture. In this text these fractures will be considered type IV tibial tubercle fractures as the mechanism of injury (jumping), treatment, and prognosis are closer to tibial tubercle fractures than proximal tibial physeal fracture.

TABLE 23-8 Frequency of Types of Fracture-Separation of the Proximal Tibial Epiphysis

Salter-Harris Classification	Aitken[a]	Burkhart[b]	Shelton[c]	Total
I	—	3	9	12 (15%)
II	9	9	17	35 (43%)
III	2	6[d]	10[d]	18 (22%)
IV	3	8[e]	3	14 (27%)
V	—	2	—	2 (3%)
				81

[a] Aitken AP. Fractures of the proximal tibial epiphyseal cartilage. *Clin Orthop* 1965;41:92–97.
[b] Burkhart SS, Peterson HA. Fractures of the proximal tibial epiphysis: *J Bone Joint Surg Am* 1979;61:996–1002.
[c] Shelton WR, Canale ST. Fractures of the tibia through the proximal tibial epiphyseal cartilage. *J Bone Joint Surg Am* 1979;61:167–173.
[d] Includes avulsion fractures of the tubercle extending up into the proximal tibial epiphysis.
[e] Includes five open injuries from rotary lawn mowers.

Surgical and Applied Anatomy

Bony Anatomy

The ossific nucleus of the proximal tibial epiphysis appears by 2 months of age. It lies in the center of the cartilaginous anlage, somewhat closer to the metaphysis than to the articular surface. Occasionally, the ossification center is double. The secondary center in the tubercle appears between the 9th and 14th years. By the 15th year, the upper epiphysis unites with the tubercle and is almost completely ossified.

The distal surface of the epiphysis is concave to match the convex upper surface of the metaphysis. In the posterolateral corner, the physeal surface is immediately inferior to the upper tibiofibular joint. On the medial side, the physis is proximal to the insertion of the superficial MCL. In the midline anteriorly, the physis dips down underneath the tibial tubercle.

The lateral edge of the physis is separated from the proximal tibiofibular joint by a thin layer of joint capsule. Hemorrhage from a separation may extend into the adjacent joint cavity and through it into the knee joint itself (69). The physis closes slightly earlier posteriorly than anteriorly (70).

Soft-Tissue Anatomy

The synovium and the capsule of the knee joint insert into the proximal tibial epiphysis well above the physis. There is a defect in the capsule where the popliteus tendon runs over the posterolateral corner of the tibia. The capsular ligament anchors the menisci to the tibial epiphysis medially and laterally. The lateral collateral ligament (LCL) of the knee inserts into the fibula (Fig. 23-23). The MCL inserts beyond the physis into the upper metaphysis of the tibia. The patellar ligament inserts, for the most part, into the secondary ossification center of the tubercle, al-

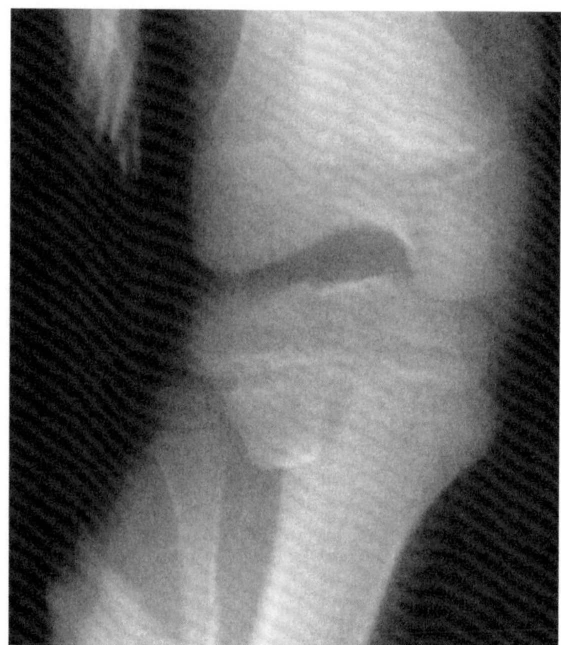

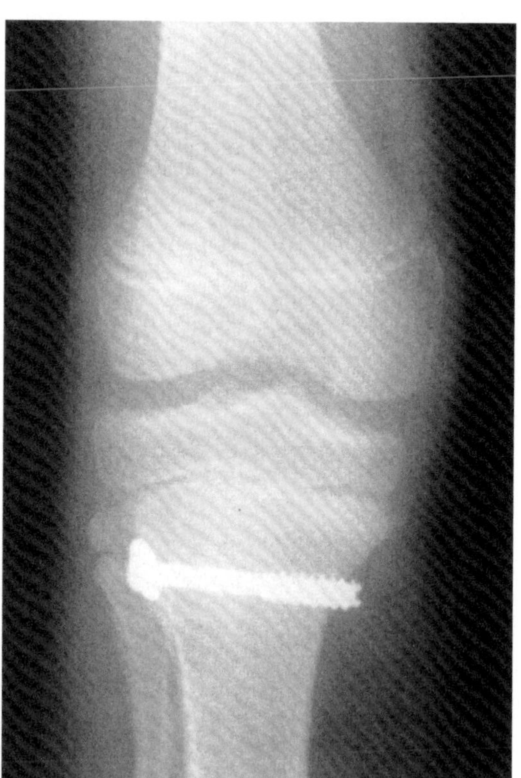

FIGURE 23-21 **A.** Salter-Harris type II separation of the proximal tibial metaphysis, with medial displacement of the proximal tibial metaphysis and complete fracture of the upper third of the fibula. **B.** After reduction and percutaneous fixation with a 4.5-mm cannulated screw.

though some fibers extend beyond the physis into the anterior aspect of the upper tibial diaphysis.

Vascular Anatomy

The distal portion of the popliteal artery lies close to the posterior aspect of the upper tibia. Firm connective tissue septa hold the vessel against the knee capsule. The popliteus muscle intervenes between the artery and bone (Fig. 23-23). The lateral inferior geniculate artery runs across the surface of the popliteus muscle, anterior to the lateral head of the gastrocnemius, and turns forward underneath the LCL. The medial inferior geniculate artery passes along the proximal border of the popliteus muscle, anterior to the medial head of the gastrocnemius, and extends forward along the medial aspect of the upper tibia. Beneath the soleal arch, the popliteal artery divides into the anterior tibial and posterior tibial branches.

The proximal tibial epiphysis derives much of its blood supply from an anastomosis between the geniculate arteries. The diffuse extra-articular blood supply to this epiphysis makes it less vulnerable to ischemia from injury.

Current Treatment Options

Closed Reduction and Immobilization

Type I and II fractures are usually amenable to closed treatment. Traction is important here as in all physeal fractures during reduction. Hyperextension fractures are reduced with traction in combination with flexion.

An abduction fracture with valgus angulation usually can be reduced by adducting the leg on the extended knee. This should be a gentle manipulation to decrease the risk of injury to the peroneal nerve. After reduction, a long leg cast with varus molding is applied with the knee in slight flexion.

Closed Reduction and Fixation

Separations of the proximal tibial epiphysis may be surprisingly unstable. Reducible but unstable type I and II fractures may be held in place with smooth pins inserted percutaneously, crossing distal to the physis to maintain reduction. In type II fractures, compression screws distal to the epiphysis, if the metaphysis is of adequate size, are sufficient (Fig. 23-21).

Open Reduction

Salter II fractures with significant residual deformity following attempted closed reduction require open reduction for removal of soft-tissue interposition. The pes anserinus and periosteum (35,62,71) have both been reported interposed in irreducible Salter II fractures. Open reduction is indicated for displaced Salter-Harris type III and IV injuries. An anterior incision is

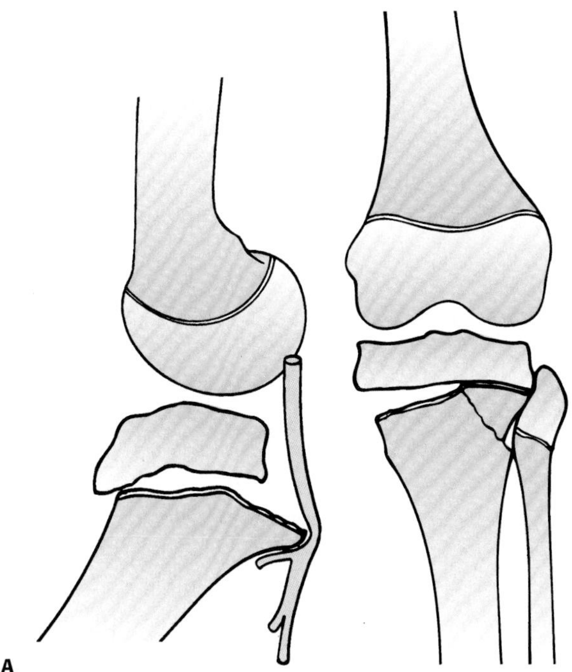

FIGURE 23-22 Classification of proximal tibial physeal fractures by direction of displacement. **A.** Type I: hyperextension type usually caused by direct force. Risk of vascular damage exists. **B.** Type II: varus or valgus type. Vascular injury is uncommon. Reduction may be inhibited by interposition of pes anserinus or periosteum.

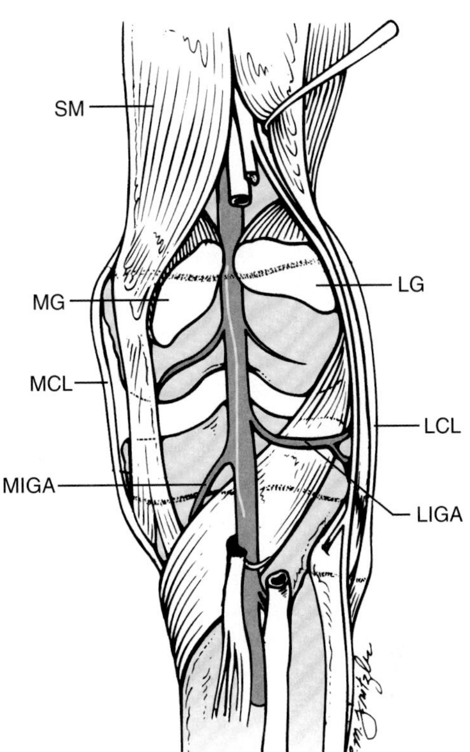

FIGURE 23-23 Posterior anatomy of the right popliteal region. Note that the popliteal vessels are protected from bone (especially the tibia) only by the popliteus muscle. The vessels are tethered by the geniculate branches and by the trifurcation of the popliteal artery into the peroneal, posterior tibial, and anterior tibial arteries. Note that the anterior tibial artery passes anteriorly between the proximal tibia and fibula, thus causing the popliteal artery to press against a posteriorly displaced tibial metaphysis. MG and LG, medial and lateral gastrocnemius heads; SM, semimembranosus; MCL, medial collateral ligament; LCL, lateral collateral ligament; MIGA, medial inferior geniculate artery; LIGA, lateral inferior geniculate artery; ATA, anterior tibial artery.

used to allow inspection of the articular surface. Anatomic reduction is performed, using the joint surface as a guide. A pin may be inserted in the displaced fragment to assist in reduction if needed. Smooth pins or screws are then inserted horizontally across the epiphysis in type III fractures, and possibly across both the epiphysis and metaphysis in type IV fractures. If there is a tear of the meniscus overlying the injured condyle, repair is performed.

Operative fixation of a hyperextension injury may be indicated if an associated popliteal artery injury needs repair. A direct posterior approach to the popliteal fossa may be made followed by fracture stabilization with fixation to prevent avulsion of the vascular repair. Most cases of vascular insufficiency resolve with fracture reduction and do not require vascular repair. Immediate exploration is not indicated for symptoms of peroneal nerve injury. Peroneal neuropathy associated with a separation of the proximal tibial epiphysis usually recovers spontaneously with time.

Timing. Given the high risk of vascular compromise, displaced proximal tibial fractures should be considered for urgent reduction. In an animal model of Salter I fractures of the proximal tibia in rats were reduced immediately or up to 48 hours after injury. Delayed reduction showed no evidence of physeal damage, physeal growth disturbance, or radiographic bar formation (72). Translation of this study to clinical medicine is unclear (Table 23-9).

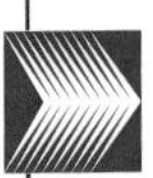

AUTHOR'S PREFERRED TREATMENT

Surgical Procedure

If a proximal tibial epiphyseal facture is nondisplaced, we place the patient in a long leg cast with the knee flexed 20 to 30 degrees. One-half-inch thick foam is placed along the knee and calf and/or the cast is bivalved to permit swelling. In most instances, the child is admitted to the hospital for observation and gentle elevation, given the high incidence of vascular injury. Anteroposterior and lateral x-rays are repeated 1 week after injury to confirm acceptable position. The cast is removed 6 weeks after injury if the fracture is radiographically and clinically healed. Return to normal activities is generally permitted in 3 to 6 weeks following cast removal.

TABLE 23-9 Methods of Treatment for Proximal Tibial Epiphyseal Fractures

	Pros	Cons	Indications
Closed reduction and immobilization	Avoids anesthesia	High risk of loss of reduction. May require significant knee flexion for hyperextension injuries.	Nondisplaced, stable fractures
Closed reduction and smooth pin or screw fixation	Minimal dissection	Intra-articular pins may lead to joint infection or require later removal.	Reducible fractures
Open reduction and screws and/or pins	Anatomic reduction	Stiffness	Nonreducible Salter I and II fractures, displaced Salter III and IV fractures

Before reducing a Salter-Harris type I hyperextension injury, we check for signs of neurologic or circulatory impairment. If there are signs of poor circulation the child is brought urgently to the operating room, or if this is not possible a closed reduction may be performed in the emergency department with sedation. With the patient supine, the fracture is reduced by flexing the hip and knee to 45 degrees while applying longitudinal traction. For all closed reductions the principal of 90% traction and 10% leverage is used. The upper leg is grasped behind the calf. The distal tibia is stabilized in the surgeons axilla, and the proximal metaphysis is pulled gently anteriorly. Reduction is confirmed by fluoroscopy. If the reduction is stable through a gentle range of knee motion, a cast is applied. If the reduction is not stable, percutaneous smooth pin fixation is used, so excessive knee flexion is not needed. With or without internal fixation, a long leg fiberglass cast is applied with ½ in. sterile foam directly on the skin to allow for swelling in 20 to 30 degrees of extension. The child is admitted for observation and slight elevation. X-rays are obtained the next day and 1 week later. The cast is removed 6 weeks after injury if the fracture is radiographically and clinically healed. Return to normal activities is generally permitted in 4 to 8 weeks following cast removal.

For an abduction injury with valgus angulation, under general anesthesia or sedation, we aspirate any significant knee effusion under sterile precautions, and test carefully for a concomitant tear of the MCL or cruciate ligament with fluoroscopy. Valgus angulation is corrected by putting manual longitudinal traction on the leg. The knee is held in almost full extension. With an assistant stabilizing the distal thigh and knee, the valgus angulation is corrected by guiding the leg into adduction. Traction is not released until reduction is accomplished. If imaging confirms reduction, the extremity is immobilized in a long leg cast as previously described, molded into varus, with the knee flexed 15 to 20 degrees. Neurovascular status is checked before and after reduction.

For flexion injuries, reduction usually is obtained by applying longitudinal traction with the knee in full extension. An extension cast is worn for 4 to 6 weeks. If a Salter-Harris type I or II fracture is unstable after reduction, percutaneous crossed smooth pins are used for fixation, preferably exiting the skin distally to prevent pin tract infections becoming intra-articular. The cast is removed 6 weeks after injury if the fracture is radiographically and clinically healed, and pins may be removed as early as 3 weeks if needed. Return to normal activities is generally permitted in 4 to 8 weeks following cast removal.

For nondisplaced Salter-Harris type III separations, a long leg cast is worn for 6 to 8 weeks. If displacement exceeds 2 mm, we perform closed or open reduction and fixation with cannulated screws or smooth pins. A smooth pin may be inserted into the fragment and used to guide the fragment into position with the help of an image intensifier. After reduction, one or two smooth pins or small cannulated screws are inserted transversely across the epiphysis, taking care not to cross the physis in a young child. After internal fixation has been obtained, the knee is again carefully stressed into valgus to see if the MCL is intact. Similarly, a gentle Lachman's test is done to ensure ACL/tibial spine integrity. An MCL injury should heal with immobilization of the fracture, however an ACL/tibial spine injury may require repair.

A similar technique is used for reduction and fixation of Salter-Harris type IV separations. If closed reduction is not anatomic, we perform an open reduction under direct vision. Screws or pins may stabilize the fracture, in the metaphysis and/or epiphysis, with the fixation parallel to the physis and not crossing the physis. If the fracture is open and the fragment is devitalized (i.e., lawn mower injury), the avascular piece is removed. Depending on the quality of fixation, non–weight-bearing is considered during healing of Salter-Harris type III and IV injuries, but active range-of-motion exercises should be started immediately after removal of the cast.

The patient is followed for 2 years to watch for signs of angular deformity or persistent instability.

Pearls

- Make a concerted effort to look for this fracture (proximal tibial physis) in children with high-force injuries about the knee. It is frequently minimally displaced, and easy to overlook.

Pitfalls

- Unrecognized or late presentation of arterial injury.
  - Even minimally displaced fractures may have arterial injury from displacement at time of injury.
- Compartment syndrome.
- Medial collateral ligament (MCL) injury—as the ligament attaches on the metaphysis, any significant opening of the medial side along the physis suggests the ligament is not in continuity.
- Intra-articular pins leading to a septic joint.
- Unrecognized ACL/tibial spine avulsion with late instability.

Complications

It is notable that a small series published in 2000 of 6 epiphyseal fractures treated with open reduction and internal fixation reported no major complications (Table 23-10) (73).

Loss of Reduction

Separations of the proximal tibial epiphysis are surprisingly unstable, regardless of the Salter-Harris type. It is wise to obtain x-rays 1 week after injury to check reduction. At that point, it still is not too late to remanipulate the extremity if necessary. This complication can usually be avoided by using screw or smooth pin fixation following fracture reduction in the operating room.

Compartment Syndrome

Compartment syndrome may occur following proximal tibial physeal fractures because of mechanical blockage of the vascular structures from a displaced fracture, damage to the popliteal artery, or collateral damage to soft tissues at time of a large force injury. It is important to remember in this injury that even a small posterior displacement of the metaphysis may obstruct popliteal blood flow as the artery is tethered anteriorly against the metaphysis by the anterior tibial artery (Fig. 23-24; see also Figs. 23-20E and 23-23). Burkhart and Peterson (65) reported a patient with vascular occlusion. A 12-year-old hurdler sustained a closed Salter-Harris type III injury that was treated with closed reduction and a long leg cast. Increased pressure in both the anterior and posterior muscle compartments caused narrowing of the terminal branches of the popliteal artery, although arteriography showed that the popliteal artery itself remained patent. Fasciotomies and a sympathectomy failed to save the leg.

Growth Disturbance

Similar to separations of the distal femoral epiphysis, injuries to the proximal tibial epiphysis may cause shortening or angulation from subsequent growth inhibition. This inhibition can occur after all types of Salter-Harris type injuries. The amount of angulation depends on the proximity of the area of growth arrest to the periphery of the physis and the years left for growth after injury. In two recent series 2/6 (74) and 0/6 (73) patients had growth disturbances. In the series with no growth disturbances open reduction and internal fixation was performed in all fractures.

If the area of growth arrest is localized to less than a third of the total area of the physis and at least 2 years of growth remain, resection of the bony bridge may be attempted. Alternatively, epiphysiodesis or stapling of the side of the physis opposite a peripheral bar may stop progression of the deformity (75). Existing deformity at the time of surgery may require proximal tibial osteotomy. If there is significant valgus deformity, an opening-wedge osteotomy to correct valgus deformity and gain

TABLE 23-10 Complications of Proximal Tibial Physeal Fractures*

	Patients	Compartment Syndrome	Arterial Injury	Peroneal Nerve Injury	Angular Growth Disturbance	Leg-Length Discrepancy
Burkhart, 1979	28	1	2	1	7	4
Shelton, 1979	34	1	2	2	9	3
Totals	62	3%	6%	5%	26%	11%

See section on associated injuries for discussion of vascular and nerve injuries.

* Includes 10 cases of tibial tubercle avulsion with intra-articular extension as type III fractures.

From Burkhart SS, Peterson HA. Fractures of the proximal tibial epiphysis. *J Bone Joint Surg Am* 1979;61:996–1002; Shelton WR, Canale ST. Fractures of the tibia through the proximal tibial epiphyseal cartilage. *J Bone Joint Surg Am* 1979;61:167–173.

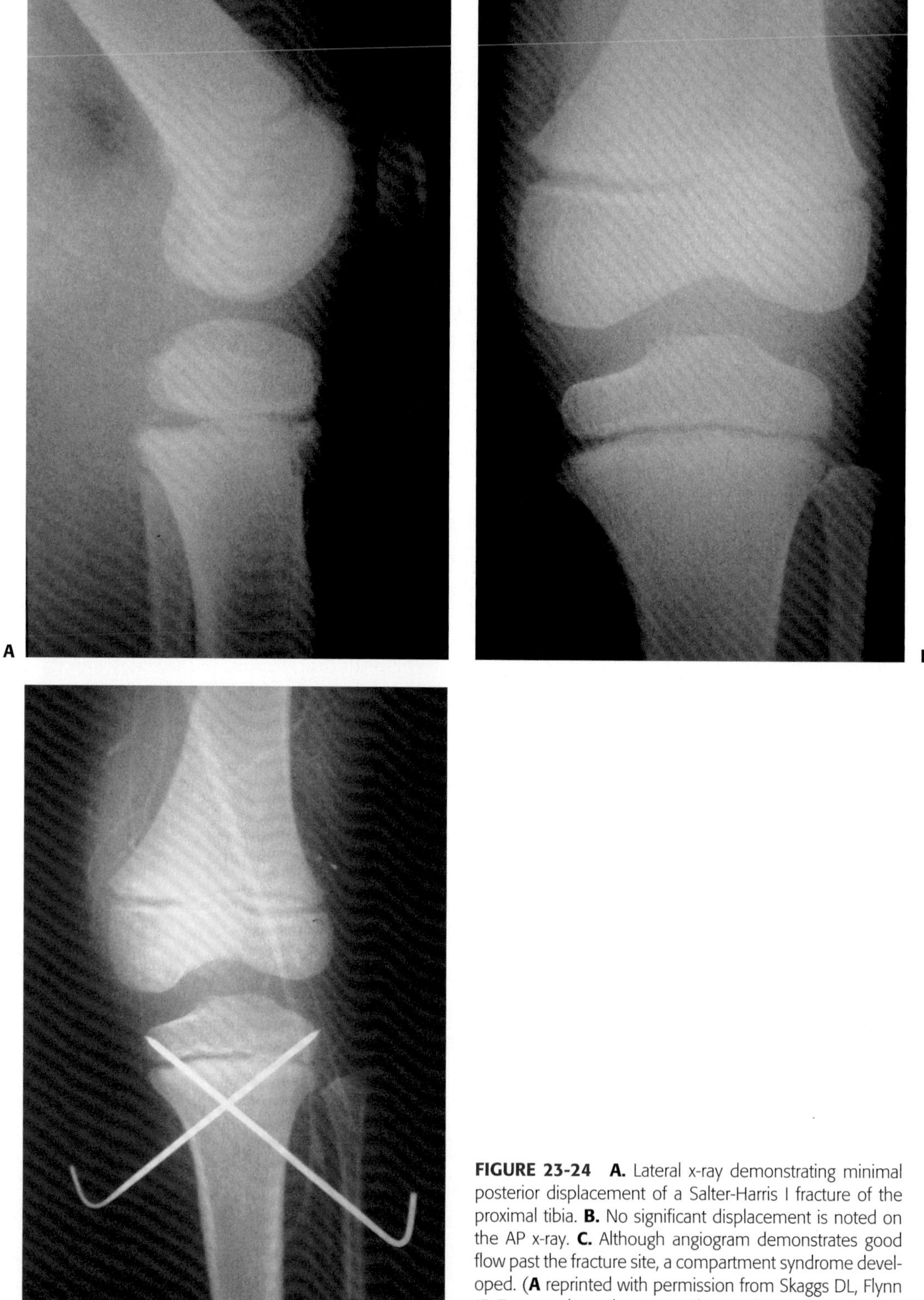

FIGURE 23-24 **A.** Lateral x-ray demonstrating minimal posterior displacement of a Salter-Harris I fracture of the proximal tibia. **B.** No significant displacement is noted on the AP x-ray. **C.** Although angiogram demonstrates good flow past the fracture site, a compartment syndrome developed. (**A** reprinted with permission from Skaggs DL, Flynn JF. Trauma about the Knee, Tibia, and Foot. In Skaggs DL, Flynn JF, eds. *Staying out of trouble in pediatric orthopaedics*. Philadelphia: Lippincott Williams & Wilkins, 2006.)

length may injure the peroneal nerve. Slow correction after corticotomy, with guided lengthening using an external fixator by surgeons familiar with this technique, is an option in patients close to skeletal maturity who have severe angular deformity and a large leg-length discrepancy.

Leg-Length Discrepancy

The proximal tibial physis grows approximately 6 mm per year. If complete growth arrest follows an epiphyseal separation at this level and the patient is within 3 years of the end of growth, an equalization procedure may be unnecessary. If more years of growth remain, epiphysiodesis of the opposite extremity may be considered or leg lengthening at a later stage may be indicated depending on the expected final leg length discrepancy.

Knee Instability/Degenerative Changes

In a series of 10 patients with type III and IV injuries, Paulsen et al reported a mean of 7 years follow-up, that 2 patients had symptomatic instability and another 2 patients had asymptomatic anterior laxity. In the same series, radiographic degenerative changes were noted in 2 patients with varus deformity (64). Bertin and Goble reported 8 cases of ligamentous laxity in 13 patients with proximal tibial physeal fractures, with 5 having anterior laxity and 4 having valgus laxity (13). Most other series do not report on late instability or degenerative changes, and I suspect this may be under reported for type III and IV fractures.

AVULSION OF THE TIBIAL TUBERCLE

Principles of Management

Mechanism of Injury

The majority of acute traumatic avulsions of the tibial tubercle occur in adolescents during jumping sports such as basketball, particularly during eccentric loading while landing (76–78). Tibial tuberosity fractures are reported almost exclusively in males, with only 2 of 89 cases reported to occur in females in 13 series. (76–88). For example, Christie and Dvonch (77) reported 8 injuries that occurred in boys aged 13 to 17 years while playing basketball.

Avulsion of the tibial tubercle occurs when the patellar ligament traction exceeds the combined strength of the physis underlying the tubercle, the surrounding perichondrium, and the adjacent periosteum. There are two mechanisms of injury: violent contraction of the quadriceps muscle against a fixed tibia as occurs in jumping, or acute passive flexion of the knee against the contracted quadriceps. A study of two adolescent gymnasts with tibial tuberosity fractures found extension strength of the contralateral and injured knee was greater than nonathletic controls and their gymnastic peers. The authors hypothesized that the greater-than-usual strength of the quadriceps was able to overcome the strength of the tibial tuberosity (89).

Signs and Symptoms

Swelling and tenderness are centered over the anterior aspect of the proximal tibia. Joint effusion and tense hemarthrosis may be present. A freely movable triangular fragment of bone may be palpated subcutaneously between the proximal tibia and the femoral condyles. This fragment may have rotated so that the distal end projects forward, tenting the overlying skin. A palpable defect on the anterior aspect of the tibia at the upper end of the anterior border of the diaphysis represents the bed from which the fragment was avulsed.

The injured knee may be held in mild flexion by hamstring spasm. The amount of patella alta is proportional to the severity of displacement of the tibial tubercle, and may be up to 10 cm. With a type I avulsion, the patient may actively extend the knee through remaining soft-tissue attachments, although not completely. With type II and III lesions, full extension is impossible.

Radiographic Findings

Because the tubercle lies just lateral to the midline of the tibia, the best profile can be obtained by a lateral projection, with the tibia rotated slightly internally. In this view the size and degree of displacement of the fragment are best seen. In children and adolescents 9 to 17 years of age, the normal tubercle is ossified to varying degrees. One or more secondary ossification centers does not represent an abnormality.

Patella alta is expected with a displaced tibial tuberosity avulsion, with the patella displacing proximally the same distance as the tibial tuberosity is displaced (Fig. 23-25). However, in the "sleeve" fracture avulsion fracture of the tibial tubercle, in which a fracture through bone is not present, patella alta may be an important radiographic finding. Patella alta can be determined by one of several radiographic methods (90–92).

Associated Injuries

Possible associated injuries include patellar and quadriceps avulsions, collateral and cruciate ligament tears, coronary ligament tears, meniscal damage, and a lateral plateau rim fracture (85,93,94).

Diagnosis and Classification

Avulsion fractures of the tibial tuberosity are differentiated from Osgood-Schlatter (OS) disease by anatomic pathology and clinical presentation. OS is a chronic avulsion of the anterior ossicle of the tuberosity with no involvement of the physis (Fig. 23-26) (17). Ogden and Southwick (81) observed new bone formation anterior to the secondary ossification center in OS and concluded that the weak link that failed under tension was the developing ossification center with overlying hyaline cartilage rather than the cartilage at the base of the tubercle apophysis, which is seen in tibial tuberosity avulsion fractures. A prospective study (95) of OS lesions done with serial MRI, CT, and bone scans showed that the most striking feature was soft-tissue inflammation, not bony avulsion. An ossicle was seen anterior to the tibial tubercle in only one third of the patients. There

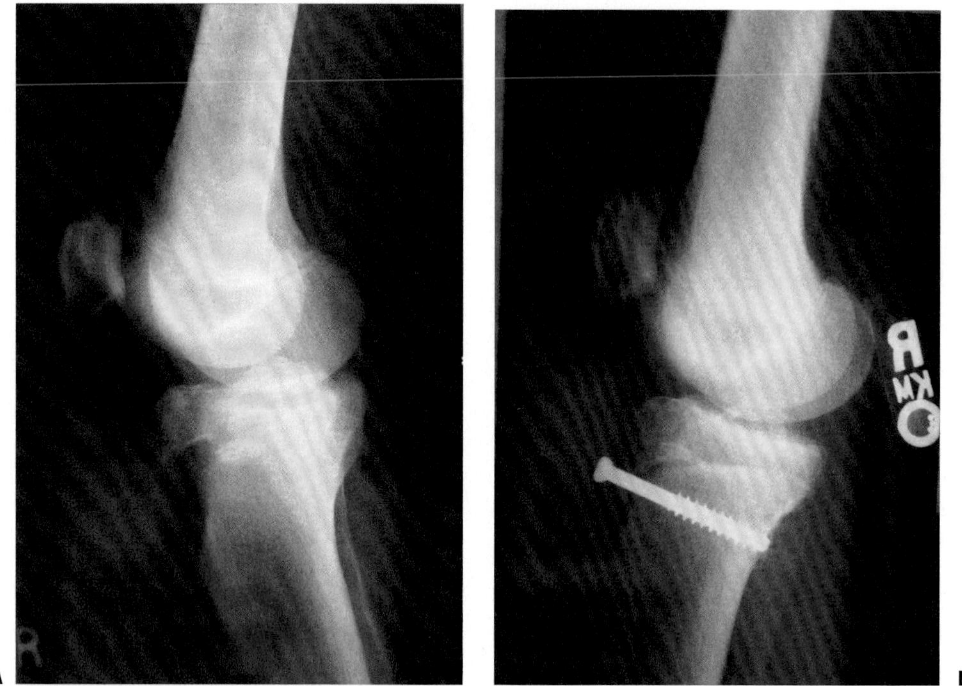

FIGURE 23-25 Type III tibial fracture with intra-articular extension. **A.** Lateral view demonstrates fracture and patella alta. **B.** Fracture was treated with open reduction and internal fixation with one 7.3 mm cannulated screw. Alternatively, multiple smaller screws could have been used.

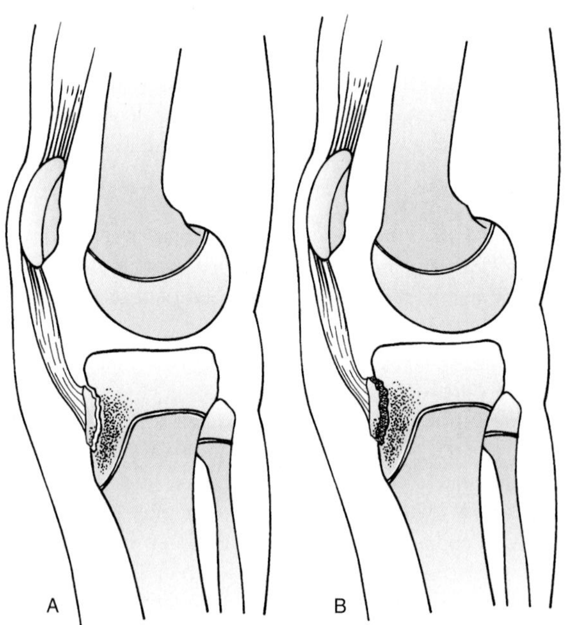

FIGURE 23-26 Development of Osgood-Schlatter lesion. **A.** Avulsion of osteochondral fragment that includes surface cartilage and a portion of the secondary ossification center of the tibial tubercle. This may be clearly differentiated from a tibial tuberosity fracture, which occurs along the apophysial cartilage. **B.** New bone fills in the gap between the avulsed osteochondral fragment and the tibial tubercle.

are clear differences in presentation as well. Avulsion of the tibial tubercle occurs acutely, with a specific injury, whereas the patient with an OS lesion usually presents with a gradual onset of symptoms characteristic of an overuse injury. An adolescent with a displaced acute avulsion of the tibial tubercle is immediately unable to stand or walk, however, an adolescent with OS disease often tries to continue sports and play activities despite discomfort. Although there has been speculation that OS may predispose children to a tibial tuberosity fracture (81), convincing scientific evidence is absent.

Classification. There is some overlap in reporting of tibial tuberosity fractures with extension into the joint, with Salter-Harris type III separations of the anterior tibial epiphysis. For example, Shelton and Canale (66) and Burkhart and Peterson (65) included tubercle avulsions in their reviews of proximal tibial physeal separations. As the mechanism of injury, associated injuries, and treatment of tibial tubercle avulsions with intra-articular extension are more similar to tibial avulsion fractures than proximal epiphyseal Salter fractures, we will consider this type of fracture as tibial tuberosity fractures.

Watson-Jones (96) described three types of avulsion fractures of the tibial tubercle with subsequent modifications by Ogden and associates (81) who noted the degree of displacement depends on the severity of injury to adjacent soft-tissue attachments (Fig. 23-27). Ryu (84) and Inoue (87) proposed a type IV fracture in which the physeal separation occurs through the tibial tuberosity, and extends posteriorly into the horizontal

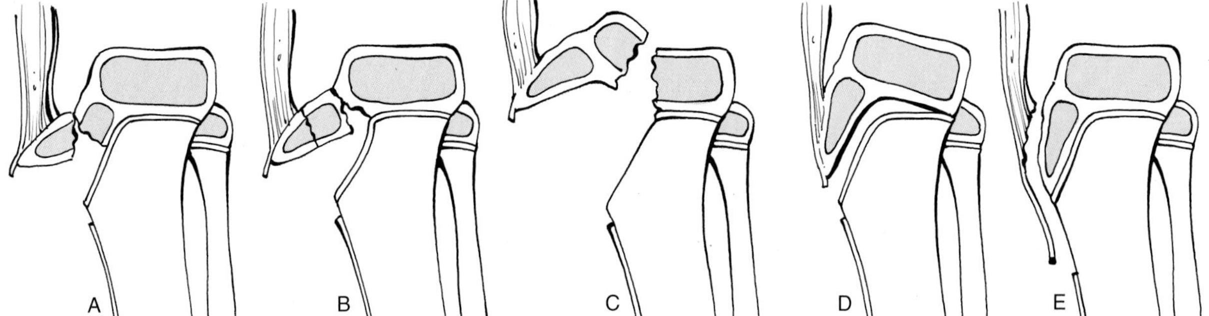

FIGURE 23-27 **A.** Type I—The physeal separation occurs through the tubercle apophysis. The fracture of tubercle is distal to the junction of the ossification centers of the tibial tubercle and the proximal tibial epiphysis. **B.** Type II—The physeal separation occurs through the tubercle apophysis. The fracture extends anteriorly through the area bridging the ossification centers of the tibial tubercle and the proximal tibial epiphysis. **C.** Type III—The physeal separation occurs through the tubercle apophysis. The fracture propagates through the proximal tibial epiphysis into the knee joint under the anterior attachments of the menisci. **D.** Type IV—The physeal separation occurs through the tubercle apophysis and propagates posteriorly through the horizontal proximal tibial epiphysis. The fracture may exit posteriorly through the physis, as a Salter I equivalent, or through the metaphyseal, as a Salter II equivalent. **E.** Type V—Avulsion of a large area of periosteal attachment of the patellar tendon associated with small subchondral fragments of bone. Not a true physeal fracture.

tibial physis. The two reports describe six 15- to 16-year-old boys in which the fracture occurred during jumping. Sleeve avulsion fractures of the tibial tuberosity extending over the anterior metaphyseal area of the tibia have been recently described in 4 children, aged 10 to 15 years (86,97). These injuries are similar to patellar sleeve fractures, in that initial x-rays may show no more than small subchondral fragments of bone. Open reduction and fixation was recommended. I will adopt Davidson and Letts recommendation that this distinct fracture pattern may be added to the Watson-Jones system as a Type V. Fractures may be comminuted or have multiple fracture lines not easily classifiable (Fig. 23-28).

Surgical and Applied Anatomy

Bony Anatomy

In its final adult form, the tibial tubercle is a bony prominence on the anterior aspect of the proximal tibia. It lies approximately one to two fingerbreadths distal to the proximal articular surface of the tibia and forward of the anterior rim of the proximal articular surface.

Ehrenborg (98) divided the postnatal development of the tibial tubercle into four stages. The cartilaginous stage occurs before the secondary ossification center appears and persists in girls until 9 years and in boys until 10 years of age. The apophyseal stage, in which the ossification center appears in the tongue of cartilage, occurs between 8 and 12 years in girls and between 9 and 14 years of age in boys. The epiphyseal stage, in which the secondary ossification centers coalesce to form a tongue of bone continuous with the proximal tibial epiphysis, occurs in girls between 10 and 15 years and in boys between 11 and 17 years of age. In the final bony stage, the epiphyseal line is closed between the fully ossified tuberosity and the tibial metaphysis.

Soft-Tissue Anatomy

The patellar ligament, which lies between the distal pole of the patella and the tibial tubercle, is the terminal portion of the inserting tendon of the powerful quadriceps muscle. During the apophyseal stage of development of the tubercle, the patellar ligament inserts into an area approximately 10 mm long, corresponding to the fibrous cartilage proximal and anterior to the secondary ossification center. The main attachment is in the proximal area of this insertion zone, at the level of the cartilage lying between the secondary ossification centers of the tubercle and the main portion of the proximal tibial epiphysis. The fibrocartilaginous tissue lying anterior to the secondary ossification center receives only the distal part of the insertion. During the epiphyseal stage, the patellar ligament inserts through fibrocartilage on the anterior aspect of the downward-projecting tongue of the proximal tibial epiphysis. The inserting fibers merge distally into deep fascia after spanning the physis. With traumatic avulsion of the tibial tubercle in this stage of development, a broad flap of adjacent periosteum is attached to the displaced fragment. In the final bony stage, the tendon fibers insert directly into bone. After physiologic epiphysiodesis has occurred, the tibial tubercle rarely is avulsed if the patient has normal bone.

Although the patellar ligament represents the main insertion of the quadriceps muscle onto the leg beyond the knee joint, it is reinforced by retinacular fibers radiating from the medial and lateral margins of the patella obliquely down to the respective tibial condyles. After traumatic avulsion of the tibial tuberosity, a limited amount of active extension of the knee still is possible through the retinacular extensions of the extensor mechanism. However, patella alta and an extensor lag are present. The anatomic position of the tibial tubercle is biomechani-

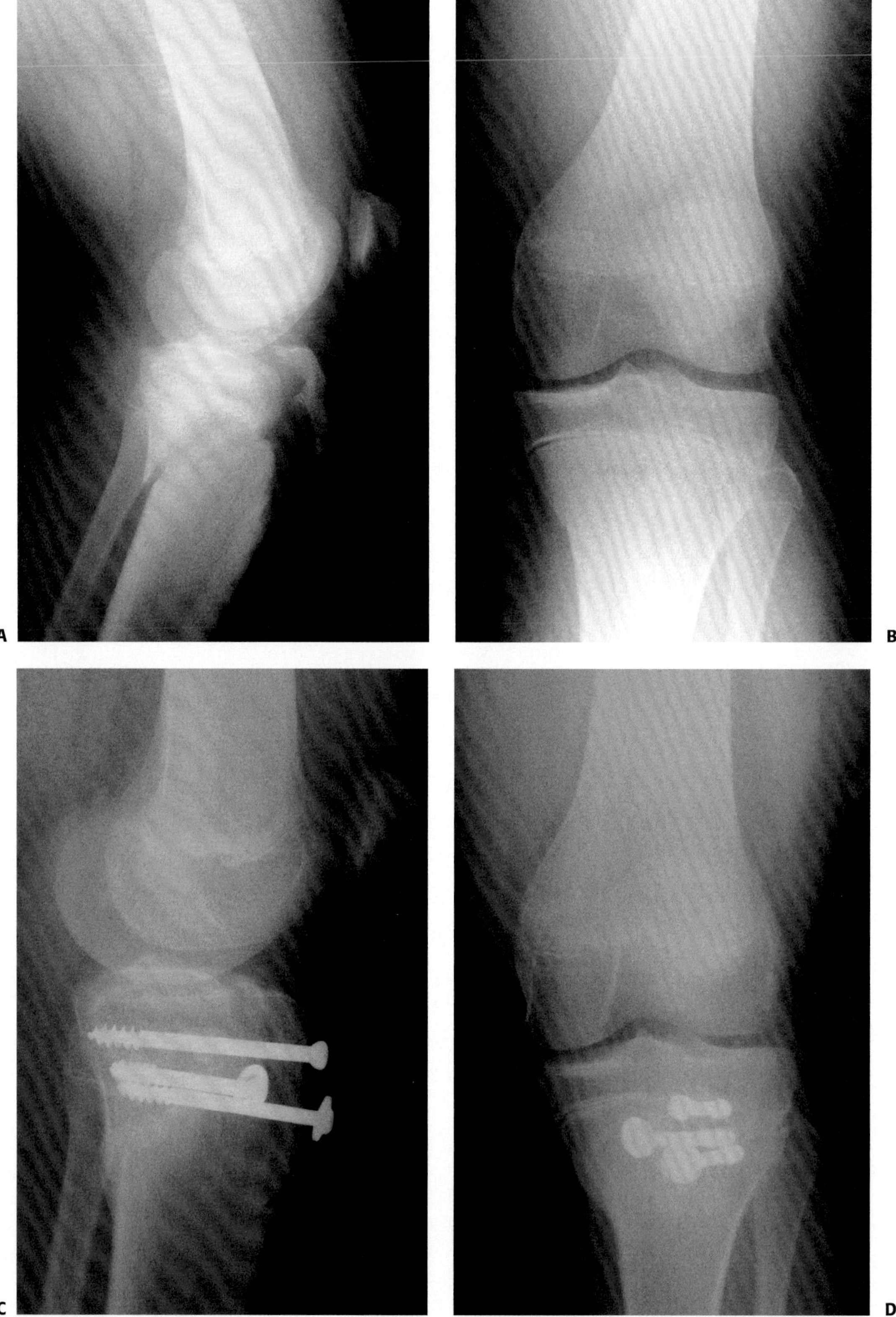

FIGURE 23-28 **A.** Lateral x-ray demonstrating a complex tibial tuberosity fracture extending into the joint, as seen in a type III fracture, as well as posterior along the physis and out the epiphysis. **B.** AP x-ray. **C.** Lateral view 3 months after surgery. **D.** AP view 3 months after surgery. (Courtesy of Robert Kay, MD.)

cally important in terms of patella tracking and patella femoral forces.

Vascular Anatomy

The tibial tubercle receives its main blood supply from an anastomosis behind the quadriceps tendon. In particular, a prominent leash of vessels bilaterally arises from the anterior tibial recurrent artery and may be torn with this fracture (Fig. 23-29) (82,83). Several small branches extend down into the secondary ossification center. A smaller part of the blood supply enters the superficial surface of the tubercle from adjacent periosteal vessels.

Current Treatment Options

Closed Reduction and Immobilization

It is important to remember that the tibial tubercle is an apophysis, with the force of the quadriceps pulling the fracture into more displacement. Minimally displaced, small avulsion fragments have been treated successfully by closed methods. In 1981, Christie and Dvonch (77) reported on two type I fractures and one type II fracture that were successfully treated with closed reduction and casting. The authors recommended an attempt at closed reduction, even in severely displaced fractures, before resorting to open reduction and internal fixation. They caution that persistence of even a small gap between the distal end of the tubercle and the adjacent metaphysis may indicate an interposed flap of periosteum.

The leg is positioned with the knee extended, but even with a long leg cast, a straight leg raise can place tension on the fracture. Molding above the proximal pole of the patella has been suggested to help maintain reduction.

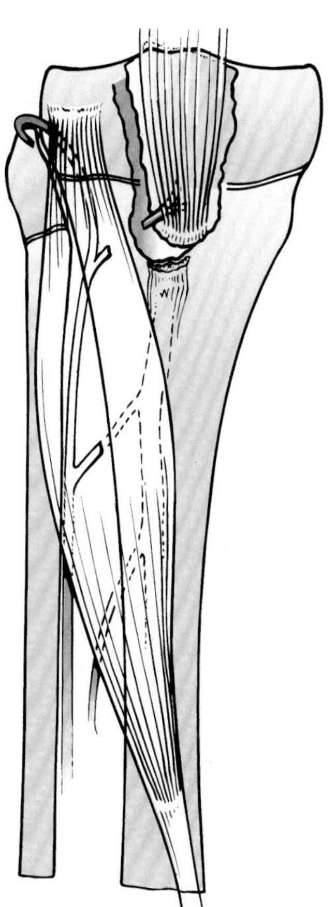

FIGURE 23-29 Probable mechanism of development of compartment syndrome after tibial tubercle avulsion. The anterior tibial recurrent artery, and possibly its branches, is torn and retracts into the anterior compartment musculature.

Operative Treatment

Most series recommend open reduction and internal fixation for all displaced fractures. A midline vertical incision is recommended to facilitate any possible knee surgery in the future. The fracture bed is carefully cleared of debris. A periosteal flap is frequently an impediment to reduction (77,80) which is extracted while the fragment is reduced with the knee extended. Depending on the size of the avulsion fragment and the patient's age, fixation is obtained with transfixing pins or screws and is reinforced by repair of the torn periosteum. A lateral parapatellar incision has been recommended as a more direct approach to this fracture that is less likely to injure the infrapatellar branch of the saphenous nerve (99).

For type III fractures arthroscopic visualized anatomic reduction with restoration of the articular surface has been reported (100). We have concerns over fluid extravasation outside of the knee joint during arthroscopy with this technique.

Davidson and Letts report fixation of the type V sleeve avulsion fracture is challenging because of a lack of a large bony fragment. They recommend fixation with small-diameter screws and heavy nonabsorbable sutures between the intact periosteum or bone and the large avulsed segment of periosteum. Because fixation is largely soft-tissue, protection of the limb in a cylinder cast for about 6 weeks is recommended, followed by gradual rehabilitation (86).

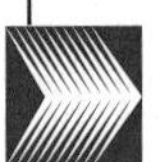

AUTHOR'S PREFERRED TREATMENT

Surgical Procedure

Closed Reduction and Immobilization. Closed treatment is used only if fractures are displaced less than 2 mm and if the knee can be actively extended to 0 degrees. A long leg cast is applied, and straight leg raising discouraged. X-rays are repeated at 1 week to verify reduction. Treatment is 6 to 8 weeks of immobilization followed by at least a month of activity restriction.

Operative Treatment. For open reduction, we prefer a vertical incision just lateral to the tibial tubercle to minimize the potential for scar discomfort over prominent bone. The gap between the displaced fragment and its bed is cleared of any soft-tissue interposition. A tourniquet may be used high on the thigh, but may need to be removed if hindering reduction of displaced fracture by limiting quadriceps motion. If the reduced fragment is large enough, we prefer to use cancellous screws in compression, extending through the tubercle, parallel to the joint into the metaphysis. Fixation across the posterior cortex is not essential, as the cortex is quite thin at this level. If large screw heads are a concern for later discomfort in thin patients, or if bone fragments are small and/or comminuted, multiple 4.5 mm screws are used (Fig. 23-30) instead of a larger 6.5 or 7.3 mm screw (Fig. 23-25B). If the patient is more than 3 years from skeletal maturity, which is uncommon for this fracture, smooth pins are used. A strong, tension-holding suture though the patella tendon, possibly combined with sutures or suture anchors in the proximal tibia may be used if the fracture fragments

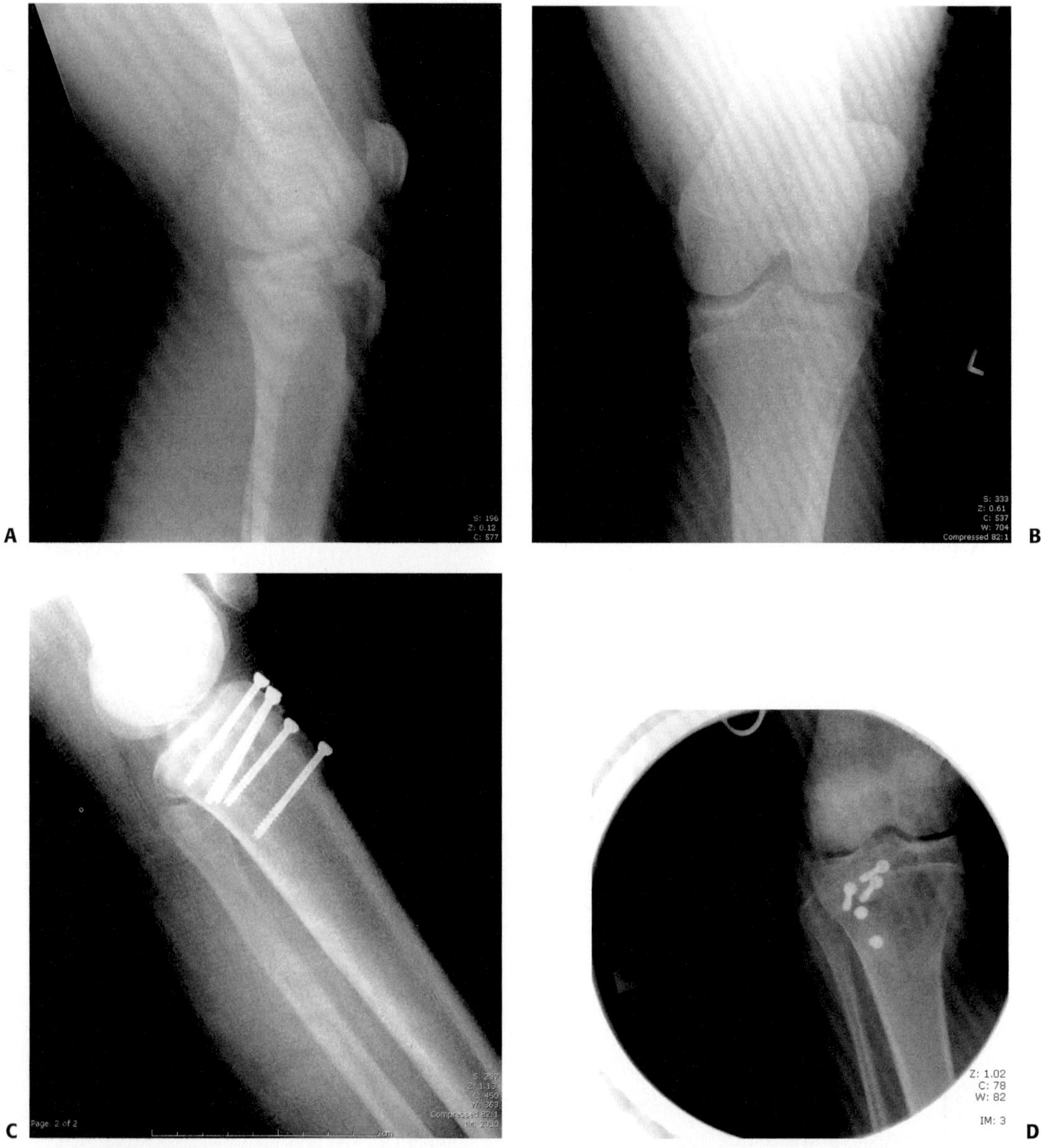

FIGURE 23-30 Type III tibial tuberosity avulsion in a 14-year-old girl sustained while landing after a jump in basketball. This is a very common mechanism of injury. **A.** Lateral view at injury. **B.** AP view at injury. **C.** Lateral view following open reduction and internal fixation with cannulated 4.5 mm screws. Note that screws are in compression with threads not crossing the fracture site. There is no significant growth left in this patient, so screw placement relative to the proximal tibial physis was not of concern. **D.** AP view of fixation. Note that screws are placed perpendicular to the plane of the fracture, which often leads to the screws directed laterally.

are small and the quality of screw fixation is questionable. Sutures also may be used in the periosteum. During an open reduction, release of the anterior compartment fascia is done to prevent compartment syndrome. After wound closure, a long leg or cylinder cast is applied in full knee extension, and the patient is observed in gentle elevation overnight.

With type III fractures, the articular surface is visualized as a guide to fracture reduction, and the menisci should be inspected for tears. For type V fractures I defer to the experience of Davidson and Letts as previously described (86).

Pitfalls

- In minimally displaced fracture, recognition of fracture
- Compartment syndrome
- Missing a sleeve fracture
- Use of tourniquet may bind quadriceps and hinder reduction of displaced fracture

Complications

Of the physeal fractures about the knee, tibial tuberosity fractures appear to have the best prognosis with the fewest complications. Many series report no complications resulting from the fracture other than prominent screws (73,80,87,99). The great majority of patients return to full athletics without residual sequelae (Fig. 23-30) (77,78,80,81,83,99).

Growth Disturbance

Premature closure of the tibial tubercle could lead to genu recurvatum in the growing child. As the great majority of these injuries occur in adolescents near the end of growth, this complication is rarely of concern.

Compartment Syndrome

Compartment syndrome has been reported in seven patients with displaced fractures, presumably because of tearing of anterior tibial recurrent vessels, which fan out at the tubercle but retract into the anterior compartment when torn (Fig. 23-29) (82,82). Close monitoring is necessary for patients treated nonoperatively and careful inspection, possibly with prophylactic anterior fasciotomy, is recommended for patients treated operatively (82,83).

Prominent Screw Heads

Wiss reported 5 of 15 patients with bursitis over prominent screw heads, 4 of whom had 6.5 mm screws. Overall, 8 of the 15 patients underwent screw removal (83). We prefer multiple smaller 4.5 mm screws in most patients to avoid this complication.

Others

Christie and Dvonch (77) reported a patient with persistent loss of 25 degrees of knee flexion 19 months after a type III injury.

TABLE 23-11 Complications of Tibial Tubercle Avulsion Fracture

Common
Screw prominence
Uncommon
Compartment syndrome
Rare
Loss of motion
Refracture
Genu recurvatum

Hand et al (80) reported a patient with persistent quadriceps atrophy. Wiss reported 1 case of refracture of a child who returned to sports 4 weeks after injury (83). Stiffness and extensor lag has been reported resulting from a malunion (85). To this short list could be added the expected complication of patella alta if a displaced tibial tubercle is not reduced adequately (Table 23-11).

FRACTURES OF THE PATELLA

Patellar fractures are much less common in children than in adults, with estimates ranging from 1% to 6% of all patella fractures (101,102). Avulsive patella fractures are more likely to occur in children than adults. Diagnoses of patella fractures in children are prone to delay in diagnosis (103). Primary osseous fractures of the patella in children are treated similarly to adults, with internal fixation of displaced fractures.

Principles of Management

Mechanism of Injury

As in adults, fractures of the patella in children result from a direct blow (most common), sudden contraction of the extensor mechanism, or a combination of both. Direct impact may cause a linear or comminuted fracture pattern.

Avulsion of the distal pole of the patella can occur from tensile loading, usually in the absence of a direct blow (104). Rosenthal and Levine (105) found fragmentation of the distal pole of the patella in seven patients with spastic cerebral palsy involving the lower extremities. They believed that the fragmentation represented stress fractures caused by excessive tension in the muscle associated with a flexed-knee gait. Three of the fragmented patellae healed after hamstring lengthening. Kaye and Freiberger (106) found either elongation or fragmentation of the patella in nearly a third of patients with cerebral palsy and fragmentation of the patella in a patient with arthrogryposis. The patella is vulnerable to osteochondral fracture or avulsion of the medial margin associated with lateral patellar dislocation (107). Patella fracture following ACL repair in an adolescent has been reported (108).

Signs and Symptoms

The injured knee is swollen and tender, often with tense hemarthrosis. Active knee extension is limited and may be painful, and weight-bearing often is impossible. Palpation may reveal a high-riding patella or a palpable defect in the extensor mechanism. If the distal pole is avulsed, voluntary contraction of the quadriceps muscle draws the patella upward, but the patellar ligament remains lax.

With marginal fractures, there may be little more than tenderness and localized swelling over the lateral or medial margin of the patella, and straight-leg raising may be possible. An avulsion fragment adjacent to the medial margin of the patella may indicate that an acute lateral dislocation of the patella has occurred. The patella may have reduced spontaneously after the injury. If dislocation has occurred, the apprehension test is positive. The patient either resists passive manipulation by contracting the quadriceps or may even grasp the examiner's hand to prevent further passive displacement.

Radiographic Findings

Transverse fractures are best seen on lateral x-rays. In a child, the major fragments may tilt away from one another, with the maximal gap anteriorly and minimal gap posteriorly (109). This may signify that the articular cartilage remains intact, even with a complete fracture through the bony portion of the patella (Fig. 23-31). The extent of displacement may not be fully appreciated unless the knee is flexed to 30 degrees when the x-ray is made.

Longitudinally oriented marginal fractures are best seen on axial or skyline views. It is important to differentiate a medial marginal fracture that traverses the entire thickness of the bone from a medial tangential osteochondral fracture. CT scan may help differentiate the two. An osteochondral fracture may include a substantial amount of cartilage not visible on plain x-rays.

Small flecks of bone adjacent to the distal pole may be noteworthy. If the fragment is scale-like and closely approximated to the anterior surface of the patella, it may represent an accessory ossification center. A symptomatic, small, visible radiodensity on the inferior pole of the patella may represent a Sinding-Larsen–Johansson lesion (110). Fragmentation or elongation of the distal pole associated with patella alta in a child with cerebral palsy indicates long-standing extensor mechanism stress.

The radiographic appearance of a sleeve fracture is often not appreciated at first presentation to an emergency room. A barely visible fleck of bone proximal to the patella may be the only radiographic abnormality appreciated in a superior patella sleeve fracture (Fig. 23-32). In an inferior patella sleeve fracture, there may be patella alta in addition to a fleck of bone distal to the patella (Fig. 23-33).

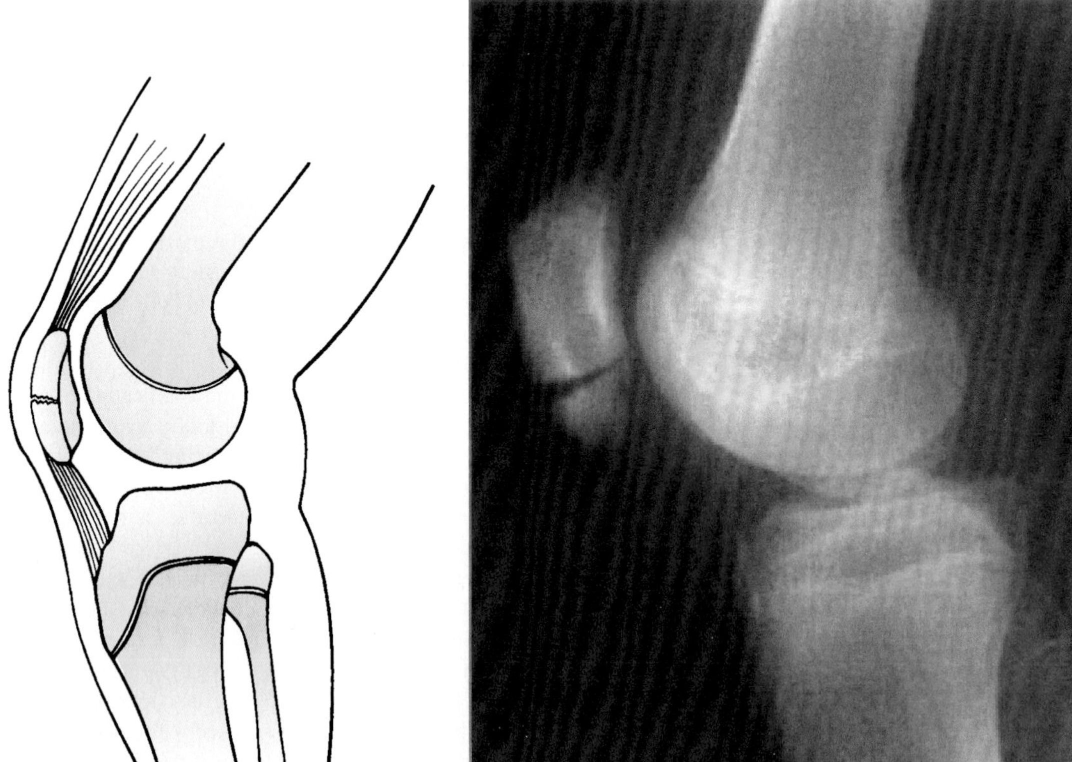

FIGURE 23-31 **A.** Incomplete transverse fracture of the patella. The articular cartilage of the patella remains intact, but the fracture gaps anteriorly. **B.** Lateral x-ray shows incomplete transverse fracture of the patella.

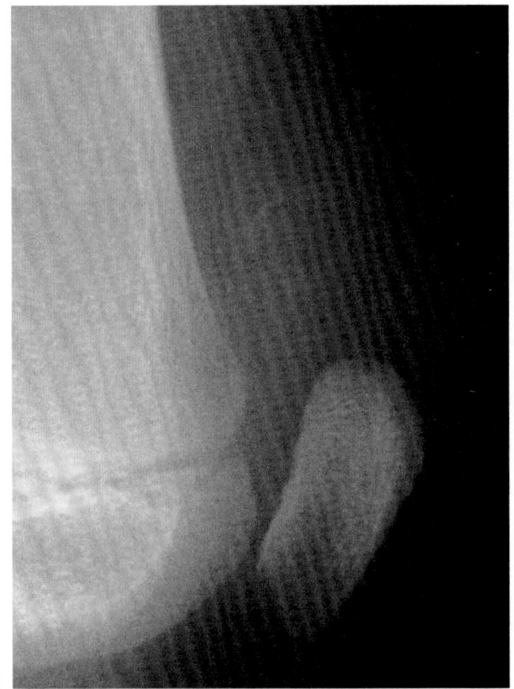
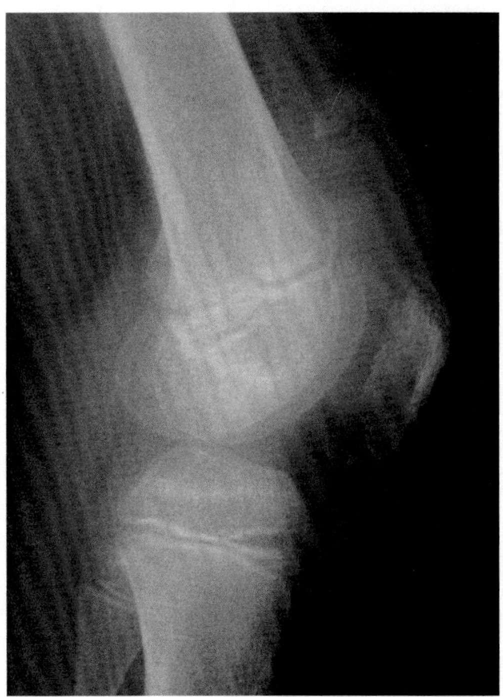

FIGURE 23-32 **A.** Lateral view of a child's knee with a superior patella sleeve fracture. The fracture was initially unrecognized at presentation. **B.** Two weeks later, ossification of the fracture is evident. Open reduction was necessary.

A bipartite patella is best seen on the anteroposterior x-ray, which shows a crescent-shaped radiolucent line in the superolateral quadrant of the patella and rounded margins of the accessory ossicle. If symptoms are confusing, comparison x-rays of the opposite knee may be helpful. A similar radiographic appearance of the contralateral patella supports the diagnosis of bipartite patella.

Associated Injuries

Medial avulsion fractures of the patella may be associated with lateral dislocation of the patella.

Diagnosis and Classification

The greatest difficulty with fractures of the patella in children is diagnosis. Developmental anomalies may be confused with fractures, and the size of fracture fragments, especially in sleeve fractures, may be underestimated in a growing child because the patella is partly cartilaginous (111). Belman and Neviaser (109) pointed out that it is not uncommon for the diagnosis of patellar fracture in a child to be missed or substantially delayed. A high riding patella without evidence of bony fragments suggests a sleeve fracture of the inferior patella, or tibial tubercle (Fig. 23-33). A palpable defect along the extensor mechanism, or inability to actively extend the knee is consistent with a patella fracture.

Classification

Primary Osseous Fractures. Typically transverse, though may be vertical or comminuted. Similar to adult injury patterns.

Avulsion Fractures. Avulsion fractures of bone without a significant portion of articular cartilage deplaced with the fracture fragment should be thought of differently from sleeve fractures. Avulsion fractures of the patella are classified according to location (Fig. 23-34) (104). A superior avulsion involves the superior pole of the patella and appears to be the least common pattern. An inferior avulsion involves the lower pole of the patella and is the most common pattern. An inferior avulsion should be distinguished from a Sinding-Larsen–Johansson lesion (110), an incomplete avulsion caused by repetitive cyclic stress. A medial avulsion involves most of the medial margin of the patella and accompanies acute lateral dislocation of the patella (104). Lateral avulsion fracture usually involves the superolateral margin of the patella and may be difficult to distinguish from a symptomatic bipartite patella (112).

An acute bipartite patella fracture is an uncommon injury. A bone scan can be helpful in confirming the diagnosis and treatment with excision has been recommended (113,114).

Sleeve Fractures. In a patella sleeve fracture there is an avulsion fracture of a small bony fragment from the patella, accompanied by a large portion of articular cartilage (Fig. 23-35) (102,104).

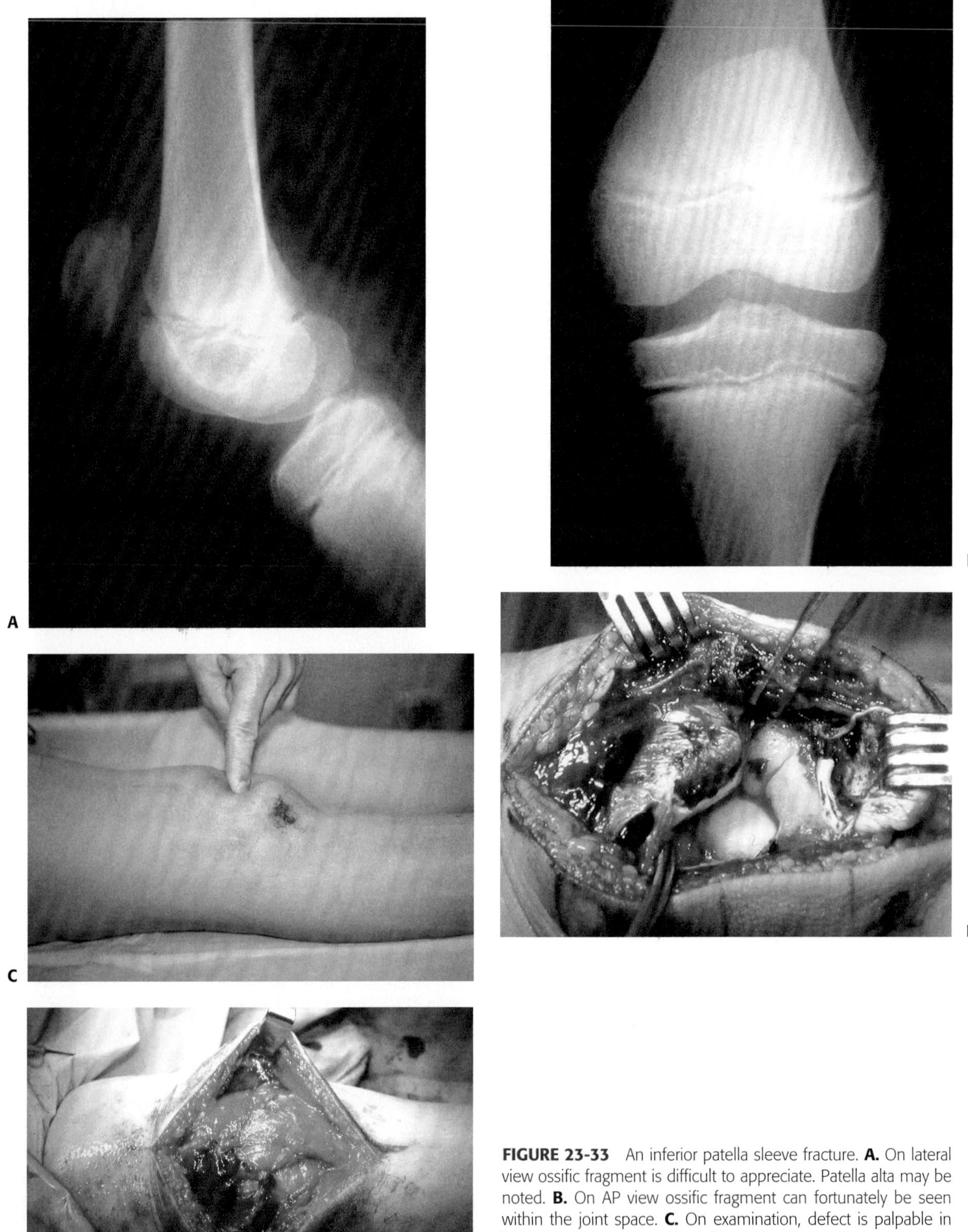

FIGURE 23-33 An inferior patella sleeve fracture. **A.** On lateral view ossific fragment is difficult to appreciate. Patella alta may be noted. **B.** On AP view ossific fragment can fortunately be seen within the joint space. **C.** On examination, defect is palpable in between the patella and patella tendon. **D.** Intraoperative exposure. **E.** Repair of transverse retinacular tears and patella sleeve fracture with sutures. (Courtesy of Robert Kay, MD.)

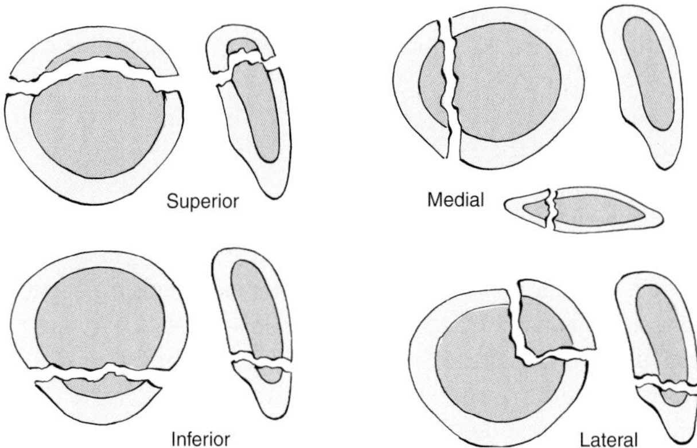

FIGURE 23-34 Patterns of superior, medial, and inferior avulsion fractures and the chronic lateral lesion of a bipartite patella.

A sleeve fracture appears to be reported even more commonly in children than a primarily osseous fracture. This is classified by the location of avulsion, with inferior being more common than superior (104). The distal pole of the patella, together with a sleeve of articular cartilage, periosteum, and retinaculum pulled off the remaining main body of the patella. The extent of injury is often not appreciated on initial x-rays (Fig. 23-32).

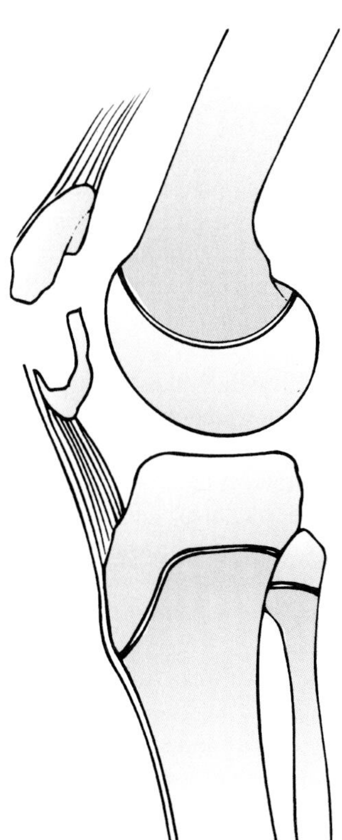

FIGURE 23-35 Sleeve fracture of the patella. A small segment of the distal pole of the patella is avulsed with a relatively large portion of the articular surface.

If allowed to heal without reduction and fixation, this gap may fill in completely or partially with bone and fibrous tissue, with enlargement of the patella. This injury has been reported in children 8 to 12 years of age (111).

Surgical and Applied Anatomy

Bony Anatomy

At birth, the shape is well defined in cartilage form. Ossification of the cartilaginous anlage begins between 3 and 6 years of age. Often there is more than one central ossicle—there may be as many as six irregular centers. Gradually, the ossicles coalesce, and ossification proceeds peripherally until all but the articular surface is replaced by bone. Until ossification is complete, the edges of the enlarging ossific nucleus may appear irregular on an x-ray. The pattern of bony development is similar in this respect to the growing epiphysis of the distal femur (Fig. 23-36). Ossification of the patella usually is complete by the beginning of the second decade.

Congenital absence (115) and congenital hypoplasia (116) of the patella are uncommon. Although these variations in development have been reported as isolated findings, they also occur as part of the hereditary symptom complex onychoosteodysplasia or nail-patella syndrome (115).

An unossified patella may be bipartite or multipartite. The overall incidence of bipartite patella in adolescents is reported

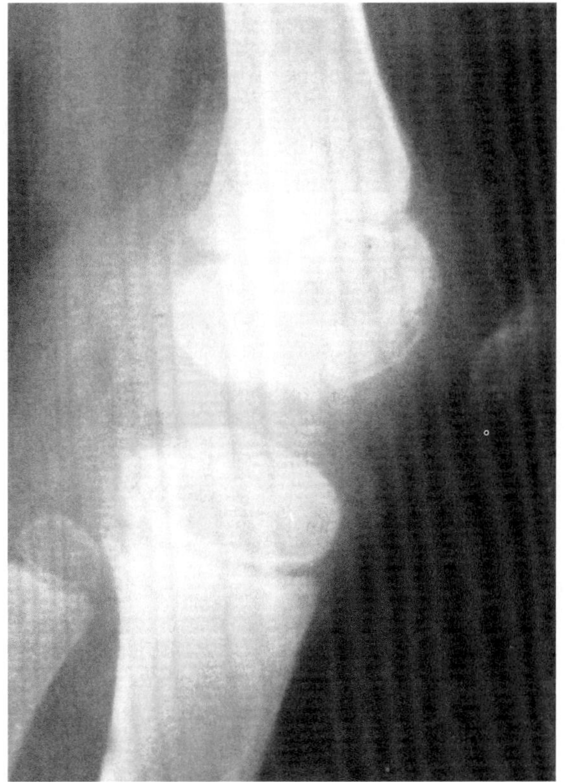

FIGURE 23-36 Normal knee in a 6-year-old child. Note irregular ossification of the patella and the distal femoral condyle.

to range from 0.2% to 6%. It is more common in boys than in girls. Green (117) found that 57% of his patients had unilateral bipartite patella. Partition of the patella into almost equal anterior and posterior portions has been reported in patients, mostly with multiple epiphyseal dysplasia (118).

Vascular Anatomy

Scapinelli (119) studied the blood supply to the human patella in specimens ranging from birth to old age. Because neither he nor Crock (120) noted differences between immature and mature specimens, it is presumed that the pattern of blood supply in children is similar to that in adults. An anastomotic circle surrounds the patella, with contributions from the paired superior and inferior geniculate arteries, as well as the anterior tibial recurrent artery. From the anastomotic ring, branches converge centripetally toward the anterior surface of the patella and enter through foramina in the middle third of this surface. Additional blood supply to the patella enters the distal pole behind the patellar ligament. Thus, virtually the entire blood supply to the patella comes from the anterior surface or distal pole, with essentially no penetration of vessels from the medial, proximal, or lateral margins of the patella. Scapinelli (119) noted that these findings correlate with the fact that marginal fractures of the patella rarely unite. Also, injury to blood vessels entering the anterior aspect of the patella may lead to osteonecrosis of the proximal pole.

Current Treatment Options

Closed treatment is recommended for nondisplaced fractures. Aspiration of a tense hemarthrosis may relieve pain. A cylinder cast in extension is applied, and progressive weight-bearing is permitted. Immobilization may be continued for 6 weeks.

Operative Versus Conservative Treatment

Indications for open treatment of fractures of the patella in children are essentially the same as for fractures of the patella in adults. An inability voluntarily to extend the knee fully indicates an associated tear of the retinaculum. Surgical repair of the retinaculum has been recommended, though I am not aware of evidence for this opinion. Operative is generally indicated for displaced fractures that exhibit 2 to 3 mm or more of articular displacement in a force-bearing area.

Operative Repair. Reduction and internal fixation are preferable to patellectomy, which is rarely indicated in children. Fixation techniques include a circumferential wire loop, nonabsorbable sutures through longitudinally drilled holes, the AO tension-band technique, or screws or pins. An experimental study by Weber et al (121) supported fixation by either modified tension-band wiring or by the Magnusson wiring method. The former consists of a wire loop passed beyond the tips of two longitudinal fixation wires and over the anterior surface of the patella (Fig. 23-37). The Magnusson technique consists of a wire loop passed through longitudinal drill holes in the two apposed fragments. The use of an absorbable suture for the fixation of a patella fracture in a child has been used successfully, which obviates the need for a second operation to remove the fixation material (122). Repair of any adjacent retinacular tear should be performed at the time of fixation of bony fragments.

Grogan et al recommend flexion/extension lateral films should be made in superior and inferior sleeve avulsion fractures to assess intrinsic soft-tissue stability. Widening of the fracture gap usually indicates a need for surgical stabilization (104). Sleeve fractures require careful approximation of the patella to prevent persistent deformity and extensor lag. Modified tension-band wiring around two longitudinal Kirschner wires helps centralize fixation in the small fragment. The extensor retinaculum should be repaired.

For medial marginal fractures, Rorabeck and Bobechko (107) advised excising the osteochondral fragment and repairing the extensor apparatus in acute dislocation of the patella. Griswold (38) suggested that marginal fractures of the patella do best with surgery. He advised excision because fibrous union can cause persistent pain. Peterson and Stener (123) described treatment of concurrent avulsions of the medial and lateral margins of the patella in a 12-year-old boy; a good result was obtained with operative repair.

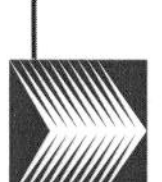

AUTHOR'S PREFERRED TREATMENT

We advise closed treatment if the fracture is not displaced. A cylinder or long leg cast is applied to hold the knee in full extension. Partial weight-bearing is allowed as soon as symptoms permit, usually within the first several days. I am are hesitant to recommend early straight leg raising as this necessarily places a tension force across the extensor mechanism.

A longitudinal midline incision is preferred to facilitate possible future surgery about the knee. The retinaculum on both the medial and lateral sides is repaired meticulously from outward in toward the margins of the patella. For displaced transverse fractures, either tension banding with smooth wires or use of compression screws both work well. I perform open reduction with internal fixation using the modified tension-band technique with a strong suture (such as Fiberwire braided polyblend suture with Kevlar woven into it, size no. 2, Arthrex, Naples, Florida) looped over parallel smooth wires. We have found that steel wire frequently causes irritation and requires further surgery, where strong suture is less irritating and provides sufficient fixation. As knee stiffness is not so much of a concern in children as in adults, immediate motion in not necessary in children, and the repair may be protected by immobilization. If osseous patella fragments are of adequate size, compression screws may be used.

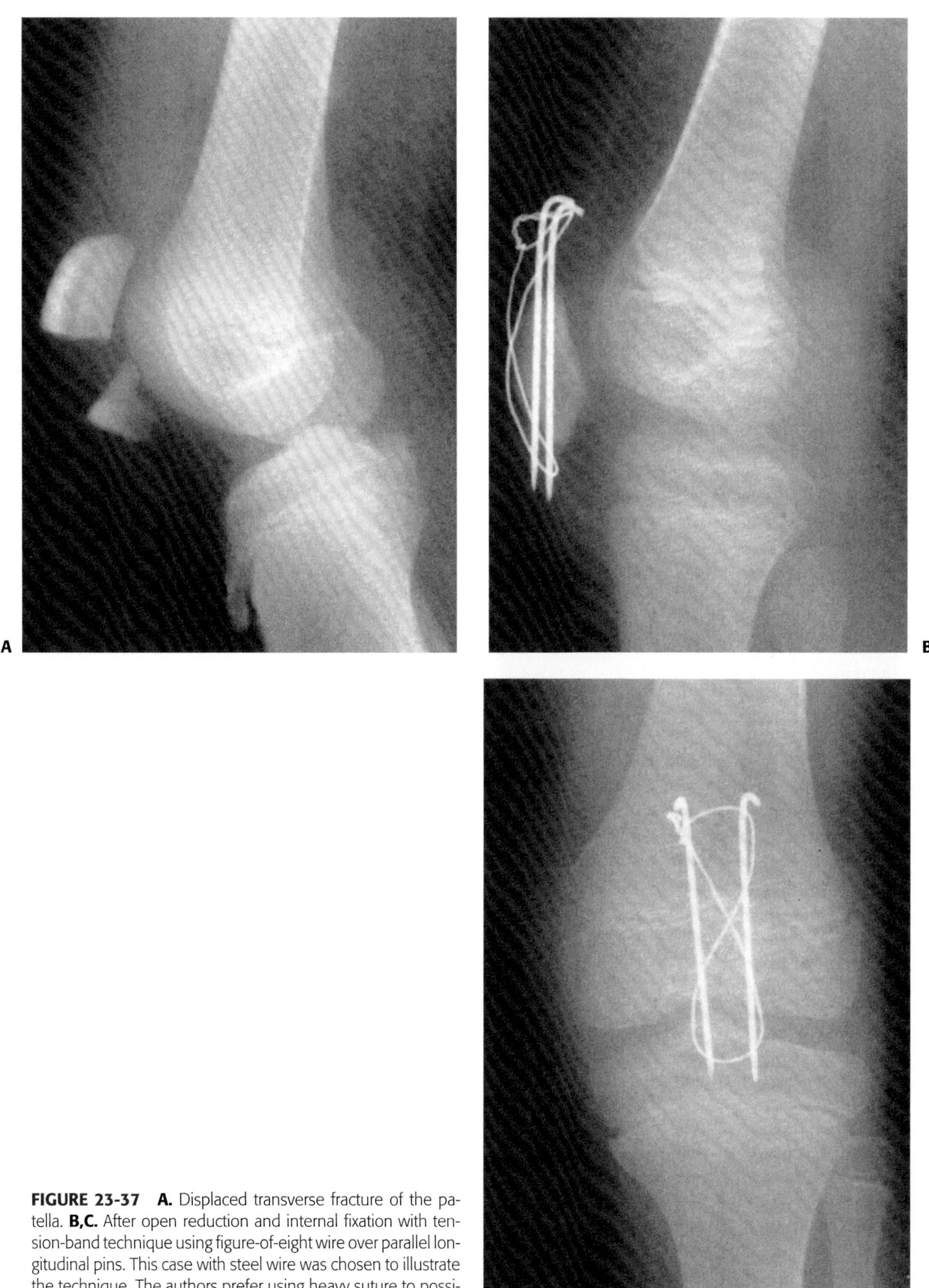

FIGURE 23-37 **A.** Displaced transverse fracture of the patella. **B,C.** After open reduction and internal fixation with tension-band technique using figure-of-eight wire over parallel longitudinal pins. This case with steel wire was chosen to illustrate the technique. The authors prefer using heavy suture to possibly avoid the need for future hardware removal.

We advise excising displaced marginal fractures, whether they are on the medial or lateral margin. The exception is a marginal fracture that includes a significant part of the articular surface. A lesion with articular surface larger than 1 cm should be replaced and fixed by Herbert screws if the screw head may otherwise contact an articular surface. A special case is a nonarticular avulsive patella fracture, not in the superior or inferior pole, less than 5 mm in size, in a child with full active extension of the leg. CT scan may be used to confirm that the fragment is not intra-articular, and that the fragment is not from the lateral femoral condyle in association with a patella dislocation. We treat this fracture with immobilization for 4 to 6 weeks. Later excision can be performed in the unlikely scenario that the patient is symptomatic. Small intra-articular fragments must be removed arthroscopically or via open reduction.

In cases of suspected patella sleeve fractures, if there is obvious displacement, or the patient cannot actively extend the knee, operative repair is indicated. If displacement is questionable, I recommend lateral x-rays of the knee in flexion and extension. If more than 2 to 3 mm of displacement, I proceed with operative exploration and reduction, as there may be significant articular cartilage avulsion not appreciated on plain x-rays. Retinacular repair as described above is performed. If necessary, sutures securing the patella tendon or quadriceps tendon may be passed through drill holes through the patella for fixation.

Postoperative and Postfracture Care

Immobilization in knee extension in a cylinder cast or knee immobilizer (depending on expected patient compliance and strength of repair) is continued for 4 to 6 weeks after either closed treatment or open reduction and internal fixation. After this time, quadriceps-strengthening exercises and range-of-motion exercises are begun.

Pearls and Pitfalls

- When repairing the retinaculum, place all the sutures first without tying them. If the sutures are tied as they are placed, it becomes increasingly difficult to visualize the torn retinaculum and fracture.
- If closing the gap of the extensor mechanism is difficult:
  - Consider letting down the tourniquet, which may be tethering the quadriceps.
  - If the fracture is not acute, quadriceps contraction may have occurred, in which case judicious musculotendinous lengthening of the quadriceps complex may be needed.
- Late recognition of patella sleeve fractures is not uncommon—consider this diagnosis in any patient who does not have full active extension of their knee.

Complications

Complications of unreduced displaced fractures include patella alta, extensor lag, decreased range of motion, patella femoral pain, and quadriceps atrophy. Sleeve fractures in particular if unrecognized, or inadequately reduced and fixed can lead to extensor lag (111,124).

REFERENCES

1. Peterson HA, Madhok R, Benson JT, et al. Physeal fractures: Part 1. Epidemiology in Olmsted County, Minnesota, 1979–1988. *J Pediatr Orthop* 1994;14:423–430.
2. Mann DC, Rajmaira S. Distribution of physeal and nonphyseal fractures in 2,650 long-bone fractures in children aged 0–16 years. *J Pediatr Orthop* 1990;10:713–716.
3. Skak SV. A case of partial physeal closure following compression injury. *Arch Orthop Trauma Surg* 1989;108:185–188.
4. Riseborough EJ, Barrett IR, Shapiro F. Growth disturbances following distal femoral physeal fracture-separations. *J Bone Joint Surg Am* 1983;65:885–893.
5. Hresko MT, Kasser JR. Physeal arrest about the knee associated with non-physeal fractures in the lower extremity. *J Bone Joint Surg Am* 1989;71:698–703.
6. Beals RK. Premature closure of the physis following diaphyseal fractures. *J Pediatr Orthop* 1990;10:717–720.
7. Navascues JA, Gonzalez-Lopez JL, Lopez-Valverde S, et al. Premature physeal closure after tibial diaphyseal fractures in adolescents [see comment]. *J Pediatr Orthop* 2000; 20:193–196.
8. Diamond LS, Alegado R. Perinatal fractures in arthrogryposis multiplex congenita. *J Pediatr Orthop* 1981;1:189–192.
9. Edvardsen P. Physeo-epiphyseal injuries of lower extremities in myelomeningocele. *Acta Orthop Scand* 1972;43:550–557.
10. Rodgers WB, Schwend RM, Jaramillo D, et al. Chronic physeal fractures in myelodysplasia: magnetic resonance analysis, histologic description, treatment, and outcome. *J Pediatr Orthop* 1997;17:615–621.
11. Lim JK, Lee EH, Chhem RK. Physeal injury in a lightning strike survivor. *J Pediatr Orthop* 2001;21:608–612.
12. Trier H. [Epiphysiolysis in the distal femur as a birth injury in Cesarean section]. *Ugeskrift for Laeger* 1992;154:1574–1575.
13. Bertin KC, Goble EM. Ligament injuries associated with physeal fractures about the knee. *Clin Orthop Rel Res* 1983:188–195.
14. Eid AM, Hafez MA. Traumatic injuries of the distal femoral physis. Retrospective study on 151 cases. *Injury* 2002;33:251–255.
15. Brone LA, Wroble RR. Salter-Harris type III fracture of the medial femoral condyle associated with an anterior cruciate ligament tear. Report of three cases and review of the literature. *Am J Sports Med* 1998;26:581–586.
16. Thomson J, Stricker S, Williams M. Fractures of the distal femoral epiphyseal plate. *J Pediatr Orthop* 1995;15:474–478.
17. Beaty JH, Kumar A. Fractures about the knee in children. *J Bone Joint Surg Am* 1994; 76:1870–1880.
18. Lombardo SJ, Harvey JP Jr. Fractures of the distal femoral epiphyses. Factors influencing prognosis: a review of thirty-four cases. *J Bone Joint Surg Am* 1977;59:742–751.
19. Starr AJ, Hunt JL, Reinert CM. Treatment of femur fracture with associated vascular injury. *J Trauma* 1996;40:17–21.
20. Braten M, Helland P, Myhre HO, et al. 11 femoral fractures with vascular injury: good outcome with early vascular repair and internal fixation. *Acta Orthop Scand* 1996;67: 161–164.
21. Stephens DC, Louis E, Louis DS. Traumatic separation of the distal femoral epiphyseal cartilage plate. *J Bone Joint Surg Am* 1974;56:1383–1390.
22. Salter R, Harris W. Injuries involving the epiphyseal plate. *J Bone Joint Surg Am* 1963; 45:587–622.
23. Torg JS, Pavlov H, Morris VB. Salter-Harris type-III fracture of the medial femoral condyle occurring in the adolescent athlete. *J Bone Joint Surg Am* 1981;63:586–591.
24. Loder RT, Swinford AE, Kuhns LR. The use of helical computed tomographic scan to assess bony physeal bridges. *J Pediatr Orthop* 1997;17:356–359.
25. White PG, Mah JY, Friedman L. Magnetic resonance imaging in acute physeal injuries. *Skel Radiol* 1994;23:627–631.
26. Robert M, Moulies D, Longis B, et al. [Traumatic epiphyseal separation of the lower end of the femur]. *Revue Chir Orthop Reparatrice Appar Mot* 1988;74:69–78.
27. Cole PA, Ehrlich MG. Management of the completely stiff pediatric knee. *J Pediatr Orthop* 1997;17:67–73.
28. Ecklund K, Jaramillo D. Patterns of premature physeal arrest: MR imaging of 111 children. *AJR. Am J Roentgenol* 2002;178:967–972.
29. Close BJ, Strouse PJ. MR of physeal fractures of the adolescent knee. *Pediatr Radiol* 2000;30:756–762.
30. Anderson M, Green WT, Messner MB. Growth and predictions of growth in the lower extremities. *J Bone Joint Surg Am* 1963;45:1–14.
31. Wattenbarger JM, Gruber HE, Phieffer LS. Physeal fractures, part I: histologic features of bone, cartilage, and bar formation in a small animal model. *J Pediatr Orthop* 2002; 22:703–709.
32. Netter F. *The Ciba collection of medical illustrations*, vol. 8, part 1. Summit, New Jersey: Ciba-Geigy Corporation, 1987.

33. Gray H. *Anatomy of the human body,* 20th ed. Philadelphia and New York: Lea & Febiger, 1918.
34. Flynn JM, Skaggs DL, Sponseller PD, et al. The surgical management of pediatric fractures of the lower extremity. *Instr Course Lect* 2003;52:647–659.
35. Thompson GH, Gesler JW. Proximal tibial epiphyseal fracture in an infant. *J Pediatr Orthop* 1984;4:114–117.
36. Graham JM, Gross RH. Distal femoral physeal problem fractures. *Clin Orthop Rel Res* 1990;255:51–53.
37. Janarv PM, Wikstrom B, Hirsch G. The influence of transphyseal drilling and tendon grafting on bone growth: an experimental study in the rabbit. *J Pediatr Orthop* 1998; 18:149–154.
38. Griswold A. Early motion in the treatment of separation of the lower femoral epiphysis. *J Bone Joint Surg Am* 1928;10:75–77.
39. Czitrom AA, Salter RB, Willis RB. Fractures involving the distal epiphyseal plate of the femur. *Int Orthop* 1981;4:269–277.
40. Makela EA, Vainionpaa S, Vihtonen K, et al. Healing of physeal fracture after fixation with biodegradable self-reinforced polyglycolic acid pins. An experimental study on growing rabbits. *Clin Mater* 1990;5:1–12.
41. Gruber HE, Phieffer LS, Wattenbarger JM. Physeal fractures, part II: fate of interposed periosteum in a physeal fracture. *J Pediatr Orthop* 2002;22:710–716.
42. Abraham E, Ansari A, Huang TL. Fracture of distal medial femoral epiphysis with subluxation of the knee joint. *J Trauma* 1980;20:339–341.
43. Shindell R, Lippiello L, Connolly JF. Uncertain effect of indomethacin on physeal growth injury. Experiments in rabbits. *Acta Orthop Scand* 1988;59:46–49.
44. Tolo VT. External skeletal fixation in children's fractures. *J Pediatr Orthop* 1983;3: 435–442.
45. Smith BG, Rand F, Jaramillo D, et al. Early MR imaging of lower-extremity physeal fracture-separations: a preliminary report. *J Pediatr Orthop* 1994;14:526–533.
46. Sasaki T, Ishibashi Y, Okamura Y, et al. MRI evaluation of growth plate closure rate and pattern in the normal knee joint. *J Knee Surg* 2002;15:72–76.
47. Carey J, Spence L, Blickman H, et al. MRI of pediatric growth plate injury: correlation with plain film radiographs and clinical outcome. *Skel Radiol* 1998;27:250–255.
48. Peterson HA. Partial growth plate arrest and its treatment. *J Pediatr Orthop* 1984;4: 246–258.
49. Gomes LS, Volpon JB. Experimental physeal fracture-separations treated with rigid internal fixation. *J Bone Joint Surg Am* 1993;75:1756–1764.
50. Kasser JR. Physeal bar resections after growth arrest about the knee. *Clin Orthop Rel Res* 1990;255:68–74.
51. Roberts JM. Operative treatment of fractures about the knee. *Orthop Clin North Am* 1990;21:365–379.
52. Langenskiold A. Surgical treatment of partial closure of the growth plate. *J Pediatr Orthop* 1981;1:3–11.
53. Carlson WO, Wenger DR. A mapping method to prepare for surgical excision of a partial physeal arrest. *J Pediatr Orthop* 1984;4:232–238.
54. Hasler CC, Foster BK. Secondary tethers after physeal bar resection: a common source of failure? *Clin Orthop* 2002;405:242–249.
55. Futami T, Foster BK, Morris LL, et al. Magnetic resonance imaging of growth plate injuries: the efficacy and indications for surgical procedures. *Arch Orthop Trauma Surg* 2000;120:390–396.
56. Scheffer MM, Peterson HA. Opening-wedge osteotomy for angular deformities of long bones in children. *J Bone Joint Surg Am* 1994;76:325–334.
57. Paley D. Current techniques of limb lengthening. *J Pediatr Orthop* 1988;8:73–92.
58. Morrissy W. *Lovell and Winters's pediatric orthopedics*, 5th ed. Philadelphia: Lippincott, Williams & Wilkins, 2001.
59. Skaggs D, Flynn JM. *Staying out of trouble in pediatric orthopaedics*. Philadelphia: Lippincott Williams & Wilkins, 2005.
60. Simonian PT, Staheli LT. Periarticular fractures after manipulation for knee contractures in children. *J Pediatr Orthop* 1995;15:288–291.
61. Stanitski CL. Stress view radiographs of the skeletally immature knee: a different view. *J Pediatr Orthop* 2004;24:342.
62. Wood KB, Bradley JP, Ward WT. Pes anserinus interposition in a proximal tibial physeal fracture. A case report. *Clin Orthop Rel Res* 1991;264:239–242.
63. Welch P, Wynne GJ. Proximal tibial epiphyseal fracture-separation: case report. *J Bone Joint Surg Am* 1963;45:782–784.
64. Poulsen TD, Skak SV, Jensen TT. Epiphyseal fractures of the proximal tibia. *Injury* 1989;20:111–113.
65. Burkhart SS, Peterson HA. Fractures of the proximal tibial epiphysis. *J Bone Joint Surg Am* 1979;61:996–1002.
66. Shelton WR, Canale ST. Fractures of the tibia through the proximal tibial epiphyseal cartilage. *J Bone Joint Surg Am* 1979;61:167–173.
67. Patari SK, Lee FY, Behrens FF. Coronal split fracture of the proximal tibia epiphysis through a partially closed physis: a new fracture pattern. *J Pediatr Orthop* 2001;21: 451–455.
68. Keret D, Mendez AA, Harcke HT, et al. Type V physeal injury: a case report. *J Pediatr Orthop* 1990;10:545–548.
69. Resnick DNG. *Diagnosis of bone and joint disorders, with emphasis on articular abnormalities*. Philadelphia: WB Saunders, 1981.
70. Blanks RH, Lester DK, Shaw BA. Flexion-type Salter II fracture of the proximal tibia. Proposed mechanism of injury and two case studies. *Clin Orthop Rel Res* 1994;301: 256–259.
71. Ciszewski WA, Buschmann WR, Rudolph CN. Irreducible fracture of the proximal tibial physis in an adolescent. *Orthop Rev* 1989;18:891–893.
72. Egol KA, Karunakar M, Phieffer L, et al. Early versus late reduction of a physeal fracture in an animal model. *J Pediatr Orthop* 2002;22:208–211.
73. Rhemrev SJ, Sleeboom C, Ekkelkamp S. Epiphyseal fractures of the proximal tibia. *Injury* 2000;31:131–134.
74. Gautier E, Ziran BH, Egger B, et al. Growth disturbances after injuries of the proximal tibial epiphysis. *Arch Orthop Trauma Surg* 1998;118:37–41.
75. Bylander B, Hagglund G, Selvik G. Stapling for tibial-growth deformity. A case report on roentgen stereophotogrammetric analysis. *Acta Orthop Scand* 1989;60:487–490.
76. Ergun M, Taskiran E, Ozgurbuz C. Simultaneous bilateral tibial tubercle avulsion fracture in a basketball player. *Knee Surg Sports Traumatol Arthrosc* 2003;11:163–166.
77. Christie MJ, Dvonch VM. Tibial tuberosity avulsion fracture in adolescents. *J Pediatr Orthop* 1981;1:391–394.
78. Levi JH, Coleman CR. Fracture of the tibial tubercle. Am J Sports Med 1976;4:254–263.
79. Deliyannis S. Avulsion of the tibial tuberosity. *Injury* 1973;4:341–344.
80. Hand W, Hand C, Dunn AW. Avulsion fractures of the tibial tubercle. *J Bone Joint Surg Am* 1971;53:1579–1583.
81. Ogden JA, Tross RB, Murphy MJ. Fractures of the tibial tuberosity in adolescents. *J Bone Joint Surg Am* 1980;62:205–215.
82. Pape JM, Goulet JA, Hensinger RN. Compartment syndrome complicating tibial tubercle avulsion. *Clin Orthop Rel Res* 1993;295:201–204.
83. Wiss DA, Schilz JL, Zionts L. Type III fractures of the tibial tubercle in adolescents. *J Orthop Trauma* 1991;5:475–479.
84. Ryu RK, Debenham JO. An unusual avulsion fracture of the proximal tibial epiphysis. Case report and proposed addition to the Watson-Jones classification. *Clin Orthop Rel Res* 1985;194:181–184.
85. Bolesta MJ, Fitch RD. Tibial tubercle avulsions. *J Pediatr Orthop* 1986;6:186–192.
86. Davidson D, Letts M. Partial sleeve fractures of the tibia in children: an unusual fracture pattern. *J Pediatr Orthop* 2002;22:36–40.
87. Inoue G, Kuboyama K, Shido T. Avulsion fractures of the proximal tibial epiphysis. *Br J Sports Med* 1991;25:52–56.
88. Donahue JP, Brennan JF, Barron OA. Combined physeal/apophyseal fracture of the proximal tibia with anterior angulation from an indirect force: report of 2 cases. *Am J Orthop* 2003;32:604–607.
89. Maffulli N, Grewal R. Avulsion of the tibial tuberosity: muscles too strong for a growth plate. *Clin J Sport Med* 1997;7:129–132; discussion 132–133.
90. Blackburne J, Peel T. A new method of measuring patellar height. *J Bone Joint Surg Br* 1977;59:241–242.
91. Blumensaat C. Die Lageabweichungen und Verrenkungen der Kniescheibe. *Ergeb Chir Orthop* 1938;31:149–223.
92. Insall J, Salvati ER. Patella position in the normal knee joint. *Radiology* 1971;101: 101–104.
93. McKoy BE, Stanitski CL. Acute tibial tubercle avulsion fractures. *Orthop Clin North Am* 2003;34:397–403.
94. Ozer H, Turanli S, Baltaci G, et al. Avulsion of the tibial tuberosity with a lateral plateau rim fracture: case report. *Knee Surg Sports Traumatol Arthrosc* 2002;10:310–312.
95. Rosenberg Z, Kawelblum M, Cheung YY, et al. Osgood-Schlatter lesion: fracture or tendonitis. Scintigraphic, CT and MR imaging features. *Radiology* 1992;185:853–858.
96. Watson-Jones R. *Fractures and joint injuries*. Edinburgh: E. & S. Livingstone, 1955–1956.
97. Bruijn JD, Sanders RJ, Jansen BR. Ossification in the patellar tendon and patella alta following sports injuries in children. Complications of sleeve fractures after conservative treatment. *Arch Orthop Trauma Surg* 1993;112:157–158.
98. Ehrenborg G. The Osgood-Schlatter lesion: a clinical and experimental study. *Acta Chir Scand Suppl* 1962;288:1–36.
99. Nimityongskul P, Montague WL, Anderson LD. Avulsion fracture of the tibial tuberosity in late adolescence. *J Trauma* 1988;28:505–509.
100. Hermus JP, Driessen MJ, Mulder H, et al. The triplane variant of the tibial apophyseal fracture: a case report and a review of the literature. *J Pediatr Orthop* Part B. 2003;12: 406–408.
101. Nummi J. Fracture of the patella. A clinical study of 707 patellar fractures. *Ann Chir Gynaecolog Fenn Supp* 1971;179:1–85.
102. Ray JM, Hendrix J. Incidence, mechanism of injury, and treatment of fractures of the patella in children. *J Trauma* 1992;32:464–467.
103. Belman DA, Neviaser RJ. Transverse fracture of the patella in a child. *J Trauma* 1973; 13:917–918.
104. Grogan DP, Carey TP, Leffers D, et al. Avulsion fractures of the patella. *J Pediatr Orthop* 1990;10:721–730.
105. Rosenthal R, Levine DB. Fragmentation of the distal pole of the patella in spastic cerebral palsy. *J Bone Joint Surg Am* 1977;59:934–939.
106. Kaye J, Freiberger R. Fragmentation of the lower pole of the patella in spastic lower extremities. *Radiology* 1971;101:97–100.
107. Rorabeck C, Bobechko W. Acute dislocation of the patella with osteochondral fracture. A review of 18 cases. *J Bone Joint Surg Br* 1976;58:237–240.
108. Hofmeister EP, Gillingham BL, Bathgate MB, et al. Results of anterior cruciate ligament reconstruction in the adolescent female. *J Pediatr Orthop* 2001;21:302–306.
109. Belman D, Neviaser R. Transverse fracture of the patella in a child. *Trauma* 1973;13: 917–918.
110. Sinding-Larsen M. A hitherto unknown affection of the patella in children. *Acta Radiol* 1922;1:171–173.
111. Houghton GR, Ackroyd CE. Sleeve fractures of the patella in children: a report of three cases. *J Bone Joint Surg Br* 1979;61-B:165–168.
112. Ogden JA, McCarthy SM, Jokl P. The painful bipartite patella. *J Pediatr Orthop* 1982; 2:263–269.

113. Canizares GH, Selesnick FH. Bipartite patella fracture. *Arthroscopy* 2003;19:215–217.
114. Ireland ML, Chang JL. Acute fracture bipartite patella: case report and literature review. *Med Sci Sports Exer* 1995;27:299–302.
115. Bernhang A, Levine S. Familial absence of the patella. *J Bone Joint Surg Am* 1973;55: 1088–1090.
116. Schoenbauer H. Bruche der Kniescheibe. *Ergeb Chir Orthop* 1959;42:56–79.
117. Green WJ. Painful bipartite patellae. *Clin Orthop* 1975;110:197–200.
118. Sheffield EG. Double-layered patella in multiple epiphyseal dysplasia: a valuable clue in the diagnosis. *J Pediatr Orthop* 1998;18:123–128.
119. Scapinelli R. Blood supply of the human patella: its relation to ischaemic necrosis after fracture. *J Bone Joint Surg Br* 1967;49:563–570.
120. Crock H. The arterial supply and venous drainage of the bones of the human knee joint. *Anat Rec* 1962;144:199–217.
121. Weber M, Janecki C, McLeod P. Efficacy of various forms of fixation of transverse fractures of the patella. *J Bone Joint Surg Am* 1980;62:215–220.
122. Sturdee SW, Templeton PA, Oxborrow NJ. Internal fixation of a patella fracture using an absorbable suture [see comment]. *J Orthop Trauma* 2002;16:272–273.
123. Peterson L, Stener B. Distal disinsertion of the patellar ligament combined with avulsion fractures at the medial and lateral margins of the patella. *Acta Orthop Scand* 1976;47: 680–685.
124. Wu CD, Huang SC, Liu TK. Sleeve fracture of the patella in children. A report of five cases. *Am J Sports Med* 1991;19:525–528.

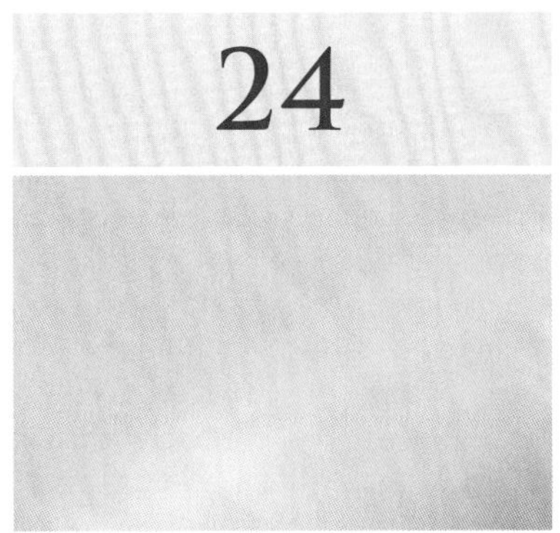

24

INTRA-ARTICULAR INJURIES OF THE KNEE

Mininder S. Kocher

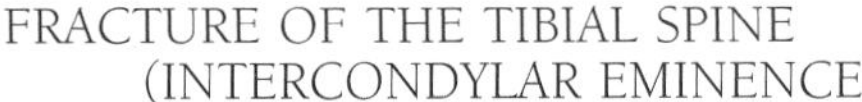

FRACTURE OF THE TIBIAL SPINE (INTERCONDYLAR EMINENCE)

Fractures of the tibial eminence occur as a result of chondroepiphyseal avulsion of the anterior cruciate ligament insertion on the anteromedial tibial eminence (1,2). Tibial eminence fractures were once thought to be the pediatric equivalent of midsubstance ACL tears in adults (3–15).

Avulsion fracture of the tibial spine is a relatively uncommon injury in children: Skak et al (16) reported that it occurred in 3 per 100,000 children each year. The most common causes of these fractures are bicycle accidents and athletic activities (17).

Historically, treatment has evolved from closed treatment of all fractures to operative treatment of certain fractures. Garcia and Neer (18) reported 42 fractures of the tibial spine in patients ranging in age from 7 to 60 years, 6 of whom had positive anterior drawer signs. They reported successful closed management in half their patients. Meyers and McKeever (19), however, recommended arthrotomy and open reduction for all displaced fractures, followed by cast immobilization with the knee in 20 degrees of flexion rather than hyperextension, believing that hyperextension aggravated the injury in one of their patients. Gronkvist et al (6) reported late instability in 16 of 32 children with tibial spine fractures and recommended surgery for all displaced tibial spine fractures, especially in children older than 10 years because "the older the patient the more the demand on the anterior cruciate ligament–tibial spine complex." Baxter and Wiley (3) noted mild to moderate knee laxity at follow-up in 45 patients, even after anatomic reduction of the tibial spine. McLennan (25) reported 10 patients with type III intercondylar eminence fractures treated with closed reduction and with arthroscopic reduction with or without internal fixation. At second-look arthroscopy 6 years after the initial injury, those treated with closed reduction had more knee laxity than those treated arthroscopically.

Modern treatment is based on fracture type. Nondisplaced fractures and hinged or displaced fractures that are able to be reduced can be treated closed. Hinged and displaced fractures that do not reduce require open or arthroscopic reduction with internal fixation. A variety of treatment options have been reported, including cast immobilization (9,21), closed reduction with immobilization (12,15), open reduction with immobilization (21), open reduction with internal fixation (12,22), arthroscopic reduction with immobilization (20), arthroscopic reduction with suture fixation (9,10,11,23), and arthroscopic reduction with wire (24) or screw fixation (4,9,20).

The prognosis for closed treatment of nondisplaced and reduced tibial spine fractures and for operative treatment of displaced fractures is good. Most series report healing with an excellent functional outcome despite some residual knee laxity (2–4,7,9–11,14–16,21,23–27). Potential complications include nonunion, malunion, arthrofibrosis, residual knee laxity, and growth disturbance (2–4,7,9–11,14–16,21,23–27).

Principles of Management

Mechanism of Injury

Historically, the most common mechanism of tibial eminence fracture in children has been a fall from a bicycle (17,28). However, with increased participation in youth sports at earlier ages and at higher competitive levels, tibial spine fractures resulting from sporting activities are being seen with increased frequency. The most common mechanism of tibial eminence fracture is forced valgus and external rotation of the tibia, although tibial spine avulsion fractures can also occur from hyperflexion, hyperextension, or tibial internal rotation. As with anterior cruciate ligament injury, tibial eminence fractures in sport may result from both contact and noncontact injuries.

Tibial eminence fractures occur as a result of a chondroepiphyseal avulsion of the anterior cruciate ligament insertion on the anteromedial tibial eminence. In a cadaver study by Roberts and Lovell (28,29), fracture of the anterior intercondylar eminence was simulated by oblique osteotomy beneath the eminence and traction on the anterior cruciate ligament. In each specimen, the displaced fragment could be reduced into its bed by extension of the knee. In adults, the same stress might cause an isolated tear of the anterior cruciate ligament, but in children the incompletely ossified tibial spine is generally weaker to tensile stress than the ligament, so failure occurs through the cancellous bone beneath the subchondral bone of the tibial spine.

In addition, loading conditions may result in different injury patterns. In experimental models, midsubstance anterior cruciate ligament injuries tend to occur under rapid loading rates, whereas tibial eminence avulsion fractures tend to occur under slower loading rates (1,2).

Intercondylar notch morphology may also influence injury patterns. In a retrospective case-control study of 25 skeletally immature patients with tibial spine fractures compared to 25 age- and sex-matched skeletally immature patients with midsubstance anterior cruciate ligament injuries, Kocher et al (30) found narrower intercondylar notches in those patients sustaining midsubstance anterior cruciate ligament injuries.

Signs and Symptoms

Patients typically present with a painful, swollen knee after an acute traumatic event. They are unable to bear weight on the affected extremity.

On physical examination, there is often a large hemarthrosis because of the intra-articular fracture and limited motion resulting from effusion. Sagittal plane laxity is often present, but the contralateral knee should be assessed for physiologic laxity. Gentle stress testing should be performed to detect any tear of the medial collateral ligament or lateral collateral ligament or physeal fracture of the distal femur or proximal tibia.

Patients with late malunion of a displaced tibial spine fracture may lack full extension because of a mechanical bony block. Patients with late nonunion of a displaced tibial spine fracture may have increased knee laxity, with a positive Lachman examination and pivot-shift examination.

Imaging

X-rays typically demonstrate the fracture, seen best on the lateral and tunnel views. The lateral x-ray is most useful in fracture classification. X-rays should be carefully scrutinized because the avulsed fragment may be mostly nonossified cartilage with only a small, thin ossified portion visible on the lateral view.

To guide treatment, important information to ascertain from the x-ray includes the classification type, amount of displacement, size of the fracture fragment, comminution of the fracture fragment, and status of the physes.

Magnetic resonance imaging (MRI) is not typically needed in the diagnosis and management of tibial eminence fractures in children. MRI may be helpful to confirm the diagnosis in cases with a very thin ossified portion of the avulsed fragment. MRI may also be useful to evaluate for associated collateral ligament or distal femoral physeal injury; however, these are uncommon.

Associated Injuries

Associated intra-articular injuries are uncommon. In a series of 80 skeletally immature patients who underwent surgical fixation of tibial eminence fractures, Kocher et al (31) found no associated chondral injuries and associated meniscal tear in only 3.8% (3/80) of patients (Fig. 24-1). Associated collateral ligament injury or proximal anterior cruciate ligament avulsion are uncommon, but they have been reported (32,33).

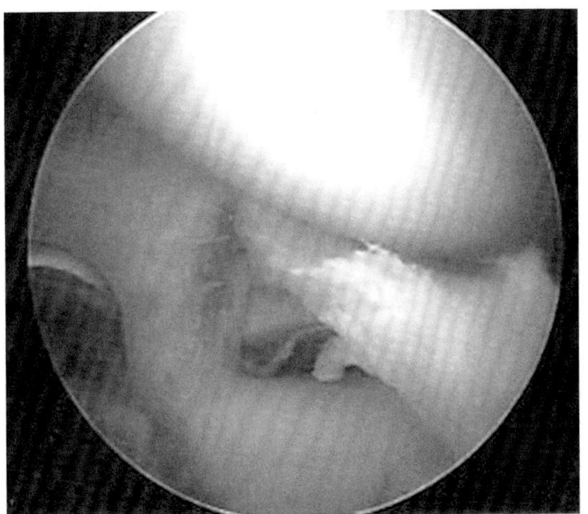

FIGURE 24-1 Longitudinal meniscal tear associated with tibial eminence fracture.

Classification

The classification system of Meyers and McKeever (17) based on the degree of displacement is widely used to classify fractures and to guide treatment (Fig. 24-2):

1. Type 1: minimal displacement of the fragment from the rest of the proximal tibial epiphysis
2. Type 2: displacement of the anterior third to half of the avulsed fragment, which is lifted upward but remains hinged on its posterior border in contact with the proximal tibial epiphysis
3. Type 3: complete separation of the avulsed fragment from the proximal tibial epiphysis, with upward displacement and rotation

X-rays of these fracture types are shown in Figure 24-3. The interobserver reliability between type 1 and types 2 and 3

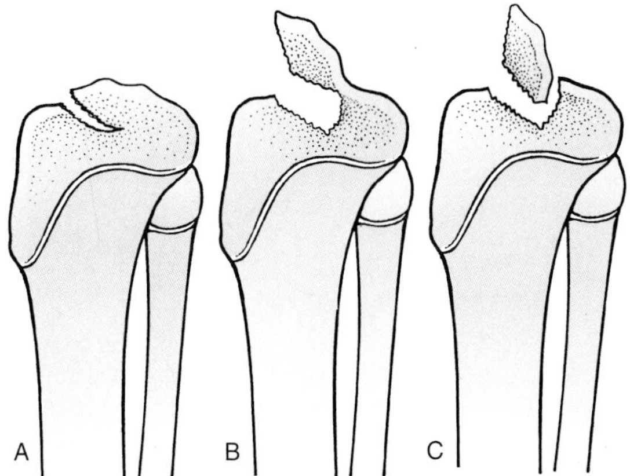

FIGURE 24-2 Classification of tibial spine fractures. **A.** Type 1—minimal displacement. **B.** Type 2—hinged posteriorly. **C.** Type 3—complete separation.

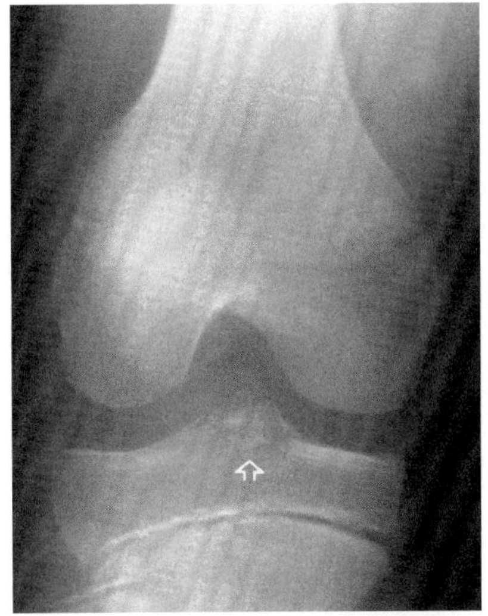

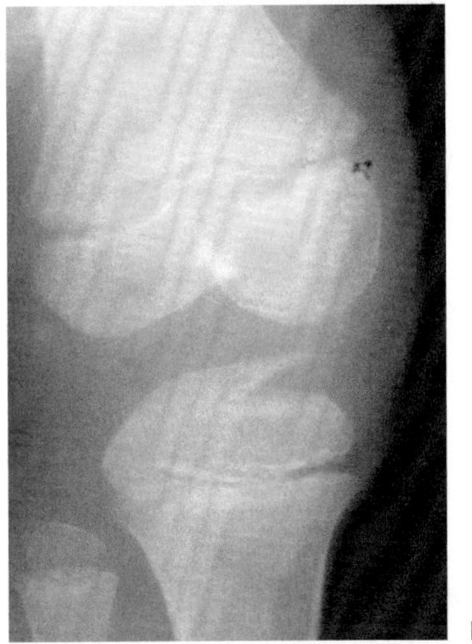

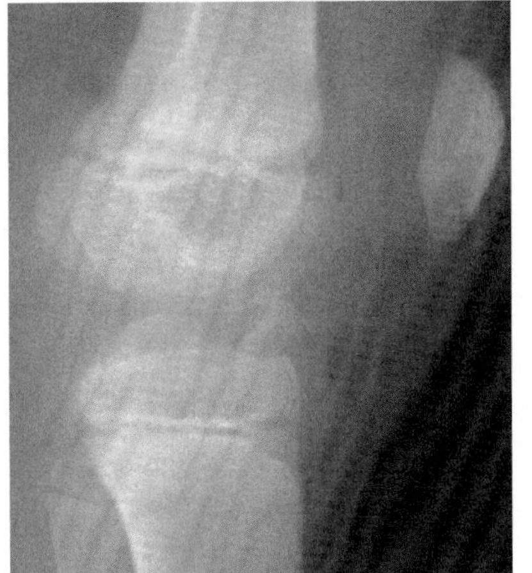

FIGURE 24-3 Stages of displacement of tibial spine fractures. **A.** Type 1 fracture, minimal displacement (*open arrow*). **B.** Type 2 fracture, posterior hinge intact. **C.** Type 3 fracture, complete displacement and proximal migration.

fractures is good; however, differentiation between types 2 and 3 fractures may be difficult (30).

Zaricznyj further classified a type 4 fracture to describe comminution of the tibial eminence fragment (34).

Surgical and Applied Anatomy

The intercondylar eminence is that part of the tibial plateau lying between the anterior poles of the menisci forward to the anterior tibial spine. It is triangular, with its base at the anterior border of the proximal tibia. In the immature skeleton, the proximal surface of the eminence is covered entirely with cartilage. The anterior cruciate ligament attaches distally to the anterior tibial spine with separate slips anterior and lateral as well (Fig. 24-4). The ligament originates off the posterior margin of the lateral aspect of the intercondylar notch. The anterior horn of the lateral meniscus is typically attached in the region of the intercondylar eminence at the anterior cruciate ligament insertion. In 12 patients with displaced tibial spine fractures that did not reduce closed, Lowe et al (35) reported that the anterior horn of the lateral meniscus consistently remained attached to the tibial eminence fracture fragment. The posterior cruciate ligament originates off the medial aspect of the intercondylar notch and inserts on the posterior aspect of the proximal tibia, distal to the joint line.

Meniscal or intermeniscal ligament entrapment under the displaced tibial eminence fragment has been reported and may be a rationale for considering arthroscopic or open reduction in displaced tibial spine fractures (Fig. 24-5) (31,36–38). Meniscal entrapment prevents anatomic reduction of the tibial spine fragment, which may result in increased anterior laxity or a block to extension (6,7,12,14,26). Furthermore, meniscal entrapment itself may cause knee pain after fracture healing (37). Falstie-Jensen and Sondergard Petersen (38), Burstein et al (36), and Chandler and Miller (37) have all reported cases of meniscal incarceration blocking reduction of type 2 or 3 tibial spine fractures in children. The prevalence of meniscal entrapment in tibial spine fractures may be common for displaced fractures. As aforementioned, the anterior horn of the lateral meniscus typically remains attached to the tibial eminence fracture fragment. However, the anterior horn of the medial meniscus or the intermeniscal ligament may become incarcerated. Mah et al (10) found medial meniscal entrapment preventing reduction in 8 of 10 children with type 3 fractures undergoing arthroscopic management. In a consecutive series of 80 skeletally immature patients who underwent surgical fixation of hinged or displaced tibial eminence fractures that did not reduce in extension, Kocher et al (31) found entrapment of the anterior horn medial meniscus (36), intermeniscal ligament (6), or anterior horn lateral meniscus (1) in 26% (6/23) of hinged (type 2) fractures and 65% (37/57) of displaced (type 3) fractures. The entrapped meniscus can typically be extracted with an arthroscopic probe and retracted with a retaining suture (Fig. 24-6).

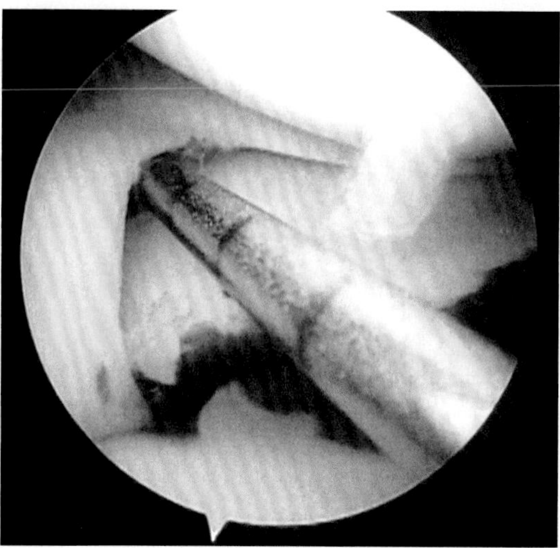

FIGURE 24-5 Meniscal entrapment under a tibial eminence fracture.

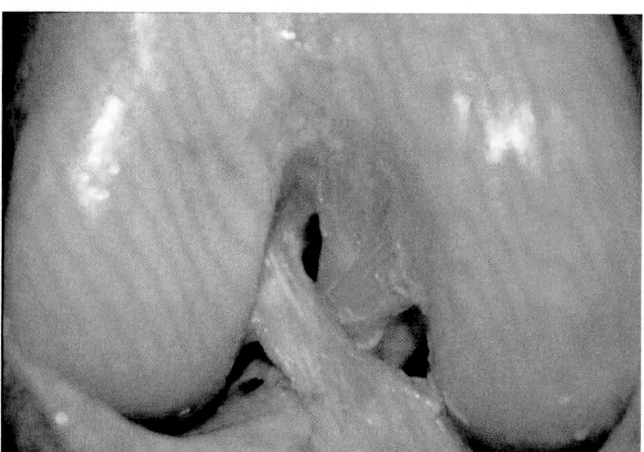

FIGURE 24-4 Anterior cruciate ligament insertion on the tibial eminence.

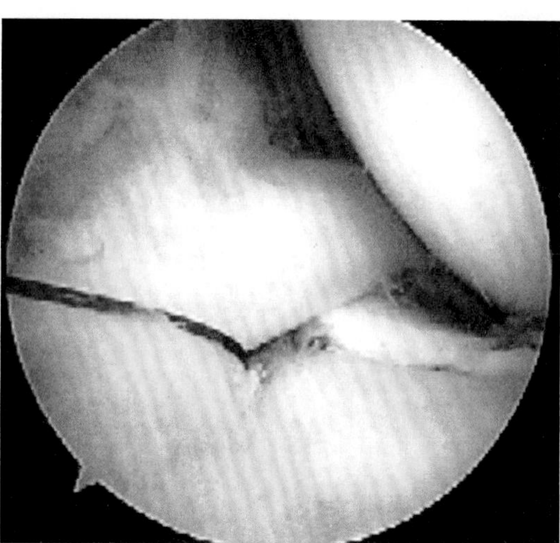

FIGURE 24-6 Retraction of an entrapped anterior horn medial meniscus using a retaining suture.

Current Treatment Options

Treatment options include cast immobilization (9,21), closed reduction with immobilization (12,15), open reduction with immobilization (21), open reduction with internal fixation (12,22), arthroscopic reduction with immobilization (20), arthroscopic reduction with suture fixation (9–11,23), and arthroscopic reduction with wire (24) or screw fixation (4,9,20).

Closed treatment is typically used for type 1 fractures and for type 2 or 3 fractures that can be reduced closed. Closed reduction is usually performed after aspiration of the hematoma with placement of the knee in full extension or 20 to 30 degrees of flexion. X-rays are used to assess adequacy of reduction. If the fracture fragment extends into the medial or lateral tibial plateau, extension may affect a reduction through pressure applied by medial or lateral femoral condyle congruence (Fig. 24-7). Fractures confined within the intercondylar notch, however, will not reduce in this manner. Portions of the anterior cruciate ligament are tight in all knee flexion positions; therefore there may not be any one position without traction being applied by the anterior cruciate ligament. Interposition of the anterior horn of the medial meniscus or intermeniscal ligament may further block reduction.

Closed reduction can be successful for some type 2 fractures, but is infrequently successful in type 3 fractures. Kocher et al (31) reported successful closed reduction in approximately 50% of type 2 fractures (26/49). However, no type 3 fractures were able to be reduced closed (0/57). Bakalim and Wilpulla (39) reported successful closed reduction in 10 patients. Smillie (40) suggested that closed reduction by hyperextension can be accomplished only with a large fragment. Meyers and McKeever (19) recommended cast immobilization with the knee in 20 degrees of flexion for all type 1 and 2 fractures and open reduction or arthroscopic treatment of all type 3 fractures.

Arthroscopic or open reduction with internal fixation of type 2 and 3 tibial eminence fractures that do not reduce has been advocated because of the potential for meniscal entrapment under the fractured tibial eminence preventing anatomic closed reduction (10,36–38), the potential for instability and loss of extension associated with closed reduction and immobilization (6,7,12,26), the ability to evaluate and treat associated intra-articular meniscal or osteochondral injuries, and the opportunity for early mobilization. For displaced fractures, Wiley and Baxter (14) found a correlation between fracture displacement at healing with knee laxity and functional outcome.

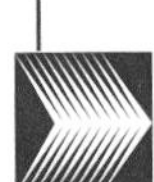

AUTHOR'S PREFERRED TREATMENT

The author's algorithm for decision making is shown in Figure 24-8.

Type 1 fractures are treated with cast immobilization. Aspiration of hematoma and injection of local anesthetic are performed under sterile conditions if the patient is in severe

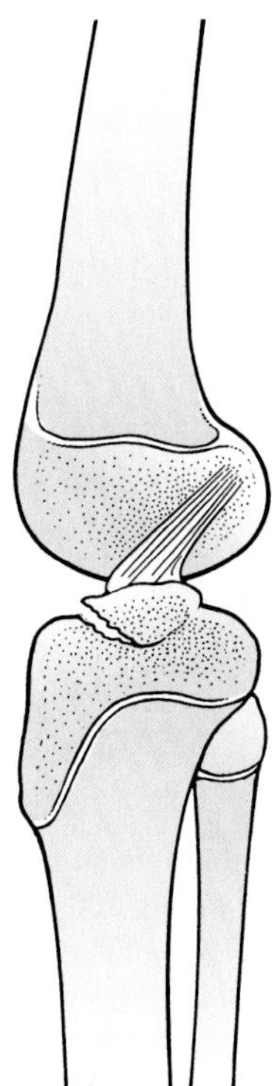

FIGURE 24-7 Reduction of type II tibial fracture with knee in 10 to 20 degrees of flexion.

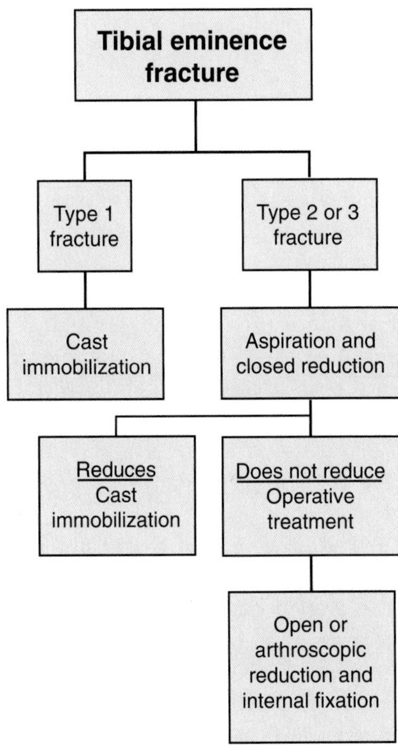

FIGURE 24-8 Algorithm for the management of tibial eminence fractures in children.

pain. A long leg cast is applied in 0 to 20 degrees of flexion. The patient and family are cautioned to elevate the leg to avoid swelling. X-rays are repeated in 1 to 2 weeks to ensure that the fragment has not displaced. The cast is removed 6 weeks after injury. A hinged knee brace is then used and physical therapy initiated to regain motion and strength. Patients are typically allowed to return to sports at 3 months after injury if they demonstrate fracture healing and adequate motion and strength.

Type 2 fractures are treated with attempted closed reduction. The hematoma is aspirated, and local anesthetic is injected into the knee under sterile conditions. Reduction is attempted at both full extension and 20 degrees of flexion. X-rays are taken to assess reduction. If anatomic reduction is obtained, a long leg cast is applied in the position of reduction. Follow-up x-rays are performed at 1 and 2 weeks post-reduction to ensure maintenance of reduction. Length of casting and postcasting management is similar to type 1 fractures. If the fracture does not reduce anatomically or if the fracture later displaces, operative treatment is performed.

Type 3 fractures may be treated with attempted closed reduction; however this is usually unsuccessful. Operative treatment is typically performed.

The author's preferred operative treatment is arthroscopic reduction with internal fixation. However, open reduction through a medial parapatellar incision can also be used according to surgeon preference and experience or if arthroscopic visualization is difficult. The author's preferred fixation is epiphyseal cannulated screws if the fragment is large or suture fixation if the fragment is small or comminuted.

Arthroscopic Reduction with Internal Fixation with Epiphyseal Cannulated Screws

General anesthesia is typically used. The patient is positioned supine on the operating room table. A lateral breakaway post is used. Alternatively, a circumferential post can be used. A standard arthroscope is used in most patients. A small (2.7 mm) arthroscope is used in younger children. An arthroscopic fluid pump is used at 35 torr. A tourniquet is routinely used. Standard anteromedial and anterolateral portals are used. Accessory superomedial and superolateral portals are used for screw insertion. Before insertion of the arthroscope through the arthroscopic cannula, the large hematoma is evacuated.

Thorough arthroscopic examinations of the patellofemoral joint, medial compartment, and lateral compartment are essential to evaluate for concomitant injuries. Usually, some anterior fat pad must be excised with an arthroscopic shaver for complete visualization of the intercondylar eminence fragment. Entrapped medial meniscus or intermeniscal ligament is extracted with an arthroscopic probe and retracted with a retention suture (see Fig. 24-5). The base of the tibial eminence fragment is elevated (Fig. 24-9A) and the fracture bed debrided with an arthroscopic shaver and hand curette (Fig. 24-9B). Anatomic reduction is obtained using an arthroscopic probe or microfracture pick with the knee in 30 to 90 degrees of flexion (Fig. 24-9C). Cannulated guide wires are placed through portals just off the superomedial and superolateral borders of the patella. A spinal needle can be helpful for the localization of these portals. The guide wires are placed into the intercondylar eminence at the base of the anterior cruciate ligament. Fluoroscopic assistance is used to confirm anatomic reduction, to guide correct wire orientation, and to avoid guide wire protrusion across the proximal tibial physis. A cannulated drill is used over the guide wires, and one or two screws are placed based on the size of the tibial eminence fragment (Fig. 24-9D). Partially threaded 3.5-mm-diameter screws (Fig. 24-9E) are used in children, and 4.5-mm-diameter screws are used in adolescents. The knee is brought through a range of motion to ensure rigid fixation without fracture displacement and to evaluate for impingement of the screw heads in extension.

Postoperatively, patients are placed in a hinged knee brace and maintained touch-down weight-bearing for 6 weeks. Motion is restricted to 0 to 30 degrees for the first 2 weeks, 0 to 90 degrees for the next 2 weeks, and then full range of motion. The brace is kept locked in extension at night. X-rays are obtained to evaluate maintenance of reduction and fracture healing (Fig.24-10). Cast immobilization for 4 weeks postoperatively may be necessary in younger children unable to comply with protected weight-bearing and brace immobilization. Physical therapy is routinely used to achieve motion, strength, and sport specific training. Patients are typically allowed to return to sports at 12 to 16 weeks postoperatively depending on knee function. Screws are not routinely removed. Functional anterior cruciate ligament bracing is used if there is residual knee laxity.

Arthroscopic Reduction with Internal Fixation with Suture

Arthroscopic setup and examination are similar to the technique described for epiphyseal screw fixation. Accessory superomedial and superolateral portals are not used. The fracture is elevated (Fig. 24-11A) and the fracture base debrided (Fig. 24-11B). The fracture is reduced. A suture is passed through the base of the anterior cruciate ligament using a suture punch (Fig. 24-11C) or a suture passer. Two guide wires are placed using the tibial anterior cruciate ligament guide system from a small incision made just below the tibial tubercle. The guide wires are placed through the base of the intercondylar eminence fragment (Fig. 24-11D). Suture retrievers are placed through the guide wire tracks, the sutures are retrieved (Fig. 24-11E), and the sutures are tied down onto the tibia (Fig. 24-11F). The procedure may be repeated for additional sutures. Heavy nonabsorbable braided sutures or fiber wire is used.

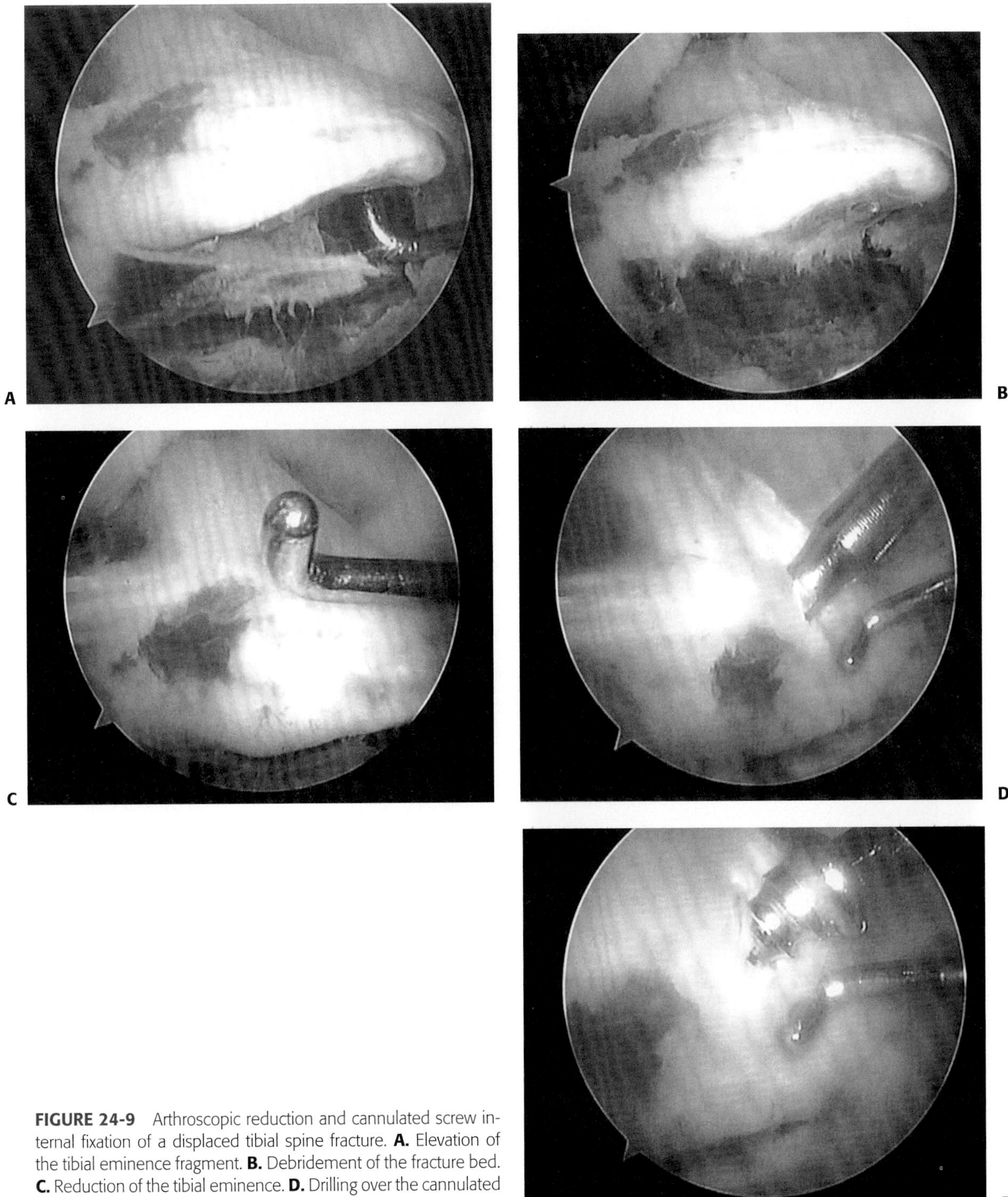

FIGURE 24-9 Arthroscopic reduction and cannulated screw internal fixation of a displaced tibial spine fracture. **A.** Elevation of the tibial eminence fragment. **B.** Debridement of the fracture bed. **C.** Reduction of the tibial eminence. **D.** Drilling over the cannulated screw guide wire. **E.** Cannulated screw fixation.

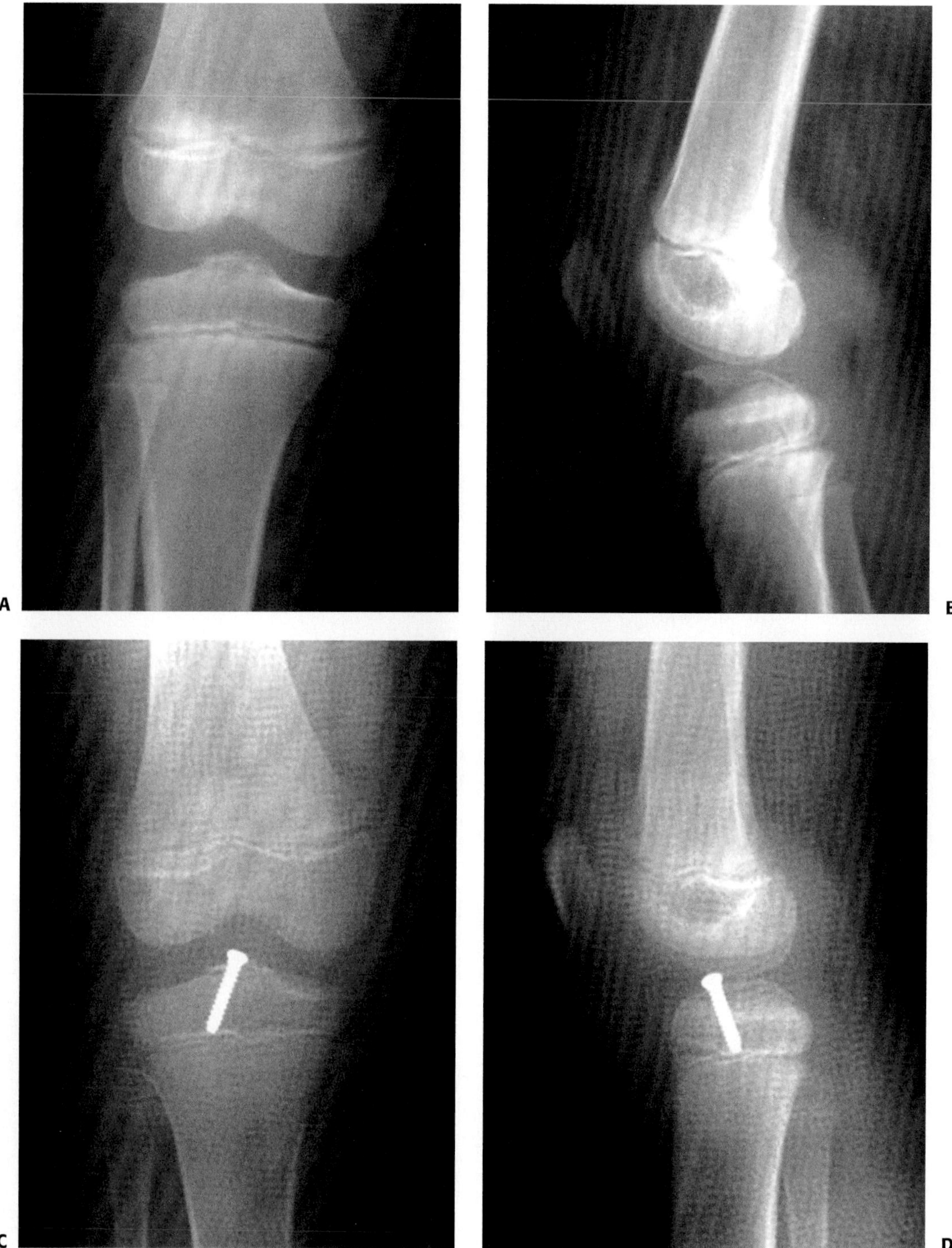

FIGURE 24-10 Type 3 tibial spine fracture in an 11-year-old boy treated with arthroscopic reduction and 3.5-mm cannulated screw fixation. Preoperative anteroposterior (AP) **(A)** and lateral **(B)** x-rays. Postoperative AP **(C)** and lateral **(D)** x-rays.

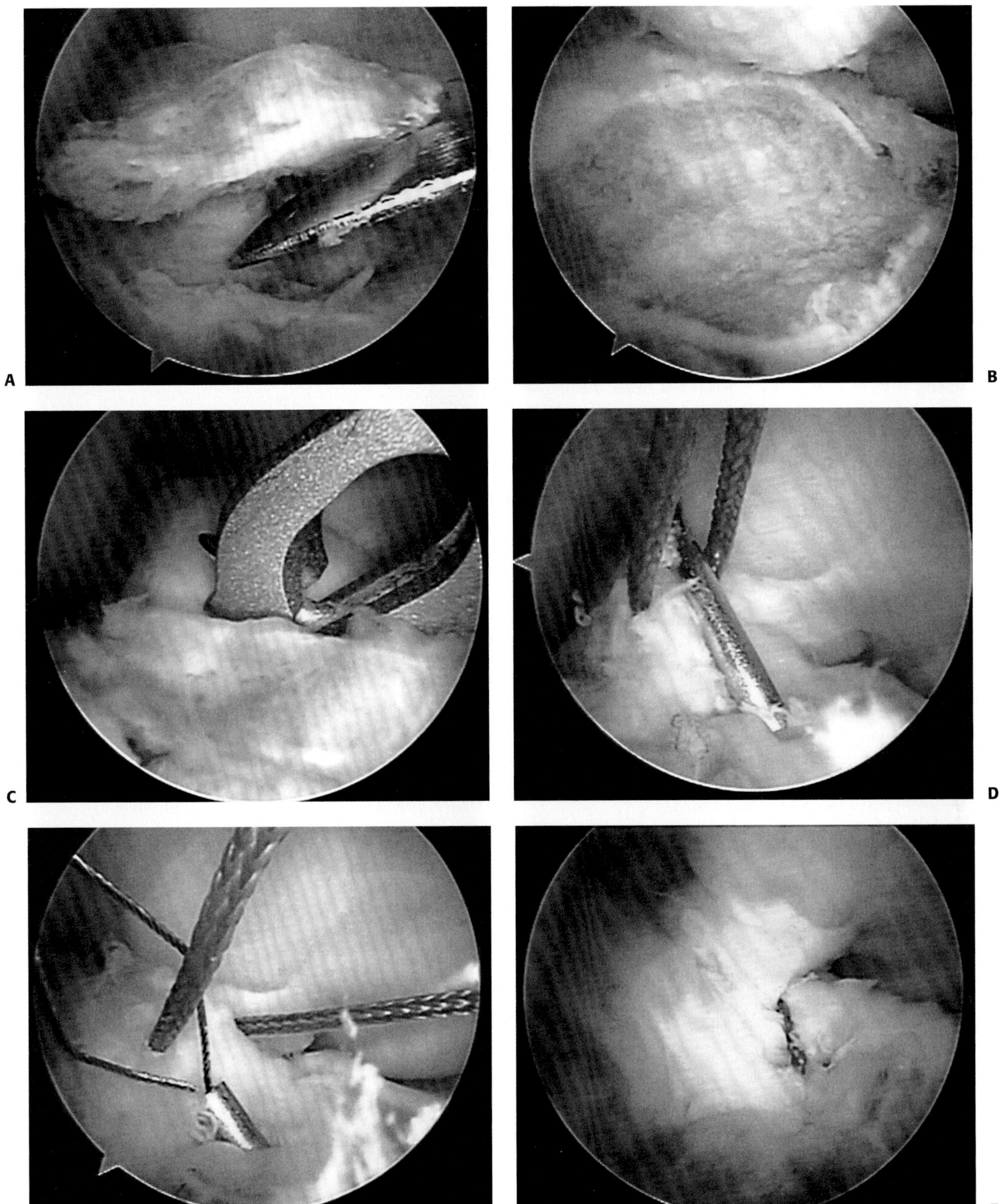

FIGURE 24-11 Arthroscopic reduction and suture fixation of a displaced tibial spine fracture. **A.** Elevation of the tibial eminence. **B.** Debridement of the fracture bed. **C.** Suture passing through the base of the anterior cruciate ligament using a suture punch. **D.** Drilling of a tibial tunnel into the tibial eminence fragment using the anterior cruciate ligament tibial guide. **E.** Retrieval of sutures using a suture passer. **F.** Appearance after suture fixation.

Pearls and Pitfalls

In the closed management of tibial eminence fractures, follow-up x-rays must be obtained at 1 and 2 weeks postinjury to verify maintenance of reduction. Late displacement and malunion can occur, particularly for type 2 fractures. Aspiration of hemarthrosis and injection of local anesthetic under sterile conditions can be helpful to minimize pain and allow full knee extension for attempted closed reduction.

During arthroscopic reduction and fixation of tibial spine fractures, arthroscopic visualization can be difficult unless the large hematoma is evacuated before introduction of the arthroscope. Adequate inflow and outflow are essential for proper visualization. Careful attention to preparation of the fracture bed is important to provide optimal conditions for bony healing. Attempted epiphyseal cannulated screw fixation of small or comminuted tibial eminence fragments can fail because the screw may further comminute the fragment. In these cases, suture fixation is a better method. If epiphyseal cannulated screw fixation is used, fluoroscopy is necessary to ensure that the screw does not traverse the proximal tibial physis, which may result in a proximal tibial physeal growth arrest.

Early mobilization is helpful to avoid arthrofibrosis, which can occur with immobilization. However, in younger children (<7 years old), compliance with protected weight-bearing and brace use can be problematic.

Prognosis and Complications

The prognosis for closed treatment of nondisplaced and reduced tibial spine fractures and for operative treatment of displaced fractures is good. Most series report healing with an excellent functional outcome despite some residual knee laxity (3,4, 9–11,14,15,20–23,26,27). Potential complications include nonunion, malunion, arthrofibrosis, residual knee laxity, and growth disturbance (3,4,9–11,14,15,20–23,26,27).

Mild residual knee laxity is seen frequently, even after anatomic reduction and healing of tibial eminence fractures. Baxter and Wiley (3,14) found excellent functional results without symptomatic instability in 17 pediatric knees with displaced tibial spine fractures, despite a positive Lachman examination in 51% of patients and increased mean instrumented knee laxity of 3.5 mm. After open reduction with internal fixation of type 3 fractures in 13 pediatric knees, Smith (27) found instability symptoms, in only 2 patients despite a positive Lachman examination in 87% of patients. In a group of 50 children after closed or open treatment, Willis et al (15) found excellent clinical results, despite a positive Lachman examination in 64% of patients and instrumented knee laxity of 3.5 mm for type 2 fractures and 4.5 mm for type 3 fractures. Similarly, Janarv et al (7) and Kocher et al (25) found excellent functional results, despite persistent laxity even in anatomically healed fractures.

Persistent laxity despite anatomic reduction and healing of tibial spine fractures in children is likely related to plastic deformation of the anterior cruciate ligament with tibial spine fracture. At the time of tibial spine fixation, the anterior cruciate ligament often appears hemorrhagic within its sheath, but grossly intact and in continuity. In a primate animal model, Noyes et al (1) found frequent elongation and disruption of ligament architecture, despite gross ligament continuity in experimentally produced tibial spine fractures at both slow and fasting loading rates. This persistent anteroposterior laxity despite anatomic reduction may be avoided by countersinking the tibial spine fragment within the epiphysis at the time of reduction and fixation. However, anterior cruciate ligament injury after previous tibial spine fracture is rare.

Poor results may occur after all types of eminence fractures associated with unrecognized injuries of the collateral ligaments or complications from associated physeal fracture (27,41,42). In addition, hardware across the proximal tibial physis may result in growth disturbance with recurvatum deformity or shortening (43).

Malunion of type 2 and 3 fractures may cause mechanical impingement of the knee during full extension (Fig. 24-12) (10,11,44). For symptomatic patients, this can be corrected by excision of the malunited fragment and anatomic reinsertion of the anterior cruciate ligament. Alternatively, excision of the fragment and anterior cruciate ligament reconstruction can be considered in adults and older adolescents.

Nonunion of type 2 and 3 tibial spine fractures treated closed can usually be managed by arthroscopic or open reduction with internal fixation (45,46). Technically, debridement of the fracture bed and the fracture fragment to fresh, bleeding bone is essential to optimize bony healing. Bone graft may be required in cases of chronic nonunion. Again, excision of the fragment and anterior cruciate ligament reconstruction can be alternatively considered in adults and older adolescents.

Stiffness and arthrofibrosis can be a challenging problem after both nonoperative and operative management of tibial eminence fractures. The milieu of a major traumatic intra-articular injury, a large hemarthrosis, and immobilization can predispose

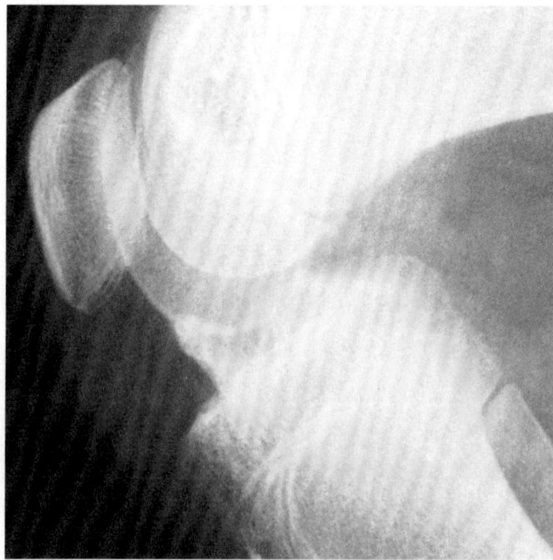

FIGURE 24-12 Lateral x-ray of a malunited displaced fracture of the intercondylar eminence of the tibia with an extension block.

to arthrofibrosis. Avoidance of cast immobilization with early mobilization using physical therapy can minimize the risk of arthrofibrosis. Dynamic splinting and aggressive physical therapy can be used during the first 3 months after fracture if stiffness is present. If significant stiffness remains after 3 months, patients should be managed with manipulation under anesthesia and arthroscopic lysis of adhesions. Overly vigorous manipulation should be avoided to prevent proximal tibial or distal femoral physeal fracture.

OSTEOCHONDRAL FRACTURES

Osteochondral fractures in skeletally immature patients are more common than once thought. They are typically associated with acute lateral patellar dislocations. The most common locations for these fractures are the medial patellar facet and the lateral femoral condyle (Fig. 24-13). The osteochondral fracture fragments may range from small, incidental loose bodies to large portions of the entire articular surface. The prevalence of osteochondral fractures associated with acute patellar dislocation ranges from 25% to 50% (47–52). Matelic et al (50) found 67% of children presenting with an acute hemarthrosis of the knee had an osteochondral fracture.

The diagnosis can be difficult because even a large osteochondral fragment may contain only a small ossified portion that is visible on plain x-rays. MRI may be useful in identifying associated osteochondral fractures in cases of traumatic patellar dislocation. Acute osteochondral fractures must be differentiated from acute chondral injuries, which do not involve subchondral bone, and osteochondritis dissecans (53,54), which is a repetitive overuse lesion of the subchondral bone that may result in a nonhealing stress fracture that can progress to fragment dissection.

Treatment of osteochondral fractures includes removal of small loose bodies and fixation of larger osteochondral fragments. In cases associated with patellar dislocation, lateral retinacular release, medial retinacular repair, and medial patellofemoral ligament repair may be performed adjunctively.

Principles of Management

Mechanism of Injury

There are two primary mechanisms for production of an osteochondral fracture (47,49–52,55). First, a direct blow to the knee with a shearing force applied to either the medial or lateral femoral condyle can create an osteochondral fracture. The second mechanism involves a flexion-rotation injury of the knee in which an internal rotation force is placed on a fixed foot, usually coupled with a strong quadriceps contraction. The subsequent contact between the tibia and femur or patella and lateral femoral condyle causes the fracture. This occurs during an acute patellar dislocation. As the patella dislocates, the medial retinaculum tears but the remaining quadriceps muscle-patellar ligament complex still applies significant compressive forces as the patella dislocates laterally and shears across the lateral femoral condyle. The medial border of the patella then temporarily becomes impacted on the prominent edge of the lateral femoral condyle before it slides back tangentially over the surface of the lateral femoral condyle because of pull of the quadriceps. Either the dislocation or the relocation phase of this injury can cause an osteochondral fracture to the lateral femoral condyle, the medial facet of the patella, or both (Fig. 24-14). Interestingly, osteochondral fractures are uncommon with chronic, recurrent subluxation or dislocation of the patella. In this situation, the laxity of the medial knee tissues and decreased compressive forces between the patella and the lateral femoral condyle prevents development of excessive shear forces.

Ahstrom (59) reported 18 osteochondral fractures; 14 occurred during sports-related activities. Most patients give a history of a twisting injury consistent with acute patellar dislocation, but a few report a direct blow to the lateral or medial femoral condyle, accounting for a shear injury. The prevalence of osteochondral fractures associated with acute patellar dislocation ranges from 25% to 50% in the literature (47,49–52,55). Nietosvaara et al (51) reported that of 69 acute patellar dislocations in children and adolescents, 62 (90%) occurred in falls; 39% also had osteochondral fractures.

Signs and Symptoms

Acutely, osteochondral fractures cause severe pain, swelling, and difficulty weight-bearing (51,56,58–79). On examination, tenderness to palpation over the medial femoral condyle, lateral femoral condyle (Fig. 24-15), or medial patella is exhibited. The patient will usually resist attempts to flex or extend the knee and may hold the knee in 15 to 20 degrees of flexion for comfort. The large hemarthrosis is due to an intra-articular fracture of the highly vascular subchondral bone. Joint aspiration may reveal a supernatant layer of fat if allowed to stand

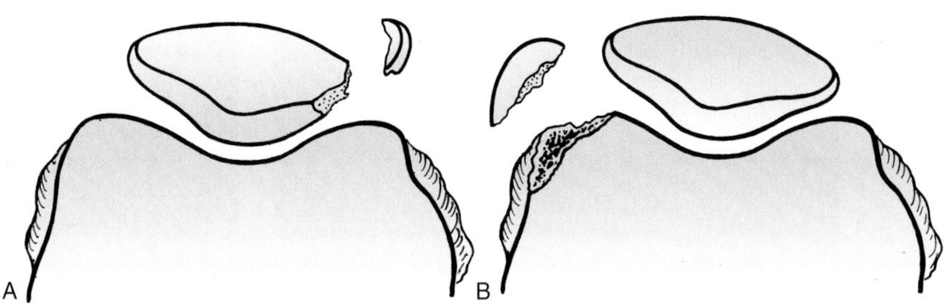

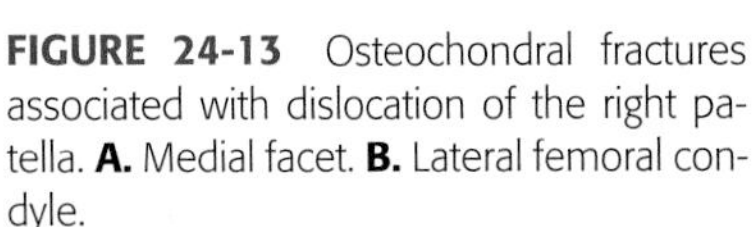

FIGURE 24-13 Osteochondral fractures associated with dislocation of the right patella. **A.** Medial facet. **B.** Lateral femoral condyle.

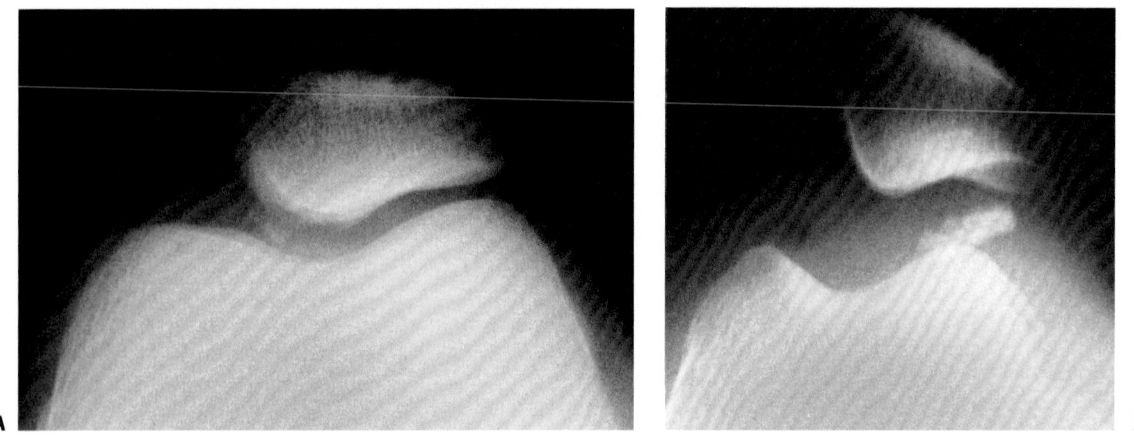

FIGURE 24-14 Osteochondral fractures associated with dislocation of the patella. **A.** Medial facet of patella. **B.** Lateral femoral condyle.

for 15 minutes, indicating an intra-articular fracture. Late examination findings may be similar to those of a loose body with intermittent locking or catching of the knee.

Imaging

X-ray visualization of the osteochondral fracture should begin with anteroposterior, lateral, and skyline plain films. However, an x-ray diagnosis can be difficult because even a large osteochondral fragment may contain only a small ossified portion that is visible on plain films. A tunnel view may help locate a fragment in the region of the intercondylar notch. Because the osteochondral fragment may be difficult to see on plain films, x-rays must be carefully assessed for even the smallest ossified fragment (see Fig. 24-20).

Matelic et al (50) reported that standard x-rays failed to identify the osteochondral fracture in 36% of children who had an osteochondral fracture found during arthroscopy. For this reason, supplemental studies such as MRI or computed tomography (CT) arthrography may be necessary in cases in which there is high suspicion of osteochondral fracture despite negative x-rays (80–82). Such cases would include an acute traumatic patellar dislocation in a patient with a large hemarthrosis.

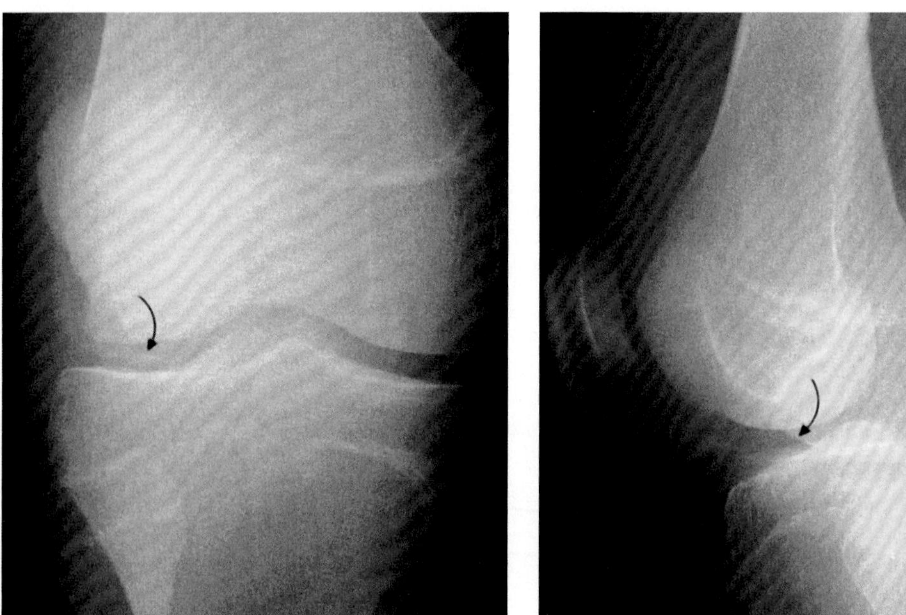

FIGURE 24-15 Osteochondral fracture of lateral femoral condyle after patellar dislocation. **A.** Fragment seen in lateral joint space. **B.** Lateral view.

Ligamentously lax patients with chronic, recurrent, atraumatic patellar instability are less likely to sustain osteochondral fractures. A high-riding patella may also have a protective effect against associated intra-articular osteochondral fractures. Patients with an Insall index greater than 1.3 have a decreased chance of sustaining an osteochondral fracture compared with patients who have an Insall index within normal limits (80). An arthrogram effect is usually present during MRI given the large hemarthrosis. Arthroscopic examination can also be done as the definitive diagnostic (and potentially therapeutic) test.

Classification

The classification of osteochondral fractures of the knee is based on the site, the type, and the mechanism of injury. The classification outlined in Table 24-1 is based on the descriptions of osteochondral fractures by Kennedy (58) and Smillie (76).

TABLE 24-1 Mechanism of Osteochondral Fractures

Site	Mechanism
Medial femoral condyle	Direct blow (fall) Compression and rotation (tibiofemoral)
Lateral condyle	Direct blow (kick) Compression and rotation (tibiofemoral) Acute patellar dislocation
Patella (medial margin)	Acute patellar dislocation

Surgical and Applied Anatomy

The patella tracks in the intercondylar notch between the medial and lateral femoral condyles during flexion and extension of the knee (64,67). With increasing knee flexion, the contact area on the articular surface of the patella moves to the proximal patella. Between 90 and 135 degrees of flexion, the patella glides into the intercondylar notch between the femoral condyles. The two primary areas of contact are the medial patellar facet with the medial femoral condyle and the superolateral quadrant of the lateral patellar facet with the lateral femoral condyle. Soft tissue support for the patellofemoral joint includes the quadriceps muscle, the medial patellofemoral ligament, the patellar tendon, and the vastus medialis and lateralis muscles.

Dislocation of the patella may tear the medial retinaculum, but the rest of the quadriceps muscle–patellar ligament complex continues to apply significant compression forces as the patella dislocates laterally. These forces are believed to cause fracture of the medial patellar facet, the lateral femoral condyle articular rim, or both (58,71,73) (see Fig. 24-13). Osteochondral fractures are uncommon with chronic recurrent subluxation or dislocation of the patella because of laxity of the medial retinaculum and lesser compressive forces on the patella and the lateral femoral condyle.

A histopathologic study by Flachsmann et al (57) helps to explain the occurrence of osteochondral fractures in the skeletally immature at an ultrastructural level. They noted that in the joint of a juvenile, interdigitating fingers of uncalcified cartilage penetrate deep into the subchondral bone, providing a relatively strong bond between the articular cartilage and the subchondral bone. In adults, the articular cartilage is bonded to the subchondral bone by the well-defined calcified cartilage layer, the cement line. When shear stress is applied to the juvenile joint, the forces are transmitted into the subchondral bone by the interdigitating cartilage, with the resultant bending forces causing the open pore structure of the trabecular bone to fail. In mature tissue, the plane of failure occurs between the deep and calcified layers of the cartilage, the tidemark, leaving the osteochondral junction undisturbed. Although the juvenile and adult tissue patterns are different, they both provide adequate fracture toughness to the osteochondral region. As the tissue transitions, however, from the juvenile to the adult pattern during adolescence, the fracture toughness is lost. The calcified cartilage layer is only partially formed, and the interdigitating cartilage fingers are progressively replaced with calcified matrix. Consequently, the interface between the articular cartilage and the subchondral bone becomes a zone of potential weakness in the joint, which may explain why osteochondral fractures are seen frequently in adolescents and young adults.

Current Treatment Options

The recommended management of acute osteochondral fractures of the knee is either surgical removal of the fragment or fixation of the fragment (8).

If the lesion is large (>1 cm), easily accessible, involves a weight-bearing area, and has adequate cortical bone attached to the chondral surface, then fixation should be attempted (58,76–79,83). This can be done via arthroscopy or arthrotomy. Fixation options include Kirschner wires (K-wires), Steinmann pins, cannulated screws, and variable-pitch headless screws. Hardware removal is typically performed after fracture healing. Lewis and Foster (69) reported good results in eight osteochondral fractures after fixation with Herbert bone screws, without need for hardware removal. More recently, bioabsorbable fixation devices are available, which may eliminate the need for hardware removal.

If the fracture fragment is small (<1 cm), chronic, or from a non-weight-bearing region of the knee, removal of loose bodies is recommended (60,66,68,73,75). The fragment's crater should be debrided to stable edges, and the underlying subchondral bone should be perforated to encourage fibrocartilage formation.

In patients with an osteochondral fracture after acute patellar dislocation, concomitant repair of the medial retinaculum and medial patellofemoral ligament at the time of fragment excision or fixation may decrease the risk of recurrent patellar instability (48,72).

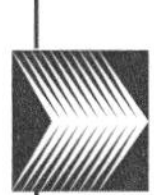

AUTHOR'S PREFERRED TREATMENT

The author's algorithm for decision making is shown in Figure 24-16.

In patients with an acute, traumatic patellar dislocation with a large hemarthrosis, MRI is performed if initial x-rays do not show any associated osteochondral fracture. If MRI does not reveal any associated osteochondral fracture, these patients are treated with a brief (1 to 2 weeks) period of immobilization, followed by patellofemoral bracing and physical therapy emphasizing patellar mobilization, straight leg raises, progressive resistance exercises, and vastus medialis strengthening. Routine diagnostic arthroscopy and routine medial patellofemoral ligament repair are not performed for initial patellofemoral dislocations. Patients are allowed to return to sports 6 to 12 weeks after dislocation, depending on their patellar alignment and rehabilitation.

Patients with small (<1 cm) osteochondral fractures, chronic loose bodies, and fractures involving non–weight-bearing areas are treated with arthroscopic removal of loose bodies. The fragment's crater is debrided to stable edges to prevent further loose bodies, and the underlying subchondral bone should be perforated to encourage fibrocartilage formation. Lateral retinacular release with medial retinacular or patellofemoral ligament repair is performed adjunctively in cases of traumatic patellofemoral dislocation to decrease the risk of recurrent patellofemoral instability.

Patients with large (>1 cm) osteochondral fractures involving weight-bearing areas with adequate subchondral bone are treated with fragment fixation. At times, these osteochondral fracture fragments can be very large, involving nearly the entire weight-bearing surface of the medial patellar facet (Fig. 24-17) or lateral femoral condyle (Fig. 24-18). Medial patellar facet osteochondral fractures can be fixed through an open lateral retinacular release by manually tilting the patella (see Fig. 24-17). Lateral femoral condyle osteochondral fractures typically require an oblique lateral arthrotomy for fragment fixation (see Fig. 24-18). Z-knee retractors are helpful for exposure, and the knee is flexed or extended to optimize visualization of the fracture bed. The osteochondral fracture fragment and the fracture bed are debrided of fibrous tissue to healthy bone. The fragment is replaced anatomically. Countersunk cannulated screws (3.5 or 4.5 mm) or Herbert screws are preferred for fixation because of the strength of fixation, which allows for fragment compression and early mobilization. Lateral retinacular release with medial retinacular or patellofemoral ligament repair is performed adjunctively in cases of traumatic patellofemoral dislocation to decrease the risk of recurrent patellofemoral instability.

Postoperatively, patients treated by excision of the fragment can begin range-of-motion exercises immediately. Crutches may be necessary in the immediate postoperative period, but patients can progress to weight-bearing as tolerated. After osteochondral fracture fixation, patients are treated with touch-down weight-bearing in a postoperative brace until fracture healing. Range of motion movement is allowed from 0 to 30 degrees for the first 2 weeks, followed by 0 to 90 degrees until fracture healing. The fracture is typically healed by 6 to 8 weeks postoperatively, and arthroscopy is then performed to confirm fragment healing, remove hardware, and assess the integrity of the articular surface. Return to athletic activities is permitted when full range of motion is recovered and strength is symmetric.

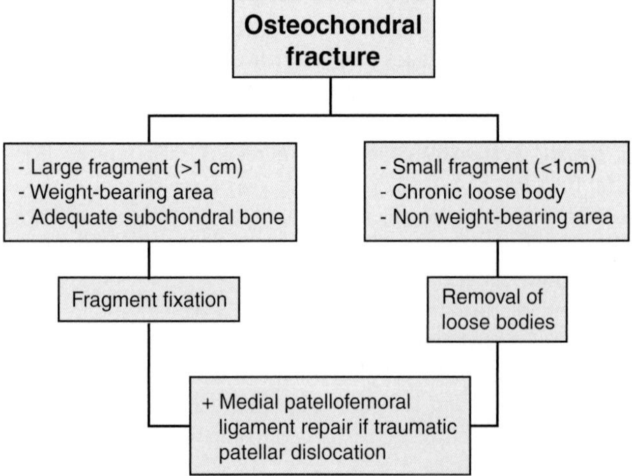

FIGURE 24-16 Algorithm for the management of osteochondral fracture in children.

Pearls and Pitfalls

An important pitfall to avoid is the failure to diagnose osteochondral fractures associated with acute, traumatic patellar dislocations. X-rays should be scrutinized for small osseous fragments, and an MRI scan should be obtained in cases with negative x-rays despite a high clinical suspicion for osteochondral fracture.

In cases of arthroscopic removal of loose bodies associated with acute, traumatic patellar dislocation, strong consideration should be given to repair of the medial structures (medial retinaculum and medial patellofemoral ligament), to decrease the risk of recurrent patellar instability.

In cases of osteochondral fracture fixation, adequate internal fixation must be obtained to allow for early motion. Screw heads should be countersunk or headless, variable-pitch screws should be used to avoid scuffing of articular surfaces. In children or adolescents with growth remaining, care must be taken to avoid crossing the distal femoral physis with hardware.

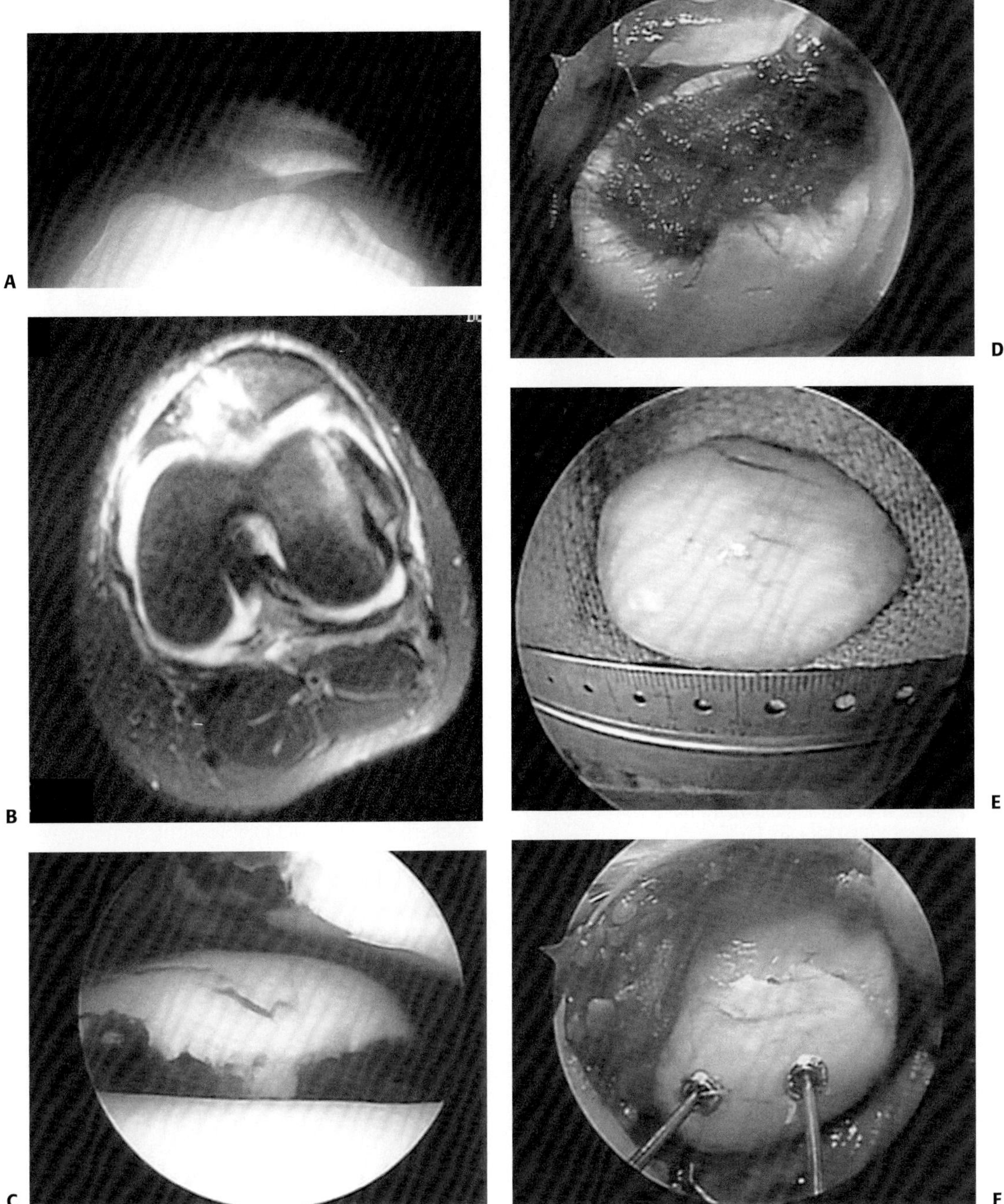

FIGURE 24-17 Fixation of a medial patellar facet osteochondral fracture in an adolescent male athlete. **A.** Skyline x-ray demonstrating a fracture of the medial patellar facet with the fragment in the lateral recess. **B.** Axial MRI scan demonstrating medial facet fracture and loose fragment. **C.** Arthroscopic view of osteochondral fragment in the lateral recess. **D.** Open view of patella. **E.** Open view of osteochondral fragment. **F.** Open view of reduction and cannulated screw fixation of medial patellar facet. (*continues*)

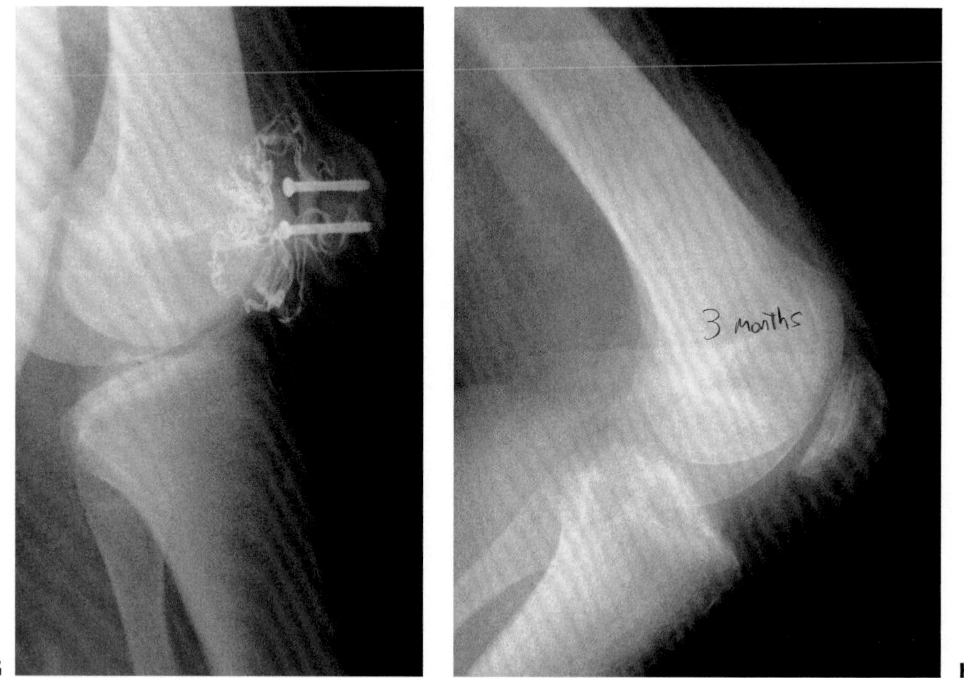

FIGURE 24-17 *(continued)* **G.** Intraoperative lateral view after fracture fixation. **H.** Lateral x-ray 3 months after fracture fixation and 6 weeks after screw removal demonstrating healing.

Prognosis and Complications

Osteochondral fractures with small fragments not involving the weight-bearing portion of the joint usually have a good prognosis after removal of loose bodies.

The prognosis for larger osteochondral fractures involving the weight-bearing surfaces is more variable. Excision of large fragments involving the weight-bearing articular surfaces predictably leads to the development of degenerative changes (84). Fracture fixation resulting in fragment healing with a congruous articular surface offers the best long-term prognosis; however, even these cases may develop crepitus, stiffness, and degenerative changes (59).

Complications include recurrent patellar instability with further osteochondral injury after both excision of loose bodies and fracture fixation. Concomitant medial patellofemoral ligament repair appears to decrease the risk of recurrent instability (62,72). Stiffness may occur, particularly after fracture fixation. Adequate internal fixation is necessary to allow for early motion, which decreases the risk of loss of motion. Stiffness may be treated with aggressive therapy and dynamic splinting during the first 3 to 4 months after injury. Beyond this time frame, manipulation under anesthesia with arthroscopic lysis of adhesions is typically required. Nonunion after fragment fixation may also occur, necessitating further attempts at fracture fixation or fracture excision. Excision of larger osteochondral fractures involving the weight-bearing articular surfaces requires associated chondral resurfacing, such as marrow stimulation procedures (microfracture), osteochondral grafting (mosaicplasty), or autologous chondrocyte implantation (74,85–87). Complications related to hardware for fracture fixation may also occur. Proud screw heads may scuff articular surfaces. Bioabsorbable implants may result in synovitis with sterile effusions.

PATELLAR DISLOCATION

Patellar instability is relatively common in children if all subluxations and dislocations from varying causes are considered. Patellar instability involves cases ranging from acute, traumatic patellar dislocation to chronic, recurrent patellar subluxation in a patient with ligamentous laxity.

Acute, traumatic patellar dislocation typically occurs in adolescents. Acute patellar dislocations in younger children usually occur in the context of underlying patellofemoral dysplasia (88). Chronic, atraumatic, recurrent patellofemoral instability occurs most often in adolescent females, with underlying laxity and alignment risk factors.

Acute, traumatic patellar dislocations without associated osteochondral fracture are treated with a short period of immobilization followed by patellofemoral bracing and rehabilitation. Acute, traumatic patellar dislocations with osteochondral fractures are treated as discussed in the previous section, with removal of loose bodies or fracture fixation. Chronic, recurrent, atraumatic patellofemoral instability is typically treated with patellofemoral bracing, rehabilitation, and orthotics if needed. Recurrent patellofemoral instability that has been recalcitrant to

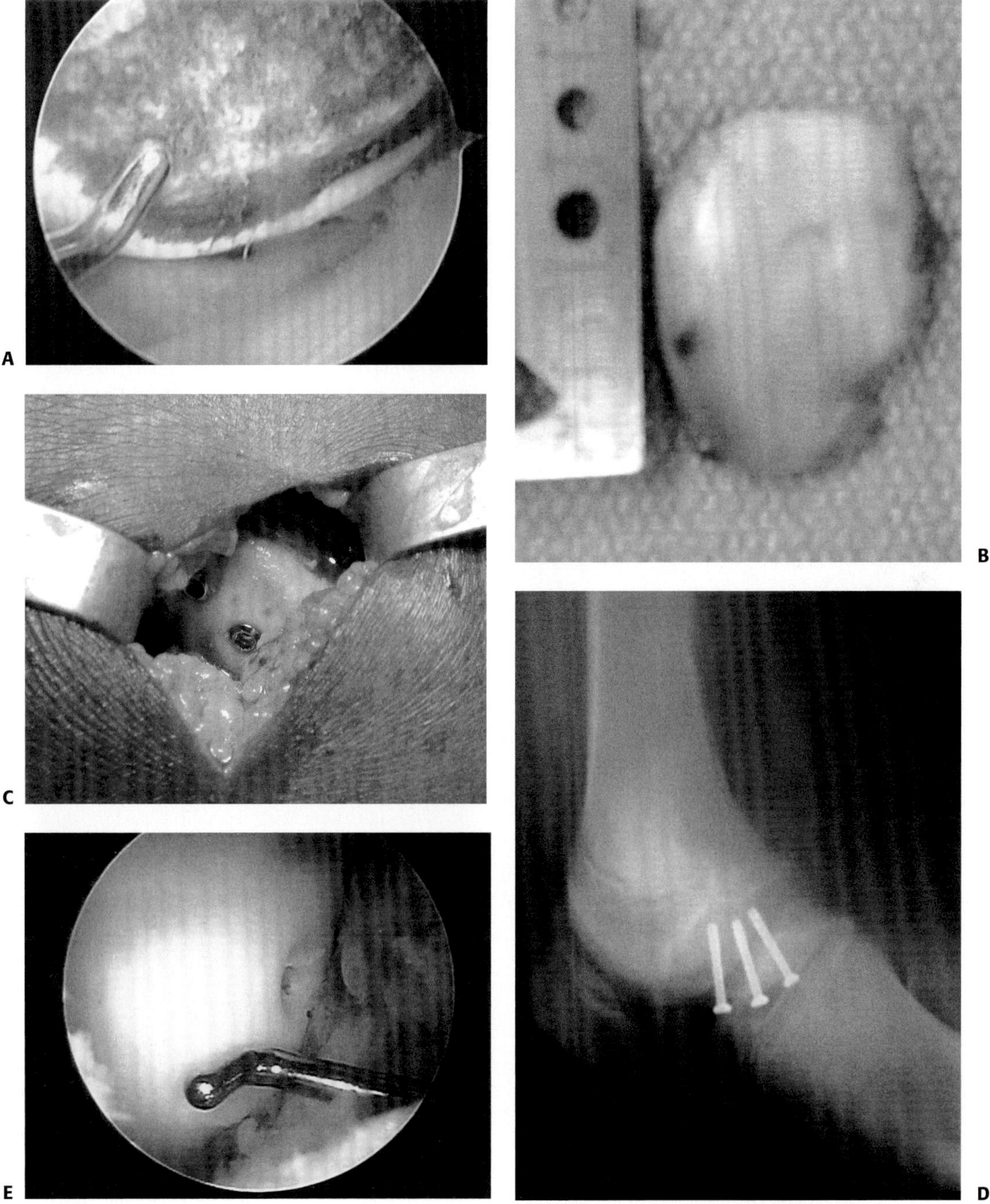

FIGURE 24-18 Fixation of a lateral femoral condyle osteochondral fracture in an adolescent female athlete. **A.** Arthroscopic view of the lateral femoral condyle. **B.** Open view of the fracture fragment. **C.** Open view of fracture fixation using cannulated screws through a limited lateral arthrotomy. **D.** Six weeks postoperative lateral x-ray demonstrating fracture healing. **E.** Arthroscopic appearance at the time of screw removal 6 weeks postoperatively.

nonoperative treatment can be managed with a variety of proximal and distal realignment procedures.

Principles of Management

Mechanism of Injury

Patellar dislocations usually occur because of a flexion-rotation injury of the knee in which an internal rotation force is placed on a fixed foot, usually coupled with a strong quadriceps contraction. As the patella dislocates, the medial retinaculum and medial patellofemoral ligament tear but the remaining quadriceps muscle-patellar ligament complex still applies significant compressive forces as the patella dislocates laterally and shears across the lateral femoral condyle. This may result in associated osteochondral fracture.

Less commonly, patellar dislocation can be caused by a direct blow to the medial aspect of the patella. Larsen and Lauridsen (89) found that a direct blow accounted for only 10% of the acute patellar dislocations in their series. Spontaneous reduction often occurs as the knee is extended.

Patellar dislocations are more likely to be caused by falls, gymnastics, dancing, cheerleading, and a wide variety of other activities. Acute patellar dislocation also should be considered in the evaluation of all athletic injuries in adolescents and young adults.

Signs and Symptoms

Patients with an acute, traumatic patellar dislocation often give a history of a twisting injury. Patients may remember feeling or seeing the patella in a laterally displaced position. Most acute patellar dislocations spontaneously reduce or reduce with incidental knee extension. It is more unusual to see a patient with an unreduced patellar dislocation (Fig. 24-19). Patients may report a "pop" associated with dislocation and a second "pop" associated with spontaneous reduction.

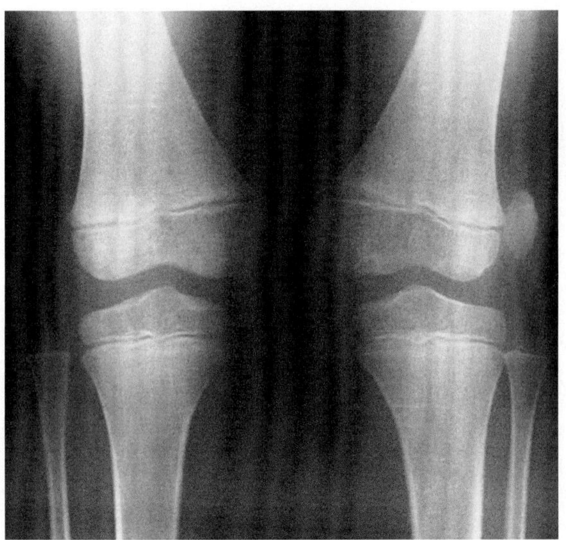

FIGURE 24-19 Acute dislocation of the left patella in a 6-year-old boy.

Symptoms include diffuse parapatellar tenderness and pain with any attempt passively to displace the patella. Patients may have a positive apprehension test with lateral translation of the patella. A defect may be palpable in the medial attachment of the vastus medialis obliquus to the patella if the medial retinaculum is completely avulsed. Tenderness on the lateral aspect of the knee usually is not as severe as on the medial side. Hemorrhage into the joint may cause hemarthrosis, and severe hemarthrosis should suggest the possibility of an osteochondral fracture (90). Nietosvaara et al (51) reported that of 72 patients with acute patellar dislocations, 28 (39%) had associated osteochondral fractures. These fractures included 15 capsular avulsions of the medial patellar margin and 15 loose intraarticular fragments detached from the patella, the lateral femoral condyle, or both. All knee ligaments should be carefully evaluated because the mechanism of patellar dislocation may cause associated ligamentous injuries.

Imaging

X-rays after acute dislocation are obtained primarily to detect any associated osteochondral fracture. Occasionally, an osteochondral fragment from the medial aspect of the patella or the lateral femoral condyle is visible on the anteroposterior or lateral view. The classic "sunrise" view is difficult to obtain in a child after acute dislocation because the required positioning of the knee causes pain. Rarely, stress x-rays may be obtained for evaluation of suspected physeal fracture or ligamentous injury. CT or MRI may be valuable to check for an osteochondral fracture.

Classification

Although there is no specific classification of patellar dislocations in children, acute dislocation should be distinguished clinically from chronic patellar subluxation or dislocation (91–94). Approximately 15% of children with acute patellar dislocations experience recurrent dislocations. Cash and Hughston (95) reported a 60% incidence of redislocation in patients 11 to 14 years of age, 30% in patients 19 to 28 years of age, and in only one patient older than 28 years of age.

Surgical and Applied Anatomy

The patella is a sesamoid bone in the quadriceps mechanism. As the insertion site of all muscle components of the quadriceps complex, it serves biomechanically to provide an extension moment during range of motion of the knee joint. The trochlear shape of the distal femur stabilizes the patella as it tracks through a range of motion. The hyaline cartilage of the patella is the thickest in the body.

At 20 degrees of knee flexion, the inferior pole of the patella contacts a relatively small area of the femoral groove. With further flexion, the contact area moves superiorly and increases in size. The medial facet of the patella comes in contact with the femoral groove only when flexion reaches 90 to 130 degrees.

The average adult trochlear femoral groove height is 5.2 mm and lateral femoral condyle height is 3.4 mm. The patellar articular cartilage is 6 to 7 mm deep, the thickest articular cartilage in the body and a reflection of the joint's inherent incongruity.

The usual normal lateral alignment of the patella is checked by the medial quadriceps expansion and focal thickening of the capsule in the areas of the medial patellofemoral and medial meniscopatellar ligaments (96). Dynamic stability depends on muscle forces, primarily the quadriceps and hamstrings acting through an elegant lower extremity articulated lever system that creates and modulates forces during gait. The quadriceps blends with the joint capsule to provide a combination of dynamic and static balance. Tightness or laxity of any of the factors involved with maintenance of the balance leads to varying levels of instability. Acute patellar dislocation almost always is in a lateral direction unless it is due to a medially oriented direct blow or follows over vigorous lateral retinacular release. Sallay et al (97) demonstrated avulsions of the medial patellofemoral ligament from the femur in 94% (15 of 16) of patients during surgical exploration after acute patellar dislocation. Desio et al (96), using a cadaveric serial cutting model, found that the medial patellofemoral ligament provided 60% of the resistance to lateral patellar translation at 20 degrees of knee flexion. The medial patellomeniscal ligament accounted for an additional 13% of the medial quadrant restraining force. If the deficit produced by attenuation of the medial vectors after acute dislocation is not eliminated, patellofemoral balance is lost, resulting in feelings of giving way and recurrent dislocation.

The patella is under significant biomechanical compressive load during activity. It has been estimated that at 60 degrees of knee flexion, the forces across the patellofemoral articulation are three times the body weight and increase to over seven times the body weight during full knee flexion.

The quadriceps mechanism is aligned in a slightly valgus position in relation to the patellar tendon. This alignment can be approximated by a line drawn from the anterosuperior iliac spine to the center of the patella. The force of the patellar tendon is indicated by a line drawn from the center of the patella to the tibial tubercle. The angle formed by these two lines is called the *quadriceps angle* or *Q angle* (Fig. 24-20). As this angle increases, the pull of the extensor mechanism tends to sublux the patella laterally. Recurrent patellar dislocation is most likely associated with some congenital or developmental deficiency of the extensor mechanism, such as patellofemoral dysplasia, deficiency of the vastus medialis obliquus, or an increased Q angle with malalignment of the quadriceps–patellar tendon complex.

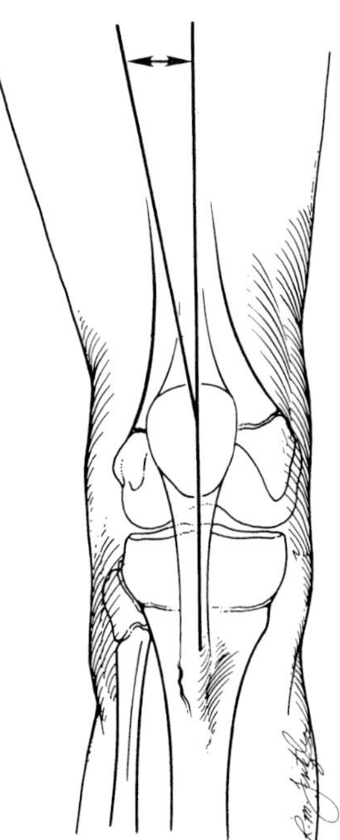

FIGURE 24-20 The Q angle. Normal valgus alignment of the quadriceps mechanism: line drawn from the anterosuperior iliac spine to center of the patella, line drawn from center of the patella to tibial spine.

Current Treatment Options

Most acute patellar dislocations in children reduce spontaneously; if not, reduction usually can be easily obtained. After appropriate sedation, reduction is done by flexing the hip to relax the quadratus femoris, gradually extending the knee, and gently pushing the patella medially back into its normal position. Gentle reduction should be emphasized to avoid the risk of osteochondral fracture associated with patellar relocation.

Surgery is usually not indicated for acute patellar dislocations in children (62,89,98). Most patellar dislocations are treated nonoperatively with immobilization, followed by patellofemoral bracing and rehabilitation. Surgical repair may be indicated if the vastus medialis obliquus is completely torn from the medial aspect of the patella, leaving a large, palpable soft tissue gap. If osteochondral fracture has occurred, arthroscopy or arthrotomy may be indicated for removal or repair of an osteochondral loose body as discussed in the previous section.

Recurrent instability of the patella that has been recalcitrant to nonoperative treatment is typically managed through various proximal or distal patellofemoral realignment procedures.

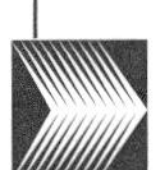

AUTHOR'S PREFERRED TREATMENT

Most acute patellar dislocations in children without osteochondral fracture are treated by closed methods with satisfactory results. A cylinder cast or knee immobilizer is used for 2 weeks. Patients are allowed full weight-bearing as tolerated. After immobilization, the patient is placed in a patellofemoral brace with a lateral bolster. Physical therapy is begun, emphasizing straight leg raises, progressive resistance exercises, patellar mobilization, and vastus medialis strengthening. Structural risk factors such as lateral patellar tightness and pes planus with pronation are addressed. Patients are allowed to return to sports 6 to 12 weeks after injury, depending on their patellofemoral mechanics and rehabilitation.

Acute surgical intervention is indicated most commonly for an associated osteochondral fracture. Removal of loose bodies or fracture fixation is performed. Adjunctive medial patellofemoral ligament repair is usually also performed to reduce the risk of recurrent patellar instability.

Chronic patellar subluxation or dislocation is common in adolescents, especially girls. Several risk factors have been identified in children likely to have chronic subluxation or dislocation, including age younger than 16 years, x-ray evidence of dysplasia of the patella or lateral femoral condyle, significant atrophy of the vastus medialis obliquus, hypermobility of the patella, and multiple previous dislocations (Fig. 24-21). Initial treatment of chronic patellar subluxation or dislocation in adolescents is immobilization followed by aggressive physical therapy for rehabilitation of the vastus medialis obliquus and quadriceps muscles. Surgical intervention is warranted in children with several risk factors who do not respond to this treatment regimen and continue to have subluxation or dislocation (99–102). Micheli and Stanitski (103) reviewed 33 skeletally immature patients with lateral retinacular releases and found that the procedure did not interfere with permanent alignment of the extensor mechanism. They recommended the technique for children who do not respond to an aggressive physical therapy program. The author usually performs medial retinaculum or medial patellofemoral ligament repair with lateral retinacular release for cases of patellar instability (Fig. 24-22A).

If subluxation or dislocation persists after adequate lateral release and medial repair, further correction of the medial deficiency is indicated. Galeazzi transfer of the semitendinosus through the inferior pole of the patella also has been reported in skeletally immature patients (Fig. 24-22B) (104). This may be indicated in adolescents with continued instability after lateral release and medial realignment or in children with associated connective tissue disorders. In skeletally mature patients with a significantly abnormal Q angle, tibial tubercle osteotomy usually achieves good results. This technique displaces the anterior tibial tubercle medially to decrease the Q angle and anteriorly to reduce the patellofemoral contact forces (Fig. 24-22C). Tibial tubercle osteotomy

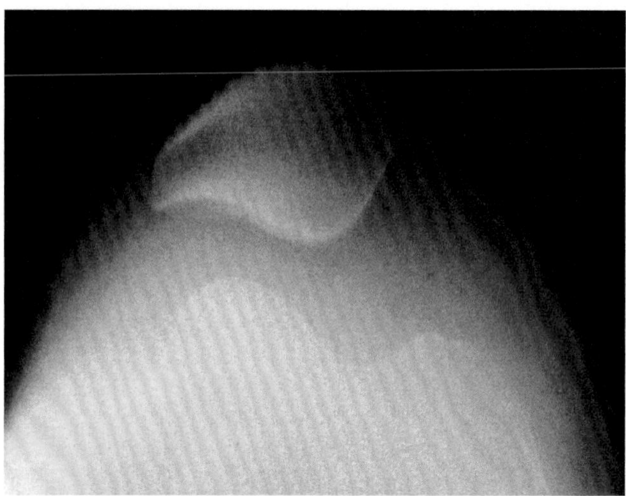

FIGURE 24-21 Chronic lateral patellar subluxation in 13-year-old girl.

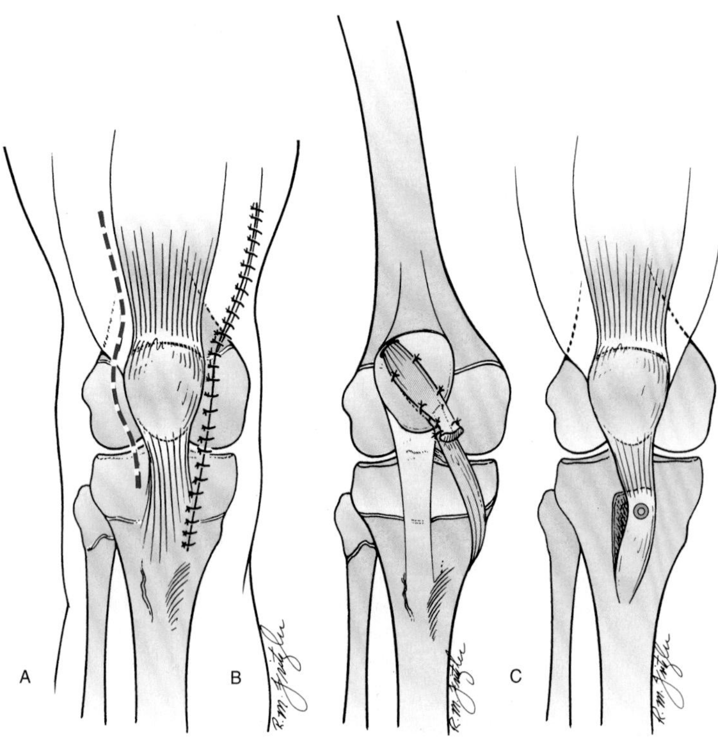

FIGURE 24-22 Surgical technique for treatment of chronic patellar subluxation or dislocation. **A.** Lateral retinacular release and medial imbrication. **B.** Semitendinosus tenodesis. **C.** Elmslie-Trillat procedure.

is contraindicated in patients with open physes because of the possibility of growth disturbance of the anterior tibial tubercle, with resulting genu recurvatum.

Peals and Pitfalls

Unrecognized associated osteochondral fractures may present later as loose bodies. Unrecognized associated ligamentous injury can present later as knee instability. Aggressive nonoperative treatment should be pursued for cases of patellofemoral instability before considering surgical management. Patients with recurrent patellar instability, particularly children, should be evaluated for underlying patellofemoral dysplasia. Overzealous and injudicious use of lateral retinacular release may result in iatrogenic medial patellar instability.

Prognosis and Complications

The prognosis of patellar dislocations in children is generally good. Approximately one in six children with acute patellar dislocations experiences recurrent dislocations. Patients with a younger age at first dislocation are at higher risk for recurrent instability. Cash and Hughston (95) noted 75% satisfactory results after nonoperative treatment in carefully selected patients.

Recurrent patellar dislocations with associated osteochondral injuries may lead to osteoarthritis of the patellofemoral joint.

Complications may occur after surgery for patellar instability. Lateral release alone without medial retinaculum or medial patellofemoral ligament repair may not adequately prevent recurrent dislocation. Stiffness, with lack of knee flexion, may occur after Galeazzi tenodesis, if the graft is overly tensioned. After tibial tubercle osteotomy, nonunion, hardware failure, neurovascular injury, and compartment syndrome have been reported.

MENISCAL INJURIES

Meniscal injuries in the pediatric athlete are being seen with increased frequency (105–126). Meniscal disorders include meniscal tears, discoid meniscus, and meniscal cysts. The exact incidence of meniscal injuries in children and adolescents is unknown. King (116) reported 52 patients younger than 15 years of age who had undergone arthrotomy because of suspected meniscal injuries, and Fowler (113) reported 117 meniscectomies in patients 12 to 16 years of age. Meniscal injuries in children under the age of 10 are rare, unless associated with a discoid meniscus (117,127–159). The incidence of meniscal and other intra-articular disorders increases with age (160). With adolescence, increased size and speed, and increased athletic demands, come higher energy injuries and an increase of intra-articular lesions.

Meniscal injury patterns differ in children compared to adults. It is estimated that longitudinal tears comprise 50% to 90% of meniscal tears in children and adolescents (117). Bucket-handle displaced tears are not uncommon (see Fig. 24-1). Also in these age-groups, meniscal injuries are commonly associated with anterior cruciate ligament injuries (118, 161–163). Cannon estimated that repairable meniscal tears occur in 30% of all knees with acute anterior cruciate ligament rupture and in 30% of patients under 20 years of age (161). Approximately two thirds of repairable meniscal tears are associated with anterior cruciate ligament rupture, with the majority of these tears limited to the posterior horn.

The incidence of medial meniscal tears is greater than lateral meniscal tears in the pediatric and especially the adolescent age-group (164). There appears to be a relatively increased incidence of lateral tears in the preadolescent age-group, which may be due to the existence of lateral discoid menisci (117).

Principles of Management

Mechanism of Injury

Injury to the nondiscoid meniscus is virtually always traumatic in nature in children and adolescents. Multiple studies have shown that between 80% to 90% of meniscal injuries in children and adolescents are sustained during sporting activities (118,127,164–166). These numbers may be lower in the preadolescent age-group. Meniscal tears most commonly occur with twisting motions, associated frequently with football, soccer, and basketball.

Meniscal tears are most commonly produced by rotation as the flexed knee moves toward extension. This rotational force with the knee partially flexed changes the relation of the femoral condyles to the menisci, and forces the menisci toward the center of the joint, where they are likely to be injured. These twisting mechanisms occur primarily in sports and may cause associated ligamentous injuries. Meniscal injuries also may be associated with degenerative changes, cyst formation, or congenital anomalies (113).

Signs and Symptoms

Pain and swelling are the most common chief complaint. Other complaints include mechanical symptoms such as snapping, catching, and locking. A bucket-handle tear that is displaced into the intercondylar notch may present with a locked knee or a knee unable to fully extend.

The differential diagnosis of acute meniscal tear in the pediatric patient includes conditions resulting in a traumatic effusion such as ligamentous injury, osteochondral fracture, chondral injury, and patellofemoral dislocation. In addition, conditions causing joint line pain must be distinguished from meniscal tears, such as plica syndrome, iliotibial friction band syndrome, osteochondritis dissecans, and bone bruises (117).

The diagnosis of meniscal tear in children and adolescents can be difficult to make. Because of the diversity of pathology and the difficulty of examination of children, diagnostic accuracy of clinical examination for meniscus tear has been shown to be as low as 29% to 59% (117,167). An accurate history may be difficult to obtain in a very young child. The older the patient, the more likely is a history of specific injury. The patient usually relates feeling or hearing a "pop" at the time of injury, with frequent popping and giving way after injury. Pain is reported by approximately 85% of patients, with tenderness over the affected joint line. More than half report giving way and effusion of the knee joint. McMurray and Apley tests may be helpful in the diagnosis of a chronic lesion, but with acute injury the knee usually is too painful to allow these maneuvers (168).

The most common findings, similar to adults, are joint line tenderness and effusion (108,119). However, some patients may have minimal findings on physical examination. In Vahvanen and Aolto's series of patients with documented meniscal tears (124), almost one third of the patients had no significant findings on physical examination. The classic McMurray test may be of little value in this age-group, whose tears are peripheral and not degenerative posterior horn lesions (117). The most accurate physical findings are joint line tenderness (especially middle to posterior) and exacerbation of the pain with varus (medial) and valgus (lateral) and rotation stress (internal, medial; external, lateral) at 30 to 40 degrees of knee flexion. Two recent studies, by examiners with pediatric sports medicine experience, have shown the diagnostic accuracy of clinical examination to be 86.3% and 93.5% overall (167,169). When medial meniscal tears were considered alone, the sensitivity and specificity of clinical examination were 62.1% and 80.7%, respectively (167). The sensitivity and specificity for lateral meniscal tears were 50% and 89.2%, respectively (167).

Imaging

Routine x-rays are obtained primarily to eliminate other sources of knee pain. Arthrography (170) may help delineate meniscal tears, but has been used less frequently since the advent of arthroscopy and MRI (121,171).

MRI is the preferred imaging method for evaluating meniscal injuries in children. MRI's accuracy rates reportedly range from 45% to 90% in the diagnosis of meniscal tears (172–175). Sensitivity and specificity of 83% and 95%, respectively, have been shown in skeletally immature patients (167,169). Kocher et al (167) showed that for medial meniscal tears the sensitivity and specificity for MRI diagnosis were 79% and 92%, respectively. For lateral meniscal tears, these numbers were 67% and 83%, respectively (167).

MRI should not be used as a screening procedure because of significant limitations of the technique in this age-group (174,176,177). Only the specificity for medial meniscal tears was significantly higher with MRI compared to clinical examination (167). The sensitivity and specificity of MRI decrease in younger children compared with older adolescents (167,169). In recent studies that compared the diagnostic accuracy of physical examination to MRI, clinical examination rates were equivalent or superior to those with MRI (167,169). These authors recommended judicious use of MRI in evaluating intra-articular knee disorders.

Normal MRI signal changes exist in the posterior horn of the medial and lateral meniscus in children and adolescents (167,169,178,179). These signal changes do not extend to the superior or inferior articular surfaces of the meniscus and likely represent vascular developmental changes (117). Takeda et al (180) reviewed the MRI signal intensity and pattern in the menisci of 108 knees in 80 normal children 8 to 15 (average 12.2) years of age using the classification of Zobal et al (179), which allows for equivocation for type 3 signals. Using tibial tubercle maturity as a definition of skeletal maturity, Takeda et al (180) found signal intensity to be proportional to age, with high signal (grades II and III) evident in 80% of patients 10 years of age or younger, 65% by 13 years of age, and 33% at 15 years of age, similar to the false-positive rate of 29% reported in asymptomatic adults (177,181). Overall, two thirds of the patients had positive findings (grades II or III), often grade IIIA, which is equivocal extension through the surface of the meniscus. Takeda et al suggested that the decrease in signal intensity was proportional to diminution of peripheral vascularity, especially in the posterior horn of the meniscus. These investigators cautioned against misinterpretation of pediatric knee MRIs and emphasized the necessity for correlation of the clinical findings with any imaging study results. When interpreting an MRI of the developing knee, care must be taken to identify a meniscal tear only when linear signal changes extend to the articular surface. As with any test, clinical correlation is mandatory before treatment decisions are made.

Classification

Classification is based on the meniscus involved (medial versus lateral), the location of the tear (posterior horn, body, anterior horn), the chronicity of the tear (acute [<3 weeks], chronic [>3 weeks]), and the tear pattern (peripheral, bucket handle, horizontal cleavage, transverse, or complex) (Fig. 24-23). Other important factors include site of the tear (outer third, middle third, inner third), stability, and associated ligamentous and chondral injuries.

Surgical and Applied Anatomy

The menisci become clearly defined by as early as 8 weeks of embryologic development (142). By week 14, they assume the normal mature anatomic relationships. At no point during their embryology are the menisci discoid in morphology (142). Thus, the discoid meniscus represents an anatomic variant, not a vestigial remnant. The developmental vasculature of the menisci has been studied extensively by Clark (112). The blood supply arises from the periphery and supplies the entire meniscus. This vascular pattern persists through birth. During postpartum development, the vasculature begins to recede and by the 9th month, the central third is avascular. This decrease in vasculature continues until approximately age 10, when the menisci attain their adult vascular pattern. Injection dye studies by Arnoczky have shown that only the peripheral 10% to 30% of the medial and 10% to 25% of the lateral meniscus receive vascular nourishment (182).

The medial meniscus is C shaped. The posterior horn is

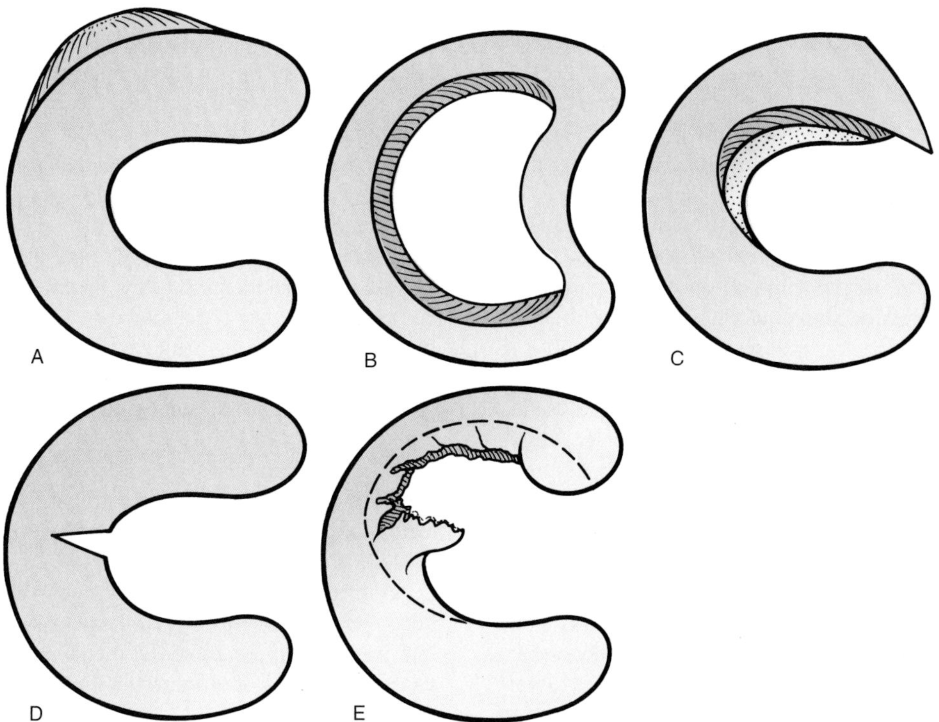

FIGURE 24-23 Meniscal tears in adolescents. **A.** Peripheral. **B.** Bucket-handle. **C.** Horizontal cleavage. **D.** Radial. **E.** Complex.

larger in anteroposterior width than the anterior horn. The medial meniscus covers approximately 50% of the medial tibial plateau. The medial meniscus is attached firmly to the medial joint capsule through the meniscotibial or coronary ligaments. There is a discrete capsular thickening at its midportion that constitutes the deep medial collateral ligament. The inferior surface is flat and the superior surface concave so that the meniscus conforms to its respective tibial and femoral articulations. To maintain this conforming relationship, the medial meniscus translates 2.5 mm posteriorly on the tibia as the femoral condyle rolls backward during knee flexion (165,166).

The lateral meniscus is more circular in shape and covers a larger portion, approximately 70%, of the lateral tibial plateau. The lateral meniscus is more loosely connected to the lateral joint capsule. There are no attachments in the area of the popliteal hiatus, and the fibular collateral ligament does not attach to the lateral meniscus. Accessory meniscofemoral ligaments exist in up to a third of cases. These arise from the posterior meniscus. If this ligament inserts anterior to the posterior cruciate ligament, it is known as the ligament of Humphrey; if it inserts posterior to the posterior cruciate ligament, it is termed the ligament of Wrisberg. Because of the lack of restraining forces, the lateral meniscus is able to translate 9 to 11 mm on the tibia with knee flexion. This may account for the lower incidence of lateral meniscal tears. Both menisci are attached anteriorly via the anterior transverse meniscal ligament (165,166).

The blood supply arises from the superior and inferior medial and lateral geniculate arteries. These vessels form a perimeniscal synovial plexus. There may be some contribution from the middle geniculate artery. King (183), in the 1930s, published classic research indicating that the peripheral meniscus did communicate with the vascular supply and thus was capable of healing. It is believed that the inner two thirds of the meniscus receives its nutrition through diffusion and mechanical pumping.

The menisci are composed primarily of type I collagen, which makes up 60% to 70% of their dry weight. Lesser amounts of types II, III, and VI collagen are also present. The collagen fibers are oriented primarily in a circumferential pattern, parallel with the long access of the meniscus (165,166). There are also radial, oblique, and vertically oriented fibers. Proteoglycans and glycoproteins are present in smaller concentrations than in articular cartilage. The menisci also contain neural elements, including mechanoreceptors and type I and II sensory fibers. In a sensory mapping study, Dye et al (184) demonstrated that the probing of the peripheral meniscus led to pain, whereas stimulation of the central meniscus elicited little or no discomfort.

Our understanding of the functional importance of the meniscus has evolved. In 1897, Bland-Sutton (185) characterized the menisci as "functionless remnants of intra-articular leg muscles." The sentiment was held onto through the 1970s, when menisci were routinely excised. Fairbanks (186), in 1948, published the first long term follow-up of patients after total meniscectomy. His article warned that degenerative changes followed meniscectomy in a substantial proportion of patients. Now, several reports have established the deleterious consequences of total and even partial meniscectomy (117–119,124,126,127, 150,156,157,162,187). Nowhere are these facts more important than in children and adolescents, in whom the long-term effects of meniscectomy will be magnified by the activity level and longevity.

It is now realized that the menisci have many functions. The menisci serve to increase contact area and congruency of the femoral tibial articulation. This allows the menisci to participate in load sharing and reduces the contact stresses across the knee joint. It is estimated that the menisci transmit up to 50% to 70% of the load in extension and 85% of the load in 90 degrees of flexion (188). Baratz et al (189) showed that after total meniscectomy contact area may decrease by 75% and contact stresses increase by 235%. They also documented the deleterious effects of partial meniscectomy, demonstrating that the contact stresses increased in proportion to the amount of meniscus removed. Excision of small bucket-handle tears of the medial meniscus increased contact stress by 65%, and resecting 75% of the posterior horn increased contact stress equivalent to that after total meniscectomy (189). Repair of meniscal tears, by either arthroscopic or open techniques, reduced the contact stresses to normal. Multiple other studies have corroborated the mechanical importance of the meniscus (165,166).

Meniscal tissue is about half as stiff as articular cartilage, allowing it to participate in shock absorption. Shock absorption capacity in the normal knee is 20% higher than in the meniscectomized knee (190,191). The menisci also have a role in joint stability. In the anterior cruciate ligament–deficient knee the posterior horn of the medial meniscus plays a very important passive stabilizing role. In the anterior cruciate ligament–deficient knee, medial meniscectomy leads to a 58% increase in anterior translation at 90 degrees of flexion (190,192). Given the presence of neural elements within their substance, it is also theorized that the menisci may have a role in proprioception.

Current Treatment Options

Some small, nondisplaced meniscal tears in the outer vascular region of the meniscus may heal or may become asymptomatic (117,165,166). Nonoperative treatment usually consists of rehabilitation of the injured knee with the avoidance of pivoting and sports for 12 weeks. However, the majority of meniscal tears in pediatric patients are larger and require surgical treatment (117,165,166). Arthroscopic management is standard, with either partial meniscectomy using motorized shavers and baskets or meniscal repairs using outside-in, all inside, or inside-out techniques (165,166,193).

The traditional treatment of a torn meniscus has been meniscectomy, but numerous reports (110,116–119,124,127,136, 150,156,157,162,187,194–197) indicating the poor long-term results of meniscectomy in children have made this less common. Up to 60% to 75% of patients have degenerative changes after meniscectomy. Manzione et al (118) reported 60% poor results in 20 children and adolescents after meniscectomy. In cadaver studies, Baratz et al (189) showed that the contact stresses on the tibiofemoral articulation increase in proportion to the amount of the meniscus removed and the degree of disruption of the meniscal structure. Clearly, as much of the meniscus should be preserved as possible.

The exact meniscal injury and potential for repair can be determined arthroscopically to help formulate treatment plans. Zaman and Leonard (198) recommended observation of small peripheral tears, repair of larger peripheral tears, and, when necessary, partial meniscectomy, leaving as much of the meniscus as possible; they concluded that total meniscectomy is contraindicated in young patients. In general, peripheral tears, which are most common in children, and longitudinal tears are good candidates for repair, with success rates of up to 90% reported (121,195,199–201).

Although King (183) suggested over 6 decades ago that, based on experimental evidence in dogs, longitudinal meniscal tears could heal if communication with peripheral blood supply existed, it was not until the work of Arnoczky and Warren (202) in the 1980s that meniscal repairs were begun based on documentation of the meniscal blood supply. They believed that tears within 3 mm of the meniscosynovial junction were vascularized, and ones more than 5 mm away were avascular unless bleeding was seen at surgery. Tears in the 3- to 5-mm range had inconsistent vascularity. Children and adolescents may have greater healing potential for meniscal repair. In adults, meniscal repair is indicated for tears involving the outer third. In children and adolescents, repair of tears in the middle third zone typically heal as well (121,195,199–201).

Meniscal tears may be seen with an underlying discoid lateral meniscus, particularly in younger children. The discoid lateral meniscus represents an anatomic variant of meniscal morphology. The incidence is thought to be 3% to 5% in the general population (117,133,140,141) and slightly higher in Asian populations (117,133,140,141). Discoid morphology almost exclusively occurs within the lateral meniscus, but medial discoid menisci have also been reported (117,133,140,141). The incidence of bilateral abnormality has been reported to be as high as 20% (128,130,149,153). Discoid menisci are classified based on the system of Watanabe (203): complete morphology (type I), incomplete morphology (type II), and any morphology that lacks peripheral attachments (type III). Although often synonymous with so-called "snapping knee syndrome," discoid lateral menisci may manifest in a variety of ways. Symptoms are often related to the type of discoid meniscus present, peripheral stability of the meniscus, and the presence or absence of an associated meniscal tear (129,133,134,140,146,151,158). Stable discoid menisci without associated tears will often remain asymptomatic, identified only as incidental findings during MRI or arthroscopy. Unstable discoid menisci more commonly present in younger children and often produce the so-called "snapping knee syndrome." In such instances, a painless and palpable, audible or visible snap is produced with knee range of motion, especially near terminal extension. In children with stable discoid lateral menisci, symptoms often present when an associated tear is present. Unlike acute meniscal tears, such symptoms may present insidiously without previous trauma. Signs and symptoms of a meniscal tear may exist, including pain, swelling, catching, locking, and limited motion. On physical examination, there may be joint line tenderness, popping, limited motion, effusion, terminal motion pain, and positive provocative tests (McMurray maneuvers, Apley test). Degenerative horizontal cleavage tears are the most common type of tear seen, reported in the largest series to occur in 58% to 98% of symptomatic discoid menisci (128,130,149). Several treatment options exist if the diagnosis of a discoid lateral meniscus is confirmed. For asymptomatic discoid lateral menisci, even if found incidentally on arthroscopy, conservative treatment is indicated. For stable, complete or incomplete discoid menisci, partial meniscectomy, "saucerization," is the treatment of choice (Fig. 24-24). If meniscal instability with detachment also exists, meniscal repair can be performed. Traditionally, complete meniscectomy via open or arthroscopic means was suggested for such lesions. However, the long-term results of complete meniscectomy and near-total meniscectomy in children are poor, with early degenerative changes (117–119,124,126,127,150,157, 187). Although there may be a rare instance in which salvage of a discoid meniscus may seem unobtainable, better arthroscopic technology and techniques have made meniscal preservation the ideal treatment through saucerization and repair.

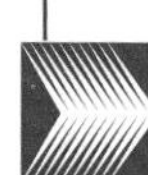

AUTHOR'S PREFERRED TREATMENT

The author's treatment algorithm is shown in Figure 24-25. Treatment is based on size, site, shape, and stability of the tear, acuity of the lesion, and knee stability.

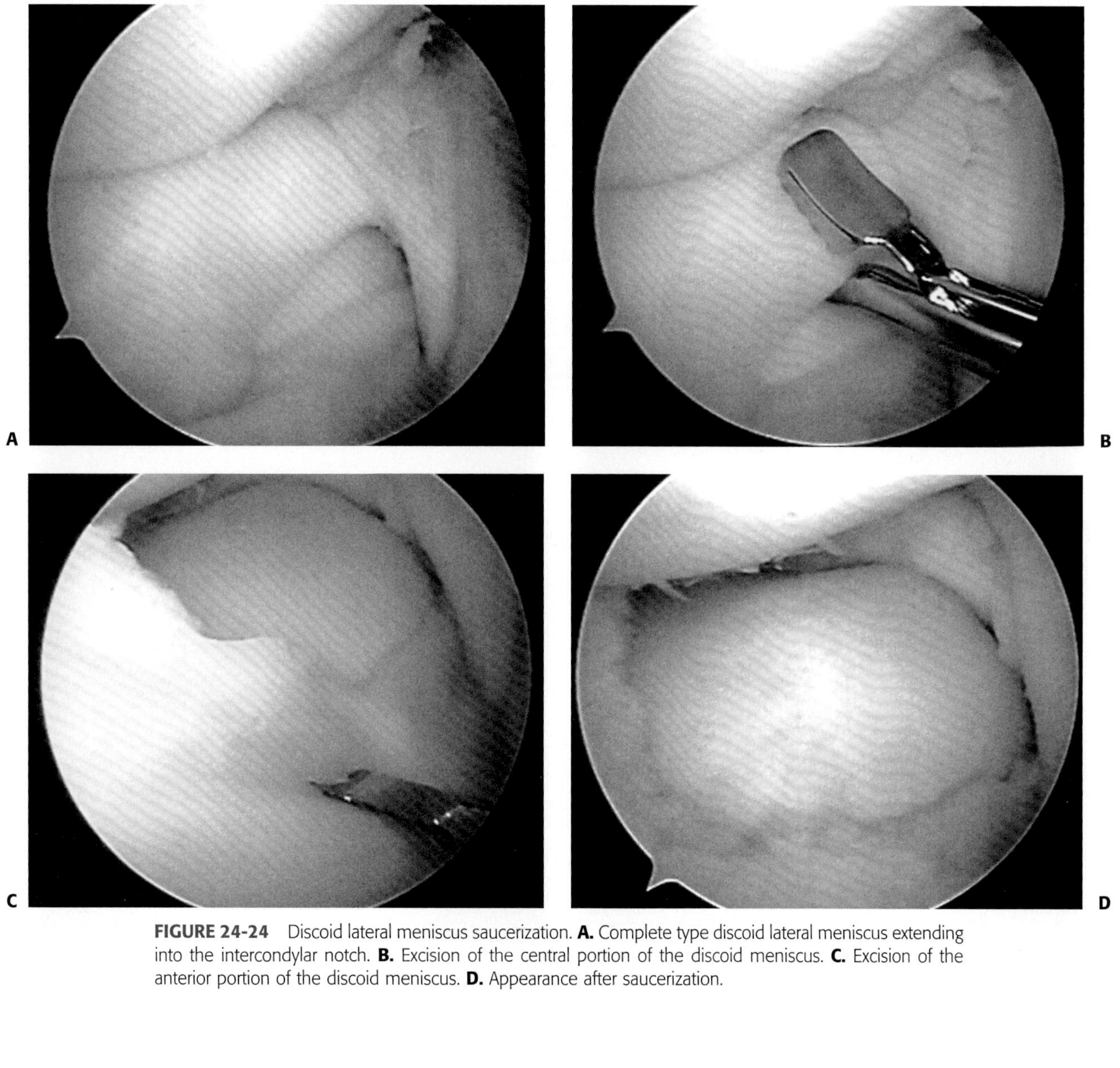

FIGURE 24-24 Discoid lateral meniscus saucerization. **A.** Complete type discoid lateral meniscus extending into the intercondylar notch. **B.** Excision of the central portion of the discoid meniscus. **C.** Excision of the anterior portion of the discoid meniscus. **D.** Appearance after saucerization.

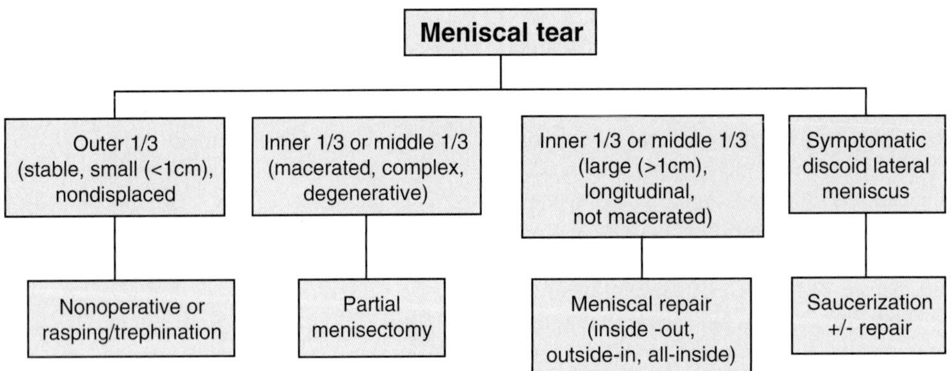

FIGURE 24-25 Algorithm for the management of meniscal tears in children and adolescents.

In a stable knee with an acute, arthroscopically documented outer third peripheral tear that is less than 1 cm long and cannot be displaced more than 3 mm, the tear is allowed to heal. For a similar tear in a chronic setting, we arthroscopically rasp or trephinate the interface between the meniscal edges and allow the tear to heal. Protected weight-bearing and limitation of flexion beyond 90 degrees is prescribed for 4 weeks. Healing can be assessed based on physical examination. Return to sports and activities is based on the absence of physical examination findings and adequate rehabilitation, usually at 2 to 3 months postoperatively.

For larger tears involving the outer third or middle third, which are longitudinal with a noncomminuted inner segment that can be reduced anatomically, meniscal repair is performed. In the chronic setting, rasping of the fragment edge, trephination, and use of a fibrin clot may enhance healing. Patients are protected postoperatively to allow for meniscal healing. Our postoperative protocol for isolated meniscal repair involves touch-down weight-bearing for 6 weeks postoperatively. Range of motion is restricted from 0 to 30 degrees for the first 2 weeks, followed by 0 to 90 degrees for the next 6 weeks. Progressive mobilization, strengthening, and sports-specific therapy are performed under the direction of a physical therapy protocol. Return to sports is allowed at 3 months postoperatively, if there is full range of motion, adequate strength, no symptoms (pain, swelling, locking), and resolution of physical examination findings (joint line tenderness, McMurray maneuvers, terminal range joint line pain). Follow-up MRI is performed only in patients with persistent symptoms or physical examination findings. Return to sports is typically 3 to 4 months after meniscal repair.

Partial meniscectomy is performed for tears involving the inner-third or middle-third tears that are macerated, horizontal, degenerative, or complex. Care should be taken to preserve as much tissue as possible (Fig. 24-26). With horizontal tears, the smaller of the two leaves is resected. Rehabilitation after partial meniscectomy includes weight-bearing

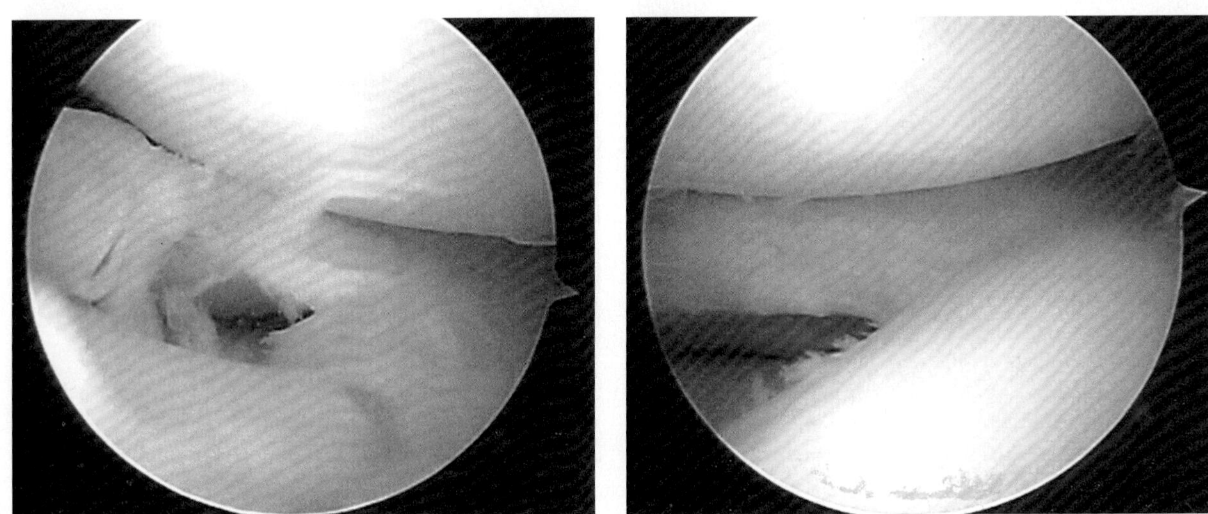

FIGURE 24-26 Complex inner-third tear of the meniscus **(A)** treated with partial meniscectomy **(B)**.

as tolerated, range of motion, and strengthening. Return to sports and activities is based on the absence of physical examination findings and adequate rehabilitation, usually at 2 to 3 months postoperatively. Patients who have undergone complete or near-total meniscectomy should be followed longer term to assess the development of degenerative changes. In symptomatic patients or those developing degenerative changes, replacement with an allograft meniscus or synthetic scaffold may be considered.

In children and adolescents, the emphasis should be on meniscal repair over meniscectomy whenever possible because of greater healing potential in this age-group, the long life span of these patients, the poor results of total and near-total meniscectomy, and the lack of longer-term results of partial meniscectomy. Meniscal repair techniques include inside-out techniques, outside-in techniques, and all-inside techniques. Outside-in techniques can be useful for anterior horn medial or lateral meniscal tears. For body and posterior horn tears, the traditional technique of meniscal repair has been inside-out repair with vertical or horizontal sutures (Fig. 24-27). Zone-specific cannulae are helpful to direct the flexible suture needles to the appropriate position to avoid neurovascular structures. In addition, we routinely make an incision posteromedially or posterolaterally to retrieve the suture needles and tie the sutures onto the joint capsule, thus protecting the saphenous nerve and vein medially and the peroneal nerve laterally. Newer all-inside devices have eased the technique of meniscal repair (Fig. 24-28). However, reports of articular cartilage damage from the heads of bioabsorbable arrows and darts exist (165,166). In addition, many of the available devices extend too far through the capsule in the small pediatric knee, with potential for neurovascular injury. We prefer more recent all-inside suture devices with a low profile in the joint. We tend to use these for posterior horn tears in adolescent knees. For smaller tears without substantial displacement, we use these alone. For larger tears with displacement such as displaced bucket-handle tears, we use these in a hybrid manner with inside-out sutures.

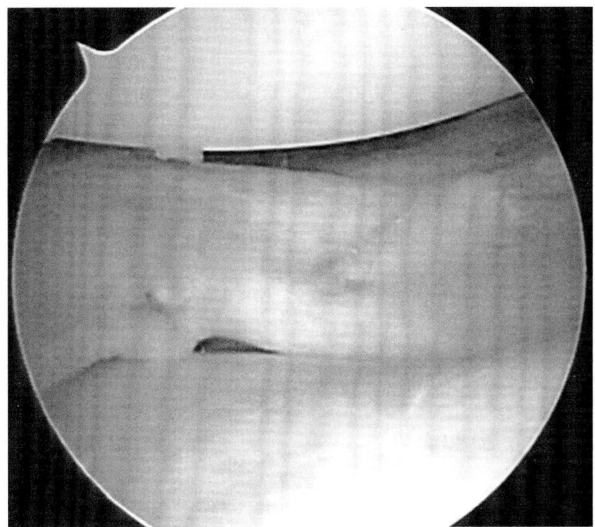

FIGURE 24-28 Longitudinal tear of the outer third of the posterior horn meniscus treated with all-inside fixation devices.

Bucket-handle displaced tears with a locked knee are treated urgently to allow for reduction and meniscal repair, and to avoid further injury to the meniscus. Meniscal tears in association with anterior cruciate ligament injuries are usually treated concurrently with anterior cruciate ligament reconstruction. Reconstruction is essential to provide a stable environment for meniscal healing and prevention of

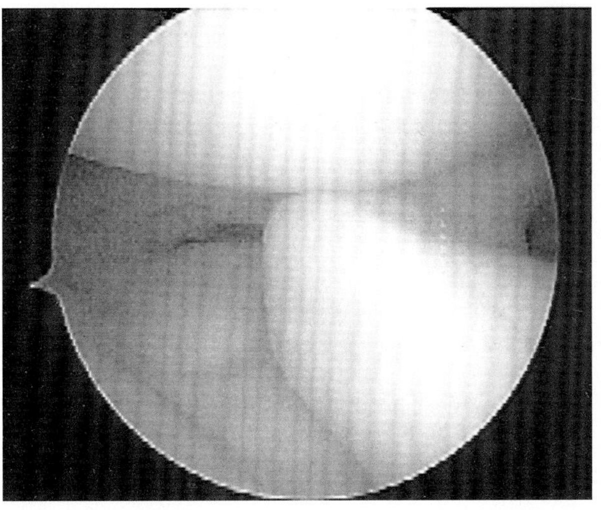

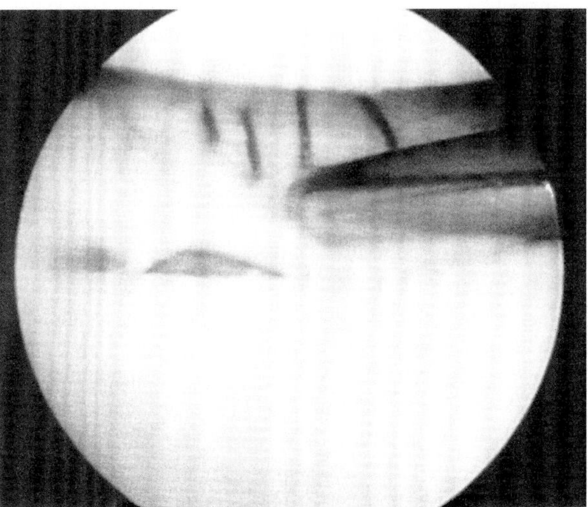

FIGURE 24-27 Longitudinal middle-third tear of the meniscus **(A)** treated with inside-out meniscal repair **(B)**.

further meniscal tears. Healing rates are high with concurrent anterior cruciate ligament reconstruction, perhaps because of the healing environment of the associated postoperative hemarthrosis. For meniscal repair in association with anterior cruciate ligament reconstruction, return to sports is dictated by the anterior cruciate ligament reconstruction, usually at 6 months postoperatively. For large, unstable meniscal tears requiring a more involved repair, staging of the anterior cruciate ligament reconstruction approximately 3 months after meniscal repair can be considered. This may result in a lower risk of arthrofibrosis, rehabilitation focused on meniscal repair, and arthroscopic assessment of meniscal healing at the time of reconstruction.

Pearls and Pitfalls

Making the diagnosis of a meniscal tear can be difficult in the child or adolescent. The differential diagnosis is varied and includes other injuries and disorders that cause pain and swelling or that cause joint line pain. Physical examination findings are variable. MRI scans must be carefully scrutinized because of the relatively high prevalence of normal signal changes in the posterior horns. Extension of the meniscal signal to the superior or inferior edge of the meniscal must be confirmed before considering the MRI diagnostic of a meniscal tear.

Total or near-total meniscectomy should be avoided in children and adolescents if at all possible, to avoid the development of degenerative changes. Patients who have had near total or total meniscectomy should be counseled regarding the risk of arthritis and the potential for meniscal replacement with allograft or synthetic scaffolds.

Several technical pitfalls exist during meniscal repair. During inside-out meniscal repair, a posterolateral incision should be made for lateral meniscal repair to avoid iatrogenic injury to the peroneal nerve, and a posteromedial incision should be made for medial meniscal repair to avoid iatrogenic injury to the saphenous vein or nerve. During all-inside repair with meniscal repair devices, consideration must be given to the size of the implant relative to the pediatric knee. Implants that protrude too far may injure neurovascular structures or cause local irritation or cysts. Implants that are high profile or protrude may damage the articular surface of the femoral condyle. Sterile effusions and synovitis may occur with bioabsorbable implants.

Prognosis and Complications

The prognosis after complete or near-total meniscectomy is poor, with numerous reports (110,116–119,124,126,127, 150,157,186,187,194,196,197,204) indicating poor long-term results with degenerative changes.

The prognosis of meniscal repair in appropriately selected cases is good. Mintzer and Richmond (120) reported on meniscal repair in 29 patients under the age of 18 (25 had closed physes and 17 underwent concomitant anterior cruciate ligament reconstruction). They reported 100% clinical healing at an average follow up of 5 years. Noyes and Barber-Westin (122) and Rubman et al (205) studied meniscal tears extending into the avascular zone in patients younger than 20 years old. Skeletal maturity had been reached in 88%. Their success rate in this group was 75%. This study showed a higher rate of healing with concomitant anterior cruciate ligament reconstruction. Eggli (162) found an overall healing rate for repair of isolated meniscal tears of 88% in patients younger than 30 years of age compared to 67% in patients over age 30. Johnson et al showed a 76% healing rate at an average follow up of greater than 10 years in a population that averaged 20 years old at the time of surgery (206). Factors that have been shown to correlate with increased healing of meniscal repairs include: younger age, decreased rim width (peripheral tears), repairs of the lateral meniscus, concomitant anterior cruciate ligament reconstruction, time from injury to surgery of less than 8 weeks, and tear length of less than 2.5 cm (161,162,165,166,206–208).

Complications after either arthroscopic or open repair may include hemorrhage, infection, persistent effusion, stiffness, and neuropathy. Both the popliteal artery and inferior geniculate branches are close to the posterior capsule can be easily lacerated. Postoperative infection should be suspected if swelling or pain persists with an elevated temperature. Swelling is best treated with external compression dressings, and stiffness is best prevented by appropriate postoperative rehabilitation. Neuroma formation rarely causes significant symptoms, but occasionally persistent localized tenderness may warrant excision.

LIGAMENT INJURIES

Ligamentous injuries of the knee in children and adolescents were once considered rare (209,210). Tibial eminence avulsion fractures were considered the pediatric anterior cruciate ligament injury equivalent (210–213). However, major ligamentous injuries are being seen with increased frequency and have received increased attention (214–251). The increased frequency of diagnosis of knee ligament injuries in children is likely related to increased participation in youth sports at higher competitive levels, the advent of arthroscopy and MRI, and an increased awareness of injuries in this age-group.

Anterior cruciate ligament injury has been reported in 10% to 65% of pediatric knees with acute traumatic hemarthroses in series ranging from 35 to 138 patients (227,233,250–252). Stanitski et al (253) reported 70 children and adolescents with acute traumatic knee hemarthroses; arthroscopic examination revealed anterior cruciate ligament injuries in 47% of those 7 to 12 years of age and in 65% of those 13 to 18 years of age. They determined that boys 16 to 18 years of age engaged in organized sports and girls 13 to 15 years of age engaged in unorganized sports had the highest risk for complete anterior cruciate ligament tears; 60% of these patients had isolated anterior cruciate ligament tears.

Injury patterns in the skeletally immature knee are dependent on the loading conditions and the developmental anatomy. Fractures of the epiphyses or physes about the knee are more common than ligamentous injuries alone. Isolated knee ligament injury in children younger than 14 years of age tends to be rare because of the relative strength of the ligaments compared to the physes (254–257). The inherent ligamentous laxity in children also may offer some protection against ligament injury, but this decreases as the adolescent approaches skeletal maturity. Faster loading conditions favor ligamentous injuries, whereas slower loading conditions favor fracture. Narrowing of the intercondylar notch during skeletal development may also predispose to ligamentous injury (212). Fractures and ligamentous injuries may occur concurrently. Bertin and Goble (258), after reviewing 29 fractures, concluded that physeal fractures about the knee are associated with a higher incidence of ligamentous injury. In addition, tibial eminence fractures, even after anatomic fixation and healing, tend to demonstrate persistent anterior cruciate ligament laxity (211).

Before the 1990s, reports of ligamentous injuries in children were isolated case reports, and most recommendations were for conservative treatment. More recent reports have indicated an increased awareness of ligament injury in association with physeal fractures (209), as well as isolated ligament injuries, and a more aggressive approach, especially in adolescents approaching skeletal maturity (225,226,259–262). Management of some of these injuries, particularly anterior cruciate ligament injuries in skeletally immature patients, is controversial. Nonreconstructive treatment of complete tears typically results in recurrent functional instability with risk of injury to meniscal and articular cartilage. A variety of reconstructive techniques have been used, including physeal sparing, partial transphyseal, and transphyseal methods using various grafts. Conventional adult anterior cruciate ligament reconstruction techniques risk potential iatrogenic growth disturbance as a result of physeal violation. Growth disturbances after reconstruction in skeletally immature patients have been reported.

Principles of Management

Mechanism of Injury

The mechanism of ligamentous injury varies with the child's age. In younger children, ligamentous injury typically is associated with significant polytrauma. Clanton et al (221) reported that five of nine children with acute knee ligament injuries were struck by automobiles. In contrast, adolescents are more likely to sustain ligamentous injury during contact sports or sports that require "cutting" maneuvers while running. As exact a description as possible of the mechanism of injury should be obtained, including the position of the knee at the time of injury, the weight-supporting status of the injured knee, whether the force applied was direct or indirect (generated by the patient's own momentum), and the position of the extremity after injury. Older adolescents may describe the knee as buckling or "jumping out of place" and can usually relate the location and severity of their pain as well as the time between injury and onset of pain and swelling. Rapid intra-articular effusion within 2 hours of injury suggests hemarthrosis, usually from injury to the anterior cruciate ligament.

Palmer (263) described four mechanisms capable of producing disruption of the ligamentous structures about the knee: abduction, flexion, and internal rotation of the femur on the tibia; adduction, flexion, and external rotation of the femur on the tibia; hyperextension; and anteroposterior displacement. The most common mechanism in adolescents is abduction, flexion, and internal rotation of the femur on the tibia occurring during athletic competition when the weight-bearing extremity is struck from the lateral side. The classic abduction, flexion, and internal rotation injury in the adolescent may cause the "unhappy triad" of O'Donoghue: tears of the medial collateral ligament and anterior cruciate ligament and injury to the medial meniscus.

Isolated injury of the lateral collateral ligament is rare in children, but a direct blow to the medial aspect of the knee may tear the lateral collateral ligament, usually with avulsion from the fibula or a physeal injury through the distal femur (264). Isolated injuries of the anterior and posterior cruciate ligaments have been reported (256,265,266). Disruption of the anterior cruciate ligament with minimal injury to other supporting structures may be caused by hyperextension, marked internal rotation of the tibia on the femur, and pure deceleration. In contrast, isolated injury of the posterior cruciate ligament most often is caused by a direct blow to the front of the tibia with the knee in flexion.

Signs and Symptoms

Both lower extremities are examined for comparison. Large areas of ecchymosis and extensive effusion are easily identified, but smaller areas may require careful palpation. In general, acute hemarthrosis suggests rupture of a cruciate ligament, an osteochondral fracture, a peripheral tear in the vascular portion of a meniscus, or a tear in the deep portion of the joint capsule (267,268). The absence of hemarthrosis is not, however, an indication of a less severe ligament injury, because with complete disruption the blood in the knee joint may escape into the soft tissues rather than distend the joint. The range of motion of the injured knee, especially extension, is compared with that of the uninjured knee. If significant effusion prevents full extension, sterile aspiration can be performed. If complete knee extension is impossible after aspiration, the diagnosis of an entrapped meniscus should be considered.

Palpation of the collateral ligaments and their bony origins and insertions should locate tenderness at the site of the ligament injury. A defect in the collateral ligaments often can be felt if the medial collateral ligament is avulsed from its insertion on the tibia or if the lateral collateral ligament is avulsed from the fibular head. If the neurovascular status is normal, stability should be evaluated by stress testing.

Stress testing for ligament injury in children (269,270), with or without concomitant fracture, is very subjective, and its usefulness depends on the knowledge and experience of the examiner. Stress testing may be done immediately after injury in cooperative adolescents who do not have other significant injuries, but sedation or general anesthesia may be required for accurate diagnosis. In nonemergent situations, beginning the

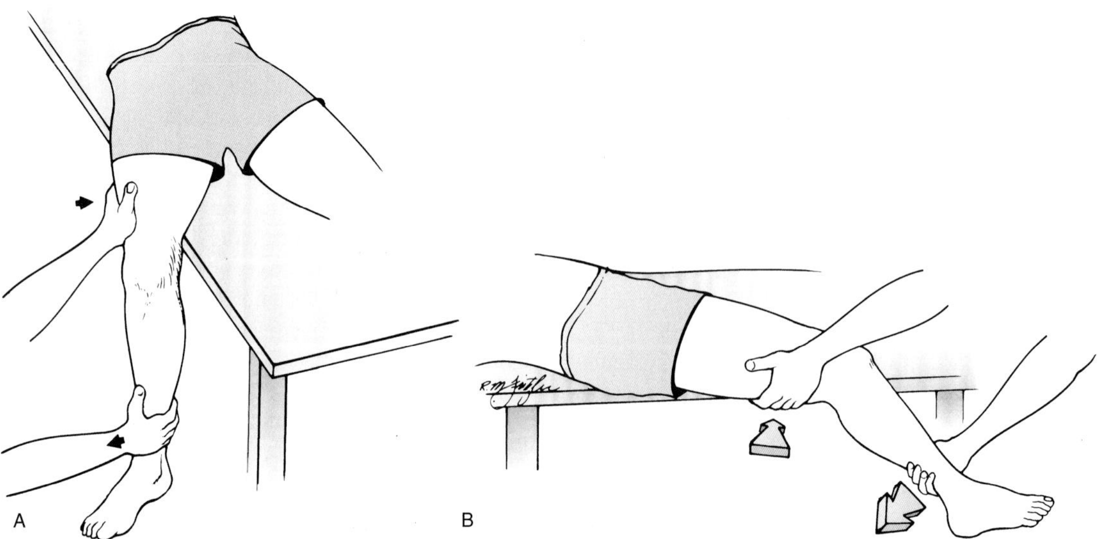

FIGURE 24-29 Valgus stress test of medial collateral ligament. Extremity is abducted off table, knee is flexed to 20 degrees, and valgus stress is applied. **A.** Frontal view. **B.** Lateral view.

examination by testing the uninjured knee often calms patients and makes them more cooperative; it also establishes a baseline for assessing the ligamentous stability of the injured knee. In the standard stress tests of specific collateral and cruciate ligaments of the knee described in the following sections, the uninjured knee should be examined first.

Valgus Stress Test of Medial Collateral Ligament. The valgus or abduction stress test is done with the child supine on the examining table and the knee to be examined on the side of the table closest to the examiner. The extremity is abducted off the side of the table, and the knee is flexed approximately 20 degrees (Fig. 24-29). With one hand about the lateral aspect of the knee and the other supporting the ankle, the examiner applies gentle abduction or valgus stress to the knee while the hand at the ankle gently externally rotates the leg. Stability of the knee is noted at 20 degrees of flexion and again at neutral.

Varus or Adduction Stress Test of Lateral Collateral Ligament. The varus or adduction stress test is done in a manner similar to the valgus stress test. It should be done with the knee in full extension and in 20 degrees of flexion. The lateral collateral ligament may be palpable as a taut structure on the lateral aspect of the knee.

The stability of the collateral ligaments may be different when tested in extension and in flexion. If a collateral ligament is torn but the cruciate ligaments and posterior capsule are intact, little instability can be detected with the knee extended. Flexion of the knee relaxes the capsule, and more instability is evident with the same degree of ligamentous injury. Significant instability with varus or valgus stress testing with the knee in full extension usually indicates a cruciate as well as a collateral ligament disruption.

Stress Testing of Anterior Cruciate Ligament. The anterior drawer test, as described by Slocum, is the classic maneuver for testing the stability of the anterior cruciate ligament (Fig. 24-30). The Lachman and pivot-shift tests, however, are considered more sensitive for evaluating anterior cruciate ligament injury when the examination can be done in a relaxed, cooperative

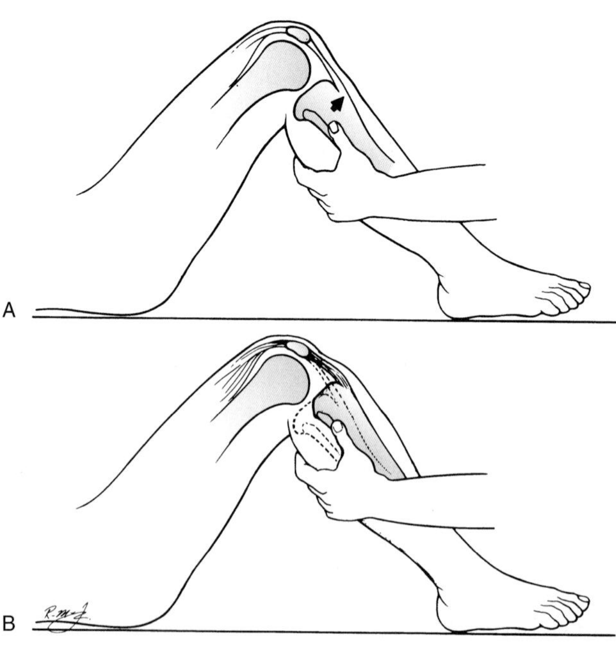

FIGURE 24-30 Anterior drawer test of anterior cruciate ligament. Foot is positioned in internal, external, and neutral rotation during examination. With anterior cruciate insufficiency, an anterior force **(A)** displaces the tibia forward **(B)**.

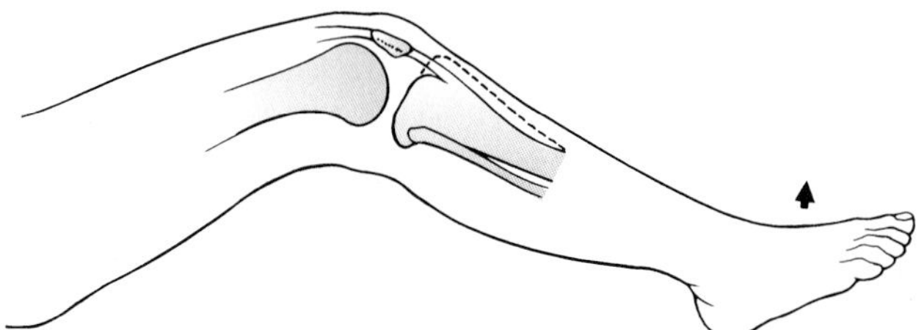

FIGURE 24-31 Lateral pivot-shift test of anterior cruciate ligament.

adolescent (Fig. 24-31). To perform the Lachman test, the examiner firmly stabilizes the femur with one hand while using the other hand to grip the proximal tibia, with the thumb placed on the anteromedial joint margin. An anteriorly directed lifting force applied by the palm and fingers causes anterior translation of the tibia in relation to the femur that can be palpated by the thumb; a soft or mushy end point indicates a positive test. When the anterior cruciate ligament is disrupted, the normal patellar ligament slope is obliterated.

Stress Testing of Posterior Cruciate Ligament. The posterior drawer test for evaluation of the posterior cruciate ligament is done with the patient supine. With the patient's foot secured to the table and the hip flexed 90 degrees, a posterior force is applied to the proximal tibia. Posterior movement of the tibia on the femur greater than in the uninjured extremity indicates posterior instability (Fig. 24-32).

Imaging

Anteroposterior and lateral x-rays are obtained when any ligament injury of the knee is suspected in children. The films are carefully inspected for evidence of occult epiphyseal or physeal fractures or bony avulsions. The intercondylar notch, especially, is inspected to detect a tibial spine fracture, which is confirmed by anterior or posterior instability on physical examination. Occasionally, a small fragment of bone avulsed from the medial femur or proximal tibia indicates injury to the medial collateral ligament. Similarly, avulsion of a small fragment of bone from the proximal fibular epiphysis or the lateral aspect of the distal femur may indicate lateral collateral ligament injury.

In children with open physes, stress x-rays may be helpful to evaluate medial and lateral instability associated with physeal fractures. Gentle stress views may be obtained with sedation, but general anesthesia may be required if the diagnosis is unclear. Stress must be performed carefully to avoid further physeal injury that may lead to physeal arrest. There are no accepted guidelines correlating joint space widening medially or laterally with knee joint instability in children, and stress views of the opposite knee may be required for comparison. If plain x-rays show a fracture of the distal femoral or proximal tibial physis, stress views may be obtained only to evaluate suspected ligamentous instability. Conversely, if the initial films appear normal but there is significant effusion about the knee, stress views may be obtained to rule out a fracture of the physis of the distal femur or proximal tibia.

Other x-ray findings include avulsion of the anterior or posterior tibial spine, indicative of injury to the anterior or posterior cruciate ligaments, widening of the joint space, and posterior subluxation of the tibia on the femur. Clanton et al (221) consider a joint space of 8 mm or wider to be a definitive indication of ligament injury. Sanders et al (266) reported 1.8 cm of posterior subluxation of the tibia on the anteroposterior stress view in a 6-year-old child with complete posterior cruciate ligament disruption.

MRI is frequently used to further delineate ligamentous injuries in the knee. It should be used to confirm an uncertain diagnosis or to gain further information that may affect treat-

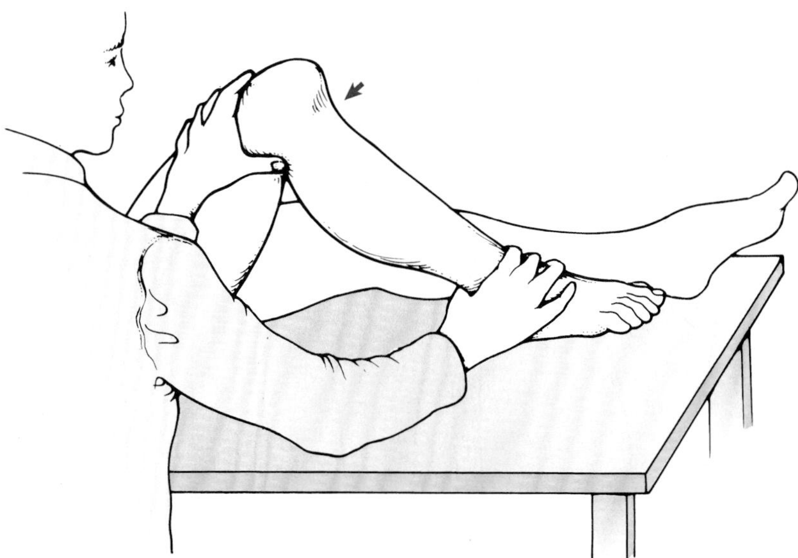

FIGURE 24-32 Posterior cruciate ligament injury. Note posterior sagging of the tibia with posterior cruciate injury.

TABLE 24-2 Anatomic Classification of Ligament Injuries, Indicating Exact Location of the Disruption

A. Medial collateral ligament insufficiency (see Fig. 24-33)
   1. Femoral origin
   2. Middle portion
   3. Tibial insertion

B. Anterior cruciate ligament insufficiency
   1. Femoral origin
   2. Interstitial
   3. Tibial insertion
      a. Without avulsion of the intercondylar eminence
      b. With avulsion of the intercondylar eminence

C. Lateral collateral ligament insufficiency (see Fig. 24-34)
   1. Femoral origin
   2. Middle portion
   3. Fibular insertion

D. Posterior cruciate ligament insufficiency
   1. Femoral origin
   2. Interstitial
   3. Tibial insertion
      a. Without avulsion fracture
      b. With avulsion fracture

ment. Conventional MRI can give information regarding medial collateral ligament injury, lateral collateral ligament injury, anterior cruciate ligament injury, posterior cruciate ligament injury, posterolateral corner injury, bone bruising, chondral injury, and meniscal injury.

Classification

Classification of knee ligament injuries is based on the severity of the injury, the specific anatomic location of the injury, and the direction of the subsequent instability caused by an isolated ligament injury or combination of ligament injuries.

A first-degree ligament sprain is a tear of a minimal number of fibers of the ligament with localized tenderness but no instability. A second-degree sprain is disruption of more ligamentous fibers, causing loss of function and more joint reaction but no significant instability. A third-degree sprain is complete disruption of the ligament, resulting in instability. Although difficult to assess clinically, the degree of sprain also is determined during stress testing by the amount of separation of the joint surfaces: first-degree sprain, 5 mm or less; second-degree sprain, 5 to 10 mm; and third-degree sprain, more than 10 mm.

Table 24-2 outlines the anatomic classification of ligament injuries that describes the exact location of the disruption (Figs. 24-33 and 24-34) (271).

Finally, the instability of the knee joint caused by the ligament disruption is classified is outlined in Table 24-3 (272,273).

Using this classification, one-plane medial instability, for example, means that the tibia moves abnormally away from the

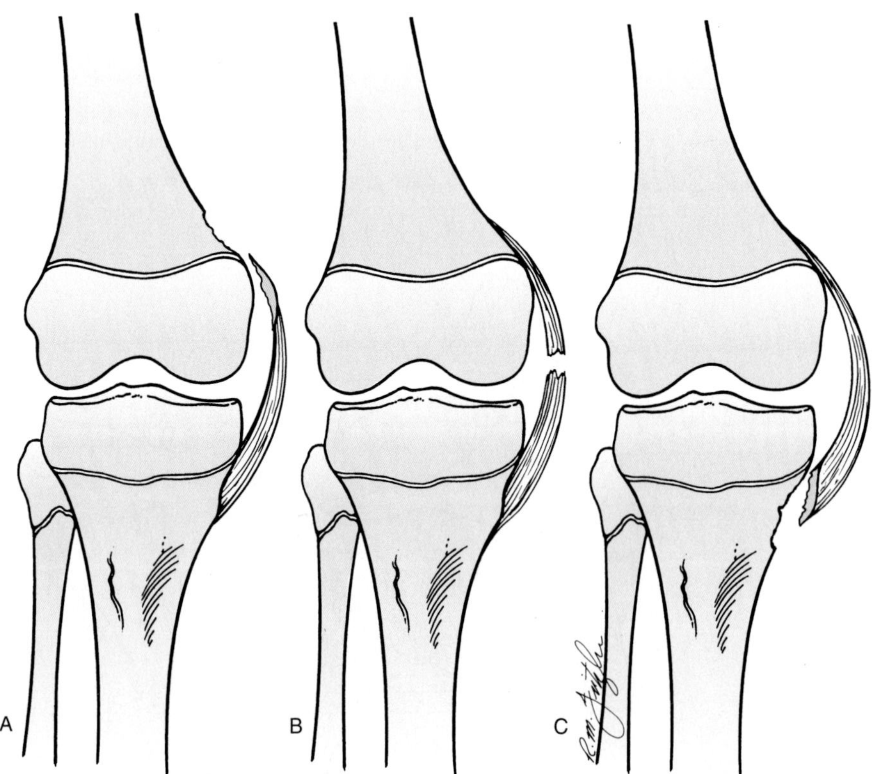

FIGURE 24-33 Medial collateral ligament injury. **A.** Femoral origin. **B.** Middle portion. **C.** Tibial insertion.

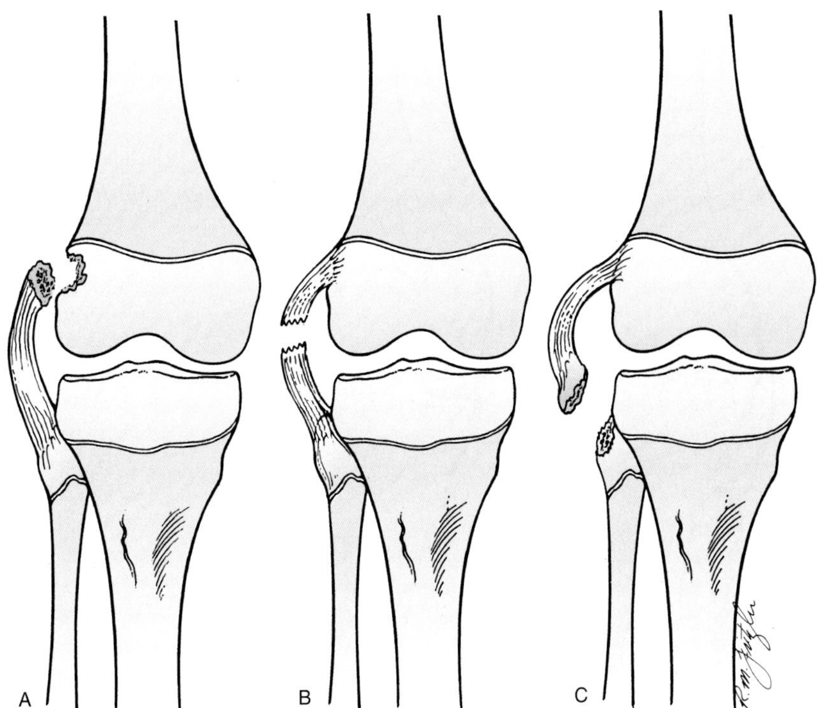

FIGURE 24-34 Lateral collateral ligament injury. **A.** Femoral origin. **B.** Middle portion. **C.** Fibular insertion.

femur on the medial side. In anteromedial rotary instability, the tibia rotates anteriorly and externally and moves away from the femur on the medial side. The classification becomes more complex as more significant ligamentous injuries involving more anatomic locations are included, but determining the type of instability resulting from the injury is helpful in planning treatment.

TABLE 24-3 Classification of Instability of the Knee Joint Caused by Ligament Disruption

A. One-plane instability (simple or straight)
   1. One-plane medial
   2. One-plane lateral
   3. One-plane posterior
   4. One-plane anterior

B. Rotary instability
   1. Anteromedial
   2. Anterolateral
      a. In flexion
      b. Approaching extension
   3. Posterolateral
   4. Posteromedial

C. Combined instability
   1. Anterolateral–posterolateral
   2. Anterolateral–anteromedial
   3. Anteromedial–posteromedial

Surgical and Applied Anatomy

The medial and lateral collateral ligaments of the knee originate from the distal femoral epiphysis and insert into the proximal tibial and fibular epiphyses, except for the superficial portion of the medial collateral ligament, which inserts into the proximal tibial metaphysis distal to the physis (Fig. 24-35). In children, these ligaments are stronger than the physes, and significant tensile stresses usually produce epiphyseal or physeal fractures rather than ligamentous injury. The anterior cruciate ligament originates from the posterolateral intercondylar notch and inserts into the tibia slightly anterior to the intercondylar eminence. The posterior cruciate ligament originates from the posteromedial aspect of the intercondylar notch and attaches on the posterior aspect of the proximal tibial epiphysis. The anterior cruciate ligament in children has collagen fibers continuous with the perichondrium of the tibial epiphyseal cartilage; in adults, the ligament inserts directly into the proximal tibia by way of Sharpey's fibers. This anatomic difference probably accounts for the fact that fracture of the anterior tibial spine occurs more frequently in children than does anterior cruciate ligament injury.

Current Treatment Options

Isolated collateral ligament injuries are usually successfully treated with bracing and rehabilitation.

Controversy exists regarding the management of anterior cruciate ligament injuries in patients with open physes. Nonoperative management of partial tears may be successful in some patients (235). However, nonoperative management of com-

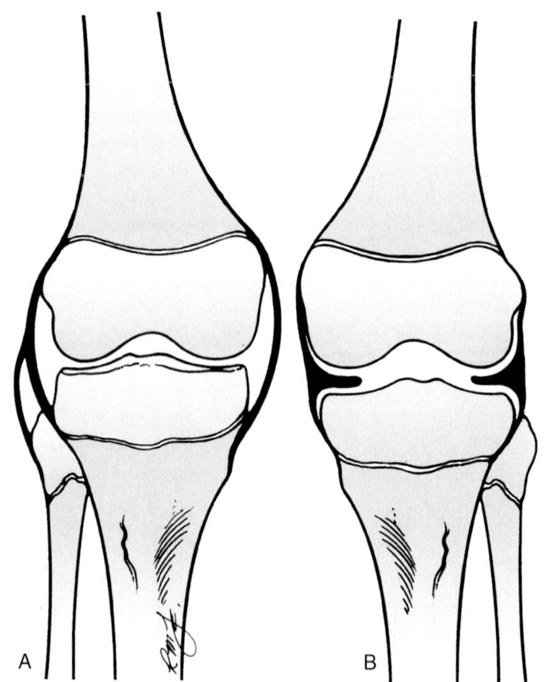

FIGURE 24-35 Anatomy of medial and collateral ligaments of the knee in the adolescent. **A.** Superficial origins and insertions. **B.** Capsular and meniscal attachments.

plete tears in skeletally immature patients generally has a poor prognosis with recurrent instability leading to further meniscal and chondral injury, which has implications in terms of development of degenerative joint disease (214,229,232,244–246,274). Graf et al (229), Mizuta et al (245), and Janarv et al (232) have reported instability symptoms, subsequent meniscal tears, decreased activity level, and need for anterior cruciate ligament reconstruction in the majority of skeletally immature patients treated nonoperatively in series of 8, 18, and 23 patients, respectively. Similarly, when comparing the results of operative versus nonoperative management of complete anterior cruciate ligament injuries in adolescents, McCarroll et al (274) and Pressman et al (246) found that those managed by anterior cruciate ligament reconstruction had less instability, higher activity and return to sport levels, and lower rates of subsequent reinjury and meniscal tears.

Conventional surgical reconstruction techniques risk potential iatrogenic growth disturbance as a result of physeal violation. Cases of growth disturbance have been reported in animal models (224,230,275) and clinical series (236–238). Animal models have demonstrated mixed results regarding growth disturbances from soft tissue grafts across the physes. In a canine model with iliotibial band grafts through 5/32-inch tunnels, Stadelmeier et al (249) found no evidence of growth arrest in the four animals with soft tissue graft across the physis, whereas the four animals with drill holes and no graft demonstrated physeal arrest. In a rabbit model using a semitendinosus graft through 2-mm tunnels, Guzzanti et al (230) did have cases of growth disturbance; however, these were not common: 5% shortening (1/21) and 10% distal femoral valgus deformity (2/21). Examining the effect of a tensioned soft tissue graft across the physis, Edwards et al (224) found a substantial rate of deformity. In a canine model with iliotibial band graft tensioned to 80 N, these investigators found significant increases compared to the nonoperated control limb in distal femoral valgus deformity and proximal tibial varus deformity, despite no evidence of a bony bar. Similarly, Houle et al (275) reported growth disturbance after a tensioned tendon graft in a bone tunnel across the rabbit physis.

Clinical reports of growth deformity after anterior cruciate ligament reconstruction are unusual. Lipscomb and Anderson (238) reported one case of 20-mm shortening in a series of 24 skeletally immature patients reconstructed with transphyseal semitendinosus and gracilis grafts. This was associated with staple graft fixation across the physis. Koman and Sanders (236) reported a case of distal femoral valgus deformity requiring osteotomy and contralateral epiphyseodesis after transphyseal reconstruction with a doubled semitendinosus graft. This case was also associated with fixation across the distal femoral physis. Kocher et al (237) reported an additional 15 cases of growth disturbances gleaned from a questionnaire of expert experience, including 8 cases of distal femoral valgus deformity with an arrest of the lateral distal femoral physis, 3 cases of tibial recurvatum with an arrest of the tibial tubercle apophysis, 2 cases of genu valgum without arrest resulting from a lateral extra-articular tether, and 2 cases of leg length discrepancy (1 shortening and 1 overgrowth). Associated factors included fixation hardware across the lateral distal femoral physis in 3 cases, bone plugs of a patellar tendon graft across the distal femoral physis in 3 cases, large (12 mm) tunnels in 2 cases, lateral extra-articular tenodesis in 2 cases, fixation hardware across the tibial tubercle apophysis in 2 cases, over-the-top femoral position in one case, and suturing near the tibial tubercle apophysis in 1 case.

Surgical techniques to address anterior cruciate ligament insufficiency in skeletally immature patients include primary repair, extra-articular tenodesis, transphyseal reconstruction, partial transphyseal reconstruction, and physeal sparing reconstruction. Primary ligament repair (221,276) and extra-articular tenodesis alone (229,274) have had poor results in children and adolescents, similar to results in adults. Transphyseal reconstructions with tunnels that violate both the distal femoral and proximal tibial physes have been performed with hamstring autograft, patellar tendon autograft, and allograft tissue (214,217,218,223,228,241,242,247,248,250,274,277). Partial transphyseal reconstructions violate only one physis with a tunnel through the proximal tibial physis and over-the-top positioning on the femur or a tunnel through the distal femoral physis with an epiphyseal tunnel in the tibia (216,219,239,278). A variety of physeal-sparing reconstructions have been described to avoid tunnels across either the distal femoral or proximal tibial physis (215,220,222,231–234,251,252,279).

In prepubescent patients, physeal sparing techniques have

been described that use hamstring tendons under the intermeniscal ligament and over-the-top on the femur, through all-epiphyseal femoral and tibial tunnels, and with a femoral epiphyseal staple (215,220,222,231–234,251,252,279). In adolescent patients with growth remaining, transphyseal reconstructions have been performed with hamstring autograft, patellar tendon autograft, and allograft tissue (214,217,218, 223,228,241,242,247,248,274,277).

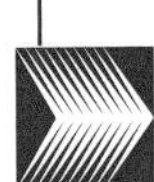

AUTHOR'S PREFERRED TREATMENT

Medial Collateral Ligament

Isolated grade I or II sprains of the medial collateral ligament are treated with crutches or a hinged knee brace for 1 to 3 weeks, depending on resolution of symptoms. Return to athletic activities is allowed when a full, painless range of motion is achieved and the patient can run and cut without pain. Isolated complete (grade III) disruption of the medial collateral ligament can be treated with 6 weeks of immobilization in a hinged knee brace followed by rehabilitation of the quadriceps muscles and knee motion provided this is an isolated injury. The physician must ensure that there is no associated injury to the anterior cruciate ligament before using nonoperative treatment for a grade III medial collateral ligament injury. Grade III disruptions of the medial collateral ligament in adolescents associated with injury of the anterior cruciate ligament are usually treated with anterior cruciate ligament reconstruction without formal medial collateral ligament repair. The medial collateral ligament is protected with a hinged knee brace and allowed to heal.

Anterior Cruciate Ligament

A torn anterior cruciate ligament does not constitute a surgical emergency, despite the image projected by celebrity athletes and their urgent care. A frank discussion must be held with the parents and the patient concerning future vocation, sport demands, treatment options, outcomes, and risks involved with return to current sport activity. The orthopaedic surgeon must assume the role of a "knee counselor," particularly with patients with a history of chronic knee abuse. All treatment algorithms are based on an accurate and complete diagnosis, which is achieved by clinical, imaging, and, if necessary, arthroscopic means. The treatment goal is a functional knee without progressive intra-articular damage or predisposition to premature osteoarthrosis.

All skeletally immature patients are not the same. Some have a tremendous amount of growth remaining, whereas others are essentially done growing. The consequences of growth disturbance in the former group would be severe, requiring osteotomy or limb lengthening. However, the consequences of growth disturbance in the latter group would be minimal. When treating a skeletally immature athlete with an anterior cruciate ligament injury, it is important to know his chronologic age, skeletal age, and physiologic age. Skeletal age can be determined from an anteroposterior x-ray of the left hand and wrist per the atlas of Greulich and Pyle (280). Alternatively, skeletal age can be estimated from knee x-rays per the atlas of Pyle and Hoerr (281). Physiologic age is established using the Tanner staging system (Table 24-4) (282). In the office, the patient can be informally staged by questioning. In the operating room, after the induction of anesthesia, Tanner staging can be confirmed. The vast majority of anterior cruciate ligament injuries in skeletally immature patients occur in adolescents. The management of these injuries in preadolescent children is particularly vexing, given the poor prognosis with nonoperative management, the substantial growth remaining, and the consequences of potential growth disturbance.

Nonsurgical treatment does not indicate nontreatment. The goal of this program is defined from the outset: it is a temporizing measure until the patient becomes mature enough for an adult-type anterior cruciate ligament reconstruction, or it is the definitive choice for a patient willing to accept the functional limitations. We use a three-phase approach. Phase one begins shortly after injury and lasts 7 to 10 days. Brief immobilization (3 to 5 days) with a knee immobilizer for comfort is followed by daily out-of-brace exercises with active knee flexion and passive knee extension. Ambulation is with crutch-protected partial weight-bearing. During this time, we reinforce patient education on the consequences of imprudent return to high-level sports. Phase two focuses on rehabilitation of the lower extremity and lasts approximately 6 weeks. Emphasis is placed on restoration of full knee motion, flexibility, strength, and endurance, with particular attention to regaining the normal quadriceps/hamstring strength ratio. As the ratio is normalized, crutch use is decreased and then eliminated. The role of functional bracing has not been defined in children and issues of fit, size, and cost need to be considered. Phase three continues the rehabilitation, incorporates the use of a functional brace for sports, and allows return to low- and moderate-demand sports when quadriceps and hamstring strength and endurance are equal to those of the opposite, noninjured side as determined by isokinetic testing at functional speeds (>260 degrees/second). In the final part of this phase, sports readiness tasks are done at less than full speed. Monthly follow-up evaluates program compliance and rules out any further knee changes in function. Compliance with a nonoperative program designed to be a temporizing measure often is quite difficult for an emerging athlete who is surrounded by peer, coaching, and, often, parental pressures to return to high-demand sports.

Our algorithm for anterior cruciate ligament reconstruction in the skeletally immature patient is based on physio-

TABLE 24-4 Tanner Staging Classification of Secondary Sexual Characteristics

Tanner Stage		Male	Female
Stage 1 (prepubertal)	Growth Development	5 to 6 cm/yr Testes <4 mL or <2.5 cm No pubic hair	5 to 6 cm/yr No breast development No pubic hair
Stage 2	Growth Development	5 to 6 cm/yr Testes 4 mL or 2.5 to 3.2 cm Minimal pubic hair at base of penis	7 to 8 cm/yr Breast buds Minimal pubic hair on labia
Stage 3	Growth Development	7 to 8 cm/yr Testes 12 mL or 3.6 cm Pubic hair over pubis Voice changes Muscle mass increases	8 cm/yr Elevation of breast; areolae enlarge Pubic hair of mons pubis Axillary hair Acne
Stage 4	Growth Development	10 cm/yr Testes 4.1 to 4.5 cm Pubic hair as adult Axillary hair Acne	7 cm/yr Areolae enlarge Pubic hair as adult
Stage 5	Growth Development	No growth Testes as adult Pubic hair as adult Facial hair as adult Mature physique	No growth Adult breast contour Pubic hair as adult
Other		Peak height velocity: 13.5 years	Adrenarche: 6 to 8 years Menarche: 12.7 years Peak height velocity: 11.5 years

logic age (Fig. 24-36). In prepubescent patients, we perform a physeal-sparing, combined intra-articular and extra-articular reconstruction using autogenous iliotibial band. In adolescent patients with significant growth remaining, we perform transphyseal anterior cruciate ligament reconstruction with autogenous hamstring tendons with fixation away from the physes. In older adolescent patients approaching skeletal maturity, we perform conventional adult anterior cruciate ligament reconstruction with interference screw fixation using either autogenous central third patellar tendon or autogenous hamstrings.

In skeletally immature patients as in adult patients, acute anterior cruciate ligament reconstruction is not performed within the first 3 weeks after injury to minimize the risk of arthrofibrosis. Prereconstructive rehabilitation is performed to regain range of motion, decrease swelling, and resolve the reflex inhibition of the quadriceps. Anterior cruciate ligament reconstruction may be staged in some cases if there is a displaced, bucket-handle tear of the meniscus that requires extensive repair to protect the meniscal repair from the early mobilization prescribed by anterior cruciate ligament reconstruction. Skeletally immature patients must be emotionally mature enough to actively participate in the extensive rehabilitation required after anterior cruciate ligament reconstruction.

Prepubescent Patient: Physeal-Sparing Anterior Cruciate Ligament Reconstruction. In the prepubescent patient with a complete anterior cruciate ligament tear without concurrent chondral or repairable meniscal injury, we first attempt nonreconstructive treatment with a program of rehabilitation, functional bracing, and return to non-high-risk activities. Although the results of nonreconstructive treatment are generally poor, with subsequent functional instability and risk of injury to meniscal and articular cartilage, surgical reconstruction poses the risk of growth disturbance. Furthermore, some patients are able to cope with their anterior cruciate ligament insufficiency or modify their activities, allowing for further growth and aging such that an adolescent-type reconstruction can be performed with transphyseal hamstring tendons in a more anatomic manner.

For those prepubescent patients with concurrent chon-

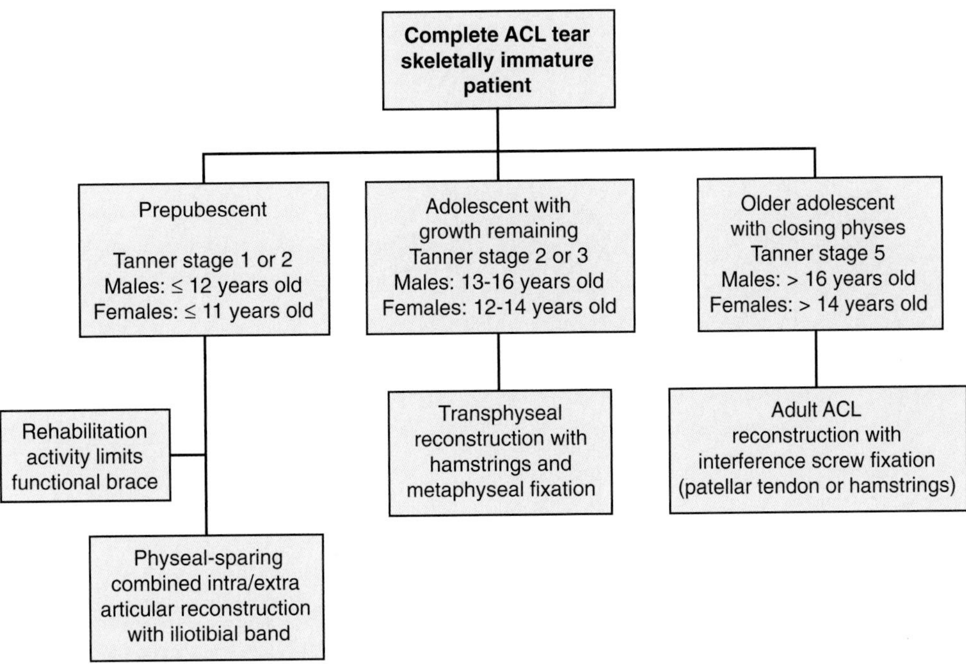

FIGURE 24-36 Algorithm for anterior cruciate ligament reconstruction in skeletally immature patients.

dral or repairable meniscal injury, or those with functional instability after nonreconstructive treatment, we perform a physeal-sparing, combined intra-articular and extra-articular reconstruction using autogenous iliotibial band (Fig. 24-37). This procedure is a modification of the combined intra-articular and extra-articular reconstruction described by MacIntosh (273). Our rationale for use of this technique is to provide knee stability and improve function in prepubescent skeletally immature patients with complete intrasubstance anterior cruciate ligament injuries while avoiding the risk of iatrogenic growth disturbance by violating the distal femoral and proximal tibial physes. In our opinion, the consequences of potential iatrogenic growth disturbance caused by transphyseal reconstruction in these young patients is prohibitive. Recognizing that this reconstruction is nonanatomic, we counsel patients and families that they may require revision reconstruction if they develop recurrent instability, but that this procedure may temporize for further growth such that they may then undergo a more conventional reconstruction with drill holes.

The procedure is performed under general anesthesia as an overnight observation procedure. Local anesthesia with sedation may not be reliable in prepubescent children with the potential for a paradoxical effect of sedation. The child is positioned supine on the operating table with a pneumatic tourniquet about the upper thigh, which is used routinely. Examination under anesthesia is performed to confirm anterior cruciate ligament insufficiency.

First, the iliotibial band graft is obtained. An incision of approximately 6 cm is made obliquely from the lateral joint line to the superior border of the iliotibial band (Fig. 24-38A). Proximally, the iliotibial band is separated from subcutaneous tissue using a periosteal elevator under the skin of the lateral thigh. The anterior and posterior borders of the iliotibial band are incised and the incisions carried proximally under the skin using curved meniscotomes (see Fig. 24-38A). The iliotibial band is detached proximally under the skin using a curved meniscotome or an open tendon stripper. Alternatively, a counter incision can be made at the upper thigh to release the tendon. The iliotibial band is left attached distally at Gerdy's tubercle. Dissection is performed distally to separate the iliotibial band from the joint capsule and from the lateral patellar retinaculum (Fig. 24-38B). The free proximal end of the iliotibial band is then tubularized with a no. 5 Ethibond whip stitch.

Arthroscopy of the knee is then performed through standard anterolateral viewing and anteromedial working portals. Management of meniscal injury or chondral injury is performed if needed. The anterior cruciate ligament remnant is excised. The over-the-top position on the femur and the over-the front position under the intermeniscal ligament are identified. Minimal notchplasty is performed to avoid iatrogenic injury to the perichondrial ring of the distal femoral physis which is in very close proximity to the over-the-top position (284). The free end of the iliotibial band graft is brought through the over-the-top position using a full-length clamp (Fig. 24-38C) or a two-incision rear-entry guide (see Fig. 24-37) and out the anteromedial portal (Fig. 24-38D).

A second incision of approximately 4.5 cm is made over the proximal medial tibia in the region of the pes anserinus

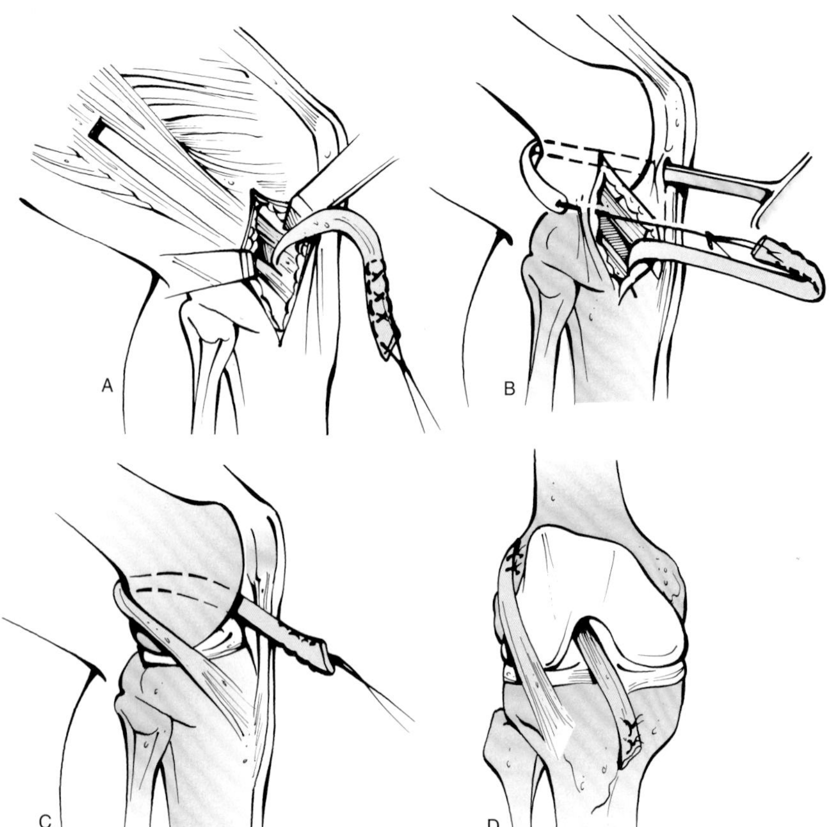

FIGURE 24-37 Physeal-sparing, combined intra-articular and extra-articular reconstruction using autogenous iliotibial band for prepubescents. **A.** The iliotibial band graft is harvested free proximally and left attached to Gerdy's tubercle distally. **B.** The graft is brought through the knee in the over-the-top position posteriorly. **C.** The graft is brought through the knee and under the intermeniscal ligament anteriorly. **D.** Resulting intra-articular and extra-articular reconstruction.

insertion. Dissection is carried through the subcutaneous tissue to the periosteum. A curved clamp is placed from this incision into the joint under the intermeniscal ligament (Fig. 24-38E). A small groove is made in the anteromedial proximal tibial epiphysis under the intermeniscal ligament using a curved rat-tail rasp to bring the tibial graft placement more posterior. The free end of the graft is then brought through the joint (Fig. 24-38F), under the intermeniscal ligament in the anteromedial epiphyseal groove, and out the medial tibial incision (Fig. 24-38G). The graft is fixed on the femoral side through the lateral incision with the knee at 90 degrees flexion and 15 degrees external rotation using mattress sutures to the lateral femoral condyle at the insertion of the lateral intermuscular septum to effect an extra-articular reconstruction (Fig. 24-38H). The tibial side is then fixed through the medial incision with the knee flexed 20 degrees and tension applied to the graft. A periosteal incision is made distal to the proximal tibial physis as confirmed with fluoroscopic imaging. A trough is made in the proximal tibial medial metaphyseal cortex, and the graft is sutured to the periosteum at the rough margins with mattress sutures (see Fig. 24-37).

Postoperatively, the patient is maintained on touch-down weight-bearing for 6 weeks. Range of motion is limited from 0 to 90 degrees for the first 2 weeks, followed by progressive full range of motion. Continuous passive motion from 0 to 90 degrees and cryotherapy are used for 2 weeks postoperatively. A protective postoperative brace is used for 6 weeks postoperatively.

Skeletally Immature Adolescent Patient: Transphyseal Anterior Cruciate Ligament Reconstruction. For adolescent patients with growth remaining who have a complete anterior cruciate ligament tear, we do not advocate initial nonreconstructive treatment because the risk of functional instability with injury to the meniscal and articular cartilage is high. The risk and consequences of growth disturbance from anterior cruciate ligament reconstruction are less, and our transphyseal technique is an anatomic reconstruction. In these patients, we perform transphyseal anterior cruciate ligament reconstruction with autogenous hamstring tendons with fixation away from the physes.

The procedure is performed under general anesthesia as an overnight observation procedure. Local anesthesia with sedation may be performed in the emotionally mature adolescent child. The patient is positioned supine on the operating table with a pneumatic tourniquet about the upper thigh, which is not used routinely. Examination under anesthesia is performed to confirm anterior cruciate ligament insufficiency.

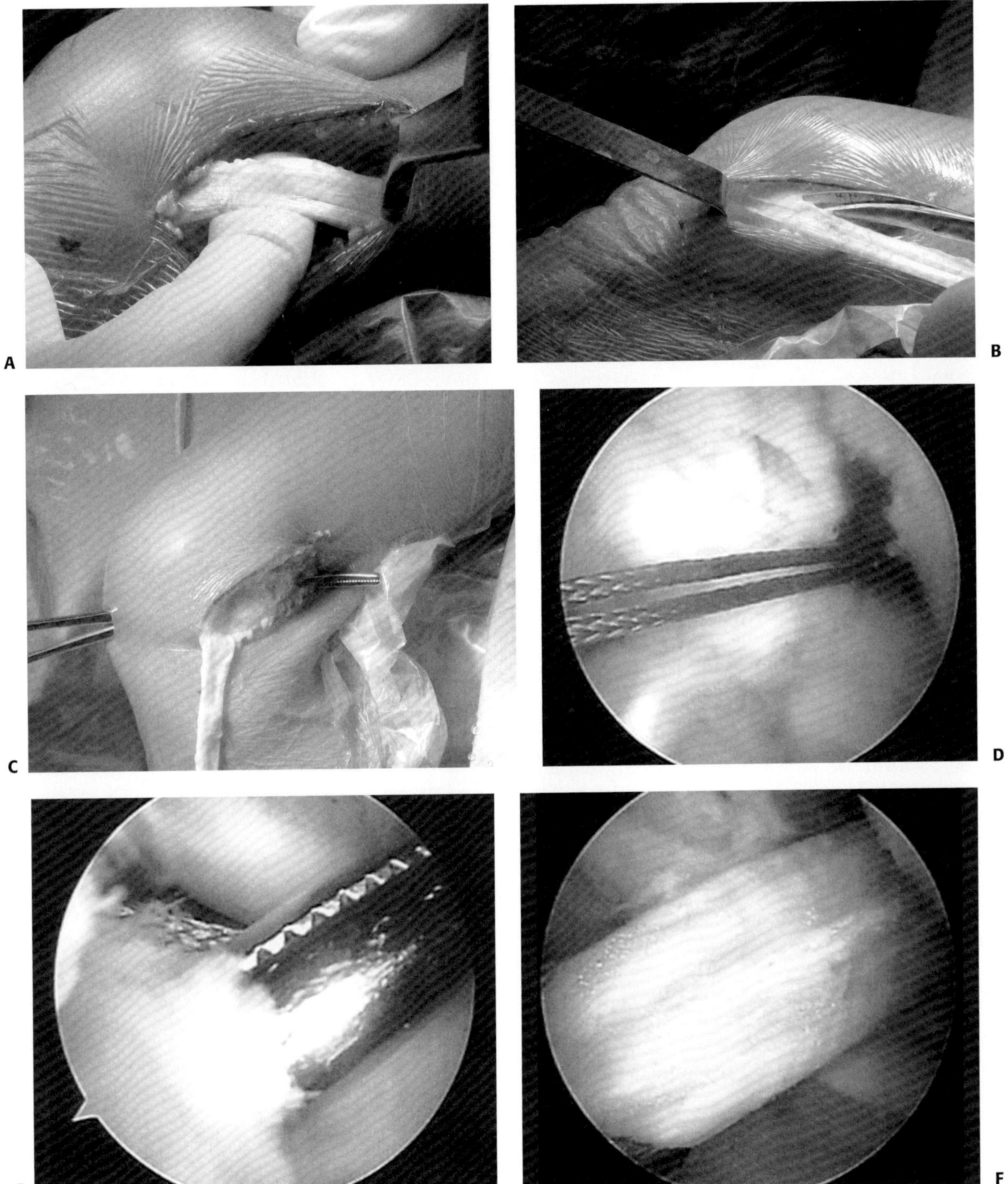

FIGURE 24-38 Technique of physeal sparing combined intra-articular and extra-articular anterior cruciate ligament reconstruction using iliotibial band. **A.** The iliotibial band is harvested through an oblique lateral knee incision. **B.** The iliotibial band graft is detached proximally, left attached distally, and dissected free from the lateral patellar retinaculum. **C.** The iliotibial band graft is brought through the knee using a full-length clamp placed from the anteromedial portal through the over-the-top position into the lateral incision. **D.** The graft is then brought through the over-the top position. **E.** A clamp is placed from a proximal medial leg incision under the intermeniscal ligament. A groove is made in the anteromedial tibial epiphysis using a rasp. **F.** The graft is brought through the knee in the over-the-top position and under the intermeniscal ligament. (*continues*)

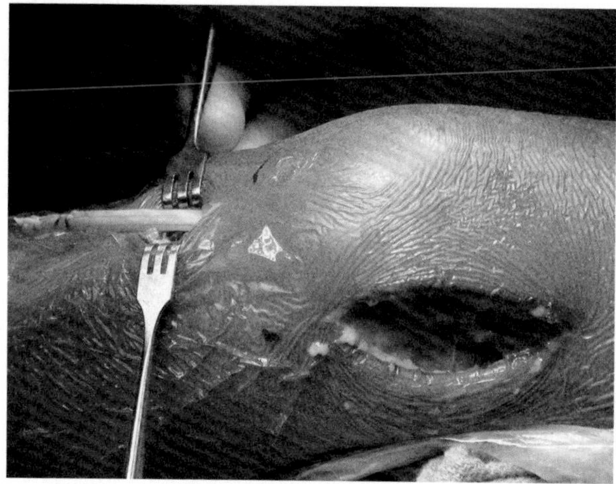

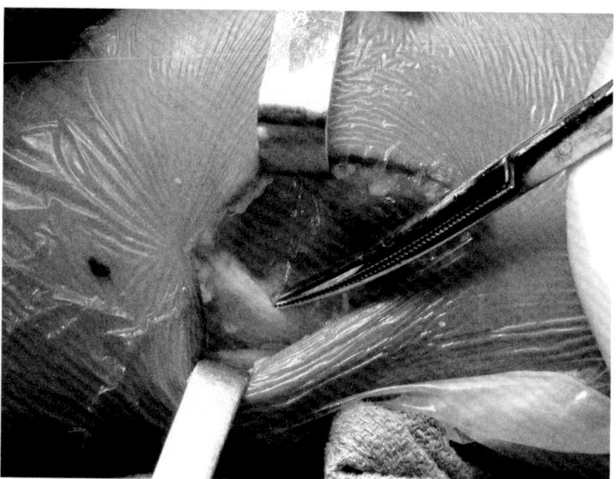

G H

FIGURE 24-38 (*continued*) **G,H.** The graft is brought out the proximal medial leg incision. It is sutured to the intermuscular septum and periosteum of the lateral femoral condyle through the lateral knee incision and it is sutured in a trough to the periosteum of the proximal medial tibial metaphysis.

First, the hamstring tendons are harvested. If the diagnosis is in doubt, arthroscopy can be performed first to confirm anterior cruciate ligament tear. A 4-cm incision is made over the palpable pes anserinus tendons on the medial side of the upper tibia (Fig. 24-39A). Dissection is carried through skin to the sartorius fascia. Care is taken to protect superficial sensory nerves. The sartorius tendon is incised longitudinally and the gracilis and semitendinosus tendons are identified. The tendons are dissected free distally and their free ends whip-stitched with no. 2 or 5 Ethibond suture. They are dissected proximally using sharp and blunt dissection. Fibrous bands to the medial head of gastrocnemius should be sought and released. A closed tendon stripper is used to dissect the tendons free proximally. Alternatively, the tendons can be left attached distally, and an open tendon stripper used to release the tendons proximally. The tendons are taken to the back table, where excess muscle is removed and the remaining ends are whip-stitched with no. 2 or 5 Ethibond sutures. The tendons are folded over a closed-loop endobutton. The graft diameter is sized and the graft is placed under tension.

Arthroscopy of the knee is then performed through standard anterolateral viewing and anteromedial working portals. Management of meniscal injury or chondral injury is performed if needed. The anterior cruciate ligament remnant is excised. The over-the-top position on the femur is identified. Minimal notchplasty is performed to avoid iatrogenic injury to the perichondrial ring of the distal femoral physis, which is in very close proximity to the over-the-top position (284).

A tibial tunnel guide (set at 55 degrees) is used through the anteromedial portal (Fig. 24-39B). A guide wire is drilled through the hamstring harvest incision into the posterior aspect of the anterior cruciate ligament tibial footprint. The guide wire entry point on the tibia should be kept medial to avoid injury to the tibial tubercle apophysis. The guide wire is reamed with the appropriate-diameter reamer. Excess soft tissue at the tibial tunnel is excised to avoid arthrofibrosis. The transtibial over-the-top guide of the appropriate offset to ensure a 1- or 2-mm back wall is used to pass the femoral guide pin (Fig. 24-39C). The femoral guide pin is overdrilled with the endobutton reamer. Both are removed in order to use the depth gauge to measure the femoral tunnel length. The guide pin is replaced and brought through the distal lateral thigh. The femur is reamed to the appropriate depth (femoral tunnel length − endobutton length + 8 mm to flip the endobutton).

The no. 5 Ethibond sutures on the endobutton are placed in the slot of the guide wire and pulled through the tibial tunnel, through the femoral tunnel, and out the lateral thigh. These are then pulled to bring the endobutton and graft through the tibial tunnel and into the femoral tunnel. One set of sutures is used to "lead" the endobutton while the other set of sutures is used to "follow." Once the graft is fully seated in the femoral tunnel, the "follow" sutures are pulled to flip the endobutton (Fig. 24-39D). The flip can be palpated in the thigh, and tension is applied to the graft to ensure no graft slippage. The knee is then extended to ensure no graft impingement. The knee is then cycled approximately 10 times with tension applied to the graft. The graft is fixed on the tibial side with the knee in 20 to 30 degrees of flexion, tension applied to the graft, and a posterior force placed on the tibia. On the tibial side, the graft is either fixed with a soft tissue interference screw if there is adequate tunnel distance (at least 30 mm) below the physis to ensure metaphyseal placement of the screw or with a post and spiked washer. Fluoroscopy can be used to ensure that the fixation is away from the physes. Postoperative x-rays are shown in Figure 24-40.

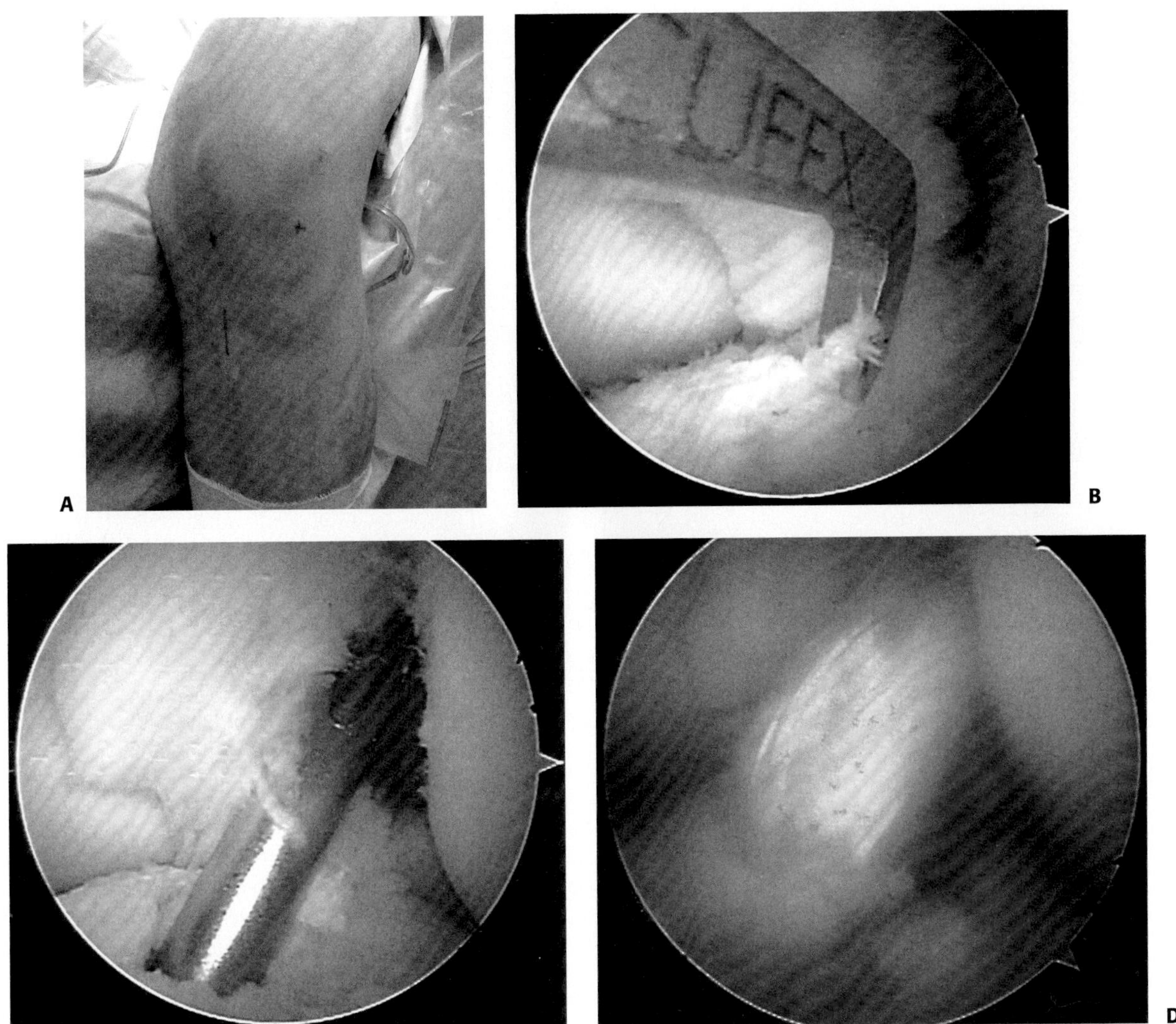

FIGURE 24-39 Transphyseal reconstruction with autogenous hamstrings for adolescents with growth remaining. **A.** The gracilis and semitendinosus tendons are harvested through an incision over the proximal medial tibia. **B.** The tibial guide is used to drill the tibial tunnel. **C.** The transtibial over-the-top offset guide is used to drill the femoral tunnel. **D.** Hamstring graft after fixation.

Postoperatively, the patient is maintained on touch-down weight-bearing for 4 weeks. Range of motion is limited from 0 to 90 degrees for the first 2 weeks, followed by progressive full range of motion. Continuous passive motion from 0 to 90 degrees and cryotherapy are used for 2 weeks postoperatively. A protective postoperative brace is used for 6 weeks postoperatively.

Lateral Collateral Ligament

Grade III injuries of the lateral collateral ligament are rare in children. Occasionally, the lateral capsular sign is seen on x-rays obtained for evaluation of knee injury. Most often, the lateral collateral ligament is avulsed from the proximal fibular epiphysis; proximal and midsubstance tears are uncommon. This injury is treated in the same manner as injury to the medial collateral ligament. For isolated grade III injuries, a 6-week period of immobilization in a hinged knee brace is recommended. If anterior cruciate ligament injury is associated with lateral collateral ligament injury, treatment is as described for combined injuries of the two ligaments. In young children, the lateral collateral ligament is repaired and the anterior cruciate ligament is left untreated. If instability persists as the adolescent nears skeletal maturity, intra-articular reconstruction can be done at that time. In adolescents near skeletal maturity at the time of injury, we prefer to repair both the anterior cruciate ligament and lateral collateral ligament.

Posterior Cruciate Ligament

In general, posterior cruciate ligament injuries in children are associated with a bony avulsion (286–288). If nondisplaced,

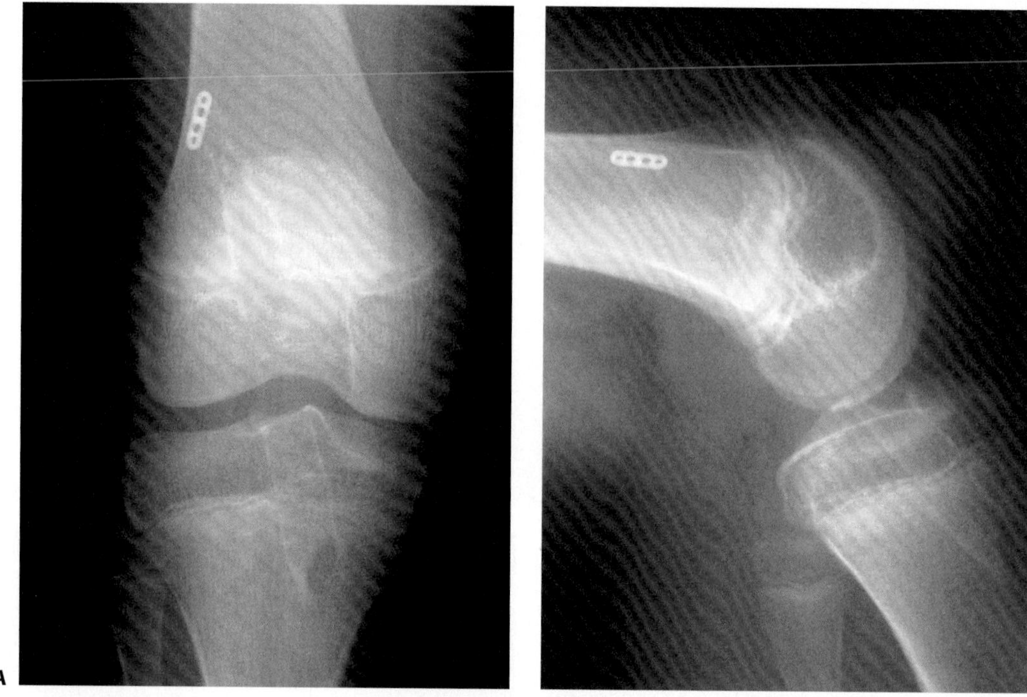

FIGURE 24-40 Transphyseal reconstruction with autogenous hamstrings for adolescents with growth remaining. Postoperative anteroposterior **(A)** and lateral **(B)** x-rays.

they should be treated with immobilization; if displaced, they should be treated with open reduction with internal fixation.

Isolated grade III injury of the posterior cruciate ligament in children and adolescents can be treated with 6 weeks of immobilization in a cast brace or hinged knee brace. If significant functional symptoms persist in an adolescent, the posterior cruciate ligament can be reconstructed at or near skeletal maturity. In a young child with grade III medial or lateral collateral ligament injury in addition to posterior cruciate ligament injury, the collateral ligament can be surgically repaired to convert the multiplane instability to single-plane instability. Posterior cruciate ligament injury may be associated with anterior cruciate ligament injury, primarily in knee dislocations, and surgical intervention usually is appropriate for this combination of injuries, especially in patients nearing skeletal maturity (288).

Knee Dislocation

Acute dislocations of the knee are uncommon in children because the forces required to produce dislocation are more likely to fracture the distal femoral or proximal tibial epiphysis (289). Acute knee dislocation usually involves major injuries of associated soft tissues and ligaments and often neurovascular injuries. Injuries typically occur in older, skeletally mature adolescents from high-energy trauma, such as motor vehicle injuries, pedestrian versus motor vehicle injury, bicycle versus motor vehicle injury, trampoline injuries, and high-energy contact sports.

Adequate follow-up studies of acute knee dislocations in children younger than 10 years of age are few (290), and most information has been obtained from reports of knee dislocations in adults. Because of the potential for associated vascular injury, acute knee dislocations in children may be emergent situations. The dislocation causes obvious deformity about the knee. With anterior dislocation, the tibia is prominent in an abnormal anterior position (Fig. 24-41). With posterior dislocation, the femoral condyles are abnormally prominent anteriorly.

After the dislocation is reduced, the stability of the knee should be evaluated with gentle stress testing. For isolated anterior or posterior dislocations, the integrity of the collateral ligaments should be carefully evaluated. Some knees may spontaneously reduce after dislocation or reduce with manipulation of the leg for transport.

The neurovascular status of the extremity should be carefully evaluated both before and after reduction, especially the dorsalis pedis and posterior tibial pulses and peroneal nerve function. Any abnormal vascular findings, either before or after reduction, require arteriography and, if necessary, arterial exploration. Popliteal artery laceration or intimal tear may occur in 20% to 35% of cases (289–293). Arteriography is unnecessary when pulses are normal before and after reduction; however, the vascular status should be carefully monitored for 48 to 72 hours after reduction. Vas-

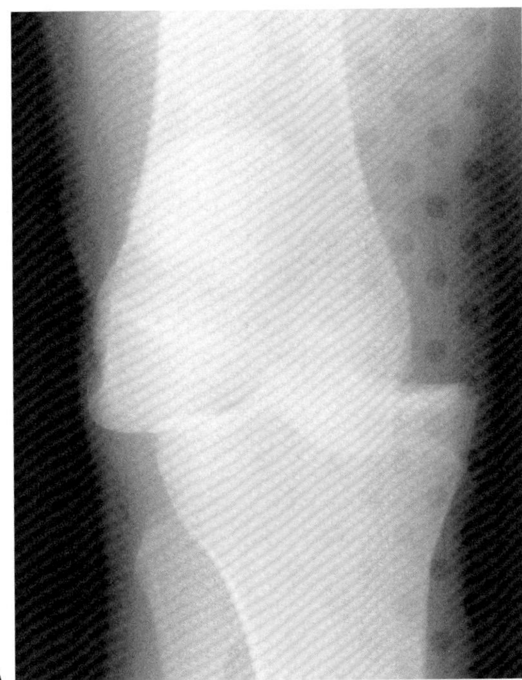

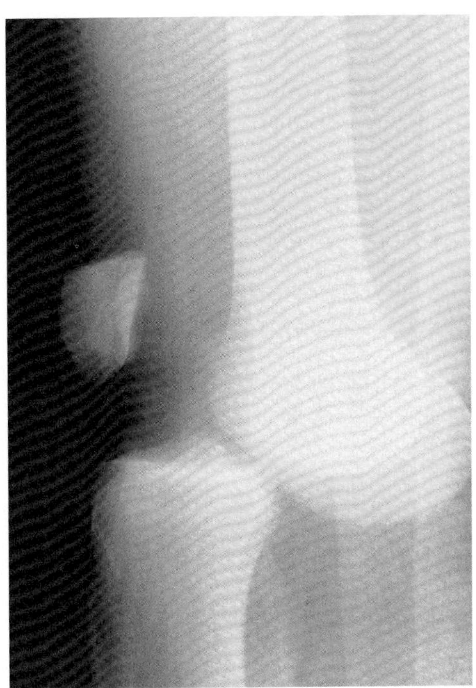

FIGURE 24-41 Dislocation of the knee. **A,B.** Anteromedial dislocation of the knee in a 14-year-old girl.

cular status may also be assessed with ultrasonography or magnetic resonance angiography. Abnormalities in the sensory or motor function of the foot and distribution of the peroneal nerve function should be noted. Peroneal nerve injury has been reported in 16% to 40% of cases (289–293). MRI is usually performed to assess the integrity of the cruciate and collateral ligaments, the posterolateral and posteromedial corners, the menisci, and the articular surfaces.

Knee dislocation usually occurs with disruption of both cruciate ligaments. With direct anterior or posterior dislocation, the collateral ligaments and the soft tissues may be retained because the femoral condyles are stripped out of their capsular and collateral ligament attachments and, when reduced, slip back inside them. Associated medial displacement is often accompanied by lateral collateral ligament disruption. Associated lateral displacement is often accompanied by medial collateral ligament disruption. Knee dislocations in adolescents have been associated with tibial spine fractures, osteochondral fractures of the femur or tibia, meniscal injuries, and peroneal nerve injuries (291).

Treatment of knee dislocations includes both acute and reconstructive management. Acutely, the knee is reduced under anesthesia. The knee should then be examined to assess the ligamentous injuries. The neurovascular status of the extremity is carefully assessed prereduction and postreduction. Vascular imaging is performed if indicated. Arterial exploration and repair or bypass grafting are performed by a vascular surgeon if indicated. If emergent vascular repair is performed, fasciotomies are usually also performed; however, ligamentous reconstruction is typically delayed. An MRI scan is obtained to document the injured structures. The knee is braced with protected weight-bearing and limited motion.

Reconstruction is delayed approximately 2 to 3 weeks after injury. Primary ligament repairs become more difficult after this period of time because of scarring and lack of definition of tissues. Reconstructions may be staged or performed at one setting. Surgery often combines arthroscopic and open techniques. General principles include ligament repair for collateral ligament injuries, ligament repair for cruciate ligament avulsions, ligament reconstruction for midsubstance cruciate ligament injuries, and meniscal repair. Allograft tissue is often used because of the multiligamentous nature of the injury. Posterior cruciate ligament reconstruction can be performed with tibial inlay techniques or arthroscopic techniques with a tibial tunnel and one or two femoral tunnels. Medially, the medial collateral ligament can be primarily repaired or reattached if avulsed. The medial meniscus may be torn if the medial collateral ligament is torn in its midsubstance. Laterally, the lateral collateral ligament, popliteofibular ligament, popliteus, and posterolateral capsule may require repair. The peroneal nerve should be decompressed and protected during repair.

Prolonged immobilization should be avoided because of the substantial risk of stiffness after knee dislocation surgery. Limited motion in a hinged knee brace and protected weight-bearing are used, followed by mobilization and strengthening.

Pearls and Pitfalls

With nonoperative treatment of complete anterior cruciate ligament tears in children and adolescents, sufficient counseling must be performed so that the patient and the family understand the relative risks and benefits of nonoperative treatment versus anterior cruciate ligament reconstruction. Compliance with bracing and activity restriction must be monitored. Careful regular follow-up is necessary to evaluate for instability episodes and further meniscal or chondral injury. Once further meniscal or chondral injury occurs, anterior cruciate ligament reconstruction should be advised because of the risk of degenerative joint disease associated with injury episodes.

Pitfalls to avoid with the physeal-sparing iliotibial band reconstruction in prepubescents include harvesting a short graft insufficient to reach the medial tibial incision, difficulty passing the graft through the posterior joint capsule, and difficulty passing the graft under the intermeniscal ligament. Pitfalls to avoid with the transphyseal hamstring reconstruction in adolescents with growth remaining include amputation of the hamstring grafts, poor tunnel placement, and graft impingement.

Based on the 15 cases of growth disturbance after anterior cruciate ligament reconstruction in skeletally immature patients that we reported, we recommend careful attention to technical details during reconstruction in skeletally immature patients, particularly the avoidance of fixation hardware across the lateral distal femoral epiphyseal plate (237). Care should also be taken to avoid injury to the vulnerable tibial tubercle apophysis. Given the cases of growth disturbances associated with transphyseal placement of patellar tendon graft bone blocks, we recommend the use of soft tissue grafts. Large tunnels should likely be avoided because the likelihood of arrest associated with lateral extra-articular tenodesis raises additional concerns about the effect of tension on physeal growth. Finally, care should be taken to avoid dissection or notching around the posterolateral aspect of the physis during over-the-top nonphyseal femoral placement to avoid potential injury to the perichondrial ring and subsequent deformity.

Prognosis and Complications

The prognosis of nonoperative management of complete tears of the anterior cruciate ligament in skeletally immature patients is generally poor, with recurrent instability leading to further meniscal and chondral injury, which has implications in terms of development of degenerative joint disease (214,229,232, 244–246).

The prognosis of anterior cruciate ligament reconstruction depends on the surgical procedure. Several case series exist regarding anterior cruciate ligament reconstruction in skeletally immature patients. However, most series are small and variably report the patients' skeletal age and growth remaining. Primary ligament repair (221,276) and extra-articular tenodesis alone (229,274) have had poor results in children and adolescents, similar to results in adults. Transphyseal reconstructions with tunnels that violate both the distal femoral and proximal tibial physes have been performed with hamstring autograft, patellar tendon autograft, and allograft tissue (214,217,218,223,227, 241,242,248,250,273,277). These anatomic anterior cruciate ligament reconstruction procedures have high success rates, as in adult patients; however, they risk injury to the physis, particularly in prepubescent patients. Partial transphyseal reconstructions violate only one physis with a tunnel through the proximal tibial physis and over-the-top positioning on the femur or a tunnel through the distal femoral physis with an epiphyseal tunnel in the tibia (216,219,278). These procedures are also near anatomic with good clinical results; however, the potential for growth disturbance exists. A variety of physeal-sparing reconstructions have been described to avoid tunnels across either the distal femoral or proximal tibial physis (215,220,222, 231–233,243,251,279). In general these procedures are nonanatomic and have some persistent knee laxity; however, they avoid physeal violation. In a follow-up outcome study of 44 skeletally immature prepubescent children who were Tanner stage 1 or 2 (mean chronologic age: 10.3 years old; range: 3.6 to 14.0 years old) who underwent the physeal sparing combined intra-articular and extra-articular anterior cruciate ligament reconstruction technique using autogenous iliotibial band that we describe above, we found a revision anterior cruciate ligament reconstruction rate of 4.5% with excellent functional outcome, return to competitive sports, and no cases of growth disturbance (294).

Complications after ligament injury in children are similar to those in adults: arthrofibrosis, persistent instability, unrecognized concomitant injury, infection, graft failure, neurovascular injury, and donor site morbidity. In skeletally immature patients, growth disturbance can occur from iatrogenic physeal injury, as previously discussed.

REFERENCES

1. Noyes FR, Delucas JL, Torvik PJ. Biomechanics of ACL failure: an analysis of strain-rate sensitivity and mechanisms of failure in primates. *J Bone Joint Surg Am* 1974;56: 236–253.
2. Woo SL-Y, Hollis JM, Adams DJ, et al. Tensile properties of the human femur-anterior cruciate ligament-tibia complex: the effects of specimen age and orientation. *Am J Sports Med* 1991;19:217–225.
3. Baxter MP, Wiley JJ. Fractures of the tibial spine in children: an evaluation of knee stability. *J Bone Joint Surg Br* 1988;70:228–230.
4. Berg EE. Pediatric tibial eminence fractures: arthroscopic cannulated screw fixation. *Arthroscopy* 1995;11:328–331.
5. Clanton TO, DeLee JC, Sanders B, et al. Knee ligament injuries in children. *J Bone Joint Surg Am* 1979;61:195–1201.
6. Gronkvist H, Hirsch G, Johansson L. Fracture of the anterior tibial spine in children. *J Pediatr Orthop* 1984;4:465–468.
7. Janarv PM, Westblad P, Johansson C, et al. Long-term follow-up of anterior tibial spine fractures in children. *J Pediatr Orthop* 1995;15:63–68.
8. Kocher MS, Micheli LJ. The pediatric knee: Evaluation and treatment. In: Insall JN, Scott WN, eds. *Surgery of the Knee,* 3rd ed. New York: Churchill-Livingstone; 2001: 1356–1397.
9. Lee YH, Chin LS, Wang NH, et al. Anterior tibial spine fracture in children: follow-up evaluation by biomechanical studies. *Chung Hua I Hsueh Tsa Chih* 1996;58:183–189.
10. Mah JY, Adili A, Otsuka NY, et al. Follow-up study of arthroscopic reduction and fixation of type III tibial eminence fractures. *J Pediatr Orthop* 1998;18:475–477.
11. Mah JY, Otsuka NY, McLean J. An arthroscopic technique for the reduction and fixation of tibial-eminence fractures. *J Pediatr Orthop* 1996;16:119–121.
12. Oostvogel HJ, Klasen HJ, Reddingius RE. Fractures of the intercondylar eminence in children and adolescents. *Arch Orthop Trauma Surg* 1988;107:242–247.
13. Pellaci F, Mignani G, Valdiserri L. Fractures of the intercondylar eminence of the tibia in children. *Ital J Orthop Traumatol* 1986;12:441–446.
14. Wiley JJ, Baxter MP. Tibial spine fractures in children. *Clin Orthop* 1990;255:54–60.
15. Willis RB, Blokker C, Stoll TM, et al. Long-term follow-up of anterior tibial eminence fractures. *J Pediatr Orthop* 1993;13:361–364.

16. Skak SV, Jensen TT, Poulsen TD, et al. Epidemiology of knee injuries in children. *Acta Orthop Scand* 1987;58:78–81.
17. Meyers MH, McKeever FM. Fracture of the intercondylar eminence of the tibia. *J Bone Joint Surg Am* 1959;41:209–222.
18. Garcia A, Neer CS II. Isolated fractures of the intercondylar eminence of the tibia. *Am J Surg* 1958;95:593–598.
19. Meyers MH, McKeever FM. Follow-up notes: fracture of the intercondylar eminence of the tibia. *J Bone Joint Surg Am* 1970;52:1677–1684.
20. McLennan JG. The role of arthroscopic surgery in the treatment of fractures of the intercondylar eminence of the tibia. *J Bone Joint Surg Br* 1982;64:477–480.
21. Molander ML, Wallin G, Wikstad I. Fractures of the intercondylar eminence of the tibia: a review of 35 patients. *J Bone Joint Surg Br* 1981;63:89–91.
22. Mulhall KJ, Dowdall J, Grannell M, et al. Tibial spine fractures: an analysis of outcome in surgically treated type III injuries. *Injury* 1999;30:289–292.
23. Jung YB, Yum JK, Koo BH. A new method for arthroscopic treatment of tibial eminence fractures with eyed Steinman pins. *Arthroscopy* 1999;15:672–675.
24. Bale RS, Banks AJ. Arthroscopically guided Kirschner wire fixation for fractures of the intercondylar eminence of the tibia. *J R Coll Surg Edinb* 1995;40:260–262.
25. Kocher MS, Foreman ES, Micheli LJ. Laxity and functional outcome after arthroscopic reduction and internal fixation of displaced tibial spine fractures in children. *Arthroscopy* 2003;19:1085–1090.
26. McLennan JG. Lessons learned after second-look arthroscopy in type III fractures of the tibial spine. *J Pediatr Orthop* 1995;15:59–62.
27. Smith JB. Knee instability after fractures of the intercondylar eminence of the tibia. *J Pediatr Orthop* 1984;4:462–464.
28. Roberts JM, Lovell WW. Fractures of the intercondylar eminence of the tibia. *J Bone Joint Surg Am* 1970;52:827.
29. Roberts JM. Fractures of the condyles of the tibia: an anatomical and clinical end-result study of 100 cases. *J Bone Joint Surg Am* 1968;50:1505–1521.
30. Kocher MS, Mandiga R, Klingele KE, et al. Anterior cruciate ligament injury versus tibial spine fracture in the skeletally immature knee: a comparison of skeletal maturation and notch width index. *J Pediatr Orthop* 2004;24:185–188.
31. Kocher MS, Micheli LJ, Gerbino PG, et al. Tibial eminence fractures in children: prevalence of meniscal entrapment. *Am J Sports Med* 2003;31:404–407.
32. Hayes JM, Masear VR. Avulsion fracture of the tibial eminence associated with severe medial ligamentous injury in an adolescent: a case report and review of the literature. *Am J Sports Med* 1984;12:330–333.
33. Robinson SC, Driscoll SE. Simultaneous osteochondral avulsion of the femoral and tibial insertion of the anterior cruciate ligament: report of a case in a 13-year-old boy. *J Bone Joint Surg Am* 1981;63:1342–1343.
34. Zaricznyj B. Avulsion fracture of the tibial eminence: treatment by open reduction and pinning. *J Bone Joint Surg Am* 1977;59:1111–1114.
35. Lowe J, Chaimsky G, Freedman A, et al. The anatomy of tibial eminence fractures: arthroscopic observations following failed closed reduction. *J Bone Joint Surg Am* 2002; 84:1933–1938.
36. Burstein DB, Viola A, Fulkerson JP. Entrapment of the medial meniscus in a fracture of the tibial eminence arthroscopy. *Arthroscopy* 1988;4:47–50.
37. Chandler JP, Miller TK. Tibial eminence fracture with meniscal entrapment. *Arthroscopy* 1995;11:499–502.
38. Falstie-Jensen S, Sondergard Petersen PE. Incarceration of the meniscus in fractures of the intercondylar eminence of the tibia in children. *Injury* 1984;15:236–238.
39. Bakalim G, Wilpulla E. Closed treatment of fracture of the tibial spines. *Injury* 1974; 5:210–212.
40. Smillie IS. *Injuries of the Knee Joint,* 5th ed. Edinburgh: Churchill-Livingstone; 1978.
41. Meyers MH. Isolated avulsion of the tibial attachment of the posterior cruciate ligament of the knee. *J Bone Joint Surg Am* 1975;57:669–672.
42. Sullivan DJ, Dines DM, Hershon SJ, et al. Natural history of a type III fracture of the intercondylar eminence of the tibia in an adult: a case report. *Am J Sports Med* 1989; 17:132–133.
43. Mylle J, Reynders R, Broos P. Transepiphyseal fixation of anterior cruciate avulsion in a child: report of a complication and review of the literature. *Arch Orthop Trauma Surg* 1993;112:101–103.
44. Fyfe IS, Jackson JP. Tibial intercondylar fractures in children: a review of the classification and the treatment of malunion. *Injury* 1981;13:165–169.
45. Keys GW, Walters J. Nonunion of intercondylar eminence fracture of the tibia. *J Trauma* 1988;28:870–871.
46. Lombardo SJ. Avulsion of a fibrous union of the intercondylar eminence of the tibia: a case report. *J Bone Joint Surg Am* 1994;76:1565–1567.
47. Alleyne KR, Galloway MT. Management of osteochondral injuries of the knee. *Clin Sports Med* 2001;20:343–363.
48. Coleman HM. Recurrent osteochondral fracture of the patella. *J Bone Joint Surg Br* 1948; 30:153–157.
49. Farmer JM, Martin DF, Boles CA, et al. Chondral and osteochondral injuries. *Clin Sports Med* 2001;20:299–319.
50. Matelic TM, Aronsson DD, Boyd DW, et al. Acute hemarthrosis of the knee in children. *Am J Sports Med* 1995;23:668–671.
51. Nietosvaara Y, Aalto K, Kallio PE. Acute patellar dislocation in children: incidence and associated osteochondral fractures. *J Pediatr Orthop* 1994;14:513–515.
52. Stanitski CL, Paletta GA. Articular cartilage injury with acute patellar dislocation in adolescents. *Am J Sports Med* 1998;26:52–55.
53. Flynn JM, Kocher MS, Ganley T. Osteochondritis dissecans of the knee. *J Pediatr Orthop* 2004;24:434–443.
54. Kocher MS, Micheli LJ, Yaniv M, et al. Functional and radiographic outcome of juvenile osteochondritis dissecans of the knee treated with transarticular drilling. *Am J Sports Med* 2001;29:562–566.
55. Birk GT, DeLee JC. Osteochondral injuries. *Clin Sports Med* 2001;20:279–287.
56. Cofield RH, Bryan RS. Acute dislocations of the patella: results of conservative treatment. *J Trauma* 1977;17:526–531.
57. Flachsmann R, Broom ND, Hardy AE, et al. Why is the adolescent joint particularly susceptible to osteochondral shear fracture? *Clin Orthop Rel Res* 2000;381:212–221.
58. Kennedy JC. *The Injured Adolescent Knee.* Baltimore: Williams & Wilkins; 1979.
59. Ahstrom JP. Osteochondral fracture in the knee joint associated with hypermobility and dislocation of the patella: report of 18 cases. *J Bone Joint Surg Am* 1965;47:1491–1502.
60. Aichroth PM. Osteochondral fractures and osteochondritis dissecans in sportsmen's knee injuries (Abstract). *J Bone Joint Surg Br* 1977;59:108.
61. Bailey WH, Blundell GE. An unusual abnormality affecting both knee joints in a child. *J Bone Joint Surg Am* 1974;56:814–816.
62. Bassett FH III. Acute dislocation of the patella, osteochondral fractures, and injuries to the extensor mechanism of the knee. *Instr Course Lect* 1976;25:40–49.
63. Edwards DH, Bentley G. Osteochondritis dissecans patellae. *J Bone Joint Surg Br* 1977; 59:58–63.
64. Goodfellow J, Hungerford DS, Zindel M. Patellofemoral joint mechanics and pathology. I. Functional anatomy of the patellofemoral joint. *J Bone Joint Surg Br* 1976;58:287–290.
65. Henderson NJ, Houghton GR. Osteochondral fractures of the knee in children. In: Houghton GR, Thompson GH, eds. *Problematic Musculoskeletal Injuries in Children.* London: Butterworth; 1983.
66. Hughston JC, Hergenroeder PT, Courtenay BG. Osteochondritis dissecans of the femoral condyles. *J Bone Joint Surg Am* 1984;66:1340–1348.
67. Hungerford DS, Barry M. Biomechanics of the patellofemoral joint. *Clin Orthop* 1979; 144:9–15.
68. Johnson EW, McLeod TL. Osteochondral fragments of the distal end of the femur fixed with bone pegs: report of two cases. *J Bone Joint Surg Am* 1977;59:677–679.
69. Lewis PC, Foster BK. Herbert screw fixation of osteochondral fractures about the knee. *Aust N Z J Surg* 1990;60:511–513.
70. McManus F, Rang M, Heslin DJ. Acute dislocation of the patella in children: the natural history. *Clin Orthop* 1979;139:88–91.
71. Ogden JA. *Skeletal Injury in the Child,* 2nd ed. Philadelphia: Lea & Febiger; 1989.
72. Rorabeck CH, Bobechko WP. Acute dislocation of the patella with osteochondral fracture: review of 18 cases. *J Bone Joint Surg Br* 1976;58:237–240.
73. Rosenberg NJ. Osteochondral fractures of the lateral femoral condyle. *J Bone Joint Surg Am* 1964;46:1013–1026.
74. Peterson L, Minas T, Brittberg M, et al. Treatment of osteochondritis dissecans of the knee with autologous chondrocyte transplantation: results at two to ten years. *J Bone Joint Surg Am* 2003;85(suppl 2):17–24.
75. Seitz WH Jr, Bibliani LU, Andrews DL, et al. Osteochondritis dissecans of the knee: a surgical approach. *Orthop Rev* 1985;14:56–63.
76. Smillie IS. *Injuries of the Knee Joint,* 5th ed. Edinburgh: Churchill-Livingstone; 1978.
77. Stanitski C, Cannon WD, eds. Patellar instability in the school-age athlete. *Instr Course Lect* 1998;47:345–350.
78. Wombwell JH, Nunley JA. Compressive fixation of osteochondritis dissecans fragments with Herbert screws. *J Orthop Trauma* 1987;1:74–77.
79. Woo R, Busch M. Management of patellar instability in children. *Oper Tech Sports Med* 1998;6:247–258.
80. Bohndorf K. Imaging of acute injuries of the articular surfaces (chondral, osteochondral, and subchondral fractures). *Skeletal Radiol* 1999;28:545–560.
81. Kocher MS, DiCanzio J, Zurakowski D, et al. Diagnostic performance of clinical examination and selective magnetic resonance imaging in the evaluation of intra-articular knee disorders in children and adolescents. *Am J Sports Med* 2001;29:292–296.
82. Wessel LM, Scholz S, Rusch M, et al. Hemarthrosis after trauma to the pediatric knee joint: what is the value of magnetic resonance imaging in the diagnostic algorithm? *J Pediatr Orthop* 2001;21:338–342.
83. Benz G, Roth H, Zachariou Z. Fractures and cartilage injuries of the knee joint in children. *Z Kinderchir* 1986;41:219–226.
84. Anderson AF; Pagnani MJ. Osteochondritis dissecans of the femoral condyles: long-term results of excision of the fragment. *Am J Sports Med* 1997;25:830–834.
85. Bentley G, Biant LC, Carrington RW, et al. A prospective, randomised comparison of autologous chondrocyte implantation versus mosaicplasty for osteochondral defects in the knee. *J Bone Joint Surg Br* 2003;85:223–230.
86. Berlet GC, Mascia A, Miniaci A. Treatment of unstable osteochondritis dissecans lesions of the knee using autogenous osteochondral grafts mosaicplasty. *Arthroscopy* 1999;15: 312–316.
87. Steadman JR, Briggs KK, Rodrigo JJ, et al. Outcomes of microfracture for traumatic chondral defects of the knee: average 11-year follow-up. *Arthroscopy* 2003;19:477–484.
88. McManus F, Rang M, Heslin DJ. Acute dislocation of the patella in children: a natural history. *Clin Orthop* 1979;139:88–91.
89. Larsen E, Lauridsen F. Conservative treatment of patellar dislocations. *Clin Orthop* 1982;171:131–136.
90. Rorabeck CH, Bobechko WP. Acute dislocation of the patella with osteochondral fracture. *J Bone Joint Surg Br* 1976;58:237–240.
91. Brady TA, Russell D. Interarticular horizontal dislocation of the patella: a case report. *J Bone Joint Surg Am* 1965;47:1393–1396.
92. Donelson RG, Tomaiuoli M. Intra-articular dislocation of the patella. *J Bone Joint Surg Am* 1979;61:615–616.
93. Frangakis EK. Intra-articular dislocation of the patella: a case report. *J Bone Joint Surg Am* 1974;56:423–424.
94. Goletz TH, Brodhead WT. Intra-articular dislocation of the patella: a case report. *Orthopaedics* 1981;4:1022–1024.

95. Cash JD, Hughston JC. Treatment of acute patellar dislocation. *Am J Sports Med* 1988; 16:244–249.
96. Desio S, Burks R, Bachus K. Soft tissue restraints to lateral patellar translation in the human knee. *Am J Sports Med* 1998;26:59–65.
97. Sallay P, Poggi J, Speer K, et al. Acute dislocation of the patella. *Am J Sports Med* 1996; 24:52–60.
98. Cofield RH, Bryan RS. Acute dislocation of the patella: results of conservative treatment. *J Trauma* 1977;17:526–531.
99. Betz RR, Longergan R, Patterson R, et al. The percutaneous lateral retinacular release. *Orthopaedics* 1982;5:57–62.
100. Hejgaard N, Skive L, Perrild C. Recurrent dislocation of the patella. *Acta Orthop Scand* 1980;51:673–678.
101. Larson RL. The unstable patella in the adolescent and preadolescent. *Orthop Rev* 1985; 14:156–162.
102. Madigan R, Wissinger AH, Donaldson WF. Preliminary experience with a method of quadriceps plasty in recurrent subluxation of the patella. *J Bone Joint Surg Am* 1975; 57:600–607.
103. Micheli LJ, Stanitski CL. Lateral patellar retinacular release. *Am J Sports Med* 1981;9: 330–336.
104. Hall JE, Micheli LJ, McManana GB. Semitendinosus tenodesis for recurrent subluxation or dislocation of the patella. *Clin Orthop* 1979;144:31–35.
105. Kocher MS, Klingele KE, Rassman S. Meniscal disorders: normal, discoid, and cysts. *Orthop Clin North Am* 2003,34:329–340.
106. Abrams RC. Meniscus lesions in the knee in young children. *J Bone Joint Surg Am* 1957; 39:194–195.
107. Abdou P, Bauer M. Incidence of meniscal lesions in children. *Acta Orthop Scand* 1989; 60:710–711.
108. Andrish JT. Meniscal injuries in children and adolescents: diagnosis and management. *J Am Acad Orthop Surg* 1996;4:231–237.
109. Andrish J. The diagnosis and management of meniscus injuries in skeletally immature athlete. *Oper Tech Sports Med* 1998;6:186–196.
110. Bhaduri T, Glass A. Meniscectomy in children. *Injury* 1972;3:176–178.
111. Busch MT. Meniscal injuries in children and adolescents. *Clin Sports Med* 1990;9: 661–680.
112. Clark CR, Ogden JA. Development of the menisci of the human knee joint: morphological changes and their potential role in childhood meniscal injury. *J Bone Joint Surg Am* 1983;65:538–547.
113. Fowler PJ. Meniscal lesions in the adolescent: the role of arthroscopy in the management of adolescent knee problems. In: Kennedy JC, ed. *The Injured Adolescent Knee.* Baltimore: Williams & Wilkins; 1979:43–76.
114. Harway RA, Handler S. Internal derangement of the knee in an infant. *Contemp Orthop* 1988;17:49–51.
115. Juhl M, Boe S. Arthroscopy in children, with special emphasis on meniscal lesions. *Injury* 1986;17:171–173.
116. King AG. Meniscal lesions in children and adolescents: a review of the pathology and clinical presentation. *Injury* 1983;15:105–108.
117. Kocher MS, Micheli LJ. The pediatric knee: evaluation and treatment. In: Insall JN, Scott WN, eds. *Surgery of the Knee,* 3rd ed. New York: Churchill-Livingstone; 2001: 1356–1397.
118. Manzione M, Pizzutillo PD, Peoples AB, et al. Meniscectomy in children: a long-term follow-up study. *Am J Sports Med* 1983;11:111–115.
119. Medlar RC, Manidberg JJ, Lyne ED. Meniscectomies in children-report of long term results. *Am J Sports Med* 1980;8:87–92.
120. Mintzer CM, Richmond JC, Taylor J. Meniscal repair in the young athlete. *Am J Sports Med* 1998;26:630–633.
121. Morrissy RT, Eubanks RG, Park JP, et al. Arthroscopy of the knee in children. *Clin Orthop* 1982;162:103–107.
122. Noyes FR, Barber-Westin SD. Arthroscopic repair of meniscal tears extending into the avascular zone in patients younger than twenty years of age. *Am J Sports Med* 2002; 30:589–600.
123. Saddawi ND, Hoffman BK. Tear of the attachment of a normal meniscus of the knee in a 4-year-old child. *J Bone Joint Surg Am* 1970;52:809–811.
124. Vahvanen V, Aolto K. Meniscotomy in children. *Acta Orthop Scand* 1979;50:791–795.
125. Volk H, Smith FM. "Bucket-handle" tear of the medial meniscus in a 5-year-old boy. *J Bone Joint Surg Am* 1953;35:234–236.
126. Wroble RR, Henderson RC, Campion ER, et al. Meniscectomy in children and adolescents: a long term follow-up study. *Clin Orthop* 1992;279:180–189.
127. Aglietti P, Bertini FA, Buzzi R, et al. Arthroscopic meniscectomy for discoid lateral meniscus in children and adolescence: a ten year followup. *Am J Knee Surg* 1999,12: 83–87.
128. Aichroth PM, Patel DV, Marx CI. Congenital discoid lateral meniscus in children: a followup study and evaluation of management. *J Bone Joint Surg Br* 1991;73:932–939.
129. Albertsson M, Gillquist S. Discoid lateral meniscus: a report of 29 cases. *Arthroscopy* 1998;4:211–214.
130. Bellier G, Dupont JY, Larrain M, et al. Lateral discoid meniscus in children. *Arthroscopy* 1989;5:52–56.
131. Dashefsky JH. Discoid lateral meniscus in three members of a family. *J Bone Joint Surg Am* 1971;53:1208–1210.
132. Dickason JM, del Pizzo W, Blazina ME, et al. A series of 10 discoid medial menisci. *Clin Orthop* 1982;168:75–79.
133. Dickhaut SC, DeLee JC. The discoid lateral meniscus syndrome. *J Bone Joint Surg Am* 1982;64:1068–1073.
134. Fleissner PR, Eilert RF. Discoid lateral meniscus. *Am J Knee Surg* 1999,12:125–131.
135. Fujikawa K, Iseki F, Mikura Y. Partial resection of the discoid meniscus in the child's knee. *J Bone Joint Surg Br* 1981;63:391–395.
136. Hamada M, Shino K, Kawano K, et al. Usefulness of MRI for detecting intrasubstance tear and/or degeneration of lateral discoid meniscus. *Arthroscopy* 1994;10:645–653.
137. Hayashi LK, Yamaga H, Ida K, et al: Arthroscopic meniscectomy for discoid lateral meniscus in children. *J Bone Joint Surg Am* 1988;70:1495–1500.
138. Ikeuchi H. Arthroscopic treatment of lateral discoid meniscus: technique and long term results. *Clin Orthop* 1982;167:19–28.
139. Johnson RG, Simmons EH. Discoid medial meniscus. *Clin Orthop* 1982;167:176–179.
140. Jordan M. Lateral meniscal variants: evaluation and treatment. *J Am Acad Orthop Surg* 1996;4:191–200.
141. Jordan M, Duncan J, Bertrand S. Discoid lateral meniscus: a review. *South Orthop J* 1993;2:239–253.
142. Kaplan EB. Discoid lateral meniscus of the knee joint. *Bull Hosp Joint Dis* 1955;16: 111–124.
143. Kaplan EB. Discoid lateral meniscus of the knee joint: nature, mechanism, and operative treatment. *J Bone Joint Surg Am* 1957;39:77–87.
144. Klingele KE, Kocher MS, Hresko MT, et al. Discoid lateral meniscus: prevalence of peripheral riminstability. *J Pediatr Orthop* 2004;24:79–82.
145. Nathan PA, Cole SC. Discoid meniscus: a clinical and pathological study. *Clin Orthop* 1969;64:107–113.
146. Neuschwander DC, Drez D, Finney TP. Lateral meniscal variant with absence of posterior coronary ligament. *J Bone Joint Surg Am* 1992;74:1186–1190.
147. Ogata K. Arthroscopic technique: two piece excision of discoid meniscus. *Arthroscopy* 1997;13:666–670.
148. Patel D, Dimakopoulos P, Penoncourt P. Bucket handle tear of a discoid meniscus: arthroscopic diagnosis and partial excision. *Orthopaedics* 1986;9:607–608.
149. Pellacci F, Montanari G, Prosperi P, et al. Lateral discoid meniscus: treatment and results. *Arthroscopy* 1992;8:526–530.
150. Raber DA, Friederich NF, Buzzi R, et al. Discoid lateral meniscus in children: long term followup after total meniscectomy. *J Bone Joint Surg Am* 1998;8:1579–1586.
151. Rosenberg TD, Paulos LE, Parker RD, et al. Discoid lateral meniscus: case report of arthroscopic attachment of a symptomatic Wrisberg-ligament type. *Arthroscopy* 1987; 3:277–282.
152. Schlonsky J, Eyring EJ. Lateral meniscus tears in young children. *Clin Orthop* 1973; 97:117–118.
153. Smillie I. The congenital discoid meniscus. *J Bone Joint Surg Br* 1948;30:671–682.
154. Stilli S, DiGennaro GL, Marchiodi L, et al. Arthroscopic surgery of the discoid meniscus during childhood. *Chir Degli Org Mov* 1997;82:335–339.
155. Sugawara O, Miyatsu M, Yamashita I, et al. Problems with repeated arthroscopic surgery in the discoid meniscus. *Arthroscopy* 1991;7:68–71.
156. Vandermeer R, Cunningham F. Arthroscopic treatment of the discoid lateral meniscus: results of long term followup. *Arthroscopy* 1989;5:101–109.
157. Washington ER, Root L, Lierner U, et al. Discoid lateral meniscus in children: long term followup after excision. *J Bone Joint Surg Am* 1995;77:1357–1361.
158. Woods GW, Whelan JM. Discoid meniscus. *Clin Sports Med* 1990;9:695–706.
159. Young RB. The external semilunar cartilage as a complete disc. In: Cleland J, Mackey JY, Young RB, eds. *Memoirs and Memoranda in Anatomy,* London: Williams and Norgate; 1889:179.
160. Dehaven KE, Linter DM. Athletic injuries: comparison by age, sport, gender. *Am J Sports Med* 1986;14:218–224.
161. Cannon WD, Vittori JM. The incidence of healing in arthroscopic meniscal repairs in the anterior cruciate ligament-reconstructed knee versus stable knees. *Am J Sports Med* 1992;20:176–181.
162. Eggli S. Long-term results of arthroscopic meniscal repair: an analysis of isolated tears. *Am J Sports Med* 1995;23:715–720.
163. Kocher MS, Micheli LJ, Gerbino PG, et al. Tibial eminence fractures in children: prevalence of meniscal entrapment. *Am J Sports Med* 2003;31:404–407.
164. Stanitski CL, Harvell JC, Fu F. Observations on acute knee hemarthrosis in children and adolescents. *J Pediatr Orthop* 1993;13:506–510.
165. Greis PE, Bardana DD, Holstrom MC, et al. Meniscal injury: basic science and evaluation. *J Am Acad Orthop Surg* 2002;10:168–176.
166. Greis PE, Holstrom MC, Bardana DD, et al. Meniscal injury. II. Management. *J Am Acad Orthop Surg* 2002;10:177–187.
167. Kocher MS, DiCanzio J, Zurakowski D, et al. Diagnostic performance of clinical examination and selective magnetic resonance imaging in the evaluation of intraarticular knee disorders in children and adolescents. *Am J Sports Med* 2001;29:292–296.
168. DeHaven KE. Diagnosis of acute knee injuries with hemarthrosis. *Am J Sports Med* 1980;8:9–14.
169. Stanitski CL. Correlation of arthroscopic and clinical examinations with magnetic resonance imaging findings of injured knees in children and adolescents. *Am J Sports Med* 1998;26:2–6.
170. Dalinka MK, Brennan RE, Canino C. Double-contrast knee arthrography in children. *Clin Orthop* 1977;125:88–93.
171. Noyes FR, Bassett RW, Grood ES, et al. Arthroscopy in acute traumatic hemarthrosis of the knee: incidence of anterior cruciate tears and other injuries. *J Bone Joint Surg Am* 1980;62:687–695.
172. Boger DC, Kingston S. MRI of the normal knee. *Am J Knee Surg* 1988;1:99–103.
173. Jackson DW, Jennings LD, Maywood RM, et al. MRI of the knee. *Am J Sports Med* 1988;16:29–38.
174. Polly DW, Callaghan JJ, Sikes RA, et al. The accuracy of selective MRI compared to the findings of arthroscopy of the knee. *J Bone Joint Surg Am* 1988;70:192–198.
175. Silva I, Silver DM. Tears of the meniscus as revealed by MRI. *J Bone Joint Surg Am* 1988;70:199–202.

176. Boden S, Davis D, Dina T, et al. A prospective and blinded investigation of magnetic resonance imaging of the knee: abnormal findings in asymptomatic subjects. *Clin Orthop* 1992;282:177–185.
177. LaPrade R, Burnett Q, Veenstra M, et al. The prevalence of abnormal magnetic resonance imaging findings in asymptomatic knees: with correlation of magnetic resonance imaging arthroscopic findings in symptomatic knees. *Am J Sports Med* 1994;22: 739–745.
178. King SL, Carty HML, Brady O. Magnetic resonance imaging of knee injuries in children. *Pediatr Radiol* 1996;26:287–290.
179. Zobel MS, Borrello JA, Siegel MJ et al. Pediatric knee MR imaging: pattern of injury in the immature skeleton. *Radiology* 1994;190:397–401.
180. Takeda Y, Ikata T, Yoshida S, et al. MRI high signal intensity in the menisci of asymptomatic children. *J Bone Joint Surg Br* 1998;80:463–467.
181. Gelb H, Glasgow S, Sapega A, et al. Magnetic resonance imaging of knee disorders: clinical value and cost effectiveness in a sports medicine practice. *Am J Sports Med* 1996;24:99–103.
182. Arnoczky SP, Warren RF. Microvasculature of the human meniscus. *Am J Sports Med* 1982;2:90–95.
183. King D. The healing of semilunar cartilage. *J Bone Joint Surg* 1936;18:333–342.
184. Dye SF, Vaupel GL, Dye CC. Conscious neurosensory mapping of the internal structures of the human knee without intraarticular anesthesia. *Am J Sports Med* 1998;26: 773–777.
185. Bland-Sutton J, ed. *Ligaments: Their Nature and Morphology*, 2nd ed. London, UK: JK Lewis; 1897.
186. Fairbank TJ. Knee joint changes after meniscectomy. *J Bone Joint Surg Br* 1948;30: 664–670.
187. Rangger C, Klesti T, Gloetzer W, et al. Osteoarthritis after arthroscopic partial meniscectomy. *Am J Sports Med* 1995;23:230–244.
188. Ahmed AM, Burke DL. In-vitro measurement of static pressure distribution in synovial joints. I. Tibial surface of the knee. *J Biomech Eng* 1983;105:216–225.
189. Baratz ME, Fu FH, Mentago R. Meniscal tears: the effect of meniscectomy and of repair on intraarticular contact areas and stress in the human knee. *Am J Sports Med* 1986; 14:270–274.
190. Levy IM, Torzilli PA, Warren RF. The effect of medial meniscectomy on anterior-posterior motion of the knee. *J Bone Joint Surg Am* 1982;64:883–888.
191. Voloshin AS, Wosk J. Shock absorption of the meniscectomized and painful knees: a comparative in vivo study. *J Biomed Eng* 1983;5:157–161.
192. Shoemaker SC, Markolf KL. The role of the meniscus in the anterior-posterior stability of the loaded cruciate deficient knee: effect of partial versus total excision. *J Bone and Joint Surg Am* 1988;68:71–79.
193. DeHaven KE, Arnoczky SP. Meniscus repair: basic science, indications for repair, and open repair. *Instr Course Lect* 1994;43:65–74.
194. Appel H. Late results after meniscectomy in the knee joint: a clinical and roentgenologic follow-up investigation. *Acta Orthop Scand Suppl* 1970;133.
195. Hamberg P, Gillquist J, Lysholm J. Suture of new and old peripheral meniscus tears. *J Bone Joint Surg Am* 1983;65:193–197.
196. Krause WR, Pope MH, Johnson RJ, et al. Mechanical changes in the knee after meniscectomy. *J Bone Joint Surg Am* 1976;58:599–604.
197. Tapper EM, Hoover NW. Late results after meniscectomy. *J Bone Joint Surg Am* 1969; 51:517–526.
198. Zaman M, Leonard MA. Meniscectomy in children: a study of 59 knees. *J Bone Joint Surg Br* 1978;60:436–437.
199. DeHaven KE. Meniscus repair in the athlete. *Clin Orthop* 1985;98:31–35.
200. Henning CE, Lynch MA, Clark JR. Vascularity for healing of meniscus repairs. *Arthroscopy* 1987;3:13–18.
201. Marshall SC. Combined arthroscopic/open repair of meniscal injuries. *Contemp Orthop* 1987;14:15–24.
202. Arnoczky SP, Warren RF, Spivak JM. Meniscal repair using an exogenous fibrin clot: an experimental study in dogs. *J Bone Joint Surg Am* 1988;70:1209–1217.
203. Watanabe M, Takada S, Ikeuchi H. *Atlas of Arthroscopy*. Tokyo: Igaku-Shoin; 1969.
204. Huckell JR. Is meniscectomy a benign procedure? A long-term follow-up study. *Can J Surg* 1965;8:254–260.
205. Rubman MH, Noyes FR, Barber-Westin SD. Arthroscopic repair of meniscal tears that extend into the avascular zone: a review of 198 single and complex tears. *Am J Sports Med* 1998;26:87–95.
206. Johnson MJ, Lucas GL, Dusek JK, et al. Isolated arthroscopic meniscal repair: a long term outcome study (more than 10 years). *Am J Sports Med* 1999;27:44–49.
207. Busek MS, Noyes FR. Arthroscopic evaluation of meniscal repairs after anterior cruciate ligament reconstruction and immediate motion. *Am J Sports Med* 1991;19:489–494.
208. Tenuta JJ, Arciero RA. Arthroscopic evaluation of meniscal repairs: factors that effect healing. *Am J Sports Med* 1994;22:797–802.
209. Crawford AH. Fractures about the knee in children. *Orthop Clin North Am* 1976;7: 639–656.
210. Rang M. *Children's Fractures*, 2nd ed. Philadelphia: Lippincott; 1983.
211. Kocher MS, Foreman ES, Micheli LJ. Laxity and functional outcome after arthroscopic reduction and internal fixation of displaced tibial spine fractures in children. *Arthroscopy* 2003;19:1085–1090.
212. Kocher MS, Mandiga R, Klingele KE, et al. Anterior cruciate ligament injury versus tibial spine fracture in the skeletally immature knee: a comparison of skeletal maturation and notch width index. *J Pediatr Orthop* 2004;24:185–188.
213. Kocher MS, Micheli LJ, Gerbino P, et al. Tibial eminence fractures in children: prevalence of meniscal entrapment. *Am J Sports Med* 2003;31:404–407.
214. Aichroth PM, Patel DV, Zorrilla P. The natural history and treatment of rupture of the anterior cruciate ligament in children and adolescents: a prospective review. *J Bone Joint Surg Br* 2002;84:618–619.
215. Anderson AF. Transepiphyseal replacement of the anterior cruciate ligament in skeletally immature patients: a preliminary report. *J Bone Joint Surg Am* 2003;85:1255–1263.
216. Andrews M, Noyes FR, Barber-Westin SD. Anterior cruciate ligament allograft reconstruction in the skeletally immature athlete. *Am J Sports Med* 1994;22:48–54.
217. Angel KR, Hall DJ. Anterior cruciate ligament injury in children and adolescents. *Arthroscopy* 1989;5:197–200.
218. Aronowitz ER, Ganley TJ, Goode JR, et al. Anterior cruciate ligament reconstruction in adolescents with open physes. *Am J Sports Med* 2000;28:168–175.
219. Bisson LJ, Wickiewicz T, Levinson M, et al. ACL reconstruction in children with open physes. *Orthopedics* 1998;21:659–663.
220. Brief LB. Anterior cruciate ligament reconstruction without drill holes. *Arthroscopy* 1991;7:350–357.
221. Clanton TO, DeLee JC, Sanders B et al. Knee ligament injuries in children. *J Bone Joint Surg Am* 1979;61:1195–1201.
222. DeLee J, Curtis R. Anterior cruciate ligament insufficiency in children. *Clin Orthop* 1983;172:112–118.
223. Edwards PH, Grana WA. Anterior cruciate ligament reconstruction in the immature athlete: long-term results of intra-articular reconstruction. *Am J Knee Surg* 2001;14: 232–237.
224. Edwards TB, Greene CC, Baratta RV, et al. The effect of placing a tensioned graft across open growth plates: a gross and histologic analysis. *J Bone Joint Surg Am* 2001;83: 725–734.
225. Eilert R. Arthroscopy of the knee joint in children. *Orthop Rev* 1976;5:61–65.
226. Eiskjaer S, Larsen ST. Arthroscopy of the knee in children. *Acta Orthop Scand* 1987; 58:273–276.
227. Eiskjaer S, Larsen ST, Schmidt MB. The significance of hemarthrosis of the knee in children. *Arch Orthop Trauma Surg* 1988;107:96–98.
228. Fuchs R, Wheatley W, Uribe JW, et al. Intra-articular anterior cruciate ligament reconstruction using patellar tendon allograft in the skeletally immature patient. *Arthroscopy* 2002;18:824–828.
229. Graf BK, Lange RH, Fujisaki CK, et al. Anterior cruciate ligament tears in skeletally immature patients: meniscal pathology at presentation and after attempted conservative treatment. *Arthroscopy* 1992;8:229–233.
230. Guzzanti V, Falciglia F, Gigante A, et al. The effect of intra-articular ACL reconstruction on the growth plates of rabbits. *J Bone Joint Surg Br* 1994;76:960–963.
231. Guzzanti V, Falciglia F, Stanitski CL. Physeal-sparing intraarticular anterior cruciate ligament reconstruction in preadolescents. *Am J Sports Med* 2003;31:949–953.
232. Janarv PM, Nystrom A, Werner S, et al. Anterior cruciate ligament injuries in skeletally immature patients. *J Pediatr Orthop* 1996;16:673–677.
233. Kim SH, Ha KI, Ahn JH, et al. Anterior cruciate ligament reconstruction in the young patient without violation of the epiphyseal plate. *Arthroscopy* 1999;15:792–795.
234. Kloeppel-Wirth S, Koltai JL, Dittmer H. Significance of arthroscopy in children with knee joint injuries. *Eur J Pediatr Surg* 1992;2:169–172.
235. Kocher MS, Micheli LJ, Zurakowski D, et al. Partial tears of the anterior cruciate ligament in children and adolescents. *Am J Sports Med* 2002;30:697–703.
236. Koman JD, Sanders JO. Valgus deformity after reconstruction of the anterior cruciate ligament in a skeletally immature patient: a case report. *J Bone Joint Surg Am* 1999;81: 711–715.
237. Kocher MS, Saxon HS, Hovis WD, et al. Management and complications of anterior cruciate ligament injuries in skeletally immature patients: survey of the Herodicus Society and The ACL Study Group. *J Pediatr Orthop* 2002;22:452–457.
238. Lipscomb AB, Anderson AF. Tears of the anterior cruciate ligament in adolescents. *J Bone Joint Surg Am* 1986;68:19–28.
239. Lo IK, Kirkley A, Fowler PJ, Miniaci A. The outcome of operatively treated anterior cruciate ligament disruptions in the skeletally immature child. *Arthroscopy* 1997;13: 627–634.
240. Luhmann SJ. Acute traumatic knee effusions in children and adolescents. *J Pediatr Orthop* 2003;23:199–202.
241. Matava MJ, Siegel MG. Arthroscopic reconstruction of the ACL with gracilis-gracilis autograft in skeletally immature adolescent patients. *Am J Knee Surg* 1997;10:60–69.
242. McCarroll JR, Shelbourne KD, Porter DA, et al. Patellar tendon graft reconstruction for midsubstance anterior cruciate ligament rupture in junior high school athletes: an algorithm for management. *Am J Sports Med* 1994;22:478–484.
243. Micheli LJ, Rask B, Gerberg L. Anterior cruciate ligament reconstruction in patients who are prepubescent. *Clin Orthop* 1999;364:40–47.
244. Millett PJ, Willis AA, Warren RF. Associated injuries in pediatric and adolescent anterior cruciate ligament tears: does a delay in treatment increase the risk of meniscal tear? *Arthroscopy* 2002;18:955–999.
245. Mizuta H, Kubota K, Shiraishi M, et al. The conservative treatment of complete tears of the anterior cruciate ligament in skeletally immature patients. *J Bone Joint Surg Br* 1995;77:890–894.
246. Pressman AE, Letts RM, Jarvis JG. Anterior cruciate ligament tears in children: an analysis of operative versus nonoperative treatment. *J Pediatr Orthop* 1997;17:505–511.
247. Shelbourne KD, Gray T, Wiley BV. Results of transphyseal anterior cruciate ligament reconstruction using patellar tendon autograft in Tanner stage 3 or 4 adolescents with clearly open growth plates. *Am J Sports Med* 2004;32:1218–1222.
248. Simonian PT, Metcalf MH, Larson RV. Anterior cruciate ligament injuries in the skeletally immature patient. *Am J Orthop* 1999;28:624–628.
249. Stadelmaier DM, Arnoczky SP, Dodds J, et al. The effect of drilling and soft tissue grafting across open growth plates: a histologic study. *Am J Sports Med* 1995;23: 431–435.

250. Stanitski CL. Anterior cruciate ligament injury in the skeletally immature patient: diagnosis and treatment. *J Am Acad Orthop Surg* 1995;3:146–158.
251. Vahasarja V, Kinnuen P, Serlo W. Arthroscopy of the acute traumatic knee in children: prospective study of 138 cases. *Acta Orthop Scand* 1993;64:580–582.
252. Kocher MS, DiCanzio J, Zurakowski D, et al. Diagnostic performance of clinical examination and selective magnetic resonance imaging in the evaluation of intraarticular knee disorders in children and adolescents. *Am J Sports Med* 2001;29:292–296.
253. Stanitski CL, Harvell JC, Fu F. Observations on acute knee hemarthrosis in children and adolescents. *J Pediatr Orthop* 1993;13:506–510.
254. Eady JL, Cardenas CD, Sopa D. Avulsion of the femoral attachment of the anterior cruciate ligament in a 7-year-old child. *J Bone Joint Surg Am* 1982;64:1376–1378.
255. Joseph KN, Pogrund H. Traumatic rupture of the medial ligament of the knee in a 4-year-old boy: a case report and review of the literature. *J Bone Joint Surg Am* 1978;60: 402–403.
256. Mayer PJ, Micheli LJ. Avulsion of the femoral attachment of the posterior cruciate ligament in an 11-year-old boy: a case report. *J Bone Joint Surg Am* 1979;61:431–432.
257. Waldrop JI, Broussard TS. Disruption of the anterior cruciate ligament in a 3-year-old child. *J Bone Joint Surg Am* 1984;66:1113–1114.
258. Bertin KC, Goble EM. Ligament injuries associated with physeal fractures about the knee. *Clin Orthop* 1983;177:188–195.
259. Bergstrom R, Gillquist J, Lysholm J, et al. Arthroscopy of the knee in children. *J Pediatr Orthop* 1984;4:542–545.
260. Morrissy RT, Eubanks RG, Park JP, et al. Arthroscopy of the knee in children. *Clin Orthop* 1982;162:103–107.
261. Sigge W, Ellebrecht T. Arthroscopy of the injured knee in children. *Z Kinderchir* 1988; 43(suppl 1):68–70.
262. Suman RK, Stother IG, Illingworth G. Diagnostic arthroscopy of the knee in children. *J Bone Joint Surg Br* 1984;66:535–537.
263. Palmer L. On the injuries to the ligaments of the knee: a clinical study. *Acta Chir Scand Suppl* 1938;81:53.
264. Indelicato PA. Nonoperative treatment of complete tears of the medial collateral ligaments of the knee. *J Bone Joint Surg Am* 1983;65:323–329.
265. Hughston JC, Bowden JA, Andrews JR, et al. Acute tears of the posterior cruciate ligament. *J Bone Joint Surg Am* 1980;62:438–450.
266. Sanders WE, Wilkins KE, Neidre A. Acute insufficiency of the posterior cruciate ligament in children. *J Bone Joint Surg Am* 1980;62:129–130.
267. DeHaven KE. Diagnosis of acute knee injuries with hemarthrosis. *Am J Sports Med* 1980;8:9.
268. DeHaven KE, Collins HR. Diagnosis of internal derangement of the knee. *J Bone Joint Surg Am* 1975;57:802–810.
269. Fetto JF, Marshall JL. The natural history and diagnosis of anterior cruciate ligament insufficiency. *Clin Orthop* 1980;147:29–38.
270. Fetto JF, Marshall JL. Injury to the anterior cruciate ligament producing the pivot-shift sign. *J Bone Joint Surg Am* 1979;61:710–714.
271. Fowler PJ. The classification and early diagnosis of knee joint instability. *Clin Orthop* 1980;147:15–21.
272. Hughston JC, Andrews JR, Cross MJ, et al. Classification of knee ligament instabilities. I. The medial compartment and cruciate ligaments. *J Bone Joint Surg Am* 1976;58:159–172.
273. Sisk TD. Knee injuries. In: Crenshaw AH, ed. *Campbell's Operative Orthopaedics*, 7th ed, vol 3. St. Louis: Mosby; 1987:2336–2338.
274. McCarroll JR, Rettig AC, Shelbourne KD. Anterior cruciate ligament injuries in the young athlete with open physes. *Am J Sports Med* 1988;16:44–47.
275. Houle JB, Letts M, Yang J. Effects of a tensioned tendon graft in a bone tunnel across the rabbit physis. *Clin Orthop* 2001;391:275–281.
276. Engebretsen L, Svenningsen S, Benum P. Poor results of anterior cruciate ligament repair in adolescents. *Acta Orthop Scand* 1988;59:684–686.
277. Volpi P, Galli M, Bait C. Surgical treatment of anterior cruciate ligament injuries in adolescents using double-looped semitendinosus and gracilis tendons: supraepiphysary femoral and tibial fixation. *Arthroscopy* 2004;20:447–449.
278. Guzzanti V, Falciglia F, Stanitski CL. Preoperative evaluation and anterior cruciate ligament reconstruction technique for skeletally immature patients in Tanner stages 2 and 3. *Am J Sports Med* 2003;31:941–948.
279. Parker AW, Drez D, Cooper JL. Anterior cruciate ligament injuries in patients with open physes. *Am J Sports Med* 1994;22:44–47.
280. Greulich WW, Pysle SI. *Radiographic Atlas of Skeletal Development of the Hand and Wrist*. 2nd ed. Stanford: Stanford University Press; 1959.
281. Pyle SI, Hoerr NL. *A Radiographic Standard of Reference the Growing Knee*. Springfield, IL: Charles C Thomas; 1969.
282. Tanner JM, Whitehouse RH. Clinical longitudinal standards for height, weight, height velocity, and stages of puberty. *Arch Dis Child* 1976;51:170–179.
283. MacIntosh DL. Lateral substitution reconstruction in proceedings and reports of universities, colleges, councils, and associations. *J Bone Joint Surg Br* 1976;58:142.
284. Behr CT, Potter HG, Paletta GA Jr. The relationship of the femoral origin of the anterior cruciate ligament and the distal femoral physeal plate in the skeletally immature knee. An anatomic study. *Am J Sports Med* 2001;29:781–787.
285. Goodrich A, Ballard A. Posterior cruciate ligament avulsion associated with ipsilateral femur fracture in a 10-year-old child. *J Trauma* 1988;28:1393–1396.
286. Ross AC, Chesterman PJ. Isolated avulsion of the tibial attachment of the posterior cruciate ligament in childhood. *J Bone Joint Surg Br* 1986;68:747.
287. Torisu T. Isolated avulsion fracture of the tibial attachment of the posterior cruciate ligament. *J Bone Joint Surg Am* 1977;59:68–72.
288. Clancy WG, Shelbourne KD, Zoellner GB, et al. Treatment of knee joint instability secondary to rupture of the posterior cruciate ligament: report of a new procedure. *J Bone Joint Surg Am* 1983;65:310–322.
289. Gartland JJ, Brenner JH. Traumatic dislocations in the lower extremity in children. *Orthop Clin North Am* 1976;7:687–700.
290. DeLee JC. Complete dislocation of the knee in a 9-year-old. *Contemp Orthop* 1979;1: 29–32.
291. Dart CH Jr, Braitman HE. Popliteal artery injury following fracture or dislocation at the knee: diagnosis and management. *Arch Surg* 1977;112:969–973.
292. Green NE, Allen BL. Vascular injuries associated with dislocation of the knee. *J Bone Joint Surg Am* 1977;59:236–239.
293. Kennedy JC. Complete dislocation of the knee joint. *J Bone Joint Surg Am* 1963;45: 889–904.
294. Kocher MS, Garg S, Micheli LJ. Growth plate sparing combined intra-articular and extra-articular anterior cruciate ligament reconstruction with iliotibial band in skeletally immature preadolescent children. *J Bone Joint Surg* (in press).

FRACTURES OF THE SHAFT OF THE TIBIA AND FIBULA

Stephen D. Heinrich and James F. Mooney, III

EPIDEMIOLOGY

Tibial and fibular fractures are the third most common pediatric long bone injuries (15%) after femoral and radial/ulnar fractures (1,2). The prevalence of tibial fractures in both boys and girls has increased since 1950 (3). The average age of occurrence is 8 years, and the frequency of occurrence does not change significantly with age (4). Seventy percent of pediatric tibial fractures are isolated injuries; ipsilateral fibular fractures occur with 30% of tibial fractures (2,5,6). Fifty to 70% of tibial fractures occur in the distal third, and 19% to 39% in the middle third. The least commonly affected portion of the tibia is the proximal third, yet these may be most problematic. Thirty-five percent of pediatric tibial fractures are oblique, 32% comminuted, 20% transverse, and 13% spiral (1). Tibial fractures in children under 4 years of age usually are isolated spiral or sharp oblique fractures in the distal and the middle one third of the bone. Most tibial fractures in older children and adolescents are at the ankle. Rotational forces produce an oblique or a spiral fracture and are responsible for approximately 81% of all tibial fractures without fibular fractures (1,5,7–9). Bicycle spoke injuries occur in children 1 to 4 years of age, whereas most tibial fractures in children 4 to 14 years of age occur in sporting or traffic accidents (1,3–5,7,9). Over 50% of ipsilateral tibial and fibular fractures result from vehicular trauma. Most isolated fibular fractures result from a direct blow (1,4). The tibia is the second most commonly fractured bone in abused children. Approximately 16% to 26% of all abused children with a fracture have an injured tibia (10,11).

Approximately 9% of pediatric tibial fractures are open. Concomitant fractures of the ankle and foot are the most common injuries associated with fractures of the tibia and fibula, followed by humeral, femoral, and radial/ulnar fractures (12). The average index severity score of a child with a tibial fracture is 10 (range, 0–45) with an average hospital stay of 6.5 days (range, 1–50 days) (12).

SURGICAL ANATOMY

Bony Structure

The tibia ("flute") is the second largest bone in the body. There are two concave condyles at the proximal aspect of the tibia. The medial condyle is larger, deeper, and narrower than the lateral condyle. An elevated process, the tibial tubercle, located between the two condyles is the site of attachment of the patellar tendon. The shaft of the tibia is prismoid, with a broad proximal extent that decreases in size until the distal third, where it gradually increases in size. The tibial crest is prominent medially from the tibial tubercle to the tibial plafond and is subcutaneous without any overlying muscles (8).

The tibia develops from three ossification centers: one in the shaft and one in each epiphysis. The tibial diaphysis ossifies at 7 weeks of gestation and expands both proximally and distally. The proximal epiphyseal center appears shortly after birth and unites with the shaft between 14 and 16 years of age. The distal epiphyseal ossification center appears in the second year of life, and the distal tibial physis closes between 14 and 15 years of age. Additional ossification centers are occasionally found in the medial malleolus and in the tibial tubercle (8).

The tibia articulates with the condyles of the femur proximally, with the fibula at the knee and the ankle, and with the talus distally (8). Twelve muscles have either their origin or insertion on the tibia (Table 25-1).

The fibula articulates with the tibia and the talus. The fibular diaphysis ossifies at about 8 weeks of gestation. The distal epiphysis is visible at 2 years of age, and the proximal secondary ossification center at 4 years. The distal fibular physis closes at approximately 16 years; the proximal physis closes later, between the age of 15 and 18 years (8). Nine muscles have either their origin or insertion on the fibula (Table 25-2) (8).

TABLE 25-1 Muscle Origins and Insertions on the Tibia

Muscle	Origin/Insertion
Semimembranosus	Inserts on inner tuberosity of the proximal tibia
Tibialis anterior, extensor digitorum longus, biceps femoris	Attach to the lateral condyle of the tibia
Sartorius, gracilis, semitendinosus	Insert on the proximal medial surface of the tibial metaphysis
Tibialis anterior	Arises on the lateral surface of the tibial diaphysis
Popliteus, soleus, flexor digitorum longus, tibialis posterior	Attach to the posterior diaphysis of the tibia
Patellar tendon	Inserts into the tibial tubercle
Tensor fascia lata	Attaches to Gerdy's tubercle, the lateral aspect of the proximal tibial metaphysis
Secondary slip of fascia lata	Occasionally inserts into the tibial tubercle

Reprinted from Gray H. Anatomy: descriptive and surgical. In: Pick TP, Howden R, eds. *Anatomy: descriptive and surgical.* New York: Bounty Books, 1977:182; with permission.

TABLE 25-2 Muscle Origins and Insertions on the Fibula

Muscle	Origin/Insertion
Soleus, flexor hallucis longus	Arise from the posterior aspect of the diaphysis
Peroneus longus, peroneus brevis	Arise from the lateral aspect of the fibular diaphysis
Biceps femoris, soleus, peroneus longus	Attach to the head of the fibula
Extensor digitorum longus, peroneus tertius, extensor hallucis longus	Attach to the anterior surface of the fibular shaft
Tibialis posterior	Arises from the medial aspect of the fibular diaphysis

Reprinted from Gray H. Anatomy: descriptive and surgical. In: Pick TP, Howden R, eds. *Anatomy: descriptive and surgical.* New York: Bounty Books, 1977:182; with permission.

VASCULAR ANATOMY

The popliteal artery descends vertically between the condyles of the femur and passes between the two heads of the gastrocnemius muscle. It ends at the distal border of the popliteus muscle, where it divides into the anterior and posterior tibial arteries. The anterior tibial artery passes between the tibia and the fibula over the proximal aspect of the intraosseous membrane. The posterior tibial artery divides several centimeters distal to this point, giving rise to the peroneal artery (Fig. 25-1) (8).

Nerves

The posterior tibial nerve runs adjacent and posterior to the popliteal artery in the popliteal fossa. The common peroneal nerve passes around the proximal neck of the fibula. It divides into the deep and superficial branches, passing into the anterior and the lateral compartments of the lower leg (8), respectively. Each branch innervates the muscles within its compartment. The deep peroneal nerve provides sensation to the first web space. The superficial branch is responsible for sensation across the dorsal surface of the foot.

Fascial Compartments

The lower leg has four fascial compartments (Fig. 25-2). The anterior compartment contains the extensor digitorum longus, the extensor hallucis longus, and the tibialis anterior muscles; the anterior tibial artery and deep peroneal nerve run in this compartment. The lateral compartment contains the peroneus longus and brevis muscles. The superficial peroneal nerve runs through this compartment. The superficial posterior compartment contains the soleus and gastrocnemius muscles. The deep posterior compartment contains the flexor digitorum longus, the flexor hallucis longus, and the tibialis posterior muscles. The posterior tibial artery, peroneal artery, and tibial nerve run in this compartment (8).

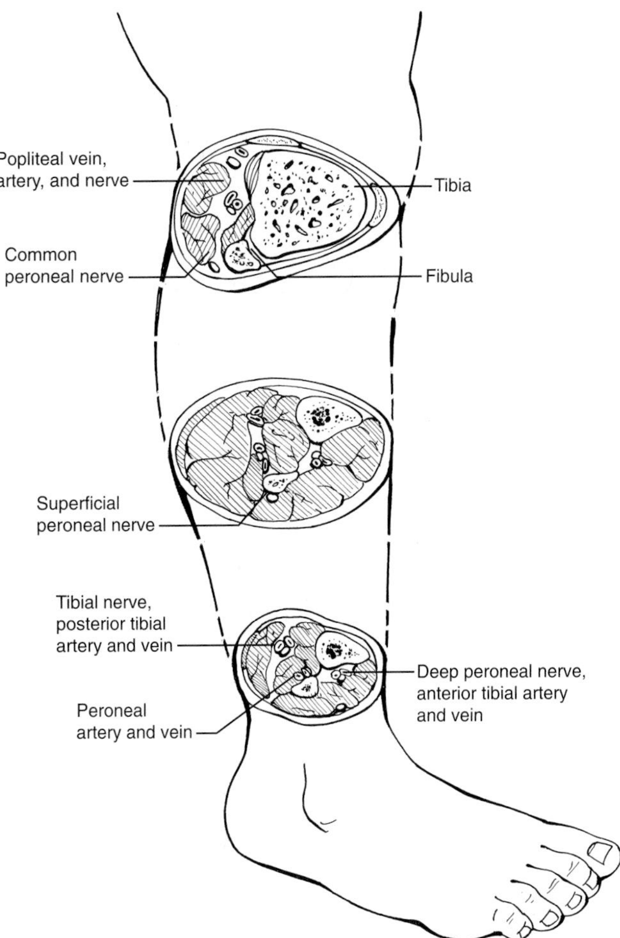

FIGURE 25-2 Fibrosseous compartments of the leg.

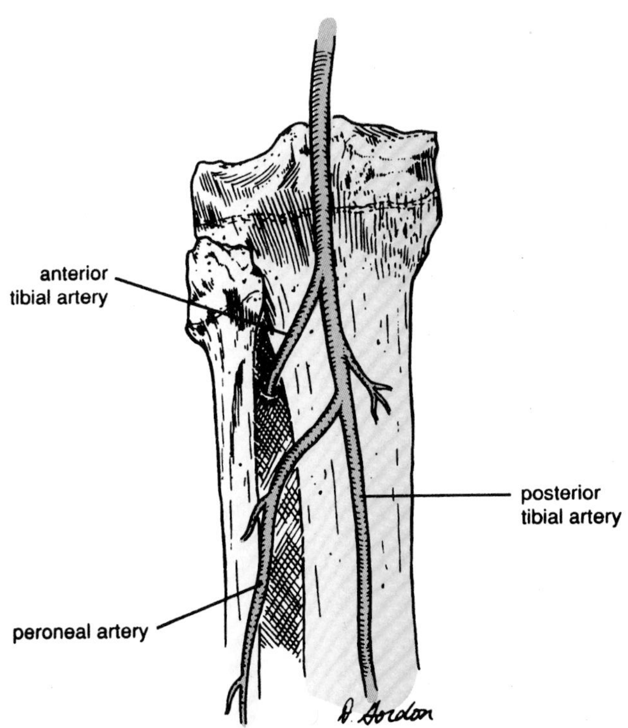

FIGURE 25-1 Vascular anatomy of the proximal tibia.

CLASSIFICATION

Nonphyseal injuries of the tibia and the fibula can be classified into three major categories based on the combination of bones fractured and the location of the injuries.

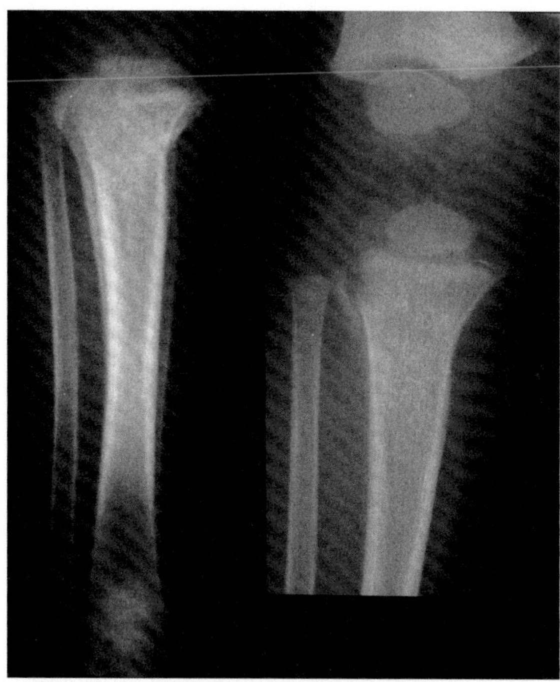

FIGURE 25-3 Anteroposterior x-rays of the knee in a 9-month-old child who was abused shows a proximal tibial metaphyseal corner fracture with extension into the physis (*right*). The follow-up x-ray on the *left* demonstrates marked new bone function, which suggests the degree of periosteal stripping that occurred at the time of the injury.

FRACTURES OF THE PROXIMAL TIBIAL METAPHYSIS

The peak incidence for proximal tibial metaphyseal fractures is between the ages of 3 and 6 years. The most common mechanism of injury is a force applied to the lateral aspect of the extended knee. The cortex of the medial tibial metaphysis fails in tension, often resulting in an incomplete fracture. The fibula ordinarily escapes injury, although plastic deformation may occur (13–28). Occasionally, a proximal tibial metaphyseal fracture can occur as the result of abuse (Fig. 25-3).

Children with proximal tibial metaphyseal fractures present with pain, swelling, and tenderness in the region of the fracture. Motion of the knee causes moderate pain, and the child will not walk. Crepitance is seldom identified on physical examination, especially if the fracture is incomplete (13–20,23–29).

X-rays usually show a complete or incomplete fracture of the proximal tibial metaphysis. The medial aspect of the fracture often is open, producing a valgus deformity (13–19, 22–28).

The most common sequela of proximal tibial metaphyseal fractures is a valgus deformity (Fig. 25-4). In 1953, Cozen (16) reported four patients with valgus deformities after fractures of the proximal tibial metaphysis. Since that time, many other investigators (2,14,15,17–20,25,26,29,30) have reported tibia valga after proximal tibial metaphyseal fractures.

Many theories have been proposed to explain the development of a valgus deformity after a proximal metaphyseal fracture (Table 25-3). Proximal tibia valga can be caused by an inadequate reduction or the loss of a satisfactory reduction in the weeks following the manipulation (23,27). Lehner and Dubas suggested that an expanding medial callus produced a valgus deformity (30), whereas Goff (31) and Keret et al (20) believed that the lateral aspect of the proximal tibial physis was injured (Salter-Harris type V fracture), resulting in asymmetric growth. Taylor (25) believed that the valgus deformity was secondary to postfracture stimulation of the tibial physis without a corresponding stimulation of the fibular physis. Pollen (32) suggested that premature weight-bearing produced an angular deformity of the fracture before union. Rooker and Salter (33) believed that the periosteum was trapped in the medial aspect of the fracture, producing an increase in medial physeal growth and a developmental valgus deformity.

A recently suggested etiology for postfracture tibia valgus is an injury to the pes anserinus tendon plate. The pes anserinus tethers the medial aspect of the physis just as the fibula tethers the lateral aspect of the proximal tibial physis. The proximal tibial fracture disrupts the pes anserinus tendon plate, producing a loss of the tethering affect. This leads to medial physeal overgrowth and a functional hemi-chondrodiastasis (14,26, 28,34,35). Exploration of the fracture followed by removal and repair of the infolded periosteum that forms the foundation of the pes anserinus tendon plate has been suggested to decrease the risk of a developmental varus deformity.

Another theory postulates that the progressive valgus deformity occurs because vascular flow to the proximal tibial physis increases after fracture, producing an asymmetric physeal response that causes increased medial growth (19). Support for this theory includes quantitative bone scans performed months after proximal tibial metaphyseal fractures that have shown increased tracer uptake in the medial aspect of the physis compared with the lateral aspect (27). Developmental tibia valga has been reported to occur after simple excision of a bone graft from the proximal tibial metaphysis (25), tibial osteotomy (13,18), and osteomyelitis of the proximal tibial metaphysis (13,25). Ogden (21) identified an increase in the collateral geniculate vascularity to the medial proximal tibia in a cadaver angiography study of a 5-year-old child. This also supports the theory that medial overgrowth occurs secondary to an increase in the blood flow supplying the medial aspect of the proximal tibia following injury (36). The overgrowth of the tibia that occurs in many children with tibial valgus deformity after fracture is further evidence of an abnormality in the response of the proximal tibial physis to fracture (18,25). A tibia valga deformity can occur after healing of a nondisplaced fracture and can recur after corrective tibial osteotomy, further supporting the premise that asymmetric physeal growth is the cause of most posttraumatic tibia valga deformities (27).

Robert et al (37), in an analysis of 25 patients with proximal tibial fractures, identified three groups of patients. Twelve chil-

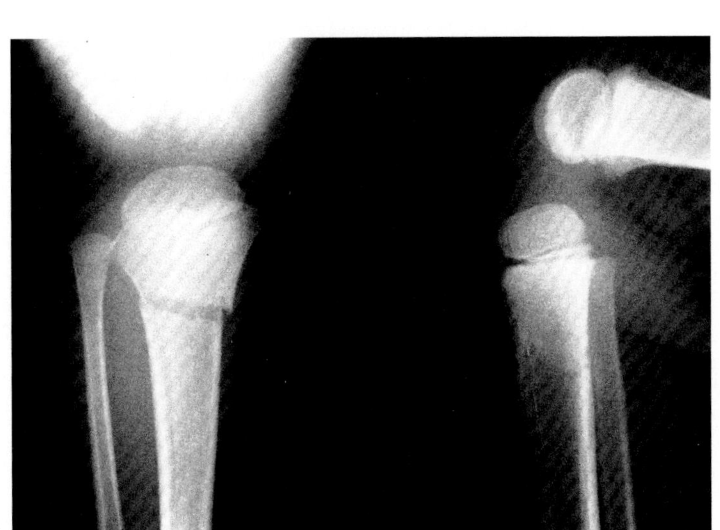
A

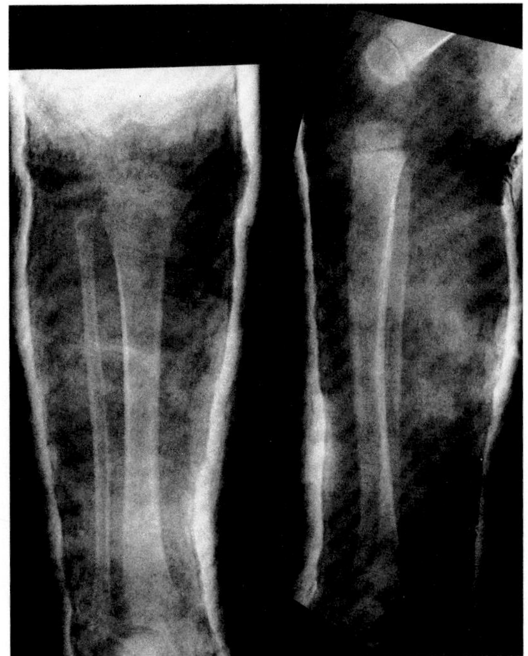
B

C

FIGURE 25-4 **A.** Anteroposterior and lateral x-rays of the proximal tibial metaphyseal fracture with an intact fibula in a 3-year-old child. **B.** Anteroposterior and lateral x-rays in the initial long leg cast demonstrate an acceptable alignment. **C.** Posttraumatic tibia valga is present 1 year after fracture union. (Reprinted from Sharps CH, Cardea JA. Fractures of the shaft of the tibia and fibula. In: MacEwen GD, Kasser JR, Heinrich SD, eds. *Pediatric fractures: a practical approach to assessment and treatment.* Baltimore: Williams & Wilkins, 1993:321; with permission.)

TABLE 25-3 Proposed Etiologies of Trauma-Induced Tibia Valgus

Asymmetric activity of medial portion of proximal tibial physis (overgrowth)
Tethering effect; fibula
Inadequate reduction
Interposed soft tissue (pes anserinus); medial collateral ligament
Loss of tethering effect of the pes anserinus
Early weight-bearing producing developmental valgus
Physeal arrest of the lateral aspect of the proximal tibial physis

dren with a greenstick or a complete fracture developed valgus deformities. No child with a torus fracture developed a valgus deformity. Altered growth at the distal tibial physis compensated for the compromised tibia valga in three children. Corrective osteotomies were performed in four children. The valgus deformity recurred in two of these four children, and two had iatrogenic compartment syndromes. This study supports the recommendation that developmental tibia valga should not be corrected until the child reaches puberty. At that point, a proximal tibial medial epiphysiodesis can be performed to allow the tibia to correct slowly (7,24,25,29,37).

Support for a "wait and see" attitude also was provided by Zionts and MacEwen (28), who followed seven children with progressive valgus deformities of the tibia for an average of 39 months after metaphyseal fractures. Most of the deformity developed during the first year after injury. The tibia continued to angulate at a slower rate for up to 17 months after injury. Six of their seven patients had spontaneous clinical corrections. At follow-up, all children had less than a 10-degree deformity.

Treatment

Nondisplaced proximal tibial metaphyseal fractures are stabilized with a long leg cast with the knee in nearly full extension and a varus mold (Fig. 25-5).

Displaced proximal tibial fractures require closed reduction with general anesthesia in the operating room or in an emergency room setting with adequate sedation. An anatomic reduction or slight varus positioning should be verified with x-rays. If closed reduction to an anatomic or slight varus position cannot be obtained, an open reduction is indicated. Interposed soft tissue is removed from the fracture, and the pes anserinus plate is repaired if ruptured. The child is placed into a long-leg, straight-knee cast after reduction, and the alignment is checked once again with x-rays. The goal is anatomic reduction or slight varus position. Frequent follow-up visits are required to verify maintenance of the reduction. The cast is removed approximately 6 weeks after injury. The child may return to normal activities after recovery of normal knee and ankle range of motion. Long-term follow-up with a warning to the family of possible growth abnormality is mandatory.

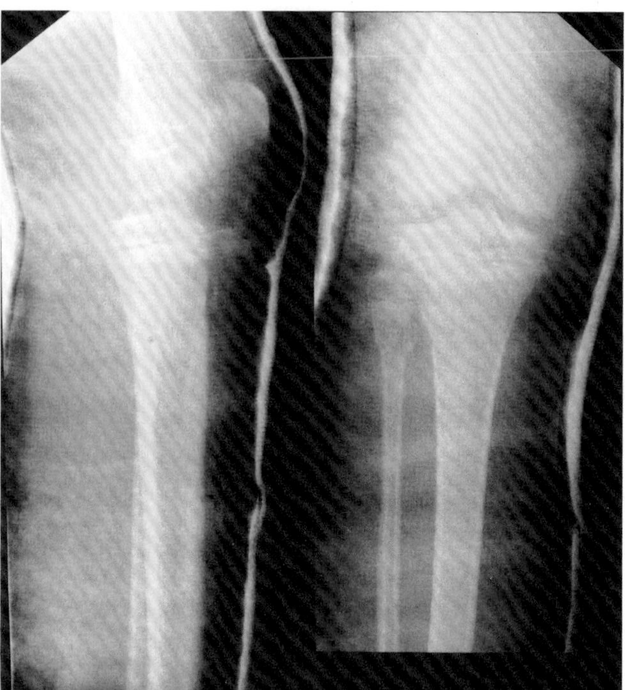

FIGURE 25-5 Anteroposterior and lateral x-rays of the proximal tibia and distal femur in a child who sustained a nondisplaced fracture of the proximal tibial metaphysis. The knee is casted in extension which facilitates accurate measurements of fracture alignment.

A child with a posttraumatic valgus deformity is followed until spontaneous correction occurs or until the child is old enough for surgical intervention. Tibial osteotomies rarely are indicated and generally should be delayed until adolescence (Fig. 25-6). A proximal tibial medial hemi-epiphysiodesis can produce a more anatomic alignment without many of the risks of osteotomy. Hemi-epiphysiodesis may be accomplished through a variety of methods including open grafting techniques or utilizing either staples or screws (Fig. 25-7) (24,36). Orthotic devices do not alter the natural history of posttraumatic tibia valga and are not recommended. However, because the valgus deformity usually is associated with overgrowth, a contralateral shoe lift of appropriate size may make the deformity less apparent.

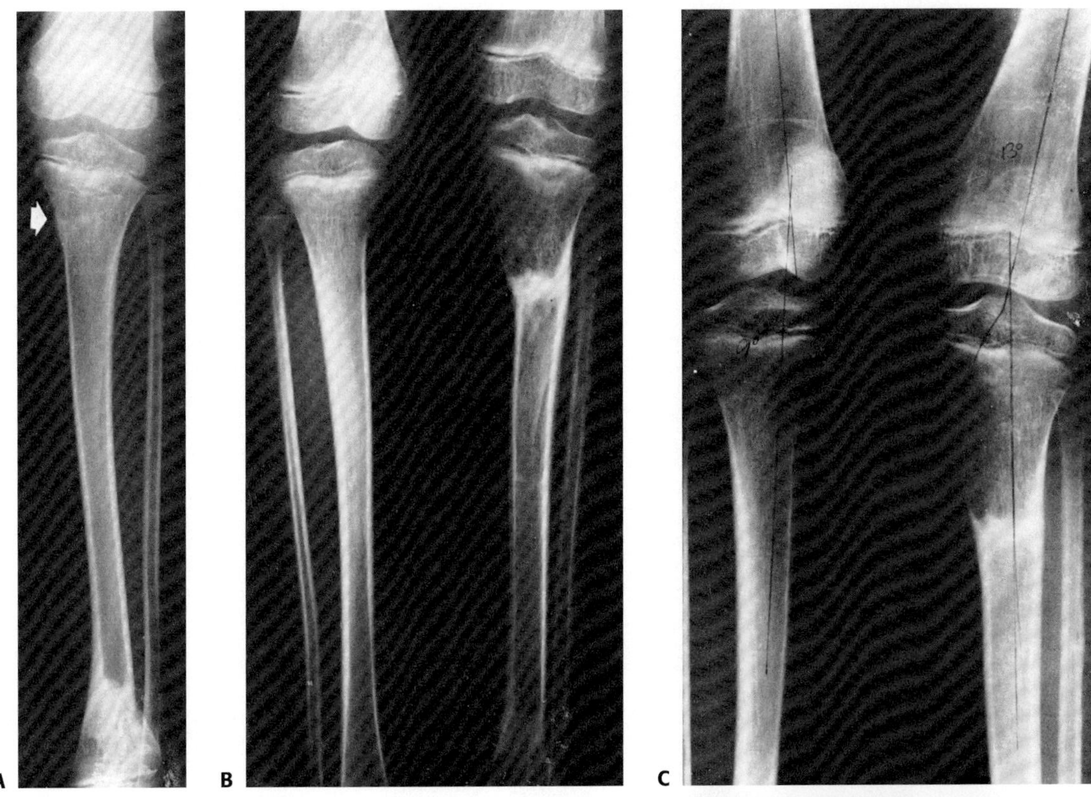

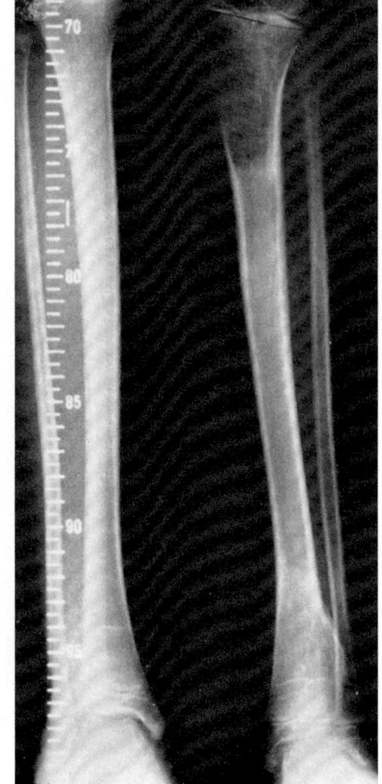

FIGURE 25-6 Developmental valgus after a proximal tibial metaphyseal fracture and subsequent corrective osteotomy. **A.** X-ray taken 6 months after a fracture of the proximal tibial injury was nondisplaced. The scar from the initial proximal metaphyseal fracture is still seen (*arrow*). This child developed a moderate valgus deformity of the tibia within 6 months of fracture. **B.** A proximal tibial corrective osteotomy was performed. **C.** Two months postoperatively the osteotomy was healed and the deformity corrected. **D.** Five months later there was a recurrent valgus deformity of 13 degrees. (Courtesy of John J.J. Gugenheim, MD.)

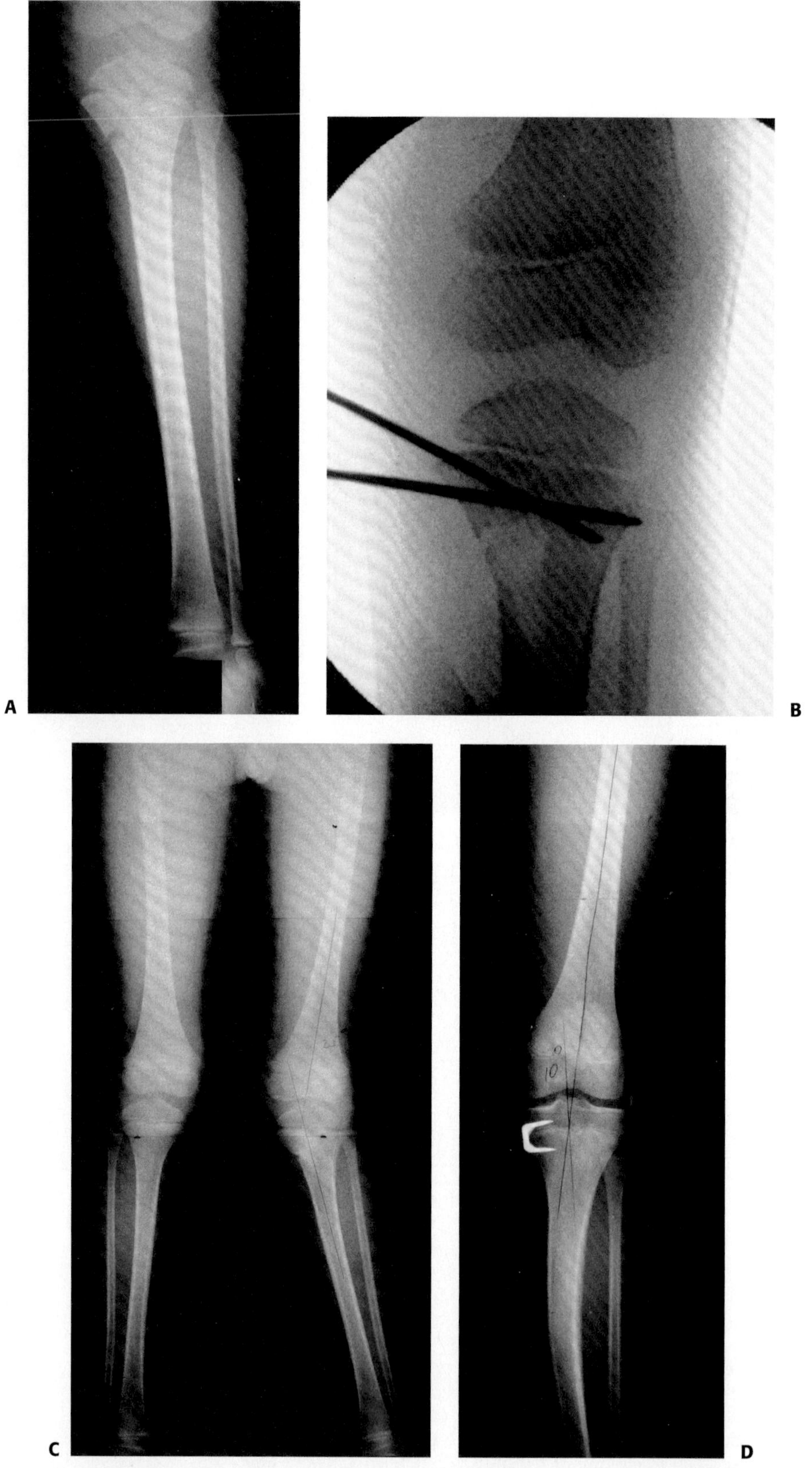

FIGURE 25-7 **A.** Anteroposterior image of a Salter-Harris type II fracture of the proximal tibia. Notice the valgus alignment. **B.** This fracture was treated with percutaneous pin fixation after reduction. **C.** This patient developed tibia valga over a period of approximately 2 years following the injury. **D.** A medial proximal tibial hemiepiphyseodesis using a staple was performed.

DIAPHYSEAL FRACTURES OF THE TIBIA AND FIBULA

Seventy percent of pediatric tibial fractures are isolated injuries (1,6,38). The fractures can be incomplete (torus, greenstick) or complete. Most tibial fractures in children under 11 years of age are caused by a torsional force and are located in the distal third of the tibia. These oblique and spiral fractures occur when the body rotates with the foot in a fixed position on the ground. The fracture line starts in the distal anteromedial aspect of the bone and propagates proximally in a posterolateral direction. Although the intact fibula prevents significant shortening of the tibia, varus angulation develops in approximately 60% of isolated tibial fractures within the first 2 weeks after injury (38) (Fig. 25-8). The force of contraction of the long flexor muscles of the lower leg are converted into an angular moment by the intact fibula producing the varus malalignment (Fig. 25-9A). Isolated transverse and comminuted fractures of the tibia are caused by direct trauma. Transverse fractures of the tibia with an intact fibula seldom displace (39,40). Comminuted fractures drift into varus alignment like oblique and spiral fractures (39,40,38).

Approximately 30% of pediatric tibial diaphyseal fractures have an associated fibular fracture (1,6,38). Plastic deformation of the fibula may produce valgus malalignment of the tibia (Fig. 25-10). The fibular injury must be identified to prevent recurrence of the malalignment after reduction (Fig. 25-11A–C). An associated complete fracture of the fibula usually results in valgus malalignment because of the action of the muscles in the anterolateral aspect of the leg (Fig. 25-9B).

An isolated fracture of the fibular shaft is rare in children and most commonly results from a direct blow to the lateral aspect of the leg (Fig. 25-12). Most isolated fractures of the fibular shaft are nondisplaced and heal quickly with symptomatic care (Fig. 25-13). Rarely, compartment syndrome may accompany this injury, and observation for this associated problem is mandatory.

Signs and Symptoms

The signs and symptoms associated with tibial and fibular diaphyseal fractures vary with the severity of the injury and the mechanism by which it was produced. Pain is the most common symptom. An isolated fibular fracture normally produces mild pain, whereas tibial fractures produce more severe pain. Children with stress fractures of the tibia or fibula complain of pain on weightbearing, but rarely have pain at rest.

Children with fractures of the tibia or fibula have swelling at the fracture site, and the area is tender to palpation. Young

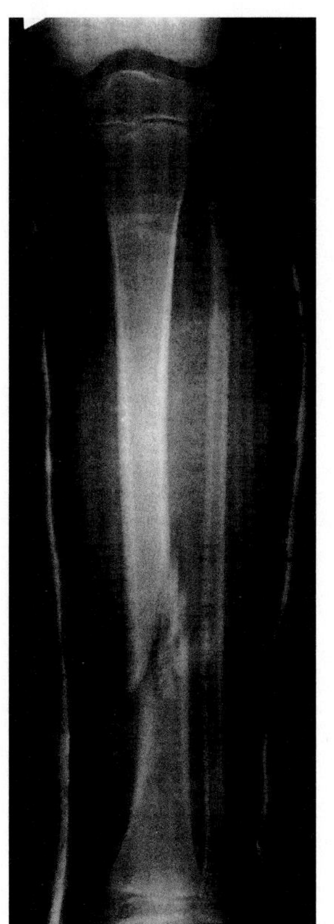

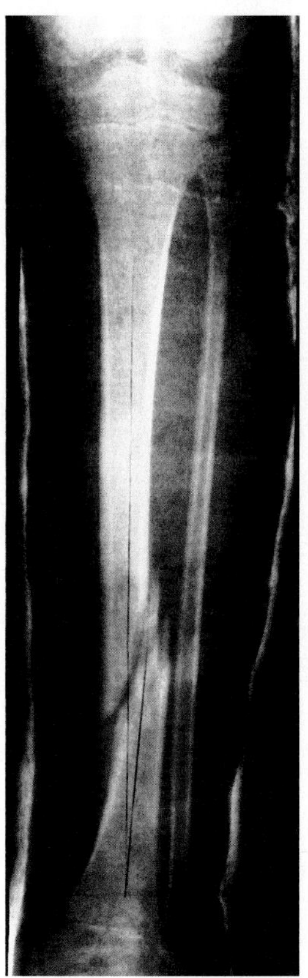

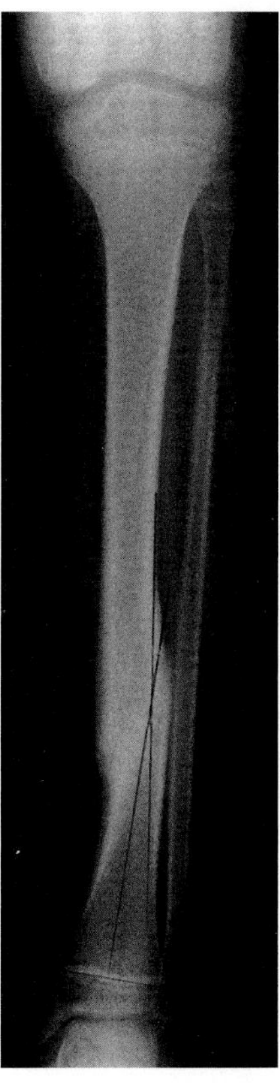

FIGURE 25-8 Anteroposterior x-ray of a distal one-third tibial fracture without concomitant fibular fracture in a 10-year-old child. **A.** The alignment in the coronal plane is acceptable (note that the proximal and distal tibial growth physes are parallel). **B.** A varus angulation developed within the first 2 weeks after injury. **C.** A 10-degree varus angulation was present after union.

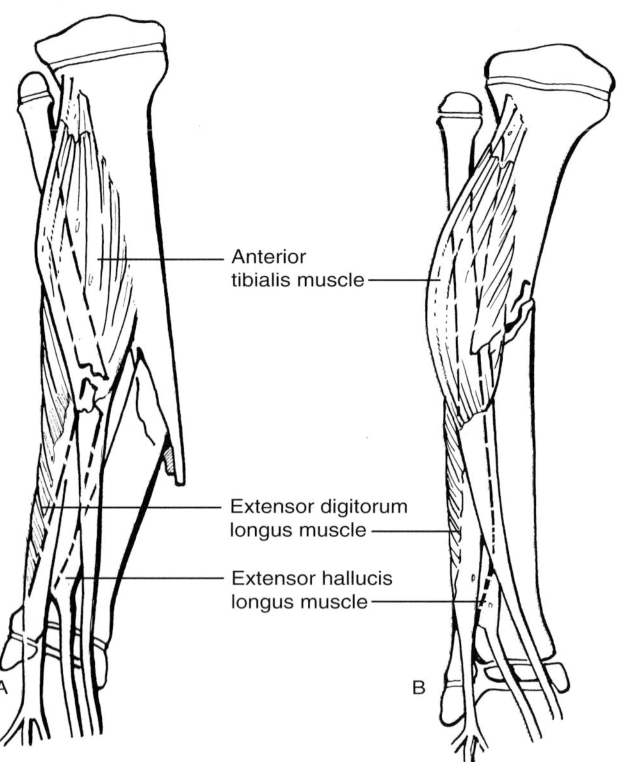

FIGURE 25-9 **A.** Fractures of the middle of the tibia without an associated fibular fracture tend to shift into varus due to the force created by the anterior compartment musculature of the lower leg and the tethering effect of the intact fibula. **B.** Fractures involving the mid-third of the tibia and fibula may shift into valgus alignment due to the activity of the muscles in the anterior and the lateral compartments of the lower leg.

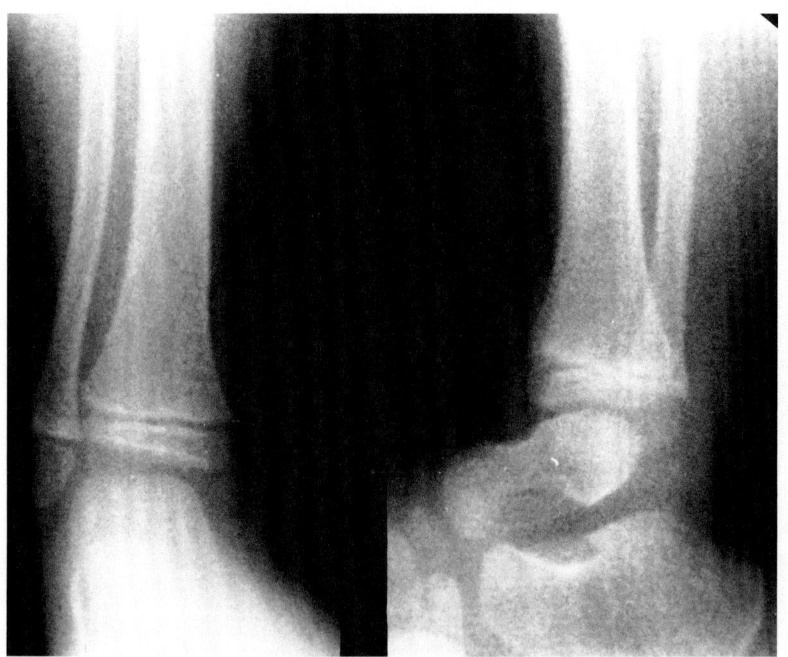

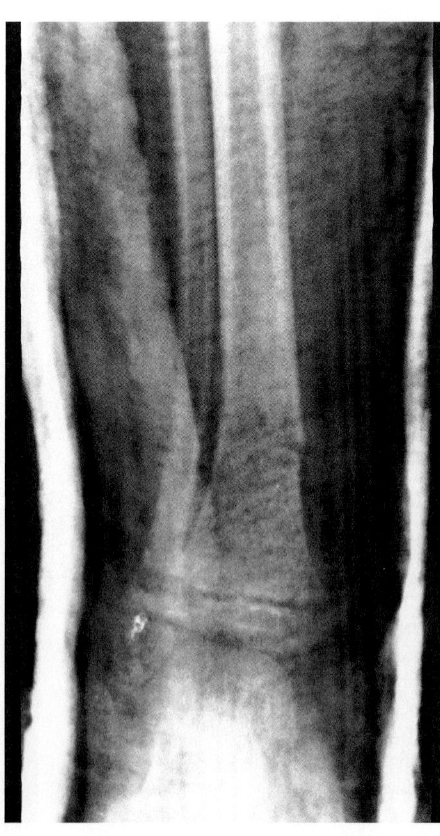

FIGURE 25-10 **A.** Plastic deformation of fibula secondary to a direct blow to the lateral aspect. Note medial nondisplaced fracture of the tibia. **B.** The tibial fracture displaced in the cast a week later from the force exerted by the plastically deformed fibula.

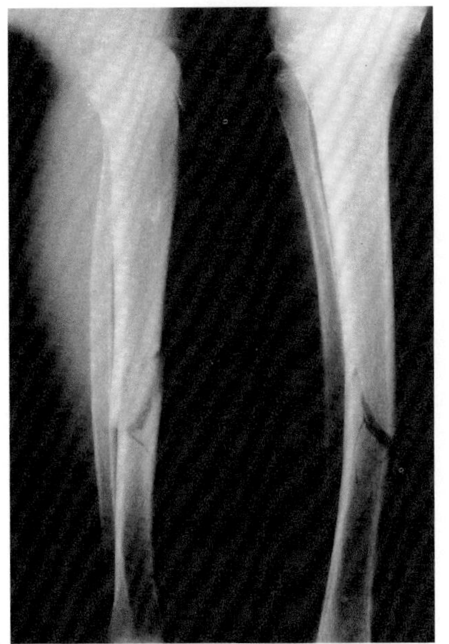

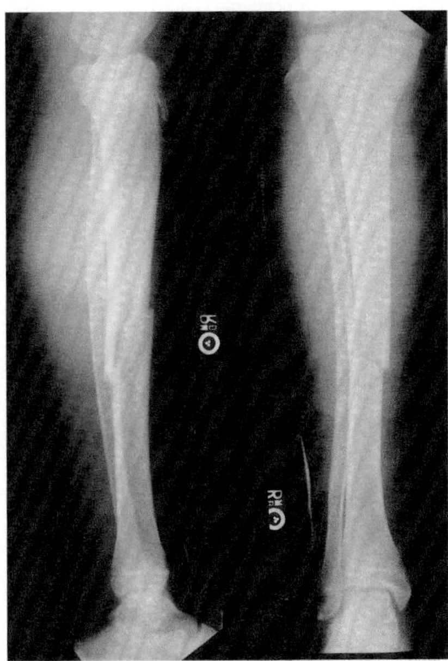

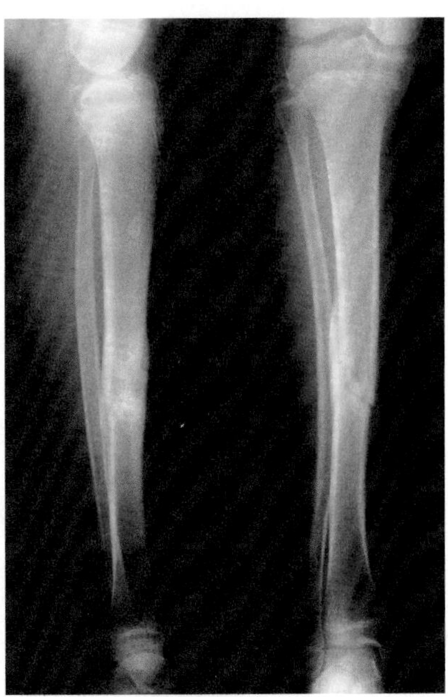

FIGURE 25-11 **A.** Anteroposterior and lateral x-ray of the lower leg in a 12-year-old child showing a comminuted tibial fracture with a concomitant plastic deformation of the fibula. Note the valgus alignment in the tibia. **B.** This patient had a closed manipulation and casting correcting the valgus alignment in the tibia and partially correcting the plastic deformation of the fibula. **C.** At union, there is an anatomic alignment of the tibia and the fibula has mild correction.

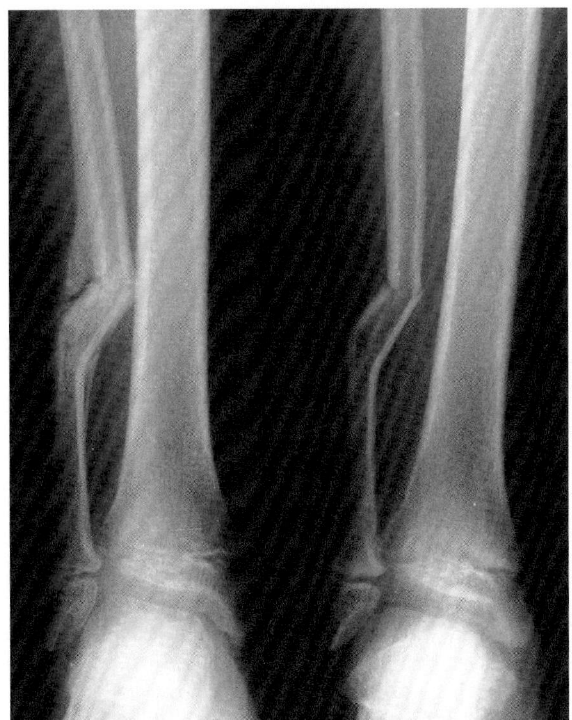

FIGURE 25-12 Distal one-third fibular fracture in an 8-year-old who was struck on the lateral side of the leg (*right*). There is moderate new bone formation 6 weeks after injury (*left*).

children with nondisplaced fractures may refuse to walk. If there is significant injury to the periosteum, a bony defect or prominence may be palpable in patients with a complete fracture. Neurologic impairment is rare except with fibular neck fractures caused by direct trauma.

Although arterial disruption is uncommon in pediatric tibial and fibular diaphyseal fractures, both the dorsalis pedis and the posterior tibial pulses should be checked, and a Doppler examination should be performed if they are not palpable. Capillary refill, sensation, and pain response patterns, particularly pain with passive motion, should be monitored.

Concomitant soft tissue injuries must be evaluated carefully. Open fractures must be treated aggressively to reduce the risk of late complications.

Radiographic Evaluation

Anteroposterior and lateral x-rays that include the knee and ankle joints (Fig. 25-14) should be obtained whenever a tibial or fibular shaft fracture is suspected. Comparison views of the uninvolved leg normally are not necessary. Children with suspected fractures not apparent on the initial x-rays may need to be treated with supportive casting to control symptoms associated with the injuries. Technetium radionuclide scans obtained at least 3 days after injury are useful to identify fractures that are unapparent on x-rays; however, in most cases, patients with clinical findings consistent with a fracture are treated as though a fracture is present. Periosteal new bone formation on plain x-rays obtained 10 to 14 days after injury confirms the diagnosis.

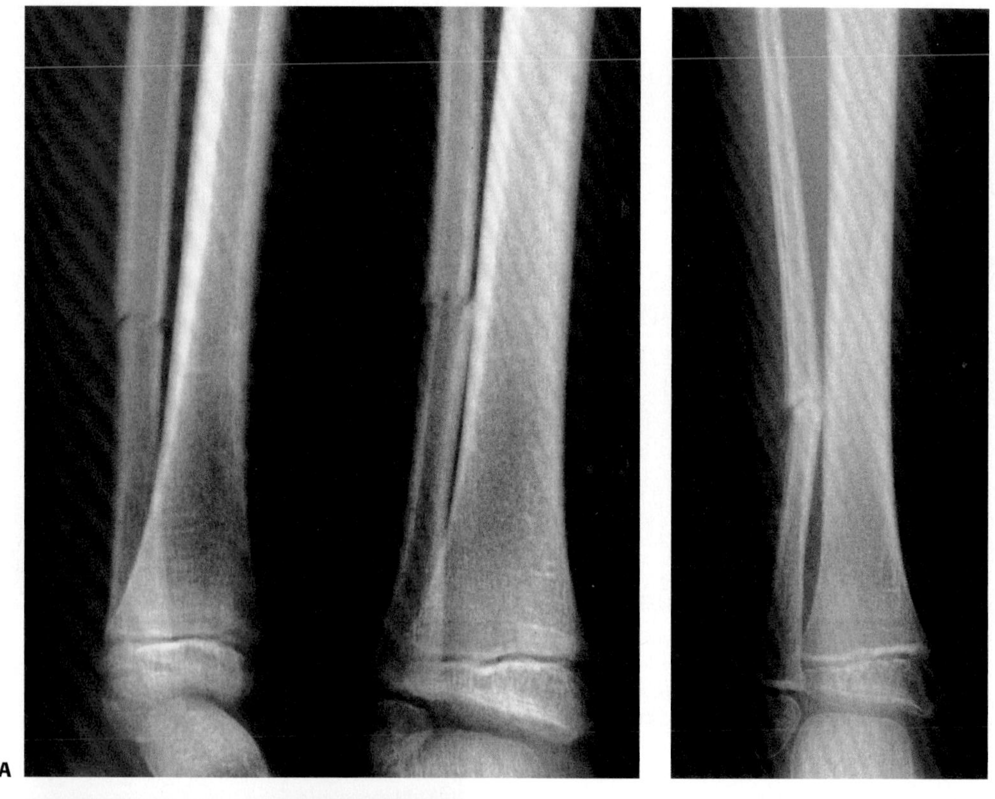

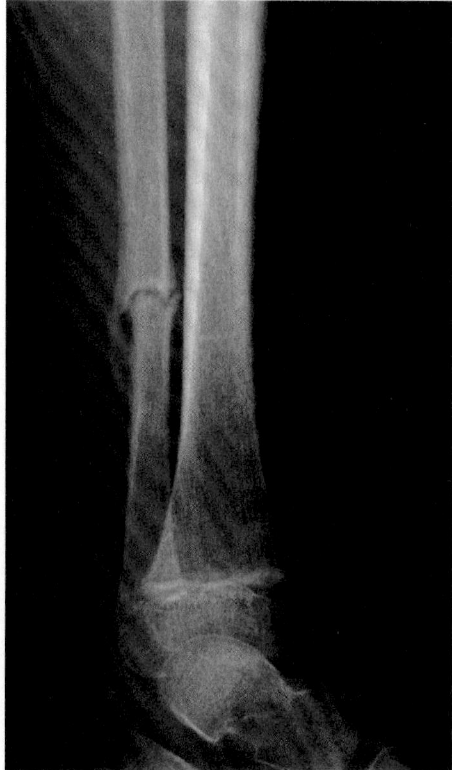

FIGURE 25-13 **A.** Anteroposterior and lateral x-rays of a 7-year-old child with an isolated open fibula fracture secondary to a bite by a pit bull. **B.** Anteroposterior x-ray 6 weeks after injury demonstrating consolidation at the fracture site. **C.** Lateral x-ray showing bridging callus 6 weeks after injury.

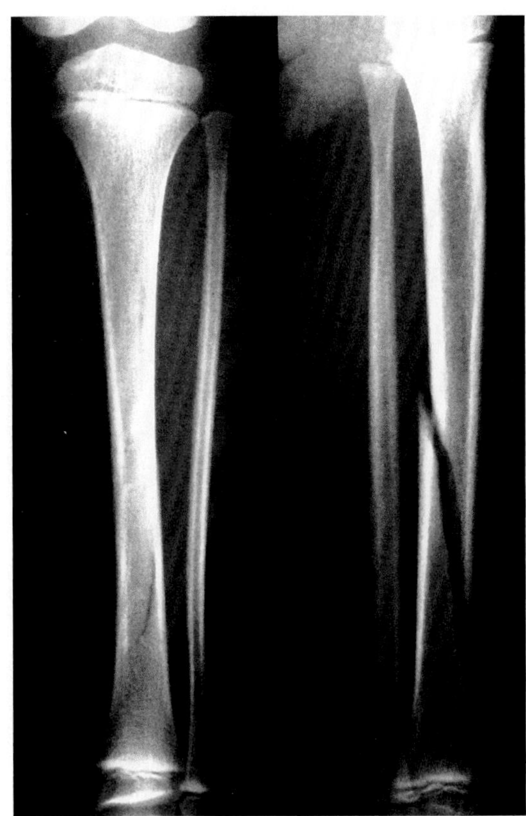

FIGURE 25-14 *Left.* Spiral fracture of the distal tibia. The fracture is difficult to identify on the anteroposterior x-ray. *Right.* The fracture is easily identified on the lateral x-ray.

TREATMENT

Cast Immobilization

Uncomplicated pediatric tibial and fibular shaft fractures can be treated by manipulation and cast application in most of patients (41). Fractures of the tibial shaft without concomitant fibular fracture may develop varus malalignment. Valgus angulation and shortening can present a significant problem in children who have complete fractures of both the tibia and the fibula. A recurvatum deformity also may develop.

Displaced fractures should be managed with reduction under appropriate sedation, using fluoroscopic assistance when available. This can be done in the emergency room, or more formally, in the operating room. The child's ankle initially may be left in some plantar flexion (20 degrees for fractures of the middle and distal thirds, 10 degrees for fractures of the proximal third) to prevent posterior angulation at the fracture. There is little risk of developing an equinus contracture.

A reduction plan should be made before manipulation based on review of the deforming forces apparent on the injury x-rays. A short-leg cast is applied with the foot in the appropriate position with either a varus or valgus mold, depending on the fracture pattern and alignment. The cast material is taken to the inferior aspect of the patella anteriorly and to a point 2 cm distal to the popliteal flexion crease posteriorly. It may be best to use plaster for the initial cast because of its ability to mold to the contour of the leg and the ease with which it can be manipulated while setting. The alignment of the fracture is rechecked after the short leg cast has been applied. The cast is then extended to the proximal thigh with the knee flexed. Most children with complete, unstable diaphyseal tibial fractures are placed into a bent-knee (45 degrees) long-leg cast to control rotation at the fracture site and to assist in maintaining nonweightbearing status during the initial healing phase.

The alignment of the fracture must be checked weekly during the first 3 weeks after the cast has been applied. Muscle atrophy and a reduction in tissue edema may allow the fracture to drift into unacceptable alignment. Some children require a second cast application with remanipulation of the fracture under general anesthesia several weeks after injury. Acceptable position is somewhat controversial. Remodeling of angular deformity is limited. No absolute number can be given, but the following general principles may be beneficial in decision making.

1. Varus and valgus deformity in the upper and mid-shaft tibia remodel slowly if at all. Up to 5 degrees of deformity can be accepted, but not more than 10 degrees.
2. Moderate translation of the shaft of the tibia in a young child is satisfactory, whereas in an adolescent, at least 50% apposition should be obtained.
3. Up to 10 degrees of anterior angulation may be tolerated, although remodeling is slow.
4. Little posterior angulation can be accepted because this forces the knee into extension at heel strike during walking and can produce pain.
5. No more than 1 cm of shortening is acceptable, because overgrowth is minimal.

Cast Wedging

Loss of fracture reduction may require the cast to be "wedged." The fracture alignment in the cast can be changed by creating a closing wedge, an opening wedge, or a combination of wedges. The location for the wedge manipulation is determined by evaluating the child's leg under fluoroscopy and marking the midpoint of the tibial fracture on the outside of the cast. If fluoroscopy is not available, a series of paper clips are placed at 2-cm intervals on the cast. Anteroposterior and lateral radiographs are then taken. The paper clips define the location of the fracture and the location most suitable for cast manipulation.

Closing Wedge Technique

A wedge of cast material encompassing 90% of the circumference of the leg with its base over the apex of the fracture is removed. The cast is left intact opposite the apex of the fracture. The edges of the cast are brought together to correct the angulation at the fracture. This wedging technique produces mild fracture shortening and may pinch the skin at the location the wedge is removed. It can also increase exterior constrictive pressure because the total volume of the cast is reduced. In light of these concerns, it may be preferable to use the opening wedge technique whenever possible.

Opening Wedge Technique

The side of the cast opposite the apex of the fracture is cut perpendicular to the long axis of the bone. A small segment of the cast is left intact directly over the apex of the malaligned tibia (~25%). A cast spreader is used to "jack" the cast open. Plastic blocks (Fig. 25-15) or a stack of tongue depressors of the appropriate size are placed into the open segment and the cast is wrapped with new casting material after the alignment has been checked on x-rays (Fig. 25-16). When using stacked tongue depressors, care must be taken to ensure that the edges do not protrude into the cast padding or cause pressure on the skin. This wedging technique lengthens the tibia while correcting the malalignment (Figs. 25-17 and 25-18).

Combination Technique

Approximately 45% of the cast opposite the apex of the malaligned fracture is cut perpendicular to the shaft of the tibia. Two vertical cuts separated by approximately 0.5 cm are made 90 degrees from the first cut in both directions directly over the fracture. A wedge of casting material is removed from the apex side of the malaligned fracture and the cast opposite the apex of the fracture is opened. This closes the defect in the cast over the apex of the fracture and produces a change in the angular alignment of the bone without a significant change in the length of the bone.

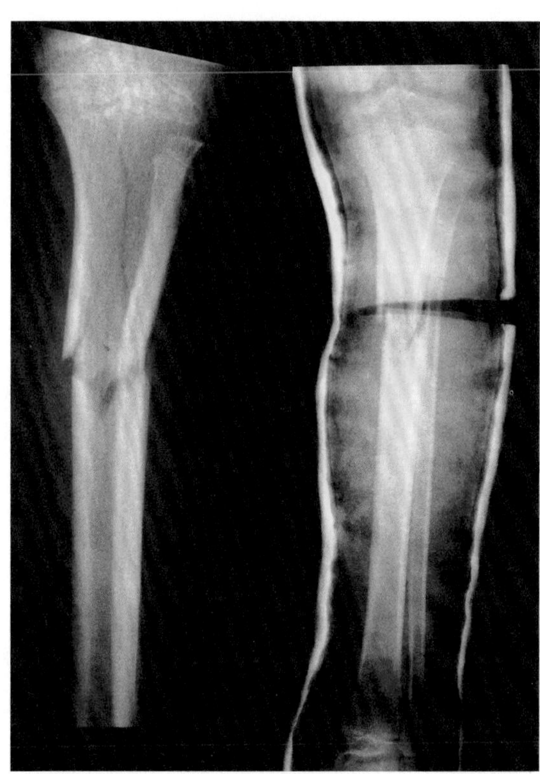

FIGURE 25-16 Comminuted fracture of the tibia and fibula in a 12-year-old boy struck by a car (*left*). Notice the extension of the fracture into the metaphysis from the diaphyseal injury. The fracture is in a valgus alignment. The fracture could not be maintained in an acceptable alignment (*right*). The cast was wedged with excellent result.

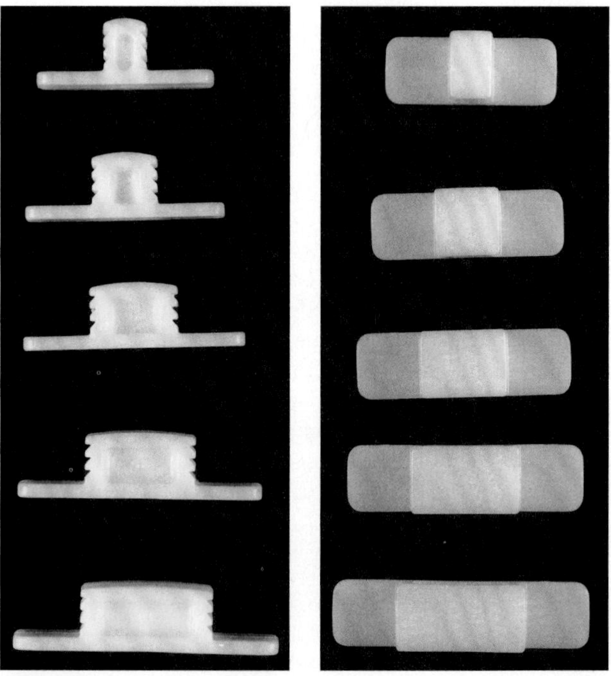

FIGURE 25-15 A,B. Blocks used to hold casts open after wedge corrections of malaligned fractures. The wings on the blocks prevent the blocks from migrating toward the skin.

Operative Treatment

In general, operative treatment is rarely needed for tibial fractures in children. Weber et al (6) reported that only 29 (4.5%) of 638 pediatric tibial fractures required surgical intervention. The indications for operative treatment include open fractures, fractures with an associated compartment syndrome, fractures in children with spasticity (head injury or cerebral palsy), fractures in which open treatment facilitates nursing care (floating knee, multiple long bone fractures, multiple system injuries), and unstable fractures that fail closed manipulation and casting (42–56).

Common methods of fixation include percutaneous metallic pins, bioabsorbable pins (57), external fixation, and plates with screws. Use of flexible intramedullary nails or even intramedullary Steinman pins is increasingly common (58).

OPEN FRACTURES

Open tibial fractures in children are treated similar to comparable injuries in adults, and they are classified by the Gustillo

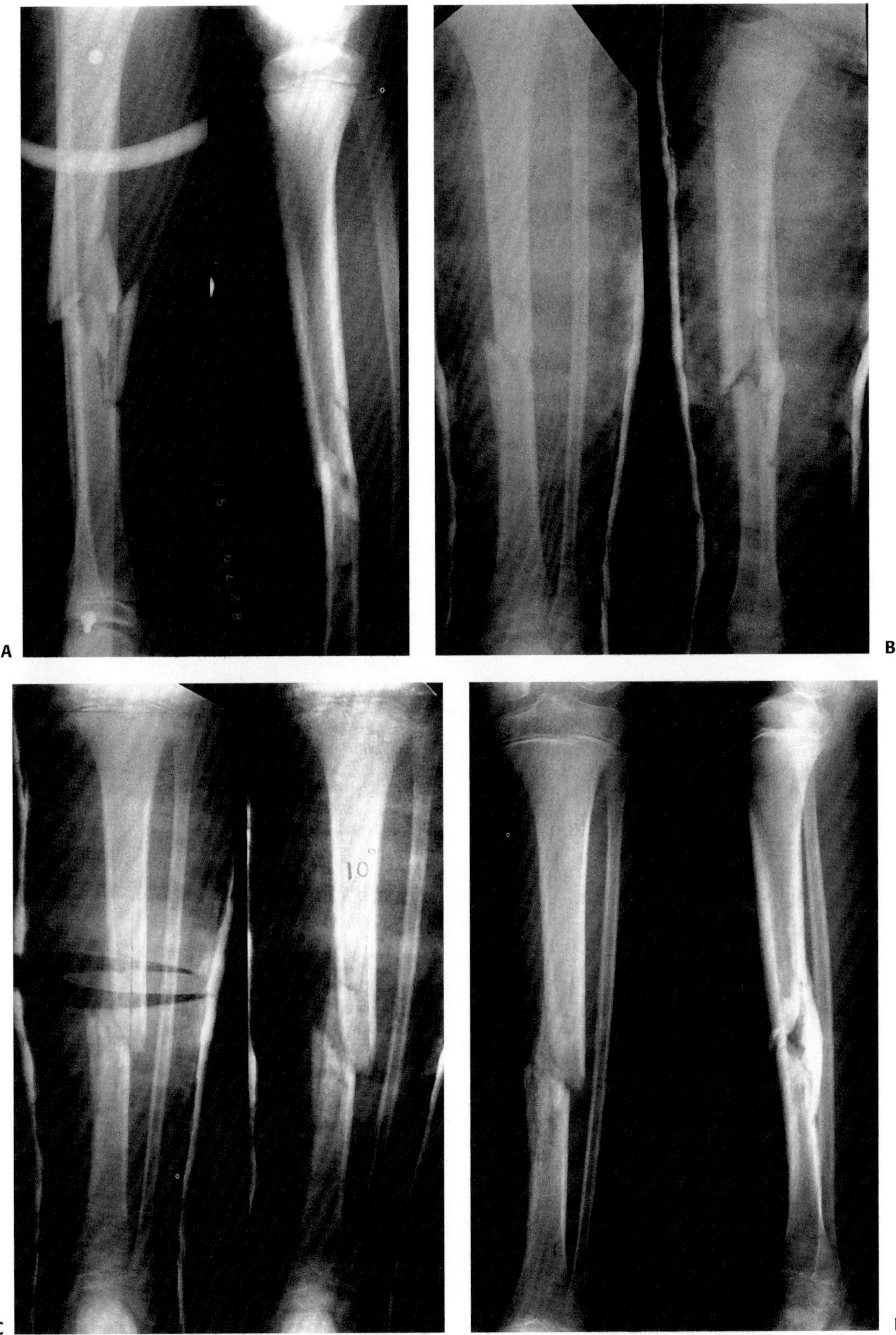

FIGURE 25-17 **A.** Anteroposterior and lateral tibial x-rays of an 11-year-old boy who was struck by an automobile, sustaining a markedly comminuted tibial fracture without concomitant fibular fracture. **B.** Despite the comminution, length and alignment were maintained in a cast. **C.** The patient's fracture shifted into a varus malalignment that measured 10 degrees (*right*). The cast was wedged, resulting in the reestablishment of an acceptable coronal alignment (*left*). **D.** The patient's fracture healed without malunion.

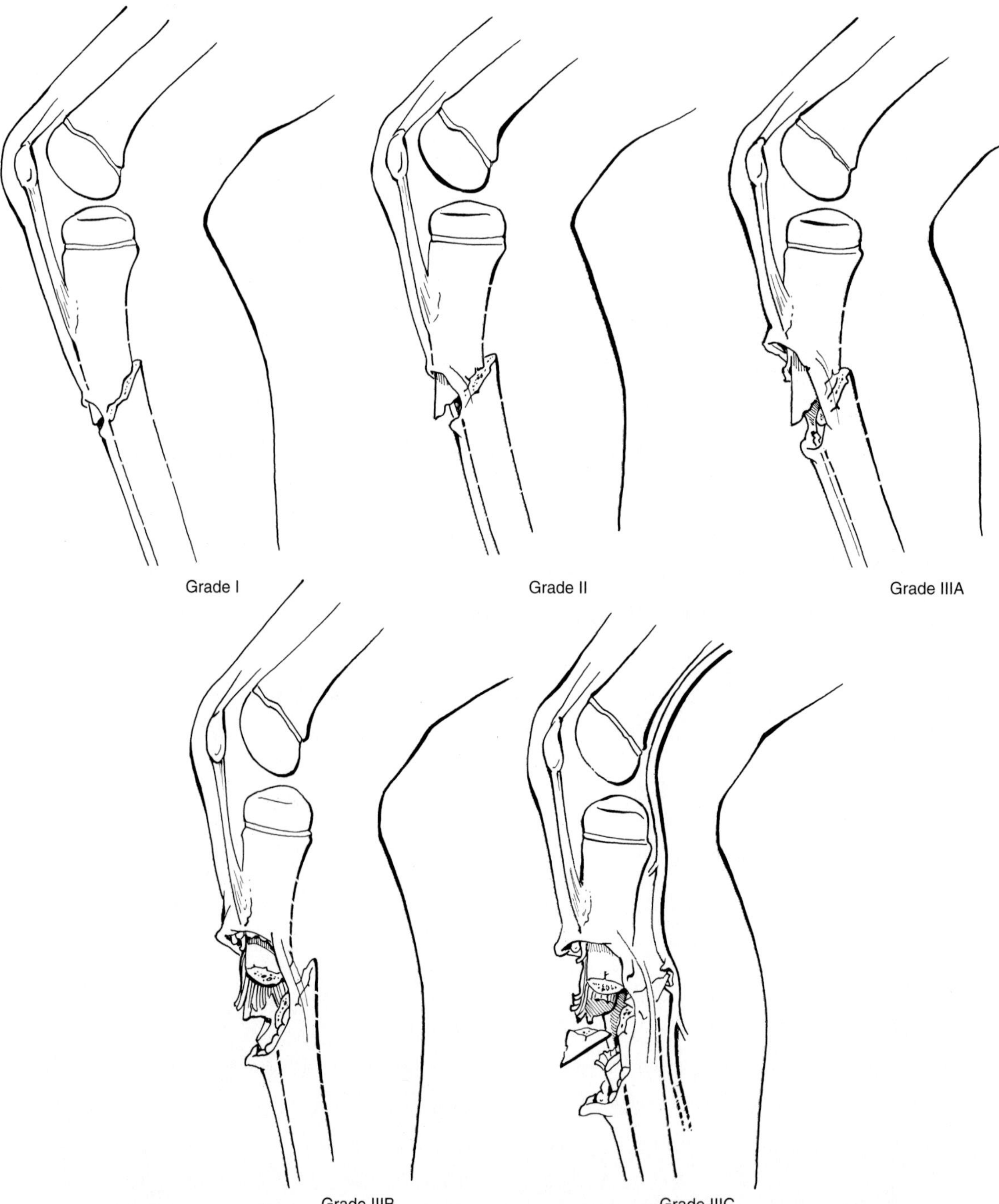

FIGURE 25-18 Gustillo and Anderson classification of open fractures. **Grade I:** The skin wound measures less than 1 cm long, usually from within, with little or no skin contusion. **Grade II:** The skin wound measures more than 1 cm long, with skin and soft tissue contusion but no loss of muscle or bone. **Grade IIIA:** There is a large severe skin wound with extensive soft tissue contusion, muscle crushing or loss, and severe periosteal stripping. **Grade IIIB:** Like grade IIIA but with bone loss and nerve or tendon injury. **Grade IIIC:** Like grade IIIA or B with associated vascular injury. (Redrawn after Alonso JE. The initial management of the injured child: musculoskeletal injuries. In: MacEwen GD, Kasser J, Heinrich SD, eds. *Pediatric fractures: a practical approach to assessment and treatment.* Baltimore: Williams & Wilkins, 1993:32; with permission.)

TABLE 25-4 Classification of Open Fractures

Grade I
- Low-energy wound, <1 cm in length
- Bone piercing skin from inside/out
- Minimal muscle damage

Grade II
- Wound >1 cm in length
- Moderate soft tissue injury

Grade III
- High-energy wound
- Usually >10 cm in length
- Extensive muscle devitalization
- Bone widely displaced or comminuted

Special cases
- Shotgun wound
- High-velocity gunshot (>2,000 ft/s)
- Segmental fracture
- Segmental diaphyseal loss
- Farmyard environment
- Associated vascular injury

Reprinted from Gustillo RB, Anderson JT. Prevention of infection in the treatment of one thousand and twenty-five fractures of long bones. *J Bone Joint Surg [Am]* 1976;58:453; with permission.

and Anderson System (Table 25-4; Fig. 25-18) (59). Most open fractures of the tibia result from high-velocity injuries.

Treatment Principles

Management principles for open tibial fractures include:

- Rapid debridement, irrigation, and appropriate antibiotic therapy
- Fracture reduction followed by stable fixation device
- Intraoperative angiography (after rapid fracture stabilization) and management of possible elevation of compartment pressure when sufficiency of the vascular perfusion is unclear
- Open wound treatment with loose gauze packing or other methods once the soft tissue base is stable (60)
- Staged debridement of necrotic soft tissue and bone in the operating room every 24 to 72 hours until a good granulation base develops
- Delayed closure or application of a split-thickness skin graft when necessary; delayed myocutaneous flap as needed
- Closed cancellous bone grafting for bone defects or delayed union after maturation of soft tissue coverage

The principles of treatment for open tibial fractures in adults have been modified by the unique characteristics of the pediatric skeleton. These differences include the following (42,44,61,62):

- Comparable soft tissue and bony injuries heal better in children than in adults, particularly in patients less than 11 years of age.
- Devitalized uncontaminated bone that can be covered with soft tissue may incorporate into the fracture callus, and in some cases may be left within the wound.
- External fixation can be maintained, when necessary, until fracture consolidation.
- Periosteum can reform bone even after segmental bone loss in younger children.
- Some uncontaminated grade I open wounds may be closed primarily.

Buckley et al (63) reported 41 children with 42 open fractures of the tibia (18 grade II, 6 grade IIIA, 4 grade IIIB, and 2 grade IIIC). Twenty-two (52%) of the fractures were comminuted. All wounds were irrigated and debrided, and antibiotics were administered for at least 48 hours. Twenty-two fractures were treated with reduction and cast application, and 20 with external fixation. Three children had early infections, and one of them developed late osteomyelitis. All infections had resolved at last follow-up. The average time to union was 5 months (range, 2–21 mo). The time to union was directly proportional to the severity of the soft tissue injury. Fracture pattern also had an effect on time to union. Segmental bone loss, infection, and the use of an external fixation device were associated with delayed union. Four angular malunions of more than 10 degrees occurred, three of which spontaneously corrected. Four children had more than 1 cm of overgrowth (63).

In a series of 40 open lower extremity diaphyseal fractures in 35 children, Cramer et al (64) reported 22 tibial fractures (1 grade I, 10 grade II, and 11 grade III). External fixation was used for 15 fractures, casting for five, and internal fixation for two. Two children required early amputation, four required soft tissue flaps, and 13 children had skin grafts. Two additional children required fasciotomy for compartment syndrome and were included in the group of open tibial fractures. Ten of the 24 injuries healed within 24 weeks. Five children required bone grafting before healing.

Hope and Cole (65) reported the results of open tibial fractures in 92 children (22 grade I, 51 grade II, and 19 grade III). Irrigation and debridement were performed on admission, antibiotics were given for 48 hours, and tetanus prophylaxis was administered as needed. Primary closure was performed in 51 children, and 41 fractures were left open. Eighteen soft tissue injuries healed secondarily, and 23 required either a split-thickness skin graft or a tissue flap. Sixty-five (71%) of the 92 fractures were stable and were reduced and immobilized in an above-the-knee plaster cast. External fixation was used for unstable fractures, injuries with significant soft tissue loss, and fractures in patients with multiple system injuries. Early complications of open tibial fractures in these children were compara-

TABLE 25-5 Early Complications Associated with Open Pediatric Tibial Fractures

Complication	Grade I	II	III	Combined
Delayed union	18%	12%	26%	16%
Nonunion	5%	6%	16%	7.5%
Malunion	9%	4%	11%	6.5%
Infection	–	12%	21%	11%
Compartment syndrome	9%	2%	5%	4%
Physeal arrest	–	2%	5%	–
Weeks to union	13	12	17	13.5

Reprinted from Hope PG, Cole WG. Open fractures of the tibia in children. *J Bone Joint Surg [Br]* 1992;74:546; with permission.

TABLE 25-6 Late Complications Associated with Open Pediatric Tibia Fractures

Complication	Grade I	II	III	Combined
Pain	38%	48%	65%	–
Decreased athletic activity	19%	15%	47%	–
Decreased mobility (stiffness)	19%	20%	35%	–
Cosmetic complaints	6%	17%	53%	–
Leg length				
Short (0.5–2 cm)	22%	23%	40%	27%
Equal	14%	46%	33%	36%
Long (5.0–2 cm)	64%	31%	27%	37%

Reprinted from Hope PG, Cole WG. Open fractures of the tibia in children. *J Bone Joint Surg [Br]* 1992;74:546; with permission.

ble with those in adults (Table 25-5) (43,63,66–75). Primary closure did not increase the risk of infection if the wound was small and uncontaminated (42,44,71). At reevaluation 1.5 to 9.8 years after injury, Hope and Cole (65) found that 50% of the patients complained of pain at the fracture site; 23% reported decreased abilities to participate in sports, joint stiffness, and cosmetic defects; and 64% had leg length inequalities (Table 25-6). Levy et al (53) found comparable late sequelae after open tibial fractures in children, including a 25% prevalence of nightmares surrounding the events of the accident. Blasier and Barnes (76) and Song et al (62) found that most late complications associated with pediatric open tibial fractures occurred in children over the age 12 and 11 years, respectively.

Skaggs et al reviewed their experience on open tibial fractures and found no increased incidence of infection in patients initially debrided more than 6 hours after injury when compared to children treated less than 6 hours after fracture. It appears that fractures with more severe soft tissue injuries were more likely to receive more expedient treatment. This apparent bias has limited overall usefulness of the data (77).

Soft Tissue Closure

The timing of soft tissue closure after an open tibial fracture that cannot be closed primarily is important in decreasing the morbidity associated with this injury (78,79). Most of the literature addressing this subject involves adult patients, and as such, must be extrapolated to pediatric fracture management. In a series of 168 open tibial fractures with late secondary wound closure, Small and Mollan (80) found increased complications with early fasciocutaneous flaps and late free flaps, but no complications with fasciocutaneous flaps created more than 1 month after injury. Complications associated with free flaps were decreased if the procedure was performed within 7 days of injury. Hallock et al reviewed 11 free flaps for coverage in pediatric patients. They reported a 91% success rate, which was similar to their rate in adults. However, they reported a significant rate of complications at both the donor and the recipient sites (81). Ostermann et al (82) reported 115 grade II and 239 grade III tibial fractures in a series of 1,085 open fractures. All patients were treated with early broad-spectrum antibiotics, serial debridements, and the application of an external fixation device. Tobramycin-impregnated polymethylmethacrylate was placed into the wounds, and dressings were changed every 48 to 72 hours until the wounds spontaneously closed, or had delayed primary closure or a flap. No infections occurred in grade I fractures; approximately 3% of grade II fractures and 8% of grade III fractures became infected. No infections occurred in patients who had the wound closed by 8 days after injury. On the basis of this and other analyses, it now is recommended that wounds associated with open tibial fractures be covered within 7 days of injury whenever possible (3,66,82–86). A delayed primary closure can be performed if the wound is clean and does not involve significant muscle loss. Closure under tension must be avoided.

Vascular Injuries

Vascular injuries have been reported in approximately 5% of children with open tibial fractures. Arterial injuries associated with open tibial fractures include those to the popliteal artery, the posterior tibial artery, the anterior tibial artery, and the peroneal artery. Complications are common in patients with open tibial fractures and associated vascular injuries. Amputation rates as high as 21% have been reported with grade IIIB fractures and as high as 79% with grade IIIC fractures. Isolated anterior tibial and peroneal artery injuries have a good prognosis, whereas injuries of the posterior tibial and popliteal arteries have a poor prognosis (71,87,88). Patients with open tibial fractures and vascular disruption may benefit from an arterial and possibly venous shunt before the bony reconstruction is performed. This allows a meticulous repair of the fracture and maintains limb perfusion until the primary vascular repair is performed (47). However, in most cases, rapid stabilization of the fracture, usually using external fixation, can be performed prior to vascular reconstruction without the need for temporary shunts.

Compartment Syndrome

The prevalence of compartment syndromes in adults with open tibial fractures ranges from 6% to 9% (43,68,72). Compartment syndromes occur in approximately 5% of children with open tibial fractures. Normal compartment tissue pressure in the lower leg is approximately 0 mm Hg. Compartment blood inflow is decreased at 20 mm Hg, and prolonged pressures of 30 to 40 mm Hg or within 30 mm Hg of diastolic blood pressure may cause severe nonreversible injury to the muscles within a fascial compartment.

Symptoms and signs associated with compartment syndrome include pain out of proportion to the injury, burning, throbbing, pain increased by passive muscle stretch, and nerve dysfunction. The compartment feels tense when palpated. Because tissue pressures can be elevated enough to produce an ischemic injury, but not high enough to occlude arterial inflow, the presence of peripheral pulses is unreliable evidence of adequate tissue perfusion.

Compartment pressure measurements are mandatory in any patient suspected of having a compartment syndrome. Historically, pressure measurements have required use of a needle manometer and/or wick catheter. More recently, small portable, handheld devices, or even arterial monitoring setups in the operating room, are used most commonly. Fasciotomy is indicated for any patient with a significant elevation of compartment pressures or, more importantly, symptoms suggestive of a compartment syndrome. When measuring compartment pressure in the leg after a tibial fracture, accurate placement of the needle is essential. Multiple measurements should be performed at different sites and depths within each compartment, due to apparent variations of pressure through the compartment.

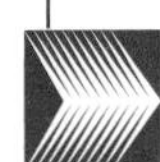

AUTHORS' PREFERRED TREATMENT

Diaphyseal Fractures

Simple pediatric diaphyseal tibial fractures unite quickly, and cast immobilization can be used without affecting the long-term range of motion in the knee and the ankle. A bent-knee, long-leg cast provides maximal comfort to the patient and controls rotation of the fractured fragments. Children with nondisplaced or minimally displaced fractures that do not require manipulation generally do not need to be admitted to the hospital. Children with more extensive injuries should be admitted for neurovascular observation and teaching of wheelchair, crutch, or walker use.

Significantly displaced fractures disrupt the surrounding soft tissues and produce a large hematoma in the fascial compartments of the lower leg. Circulation, sensation, and both active and passive movement of the toes should be monitored carefully after injury. The child should be admitted to the hospital, and reduction should be performed with adequate sedation and fluoroscopy if available. Most fractures are casted after reduction. The cast may be bivalved or split to allow swelling. The fracture must be checked within a week of manipulation to verify maintenance of the reduction. The cast can be wedged to correct minor alignment problems. Significant loss of reduction requires repeat reduction with general anesthesia (Table 25-7) or utilization of a more rigid fixation method. The long-leg cast may be changed to a short-leg, weight-bearing cast at 4 to 6 weeks after injury. Children over 11 years of age may be placed into a patellar tendon–bearing cast after removal of the long leg cast (75). Weight-bearing immobilization is maintained until sufficient callus is apparent.

Fractures in patients with complicating factors including spasticity, a floating knee, multiple long-bone fractures, extensive soft tissue damage, or multiple system injuries may be stabilized with a more rigid fixation method, such as

TABLE 25-7 Acceptable Alignment of a Pediatric Diaphyseal Tibial Fracture

Patient Age	<8 Years	≥8 Years
Valgus	5°	5°
Varus	10°	5°
Angulation anterior	10°	5°
Posterior angulation	5°	0°
Shortening	10 mm	5 mm
Rotation	5°	5°

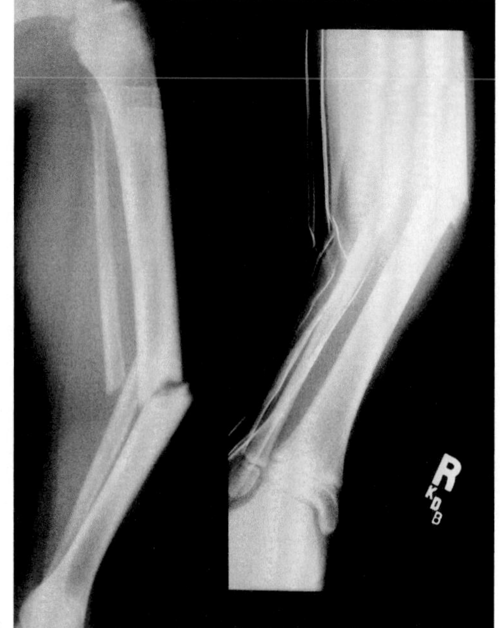

A

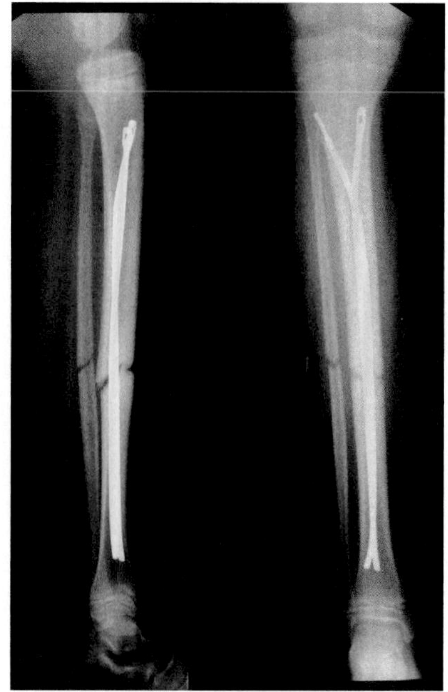

B

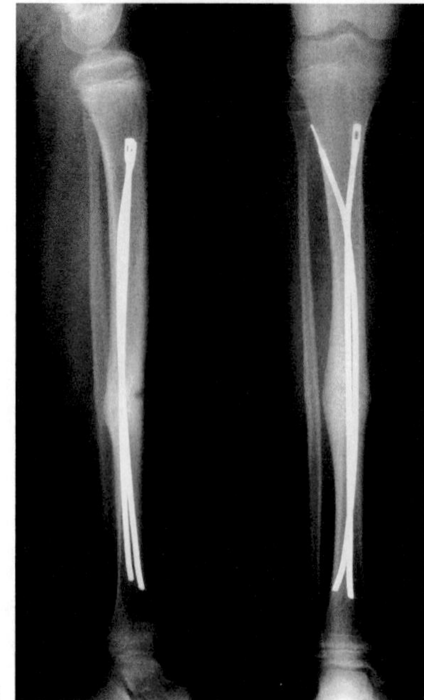

C

FIGURE 25-19 **A.** Anteroposterior and lateral x-rays of a 12-year-old who was involved in a motor-vehicle accident sustaining a grade I open middle one-third tibial and fibular fractures. **B.** This injury was treated with intramedullary nail fixation. **C.** At union, the patient has an anatomic alignment and no evidence of a growth disturbance.

external fixation, percutaneous Kirschner wires, or flexible intramedullary nails (Figs. 25-19 and 25-20).

Open Fracture Treatment

Open tibial fractures of any grade should have thorough irrigation and debridement of the wound as soon as possible, although there is some evidence that the infection rate is similar in injuries managed at less than 6 hours after injury and those treated later (77). The patient's tetanus status is determined, and prophylaxis is administered as needed. Appropriate IV antibiotic treatment is initiated as soon as possible and maintained as required based on the severity of the open fracture. The soft tissue wounds can be extended to be certain that the area is cleansed and debrided of all nonviable tissue and foreign material. Devitalized bone can be left in place if it is clean and can be covered by soft tissue. The operative wound extension may be closed along with the open segment in clean grade I injuries. The wound is allowed to heal by secondary intention if there is moderate contami-

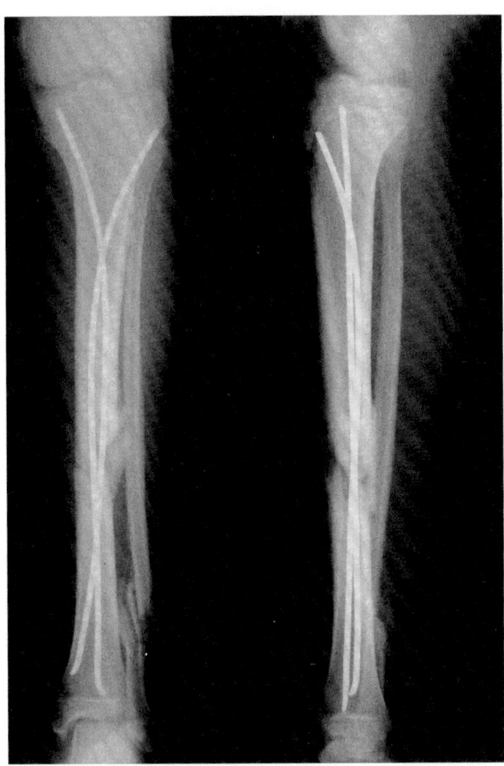

FIGURE 25-20 Anteroposterior x-ray of a 14-year-old who was involved in a motor-vehicle accident sustaining a distal one-third tibial fracture and comminuted distal fibular fracture. This was stabilized with titanium elastic nails.

nation after irrigation and debridement. Grade II and III wounds are debrided of devitalized tissue and foreign material. Patients with uncomplicated grade I fractures can be placed in a splint or a cast, or simple smooth pin fixation will prevent displacement of many unstable fractures (Fig. 25-21), but requires supplemental splinting or casting. A wide variety of internal and external fixation systems are available. Most children with grade II and all children with grade III wounds require more rigid fracture stabilization, usually with external fixation, although intramedullary nails may be used as well. More rigid fixation precludes the need for significant external splinting, thereby allowing better access for wound care and sequential compartment evaluation as needed.

The most versatile external fixation device for open pediatric tibial fractures is a unilateral frame (Fig. 25-22). The unilateral frame is easy to apply and allows minor corrections in angular alignment and length. Secondary pins can be used for added support (Fig. 25-23); these are connected to the standard pins or the body of the external fixation device. This allows control of segmental fragments. Fracture reduction clamps can be applied to the pin clamps to assist in manipulating the fracture. A small-pin or thin-wire circular frame can be used for complicated fractures adjacent to the joint, although unilateral frames may be placed to span the joint in question so as to use ligamentotaxis to establish or maintain alignment (Fig. 25-24).

External fixation pins are placed no closer than 1 cm to the physis. The external fixation device is applied, and a reduction maneuver is performed. All of the connections in

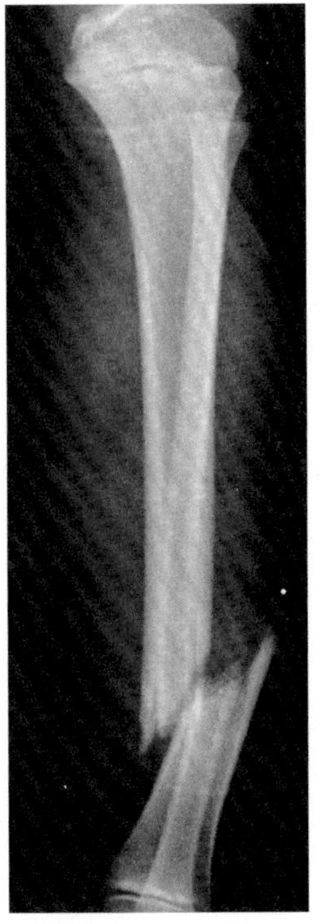

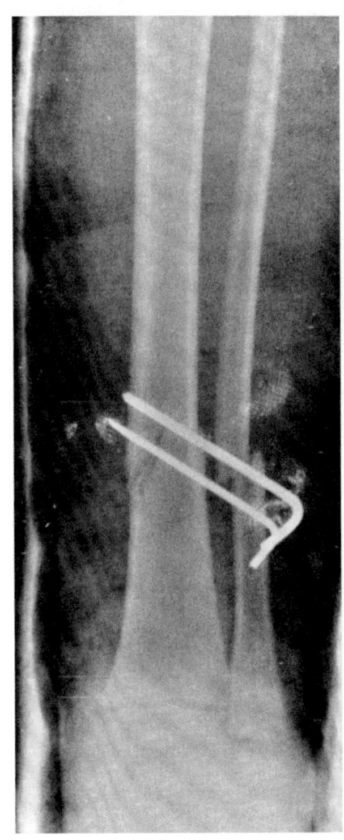

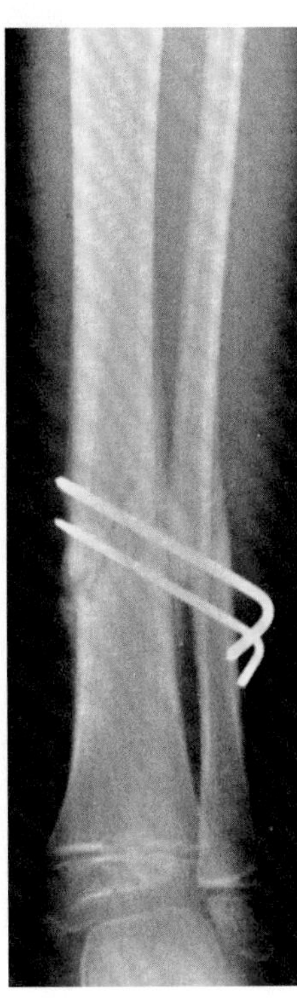

FIGURE 25-21 **A.** Anteroposterior x-ray of a grade I open distal one-third tibial fracture in a 7-year-old child. **B.** Two percutaneous pins were used to stabilize this fracture after irrigation and debridement. **C.** Good fracture callus was present and the pins were removed 4 weeks after injury.

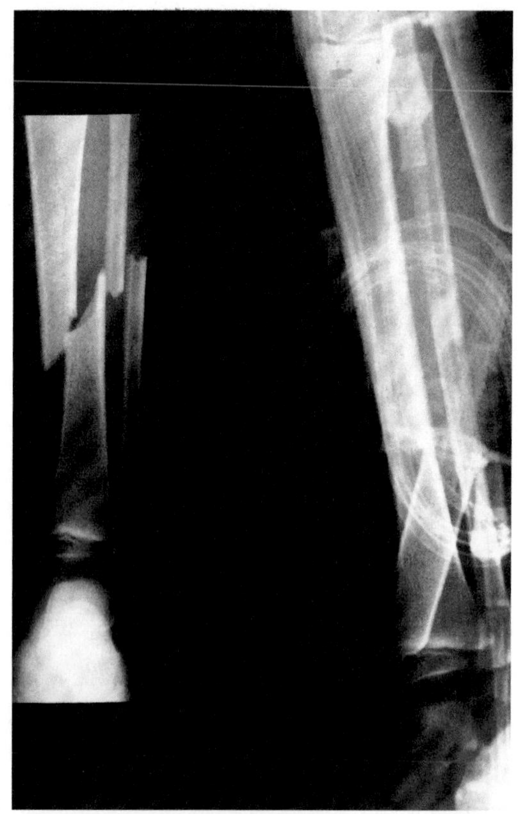

A

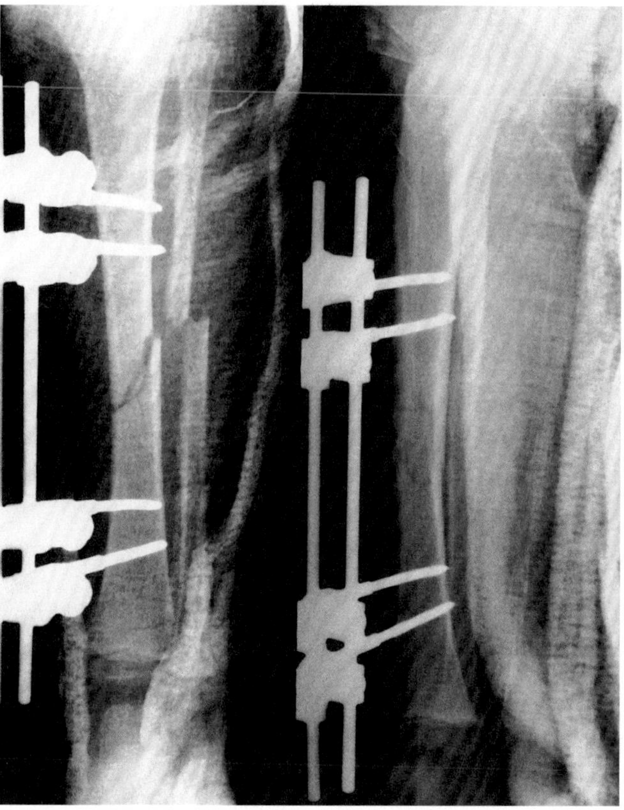

B

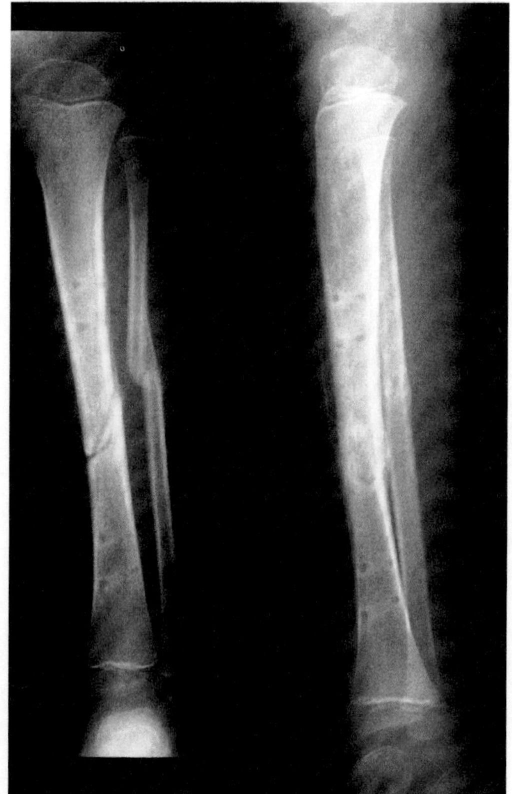

C

FIGURE 25-22 **A,B.** Type II open fracture of the tibia in a 5-year-old boy treated with debridement, unilateral external fixation, and split-thickness skin graft. **C.** Four months after removal of the external fixation.

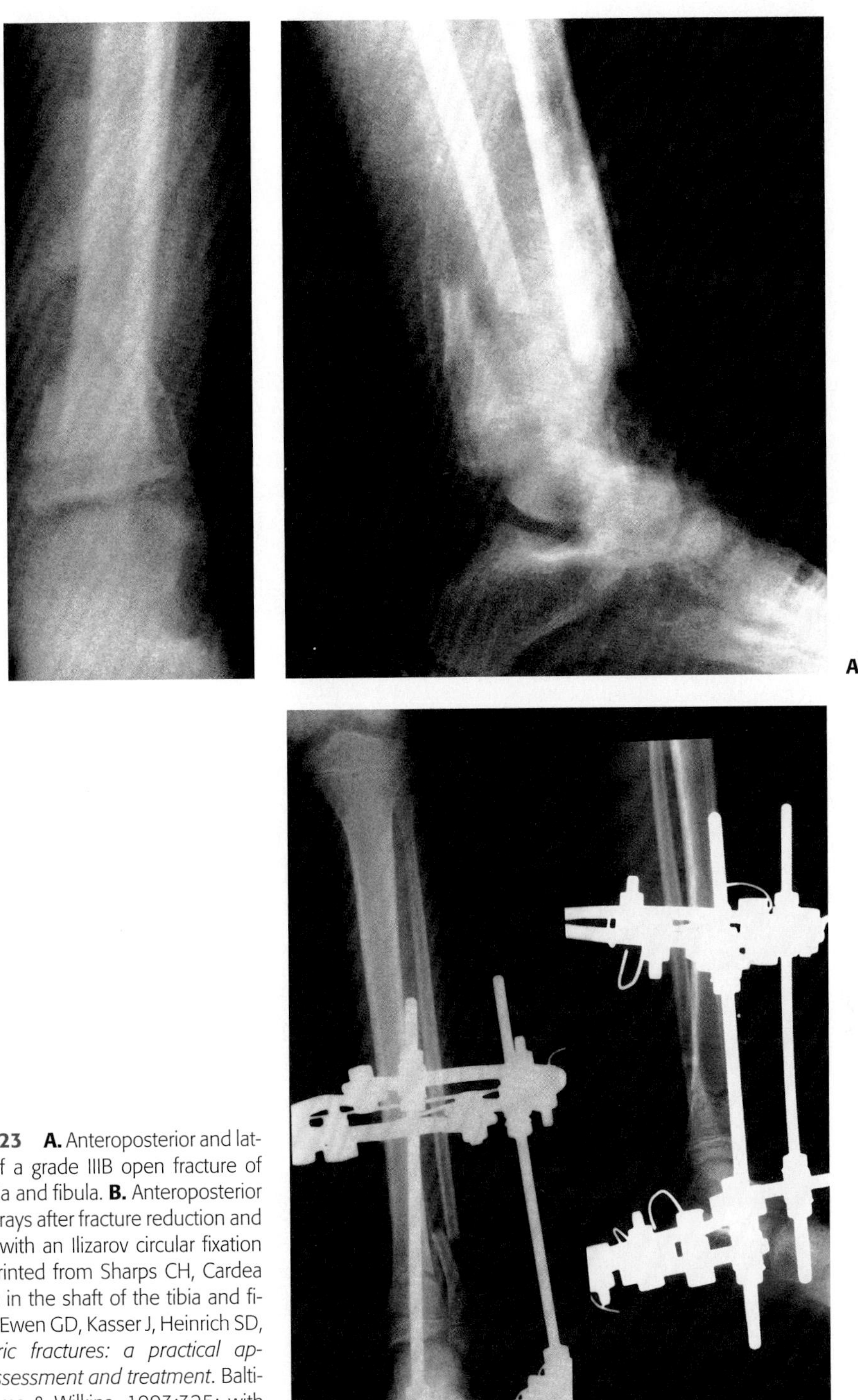

FIGURE 25-23 A. Anteroposterior and lateral x-rays of a grade IIIB open fracture of the distal tibia and fibula. **B.** Anteroposterior and lateral x-rays after fracture reduction and stabilization with an Ilizarov circular fixation frame. (Reprinted from Sharps CH, Cardea JA. Fractures in the shaft of the tibia and fibula. In: MacEwen GD, Kasser J, Heinrich SD, eds. *Pediatric fractures: a practical approach to assessment and treatment*. Baltimore: Williams & Wilkins, 1993:325; with permission.)

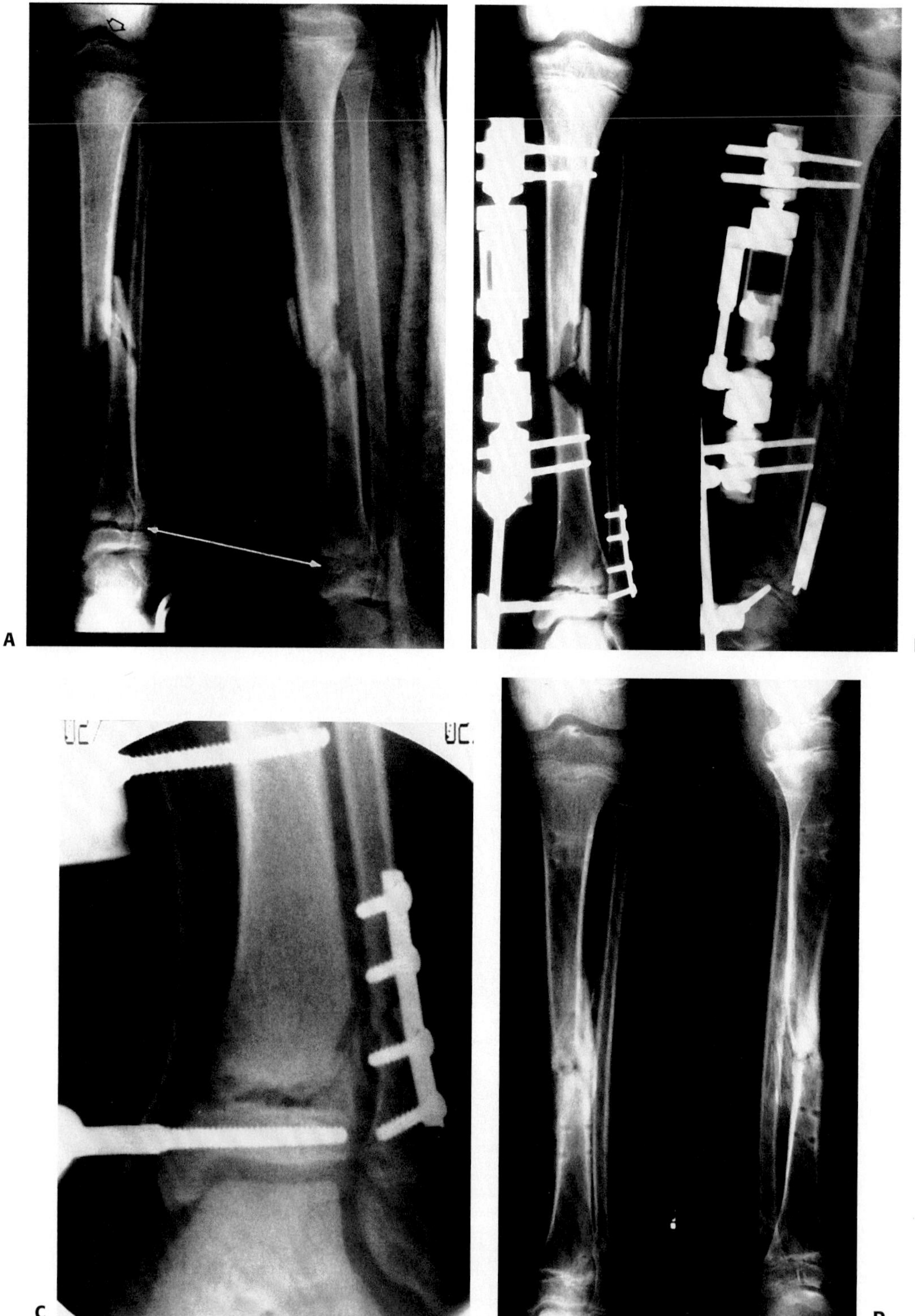

FIGURE 25-24 **A.** Anteroposterior and lateral x-rays of the tibia of a 12-year-old boy who was struck by a car. This child sustained a grade IIIB open middle one-third tibial fracture, a Salter-Harris type II fracture of the distal tibial physis with associated distal fibular fracture (*closed arrows*), and a tibial eminence fracture (*open arrow*). **B.** Irrigation and debridement and application of an external fixation device, were performed. **C.** The fracture of distal tibial physis was stabilized with a supplemental pin attached to the external fixation device. Open reduction and internal fixation of the fibula were performed to enhance the stability of the external fixator in the distal tibia. **D.** Anteroposterior and lateral x-rays of the tibia approximately 9 months after injury demonstrate healing of the tibial eminence fracture, the comminuted middle one-third tibial fracture, and the distal tibial physeal fracture. The distal tibial physis remains open at this time.

the external fixation device are tightened after reduction has been obtained. Secondary pins to improve fracture stability are placed at this time. Limited internal fixation of the fracture can be used to aid in controlling fracture alignment. A posterior splint can be applied to prevent the foot from dropping into plantar flexion. This splint is easy to remove during subsequent pin care and dressing changes of the open injury. Splinting can be avoided by external fixation, be it unilateral or circular, to the forefoot.

Intramedullary fixation may be accomplished using stainless steel prebent Enders nails, flexible titanium nails, or even simple Steinman pins. The implants are placed in a proximal to distal fashion from medial and lateral proximal points. Fluoroscopy is required for accurate placement. Care must be taken to avoid injury to the proximal tibial physes, including the tibial tubercle apophysis. Use of supplemental external splinting is at the discretion of the treating surgeon.

Immobilization

The length of immobilization varies with the child's age and the type of fracture. The duration of immobilization was 8 to 10 weeks in the Steinert and Bennek series (89). Hansen et al (4) found that healing time ranged from 5 to 8 weeks for "fissures and infractions" and from 5 to 13 weeks for oblique, transverse, and comminuted fractures. Hoaglund and States (70) reported that in 43 closed fractures in children, the average time in a cast was 2.5 months (range, 1.5–5.5 mo), whereas the five children with open fractures were immobilized for 3 months.

Kreder and Armstrong (51) found an average time to union of 5.4 months (range, 1.5–24.8 months) in a series of 56 open tibial fractures in 55 children. The factor with the most effect on union time was the age of the patient. Grimard et al (61) reported that the age of the patient and the grade of the fracture were significantly associated with union time. Blasier and Barnes (76) found that children under 12 years of age required less aggressive surgical treatment and healed faster than older children. They also found that younger children were more resistant to infection and had fewer complications than older children.

Rehabilitation

Most children with a tibial fracture do not require extensive rehabilitation. Children's normal walking and running activities serve as therapy. Most children limp with an out-toeing rotation gait on the involved extremity for several weeks to a month after the cast is removed. This usually is due to muscle weakness and joint stiffness rather than a malalignment of the fracture. As the muscle atrophy and weakness resolve, so does the limp.

Active physical therapy may be beneficial in treating some children with a tibial fracture. In an older child progressing from a bent knee cast to weight-bearing on a short-leg cast, knee range of motion exercises and quadriceps strengthening are useful. Progressive weight-bearing on a short-leg cast requires the patient to wean off crutches or a walker. In some children, this requires supervision. After removal of the cast, toe rises for strength should be performed. The child may return to sports when the fracture is healed and the patient has regained strength comparable to that of the uninjured leg.

Fractures of the Distal Tibial Metaphysis

Fractures of the distal tibial metaphysis are often greenstick injuries. The anterior cortex is impacted while the posterior cortex is displaced, with a tear of the overlying periosteum. A recurvatum deformity may occur (Fig. 25-25). Reduction of these injuries should be performed with adequate sedation and maintained with a long-leg cast. The foot should be in moderate plantar flexion to prevent recurvatum at the fracture site. The foot is brought up to neutral after 3 to 4 weeks, and a short-leg walking cast is applied. Unstable injuries can be treated with percutaneous pins (Fig. 25-26) or with open reduction and internal fixation as needed (Fig. 25-27).

COMPLICATIONS ASSOCIATED WITH DIAPHYSEAL TIBIAL AND FIBULAR FRACTURES

Compartment Syndrome

A compartment syndrome may occur after either a minor closed fracture or a severe injury in which the interosseus membrane is disrupted (52). Schrock (90) also described compartment syndromes after derotational osteotomies of the tibia in children. Compartment syndromes may occur in any or all of the four compartments of the lower leg after trauma. Hemorrhage and soft tissue edema produce an elevation in the pressure within the myofascial compartment that impairs venous outflow. The small arterioles leading into the compartment become less efficient in delivering blood as venous outflow becomes occluded. The arterioles and capillaries close when the pressure in the compartment exceeds the pressure in the vessels. Ischemia soon follows.

Patients with a compartment syndrome may complain of pain out of proportion to the severity of the injury. The compartment is firm to palpation. The patient may have a sensory defect in the distribution of the nerves that run through the compartment. Weakness of the muscles within the involved compartment and pain on passive motion of the toes also are common. Paralysis of the muscles in the involved compartment is a late finding. Pain with passive range of motion appears to be an early and strong clinical finding.

Patients with a compartment syndrome involving the deep posterior compartment have severe pain that increases with passive extension of the toes, plantar hyperesthesias, and weakness of toe flexion (91). Late complications of untreated compartment syndrome include clawed toes and limited subtalar motion secondary to a fibrous contracture of the muscles in the deep posterior compartment (92).

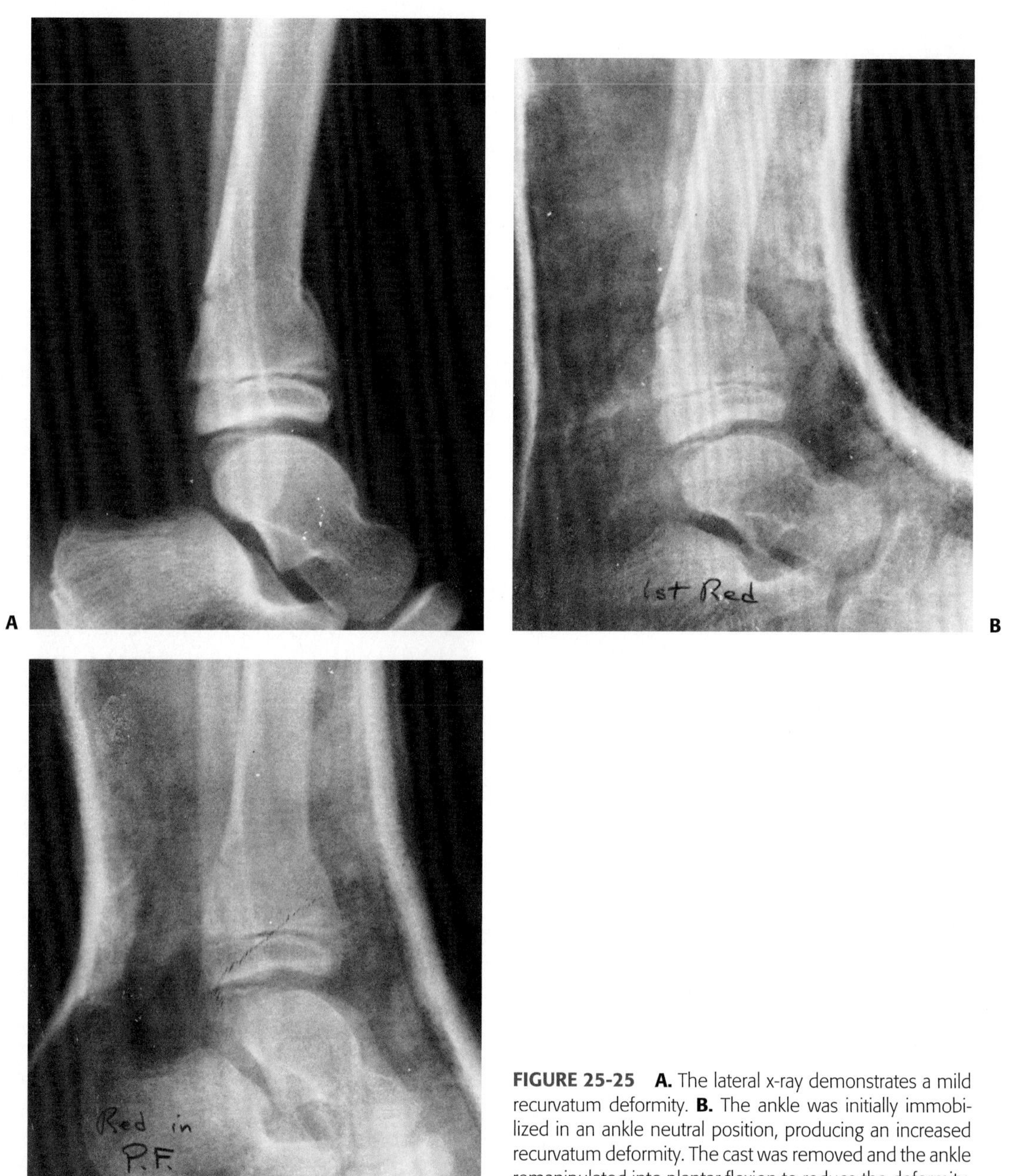

FIGURE 25-25 **A.** The lateral x-ray demonstrates a mild recurvatum deformity. **B.** The ankle was initially immobilized in an ankle neutral position, producing an increased recurvatum deformity. The cast was removed and the ankle remanipulated into plantar flexion to reduce the deformity. **C.** The ankle was then immobilized in plantar flexion, which is the proper position for this type of fracture.

Diagnosis

Direct intracompartmental pressure measurements at the level of the fracture provide an accurate assessment of compartment conditions and allow early fasciotomy to reduce the pressure. Whitesides et al (93) designed an inexpensive apparatus that permits accurate measurement of compartment tissue pressure (Fig. 25-28). Other devices also are available to measure compartment pressures. Normal tissue pressures are about 0 mm Hg. Vascular flow ceases in the microcirculation of an extremity by the time tissue pressures within a closed compartment reach the diastolic pressure. Compartment release should be performed when the pressures are within 20 to 30 mm Hg of the diastolic pressure. This is especially critical in a hypotensive polytrauma patient.

Treatment

Any cast should be bivalved and the padding divided in a patient with increased or increasing pain. If after removal of

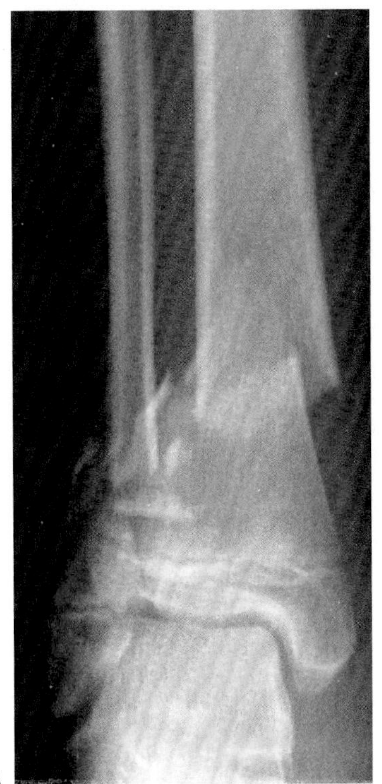
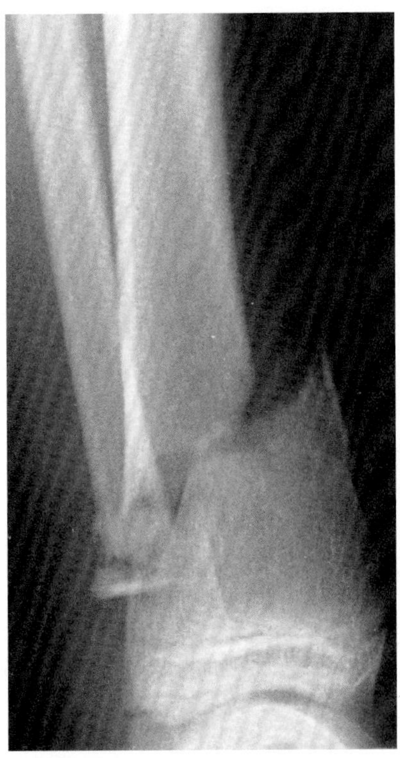
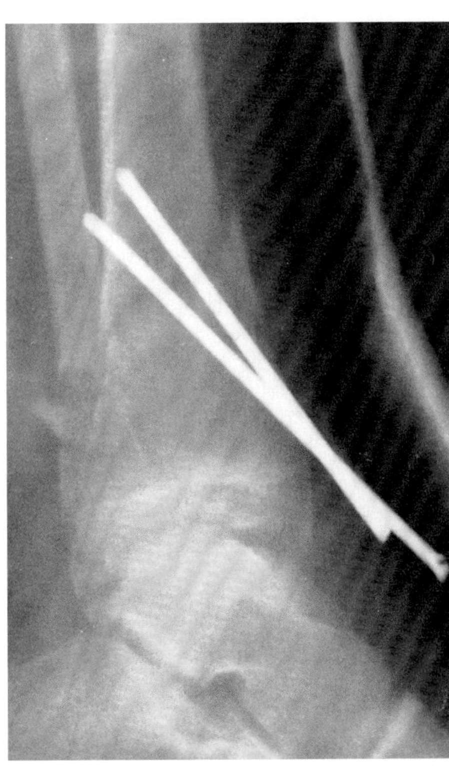

FIGURE 25-26 A,B. Unstable distal metadiaphyseal fractures of the tibia and fibula in a 15-year-old girl. **C.** This fracture was stabilized with percutaneous pins because of marked swelling and fracture instability.

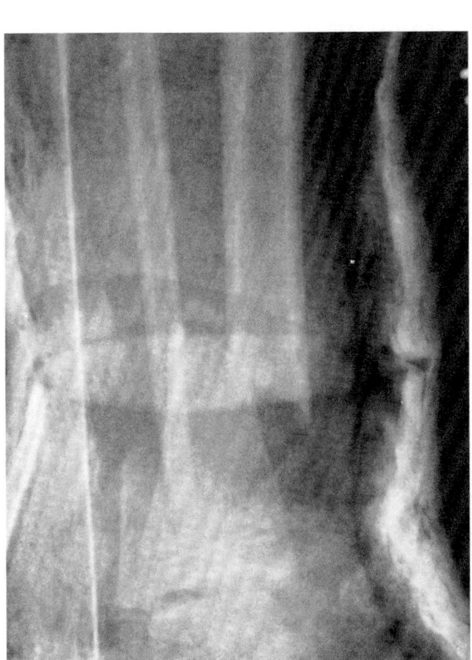
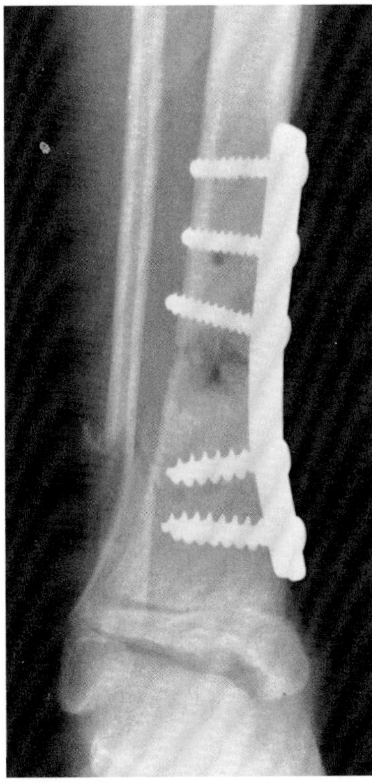

FIGURE 25-27 A. Anteroposterior x-ray of a distal one-third tibial and fibular fractures in a 9-year-old girl with a closed head injury and severe spasticity. The initial reduction in a cast could not be maintained. **B.** Open reduction and internal fixation with a medial buttress plate were used to achieve and maintain the alignment.

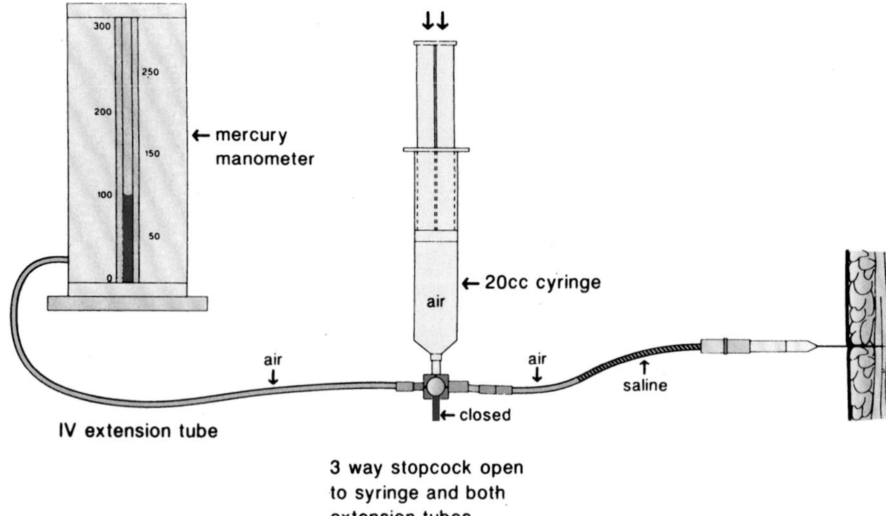

FIGURE 25-28 Whitesides' technique for measuring intracompartmental pressure. (Reprinted from Whitesides TE, Hanley TC, Morinotok K, et al. Tissue pressure measurement as a determinant for the need for fasciotomy. *Clin Orthop* 1975;113:43; with permission.)

circular wraps there is no relief, compartment syndrome should be considered. Any child who has objective or subjective evidence of a compartment syndrome should undergo an emergent fasciotomy. While there is some controversy in the literature, patients with compartment pressures greater than 30 mm Hg, with or without significant symptoms, should be managed with fasciotomy (94,95). Patients with altered mental status and borderline pressures should undergo either release or sequential pressure testing due to difficulty in obtaining adequate serial examinations. The two-incision technique is preferred, although a single incision, perifibular release is used at some centers (Fig. 25-29A,B). One incision is anterolateral and the second posteromedial. The fascia surrounding each of the four compartments should be opened from proximal to distal. The wound is left open and a delayed closure is performed. Fibulectomy should not be performed for decompression of a compartment syndrome in a skeletally immature patient because subsequent fibular shortening can produce a valgus deformity at the ankle and may result in external tibial torsion and a significant gait impairment (16,96). Adequate decompression of all four compartments can also be achieved through a single lateral approach (97). Decompression is an operative emergency as irreversible injury to muscles and nerves begins after approximately 5 hours of

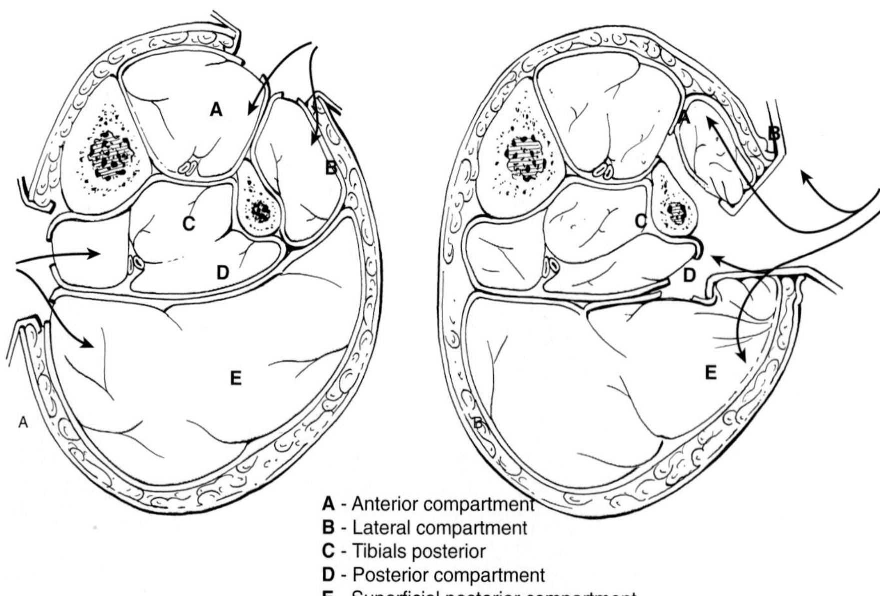

FIGURE 25-29 **A.** Decompressive fasciotomies through a two incision approach. The anterior lateral incision allows decompression of the anterior and lateral compartments. The medial incision allows decompression of the superficial posterior and the deep posterior compartments. **B.** A one-incision decompression fasciotomy can be performed through a lateral approach which allows a dissection of all four compartments.

ischemia (98). Ninety percent of muscle fibers show evidence of injury after 8 hours of ischemia (99). Hyperesthesia, motor defects, and decreased pulses are late changes and denote significant tissue injury. They occur only after the ischemia has been well established and the injury is permanent (92,93).

Vascular Injuries

Vascular injuries associated with tibial fractures are uncommon in children; however, when they do occur, the sequelae can be devastating. In an evaluation of 14 patients with lower extremity fractures and concomitant vascular injuries, Allen et al (87) noted that only three children returned to normal function. One factor leading to a poor outcome was a delay in diagnosis. Evaluation for vascular compromise is imperative (during the primary and secondary trauma surveys) in all children with tibial fractures.

The tibial fracture most frequently associated with vascular injury is that of the proximal metaphysis. The anterior tibial artery is in close proximity to the proximal tibia as it passes over the interosseous membrane into the anterior compartment (71,88). Distal tibial fractures also are associated with injuries to the anterior tibial artery. The vessels are injured when the distal fragment is translated posteriorly. Posterior tibial artery injuries are rare, except in fractures caused by heavy machinery or gunshots.

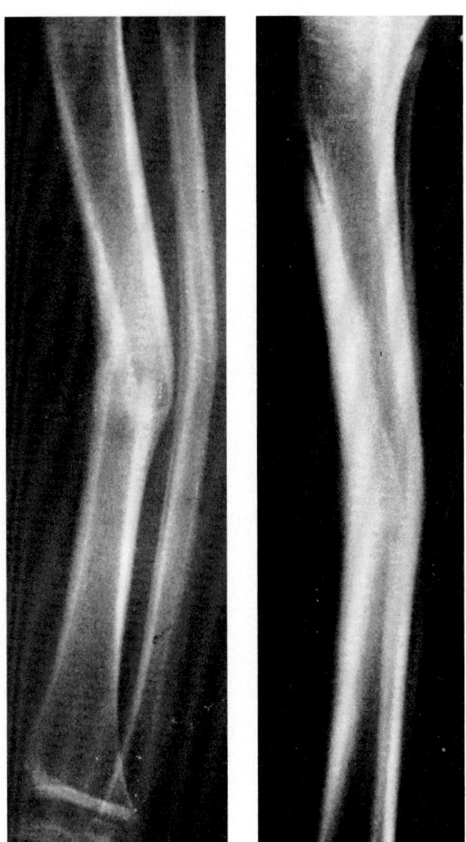

FIGURE 25-30 Four-year, two-month-old child with a middle one-third transverse tibial fracture and a plastically deformed fibular fracture. **A.** Lateral view shows 20-degree posterior angulation. **B.** The deformity is still 15 degrees 4 years after the injury.

Angular Deformity

Spontaneous correction of axial malalignment after a diaphyseal fracture of a child's forearm or femur is common. Remodeling of a malaligned tibial fracture, however, often is incomplete (Fig. 25-30) (100). As such, the goal of treatment should be to obtain as close to an anatomic alignment as possible.

Swaan and Oppers (101) evaluated 86 children treated for fractures of the tibia. The original angulation of the fracture was measured on x-rays in the sagittal and frontal projections. Girls 1 to 8 years of age and boys 1 to 10 years of age demonstrated moderate spontaneous correction of residual angulation after union. In girls 9 to 12 years of age and boys 11 to 12 years of age, approximately 50% of the angulation was corrected. No more than 25% of the deformity was corrected in children over 13 years of age. Bennek and Steinert (102) found that recurvatum malunion of more than 10 degrees did not correct completely. Twenty-six of 28 children with varus or valgus deformities at union had significant residual angular deformities at follow-up. Valgus deformities had a worse outcome because the tibiotalar joint was left in a deficient position.

Weber et al (6) demonstrated that a fracture with varus malalignment of 5 to 13 degrees completely corrected at the level of the physis. Most children with valgus deformities of 5 to 7 degrees did not have a full correction.

Hansen et al (4) reported 102 pediatric tibial fractures, 25 of which had malunions of 4 to 19 degrees. Angular malunions ranged from 3 to 19 degrees at follow-up, without a single patient having a complete correction. The spontaneous correction was approximately 13.5% of the total deformity. Shannak (1) reviewed the results of treatment of 117 children with tibial shaft fractures treated in above-the-knee casts. Deformities in two planes did not remodel as completely as those in a single plane. The least correction occurred in posteriorly angulated fractures, followed by fractures with a valgus malalignment (Fig. 25-31). Spontaneous remodeling of malunited tibial fractures in children has been reported to end at approximately 18 months after fracture (4).

Malrotation

Because rotational malalignment of the tibia does not spontaneously correct with remodeling (4), any malrotation should be avoided. A computerized tomographic evaluation of tibial rotation can be performed if there is any question about the rotational alignment of the fracture.

Rotational malalignment of more than 10 degrees may produce significant functional impairment and necessitate a late derotational osteotomy of the tibia. The derotational osteotomy should be performed in the supramalleolar aspect of the distal tibia. The tibia is osteotomized and internally fixed. The fibula

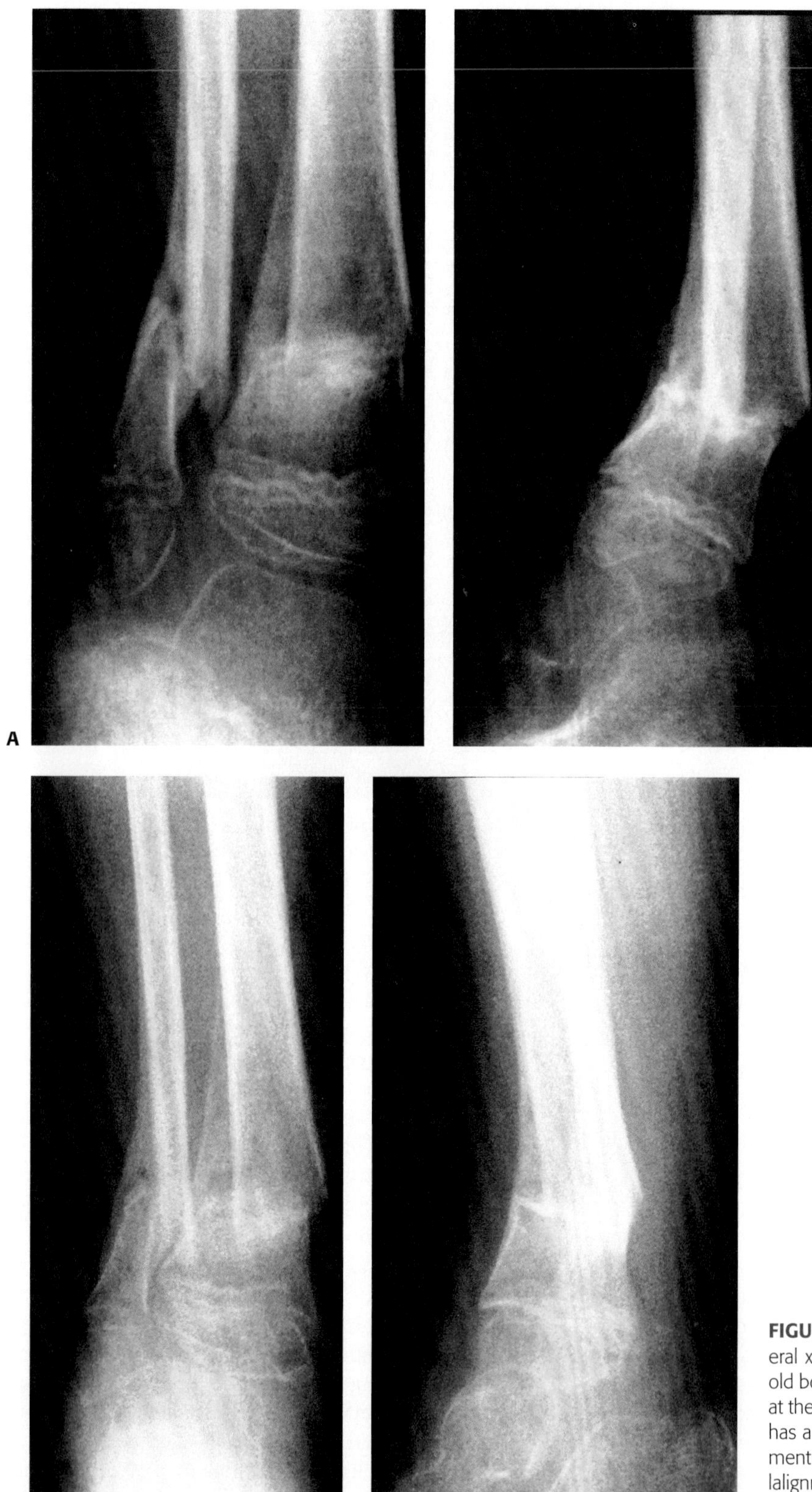

FIGURE 25-31 **A.** Anteroposterior and lateral x-rays 2 months after injury in a 6-year-old boy reveal a valgus and anterior malunion at the fracture. **B.** One year later, the child still has a moderate valgus and anterior malalignment of the distal fractured segment. This malalignment produced painful hyperextension of the knee at heel strike during ambulation.

may be left intact, particularly for planned derotation of less than 20 degrees.

Leg Length Discrepancy

Hyperemia associated with fracture repair may stimulate the physes in the involved leg, producing growth acceleration. Tibial growth acceleration after fracture is less than that seen after femoral fractures in children of comparable ages. Shannak (1) showed that the average growth acceleration of a child's tibia after fracture is approximately 4.5 mm. Comminuted fractures have the greatest risk of accelerated growth and overgrowth.

Swaan and Oppers (101) reported that young children have a greater chance for overgrowth than older children. Accelerated growth after tibial fracture occurs in children under 10 years of age, whereas older children may have a mild growth inhibition associated with the fracture (4). The amount of fracture shortening also has an effect on growth stimulation. Fractures with significant shortening have more physeal growth after fracture union than injuries without shortening at union (9). The presence of angulation at union does not affect the amount of overgrowth (48).

Anterior Tibial Physeal Closure

Morton and Starr (79) reported closure of the upper tibial physis after fracture in two children. Both patients sustained a comminuted fracture of the tibial diaphysis without a concomitant injury of the knee. Both fractures were reduced and stabilized with Kirschner wires placed distal to the tibial tubercle. A genu recurvatum deformity developed after premature closure of the anterior physis.

Smillie (103) reported one child who had an open tibial fracture complicated by a second fracture involving the supracondylar aspect of the femur. This patient also developed a recurvatum deformity secondary to closure of the anterior proximal tibial physis. At present, no universally acceptable explanation can be given for this phenomenon. Some patients have demonstrated apparently iatrogenic closure after placement of a proximal tibial traction pin, the application of pins and plaster, or the application of an external fixation device. Other children have an undiagnosed injury of the tibial physis at the time of the ipsilateral tibial diaphyseal fracture (104). Regardless of etiology, premature closure of the physis produces a progressive recurvatum deformity and loss of the normal anterior to posterior slope of the proximal tibia as the child grows.

Delayed Union and Nonunion

Delayed union and nonunion are uncommon after tibial fractures in children. The use of an external fixation device may lengthen the time to union in some patients, particularly those with open fractures resulting from high energy injury. Inadequate immobilization that allows patterned motion also can slow the rate of healing in patients with delayed union or nonunion; a fibulectomy approximately 4 cm from the tibial fracture allows compression at the delayed union or nonunion site and induces healing (Fig. 25-32). A posterolateral bone graft also is an excellent technique to produce union in younger children (Fig. 25-33). Adolescents near skeletal maturity can be treated with a reamed intramedullary nail, with a concomitant fibular osteotomy and correction of angulation at the nonunion site as necessary (Fig. 25-34).

SPECIAL FRACTURES

Toddler's Fractures

External rotation of the foot with the knee fixed in an infant or toddler can produce a spiral fracture of the tibia without a concomitant fibular fracture (Fig. 25-35). This fracture pattern was first reported by Dunbar et al (105) in 1964. The traumatic episode often is unwitnessed by the adult caretaker. Of those injuries that are witnessed, most caregivers report a seemingly minor, twisting mechanism. Most children with this injury are under 6 years of age. Sixty-three of 76 such fractures reported by Dunbar et al were in children under $2\frac{1}{2}$ years of age. Spiral tibial fractures occur in boys more often than in girls and in the right leg more often than in the left. The average age at injury in one study was 27 months. Most children report tripping or twisting their ankles. Occasionally, a child sustains a toddler's fracture in a fall from a height (106,107).

Oujhane et al (108) analyzed the x-rays of 500 acutely limping toddlers and identified 100 in whom a fracture was the etiology of the gait disturbance. The most common site of fracture was the distal metaphysis of the tibia. The fibula was fractured with the tibia in 12 of the 56 tibial fractures. Only one physeal injury was noted.

The examination of a child with an acute limp begins with an evaluation of the uninvolved side. This serves as a control for the symptomatic extremity. The examination begins at the hip and proceeds to the thigh, knee, lower leg, ankle, and foot. It is important to note the areas of point tenderness, an increase in local temperature, and any swelling or bruising of the leg (107).

X-rays of the tibia and fibula should be obtained in both anteroposterior and lateral projections. An internal oblique view can be helpful in identifying a nondisplaced toddler's fracture. Fluoroscopy also may assist in the identification of subtle fractures. Occasionally, a fracture line cannot be identified, and the first evidence of fracture becomes apparent on x-ray when periosteal new bone forms 7 to 10 days after the injury (Fig. 25-36). Technetium radionuclide imaging can assist in the diagnosis of unapparent fractures, but are used rarely. Bone scan of a patient with such a spiral fracture of the tibia will demonstrate diffuse increased uptake of tracer throughout the affected bone ("black tibia"). This can be differentiated from infection because infection tends to produce a local area of increased tracer uptake (105).

A child with a toddler's fracture should be immobilized in a bent-knee, long-leg cast for approximately 3 weeks. Most children require an additional 2 weeks of immobilization in a

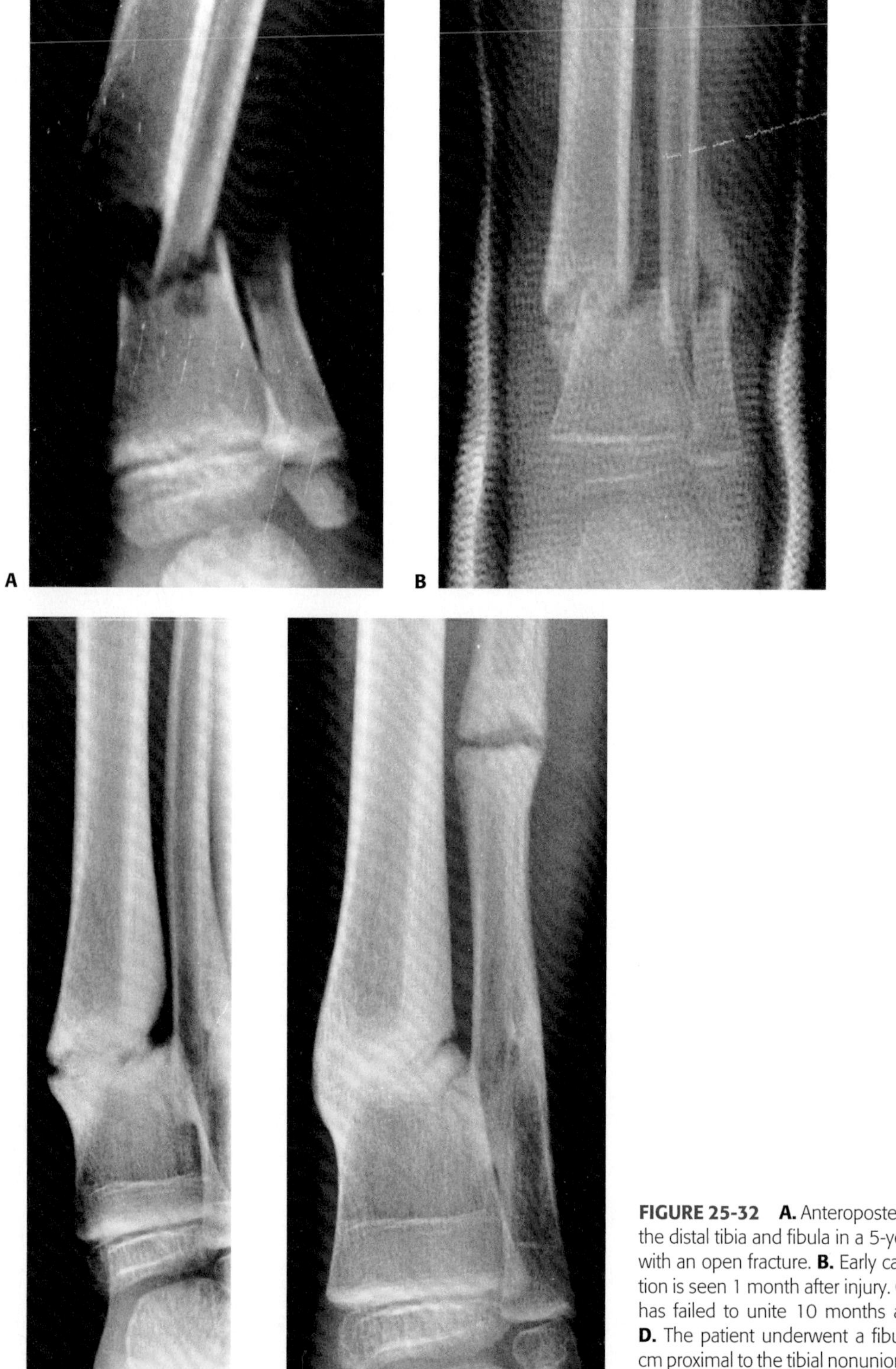

FIGURE 25-32 **A.** Anteroposterior x-ray of the distal tibia and fibula in a 5-year-old boy with an open fracture. **B.** Early callus formation is seen 1 month after injury. **C.** The tibia has failed to unite 10 months after injury. **D.** The patient underwent a fibulectomy 4 cm proximal to the tibial nonunion. The tibial fracture united 8 weeks after surgery.

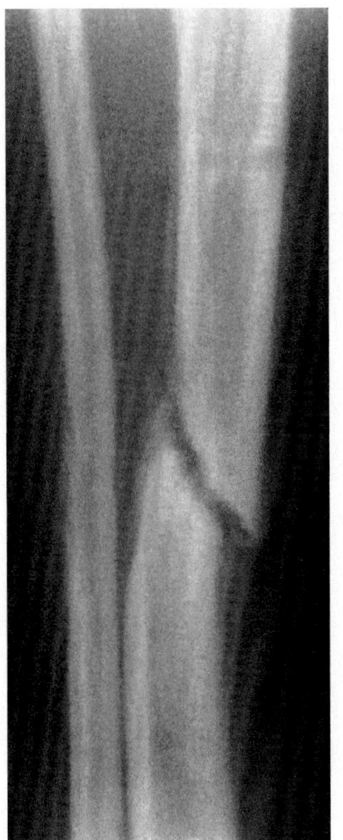

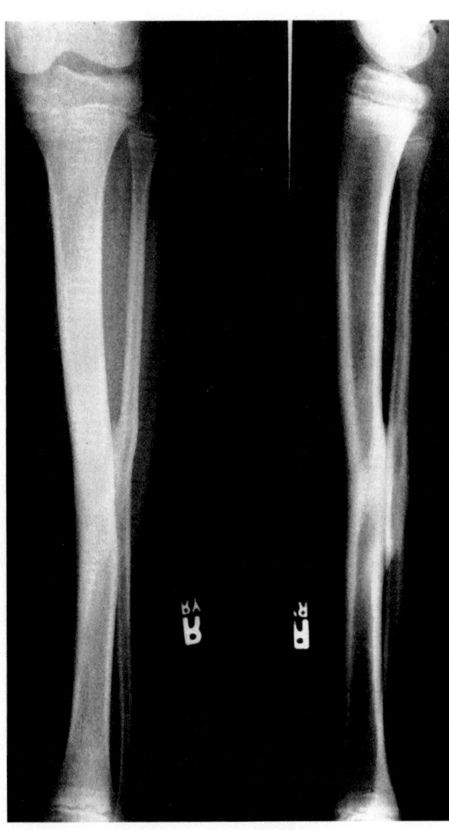

FIGURE 25-33 **A.** Nonunion of an open tibial fracture. **B.** After posterolateral tibial bone graft.

below-the-knee walking cast once the above-the-knee cast is removed.

Bicycle Spoke Injuries

Bicycle spoke injuries normally occur when a child's foot is thrust forcibly between the spokes of a turning bicycle wheel. This produces a severe compression or crushing injury to the soft tissues of the foot and ankle. An oblique or spiral fracture of the tibia also can occur. The injury to the foot, ankle, and lower leg can be compounded when the child's foot is extracted forcibly from the spokes of the bicycle. This scenario occurs most commonly when two children are riding a bicycle designed for one, with the injured passenger riding on the handlebars or the rear fender (109,110).

Izant et al (111) reviewed 60 bicycle spoke injuries in children under 14 years of age. The most common age range of injury was 2 to 8 years. The initial appearance of the extremity in a child with a bicycle spoke injury may be deceiving. The foot often appears normal or may show only minor skin abrasions. The patient often presents 24 to 48 hours after the accident complaining of a painful swollen foot and leg. This injury is similar to a "wringer" injury of the arm because the initial examination may not reveal the true extent of the injury. Izant et al (111) identified three components to this trauma: (a) a laceration of the tissue from the knifelike action of the spoke, (b) a crushing from the impingement between the wheel and the frame of the bicycle, and (c) a shearing injury from the coefficient of these two forces. The laceration created by this injury often involves the malleoli, the Achilles tendon area of the heel, and the dorsum of the foot. A child with a bicycle spoke injury may require multiple debridements, and definitive treatment must await delineation of the necrotic area.

A child with a bicycle spoke injury should be admitted to the hospital because the extent of the damage may not be identified initially. Initial therapy consists of a mild compression dressing with a multilayered cotton bandage. The extremity is elevated and the child is kept at bedrest during the first 24 hours. A long-leg splint is applied if a tibial fracture is present. The child may ambulate with crutches non-weightbearing after that. Frequent inspection of the extremity must be made during the subsequent 48 hours. Debridement of devitalized tissue is performed as necrosis becomes apparent. Large areas of hematoma formation are treated with aspiration to prevent further elevation of the overlying skin. Wound closure with a split-thickness skin graft is performed if full-thickness skin loss occurs. Occasionally, a free flap may be required, but this is rare. Most patients regain normal function of the foot and ankle. The average time for complete healing may be 5 to 6 weeks (109–111). A child with a concomitant tibial fracture is placed in an above-the-knee non-weightbearing cast at the completion of care for the foot injury (109). The tibial fracture may need to be stabilized with an external fixation device if the soft tissue loss on the foot and ankle is severe.

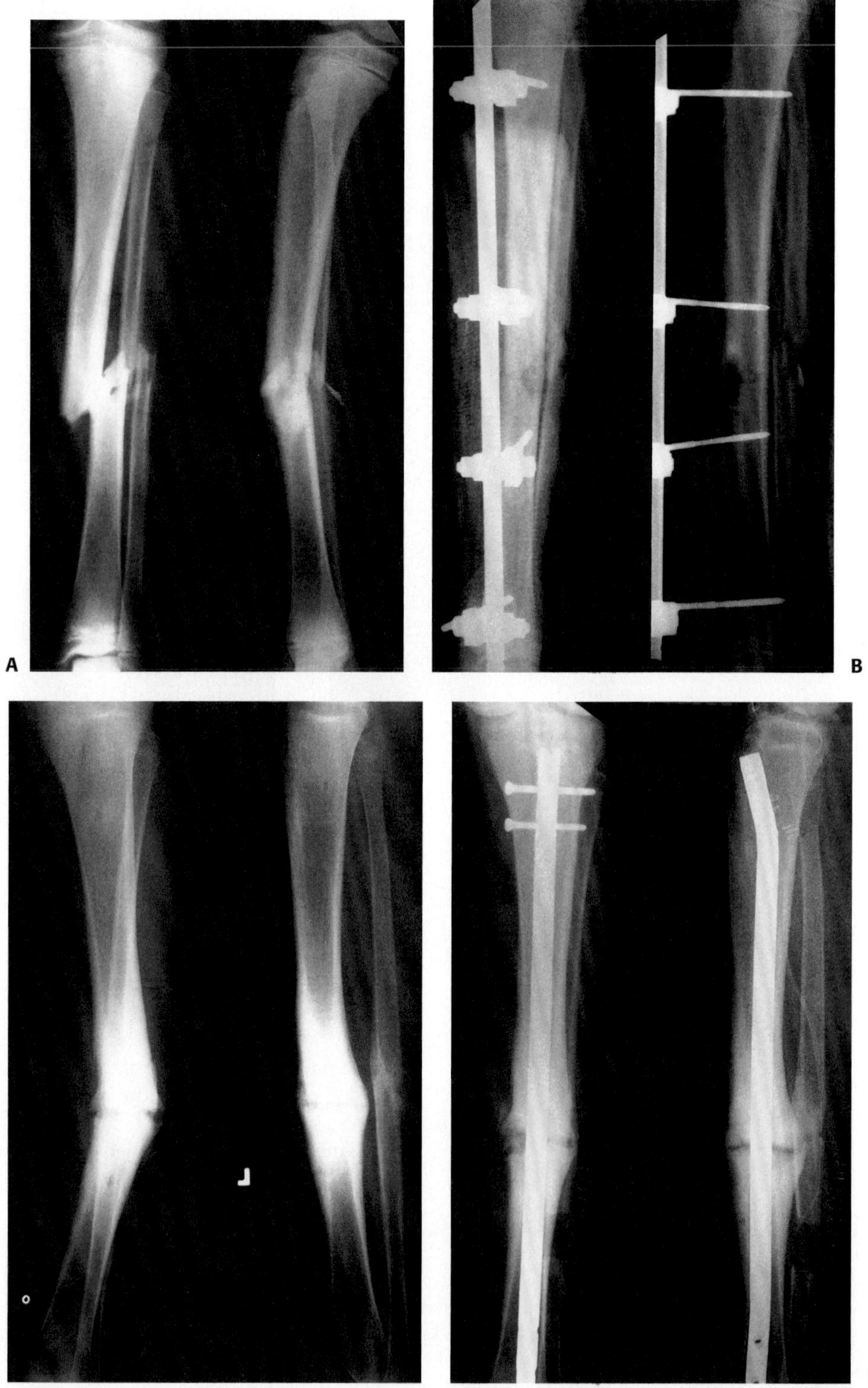

FIGURE 25-34 **A.** Anteroposterior and lateral x-rays of a 14-year-old adolescent who was struck by a car, sustaining a grade IIIB open fracture of the tibia. **B.** Anteroposterior and lateral x-rays of the tibia after irrigation and debridement, and application of an external fixation device. **C.** The patient developed a nonunion at the tibia, which progressively deformed into an unacceptable varus alignment. **D.** The nonunion was treated with a fibular osteotomy followed by a closed angular correction of the deformity and internal fixation with a reamed intramedullary nail.

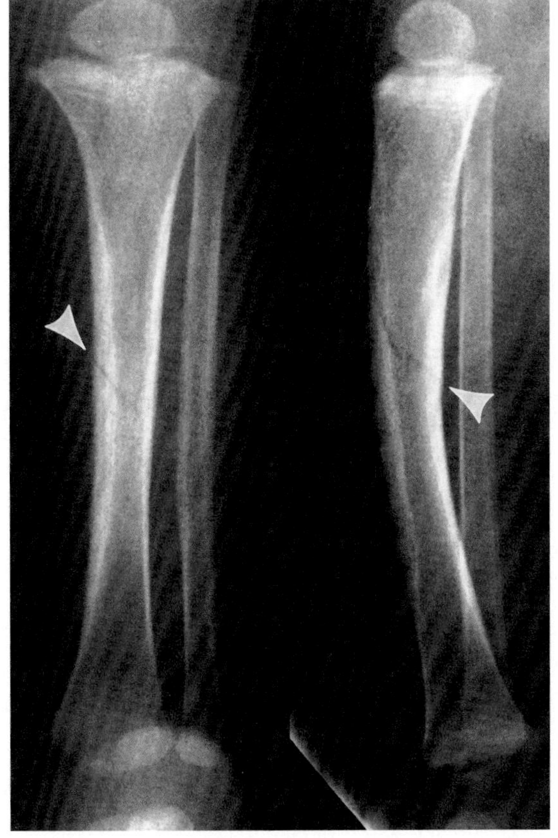

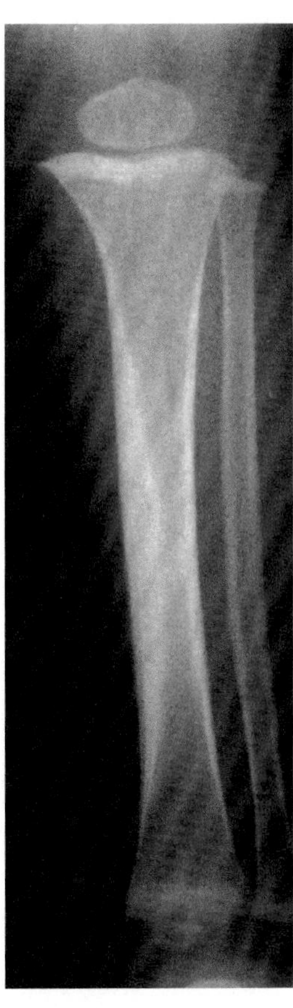

FIGURE 25-35 **A.** Anteroposterior and lateral x-rays of an 18-month-old child who presented with refusal to bear weight on her leg. Note the spiral middle one-third "toddler's" fracture (*arrows*). **B.** This fracture healed uneventfully after 4 weeks of immobilization in a cast.

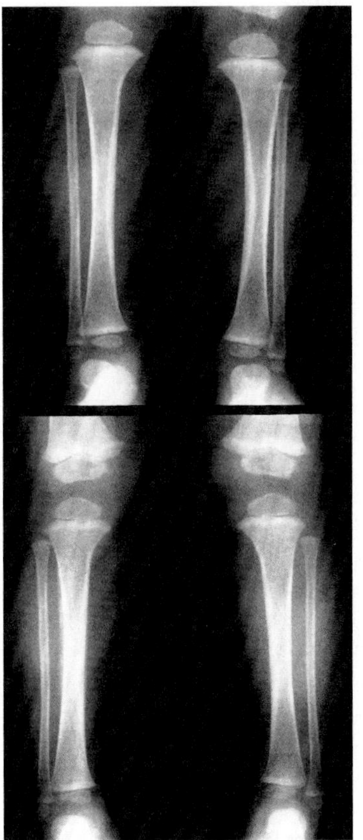

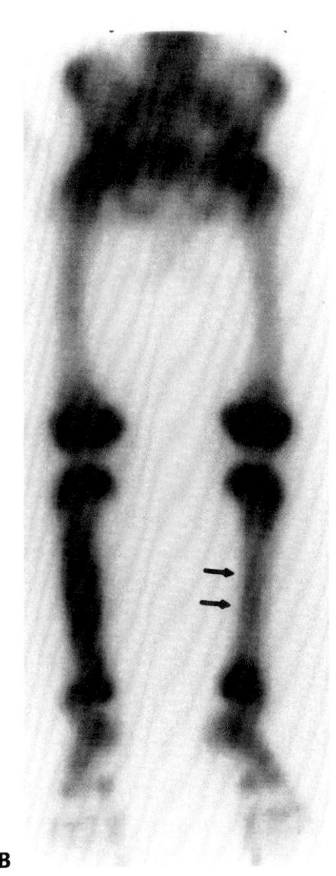

FIGURE 25-36 **A.** Anteroposterior x-ray of the tibia in a 3-year-old child who refused to bear weight on the right leg 3 weeks before presentation. The history of obvious trauma was absent. The x-rays revealed periosteal new bone formation in the mid-shaft of the right tibia. There was also tenderness to palpation in the mid-left tibia as well despite normal x-rays. **B.** A bone scan showed increased uptake in both the left and right tibia. There was significantly less uptake on the left side, the more recent injury.

Floating Knee

Significant trauma can cause fractures involving both the femur and the tibia. In the past, these injuries often were treated with traction and casting (Fig. 25-37). The extent of the injuries often left permanent functional deficits when not aggressively managed (100,112).

Most children between 2 and 4 years of age with ipsilateral femoral and tibial fractures are treated with operative stabilization of the femur and either cast immobilization of the tibia after reduction or external fixation. In children 2 to 6 years of age, the femoral fracture can be stabilized with a unilateral external fixator, plate with screws, or flexible nails; children 6 years of age and older may be stabilized with flexible intramedullary nails or an external fixator. Open reduction and plate fixation is used for fractures in the subtrochanteric or supracondylar area of the femur in adolescents, although external fixation may be useful in these areas as well. The tibial fracture is reduced and stabilized after the femoral fracture has been stabilized. Open tibial fractures associated with a femoral fracture are stabilized with a unilateral external fixator or flexible intramedullary nails (Fig. 25-38). If adequate closed reduction is not achieved, open reduction with internal or external fixation is indicated.

Tibial Fracture in Paraplegic Children

Motor paralysis from poliomyelitis was once the most common cause of lower extremity weakness in children. Because these patients have sensation, fractures are identified early. Disease trends have changed, however. As late as 1958, 90% to 95% of children with myelomeningocele died in the first year of life, usually from a neurosurgical complication. Recent advances in neurosurgery and urology have significantly increased the life span of children with myelomeningocele. The mortality rate for these children is now 3% to 5%. Currently, pediatric orthopaedic surgeons manage a large number of paraplegic children who have sensory and/or motor deficits (113–115).

Tibial fractures in children without sensation require special attention. Gillies and Hartung (115) are the first to report children with myelomeningocele who sustained pathologic fractures of the proximal tibia. These two children had tense hyperemic skin and x-ray evidence of exuberant new bone formation, suggesting a malignant tumor (Fig. 25-39). Both children had a biopsy because of this x-ray finding.

Soutter (116) stressed that clinical findings such as swelling, warmth, and erythema are common in paraplegic children with a fracture. He stated that "fractures to the growth plate in paraplegic children often resemble osteomyelitis."

Fractures around the knee are common in children with paraplegia because of the length of the lower extremity and the association with joint contractures (117). These fractures are more common in children with flaccid paralysis than those with spastic paralysis (118,119).

James (118) reported 44 fractures in 22 children in a population of 122 children with myelomeningocele. The most common age range at fracture was 3 to 6 years. These fractures were more common in a flail limb. Only 6.6% of the patients with quadriceps activity had fractures, whereas 19% of those with no active muscle contraction (flail limb) had fractures. This incidence decreased to 12.5% in a group of children with spastic paralysis. The tibia and femur were the most common bones affected. The most common locations for tibial fractures were the distal diaphysis and distal metaphysis.

Parsch and Rossak (120) reported 31 fractures in 120 patients with myelomeningocele. They emphasized treatment with a wrap and splint until early fracture consolidation. To prevent "fracture disease," they stressed early standing and walking to help reduce the degree of osteopenia these children develop.

Drennan and Freehafer (113) reported 58 fractures in 25 patients among 84 children with myelomeningocele. Ten fractures were in the tibia. Eleven of the 58 fractures occurred after the removal of a spica cast, suggesting that immobilization worsened osteopenia and increased the risk of subsequent fracture.

Complications in patients with paralysis and a tibial fracture are rare and usually are related to pressure sores produced by poorly padded casts. Early physeal arrest can occur, producing a leg length discrepancy, and physeal involvement is common in paralytic children with fractures (116). Golding (117) reported one physeal injury to the distal tibia in a child with myelomeningocele. Gyepes et al (121) reported seven metaphyseal and physeal injuries in patients with myelomeningocele. X-rays were characterized by an irregular, dense, widened physis and adjacent subperiosteal new bone formation. Stern et al (122) reported bilateral distal tibial and fibular physeal injuries in a child with myelomeningocele.

Incidental trauma probably is the primary factor producing the complex x-ray findings associated with a tibial fracture in a paralytic child (121). Repeated microtrauma can lead to a metaphyseal infraction, subperiosteal hemorrhage, and, perhaps, physeal hemorrhage. Subsequent healing produces endosteal and periosteal callus formation and some generalized osteopenia secondary to the immobilization. The widening of the physis most likely is secondary to a disturbance of the normal reabsorption mechanism during bone development at the metaphysis. This results from frequent subclinical metaphyseal infractions. It also could be produced by hemorrhage into the physis itself.

Fracture of the tibia in a paralytic child can occur with minor trauma. Many fractures are nondisplaced, and nonoperative therapy is indicated. Displaced fractures are reduced closed and immobilized for 3 to 4 weeks in a bulky dressing or a posterior, molded, well-padded splint. The child should be fitted with an orthosis or placed back into his or her pre-fracture orthosis after the immobilization is discontinued.

Physeal injuries may require prolonged periods of immobilization. Healing is determined by the absence of local warmth and swelling and the reconstitution of the width of the physis on x-ray (123).

Stress Fractures of the Tibia and Fibula

Roberts and Vogt (124) in 1939 reported an "unusual type of lesion" in the tibia of 12 children. All of these were determined

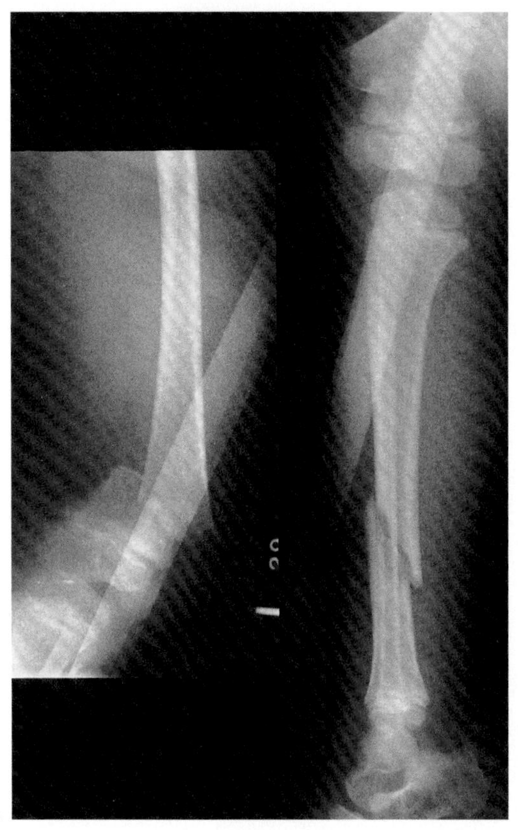
A

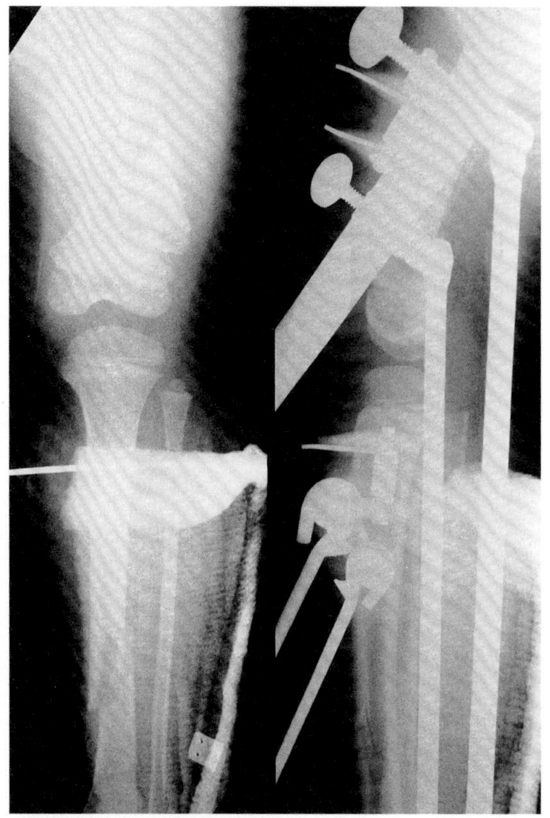
B

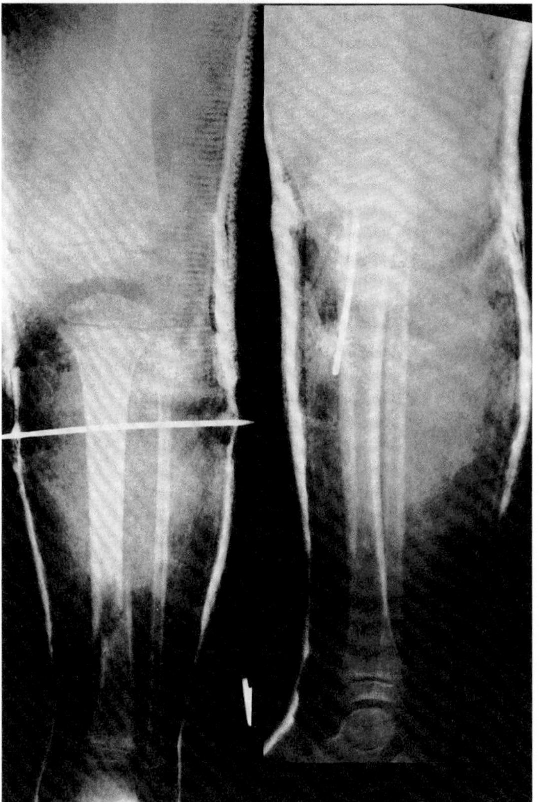
C

FIGURE 25-37 **A.** Ipsilateral fractures of the distal femur and tibia without an ipsilateral fibular fracture in a 5-year-old. **B.** The child was treated with tibial pin traction for the femoral injury (pin applied below the tibial tubercle) and a short leg splint for the tibial fracture initially. **C.** The child was placed into a spica cast after 2 weeks of traction. The tibial traction pin was used to help stabilize both fractures.

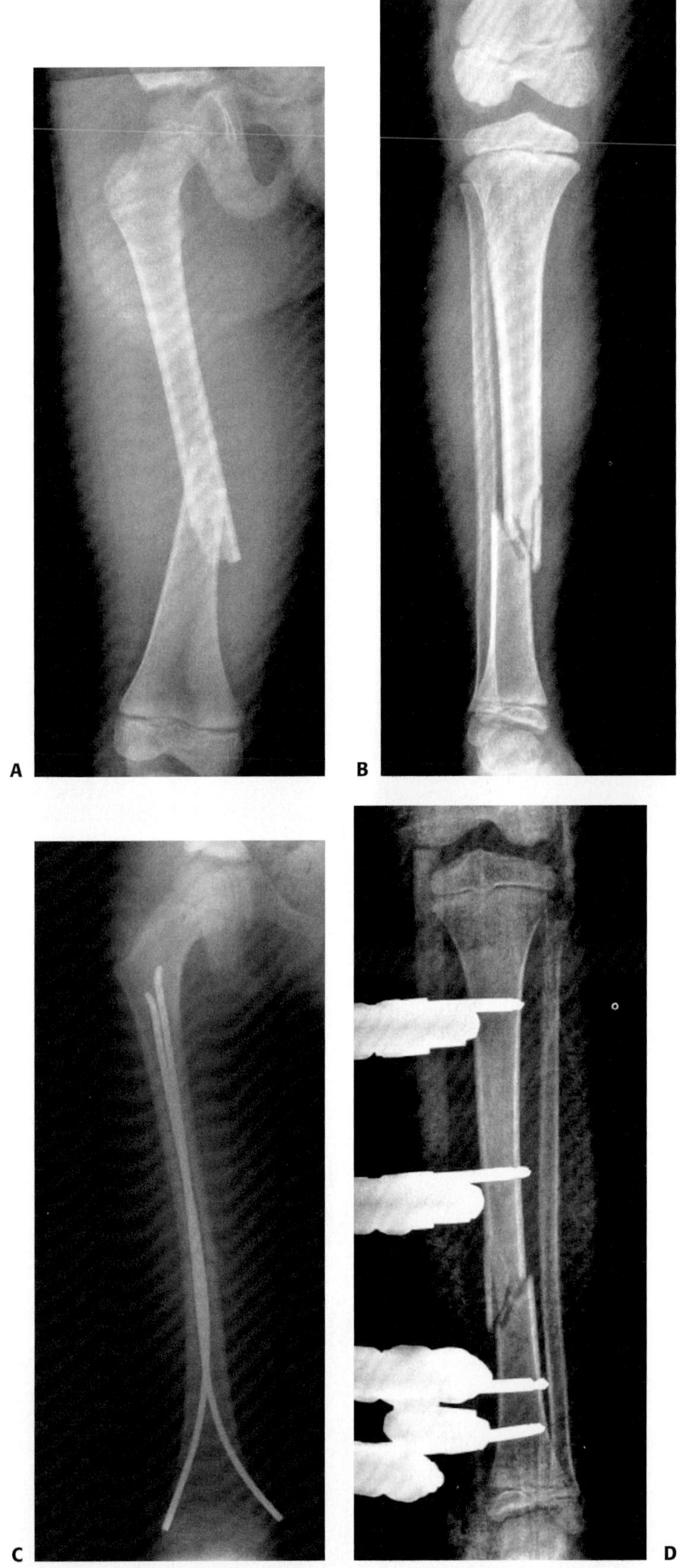

FIGURE 25-38 **A,B.** Floating knee injury in a 7-year-old boy. **C.** Femoral fracture was fixed with flexible intramedullary nails. **D.** Tibial fracture was stabilized with external fixation.

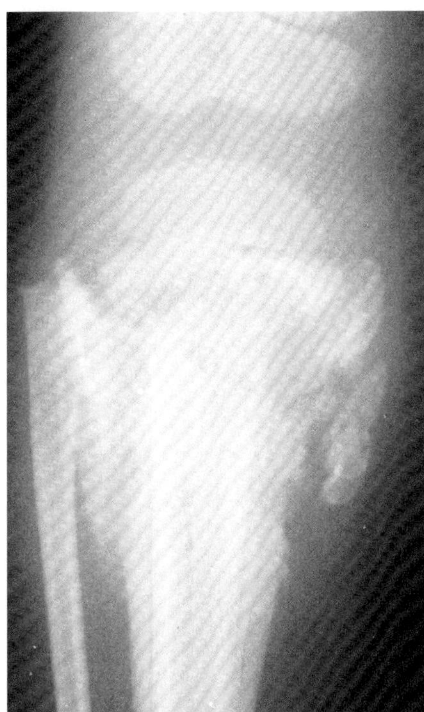

FIGURE 25-39 An undisplaced fracture of the proximal tibial metaphysic in a child with myelodysplasia. Note the exuberant new bone formation.

to be stress fractures involving the upper third of the tibial shaft. Since then, numerous reports of stress fractures involving the tibia and the fibula have been published (45,125–137).

The pattern of stress fractures in children differs from that in adults (126,138,139). In adults, the fibula is involved in stress fractures twice as often as the tibia; in children the tibia is affected more often than the fibula (Fig. 25-40). The prevalence of stress fractures in boys and girls is equal.

A child with a stress fracture usually has an insidious onset of symptoms (126,138). There is evidence of local tenderness that worsens with activity. The child may have a painful limp. A toddler with a stress fracture will not bear weight on the involved extremity. The pain tends to be worse in the day and to improve at night and with rest. The knee and the ankle have full ranges of motion. Usually, there is minimal, if any, swelling at the fracture site (85,126,127,138,140,141).

X-rays reveal changes consistent with a stress fracture approximately 2 weeks after the onset of symptoms (126). X-ray evidence of fracture repair can manifest in one of three ways: localized periosteal new bone formation, endosteal thickening, or, rarely, a radiolucent cortical fracture line (Fig. 25-41) (85,113,126,136,138).

Technetium radionuclide bone imaging reveals a local area of increased tracer uptake at the site of the fracture (Fig. 25-42). Computerized tomography rarely demonstrates the fracture line, but delineates increased marrow density and endosteal and periosteal new bone formation. It also may show soft tissue edema. Magnetic resonance (MR) imaging (85,141) shows a localized band of very low signal intensity continuous with the cortex. MR signaling can be diagnostic of stress fracture and differentiate it from malignancy obviating the need for biopsy.

Stress fractures occur when the force applied to a bone is exceeded by the bone's capacity to withstand it. Initially, osteoclastic tunnel formation increases. These tunnels normally fill with mature bone. With continued force, cortical reabsorption accelerates. New bone is produced to splint the weakened cortex. This bone is immature, however, and does not have the strength of the bone it replaces. A fracture occurs when bone reabsorption outstrips bone production. When the offending force is reduced or eliminated, bone production exceeds bone reabsorption. This produces cortical and endosteal widening with dense repair bone that later remodels to mature bone (108,142,143).

Tibia

The most common location for a tibial stress fracture is in the upper third. The child normally has a painful limp of gradual onset with no history of a specific injury. The peak incidence of tibial stress fractures in children is between 10 and 15 years of age. Pain is relieved with rest. The pain is described as dull, occurring in the calf near the upper end of the tibia on its medial aspect, and occasionally is bilateral. Physical findings include local tenderness on one or both sides of the tibial crest with a varying degree of swelling.

The treatment of a child with a stress fracture of the tibia (or fibula) begins with activity modification. An active child can rest in a long leg walking cast for 4 to 6 weeks followed by gradual increase in activity. Nonunions of stress fractures of the tibia have been described. Green (17) reported six nonunions, three of which were in children. Two required excision of the nonunion site with iliac crest bone grafting. The third was treated by electromagnetic stimulation. In all three, the stress fractures occurred in the middle third of the tibia.

Fibula

Pediatric fibular stress fractures normally occur between the ages of 2 and 8 years (144). The fractures are normally localized to the distal third of the fibula.

The child presents with a limp and may complain of pain. Tenderness is localized to the distal half of the fibular shaft. Swelling normally is not present. The obvious bony mass commonly seen in a stress fracture of the fibula in an adult is normally not seen in a comparable fracture in a child.

No x-ray abnormalities are identified in the first 10 days to 2 weeks after the symptoms begin. The earliest sign of a stress fracture of the fibula is the presence of "eggshell" callus along the shaft of the fibula (140). The fracture itself cannot always be seen because the periosteal callus may obscure the changes in the narrow canal. Radionuclide bone imaging can help to identify stress fractures before the presence of x-ray changes (Fig. 25-43).

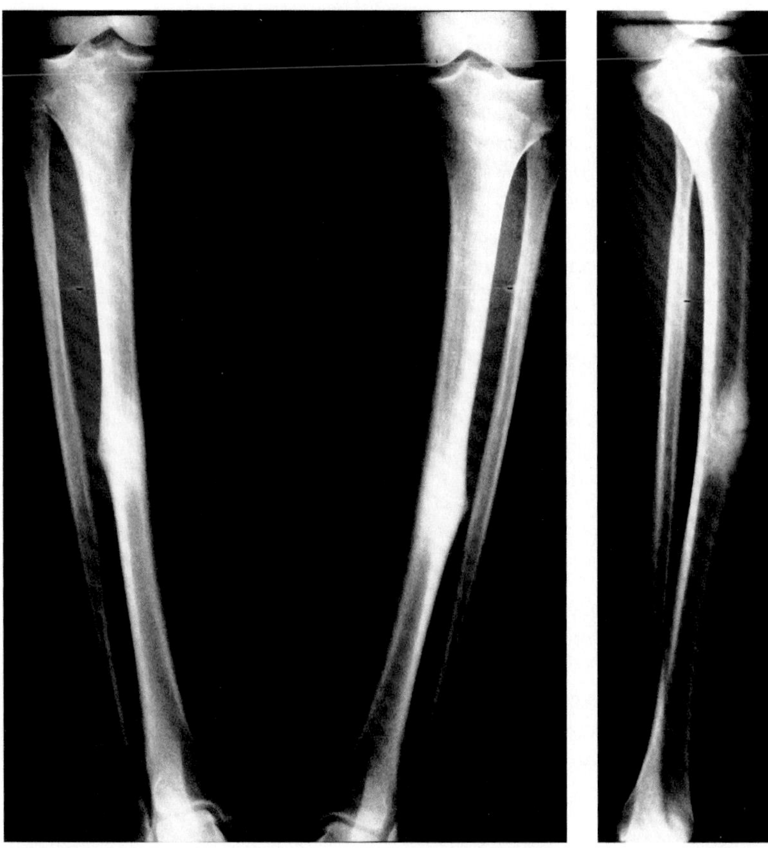

FIGURE 25-40 Bilateral mid-tibial stress fractures in an adolescent with genu varus.

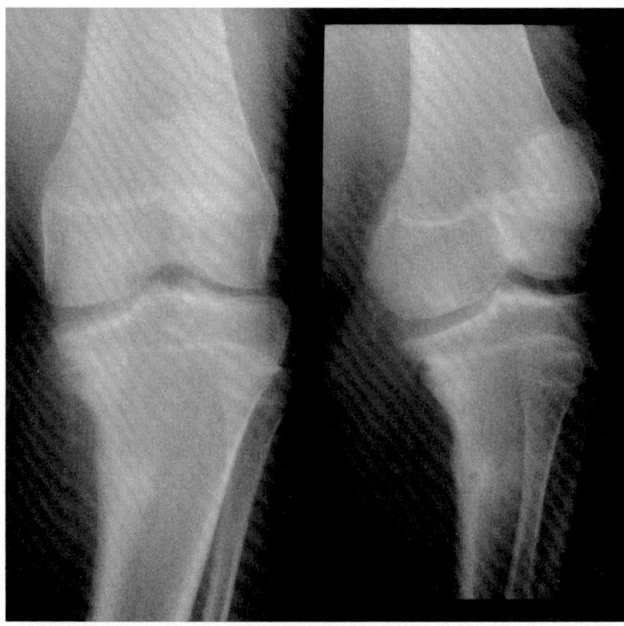

FIGURE 25-41 Anteroposterior and lateral x-rays of the knee of a 15-year-old with adolescent onset tibia vara. Note the posteromedial stress fracture.

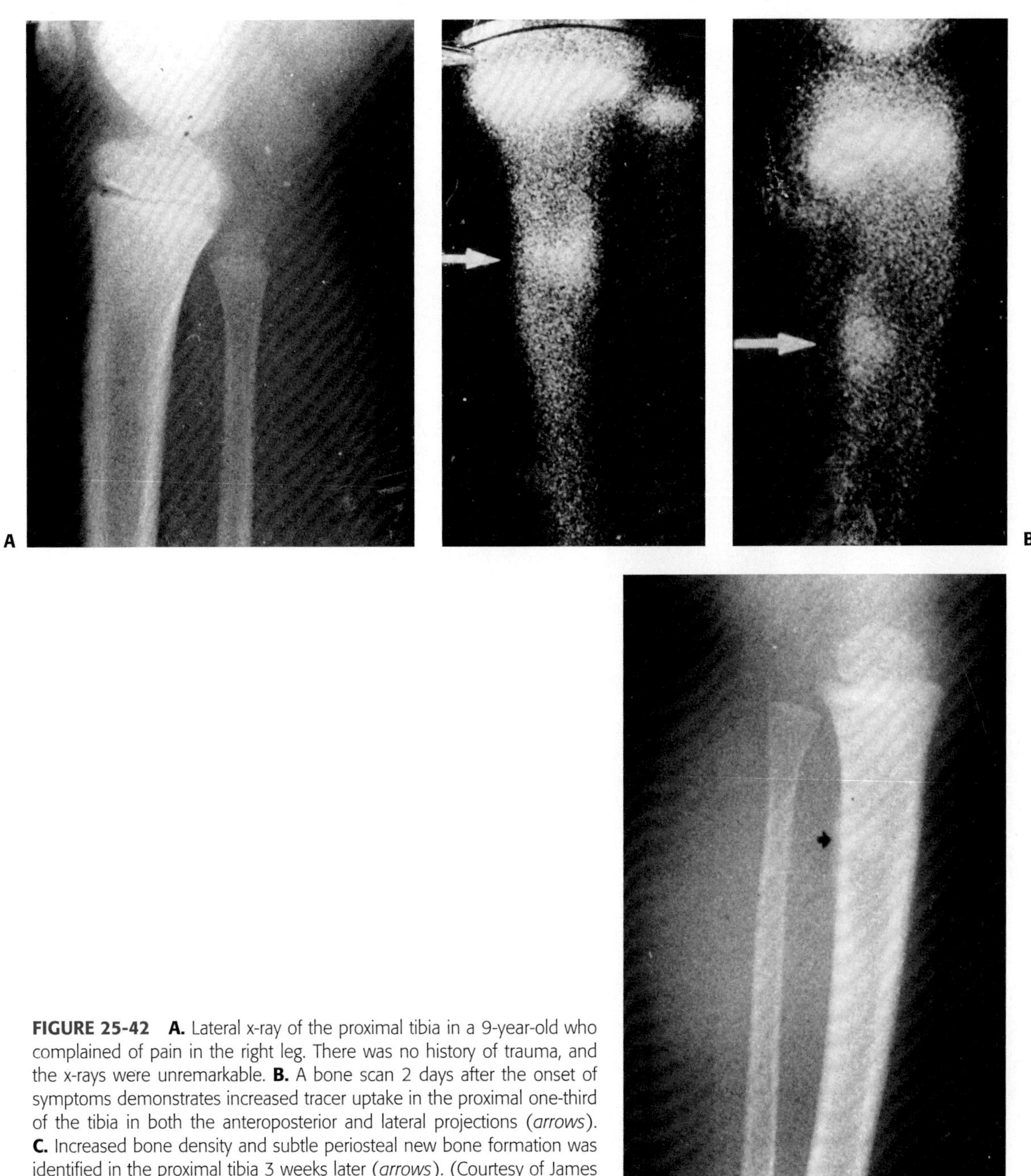

FIGURE 25-42 **A.** Lateral x-ray of the proximal tibia in a 9-year-old who complained of pain in the right leg. There was no history of trauma, and the x-rays were unremarkable. **B.** A bone scan 2 days after the onset of symptoms demonstrates increased tracer uptake in the proximal one-third of the tibia in both the anteroposterior and lateral projections (*arrows*). **C.** Increased bone density and subtle periosteal new bone formation was identified in the proximal tibia 3 weeks later (*arrows*). (Courtesy of James Conway, MD.)

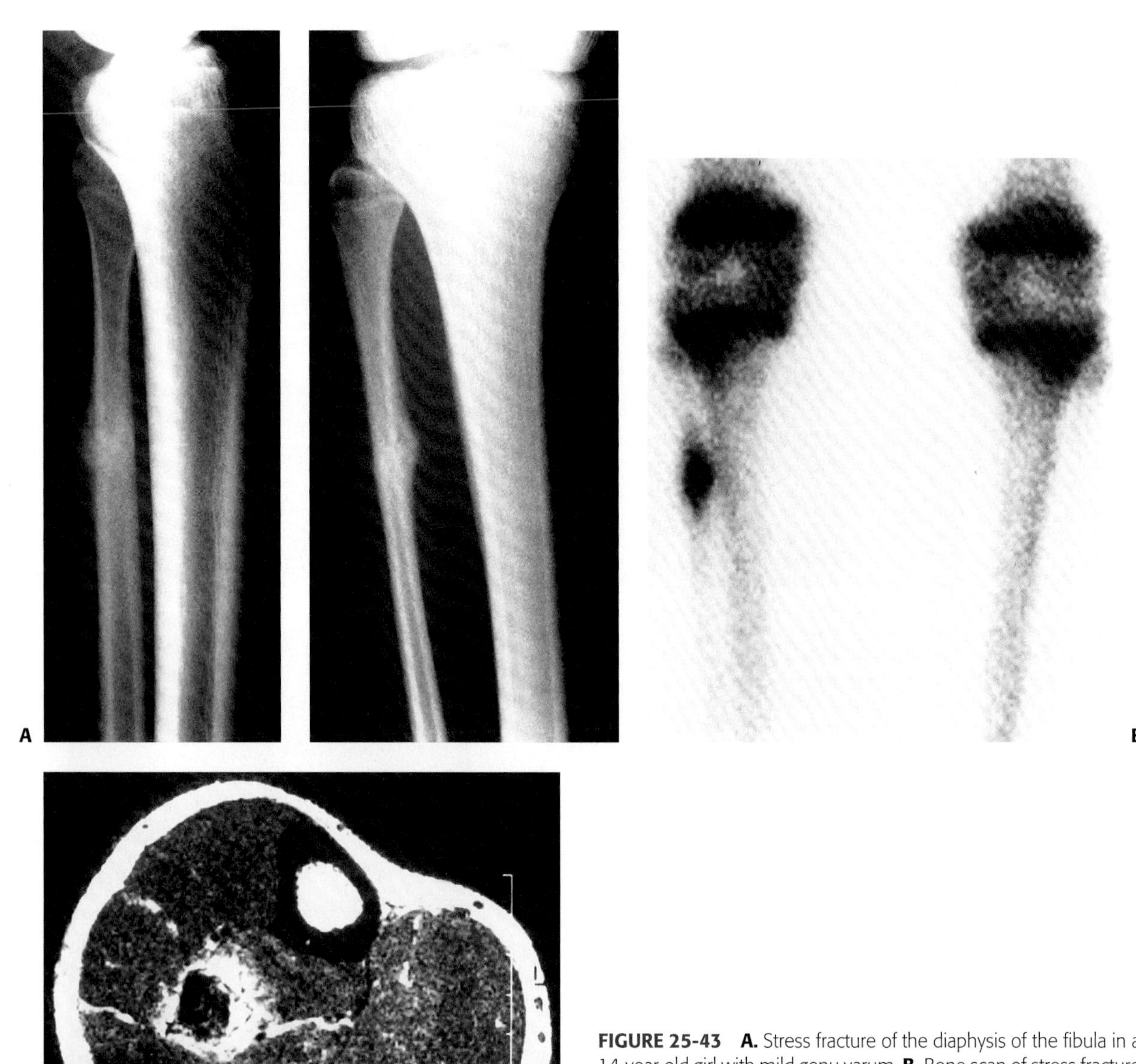

FIGURE 25-43 **A.** Stress fracture of the diaphysis of the fibula in a 14-year-old girl with mild genu varum. **B.** Bone scan of stress fracture showing marked increased tracer uptake. **C.** Magnetic resonance image demonstrates new central bone formation and an inflammatory zone around the fibular cortex. (Reprinted from Sharps CH, Cardea JA. Fractures of the shaft of the tibia and fibula. In: MacEwen GD, Kasser JR, Heinrich SD, eds. *Pediatric fractures: a practical approach to assessment and treatment*. Baltimore: Williams & Wilkins, 1993:324; with permission.)

The differential diagnosis includes sarcoma of bone, osteomyelitis, and a soft tissue injury without accompanying bony injury. Treatment consists of rest or, in a very active child, a short leg-walking cast for 4 to 6 weeks.

REFERENCES

1. Shannak AO. Tibial fractures in children: follow-up study. *J Pediatr Orthop* 1988;8:306.
2. Steinert VV, Bennek J. Unterschenkelfrakturen in kindesalter. *Zentralbl Chir* 1966;91:1387.
3. Karrholm J, Hansson LI, Svensson K. Incidence of tibio-fibular shaft and ankle fractures in children. *J Pediatr Orthop* 1982;2:386.
4. Hansen BA, Greiff S, Bergmann F. Fractures of the tibia in children. *Acta Orthop Scand* 1976;47:448.
5. Cheng JCY, Shen WY. Limb fracture pattern in different pediatric age groups:a study of 3,350 children. *J Orthop Trauma* 1993;7:15–22.
6. Weber BG, Brunner C, Freuner F, eds. *Treatment of fractures in children and adolescents.* Berlin: Springer-Verlag, 1980.
7. Blount WP. *Fractures in children.* Baltimore: Williams & Wilkins, 1955.
8. Gray H. Anatomy: descriptive and surgical. In: Pick TP, Howden R, eds. *Anatomy: descriptive and surgical.* New York: Bounty Books, 1977:182.
9. Mellick LB, Reesor K, Demers D, et al. Tibial fractures of young children. *Pediatr Emerg Care* 1988;4:97.
10. King J, Defendorf D, Apthorp J, et al. Analysis of 429 fractures in 1889 battered children. *J Pediatr Orthop* 1988;8:585.

11. Loder RT, Bookout C. Fracture patterns in battered children. *J Ortho Trauma* 1991;5: 428–433.
12. Buckley SL, Gotschall C, Robertson W, et al. The relationship of skeletal injuries with trauma score, injury severity score, length of hospital stay, hospital charges and mortality in children admitted to a regional pediatric trauma center. *J Pediatr Orthop* 1994; 14:449.
13. Balthazar DA, Pappas AM. Acquired valgus deformity of the tibia in children. *J Pediatr Orthop* 1984;4:538.
14. Bassey LO. Valgus deformity following proximal metaphyseal fractures in children: experiences in the African tropics. *J Trauma* 1990;30:102.
15. Coates R. Knock-knee deformity following upper tibial "greenstick" fractures. *J Bone Joint Surg [Br]* 1977;59:516.
16. Cozen L. Fracture of the proximal portion of the tibia in children followed by valgus deformity. *Surg Gynecol Obstet* 1953;97:183.
17. Green NE. Tibia valga caused by asymmetrical overgrowth following a nondisplaced fracture of the proximal tibia metaphysis. *J Pediatr Orthop* 1983;3:235.
18. Jackson DW, Cozen L. Genu valgum as a complication of proximal tibial metaphyseal fractures in children. *J Bone Joint Surg [Am]* 1971;53:1571.
19. Jordan SE, Alonso JE, Cook FF. The etiology of valgus angulation after metaphyseal fractures of the tibia in children. *J Pediatr Orthop* 1987;7:450.
20. Keret D, Harcke HT, Bowen JR. Tibia valga after fracture: documentation of mechanism. *Arch Orthop Trauma Surg* 1991;110:216–219.
21. Ogden JA. Tibia and fibula. In: *Skeletal injury in the child.* Philadelphia: Lea & Febiger, 1982:587.
22. Salter RB, Best T. The pathogenesis and prevention of valgus deformity following fractures of the proximal metaphyseal region in the tibia in children. *J Bone Joint Surg [Am]* 1973;55:1324.
23. Skak S. Valgus deformity following proximal tibial metaphyseal fracture in children. *Acta Orthop Scand* 1982;53:141.
24. Steel HH, Sandrow RE, Sullivan PD. Complications of tibial osteotomy in children for genu varum or valgum. *J Bone Joint Surg [Am]* 1971;53:1629.
25. Taylor SL. Tibial overgrowth: a cause of genu valgum. *J Bone Joint Surg [Am]* 1963;45: 659.
26. Weber BG. Fibrous interposition causing valgus deformity after fracture of the upper tibial metaphysis in children. *J Bone Joint Surg [Br]* 1977;59:290.
27. Zionts LE, Harcke HT, Brooks KM, et al. Post traumatic tibia valga: a case demonstrating asymmetric activity at the proximal growth plate on technetium bone scan. *J Pediatr Orthop* 1977;7:458.
28. Zionts LE, MacEwen GD. Spontaneous improvement of post traumatic tibia valga. *J Bone Joint Surg [Am]* 1986;68:680.
29. Ogden JA, Ogden DA, Pugh L, et al. Tibia valga after proximal metaphyseal fracture in childhood: a normal biologic response. *J Pediatr Orthop* 1995;15:489–494.
30. Lehner A, Dubas J. Sekundare Deformierungen nach Epiphysenlosungen und Epiphysenliniennahen Fraktunen. *Helv Chir Acta* 1954;21:388.
31. Goff CW. *Surgical treatment of unequal extremities.* Springfield, IL: Charles C Thomas, 1960:135–136.
32. Pollen AG. *Fractures and dislocations in children.* Baltimore: Williams & Wilkins, 1973: 179.
33. Rooker G, Salter R. Presentation of valgus deformity following fracture of the proximal metaphysis of the tibia in children. *J Bone Joint Surg [Br]* 1980;62:527.
34. DeBastiani G, Aldegheiri R, Renzi-Brivio L, et al. Limb lengthening by distraction of the epiphyseal plate. *J Bone Joint Surg [Br]* 1986;68:545.
35. DeBastiani G, Aldegheiri R, Renzi-Brivio LR, et al. Chondrodiastasis-controlled symmetrical distraction of the epiphyseal plate. *J Bone Joint Surg [Br]* 1986;68:550.
36. Metaizeau JP, Wong-Chung J, Bertrand H, et al. Percutaneous Epiphysiodesis using transphyseal screws (PETS). *J Pediatric Ortho* 1998;18:363–369.
37. Robert M, Khouri N, Carlioz H, et al. Fractures of the proximal tibial metaphysis in children: review of a series of 25 cases. *J Pediatr Orthop* 1987;7:444.
38. Yang J, Letts M. Isolated fractures of the tibia with intact fibula in children: a review of 95 patients. *J Pediatr Orthop* 1997;17:347–351.
39. Karlsson MK, Nilsson BE, Obrant KJ. Fracture incidence after tibial shaft fractures: a 30-year follow-up study. *Clin Orthop* 1993;287:87.
40. Briggs TWR, Orr MM, Lightowler CDR. Isolated tibial fractures in children. *Injury* 1992;23:308.
41. Holderman WD. Results following conservative treatment of fractures of the tibial shaft. *Am J Surg* 1959;98:593.
42. Bartlett GS III, Weiver LS, Yang EC. Treatment of type II and type III open tibia fractures in children. *J Orthop Trauma* 1997;11:357–362.
43. Blick SS, Brumback RJ, Poka A, et al. Compartment syndrome in open tibial fractures. *J Bone Joint Surg [Am]* 1986;68:1348.
44. Cullen MC, Roy DR, Crawford AH, et al. Open fractures of the tibia in children. *J Bone Joint Surg [Am]* 1996;78:1039–1047.
45. Edwards CC. Staged reconstruction of complex open tibial fractures using Hoffmann external fixation. *Clin Orthop* 1983;178:130.
46. Evanoff M, Strong ML, MacIntosh R. External fixation maintained until fracture consolidation in the skeletally immature. *J Pediatr Orthop* 1983;13:98.
47. Gates JD. The management of combined skeletal and arterial injuries of the lower extremity. *Am J Orthop* 1995;24:674–680.
48. Greiff J, Bergmann F. Growth disturbance following fracture of the tibia in children. *Acta Orthop Scand* 1980;15:315.
49. Hull JB, Sanderson PL, Rickman M, et al. External fixation of children's fractures: Use of the Orthofix Dynamic Axial Fixator. *J Pediatr Orthop* 1997;6:203–206.
50. Katzman SS, Dickson K. Determining the prognosis for limb salvage in major vascular injuries with associated open tibial fractures. *Orthop Rev* 1992;21:195.
51. Kreder HJ, Armstrong P. A review of open tibia fractures in children. *J Pediatr Orthop* 1995;15:482–488.
52. Leach RE, Hammond G, Stryker WS. Anterior tibial compartment syndrome. *J Bone Joint Surg [Am]* 1967;49:451.
53. Levy AS, Wetzlan M, Lewars M, et.al. The orthopaedic and social outcome of open tibia fractures in children. *Orthopaedics* 1997;20:593–598.
54. Robertson P, Karol LA, Rab GT. Open fractures of the tibia and femur in children. *J Pediatr Orthop* 1996;16:621–626.
55. Siegmeth A, Wruhs O, Vecsei V. External fixation of lower limb fractures in children. *Eur J Pediatr Surg* 1998;8:35–41.
56. Wood D, Hoffer MH. Tibial fractures in head injured children. *J Trauma* 1987;27:65.
57. Benz G, Kallieris D, Seebock T, et al. Bio-reabsorbable pins and screws in pediatric traumatology. *Eur J Pediatr Surg* 1994;4:103–107.
58. Qidwai SA. Intramedullary Kirschner wiring for tibia fractures in children: *JPO* 2001; 21:294–297.
59. Gustillo RB, Anderson JT. Prevention of infection in the treatment of one-thousand and twenty-five fractures of long bones. *J Bone Joint Surg [Am]* 1976;58:453.
60. Mooney JF III, Argenta LC, Marks MW, et al. Treatment of soft tissue defects in pediatric patients using the VAC™ system. CORR 376;2000:26–31.
61. Grimard G, Navdie D, Laberge LC, et al. Open fractures of the tibia in children. *Clin Orthop* 1996;332:62–70.
62. Song KM, Sangeorzan B, Benirschke S, et al. Open fractures of the tibia in children. *J Pediatr Orthop* 1996;16:635–638.
63. Buckley SL, Smith G, Sponseller PD, et al. Open fractures of the tibia in children. *J Bone Joint Surg [Am]* 1990;72:1462.
64. Cramer KE, Limbird TJ, Green NE. Open fractures of the diaphysis of the lower extremity in children. *J Bone Joint Surg [Am]* 1992;74:218.
65. Hope PG, Cole WG. Open fractures of the tibia in children. *J Bone Joint Surg [Br]* 1992; 74:546.
66. Caudle RJ, Stern PJ. Severe open fractures of the tibia. *J Bone Joint Surg [Am]* 1987;69: 801.
67. Clancey GJ, Hansen ST Jr. Open fractures of the tibia: a review of one hundred and two cases. *J Bone Joint Surg [Am]* 1978;60:118.
68. DeLee JC, Strehl JB. Open tibia fracture with compartment syndrome. *Clin Orthop* 1981;160:175.
69. Gustillo RB, Mendoza RM, Williams PN. Problems in the management of type III (severe) open fractures: a new classification of type III open fractures. *J Trauma* 1984; 24:742.
70. Hoaglund FT, States JD. Factors influencing the rate of healing in tibial shaft fractures. *Surg Gynecol Obstet* 1967;124:71.
71. Hoover NW. Injuries of the popliteal artery associated with fractures and dislocations. *Surg Clin North Am* 1961;41:1099.
72. Larsson K, van der Linden W. Open tibial shaft fractures. *Clin Orthop* 1983;180:63.
73. Nicoll EA. Fractures of the tibial shaft, a survey of 705 cases. *J Bone Joint Surg [Br]* 1964;46:373.
74. Patzakis MJ, Wilkins J, Moore TM. Used antibiotics in open tibial fractures. *Clin Orthop* 1983;118:31.
75. Sarmiento A. A functional below-the-knee cast for tibial fractures. *J Bone Joint Surg [Am]* 1967;49:855.
76. Blasier RD, Barnes CL. Age as a prognostic factor in open tibial fractures in children. *Clin Orthop* 1996;331:261–264.
77. Skaggs DL, Kautz SM, Kay RM, et al. Effects of delay on surgical treatment on rate of infection in open fractures in children. J Pediatric Ortho 2000;20:19–22.
78. Klein DM, Caligiuri DA, Katzman BM. Local-advancement soft-tissue coverage in a child with ipsilateral grade IIIB open tibial and ankle fractures. *J Orthop Trauma* 1996; 10:577–580.
79. Morton KS, Starr DE. Closure of the anterior portion of the upper tibial epiphysis as a complication of tibial-shaft fracture. *J Bone Joint Surg [Am]* 1964;46:570.
80. Small JO, Mollan RAB. Management of the soft tissues in open tibial fractures. *Br J Plast Surg* 1992;45:571.
81. Hallock GG. Efficacy of free flaps for pediatric trauma patients. *J Reconstructive Microsurgery* 1995;11:169–174.
82. Ostermann PAW, Henry SL, Seligson D. Timing of wound closure in severe compound fractures. *Orthopedics* 1994;17:397.
83. Byrd HS, Spicer PJ, Cierney G. Management of open tibial fractures. *Plast Reconstr Surg* 1985;76:719.
84. Cierny G, Byrd HS, Jones RE. Primary versus delayed tissue coverage for severe open tibial fractures: a comparison of results. *Clin Orthop* 1983;178:54.
85. Kozlowski K, Azouz M, Barrett IR, et al. Midshaft tibial stress fractures in children. *Aust Radiol* 1992;36:131–134.
86. Van der Werkon C, Meevwis JD, et al. The simple fix: external fixation of displaced isolated tibial fractures. *Injury* 1993;24:46.
87. Allen MJ, Nash JR, Ioannidies TT, et al. Major vascular surgeries associated with orthopaedic injuries to the lower limb. *Ann R Coll Surg Engl* 1984;66:101.
88. Haas LM, Staple TW. Arterial injuries associated with fractures of the proximal tibia following blunt trauma. *South Med J* 1969;62:1439.
89. Steinert VV, Bennek J. Unterschenkelfrakturen im Kindesalter. *Zentralbl Chir* 1966;91: 1387.
90. Schrock RD. Peroneal nerve palsy following derotation osteotomies for tibial torsion. *Clin Orthop* 1969;62:172.
91. Matsen FA III, Clawson DK. The deep posterior compartmental syndrome of the leg. *J Bone Joint Surg [Am]* 1975;57:34.
92. Karlstrom G, Lonnerholm T, Olerud S. Cavus deformity of the foot after fracture of the tibial shaft. *J Bone Joint Surg [Am]* 1975;57:893.

93. Whitesides TE Jr, Haney TC, Morimoto K, et al. Tissue pressure measurements as a determinant for the need of fasciotomy. Clin Orthop 1975;113:43.
94. Janzing HMJ, Boaos PLO. Routine monitoring of compartment pressures in patients with tibial fractures: beware of over treatment. *Injury* 2001;32:415–421.
95. Mars M, Hadley GP. Raised compartmental pressures in children: A basis for treatment: *Injury* 1998;24:183–185.
96. Dias LS. Ankle valgus in children with myelomeningocele. *Dev Med Child Neurol* 1978; 20:627.
97. Matsen FA III, Winquist RA, Krugmire RTS. Diagnosis and management of compartment syndromes. *J Bone Joint Surg [Am]* 1980;62:286–291.
98. Scully RE, Shannon JM, Dickerson JR. Factors involved in recovery from experimental skeletal ischemia in dogs. *Am J Pathol* 1961;39:721.
99. Harman JW, Guinn RP. The recovery of skeletal muscle fibers from acute ischemia as determined by histologic and chemical methods. *Am J Pathol* 1948;25:751.
100. Bohn WW, Durbin RA. Ipsilateral fractures of the femur and tibia in children and adolescents. *J Bone Joint Surg [Am]* 1991;73:429.
101. Swaan JW, Oppers VM. Crural fractures in children. *Arch Chir Neerl* 1971;23:259.
102. Bennek J, Steinert V. Knochenwachstam kindern. *Zentralbl Chir* 1966;91:633.
103. Smillie IS. *Injuries of the knee joint,* 2nd ed. Baltimore: Williams & Wilkins, 1951.
104. Knight JL. Genu recurvatum deformity secondary to partial proximal tibial epiphyseal arrest. *Am J Knee Surg* 1998;11:111–115.
105. Dunbar JS, Owen HF, Nogrady MB, et al. Obscure tibial fracture of infants—the toddler's fracture. *J Can Assoc Radiol* 1964;25:136.
106. DeBoeck K, van Eldere, DeVos P, et al. Radionuclide bone imaging in toddler's fracture. *Eur J Pediatr* 1991;150:166.
107. Tenebein M, Reed MH. The Toddler's fracture revisited. *Am J Emerg Med* 1990;8:208.
108. Oujhane K, Newman B, Oh KS, et al. Occult fractures in pre-school children. *Trauma* 1988;28:858.
109. Felman AH. Bicycle spoke fractures. *J Pediatr* 1973;82:302.
110. Mellick LB, Reesor K. Spiral tibial fractures of children: a commonly accidental spiral long bone fracture. *Am J Emerg Med* 1990;8:234.
111. Izant RJ, Rothman BF, Frankel V. Bicycle spoke injuries of the foot and ankle in children: an underestimated "minor" injury. *J Pediatr Surg* 1969;4:654.
112. Letts M, Vincent M. The "floating knee" in children. *J Bone Joint Surg [Br]* 1986;68: 442.
113. Drennan JC, Freehafer AA. Fractures of the lower extremities in paraplegic children. *Clin Orthop* 1971;77:211.
114. Freehafer AA, Mast WA. Lower extremity fractures in patients with spinal-cord injury. *J Bone Joint Surg [Am]* 1965;47:683.
115. Gillies CL, Hartung W. Fracture of the tibia in spina bifida vera. *Radiology* 1938;31: 621.
116. Soutter FE. Spina bifida and epiphyseal displacement. *J Bone Joint Surg [Br]* 1962;44: 106.
117. Golding C. Museum pages. III: spina bifida and epiphyseal displacement. *J Bone Joint Surg [Br]* 1960;42:387.
118. James CCM. Fractures of the lower limbs in spina bifida cystica: a survey of 44 fractures in 122 children. *Dev Med Child Neurol Suppl* 1970;22:88.
119. Robin G. Fracture in childhood paraplegia. *Paraplegia* 1966;3:165.
120. Parsch K, Rossak K. Die Pathologischen Frakturen Bei Spina Bifida. *Arch DeVecchi Anat Pat* 1968;53:165.
121. Gyepes MT, Newbern DH, Neuhauser EBD. Metaphyseal and physeal injuries in children with spina bifida and meningomyeloceles. *AJR* 1965;95:168.
122. Stern MB, Grant SS, Isaacson AS. Bilateral distal tibial and fibular epiphyseal separation associated with spina bifida. *Clin Orthop* 1967;50:191.
123. Kumar SJ, Lowell HR, Townsend P. Physeal, metaphyseal and diaphyseal injuries of the lower extremities in children with myelomeningocele. *J Pediatr Orthop* 1984;4:25.
124. Roberts SM, Vogt EC. Pseudofracture of the tibia. *J Bone Joint Surg* 1939;21:891.
125. Berkebile RD. Stress fracture of the tibia in children. *AJR* 1964;91:588.
126. Devas MB, Sweetman R. Stress fracture of the fibula. *J Bone Joint Surg [Br]* 1956;38: 818.
127. Engh CA, Robinson RA, Milgram J. Stress fractures in children. *J Trauma* 1970;10: 532.
128. Hartley JB. Fatigue fracture of the tibia. *Br J Surg* 1942;30:9.
129. Ingersoll CF. Ice skater's fracture. A form of fatigue fracture. *AJR* 1943;50:469.
130. Kozlowski K, Urbonaviciene A. Stress fracture of the fibula in the first few years of life (report of six cases). *Aust Radiol* 1996;40:261–263.
131. Matin P. The appearance of bone scans following fractures, including immediate and long-term studies. *J Nucl Med* 1979;20:1227.
132. Meurman KOA, Elfving S. Stress fracture in soldiers: a multifocal bone disorder. *Radiology* 1980;134:483.
133. Micheli LJ, Gerbino PG. Etiologic assessment of stress fractures of the lower extremity in young athletes. *Orthop Trans* 1980;4:1.
134. Prather JL, Nusynowitz ML, Snowdy HA, et al. Scintigraphic findings in stress fractures. *J Bone Joint Surg [Am]* 1977;59:869.
135. Roub LW, Gumerman LW, Hanley EN, et al. Bone stress: a radionuclide imaging perspective. *Radiology* 1979;132:431.
136. Savoca CJ. Stress fractures. A classification of the earliest radiographic signs. *Radiology* 1971;100:519.
137. Taunton JE, Clement DB, Webber D. Lower extremity stress fractures in athletes. *J Sports Med Phys Fitness* 1981;9:77.
138. Devas MB. Stress fractures in children. *J Bone Joint Surg [Br]* 1963;45:528.
139. Sawmiller S, Michener WM, Hartman JT. Stress fracture in childhood. *Cleveland Clin Q* 1965;32:119.
140. Burrows HJ. Fatigue fractures of the fibula. *J Bone Joint Surg [Br]* 1948;30:266.
141. Horev G, Korenreich L, Ziv N, et al. The enigma of stress fractures in the pediatric age: clarification or confusion through the new imaging modalities. *Pediatr Radiol* 1990; 20:469.
142. Elton RL. Stress reaction of bone in army trainees. *JAMA* 1968;204:314.
143. Johnson LC. Morphologic analysis. In: Frost HM, ed. *Pathology in bone biodynamics.* Boston: Little, Brown, 1963.
144. Griffiths AL. Fatigue fracture of the fibula in childhood. *Arch Dis Child* 1952;27:552.

DISTAL TIBIAL AND FIBULAR FRACTURES

R. Jay Cummings

INCIDENCE, PREVALENCE, AND DEMOGRAPHICS

Injuries to the distal tibial and fibular physes generally are reported to account for 25% to 38% of all physeal fractures (1). Peterson et al (2) reported that phalangeal physeal fractures were most common, followed by physeal injuries of the radius and ankle. In skeletally immature individuals, physeal ankle fractures are slightly more common than fractures of the tibial or fibular diaphysis (3).

Up to 58% of physeal ankle fractures occur during sports activities (4,5) and account for 10% to 40% of all injuries to skeletally immature athletes (6–8). Ankle fractures occur more commonly with basketball than any other sport (9). Recently popularized recreational activities such as inline skating (10) and motorized scooters (3) have been found to cause significant numbers of ankle injuries in skeletally immature individuals.

Physeal ankle fractures are more common in boys than in girls (11). Tibial physeal fractures most commonly occur between the ages of 8 and 15 years and fibular fractures between the ages of 8 and 14 years (11). Patients who sustain Salter-Harris I and II injuries of the distal tibia frequently have excessive external tibial torsion, and it has been theorized that such individuals may be predisposed to injury (12).

HISTORY

Although Foucher (13) reported the first pathologic study of these injuries in 1863, Poland's 1898 monograph (14) generally is recognized as the most extensive early study of physeal ankle fractures. He stated that in children ligaments are stronger than physeal cartilage; forces that result in ligament damage in adults cause fractures of the physes in children. In 1922, Ashhurst and Bromer (15) published a thorough review of the literature and the results of their own extensive investigations and described a classification of ankle injuries based on the mechanism of injury. This classification did not differentiate between ankle injuries in adults and those in children. Bishop (16) in 1932 classified 300 ankle fractures according to Ashhurst and Bromer's system; 33 fractures were physeal injuries, and the grouping of these injuries according to mechanism of injury represents one of the first attempts to classify physeal ankle injuries.

Aitken's (17) study of 21 physeal ankle injuries in 1936 is one of the first to attempt to determine the results of treatment of these injuries; he also outlined an anatomic classification. Only one of his patients (5%) had a deformity after fracture, in contrast to findings by McFarland (18), who in 1932 reported deformities in 40% of a larger series of patients. In 1955, Caruthers and Crenshaw (19) reported 54 physeal ankle fractures, which were classified according to their modification of Ashhurst and Bromer's system. They confirmed that growth-related deformities were frequent after adduction (Salter-Harris type III and IV injuries) fractures and infrequent after fractures caused by external rotation, abduction, and plantarflexion (Salter-Harris type II injuries). Spiegel et al (11), in a 1978 review of 237 physeal ankle fractures, reported a high rate of growth abnormalities after Salter-Harris type III and IV injuries but also found complications in 11 (16.7%) of 66 patients with Salter-Harris type II fractures. Most of these patients had only mild shortening, but 6 had angular deformities that did not correct with growth. Based on the results of 65 physeal ankle fractures, Kling et al (20) concluded in 1984 that the frequency of growth-related deformities could be reduced by open reduction and internal fixation of Salter-Harris III and IV fractures.

A separate group of physeal ankle fractures occurring in adolescents, known as transitional fractures, has been identified. The fractures included in this group are juvenile Tillaux and triplane fractures described by Kleiger and Mankin (21), Marmor (22), Cooperman et al (23), Karrholm et al (24), and Denton and Fischer (25). Recently, two new types of transitional fractures have been identified: the adolescent pilon fracture described by Letts et al (26) and the incisural fracture described by Cummings and Hahn (27).

PRINCIPLES OF MANAGEMENT

Mechanism of Injury and Classification

Classifications of ankle fractures are of two broad types: anatomic (11,17,28–30) and mechanism-of-injury (15,16,31). Anatomic classifications divide fractures into groups based on the parts of the epiphyses or metaphyses that make up the fracture fragments. Mechanism-of-injury classifications are based on the nature of the force that creates the fractures and often include the position of the foot at the time the force is applied. Most mechanism-of-injury classifications include the anatomic type of injury produced by a particular mechanism.

Anatomic classifications (Fig. 26-1) are effective for rapid communication because most have few groups without multiword titles that require visualization of movements that sometimes seem incompatible with the position of the foot on the ground. Because they are applicable to all physes, anatomic classifications are used more frequently and are easier to recall than mechanism-of-injury classifications. Mechanism-of-injury classifications are considered by some to be more precise because they reflect not only the anatomic fracture pattern but also the position of the fragments in relation to each other. This increased precision, however, may result in less rapid and possibly more confusing communication.

The prognoses for growth and deformity have been predicted on the basis of both types of classification (32–34). A theoretical advantage of mechanism-of-injury classifications is that identification of the force producing the injury might give even more information about the possible development of growth arrest than anatomic classifications. For example, a Salter-Harris type III or IV fracture of the tibia produced by a shearing or crushing force (Fig. 26-2) might be more likely to result in growth arrest than a similar injury produced by an avulsion force. However, it is difficult to establish that one type of classification is superior

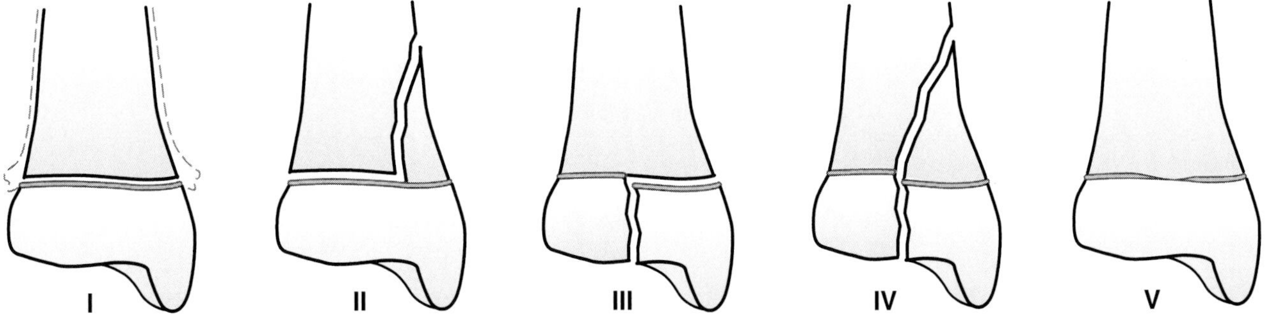

FIGURE 26-1 Salter-Harris anatomic classification as applied to injuries of the distal tibial epiphysis.

to the other in this regard because of the relatively small numbers of patients reported, the varying ages of patients in most series, and questions about the reproducibility of various classifications.

Both anatomic and mechanism-of-injury classifications can provide information useful for determining appropriate treatment. An important benefit of mechanism-of-injury classifications (Table 26-1) is that they provide clues that may be helpful in planning closed reduction: the mechanism of injury is simply reversed to reduce the fracture. Surgeons who rely on anatomic classifications usually attempt to obtain reduction by returning the displaced fragments directly to their proper anatomic locations.

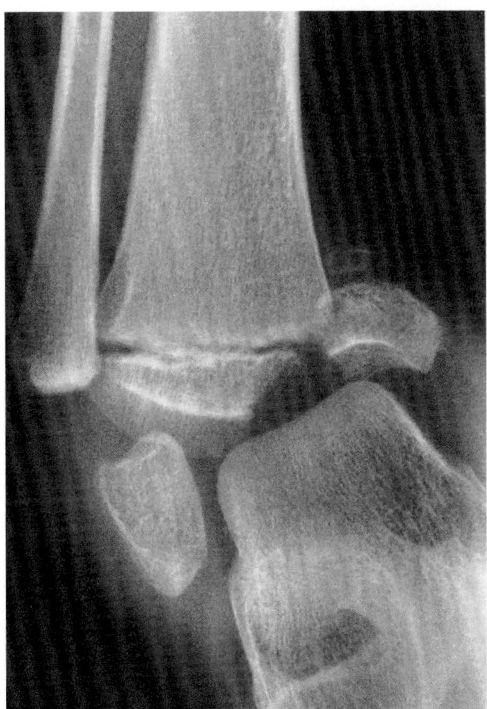

FIGURE 26-2 Comminuted Salter-Harris type IV fracture of the distal tibia and displaced Salter-Harris type I fracture of the distal fibula produced by an inversion (shearing) mechanism in a 10-year-old girl.

Any classification system that cannot be easily remembered and reproducibly applied will ultimately prove to be less than useful. Thomsen et al (35) studied the reproducibility of the Lauge-Hansen (mechanism-of-injury) and Weber (anatomic) classifications in a series of ankle fractures in adults. After all investigators in the study had received a tutorial on both systems and their application, they were asked to classify 94 fractures. On the first attempt, only the Weber classification produced an acceptable level of interobserver agreement. On a second attempt, the Weber classification and most of the Lauge-Hansen classification achieved an acceptable level of interobserver agreement. These investigators concluded that all fracture classification systems should have demonstrably acceptable interobserver agreement rates before they are adopted. The same argument was made even more forcefully in an editorial by Burstein (36). Vahvanen and Aalto (37) compared their ability to classify 310 ankle fractures in children with the Weber, Lauge-Hansen, and Salter-Harris classifications. They found that they were "largely unsuccessful" using the Weber and Lauge-Hansen classifications but could easily classify the fractures using the Salter-Harris system.

The most widely accepted mechanism-of-injury classification of ankle fractures in children is that described by Dias and Tachdjian (Fig. 26-3) (38), who modified the Lauge-Hansen classification based on their review of 71 physeal ankle fractures. Their original classification (1978) consisted of four types in which the first word refers to the position of the foot at the time of injury and the second word refers to the force that produces the injury.

Four other types, axial compression, juvenile Tillaux, triplane, and other physeal injuries, were subsequently added (39). Although these are designated differently, the first three have identifiable mechanisms of injury. Axial compression injury describes the mechanism of injury but not the position of the foot. Juvenile Tillaux and triplane fractures are believed to be caused by external rotation. As mentioned earlier, juvenile Tillaux and triplane fractures belong to a group of fractures known as transitional fractures. The incisural fracture, which recently has been added to this group, also is believed to be caused by external rotation. The final category, other physeal

TABLE 26-1 **Representative Mechanism of Injury Classifications**

	Applied Force						
Ashhurst-Bromer (adult) External rotation	Abduction	Adduction	–	Compression	–		
Carothers-Crenshaw (child) External rotation	Abduction	Adduction	Plantarflexion	Compression	–		
Lauge-Hansen (adult) Supination Eversion (external rotation)	Pronation Abduction	Supination Adduction	–	– Compression	Pronation Eversion (external rotation)		
Dias-Tachdjian (child) Supination External rotation	Pronation (eversion abduction) External rotation	Supination Inversion (adduction)	Supination Plantarflexion	Axial compression		Juvenile tillaux	Triplane

Lauge-Hansen pronation: external rotation of foot, abduction of hindfoot, and eversion of forefoot. Lauge-Hansen supination: external rotation of foot, adduction of hindfoot, and inversion of forefoot.

injuries, includes diverse injuries, many of which have no specific mechanism of injury.

Classification of Ankle Fracture in Children (Dias-Tachdjian)

Supination–Inversion. In grade I the adduction or inversion force avulses the distal fibular epiphysis (Salter-Harris type I or II fracture). Occasionally, the fracture is transepiphyseal; rarely, the lateral ligaments fail. In grade II (Fig. 26-4), further inversion produces a tibial fracture, usually a Salter-Harris type III or IV and, rarely, a Salter-Harris type I or II injury, or the fracture passes through the medial malleolus below the physis (Fig. 26-5).

Supination–Plantarflexion. The plantarflexion force displaces the epiphysis directly posteriorly, resulting in a Salter-Harris type I or II fracture. Fibular fractures were not reported with

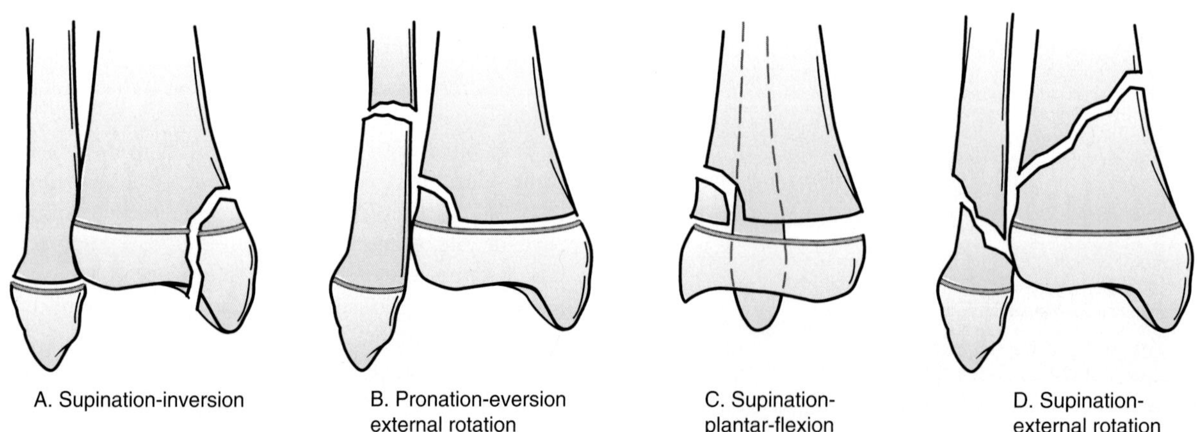

FIGURE 26-3 Dias-Tachdjian classification of physeal injuries of the distal tibia and fibula.

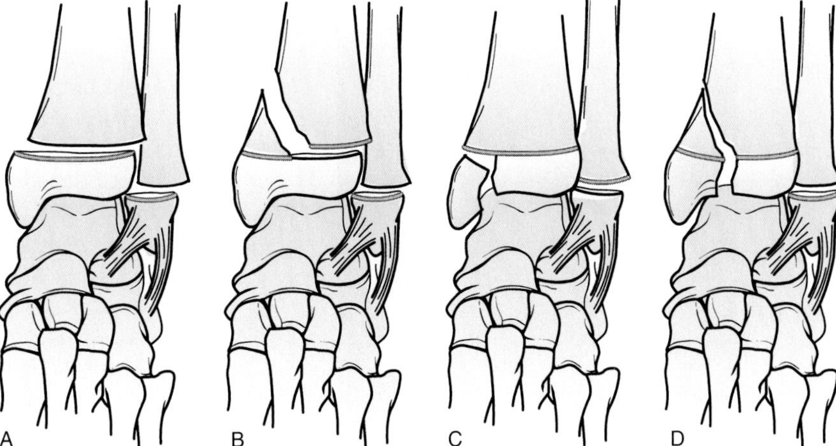

FIGURE 26-4 Variants of grade II supination–inversion injuries (Dias-Tachdjian classification). **A.** Salter-Harris I fracture of the distal tibia and fibula. **B.** Salter-Harris I fracture of the fibula, Salter-Harris II tibial fracture. **C.** Salter-Harris I fibular fracture, Salter-Harris III tibial fracture. **D.** Salter-Harris I fibular fracture, Salter-Harris IV tibial fracture.

this mechanism. The tibial fracture usually is difficult to see on anteroposterior x-rays (Fig. 26-6).

Supination–External Rotation. In grade I the external rotation force results in a Salter-Harris type II fracture of the distal tibia (Fig. 26-7). The distal fragment is displaced posteriorly, as in a supination–plantarflexion injury, but the Thurston-Holland fragment is visible on an anteroposterior x-ray, with the fracture line extending proximally and medially. Occasionally, the distal tibial epiphysis is rotated but not displaced. In grade II, with further external rotation, a spiral fracture of the fibula is produced, running from anteroinferior to posterosuperior (Fig. 26-8).

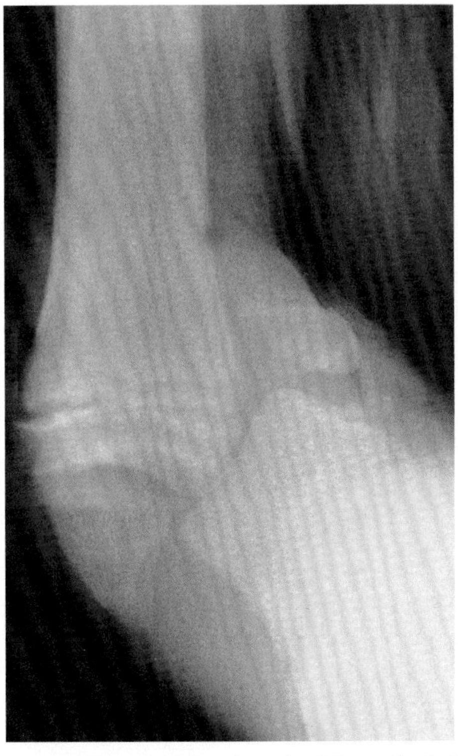

FIGURE 26-5 Severe supination–inversion injury with displaced fracture of the medial malleolus distal to the physis of the tibia.

Pronation–Eversion–External Rotation. A Salter-Harris type I or II fracture of the distal tibia occurs simultaneously with a transverse fibular fracture. The distal tibial fragment is displaced laterally, and the Thurston-Holland fragment, when present, is lateral or posterolateral (Fig. 26-9). Less frequently, a transepiphyseal fracture occurs through the medial malleolus (Salter-

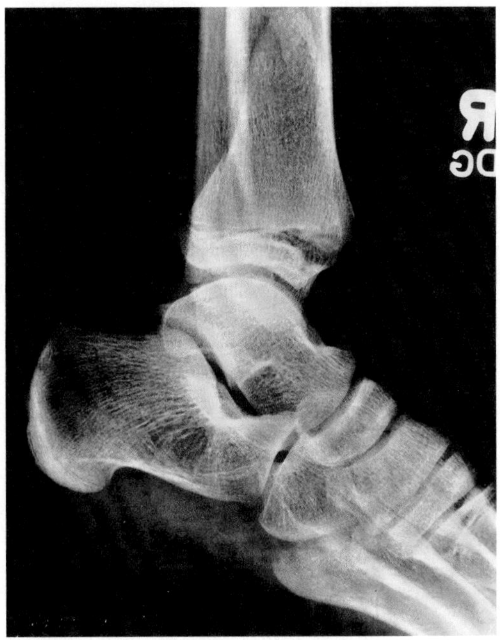

FIGURE 26-6 Lateral view of a supination plantarflexion injury.

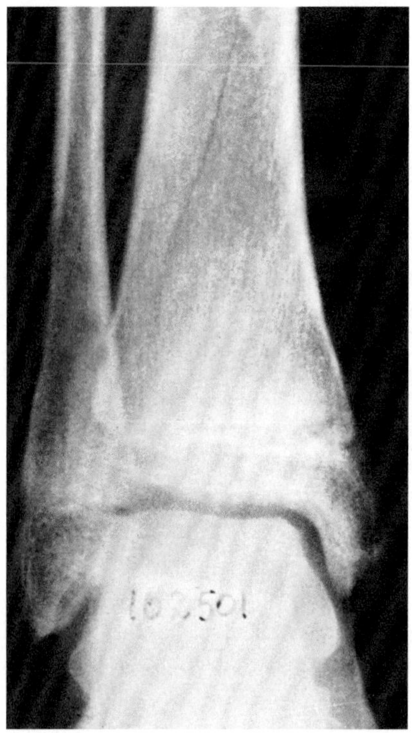

FIGURE 26-7 Stage I supination–external rotation injury in a 10-year-old child; the Salter-Harris type II fracture begins laterally.

Harris type II). Such injuries may be associated with diastasis of the ankle joint, which is uncommon in children.

Axial Compression. Axial compression is a Salter-Harris type V injury of the distal tibial physis. Initial x-rays usually show no abnormality, and the diagnosis is established when growth arrest is demonstrated on follow-up x-rays.

Transitional Fractures

Because the distal tibial physis closes in an asymmetric pattern over a period of about 18 months, injuries sustained during this period can produce fracture patterns that are not seen in younger children with completely open physes (40). This group of fractures has been labeled transitional fractures because they occur during the transition from a skeletally immature ankle to a skeletally mature ankle.

Juvenile Tillaux Fracture

The juvenile Tillaux facture is a Salter-Harris type III fracture involving the anterolateral distal tibia. The portion of the physis not involved in the fracture is closed (Fig. 26-10).

Triplane Fracture

The triplane fracture has the appearance of a Salter-Harris type III fracture on an anteroposterior x-ray and of a Salter-Harris type II fracture on a lateral x-ray (Fig. 26-11). Classification of juvenile Tillaux and triplane fractures is even more confusing

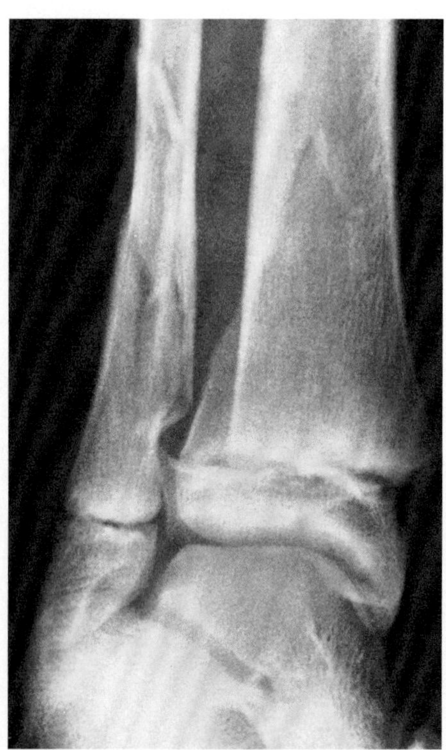

A

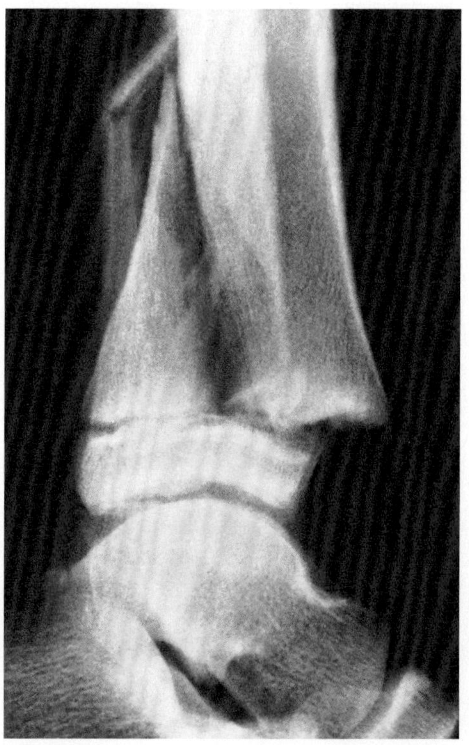

B

FIGURE 26-8 Stage II supination–external rotation injury. **A.** Oblique fibular fracture also is visible on anteroposterior view. **B.** Lateral view shows the posterior metaphyseal fragment and posterior displacement.

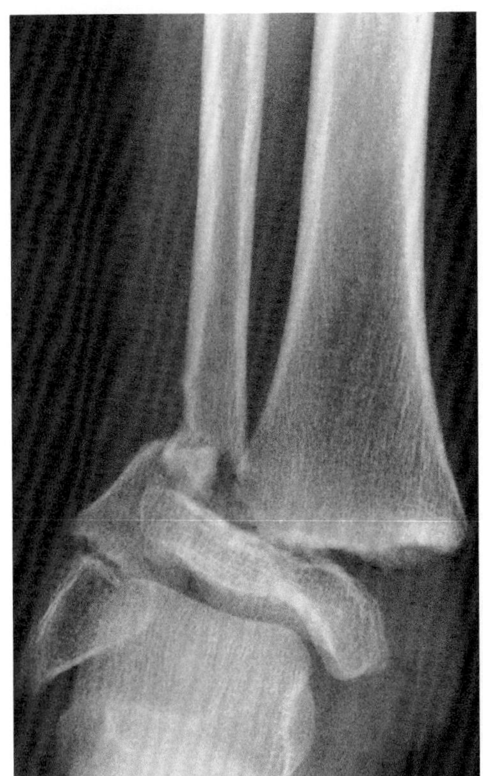

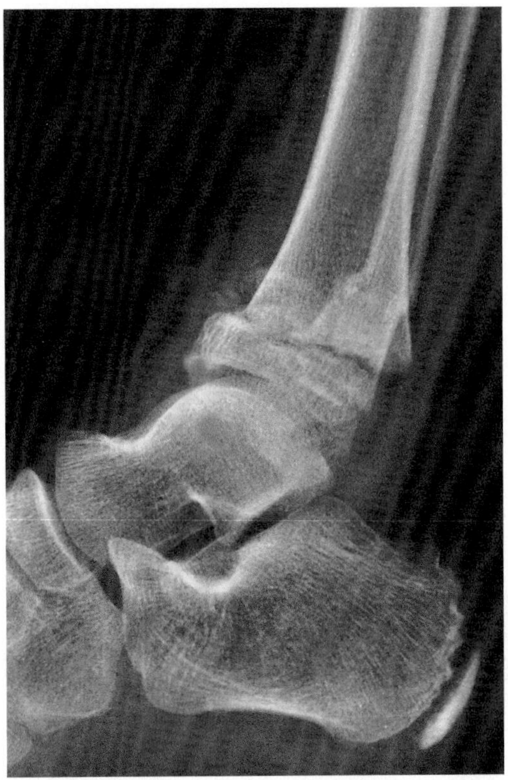

FIGURE 26-9 **A.** According to the Dias-Tachdjian classification, this injury in a 12-year-old boy would be considered a pronation–eversion–external rotation injury resulting in a Salter-Harris type II fracture of the distal tibia and a transverse fibular fracture. **B.** The anterior displacement of the epiphysis, visible on the lateral view, however, makes external rotation an unlikely component of the mechanism of injury; the mechanism is more likely pronation–dorsiflexion.

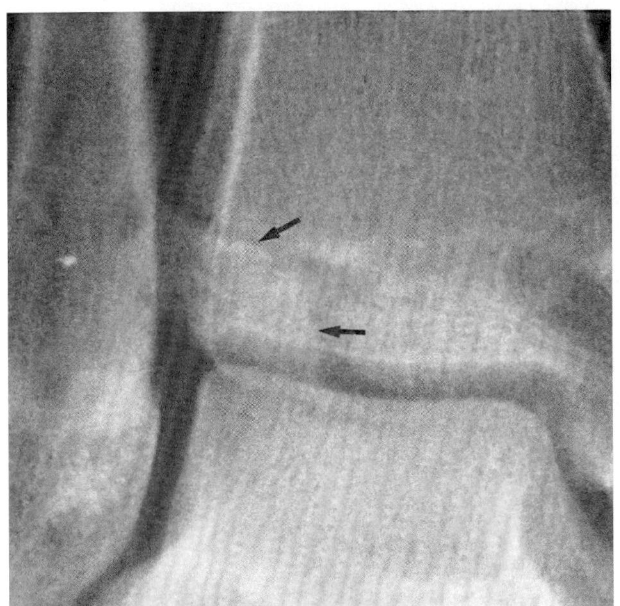

FIGURE 26-10 Salter-Harris type III fracture (juvenile Tillaux) (*arrows*) of the anterolateral portion of the distal tibial epiphysis in a 13-year-old girl.

than that of other distal tibial fractures. Advocates of mechanism-of-injury systems agree that most juvenile Tillaux and triplane fractures are caused by external rotation, but they disagree as to the position of the foot at the time of the injury (41–43). Some researchers (42) classify juvenile Tillaux fractures as stage I injuries, with further external rotation causing triplane fractures, and still further external rotation causing fibular fractures. Others emphasize the extent of physeal closure as the only determinant of fracture pattern (44).

Advocates of anatomic classifications are handicapped by the different anatomic configurations triplane fractures may exhibit on different x-ray projections, making tomography, CT scanning, or examination at open reduction necessary to determine fracture anatomy and number of fragments. Because these fractures occur near the end of growth, growth disturbance rarely is significant. Therefore, anatomic classification is more useful for descriptive purposes than for prognosis.

Adolescent Pilon Fractures

The pediatric pilon fracture (26) is defined as "any fracture of the tibial plafond with articular and physeal involvement, variable talar and fibular involvement, variable comminution, and greater than 5 mm of displacement" (Fig. 26-12). After review-

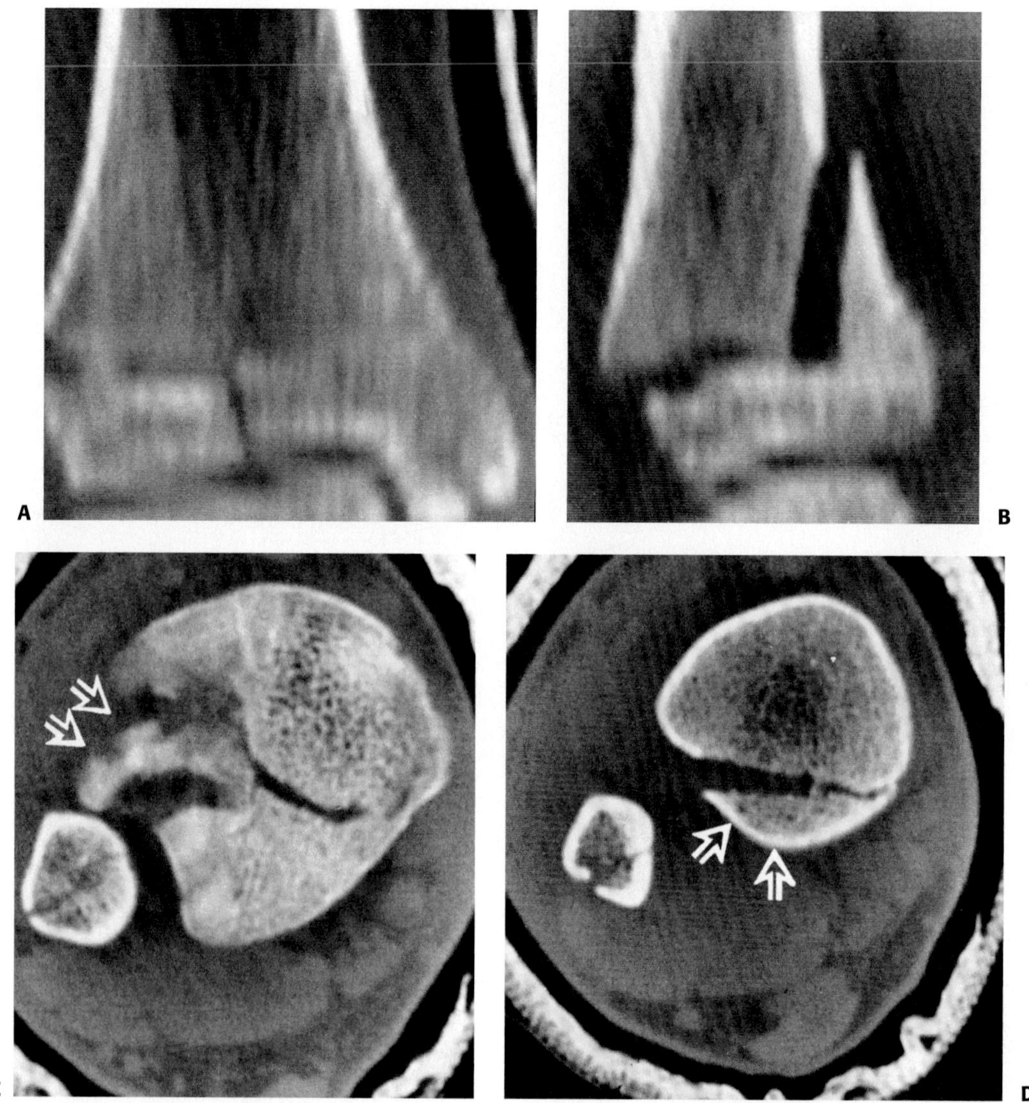

FIGURE 26-11 Computed tomography scanning of a three-part triplane fracture. **A.** Coronal cut shows lateral epiphyseal fragment. **B.** Sagittal cut shows posterior displacement of the epiphyseal–metaphyseal fragment. **C.** Horizontal cut through the epiphysis shows displacement of the lateral epiphyseal fragment (*arrows*). **D.** Horizontal cut through the metaphysis shows the fibular fracture and the displaced metaphyseal fragment (*arrows*).

ing seven patients with eight fractures treated at their institution, Letts et al (27) developed a three-part classification. Type I fractures have minimal comminution and no physeal displacement. Type II fractures have marked comminution and less than 5 mm of physeal displacement. Type III fractures have marked comminution and more than 5 mm of physeal displacement. Because of the small number of patients in their study, it is not possible to draw conclusions as to preferred treatment or expected outcomes based on their classification.

Incisural Fractures

Incisural fractures are fractures that on anteroposterior and mortise views appear to be Tillaux fractures, with the fractured piece appearing smaller than usual and essentially nondisplaced (Fig. 26-13). On CT scan the fracture line does not extend through the anterior cortex, as is seen in a typical Tillaux fracture (Fig. 26-14). It appears, therefore, that the fragment is not the result of avulsion by the anterior tibiofibular ligament, the accepted mechanism of injury for a Tillaux fracture, but rather that the fragment is avulsed by the intraosseous ligament and represents the pediatric equivalent of an adult diastasis injury.

Other Physeal Injuries

The group referred to as other physeal injuries are the fractures that do not fit into any of the other seven types (such as injuries to the perichondral ring and stress fractures) (Fig. 26-15).

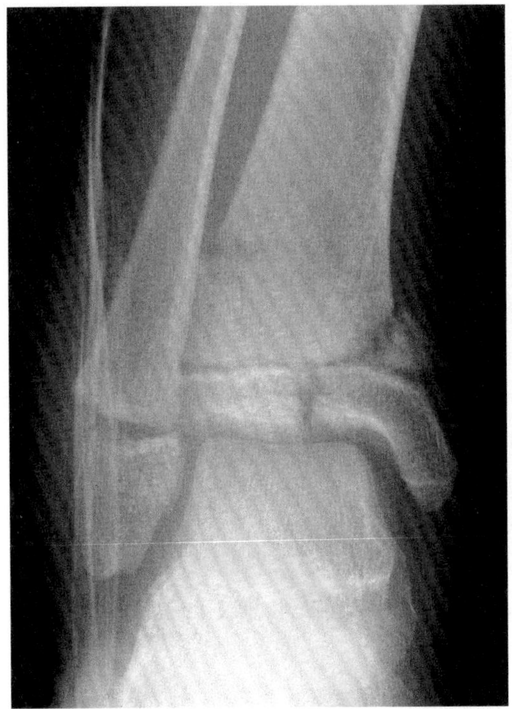

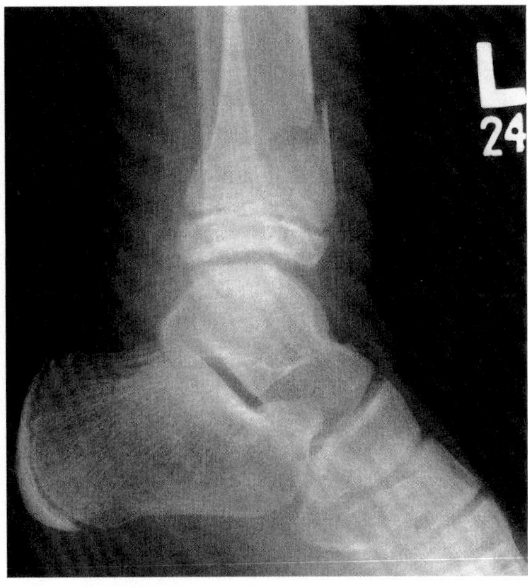

FIGURE 26-12 Anterior posterior and lateral x-rays of an adolescent pilon fracture.

Signs and Symptoms

Patients with significantly displaced fractures have severe pain and obvious deformity. The position of the foot relative to the leg may provide important information about the mechanism of injury (Fig. 26-16) and should be considered in planning reduction. The status of the skin, pulses, and sensory and motor function should be determined and recorded. Tenderness, swelling, and deformity in the ipsilateral leg and foot should be noted. Jarvis and Miyanji (45) reported six patients with ipsilateral tibial shaft and triplane fractures. The triplane fracture initially was overlooked in two patients (45). Navascues et al (46) reported four patients who developed premature closure of their distal tibial physes after diaphyseal fractures of the tibia that had no evidence of physeal injury. It is therefore important in patients with tibial shaft fractures to carefully evaluate the ipsilateral ankle clinically and by x-ray.

Diagnosis

Imaging Studies

Patients with nondisplaced or minimally displaced ankle fractures often have no deformity, minimal swelling, and moderate pain. Because of their benign clinical appearance, such fractures may be easily missed if x-rays are not obtained. Petit et al (47) studied 2,470 children in whom x-rays were obtained in pediatric emergency rooms. They found that the rate of abnormal x-ray findings for ankle injuries was only 9%. Because all physicians have an obligation to try to minimize unnecessary x-rays, both to avoid unnecessary irradiation of patients and for cost containment, objective criteria for determining when ankle x-rays are indicated when evaluating traumatized ankles would be useful. Guidelines known as the Ottawa Ankle Rules have been established for adults to try to determine which injuries require x-rays (34). The indications for x-ray according to the guidelines are complaints of pain near a malleolus with either inability to bear weight or tenderness to palpation at the malleolus. Chande (48) prospectively studied 71 children with acute ankle injuries to determine if these guidelines could be applied to pediatric patients with ankle injuries. He determined that if x-rays were obtained only in children who had tenderness over the malleoli and an inability to bear weight, a 25% reduction in x-ray examinations could be achieved without missing any fractures. Chande's conclusions were supported by a much larger, recent study by Karpas et al (49). In a study of a similar number of children, however, Clark et al (50) found the sensitivity of the Ottawa Ankle Rules to be only 83% in children.

For patients with obvious deformities, anteroposterior and lateral x-rays centered over the ankle may provide sufficient information to plan treatment. Although obtaining views of the joint above and below is recommended for most fractures, obtaining a film centered over the mid-tibia to include the knee and ankle joints on the x-ray significantly decreases the quality of ankle views and is not recommended.

For patients without obvious deformities, a high-quality mortise view of the ankle is essential in addition to anteroposterior and lateral views. On a standard anteroposterior view, the lateral portion of the distal tibial physis usually is partially obscured by the distal fibula. The vertical component of a triplane or Tillaux fracture can be hidden behind the overlying fibular

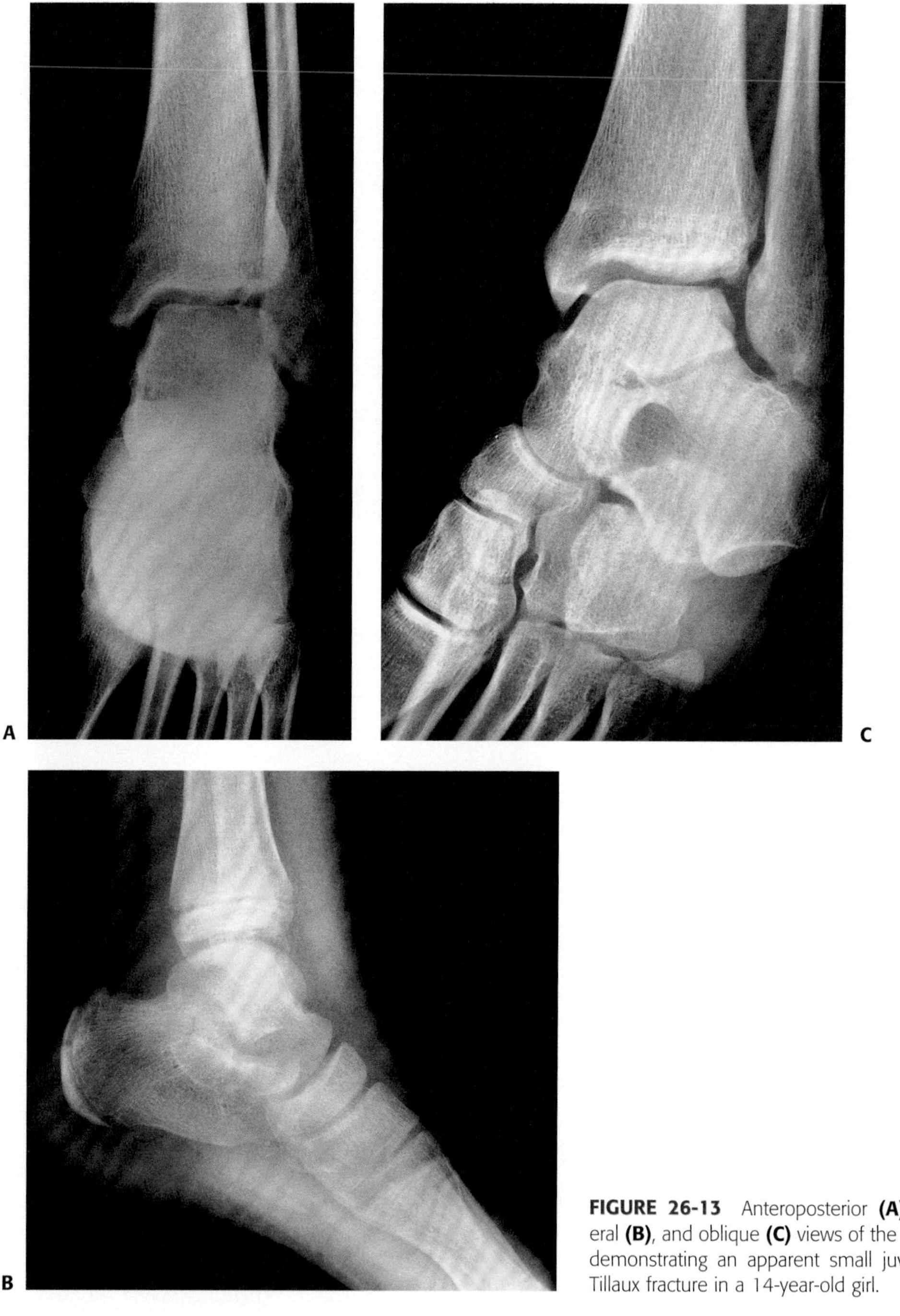

FIGURE 26-13 Anteroposterior **(A)**, lateral **(B)**, and oblique **(C)** views of the ankle demonstrating an apparent small juvenile Tillaux fracture in a 14-year-old girl.

cortical shadow (51). A study by Vangsness et al (52) found that diagnostic accuracy was essentially equal when using anteroposterior, lateral, and mortise views compared with using only mortise and lateral views. Therefore, if only two views are to be obtained, the anteroposterior view can be omitted and lateral and mortise views obtained.

Haraguchi et al (53) described two special views designed to detect avulsion fractures from the lateral malleolus that are not visible on routine views and to distinguish whether they represent avulsions of the anterior tibiofibular ligament or the calcaneofibular ligament attachments. The anterior tibiofibular ligament view is made by positioning the foot in 45 degrees of plantar flexion and elevating the medial border of the foot 15 degrees. The calcaneofibular ligament view is obtained by rotating the leg 45 degrees inward. Stress views occasionally may be needed to rule out ligamentous instability (Fig. 26-17). Stress

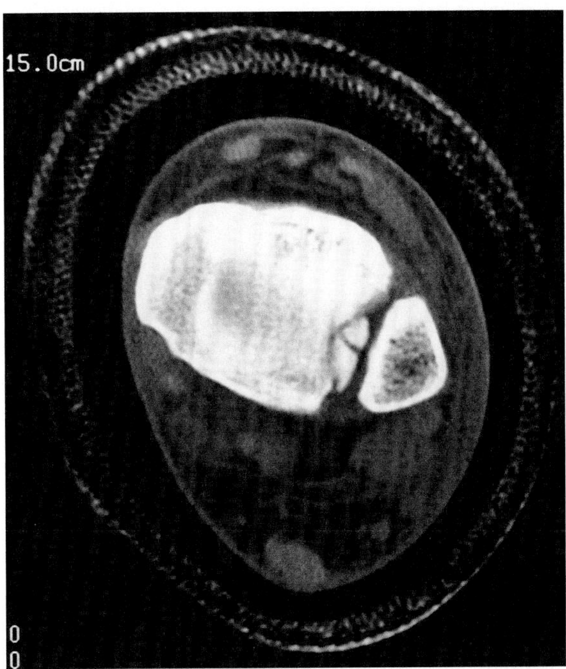

FIGURE 26-14 Computed tomography scan at the level of the tibiotalar joint demonstrates that the fracture fragment does not include the attachment of the anterior inferior tibiofibular ligament.

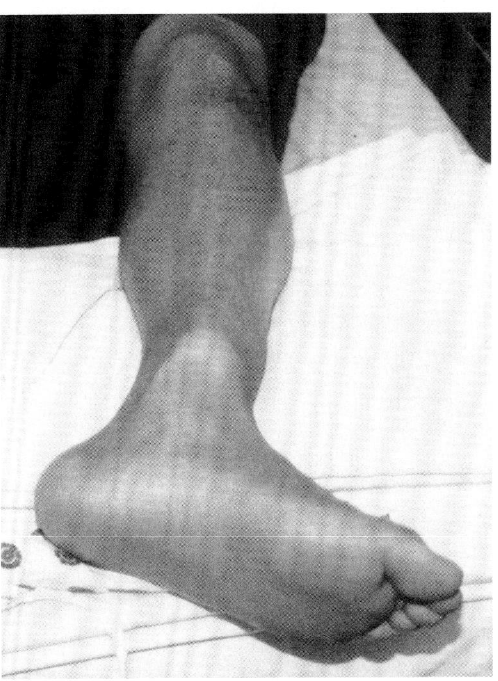

FIGURE 26-16 Severe clinical deformity in a 14-year-old boy with an ankle fracture. It is obvious without x-rays that internal rotation will be needed to reduce this fracture.

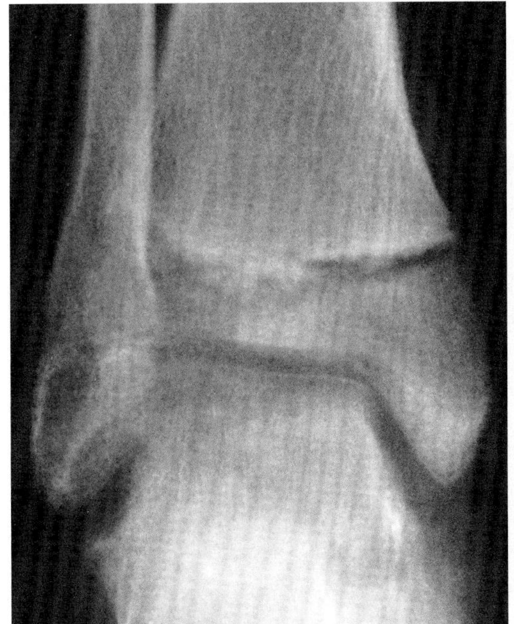

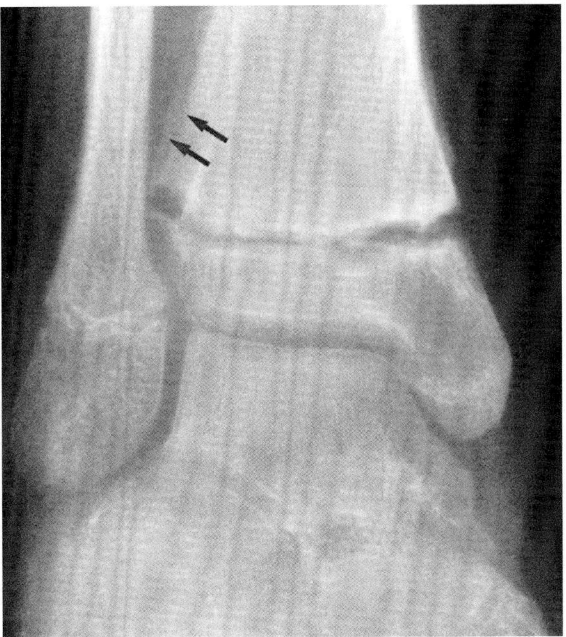

FIGURE 26-15 Stress fracture of the distal tibia in normal 13-year-old child who complained of pain in his ankle after running. **A.** Initial x-rays were interpreted as being normal, although abnormal widening of the tibial physis was present. The ankle was immobilized for 10 days. **B.** Six weeks later, pain persisted and x-rays showed further widening and irregularity of the physis, with a faint periosteal new bone formation (*arrows*) around the distal tibial metaphysis.

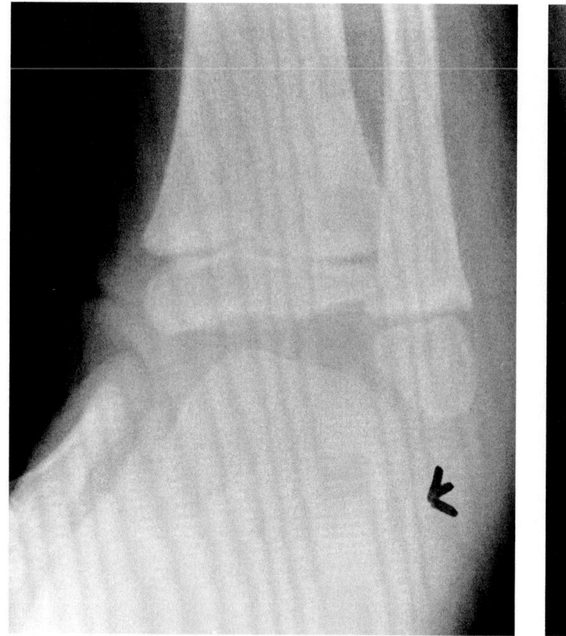

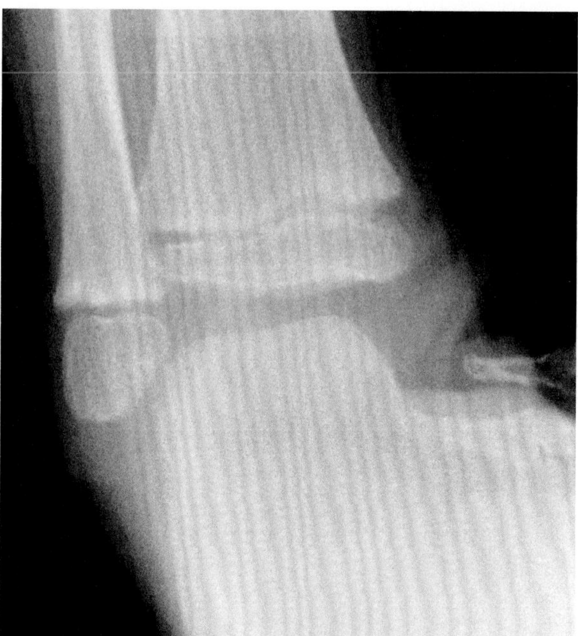

FIGURE 26-17 **A.** Stress x-ray showing abnormal varus tilt in a 5-year-old who had sustained a left ankle injury. Note the small avulsion fracture from the talus (*arrow*) and soft tissue swelling laterally. **B.** Comparative stress x-ray of the right ankle.

views may be considered to document a Salter-Harris type I fracture, but a patient with clinical signs of this fracture should be treated appropriately, regardless of stress view findings. Stress views may help document lack of motion at the fracture in an apparent nonunion (Fig. 26-18).

To aid in diagnosis of distal tibiofibular syndesmotic injury in children, Bozic et al (54) studied the age at which the x-ray appearance of the incisura fibularis, tibiofibular clear space, and tibiofibular overlap develop in children. They found that the incisura became detectable at a mean age of 8.2 years in girls and 11.2 years in boys. The mean age at which tibiofibular overlap appeared on the anteroposterior view was 5 years in

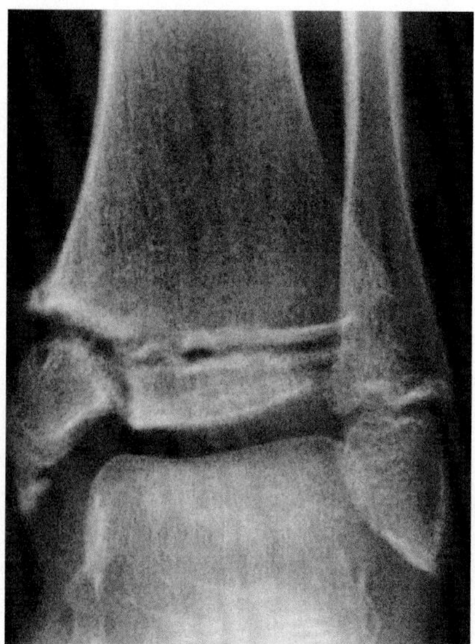

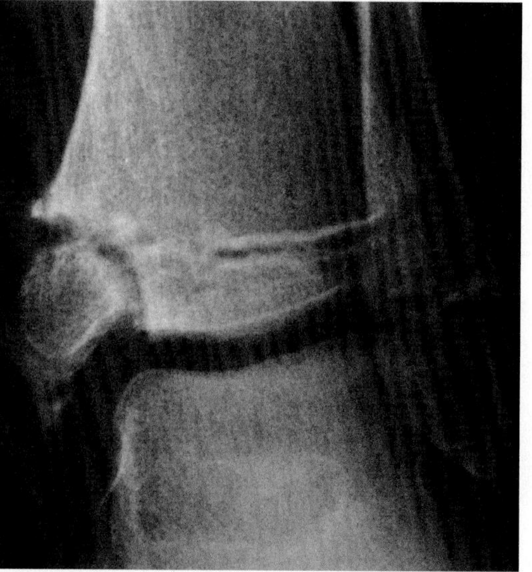

FIGURE 26-18 **A.** Anteroposterior x-ray of a 10-year-girl after 12 weeks of immobilization for an initially nondisplaced Salter-Harris type III fracture of the distal tibia. **B.** Stress view showing no motion at the fracture site with articular and physeal malunion.

both sexes; on the mortise view, it was 10 years in girls and 16 years in boys. The range of clear space measurements in normal children was 2 to 8 mm, with 23% of children having a clear space of more than 6 mm, a distance considered abnormal in adults.

Computed tomography (CT) is useful in the evaluation of intra-articular fractures, especially juvenile Tillaux and triplane fractures (Fig. 26-19) (55–57). Horn et al studied the accuracy of plain films and CT scans in a cadaver model. They found that plain films and CT scans were accurate within 1 mm 50% of the time. CT scans were more sensitive than plain films in detecting fractures with more than 2 mm of displacement (58). Cuts generally are made in the transverse plane. With thin cuts localized to the joint, it is possible to generate high-quality reconstructions that allow evaluation in the coronal and sagittal planes without repositioning the ankle. Three-dimensional CT reconstructions rarely add further useful information. Other indications for CT scanning are described in the discussion of treatment.

Magnetic resonance imaging (MRI) also may be useful for evaluating both intraarticular and extraarticular physeal ankle fractures. Smith et al (59) found that of four patients with acute (3 to 10 days) physeal injuries, MRI showed that three had more severe fractures than indicated on plain films (Fig. 26-20). Early MRI studies (3 to 17 weeks after injury) not only added information about the pattern of physeal disruption but also supplied early information about the possibility of growth abnormality.

Carey et al (60) obtained MRI studies on 14 patients with known or suspected physeal injuries. The MRI detected five radiographically occult fractures in the 14 patients, changed the Salter-Harris classification in 2 patients, and resulted in a change in treatment plan in 5 patients. Iwinska-Zelder et al (61) found that MRI changed the therapeutic management in 4 of 10 children with ankle fractures visible on plain x-rays. Seifert et al (62) evaluated 12 patients who sustained triplane fractures with both plain films and MRI and found that plain films missed rotational dislocations in 2 patients and two fractures were in-

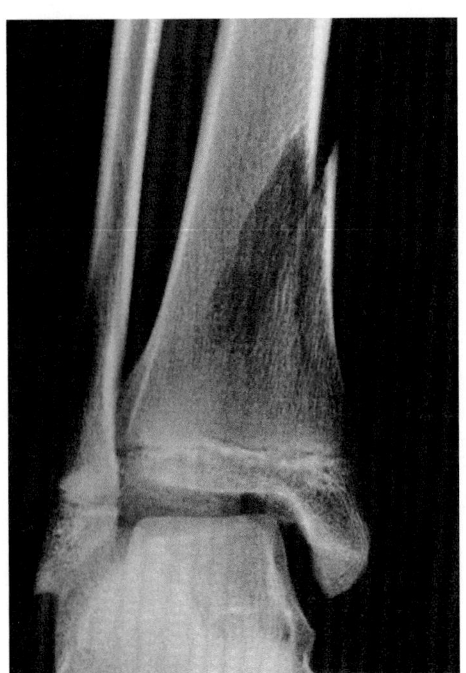

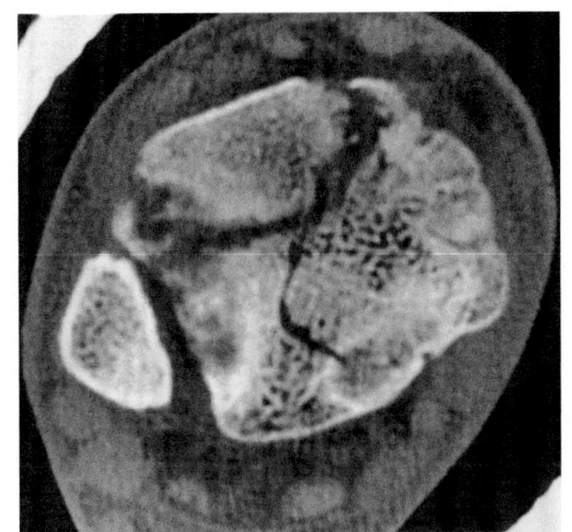

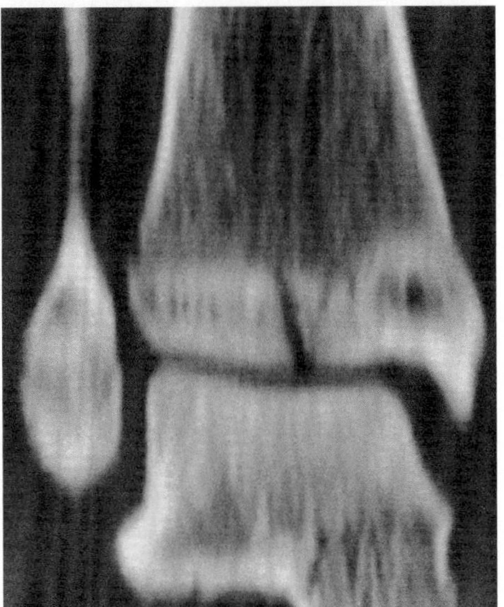

FIGURE 26-19 A. Anteroposterior view of a 13-year-old boy with a tibial fracture extending into the ankle joint. It is unclear on this view whether the metaphyseal fracture is a separate injury or part of the intra-articular fracture. **B.** Transverse CT scan a few millimeters above the ankle joint confirmed the triplane nature of this injury. **C.** Anteroposterior reconstruction from the CT scan shows 3 mm of displacement at the fracture site in the tibial epiphysis.

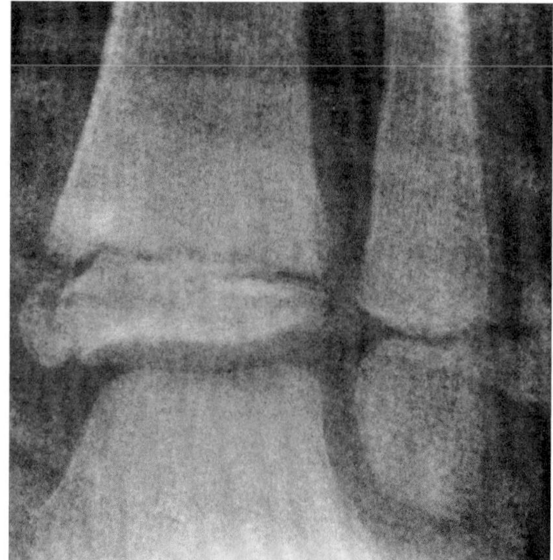

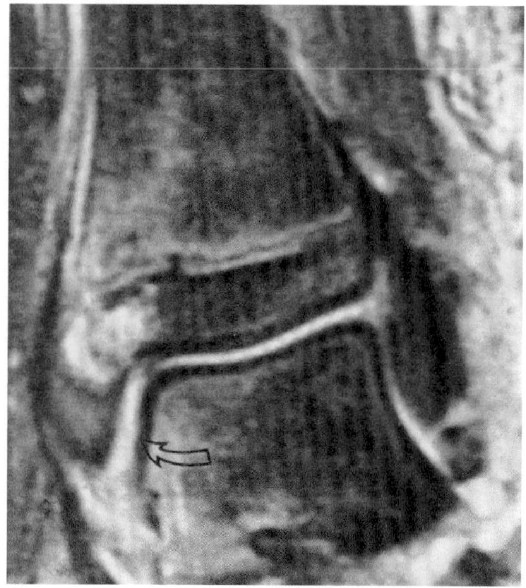

FIGURE 26-20 **A.** Follow-up x-ray of a 7-year-old boy 1 week after an initially nondisplaced Salter-Harris type III fracture from a supination–inversion injury of the distal tibia. **B.** Because of the incomplete ossification of this area and concern that the fracture might have displaced, magnetic resonance imaging was performed. Note that the distance between the medial malleolus and the talus is greater than the distance between the talus and the distal tibia or lateral malleolus, confirming displacement of the fracture.

correctly classified as to fracture type. On an average, plain films underestimated fracture displacement by 0.5 mm.

In a series of 29 patients, Petit et al (63) found only 1 patient in whom MRI revealed a diagnosis different from that made from plain films. More recently, Lohman et al (64) studied 29 children with a clinical diagnosis of lateral ligament injury and 31 patients with a clinical diagnosis of physeal ankle fracture with both plain films and MRI. Even though the false negative rate for plain films was 18%, in no case was treatment altered by the MRI findings, leading them to conclude that plain x-rays were still the diagnostic study of choice for pediatric ankle injuries (64). It would appear, therefore, that the usefulness of routine MRI evaluation of acute pediatric ankle fractures remains debatable.

MRI scans obtained 6 months or longer after fracture have been reported useful for mapping physeal bars (65,66). MRI also has been reported to be occasionally helpful in the identification of osteochondral injuries to the joint surfaces in children with ankle fractures (67).

Pitfalls in Diagnosis

Accessory ossification centers and normal anatomic variations may cause confusion in the interpretation of plain films of the ankle (Fig. 26-21). In a group of 100 children between the ages of 6 and 12 years, Powell (68) found accessory ossification centers on the medial side (os subtibiale) in 20% and on the lateral side (os subfibulare) in 1%. If they are asymptomatic on clinical examination, these ossification centers are of little concern, but tenderness localized to them may indicate an injury. Stress views to determine motion of the fragments or bone scanning occasionally may be considered if an injury to an accessory ossification center is suspected.

Clefts in the lateral side of the tibial epiphysis may simulate juvenile Tillaux fractures, and clefts in the medial side may simulate Salter-Harris type III fractures (69). The presence of these clefts on an x-ray of a child with an ankle injury may

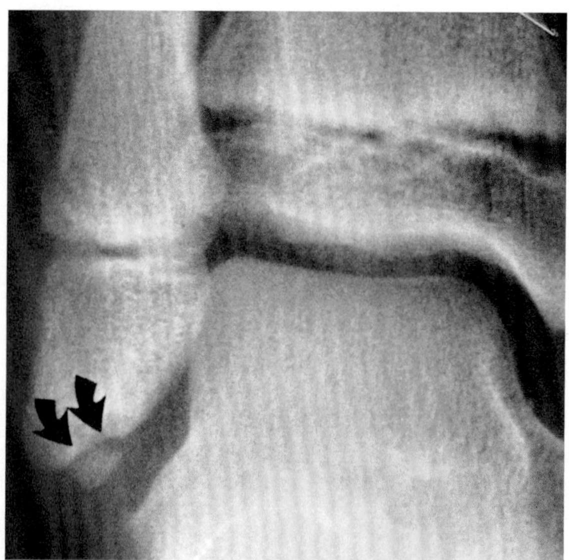

FIGURE 26-21 Secondary ossification center in the lateral malleolus (*arrows*) of a 10-year-old girl. Note the smooth border of the fibula and the ossification center. She also has a secondary ossification center in the medial malleolus.

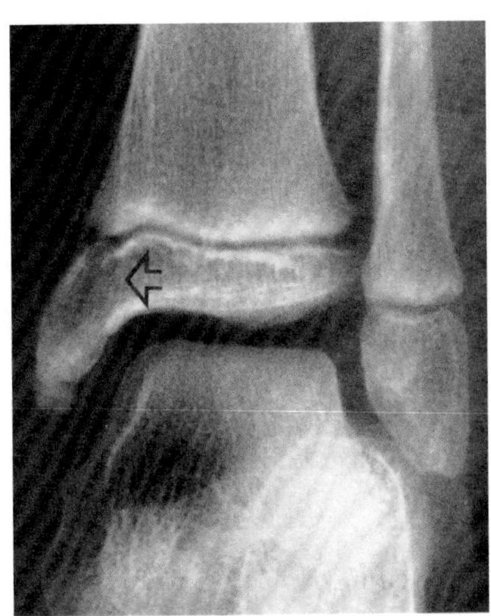

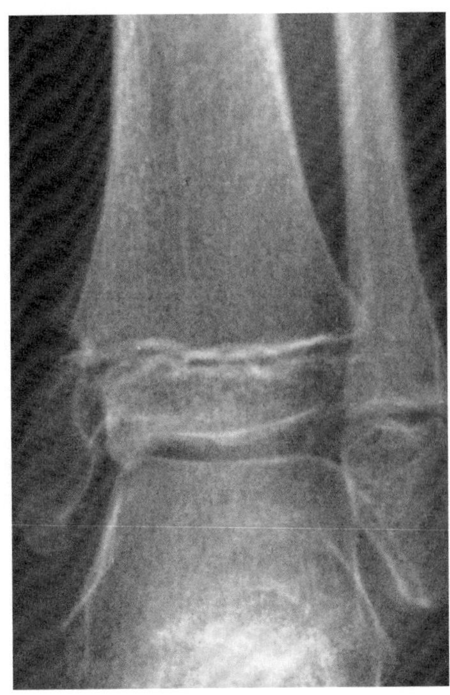

FIGURE 26-22 **A.** Mortise view of the ankle of a 10-year-old girl who had slight swelling and tenderness at the medial malleolus after an "ankle sprain." The ossicle at the tip of the medial malleolus was correctly identified as an os subtibiale. A subtle line extending from the medial physis to just distal to the medial tibial plafond (*arrow*) was believed to also be an anatomic variant. **B.** Four weeks after injury, soreness persisted and x-ray clearly demonstrated a displaced Salter-Harris type III fracture.

result in overtreatment if they are misdiagnosed as a fracture. Conversely, attributing a painful irregularity in these areas to anatomic variation may lead to undertreatment (Fig. 26-22). Other anatomic variations include a bump on the distal fibula that simulates a torus fracture and an apparent offset of the distal fibular epiphysis that simulates a fracture.

SURGICAL AND APPLIED ANATOMY

The ankle is the joint that most closely approximates a hinge joint. It is the articulation between the talus and the ankle mortise, which is a syndesmosis consisting of the distal tibial articular surface, the medial malleolus, and the distal fibula or lateral malleolus.

Ligamentous structures bind the distal tibia and fibula into the ankle mortise (Fig. 26-23). The anterior and posterior inferior tibiofibular ligaments course inferiorly from the anterior and posterior surfaces of the distal lateral tibia to the anterior and posterior surfaces of the lateral malleolus. The anterior ligament is important in the pathomechanics of transitional ankle fractures. Just anterior to the posteroinferior tibiofibular ligament is the broad, thick inferior transverse ligament, which extends down from the lateral malleolus along the posterior border of the articular surface of the tibia, almost to the medial malleolus. This ligament serves as a part of the articular surface for the talus. Between the anterior and posterior inferior tibiofibular ligaments, the tibia and fibula are bound by the interosseous ligament, which is continuous with the interosseous membrane above. This ligament may be important in the pathomechanics of incisural fractures.

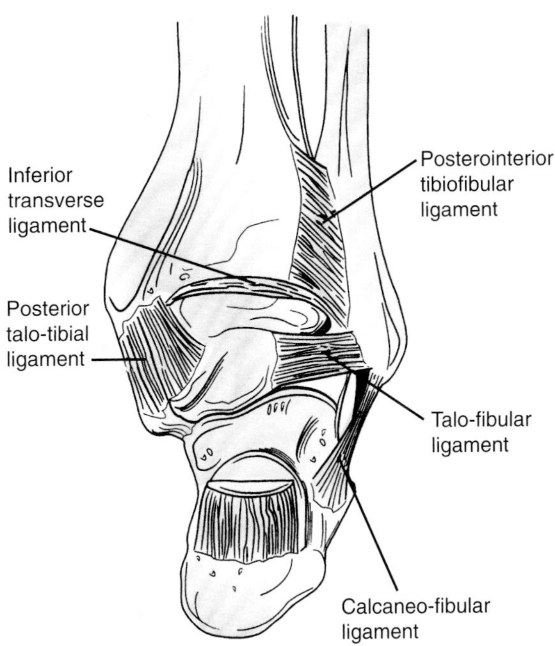

FIGURE 26-23 Posterior view of the distal tibia and fibula and the ligaments making up the ankle mortise.

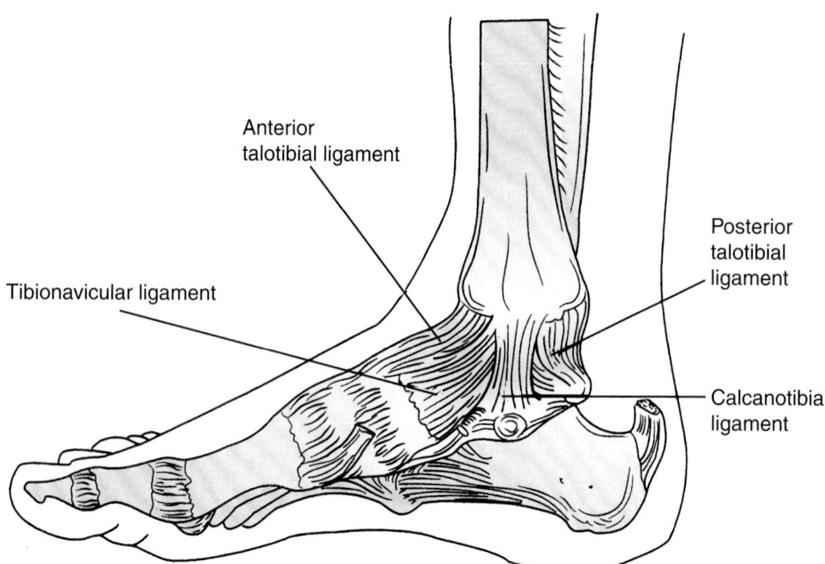

FIGURE 26-24 Medial view of the ankle demonstrating the components of the deltoid ligament.

On the medial side of the ankle, the talus is bound to the ankle mortise by the deltoid ligament (Fig. 26-24). This ligament arises from the medial malleolus and divides into superficial and deep layers. Three parts of the superficial layer are identified by their attachments: tibionavicular, calcaneotibial, and posterior talotibial ligaments. The deep layer is known as the anterior talotibial ligament, again reflecting its insertion and origin. On the lateral side, the anterior and posterior talofibular ligaments, with the calcaneofibular ligaments, make up the lateral collateral ligament (Fig. 26-25).

In children, all of the ligamentous structures that bind the medial and lateral malleoli to the talus and the distal tibial epiphysis to the distal fibular epiphysis are attached to the malleoli distal to the physes. Because the ligaments are stronger than the physes, physeal fractures are more common than ligamentous injuries in children. When they accompany distal tibial physeal injuries, displaced diaphyseal fibular fractures usually are associated with injuries to and displacement of the entire distal tibial epiphysis rather than with injuries to the ligaments, making diastasis of the ankle uncommon in children (Fig. 26-26).

The distal tibial ossification center generally appears at 6 to 24 months of age. Its malleolar extension begins to form around the age of 7 years and is mature or complete at the age of 10 years. The physis usually closes around the age of 15 years in girls and 17 years in boys. This process takes approximately 18 months and occurs first in the central part of the physis, extend-

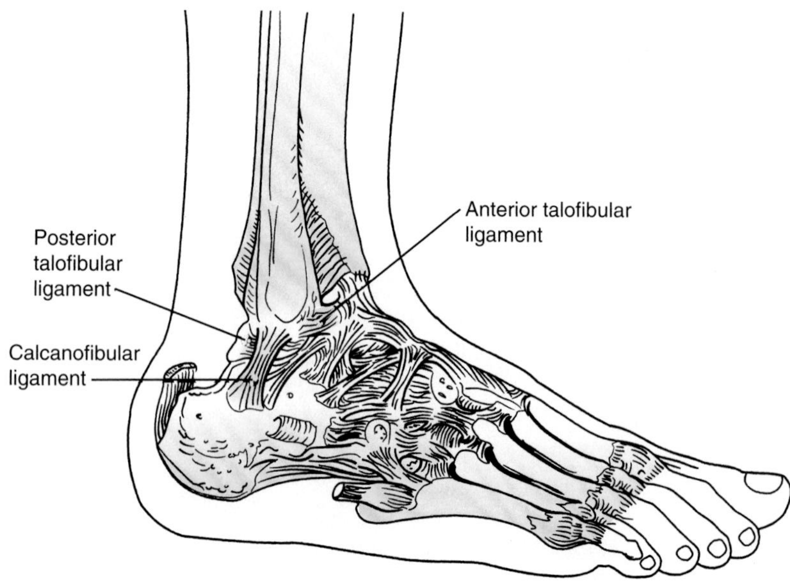

FIGURE 26-25 Lateral view of the ankle demonstrating the anterior and posterior talofibular ligaments and the calcaneofibular ligament.

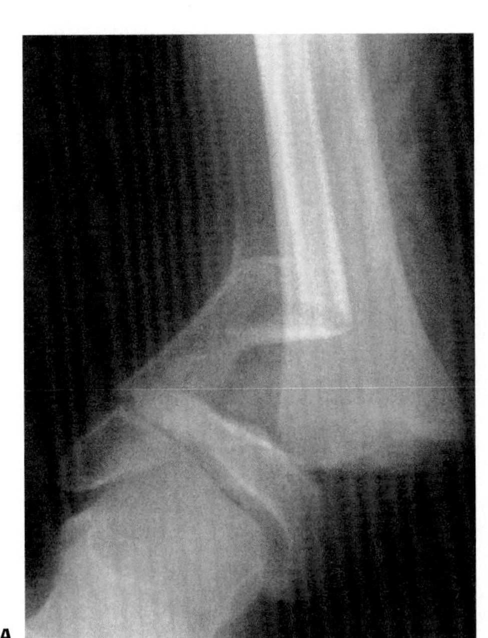

A

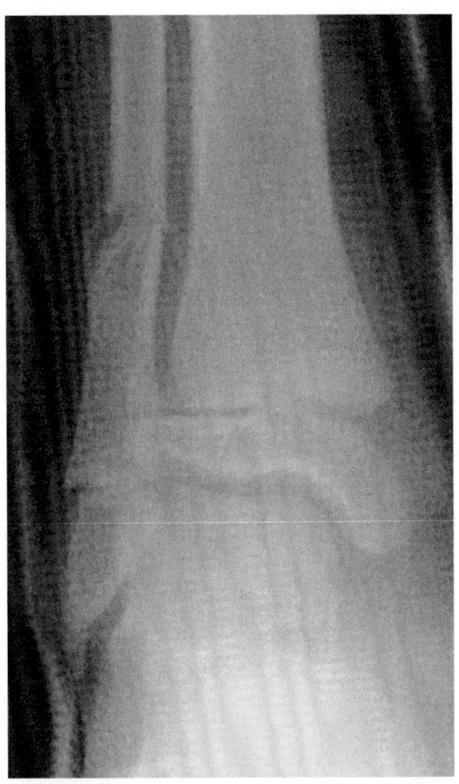

B

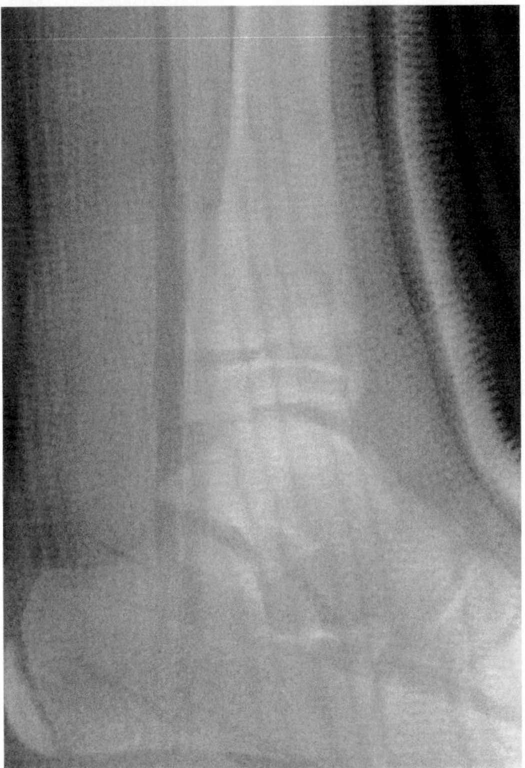

C

FIGURE 26-26 **A.** Pronation–external rotation injury resulting in a Salter-Harris type I fracture of the distal tibial physis. **B,C.** Anteroposterior and lateral x-rays demonstrate satisfactory closed reduction.

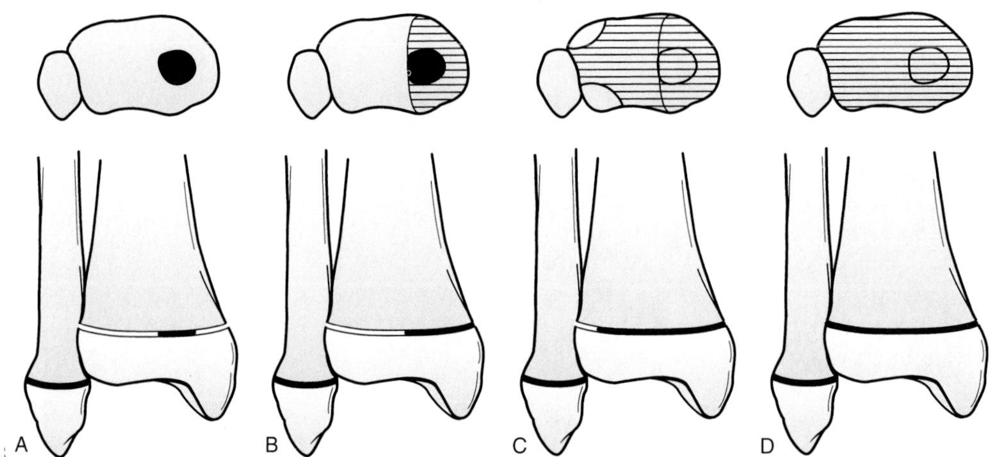

FIGURE 26-27 Closure of the distal tibial physis begins centrally **(A)**, and extends medially **(B)** and then laterally **(C)** before final closure **(D)**.

ing next to the medial side, and finally ending laterally. This asymmetric closure sequence is an important anatomic feature of the growing ankle and is responsible for certain fracture patterns in adolescents (Fig. 26-27).

The distal fibular ossification center appears around the age of 9 to 24 months. Its physis is located at the level of the ankle joint. Closure of this physis generally follows closure of the distal tibial physis by 12 to 24 months.

CURRENT TREATMENT OPTIONS: GENERAL PRINCIPLES

Appropriate treatment of ankle fractures in children depends on the location of the fracture, the degree of displacement, and the age of the child (Table 26-2). Nondisplaced fractures may be simply immobilized. Closed reduction and cast immobilization may be appropriate for displaced fractures; if the closed reduction cannot be maintained with casting, skeletal fixation is necessary. If closed reduction is not possible, open reduction is indicated, provided there is significant physeal or articular displacement, followed by internal fixation or cast immobilization.

The anatomic type of the fracture (usually defined by the Salter-Harris classification), the mechanism of injury, and the amount of displacement of the fragments are important considerations. When the articular surface is disrupted, the amount of articular step-off or separation must be measured. The neurovascular status of the limb or the status of the skin may require emergency treatment of the fracture and associated problems. The general health of the patient and the time since injury also must be considered.

TABLE 26-2 Current Treatment Options

	Advantages	Disadvantages
Short versus long cast (nondisplaced fractures)	Short casts result in less knee stiffness and quad weakness	Greater chance of subsequent displacement
Local anesthesia/sedation versus general anesthesia (closed reduction displaced fractures)	Local sedation may be more expeditious, less expensive	May increase risk of further damage to the physis
Minimally invasive versus traditional surgical exposure (open reduction displaced fractures)	Minimally invasive exposure leaves a smaller scar, possibly more rapid recovery	May compromise adequacy of restoration of the articular surface and realignment of the physeal line
Bioabsorbable versus metal internal fixation devices	Bioabsorbable pins do not require removal for later CT/MRI evaluations of the physis	May cause local inflammatory reaction and provide less secure fixation

Distal Tibial Physeal Fractures

Salter-Harris Type I and II Fractures

According to Dias and Tachdjian (38,39), Salter-Harris type I fractures of the distal tibia can be caused by any of four mechanisms: supination–inversion, supination–plantarflexion, supination–external rotation, or pronation–eversion–external rotation. Spiegel et al (11) reported that these fractures accounted for 15.2% of 237 ankle injuries in their series and occurred in children significantly younger (average age, 10.5 years) than those with other Salter-Harris types of fractures.

Salter-Harris type II fractures also can be caused by any of the four mechanisms of injury described by Dias and Tachdjian (38). In the series of Spiegel et al (11), Salter-Harris type II fractures were the most common injuries (44.8%).

The mechanism of injury for Salter-Harris I fractures is deduced primarily by the direction of displacement of the distal tibial epiphysis; for example, straight posterior displacement indicates a supination–plantarflexion mechanism. The type of associated fibular fracture also is indicative of the mechanism of injury; for example, a high, oblique, or transverse fibular fracture indicates a pronation–eversion–external injury, whereas a lower spiral fibular fracture indicates a supination–external rotation injury. Lovell (70), Broock and Greer (71), and Nevelos and Colton (72) reported unusual Salter-Harris type I fractures in which the distal tibial epiphysis was externally rotated 90 degrees without fracture of the fibula or displacement of the tibial epiphysis in any direction in the transverse plane.

In addition to the direction of displacement of the distal tibial epiphysis and the nature of any associated fibular fracture, the location of the Thurston-Holland fragment is helpful in determining the mechanism of injury for Salter-Harris II fractures. For example, a lateral fragment indicates a pronation-eversion-external rotation injury; a posteromedial fragment, a supination-external rotation injury; and a posterior fragment, a supination-plantar flexion injury (Fig. 26-28).

Cast immobilization is generally sufficient treatment for nondisplaced Salter-Harris type I and II fractures of the distal tibia. Recommended treatment ranges from a below-knee cast worn for 4 weeks to a long non–weight-bearing cast worn for 3 weeks, followed by 3 weeks of immobilization in a short-leg walking cast.

Most authorities agree that closed reduction of significantly displaced Salter-Harris I and II fractures should be attempted. Because of fears of iatrogenic damage to the distal tibial physis during closed reduction, many researchers recommend the use of general anesthesia with adequate muscle relaxation for all patients with Salter-Harris I and II distal tibial fractures. However, no study has compared the frequency of growth abnormalities in patients with these fractures reduced under sedation and local analgesia to those with fractures reduced with the use of general anesthesia. I compared nine patients who underwent closed reduction in the emergency department with the use of sedation and hematoma block to nine patients who had closed reduction in the operating room with the use of general anesthesia. All fractures were reduced with a single manipulation, except for one in the emergency department group that required repeat manipulation. One patient in each group had a growth alteration.

When closed reductions are not done with general anesthesia, they usually are done with intravenous sedation. Etomidate recently has been found to be effective and safe for sedation for reduction of pediatric ankle fractures (73). Furia et al (74) demonstrated significantly improved pain relief with hematoma block for ankle fractures in a study comparing patients treated with intravenous sedation to patients receiving hematoma block. Intravenous regional anesthesia or Bier block also has been reported to be effective for pain relief in patients with lower extremity injuries (75).

Opinions differ as to what degree of residual displacement or angulation is unacceptable and requires open reduction. Based on follow-up of 33 Salter-Harris type II ankle fractures, Caruthers and Crenshaw (19) concluded that "accurate reposition of the displaced epiphysis at the expense of forced or repeated manipulation or operative intervention is not indicated since spontaneous realignment of the ankle occurs even late in the growing period." They found no residual angulation at follow-up in patients who had up to 12 degrees of valgus tilt after reduction, even in patients as old as 13 years at the time of injury. Spiegel et al (11), however, reported complications at follow-up in 11 of 16 patients with Salter-Harris type II ankle fractures. Because 6 of these 11 patients had angular deformities that were attributed to lack of adequate reduction of the fracture, Spiegel et al recommended "precise anatomic reduction."

Incomplete reduction usually is caused by interposition of soft tissue between the fracture fragments. Grace (76) reported three patients in whom the interposed soft tissue included the neurovascular bundle, resulting in circulatory embarrassment when closed reduction was attempted. In this situation, open reduction and extraction of the soft tissue obviously are required (Fig. 26-29).

A less definitive indication for open reduction is interposition of periosteum, which causes physeal widening with no angulation or with minimal angulation. Good results have been reported after open reduction and extraction of the periosteal flap (77). It is not clear, however, that failure to extract the periosteum in such cases results in problems sufficient to warrant operative treatment.

Pfeiffer et al (78) studied the effects of interposed periosteum in experimental physeal fractures in a rat model. They found that in some animals the periosteum was degraded by giant cells and in others the physis grew around it (78). Both animals without and animals with periosteum interposed were observed to frequently develop small physeal bars. The presence of these small physeal bars was not always associated with the development of a leg length inequality. For those animals with leg length discrepancy, the magnitude was small, averaging 0.5% of the contralateral leg for those animals with physeal fractures with-

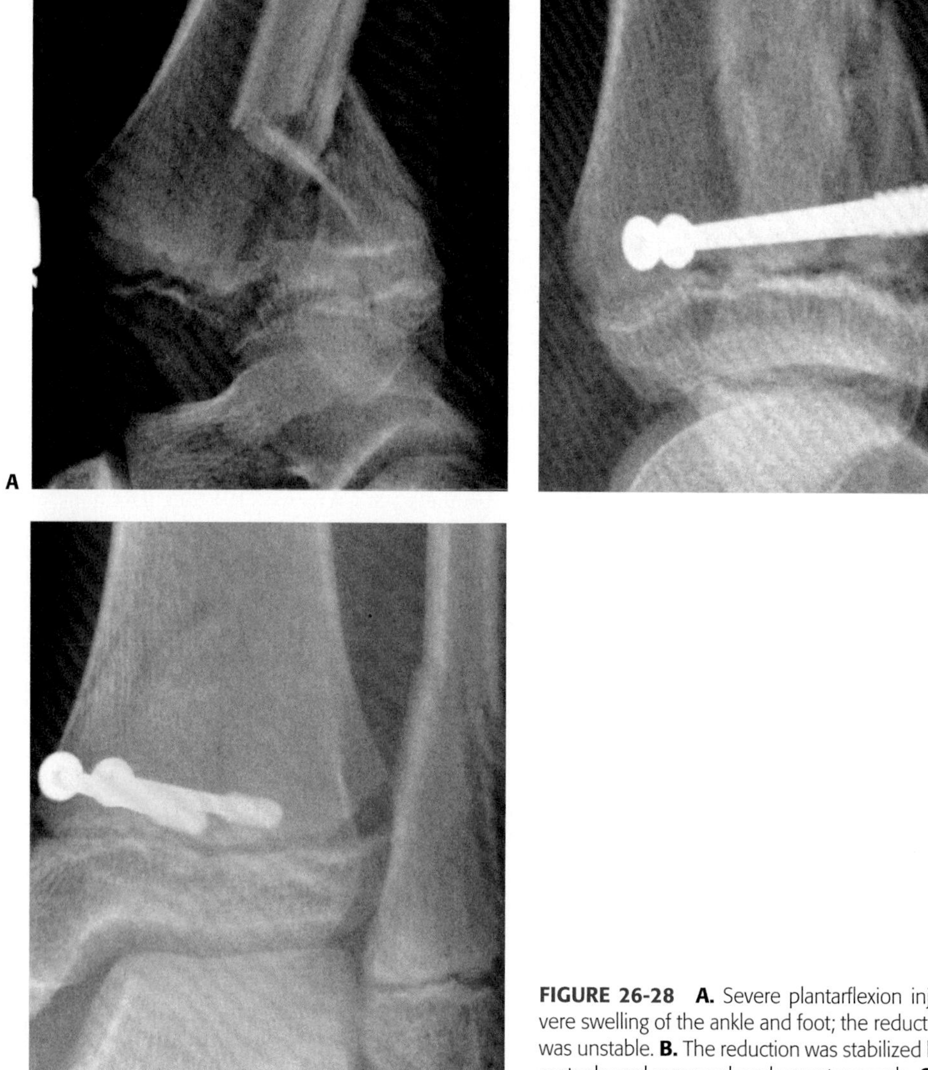

FIGURE 26-28 **A.** Severe plantarflexion injury with severe swelling of the ankle and foot; the reduction obtained was unstable. **B.** The reduction was stabilized by two transmetaphyseal screws placed percutaneously. **C.** Anteroposterior view confirms an anatomic reduction.

out periosteal interposition to 2% of the contralateral leg for those with interposition (79).

Barmada et al (80) reviewed their experience with 44 Salter-Harris I and II fractures. They found that in patients with less than 3 mm of residual physeal widening after closed reduction, a diagnosis of premature partial growth arrest could be made in 17% at follow-up. In patients with more than 3 mm of residual physeal widening, the frequency increased to 60% (Fig. 26-30). Based on their findings, they recommended open reduction and removal of entrapped periosteum for residual physeal widening of more than 3 mm. They were unable, however, to show a significant decrease in the chance of partial growth arrest in the patients treated with surgery when compared to the patients treated without surgery (80).

Salter-Harris Type III and IV Fractures

Salter-Harris type III and IV fractures share the same mechanism of injury (supination–inversion), and their treatment and prognosis are similar. In the series of Spiegel et al. (11), 24.1% of the fractures were Salter-Harris type III injuries and 1.4% were type IV. These injuries usually are produced by the medial corner of the talus being driven into the junction of the distal tibial articular surface and the medial malleolus. As the talus shears off the medial malleolus, the physis also may be damaged (Fig. 26-31).

Nondisplaced Salter-Harris type III and IV fractures can be treated with above-knee cast immobilization, but care must be taken to be sure no displacement is present, which may require CT evaluation, and that no displacement occurs after casting,

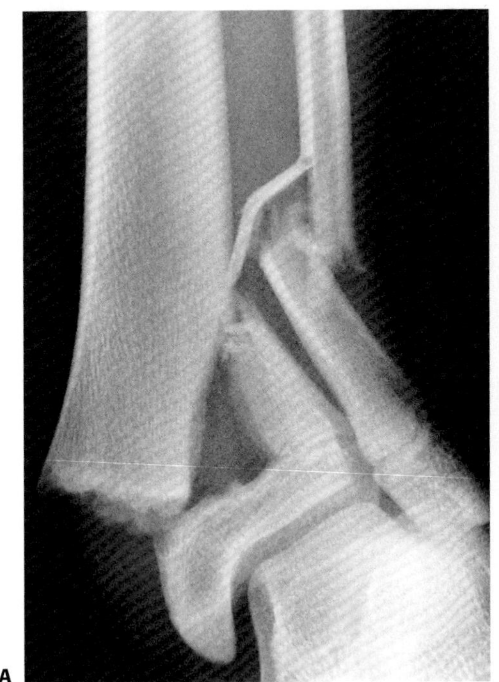

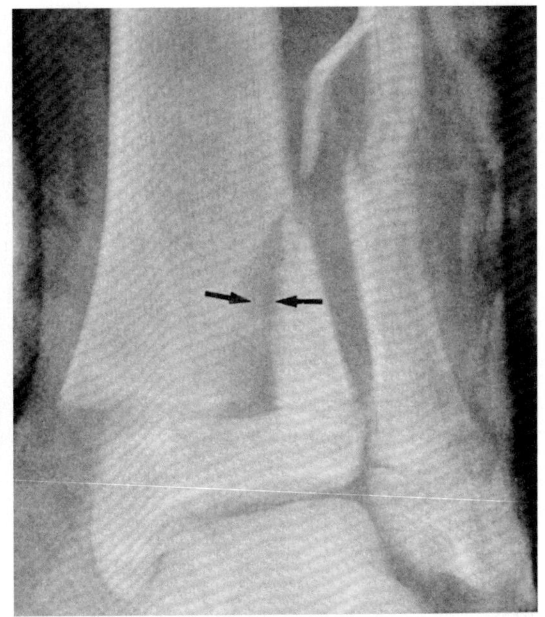

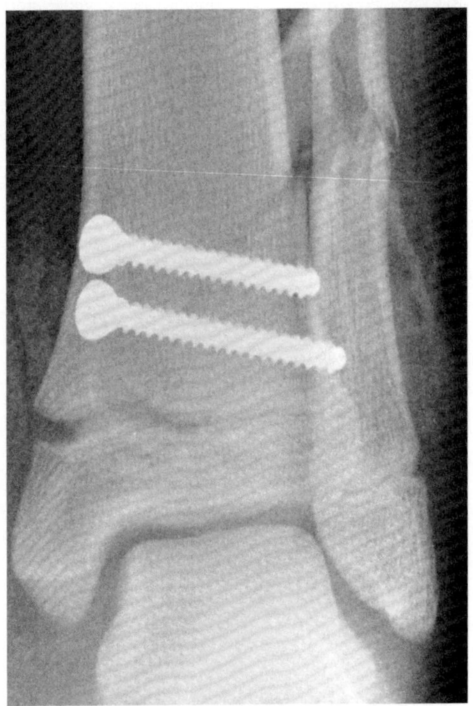

FIGURE 26-29 A. Severely displaced pronation–eversion–external rotation injury. **B.** Closed reduction was unsuccessful, and a valgus tilt of the ankle mortise was noted. At surgery, soft tissue was interposed laterally (*arrows*). **C.** Reduction completed and stabilized with two cancellous screws placed above the physis.

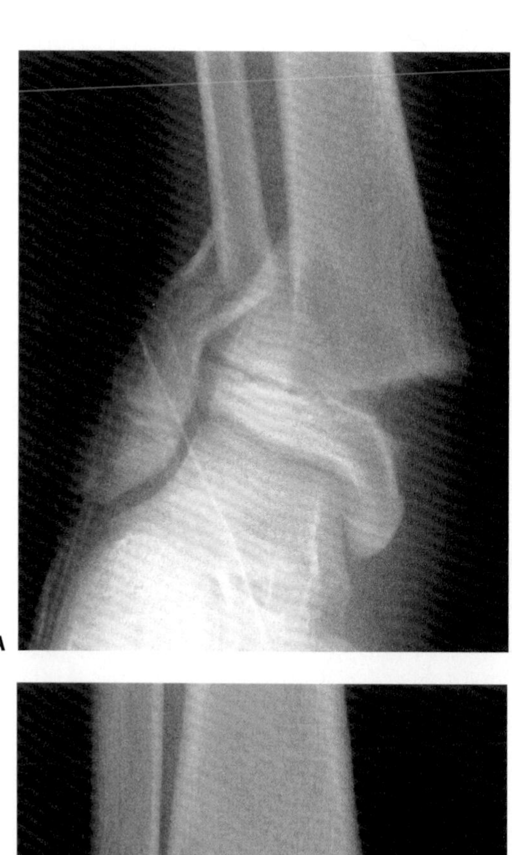

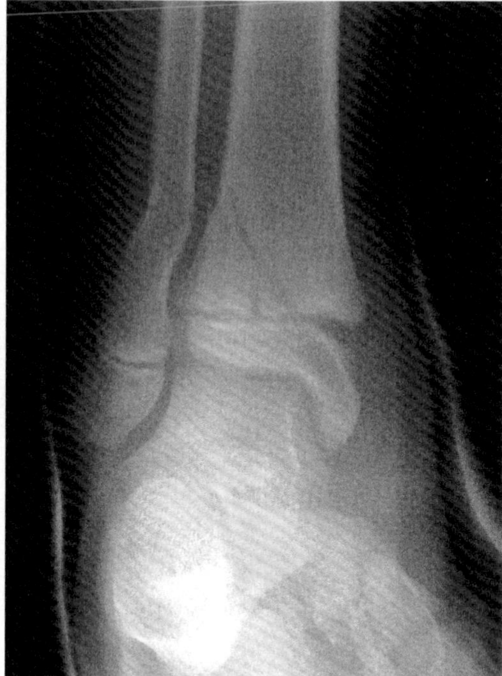

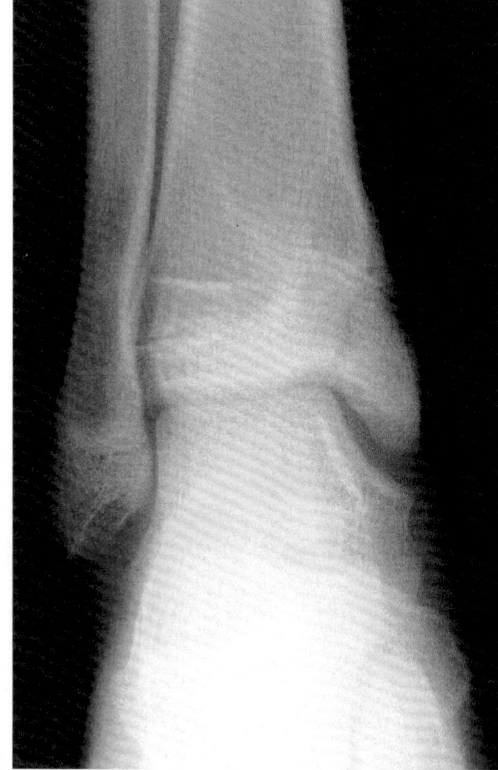

FIGURE 26-30 **A.** Anteroposterior view of a patient with a pronation-eversion external rotation fracture. **B.** Postreduction view shows residual gapping of physis suggesting periosteal interposition. **C.** Anteroposterior view obtained for a new injury (medial malleolar fracture) shows premature closure of the physis.

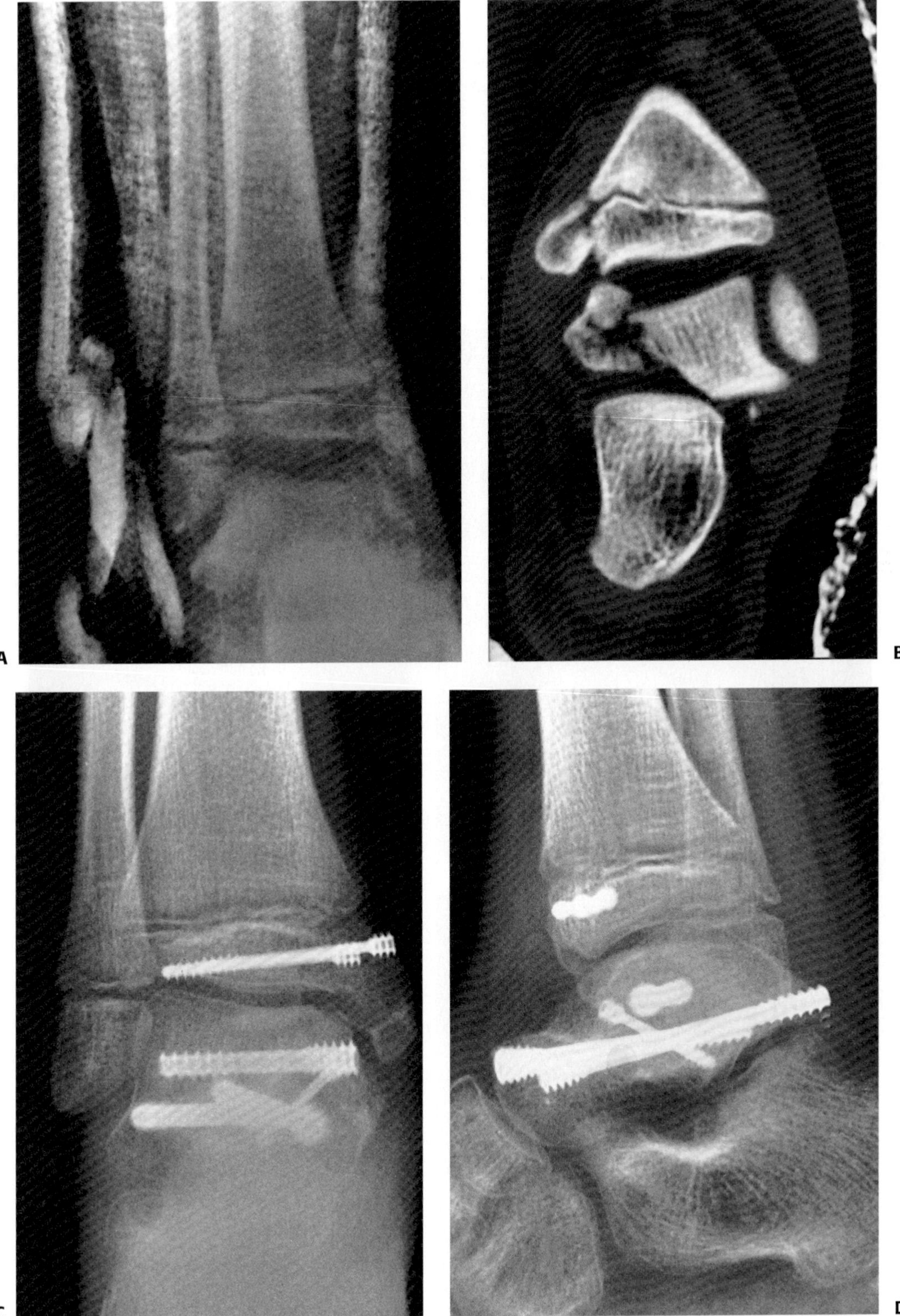

FIGURE 26-31 **A.** Severe ankle injury sustained by an 8-year-old involved in a car accident. The anteroposterior view in the splint does not clearly show the Salter-Harris type IV fracture of the tibia. The dome of the talus appears abnormal. **B.** Computed tomography scan shows the displaced Salter-Harris type IV fracture of the medial malleolus and a severe displaced intraarticular fracture of the body of the talus. **C,D.** Open reduction of both fractures was performed, and Herbert screws were used for internal fixation. (Courtesy Armen Kelikian, MD.)

which requires weekly x-ray evaluation for the first 2 weeks after casting.

Displaced fractures require as anatomic a reduction as possible. Failure to obtain anatomic reduction frequently results in articular incongruity and post-traumatic arthritis, which often becomes symptomatic 5 to 8 years after skeletal maturity (Fig. 26-32) (81). The risk of growth arrest also has been linked to the accuracy of reduction (20). Closed reduction may be attempted but is likely to succeed only in minimally displaced fractures. If closed reduction is obtained, it can be maintained with a cast or with percutaneous pins or screws supplemented by a cast.

If anatomic reduction cannot be obtained by closed methods, open reduction with internal fixation should be performed. Beaty and Linton (82) reported a Salter-Harris type III fracture with an intra-articular fragment (Fig. 26-33); these fractures also require open reduction for inspection of the joint and replacement or removal of loose osteochondral fragments.

Lintecum and Blasier described a technique of open reduction through a limited exposure of the fracture with the incision

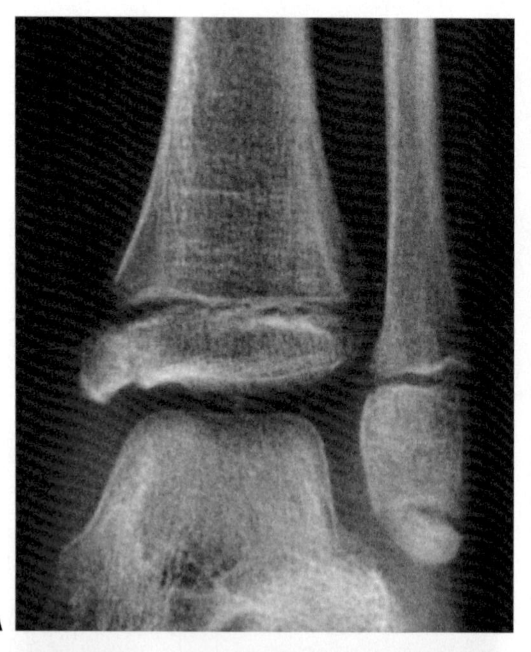

A

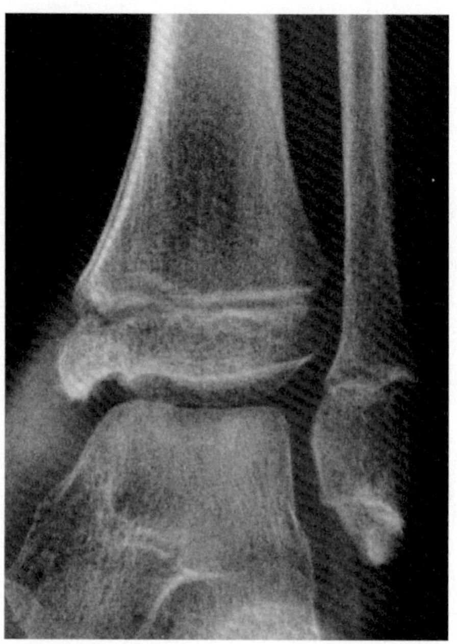

B

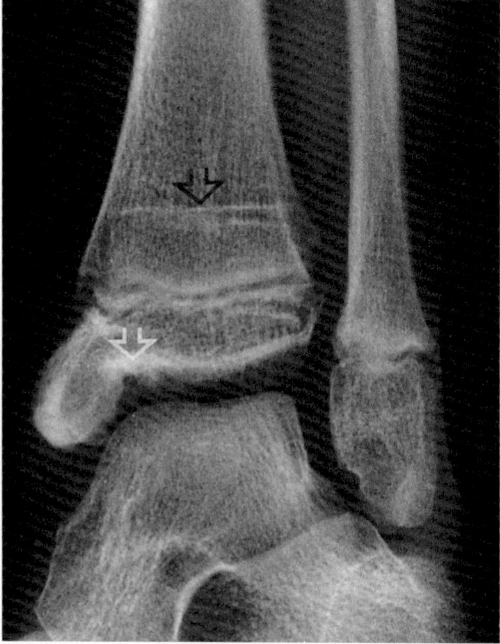

C

FIGURE 26-32 **A.** Displaced Salter-Harris type III supination–inversion fracture in an 8-year-old girl who presented for treatment 2 weeks after injury. **B.** After cast removal 6 weeks after injury. **C.** Two years after injury. Although the injury does not seem to have interfered with growth, as evidenced by the Park-Harris growth arrest line parallel to the physis (*black arrow*), her articular incongruity (*white arrow*) is associated with occasional mild ankle pain.

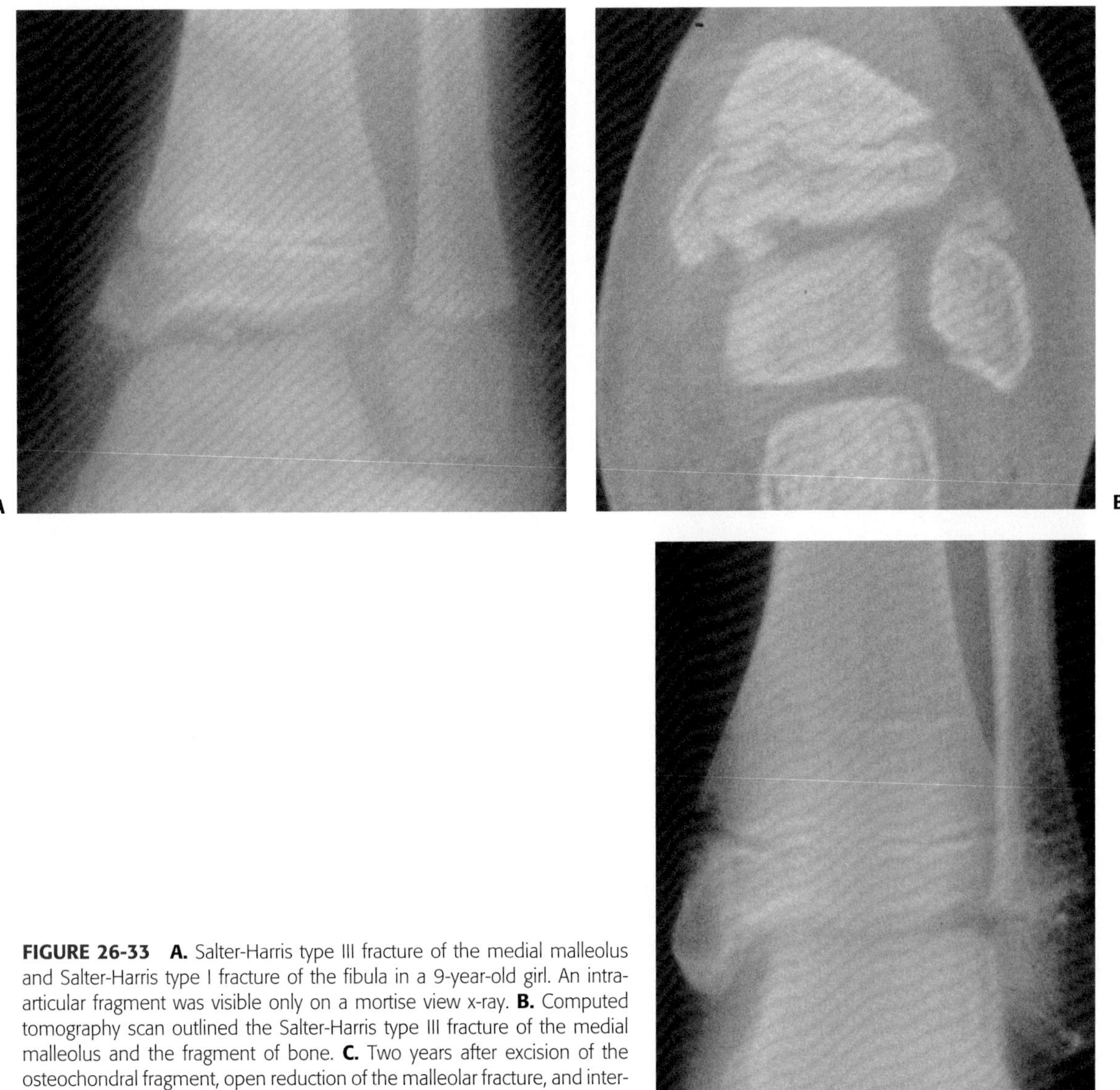

FIGURE 26-33 **A.** Salter-Harris type III fracture of the medial malleolus and Salter-Harris type I fracture of the fibula in a 9-year-old girl. An intra-articular fragment was visible only on a mortise view x-ray. **B.** Computed tomography scan outlined the Salter-Harris type III fracture of the medial malleolus and the fragment of bone. **C.** Two years after excision of the osteochondral fragment, open reduction of the malleolar fracture, and internal fixation. (**A** and **B** reprinted from Beaty JH, Linton RC. Medial malleolar fracture in a child: a case report. *J Bone Joint Surg Am* 1988;70: 1254–1255; with permission.)

centered over the fracture site combined with percutaneous cannulated screw fixation (16). This technique was used in 13 patients: 8 with Salter-Harris IV fractures, 4 with Salter-Harris III fractures, and 1 with a triplane fracture. The investigators reported 1 growth arrest at follow-up averaging 12 months.

Internal fixation devices should be inserted within the epiphysis, parallel to the physis, and should avoid the physis and ankle joint (Fig. 26-34).

Options for internal fixation include smooth Kirschner wires (K-wires), small fragment cortical and cancellous screws, and 4-mm cannulated screws (Fig. 26-35). Several reports (83–85) have advocated the use of absorbable pins for internal fixation of ankle fractures. Benz et al (83) reported no complications or growth abnormalities after the use of absorbable pins with metal screw supplementation for fixation of five ankle fractures in patients between the ages of 5 and 13 years. In reports of the use of absorbable pins without supplemental metal fixation in adults (86–89), complications have included displacement (14.5%), sterile fluid accumulation requiring incision and drainage (8.1%), pseudarthrosis (8%), distal tibiofibular synostosis (3.8%), and infection (1.6%). Bucholz et al (85) reported few complications in a series of fractures in adults fixed with absorbable screws made of polylactide and suggested that complications in earlier series might be related to the fact that those pins were made of polyglycolide. A report in 1993 by Bostman et al (84), however, included few complications in a series of frac-

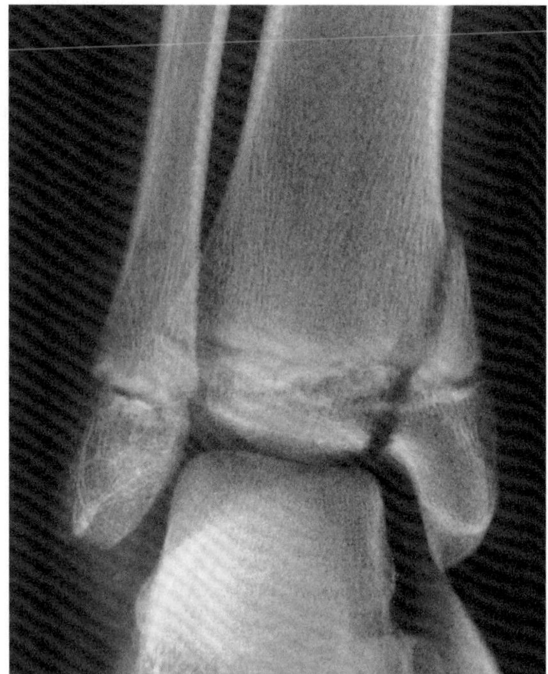
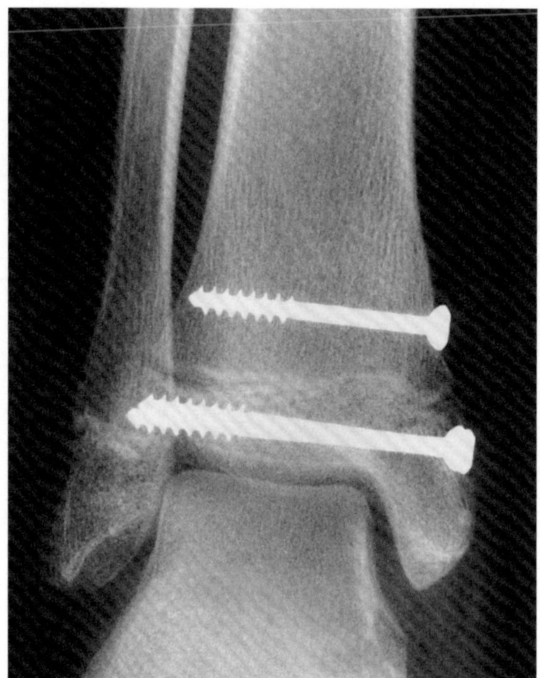

FIGURE 26-34 **A.** Grade II supination–inversion injury in a 12-year-old girl, resulting in a displaced Salter-Harris type IV fracture of the distal tibia and a nondisplaced Salter-Harris type I fracture of the distal fibula. **B.** After anatomic open reduction and stable internal fixation.

tures in children fixed with polyglycolide pins. A follow-up report by Rokkanen et al (90) in 1996 reported a 3.6% rate of infection and a 3.7% rate of failure of fixation. Fibrin glue has been used for fixation of fractures in patients with slightly displaced distal tibial/fibular fractures, but fibrin glue is not very firm and the added support of cast immobilization is required (91).

The main advantage of absorbable pins and screws is that hardware removal is avoided. Böstman (92) compared the cost effectiveness of absorbable implants in 994 patients to metallic implants in 1,173 patients. According to his cost analysis, the "break-even" point would be attained at removal rates ranging from 19% for metacarpal fractures to 54% for trimalleolar fractures. He concluded that the use of absorbable devices would be more cost effective only at higher removal rates for the metallic implants.

Salter-Harris Type V Fractures

Salter-Harris type V fractures of the ankle are believed to be caused by severe axial compression and crushing of the physis (Fig. 26-36). As originally described, these injuries are not associated with displacement of the epiphysis relative to the metaphysis, which makes diagnosis of acute injury impossible from plain x-rays; the diagnosis can be made only on follow-up x-rays when premature physeal closure is evident. Spiegel et al (11) designated comminuted fractures that are otherwise unclassifiable as Salter-Harris type V injuries.

The incidence of Salter-Harris type V ankle fractures is difficult to establish because of the difficulty of diagnosing acute injuries. Spiegel et al (11) included two type V fractures in their series, but both were comminuted fractures rather than the classic crush injury.

Because of the uncertain nature of this injury, no specific treatment recommendations have been formulated. Treatment usually is directed primarily toward the sequelae of growth arrest that invariably follow Salter-Harris type V fractures. Perhaps more sophisticated scanning techniques will eventually allow identification and localization of areas of physeal injury so that irreparable damaged cells can be removed and replaced with interposition materials to prevent growth problems, but at present this diagnosis is made only several months after injury.

Other Fractures of the Distal Tibia

Accessory ossification centers of the distal tibia (os subtibiale) are common and may be injured. Treatment usually consists of cast immobilization for 3 to 4 weeks. Ogden and Lee (93) reported good results after cast immobilization in 26 of 27 patients with injuries involving the medial side of the tibia; only 1 patient required surgery.

Injuries to the perichondral ring of the distal tibial and fibular physes, with physeal disruption, have been described. Most of these injuries are caused by skiving of the bone by machinery such as lawnmowers. They may result in growth arrest or retardation and in angular deformities (see the discussion of open fractures and lawnmower injuries).

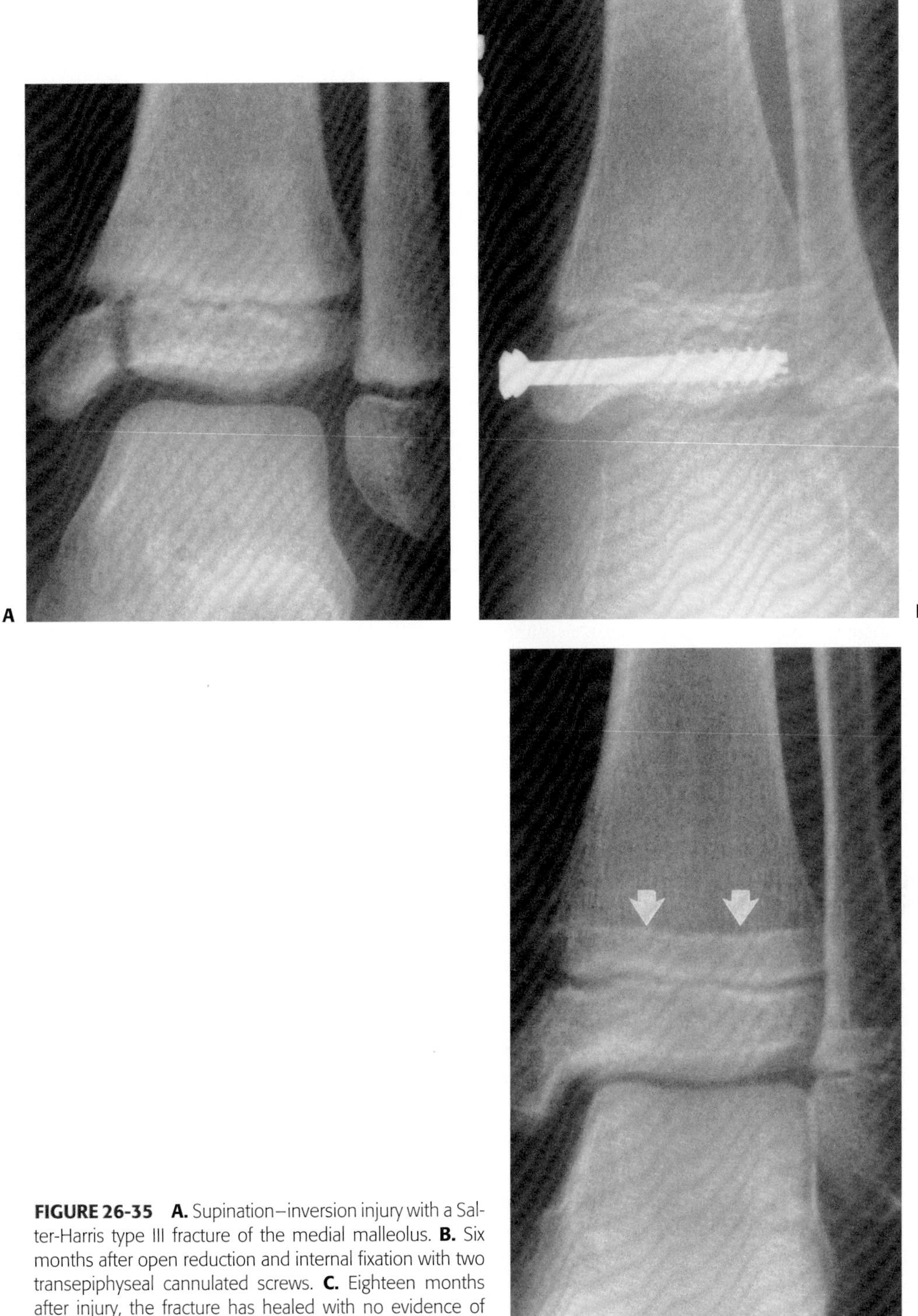

FIGURE 26-35 **A.** Supination–inversion injury with a Salter-Harris type III fracture of the medial malleolus. **B.** Six months after open reduction and internal fixation with two transepiphyseal cannulated screws. **C.** Eighteen months after injury, the fracture has healed with no evidence of growth arrest or angular deformity. *Arrows* note normal, symmetric Park-Harris growth arrest line.

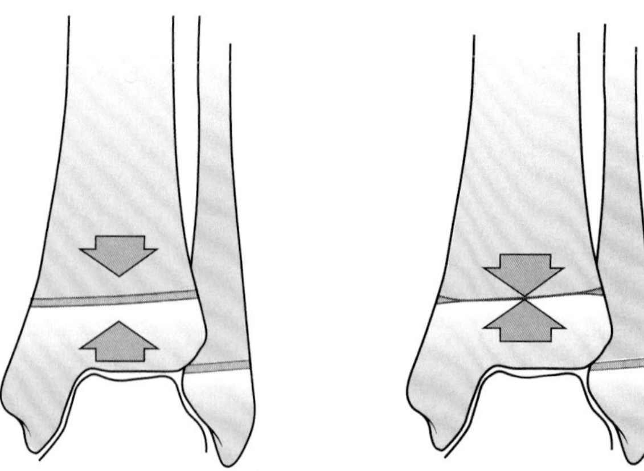

FIGURE 26-36 Compression-type injury of the tibial physis. Early physeal arrest can cause leg length discrepancy.

Juvenile Tillaux Fractures

Juvenile Tillaux fracture is the adolescent counterpart of the fracture described in adults by the French surgeon Tillaux. It occurs when, with external rotation of the foot, the anteroinferior tibiofibular ligament through its attachments to the anterolateral tibia avulses a fragment of bone corresponding to the portion of the distal tibial physis that is still open (Fig. 26-37). In the series of Spiegel et al (11), these fractures occurred in 2.9% of patients.

Tillaux fractures may be isolated injuries or may be associated with ipsilateral tibial shaft fractures (94). The fibula usually prevents marked displacement of the fracture, and clinical deformity generally is absent. Swelling usually is slight, and local tenderness is at the anterior lateral joint line, in contrast to ankle sprains, in which the tenderness tends to be below the level of the ankle joint.

A mortise view is essential to obtain a view of the distal tibial epiphysis that is unobstructed by the fibula (Fig. 26-38). Steinlauf et al reported a patient in whom the Tillaux fragment became entrapped between the distal tibia and fibula, producing apparent diastasis of the ankle joint (95). To allow measurement of displacement from plain films, the x-ray beam would have to be directly in line with the fracture site, which makes CT confirmation of reduction mandatory after all closed reductions of these fractures.

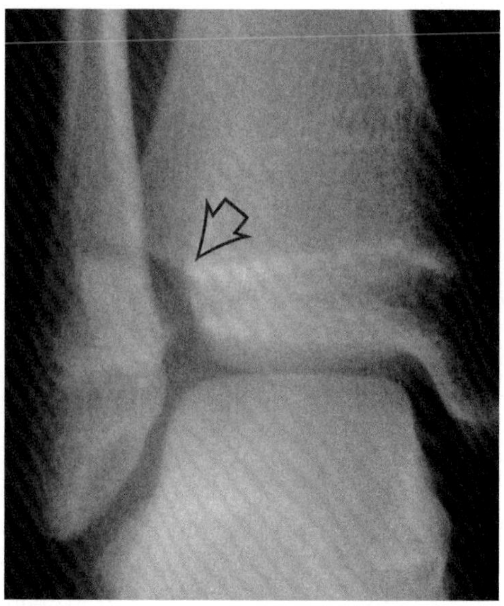

FIGURE 26-38 Anteroposterior mortise view of a 14-year-old who sustained a juvenile Tillaux fracture.

Both below-knee and above-knee casts have been used for immobilization of nondisplaced juvenile Tillaux and triplane fractures. Fractures with more than 2 mm of displacement require closed or open reduction. Closed reduction is attempted by internally rotating the foot and applying direct pressure over the anterolateral tibia. If necessary, percutaneous pins can be used for stabilization of the reduction. If closed reduction is not successful, open reduction is required. Occasionally, percutaneously inserted pins can be used to manipulate the displaced fragment into anatomic position and then advanced to fix the fragment in place (96). Leetun and Ireland (97) described arthroscopic-assisted reduction and fixation in juvenile Tillaux fractures.

Triplane Fractures

Karrholm attributed the original description of this injury to Bartl (98), in 1954, and noted that Gerner-Smidt (99), in 1963,

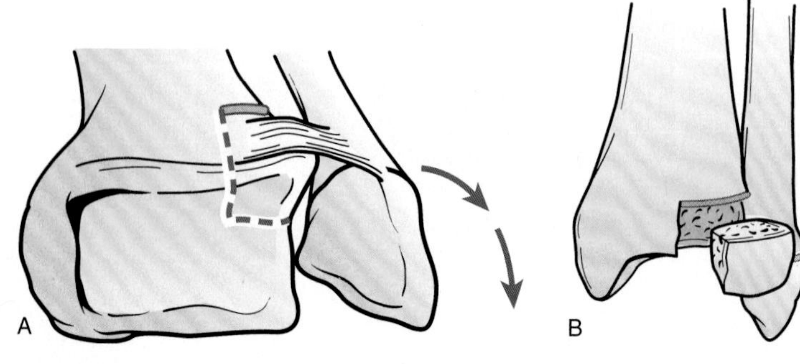

FIGURE 26-37 Juvenile Tillaux fracture. Mechanism of injury, the anteroinferior tibiofibular ligament avulses a fragment of the lateral epiphysis **(A)** corresponding to the portion of the physis that is still open **(B)**.

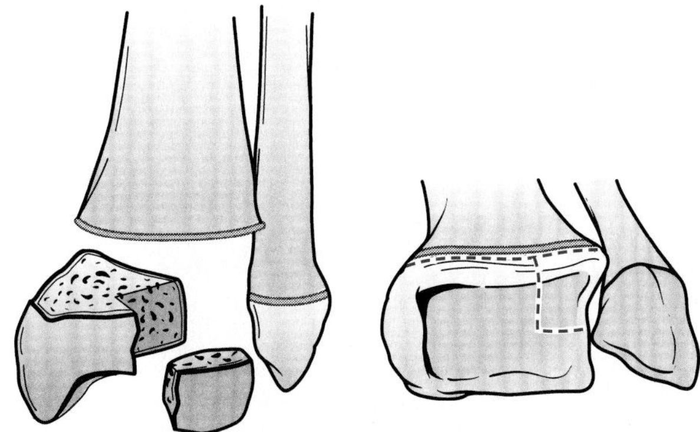

FIGURE 26-39 Anatomy of a three-part lateral triplane fracture (left ankle). Note the large epiphyseal fragment with its metaphyseal component and the smaller anterolateral epiphyseal fragment.

described triplane and Tillaux fractures as different stages of the same injury. In 1957, Johnson and Fahl (100) described a triplane fracture in their report of 27 physeal ankle injuries and reported that they had seen 10 such fractures. Despite these earlier reports, the nature of triplane fractures was not appreciated until Marmor's (22) report in 1970 of an irreducible ankle fracture that at surgery was found to consist of three parts (Fig. 26-39). Two years after Marmor's report, Lynn (40) reported two additional such fractures and coined the term triplane fracture. He described the fracture as consisting of three major fragments: (a) the anterolateral quadrant of the distal tibial epiphysis, (b) the medial and posterior portions of the epiphysis in addition to a posterior metaphyseal spike, and (c) the tibial metaphysis. However, in their 1978 report of 15 such fractures, Cooperman et al (23) concluded that, based on tomographic studies, most were two-part fractures produced by external rotation (Fig. 26-40). Variations in fracture patterns were attributed to the extent of physeal closure at the time of injury. Karrholm et al (32) reported that CT evaluation of adolescents with triplane fractures confirmed the existence of two-part and three-part

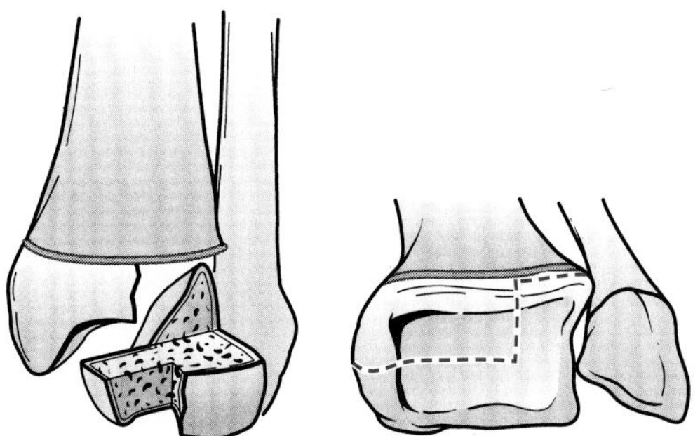

FIGURE 26-40 Anatomy of a two-part lateral triplane fracture (left ankle). Note the large posterolateral epiphyseal fragment with its posterior metaphyseal fragment. The anterior portion of the medial malleolus remains intact.

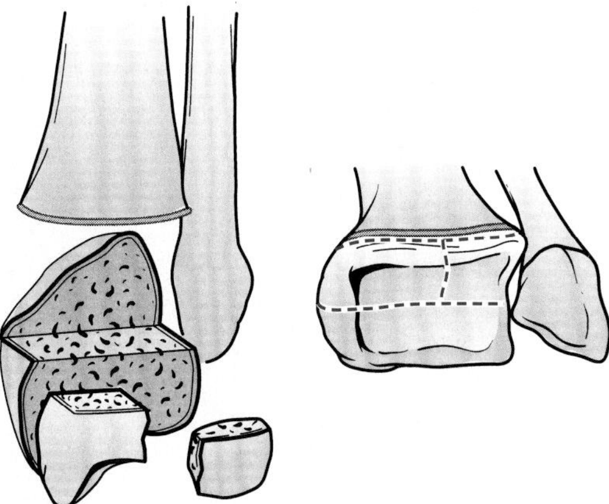

FIGURE 26-41 Anatomy of a four-part lateral triplane fracture (left ankle). The anterior epiphysis has split into two fragments, and the posterior epiphysis is the larger fragment with its metaphyseal component.

fractures and also revealed four-part fractures (Fig. 26-41). Denton and Fischer (25) described a two-part medial triplane fracture that they believed was caused by adduction and axial loading, and Peiro et al (101) reported a three-part medial triplane fracture.

El-Karef et al (102) prospectively studied 21 triplane fractures. Nineteen were lateral triplane fractures and two were medial triplane fractures. Twelve were two-part fractures, 6 were three-part fractures, and 3 were four-part fractures (102).

Von Laer (103) described a subgroup of two-part and three-part triplane fractures in which the fracture line on the anteroposterior x-ray did not extend into the ankle joint but into the medial malleolus instead (Fig. 26-42). Feldman et al. also reported an extraarticular triplane fracture in a skeletally immature patient (44). Shin et al. reported five patients with intramalleolar triplane variants (105). They divided these into three types: type I, an intramalleolar intraarticular fracture: type II, an intramalleolar, intraarticular fracture outside the weight-bearing surface; and type III, an intramalleolar, extraarticular fracture (Fig. 26-43). These researchers found that CT scans were helpful in determining displacement and deciding if surgery is indicated.

In the series of physeal ankle fractures reported by Spiegel et al (11), 7.3% were triplane fractures. Karrholm (106) reviewed 209 patients with triplane fractures and found that the mean age at the time of injury was 14.8 years for boys and 12.8 years for girls. This type of injury did not occur in children under 10 or over 16.7 years. Patients with triplane fractures may have completely open physes. Swelling usually is more severe than with Tillaux fractures, and deformity may be more severe, especially if the fibula is also fractured. X-ray views should include anteroposterior, lateral, and mortise views. Rapariz et al (107) found that 48% of triplane fractures were associated with fibular fractures and 8.5% were associated with ipsilateral tibial shaft fractures. Healy et al (108) reported a triplane

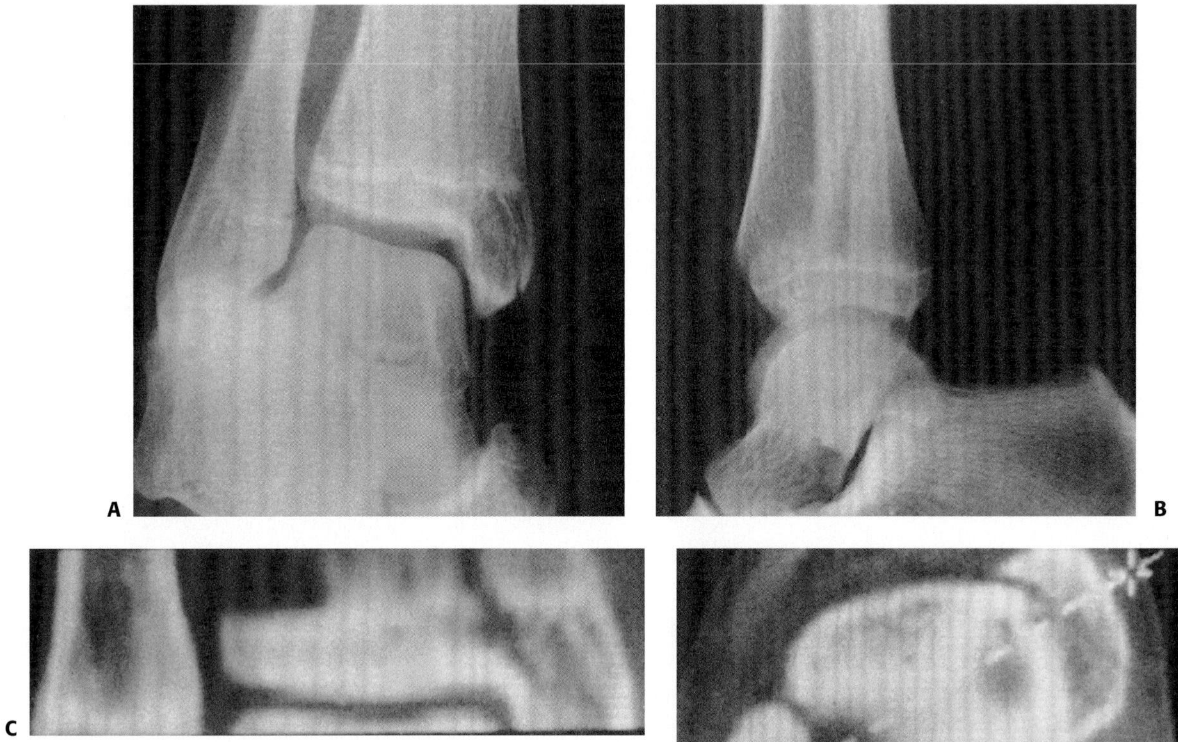

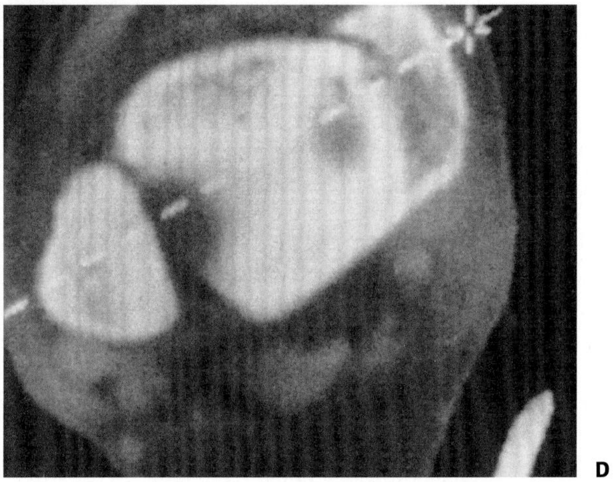

FIGURE 26-42 **A,B.** Anteroposterior and lateral x-rays of an "intramalleolar" variant triplane fracture in a 14-year-old boy. **C,D.** CT scans demonstrate extraarticular nature of the fracture.

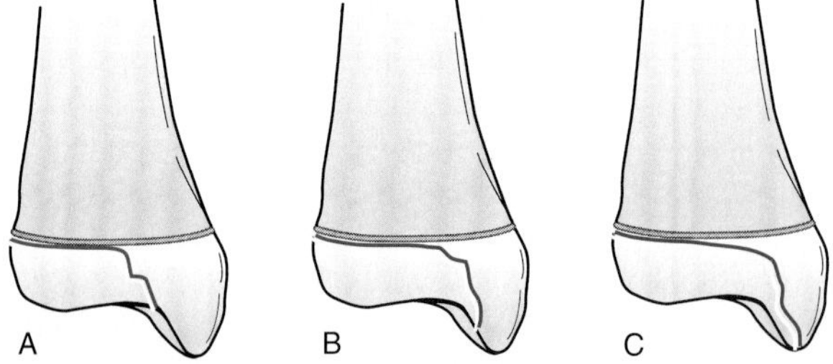

FIGURE 26-43 Schematic drawing of the immature distal tibial physis demonstrating types I, II, and III intramalleolar triplane fractures. **A.** Type I intramalleolar, intra-articular fracture at the junction of the tibial plafond and the medial malleolus. **B.** Type II intramalleolar, intra-articular fracture outside the weight-bearing zone of the tibial plafond. **C.** Type III intramalleolar, extraarticular fracture. (Adapted from Shin A, Moran ME, Wenger DR. Intramalleolar triplane fractures. *J Pediatr Orthop* 1997;17:352–355; with permission.)

fracture associated with a proximal fibular fracture and syndesmotic injury (Masionneuve equivalent). Failure to detect such injury may lead to chronic instability. Therefore, tenderness proximal to the ankle should be sought; if found, it is certainly an indication for x-ray of the proximal leg. CT has largely replaced plain tomography for evaluation of the articular surface and the fracture anatomy and should be routinely used.

Nondisplaced triplane fractures (those with less than 2 mm of displacement) and extra-articular triplane fractures can be treated with long-leg cast immobilization with the foot in internal rotation for lateral fractures and in eversion for medial fractures. Fractures with more than 2 mm of displacement (65% of the injuries in Karrholm's series) require reduction; this can be attempted in the emergency department or in the operating room with the use of general anesthesia. Closed reduction of lateral triplane fractures is attempted by internally rotating the foot. Based on the mechanism of injury, the most logical maneuver for reduction of medial triplane fractures is abduction. If closed reduction is shown to be adequate by fluoroscopic examination, as is the case about half the time, a long-leg cast is applied or percutaneous screws are inserted for fixation if necessary. If closed reduction is unsuccessful, open reduction is required. This can be accomplished through an anterolateral approach for lateral triplane fractures or through an anteromedial approach for medial triplane fractures.

Whipple et al (109) described arthroscopic reduction of two-part triplane fractures in two patients. With the arthroscope in an anterolateral portal and an anteromedial portal used for inflow, two pins were inserted laterally into the epiphyseal fragment and used to maneuver it into proper position under direct arthroscopic vision. The pins were then advanced for fixation of the fragment.

Pilon Fractures

Soft tissue complications are frequent problems during surgical treatment of these injuries. The more soft tissue edema that is present at the time of surgery, the more often it is that these complications occur. It is therefore recommended that open surgical procedures be done either before significant swelling is present (within 12 hours of injury) or after it subsides (usually after 5 to 7 days).

Open reduction with internal fixation of adult pilon fractures has been reported to have poor results and a high complication rate (56). All seven of the adolescent patients in the series of Letts et al (26) were managed with open reduction and internal fixation (Fig. 26-44). Only two of their patients developed posttraumatic osteoarthritis and none had any other complications, leading the authors to conclude that open reduction with internal fixation was more effective in this age-group than in adults. No studies describing the outcomes of other treatment alternatives, such as skeletal traction or external fixation with or without limited open reconstruction of the articular surface, have been reported in this age-group.

Fractures of the Incisura

We have seen two patients with this injury who were initially treated elsewhere with cast immobilization. After 12 weeks of casting, the patients demonstrated no bony healing. Cast immobilization was discontinued and rehabilitation begun. Both were symptom free 2 years postinjury despite lack of bony union. Since the last edition of this text, one of these patients returned for follow-up and complained of occasional pain in the involved ankle. It is my current opinion that if syndesmotic instability can be demonstrated in patients with this injury, open reduction of this fracture and the insertion of a syndesmotic screw should be considered (32).

OPEN FRACTURES AND LAWNMOWER INJURIES

Severe open ankle fractures often are produced by high-velocity motor vehicle accidents or lawnmower injuries (Fig. 26-45) (110,111). Approximately 25,000 lawnmower injuries occur each year, 20% of which are in children. Riding lawnmowers are associated with the most severe injuries, requiring more surgical procedures and resulting in more functional limitations (13,112–116). Loder et al (117) reviewed 144 children injured by lawnmowers. The average age at the time of injury was 7 years. The child was a bystander in 84 cases. Sixty-seven children required amputation. Soft tissue infection occurred in 8 of 118 and osteomyelitis in 6 of 117.

Principles of treatment are the same as in adults: copious irrigation and debridement, tetanus toxoid, and intravenous antibiotics. Gaglani et al (118) reported the bacteriologic findings in three children with infections secondary to lawnmower injuries. They found that organisms infecting the wounds frequently were different from those found on initial debridement. Gram-negative organisms were common, and some patients were infected with fungi as well. In children with lawnmower injuries, grass, dirt, and debris are blown into the wound under pressure, and removal of these embedded foreign objects requires meticulous mechanical debridement.

In most patients, the articular surface and physis should be aligned and fixed with smooth pins that do not cross the physis at the time of initial treatment. Exposed physeal surfaces should be covered with local fat to help prevent union of the metaphysis to the epiphysis. An external fixator may be used if necessary, but small pins should be used through the metaphysis and epiphysis, avoiding the physis (119–123). Wound closure may be a problem in patients with significant soft tissue injury and exposed bone. Skin coverage with local tissue is ideal, but if local coverage is not possible, split-thickness skin grafting generally is the next choice. Free vascular flaps and rotational flaps may be required for adequate coverage. Klein et al (124) reported two patients who had associated vascular injury precluding such flaps. The injury was covered successfully with local advancement flaps made possible by multiple relaxing incisions. Mooney et al (125) reported the use of cross-extremity flaps for such cases. They found external fixation for linkage of the lower extremities during the procedure to be valuable. After fixator removal, range of motion returned.

Vosburgh et al (116) reported 33 patients with lawnmower injuries to the foot and ankle. They found that the most severe injuries were to the posterior–plantar aspect of the foot and ankle. Of their patients, 5 required split-thickness skin grafts and 1 required a vascularized flap for soft-tissue coverage. Two ultimately required Syme amputations. Four of the patients had complete disruption of the Achilles tendon. Three had no repair or reconstruction of the triceps surae tendon, and 1 had delayed reconstruction 3 months after injury. Vosburgh et al (116) speculated that dense scarring in the posterior ankle results in a "physiologic tendon" and that extensive reconstructive surgery is not always necessary for satisfactory function. Boyer et al reported a patient with deltoid ligament loss due to a severe grinding injury that required a free plantaris tendon graft to reconstruct the ligament (126). Soft tissue coverage was achieved using a free muscle transfer.

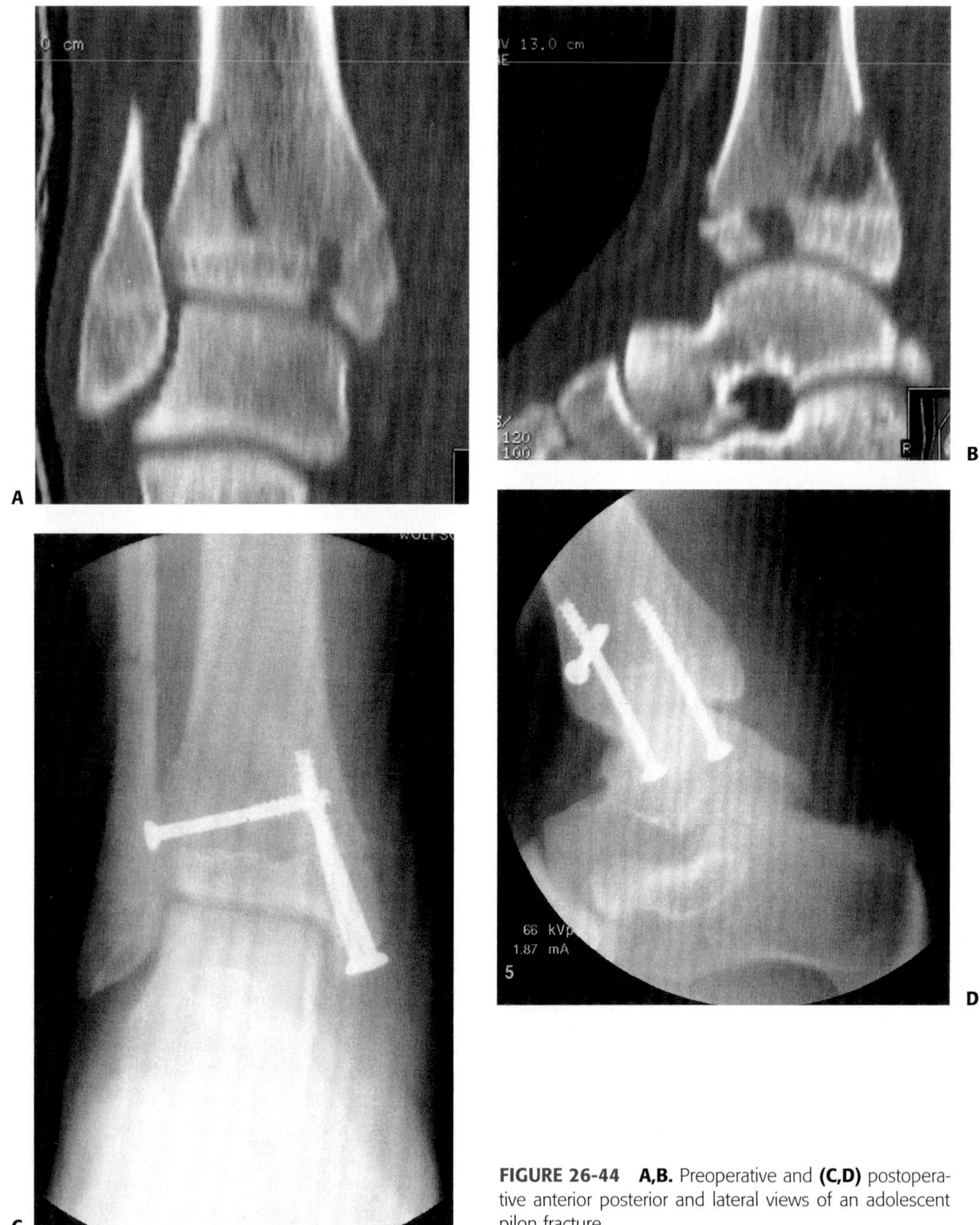

FIGURE 26-44 **A,B.** Preoperative and **(C,D)** postoperative anterior posterior and lateral views of an adolescent pilon fracture.

DISTAL FIBULAR FRACTURES

Fractures involving the fibular physis are most commonly Salter-Harris type I or II fractures that are caused by a supination–inversion injury. Isolated fibular fractures usually are minimally displaced and can be treated with immobilization in a below-knee cast for 4 to 6 weeks. Significantly displaced fibular fractures accompany Salter-Harris type III and IV tibial fractures and usually reduce when the tibial fracture is reduced. Internal fixation of the tibial fracture generally results in stability of the fibular fracture such that cast immobilization is sufficient. If the fibular fracture is unstable after reduction and fixation of the tibial fracture, fixation with a smooth intramedullary or obliquely inserted K-wire is recommended. In older adolescents in whom growth is not a consideration, an intramedullary rod or plate-and-screw device can be used as in adults (Fig. 26-46).

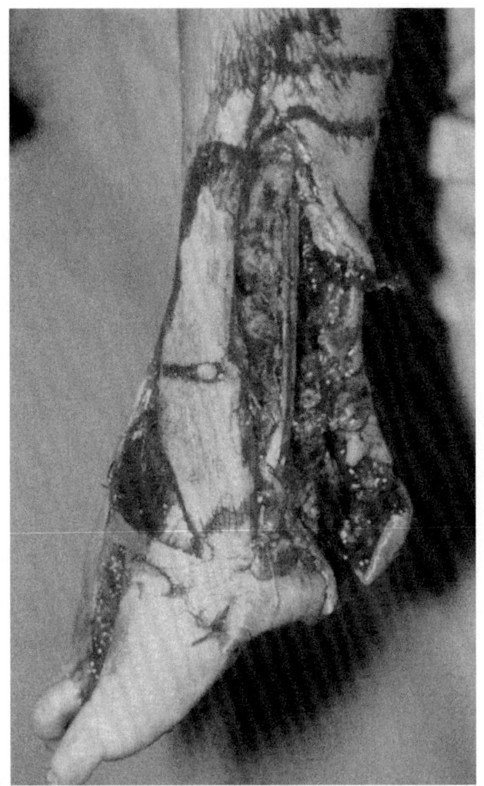

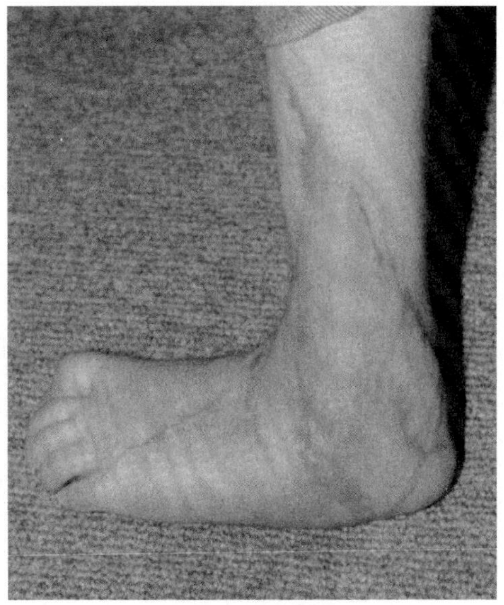

FIGURE 26-45 **A.** Severe lawn mower injury in a 5-year-old boy. **B.** One year after initial treatment with debridement, free flap, and skin graft coverage.

Avulsion fractures from the lateral malleolus occur in children with inversion sprain-type injuries to the ankle. These may fail to unite with cast immobilization. Patients with such nonunions may have pain without associated instability. In such patients, simple excision of the ununited fragment usually relieves their pain (127,128). When the nonunions are associated with instability, reconstruction of one or more of the lateral ankle ligaments is required (see section on Lateral Ankle Sprains).

Avulsion fracture of accessory ossification centers of the distal fibula (os subfibulare) also are common. In the series reported by Ogden and Lee (93), 5 of 11 patients with injuries treated with cast immobilization had persistent symptoms and required excision.

LATERAL ANKLE SPRAINS

In 1984, Vahvanen published a prospective study of 559 children who presented with severe supination injuries or sprains of the ankle (129). Forty patients, 28 boys and 12 girls, with an average age of 12 years (range 5 to 14) were surgically explored. The indications for surgery included swelling, pain over the anterior talofibular ligament, limp, clinical instability, and displaced avulsion fracture. Such fractures were visible on x-rays in only 8 patients but were found at surgery in 19. Thirty-six ankles were found to have injury of the anterior talofibular ligament at surgery. Only 16 of these had either a positive lateral or anterior drawer stress test. At follow-up all patients were pain-free and none complained of instability. Based on the incidence of residual disability after such injuries in adults reported in the literature (21% to 58%), these researchers suggested primary surgical repair.

Busconi and Pappas (130) reported 60 skeletally immature children with chronic ankle pain and instability. Fifty of these children responded to rehabilitation, but 10 had persistent symptoms. Although 3 of these patients' initial x-rays were within normal limits, all patients with persistent symptoms eventually were found to have ununited osteochondral fractures of the fibular epiphysis. All 10 patients with persistent symptoms were treated with excision of the ununited osteochondral fracture and a Broström reconstruction of the lateral collateral ligament. All were able to return to activities, and none reported further pain or instability.

ANKLE DISLOCATIONS

Nusem et al (131) reported a 12-year-old girl with a posterior dislocation of the ankle without associated fracture (Fig. 26-47). This was a closed injury and resulted from forced inversion of a maximally plantarflexed foot. The dislocation was reduced under intravenous sedation and the ankle was immobilized in a short-leg cast for 5 weeks. The patient was asymptomatic at

FIGURE 26-46 **A.** Salter-Harris type II fracture of the distal fibula in a 15-year-old. **B.** Lateral view shows the fibular metaphyseal fragment (*arrow*). Considerable soft-tissue swelling was noted in the medial aspect of the ankle. **C.** Stress films showed complete disruption of the deltoid ligament. **D.** The fibular fracture was fixed with a cannulated screw; the deltoid ligament was not repaired.

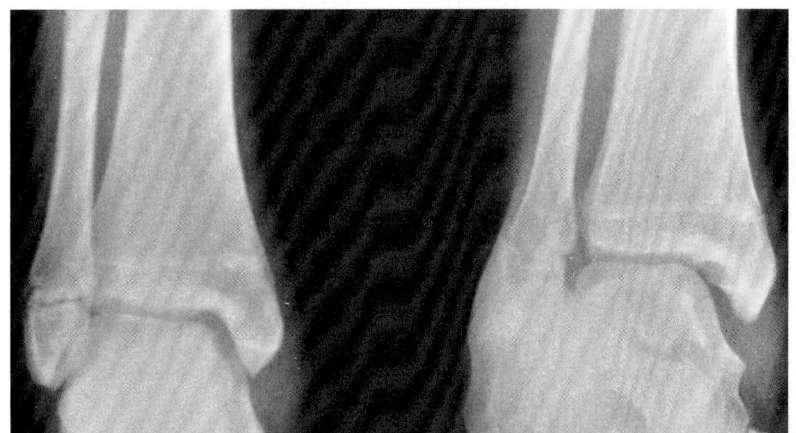

A

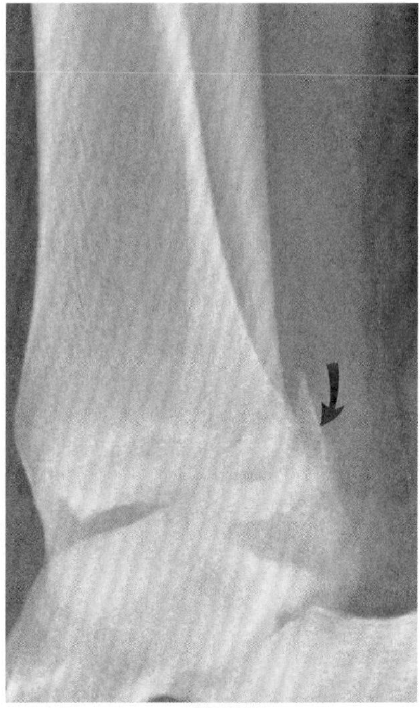

B

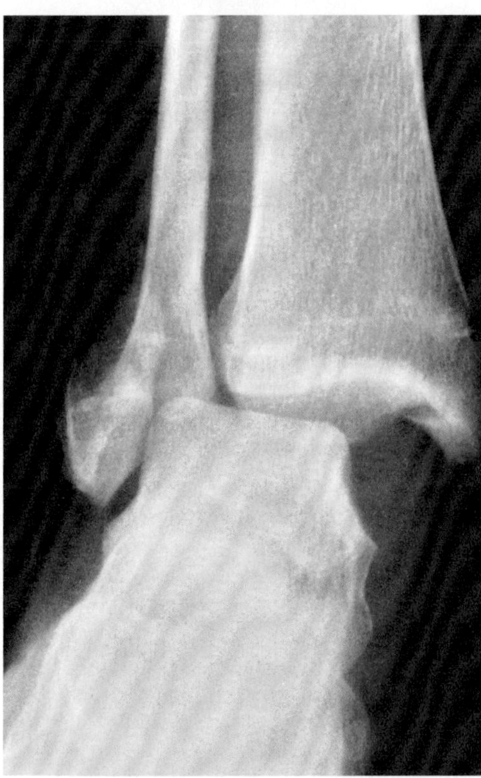

C

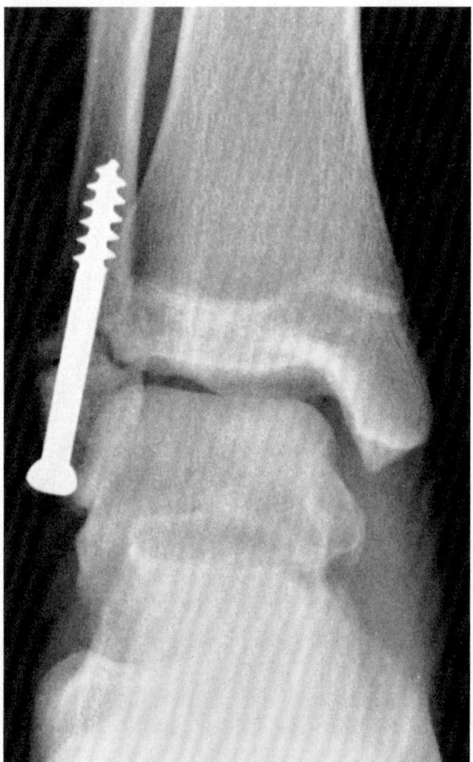

D

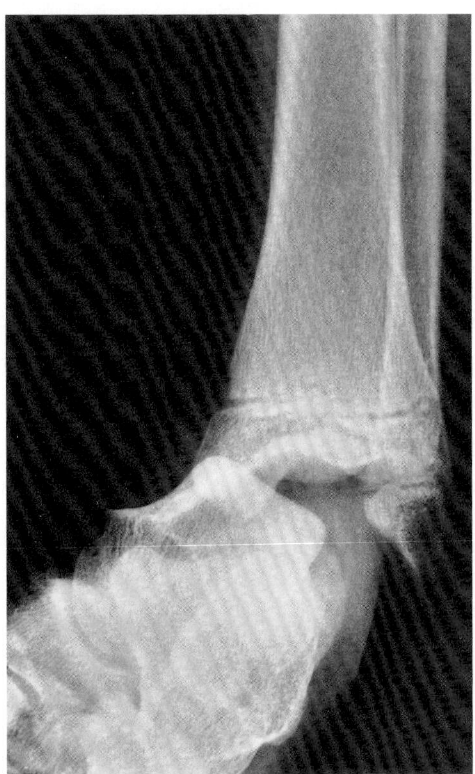

FIGURE 26-47 Anteroposterior x-ray of child with tibiotalar dislocation without fracture.

follow-up 4 years after injury. The inversion stress views at that time revealed only a 3-degree increase in laxity compared with the uninjured side. The anterior drawer sign was negative. There was no evidence of osteonecrosis of the talus on follow-up x-rays.

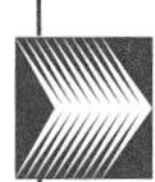

AUTHOR'S PREFERRED TREATMENT

Salter-Harris Type I and II Fractures of the Distal Tibia

I treat most nondisplaced Salter-Harris type I and II fractures initially with above-knee cast immobilization. Non–weight-bearing is continued for 3 to 4 weeks after injury, when the cast is changed to a below-knee walking cast that is worn for an additional 3 to 4 weeks. Follow-up x-rays are obtained every 6 months for at least 2 years and preferably until skeletal maturity,

For displaced fractures in children with at least 2 years of growth remaining, my objective is to accept no more than 15 degrees of anterior angulation for posteriorly displaced fractures, 10 degrees of valgus for laterally displaced fractures, and 0 degrees of varus for medially displaced fractures (Fig. 26-48). For children with 2 years or less of growth remaining, the amount of angulation I accept is less than 5 degrees. When possible I attempt reduction of markedly displaced fractures with the use of general anesthesia with good muscle relaxation and fluoroscopic control. In children with significantly displaced fractures, if anesthesia is not going to be available for many hours, I make one attempt

A
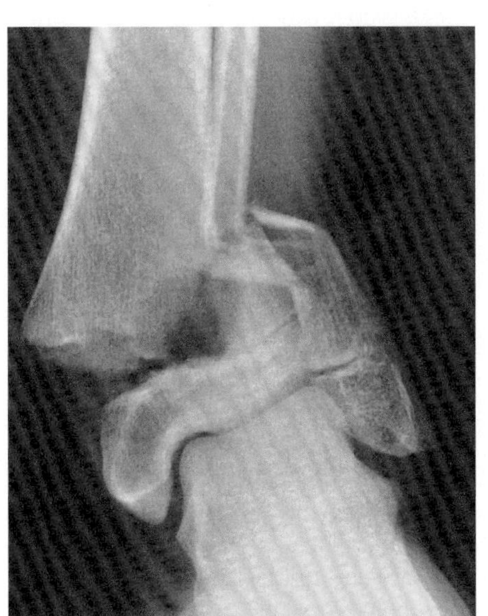

B
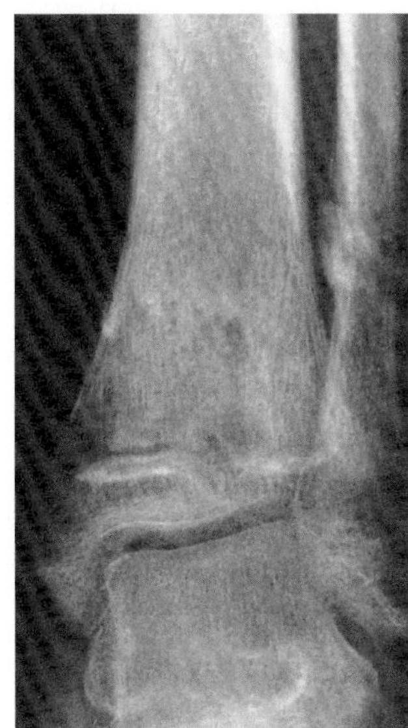

C
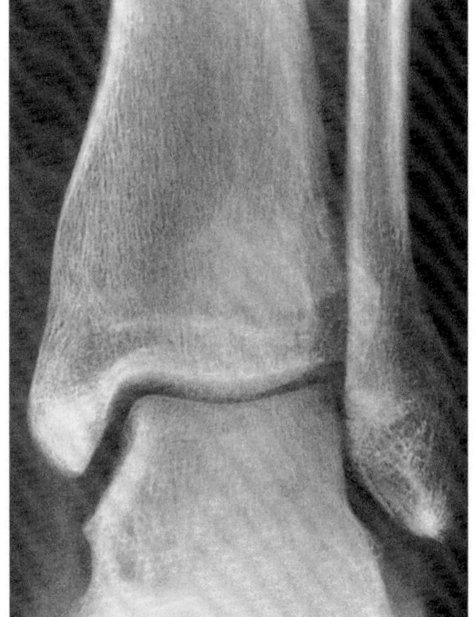

FIGURE 26-48 **A.** Displaced pronation–eversion–external rotation fracture of the distal tibia in a 12-year-old boy was treated with closed reduction and cast immobilization. **B.** After cast removal a 10-degree valgus tilt was present. **C.** At maturity, the deformity has completely resolved.

at gentle closed reduction under a hematoma block supplemented as needed by well-monitored intravenous sedation. Once adequately reduced, the fractures usually are stable and a long-leg cast can be used for immobilization. Rarely, for markedly unstable fractures or severe soft tissue injuries that require multiple debridements, percutaneous screws are used when the Thurston-Holland fragment is large enough to allow screw fixation. When the fragment is too small, smooth wire fixation across the physis is the only alternative. It has been suggested that repeated attempts at closed manipulation of these fractures may increase the risk of growth abnormality and should be avoided. In patients with fractures that are not seen until 7 to 10 days after injury, moderate residual displacement probably is best accepted. If growth does not sufficiently correct malunion, corrective osteotomy can be done later.

I have found that open reduction of these fractures is infrequently indicated. The exception usually has been pronation–eversion–external rotation fractures with interposed soft tissue. For fractures with lateral and posterior displacement, an anterior incision is made and any interposed soft tissues, such as periosteum or tendons, are extracted before the fracture is reduced. Even though reduction usually is stable, I generally use internal fixation through the metaphyseal fragment, avoiding fixation across the physis if possible.

Salter-Harris Type III and IV Fractures of the Distal Tibia

Treatment of nondisplaced Salter-Harris type III and IV fractures is the same as for nondisplaced type I and II fractures, with two modifications. First, after cast application I confirm the reduction of the fracture fragments with CT scanning. Second, these patients are examined more frequently (once a week) for the first 3 weeks after cast application to ensure that the fragments do not become displaced.

Generally, only truly nondisplaced Salter-Harris type III and IV fractures, or those with 1 mm or less of displacement, can be treated closed. Fractures with 2 mm or more of displacement require open reduction and internal fixation with anatomic alignment of the physis and fracture fragments.

For fractures with 2 mm or less of displacement, closed reduction is attempted in the operating room with the use of general anesthesia. After the extremity is prepared and draped, gentle longitudinal traction is applied to the foot, followed by eversion of the foot and direct digital pressure over the medial malleolus. If fluoroscopic examination confirms anatomic reduction, the fracture can be fixed with 2 percutaneous smooth wires placed in the epiphysis parallel to the physis. Cannulated screws can be inserted if the epiphysis is large enough. For a patients with fractures that are seen more than 7 days after injury, I have accepted up to 2 mm of displacement without attempting closed or open reduction (Fig. 26-49). Reliable patients whose fractures are fixed with screws can be immobilized in below-knee casts. Above-knee casts are used for all other patients.

Fractures with moderate displacement should be reduced, regardless of whether the fracture is acute or not. Closed reduction can be attempted, but these fractures usually require open reduction.

Open Reduction with Internal Fixation of Salter-Harris Type III or IV Fractures of the Distal Tibia

The patient is placed supine on an operating table that is radiolucent at the lower extremity. After exsanguination of the extremity and inflation of the tourniquet, a hockey stick incision is made, extending from approximately 4 cm above the ankle joint to 1 cm posterior to the tip of the medial malleolus. Alternatively, if more anterior exposure is required, a 4- to 6-cm transverse incision is made from the posterior aspect of the medial malleolus to the anterior aspect of the ankle. The saphenous vein is identified, dissected free, and retracted. The fracture site is identified, and an anteromedial capsulotomy of the ankle joint is performed. The arthrotomy is continuous with the fracture line and the traumatic disruption of periosteum and perichondral ring. The fracture surfaces are exposed and gently cleaned with irrigation and forceps (curettage is not used).

For Salter-Harris type IV fractures, the periosteum may be elevated several millimeters from the metaphyseal fracture edges. I prefer not to excise the metaphyseal portion of a Salter-Harris type IV fragment. The epiphyseal edges and joint surfaces are examined through the arthrotomy. The perichondral ring should not be elevated from the physis. For Salter-Harris type III fractures, the reduction is evaluated by checking the joint surface and epiphyseal fracture edges through the arthrotomy. The epiphyseal fragment is grasped with a small towel clip or reduction forceps, and the fracture is reduced. Internal fixation is inserted under direct vision and fluoroscopic control. It is important to view both the lateral and anteroposterior projections because of the curved shape of the distal tibial articular surface. If the fragment is large enough, 4-mm cannulated lag screws are inserted through the epiphyseal fragment (Fig. 26-50); if the fragment is too small for screws, smooth K-wires are used. The reduction and the position of the internal fixation are checked through the arthrotomy. In fractures with a significant Thurston-Holland fragment, a metaphyseal screw can be used if a gap exists after the epiphyseal screws are inserted. After reduction of the tibial fracture, the associated Salter-Harris type I or II fibular fracture usually reduces and is stable. If it is not, closed reduction and fixation with percutaneous oblique smooth K-wires are performed. The wound is closed using a subcuticular suture for the skin. A well-padded above-knee cast is applied.

The patient is kept non–weight-bearing for 3 weeks, and then the cast is changed to a below-knee walking cast, which

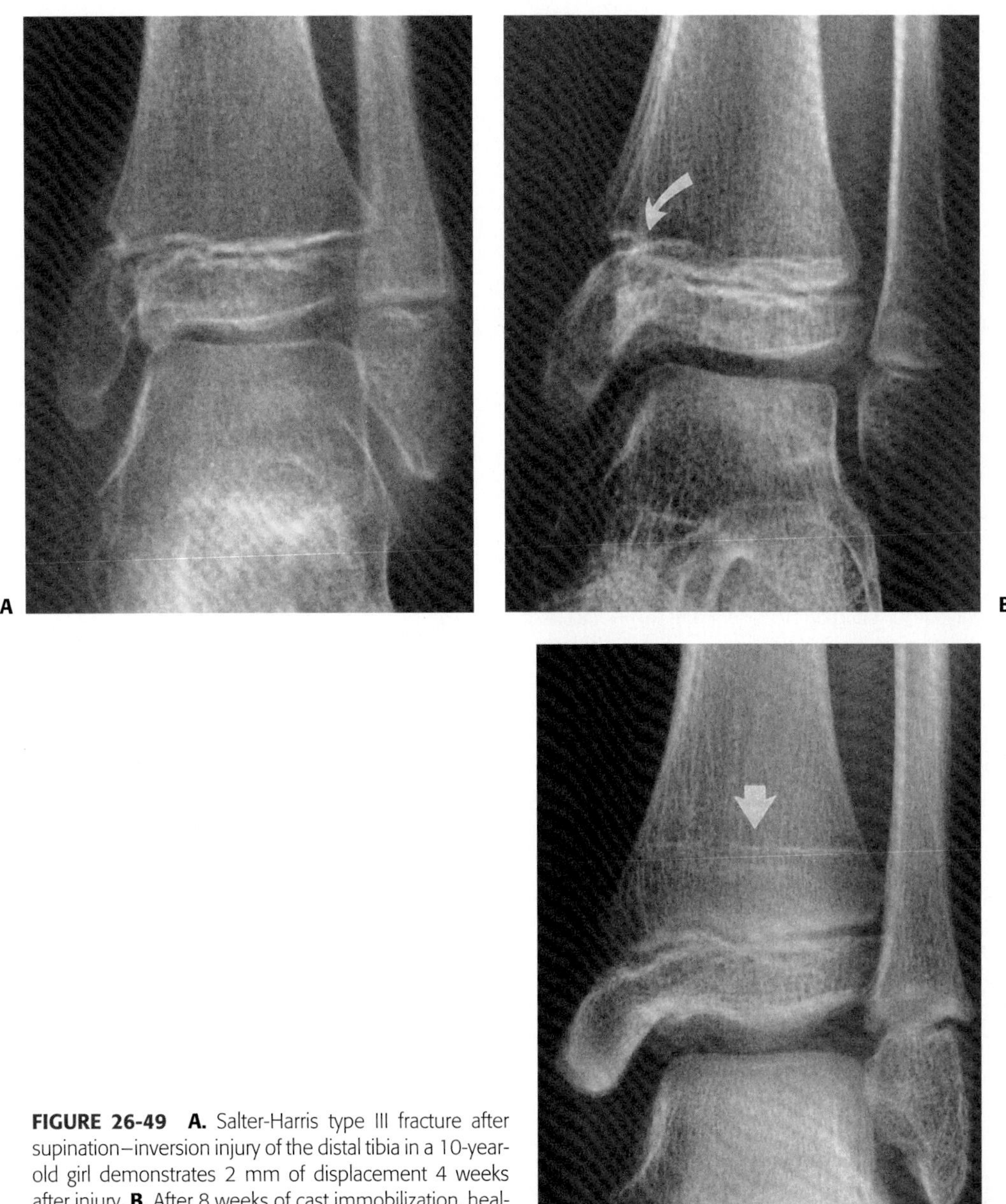

FIGURE 26-49 **A.** Salter-Harris type III fracture after supination–inversion injury of the distal tibia in a 10-year-old girl demonstrates 2 mm of displacement 4 weeks after injury. **B.** After 8 weeks of cast immobilization, healing is apparent but there is a suggestion of early physeal bar formation. **C.** Nine months later, growth is normal, as evidenced by the Park-Harris growth arrest line parallel to the physis.

is worn for an additional 3 weeks. Frequent follow-up evaluations (every 3 months for the first year and yearly thereafter) are necessary to detect growth abnormalities until skeletal maturity.

Juvenile Tillaux Fractures

For nondisplaced fractures and fractures displaced less than 2 mm, I prefer immobilization in an above-knee cast with the knee flexed 30 degrees and the foot internally rotated. If the position appears acceptable on plain films, CT scanning in the transverse plane with coronal and sagittal reconstructions is used to confirm acceptable reduction. For fractures with more than 2 mm of initial displacement, manipulation can be attempted by internal rotation of the foot and application of direct pressure over the anterolateral joint line. If reduction is not obtained with this maneuver, reduction can be attempted by dorsiflexing the pronated foot and then internally rotating the foot (132). If successful closed reduction is obtained in the operating room, percuta-

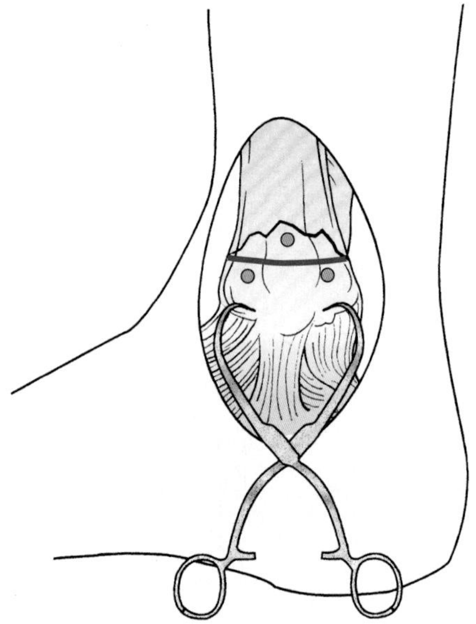

FIGURE 26-50 Technique for reduction of a Salter-Harris type IV fracture of the distal tibia.

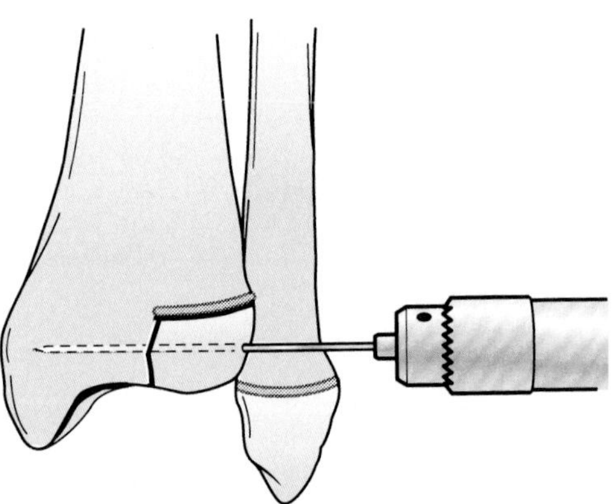

FIGURE 26-52 Advancement of pin after reduction of juvenile Tillaux fracture.

neous pins or screws are inserted and a short-leg cast is applied. If reduction is done outside the operating room and appears adequate, a long-leg cast with the knee flexed and the foot internally rotated is applied. A CT scan is then obtained to confirm adequate reduction of the fracture.

If closed reduction is unsuccessful but residual displacement is not severe, I occasionally insert 1 or 2 smooth pins into the Tillaux fragment under fluoroscopic control (Fig. 26-51) and use them to attempt to guide the fragment into proper position (Fig. 26-52). Cannulated screw guide pins may not be stiff enough for this purpose, and a larger pin may be required. If successful, the pins are advanced and 1 or 2 screws are inserted (Fig. 26-53). Because preservation of growth is not a concern, the screw does not have to be intraepiphyseal. If reduction is not successful, open reduction is done.

Open Reduction with Internal Fixation of Juvenile Tillaux Fractures

The patient is placed supine on an operating table that is radiolucent at the lower extremity. After the extremity is prepared and draped, it is exsanguinated. The location of the fracture line is determined with intraoperative fluoroscopy, and a 2- to 3-cm incision is made directly over it. Care is taken to avoid the superficial peroneal nerve. Dissection is carried down to the fracture site. Interposed soft tissue is extracted, and the fracture surfaces are cleaned. The fracture gap then usually can be closed by direct pressure on the Tillaux fragment. If more exposure is required, the incision can be extended distally, curving it under the tip of the

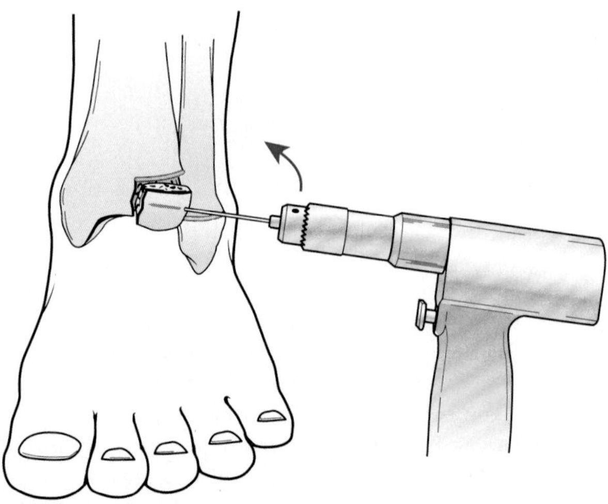

FIGURE 26-51 Technique of placement of percutaneous pins for manipulation of a juvenile Tillaux fracture.

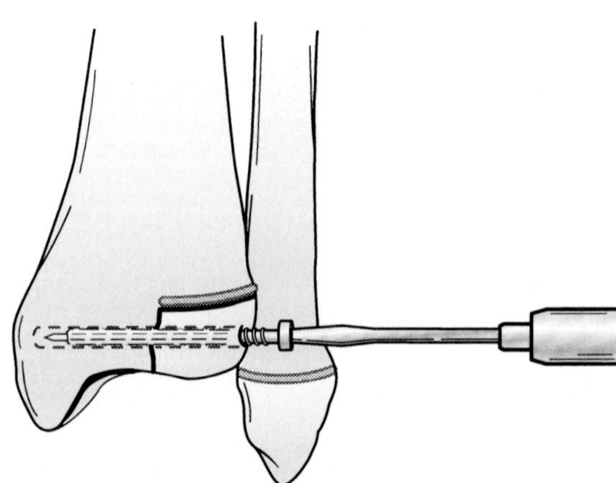

FIGURE 26-53 Percutaneous insertion of 4-mm cannulated screw over pin that has been advanced into the medial distal tibia after reduction of the juvenile Tillaux fracture fragment.

fibula. After the fracture is reduced, the articular surface is inspected through a capsulotomy incision. Once satisfactory reduction is confirmed, fixation is obtained by placing a 4-mm cannulated screw across the fracture site (Fig. 26-54). The wound is closed with a subcuticular suture and a well-padded short-leg cast is applied. The patient is kept non-weight-bearing for 3 weeks, at which time a short-leg walking cast is applied and worn for an additional 3 weeks.

Triplane Fractures

For nondisplaced or minimally displaced (<2 mm) fractures, I prefer immobilization in a long-leg cast with the knee flexed 30 to 40 degrees. The position of the foot is determined by whether the fracture is lateral (internal rotation) or medial (eversion). A CT scan is obtained immediately after casting to document adequate reduction. A CT scan is obtained approximately 7 days after cast application to verify that displacement has not recurred. At 3 to 4 weeks, the cast is changed to a below-knee walking cast, which is worn another 3 to 4 weeks.

For fractures with more than 2 mm of displacement, I usually attempt closed reduction with sedation in the emergency department. An above-knee cast is applied. If plain x-rays show satisfactory reduction, a CT scan is obtained. If

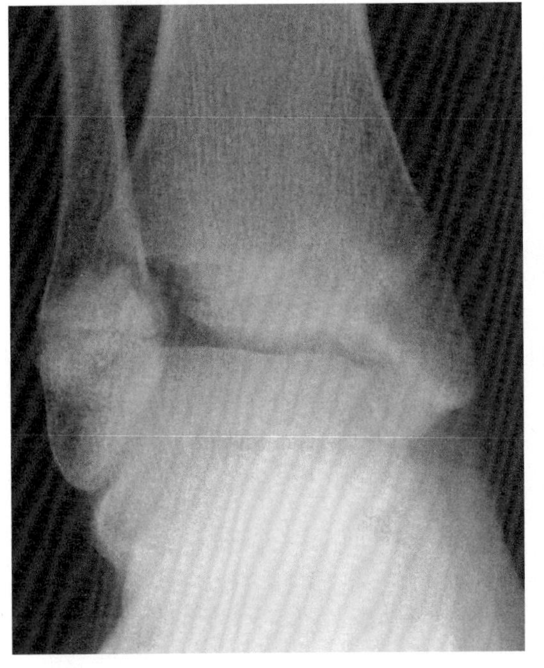

A

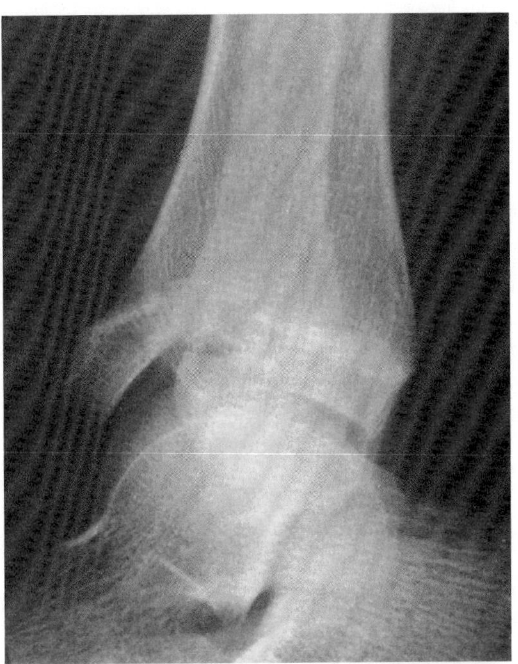

B

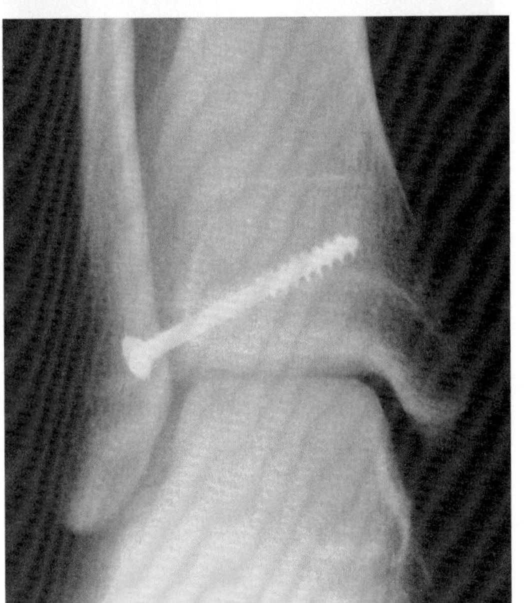

C

FIGURE 26-54 A,B. Displaced juvenile Tillaux fracture. Closed reduction was not successful. **C.** After open reduction with internal fixation with a small fragment screw.

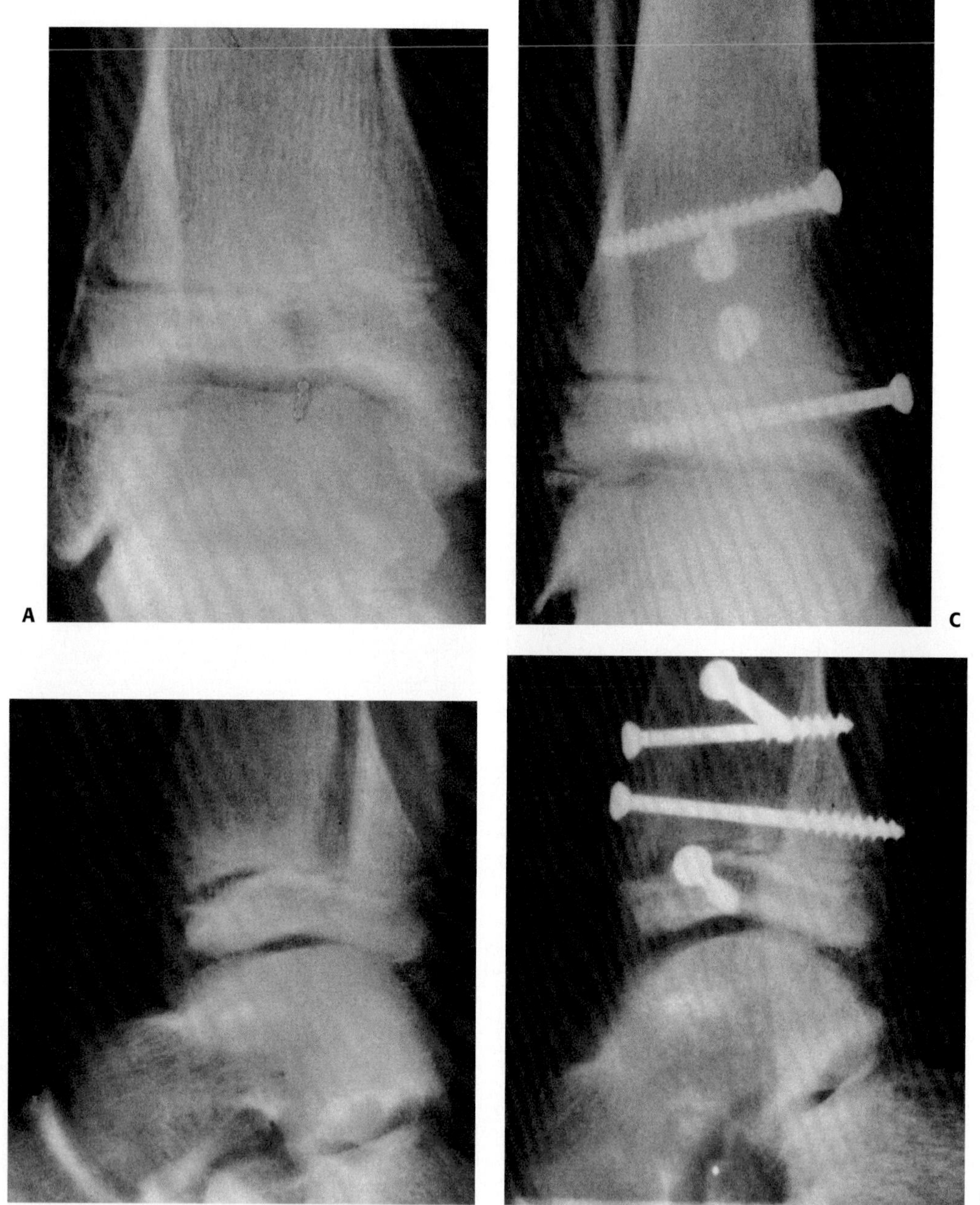

FIGURE 26-55 **A,B.** Irreducible three-part triplane fracture in a 13-year-old girl. **C,D.** After open reduction with internal fixation. Note anterior-to-posterior and medial-to-lateral screw placement that avoids the physis.

reduction is acceptable, treatment is the same as for nondisplaced fractures. If the reduction is unacceptable, closed reduction is attempted in the operating room with the use of general anesthesia. If fluoroscopy shows an acceptable reduction, percutaneous screws are inserted, avoiding the physis, and a short-leg cast is applied. If closed reduction is unacceptable, open reduction is performed. Preoperative CT scanning may be helpful for evaluating the position of the fracture fragments in the anteroposterior and lateral planes and for determining the appropriate skin incisions.

Open Reduction of Triplane Fracture

The patient is placed supine on a radiolucent operating table with padded elevation behind the hip on the affected side. The surgical approach depends on the fracture anatomy as determined by the preoperative CT scan. I prefer to approach a two-part medial triplane fracture through a hockey stick anteromedial incision. The fracture fragments are irrigated to remove debris, and any interposed periosteum is removed. The fracture is reduced, and reduction is confirmed by direct observation through an anteromedial arthrotomy and by fluoroscopic examination. Two 4-mm cancellous screws are inserted from medial to lateral or from anterior to posterior or both, depending on the fracture pattern (Fig. 26-55). Anterior-to-posterior screw placement may require an additional anterolateral incision, or the screws may be inserted percutaneously.

For two-part lateral triplane fractures, I prefer a hockey stick anterolateral approach. The fracture is reduced and stabilized with two screws placed from lateral to medial or from anterior to posterior or both, and reduction is confirmed through direct observation and by fluoroscopic examination. Fractures with three or more parts may occasionally require more exposure for reduction and internal fixation. If the fibula is fractured, posterior exposure of the tibial fracture can be readily obtained by detaching the anterior and posterior inferior tibiofibular ligaments and turning down the distal fibula on the lateral collateral ligament (Fig. 26-56). If the fibula is not fractured, a fibular osteotomy can be done. Careful dissection is necessary to avoid iatrogenic fractures through the physis of the fibula. Medial exposure is obtained through an anteromedial or posteromedial incision. Reduction and internal fixation are performed in a stepwise fashion. For typical three-part fractures, I prefer to reduce the Salter-Harris type II fracture first and provisionally fix it to the distal tibia through the metaphyseal fragment. Usually, the Salter-Harris type III fragment can then be reduced and provisionally fixed to the stabilized type II fragment (Fig. 26-57). Occasionally, the order of reduction and fixation should be reversed. Fractures with four or more fragments require additional steps, but I have found it easier to fix the Salter-Harris type II or IV fragment through the metaphysis to the distal tibia before attaching the Salter-Harris type III fragment or fragments (Fig. 26-58). After reduction, reliable patients can be treated with immobilization in a short-leg cast for 6 to 8 weeks, with weight-bearing allowed at 3 to 4 weeks.

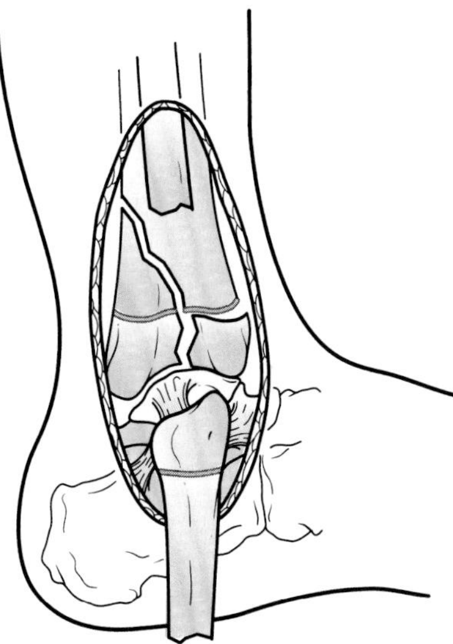

FIGURE 26-56 Transfibular approach to a complex lateral triplane fracture.

Pearls and Pitfalls: Open Reduction with Internal Fixation of Physeal Ankle Fractures

Soft Tissue Healing Problems

Under ideal circumstances, open reduction with internal fixation of ankle fractures is best done before excessive swelling occurs. Markedly swollen ankles often develop fracture blisters, which may become infected. The integrity of skin closure and, even more important, the vascularity of the wound edges also are threatened by excessive soft tissue swelling. When marked soft tissue swelling develops before surgery can be performed, elevation of the extremity in a soft compression bandage until swelling begins to subside is recommended.

Partially Healed or Comminuted Physis

On occasion, inspection of the fractured fragments at the time of open reduction and internal fixation reveals comminution at the physeal line. In such cases, debridement of loose fragments back to normal-appearing physis and the insertion of a fat graft into the resulting void are recommended. This technique also can be useful for fractures that present for treatment a week or more after injury. Early callus that prevents the apposition of healthy physeal tissue at the fracture site is debrided and a fat graft is inserted (Fig. 26-59).

Fibular Fractures

I usually treat nondisplaced fibular physeal fractures with immobilization in a below-knee walking cast for 3 to 4 weeks. I

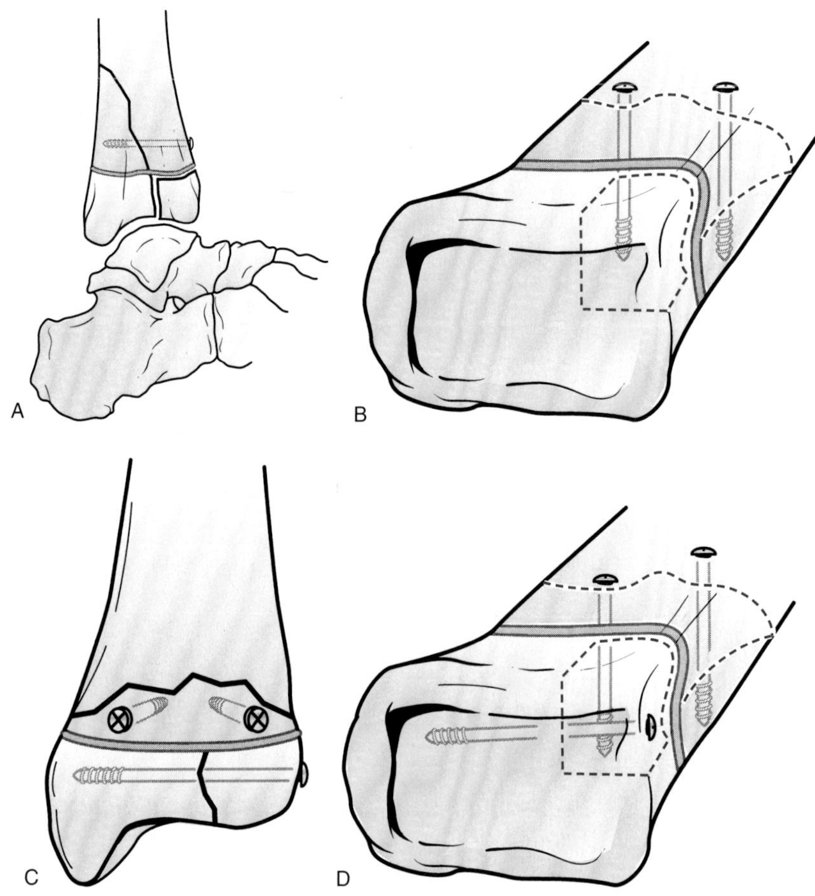

FIGURE 26-57 Open reduction with internal fixation of a three-part lateral triplane fracture. **A,B.** Reduction and fixation of the Salter-Harris type II fragment to the metaphysis. **C,D.** Reduction and internal fixation of the Salter-Harris type III fragment to the Salter-Harris type II fragment.

have attempted closed reduction of displaced Salter-Harris types I and II fibular fractures, but when reduction was unsuccessful, I have accepted up to 50% displacement without problems at long-term follow-up (Fig. 26-60). Dias (41), however, reported a patient with a symptomatic spike that required excision after inadequate reduction. I have not found open reduction of isolated physeal fibular fractures necessary but would not hesitate to perform open reduction of a displaced Salter-Harris type III or IV fracture if necessary.

Lateral Ankle Sprains

It is my opinion that the diagnosis of an acute ankle sprain in a child with an open fibular physis is reasonable when the child has tenderness well localized to the tip of the fibula or over the anterior talofibular ligament with little or no tenderness over the open fibular physis. The presence on an otherwise normal x-ray of an avulsion fracture of either the tip of the fibula or the lateral aspect of the talus also is consistent with this diagnosis. When routine views fail to demonstrate such avulsion fractures, the views described by Haraguchi et al may be helpful (53).

Because chronic pain and instability do not always complicate such injuries, I treat these injuries nonoperatively when they are seen acutely. Patients who have persistent complaints after adequate rehabilitation are treated with excision of any ununited fragments and Broström reconstruction as necessary. Letts et al (133) also reported satisfactory results in this age-group with nonanatomic reconstructions (Evans, Watson-Jones, Chrisman, and Snook).

REHABILITATION

For patients treated with cast immobilization, quadriceps, hamstring, and abductor exercises are begun as soon as pain and swelling allow. Usually a below-knee cast is worn during the last 2 to 3 weeks of immobilization, and weight-bearing to tolerance is allowed during this time. After immobilization is discontinued, ankle range-of-motion exercises and strengthening exercises are begun. Protective splinting or bracing usually is not required after cast removal. Running is restricted until the patient demonstrates an essentially full, painless range of ankle and foot motion and can walk without a limp.

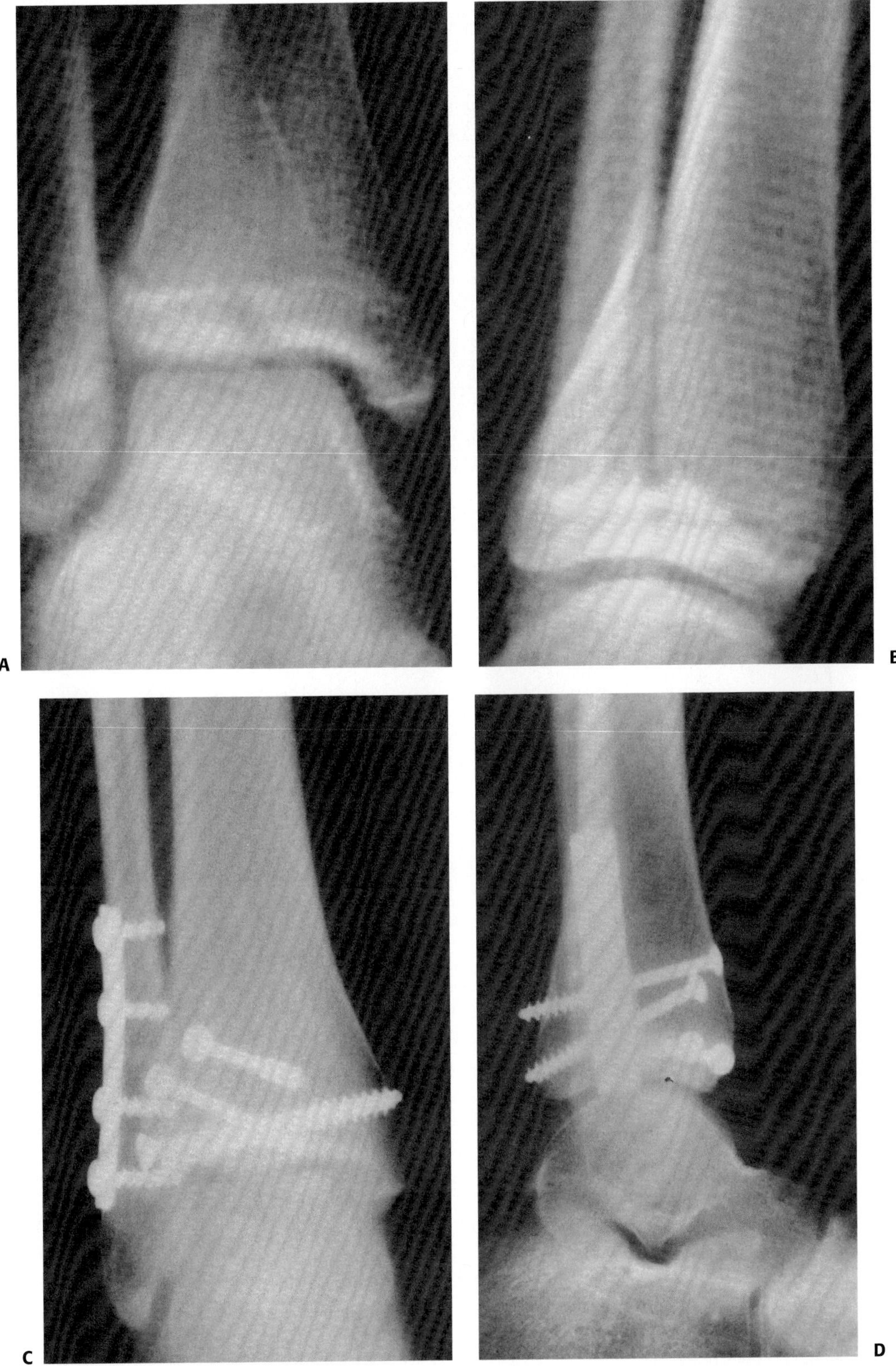

FIGURE 26-58 **A,B.** Irreducible three-part lateral triplane fracture in a 14-year-old boy. **C, D.** After open reduction through a transfibular approach and internal fixation with anterior-to-posterior and lateral-to-medial screws.

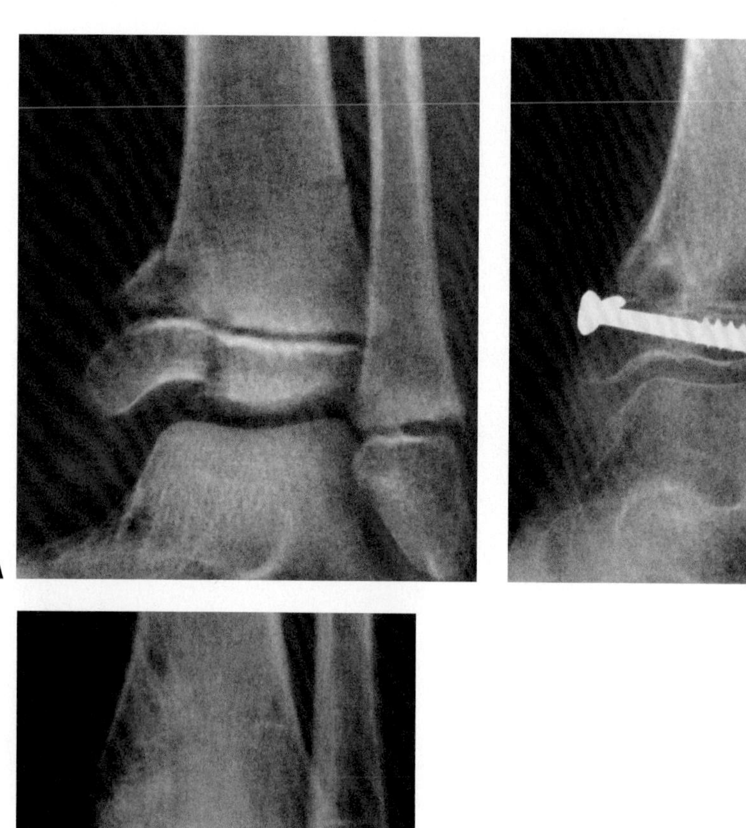

FIGURE 26-59 **A.** Eight-year-old girl who presented 10 days after a displaced Salter-Harris type IV fracture of the distal tibia. **B.** At open reduction, comminution of the physis was noted. The physis was debrided, and a fat graft was inserted before reduction and internal fixation of the fracture. **C.** Three years after injury there is no evidence of physeal bar formation or growth abnormality.

Running progresses from jogging to more strenuous running and jumping as soreness and endurance dictate. For athletes, unrestricted running and jumping ability should be achieved before return to sports. Patients should be able to hop on the injured side equal to the noninjured side. Protective measures such as taping or bracing are recommended initially for return to most sports.

Most patients with physeal ankle fractures recover quickly and require little or no formal physical therapy. For this reason, and because of compliance considerations, fractures treated with internal fixation are usually protected with below-knee casting instead of starting an early range-of-motion program in a removable splint.

Reflex sympathetic dystrophy occasionally develops after these injuries and is treated initially with an intensive formal physical therapy regimen that encourages range of motion and weight-bearing (134). For patients who do not respond quickly to such a program, I have had good success with a brief hospital admission for physical therapy in association with continuous epidural analgesia.

PROGNOSIS AND COMPLICATIONS

Delayed Union and Nonunion

Delayed union and nonunion are rare after distal tibial physeal fractures (Fig. 26-61). Dias (41) reported one patient with a

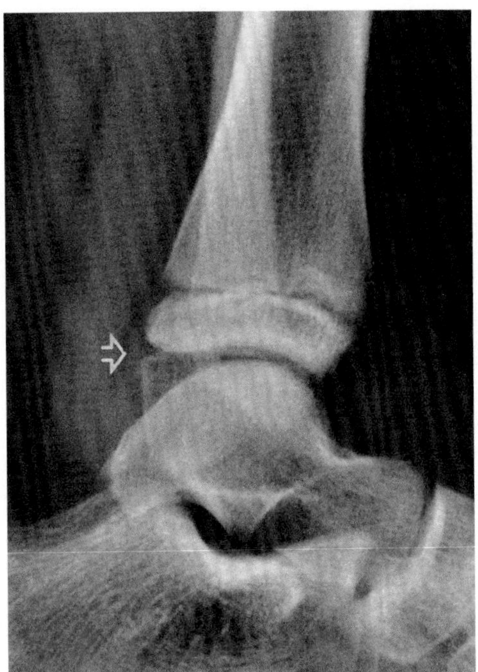

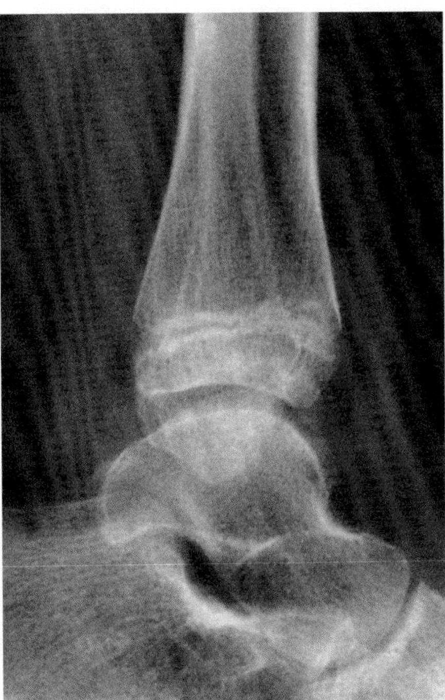

FIGURE 26-60 **A.** Lateral x-ray of a 13-year-old girl who was seen 7 days after an inversion sprain of the ankle; the Salter-Harris type I fracture of the distal fibula is displaced 50%. Closed reduction was unsuccessful. **B.** Six months after injury, remodeling is complete at the fracture site and the patient is asymptomatic.

delayed union and one patient with a previous physeal bar excision who had a nonunion that healed after open reduction, internal fixation, and bone grafting. Siffert and Arkin (135) reported nonunion in a patient with osteonecrosis of the distal tibial epiphysis. I have seen two younger patients with Salter-Harris type III fractures that appeared to be progressing to nonunion. Because neither patient had any complaints of pain or any evidence of progressive displacement of the fracture and stress views showed no instability, no treatment was undertaken. Both fractures eventually united (Fig. 26-62). I have seen one patient with a nonunion after open reduction with internal fixation in whom pin fixation and cast immobilization were discontinued prematurely. The fracture healed after repeat open reduction with internal fixation.

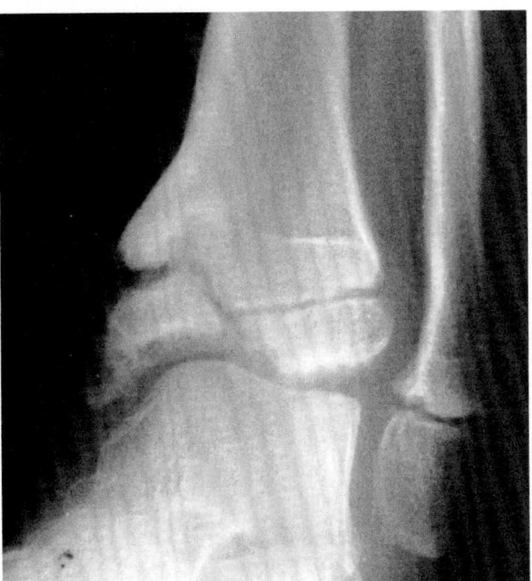

FIGURE 26-61 Complex nonunion of a Salter-Harris type III fracture of the medial malleolus in an 8-year-old boy. Note that the distal tibial epiphysis is in valgus, whereas the talus is in varus. (Courtesy Brent Broztman, MD.)

Deformity Secondary to Malunion

Rotational malunion usually occurs after triplane fractures that are either incompletely reduced or are initially immobilized in below-knee casts. Rotational malunion can also occur after Salter-Harris I and II fractures. In Phan et al's study of 23 patients with Salter-Harris I and II fractures (12), footprint analysis revealed 14 with an external rotation deformity relative to the uninjured side.

Derotational osteotomy can be used for malunited extraarticular fractures if discomfort and stiffness occur. Guille et al (136) reported a rotational malunion of a lateral malleolar fracture that led to a stress fracture of the distal fibula that went on to

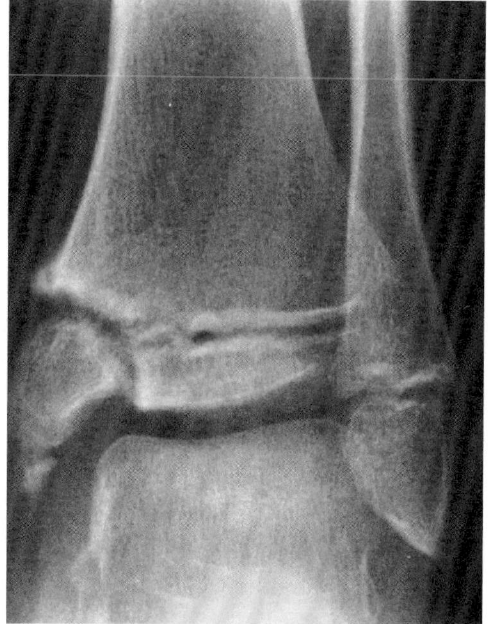
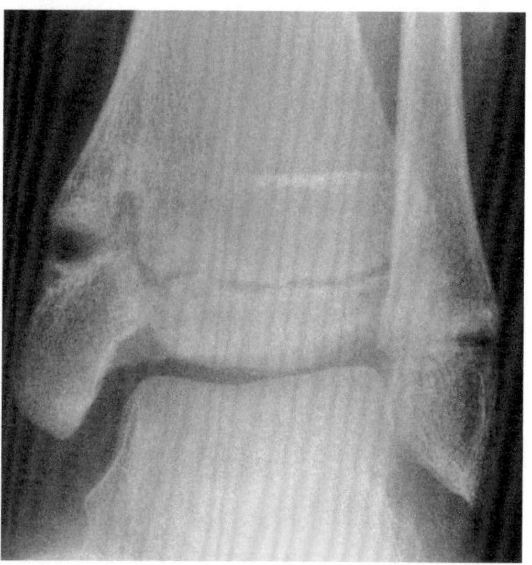

FIGURE 26-62 Nonunion and delayed union. **A.** Ten-year-old girl with incomplete healing of a supination–inversion Salter-Harris type III fracture of the distal tibia after 12 weeks of cast immobilization. **B.** Sixteen months after injury, the fracture united without further immobilization; no physeal bar formation or growth abnormality has occurred.

delayed union. Their patient required correction of the malrotated distal fibula and bone grafting of the delayed union site.

Anterior angulation or plantarflexion deformity usually occurs after supination–plantarflexion Salter-Harris type II fractures. Theoretically, an equinus deformity might occur if the angulation exceeds the range of ankle dorsiflexion before fracture, but this is rare, probably because the deformity is in the plane of joint motion and tends to remodel with growth.

Valgus deformity is most common after external rotation Salter-Harris type II fractures. The degree to which the deformity may spontaneously resolve or remodel with growth is controversial. Caruthers and Crenshaw (19) reported resolution of a 12-degree valgus deformity in a 13½-year-old boy, but Spiegel et al (11) reported persistent residual deformity in a significant number of their patients (Fig. 26-63). Varus deformity most often results from growth abnormality and infrequently is the result of simple malunion.

If significant angular deformity persists at the completion of growth, supramalleolar osteotomy should be performed. Moon et al (137) followed nine children with post-traumatic varus deformities of the ankle secondary to supination inversion injuries. These patients developed medial subluxation of their ankles with associated internal rotational deformity. Takakura et al (138) described successful opening wedge osteotomy for varus deformity in nine patients. Scheffer and Peterson (139) recommended opening wedge osteotomy if angular deformity is 25 degrees or less and limb length discrepancy is or will be 25 mm or less at maturity. Preoperative planning should include templating the

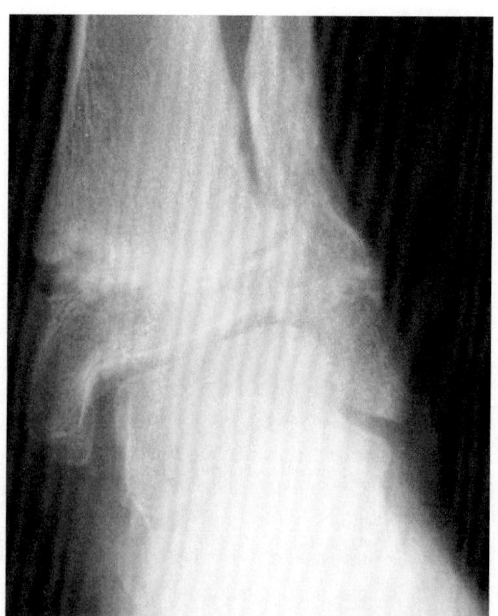

FIGURE 26-63 X-ray of a 14-year-old boy, 4 months after pronation–eversion–external rotation injury, reveals 16 degrees of valgus angulation.

various types of osteotomies to determine which technique will maintain the proper mechanical alignment of the tibia and ankle joint and will not make the malleoli unduly prominent. The effectiveness of intra-articular osteotomy for malunion of intraarticular fractures is not well established (Fig. 26-64).

Growth Arrest

Deformity caused by growth arrest usually occurs after Salter-Harris type III and IV fractures in which a physeal bar develops at the fracture site, leading to varus deformity that progresses with continued growth. Spiegel et al (11) reported growth problems in 9 of 66 patients with Salter-Harris type II fractures.

Earlier reports (19,140) attributed the development of physeal bars to crushing of the physis at the time of injury. More recent reports (20,100) claim that with anatomic reduction (open reduction with internal fixation if needed), the incidence of physeal bar formation can be decreased. For example, Kling et al (20) reported physeal bars in two of five patients treated nonoperatively and in none of three patients treated operatively in children 10 years of age and younger. The validity of this claim is difficult to determine from published reports. One problem is the small numbers of patients in all series and the even smaller numbers within each group in each series. Another problem is the age of the patients in operative and nonoperative groups in the various series; for example, many children reported to do well with a particular treatment method had so little growth remaining that treatment may have had little or no effect on growth.

Hasler and von Laer (141) found a 20% incidence of growth abnormalities after anatomic open reduction with internal fixation of distal tibial physeal fractures. This supports the conclusion of Cass and Peterson (142), Ogden (28), and others that growth problems after these injuries may not always be prevented by open reduction with internal fixation. Open reduction of displaced Salter-Harris type III and IV ankle fractures would seem advisable to restore joint congruity, regardless of whether growth potential can be preserved.

Harris growth lines have been reported to be reliable predictors of growth abnormality (1), but I have found that although lines parallel to the physis are reliable, lines that appear to diverge from the physis may be misleading (Fig. 26-65). Harcke et al reported early detection of growth arrest with bone scanning techniques (143).

Spontaneous resolution of distal tibial physeal bars has been reported (144,145), but is rare. Most patients require excision of bony bars and may require correction of significant angular deformity with osteotomy (Fig. 26-66). If bar resection is not advisable, osteotomy should be delayed until the remaining physis ceases to grow. The evaluation and treatment of physeal bars, angular deformity, and leg-length discrepancy are discussed in Chapter 5.

Karrholm et al (146) reported progressive ankle deformity caused by complete growth arrest of the distal fibula with normal growth of the tibia (Fig. 26-67). They found that continued fibular growth with complete arrest of tibial growth usually was compensated by proximal migration of the fibula so that varus deformity did not occur.

Because the amount of growth remaining in the distal tibial physis is small (approximately 0.25 inch per year) in most older patients with these injuries, the amount of leg length discrepancy resulting from complete growth arrest tends to be relatively small. Treatment may be required if the anticipated discrepancy is projected to be clinically significant.

Arthritis

Epiphyseal ankle fractures that do not extend into the joint have a low risk of post-traumatic arthritis, but injuries that extend into the joint may produce this complication. Caterini et al (81) found that 8 of 68 (12%) patients had pain and stiffness that began 5 to 8 years after skeletal maturity. Ertl et al (147) found that 18 to 36 months after injury 20 patients with triplane fractures were asymptomatic, but at 36 months to 13 years after injury only 8 of 15 patients evaluated were asymptomatic.

Ramsey and Hamilton (148) demonstrated in a cadaver study that 1 mm of lateral talar displacement decreases tibiotalar contact area by 42%, which greatly increases the stress on this weight-bearing joint. More recently, Michelson et al (149) reported that a cadaver study using unconstrained specimens suggested that some lateral talar displacement occurs with normal weight-bearing. Because of their findings, they questioned the current criterion of 2 mm of displacement for unstable ankle fractures. However, the results of Ramsey and Hamilton's study correlate well with other studies that have shown increased symptoms in patients in whom more than 2 mm of displacement was accepted (81,144,147).

Some investigators have suggested that the presence of transepiphyseal screws increases joint contact pressure. Charlton et al (150) confirmed this phenomenon in a cadaver. They found that removal of the screws led to a return of contact pressures to control levels. Their study suggests that removal of transepiphyseal screws after fracture healing might reduce the incidence of post-traumatic arthritis.

Osteonecrosis of the Distal Tibial Epiphysis

Siffert and Arkin (135), in 1950, were the first to call attention to this complication of distal tibial fractures. In their patient, the combination of nonunion of a medial malleolar fracture and osteonecrosis caused pain that required an arthrodesis 14 months after injury. Dias (41) reported a patient with this complication who did not require arthrodesis but who had a significant leg length discrepancy that required epiphysiodesis of the contralateral tibia. I have seen one patient with this complication. The patient had significant joint stiffness and developed a valgus deformity secondary to collapse. After revascularization of the epiphysis, the ankle was realigned with a supramalleolar osteotomy, and 5 years later the patient had satisfactory function without pain.

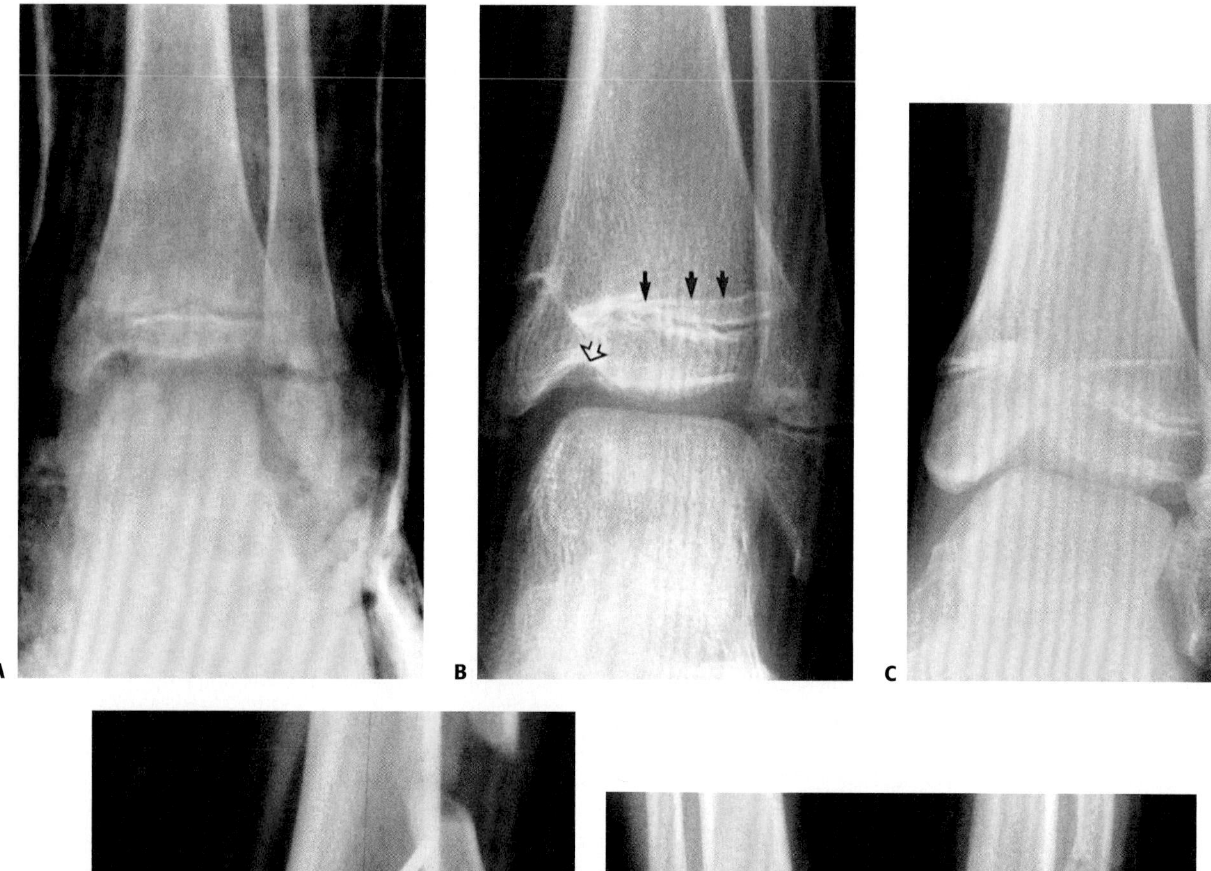

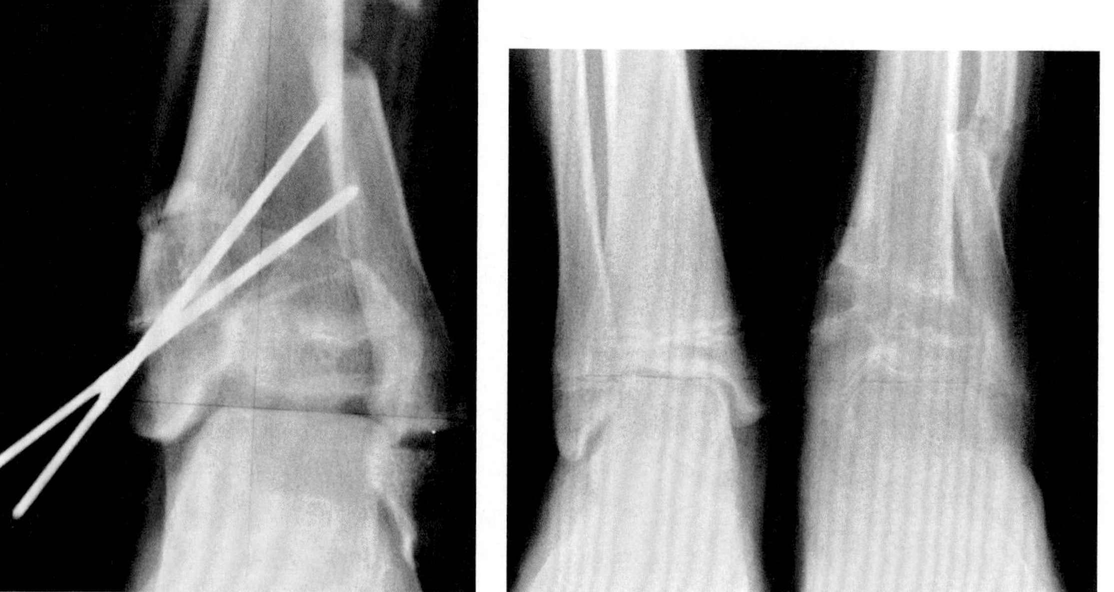

FIGURE 26-64 **A.** This apparently nondisplaced medial malleolar fracture in an 11-year-old boy was treated with immobilization in a long leg cast. **B.** Fourteen months after injury, there is a clear medial osseous bridge and asymmetric growth of the Park-Harris growth arrest lines (*black arrows*). Note the early inhibition of growth on the subchondral surface of the fracture (*open arrow*). **C.** Five years after injury, the varus deformity has increased significantly and fibular overgrowth is apparent. **D.** The deformity was treated with a medial opening-wedge osteotomy of the tibia, an osteotomy of the fibula, and epiphysiodesis of the most lateral portion of the tibial physis and fibula. **E.** Three months after surgery, the osteotomies are healed and the varus deformity is corrected; the joint surface remains irregular. (Courtesy Earl A. Stanley, Jr., MD.)

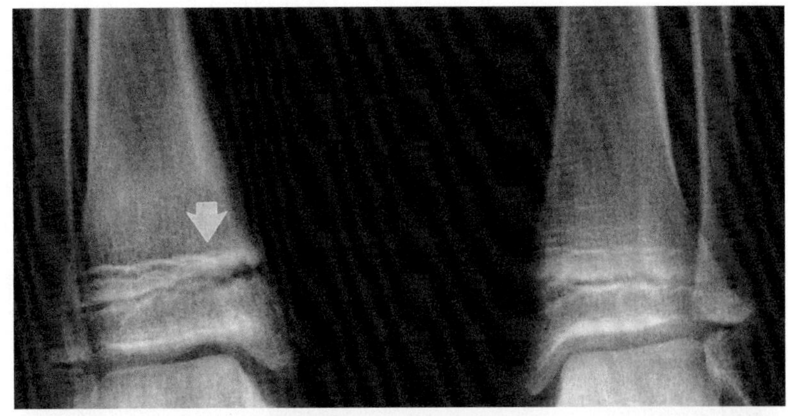

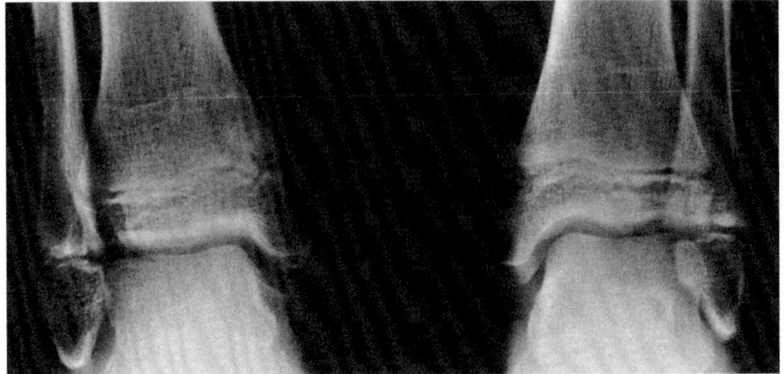

FIGURE 26-65 **A.** Six months after cast immobilization of a nondisplaced supination–inversion Salter-Harris type III fracture of the right distal tibia in an 8-year-old boy. The Park-Harris growth arrest line (*arrow*) appears to end in the physis medially and diverge from the physis laterally. **B.** Two years later, no physeal bar is present and growth is normal.

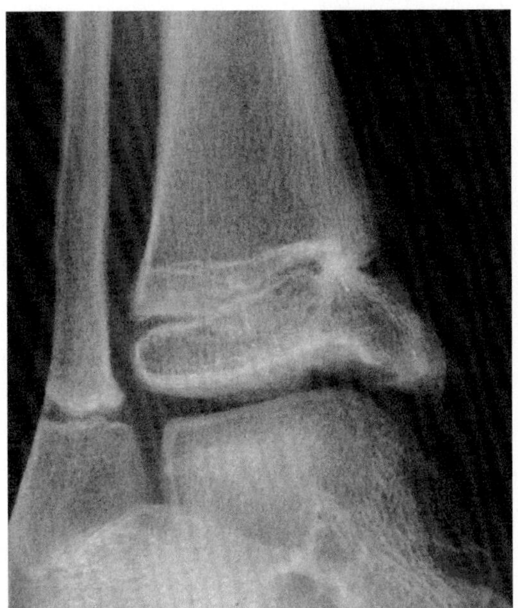

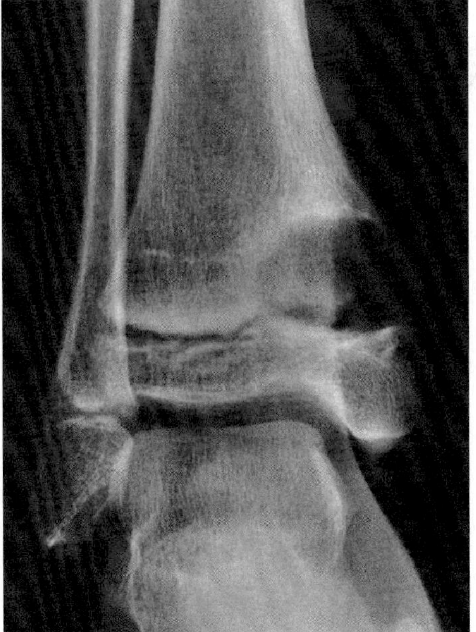

FIGURE 26-66 **A.** One year after open reduction and internal fixation of a Salter-Harris type III fracture of the distal tibia in a 7-year-old boy, varus deformity has been caused by a physeal bar. **B.** Two years after excision of the physeal bar and insertion of cranioplast, satisfactory growth has resumed and the deformity has resolved.

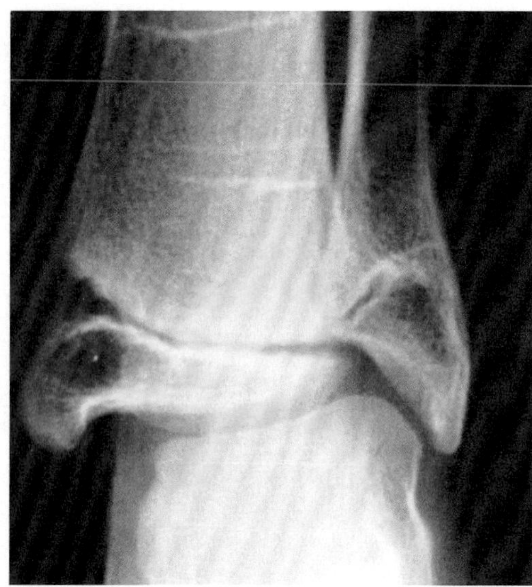

FIGURE 26-67 Valgus deformity of the ankle, lateral displacement of the talus with widening of the joint medially, and severe shortening of the fibula after early physeal arrest in a child who sustained an ankle injury at 6 years of age. (Courtesy James Roach, MD.)

Compartment Syndrome

Yeap et al (151) reported compartment syndrome involving the calf and foot secondary to distal tibial and fibular physeal fractures in a 14-year-old boy.

CONTROVERSIES AND FUTURE DIRECTIONS

Controversy still exists as to optimal diagnostic and treatment methods for physeal ankle fractures. The usefulness of the Ottawa Ankle Rules for children and the place of MRI in the evaluation of acute fractures are still debated. Periosteal interposition between fractured fragments in Salter-Harris I and II fractures does seem to increase the risk of premature physeal closure, but a large series of operatively treated Salter-Harris I and II fractures showing decreased rates of premature physeal closure after open reduction and extraction of interposed periosteum has not been reported.

It is hoped that future technologic innovations will improve our ability to identify patients who will develop premature physeal closure and modify their initial treatment so as to avoid growth problems. Various organizations are now committed to injury prevention. Although these injuries cannot be entirely eliminated, hopefully such efforts will decrease their number and severity.

REFERENCES

1. Hynes D, O'Brien T. Growth disturbance lines after injury of the distal tibial physis. *J Bone Joint Surg Br* 1988;70:231–233.
2. Peterson H, Modhok R, Benson J, et al. Physeal fractures. I. Epidemiology in Olmsted County, Minnesota, 1979–1988. *J Pediatr Orthop* 1994;14:423–430.
3. Mann DC, Rajmaira S. Distribution of physeal and nonphyseal fractures in 2,650 long-bone fractures in children aged 0–16 years. *J Pediatr Orthop* 1990;10:713–716.
4. Goldberg VM, Aadalen R. Distal tibial epiphyseal injuries: the role of athletics in fifty-three cases. *Am J Sports Med* 1978;6:263–268.
5. Zaricznyj B, Shattuck LJM, Mast TA, et al. Sports-related injuries in school age children. *Am J Sports Med* 1980;8:318–324.
6. Nilsson S, Roaas A. Soccer injuries in adolescents. *Am J Sports Med* 1978;6:358–361.
7. Orava S, Saarela J. Exertion injuries to young athletes: a follow-up research of orthopaedic problems of young track and field athletes. *Am J Sports Med* 1978;6:68–74.
8. Sullivan JA, Gross RH, Grana WA, et al. Evaluation of injuries in youth soccer. *Am J Sports Med* 1980;8:325–327.
9. Damore DT, Metzl JD, Ramundo M, et al. Patterns in childhood sports injury. *Pediatr Emerg Care* 2003;19:65–67.
10. Nguyen D, Letts M. In-line skating injuries in children: a 10-year review. *J Pediatr Orthop* 2001;21:613–618.
11. Spiegel P, Cooperman D, Laros G. Epiphyseal fractures of the distal ends of the tibia and fibula. *J Bone Joint Surg Am* 1978;60:1046–1050.
12. Phan VC, Wroten E, Yngve DA. Foot progression angle after distal tibial physeal fractures. *J Pediatr Orthop* 2002;22:31–35.
13. Foucher J. De la divulsion des epiphyses. *Cong Med France* 1867;1:63 (reprinted in English in *Clin Orthop* 1984;188:3–9).
14. Poland J. *Traumatic Separation of the Epiphysis.* London: Smith, Elder & Co, 1898.
15. Ashhurst APC, Bromer RS. Classification and mechanism of fractures of the leg bones involving the ankle. *Arch Surg* 1922;4:51–129.
16. Bishop PA. Fractures and epiphyseal separation fractures of the ankle. *Am J Roentgenol* 1932;28:49–67.
17. Aitken AP. The end results of the fractured distal tibial epiphysis. *J Bone Joint Surg* 1936;18:685–691.
18. McFarland B. Traumatic arrest of epiphyseal growth at the lower end of the tibia. *Br J Surg* 1931;19:78–82.
19. Caruthers CO, Crenshaw AH. Clinical significance of a classification of epiphyseal injuries at the ankle. *Am J Surg* 1955;89:879–889.
20. Kling T, Bright R, Hensinger R. Distal tibial physeal fractures in children that may require open reduction. *J Bone Joint Surg Am* 1984;66:647–657.
21. Kleiger B, Mankin HJ. Fractures of the lateral portion of the distal tibial epiphysis. *J Bone Joint Surg Am* 1964;46:25–32.
22. Marmor L. An unusual fracture of the tibial epiphysis. COOR 1970;73:132–135.
23. Cooperman DR, Spiegel PG, Laros GS. Tibial fractures involving the ankle in children: the so-called triplane epiphyseal fracture. *J Bone Joint Surg Am* 1978;60:1040–1046.
24. Karrholm J, Hansson LI, Laurin S. Computed tomography of intraarticular supination-eversion fractures of the ankle in adolescents. *J Pediatr Orthop* 1981;1:181–187.
25. Denton JR, Fischer SJ. The medial triplane fracture: report of an unusual injury. *J Trauma* 1981;21:991–995.
26. Letts M, Davidson D, McCaffrey M. The adolescent pilon fracture: management and outcome. *J Pediatr Orthop* 2001;21:2026.
27. Cummings RJ, Hahn GA. The incisural fracture: a case report. *Foot Ankle Int* 2004;25: 132–135.
28. Ogden JA. *Skeletal Injury in the Child.* Philadelphia: Lea & Febiger, 1982.
29. Peterson HA. Physeal fractures. III. Classification. *J Pediatr Orthop* 1994;14:439–448.
30. Salter RB. Injuries of the ankle in children. *Orthop Clin North Am* 1974;5:147–152.
31. Lauge-Hansen N. Fractures of the ankle. II. *Arch Surg* 1950;60:957–985.
32. Karrholm J, Hansson LI, Laurin S. Supination–eversion injuries of the ankle in children: a retrospective study of radiographic classification and treatment. *J Pediatr Orthop* 1982; 2:147–159.
33. Karrholm J, Hansson LI, Laurin S. Pronation injuries of the ankle in children. *Acta Orthop Scand* 1983;54:1–17.
34. Stiell IG, Greenberg GH, McKnight RD, et al. A study to develop clinical decision rules for the use of radiography in acute ankle injuries. *Ann Emerg Med* 1992;21:384–390.
35. Thomsen NO, Overgaard S, Olsen LH, et al. Observer variation in the radiographic classification of ankle fractures. *J Bone Joint Surg Br* 1991;73:676–678.
36. Burstein AH. Editorial: Fracture classification systems: do they work and are they useful? *J Bone Joint Surg Am* 1993;75:1743–1744.
37. Vahvanen V, Aalto K. Classification of ankle fractures in children. *Arch Orthop Trauma Surg* 1980;97:1–5.
38. Dias LS, Tachdjian MO. Physeal injuries of the ankle in children. *Clin Orthop* 1978; 136:230–233.
39. Tachdjian MO. *The Child's Foot.* Philadelphia: WB Saunders, 1985.
40. Lynn MD. The triplane distal tibial epiphyseal fracture. *COOR* 1972;86:187–190.
41. Dias L. Fractures of the tibia and fibula. In: Rockwood CA, Wilkins KE, King RE, eds. *Fractures in children,* 3rd ed. Philadelphia: JB Lippincott, 1991:1271–1381.
42. Dias L, Giegerich C. Fractures of the distal tibial epiphysis in adolescence. *J Bone Joint Surg Am* 1983;65:438–444.
43. Pollen AG. Fractures involving the epiphyseal plate. *Reconstr Surg Traumatol* 1979;17: 25–39.
44. Clement DA, Worlock PH. Triplane fracture of the distal tibia: a variant in cases with an open growth plate. *J Bone Joint Surg Br* 1987;69:412–415.
45. Jarvis JG, Miyanji R. The complex triplane fracture: ipsilateral tibial shaft and distal triplane fracture. *J Trauma* 2001;51:714–716.
46. Navascues JA, Gonzalez-Lopez JL, Lopez-Valverde S, et al. Premature physeal closure after tibial diaphyseal fractures in adolescents. *J Pediatr Orthop* 2000;20:193–196.
47. Petit P, Sapin C, Henry G, et al. Rate of abnormal osteoarticular radiographic findings in pediatric patients. *Am J Roentgenol* 2001;176:987–990.
48. Chande VT. Decision rules for roentgenography of children with acute ankle injuries. *Arch Pediatr Adolesc Med* 1995;149:255–258.

49. Karpas A, Hennes H, Walsh-Kelly CM. Utilization of the Ottawa Ankle Rules by nurses in a pediatric emergency department. *Acad Emerg Med* 2002;9:130–133.
50. Clark KD, Tanner S. Evaluation of the Ottawa Ankle Rules in children. *Pediatr Emerg Care* 2003;19:73–78.
51. Letts RM. The hidden adolescent ankle fracture. *J Pediatr Orthop* 1982;2:161–164.
52. Vangsness C, Carter V, Hunt T, et al. Radiographic diagnosis of ankle fractures: are three views necessary. *Foot Ankle Int* 1994;15:172–174.
53. Haraguchi N, Kato F, Hayashi H. New radiographic projections for avulsion fractures of the lateral malleolus. *J Bone Joint Surg Br* 1998;80:684–688.
54. Bozic KJ, Jaramillo D, DiCanzio J, et al. Radiographic appearance of the normal distal tibiofibular syndesmosis in children. *J Pediatr Orthop* 1999;19:14–21.
55. Herzenberg J. Computed tomography of pediatric distal tibial growth plate fractures: a practical guide. *Tech Orthop* 1989;4:53–64.
56. Jones S, Phillips N, Ali F, et al. Triplane fractures of the distal tibia requiring open reduction and internal fixation: pre-operative planning using computed tomography. *Injury* 2003;34:293–298.
57. Yao J, Huurman WW. Tomography in a juvenile Tillaux fracture. *J Pediatr Orthop* 1986; 6:349–351.
58. Horn BD, Crisci K, Krug M, et al. Radiologic evaluation of juvenile Tillaux fractures of the distal tibia. *J Pediatr Orthop* 2001;21:162–164.
59. Smith BG, Rand F, Jaramillo D, et al. Early MR imaging of lower-extremity physeal fracture-separations: a preliminary report. *J Pediatr Orthop* 1994;14:526–533.
60. Carey J, Spence L, Blickman H, et al. MRI of pediatric growth plate injury: correlation with plain film radiographs and clinical outcome. *Skel Radiol* 1998;27:250–255.
61. Iwinska-Zelder J, Schmidt S, Ishaque N, et al. Epiphyseal injuries of the distal tibia: does MRI provide useful additional information? *Radiologe* 1999;39:25–29.
62. Seifert J, Laun R, Paris S, et al. Value of magnetic resonance tomography (MRI) in diagnosis of triplane fractures of the distal tibia. *Unfallchirurg* 2001;104:524–529.
63. Petit P, Panuel M, Faure F, et al. Acute fracture of the distal tibial physis: role of gradient-echo MR imaging versus plain film examination. *Am J Radiol* 1996;166:1203–1206.
64. Lohman M, Kivisaari A, Kallio P, et al. Acute paediatric ankle trauma: MRI versus plain radiography. *Skeletal Radiol* 2001;30:504–511.
65. Gabel GT, Peterson HA, Berquist TH. Premature partial physeal arrest: diagnosis by magnetic resonance imaging in two cases. *Clin Orthop* 1991;272:242–247.
66. Havranek P, Lizler J. Magnetic resonance imaging in the evaluation of partial growth arrest after physeal injuries in children. *J Bone Joint Surg Am* 1991;73:1234–1241.
67. Kerr R, Forrester DM, Kingston S. Magnetic resonance imaging of foot and ankle trauma. *Orthop Clin North Am* 1990;21:591–601.
68. Powell H. Extra centre of ossification for the medial malleolus in children: incidence and significance. *J Bone Joint Surg Br* 1961;43:107–113.
69. Keats T. *Atlas of Normal Roentgen Variants That May Simulate Disease,* 5th ed. St. Louis: Mosby; 1992.
70. Lovell E. An unusual rotating injury of the ankle. *J Bone Joint Surg Am* 1968;50: 163–165.
71. Broock GJ, Greer RB. Traumatic rotational displacements of the distal growth plate. *J Bone Joint Surg Am* 1970;52:1666–1668.
72. Nevelos A, Colton C. Rotational displacement of the lower tibial epiphysis due to trauma. *J Bone Joint Surg Br* 1977;59:331–332.
73. Dickinson R, Singer AJ, Carrion W. Etomidate for pediatric sedation prior to fracture reduction. *Acad Emerg Med* 2001;8:74–77.
74. Furia JP, Alioto RJ, Marquardt JD. The efficacy and safety of the hematoma block for fracture reduction in closed, isolated fractures. *Orthopedics* 1997;20:423–426.
75. Lehman W, Jones W. Intravenous lidocaine for anesthesia in the lower extremity. *J Bone Joint Surg Am* 1984;66:1056–1060.
76. Grace DL. Irreducible fracture–separations of the distal tibial epiphysis. *J Bone Joint Surg Br* 1983;65:160–162.
77. Kling T. Fractures of the ankle and foot. In: Drennan J, ed. *The child's foot and ankle.* New York: Raven Press; 1992.
78. Phieffer LS, Meyer RA Jr., Gruber HE, et al. Effect of interposed periosteum in an animal physeal fracture model. *Clin Orthop* 2000;376:15–25.
79. Gruber HE, Phieffer LS, Wattenbarger JM.Physeal fractures. II. Fate of interposed periosteum in a physeal fracture. *J Pediatr Orthop* 2003;22:710–716.
80. Barmada A, Gaynor T, Mubarak SJ. Premature physeal closure following distal tibia physeal fractures: a new radiographic predictor. *J Pediatr Orthop* 2003;23:733–739.
81. Caterini R, Fursetti P, Ippolito E. Long-term follow-up of physeal injury to the ankle. *Foot Ankle* 1991;11:372–383.
82. Beaty JH, Linton RC. Medial malleolar fracture in a child: a case report. *J Bone Joint Surg Am* 1988;70:1254–1255.
83. Benz G, Kallieris D, Seebock T, et al. Bioresorbable pins and screws in paediatric traumatology. *Eur J Pediatr Surg* 1994;4:103–107.
84. Böstman OM, Makela EA, Sodergard J, et al. Absorbable polyglycolide pins in internal fixation of fractures in children. *J Pediatr Orthop* 1993;13:242–245.
85. Bucholz RW, Henry S, Henley MB. Fixation with bioabsorbable screws for the treatment of fractures of the ankle. *J Bone Joint Surg Am* 1994;76:319–324.
86. Böstman OM. Distal tibiofibular synostosis after malleolar fractures treated using absorbable implants. *Foot Ankle* 1993;14:38–43.
87. Böstman OM, Hirvensalo E, Vainionpaa S, et al. Degradable polyglycolide rods for the internal fixation of displaced bimalleolar fractures. *Int Orthop* 1990;14:1–8.
88. Frokjaer J, Moller BN. Biodegradable fixation of ankle fractures: complications in a prospective study of 25 cases. *Acta Orthop Scand* 1992;63:434–436.
89. Hirvensalo E. Fracture fixation with biodegradable rods. *Acta Orthop Scand* 1989;60: 601–606.
90. Rokkanen P, Bostman O, Vainionpaa S, et al. Absorbable devices in the fixation of fractures. j *Trauma* 1996;40(suppl):123–127.
91. Havranek P, Hajkova H. Fibrin glue osteosynthesis of epiphyseal injuries in children. *Acta Univ Carol Med (Praha)* 1978;35:266–264.
92. Böstman O. Metallic or absorbable fracture fixation devices. *Clin Orthop Rel Res* 1996; 329:233–239.
93. Ogden JA, Lee J. Accessory ossification patterns and injuries of the malleoli. *J Pediatr Orthop* 1990;10:306–316.
94. Cox PJ, Clark NJ. Juvenile Tillaux fracture of the ankle associated with a tibial shaft fracture: a unique combination. *Injury* 1996;27:221–222.
95. Steinlauf SD, Stricker SJ, Halen CA. Juvenile Tillaux fracture simulating syndesmosis separation: a case report. *Foot Ankle Int* 1998;19:332–335.
96. Schlesinger I, Wedge JH. Percutaneous reduction and fixation of displaced juvenile Tillaux fractures: a new surgical technique. *J Pediatr Orthop* 1993;13:389–391.
97. Leetun DT, Ireland ML. Arthroscopically assisted reduction and fixation of a juvenile Tillaux fracture. *Arthroscopy* 2002;18:427–429.
98. Bartl R. Die Traumatische Epiphysenlosung am Distalen Ende des Schienbeines und des Wadenbeines. *Hefte Unfallheilkd* 1957;54:228.
99. Gerner-Smidt M. *Ankelbrud Hos Born.* Copenhagen: Nytt Nordiskt Forlaz; 1963.
100. Johnson EW Jr, Fahl JC. Fractures involving the distal epiphysis of the tibia and fibula in children. *Am J Surg* 1957;93:778–781.
101. Peiro A, Aracil J, Martos F, et al. Triplane distal tibial epiphyseal fracture. *Clin Orthop* 1981;160:194–200.
102. El-Karef E, Sadek HI, Nairn DS, et al. Triplane fracture of the distal tibia. *Injury* 2000; 31:729–736.
103. Von Laer L. Classification, diagnosis, and treatment of transitional fractures of the distal part of the tibia. *J Bone Joint Surg Am* 1985;67:687–698.
104. Feldman DS, Otsuka NY, Hedden DM. Extra-articular triplane fracture of the distal tibial epiphysis. *J Pediatr Orthop* 1996;16:479–481.
105. Shin AY, Moran ME, Wenger DR. Intramalleolar triplane fractures of the distal tibial epiphysis. *J Pediatr Orthop* 1997;17:352–355.
106. Karrholm J. The triplane fracture: four years of follow-up of 21 cases and review of the literature. *J Pediatr Orthop* 1997;6:91–102.
107. Rapariz JM, Ocete G, Gonzalez-Herranz P, et al. Distal tibial triplane fractures: long term follow up. *J Pediatr Orthop* 1996;16:113–118.
108. Healy WA III, Starkweather KD, Meyer J, et al. Triplane fracture associated with a proximal third fibula fracture. *Am J Orthop* 1996;25:449–451.
109. Whipple TL, Martin DR, McIntyre LF, et al. Arthroscopic treatment of triplane fractures of the ankle. *Arthroscopy* 1993;9:456–463.
110. Farley FA, Senunas L, Greenfield ML, et al. Lower extremity lawn-mower injuries in children. *J Pediatr Orthop* 1996;16:669–672.
111. Grosfeld JL, Muse TS, Eyring EJ. Lawn mower injuries in children. *Arch Surg* 1970; 100:582–583.
112. Adler P. Ride on mower hazard analysis 1987–1990. Washington, DC: Directorate for Epidemiology, USA Consumer Product Safety Commission; 1993:1–65.
113. Alonso JE, Sanchey FL. Lawn mower injuries in children: a preventable impairment. *J Pediatr Orthop* 1995;15:83–89.
114. Dormans JP, Azzoni M, Davidson RS, et al. Major lower extremity lawn mower injuries in children. *J Pediatr Orthop* 1995;15:78–82.
115. Rougraff BT, Kernek CB. Lawn mower injury resulting in Chopart amputation in a young child. *Orthopedics* 1996;19:689–691.
116. Vosburgh CL, Gruel CR, Herndon WA, et al. Lawn mower injuries of the pediatric foot and ankle: observations on prevention and management. *J Pediatr Orthop* 1995; 15:504–509.
117. Loder RT, Brown KL, Zaleske DJ, et al. Extremity lawn-mower injuries in children: report by the Research Committee of the Pediatric Orthopaedic Society of North America. *J Pediatr Orthop* 1997;17:360–364.
118. Gaglani MJ, Friedman J, Hawking EP, et al. Infections complicating lawn mower injuries in children. *Pediatr Infect Dis J* 1996;15:452–455.
119. Horowitz JH, Nichter LS, Kenny JG, et al. Lawn-mower injuries in children: lower extremity reconstruction. *J Trauma* 1985;25:1138–1146.
120. Johnstone BR, Bennett CS. Lawn-mower injuries in children. *Aust N Z J Surg* 1989; 59:713–718.
121. Love SM, Grogan DP, Ogden JA. Lawn-mower injuries in children. *J Orthop Trauma* 1988;2:94–101.
122. Reff RB. The use of external fixation devices in the management of severe lower extremity trauma and pelvic injuries in children. *Clin Orthop Rel Res* 1984;188:21–23.
123. Ross PM, Schwentker EP, Bryan H. Mutilating lawn mower injuries in children. *JAMA* 1976;236:480–481.
124. Klein DM, Caligiuri DA, Katzman BB. Local-advancement soft-tissue coverage in a child with ipsilateral grade IIIB open tibial and ankle fractures. *J Orthop Trauma* 1996;10: 577–580.
125. Mooney JR III, DeFranzo A, Marks MW. Use of cross-extremity flaps stabilized with external fixation in severe pediatric foot and ankle trauma: an alternative to free tissue transfer. *J Pediatr Orthop* 1998;18:26–30.
126. Boyer MI, Bowen U, Weiler P. Reconstruction of a severe grinding injury to the medial malleolus and the deltoid ligament of the ankle using a free plantaris tendon graft and vascularized gracilis free muscle transfer: case report. *J Trauma* 1994;36:454–457.
127. Danielsson LG. Avulsion fracture of the lateral malleolus Manderson EL, Ollivierre CO. Closed anatomic reduction of a juvenile Tillaux fracture by dorsiflexion of the ankle. *Clin Orthop* 1992;276:262–266.in children. *Injury* 1980;12:165–167.
128. Haramati N, Roye DP, Adler PA, et al. Non-union of pediatric fibula fractures: easy to overlook, painful to ignore. *Pediatr Radiol* 1994;24:248–250.
129. Vahvanen V, Westerlund M, Nikku R. Lateral ligament injury of the ankle in children: follow-up results of primary surgical treatment. *Acta Orthop Scand* 1984;55:21–25.

130. Busconi BD, Pappas AM. Chronic, painful ankle instability in skeletally immature athletes: ununited osteochondral fractures of the distal fibula. *Am J Sports Med* 1996;24:647–651.
131. Manderson EL, Ollivierre CO. Closed anatomic reduction of a juvenile Tillaux fracture by dorsiflexion of the ankle. *Clin Orthop* 1992;276:262–266.
132. Nusem I, Ezra E, Wientroub S. Closed posterior dislocation of the ankle without associated fracture in a child. *J Trauma* 1999;46:350–351.
133. Letts M, Davidson D, Mukhtar I. Surgical management of chronic lateral ankle instability in adolescents. *J Pediatr Orthop* 2003;23:392–397.
134. Wilder RT, Berde CB, Wolohon MA, et al. Reflex sympathetic dystrophy in children. *J Bone Joint Surg Am* 1992;74:910–919.
135. Siffert R, Arkin A. Post-traumatic aseptic neurosis of the distal tibial epiphysis. *J Bone Joint Surg Am* 1950;32:691–697.
136. Guille JT, Lipton GE, Bowen JR, et al. Delayed union following stress fracture of the distal fibula secondary to rotational malunion of lateral malleolar fracture. *Am J Orthop* 1997;26:442–445.
137. Moon MS, Kim I, Rhee SK, et al. Varus and internal rotational deformity of the ankle secondary to distal tibial physeal injury. *Bull Hosp Joint Dis* 1997;56:145–148.
138. Takakura Y, Takaoka T, Tanaka Y, et al. Results of opening-wedge osteotomy for the treatment of a post-traumatic varus deformity of the ankle. *J Bone Joint Surg Am* 1998;80:213–218.
139. Scheffer MM, Peterson HA. Opening-wedge osteotomy for angular deformities of long bones in children. *J Bone Joint Surg Am* 1994;76:325–334.
140. Crenshaw AH. Injuries of the distal tibial epiphysis. *Clin Orthop* 1965;41:98–107.
141. Hasler CC, von Laer L. Pathophysiology of posttraumatic deformities of the lower limb during growth. *Orthopade* 2000;29:757–765.
142. Cass JR, Peterson HA. Salter-Harris type IV injuries of the distal tibial epiphyseal growth plate, with emphasis on those involving the medial malleolus. *J Bone Joint Surg Am* 1983;65:1059–1070.
143. Harcke HT, Macy NJ, Mandell GA, et al. Quantitative assessment of growth plate activity [Abstract]. *J Nucl Med* 1984;25:P115.
144. Bostock SH, Peach GS. Spontaneous resolution of an osseous bridge affecting the distal tibial epiphysis. *J Bone Joint Surg Br* 1996;78:662–663.
145. Chadwick L. Spontaneous resolution of varus deformity at the ankle following adduction injury of the distal tibial epiphysis. *J Bone Joint Surg Am* 1982;64:774–776.
146. Karrholm J, Hansson L, Selvik G. Changes in tibiofibular relationships due to growth disturbances after ankle fractures in children. *J Bone Joint Surg Am* 1984;66:1198–1210.
147. Ertl J, Barrack R, Alexander A, et al. Triplane fracture of the distal tibial epiphysis: long-term follow-up. *J Bone Joint Surg Am* 1988;70:967–976.
148. Ramsey P, Hamilton W. Changes in tibiotalar area of contact caused by lateral talar shift. *J Bone Joint Surg Am* 1976;58:356–357.
149. Michelson JD, Clarke HJ, Jinnah RH. The effect of loading on tibiotalar alignment in cadaver ankles. *Foot Ankle* 1990;10:280–284.
150. Charlton M, Costello R, Mooney JF 3rd, et al. Ankle joint biomechanics following transepiphyseal screw fixation of the distal tibia. *J Pediatr Orthop* 2005;25:635–640.
151. Yeap JS, Fazir M, Ezian S, et al. Compartment syndrome of the calf and foot following a displaced Salter-Harris type II fracture of the distal tibia: a review of the literature and a case report. *Med J Malaysia* 2001;56(suppl C):66–69.

FRACTURES AND DISLOCATIONS OF THE FOOT

James G. Jarvis and Paul J. Moroz

Children and adolescents today are increasingly participating in recreational activities of greater intensity and physical contact than ever before (1–4), with some children now even competing in the so-called extreme sports (motocross, all terrain vehicles, motorized dirt bike or snow-mobile racing, rock-climbing, and others) (1,5). As a result, not only are *more* musculoskeletal injuries occurring in the pediatric population but more *severe* and complex injuries are becoming frequent.

In the first textbook devoted solely to the management of pediatric fractures, Blount (6) generalized that for the most part the child's foot was so flexible and resilient that traumatic forces usually were transmitted more proximally to cause fractures above the foot, in the ankle and tibial region. Rang's popular textbook (7) of pediatric fractures, from the early 1970s, further promoted a generally minimalist approach to pediatric foot fractures: "Injuries to children's feet, despite all the little bones and joints, are remarkably uninteresting. Very few fractures will be encountered that display any subtleties or tricks; few are even displaced."

This approach is inadequate today; however, most foot fractures in children require only immobilization for treatment.

Differences between the pediatric and the adult foot need to be recognized and can make for important differences in the management of injuries. Ogden (8) noted the predominately cartilaginous nature of a very young child's developing foot with an increased elasticity of the growing cartilage and bone dissipating significant amounts of applied energy across the entire foot, leading to patterns of injuries different from those in adults.

In adolescents, fracture patterns are similar to those in adults, such as calcaneal fractures, which appear similar on computed tomography (CT) scan of adolescents and adults (9). As a result, many of the principles of management of calcaneal fractures in adults can likely be adapted to the management of similar injuries in older children and adolescents.

AN EVIDENCE-BASED APPROACH TO PEDIATRIC FOOT FRACTURES

A study examining trends of randomized controlled trials of different orthopaedic fractures in adults found that foot fractures had the fewest such trials available for analysis of treatment efficacy (10). Fractures in children, being overall fewer than in adults, are likely to have even fewer, if any, randomized controlled trials; therefore, for the purposes of this chapter, an evidence-based approach bases almost all conclusions on literature that uses the lowest levels of study efficacy: level V (expert consensus) and a few level IV studies (uncontrolled case series). No systematic reviews or meta-analyses, to our knowledge, have involved pediatric foot fractures.

It should be noted also that in the review of the current literature for this chapter, a significant number of quality papers were not in the English language. Most of these reports were published in German, a trend noted by Robert et al (10). Brunet (11), in his discussion of pediatric calcaneal fractures, also referred to a number of articles in the non–English language literature (12–14). This non-English literature is important because these articles have been among the earliest to report a more aggressive operative approach to calcaneal fractures in children, a trend that is now finding its way into the English literature.

Anatomy of the Growing Foot

Modern imaging techniques, such CT scanning and magnetic resonance imaging (MRI), have increased our ability to document injury to the pediatric foot beyond what Blount (8) and Rang (7) could appreciate on plain x-rays. A minimally displaced fracture on a plain x-ray appears much more innocuous than the extensive brightness of soft-tissue swelling, cartilaginous disruption, and subchondral bony bruising seen on a T2-weighted MRI scan.

The calcaneus and the talus usually are ossified at birth, and the cuboid ossification center usually appears at birth or shortly after (Fig. 27-1) (8,15). The navicular tarsal bone is the last of

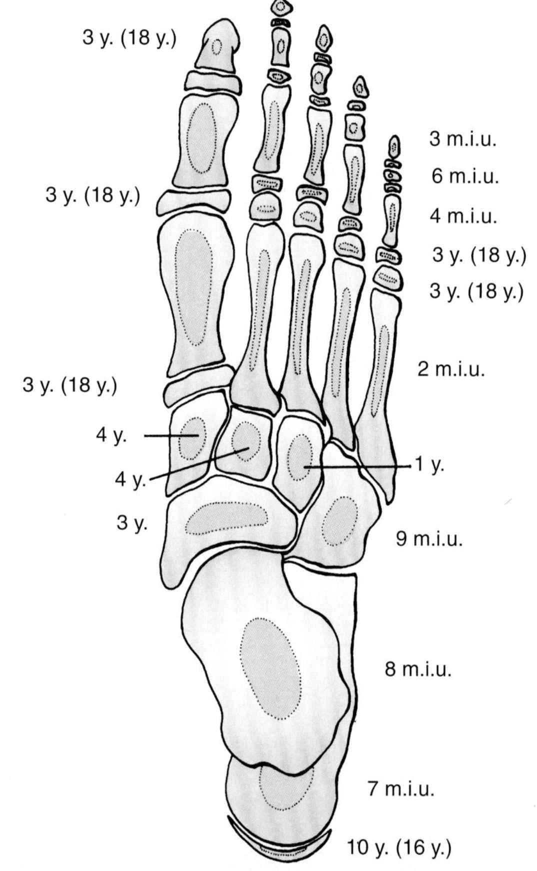

FIGURE 27-1 Appearance and fusion times of foot ossification centers, with figures in parentheses indicating the time of fusion of the primary and secondary ossification centers (y, years; m.i.u., months in utero). (From Aitken JT, Joseph J, Causey G, et al. *A Manual of Human Anatomy,* 2nd ed., vol. IV. London: E & S Livingstone; 1966:80; with permission).

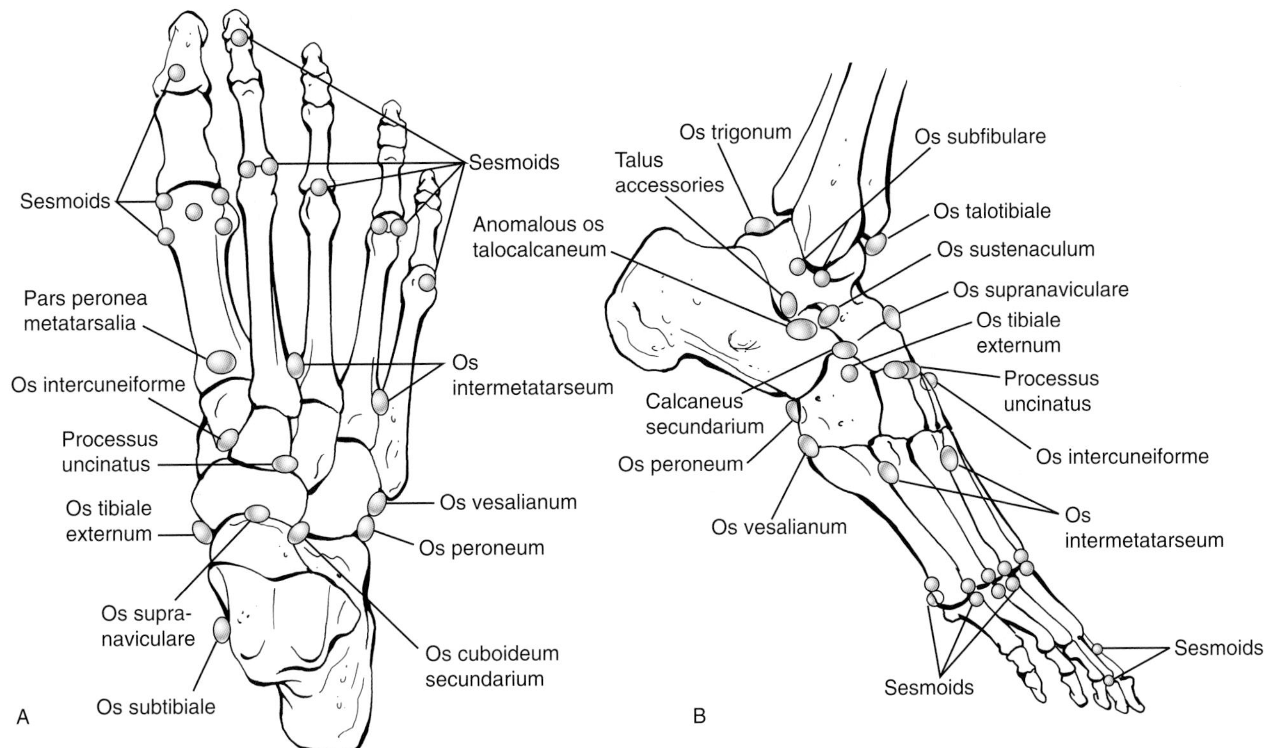

FIGURE 27-2 Diagrammatic representation of accessory ossicles and sesamoid bones about the foot and ankle. Note that the sesamoid bones can be bipartite and that accessory ossicles can be multicentric. (From Traughber PD. Imaging of the foot and ankle. In Coughlin MJ, Mann RA. *Surgery of the Foot and Ankle,* 7th ed. St. Louis: Mosby; 1999.)

the large tarsal bones to develop primary ossification, usually around 3 years of age.

The adult foot ultimately consists of 26 bones and can have a variety of sesamoids and accessory ossicles (Fig. 27-2). The foot is divided into the forefoot (5 metatarsals and 14 phalanges), which is separated from the midfoot (3 cuneiforms, navicular, and cuboid) by the tarsometatarsal joint of Lisfranc. The hindfoot (talus and calcaneus) is separated from the midfoot by the midtarsal joint of Chopart.

TALAR FRACTURES

Introduction

The talus rarely is fractured in a child or adolescent (8,16). A reported incidence between 0.01% and 0.08% (17) makes it rarer in children than in adults. However, the incidence likely is increasing because of the increasing participation of children in high-impact sports. When injury occurs to the growing talus, the diagnosis, management, and functional outcomes can differ from those in adults.

The most common talar fracture involves the talar neck. Letts and Gibeault (18) reported 12 fractures of the neck of the talus in children, 4 of which were in children under the age of 3 years. Canale and Kelly (19) reported 71 fractures of the talar neck, 12 of which were in children. As with many pediatric fractures, and in particular those of the pediatric foot, large series are rare.

Management of talar fractures in young children in general usually is conservative, with cast immobilization, because most fractures tend to be minimally displaced. In older adolescents fracture patterns and problems are similar those in adults. There is some recent evidence to suggest that complications, especially osteonecrosis, may be more common in adolescents than in adults (20).

Anatomy

The talus is a compact bone with a complex morphology that is the connecting link between the leg and the foot. Its anatomy continues to be studied in detail (21), and, with the availability of high-speed helical three-dimensional CT scanning, precise fracture reduction can be achieved (Figs. 27-3 and 27-4)

The talus consists of a head, neck, and body. The head of the talus articulates with the navicular bone and is mostly cartilaginous. Little cartilage is present on the neck, which is largely an area of vascular perforation. Under the talar neck lies the intraosseous ligament.

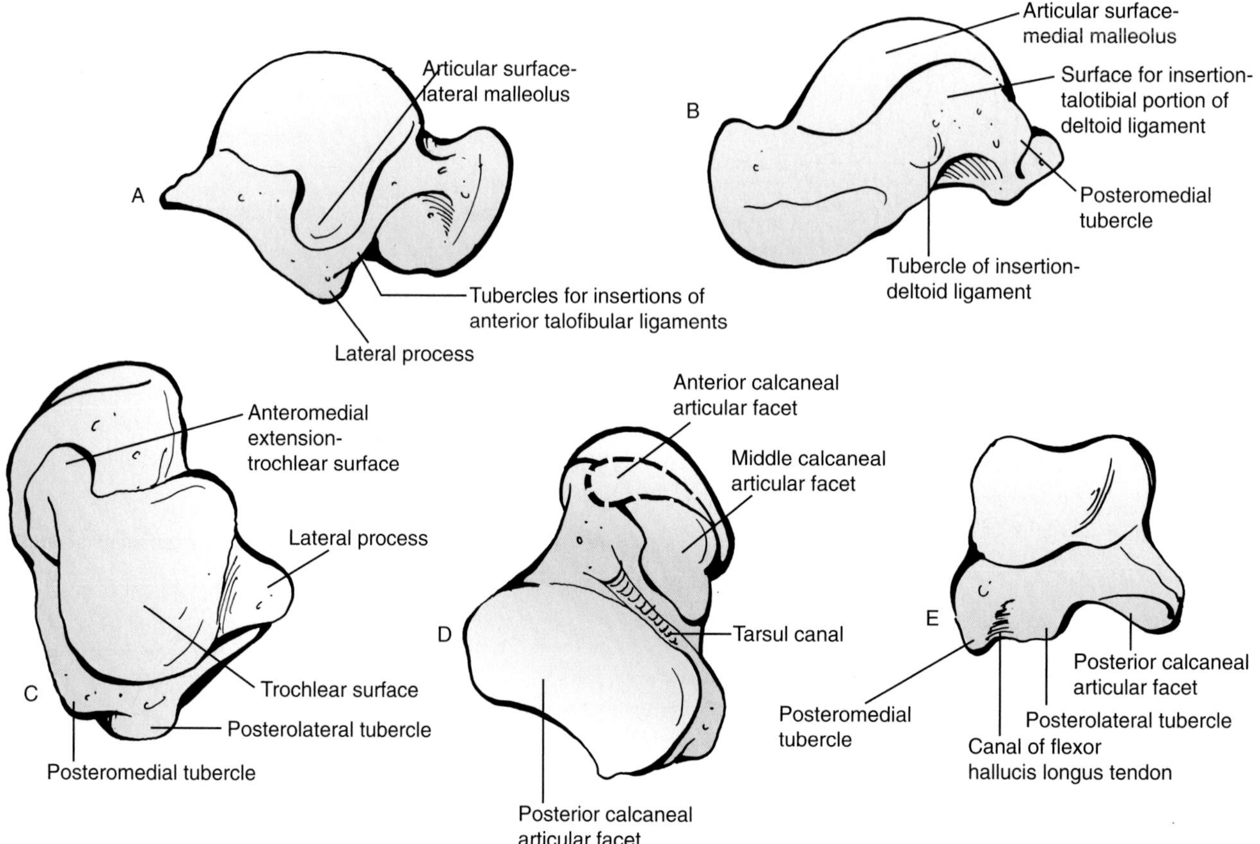

FIGURE 27-3 Anatomical details of the talus are important when correlating high-definition imaging, such as CT scans, with normal anatomy for the purposes of fracture management decision making.

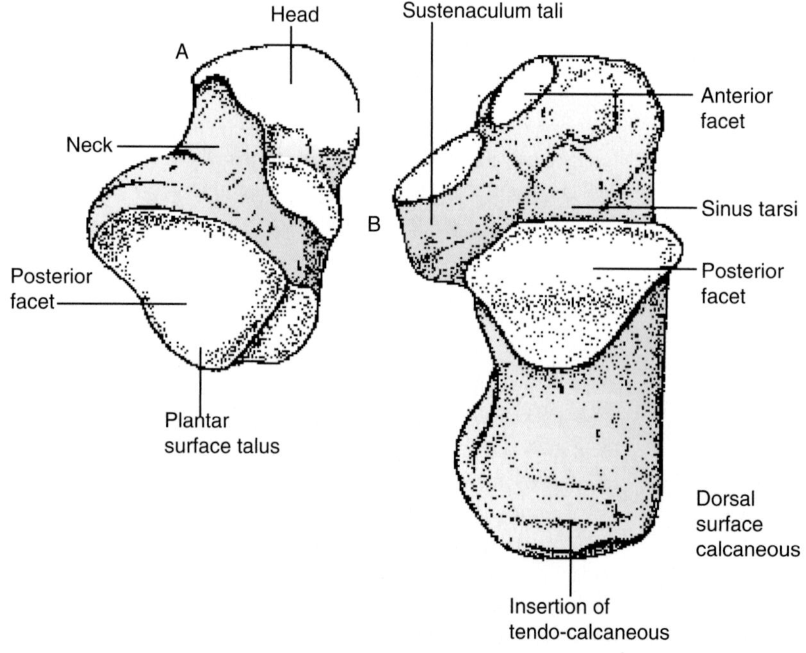

FIGURE 27-4 Subtalar joint opened such that the medial borders of the joint face each other. **A.** Plantar surface of the talus, which articulates with the dorsal surface of the calcaneus. Note the extensive area of the talus that is articular cartilage. **B.** Dorsal surface of the calcaneus with the articular facets occupying the anterior half of the calcaneus. (From Sammarco GJ. Anatomy. In: Helal B, Rowley D, Cracchiolo AC, et al, eds. *Surgery of Disorders of the Foot and Ankle.* Philadelphia: Lippincott-Raven, 1996.)

The tarsal canal is a funnel-shaped sulcus on the inferior aspect of the talus and between the talus and the calcaneus, extending in a posteromedial to anterolateral direction exiting as the laterally based conical space called the sinus tarsi. The tarsal canal accommodates the anastomosis of the artery of the sinus tarsi and the artery of the tarsal canal. The canal also contains the broad interosseous ligament joining the calcaneus and the talus.

At the end of growth, roughly two thirds of the talar surface is covered with articular cartilage and without any direct muscular attachments. The body of the talus is almost entirely cartilaginous and articulates with the ankle superiorly and with the three facets of the calcaneus inferiorly. The sides of the talar body make up facets that are wedged between the ankle malleoli.

The lateral process of the talus projects laterally as a large wedge-shaped process covered with articular cartilage and articulates with the fibula superiorly and the subtalar joint inferiorly. The origin of the lateral talocalcaneal ligament is on the lateral process (22,23).

In the growing talus ossification begins in the region of the head and neck, then extends in a retrograde fashion into the body of the talus (24,25). Normal ossification of the talus is dependent on a normally functioning blood supply. The subchondral ankle mortise section of the talus is the last region of the talus to ossify (8).

Ischemic damage to structures of the talus depends on the extent of chondro-osseous transformation that has occurred at the time of injury (8). The less ossified structures are more resistant to permanent damage and have a better chance of remodeling.

In general, it is this remarkable healing response of the nonossified talar anlage that allows conservative treatment of talar fractures in children younger than 8 years of age. After age 10 years, when much of the ossification has occurred and the amount of vascularly dependent bone mass is increased, talar fractures resemble those in adults and generally are treated similarly.

Blood Supply

Osteonecrosis is the primary reason for any long-term disability after a fracture of the talus (8), in particular displaced talar neck fractures. The frequency of osteonecrosis associated with fractures of the talus has prompted extensive study of the blood supply to the talus. Because much of the talar surface is made up of articular cartilage, it has limited vascular connections and a precarious blood supply that can be directly affected by fracture. In particular, the extent of fracture displacement can affect blood supply and lead to osteonecrosis of the talar body, which receives most of its blood supply from the head and neck. The talar neck is noncartilaginous once fully formed and is perforated with vascular foramina throughout its entire circumference.

The major blood supply to the talar body is provided by the artery of the tarsal canal (Fig. 27-5). This artery comes off of the posterior tibial artery medially and anastomoses within the subtalar canal with the artery of the tarsal sinus. This anastomosis supplies most of the talar body. Before entering the canal medially, the artery of the tarsal canal gives off a deltoid branch, which nourishes the medial quarter of the talar body. This deltoid branch also extends dorsally to anastomose around the talar neck with inferior reaching medial branches of the dorsalis pedis artery, and these branches enter the bone through talar neck perforations. The artery of the tarsal sinus, before it enters the canal laterally, is derived from an anastomosis of the posterior lateral perforating peroneal artery and lateral branches of the dorsalis pedis artery (via the lateral tarsal artery) (26).

Mechanism of Injury

Dorsiflexion of the foot in a fall from a height is the predominant mechanism of injury cited in the literature (18,27,28). The combination of dorsiflexion and axial loading would seem to direct a substantial vertical shear force against the talar neck while the talar body is fixed between the tibia and the calcaneus.

In more severe talar fractures a component of supination also may combine with the forced dorsiflexion and axial loading, which also impinges the talar neck onto the medial malleolus, leading to both comminution and subtalar joint subluxation (29).

Crushing injuries to the foot can cause fractures of talar body, and lawnmower injuries can result in open talar fractures. Ogden (8) described severely mangled legs from lawn mower injuries, often involving open gouges into the body of the talus; this has been our observation as well (see discussion on lawn mower injuries later in this chapter).

Signs and Symptoms

The signs and symptoms of fractures of the talus typically include history of forced dorsiflexion of the foot, pain and swelling in the region of the talus, and painful dorsiflexion.

Any of these should lead to careful scrutiny of foot x-rays for talar involvement. Careful examination also is required, although Letts and Gibeault (18) noted in their series that occasionally a low level of suspicion for a fracture can be drawn based solely on physical examination. Mechanism of injury is important to help guide physical examination, as a history of forced dorsiflexion should make one suspicious of talar injury.

The injured foot must be examined for vascular viability and for any sensory deficits, as well as for signs and symptoms of foot compartment syndrome. Ogden (8) remarked that with significant foot injuries "the most consistent physical finding was tense swelling of the foot," and in this scenario compartment syndrome should always be ruled out.

Compartment syndrome is discussed more fully elsewhere in this chapter. It should be noted that measuring tissue pressures is an important aide to diagnosis, but it is our belief that clinical presentation alone can be sufficient to bring a child to the operating room for decompression. We also stress, as does

Medial

1- Anterior tibial artery
2 - Medial rrecurrent tarsal artery
3 - Medial talar artery
4 - Posterior tibial artery
5 - Posterior tubercle artery
6 - Deltoid branches
7 - Artery of tarsal canal
8 - Medial plantar artery
9 - Lateral plantar artery

A

Lateral

1 - Anterior tibial artery
2 - Lateral talar artery
3 - Lateral tarsal artery
4 - Posterior recurrent branch of lateral tarsal
6 - Perforating peroneal
7 - Anterior lateral malleolar artery

B

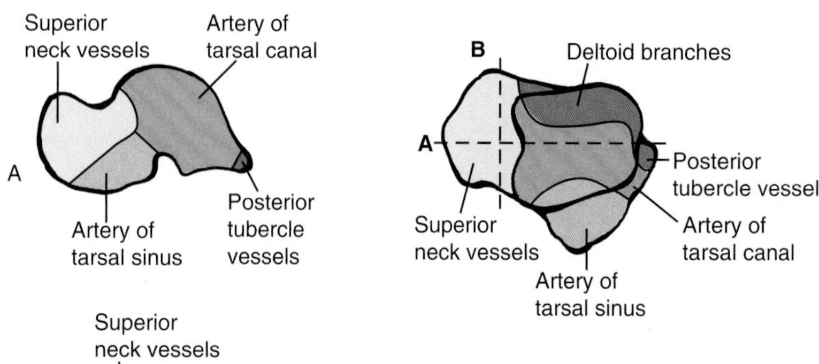

FIGURE 27-5 Arterial blood supply to the talus. **A.** Medial blood supply and **(B)** lateral blood supply. Dorsal view with sagittal cut through length (*a*) of talus and transverse cut through neck of talus (*b*). (From Gelberman RH, Mortensen WW. The arterial anatomy of the talus. *Foot Ankle* 1983;4:64–72.)

Ogden (8), that compartment syndrome of the foot in children can occur with soft tissue damage alone, without an obvious fracture. Ziv et al (30) and Ogden (8) showed that compartment syndrome can occur even with open fractures.

The status of the soft tissue should also be noted for any potential small puncture wounds or lacerations, which could represent an open fracture. This changes fracture management profoundly because such injuries must be taken immediately to the operating room for irrigation and debridement and fracture treatment.

Any patient with a foot fracture must have all bandages, splints, and casts removed in the emergency department for a close circumferential inspection of the soft tissues about the fracture and to search for punctures and lacerations. Any blood present on skin or dressings must be accounted for; a simple abrasion must be differentiated from a full-thickness breech of the dermis, which may represent an open fracture. Although removal of a splint and bandages may cause some distress to the child and parents, a gentle technique and a careful explanation quickly win parents over. Furthermore, determining the extent of soft tissue swelling can help in planning the operative approach, if indicated, or may prompt a delay in surgery if, for example, fracture blisters are present.

Pain medication for children should be carefully calculated on a per kilogram basis because undermedication can lead to confusion over an impending compartment syndrome and overmedication can cause respiratory depression.

Imaging Evaluation

Diagnosis of talar fractures can be difficult using only regular x-rays, especially in younger children with largely cartilaginous tarsal bones. The growing talus does not appear radiographically normal until the second decade of life, and the normal bony contours seen on x-rays of the talus in adults are not present in children and cannot reliably be used to assess the presence or absence of injury.

Routine x-ray views of the talus include anteroposterior (AP), lateral, and oblique views centered over the hindfoot. Canale and Kelly (19) described an x-ray technique that optimizes viewing of the position of talar neck fractures in the AP plane. The view is obtained with the ankle plantar flexed, in 15 degrees of internal rotation, and with the x-ray beam directed 75 degrees cephalad from the table. The view allows accurate assessment of talar head, neck, and body alignment and aids in avoiding varus malalignment following reduction. This is an important view on the operating table using fluoroscopy to assess quality of reduction. For preoperative purposes this x-ray view has been largely supplanted by CT scanning, with its potential for three-dimensional reconstruction.

Plain x-ray views usually are sufficient for identifying a talar fracture, and CT scanning can better delineate the talar fracture if required. Two-dimensional CT planes usually are sufficient to assess fracture comminution, displacement, and subluxation. If a talar fracture is suspected but not seen on plain films, CT scanning is best to confirm or refute the presence of a fracture.

Hawkins (31) described his experience with talar neck fractures in adults, and his classic x-ray classification has been widely accepted (Fig. 27-6). In this classification, type I fractures

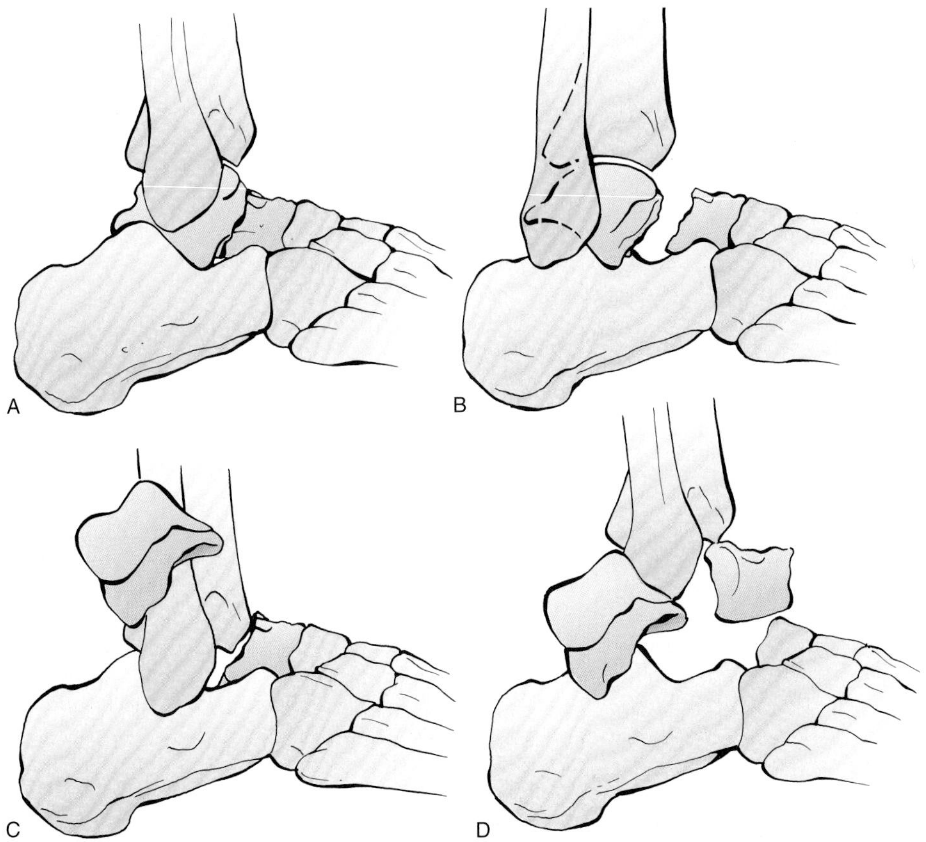

FIGURE 27-6 Hawkins classification of talar neck fractures (see text for details). **A.** Type I, nondisplaced fracture of the talar neck. **B.** Type II, displaced talar neck fracture with subluxation or dislocation of the subtalar joint. **C.** Type III, displaced talar neck fracture with associated dislocation of the talar body from both the subtalar and tibiotalar joints. **D.** Type IV, as suggested by Canale and Kelly, displaced talar neck fracture with an associated dislocation of the talar body from subtalar and tibiotalar joints and dislocation of the head and neck fragment from the talonavicular joint. (From Canale ST, Kelly FB Jr. Fractures of the neck of the talus: long-term evaluation of seventy-one cases. *J Bone Joint Surg Am* 1978;60:143–156.)

are nondisplaced talar neck fractures, type II fractures are displaced with subtalar dislocation or subluxation, and type III fractures include subluxation or dislocation of both the subtalar and ankle joints. The Hawkins sign, a subchondral osteolucency of the dome of the talus, is useful in predicting osteonecrosis because its presence confirms normal blood flow to the talus (Figs. 27-7 and 27-8). Ogden (8) pointed out that in children the talus is largely cartilage, especially in the ankle subchondral bone and, therefore, the Hawkins sign would not be easily seen here. However, the availability of MRI has largely supplanted the need for reliance on the Hawkins sign or the use of scintigraphy to look for cold spots indicative of a lack of vascularity. DeLee (32) suggested that segmental collapse of the talar body occurred in approximately one third of those with total body involvement but was rare in patients with only partial osteonecrosis.

MRI studies of cartilaginous morphology are a more reliable means than x-rays for precise determination of damage in children under the age of 10 years (8,33).

Management

Factures of the talus can be classified into three types: fractures of the talar neck, fractures of the talar body and dome, and osteochondral fractures of the talus.

Fractures of the Talar Neck

Most talar fractures in children are extra-articular and involve the talar neck. The classic x-ray description by Hawkins (31)

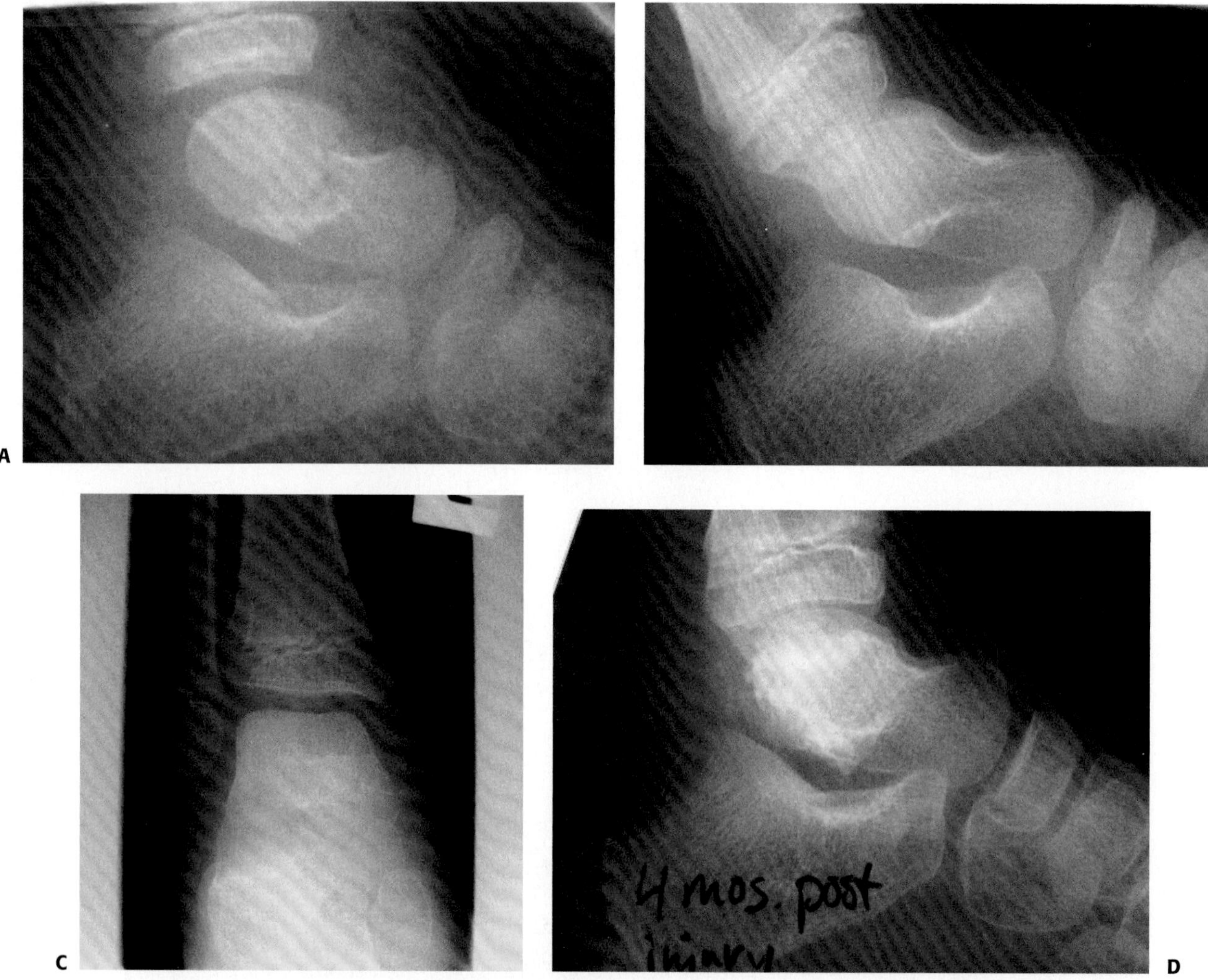

FIGURE 27-7 This 6-year-old boy fell from a height sustaining a Hawkins type I fracture of the talar neck of the left ankle **(A)**. **B.** Comparison view of uninjured right ankle. Absence of Hawkins sign **(C)** at 2 months after injury indicates impending osteonecrosis (see text). **D.** Lateral view at 4 months shows degenerative changes. (*continues*)

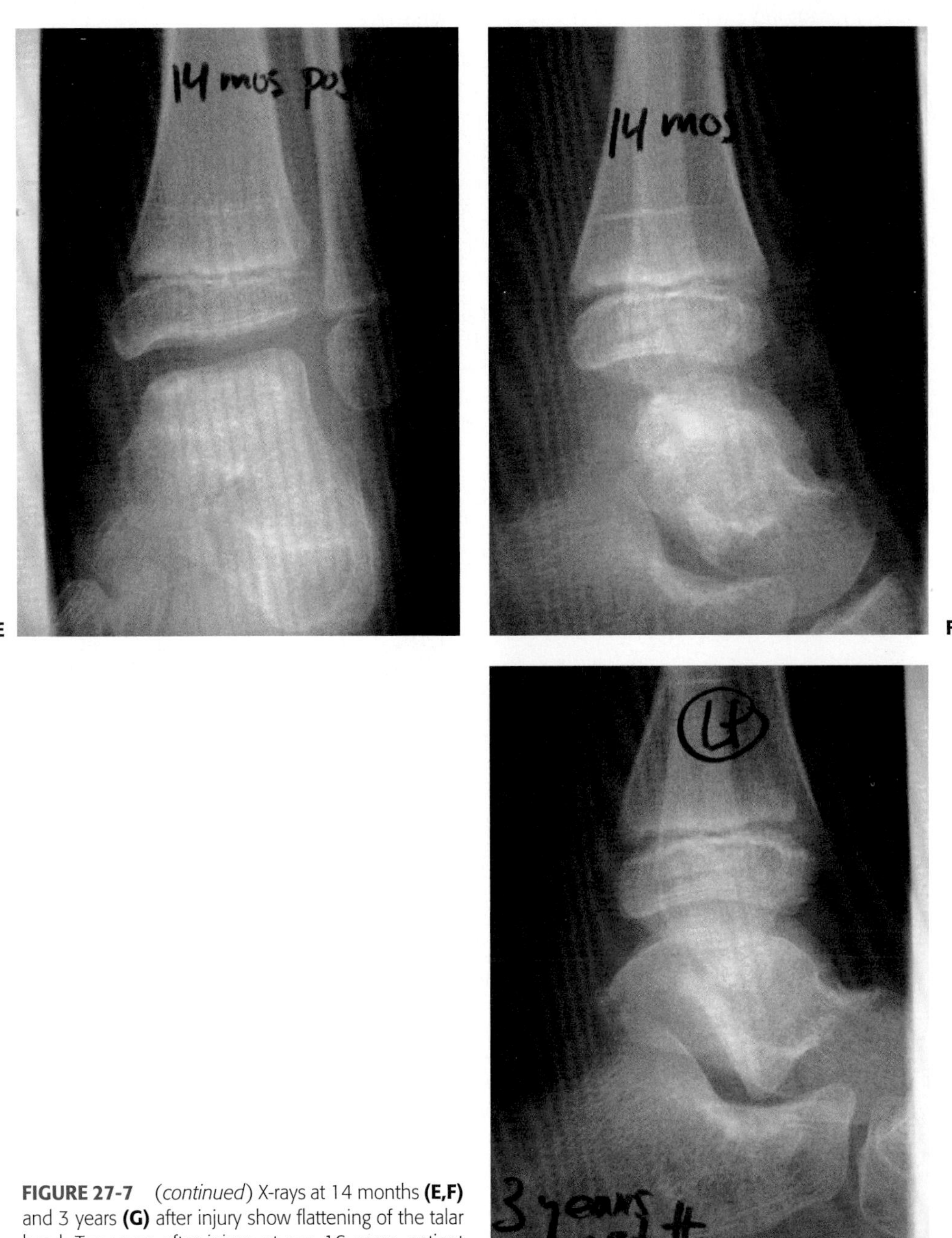

FIGURE 27-7 (*continued*) X-rays at 14 months **(E,F)** and 3 years **(G)** after injury show flattening of the talar head. Ten years after injury, at age 16 years, patient reported no pain but some decreased range of motion.

has a three-part classification based on the amount of fracture displacement. Canale and Kelly (19) later modified the classification (see Fig. 27-6) to include a rare fourth type with dislocation of the talar head from the talonavicular joint.

Malalignment of talar neck fractures alters the relationship with the inferior articular surfaces of the talus and the superior calcaneal articulations through the three facets on the calcaneus.

The management of talar neck fractures in children depends largely on the amount of fragment displacement and the Hawkins classification. In general, the approach to pediatric talar fractures is similar to that for talar fractures in adults (Table 27-1) (34).

Hawkins Type I Fractures. Management of mildly displaced Hawkins type I fractures requires a closed reduction followed by casting and a period of non–weight-bearing immobilization in a short-leg cast for 6 to 8 weeks. Most talar neck fractures in children are type I, undisplaced, and we agree with Canale

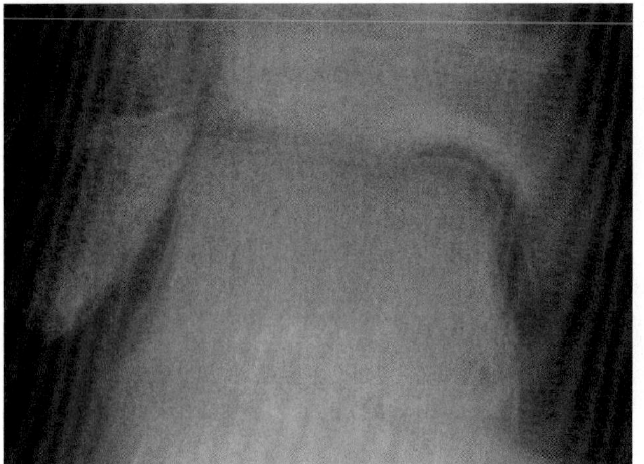

FIGURE 27-8 A 14-year-old girl with a talar neck fracture and a positive Hawkins sign. Disuse osteoporosis leads to a halolike image of the talus on the anteroposterior view denoting adequate talar dome vascularization; if there were no blood supply, there would be no blood flow to lose calcium. If this happens, the dome of the talus would become denser and more radio-opaque than the surrounding bones that are undergoing disuse osteoporosis.

(35) that acceptable guidelines for a nondisplaced fracture include displacement of 5 mm or less and a neck malalignment of 5 degrees or less, although we acknowledge that the definition of an acceptable reduction has not been established definitively (36). Children under 8 years of age with minimal displacement generally respond well to nonoperative management (18,27, 28). Weight-bearing begins after the fracture appears consolidated on serial x-rays, and this often corresponds to when the cast comes off.

Hawkins Type II Fractures. In children under 10 years of age, a displaced talar neck fracture, without subluxation of the ankle or subtalar joint, usually has a distal fragment that is dorsally and medially displaced. Closed reduction with gentle plantar flexion and pronation and the use of conscious sedation or general anesthesia should be attempted. If the reduction is successful, a long-leg cast with the foot in plantar flexion is worn for at least 4 weeks. Then the foot is brought to neutral position and placed into a below-knee cast for an additional 4 weeks of non–weight-bearing. If reduction cannot be maintained with casting because of soft tissue swelling but can be maintained by direct palpation intraoperatively, two Kirschner wires from anterior to posterior can be used to maintain the reduction (Fig. 27-9).

TABLE 27-1 Hawkins Classification of Talar Neck Fractures

Type	Description	Treatment	Affect on Blood Supply*	Osteonecrosis Rate
Type I	Stable, undisplaced vertical fracture through talar neck.	8 weeks in cast, 4 weeks in CAM cast.	Theoretical damage to only one vessel entering talar neck.	0% to 10%
Type II	Displaced fracture with subtalar joint subluxation or dislocation; normal ankle joint.	Immediate closed reduction.† A near anatomic reduction delays surgical treatment.	Two of three blood supply vessels lost: neck vessel and one entering the tarsal canal.	20% to 50%
Type III	Same as type II but with subluxation or dislocation of both the ankle and subtalar joint.	Direct to operating room for combined anteromedial and anterolateral surgical approach (see text).	All three sources of blood affected.	80% to 100%
Type IV	Very rare; basically a type III with talonavicular joint displacement.	Same as type III.	Not related to blood supply.	100%

* See text for further details of blood supply to the talus.

† Reduction maneuver: maximal plantar flexion and foot traction to realign head and body in sagittal plane. Varus/valgus with or without supination/pronation stress realigns neck in coronal plane.

CAM, Controlled active motion.

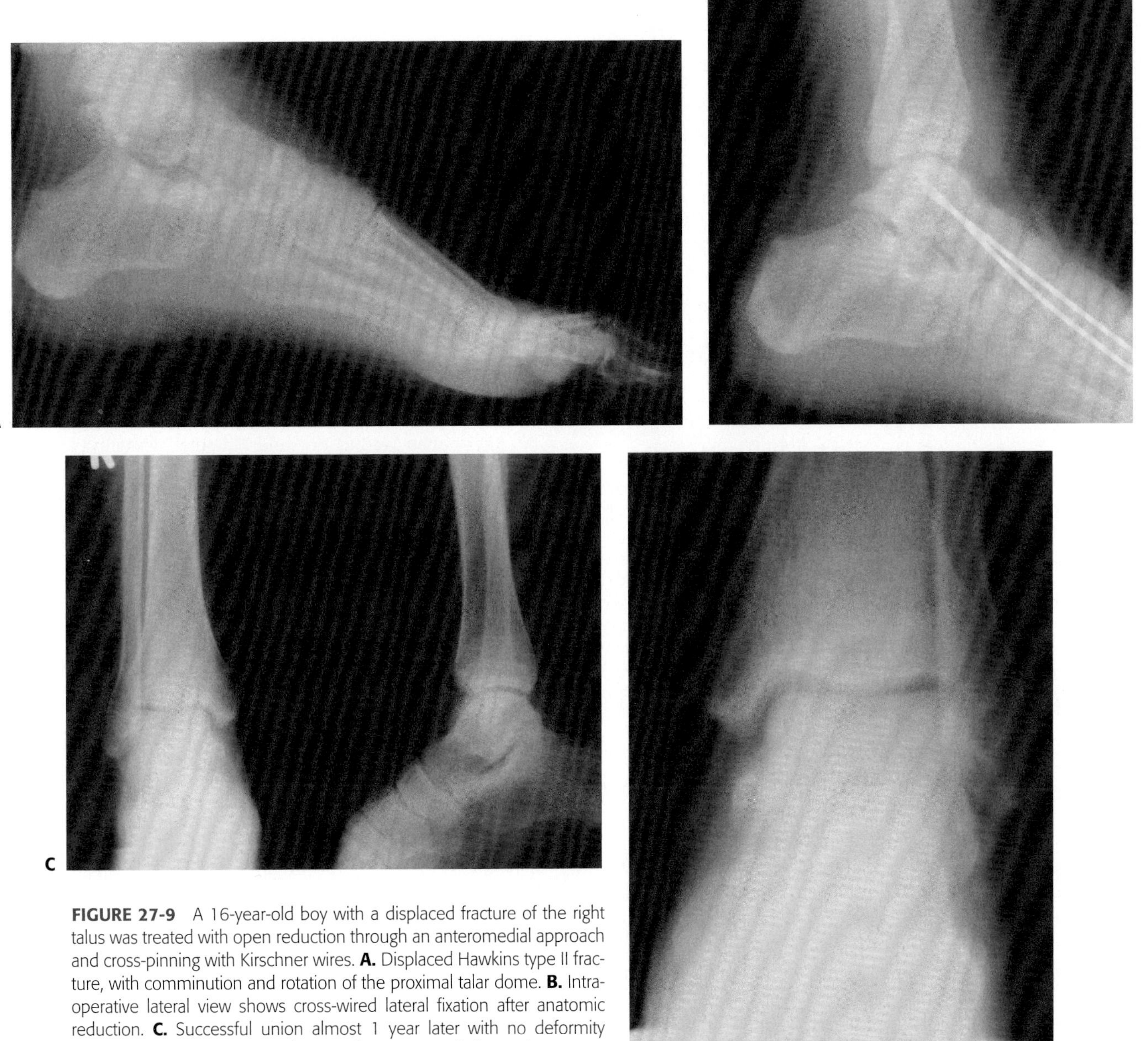

FIGURE 27-9 A 16-year-old boy with a displaced fracture of the right talus was treated with open reduction through an anteromedial approach and cross-pinning with Kirschner wires. **A.** Displaced Hawkins type II fracture, with comminution and rotation of the proximal talar dome. **B.** Intraoperative lateral view shows cross-wired lateral fixation after anatomic reduction. **C.** Successful union almost 1 year later with no deformity except for a small fragment that can be seen medially on the anteroposterior view **(D)**.

Hawkins Type III Fractures. These fractures include a talar neck fracture and dislocation of the body from both the ankle and the subtalar joints. This requires open reduction and internal fixation. Displaced fractures of the talar neck are considered an orthopaedic emergency, and management should proceed immediately.

Surgical Approaches

Three principal surgical approaches are used for open reduction of displaced talar neck fractures: posterolateral, anteromedial, and anterolateral. The approach used is determined by a number of factors, including presence or absence of open wounds or fracture blisters, fracture location, and other fractures in the region.

The posterolateral approach is commonly considered the best for fixation of talar neck fractures (Fig. 27-10). It is a safe approach, avoiding any further injury to the vascular supply of the talar head and neck that might occur with anterior approaches. Also the biomechanical superiority of posterior screws has been well established (37), and the extra-articular postero-

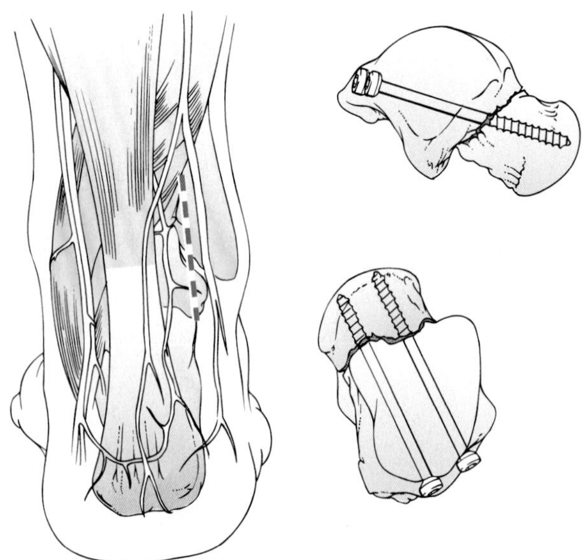

FIGURE 27-10 Posterolateral approach to the talus. Incision is based lateral to the Achilles tendon. The Achilles tendon and flexor hallucis longus are reflected medially. The posterolateral talar tubercle is the starting point for the guide pin. *Right*: Screws are directed in line with the long axis of the neck of the talus in a plantar-medial direction such that the distal threads of the screw are all in the distal fragment (talar head), beyond the fracture line to allow for compression. Combinations of two screws or one screw and one smooth pin are determined by size and anatomy. (Modified from Adelarr RS. Complex fractures of the talus. *Instr Course Lect* 1997;46:328; with permission.)

lateral approach avoids disruption of the anterior articular cartilage. The posterolateral approach is made just lateral to the Achilles tendon, with deeper dissection to the posterior capsule for exposure of the posterior talus. One or two (4.0- or 4.5-mm) partially threaded, cannulated cancellous screws are used for fixation, or a single 6.5-mm screw can be used with a single Kirschner wire (K-wire) for rotational stability. It is best to use short threaded cancellous screws and to ensure that no threads cross the actual fracture line in order to allow for compression. We recommend titanium screws, which are MRI compatible and allow MRI scanning if osteonecrosis becomes a problem.

Limited anterior approaches to ensure anatomic reduction can be combined with posterolateral approaches for fixation. Anteromedial or anterolateral approaches also can be used when the posterior approach fails to allow reduction. K-wires can be inserted, either going through the navicular into the talar head or just in the talar head. The anteromedial approach may be the most widely used despite the advantages of the posterolateral approach. The anteromedial approach begins at the anterior aspect of the medial malleolus and extends distally along the medial border of the midfoot. This incision can be extended for reduction of fractures of the medial malleolus or for osteotomy of the medial malleolus if required. Deeper dissection is medial to the anterior tibialis tendon, and the interval is between the tibialis anterior tendon and the tibialis posterior tendon. This approach exposes the medial neck of the talus and allows both reduction and application of fixation. Care must be taken to avoid disruption of the medially based deltoid branch of the posterior tibial artery during this approach, because it may be the major remaining blood supply to the talar body. In general, the anteromedial approach is less potentially harmful to the blood supply of the talus (38) than the anterolateral approach.

The anterolateral incision starts at the anterior tip of the lateral malleolus and goes to the base of the fourth metatarsal, exposing the lateral neck and giving access to the subtalar joint. Retraction using the region of the sinus tarsi should be avoided to avoid disruption of the tarsal canal vascular anastomosis. After reduction, careful inspection with fluoroscopy or x-ray is required to assess the quality of reduction. The view described by Canale and Kelly (19) to assess the true valgus-varus angle of the coronal talar neck is valuable to prevent malreduction.

After open reduction and internal fixation a short, non–weight-bearing cast is used for 6 weeks. Anteroposterior and mortise x-rays are taken 6 and 8 weeks after surgery to look for the Hawkins sign (see Fig. 27-8), which, if present, excludes the presence of osteonecrosis. When the Hawkins sign is absent and osteonecrosis is suspected (see Fig. 27-7), continued non–weight-bearing is required to help avoid talar dome collapse.

Fractures of the Talar Body and Dome

Fractures of the talar body (Fig. 27-11) are rare in children. Anatomic reduction of displaced fractures has been recommended because residual displacement of the articular surfaces leads to degenerative osteoarthritis (39). Table 27-2 lists the classification of Sneppen et al (40) for talar body fractures.

Fractures of the Lateral Process of the Talar Body

Leibner et al (35) estimated that fractures of the lateral process of the talus are initially missed in 46% of patients (22,23,42) and often are mistaken for a sprained ankle (43). Failure to diagnose and treat these injuries appropriately is believed to lead to subtalar arthrosis, although extensive evidence of this is lacking (22).

Lateral talar process fractures may be increasing in frequency because of the increasing popularity of snowboarding in adolescents (41,43,44). Kirkpatrick et al (43) found that in snowboarders 34% of fractures involved the lateral talar process. Hawkins (22) suggested that the combination of ankle dorsiflexion with inversion of the hindfoot was the mechanism of injury related to lateral process fractures. Mukherjee et al (45) reported that internal rotation views of the ankle, at approximately 20 to 25 degrees, best demonstrated this fracture; however, as Kirkpatrick et al (43) suggested, CT scanning is likely the best mode of investigation of lateral talar process fractures.

The lateral process projects laterally so that its superolateral surface articulates with the lateral malleolus and its inferolateral surface makes up part of the posterior facet of the talocalcaneal joint (41). This fracture is believed to occur with ankle

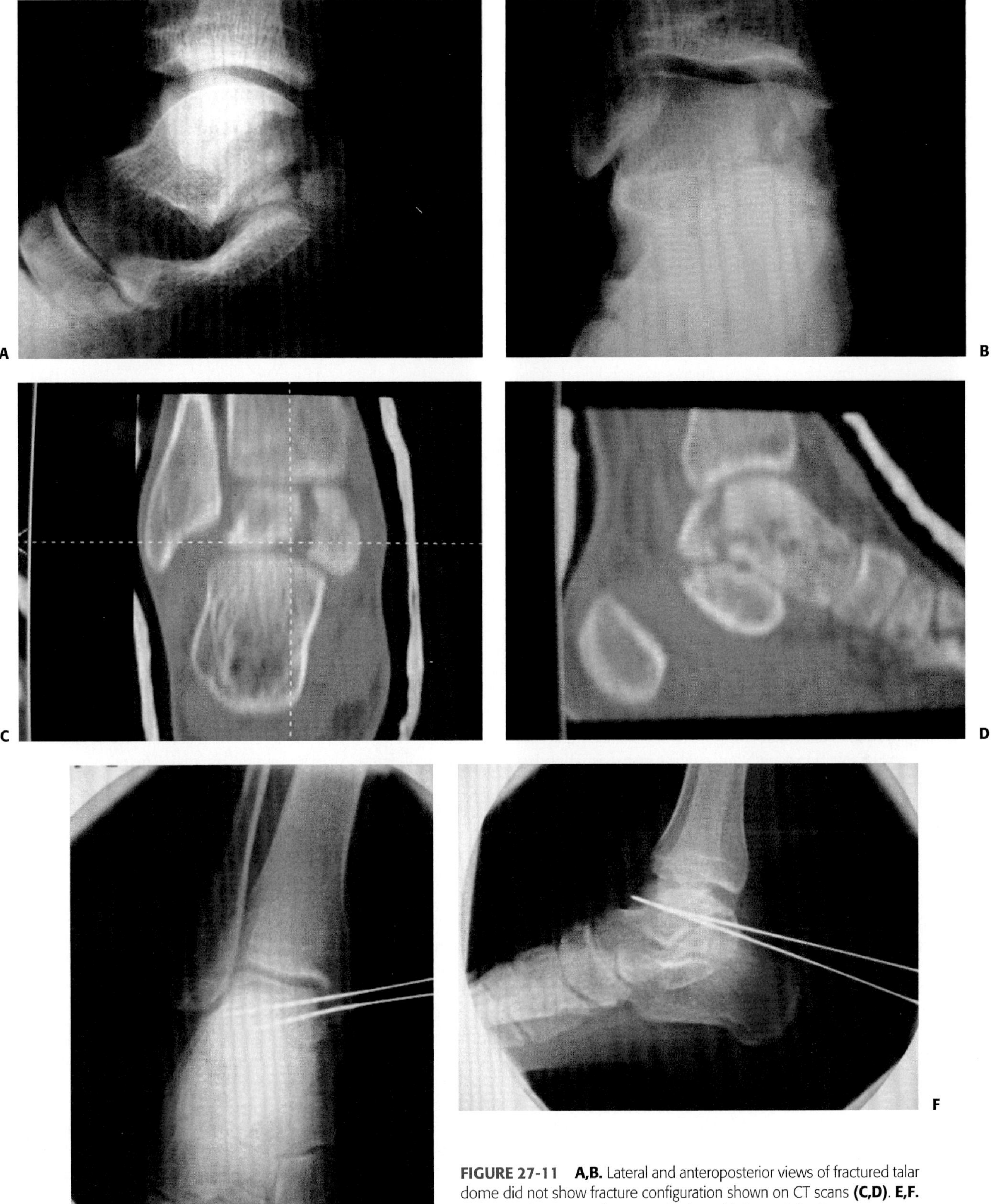

FIGURE 27-11 **A,B.** Lateral and anteroposterior views of fractured talar dome did not show fracture configuration shown on CT scans **(C,D)**. **E,F.** Intraoperative x-rays of open reduction with internal fixation.

TABLE 27-2 Sneppen Classification System of Talar Body Fractures

Sneppen Grade	Fracture Type
1	Transchondral/osteochondral
2	Coronal, sagittal, or horizontal shear
3	Posterior tubercle
4	Lateral process
5	Crush fracture

dorsiflexion and inversion (23), producing pain and tenderness largely over the anterior talofibular ligament and thus mimicking a lateral ankle sprain.

Plain x-rays are required for diagnosis, but CT scanning should be done if there is any question of the exact nature of the fracture (46).

Nondisplaced fractures are treated conservatively with a non–weight-bearing cast (23), while displaced fractures may require open reduction and internal fixation (41). Intra-articular fragments, if not recognized, can result in subtalar osteoarthritis. Nonunion of the lateral process has been managed with open reduction and internal fixation (46).

Other fractures of the talus involving the lateral or posterior processes also are rare.

Fractures of the Osteochondral Surface of the Talus

Twisting injuries to the ankle apply both shear and impaction stresses to the talar dome and can damage the osteochondral surface. Any x-rays made for evaluation of any ankle injury should be carefully reviewed for injuries of the talar dome. Talar injuries often are associated with ankle fractures, especially those of the medial malleolus (19,31,47).

Pain and swelling 6 to 8 weeks after an apparent ankle sprain should prompt careful clinical and x-ray examination to search for osteochondral lesions. Catching and locking also can occur with these lesions if the loose fragment becomes trapped within the joint. Often plain x-rays appear normal because these lesions can be purely cartilaginous, and ongoing symptoms should prompt MRI evaluation.

Berndt and Harty (48) found in their biomechanical studies that dorsiflexion and inversion produced anterolateral lesions and plantarflexion and inversion produced posteromedial lesions (Fig. 27-12).

Konig (49), in 1888, was the first to use the term "osteochondritis dissecans" to refer to an osteochondral lesion in a knee. We prefer *osteochondral defect* because this is a defect in the cartilaginous surface and its underlying subchondral bone. Even today, with arthroscopic techniques, these lesions in the talus can be challenging to treat (50).

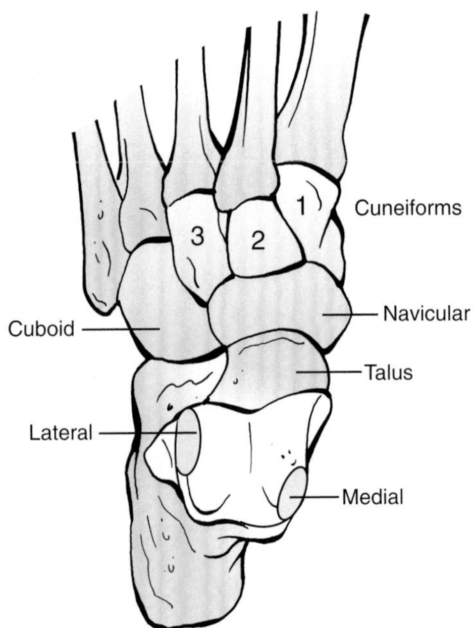

FIGURE 27-12 Typical positions of osteochondral lesions of the talus. Berndt et al (48) found that of 201 osteochondral lesions in adults 56% were on the medial side and 44% on the lateral side. Letts found medial lesions in 79% of 24 children, lateral lesions in 21%, and central lesions in 1%. (From Letts M, Davidson D, Ahmer A. Osteochondritis dissecans of the talus in children. *J Pediatr Orthop* 2003;23:617–625; with permission.)

Canale and Belding (51) described a series of osteochondral lesions of the talus mostly in teenagers; however, these lesions probably are more common in young adults in their second decade. Letts et al (39) believed that the frequency of talar osteochondral defects may be underestimated. The talus is the third most frequent anatomic site for osteochondral defects, after the knee and elbow (49,52,53).

Berndt and Harty (48) established the first classification of talar osteochondral lesions, and this has subsequently been adapted by Anderson et al (54) to include MRI-based findings (Fig. 27-13). The etiology of osteochondral defects was unknown until the classic description by Berndt and Harty (48), who supported a traumatic cause, especially for talar dome lesions (see Fig. 27-12). They found medial lesions (56%) slightly more common than lateral lesions (44%).

Letts et al (39) published the largest series of talar osteochondral defects in children. Although they noted their experience with an arthroscopic approach, they usually used arthrotomy. The development of small joint arthroscopy systems may allow arthroscopic treatment of most of these lesions.

A number of approaches to the management of these lesions currently are available and have been extensively reviewed by Giannini et al (55). Arthroscopic repair, resection, debridement, and drilling continue to be treatment options, although newer techniques are available, including osteochondral allografting, autogenous grafts, or autologous chondrocyte transplantation.

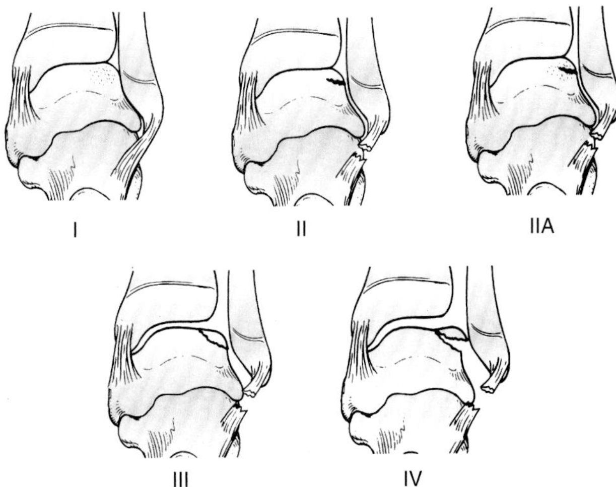

FIGURE 27-13 Adaptation of the Berndt and Hardy (1951) classification of osteochondral injuries of the talus by Anderson et al. Stage 1 is identified only by MRI scanning, which demonstrates trabecular compression of subchondral bone; stage 2 lesions have incomplete separation of the osteochondral fragment from the talus. If a subchondral cyst also is present, the lesion is designated stage 2a. Stage 3 lesions occur when the fragment is no longer attached to the talus but is undisplaced. Stage 4 indicates both complete detachment and displacement. (Adapted with permission from Alexander IF, Chrichton KI, Grattan-Smith Y, et al. Osteochondral fractures of the dome of the talus. *J Bone Joint Surg Am* 1989; 71:1143.)

These options appear to be viable alternatives, even for defects larger than 2 cm^2.

Associated Injuries

Hawkins (31) found that 64% of adults with talar fractures in his study also had an associated musculoskeletal injury. Others have shown talar fractures associated with other injuries, including calcaneal fractures (9), malleolar fractures, tibial fractures, and fractures of the lumbar spine (19,31,47,56). One reason may be, as Peterson et al (57) noted, that high forces are required to fracture the talus, a force they estimated to be twice that required to fracture the calcaneus or navicular bone. A high index of suspicion for other injuries should be present with any talar fracture.

Arthroscopic Assessment of Talar Lesions

Letts et al (39) did not find arthroscopy feasible for treatment osteochondral defects of the talus in children, stating that the small size of children and younger adolescents made it difficult. They used the arthroscope in only 3 of their 24 patients and in 2 of the 3, abandoned arthroscopy for open arthrotomy. With newer, small joint arthroscopic equipment, we have found, as have others (58), that ankle arthroscopy can be very useful in diagnosing, staging, and treating osteochondral lesions of the talus, especially those that are anterior on the dome.

Loren and Ferkel (59) reported arthroscopic identification of "treatable" articular surface injuries to the dome of the talus in a prospective series of ankle fractures in adults. These intra-articular chondral lesions would have been missed without arthroscopic examination; however, the long-term functional outcome of these lesions has not been established. Loren and Ferkel (59) found more chondral lesions on the talar side of the joint than on the tibial side and more lesions on the medial side of the talar dome than on the lateral side.

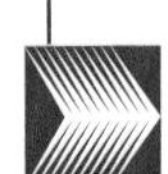

AUTHORS' PREFERRED TREATMENT

Several authors (18,27,28,36) have suggested that talar fractures in children may be best classified on the basis of the age of the injured child, with children under 8 years of age having a better prognosis than older children and in general doing well without operative management.

Although displacement of talar fractures has a critical effect on the blood supply to fracture fragments, the question of how soon following fracture is it critical to reduce displacement is unknown. Kellam et al (60) compared the outcomes of talar neck fractures in adults repaired early (within 12 hours) to those with delayed (after 12 hours) treatment and found that there were no significant differences with respect to osteonecrosis rates, ankle and subtalar joint arthrosis, minor and major complications, or need for a salvage arthrodesis. They found that other factors, such as injury severity, quality of reduction, and surgical complications, affected outcome more than timing.

We prefer to reduce talar fractures as soon as reasonably possible (within 12 to 24 hours). Although reducing simple talar neck fractures under conscious sedation with fluoroscopic control is appealing, it has been the practice at our center to reduce these fractures in the operating room with general anesthesia, where maximal sedation and muscular relaxation can be achieved and a carefully molded cast can be applied; also, if necessary, percutaneous pinning can be done.

For internal fixation we prefer posterolateral screws (see Fig. 27-10), because they are biomechanically stronger than K-wires. We use a posterolateral surgical approach, which is less likely to violate further any talar blood supply. Titanium screws allow MRI evaluation of osteonecrosis postoperatively.

Complications

Complications of talar fractures include skin necrosis, osteonecrosis, osteomyelitis, delayed union, and nonunion.

Skin Necrosis

Skin necrosis usually is related to an unreduced talar fracture pushing on the thin dorsal skin of foot. When skin appears tented and blanched, it is essential that the fracture be reduced immediately. This should be done in the emergency room if necessary because the incisions required for management of talar neck fractures often are through the compromised skin region. Alternative posterior approaches have been suggested (61,62) when the anterior skin is damaged; however, they have been considered suboptimal approaches (63). We have no experience with posterior approaches to the talus in children and have not seen these approaches described in the pediatric literature.

Osteonecrosis of the Talus

Osteonecrosis of the talus can occur in children (19,28,31) and is, as in adults, the main cause of disability after a fracture of the talus (8,27). Osteonecrosis is the most common complication of fracture of the talus in adults and possibly children (19).

Osteonecrosis usually follows some displacement of the talar neck that disturbs the blood supply to the body of the talus. Canale and Kelly (19), however, described two undisplaced talar neck fractures (type I) that developed osteonecrosis. Hawkins' original series (31) had an overall rate of osteonecrosis of 58% from all types. Osteonecrosis seems to occur within 8 weeks of injury (64).

The classic x-ray findings of talar osteonecrosis as described by Hawkins (31) (see Fig. 27-8) have been confirmed by other investigators (19,47). More recently, Tehranzadeh et al (65) introduced the concept of a "partial Hawkins sign" associated with incomplete osteonecrosis secondary to disruption of the intraosseous blood supply without subluxation or dislocation in adults. How closely pediatric talar fractures are reflective of talar fractures in adults in terms of osteonecrosis incidence is uncertain. Rammelt et al (20) described a 5-year-old child with a minimally displaced fracture of the talar neck with no subtalar or ankle joint subluxation who developed osteonecrosis 6 months after the injury. Citing an extensive literature search, they reported an osteonecrosis incidence of 16% after undisplaced talar neck fractures, considerably higher than that reported after Hawkins type I fractures in adults. Rammelt et al (20) reported that none of the children in their series who developed osteonecrosis was older than 9 years, suggesting that the immature talus may be more susceptible to it. They also reported that prolonged non–weight-bearing did not seem to influence talar fracture healing. Draijer et al (34) in the German literature described 2 children with partial osteonecrosis in their review of 11 talar fractures in children.

Hawkins' classic description (31) of talar osteonecrosis noted that about 6 to 8 weeks after injury the density of the bone in the dome of the talus should be decreased secondary to disuse osteoporosis from non–weight-bearing. This osteopenia denotes vascularization because osteoclastic loss of density occurs only if there is a blood supply. This appearance—the Hawkins sign—indicates that the talus is vascular and osteonecrosis is unlikely to occur. If the dome of the talus remains dense compared to the surrounding bone, this indicates osteonecrosis because the blood supply required for bone resorption is missing. Canale and Kelly (19), however, suggested that some patients who mobilize quickly after stable, undisplaced type I fractures may not develop disuse osteoporosis and therefore will not develop a Hawkins sign. Therefore, the absence of the Hawkins sign does not necessarily portend osteonecrosis. Canale and Kelly (19) waited 12 weeks before making their diagnosis of osteonecrosis, and one of their patients with a Hawkins sign did develop osteonecrosis. Indeed, although the Hawkins sign is highly sensitive, it is only moderately specific. If the Hawkins sign is present, it is a reliable indicator that osteonecrosis will not develop, but the absence of the Hawkins sign does not rule out the late appearance (19,29).

The management of established osteonecrosis remains controversial. Canale and Kelly (19) looked at the long-term results in their 71 patients and found that none of 22 patients with osteonecrosis had undergone surgical management at an average of 15 years after non–weight-bearing treatment. Protected weight-bearing while awaiting reossification of the talar dome can be very time consuming and frustrating, but is the standard of care. It, however, has not been compared to full weight-bearing.

Osteomyelitis

Osteomyelitis usually occurs after open fractures or surgical approaches, but it can occur after closed reduction and percutaneous pinning, especially if the pins are left out through the skin. When using K-wires, it has been our practice to bury the bent ends under the skin because the pins are left in for a minimum of 6 to 8 weeks, often under a cast, where pin surveillance or pin care cannot be carried out.

Signs and symptoms of osteomyelitis of the talus are typical of any infection, but a high index of suspicion should be maintained. The cast should be removed if there is any question of infection. If infection is suspected, we suggest culture-specific intravenous antibiotics. Incision and debridement should be done in the operating room and stable hardware retained. Progress is monitored clinically, as well as with erythrocyte sedimentation rate and C-reactive protein (CRP) blood levels.

CALCANEAL FRACTURES

Epidemiology

Calcaneal fractures have been estimated to account for only 0.005% of all fractures before the age of 15 years, in contrast to an incidence of about 1% to 2% in adults (66). The calcaneus is the most frequently fractured tarsal bone in children (8,67). Studies of calcaneal fractures in children are few because of their overall low incidence, as well as probable under-reporting because of missed diagnosis in very young patients who rapidly recover before MRI is required (68). Also, a low referral rate to surgeons because of the usual nonoperative approach may contribute to the low recorded incidence. Many studies on calcaneal fractures in children are anecdotal, with relatively small numbers and without a clear indication of the role of surgical management (11,69,70–74). Reported results of operative treatment of calcaneal fractures in young adults, however, may have some important implications for surgical decision making in the pediatric age-group. Using validated quality-of-life scales 2 to 8 years after surgery, Buckley et al (75) found that younger patients (adults under the age of 30 years) who had operative treatment had better gait satisfaction scores than those who did not have surgery. Allmacher et al (76) questioned whether short-term or intermediate results of displaced intraarticular calcaneal fractures can predict long-term functional outcome. Using validated outcome instruments, they studied adult patients treated nonoperatively and found that nonoperative treatment often led to pain and loss of function, which increased in the second decade after injury.

Many series have reported excellent outcomes with nonoperative management of pediatric calcaneal fractures (11,68,72, 77,78), although some of these had no real outcomes instrument (9,72,79). Buckingham et al (9) suggested that these studies reviewed mostly younger patients (less than 10 years) who have a higher preponderance for energy dissipation and remodeling and also might have fewer displaced intra-articular fractures, which usually are seen in older children.

The older pediatric literature suggests that most calcaneal fractures in children are extra-articular and are suitable for nonoperative treatment because the subtalar joint itself is preserved. More recent reports (80,81) indicated that intra-articular calcaneal fractures are common in the pediatric age group and recommended open reduction with internal fixation in older adolescents with displaced intra-articular fractures. Pickle et al (81) reported positive midterm clinical outcomes with few major complications in 6 children with 7 calcaneal fractures.

Several long-term pediatric calcaneal studies have been reported. Brunet (11) reported 17 children (19 calcaneal fractures) with an average 17-year follow-up and found that almost all had excellent long-term functional results with conservative management. He postulated that in children younger than 10 years of age with a damaged articular surface and depressed Bohler angle anatomic congruence is achieved through remodeling. This concept also was supported by Mora et al (80), who concluded that open reduction may be suitable only for severely displaced fractures in adolescents.

Management

Mechanism of Injury

Wiley and Profitt (78) noted that in children under 10 years of age, even a simple fall could cause a calcaneal fracture; Ogden (8) postulated that in older adolescents, as in adults, a fall from a significant height is required to fracture the calcaneus. Non–weight-bearing or limp in a toddler can be caused by a buckle-type fracture of the calcaneus that heals very quickly (8). Comminution is possible in children but is less frequent than in adults, even though in their series Buckingham et al (9) reported children falling from higher heights. Atkins et al (82) found that in adults the height fallen correlated with the degree of comminution of the calcaneus, but such a relationship has not been clearly established in children. In general, pediatric calcaneal fractures often are caused by low-energy trauma.

Care must be taken to examine for calcaneal, as well as talar, fractures in lawnmower injuries to the pediatric foot, because calcaneal fractures are frequent in this situation (83).

Surgical and Applied Anatomy

The anatomy of the various surfaces of the calcaneus (see Figs. 27-4 and 27-4) shows the intricate subtalar joint between the talus and the calcaneus. We agree with Sanders (63,84) that the coronal view (Fig. 27-15) shows details of fracture fragments with respect to the sustentaculum tali, which is exceptionally important in understanding how each individual fracture will need reconstruction.

The calcaneus, the largest of the tarsal bones, has an irregular shape consisting of six surfaces with three dorsal cartilaginous facets (anterior, middle, posterior) that articulate with the talus to make up the subtalar joint (see Fig. 27-4). The posterior facet is the largest of the three facets and is the major weight-bearing surface. The subtalar articulation with the three facets is in the anterior half of the calcaneus dorsally and the large extraarticular portion makes up the posterior tuberosity. In children, the calcaneal apophysis extends posteriorly, and this can be fractured completely or in pieces (Fig. 27-16). Secondary ossification of the calcaneal apophysis is variable between the ages of 6 and 10 years, and it can be multifocal, which can make it look on plain films like a fracture (see Fig. 27-1) (85). The Achilles tendon inserts on the dorsal posterior surface of the tuberosity.

The sustentaculum tali is another dorsal structure of the calcaneus that sits medial to the main body of the calcaneus and supports the neck of the talus (see Figs. 27-4 and 27-15). The middle facet sits on the sustentaculum tali and frequently is contiguous with the anterior facet. Underneath the sustentaculum medially runs the flexor hallucis longus. Laterally along the body of the calcaneus are two shallow grooves that house the peroneal tendons and are separated by the ridge-like peroneal trochlea (see Fig. 27-15).

The anterior surface of the calcaneus articulates with the laterally based cuboid bone in a saddle-shaped joint, which can be directly viewed or palpated with a blunt probe through an extensile lateral approach to the calcaneus.

There are multiple tendinous and ligamentous attachments to the calcaneus. It is attached to the talus inside the tarsal canal by the interosseous ligament. The deltoid ligament medially also attaches the calcaneus to the talus.

In very young children with calcaneal fractures, it should be kept in mind that the calcaneus can have dual ossification centers (86).

Signs and Symptoms

A mechanism of injury with a relatively high transfer of energy, such as a fall from a height or involvement of a motorized vehicle, either a motor-vehicle crash or a recreational vehicle, should prompt suspicion of a foot fracture, especially when

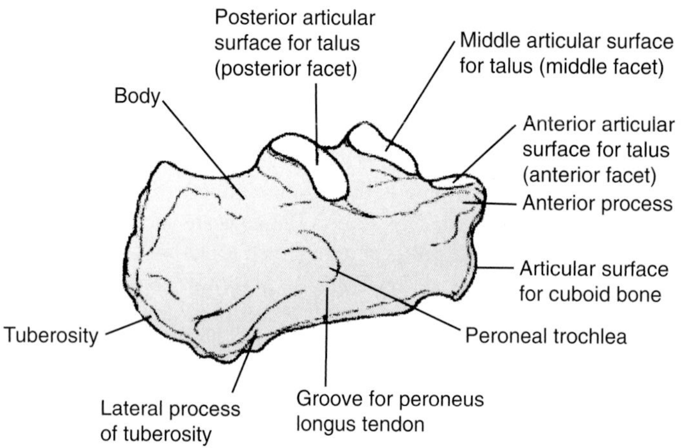

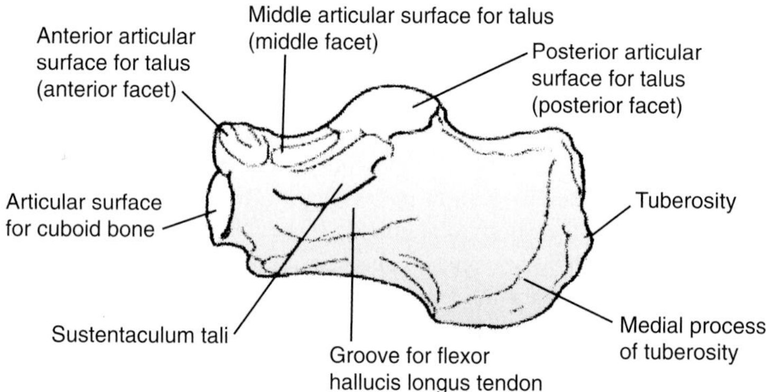

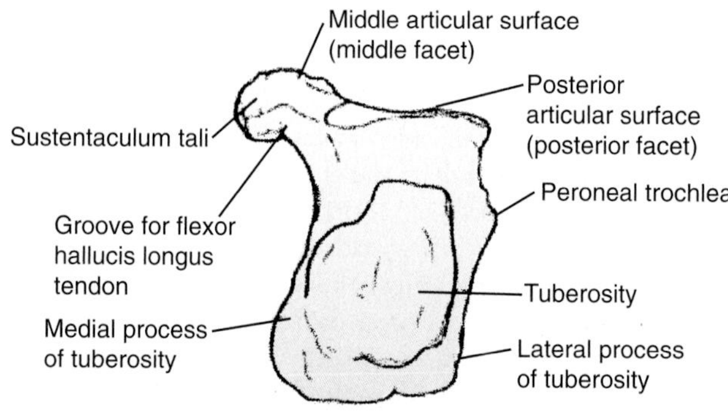

FIGURE 27-14 Anatomical details of various angles of the calcaneus including **(A)** lateral view, **(B)** medial view, and **(C)** coronal view through the level of the sustentaculum tali, which correlate with the CT scan view important in reconstruction of the posterior facet.

localized or generalized swelling, inability to ambulate, and significant pain are present. Subfascial bleeding, fracture blisters, and a prolonged inability to ambulate, in particular after 24 to 48 hours, are indicative of a foot fracture.

Minor fractures of the calcaneus probably are under-reported because they usually are difficult to diagnose, even with x-rays, and often rapidly get better with rest. Confirmation of such fractures with bone scan, CT scanning, or MRI usually is not obtained because these injuries usually are self-limiting. Many calcaneal fractures in children are initially missed and diagnosed late. Often the fracture line is not evident on the initial x-rays. Inokuchi et al (77) reported that 44% of fractures in their series were initially missed, as were 55% of those reported by Schantz and Rasmussen (68) and 44% of those reported by Wiley and Profitt (78).

Associated Injuries

Schmidt and Weiner (67) reported an association of spinal compression fractures with calcaneal fractures in children simi-

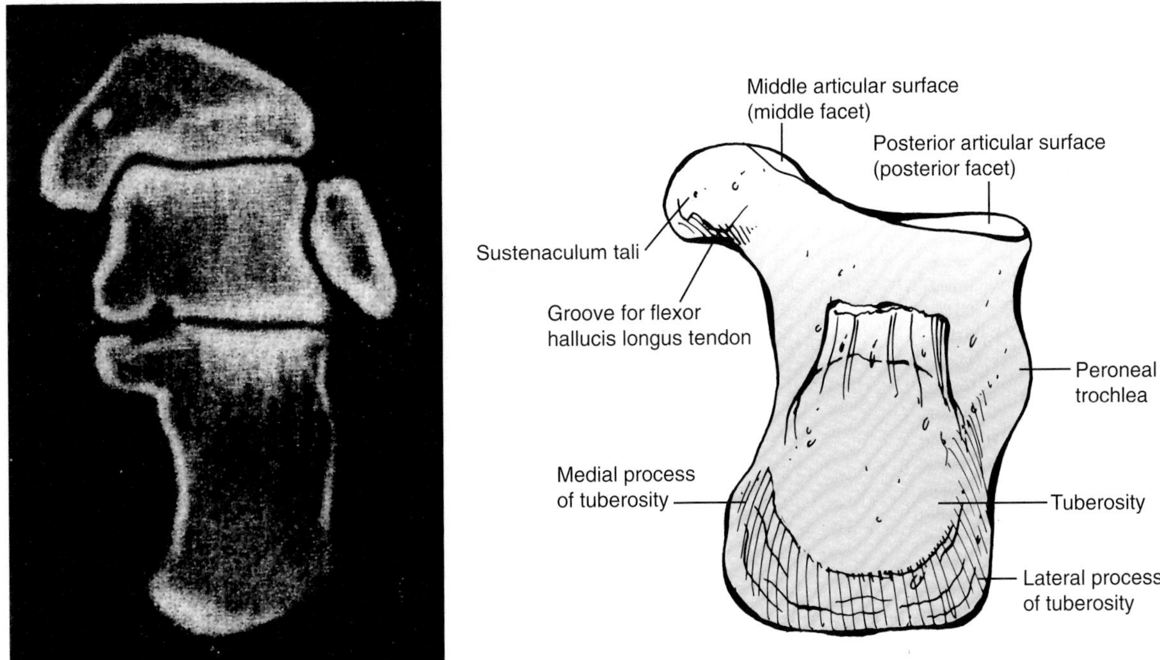

FIGURE 27-15 Anatomic correlation of anatomy with the coronal CT scan of the calcaneus. This is perhaps the most important view to assess the clinical reconstructability of the subtalar joint in displaced intra-articular fractures of the calcaneus.

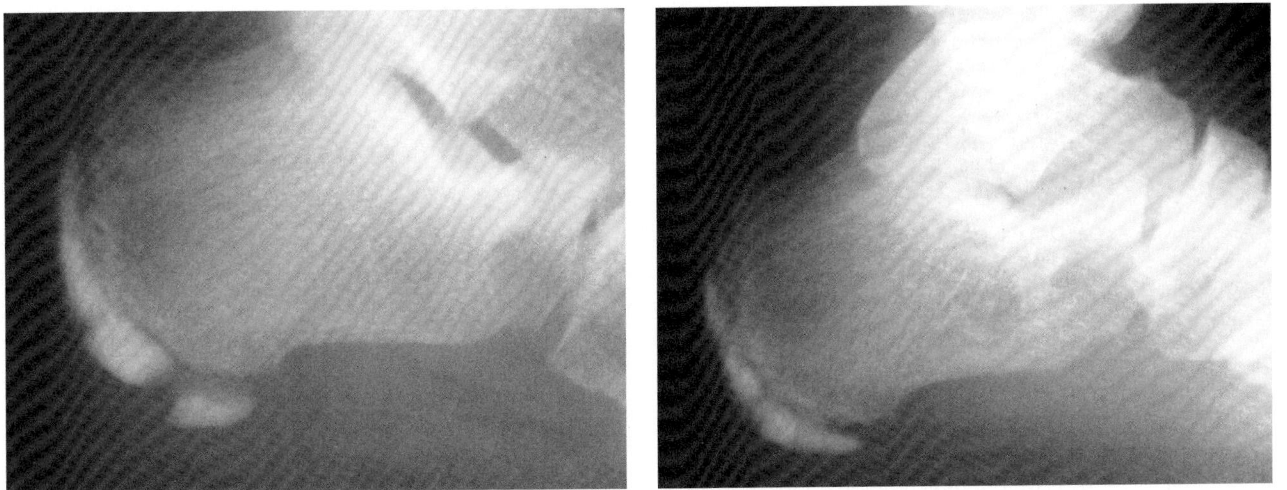

FIGURE 27-16 Calcaneal apophyseal fracture. **A.** True avulsion injury of an inferior segment of the calcaneal apophysis, which was treated in a cast for comfort. **B.** Uninjured side shows normal apophyseal segmentation.

lar to that reported in adults; Ogden (8) reported a lower association in children than in adults. Wiley and Profitt (78) reported two concomitant spine fractures with calcaneal fractures in the 32 children in their series.

Because of the high-energy mechanisms of injury involved, a child with a calcaneal fracture should have a careful and full physical examination to search for injuries elsewhere, such as the spine and tibial plateau. Talar fractures also are known to accompany calcaneal fractures (19,31). Kim and Berkowitz (79) described a 15-year-old with a calcaneal fracture associated with a talocalcaneal coalition.

Imaging Evaluation

Plain X-Rays

In children younger than 3 years of age, calcaneal fractures are difficult to view on plain x-rays (71,87,88) but often can be seen in x-rays taken subsequently (see Fig. 27-19). Initial views of calcaneal fractures may be negative, but repeat x-rays 10 to 14 days after injury may outline calcification or sclerotic lines along the extent of the fracture. Until after the age of 10 years, an x-ray of the largely cartilaginous calcaneus does not resemble that of an adult calcaneus, and the bony contours relied on in adults to generate angles such as the Bohler angle and Gissane angle cannot be used reliably (8,24,25,33). MRI shows more reliably the cartilaginous morphology of the calcaneus.

A three-view series of the calcaneus usually consists of a lateral view, a dorsoplantar view, and an axial view. Usually, initial views of the foot and ankle have been taken by the primary care physician or emergency room physician, but suitable views of the calcaneus should be obtained so that assessment of angles such as the Bohler angle can be made. Figure 27-17 shows the landmarks for calculating the Bohler angle. Joint depression is easily seen when the Bohler angle in the injured foot is compared with than in the opposite uninjured foot. In children the Bohler angle tends to be smaller than in adults.

When reviewing x-rays of children's feet, it is always important to be cognizant of the normally appearing ossification centers and accessory bones about the growing foot, which often are confused with fractures (see Figs. 27-1 and 27-2) (89).

Technetium-99m Scintigraphic Bone Scanning

The cost and exposure of bone scanning can be avoided by repeating plain x-rays 10 to 14 days after injury and while the patient's foot is immobilized in a back-slab or some other form of immobilization. Sclerotic lines can be seen on these repeat films (Fig. 27-18). If it is important to establish the presence of bony injury sooner, for example, when child abuse is suspected, bone scanning can reliably identify a fracture within 7 hours of injury. Furthermore, a negative bone scan at 72 hours after injury virtually excludes bony injury (90). Laliotis et al (87) used technetium bone scanning to identify calcaneal fractures in five of seven toddlers under 36 months of age who had no history of significant injury. Bone scanning, of course, as a diagnostic test is sensitive but not specific and can be positive in other pathologic states such as infection, some neoplasms, or other forms of bony or joint irritation. Other diagnostic tests must accompany bone scanning to improve diagnostic precision.

Computed Tomography Scanning

CT scanning is the best method of imaging of the injured pediatric foot because it identifies the key features of calcaneal fractures, including the degree of involvement of the posterior facet, the sustentaculum, or the calcaneocuboid joints (91,92). Fine cuts, 2- to 3-mm wide, can help develop two- and three-dimensional reconstructions that give unparalleled views of the damaged bone and aid in surgical reconstruction. CT scanning

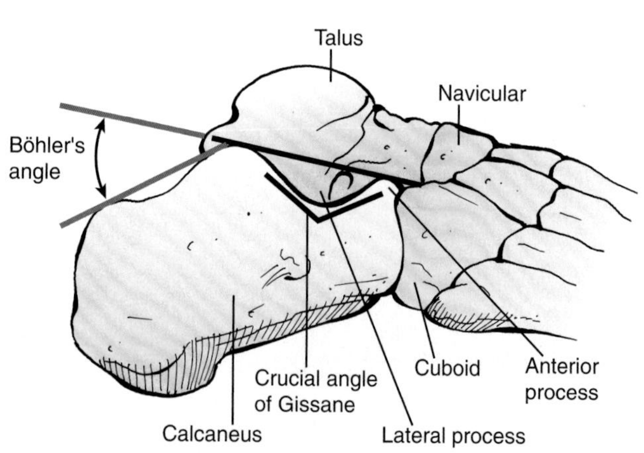

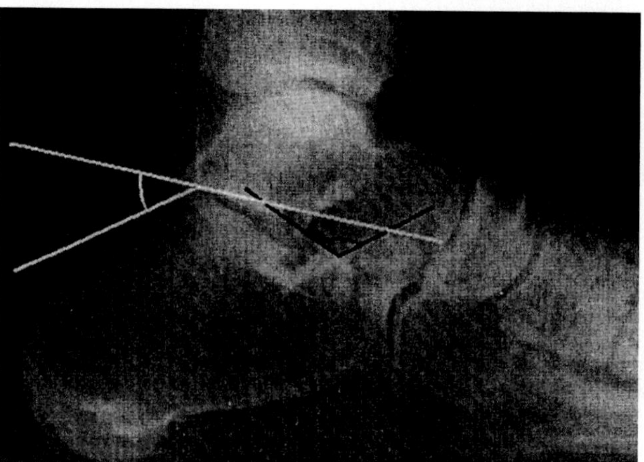

FIGURE 27-17 Diagrammatic depictions of the crucial angle of Gissane **(A)** and the Bohler angle **(B)**. The Bohler angle is more frequently used for decision making regarding fracture management. For measuring the Bohler angle, the landmarks on the lateral x-ray of the calcaneus are the anterior and posterior facets and the superior margin of the calcaneal tuberosity.

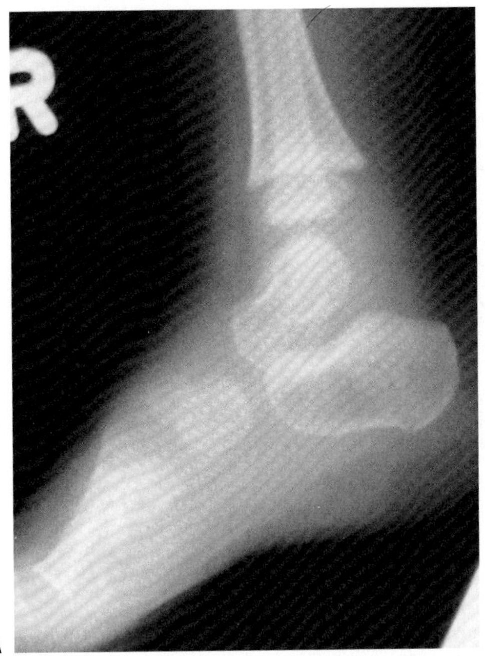

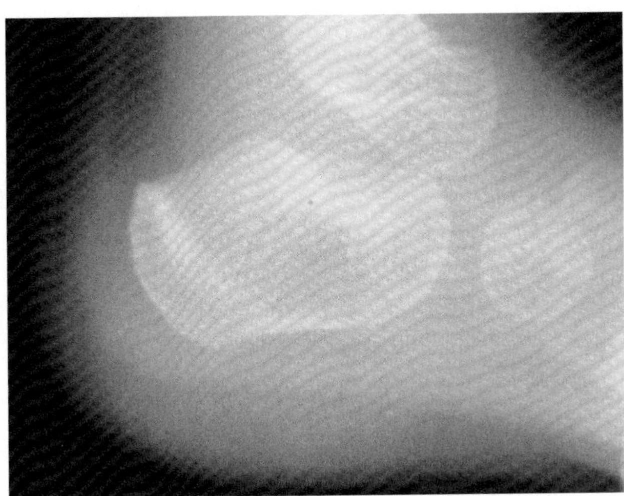

FIGURE 27-18 Fracture of the calcaneus in a toddler was not seen on the initial x-ray **(A)** but was visible on subsequent x-rays **(B)**.

protocols for evaluation of the calcaneus are well established, and almost all current fracture classifications are based on CT evaluation, with the Sanders (84) classification (Fig. 27-19) for adults being the most established.

Buckingham et al (9) are, to our knowledge, the first to compare CT scans of calcaneal fractures in children and adults. They found less comminution in children than in adults, even though the children reportedly had fallen from higher heights. Atkins et al (82) reported that in adults the height of the fall correlated with the degree of comminution. Buckingham et al (9) found that CT calcaneal fracture patterns in adolescents were similar to those in adults.

Magnetic Imaging Resonance

In children younger than 10 years of age, MRI shows osteochondral injuries better than CT scanning (54) or plain x-rays. It is likely that the reported frequency of osteochondral injuries will increase because of the improved ability to identify such injuries with MRI.

Classification

Bohler (93) in the 1930s was probably the first to accurately describe fractures of the calcaneus. In adults the Essex-Lopresti (94) and Letournel (95) classifications have been the most frequently used and have made important contributions in helping us to appreciate, for example, secondary fracture lines and other features. For children's calcaneal fractures, Schmidt et al (67) modified adult systems (94,96) to more accurately describe the pediatric patterns of fracture (Fig. 27-20). However, the Sanders

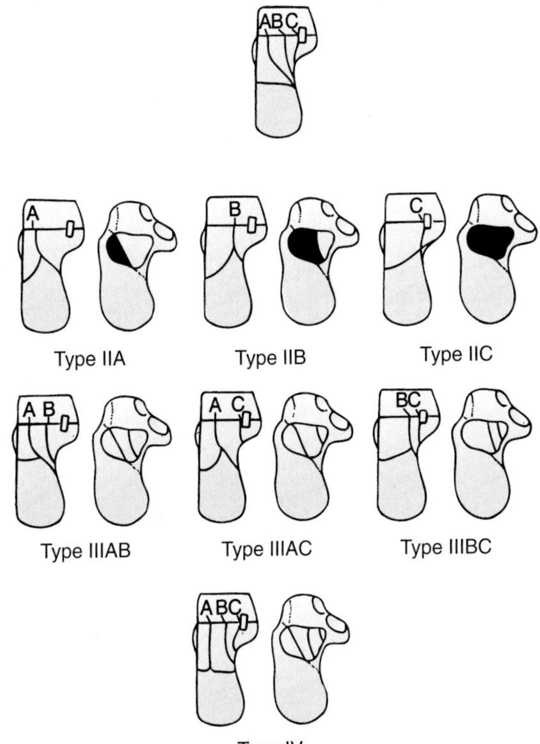

FIGURE 27-19 Sanders CT-based classification of intrarticular fractures of the calcaneus in adults. (From Sanders R. Intraarticular fractures of the calcaneus: present state of the art. *J Orthop Trauma* 1992;6:254; with permission.)

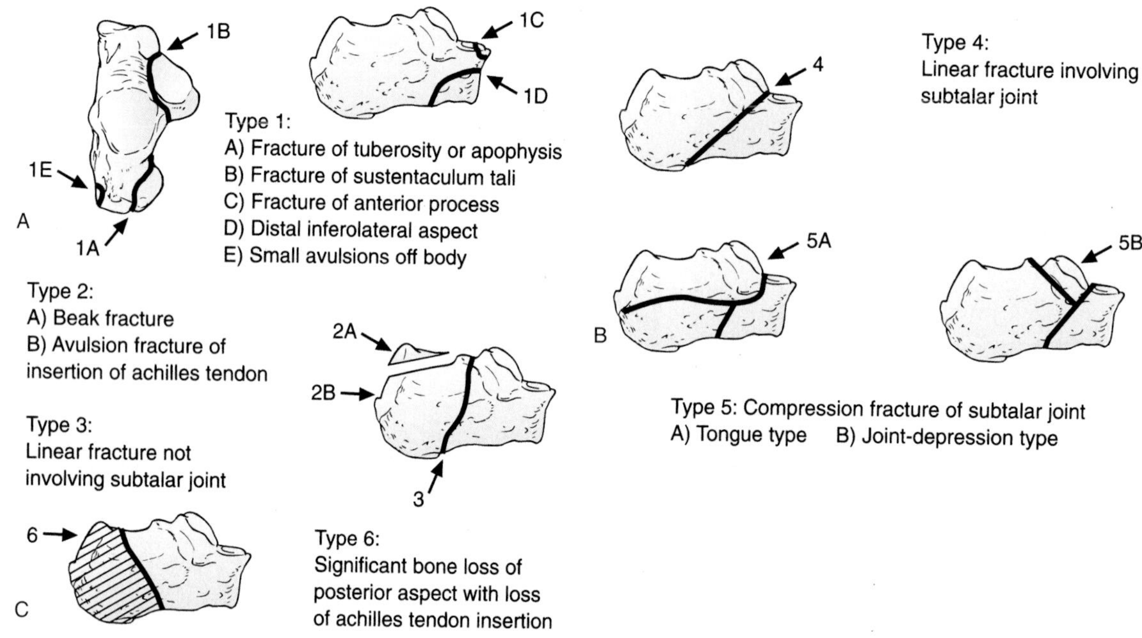

FIGURE 27-20 Schmidt classification of calcaneal fracture patterns in children. **A.** Extra-articular fractures. **B.** Intra-articular fractures. **C.** Type 6 fracture pattern with significant bone loss, soft-tissue injury, and loss of Achilles tendon insertion. (From Schmidt TL, Weiner DS. Calcaneus fractures in children: an evaluation of the nature of injury in 56 children. *Clin Orthop* 1982;171:150, with permission.)

classification (see Fig. 27-19), an adult classification system that is based on CT scans, has become more widely accepted, and its correlation with functional outcomes indicates that it may have some prognostic value.

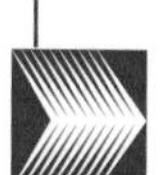

AUTHORS' PREFERRED TREATMENT

We believe that nonoperative management (non–weight-bearing cast immobilization for 4 to 6 weeks) is appropriate for calcaneal fractures in children and adolescents when CT scanning and plain x-rays show less than 4 mm of disruption of the three subtalar facets of the calcaneus, no subtalar joint subluxation secondary to widening, and no fibular impingement from the lateral cortex of the calcaneus. Nonoperative management also is indicated when there is severe soft tissue compromise about the calcaneal fracture. Multiple trauma may not warrant an extensive procedure to the foot in the first several weeks after injury.

Tongue-type fractures can be treated nonoperatively if the posterior gap is less than 1 cm and the Achilles tendon has not been significantly shortened by bringing the fragment up proximally. Occasionally, the technique described by Essex-Lopresti (94) for percutaneous reduction of tongue-type fractures (Fig. 27-21) is useful.

Pickle et al (81) reviewed the results of open reduction with internal fixation of displaced intra-articular calcaneal fractures in six adolescent patients (average age, 13 years) and found good short-term results at an average of 30 months after injury. None of the six patients (seven calcaneal fractures) developed any of the serious complications reported in adults. Four of the seven feet were completely pain-free, and three had some minor pain with sports or hard floors.

Open reduction with internal fixation of the calcaneus is a reasonable option for an older child or adolescent with a fracture pattern showing sufficient disruption on CT scan. The overall goal of surgery is the same as for adults: a functional, pain-free, plantigrade foot that fits into normal footwear. Principles for attaining these goals with operative management of calcaneal fractures in children and adolescents are essentially the same as for adults (84,97,98), including the following:

1. Restoration of the articular surface of the subtalar joint
2. Restoration of the normal height of the calcaneus
3. Restoration of the normal width of the calcaneus
4. Reduction and fixation of the calcaneocuboid and anterior and middle facets
5. Decompression of any fibular-calcaneal impingement

Occasionally not all of these goals can be obtained, with restoration of the articular surface usually being the most challenging. However, we believe that restoring the height

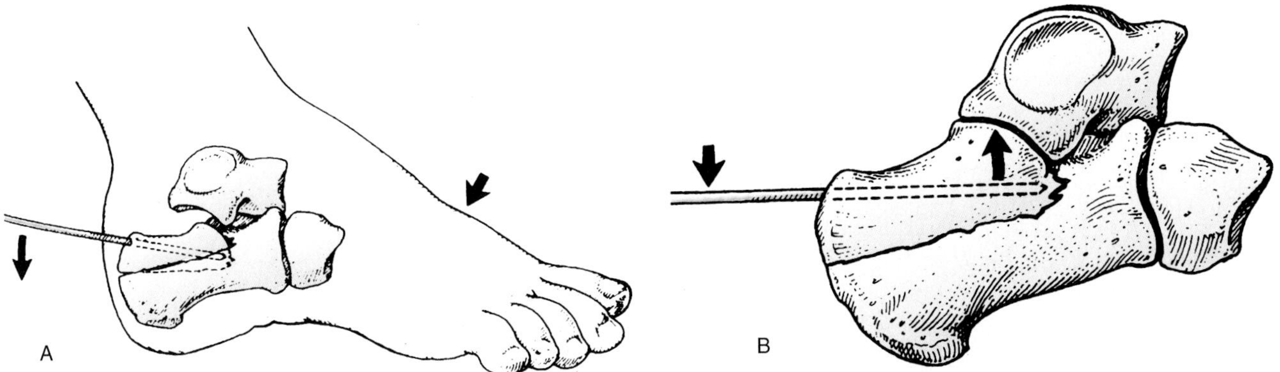

FIGURE 27-21 Percutaneous reduction technique for tongue-type fractures of the calcaneus, as described by Essex-Lopresti. This technique remains an alternative to conservative treatment and open reduction with internal fixation of displaced, tongue-type fractures. **A.** A pin is inserted into the tongue fragment and used as a joystick to manipulate the fragment into better position, usually with a downward force on the pin and the forefoot (plantarflexion). **B.** After reduction the pin is driven across the fracture to maintain reduction. (From Tornetta P, III. The Essex-Lopresti reduction for calcaneal fractures revisited. *J Orthop Trauma* 1998; 12:471, with permission.)

and reducing the width of the fractured and displaced calcaneus are important, even when reconstruction of the subtalar joint is suboptimal and could lead to premature subtalar arthritis, because this ensures a more successful subtalar fusion if needed later.

In adolescents with open physes, displaced intra-articular calcaneal fractures can be successfully reduced and fixed through standard approaches used in adults, including an L-shaped Letournel approach from the lateral side (Figs. 27-22 and 27-23).

The principles of management of calcaneal fractures are, in our opinion, the following (Table 27-3):

1. Rule out other injuries known to be associated with calcaneal fractures, such as spinal fractures in falls from heights.
2. Define the true nature and extent of the fracture with imaging.
3. Use special views and alternative imaging to aid in decision making.
4. Restore the Bohler angle and heel height.
5. Reduce the heel width to as close to normal as possible.
6. Reduce or rebuild fragments of the posterior facet of the subtalar joint, and reduce the sustentaculum tali fragment.
7. Use sufficient internal fixation.

Complications

Fracture Blisters

Very few studies of fracture blisters have been carried out, with none in children. Giordano and Koval (99) followed 53 adults over a 6-year period and identified two kinds of fracture blisters: fluid-filled and blood-filled. They also reviewed the results of a variety of treatments, from aspiration to deroofing or leaving intact, and found no significant differences in the complication rates of the different treatments. They recommended leaving fracture blisters intact; for ruptured blisters they recommended that they be deroofed and covered with nonadherent dressing. Giordano et al (100) also found a somewhat longer delay in wound healing of incisions made through blood-filled blisters, and they suggested that a blood-filled blister represented a slightly deeper injury than a clear fluid-filled blister.

Varela et al (101) found that the timing of surgery affected the occurrence of fracture blisters. Acute fractures treated with open reduction with internal fixation within 24 hours of injury had a 2% occurrence of fracture blisters, whereas if surgery was delayed more than 24 hours, the frequency rose to 8%. If surgery was done when fracture blisters were present, patient care was affected in 71% of patients, with 20% developing deep infections. They found no adverse affects if fracture blisters developed after open reduction with internal fixation.

We usually delay complicated open reduction with internal fixation of severe foot or ankle fractures if the patient is seen more than 24 hours after injury. A delay of 2 or 3 days to up to 2 weeks can be tolerated in older children and children.

Open Fractures

Thornton et al (102) reported that the risk of complications after open calcaneal fractures was related to the size and position of the traumatic wound. They found that lateral wounds had high complication rates regardless of the method of fracture stabilization and concluded that

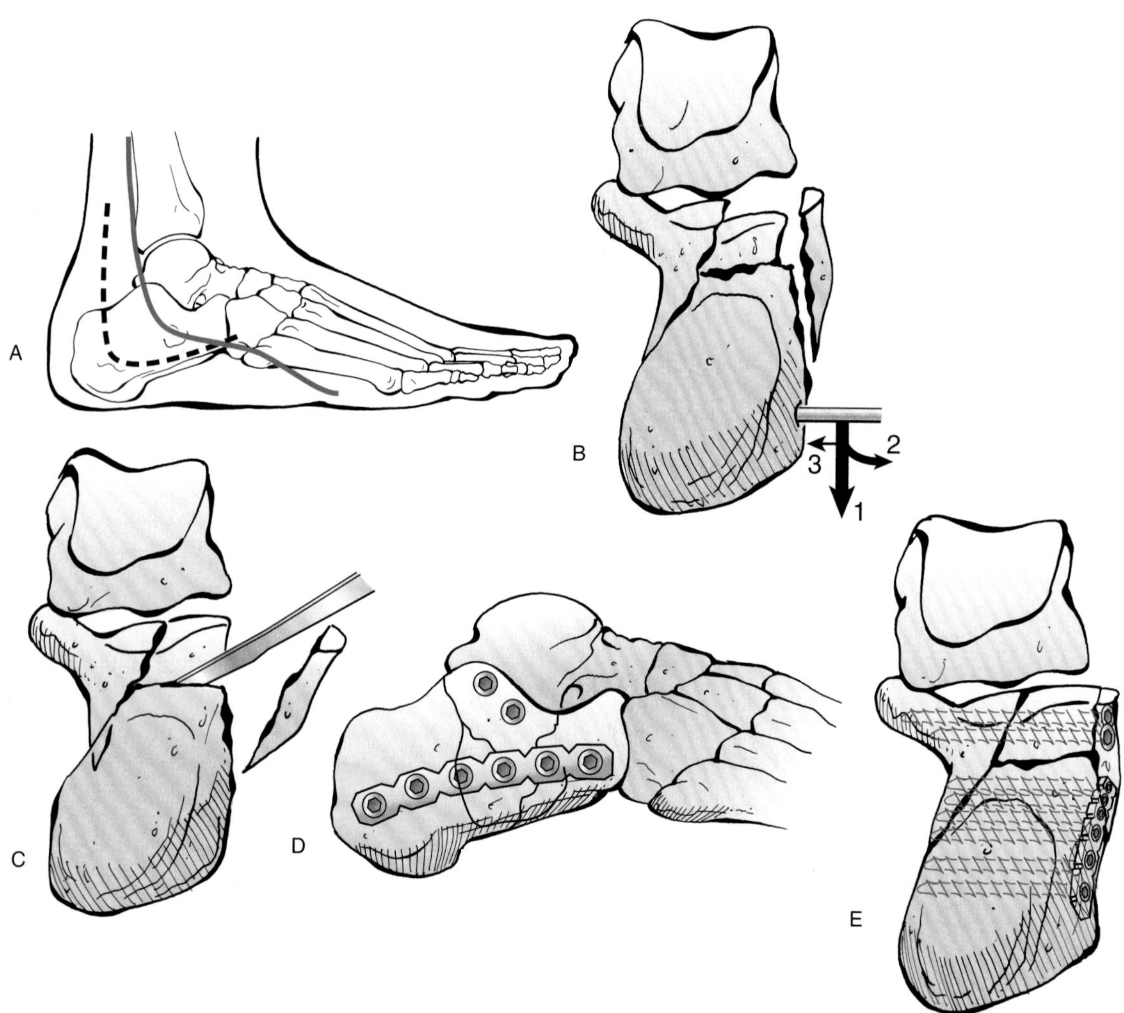

FIGURE 27-22 **A.** Lateral L-shaped approach to displaced intra-articular calcaneal fractures. The incision (*dashed line*) is laterally based, with the proximal arm approximately half the distance from the fibula to the posterior border of the foot and the distal arm halfway from the tip of the fibula to the sole of the foot. The sural nerve is illustrated. A full-thickness, subperiosteal flap exposes the entire lateral calcaneus. **B.** Reduction maneuvers 1, 2, and 3 (*densest arrow indicates greatest displacement*) with a Schantz screw are used to pull the tuberosity down and allow access to disimpact the posterior facet **(C)** after the lateral wall of the calcaneus is levered open. The posterior facet is then reduced anatomically, held provisionally with Kirschner wires, and then fixed with two partially threaded cancellous screws (outside of plate) into the sustentaculum tali. **D.** Lateral view of reduced calcaneus and **(E)** axial view of reduced fracture with hardware. (From Benirschke SK, Sangeorzan BJ. Extraarticular fractures of the foot: surgical management of calcaneal fractures [Review]. *Clin Orthop Relat Res* 1993;292:128–134; with permission.)

large or unstable wounds on the lateral side of the calcaneus should be treated with percutaneous wire fixation rather than open reduction with internal fixation. Medium-sized wounds were much less likely to develop infection than large wounds.

When wound problems occur, whether after an open or closed fracture, some recent advances can be useful. Mooney et al (103) reported excellent results with the use of vacuum assisted closure (VAC) techniques in patients from 3 days to 18 years of age with a variety of traumatic wounds and believed that 9 of their 27 patients would have required a free tissue transfer to secure wound coverage if not for the success of the VAC system.

Benirschke and Kramer (104) reviewed the literature to determine the rate of serious infection after closed and open calcaneal fractures treated with open reduction with internal fixation through an extensive lateral approach. They calculated that 1.8% of closed fractures and 7.7% of open fractures

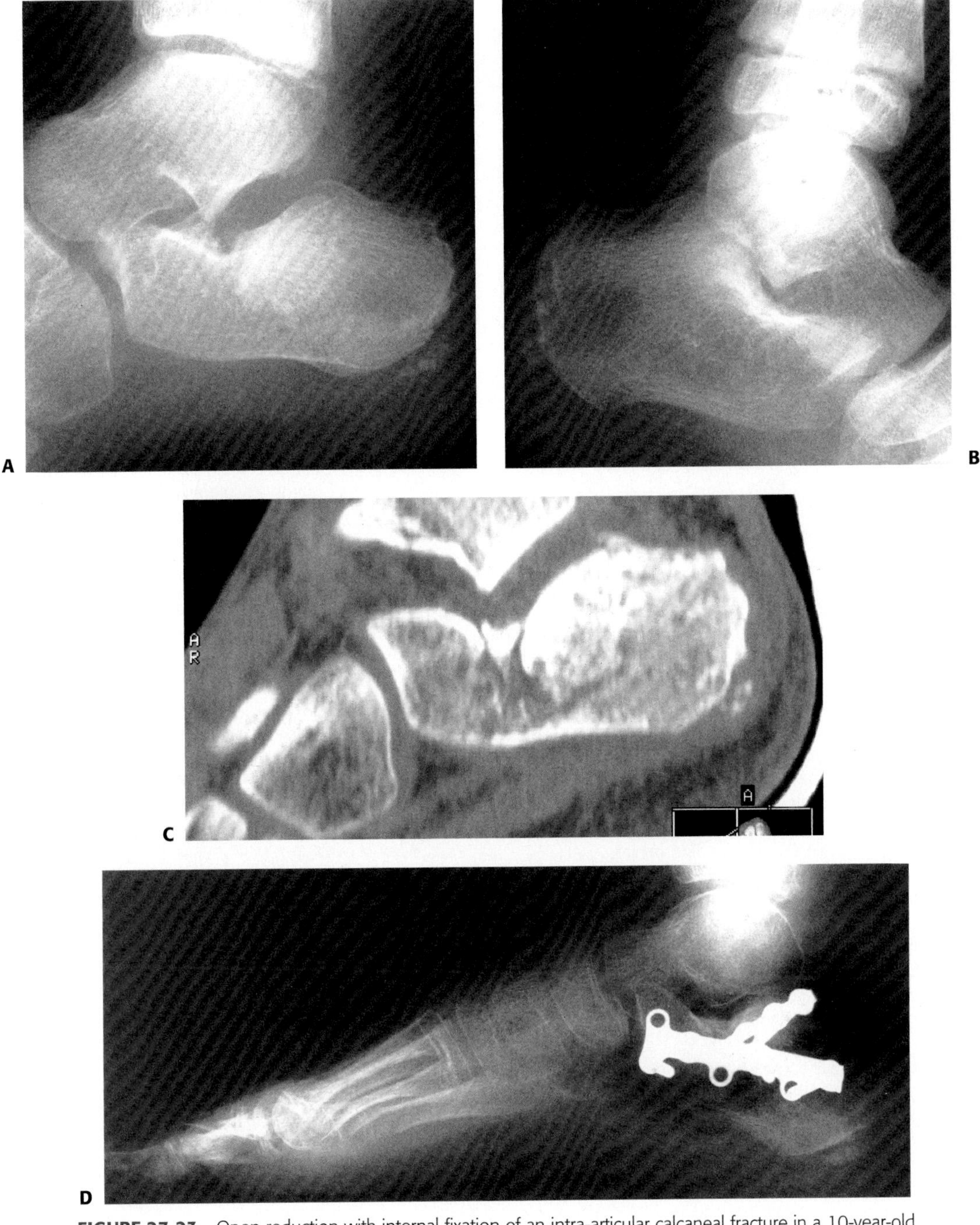

FIGURE 27-23 Open reduction with internal fixation of an intra-articular calcaneal fracture in a 10-year-old boy after injury on a trampoline. **A.** Lateral x-ray shows a severely depressed intra-articular fracture of the posterior facet of the calcaneus with a Bohler angle of 15 degrees. **B.** Lateral x-ray of opposite foot shows normal Bohler angle of 40 degrees. **C.** CT scan also indicates severe loss of the Bohler angle and the intra-articular fracture line. **D.** Lateral x-ray after open reduction with internal fixation with a calcaneal fracture plate (Synthes) through a lateral approach. No bone graft was required and an anatomic reduction was obtained. (Case courtesy of M. Kocher, MD, Children's Hospital, Boston, MA.)

TABLE 27-3 Operative Planning for Open Reduction with Internal Fixation of Intra-articular Calcaneal Fractures in Adolescents

Equipment	Radiolucent table C-arm Bean bag 30 cc of bone graft substitute (do not open unless required) 0.054-in Kirschner wires with driver Osteotomes Freer or Howarth type elevators Synthes calcaneal plates Small fragment set
Positioning	Lateral decubitus on large bean bag Unsterile tourniquet Knee and hip flexed C-arm monitor opposite operating surgeon Consider preparing for iliac crest bone graft
Incision	Lateral L-shaped incision (see Fig. 27-22) Start 2 to 3 cm superior to the tip of fibula, just anterior to Achilles tendon 90-degree turn at inferior aspect of calcaneus (smooth edge) Extend distally for 3 cm, then angle slightly dorsal to base of fifth metatarsal
Exposure	Mark out peroneus brevis and course of sural nerve Start deep dissection over tuberosity of calcaneus and go to bone Proximal dissection with scissors to avoid sural nerve Distally, go down to abductor digiti minimi Subperiosteal dissection including ankle ligament and peroneal tendons Identify peroneal tendons distally and protect Continue until subtalar joint and posterior facet of talus are reached Place two 0.054-in K-wires, one in talus and one in fibula, to hold flap back

Reduction	Consider medial approach to aid reduction
	Remove lateral wall piece with an osteotome, retain
	Clean fracture site, irrigate
	Mobilize intra-articular pieces
	Reduce tuberosity first
	Reduce posterior facet
	  Put two lateral pieces together first with K-wires
	  Reduce lateral group onto medial bone
	Check reduction with Freer, C-arm lateral (double density)
	Use K-wires to provisionally hold reduction
	Know where the sustentaculum tali fragment is

Fixation	Use 3.5-mm cortical lag screws with washers across facet
	Place first screw into sustentaculum tali (if intact)
	  Insert perpendicular to lateral margin of posterior facet
	  Angle from proximal-lateral to distal-medial
	Use two lag screws
	Apply lateral calcaneal plate
	  2 screws in tuberosity
	  2 screws in anterior calcaneus
	  2 screws in medial part of facet

Closure	Irrigate Consider small vacuum drain (rarely done) Close abductor digiti minimi fascia Use 2–0 Vicryl sutures in subdermal tissues Clamp all sutures before tying Tie from edges to apex to minimize tension Use 3–0 nylon vertical mattress sutures for skin closure
Dressing	Antibiotic gel dressing/4 × 8s Sterile Webril Two 6-in plaster slabs for U-splint 4-in elastic wraps
Postoperative	Elevate IV antibiotics for 24 hours Remove drain when less than 30 cc over 24 hours Splint non–weight-bearing Followup in 1 week for dressing change and wound check At 3 weeks, start range-of-motion movement of ankle, remove sutures, check x-rays Partial weight-bearing at 8 to 10 weeks if x-rays show healing

were followed by serious infections that required more intervention than oral antibiotics. All wounds and fractures, however, healed. They suggested that these rates were acceptable in light of the access the extensile lateral approach provides for the reconstruction of the calcaneus.

Aldridge et al (105) reported their experience of operative treatment of open calcaneal fractures in 19 patients, including 4 who were younger than 18 years of age. They found that definitive management with plates or K-wires was best after management of the soft tissue component and suggested a delay in definitive stabilization.

Reflex Sympathetic Dystrophy

Sarrail et al (106) reviewed reflex sympathetic dystrophy (RSD) in 24 children and adolescents and found that 73% had foot or ankle injuries. As in adults, RSD in children often presents with pain out of proportion to the injury along with signs of autonomic dysfunction in the affected foot. In a large series of 70 children (average age, 12.5 years) with RSD, Wilder et al (107) reported a 1-year delay from the onset of symptoms to the diagnosis; 84% of the patients were girls and 87% of injuries were in the lower extremity. At more than 3 years' follow-up, 54% of patients still had persistent symptoms of RSD. Diagnosis was based on clinical presentation and bone scanning and the mean time to diagnosis was 17.9 weeks.

Compartment Syndrome of the Foot

Approximately 10% of adults with calcaneal fractures develop increased hydrostatic pressure in the foot, and half of these develop claw toes if not treated (108). Brunet (11), however, in a long-term (more than 16 years) follow-up of 17 pediatric patients, found that none had developed claw toes or other signs of unrecognized compartment syndrome, except one who had an open fracture. We are always cautious when a child has a foot that is severely swollen and recommend measuring compartment pressure when clinical signs of compartment syndrome are present.

SUBTALAR DISLOCATION

Subtalar dislocations are unusual in children and may be missed on initial evaluation. Pain and swelling with obvious deformity usually indicate that x-rays are necessary and these usually show the subtalar dislocation.

Treatment

Closed reduction of acute dislocations should be attempted; however, when diagnosis is delayed or closed reduction is not successful, open reduction should be done, with consideration of application of K-wire to the talonavicular joint if the reduction is unstable. We prefer wire fixation of all subtalar dislocations because the initial cast becomes loose as acute swelling diminishes and the talonavicular joint may redislocate.

PERITALAR DISLOCATION

Although we have seen a number of talonavicular dislocations in children at our center, few have been described in the literature. Dimentberg and Rosman (3) only a decade ago noted that peritalar dislocation was not mentioned in the current major textbooks of children's fractures and dislocations. These injuries may have been included in studies reviewing subtalar dislocations without a discussion of the talonavicular joint. Nevertheless, this does appear to be a rare injury.

Talonavicular dislocation often is associated with fractures of the talar head and the navicular. The dislocation is a rotation deformity of the midfoot (Fig. 27-24). After closed reduction, severe joint incongruity of the talonavicular joint may require open reduction and internal fixation. Dimentberg and Rosman (3) reported that, although most talonavicular dislocations could be treated closed, open reduction was necessary if closed reduction was prevented by the toe flexors or associated impaction fractures or if the diagnosis was delayed.

MIDTARSAL INJURIES

Fractures and dislocations of the navicular, cuboid, and cuneiforms are rare pediatric foot injuries (109,110) because of children's low body mass and a relatively short lever arm across the midtarsal joint. Most tarsal fractures are avulsion or stress fractures that can be treated in a walking cast for 2 to 3 weeks.

Variabilities of ossification can occur throughout the foot, particularly in the navicular. The so-called Kohler disease is commonly seen between the ages of 2 and 5 years and can be confused with a fracture (Fig. 27-25) (111). The x-ray appearance of a sclerotic, thin, fragmented navicular may represent repetitive microtrauma or an abnormal ossification pattern.

Complete fractures of the midtarsal bones usually result from high-energy trauma and are typically associated with other injuries such as those of the Lisfranc complex. Midtarsal dislocation may be caused by forceful forefoot supination that disrupts the calcaneocuboid joint and may fracture or dislocate the navicular or cuneiform bones (112). The diagnosis should be suspected if a fracture of the midtarsal bones is detected. The calcaneocuboid joint is best shown on lateral and oblique x-rays.

Because the tarsal bones are largely intra-articular, closed or open reduction with internal fixation is usually required for displaced fractures (Fig. 27-26). As with other high-energy injuries, compartment syndrome of the foot can occur.

TARSOMETATARSAL INJURIES (LISFRANC FRACTURE-DISLOCATION)

Although tarsometatarsal (TMT) joint injuries are not unusual in adults, they are rare in children (113). Although mostly de-

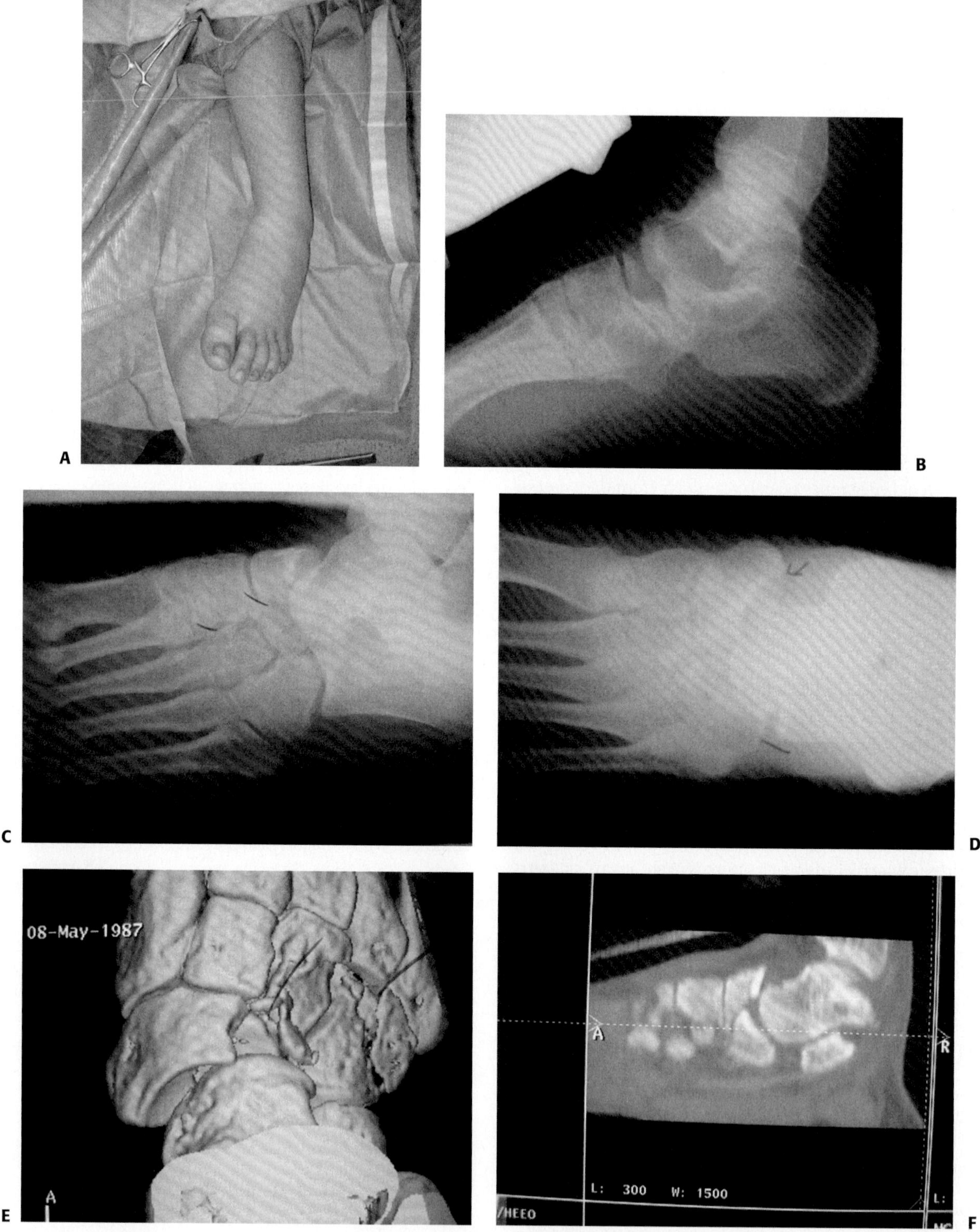

FIGURE 27-24 Peritalar dislocation with major disruption of the talonavicular joint in 16-year-old boy injured in a motocross accident. **A.** Clinical photograph shows appearance of an acquired club-foot. **B–D.** X-rays show fracture-dislocation of the talonavicular joint with the navicular dislocated medially with respect to the talar head. **E,F.** CT scans show greater detail. Even after closed reduction **(F),** severe joint incongruity between the talar head and the navicular bone required open reduction with internal fixation. See Figure 27-26 for postoperative x-rays.

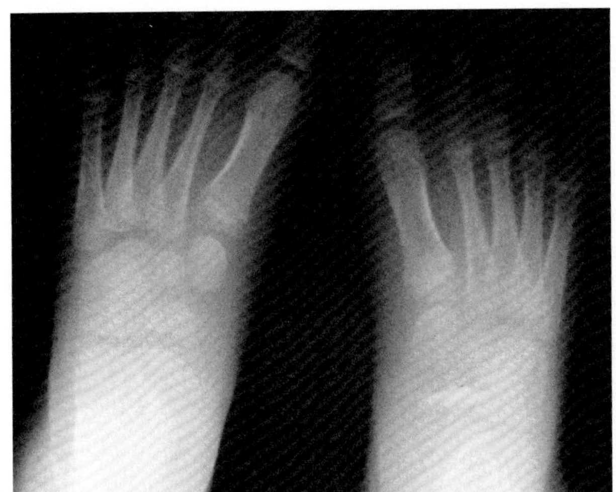
A

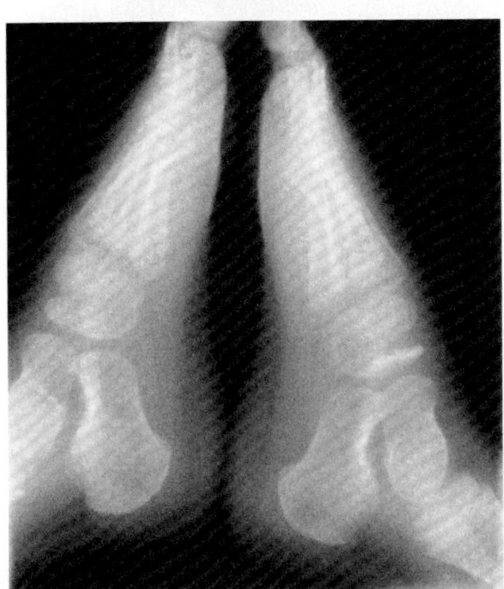
B

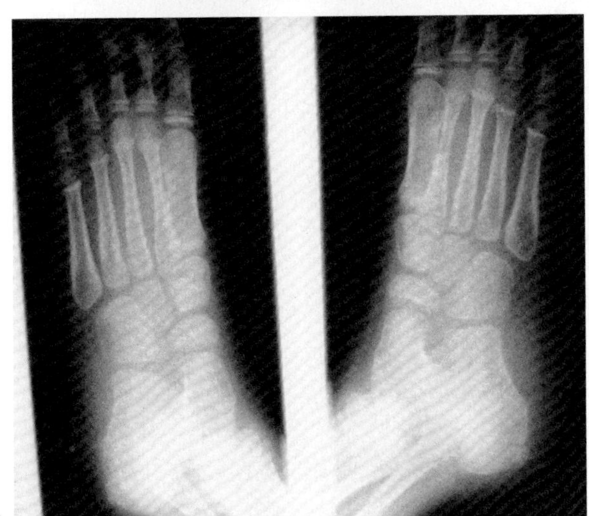
C

FIGURE 27-25 Kohler disease in a 3-year-old boy. **A,B.** Flattening, irregularity, and sclerosis are consistent with an ossification irregularity of the tarsal navicular. **C.** One year later, the area appears healed.

scribed as isolated case reports (114–116), a series of 18 TMT joint injuries in children was reported by Wiley (117) in 1981, and more recently Buoncristiani et al (118) described an additional 8 such injuries in skeletally immature patients.

Management

Mechanism of Injury

Tarsometatarsal injuries are either direct, usually secondary to an object falling on the foot, or indirect, in which the foot is either violently plantar flexed or abducted in the toe walking position or while trying to break speed or from a fall from a height. Wiley described three basic mechanisms of injury (117) (Fig. 27-27).

Traumatic Impact in the Tiptoe Position. An example of a traumatic impact injury occurring while in the tiptoe position would be jumping from a height and landing on the toes. This usually causes metatarsal joint dislocation and fracture of the base of the metatarsal.

Heel-to-Toe Compression. In this situation, the patient is in a kneeling position when the impact load strikes the heel. There may be lateral dislocation of the second, third, fourth, and fifth metatarsals and fracture of the second metatarsal base.

The Fixed Forefoot. In this situation, the patient falls backward while the forefoot is fixed to the ground by a heavy weight. The patient's heel resting on the ground becomes the fulcrum for the forefoot injury. The most common mechanism in children is a fall from a height, followed by a fall backward and heel-to-toe compression (117,119). However, in adults, these injuries usually result from motor vehicle accidents, crush injuries, and falls from a height.

Signs and Symptoms

Typically, swelling is present on the dorsum of the foot overlying the tarsometatarsal joints. However, the diagnosis of these injuries may be difficult, and in adults as many as 20% of injuries are misdiagnosed or overlooked (120,121). Most injuries either are not displaced at the time of injury or reduce spontaneously after injury. Although, with significant trauma, the entire dorsum of the foot may be swollen and localization of pain may be difficult, with milder injuries more focal swelling may allow identification of pain over the tarsometatarsal joint. Ecchymosis on the plantar aspect of the midfoot suggests trauma to the tarsometatarsal ligaments and is highly indicative of an injury to that joint (122) (Fig. 27-28).

Associated Injuries

Of course, in falls from a height and motor vehicle crashes, associated injuries such as lumbar vertebral fractures, pelvic fractures, and other lower and upper extremity fractures should be sought. With a direct mechanism of injuries, associated inju-

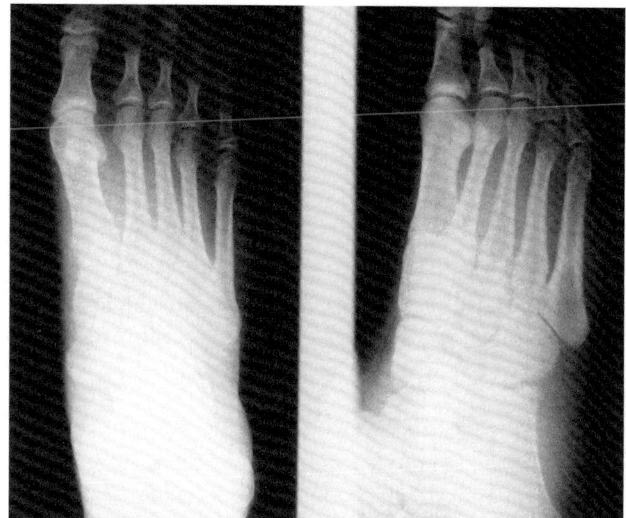

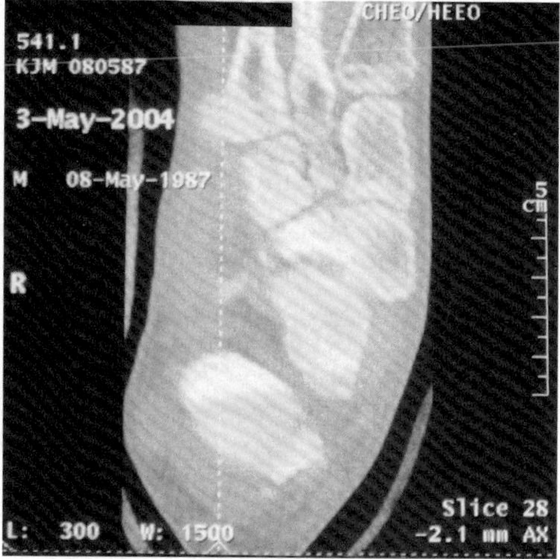

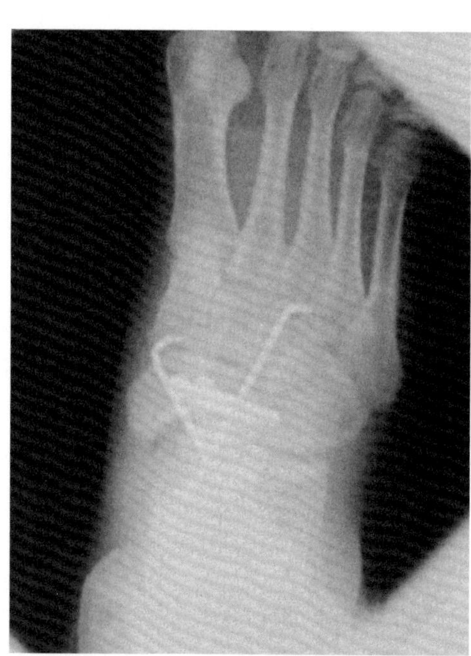

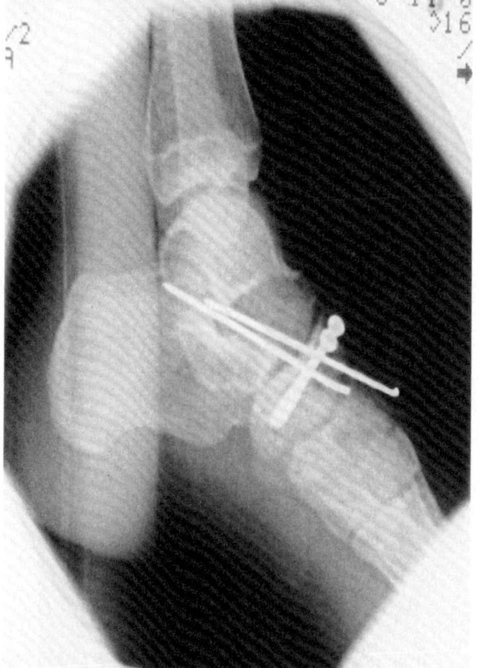

FIGURE 27-26 Fracture-dislocation of the navicular. **A.** This 16-year-old boy sustained a fracture-dislocation of the navicular in a motocross accident. **B.** CT scan shows fractures of the navicular and cuneiform. **C,D.** After open reduction with internal fixation using combined pins and screws.

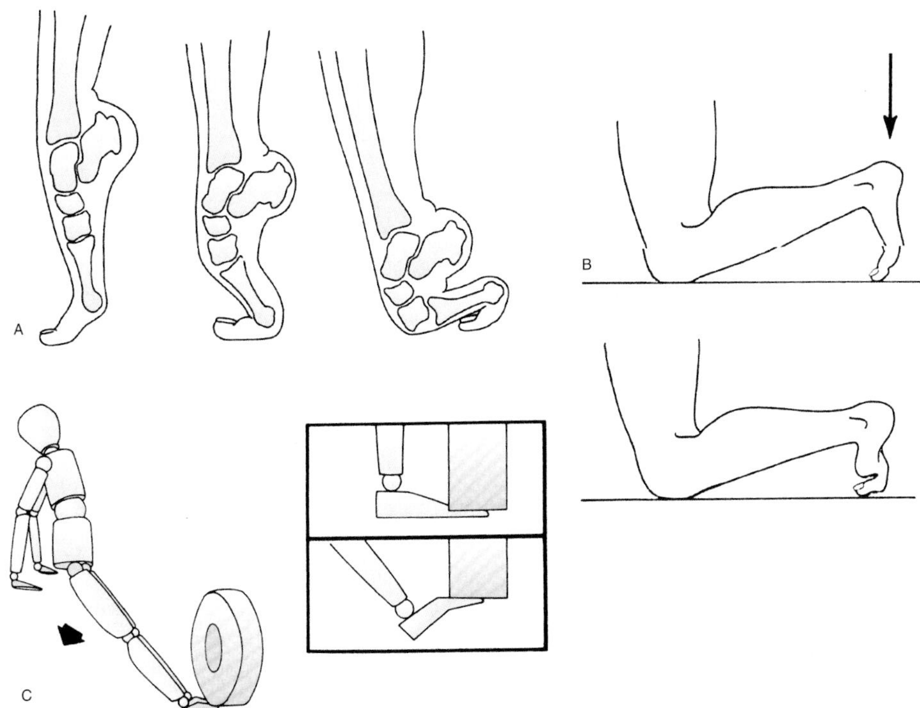

FIGURE 27-27 Mechanism of Lisfranc injuries. **A.** The most common mechanism of injury: progression from the "tiptoe" position to complete collapse of the tarsometatarsal joint. **B.** Plantar flexion injury: direct heel-to-toe compression produces acute plantar flexion of the tarsometatarsal joint. **C.** Backward fall with the forefoot pinned.

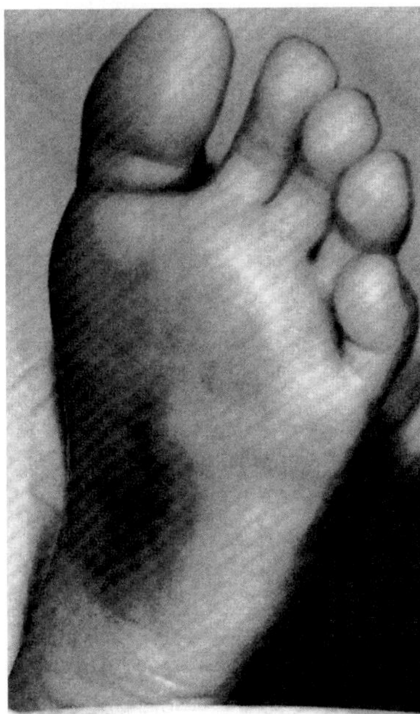

FIGURE 27-28 Plantar ecchymosis sign. Ecchymosis along the plantar aspect of the midfoot is an important clinical finding in subtle Lisfranc tarsometatarsal injuries. (From Ross G, Cronin R, Hauzenblas J, et al. Plantar ecchymosis sign: a clinical aid to diagnosis of occult Lisfranc tarsometatarsal injuries. *J Orthop Trauma* 1996;10:120.)

ries are unusual. Rare but reported concomitant injuries include cuboid compression or "nutcracker" fractures, as well as cuneiform instabilities and posterior tibial tendon injuries.

Classification

A three-part classification system devised by Hardcastle, a modification of a system described by Quenu and Kuss (123) in 1909, is simple and practical (Fig. 27-29) (123,124).

Type A: Total incongruity. There is incongruity of the entire metatarsal joint in a single plane with lateral displacement.

Type B: Partial incongruity. Only partial incongruity of the joint is seen involving either the medial or lateral aspect of the foot. The medial dislocation involves displacement of the first metatarsal from the first cuneiform because of disruption of the Lisfranc ligament or fracture at the base of the metatarsal, which remains attached to the ligament.

Type C: Divergent pattern. The first metatarsal is displaced medially; any combination of the lateral four metatarsals may be displaced laterally. This is associated with partial or total incongruity.

Most children's injuries are type B with minimal displacement, whereas types A and C are rare (117).

Imaging

Essential x-rays include anteroposterior, lateral, and oblique views of the foot. The lateral border of the first metatarsal should

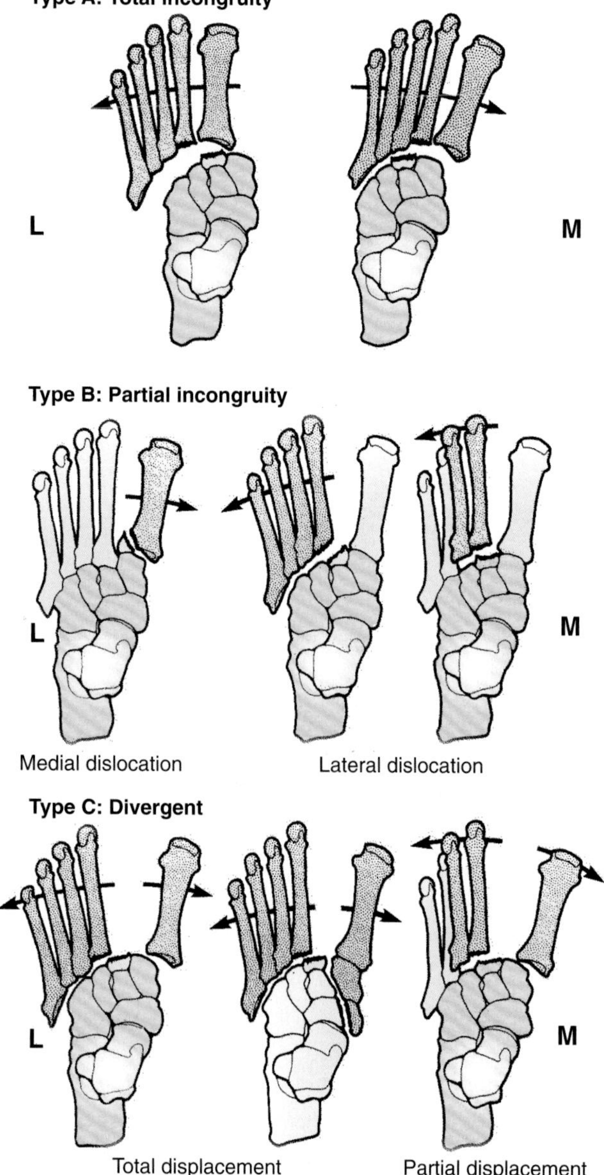

FIGURE 27-29 Classification of tarsometatarsal dislocations. *L*, lateral; *M*, medial. (Reproduced with permission from DeLee JC. Fractures and dislocations of the foot. In: Mann RA, Coughlin MJ. *Surgery of the Foot and Ankle*, 6th ed. St. Louis: Mosby; 1993:1465–1703; adapted from Hardcastle PH, Reschauer R, Kutscha-Lissberg E, et al. Injuries to the tarsometatarsal joint: incidence, classification and treatment. *J Bone Joint Surg Br* 1982;64:349–356.)

be in line with the medial cuneiform. The medial aspect of the second metatarsal should line up with the medial aspect of the middle cuneiform on the oblique x-ray. Fracture of the base of the second metatarsal should alert the examiner to the possibility of a tarsometatarsal dislocation because these injuries can spontaneously reduce. A cuboid fracture in combination with a fracture of the base of the second metatarsal indicates tarsometatarsal dislocation (Fig. 27-30).

Weight-bearing x-rays and abduction stress views of the Lisfranc joint have been advocated when routine views are normal (125,126). However, these are difficult to obtain without ankle block or general anesthesia, limiting their usefulness in children. CT scans can be useful to define the extent of injury when x-rays are not conclusive (127–129). Bone scans may be helpful to screen for injury when x-rays are normal, although they are not specific for the severity of the injury (130). MRI scans can delineate ligamentous injuries to the tarsometatarsal joint but do not offer a significant advantage in determining treatment (131).

Surgical and Applied Anatomy

Stability of the TMT joint is based on bony architecture as well as supporting ligaments. The cuneiform and tarsal bones, along with the medial three metatarsal bases, have a trapezoidal configuration that is wider on the dorsal aspect. This "Roman arch" effect aids in resisting collapse. Similarly, the second metatarsal base is recessed between the medial and lateral cuneiforms. This "keystone" mortise adds to the stability in the transverse plane. Strong plantar intertarsal ligaments at the base of the second through the fifth metatarsals add to the stability, although there is no direct link between the first and second metatarsals (Fig. 27-31) (132). A strong Lisfranc ligament traverses the base of the second metatarsal to the medial cuneiform. The less rigid relationship between the first and second metatarsals allows the frequent divergent injury.

The TMT joint can be considered in three columns. The medial column involves the first ray; the middle column, the second and third rays; and the lateral column, the fourth and fifth rays. The metatarsal joints are all in the same plane, distal to the recessed second metatarsal base. Because of this "keystone" positioning, injuries that are forceful enough to create displacement usually result in fracture of the second metatarsal. Occasionally, a subtle "fleck sign" is seen on x-rays when the Lisfranc ligament has been avulsed from the second metatarsal base (Fig. 27-32) (132).

Current Treatment Options

Successful treatment depends on obtaining and maintaining an adequate stable reduction. For minimally or nondisplaced fractures (less than 2 mm), elevation, and application of a compression dressing can be followed by application of a short-leg cast once swelling has decreased. Immobilization typically is continued for 5 or 6 weeks.

For fractures that are displaced 2 mm or more, reduction should be achieved with the use of general anesthesia. Closed reduction can be performed with longitudinal traction along the affected toes coupled with manual pressure over the dorsum of the foot to reduce any dorsal displacement. Percutaneous pinning is used to maintain the reduction. The key to reduction involves primary pinning and stabilization of the second meta-

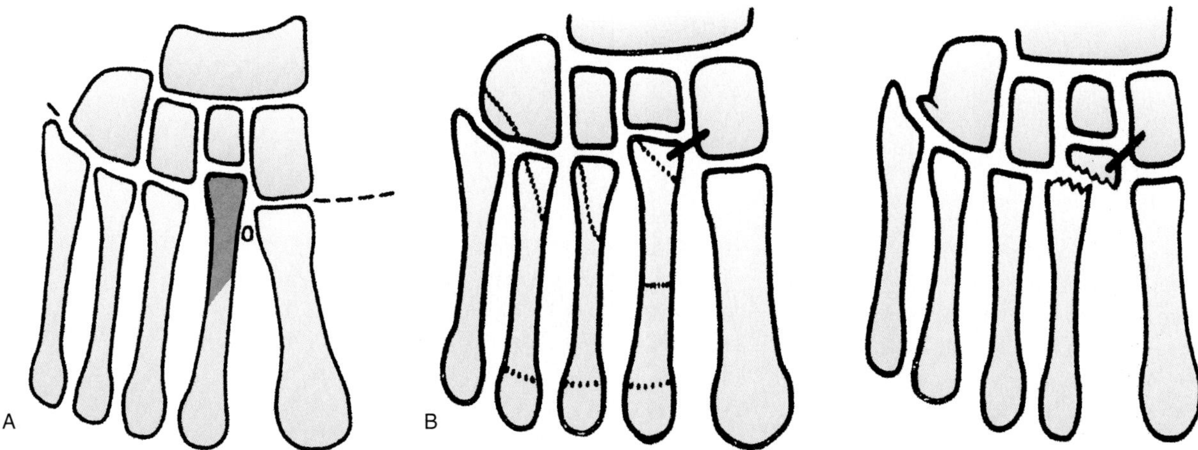

FIGURE 27-30 **A.** Second metatarsal is the "keystone" of the locking mechanism. **B.** Fractures of the cuboid and second metatarsal are pathognomonic signs of disruption of the tarsometatarsal joints.

tarsal to the medial cuneiform. Additional pins can be placed according to the fracture pattern, including medial pins to secure the first metatarsal and medial cuneiform and lateral pins to stabilize the lateral metatarsals to the second or third cuneiform or the cuboid as indicated.

Open reduction is reserved for fractures in which anatomic reduction cannot be achieved or possibly for fractures in skeletally mature patients. Longitudinal incisions over the first-second metatarsal interspace or third-fourth metatarsal interspace or both are used. The usual impediments to reduction are interposition of the tibialis anterior tendon, incongruity of the medial cuneiform–first metatarsal articulation and interposition of fracture fragments in the second metatarsal–middle cuneiform joint (Fig. 27-33) (133). In skeletally mature patients, rigid fixation with screws across the medial three TMT or intertarsal joints is coupled with percutaneous pin fixation of the fourth and fifth tarsometatarsal joints in order to preserve their mobility (Fig. 27-34) (134). Pins can be removed after 4 to 6 weeks with progressive mobilization of the foot.

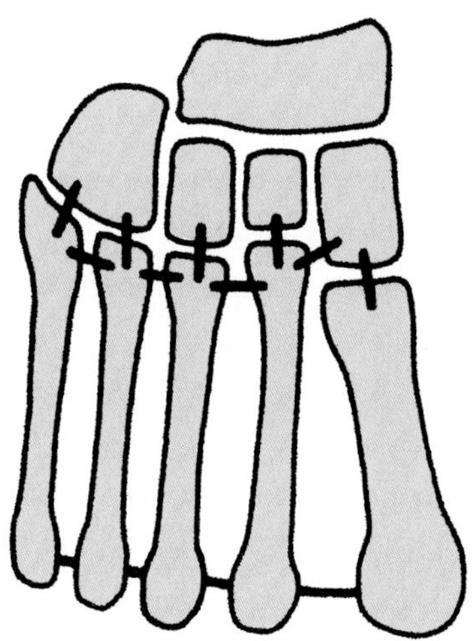

FIGURE 27-31 The ligamentous attachments at the tarsometatarsal joints. There is only a flimsy connection between the bases of the first and second metatarsals (not illustrated). The second metatarsal is recessed and firmly anchored. (From Wiley JJ. The mechanism of tarsometatarsal joint injuries. *J Bone Joint Surg Br* 1971;53:474, with permission.)

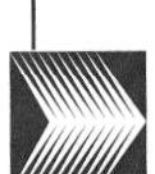

AUTHORS' PREFERRED TREATMENT

We prefer to carry out reduction with the use of general anesthesia and finger traps with the patient supine. Percutaneous pinning is accomplished under image intensifier control, as described above, with supplemental pins as necessary based on the direction of displacement. When necessary, open reduction can be obtained through dorsal incisions. We prefer to leave pins protruding through the skin at right angles and padded with felt. We have no experience with the technique of screw fixation in this injury (see Fig. 27-34).

Complications

Post-traumatic arthritis is known to occur after TMT injuries in a significant percentage of adults. Wiss et al (135), in a series of adult patients, found that no patient had a normal gait after a displaced Lisfranc fracture-dislocation. In fact, in young adult athletes, a delay in diagnosis and failure to attain anatomic reduction have been associated with a poor prognosis (136). In Wiley's series (117) of 18 patients, none of whom required open reduction, 14 patients had excellent

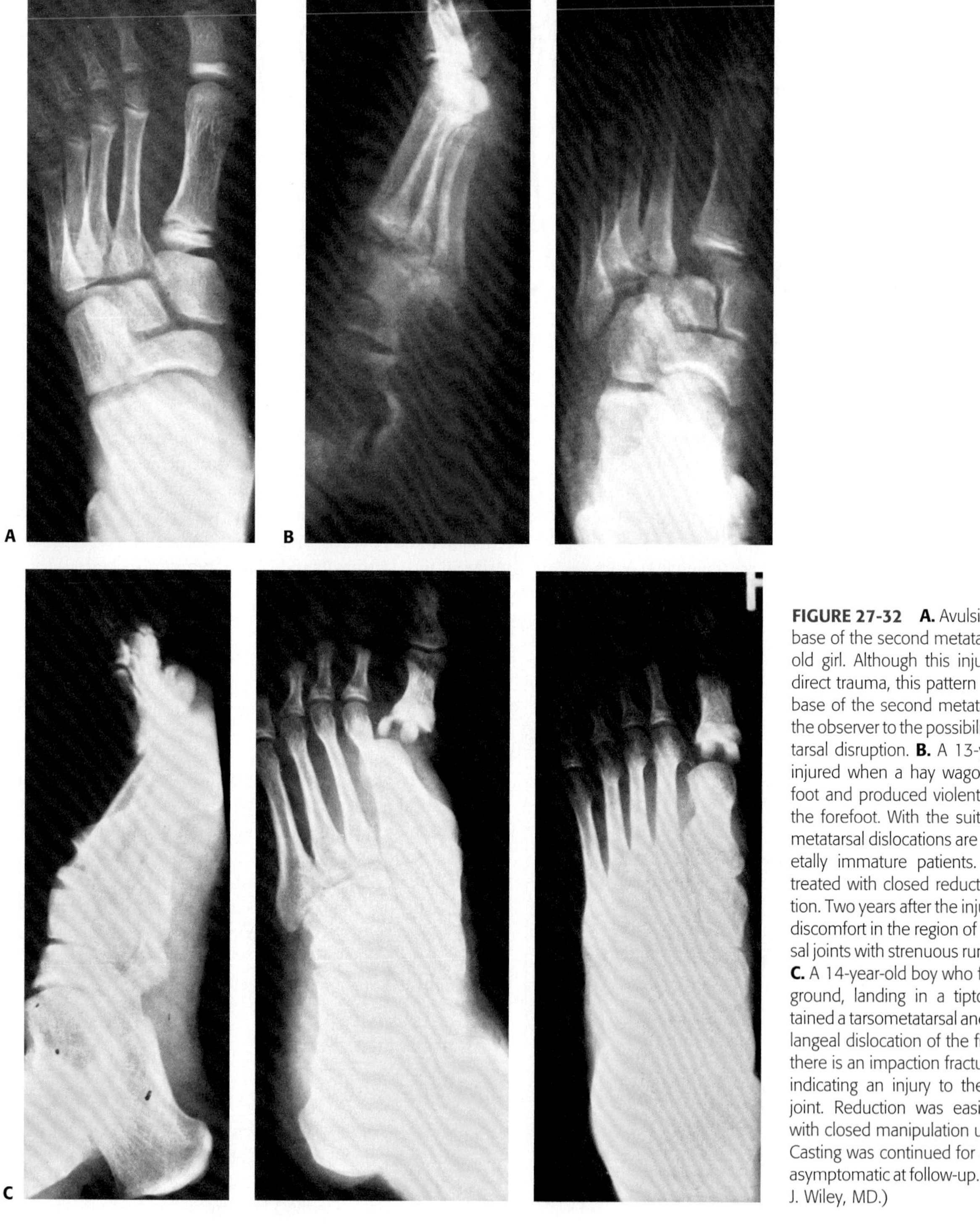

FIGURE 27-32 **A.** Avulsion fracture of the base of the second metatarsal in an 8-year-old girl. Although this injury resulted from direct trauma, this pattern of fracture of the base of the second metatarsal should alert the observer to the possibility of a tarsometatarsal disruption. **B.** A 13-year-old boy was injured when a hay wagon rolled over his foot and produced violent plantarflexion of the forefoot. With the suitable injury force, metatarsal dislocations are produced in skeletally immature patients. This injury was treated with closed reduction with pin fixation. Two years after the injury, he had minor discomfort in the region of the tarsometatarsal joints with strenuous running or climbing. **C.** A 14-year-old boy who fell 18 feet to the ground, landing in a tiptoe position, sustained a tarsometatarsal and metatarsal-phalangeal dislocation of the first ray. Note that there is an impaction fracture of the cuboid, indicating an injury to the tarsometatarsal joint. Reduction was easily accomplished with closed manipulation under anesthesia. Casting was continued for 4 weeks; he was asymptomatic at follow-up. (Courtesy James J. Wiley, MD.)

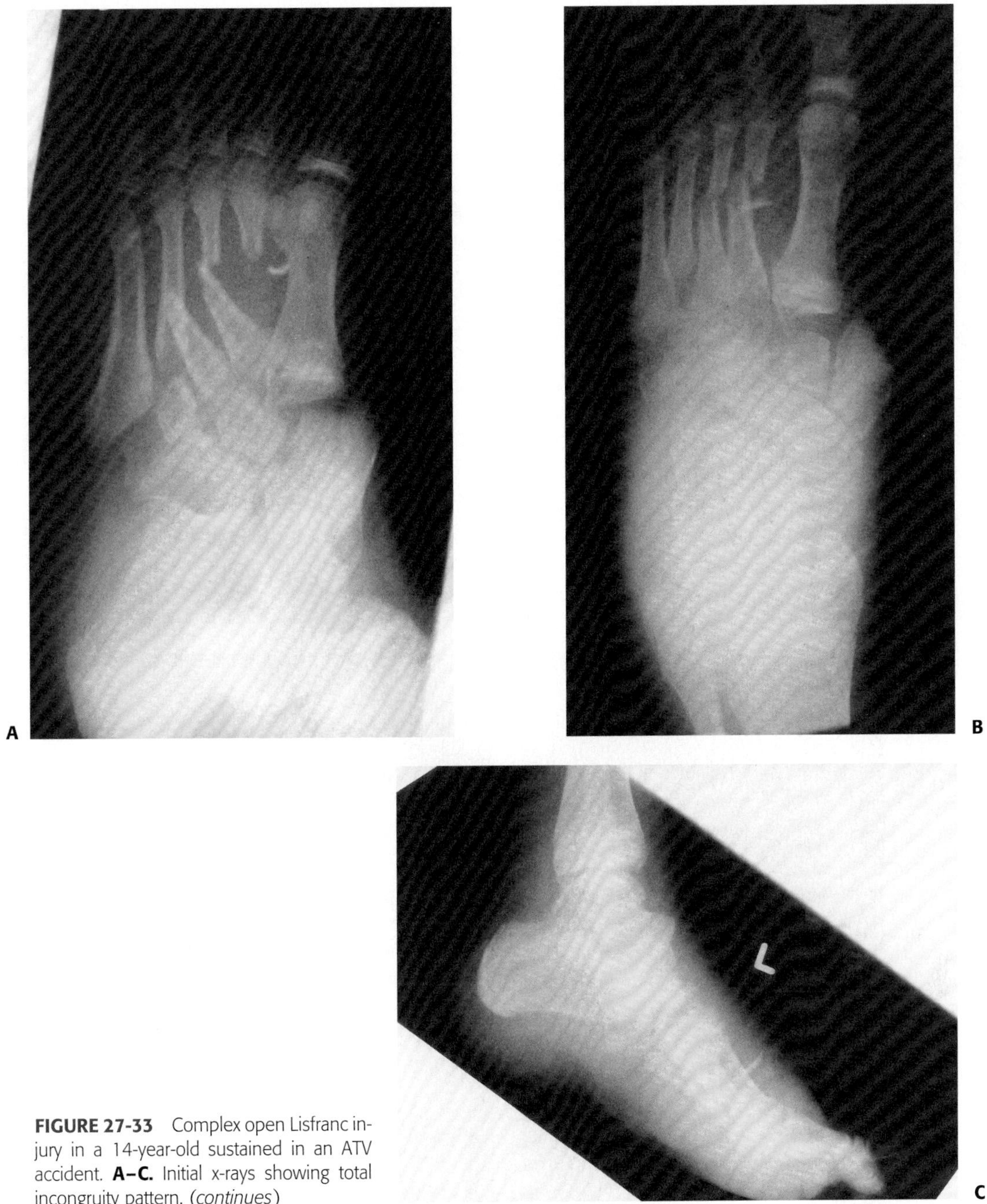

FIGURE 27-33 Complex open Lisfranc injury in a 14-year-old sustained in an ATV accident. **A–C.** Initial x-rays showing total incongruity pattern. *(continues)*

results without residual symptoms at short-term follow-up. Of the 4 patients with discomfort at 1 year follow-up, 2 had residual malunions. In 1 of these the injury had been unrecognized and in the other satisfactory closed reduction had not been obtained. One 16-year-old developed asymptomatic osteonecrosis of the second metatarsal head, but no definite connection between these conditions has been established. Of the 8 patients in the series of Buoncristiani et al (118) 7 had no limitations at 32-month follow-up. One patient had midfoot pain with light activities as well as x-ray evidence of degenerative changes across the TMT interval at 3-year follow-up. These results suggest that although indirect pediatric TMT injuries have a generally favorable prognosis, early degenerative changes can occur and may be responsible for chronic pain and activity limitation. Orthotics and stiff-soled shoes with a rocker bottom constitute conservative care of post-traumatic arthritis of the TMT joint. Arthrodesis may be required for a painful degenerative arthritic joint.

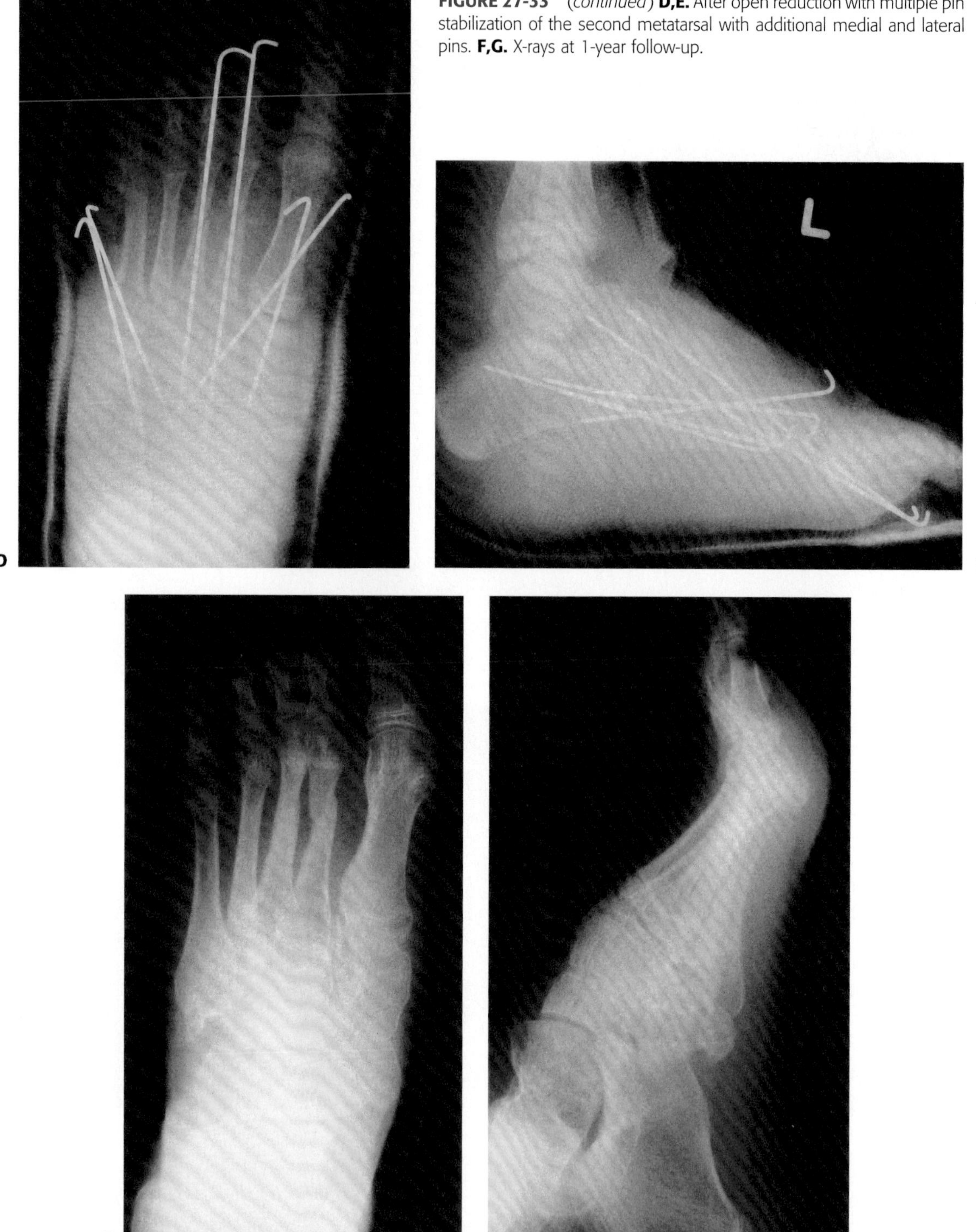

FIGURE 27-33 (*continued*) **D,E.** After open reduction with multiple pin stabilization of the second metatarsal with additional medial and lateral pins. **F,G.** X-rays at 1-year follow-up.

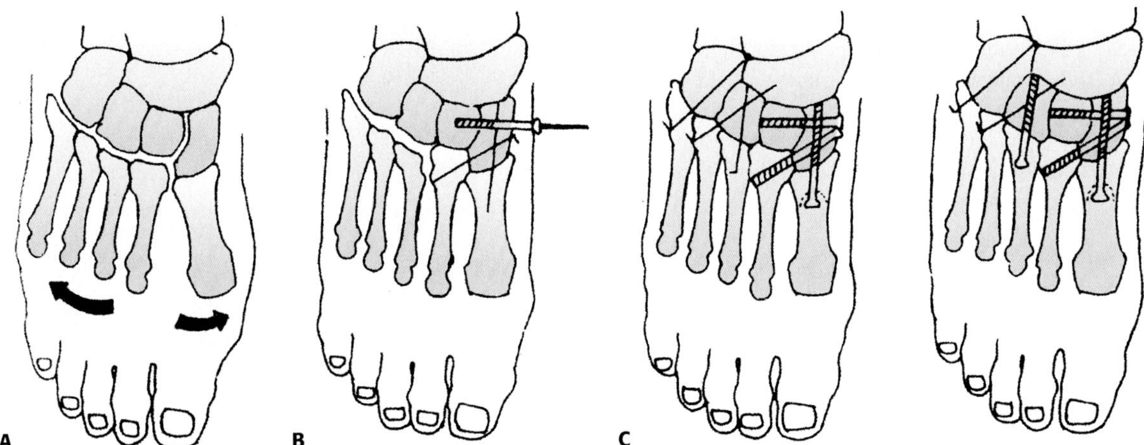

FIGURE 27-34 Sequence of repair for reduction and stabilization of tarsometatarsal fracture dislocations. **A.** Stabilization of the first ray by alignment of the metatarsal, medial cuneiform, and navicular. **B.** Stabilization of the Lisfranc ligament by accurate alignment of the second metatarsal to the medial cuneiform, as well as the medial and middle cuneiforms. **C.** Alignment and stabilization of the third through fifth metatarsal rays. Cannulated screws can be used instead of pins as needed for stability and compression. (From Trevino SG, Kodros S. Controversies in tarsometatarsal injuries. *Orthop Clin North Am* 1995;26:229–238; with permission.)

METATARSAL FRACTURES

Fractures of the metatarsals are the most common fractures of the foot in children, accounting for up to 60% of all pediatric foot fractures (137,138). In children younger than 5 years of age, 75% of metatarsal fractures involve the first metatarsal, whereas in children older than 10 years the most commonly fractured foot bone is the fifth metatarsal.

Management

Mechanism of Injury

The mechanism of metatarsal fractures may be either direct or indirect. Direct injuries result from the impact of falling objects or crush injuries typically involving bicycles or motor vehicles. Indirect injuries are caused by axial loading, inversion, rotation, or a combination of these.

Signs and Symptoms

Typically patients present with pain in the foot following a twisting injury or a direct blow. With crush injuries, swelling can be significant and the patient should be carefully evaluated for possible compartment syndrome (139). This is particularly important in patients with multiple injuries because other injuries may have taken precedence.

Associated Injuries

When fractures of the metatarsal occur proximally, rather than in the mid shaft, evaluation of the tarsal joint complex for concomitant injury is important.

Imaging Evaluation

X-ray evaluation should consist of AP, lateral, and oblique views. Occasionally, x-rays in a young child may need to be repeated in 10 to14 days to rule out a fracture. AP and oblique views generally demonstrate the fracture, but lateral views are necessary to rule out important dorsal or plantar displacement.

Classification

Fractures of the base of the fifth metatarsal can be classified according to their location into one of three zones (Fig. 27-35).

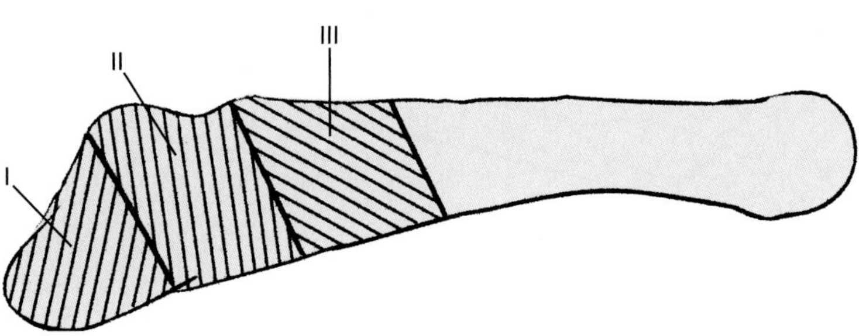

FIGURE 27-35 The three anatomic zones of the proximal fifth metatarsal.

Zone 1 is made up of the cancellous tuberosity, which includes the insertion of the peroneus brevis and abductor digiti minimi tendons and the calcaneal-metatarsal ligament of the plantar fascia. Zone 2 is the distal aspect of the tuberosity and includes dorsal and plantar ligamentous attachments to the fourth metatarsal. Zone 3 comprises the zone distal to the ligamentous attachments to approximately the mid-diaphyseal area.

Surgical and Applied Anatomy

The blood supply to the base of the fifth metatarsal is unique and is a significant factor in the risk of fracture nonunion (140–142). The nutrient artery enters the shaft along its medial border and branches proximally and distally. There is a watershed area between the proximal branch of the nutrient artery and the metaphyseal vessels. Fractures in this area (zone 2) are at risk for delayed union or nonunion (Fig. 27-36). The apophyseal growth center of the base of the fifth metatarsal appears by the age of 9 years and usually unites between the ages of 12 and 15 years. This apophyseal growth center (os vesalianum) is sagittal in orientation, which helps differentiate it from most fractures, which are oriented transversely (Fig. 27-37).

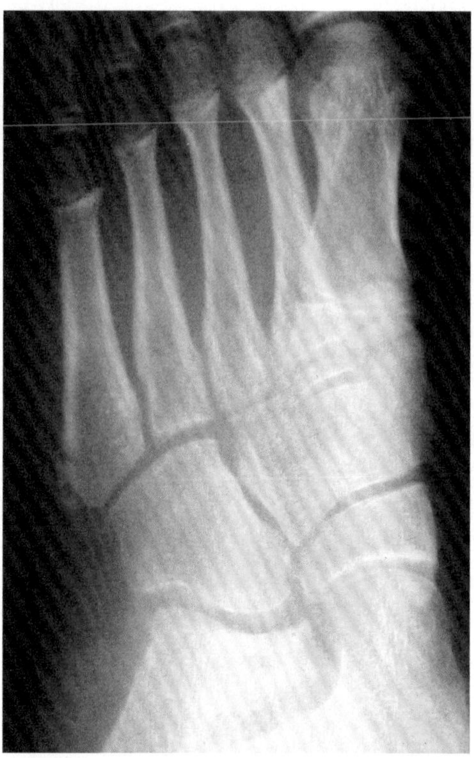

FIGURE 27-37 Orientation of the apophysis of the fifth metatarsal is parallel to the shaft and should not be confused with a fracture. (This patient also has an undisplaced, transverse fracture.)

Current Treatment Options

Most metatarsal fractures in children can be treated nonoperatively. Initial management depends on the severity of the injury. With marked swelling and soft tissue injury, compartment syndrome should be considered and treated appropriately. Significant soft tissue swelling of the foot is a contraindication to application of a circumferential cast. In this situation, a bulky dressing, posterior splint, or U-splint should be applied with the foot in equinus position and the foot should be elevated. When the swelling has diminished, a circular cast can be applied. Weight-bearing is allowed, and immobilization is continued for 3 to 6 weeks depending on the age of the child and the amount of fracture displacement.

Indications for closed reduction include completely displaced fractures in older children and fractures angled more than 20 degrees, especially apex-dorsal. Reduction is carried out with the use of conscious sedation. Chinese finger traps can be used, placing the respective toes of the injured metatarsals in the traps with counter pressure on the ankle in conjunction with manipulative reduction (143,144). The cast should be well molded over the dorsal and plantar aspects of the foot, leaving the ankle in slight plantar flexion. If the reduction is unstable, percutaneous K-wire fixation can be helpful for the first and fifth metatarsals. Considerable lateral displacement and even dorsal angulation of metatarsal necks can be accepted in younger children. Open reduction rarely is necessary. However, open reduction with internal fixation is indicated for open fractures and fractures that cannot be maintained in a cast. The standard technique is a dorsal exposure with K-wire placement in the distal fragment, exiting through the plantar skin. The fracture is then reduced and pinned retrograde. The pin is bent and cut and left out through the skin with appropriate padding and application of a short-leg non–weight-bearing cast. Pins are removed at 4 to 6 weeks, and a walking cast is worn until consolidation of the fracture (Fig. 27-38).

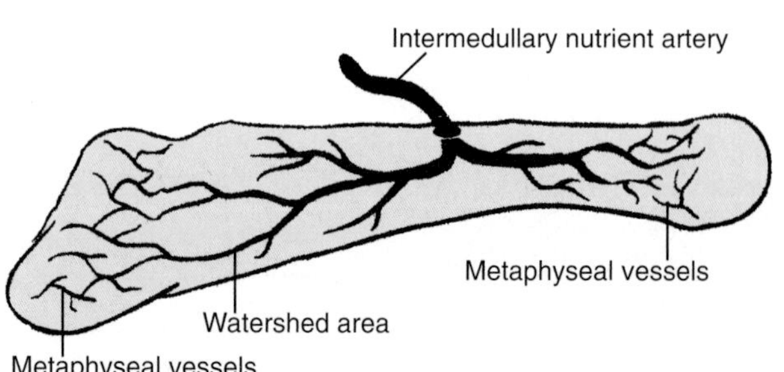

FIGURE 27-36 Blood supply of the proximal fifth metatarsal.

Fractures of the Base of the Fifth Metatarsal

Treatment of fractures of the base of the fifth metatarsal is determined by the zone of the fracture. Zone 1 injuries usually are avulsion fractures secondary to the pull of the tendinous portion

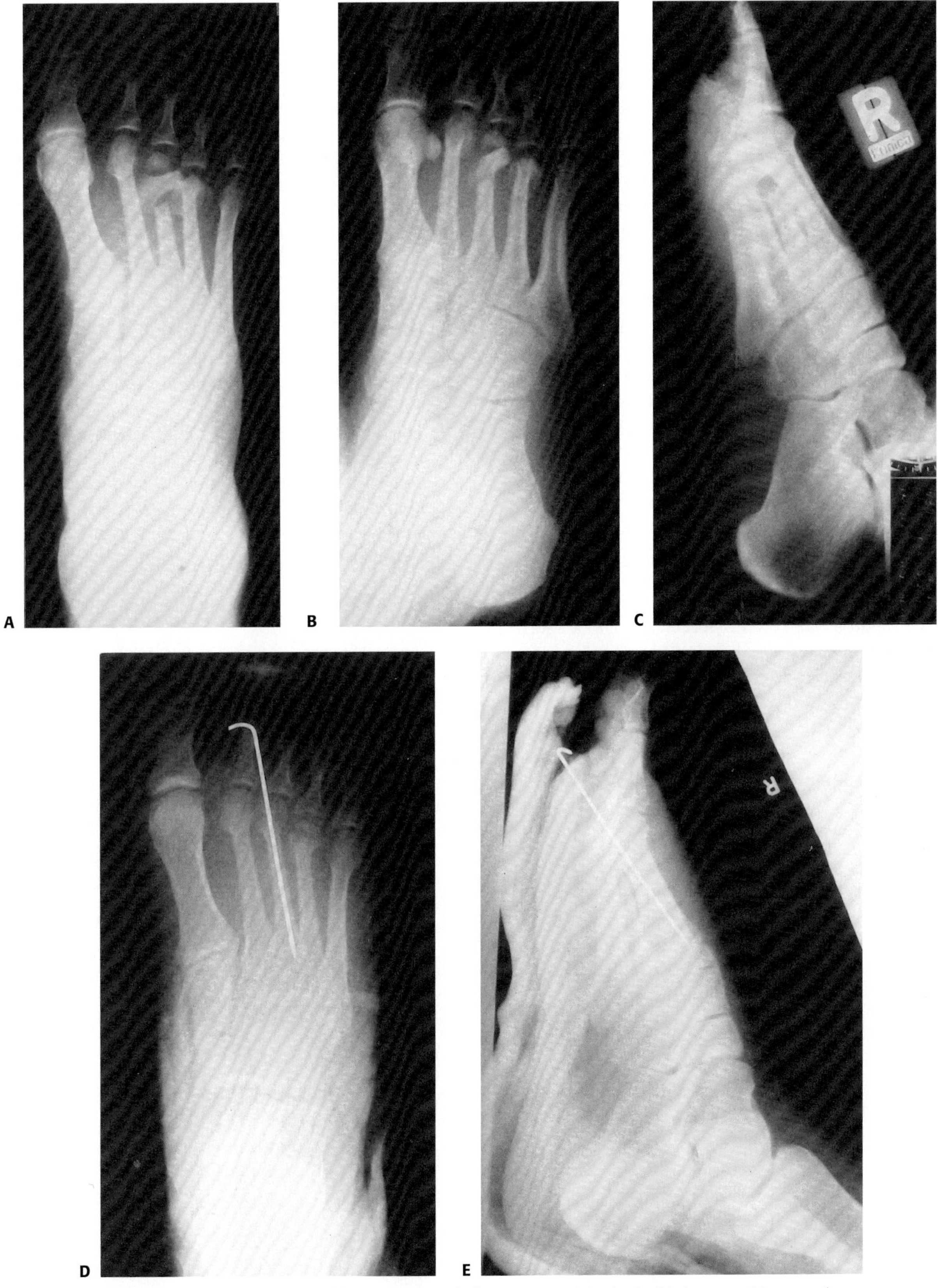

FIGURE 27-38 This 14-year-old boy jumped into shallow water sustaining irreducible fractures of the second, third, and fourth metatarsal necks. **A–C.** Initial x-rays show wide displacement. **D,E.** After open reduction and intramedullary fixation with Kirshner wires left protruding through the plantar skin.

of the abductor digiti minimi and the tough lateral cord of the plantar aponeurosis inserting into the fifth metatarsal base. Minimal treatment is required and usually involves a below-knee walking cast for 3 to 6 weeks (145). X-ray union usually lags behind resolution of symptoms, and most patients are asymptomatic after 3 weeks. Nonunion can occur but usually is asymptomatic (146). For large symptomatic nonunions, fixation with a small lag screw may be considered. Although operative fixation of acute tuberosity avulsions rarely is indicated, it may be considered for significant displacement (more than 3 mm) in young active patients.

Fractures in zone 2 include the Jones fracture. This is an oblique fracture at the proximal metaphyseal-diaphyseal junction. It typically occurs in 15- to 20-year-old adolescents and is thought to be caused by a combination of vertical loading and coronal-plane shear forces at the junction of the stable proximal metaphysis and the mobile fifth metatarsal diaphysis. Frequently, these fractures are stress injuries, usually involving athletic adolescents who present with a traumatic event superimposed on prior symptoms (144,147–151). A good history is important to determine the duration of symptoms because chronic injuries are unlikely to respond to nonoperative treatment.

Acute injuries should be immobilized in a short-leg non–weight-bearing cast for 6 weeks. Serial x-rays and examinations are necessary to determine adequate healing and further non–weight-bearing immobilization may be necessary. With evidence of callus and diminished tenderness, the patient can begin protected weight-bearing in a hard-soled shoe for an additional 4 weeks. In a series of adults, Torg et al (152) reported successful healing in 14 of 15 patients treated with non–weight-bearing casts, whereas only 4 of 10 who were allowed to bear weight went on to union (Fig. 27-39).

For chronic injuries with symptoms exceeding 3 months, healing is unlikely. Although an attempt at non–weight-bearing immobilization for 6 weeks is worthwhile, many injuries will require operative intervention. Typically this involves intramedullary fixation using a 4-mm cannulated screw coupled with bone grafting, either from the distal tibia in mature individuals or the iliac crest in skeletally immature patients (153) (Fig. 27-40).

Fractures in zone 3 often are stress fractures in active athletes. Although acute fractures may be treated with non–weight-bearing short-leg casts for approximately 6 weeks followed by protective weight-bearing, chronic injuries are likely to require intramedullary screw fixation and grafting similar to treatment of Jones fractures.

Complications

Malunion of metatarsal neck or shaft fractures can lead to pressure problems and difficulty with ambulation necessitating oste-

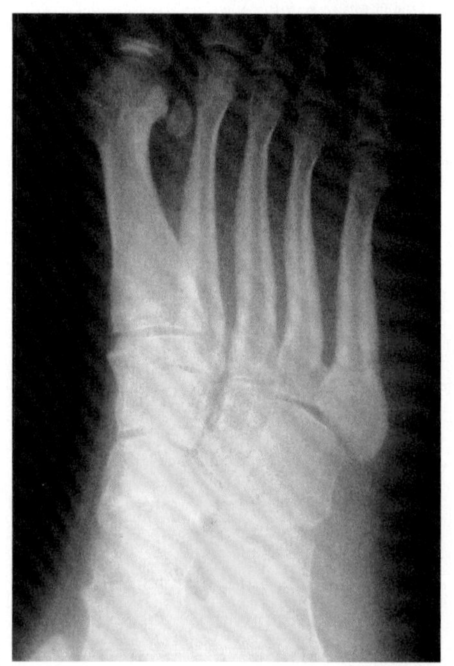
A

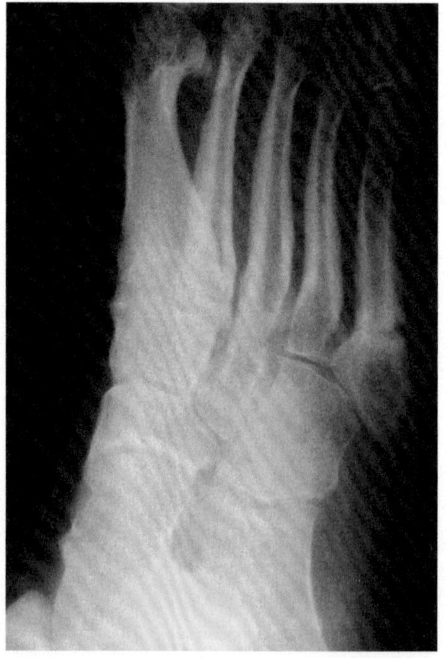
B

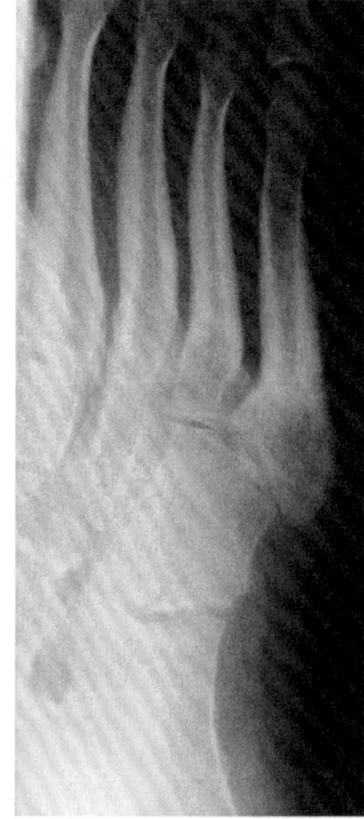
C

FIGURE 27-39 This 13-year-old girl sustained a "Jones" fracture playing basketball and was treated nonoperatively. **A.** Initial x-ray shows minimal displacement. **B.** At 3 months, there is residual lucency, but the patient is asymptomatic. **C.** At 6 months, consolidation is still delayed but patient remains asymptomatic.

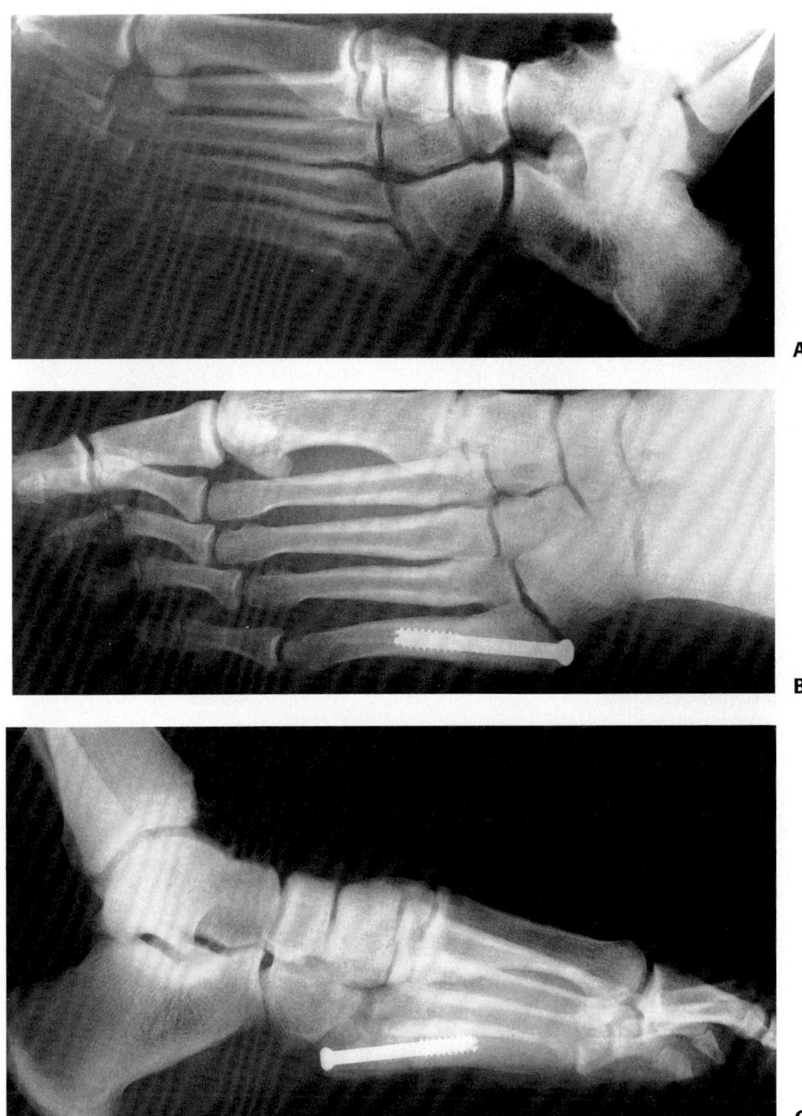

FIGURE 27-40 This 15-year-old high-level basketball player sustained a proximal fifth metatarsal fracture at the metaphyseal-diaphyseal junction. The patient chose intramedullary screw fixation because of his desire to return to sport as promptly as possible, lessen his time in immobilization, and lessen the risk of delayed union or nonunion. **A.** X-ray at time of injury. **B,C.** After intramedullary screw fixation. (Courtesy of Keith S. Hechtman, MD.)

otomy. Shortening of the first metatarsal as a result of physeal injury can result in deficiency in the longitudinal arch. We have seen growth arrest in the lesser metatarsals resulting from a high-energy crush injury (Fig. 27-41).

PHALANGEAL FRACTURES

Phalangeal fractures are relatively common in children. Many of these fractures are treated symptomatically by the patient and family or by the primary care physician. They usually result from "stubbing the toe" (indirect) or from falling objects (direct). Most phalangeal fractures are treated with buddy taping and weight-bearing in a stiff-soled shoe. Rarely, manipulative reduction with traction and taping are required. In an older child with a displaced fracture, percutaneous pin stabilization may be necessary after reduction. Pins can be removed at about 6 weeks and progressive weight-bearing allowed.

Special Circumstances

Intra-articular fractures involving the proximal phalanx of the great toe include Salter Harris types III and IV fractures. Those involving more than 30% of the joint surface and with displacement of more than 3 mm require reduction and pinning. This can be done percutaneously or through a dorsal incision when necessary. Growth arrest and stiffness are occasional complications of fractures of the great toe.

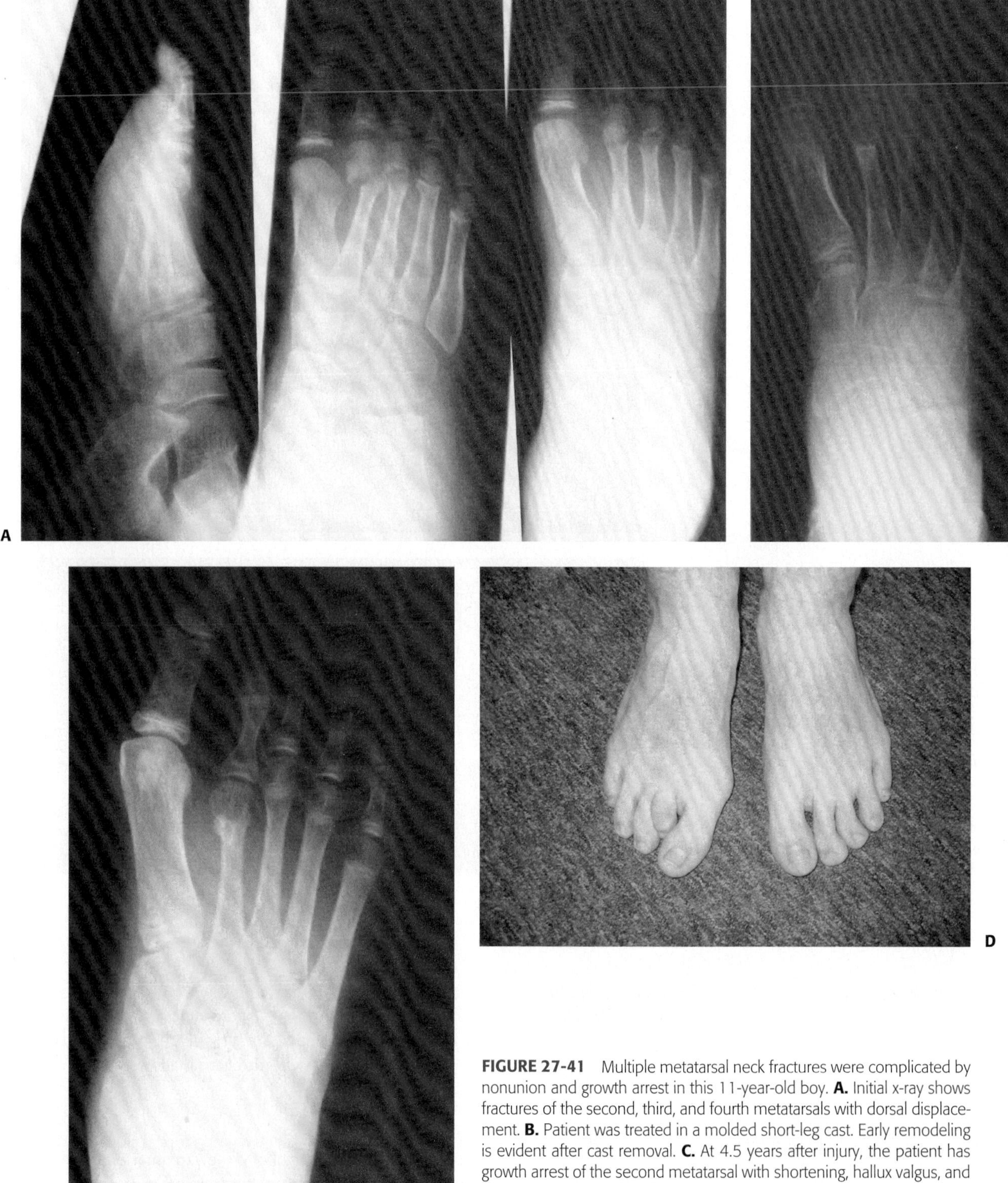

FIGURE 27-41 Multiple metatarsal neck fractures were complicated by nonunion and growth arrest in this 11-year-old boy. **A.** Initial x-ray shows fractures of the second, third, and fourth metatarsals with dorsal displacement. **B.** Patient was treated in a molded short-leg cast. Early remodeling is evident after cast removal. **C.** At 4.5 years after injury, the patient has growth arrest of the second metatarsal with shortening, hallux valgus, and clawing of the second toe. **D.** Clinical appearance.

Distal phalangeal physeal fractures of the great toe may be open because of their proximity to the nail matrix. The Seymour lesion occurs when the skin and nail fold at the dorsum of the toe are disrupted. The toe should be closely scrutinized for this open injury, which may lead to osteomyelitis. Irrigation and debridement have been recommended, along with reduction and protection by buddy taping, hard-soled shoes, or occasionally a below-knee walking cast. Prophylactic antibiotics are recommended for 7 to 10 days after this injury. Established osteomyelitis may require debridement and intravenous antibiotic therapy (Fig. 27-42).

LAWN MOWER AND OTHER MUTILATING INJURIES

Lawn mowers have been reported to cause as many as 160,000 injuries annually, including approximately 2000 that result in permanent impairment in children (154–158). These can occur to children who are passengers or operators of the lawn mower (158,159) or when the child is a bystander (157,160). Loder (161), in a report of the demographics of traumatic amputations in children in the upper midwestern United States, noted that in 235 children sustaining traumatic amputations, lawn mowers and farm machinery were most often involved. Riding lawn

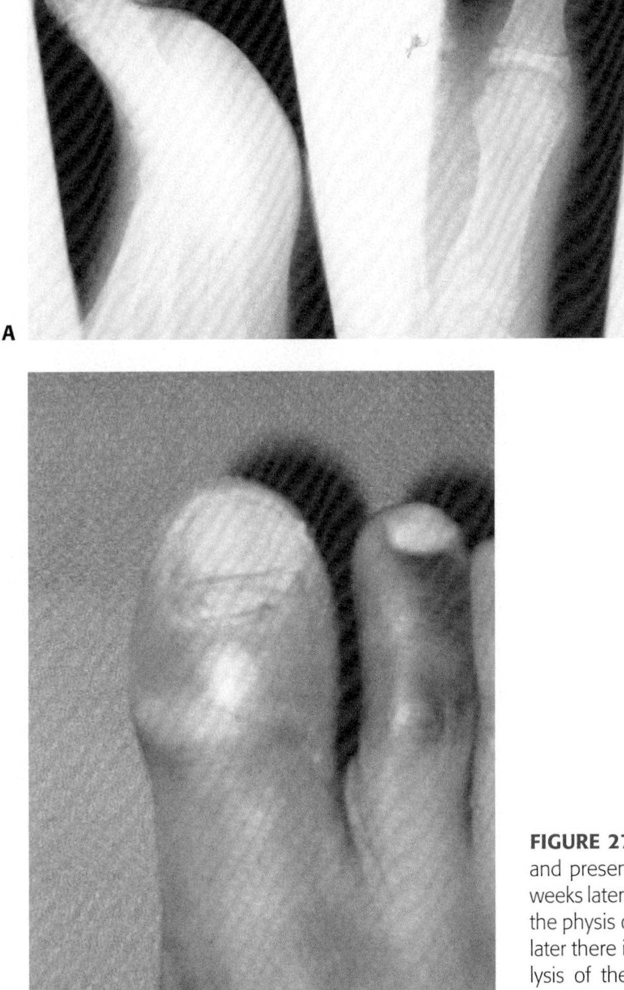

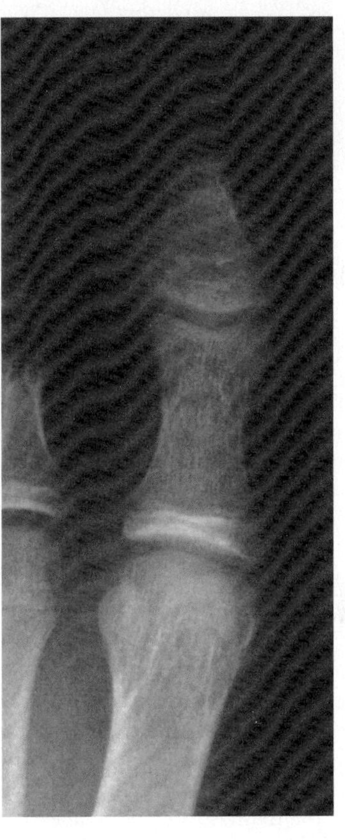

FIGURE 27-42 This 13-year-old boy "stubbed his toe" and presented with osteomyelitis of the distal phalanx 2 weeks later. **A.** Initial x-ray shows angulated fracture through the physis of the distal phalanx (mallet toe). **B.** Two weeks later there is erythema and swelling. **C.** X-rays show osteolysis of the distal phalanx consistent with osteomyelitis. *(continues)*

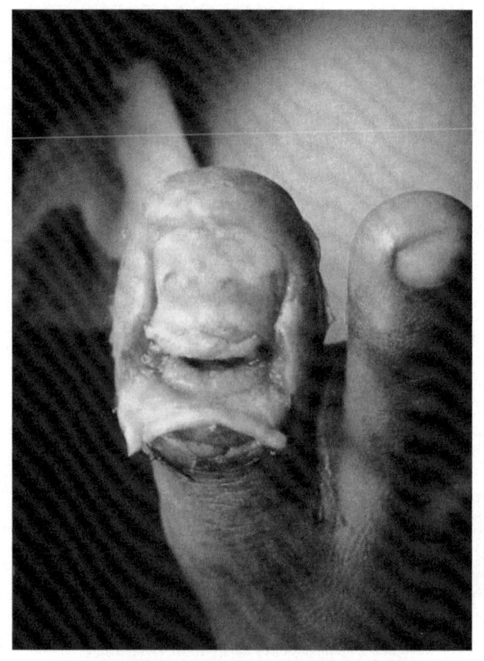

D

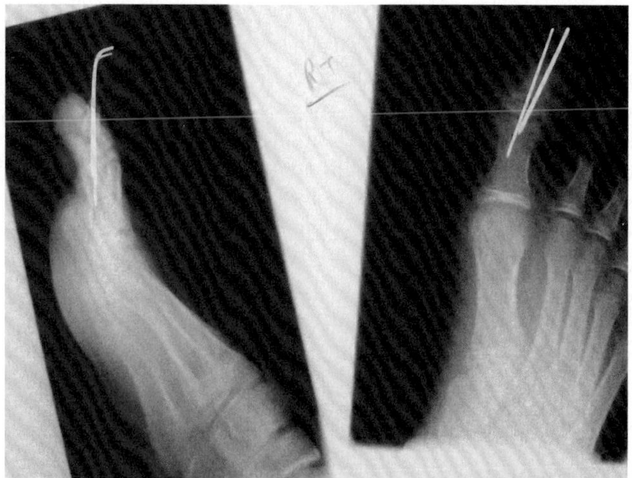

E

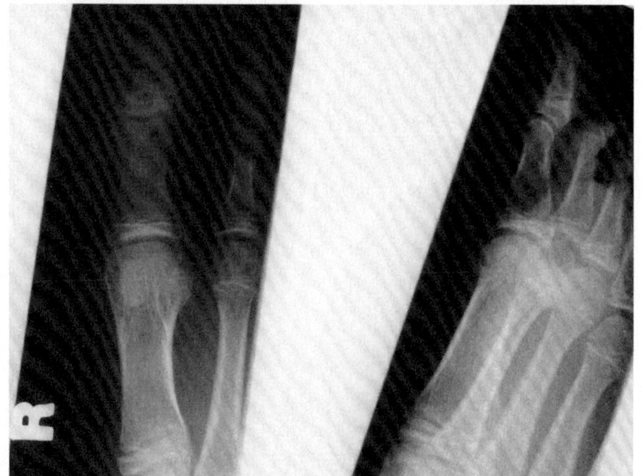

F

FIGURE 27-42 (*continued*) **D,E.** Patient had debridement of the proximal phalanx, with preservation of the nail matrix, followed by open reduction and pinning. **F.** Healed fracture 2 months later.

mowers are more often involved than push mowers and generally result in more severe injury patterns (158). Obviously, these injuries are more common in the spring and summer (161). Children under the age of 14 years are most susceptible to injury; those under the age of 6 years have the greatest risk of death (162). Not only are these the most destructive injuries to the child's foot but they also are preventable (161,163–166).

Assessment of the injured child should be thorough and prompt to allow urgent transfer to the operating room for initial irrigation and debridement. Antibiotics, including a cephalosporin, an aminoglycoside, and penicillin, should be administered in the emergency room.

Treatment

Considerable judgment is required to determine whether to amputate or save a questionable part. Multiple debridements at 48-hour intervals until viable tissue is present at all wound edges is believed to give the best chance of success because the extent of tissue damage may be difficult to assess at the time of injury (157). Jet water lavage can force foreign material under pressure into the soft tissue envelope and usually is not effective in removing small debris. Tissue of questionable viability should be preserved, and the wound should be left open. Plastic surgery consultation is advisable early in the process to allow optimal preparation for coverage procedures. Bony injuries should be stabilized using standard techniques at the initial debridement. Most of these injuries require some form of ablative procedure, and attempts should be made to preserve as much length as possible. Transdiaphyseal amputation should be avoided when possible to prevent difficulties with stump overgrowth (160,167).

Methods for soft tissue coverage of lawn mower injuries are numerous, but delayed closure or split-thickness skin grafting work well (157,158,160,168). Split-thickness skin grafts can function surprisingly well on weight-bearing surfaces in children (157,158). Microsurgical free-flap transfer can be helpful when extensive defect reconstruction is necessary (169,170). Finally, it is important to appraise the degree of injury realisti-

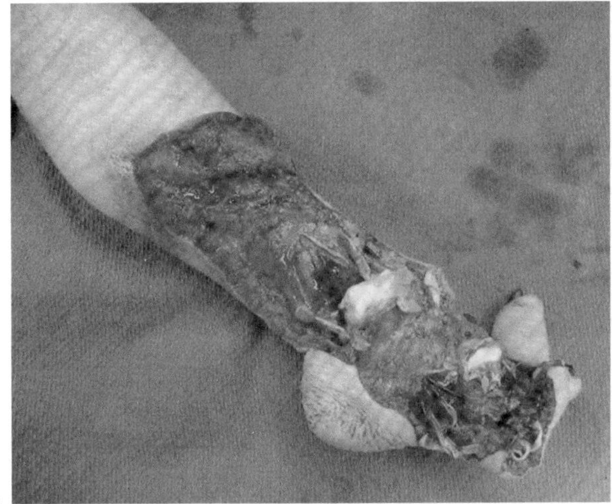

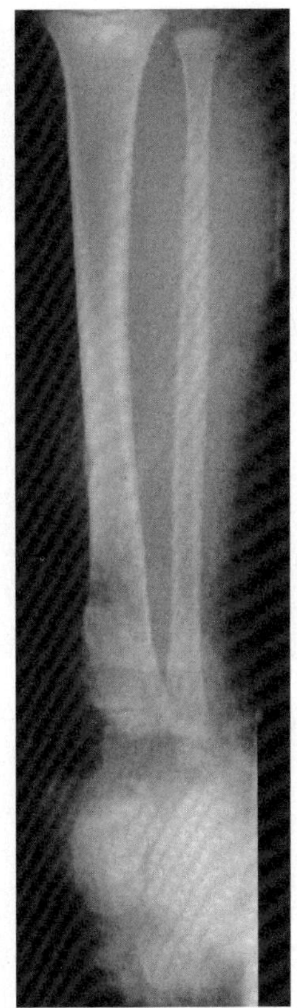

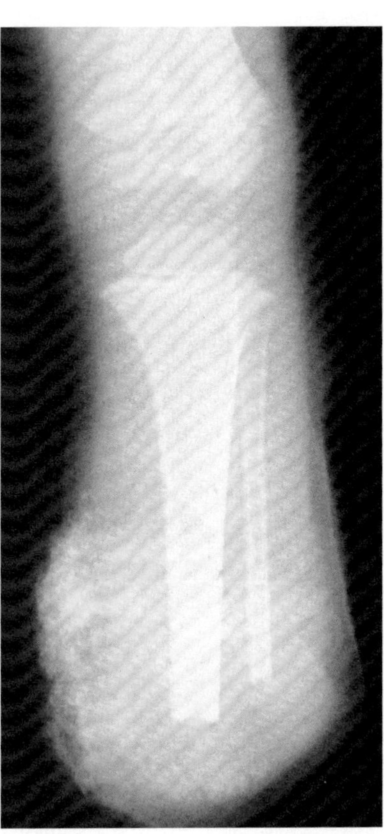

FIGURE 27-43 This 3-year-old boy fell under a riding lawn mower. **A.** Clinical photograph shows gross contamination and extensive damage. **B.** Initial x-ray. **C.** After below-knee amputation (through-ankle amputation was not possible).

cally and not pursue salvage at any cost. Formulas for determining the feasibility of salvage in adults are not directly applicable to children who have further growth potential. Soft tissue damage from lawn mower injuries is extensive, and the soft tissue envelope generally appears better on presentation than it does in the ensuing days because of the initial compromised soft tissue perfusion. There seldom is a need for an immediate decision, and the degree of tissue damage noted at subsequent debridements usually is a better determinant of the ultimate amputation level. Advances in bone transport with ring and other external fixators, including stump-lengthening procedures, now make better function with a short amputation a possibility (Fig. 27-43).

COMPARTMENT SYNDROME

Children, like adults, are susceptible to the development of compartment syndrome after severe crush injuries, significant fractures, or as a result of reperfusion following temporary loss of arterial inflow (171,172). The nine fascial compartments, containing the interossei and short plantar flexor muscles, are prone to contained swelling. Compartment syndrome should be suspected with crush injuries. Generally, examination reveals tense swelling and pain that are out of proportion to what would be expected for the musculoskeletal injuries. Pallor, pulselessness, and paresthesia are late signs and not particularly helpful in making an acute diagnosis. Although uncommon in children, late sequelae of missed compartment syndrome can lead to significant disability including claw-toe deformity, paresthesia, cavus deformity, stiffness, and residual pain (173,174).

Although clinical suspicion is the most important parameter, the diagnosis can be made objectively with the measurement of compartment pressures (Fig. 27-44). This may be particularly helpful in patients with altered mental status, when clinical signs may not be easily appreciated. Although there is no general consensus, pressures of greater than 30 mm Hg are generally believed to be an indication for fasciotomy (175,176). Medial and lateral longitudinal incisions are made over the second and fourth metatarsals for injuries of the forefoot or midfoot. A medial approach is more suitable for injuries of the hindfoot, with the incision extending from the base of the first metatarsal to the medial malleolus. The tarsal tunnel can be released through this incision (176) (Fig. 27-45).

PUNCTURE WOUNDS

Puncture wounds of the foot are very common in children and are seemingly innocuous (177,178). However, when complicated by deep pseudomonas infection, these injuries have a

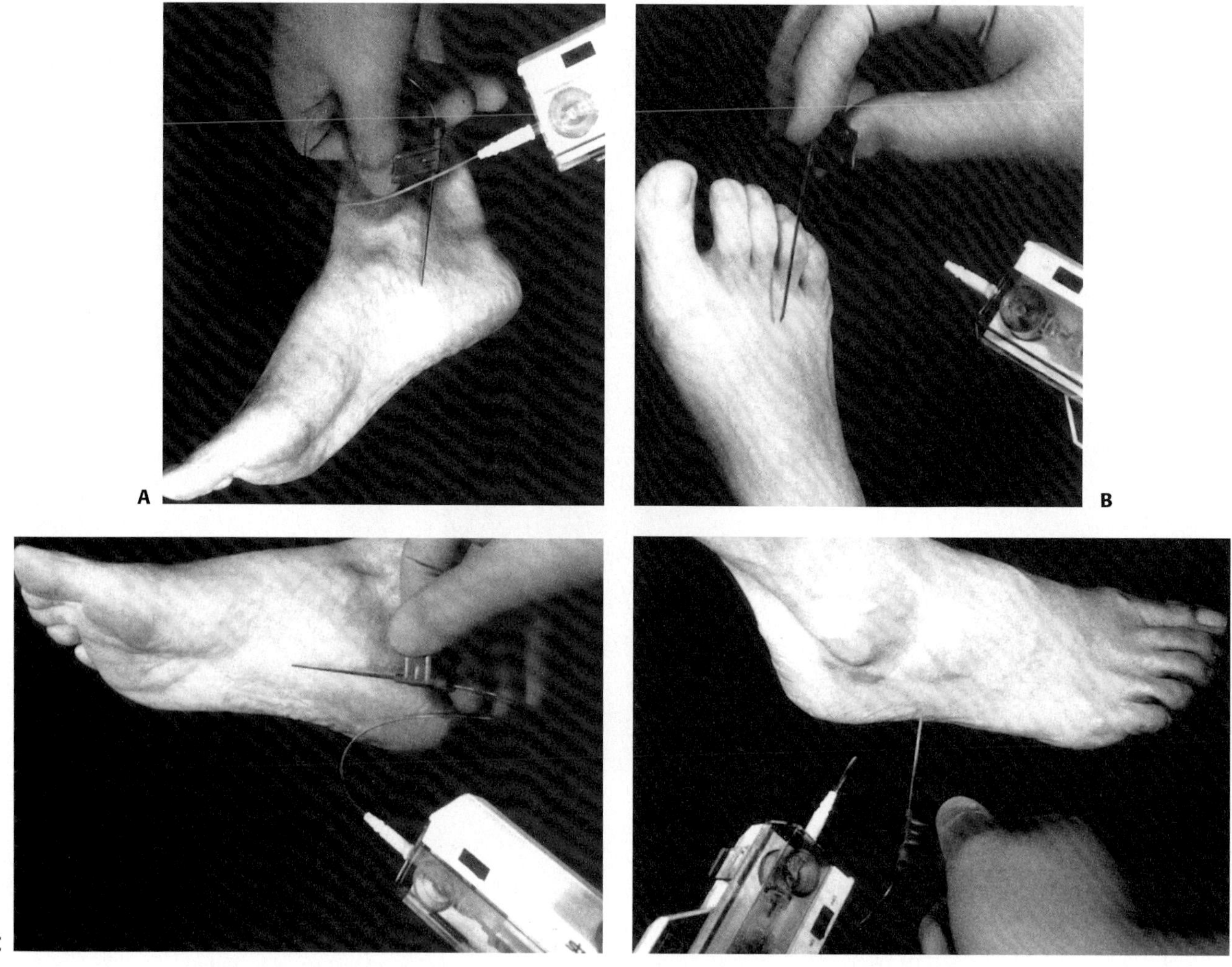

FIGURE 27-44 Compartment pressure measurement technique. **A.** The medial and calcaneal compartments are measured with the needle introduced in the medial hindfoot several centimeters below the medial malleolus. **B.** Forefoot pressures are measured with the needle in the first or second interspace measuring the respective interosseous space pressure; advancement of the needle deeper measures the adductor compartment pressure. **C.** Superficial compartment is measured in the central plantar surface of the foot. **D.** Lateral compartment measurement is just below the base of the fifth metatarsal. (From Manoli A II, Fakhouri AJ, Weber TG. Compartmental catheterization and fasciotomy of the foot. *Operative Tech Orthop* 1992;2:205, with permission.)

worse prognosis than in adults and can lead to permanent sequelae (179,180). Typically, these injuries result from stepping on a nail (181). Generally, appropriate initial care of puncture wounds of the foot consists of irrigation of the entry site with saline with the use of local anesthetic, regional block, or conscious sedation. With severe contamination, formal debridement in the operating room may be necessary. Tetanus toxoid is administered when appropriate. Prophylactic antibiotic treatment generally is not recommended and does not appear to have value in eradicating pseudomonas inoculum in routine puncture wounds.

The development of cellulitis after puncture wounds usually is due to *Staphylococcus aureus* and not pseudomonas. It can be treated with intravenous antibiotics, although occasionally surgical debridement is required.

Osteochondritis and osteomyelitis are serious complications and frequently involve the metatarsal-phalangeal area or the calcaneus (Fig. 27-46). Pseudomonas osteochondritis is believed to be caused by penetration into the cartilaginous surface at the time of the initial injury (177). Usually, there is a paucity of local inflammation followed by delayed onset of localized pain and swelling between 5 and 10 days (182,183). Systemic indicators such as temperature and white blood count often are normal, whereas erythrocyte sedimentation rate (ESR) may be

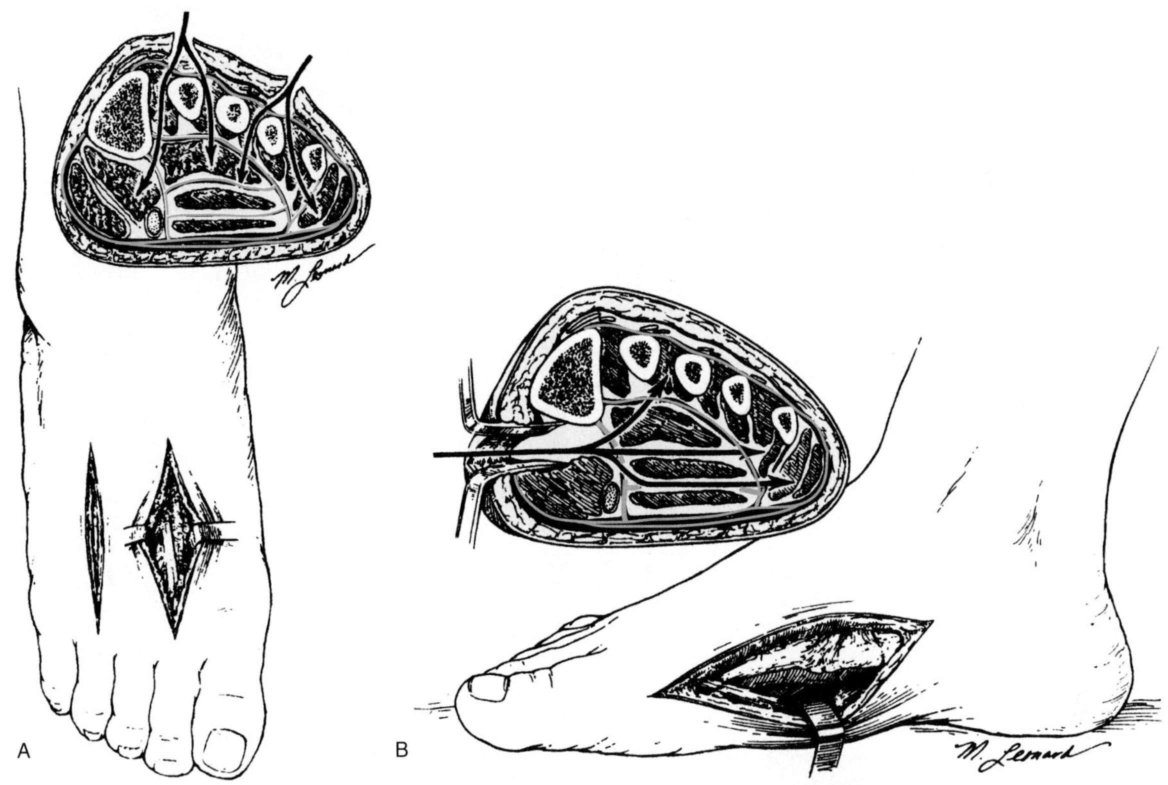

FIGURE 27-45 Surgical approaches for fasciotomy of the foot. **A.** The dorsal approach is made through an incision over the second and fourth metatarsal shafts and is more suitable for injuries of the forefoot or midfoot. **B.** The medial approach is more suitable for injuries of the hindfoot, with the incision extending from the base of the first metatarsal to the medial malleolus. A tarsal tunnel release can be done through this incision. (From Myerson MS. Experimental decompression of the fascial compartments of the foot: the basis for fasciotomy in acute compartment syndromes. *Foot Ankle* 1988;8:308–314; with permission.)

elevated (179). Several authors have postulated that footwear is the source of the pseudomonas inoculum (184,185).

X-rays often are equivocal or normal, but bone scans may show focally increased uptake. CT scanning can be helpful when there is frank osseous destruction (179); ultrasound and MRI are useful to identify nonradiopaque foreign bodies (186). Lau et al (187) found early MRI to be cost effective in the diagnosis of pseudomonas infection following puncture wounds.

Once the diagnosis of osteomyelitis or pseudomonas osteochondritis has been established, surgical debridement is indicated. Although Johanson (188) reported treatment with surgical debridement only, most authors recommend intravenous antibiotic therapy. Unfortunately, there appears to be no scientific basis for recommending duration of treatment. Typically, intravenous therapy ranges from 7 days to 3 weeks (179,189).

Although a satisfactory outcome usually can be obtained, complications of pseudomonas osteochondritis are more common in children than in adults and can include recurrence, chronic pain, and deformity. An individualized approach is required.

STRESS FRACTURES

Although probably more common in adults, stress fractures of the foot do occur in children (190). The tibia and fibula are most commonly affected, but these injuries can occur in both the tarsals and metatarsals (190–192). Stress fractures are common in children and adults who undertake a sudden increase in physical activity. This usually occurs in maturing adolescents who embark on intensive training for sports. The mechanism of injury appears to be reabsorption and demineralization at the site of stress, followed by a reparative process evidenced by periosteal layering of new bone. The bone fails when the fatigue process exceeds the reparative process. Bone failure is based on the amount of load and the degree of repetitive stress, as well as the frequency of loading.

Patients present with pain on weight-bearing but less discomfort than would be expected with an acute fracture. Swelling often is minimal, but localized tenderness is marked and discreet. Early x-rays often are not helpful but usually indicate the

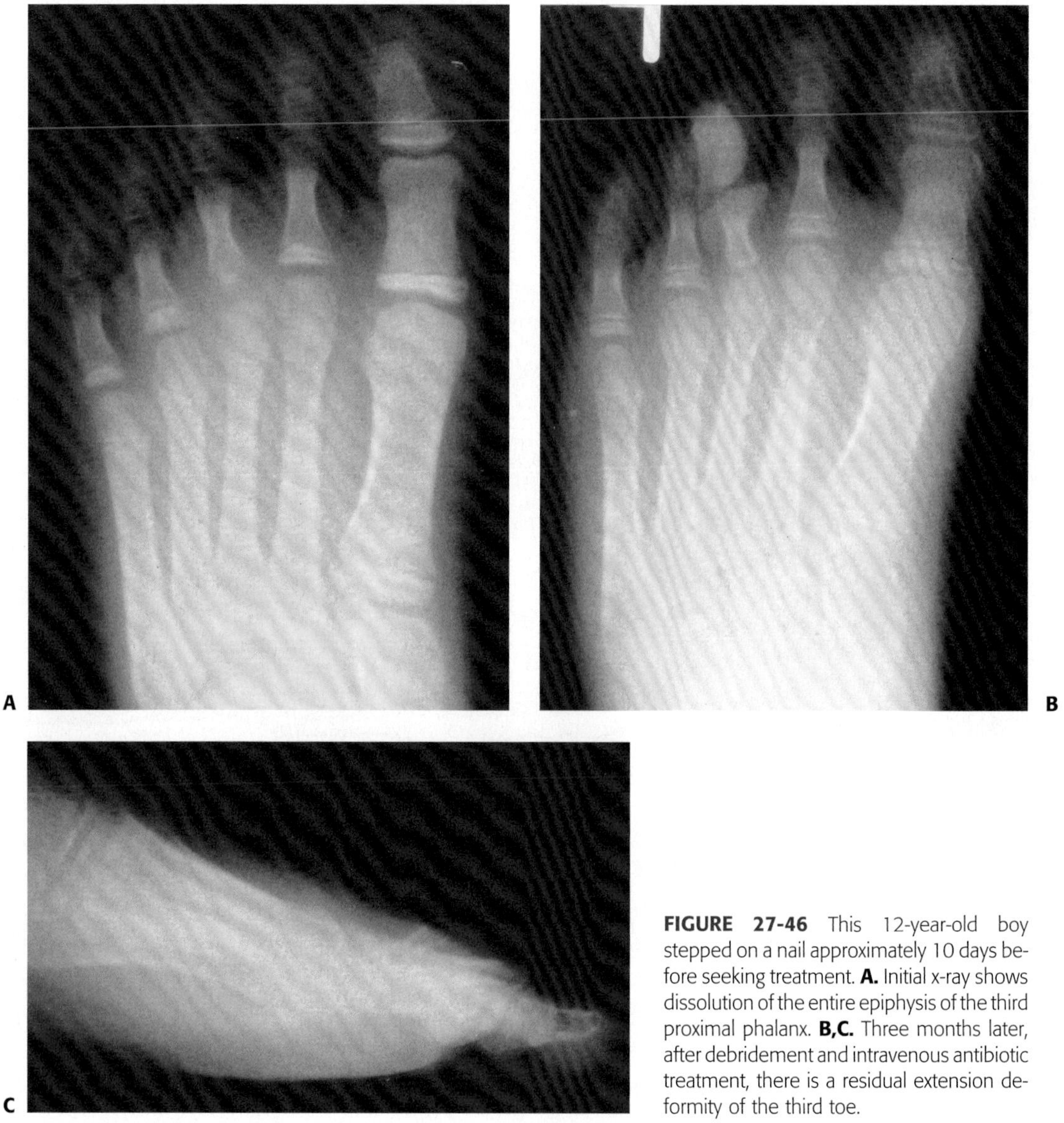

FIGURE 27-46 This 12-year-old boy stepped on a nail approximately 10 days before seeking treatment. **A.** Initial x-ray shows dissolution of the entire epiphysis of the third proximal phalanx. **B,C.** Three months later, after debridement and intravenous antibiotic treatment, there is a residual extension deformity of the third toe.

healing fracture site with callous development by 2 to 4 weeks after the onset of symptoms (Fig. 27-47). Bone scans are more sensitive but are not necessary to initiate treatment except in atypical cases (193,194).

Patients should be assessed for possible etiology of the stress fracture. Incorrect training technique is a common cause in athletes. There may have been a change in footwear or an increase in activity. The Morton foot, with a short first ray, has been implicated in stress fractures of the second and third metatarsals, but this is not universally accepted (195).

Treatment should be individualized, with reduced activity and protective footwear as the basis. In contrast to acute fractures, there is no distinct starting point for the treatment of stress fractures.

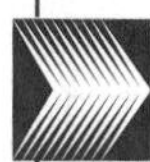

AUTHORS' PREFERRED TREATMENT

We individualize the treatment to the symptoms. If the foot is painful only during sports, relative restriction of activity according to symptoms is all that is recommended. Although shoe modifications, such as metatarsal bars, have been advocated (179), we prefer to apply a short-leg cast for about 2 weeks, followed by activity restriction. Gradual return to activity can be allowed after 8 to 12 weeks, while avoiding training errors that may have caused the problem. Although we have not encountered it, should sagittal plane angulation develop, indications for open reduction with internal fixation would be the same as for an acute fracture.

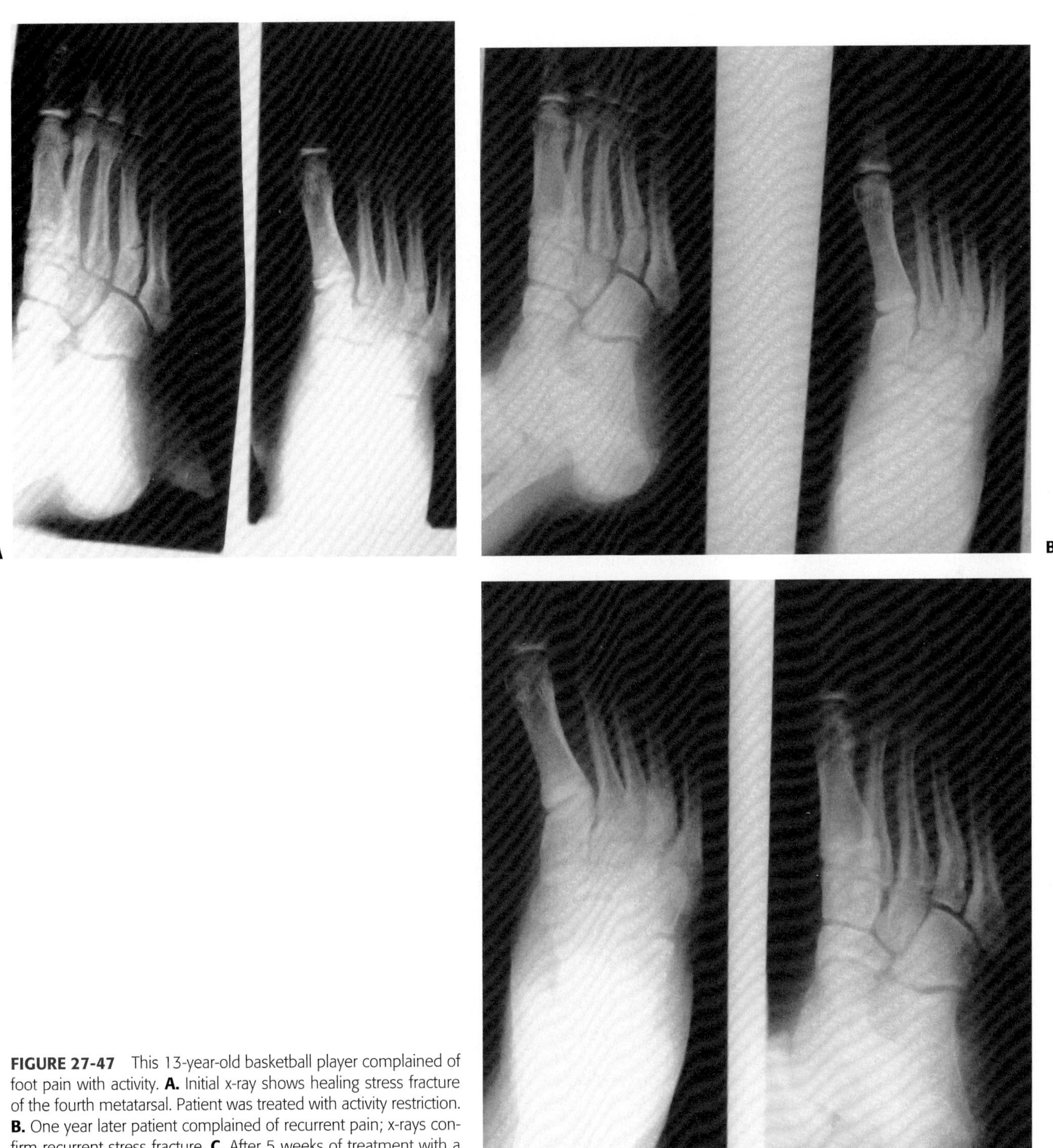

FIGURE 27-47 This 13-year-old basketball player complained of foot pain with activity. **A.** Initial x-ray shows healing stress fracture of the fourth metatarsal. Patient was treated with activity restriction. **B.** One year later patient complained of recurrent pain; x-rays confirm recurrent stress fracture. **C.** After 5 weeks of treatment with a short-leg cast, the fracture is consolidating well.

REFERENCES

1. Adirim TA, Cheng TL. Overview of injuries in the young athlete. *Sports Med* 2003;33: 75–81.
2. Damore DT, Metzl JD, Ramundo M, et al. Patterns in childhood sports injury. *Pediatr Emerg Care* 2003;19:65–67.
3. Dimentberg R, Rosman M. Peritalar dislocations in children. *J Pediatr Orthop* 1993;13: 89–93.
4. Purvis JM, Burke RG. Recreational injuries in children: incidence and prevention. *J Am Acad Orthop Surg* 2001;9:365–374.
5. Stanitski CL. Paediatric and adolescent sports injuries. *Clin Sports Med* 1997;16: 613–633.
6. Blount WP. Injuries of the foot. In: *Fractures in Children*. Philadelphia: Williams and Wilkins; 1955:195–196.
7. Rang M. The foot. In: *Children's Fractures*, 2nd ed. Philadelphia: JB Lippincott; 1974.
8. Ogden J. The foot. In. Ogden J: *Skeletal Injury in the Child*. New York: Springer Verlag; 2000.
9. Buckingham R, Jackson M, Atkins R. Calcaneal fractures in adolescents CT classification and results of operative management. *Injury* 2003;34:454–459.
10. Robert IE, Hyde CJ, Bridgman SA. Orthopaedic fractures: trends in randomized controlled trials. *Injury* 2001;32:779–782.
11. Brunet JA. Calcaneal fractures in children. *J Bone Joint Surg Br* 2000;82:211–216.
12. Hufner T, Thermann H, Schratt HE. Treatment of juvenile os calcis fracture: a long term follow-up. Proceedings 13th Annual Summer Meeting American Orthopaedic Foot and Ankle Society, 1997, 6–7.
13. Knorr P, Dietz HG, Kruger P. Bilateral calcaneus fracture in childhood: a report of experiences. *Unfallchirurg* 1992;95:106–108.
14. Rigault P, Padovani JP, Kliszowski H. Les fractures du calcaneum chez l'enfant: a propos de 26 cas. *Ann Chir Infant* 1973;14:115–134.
15. Aitken AP. Fractures of the os calcis: treatment by closed reduction. *Clin Orthop* 1963; 30:67–75.
16. Crawford AH. Fractures and dislocations of the foot and ankle. In: Green NE, Swiontkowski MF, eds. *Skeletal Trauma in Children*. Philadelphia: WB Saunders; 1993.
17. Schmidt M, Havemann D, Behrens P. Talusfrakturen bei Kindern und Jugendlichen. In: Rahmanzadeh R and Breyer H G, eds: *Verletzungen der unteren Extremitaten bei Kindern und Jugendlichen*. Berlin: Springer-Verlag; 1990:337–339.
18. Letts RM, Gibeault D. Fractures of the neck of the talus in children. *Foot Ankle* 1980; 1:74–77.
19. Canale ST, Kelly FB Jr. Fractures of the neck of the talus. *J Bone Joint Surg Am* 1978; 62:143–156.
20. Rammelt S, Zwipp H, Gavlik JM. Avascular necrosis after minimally displaced talus fracture in a child. *Foot Ankle Int* 2000;21:1030–1036.
21. Morgan A, Kim PS, Christman RA. Radiographic anatomy of the talus. *J Am Podiatr Med Assoc* 2003;93:449–480.
22. Hawkins LG. Fracture of the lateral process of the talus: a review of thirteen cases. *J Bone Joint Surg Am* 1965;47:1170–1175.
23. Heckman JD, McLean MR. Fractures of the lateral process of the talus. *Clin Orthop* 1985;199:108–113.
24. Howard CB, Benson MK. The ossific nuclei and the cartilage anlage of the talus and calcaneum. *J Bone Joint Surg Br* 1992;74:620–623.
25. Hubbard AM, Meyer JS, Davidson RS, et al. Relationship between the ossification center and cartilaginous anlage in the normal hindfoot in children: study with MR imaging. *Am J Roentgenol* 1993;161:849–853.
26. Gelberman RH, Mortensen WW. The arterial anatomy of the talus. *Foot Ankle* 1983; 4:64–72.
27. Jensen I, Wester JU, Rasmussen F, et al. Prognosis of fracture of the talus in children: 21 (7–34) year follow-up of 14 cases. *Acta Orthop Scand* 1994;65:398–400.
28. Mazel C, Rigault P, Padovani JP, et al Fractures of the talus in children: apropos of 23 cases. *Rev Chir Orthop* 1986;72:183–195.
29. Daniels TR, Smith JW. Talar neck fractures. *Foot Ankle* 1993;14:225–234.
30. Ziv I, Mosheiff R, Zelgowski A, et al. Crush injuries of the foot with compartment syndrome: immediate one-stage management. *Foot Ankle* 1989;9:285–289.
31. Hawkins LG. Fractures of the neck of the talus. *J Bone Joint Surg Am* 1970;52:991–995.
32. DeLee JC. Fracture and dislocations of the foot. In: Mann RA, Coughlin MJ, eds. *Surgery of the Foot and Ankle*. St. Louis: Mosby; 1993.
33. Vanderwilde R, Staheli LT, Chew DE, et al. Measurement on radiographs of the foot in normal infants and children. *J Bone Joint Surg Am* 1988;70:407–414.
34. Draijer F, Havemann D, Bielstein D. Injury analysis of pediatric talus fractures. *Unfallchirurg* 1995;98:130–132.
35. Canale ST. Fractures in children. In: Canale ST, ed: *Campbell's Operative Orthopaedics*, 10th ed. St. Louis: Mosby; 2003.
36. Herring JA, ed. Lower extremity injuries. In: *Tachdjian's Pediatric Orthopaedics*, 3rd ed. Philadelphia: WB Saunders; 2002:2417.
37. Swanson TV, Bray TJ, Holmes GB Jr. Fractures of the talar neck: a mechanical study of fixation. *J Bone Joint Surg Am* 1992;74:544–551.
38. Adelaar RS. Complex fractures of the talus. *Instr Course Lect* 1997;46:328.
39. Letts M, Davidson D, Ahmer A. Osteochondritis dissecans of the talus in children. *J Pediatr Orthop* 2003;23:617–625.
40. Sneppen O, Christensen SB, Krogsoe O, et al. Fracture of the body of the talus. *Acta Orthop Scand* 1977;48:317–324.
41. Leibner ED, Simanovsky N, Abu-Sneinah K, et al. Fractures of the lateral process of the talus in children. *J Pediatr Orthop* 2001;10:68–72.
42. Dimon JH. Isolated displaced fracture of the posterior facet of the talus. *J Bone Joint Surg Am* 1961;43:275–281.
43. Kirkpatrick DP, Hunter RE, Janes PC, et al. The snowboarders foot and ankle. *Am J Sports Med* 1998;26:271–277.
44. Nicholas R, Hadley J, Paul C, Janes P. 'Snowboarders fracture': fracture of the lateral process of the talus. *J Am Board Family Pract* 1994;7:130–133.
45. Mukherjee SK, Pringle RM, Baxter AD. Fracture of the lateral process of the talus: a report of thirteen cases. *J Bone Joint Surg Br* 1974;56:263.
46. Noble J, Royle SG. Fracture of the lateral process of the talus: computed tomographic diagnosis. *Br J Sports Med* 1993;26:245–246.
47. Penny JN, Davis ML. Fractures and fracture-dislocation of the neck of the talus. *J Trauma* 1980;20:1029–1037.
48. Berndt AL, Harty M. Transchondral fractures (osteochondritis dissecans) of the talus. *J Bone Joint Surg Am* 1959;41:988–1020.
49. Konig A. Uber freie korper in den Gelenken. *Dtsch Z Cir* 1888;27:90–103.
50. Hepple S, Winson IG, Glew D. Osteochondral lesions of the talus: a revised classification. *Foot Ankle* 1999;20:789–793.
51. Canale ST, Belding RH. Osteochondral lesions of the talus. *J Bone Joint Surg Am* 1980; 62:97–102.
52. Aichroth P. Osteochondrosis dissecans of the knee. *J Bone Joint Surg Br* 1971;53: 440–447.
53. Aichroth P. Osteochondral fractures and their relationship to osteochondritis dissecans of the knee. *J Bone Joint Surg Br* 1971;53:448–454.
54. Anderson IF, Crichton KJ, Grattan-Smith T, et al. Osteochondral fractures of the dome of the talus. *J Bone Joint Surg Am* 1989;71:1143–1152.
55. Giannini S, Vannin F. Operative treatment of osteochondral lesions in the talar dome: current concepts review. *Foot Ankle Int* 2004;25:168–175.
56. Pennal GF. Fractures of the talus. *Clin Orthop* 1963;30:53–63.
57. Peterson L, Romanus B, Dahlberg E. Fracture of the collum tali: an experimental study. *J Biomech* 1976;9:277–279.
58. Ferkel RD, Scranton PE. Arthroscopy of the ankle and foot. Current concepts review. *J Bone Joint Surg Am* 1993;75:1233–1242.
59. Loren GJ, Ferkel RD. Arthroscopic assessment of occult intra-articular injury in acute ankle fractures. *Arthroscopy* 2002;18:412–421.
60. Kellam JF, Bosse MJ, Obremskey WT. Timing of surgical fixation of talar neck fractures. Paper #45, Orthopedic Trauma Association Annual General Meeting, OTA meeting prospectus, Oct 9–11, 2003, Salt Lake City, Utah, p 180.
61. LeMaire RG, Bustin M. Screw fixation of fractures of the neck of the talus using a posterior approach. *J Trauma* 1980;20:669–673.
62. Szyszkowitz R, Reschauer R, Seggl W. Eighty-five talus fractures treated by ORIF with five to eight years of followup study of 69 patients. *Clin Orthop* 1985;199:97–107.
63. Sanders R. Fractures and fracture-dislocations of the calcaneus. In: Coughlin MJ, Mann RA, eds. *Surgery of the Foot and Ankle*, 7th ed. St. Louis: Mosby; 1999.
64. Coltart WD. Aviator's astralgus. *J Bone Joint Surg Br* 1952;34:546–566.
65. Tehranzadeh J, Stuffman E, Ross SD. Partial Hawkins sign in fractures of the talus: report of three cases. *Am J Roentgenol* 2003;181:1559–1563.
66. van Frank E, Ward JC, Engelhardt P. Bilateral calcaneal fracture in childhood: case report and review of the literature. *Arch Orthop Trauma Surg* 1998;118:111–112.
67. Schmidt TL, Weiner DS. Calcaneal fractures in children: an evaluation of the nature of the injury in 56 children. *Clin Orthop* 1982;171:150–155.
68. Schantz K, Rasmussen F. Good prognosis after calcaneal fracture in childhood. *Acta Orthop Scand* 1988;59:560–563.
69. De Beer JD, Maloon S, Hudson DA. Calcaneal fractures in children. *S Afr Med J* 1989; 76:53–54.
70. Dvaric DM, Schmidt EW. Irreducible fracture of the calcaneus in a child: case report. *J Orthop Trauma* 1988;2:154–157.
71. Matteri RE, Frymoyer JW. Fracture of the calcaneus in young children. *J Bone Joint Surg Am* 1973;55:1091–1094.
72. Sandermann J, Torp FT, Thomsen PB. Intraarticular calcaneal fractures in children: report of two cases and a survey of the literature. *Arch Orthop Trauma Surg* 1987;106: 129–131.
73. Schindler A, Mason DE, Allington NJ. Occult fracture of the calcaneus in toddlers. *J Pediatr Orthop* 1996;16:201–205.
74. Thomas MH. Calcaneal fracture in childhood. *Br J Surg* 1969;56:664–666.
75. Buckley RE, O'Brien J, McCormack RG, et al. Personal gait satisfaction of patients with displaced intraarticular calcaneal fractures: a 2- to 8-year follow-up. Poster Presentation #70, Orthopaedic Trauma Association Annual Meeting, Salt Lake City, Utah, October, 2003.
76. Allmacher D, Galles K, Marsh JL. Intraarticular calcaneal fractures observed sequentially for two decades. Paper #48, Orthopaedic Trauma Association annual general meeting prospectus, Oct 11, 2003, Salt Lake City, p 187.
77. Inokuchi S, Usami N, Hiraishi E, et al. Calcaneal fractures in children. *J Pediatr Orthop* 1998;18:469–474.
78. Wiley JJ, Profitt A. Fractures of the os calcis in children. *Clin Orthop* 1984;188:131–138.
79. Kim DH, Berkowitz MJ. Fracture of the calcaneus associated with talocalcaneal coalition. *Foot Ankle Int* 2004;25:426–428.
80. Mora S, Thordarson DB, Zionts LE, et al. Pediatric calcaneal fractures. *Foot Ankle Int* 2001;22:471–477.
81. Pickle A, Benaroch TE, Guy P, et al. Clinical outcome of pediatric calcaneal fractures treated with open reduction and internal fixation. *J Pediatr Orthop* 2004;24:178–180.
82. Atkins RM, Allen PE, Livingstone JA. Demographic features of intra-articular fractures of the calcaneum. *Foot Ankle Surg* 2001;7:77–84.
83. Kay RM, Tang CW. Pediatric foot fractures: evaluation and treatment. *J Am Acad Orthop Surg* 2001;9:308–319.

84. Sanders R. Intraarticular fractures of the calcaneus: present state of the art. *J Orthop Trauma* 1992;6:252–265.
85. Schopfner CE, Coin CG. Effect of weight-bearing on the appearance and development of the secondary calcaneal epiphysis. *Radiology* 1968;86:201–206.
86. Paccola CAJ, Kunioka CT. Bifid calcaneus. *The Foot* 1991;1:49–50.
87. Laliotis N, Pennie BH, Carty H, et al. Toddler's fracture of the calcaneum. *Injury* 1993; 24:169–170.
88. Starshak RJ, Simons GW, Sty JR. Occult fracture of the calcaneus: another toddler's fracture. *Pediatr Radiol* 1984:14:37–40.
89. Carroll N. Fractures and dislocations of the tarsal bones. In: Letts RM, Baxter MP, eds. *Management of Pediatric Fractures*. New York: Churchill Livingstone; 1994.
90. Rosenthall L, Hill RO, Chuang S. Observation on the use of 99mTc-phosphate imaging in peripheral bone trauma. *Radiology* 1976;119:637.
91. Forrester DM, Kerr R. Trauma to the foot. *Radiol Clin North Am* 1990;28:423–433.
92. Heckman JD, Champine MJ. New techniques in the management of foot trauma. *Clin Orthop* 1989;240:105–114.
93. Bohler L. Diagnosis, pathology and treatment of fractures of the os calcis. *J Bone J Surg* 1931;13:75.
94. Essex-Lopresti P. The mechanism, reduction technique, and results in fractures of the os calcis. *Br J Surg* 1952;39:395.
95. Letournel E. Open treatment of acute calcaneal fractures. *Clin Orthop* 1993;290:60.
96. Chapman H, Galway H. Os calcis fractures in childhood. *J Bone Joint Surg Br* 1977; 59:510.
97. Sanders R, Fortin P, DiPasquale T, Wallings A. Operative treatment in 120 displaced intra-articular calcaneal fractures. *Clin Orthop* 1993;290:87–95.
98. Sanders R. Displaced intra-articular fractures of the calcaneus. *J Bone Joint Surg Am* 2000;82:225–250.
99. Giordano CP, Koval KJ. Treatment of fracture blisters: a prospective study of 53 cases. *J Orthop Trauma* 1995;9:171–176.
100. Giordano CP, Koval KJ, Zuckerman JD, Desai P. Fracture blisters. *Clin Orthop* 1994; 307:214–221.
101. Varela CD, Vaughan TK, Carr JB, et al. Fracture blisters: clinical and pathological aspects. *J Orthop Trauma* 1993;7:417–427.
102. Thornton SJ, Cheleuitte D, Ptaszek AJ, et al. Treatment of open intraarticular calcaneal fractures: evaluation and rate of soft tissue complications for a treatment protocol based on wound location and size. Presented at Orthopaedic Trauma Association Annual Meeting, Salt Lake City, Utah, October 9–11, 2003.
103. Mooney JF, Argenta LC, Marks MW, et al. Treatment of soft tissue defects in pediatric patients using the V.A.C. system. *Clin Orthop* 2000;376:26–31.
104. Benirschke SK, Kramer PA. Wound healing complications in closed and open calcaneal fractures. *J Orthop Trauma* 2004;18:1–6.
105. Aldridge JM, Easley M, Numley JA. Open calcaneal fracture: results of operative treatment. *J Orthop Trauma* 2004;18:7–11.
106. Sarrail R, Launay F, Marez MC, et al. Reflex dystrophy in children and adolescents. *J Bone Joint Surg Br* 2004;86(suppl):23.
107. Wilder RT, Berde CB, Wolohan M, et al. Reflex sympathetic dystrophy in children: clinical characteristics and follow-up of seventy patients. *J Bone Joint Surg Am* 1992; 74:910–919.
108. Myerson M, Manoli A. Compartment syndrome in feet after calcaneal fractures. *Clin Orthop* 1993;290:142–150.
109. Crawford AH. Fractures and dislocations of the foot and ankle. In: Green NE, Swiontkowski MF, eds: *Skeletal Trauma in Children*. Philadelphia: WB Saunders; 1994: 449–516.
110. Owen RJT, Hickey FG, Finlay DB. A study of metatarsal fractures in children. *Injury* 1995;26:537–538.
111. Waugh W. The ossification and vascularization of the tarsal navicular and their relation to Kohler's disease. *J Bone Joint Surg Br* 1958;40:765–777.
112. Hosking KV, Hoffman EB. Midtarsal dislocations in children. *J Pediatr Orthop* 1999; 19:592–595.
113. Wilson DW. Injuries of the tarso-metatarsal joints. *J Bone Joint Surg Br* 1972;54: 677–686.
114. Bonnel F, Barthelemy M. (Injuries of Lisfranc's joint: severe sprains, dislocations, fractures—study of 39 personal cases and biomechanical classification). *J Chir (Paris)* 1976; 111:573.
115. Cehner J. Fractures of the tarsal bones, metatarsals, and toes. In: Weber BG, Brunner C, Freuler F, eds. *Treatment of Fractures in Children and Adolescents*. New York: Springer-Verlag; 1980.
116. Rainaut JJ, Cedard C, D'Hour JP. (Tarso-metatarsal luxations). *Rev Chir Orthop Reparatrice Appar Mot* 1966;52:449.
117. Wiley JJ. Tarso-metatarsal injuries in children. *J Pediatr Orthop* 1981;1:255–260.
118. Buoncristiani AM, Manos RE, Mills WJ. Plantar-flexion tarsometatarsal joint injuries in children. *J Pediatr Orthop* 2001;21:324–327.
119. Johnson GF. Pediatric Lisfranc injury: "bunk bed" fracture. *Am J Roentgenol* 1981;137: 1041–1044.
120. Burroughs KE, Reimer CD, Fields KB. Lisfranc injury of the foot: a commonly missed diagnosis. *Am Fam Physician* 1998;58:118.
121. Rosenberg GA, Patterson BM. Tarsometatarsal (Lisfranc's) fracture-dislocation. *Am J Orthop* 1995;2(suppl 1):7.
122. Ross G, Cronin R, Hauzenblas J, et al. Plantar ecchymosis sign: a clinical aid to diagnosis of occult Lisfranc tarsometatarsal injuries. *J Orthop Trauma* 1996;10:119–122.
123. Quénu E, Küss G. Étude sur les luxations du metataese (luxations métatarsotariennes) du diastasis entre le 1er et la 2e metatarsien. *Rev Chir* 1909;39:281–336.
124. Hardcastle PH, Reschauer R, Kitsha-Lissberg E, et al. Injuries to the tarsometatarsal joint: incidence, classification, and treatment. *J Bone Joint Surg Br* 1982;64:349–356.
125. Faciszewski T, Burks RT, Manaster BJ. Subtle injuries of the Lisfranc joint. *J Bone Joint Surg Am* 1990;72:1519–1522.
126. Shapiro MS, Wascher DC, Fireman GAM. Rupture of Lisfrancs ligament in athletes. *Am J Sports Med* 1994;22:687–691.
127. Goiney RC, Connell DG, Nichols DM. CT evaluation of tarsometatarsal fracture-dislocation injuries. *Am J Roentgenol* 1985;144:985.
128. Leenen LP, van der Werken C. Fracture-dislocations of the tarsometatarsal joint: a combined anatomical and computed tomographic study. *Injury* 1992;23:51.
129. Lu J, Ebraheim NA, Skie M, et al. Radiographic and computed tomographic evaluation of Lisfranc dislocation: a cadaver study. *Foot Ankle Int* 1997;18:351.
130. Groshar D, Alperson M, Mendes DG, et al. Bone scintigraphy findings in Lisfranc joint injury. *Foot and Ankle Int* 1995;16:710.
131. Potter HG, Deland JT, Gusmer PB, et al. Magnetic resonence imaging of the Lisfranc ligament of the foot. *Foot Ankle Int* 1998;19:438–446.
132. Wiley JJ. The mechanism of tarso-metatarsal injuries. *J Bone Joint Surg Br* 1971;53: 474–482.
133. Blair WF. Irreducible tarsometatarsal fracture-dislocations. *J Trauma* 1981;21:988.
134. Trevino SG, Kodros S. Controversies in tarsometatarsal injuries. *Orthop Clin North Am* 1995;26:229–238.
135. Wiss DA, Kull DM, Perry J. Lisfranc fracture-dislocations of the foot: a clinical-kinesiological study. *J Orthop Trauma* 1987;1:267–274.
136. Curtis MJ, Myerson M, Szura B. Tarsometatarsal joint injuries in the athlete. *Am J Sports Med* 1993;21:497–502.
137. Crawford AH. Fractures and dislocations of the foot and ankle. In Green NE, Swiontkowski MF, eds. *Skeletal Trauma in Children*. Philadelphia: WB Saunders; 1994: 449–516.
138. Owen RJT, Hickey FG, Finlay DB. A study of metatarsal fractures in children. *Injury* 1995;6:537–538.
139. Silas SI, Herzenberg JE, Myerson MS, et al. Compartment syndrome of the foot in children. *J Bone Joint Surg Am* 1995;77:356–361.
140. Carp L. Fracture of the fifth metatarsal bone with special reference to delayed union. *Ann Surg* 1927;86:308.
141. Shereff MJ, Yang QM, Kummer FJ, et al. Vascular anatomy of the fifth metatarsal. *Foot Ankle* 1991;11:350.
142. Smith JW, Arnoczky SP, Hersh A. The intraosseous blood supply of the fifth metatarsal: implications for proximal fracture healing. *Foot Ankle* 1992;13:143–152.
143. Giannestras NJ. *Medical and Surgical Management*, 2nd ed. Philadelphia: Lea & Febiger; 1973:558.
144. Sammarco GJ. The Jones fracture. *Instr Course Lect* 1993;42:201–205.
145. Dameron TB. Fractures and anatomical variations of the proximal portion of the fifth metatarsal. *J Bone Joint Surg Am* 1975;57:788–792.
146. Dameron TB. Fractures of the proximal fifth metatarsal: selecting the best treatment option. *JAAOS* 1995;3:110–114.56.
147. Byrd T. Jones fracture: relearning an old injury, *South Med J* 1992;85–748.
148. Craigen MA, Clarke NM. Bilateral "Jones" fractures of the fifth metatarsal following relapse of talipes equinovarus. *Injury* 1996;27:599.
149. Josefsson PO, Karlsson M, Redlund-Johnell I, et al. Jones fracture: surgical versus nonsurgical treatment. *Clin Orthop* 1994;299:252.
150. Josefsson PO, Karlsson M, Redlund-Johnell I, et al. Closed treatment of Jones fracture: good results in 40 cases after 11–26 years. *Acta Orthop Scand* 1994;65:545–547.
151. Lawrence SJ, Botte MJ. Jones' fractures and related fractures of the proximal fifth metatarsal. *Foot Ankle* 1993;14:358–365.
152. Torg JS, Balduini FC, Zelko RR, et al. Fractures of the base of the fifth metatarsal distal to the tuberosity: classification and guidelines for non-surgical and surgical management. *J Bone Joint Surg* 1984;66:209–214.
153. Lehman RC, Torg JS, Pavlov H, et al. Fractures of the base of the fifth metatarsal distal to the tuberosity: a review. *Foot Ankle* 1987;7:245–252.
154. Adler P. *Ride-on Mower Hazard Analysis 1987–1990: Directorate for Epidemiology*. Washington, D.C.: US Consumer Product Safety Commission; 1993.
155. Alonso JE, Sanchez FL. Lawn mower injuries in children: a preventable impairment. *J Pediatr Orthop* 1995;15:83–89.
156. David J. *Deaths Related to Ride-on Mowers: 1987–1990*. US Consumer Product Safety Commission, Washington, D.C.; 1993.
157. Dormans JP, Azzoni M, Davidson RS, et al. Major lower extremity lawn mower injuries in children. *J Pediatr Orthop* 1995;15:78–82.
158. Vosburgh CL, Gruel CG, Herndon WA, et al. Lawn mower injuries of the pediatric foot and ankle: observations on prevention and management. *J Pediatr Orthop* 1995; 15:504–509.
159. Ross PM, Schwentker EP, Bryan H. Mutilating lawn mower injuries in children. *JAMA* 1976;236:480–481.
160. Love SM, Grogan DP, Ogden JA. Lawn-mower injuries in children. *J Orthop Trauma* 1988;2:95–101.
161. Loder RT. Demographics of traumatic amputations in children: implications for prevention strategies. *J Bone Joint Surg Am* 2004;86:923–928.
162. Newman R, Miles R. *Hazard Analysis: Injuries Associated with Riding Type Mowers*. Washington, D.C.: U.S. Consumer Products Safety Commission; 1981.
163. Gruel CR, Sullivan JA. Prevention of lawnmower injuries in children. *J Okla State Med Assoc* 2003;96:187–188.
164. Letts RM, Mardirosian A. Lawnmower injuries in children. *Can Med Assoc J* 1977;116: 1151–1153.
165. Martin LI. Lawnmower injuries in children: destructive and preventable. *Plast Surg Nurs* 1990;10:69–70, 75–76.

166. Robertson WW Jr. Power lawnmower injuries. *Clin Orthop* 2003;409:37–42.
167. Abraham E, Pellicore RJ, Hamilton RC, et al: Stump overgrowth in juvenile amputees. *J Pediatr Orthop* 1986;6:66.
168. Horowitz JH, Nichter LS, Kenney JG, et al: Lawnmower injuries in children: lower extremity reconstruction. *J Trauma* 1985;25:1138.
169. Erdmann D, Lee B, Roberts CD, et al. Management of lawnmower injuries to the lower extremity in children and adolescents. *Ann Plast Surg* 2000;45:595–600.
170. Lickstein LH, Bentz ML. Reconstruction of pediatric foot and ankle trauma. *J Craniofac Surg* 2003;14:559–565.
171. Shereff M. Compartment syndromes of the foot. *Instr Course Lect* 1990;39:127–132.
172. Weber TG, Manoli A II. Compartment syndromes of the foot. *Foot Ankle Clin* 1999;4: 473–486.
173. Bibbo C, Lin SS, Cunningham FJ. Acute traumatic compartment syndrome of the foot in children. *Pediatr Emerg Care* 2000;16:244–248.
174. Swoboda B, Scola E, Zwipp H. Surgical treatment and late results of foot compartment syndrome [German]. *Unfallchirurg* 1991;94:262–266.
175. Manoli A II, Fakhouri AJ, Weber TG. Compartmental catheterization and fasciotomy of the foot. *Operative Tech Orthop* 1992;2:203–210.
176. Myerson MS. Experimental decompression of the fascial compartments of the foot: the basis for fasciotomy in acute compartment syndromes. *Foot Ankle* 1988;8:308–314.
177. Fitzgerald RH, Cowan JDE. Puncture wounds of the foot. *Orthop Clin North Am* 1975; 6:965–972.
178. Weber EJ. Plantar puncture wounds: a survey to determine the incidence of infection. *J Accid Emerg Med* 1996;13:274–247.
179. Jarvis JG, Skipper J. *Pseudomonas* osteochondritis complicating puncture wounds in children. *J Pediatr Orthop* 1994;14:755–759.
180. Siebert WT, Dewan S, Williams TW Jr. Case report: pseudomonas puncture wound osteomyelitis in adults. *Am J Med Sci* 1982;283:83–88.
181. Verdile VP, Freed H, Gerard J. Puncture wounds to the foot. *J Emerg Med* 1989;7: 193–199.
182. Eidelman M, Bialik V, Miller Y, et al. Plantar puncture wounds in children: analysis of 80 hospitalized patients and late sequelae. *Isr Med Assoc J* 2003;5:268–271.
183. Niall DM, Murphy PG, Fogarty EE, et al. Puncture wound related pseudomonas infections of the foot in children. *Ir J Med Sci* 1997;166:126–128.
184. Fisher MC, Goldsmith JF, Gilligan PH. Sneakers as a source of *Pseudomonas aeruginosa* in children with osteomyelitis following puncture wounds. *J Pediatr Orthop* 1985;106: 607–609.
185. Laughlin TJ, Armstrong DG, Caporusso J, et al. Soft tissue and bone infections from puncture wounds in children. *West J Med* 1997;166:126–128.
186. Imoisili MA, Bonwit AM, Bulas DI. Toothpick puncture injuries of the foot in children. *Pediatr Infect Dis J* 2004;23:80–82.
187. Lau LS, Bin G, Jaovisidua S, et al. Cost effectiveness of magnetic resonance imaging in diagnosing *Pseudomonas aeruginosa* infection after puncture wound. *J Foot Ankle Surg* 1997;36:36–43.
188. Johanson PH. Pseudomonas infections of the foot following puncture wounds. *JAMA* 1968;204:170–172.
189. Jacobs RF, McCarthy RE, Elser JM. *Pseudomonas* osteochondritis complicating puncture wounds of the foot in children: a 10-year evaluation. *J Infect Dis* 1989;160:657–661.
190. Yngve DA. Stress fractures in the pediatric athlete. In: Sullivan JA, Grana WA, eds. *The Pediatric Athlete.* Park Ridge, IL: American Academy of Orthopaedic Surgeons; 1990: 235–240.
191. Childress HM. March fracture in a seven year old boy. *J Bone Joint Surg* 1946;28:877.
192. Devas MD. Stress fractures in children. *J Bone Joint Surg* 1963;45:528–541.
193. Englaro EE, Gelfand MJ, Paltiel HJ. Bone scintigraphy in preschool children with lower extremity pain of unknown origin. *J Nucl Med* 1992;33:351–354.
194. Sangeorzan BJ, Hansen ST. Early and late posttraumatic foot reconstruction. *Clin Orthop* 1989;243:86–91.
195. Drez D, Young JC, Johnston RD, et al. Metatarsal stress fractures. *Am J Sports Med* 1980;8:123–125.

INDEX

Note: Page numbers followed by an "f" indicate figures; page numbers followed by a "t" indicate tables.

D

E

L

M

N

Q

R

S

T

V

W